American Psychiatric Association

Practice Guidelines for the Treatment of Psychiatric Disorders

COMPENDIUM 2006

Published by the
American Psychiatric Association
Arlington, Virginia

Manufactured in the United States of America on acid-free paper

American Psychiatric Association
1000 Wilson Boulevard
Arlington, VA 22209-3901
www.psych.org

Library of Congress Cataloging-in-Publication Data
American Psychiatric Association.
American Psychiatric Association practice guidelines for the treatment of psychiatric disorders. Compendium 2006.
p. ; cm.
Includes bibliographical references and index.
ISBN 0-89042-383-0 (hardcover : alk. paper) — ISBN 0-89042-385-7 (pbk : alk. paper)
1. Mental illness—Treatment—Handbooks, manuals, etc. 2. Mental illness—Diagnosis—Handbooks, manuals, etc.
[DNLM: 1. Mental Disorders—therapy—Practice Guideline. 2. Mental Disorders—diagnosis—Practice Guideline. WM 400 A5131a 2006] I. Title: Practice guidelines for the treatment of psychiatric disorders. II. Title: Treatment of psychiatric disorders. III. Title.
RC480.A528 2006
616.89—dc22

2006006928

British Library Cataloguing in Publication Data
A CIP record is available from the British Library.

Hardcover ISBN 0-89042-383-0, ISBN-13 [978-0-89042-383-7] 1st printing April 2006
Softcover ISBN 0-89042-385-7, ISBN-13 [978-0-89042-385-1] 1st printing April 2006

AMERICAN PSYCHIATRIC ASSOCIATION STEERING COMMITTEE ON PRACTICE GUIDELINES

John S. McIntyre, M.D.,
Chair
Sara C. Charles, M.D.,
Vice-Chair

Daniel J. Anzia, M.D.
Ian A. Cook, M.D.
Molly T. Finnerty, M.D.
Bradley R. Johnson, M.D.
James E. Nininger, M.D.
Paul Summergrad, M.D.
Sherwyn M. Woods, M.D., Ph.D.
Joel Yager, M.D.

AREA AND COMPONENT LIAISONS

Robert Pyles, M.D. (Area I)
C. Deborah Cross, M.D. (Area II)
Roger Peele, M.D. (Area III)
Daniel J. Anzia, M.D. (Area IV)
John P. D. Shemo, M.D. (Area V)
Lawrence Lurie, M.D. (Area VI)
R. Dale Walker, M.D. (Area VII)
Mary Ann Barnovitz, M.D.
Sheila Hafter Gray, M.D.
Sunil Saxena, M.D.
Tina Tonnu, M.D.

STAFF

Robert Kunkle, M.A., *Senior Program Manager*
Amy B. Albert, B.A., *Assistant Project Manager*
Laura J. Fochtmann, M.D., *Medical Editor*
Claudia Hart, *Director, Department of Quality Improvement and Psychiatric Services*
Darrel A. Regier, M.D., M.P.H., *Director, Division of Research*

For Continuing Medical Education credit for APA Practice Guidelines, visit **www.psych.org/cme**

To order the 2006 Compendium of Quick Reference Guides to the APA Practice Guidelines, visit **www.appi.org** or call **800-368-5777.**

The American Board of Psychiatry and Neurology (ABPN) has reviewed the APA Practice Guidelines CME Program and has approved this product as part of a comprehensive lifelong learning program, which is mandated by the American Board of Medical Specialties as a necessary component of maintenance of certification.

ABPN approval is time limited to 3 years for each individual Practice Guideline CME course. Refer to APA's CME web site for ABPN approval status of each course.

CONTENTS

Statement of Intent vii

Introduction ix

▶ Practice Guideline for the Psychiatric Evaluation of Adults, Second Edition 1

Guideline Watch: Practice Guideline for the Treatment of Patients With Delirium 61

▶ Practice Guideline for the Treatment of Patients With Delirium 65

Guideline Watch: Practice Guideline for the Treatment of Patients With Alzheimer's Disease and Other Dementias of Late Life 101

▶ Practice Guideline for the Treatment of Patients With Alzheimer's Disease and Other Dementias of Late Life 105

Guideline Watch: Practice Guideline for the Treatment of Patients With HIV/AIDS 169

▶ Practice Guideline for the Treatment of Patients With HIV/AIDS 187

▶ Practice Guideline for the Treatment of Patients With Substance Use Disorders, Second Edition 291

▶ Practice Guideline for the Treatment of Patients With Schizophrenia, Second Edition 565

Guideline Watch: Practice Guideline for the Treatment of Patients With Major Depressive Disorder, Second Edition 747

▶ Practice Guideline for the Treatment of Patients With Major Depressive Disorder, Second Edition . . . 763

Guideline Watch: Practice Guideline for the Treatment of Patients With Bipolar Disorder, Second Edition 841

▶ Practice Guideline for the Treatment of Patients With Bipolar Disorder, Second Edition 851

Guideline Watch: Practice Guideline for the Treatment of Patients With Panic Disorder 933

▶ Practice Guideline for the Treatment of Patients With Panic Disorder 945

▶ Practice Guideline for the Treatment of Patients With Acute Stress Disorder and Posttraumatic Stress Disorder 1003

▶ Practice Guideline for the Treatment of Patients With Eating Disorders, Third Edition 1097

Guideline Watch: Practice Guideline for the Treatment of Patients With Borderline Personality Disorder.... 1223

Practice Guideline for the Treatment of Patients With Borderline Personality Disorder.......... 1233

Practice Guideline for the Assessment and Treatment of Patients With Suicidal Behaviors 1315

Appendix: Practice Guideline Development Process 1497

Index 1505

STATEMENT OF INTENT

The American Psychiatric Association (APA) Practice Guidelines are not intended to be construed or to serve as a standard of medical care. Standards of medical care are determined on the basis of all clinical data available for an individual patient and are subject to change as scientific knowledge and technology advance and practice patterns evolve. These parameters of practice should be considered guidelines only. Adherence to them will not ensure a successful outcome for every individual, nor should they be interpreted as including all proper methods of care or excluding other acceptable methods of care aimed at the same results. The ultimate judgment regarding a particular clinical procedure or treatment plan must be made by the psychiatrist in light of the clinical data presented by the patient and the diagnostic and treatment options available.

These practice guidelines have been developed by psychiatrists who are in active clinical practice. In addition, some contributors are primarily involved in research or other academic endeavors. It is possible that through such activities some contributors, including work group members and reviewers, have received income related to treatments discussed in these guidelines. A number of mechanisms are in place to minimize the potential for producing biased recommendations due to conflicts of interest. Work group members are selected on the basis of their expertise and integrity. Any work group member or reviewer who has a potential conflict of interest that may bias (or appear to bias) his or her work is asked to disclose this to the Steering Committee on Practice Guidelines and the work group. Iterative guideline drafts are reviewed by the Steering Committee, other experts, allied organizations, APA members, and the APA Assembly and Board of Trustees; substantial revisions address or integrate the comments of these multiple reviewers. The development of the APA practice guidelines is not financially supported by any commercial organization.

More detail about mechanisms in place to minimize bias is provided in a document available from the APA Department of Quality Improvement and Psychiatric Services, "APA Guideline Development Process," which is also included in the Appendix to this volume.

INTRODUCTION

John S. McIntyre, M.D.
Sara C. Charles, M.D.
Laura J. Fochtmann, M.D.

The 2006 Compendium contains 13 practice guidelines developed by the American Psychiatric Association (APA). Each of these practice guidelines has been published in *The American Journal of Psychiatry.* The guideline on acute stress disorder and posttraumatic stress disorder is new since the publication of the previous compendium; three guidelines (psychiatric evaluation of adults, substance use disorders, and eating disorders) are revisions. Following the practice guideline on evaluation of adults, the other practice guidelines are presented in the order in which the categories of disorder appear in DSM-IV-TR. The practice guideline on suicidal behaviors, a special topic that crosses multiple disorders, appears last.

The term *practice guideline* refers to a set of patient care strategies developed to assist physicians in clinical decision making. The APA is continually developing new and revised guidelines, which are published as they are completed. Currently in development are a practice guideline on obsessive-compulsive disorder and revisions of practice guidelines for Alzheimer's disease and other dementias of late life, panic disorder, HIV/AIDS, major depressive disorder, and bipolar disorder.

APA recognizes that guideline recommendations are most useful if they are current. As a result, this compendium includes "watches" for seven guidelines published in previous compendiums (delirium, Alzheimer's disease and other dementias of late life, HIV/AIDS, major depressive disorder, bipolar disorder, panic disorder, and borderline personality disorder). Watches briefly describe major developments in the scientific literature since original guideline publication. Watches may be authored and reviewed by experts associated with the original guideline development effort and are approved for publication by APA's Executive Committee on Practice Guidelines. Thus, watches represent opinion of the authors and approval of the Executive Committee but not policy of the APA.

Readers should note that these parameters of care are indeed "guidelines" and are not intended to be "standards of care." These guidelines do not necessarily include all proper methods of care for a particular disorder. The ultimate judgment concerning the selection and implementation of a specific plan of treatment must be made by the psychiatrist in light of the clinical data presented by the patient and the diagnostic and treatment options available. Further description of the intended role of the practice guidelines can be found in the Statement of Intent (p. vii).

Although the APA has published specific recommendations about the practice of psychiatry since 1851, the commitment of resources to the practice guideline development process since 1991 represents a qualitative change in the APA's role in establishing guidelines. Such a change raises many questions.

Why Is the APA Developing Practice Guidelines?

For nearly 150 years, the APA's fundamental aim in developing practice guidelines has been to assist psychiatrists in their clinical decision making, with the ultimate goal of improving the care of patients. The explosion of knowledge in our field over the last several decades amplifies the value of these guidelines. Furthermore, the current health care climate is characterized by concerns about quality of care, access to care, and cost. Efforts to respond to these problems by exerting external control over the types and amount of care that can be provided have led to new concerns about the quality of the data on which such efforts are based and the process by which the data are used to determine "appropriate" or "reimbursable" care. The realization that both treatment and reimbursement decisions are occurring without systematic scientific and clinical input has led the APA, along with many other medical specialty societies, to accelerate the process of documenting clearly and concisely what is known and what is not known about the treatment of patients. Although there are a number of other groups, including the federal and state governments, managed care organizations, and care delivery systems, that are also developing practice guidelines, the APA has decided that the psychiatric profession should take the lead in describing the best treatments and the range of appropriate treatments available to patients with mental illnesses.

How Are Practice Guidelines Developed?

The APA practice guidelines are developed under the direction of the Steering Committee on Practice Guidelines. The process is designed to ensure the development of reliable and valid guidelines and is consistent with the recommendations of the American Medical Association and the Institute of Medicine. It is characterized by rigorous scientific review of the available literature, widespread review of iterative drafts, and ultimate approval by the APA Assembly and Board of Trustees. The APA is committed to revising the guidelines at 5-year intervals. A revision may be accelerated if there is substantial new evidence suggesting a change in preferred treatment approaches. The development process is fully described in the Appendix to this compendium. Between guideline revisions, "guideline watches" highlight significant developments relevant to specific guideline recommendations. As they are completed, watches are made available online on the Practice Guidelines page in the Psychiatric Practice section of the APA web site at http://www.psych.org. Psychiatrists who use the guidelines in this compendium are advised to check the web site periodically to stay informed about important developments that may affect how they decide to implement guideline recommendations in their clinical practice.

What Are the Potential Benefits of This Project?

Ultimately, the aim of practice guidelines is to improve patient care. Guidelines should help practicing psychiatrists determine what is known today about how best to help their patients. In addition, psychiatrists and those charged with the allocation of health care resources must try to make the best possible decisions on the basis of currently available data. Well-developed guidelines can help in these efforts.

Toward the end of helping patients, guidelines can have other beneficial effects. They are a vehicle for educating psychiatrists, other medical and mental health professionals, and the general public about appropriate and inappropriate treatments. By demonstrating that the quality of evidence for psychiatric treatments is on par with (and in many cases exceeds) that for other medical care, guidelines contribute to the credibility of the field. Guidelines identify those areas in which critical information is lacking and in which research could be expected to improve clinical decisions. Finally, guidelines can help those charged with overseeing the utilization and reimbursement of psychiatric services to develop more scientifically based and clinically sensitive criteria.

What Are the Possible Risks?

The APA reasons that the risks of this project are small and are considerably outweighed by the benefits. One risk is that the guidelines can be misinterpreted and misused by third parties in a way that will ultimately harm patients. Although this risk rightfully concerns many psychiatrists, it is the judgment of the Steering Committee, the Assembly, and the Board of Trustees that the existence of guidelines helps to clarify the sources of disagreement between treating psychiatrists and reviewers and that their use can be a great improvement over the use of criteria developed through less objective procedures. In addition, many have expressed the concern that guidelines can "homogenize" the care of patients and detract from psychiatrists' freedom to shape treatment in ways that they feel best suit their individual patients. Inevitably, there is a tension in writing guidelines between the desire for specificity and the desire to allow for the consideration of individual clinical circumstances. These concerns must be balanced in such a way that allows psychiatrists to make appropriate clinical decisions. This very important issue is addressed in the Statement of Intent that begins each individually published guideline (see p. vii of this compendium). Finally, there are concerns that the APA-approved guidelines may lead to an increase in malpractice claims. At this time, legal experts have mixed opinions about the impact of guidelines on the volume and severity of malpractice suits. However, in fact, some medical specialties that have been developing guidelines over the past two decades report that guidelines seem to have had the positive effect of fewer claims and, for at least one specialty (anesthesiology), lower malpractice insurance premiums. Since the publication of APA's first practice guideline in 1993, the Steering Committee has been monitoring the potential impact of the guidelines on malpractice actions and has not noted any trends suggesting an increase in the number or severity of malpractice claims that might be attributed to the existence of APA-approved guidelines.

How Can We Improve the Current Process?

Since the inception of the APA project in 1989, the practice guideline development process has evolved significantly. Specifically, the activities of the work groups developing the guidelines have been made more explicit, and the nature of the reviewers' input has been standardized. Also, the format of each guideline has evolved over the past several years. In guidelines developed after 1999, the recommendations covering treatment, including the formulation of a treatment plan, are presented before background information and the evidence that supports these recommendations. This change in format was based on input from psychiatrists and is designed to make the guidelines more user-friendly.

Certain principles remain crucial to further improvement. Clearly, practice guidelines should be based on objective data whenever possible. Such data are of two types: well-designed research studies and systematically identified clinical expertise. Systematic reviews of the literature are an essential part of this work. However, efforts to synthesize studies in any given area are hampered by the uneven quantity and quality of research, by problems in generalizing from a literature largely derived from tertiary care research settings to more typical clinical practice, by the inherent difficulty in conducting controlled studies of some treatments for some populations, and by the difficulty in characterizing "clinical consensus." These issues are being partially addressed through the use of the APA's Practice Research Network (PRN), which uses a panel of approximately 800 psychiatrists in the full range of practice settings to gather data for clinical research. Practice research networks are also being used in other areas of medicine (e.g., family practice and pediatrics) to gather data from practice settings of relevance to the development of guidelines. For example, data about prevailing practice patterns and patient outcomes can be systematically gathered and incorporated into the guidelines. In addition, the impact of guidelines on psychiatric practice and patient outcomes can be assessed; ultimately, it should be possible to determine whether guidelines improve patient care. Currently, a major thrust of the APA project is to explore, devise, and test educational and dissemination strategies that will increase psychiatrists' use of the guidelines in daily practice.

Quick Reference Guides

In further attempts to increase the use and usefulness of the practice guidelines, the APA now publishes with each guideline a quick reference guide. The quick reference guide is a summary of the guideline's major recommendations. The quick reference guide is designed to assist psychiatrists in using the material presented in the full-text guideline. A compendium of quick reference guides is available from American Psychiatric Publishing, Inc.

Online CME

Interactive continuing medical education programs for many of the individual practice guidelines are available on the APA's web site (www.psych.org/cme). Each program offers Category 1 CME credits that are accepted by the APA and the American Medical Association.

The American Board of Psychiatry and Neurology (ABPN) has reviewed the APA Practice Guidelines CME Program and has approved this product as part of a comprehensive lifelong learning program, which is mandated by the American Board of Medical Specialties as a necessary component of maintenance of certification.

ABPN approval is time limited to 3 years for each individual Practice Guideline CME course. Refer to APA's CME web site for ABPN approval status of each course.

Conclusions

The practice guidelines included in this volume represent an important step in the development of an "evidence-based psychiatry." The development of better research tools, the accumulation of new research data, the systematic identification of best clinical practice, and the iterative improvement of the process for developing practice guidelines will contribute to the continual development of better practice guidelines to aid psychiatrists in their clinical decision making.

PRACTICE GUIDELINE FOR THE
Psychiatric Evaluation of Adults
Second Edition

WORK GROUP ON PSYCHIATRIC EVALUATION

Michael J. Vergare, M.D., Chair

Renée L. Binder, M.D.
Ian A. Cook, M.D.
Marc Galanter, M.D.
Francis G. Lu, M.D.

This practice guideline was approved in December 2005 and published in June 2006. A guideline watch, summarizing significant developments in the scientific literature since publication of this guideline, may be available in the Psychiatric Practice section of the APA web site at www.psych.org.

CONTENTS

Development Process 5

Introduction 6

I. Purpose of Evaluation 7
   A. General Psychiatric Evaluation 7
   B. Emergency Evaluation 8
   C. Clinical Consultation 9
   D. Other Consultations 9

II. Site of the Clinical Evaluation 10
   A. Inpatient Settings 10
   B. Outpatient Settings 10
   C. General Medical Settings 11
   D. Other Settings 12

III. Domains of the Clinical Evaluation 12
   A. Reason for the Evaluation 12
   B. History of the Present Illness 12
   C. Past Psychiatric History 17
   D. History of Substance Use 17
   E. General Medical History 17
   F. Developmental, Psychosocial, and Sociocultural History 18
   G. Occupational and Military History 19
   H. Legal History 19
   I. Family History 20
   J. Review of Systems 20
   K. Physical Examination 20
   L. Mental Status Examination 21

IV. Evaluation Process 23
   A. Methods of Obtaining Information 23
   B. The Process of Assessment 35

V. Special Considerations 38
   A. Privacy and Confidentiality 38
   B. Interactions With Third-Party Payers and Their Agents 39
   C. Legal and Administrative Issues in Institutions 40
   D. Special Populations 40

VI. Future Research Needs . . . 42
A. Interviewing Approaches . . . 42
B. Rating Scales . . . 43
C. Diagnosis and Formulation . . . 43
D. Diagnostic Testing . . . 43

Individuals and Organizations That Submitted Comments . . . 44

References . . . 45

DEVELOPMENT PROCESS

This practice guideline was developed under the auspices of the Steering Committee on Practice Guidelines. The development process is detailed in a document available from the APA Department of Quality Improvement and Psychiatric Services, the "APA Guideline Development Process." Key features of this process include the following:

- A comprehensive literature review
- Development of evidence tables
- Initial drafting of the guideline by a work group that included psychiatrists with clinical and research expertise in psychiatric evaluation
- Production of multiple revised drafts with widespread review (14 organizations and 64 individuals submitted significant comments)
- Approval by the APA Assembly and Board of Trustees
- Planned revisions at regular intervals

Relevant literature was identified through a computerized search of MEDLINE, using PubMed, for the period from 1994 to 2005. The search strategy (psychiatric assessment OR psychiatric assessments OR psychiatric emergencies OR psychiatric emergency OR psychiatric evaluation OR psychiatric evaluations OR psychiatric histories OR psychiatric history OR psychiatric interview OR psychiatric interviewing OR psychiatric interviews OR psychological assessment OR psychological assessments OR psychological evaluation OR psychological interview OR mental status examination OR mental status examinations OR psychiatric rating) OR (mental disorders/diagnosis AND [laboratory findings OR laboratory techniques OR laboratory test OR laboratory tests OR radiograph OR radiographic OR radiography OR x ray OR imaging OR MRI OR tomography OR physical exam OR physical examination OR interview OR interviewing OR history taking OR evaluation OR assessment]) yielded 19,429 references, of which 7,894 were published between 1994 and 2005 in English and had associated abstracts. An additional search on history taking AND (psychiatric OR sexual OR occupational OR social OR psychosocial) yielded 1,927 references, with 731 of these published with abstracts in English between the years 1994 and 2005.

Additional, more limited searches were conducted by APA staff and individual members of the Work Group on Psychiatric Evaluation to address discrete issues outside of the primary guideline topic.

This document represents a synthesis of current scientific knowledge and rational clinical practice on the psychiatric evaluation of adults. It strives to be as free as possible of bias toward any theoretical approach.

INTRODUCTION

Psychiatric evaluations vary according to their purpose. This guideline is intended primarily for general, emergency, and consultation evaluations for clinical purposes. It is applicable to evaluations conducted by a psychiatrist with adult patients (age 18 or older), although sections may be applicable to younger patients. Other types of psychiatric evaluations (including forensic, child custody, and disability evaluations) are not the focus of this guideline; however, the general recommendations of this guideline may be applicable to other, more specialized evaluations.

The guideline presumes familiarity with basic principles of psychiatric diagnosis and treatment planning as outlined in standard, contemporary psychiatric textbooks (1–6) and taught in psychiatry residency training programs. It was developed following a review of contemporary references, and it emphasizes areas of consensus in the field.

Recommendations of this guideline are intended to be consistent with the care model endorsed in the Institute of Medicine report *Crossing the Quality Chasm* (7). This report notes that with advancements in medical science, the emphasis of health care delivery must shift to ongoing management of chronic conditions. The initial psychiatric evaluation may set the stage for such ongoing care by establishing initial treatment goals, gathering relevant baseline data, establishing a plan for systematic follow-up assessment using formal but practical and relevant measures, and ensuring longitudinal follow-up.

While there is broad agreement that each element of the extensive general evaluation described in this guideline may be relevant or even crucial in a particular patient, the specific emphasis of an evaluation will vary according to its purpose and the patient's presenting problem. Consideration of the domains outlined in this guideline is part of a general psychiatric evaluation, but the content, process, and documentation must be determined by applying the professional skill and judgment of the psychiatrist. The performance of a particular set of clinical procedures does not ensure the adequacy of a psychiatric evaluation, nor does their omission imply that the evaluation is deficient. The particular emphasis or modifications applied by the psychiatrist to the generic evaluation offered in this guideline should be consonant with the aims of the evaluation, the setting of practice, the patient's presenting problem, and the ever-evolving knowledge base concerning clinical assessment and clinical inference. Although documentation is an integral part of an evaluation, it is important to emphasize that the scope and detail of clinically appropriate documentation also will vary with the patient, setting, clinical situation, and confidentiality issues. Because of the wide variation in these factors, this guideline does not include recommendations regarding the content or frequency of documentation. Such determinations must be based on the specific circumstances of the evaluation.

To share feedback on this or other published APA practice guidelines, a form is available at http://www.psych.org/psych_pract/pg/reviewform.cfm.

I. PURPOSE OF EVALUATION

The purpose and conduct of a psychiatric evaluation depend on who requests the evaluation, why it is requested, and the expected future role of the psychiatrist in the patient's care. The outcome of the evaluation may or may not lead to a specific psychiatric diagnosis. Three types of clinical psychiatric evaluations are discussed: 1) general psychiatric evaluation, 2) emergency evaluation, and 3) clinical consultation. In addition, general principles to guide the conduct of evaluations for administrative or legal purposes are reviewed. At times there may be a conflict between the need to establish an effective working relationship with the patient and the need to obtain comprehensive information efficiently. If the psychiatrist expects to provide care directly to the patient, the establishment of an effective working relationship with the patient may take precedence over the comprehensiveness of the initial interview or interviews (8). In such a case, emphasis may be placed on obtaining information needed for immediate clinical recommendations and decisions (9).

A. GENERAL PSYCHIATRIC EVALUATION

A general psychiatric evaluation has as its central component an interview with the patient. The interview-based data are integrated with information that may be obtained through other components of the evaluation, such as a review of medical records, a physical examination, diagnostic tests, and history from collateral sources. A general evaluation usually is time intensive. The amount of time necessary generally depends on the complexity of the problem and the patient's ability and willingness to work cooperatively with the psychiatrist. Language competence needs to be assessed early in the evaluation so that the need for an interpreter can be determined. Several meetings with the patient, and in many cases appropriate family or relational network members, may be necessary. More focused evaluations of lesser scope may be appropriate when the psychiatrist is called on to address a specific, limited diagnostic or therapeutic issue.

The aims of a general psychiatric evaluation are 1) to establish whether a mental disorder or other condition requiring the attention of a psychiatrist is present; 2) to collect data sufficient to support differential diagnosis and a comprehensive clinical formulation; 3) to collaborate with the patient to develop an initial treatment plan that will foster treatment adherence, with particular consideration of any immediate interventions that may be needed to address the safety of the patient and others—or, if the evaluation is a reassessment of a patient in long-term treatment, to revise the plan of treatment in accordance with new perspectives gained from the evaluation; and 4) to identify longer-term issues (e.g., premorbid personality) that need to be considered in follow-up care.

In the course of any evaluation, it may be necessary to obtain history from other individuals (e.g., family or others with whom the patient resides; individuals referring the patient for assessment, including other clinicians). Although the default position is to maintain confidentiality unless the patient gives consent to a specific intervention or communication, the psychiatrist is justified in attenuating confidentiality to the extent needed to address the safety of the patient and others (10, 11). In addition, the psychiatrist can elicit and listen to information provided by friends or family without disclosing information about the patient to the informant.

More detailed recommendations for performing a general psychiatric evaluation are provided in Section III.

B. EMERGENCY EVALUATION

The emergency psychiatric evaluation generally occurs in response to thoughts, feelings, or urges to act that are intolerable to the patient, or to behavior that prompts urgent action by others, such as violent or self-injurious behavior, threats of harm to self or others, failure to care for oneself, bizarre or confused behavior, or intense expressions of distress. The aims and specific approaches to the emergency evaluation have been reviewed elsewhere in detail (11–15) and include the following:

1. Assess and enhance the safety of the patient and others.
2. Establish a provisional diagnosis (or diagnoses) of the mental disorder(s) most likely to be responsible for the current emergency, including identification of any general medical condition(s) or substance use that is causing or contributing to the patient's mental condition.
3. Identify family or other involved persons who can give information that will help the psychiatrist determine the accuracy of reported history, particularly if the patient is cognitively impaired, agitated, or psychotic and has difficulty communicating a history of events. If the patient is to be discharged back to family members or other caretaking persons, their ability to care for the patient and their understanding of the patient's needs must be addressed.
4. Identify any current treatment providers who can give information relevant to the evaluation.
5. Identify social, environmental, and cultural factors relevant to immediate treatment decisions.
6. Determine whether the patient is able and willing to form an alliance that will support further assessment and treatment, what precautions are needed if there is a substantial risk of harm to self or others, and whether involuntary treatment is necessary.
7. Develop a specific plan for follow-up, including immediate treatment and disposition; determine whether the patient requires treatment in a hospital or other supervised setting and what follow-up will be required if the patient is not placed in a supervised setting.

The emergency evaluation varies greatly in length and may on occasion exceed several hours. Patients who will be discharged to the community after an emergency evaluation may require more extensive evaluation in the emergency setting than those who will be hospitalized. For example, patients who have presented with intoxication or who have received medications in the emergency department may require additional observation to verify their stability for discharge. In other individuals with significant symptoms but without apparent acute risk to self or others, additional time may be needed to obtain more detailed input from family, other involved caretaking persons, and treatment providers; to verify that the proposed plan of follow-up is viable; and to communicate with follow-up caregivers about interventions or recommendations resulting from the emergency assessment.

When patients are agitated, psychotic, or uncooperative with assessment, and when their clinical presentation appears to differ from the stated factors prompting assessment, it may be especially important to obtain history from other individuals (e.g., family members, other professionals, police), keeping in mind principles of confidentiality, as described in Section I.A above and in Section V.A.

Patients presenting for emergency psychiatric evaluation have a high prevalence of combined general medical and psychiatric illness, recent trauma, substance use and substance-related conditions, and cognitive impairment (16–27). These diagnostic possibilities deserve careful consideration. General medical and psychiatric evaluations should be coordinated so that additional medical evaluation can be requested or initiated by the psychiatrist on the basis of diagnostic or therapeutic considerations arising from the psychiatric history and interview. Although issues of confidentiality are sometimes raised, in an emergency situation necessary information about the patient can be communicated with the emergency medicine department staff. In many emergency settings, patients initially are examined by a nonpsychiatric physician to exclude acute general medical problems. Such examinations usually are limited in scope and rarely are definitive (18, 19, 28–30). Furthermore, psychiatrists and emergency physicians sometimes have different viewpoints on the utility of laboratory screening for substance use or medical disorders in psychiatric emergency department patients (31, 32). Therefore, on the basis of clinical judgment and the specific circumstances of the evaluation, the psychiatrist may need to request or initiate further general medical evaluation to address diagnostic concerns that emerge from the psychiatric evaluation (12, 16, 18–27, 33–35).

C. CLINICAL CONSULTATION

Clinical consultations are evaluations requested by other physicians or health care professionals, patients, families, or others for the purpose of assisting in the diagnosis, treatment, or management of an individual with a suspected mental disorder or behavioral problem. These evaluations may be comprehensive or may be focused on a relatively narrow question, such as the preferred medication for treatment of a known mental disorder in a patient with a particular general medical condition. Psychiatric evaluations for consultative purposes use the same data sources as general evaluations. Consideration is given to information from the referring source on the specific problem leading to the consultation, the referring source's aims for the consultation, information that the psychiatrist may be able to obtain regarding the patient's relationship with the primary clinician, and the resources and constraints of those currently treating the patient. Also, in the case of a consultation regarding a mental or behavioral problem in a patient with a general medical illness, information about that illness, its treatment, and its prognosis is relevant. The patient should be informed that the purpose of the consultation is to advise the party who requested it. Permission to report findings to others, including family, needs to be clarified with the patient and other concerned parties before the evaluation begins.

The aim of the consultative psychiatric evaluation is to provide clear and specific answers to the questions posed by the party requesting the consultation (36, 37). For example, the psychiatrist may be asked to determine the patient's capacity to give consent for treatment decisions. On other occasions, the psychiatrist may be asked to assess a particular sign, symptom, or syndrome; provide a diagnosis; and recommend evaluation, treatment, or disposition at a level of specificity appropriate to the needs of the treating clinician.

In the course of the evaluation, the consultant may also identify a diagnostic or therapeutic issue that was not raised in the request for consultation but that is of concern to the patient or of relevance to treatment outcome. For example, treatment adherence may be affected by personality and countertransference issues that compromise the patient's therapeutic alliance with the referring clinician. If any conflicts between the patient and the primary clinician do emerge as an issue, positive resolution of them should be encouraged in a manner that respects the patient's relationship with the primary clinician.

If agreed to by the patient, discussion of findings and recommendations with the family or involved persons can assist with appropriate follow-up and adherence with recommendations.

D. OTHER CONSULTATIONS

Other psychiatric consultations are directed toward the resolution of specific legal, administrative, or other nonclinical questions. While the details of these evaluations, such as forensic evaluations, child custody evaluations, and disability evaluations, are beyond the scope of this guideline, several general principles apply. First, the evaluee usually is not the psychiatrist's patient, and there are limits to confidentiality implicit in the aims of the evaluation; accordingly, the aims of the evaluation and the scope of disclosure should be addressed with the evaluee at the start of the interview (38, 39). Second, questions about the evaluee's legal status and legal representation should be resolved before the assessment begins, if possible. Third, many such consultations rely heavily, or even entirely, on documentary evidence or data from collateral sources. The quality and potential biases of such data should be taken into account.

The aims of these psychiatric consultations are 1) to answer the requester's question to the extent possible with the data obtainable and 2) to make a psychiatric diagnosis if it is relevant to the question.

II. SITE OF THE CLINICAL EVALUATION

A. INPATIENT SETTINGS

The scope, pace, and depth of inpatient evaluation depend on the patient population served by the inpatient service, the goals of the hospitalization, and the role of the inpatient unit within the overall system of mental health services available to the patient (40, 41).

In addition to providing a highly structured and contained setting in which patient safety can be monitored and optimized, the inpatient setting permits intensive and continuous observation of signs and symptoms while the patient is being treated for psychiatric and general medical conditions through the collaborative efforts of the multidisciplinary treatment team (see also Section IV.A.5). Particularly for individuals with complex psychiatric presentations or multiple co-occurring disorders, the enhanced level of observation in the inpatient environment may facilitate assessment of co-occurring general medical conditions or evaluation for procedures such as electroconvulsive therapy, may aid in resolving diagnostic dilemmas, and may help in determining a patient's ability to function safely and independently in a less restrictive setting (41, 42).

Inpatient settings provide enhanced opportunity to corroborate clinical judgment and decision making, including discharge planning, through access to information from multiple sources. These include the multidisciplinary treatment team, family, friends, and individuals involved in the care of the patient outside the hospital, as well as prior hospitalization records.

From the outset, the inpatient evaluation should include assessment of the patient's access to appropriate treatment following hospitalization. The patient's living arrangements should also be assessed to determine whether they will continue to be suitable after discharge. If the posthospitalization disposition is not apparent, the evaluation should identify both patient factors and community resources that would be relevant to a viable disposition plan and should identify the problems that could impede a suitable disposition. Family involvement, when appropriate, can also be initiated, and goals for inpatient family work can be identified.

B. OUTPATIENT SETTINGS

Outpatient settings differ widely, from office-based practices to community mental health centers to intensive outpatient or partial hospital programs, among others. Nevertheless, evaluation in the outpatient setting usually differs in intensity from inpatient evaluation because of less frequent interviews and less immediate availability of laboratory services and consultants from other medical specialties. Also, the psychiatrist in the outpatient setting has substantially less opportunity to directly observe the patient's behavior and to implement protective interventions when necessary. For this reason, during the period of evaluation it is important for the psychiatrist to reassess whether the patient requires hospitalization or more intensive outpatient care (e.g., greater visit frequency, intensive outpatient or partial hospital programs, programs of assertive community treatment). Unresolved questions about the patient's general medical status may also require more rapid assessment in a more structured setting. If the patient's presentation is atypical (e.g., with respect to symptoms, symptom severity, or age at onset), a more thorough medical workup may be required or coordinated with the patient's primary care physician. Patients who do not have a primary care physician may need assistance in obtaining appropriate referrals. A decision to change the setting for evaluation will depend on the patient's current mental status and behavior as well as the patient's history of psychiatric symptoms and treatment, the status of co-occurring general medical conditions or substance use, and the availability of diagnostic resources, therapeutic resources, and sociocultural supports.

Advantages of the outpatient setting include greater patient autonomy and the potential for a more longitudinal perspective on the patient's symptoms. However, the lack of continuous direct observation of behavior limits the obtainable data on how the patient's behavior appears to others. Consequently, extended evaluation of the patient in the context of psychoeducational or time-limited groups can complement and augment observations from one-to-one interviews. With the patient's permission, involvement of family or significant others as collateral sources in the evaluation process also deserves consideration. It is also useful to be aware that family and significant others may not be supportive of the patient or of psychiatric treatment. If the patient states that family systems issues, especially marital or partner issues, are a problem, an evaluation session with the partner can provide valuable information and clarify the systems issues. When substance use is suspected, obtaining data from other involved persons (e.g., family, close friends, staff), determining blood alcohol levels, or screening for substances of abuse may be especially important.

C. GENERAL MEDICAL SETTINGS

Evaluations are also conducted in hospital emergency departments (see Section I.B) and general medical (i.e., nonpsychiatric) settings, such as inpatient units. The latter allow for some direct behavioral observation by staff and for some safeguards against self-injurious or other violent behavior by patients. However, the level of behavioral observation and potential intervention against risky behavior in these settings tends to be less than on psychiatric inpatient units. In addition, psychiatric interviews on general medical-surgical units are often compromised by interruptions and lack of privacy. These problems sometimes can be mitigated by using a space on the unit where the patient and the psychiatrist can meet privately.

Developing an ongoing relationship with staff on medical inpatient units will increase the likelihood of obtaining accurate behavioral data as well as of ensuring that staff implement recommendations. If there is prominent hostility or anxiety in interactions between the patient and hospital staff, the evaluating physician must consider interfacing with others in the hospital system to determine its contributors.

If the patient has an unclear sensorium or other cognitive impairments, it is critical to interview people in the patient's relational network to see if these symptoms were present before hospitalization or have developed since treatment was begun. In interviewing family members, it is very useful to discuss their beliefs about the patient's illness and prior treatment, the patient's record of adherence to medication treatment, and concerns about discharge planning. If family members do not perceive themselves as allies in treatment, the patient's treatment is likely to be compromised once he or she leaves the hospital (43).

Documentation of psychiatric evaluations in general medical charts should be sensitive to the standards of confidentiality of the nonpsychiatric medical sector and the possibility that charts may be read by persons who are not well informed about psychiatric issues. Information written in general medical charts should be confined to that necessary for the general medical team and should be conveyed with a level of detail and specificity that will be most helpful to the overall management of the patient. It is also important that documentation be of sufficient detail to establish a diagnosis and treatment plan.

D. OTHER SETTINGS

Evaluations conducted in other settings, such as residential treatment facilities, home care services, nursing homes, long-term care facilities, schools, and prisons, are affected by a number of factors: 1) the level of behavioral observations available and the quality of those observations, 2) the availability of privacy for conducting interviews, 3) the availability of general medical evaluations and diagnostic tests, 4) resources to conduct the evaluation safely, and 5) the degree of likelihood that information written in facility records will be understood and kept confidential.

In light of these factors, it is necessary to consider whether a particular setting permits an evaluation of adequate speed, safety, accuracy, and confidentiality to meet the needs of the patient. Factors of the setting that compromise the evaluation merit documentation.

III. DOMAINS OF THE CLINICAL EVALUATION

General psychiatric evaluations involve a systematic consideration of the broad domains described in this guideline and vary in scope and intensity. Table 1 summarizes the domains. The intensity with which each domain is assessed depends on the purpose of the evaluation and the clinical situation. An evaluation of lesser scope may be appropriate when its purpose is to answer a circumscribed question. Such an evaluation may involve a particularly intense assessment of one or more domains especially relevant to the reason for the evaluation.

Across all domains, evaluations are generally based on three sources of information: 1) observation and interview of the patient; 2) information from others (e.g., family, significant others, case managers, other clinicians [including the patient's primary care physician]) that corroborates, refutes, or elaborates on the patient's report; and 3) medical records. An awareness of how people report current symptoms and events is important to the clinical assessment process. In considering the information obtained, the patient's current mental state is relevant. Mistakes in comprehension, recall, and expression may also lead to erroneous reporting of information (44).

A. REASON FOR THE EVALUATION

The purpose of the evaluation influences the focus of the examination and the form of documentation. The reason for the evaluation usually includes (but may not be limited to) the chief complaint of the patient. It should be elicited in sufficient detail, including the patient's words, to permit an understanding of the duration of the complaint and the patient's specific goals for the evaluation. If the symptoms are of long standing, the reason for seeking treatment at this specific time is relevant; if the evaluation was occasioned by a hospitalization, the reason for the hospitalization is also relevant. If the patient did not initiate the evaluation, the reason another individual or entity may have requested or required it should be noted. The opinions of other parties, including family, can also assist in establishing a reason for evaluation. Under some circumstances (e.g., with psychotic or uncommunicative patients), input from others may be crucial.

B. HISTORY OF THE PRESENT ILLNESS

The history of the present problem or illness is a chronologically organized history of recent exacerbations or remissions and current symptoms or syndromes. These may involve descriptions of worries, changes in mood, suspicions, preoccupations, delusions, or hallucinatory ex-

TABLE 1. Domains of the Clinical Evaluation

Domain	Questions to Consider
Reason for the evaluation	What is the patient's chief complaint and its duration? What reason does the patient give for seeking evaluation at this specific time? What reasons are given by other involved parties (e.g., family, other health professionals) for seeking evaluation at this specific time?
History of the present illness	What symptoms is the patient experiencing (e.g., worries; preoccupations; changes in mood; suspicions; delusions or hallucinatory experiences; recent changes in sleep, appetite, libido, concentration, memory, or behavior, including suicidal or aggressive behaviors)? What is the severity of the patient's symptoms? Over what time course have these symptoms developed or fluctuated? Are associated features of specific psychiatric syndromes (i.e., pertinent positive or negative factors) present or absent during the present illness? What factors does the patient believe are precipitating, aggravating, or otherwise modifying the illness or are temporally related to its course? Did the patient receive prior treatment for this episode of illness? Are other clinicians who care for the patient available to comment?
Past psychiatric history	What is the chronology of past episodes of mental illness, regardless of whether such episodes were diagnosed or treated? What are the patient's previous sources of treatment, and what diagnoses were given? With respect to somatic therapies (e.g., medications, electroconvulsive therapy), what were the dose or treatment parameters, efficacy, side effects, treatment duration, and adherence? With respect to psychotherapy, what were the type, frequency, duration, adherence, and patient's perception of the therapeutic alliance and helpfulness of the psychotherapy? Is there a history of psychiatric hospitalization? Is there a history of suicide attempts or aggressive behaviors? Are past medical records available to consult?
History of alcohol and other substance use	What licit and illicit substances have been used, in what quantity, how frequently, and with what pattern and route of use? What functional, social, occupational, or legal consequences or self-perceived benefits of use have occurred? Has tolerance or withdrawal symptoms been noted? Has substance use been associated with psychiatric symptoms? Are family members available who could provide corroborating information about the patient's substance use and its consequences?

TABLE 1. Domains of the Clinical Evaluation *(continued)*

Domain	Questions to Consider
General medical history	What general medical illnesses are known, including hospitalizations, procedures, treatments, and medications? Are undiagnosed illnesses causing major distress or functional impairment? Does the patient engage in high-risk behaviors that would predispose him or her to a medical illness? Is the patient taking any prescribed or over-the-counter medications, herbal products, supplements, and/or vitamins? Has the patient experienced allergic reactions to or severe adverse effects of medications?
Developmental, psychosocial, and sociocultural history	What have been the most important events in the patient's life, and what were the patient's responses to them? What is the patient's history of formal education? What are the patient's cultural, religious, and spiritual beliefs, and how have these developed or changed over time? Is there a history of parental loss or divorce; physical, emotional, or sexual abuse; or exposure to other traumatic experiences? What strategies for coping has the patient used successfully during times of stress or adversity? During childhood or adolescence, did the patient have risk factors for any mental disorders? What has been the patient's capacity to maintain interpersonal relationships, and what is the patient's history of marital and other significant relationships? What is the patient's sexual history, including sexual orientation, beliefs, and practices? Does the patient have children? What past or current psychosocial stressors have affected the patient (including primary support group, social environment, education, occupation, housing, economic status, and access to health care)? What is the patient's capacity for self-care? What are the patient's sociocultural supports (e.g., family, friends, work, and religious and other community groups)? What are the patient's own interests, preferences, and values with respect to health care?
Occupational and military history	What is the patient's occupation, and what jobs has the patient held? What is the quality of the patient's work relationships? What work skills and strengths does the patient have? Is the patient unable to work due to disability? Regarding military service, what was the patient's status (volunteer, recruit, or draftee), did the patient experience combat, and did the patient suffer injury or trauma? Is the patient preparing for or adjusting to retirement?

TABLE 1. Domains of the Clinical Evaluation *(continued)*

Domain	Questions to Consider
Legal history	Does the patient have any past or current involvement with the legal system (e.g., warrants, arrests, detentions, convictions, probation, parole)? Do past or current legal problems relate to aggressive behaviors or substance intoxication? Has the patient had other significant interactions with the court system (e.g., family court, workers' compensation dispute, civil litigation, court-ordered psychiatric treatment)? Is past or current legal involvement a significant social stressor for the patient?
Family history	What information is available about general medical and psychiatric illnesses, including substance use disorders, in close relatives? Is there a family history of suicide or violent behavior? Are heritable illnesses present in family members that relate to the patient's presenting symptoms?
Review of systems	Is the patient having difficulty with sleep, appetite, eating patterns, or other vegetative symptoms, or with pain, neurological symptoms, or other systemic symptoms? Does the patient have symptoms that suggest an undiagnosed medical illness that may be causing or contributing to psychiatric symptoms? Is the patient experiencing side effects from medications or other treatments?
Physical examination	What is the appropriate timing, scope, and intensity of the exam for this patient, and who is the most appropriate examiner? Upon examination, are there abnormalities in the patient's general appearance, vital signs, neurological status, skin, or organ systems? Is more detailed physical examination necessary to assess the patient for specific diseases?
Mental status examination	What symptoms and signs of a mental disorder is the patient currently exhibiting? What are the patient's general appearance and behavior? What are the characteristics of the patient's speech? What are the patient's mood and affect, including the stability, range, congruence, and appropriateness of affect? Are the patient's thought processes coherent? Are there recurrent or persistent themes in the patient's thought processes? Are there any abnormalities of the patient's thought content (e.g., delusions, ideas of reference, overvalued ideas, ruminations, obsessions, compulsions, phobias)? Is the patient having thoughts, plans, or intentions of harming self or others? Is the patient experiencing perceptual disturbances (e.g., hallucinations, illusions, derealization, depersonalization)?

TABLE 1. Domains of the Clinical Evaluation *(continued)*

Domain	Questions to Consider
Mental status examination *(continued)*	What are the patient's sensorium and level of cognitive function (e.g., orientation, attention, concentration, registration, short- and long-term memory, fund of knowledge, level of intelligence, drawing, abstract reasoning, language, and executive functions)? What are the patient's level of insight, judgment, and capacity for abstract reasoning? What is the patient's motivation to change his or her health risk behaviors?
Functional assessment	What are the patient's functional strengths, and what is the disease severity? To what degree can the patient perform physical activities of daily living (e.g., eating, toileting, transferring, bathing, dressing)? To what degree can the patient perform instrumental activities of daily living (e.g., driving, using public transportation, taking medications as prescribed, shopping, managing finances, keeping house, communicating by mail or telephone, caring for dependents)? Would a formal assessment of functioning be useful (e.g., to document deficits or aid continued monitoring)?
Diagnostic tests	What diagnostic tests are necessary to establish or exclude a diagnosis, aid in the choice of treatment, or monitor treatment effects or side effects?
Information derived from the interview process	Are symptoms minimized or exaggerated by the patient or others? Does the patient appear to provide accurate information? Do particular questions evoke hesitation or signs of discomfort? Is the patient able to communicate about emotional issues? How does the patient respond to the psychiatrist's comments and behaviors?

periences as well as recent changes in sleep, appetite, libido, concentration, memory, or behavior, including suicidal or aggressive behaviors. Information gathered on the pertinent positive and pertinent negative features of the history of present illness will vary with the patient's presenting symptoms or syndrome. Temporal features relating to the onset or exacerbation of symptoms may also be relevant (e.g., onset after use of exogenous hormones, herbal products, or licit or illicit substances; variation in symptoms with the menstrual cycle; postpartum onset). Also pertinent are factors that the patient and other informants believe to be precipitating, aggravating, or otherwise modifying the illness. Available details of previous treatments and the patient's response to those treatments will be delineated as part of the history of present illness. If the patient was or is in treatment with another clinician, the effects of that relationship on the current illness, including transference and countertransference issues, are considered. Input from members of a clinical team who care for the patient can be very helpful (Section IV.A.6). For patients seen on medical-surgical units, it is important to consider the history of both the present medical-surgical illness and the present psychiatric illness (45).

C. PAST PSYCHIATRIC HISTORY

The past psychiatric history includes a chronological summary of all past episodes of mental illness, including substance use disorders, and treatment. The summary includes prior hospitalizations; suicide attempts, aborted suicide attempts, or other self-destructive behavior; psychiatric syndromes not formally diagnosed at the time; previously established diagnoses; treatments offered; and responses to and satisfaction with treatment. With respect to psychotherapy, it is important to ascertain the type (e.g., psychodynamic, cognitive, behavioral, supportive), format (e.g., group, individual, couple), frequency, duration, patient's perception of the alliance, and adherence. With respect to medications, the dose, efficacy, side effects, treatment duration, and adherence are important to ascertain while understanding that reporting errors are more likely to occur when treatment involved more than one medication (46). With respect to other somatic therapies such as electroconvulsive therapy, information on the number of treatment sessions, treatment course duration, technical parameters, efficacy, and side effects is similarly useful to obtain. When past medical records are available and readily accessible, it is important that they be consulted for ancillary information.

The chronological summary also delineates the most recent periods of stability as well as episodes when the patient was functionally impaired or seriously distressed by mental or behavioral symptoms, even if no formal treatment occurred. Such episodes frequently can be identified by asking the patient about the past use of psychotropic medications prescribed by other clinicians and otherwise unexplained episodes of social or occupational disability.

D. HISTORY OF SUBSTANCE USE

The psychoactive substance use history includes past and present use of both licit and illicit psychoactive substances, including but not limited to alcohol, caffeine, nicotine, marijuana, cocaine, opiates, sedative-hypnotic agents, stimulants, solvents, MDMA (methylenedioxymethamphetamine), androgenic steroids, and hallucinogens (47). Relevant information includes the quantity and frequency of use and route of administration; the pattern of use (e.g., episodic versus continual, solitary versus social); functional, interpersonal, or legal consequences of use; tolerance and withdrawal phenomena; any temporal association between substance use and other present psychiatric illnesses; and any self-perceived benefits of use. It is also important to inquire about prior treatments for substance use disorders as well as about periods of abstinence, including their duration, recentness, and factors that aided in sobriety or contributed to relapse. Obtaining an accurate substance use history often involves a gradual, nonconfrontational approach to inquiry that involves asking multiple questions to seek the same information in different ways and using slang terms for drugs, patterns of use, and drug effects. Patients are particularly likely to underestimate their level of substance abuse and their related functional impairments; corroboration by other family members is useful when possible. It is also helpful to inquire about patterns of substance use by others within the family or living constellation. For more extensive discussion of the assessment of substance use, abuse, and dependence, the reader is referred to the Center for Substance Abuse Treatment's *Assessment and Treatment of Patients With Coexisting Mental Illness and Alcohol and Other Drug Abuse* (48) and APA's *Practice Guideline for the Treatment of Patients With Substance Use Disorders* (49).

E. GENERAL MEDICAL HISTORY

The general medical history includes available information on known general medical illnesses (e.g., hospitalizations, procedures, treatments, and medications), allergies or drug sensitivities, and undiagnosed health problems that have caused the patient major distress or functional impairment. This includes history of any episodes of important physical injury or trauma; sexual and reproductive history; and any history of endocrinological, infectious (including but not limited to HIV, tuberculosis, and hepatitis C) (50), neurological disorders, sleep disorders (including sleep apnea), and conditions causing pain and discomfort. Of particular importance is a specific history regarding diseases and symptoms of diseases that have a high prevalence among individuals with the patient's demographic characteristics and background—for example, infectious diseases in users of intravenous drugs or pulmonary and cardiovascular disease in people who smoke. Information regarding all current and recent medications, including hormones (e.g., birth control pills, androgens), over-the-counter medications, herbal supplements, vitamins, complementary and alternative medical treatments, and medication side effects, is part of the general medical history. With all aspects of the general medical history, obtaining corroborating information (e.g., from medical records, treating clinicians, family) can be helpful, since ordinary errors in comprehension, recall, and expression can lead to errors in patient reports (51).

F. DEVELOPMENTAL, PSYCHOSOCIAL, AND SOCIOCULTURAL HISTORY

The personal history reviews the stages of the patient's life, with special attention to perinatal events, delays in physical or psychological development, formal educational history, academic performance, and patterns of response to normal life transitions and major life events, including parental loss or divorce; physical, emotional, or sexual abuse; and other trauma such as exposure to political repression, war, or a natural disaster (52–55). The childhood and adolescent history of risk factors for later psychiatric disorders (Table 2) may also be relevant. History of adaptive skills and strengths to overcome challenges is also relevant.

The patient's capacity to maintain stable and gratifying interpersonal relationships should be noted, including the patient's capacities for attachment, trust, and intimacy. A sexual history is obtained and includes consideration of sexual orientation and practices, past sexual experiences (including unwanted experiences), and cultural beliefs about sex (54). The psychosocial history also determines the patient's past and present levels of interpersonal functioning in family and social roles (e.g., marriage, parenting) (56–58). This includes a delineation of the patient's history of marital and other significant relationships. For patients with children (including biological, foster, adopted, or stepchildren), the psychosocial history will include information about these individuals and their relationship to the patient.

As part of the psychosocial history, past or current stressors are assessed and include the categories on axis IV of DSM-IV-TR: primary support group, social environment (e.g., discrimination and acculturation), education, occupation, housing, economic status, and access to health care. Specific information obtained in evaluating psychosocial stressors may include details about patients' living arrangements, access to transportation, sources of income, insurance or prescription coverage, and past or current involvement with social agencies. Assessment of the patient's self-care functioning may also include consideration of exercise behavior and money management skills, including gambling behavior.

The sociocultural history delineates the patient's migration history and past and current sociocultural context of supports and stressors as well as other important cultural and religious influences on the patient's life (59). Emphasis is given to relationships, both familial and nonfamilial, and to religion and spirituality that may give meaning and purpose to the patient's life and provide support, as described in the DSM-IV-TR Outline for Cultural Formulation (described in more detail in Section IV.B.1.a).

Patients present for a psychiatric evaluation with their own interests, preferences, and value systems pertaining to health care practice, and these are another important part of the sociocultural history. They may involve cultural factors and explanatory models of illness that affect attitudes, expectations, and preferences for professional and popular treatments, as described in the DSM-IV-TR Outline for Cultural Formulation and the 2004 Core Competencies of the American Board of Psychiatry and Neurology (60). Also important to the assessment and treatment process are other domains such as existential, moral, and interpersonal values and social

TABLE 2. Questions About Childhood Developmental History for Which Affirmative Answers May Indicate Increased Risk for Psychiatric Illness

Did the patient lose a parent at an early age?
Was there unusual or excessive separation anxiety during childhood or adolescence?
Were there significant problems with sleep?
Were there eating disturbances?
Were there problems making or keeping friends?
Was severe shyness a problem, including when interacting in peer groups?
Were there problems with being bullied or bullying?
Were there frequent disciplinary problems in school?
Were there serious difficulties with temper?
Were there many school absences for medical problems or any other problems?
Were there any delays in learning to read, write, or do math?
Were there serious problems paying attention, finishing school work, or completing homework?
Did the above problems lead to grade retention or special education intervention?

influences such as school, church, work, and community or other agencies. Attending to these factors plays a crucial role in developing a therapeutic alliance, negotiating a treatment plan, determining the outcome criteria for successful treatment, and enhancing treatment adherence. Belief systems may also influence the handling of privacy and confidentiality during the evaluation as well as influence the type and amount of information disclosed as part of any informed consent process. In addition, patients' value systems are relevant to clinical considerations at important life transitions (e.g., job and career transitions, marital transitions, genetic counseling before or during pregnancy, end-of-life planning).

G. OCCUPATIONAL AND MILITARY HISTORY

The occupational history describes the sequence and duration of jobs held by the patient, reasons for job changes, and the patient's current or most recent employment, including quality of work relationships and whether current or recent jobs have involved shift work, a noxious or perilous environment, exposure to hazardous materials, unusual physical or psychological stress, or injury or exposure to trauma while in the military or hazardous occupations (e.g., fire and rescue, law enforcement). Work skills and strengths are noted, as well as the quality of the patient's relationships with co-workers and work supervisors. Past or current experience with the workers' compensation system and patterns of recovery or disability following episodes of illness are also determined (61–64). When appropriate, a history of preparation for and adjustment to retirement is included.

Relevant data about military experience include volunteer, recruited, or draftee status; reasons for rejection at time of enlistment (if relevant); combat exposure (if any); awards; disciplinary actions; and discharge status.

H. LEGAL HISTORY

The legal history includes a description of past or current involvement with the legal system (65). This may include interactions with the police without formal arrest as well as involvement with the juvenile or criminal justice system (e.g., arrests, detentions including jail or prison confinement). Individuals may be on probation or parole or may have pending court appearances or active warrants for arrest that will influence treatment planning. A history of legal problems relating to aggressive behaviors or occurring in the context of substance intoxication is similarly relevant. Other past or current interactions with the court system (e.g., family court, workers' compensation, civil litigation, court-ordered psychiatric treatment) may serve as significant stressors for the patient and are also important to address (55, 66).

I. FAMILY HISTORY

The family history includes available information about the patient's family constellation and the strength of relationships with family members. Information obtained about close family members, including parents and, if applicable, siblings, spouse, and children, will include general information (e.g., current age or age at time of death, position in sibship, occupation), quality of relationship to the patient, and health status. General medical and psychiatric illness in close relatives is noted, including disorders that may be familial or may strongly affect the family environment. A history of adoption or foster care or disruptions in the family environment because of divorce, remarriage, prolonged absences of family members (e.g., occupational absences, hospitalization, incarceration), or deaths may be useful to elicit. Family history information will also consist of any history of psychiatric hospitalizations, illness, or significant symptoms, including suicide and attempted suicide in first- and second-degree relatives. More specific questions are important to ask depending on the patient's clinical presentation, given the heritability of psychosis; mood disorders; anxiety disorders; cognitive disorders; learning disabilities; developmental disabilities, including autism, hyperactivity, or attention deficit disorder; substance use disorders; and antisocial behavior. For family members who have experienced psychiatric symptoms, it is helpful to learn the treatment received and their response to treatment. It is also important to determine first- and second-degree relatives' history of medical disorders (67), particularly those with relevance to psychiatric illness and treatment, such as cardiac, neurological, and endocrine disorders. If family health problems are current, this may contribute psychological or financial stresses for the patient.

Construction of a formal pedigree or genogram is often helpful in delineating family relationships and identifying a family history of illness. The web sites of the American Medical Association (68), the American Society of Human Genetics (69), and the March of Dimes (70) provide additional details on the drawing of pedigrees.

J. REVIEW OF SYSTEMS

The review of systems includes current symptoms not already identified in the history of the present illness. If not already addressed in the history of present illness, sleep, appetite, eating patterns, vegetative symptoms of mood disorder, pain and discomfort, systemic symptoms such as fever and fatigue, and neurological symptoms are also relevant. In addition, common symptoms of diseases for which the patient is known to be at particular risk because of historical, genetic, environmental, or demographic factors are an important part of the review of systems. Special attention should be given to typical side effects observed with prescribed or over-the-counter medications and other treatments, including complementary or alternative therapies, that the patient is receiving.

K. PHYSICAL EXAMINATION

Evaluation of the patient's general medical status necessitates that a physical examination be performed. Although the process of the physical examination is described more fully in Section IV.A.5, specific elements assessed as part of the physical examination may include the following:

1. General appearance, height, weight, body mass index (BMI), and nutritional status
2. Vital signs
3. Head and neck, heart, lungs, abdomen, and extremities
4. Neurological status, including cranial nerves, motor and sensory function, gait, coordination, muscle tone, reflexes, and involuntary movements
5. Skin, with special attention to any stigmata of trauma, self-injury, or drug use
6. Any body area or organ system that is specifically mentioned in the history of the present illness or review of systems or that is relevant to determining the current status of problems mentioned in the past medical history

Additional items may be added to the examination to address specific diagnostic concerns or to screen a member of a clinical population at risk for a specific disease. For example, an individual with mental retardation might be assessed for the physical characteristics of a recognized syndrome.

L. MENTAL STATUS EXAMINATION

The purpose of the mental status examination is to obtain evidence of symptoms and signs of mental disorders, including dangerousness to self and others, that are present at the time of the interview. Further, evidence is obtained regarding the patient's insight, judgment, and capacity for abstract reasoning to inform decisions about treatment strategy and the choice of an appropriate treatment setting. Thus, the mental status examination is a systematic collection of data based on observation of the patient's behavior while the patient is in the psychiatrist's view during, before, and after the interview. During the mental status examination, the patient might also mention past symptoms and signs, but these should be recorded under the history of the present illness.

Responses to specific questions are an important part of the mental status examination (71, 72), particularly in the assessment of cognition. Consequently, in recording the findings of the mental status examination, it is useful to include examples that illustrate the clinical observations. For example, it would be preferable to note that the patient exhibited poor judgment in precipitously attempting to remove his intravenous line rather than simply describing the patient's judgment as impaired.

Although its precise organization may vary, the mental status examination typically contains the following elements:

1. *Appearance and general behavior.* In describing the patient's appearance, factors such as approximate age, body habitus, dress, grooming, hygiene, and distinguishing features (e.g., scars, tattoos) may be noted. The patient's general behavior, level of distress, degree of eye contact, and attitude toward the interviewer are also considered.
2. *Motor activity.* The patient's level of psychomotor activity is noted, as is the presence of any gait abnormalities or purposeless, repetitive, or unusual postures or movements (e.g., tremors, dyskinesias, akathisia, mannerisms, tics, stereotypies, catatonic posturing, echopraxia, apparent responses to hallucinations).
3. *Speech.* Characteristics of the patient's speech are described and may include consideration of rate, rhythm, volume, amount, accent, inflection, fluency, and articulation.
4. *Mood and affect.* The patient's expressions of mood and affect are noted. Although the use and definitions of the terms *mood* and *affect* vary, mood is typically viewed as referring to the patient's internal, subjective, and more sustained emotional state, whereas affect relates to the patient's externally observable and more changeable emotional state (71, 73). Affect is often described in terms of its range, intensity, stability, appropriateness, and congruence with the topic being discussed in the interview.

5. *Thought processes.* Features of the patient's associations and flow of ideas are described, such as vagueness, incoherence, circumstantiality, tangentiality, neologisms, perseveration, flight of ideas, loose or idiosyncratic associations, and self-contradictory statements.
6. *Thought content.* The patient's current thought content is assessed by noting the patient's spontaneously expressed worries, concerns, thoughts, and impulses, as well as through specific questioning about commonly observed symptoms of specific mental disorders. These symptoms include delusions (e.g., erotomania or delusions of persecution, passivity, grandeur, infidelity, infestation, poverty, somatic illness, guilt, worthlessness, thought insertion, thought withdrawal, or thought broadcasting), ideas of reference, overvalued ideas, ruminations, obsessions, compulsions, and phobias. Assessment of suicidal, homicidal, aggressive, or self-injurious thoughts, feelings, or impulses is essential for determining the patient's level of risk to self or others as part of the clinical formulation. If such features are present, details are elicited regarding their intensity and specificity, when they occur, and what prevents the patient from acting on them (11, 74–79).
7. *Perceptual disturbances.* Hallucinations (i.e., a perception in the absence of a stimulus) and illusions (i.e., an erroneous perception in the presence of a stimulus) may occur in any sensory modality (e.g., auditory, visual, tactile, olfactory, gustatory). Other perceptual disturbances that patients may experience include depersonalization and derealization.
8. *Sensorium and cognition.* Systematic assessment of cognitive functions is an essential part of the general psychiatric evaluation, although the level of detail necessary and the appropriateness of particular formal tests will depend on the purpose of the evaluation and the psychiatrist's clinical judgment. Evaluation of the patient's sensorium includes a description of the level of consciousness and its stability. Elements of the patient's cognitive status that may be assessed include orientation (e.g., person, place, time, situation), attention and concentration, and memory (e.g., registration, short-term, long-term). Arithmetic calculations may be used to assess concentration or knowledge; other aspects of the patient's fund of knowledge may also be assessed as appropriate to sociocultural and educational background. Additional aspects of the cognitive examination may include assessment of level of intelligence, language functions (e.g., naming, comprehension, repetition, reading, writing), drawing (e.g., copying a figure or drawing a clock face), abstract reasoning (e.g., explaining similarities or interpreting proverbs), and executive functions (e.g., list making, inhibiting impulsive answers, resisting distraction, recognizing contradictions).
9. *Insight.* The patient's insight into his or her current situation is typically assessed by inquiring about the patient's awareness of any problems and their implications. Patients may or may not recognize that psychosis or other symptoms may reflect an underlying illness or that their behavior affects their relationships with other individuals. They also may or may not recognize the potential benefits of treatment.

    Another element of insight involves the patient's motivation to change his or her health risk behaviors. Such motivation often fluctuates over time from denial and resistance to ambivalence to commitment, a sequence that has been referred to as "stages of change" (80–82). The stages, which are not necessarily discrete, have been labeled *precontemplation* (denial, minimization); *contemplation* (musing or thinking about doing something); *preparation* (actually getting ready to do something); *action* (implementing concrete actions to deal with the problem); and *maintenance* (acting to ensure that the changes are maintained) (83). Patients who are not quite ready to change may vacillate about modifying their behaviors before actually committing to change and acting on it. Assessing stages of change as part of the evaluative process leads to stage-appropriate educational and therapeutic interventions that attempt to help patients move to more adaptive stages in a patient-centered manner (84–86).

10. *Judgment.* The quality of the patient's judgment has sometimes been assessed by asking for the patient's responses to hypothetical situations (e.g., smelling smoke in a theater). However, in assessing judgment, it is generally more helpful to learn about the patient's responses and decision making in terms of his or her own self-care, interactions, and other aspects of his or her recent or current situation and behavior. If poor judgment is present, a more detailed explication of the patient's decision-making processes may help differentiate the potential causes of this impairment.

IV. EVALUATION PROCESS

A. METHODS OF OBTAINING INFORMATION

1. Patient interview

The psychiatrist's primary assessment tool is the direct face-to-face interview of the patient. Evaluations based solely on review of records and interviews of persons close to the patient are inherently limited by a lack of the patient's perspective. Furthermore, the clinical interview provides the psychiatrist with a sample of the patient's interpersonal behavior and emotional processes. It can either support or qualify diagnostic inferences from the history and can also aid in prognosis and treatment planning. Important information can be derived by observing the patient's general style of relating, the ways in which the patient minimizes or exaggerates certain aspects of his or her history, and whether particular questions appear to evoke hesitation or signs of discomfort. Additional observations concern the patient's ability to communicate about emotional issues, the defense mechanisms the patient uses when discussing emotionally important topics, and the patient's responses to the psychiatrist's comments and to other behavior, such as the psychiatrist's handling of interruptions or time limits.

The interview should be done in a manner that facilitates the patient's telling of his or her story, while simultaneously obtaining the necessary information. Time constraints need to be considered and adequate time allowed for the interview. High-priority tasks include an assessment of the patient's safety and the identification of signs, symptoms, or disorders requiring urgent treatment.

Opening with a discussion of the purpose of the interview offers the patient an understanding of the process. Empirical studies of the interview process suggest that the most comprehensive and accurate information emerges from a combination of 1) open-ended questioning with empathic listening and 2) structured inquiry about specific events and symptoms (87–92). When the purpose is a general evaluation, beginning with open-ended, empathic inquiry about the patient's concerns usually is best. Attention to the patient's most pressing concerns, whenever possible, will improve the therapeutic alliance and is likely to facilitate increased patient cooperation; other inquiries may be more limited initially in the service of the alliance. Patient satisfaction with open-ended inquiry is greatest when the psychiatrist provides feedback to the patient at multiple points during the interview. Structured, systematic questioning has been shown to be especially helpful in eliciting information about substance use and traumatic life events and in ascertaining the presence or absence of specific symptoms and signs of particular mental disorders (93–102) (Section IV.A.3).

Throughout the interview, useful clinical information is obtained by being sensitive to issues of development, culture, race, ethnicity, primary language, health literacy, disabilities, gender, sexual orientation, familial/genetic patterns, religious and spiritual beliefs, social class, and physical and social environment influencing the patient's symptoms and behavior. Respectful evaluation involves an empathic, nonjudgmental attitude and appropriate responses concerning the patient's cultural identity, his or her own explanation of illness and treatment pathways, sociocultural stressors and supports, and modes of interpersonal communication, both verbal and nonverbal. An awareness of one's possible biases or prejudices about patients from different subcultures and an understanding of the limitations of one's knowledge and skills in working with such patients may help one determine when it is advisable to consult with a clinician who has expertise concerning a particular subculture (103–105).

a) Use of interpreters in the interview

When available, professionally trained interpreters with mental health experience should be used for encounters involving patients with limited English proficiency and those who are deaf or have severely limited hearing and who prefer to communicate using sign language (106, 107). Bilingual and bicultural staff may also be helpful (108). With cooperative patients, over-the-phone language interpretation services can be used when other professionally trained interpreters are unavailable, although establishing rapport with the patient may be more difficult. Family members, community members, or friends should not be used unless the patient refuses to use the professional interpreter or under emergency circumstances, in which case this should be noted in the patient record. The interpreter should be instructed to translate the patient's own words and to avoid paraphrasing except as needed to translate the correct meaning of idioms and other culture-specific expressions (109–111).

b) Interviews with agitated or aggressive individuals

When evaluating individuals who are agitated or aggressive, the psychiatrist needs to give consideration to the patient interview as well as to his or her own safety (13, 77, 112–116). Establishing the presence of backup personnel and choosing an appropriate space in which to conduct the interview are useful preparations before meeting with an agitated or aggressive patient. Because such individuals may become more agitated if they feel trapped within a small room or are too closely positioned to the interviewer, a distance of several arms' length from the patient, with both psychiatrist and patient having access to the door, is generally optimal. A safe office environment should not contain potentially dangerous objects (e.g., decorative items), and the clinician should avoid clothing that can be used against him or her (e.g., neckties, scarves, prominent dangling earrings). Depending on the configuration of the office or interview room and its proximity to other staff, a mechanism for summoning assistance (e.g., a panic button) may also be indicated.

During the interview, a nonconfrontational and straightforward approach is often most effective. Attending to the patient's comfort, using reflective or active listening techniques, and showing respect for the patient's feelings and stated concerns may aid in establishing rapport. The key to calming an aggressive patient is affect management. Patients who are affectively aroused will need to ventilate their feelings, and the clinician should allow the patient to tell his or her own story. Logical or rational responses to an affectively flooded individual may further inflame the patient. Affect management involves acknowledging the patient's affect, validating the affect when appropriate, and encouraging the patient to talk about his or her feelings (116).

In some circumstances, it may be appropriate to set limits (e.g., noting that aggressive behavior cannot be permitted) while simultaneously emphasizing the need to attend to the safety of the patient and others. Throughout the interview, the clinician needs to be alert for signs that the patient's agitation is escalating (e.g., increased body movements or pacing, clenched fists, verbal threats, or increasing verbal volume); such signs may indicate a need to adjust the interview style or timing. At times, it will be best to postpone in-depth history taking or discussion of distressing topics that are not germane to the patient's current presentation.

In some instances, administration of psychotropic medications or judicious use of seclusion or restraint may be necessary to enhance the safety of the patient and others (114) or to permit essential physical examination, laboratory studies, or other diagnostic assessment. Reliance on such measures should be justified by the urgency of obtaining the diagnostic information and should be in compliance with applicable laws and regulations. The psychiatrist should consider how any special circumstances of the interview or examination may influence clinical findings. When the patient is able to cooperate, parts of the examination that cannot be completed or that are significantly influenced by the use of medication, seclusion, or restraint should be repeated if possible.

Guidelines for reducing the use of seclusion and restraint while at the same time maintaining the safety of patients and staff are available in a report developed by the APA with the American Psychiatric Nurses Association and the National Association of Psychiatric Health Systems (117). Recommendations of the report include assessing for anger management problems, identifying risk factors (e.g., pregnancy, asthma, head or spinal injury) before using restraint, identifying triggers, involving patients in treatment planning, asking patients about past experiences of seclusion and restraint, involving family, and documenting interventions attempted before using seclusion or restraint.

2. Use of collateral sources

Family members, other important people in the patient's life, and records of prior medical and psychiatric treatment are frequently useful sources of information. Collateral information is particularly important when patients have impaired insight, including when patients have substance use disorders or cognitive impairment, and is essential for treatment planning when patients require a high level of assistance or supervision because of impaired function or unstable behavior. Family members and others who know the patient well may provide important information about the patient's personality before the onset of illness, since the patient's own account may be unduly influenced by his or her mental state. Collateral sources of information may also provide essential information about the illness course (Section III.C), the current symptoms and behavior (Section III.B), and the reasons for the evaluation (Section III.A). The extent of the collateral interviews and the extent of prior record review should be commensurate with the purpose of the evaluation, the complexity of the clinical presentation, and the diagnostic and therapeutic goals. For example, in an acute inpatient or emergency setting, collateral information may be crucial to developing an understanding of the patient's clinical condition, whereas in long-term outpatient psychotherapy the impact on the treatment process of obtaining collateral information from family or others needs to be considered. Except when immediate safety concerns are paramount, the confidentiality of the patient should be respected. At the same time, it is permissible for the psychiatrist to listen to information provided by family members and other important people in the patient's life, as long as confidential information is not provided to the informant (Sections I.A, I.B, II.C, and V.A).

3. Use of structured interviews and rating scales, including functional assessments

Structured interviews, standardized data forms, questionnaires, and rating scales can be useful tools for diagnostic assessment and evaluation of treatment outcome. Table 3, while not all-inclusive, lists many of the common structured instruments in use (see also the CD-ROM from APA's *Handbook of Psychiatric Measures* [118]). Such structured instruments may be used as components for establishing a diagnosis, measuring social or occupational function, or monitoring changes in symptom severity or side effects over time during treatment.

Although most commonly used in psychiatric research, rating scales may also help psychiatrists structure a thorough line of questioning. In addition, self-report scales may be valuable in opening communication with patients about their symptoms, feelings, or experiences. At the

TABLE 3. Examples of Clinical Rating Scales

Scale	Administration (Time)	Clinical Use	Reference	Availability
Quality of life				
Quality of Life Enjoyment & Satisfaction Questionnaire (Q-LES-Q)	Self-administered questionnaire; short (16-item; 5 min) or long (60-item; 15 min) format	Assessment of degree of enjoyment and satisfaction in various areas of daily life	Endicott J, Nee J, Harrison W, et al: Quality of Life Enjoyment and Satisfaction Questionnaire: a new scale. Psychopharmacol Bull 29:321–326, 1993	Jean Endicott, Ph.D.; Dept. of Research Assessment and Training, New York State Psychiatric Institute, Unit 123; 1051 Riverside Drive; New York, NY 10032; ph 212-543-5536
Mental health status and functioning				
Clinical Global Impression (CGI) Scale	Clinician-rated scale (1–2 min after clinical information is obtained)	Global assessment of response to medication treatment	Guy W, Bonato RR (eds): Manual for the ECDEU Assessment Battery, revised 2nd ed. Chevy Chase, Md, National Institute of Mental Health, 1970, pp 12.1–12.6	Guy W: ECDEU Assessment Manual for Psychopharmacology, revised ed. Washington, DC, US Department of Health, Education, and Welfare, 1976; APA (2000) *Handbook of Psychiatric Measures*
Global Assessment of Functioning (GAF) Scale	Clinician-rated scale, ranked 0–100 (1–2 min after clinical information is obtained)	Assessment of patient functioning, monitoring of change, and selection of patients suitable for short-term treatment	American Psychiatric Association: DSM-IV-TR	DSM-IV-TR
Social and Occupational Functioning Assessment Scale (SOFAS)	Clinician-rated scale, ranked 0–100 (1–2 min after clinical information is obtained)	Assessment of patient social and occupational functioning and monitoring of change	American Psychiatric Association: DSM-IV-TR	DSM-IV-TR

TABLE 3. Examples of Clinical Rating Scales *(continued)*

Scale	Administration (Time)	Clinical Use	Reference	Availability
Adverse effects				
Abnormal Involuntary Movement Scale (AIMS)	Observer-rated 12-item anchored scale (5–10 min)	Assessment of patients who may have involuntary movement disorders (from antipsychotic medications) and may have tardive dyskinesia	Guy W (ed): ECDEU Assessment Manual for Psychopharmacology, revised ed. DHEW Publ No ADM 76-338. Washington, DC, US Department of Health, Education, and Welfare, 1976	Guy 1976; APA (2000) *Handbook of Psychiatric Measures*
Rating Scale for Extrapyramidal Side Effects or Simpson-Angus Extrapyramidal Symptom Rating Scale	Observer-rated 10-item anchored scale (10 min)	Assessment of dose-limiting side effects when antipsychotic medications are initiated, titrated, and monitored and effectiveness of anticholinergic or other agents in the treatment of extrapyramidal side effects	Simpson GM, Angus JWS: A rating scale for extrapyramidal side effects. Acta Psychiatr Scand Suppl 1970; 212:11–19	APA (2000) *Handbook of Psychiatric Measures*
Cognitive disorders				
Delirium Rating Scale Revised–98 (DRS–R98)	Clinician-administered structured exam (15–30 min)	Assessment of a broad range of delirium symptoms: the 16-item scale can be used to diagnose delirium; the 13-item severity subscale can be used to rate symptom severity	Trzepacz PT et al: Validation of the Delirium Rating Scale—Revised–98: comparison with the Delirium Rating Scale and the Cognitive Test for Delirium. J Neuropsychiatry Clin Neurosci 2001; 13:229–242; erratum, 2001; 13:433	© Paula T. Trzepacz, M.D., Lilly Research Laboratories, Indianapolis, IN 46285; PTT@lilly.com
Mini-Mental State Examination (MMSE)	Clinician-administered 30-item structured scale (5–10 min)	Detecting and tracking the progression of cognitive impairment associated with neurogenerative diseases	Folstein MF et al: "Mini-Mental State": a practical method for grading the cognitive state of patients for the clinician. J Psychiatr Res 1975; 12:189–198	Administrator of the Mini-Mental LLC, 31 St. James Avenue, Suite 1, Boston, MA 02116; ph 617-587-4215; APA (2000) *Handbook of Psychiatric Measures*

TABLE 3. Examples of Clinical Rating Scales *(continued)*

Scale	Administration (Time)	Clinical Use	Reference	Availability
Alcohol use disorders				
CAGE Questionnaire	Self-report or observer-rated 4-item questionnaire (<1 min)	Screening for alcohol problems	Ewing JA: Detecting alcoholism: The CAGE questionnaire. JAMA 1984; 252: 1905–1907	APA (2000) *Handbook of Psychiatric Measures*
Mood disorders				
Beck Depression Inventory, 2nd Revision (BDI-II)	Self-report or observer-rated 21-item questionnaire, ranked on a 0–3 scale (5–10 min)	Assessment of severity of depressive symptoms in patients with diagnosed depressive illness and monitoring of treatment effects	Beck AT et al: An inventory for measuring depression. Arch Gen Psychiatry 1961; 4:561–571	Harcourt Assessment, Inc., 19500 Bulverde Road, San Antonio, TX 78259; ph 800-211-8378; http://harcourt assessment.com/haiweb/ Cultures/en-US/default.htm
Hamilton Depression Rating Scale (Ham-D)	Observer-rated 21- or 17-item checklist, ranked on a 0–4 or 0–2 scale (15–20 min)	Assessment of severity of depressive symptoms in patients with primary depressive illness and monitoring changes with treatment	Hamilton M: A rating scale for depression. J Neurol Neurosurg Psychiatry 1960; 23:56–62	Guy W: ECDEU Assessment Manual for Psychopharmacology, revised ed. DHEW Publ No ADM 76-338. Washington, DC, US Department of Health, Education, and Welfare, 1976
Quick Inventory of Depression Symptomatology—Self-Report (QIDS-SR)	Self-report 16-item scale including the nine domains of major depressive disorder (5–7 min)	Assessment of depressive symptom severity and symptomatic changes in a time efficient manner to gauge effects of treatment	Rush AJ et al: The 16-Item Quick Inventory of Depressive Symptomatology (QIDS), Clinician Rating (QIDS-C), and Self-Report (QIDS-SR): a psychometric evaluation in patients with chronic major depression. Biol Psychiatry 2003; 54:573–583; erratum, 2003; 54:585	Trivedi MH et al: The Inventory of Depressive Symptomatology, Clinician Rating (IDS-C) and Self-Report (IDS-SR), and the Quick Inventory of Depressive Symptomatology, Clinician Rating (QIDS-C) and Self-Report (QIDS-SR) in public sector patients with mood disorders, a psychometric evaluation. Psychol Med 2004; 34:73–82

TABLE 4. Tests That May Be Indicated as Part of a Psychiatric Evaluation

Test	Notes
Basic laboratory tests (e.g., complete blood count; blood chemistries, including lipid profile, B_{12}, folate; urinalysis)	Used to screen for general medical conditions or provide baseline measures prior to treatment. Recommended frequency of screening may vary with health status and with specific ongoing treatments (e.g., second-generation antipsychotics, lithium).
Medication levels	Used to monitor therapeutic levels of medications.
Pregnancy test	Some psychiatric conditions and treatments may entail risks to a pregnant woman or her fetus.
Fasting blood glucose or hemoglobin A1c	Used to diagnose diabetes or help determine risk. Patients prescribed second-generation antipsychotics may be at increased risk of developing diabetes.
Lyme serology, syphilis serology, HIV test	May assist in evaluation of cognitive and behavioral changes. Individuals with behavioral problems such as impulsivity or drug use may be at increased risk for HIV infection.
Thyroid function tests	May be important for patients with suspected mood disorder, anxiety disorder, or dementia. Used to monitor lithium effects.
Toxicology screen, blood alcohol level	Used to screen for substance use or abuse. Individuals with a mental disorder are at increased risk for substance abuse.
Electrocardiogram	Used to assess effects of medications that may influence cardiac conduction (e.g., tricyclic antidepressants, some antipsychotics). May also be indicated depending on age and health status.
Chest X-ray	Used to diagnose cardiopulmonary disorders (e.g., pneumonia, tuberculosis) that may contribute to delirium. May also be part of a pre-ECT evaluation depending on age and health status.
Imaging studies	Structural (e.g., computed tomography [CT], magnetic resonance imaging [MRI]) and functional (e.g., positron emission tomography [PET], single photon emission computed tomography [SPECT], electroencephalogram [EEG], functional magnetic resonance imaging [fMRI]) studies may indicate regional brain abnormalities related to a psychiatric illness and its management.
Lumbar puncture	Used to diagnose central nervous system infection (e.g., meningitis, herpes, toxoplasmosis, syphilis, Lyme disease). May be important for differential diagnosis of delirium.
Polysomnography	Used to diagnose sleep disorders, including sleep apnea. May be important for differential diagnosis of depression, psychosis, or other cognitive or behavioral changes.
Psychological testing	May be requested when cognitive deficits are suspected or there is need to grade for severity or progression of symptoms over time. May also be helpful in establishing a diagnosis (e.g., dementia, mental retardation) or in delineating specific deficits that affect thought processes, treatment, or vocational planning.

persist in otherwise responsive depression (163), and working memory may remain impaired in schizophrenia independent of response of positive and negative symptoms (149, 164). Thus, for some patients, a better understanding of persistent neuropsychological impairments can aid in treatment and vocational planning.

5. Physical examination

An understanding of the patient's general medical condition is important in order to 1) properly assess the patient's psychiatric symptoms and their potential cause, 2) determine the patient's need for general medical care, and 3) choose among psychiatric treatments that can be affected by the patient's general medical status (16, 22, 25, 26, 34, 144, 165, 166). The psychiatrist also ensures that a recent medical workup with appropriate laboratory tests and monitoring is performed. The psychiatrist should be informed about the results of the medical workup and incorporate this information into the evaluation. The psychiatrist's close involvement in the patient's general medical evaluation and ongoing care can also improve the patient's care by promoting cooperation, facilitating follow-up, and permitting prompt reexamination of symptomatic areas when symptoms change.

The physical examination may be performed by the psychiatrist, another physician, or a medically trained clinician. Considerations influencing the decision of whether the psychiatrist will personally perform the physical examination include potential effects on the psychiatrist-patient relationship, the purposes of the evaluation, and the complexity of the medical condition of the patient. The timing, scope, and intensity will vary according to clinical circumstances. For example, the physical examination of an otherwise healthy patient with paranoia, or the genital-rectal examination of a patient with a history of sexual abuse, may be deferred to a more appropriate time and setting.

In most circumstances, the physical examination should be chaperoned. Particular caution is warranted in the physical examination of persons with histories of physical or sexual abuse or with other features that could increase the possibility of the patient's being distressed as a result of the examination (e.g., a patient with an erotic or paranoid transference to the psychiatrist). All but limited examinations of such patients should be chaperoned.

6. Work with multidisciplinary teams

In many settings, it has become commonplace for the care of psychiatric patients to draw on the expertise of multidisciplinary teams. In the evaluation phase of care, other members of the clinical team (e.g., nurses, psychologists, occupational therapists, social workers, case managers, peer counselors, chaplains) may gather data or perform discipline-specific assessments. The psychiatrist responsible for the patient's care reviews and integrates these assessments into the psychiatric evaluation of the patient and works with other members of the multidisciplinary team in developing and implementing a plan of care.

The opportunity to improve systematic observations of patients' behavior by staff is an advantage of controlled settings such as hospitals, partial hospital settings, residential treatment facilities, and other institutions. Several types of observations may be gathered, according to the patient's specific situation:

1. *General observations.* These are relevant to all patients in all settings and include notes on patients' behavior, statements and expressed concerns, cooperativeness with or resistance to staff, sleep/wake patterns, and self-care.
2. *Diagnosis-specific observations.* These are observations relevant to confirming a diagnosis or assessing the severity, complications, or subtype of a disorder. Examples include recording signs of withdrawal in an alcohol-dependent patient and observations during meals for patients with eating disorders.

3. *Patient-specific observations.* These are observations aimed at assessing a clinical hypothesis. An example is observation of behavior following a family meeting for a patient in whom family conflicts are suspected of having contributed to a psychotic relapse.
4. *Observations of response to treatment interventions.* Examples include systematic recording of a target behavior in a trial of behavior therapy, observations of the effects of newly prescribed medications, and nurse-completed rating scales to measure changes after behavioral or psychotherapeutic interventions.

B. THE PROCESS OF ASSESSMENT

The actual assessment process during a psychiatric evaluation usually involves the development of initial impressions and hypotheses during the interview and their continual testing and refinement on the basis of information obtained throughout the interview and from mental status examination, diagnostic testing, and other sources (167).

1. Clinical formulation

The integrative formulation aids in understanding the patient as a unique human being and allows the psychiatrist to appreciate the patient's environment, strengths, challenges, and coping skills. The formulation includes information specific to the patient that goes beyond what is conveyed in the diagnosis; it will vary in scope and depth with the purpose of the evaluation. Components of the formulation include phenomenological, neurobiological, psychological, and sociocultural issues involved in diagnosis and management (60, 168–179). As relevant to each domain, the formulation will typically include a concise synthesis of what is known about the patient (e.g., individual characteristics, genetic predispositions, general medical conditions or laboratory abnormalities, past life experiences and developmental history, extent and quality of interpersonal relationships, central conflicts and defense mechanisms) and the patient's past and current symptomatology (including childhood or subsyndromal illness and predisposing, precipitating, perpetuating, or protecting factors) as well as the responses of symptoms to treatment. Variations in phenomenology with factors such as a patient's age or gender can be relevant in determining whether or not a behavior is indicative of psychopathology (180). Thus, the formulation may also include a discussion of the diagnostic, therapeutic, and prognostic implications of the evaluation findings.

a) Cultural formulation

The DSM-IV-TR Outline for Cultural Formulation (Table 5) provides a systematic method of considering and incorporating sociocultural issues into the clinical formulation (181–185). Depending on the focus and extent of the evaluation, it may not be possible to do a complete cultural formulation based on the findings of the initial interview. However, when cultural issues emerge, they may be explored further during subsequent meetings with the patient. In addition, the information contained within the cultural formulation may be integrated with the other aspects of the clinical formulation or recorded as a separate element.

The cultural formulation begins with a review of the individual's cultural identity and includes the patient's self-construal of identity over time (186). Cultural identity involves not only ethnicity, acculturation/biculturality, and language but also age, gender, socioeconomic status, sexual orientation, religious and spiritual beliefs, disabilities, political orientation, and health literacy, among other factors.

Next, the formulation explores the role of the cultural context in the expression and evaluation of symptoms and dysfunction, including the patient's explanatory models or idioms of distress through which symptoms or needs may be communicated. These are assessed against the norms of the cultural reference group. Treatment experiences and preferences (including complementary and alternative medicine and indigenous approaches) are also identified. Cul-

TABLE 5. Components of a Cultural Formulation

Cultural identity of the individual
Cultural explanations of the individual's illness
Cultural factors related to psychosocial environment and levels of functioning
Cultural elements of the relationship between the individual and the clinician
Overall cultural assessment for diagnosis and care

Source. From DSM-IV-TR, pp. 897–898.

tural factors related to psychosocial stressors, available social supports, and levels of function or disability are also assessed; during this process, the roles of family/kin systems and religion and spirituality in providing emotional, instrumental, and informational support are highlighted.

The cultural formulation also includes specific consideration of cultural elements influencing the relationship between the individual and the clinician. In this regard, it is important for clinicians to cultivate an attitude of "cultural humility" (187) in knowing their limits of knowledge and skills rather than reinforcing potentially damaging stereotypes and overgeneralizations. Differences in language, culture, or social status, as well as difficulties in identifying and understanding the cultural significance of behaviors or symptoms, may add to the complexities of the clinical encounter. Transference and countertransference may also be influenced by cultural considerations and may either aid or interfere with the treatment relationship. Further, the potential effect of the psychiatrist's sociocultural identity on the attitude and behavior of the patient should be taken into account in the subsequent formulation of a diagnostic opinion.

The cultural formulation concludes with an overall assessment of the ways in which these varied cultural considerations will specifically apply to differential diagnosis and treatment planning.

b) Risk assessment

An additional component of the formulation involves an assessment of the patient's risk of harm to self or others. This may include consideration of suicide or homicide risk as well as other forms of self-injury (e.g., cutting behaviors, accidents), aggressive behaviors, neglect of self-care, or neglect of the care of dependents. The risk assessment is intended to identify specific factors that may increase or decrease a patient's degree of risk, thereby suggesting specific interventions that may modify particular risk factors or address the safety of the patient or others. Specific risk factors may include demographic parameters (e.g., age, gender), past behavior (e.g., suicide attempts, self-injury, aggression), psychiatric diagnoses, psychiatric symptoms (e.g., anxiety, hopelessness), co-occurring general medical conditions, sociocultural factors, psychosocial stressors, or individual strengths and vulnerabilities. For patients with suicidal behaviors, this risk assessment process is described in detail in APA's *Practice Guideline for the Assessment and Treatment of Patients With Suicidal Behaviors* (11). Although standardized rating scales of suicidal or aggressive behaviors are often used in research and may suggest helpful lines of clinical inquiry, their utility in clinical risk assessment is limited by their low predictive value (11).

For individuals with dependent children, the risk assessment also includes an evaluation of the patient's capacity to parent. In addition to considering the number and ages of any children, the assessment reviews the patient's capacity to meet the needs of dependent children, both in general and during psychiatric crises if these are likely to occur. The overall health, including mental health, of the children is also relevant, especially when the patient's psychiatric condition is likely to affect the children through genetic or psychosocial mechanisms or to impede the patient's ability to recognize and attend to the needs of a child.

2. Diagnosis

On the basis of information obtained in the evaluation, a differential diagnosis is developed. The differential diagnosis comprises conditions (including personality disorders or personality traits) described in the *Diagnostic and Statistical Manual of Mental Disorders,* Fourth Edition, Text Revision (DSM-IV-TR) (188), APA's current edition of DSM. A multiaxial system of diagnosis provides a convenient format for organizing and communicating the patient's current clinical status, other factors affecting the clinical situation, the patient's highest level of past functioning, and the patient's quality of life (188, pp. 27–33). General medical conditions are established through history, examination, diagnostic tests, medical records, and consultation.

The DSM classification and the specific diagnostic criteria are meant to serve as guidelines to be informed by clinical judgment in the categorization of the patient's condition(s) and are not meant to be applied in a rote fashion. (Other issues in the use of DSM and its application in developing a psychiatric diagnosis are discussed in DSM-IV-TR, pp. xxiii–xxxv and 1–12.) To augment the DSM multiaxial approach, some clinicians also find it helpful to identify the patient's level of defensive functioning or incorporate dimensional or other approaches into their diagnostic assessments (188, pp. 807–813; 189, 190).

3. Initial treatment plan

The initial treatment plan addresses any specific diagnoses and psychiatric needs of the patient that have been identified during evaluation. If diagnostic or other questions have been posed or additional information is necessary, these issues should be addressed in the treatment plan.

The initial treatment plan begins with a determination of the appropriate treatment setting and includes an explicit statement of the diagnostic, therapeutic, and rehabilitative goals for treatment that includes short-term as well as longer-term goals. In the case of patients who initially will be treated in an inpatient or partial hospital setting, this implies apportioning the therapeutic task between a hospital phase and a posthospital phase. Within the acute care setting, some goals may be targeted for achievement within several days, whereas other goals will be targeted for completion by the time of discharge. On the basis of the goals, the plan specifies further diagnostic tests and procedures, further systematic observations or additional information to be obtained, and specific therapeutic modalities to be applied.

A comprehensive treatment plan addresses biological, psychological, and sociocultural domains. The psychiatrist can select from a range of individual, group, and family therapies to create an integrated multimodal treatment that includes biological and sociocultural interventions (60).

Quality care involves treatment plans that are safe, timely, effective, efficient, equitable (i.e., not influenced in quality by personal characteristics such as gender, ethnicity, geographic location, and socioeconomic status), and person-centered (7). Such treatment plans encourage recovery from illness through community integration and empower patients to make choices that improve their quality of life (191). Thus, the treatment plan is ideally the result of collaboration between the patient, the psychiatrist, and other members of the treatment team as well as the primary care practitioner for patients who have an established source of primary care.

A range of potentially effective treatments is initially considered. More detailed consideration and documentation of the risks and benefits of treatment options may be needed in the following circumstances: when a relatively risky, costly, or unusual treatment is under consideration; when involved parties disagree about the optimal course of treatment; when the patient's motivation or capacity to benefit from potential treatment alternatives is in question; when the treatment would be involuntary or when other legal or administrative issues are involved; or when available treatment options are limited by external constraints (e.g., financial barriers, insurance restrictions, geographic barriers, service availability, the patient's capacity to participate in the proposed treatment). Such considerations are also relevant when considering the level of care needed to provide an individual patient with appropriate treatment. In addition, level-of-care determinations will vary with the diagnosis, the presence of co-occurring general medical or psychiatric disorders (including substance use disorders), the assessment of the patient's risk to self or others, the current severity of symptoms, the patient's prior illness course and complications, his or her psychosocial supports, his or her treatment adherence, and the strength of the therapeutic alliance, among other factors. In some circumstances, it is also important for the psychiatrist to be able to recognize the limitation of health care resources and demonstrate the ability to act as an advocate for patients within their sociocultural and financial constraints (60).

4. Decisions regarding treatment-related legal and administrative issues

Although the consideration of forensic evaluations is outside the scope of this practice guideline, there are times when the general psychiatric evaluation may need to address legal or administrative concerns (Section V.C). Examples include deciding between voluntary and involuntary admission, determining whether legally mandated treatment should be pursued in objecting patients, determining whether there is a duty to protect (e.g., by modifying the patient's treatment, increasing outpatient visit frequency, initiating hospitalization, warning the victim) if the patient is deemed a potential risk to others, and deciding on the level of observation needed to address the patient's safety (11). In situations such as these, the psychiatrist's decision making will depend on the risk assessment (Section IV.B.1.b) as well as other relevant aspects of the history, examination, symptoms, diagnosis, and clinical formulation. Assessment of the patient's decision-making capacity may also be needed as part of the informed consent process. When a patient's capacity to consent to treatment is uncertain, questioning to determine mental status should be extended to include items that test the patient's decision-making capacity (192). As with other aspects of the evaluation, it is important to document the rationales for making a particular treatment decision, including a discussion of supporting evidence from the evaluation findings.

5. Systems issues

An assessment of family, peer networks, and other support systems is an important part of the psychiatric evaluation because of the potential role of these systems in ameliorating or augmenting the patient's signs and symptoms of illness. This is particularly true when evaluating individuals with complex biopsychosocial challenges or serious psychiatric or general medical conditions. If the initial evaluation indicates that aspects of the care system have an important role in the patient's illness and treatment, goals are developed in response to these findings. Systems may be more open to considering change at times of crisis. Consequently, as well as generating goals for the patient's diagnosis and individual treatment, the evaluation may lead to goals for intervening with the family, other important people in the patient's life, other professionals (e.g., therapists), general medical providers, and governmental or social agencies (e.g., community mental health centers or family service agencies). Specific plans may be needed for addressing problems in the care system that are seen as important to the patient's illness, symptoms, function, or well-being and that appear amenable to modification. For example, a parent may be unable to attend follow-up appointments unless issues relating to care of dependents are addressed; financial issues or formulary restrictions may preclude patients from obtaining their medications; or geographic constraints may limit access to a full range of treatment options. Plans to address such systems issues should consider feasibility, the patient's wishes, and the willingness of other people to be involved.

V. SPECIAL CONSIDERATIONS

A. PRIVACY AND CONFIDENTIALITY

Considerations of privacy and confidentiality are an integral component of any psychiatric encounter. Aspects of privacy and confidentiality relating to communication with other medical

professionals and with sources of collateral information have been discussed above (Sections I.A, I.B, II.C, and IV.A.2). In general, the default position is to maintain confidentiality unless the patient gives consent to a specific intervention or communication. However, the psychiatrist is justified in attenuating confidentiality to the extent needed to address the safety of the patient and others (10, 11). This includes the ability to communicate necessary information about the patient to medical personnel in the context of an emergency situation. It is also permissible for the psychiatrist to listen to information provided by family members and other important people in the patient's life, as long as confidential information is not provided to the informant.

The Health Insurance Portability and Accountability Act (HIPAA) contains guidelines for release of the results of psychiatric evaluations. State laws may be more restrictive, and if so, state laws take precedence over HIPAA. According to HIPAA, information can be released without a specific consent form for purposes of "treatment, payment, and health care operations." Otherwise, patients must sign an authorization form that indicates the information to be used or disclosed, the purposes to which it will be put, the recipient of the information, and an expiration date. HIPAA gives special protection to psychotherapy notes if they are kept in a separate part of the medical chart (193, 194). The interpretation of HIPAA and other federal and state laws about confidentiality continues to evolve, and legal or risk management consultation should be sought if there are questions about the regulations related to release of information and protection of psychiatric records (195).

For individuals in treatment for substance use disorders, the provisions of 42 CFR §2.11 will apply (196) and will generally be more strict and supersede the provisions of HIPAA (197). As with HIPAA, necessary information may be disclosed to medical personnel in the context of treating a condition that poses an immediate threat to the health of any individual and that requires immediate medical intervention. Under such circumstances, documentation in the medical record needs to include "the name of the medical personnel to whom disclosure was made and their affiliation with any health care facility; the name of the individual making the disclosure; the date and time of the disclosure; and the nature of the emergency" (42 CFR §2.51 [196]).

Medical records may also be viewed by others in addition to the clinician writing the note (198) or other members of an interdisciplinary treatment team. These include third-party payers, quality assurance/peer review evaluators, the patient, and, in certain jurisdictions, the executor of an estate after a patient's death. Furthermore, records may be part of future or current legal or administrative hearings, including disability litigation, divorce and custody adjudication, competency determinations, and actions of medical licensing boards. Such accessing of patient's medical records needs to be taken into consideration when documenting the evaluation, formulation, diagnosis, and plan of treatment.

B. INTERACTIONS WITH THIRD-PARTY PAYERS AND THEIR AGENTS

Third-party payers and their agents frequently request data from psychiatric evaluations to make determinations about whether a hospital admission or a specific treatment modality will be covered by a particular insurance plan. Despite the blanket consents to release information to payers that most patients must sign to obtain insurance benefits, it is useful for the psychiatrist to obtain, whenever feasible, contemporaneous consent for such communications. In some instances, it may be necessary to inform the patient what specific information has been requested and obtain specific consent for the release of that information. With valid consent, the psychiatrist may release information to a third-party reviewer, supplying the third-party reviewer with sufficient information to understand the rationale for the treatment and why it was selected over potential alternatives. However, the psychiatrist may also withhold information about the patient not directly relevant to the utilization review or preauthorization decision (199, 200).

C. LEGAL AND ADMINISTRATIVE ISSUES IN INSTITUTIONS

When a patient is admitted to a hospital or other residential setting, the patient's legal status should be promptly clarified to establish whether the admission is voluntary or involuntary, whether the patient gives or withholds consent to evaluation and recommended treatment, whether the patient appears able to make treatment-related decisions, and whether an advance directive is in place. If there is a potential legal impediment to necessary treatment, action should be taken to resolve the issue.

The decision to hospitalize a patient involuntarily will depend on multiple factors, including the estimated level of risk to the patient and others, the patient's level of insight and willingness to seek care, and the legal criteria in that jurisdiction. In general, patients at risk for causing harm to themselves or others will satisfy the criteria for involuntary admission; however, the specific requirements vary from state to state (201), and in some states, willingness to enter a hospital voluntarily may preclude involuntary admission. To that end, psychiatrists need to be familiar with their specific state statutes regarding involuntary hospitalization.

Advance directives are attempts to ensure that individuals' wishes about treatment will be honored. Such directives may relate to wishes about treatment at the end of life (202) but may also relate to wishes about psychiatric treatment (203) or assignment of a durable power of attorney or health care proxy to make decisions in the event that the individual lacks capacity to do so (204). Although the specifics of advance directive regulations vary by jurisdiction, psychiatrists should include in their evaluation whether the patient has executed an advance directive—and, if so, the nature of the advance directive should be determined.

In every institution, whether public or private, fiscal and administrative considerations limit treatment options. Usually there are constraints on length of stay and on the intensity of services available. Further constraints can arise from the absence or inadequate funding of aftercare services or of a full continuum of care. The initial assessment of treatment needs should not be confounded unduly with concerns about financing or availability of services, although the actual treatment may represent a balancing of optimal treatment and external constraints. A common example is the situation in which a patient's safety requires a level of supervision not available in a given facility. Another example is when a patient requires a general medical evaluation that cannot be carried out in a free-standing psychiatric facility and requires the patient's transfer to a general hospital. If such issues result in a major negative effect on patient care, efforts should be made to find alternatives, and the patient, family, and/or third-party payer should be informed of the limitations of the current treatment setting and/or resources.

D. SPECIAL POPULATIONS

1. Elderly patients and patients with medical conditions

While advanced chronological age alone does not necessitate a change in the approach to the psychiatric evaluation, the strong association of old age with chronic disease and related impairments may increase the need for emphasis on certain aspects of the evaluation. The general medical history and evaluation, cognitive mental status examination, and functional assessment may need to be especially detailed because of the high prevalence of disease-related disability, use of multiple medications, cognitive impairment, and functional impairment in older people. The psychiatrist should attempt to identify all of the general medical and personal care clinicians involved with the patient and to obtain relevant information from them if the patient consents. It is also helpful to obtain information from the family.

The personal and social history includes coverage of common late-life issues, including the loss of a spouse or partner, the loss of friends or close relatives, residential moves, the new onset of disabilities, financial concerns related to illness or disability, and intergenerational issues,

such as informal caregiving or financial transfers between members of different generations. It is important to evaluate intergenerational strains such as midlife couples with young children who cannot care for elderly relatives or, increasingly, patients in their 90s whose children are now in their 70s and ill themselves.

The psychiatrist may need to accommodate the evaluation to patients who cannot hear adequately. Use of sign language interpreters, amplification, a quieter interview room, and enabling lip reading are possible means to do this. When an elderly patient is brought for psychiatric evaluation by a family member, special effort may be necessary to ensure that both patient and family member have an opportunity to talk to the psychiatrist alone.

2. Incarcerated persons

Increasing numbers of individuals with mental illness are incarcerated in jails, prisons, and other correctional facilities and require psychiatric evaluation (205–208). In addition, suicide is one of the leading causes of death in correctional settings, and urgent suicide assessments may be needed for individuals at risk (11, 209, 210).

The psychiatric evaluation of incarcerated individuals will include the general elements common to any psychiatric evaluation (211–213) but will place additional emphasis on aspects of the individual's alcohol and substance use history and legal history, including previous episodes of incarceration and associated behavioral changes. Psychosocial stressors, including new legal complications (e.g., denial of parole), receiving bad news about loved ones at home, and experiencing sexual assault or other trauma, are also important to assess, as these may increase the likelihood of suicidal behaviors (214). Similarly, the recentness of the incarceration (210, 214, 215) or placement in isolation (216–219) may be relevant to determination of suicide risk. Depending on the likely duration of incarceration, options for care following transfer between correctional institutions or for aftercare following release may also need to be explored as part of the evaluation.

Access to space that allows for auditory privacy and physical safety is necessary to adequately perform psychiatric evaluations in correctional settings (212).

3. Homeless persons

Evaluations of persons who are homeless may require both modifications of the evaluation process and unique interviewing skills. The disengaged lifestyle and mistrust often encountered in homeless persons may make a classically direct approach difficult if not impossible (220). As a result, the first step toward psychiatric evaluation is engagement. This process can take from days to years in nonclinical settings (e.g., on the street, under bridges, in shelters). Evaluation becomes possible when the homeless person believes that engaging with the psychiatrist will not recapitulate previous negative experiences, lost opportunities within the health care system, and encounters in jail and prison that heighten a fear of consequences from talking honestly. By necessity, then, the full psychiatric evaluation of homeless persons typically unfolds over numerous, often brief, and seemingly casual interactions.

4. Persons with mental retardation

The evaluation of individuals with mental retardation presents a number of clinical challenges. Although psychiatric illnesses occur at increased rates in those with mental retardation (221, 222), it is not always possible to establish a definitive axis I diagnosis as a cause for behavioral symptoms (223). Depending on the extent of the patient's intellectual limitations, the diagnosis of mental retardation may have been unrecognized before the behavioral symptoms began.

In interviewing individuals with mental retardation, particular attention needs to be given to the phrasing of questions so that they will be understandable to the patient. The use of general psychiatric self-report scales or other structured interview formats may be problematic in this

regard (221, 224). Behavioral observations or functional measures will often carry a greater weight in the assessment process, and patients with more severe mental retardation may be unable to report on their own mental experiences (225, 226). Thus, obtaining a comprehensive description of symptoms, signs, and aspects of history from family members, caretakers, and other professionals is often crucial. This is particularly true when persons with mental retardation present for evaluation in the context of a behavioral crisis, because otherwise minor events (e.g., changes in routine, upsetting interpersonal interactions) may be quite distressing and result in catastrophic reactions. Similar issues with evaluation may be observed in individuals with other developmental disabilities.

Evaluation for co-occurring general medical conditions is particularly important in adults with mental retardation, given higher rates of undetected medical illnesses (222, 227) as well as the tendency for atypical clinical presentations of medical illnesses (140, 227).

VI. FUTURE RESEARCH NEEDS

Psychiatric evaluation is, by necessity, highly individualized to the patient and to the treatment setting, making the development of rigorous research designs challenging. Nonetheless, a number of aspects of psychiatric interviewing and assessment may lend themselves to formal study and are discussed in further detail below. In addition, the research agenda for DSM-V (228) provides suggestions for research relating to psychiatric diagnosis, which has many areas of overlap with research on psychiatric assessment.

A. INTERVIEWING APPROACHES

Some research, predominantly conducted in primary care settings, has examined the differences between specific interviewing approaches. For example, approaches to enhancing reporting and recall of historical information have been evaluated (229, 230). Additional studies have assessed the effects of communication style and vocabulary on outcomes such as patient satisfaction (231–236). The development of new evaluation strategies could help strengthen psychiatric interviewing approaches. In addition, it will be important to expand such research across different patient subgroups (e.g., according to age, gender, sexual orientation, race, ethnicity, cultural background), to individuals with psychiatric disorders, and to collaborative models of assessment and care. Measures of outcomes will also need to be expanded to include factors such as treatment adherence and the strength of the therapeutic alliance. Furthermore, studies will need to assess whether guideline-concordant approaches to assessment are associated with improved outcomes in community-based patient samples (237).

Research has also focused on the impact of technology on information gathering and the physician-patient encounter. For example, some studies have examined differences in the information elicited by face-to-face interviews as compared with computer-aided assessments or telephone interviews (238, 239). Other studies have assessed computerized documentation by physicians at the time of evaluation and its effect on patient perceptions (240–242). Patients and family members are increasingly learning about possible diagnoses and treatments through direct-to-consumer advertising and through Internet-based educational resources, which they sometimes bring to the evaluation. Systematic study of the influences of these information sources on the assessment and treatment planning processes would be useful. It also remains unclear whether use of template-based electronic health records as compared with narrative-based health records will influence the evaluation process, the physician-patient relationship, or communi-

cation with other members of the health care team. Thus, with the increasing use of technology in medicine, including computer-based interviews and telepsychiatry, the influence of such technologies is worthy of additional study in the full range of psychiatric settings.

B. RATING SCALES

Although rating scales have been widely used in clinical research for assessment by the clinician and self-assessment, they are less often incorporated into psychiatric evaluations in clinical practice. To be most useful, rating scales need to be valid and reliable as well as demonstrate practical utility in typical clinical settings. Further study of clinical rating scales is required in clinical samples including patients with potentially confounding co-occurring disorders (243). Development and testing of rating scales also need to consider the different requirements for rating scales that are used in initial diagnostic assessments as compared with those used in monitoring of signs and symptoms over time or with treatment. The ability to use rating scales to detect prodromal or subsyndromal disorders as part of the psychiatric evaluation would be an important step in the design and testing of preventive approaches to psychiatric disorders. Ideally, research on rating scales could lead to the development of a limited set of formal systematic measures for screening and monitoring, with resulting benefits in identification and treatment of common psychiatric disorders, including substance use disorders.

C. DIAGNOSIS AND FORMULATION

An integral part of the psychiatric evaluation is the process by which the information gathered as part of the psychiatric evaluation is synthesized and integrated into the development of a multiaxial diagnosis and biopsychosocial formulation. In addition to research on the validity and reliability of specific diagnoses, further research is needed on variations in both clinical and community presentations across different patient subgroups (e.g., according to age, gender, sexual orientation, race, ethnicity, cultural background) and in the presence of co-occurring general medical and psychiatric conditions. It is anticipated that the development of DSM-V will stimulate such research across many diagnostic areas, guided by APA's systematic efforts to review existing data and provide agendas for new research (228). With the advent of electronic health records and the increasing availability of decision-support tools, computerized approaches that may permit development of differential diagnoses or formulations will need to be compared to clinician-generated assessments. Longitudinal research on the reliability and validity of approaches to the clinical formulation may aid in fine-tuning this aspect of assessment.

D. DIAGNOSTIC TESTING

With regard to diagnostic testing, neurogenetics and structural and functional neuroimaging techniques are areas of active and promising research. A burgeoning body of literature has reported associations between genetic markers (e.g., apoplipoprotein E $\varepsilon 4$ allele, dopamine D_4 allele, catechol-*O*-methyltransferase polymorphisms, promoter polymorphisms of the serotonin transporter gene) and the presence of psychiatric illnesses or symptoms (244–251). Neurogenetic approaches may ultimately be useful in distinguishing between genetic and environmental etiologies of psychiatric disorders as part of the psychiatric evaluation (252), thereby permitting greater specificity in treatment planning and outcome measurement. While some have speculated that characterization of the particular genotype of a patient will lead to "personalized medicine" by guiding treatment choices, significant support for such therapeutic guidance in psychiatric disorders is not yet substantiated by the literature. The potential for progress in this area merits continued vigilance for reports of its impact on the practice of psychiatry.

Neuroimaging techniques are currently used in identifying central nervous system processes such as infection, malformations, cerebrovascular events, and malignancy. Accumulating evidence also suggests other applications of neuroimaging in psychiatric evaluation. In cognitive disorders of late life, such as Alzheimer's disease, neuroimaging techniques have been evaluated for use as surrogate markers for the microscopic neuropathologies that characterize the illness (253–256). Functional neuroimaging with positron emission tomography or single-photon emission computed tomography has demonstrated an association between reduced regional activity (metabolism or perfusion) in temporoparietal regions and the presence and severity of Alzheimer's disease (257–264), whereas other dementing illnesses do not show this temporoparietal feature. The reproducibility of these findings has enhanced the differentiation between Alzheimer's disease and other dementing illnesses (265). Ongoing work aims to confirm the clinical utility of such information.

In patients with schizophrenia and mood and anxiety disorders, structural and functional neuroimaging studies have reported differences between patients and healthy control persons (266–288) as well as differences in some patient subgroups (289–292) and in responders and nonresponders to some treatments (293–302). Nevertheless, the clinical utility of neuroimaging techniques for planning of individualized treatment has not yet been shown. Further research is needed to demonstrate a clinical role for structural and functional neuroimaging in establishing psychiatric diagnoses, monitoring illness progression, and predicting prognoses.

INDIVIDUALS AND ORGANIZATIONS THAT SUBMITTED COMMENTS

Norman Abeles, Ph.D.
Renato D. Alarcon, M.D., M.P.H.
Mark A. Amdur, M.D.
Kamal Artin, M.D.
David Baron, M.S.Ed., D.O.
Carl C. Bell, M.D.
David W. Brook, M.D.
Beth Ann Brooks, M.D.
Karen Broquet, M.D.
R.W. Burgoyne, M.D., Ph.D.
Gabrielle A. Carlson, M.D.
Mitchell J.M. Cohen, M.D.
Paul D. Cox, M.D., C.G.P.
Larry Culpepper, M.D., M.P.H.
Glenn Currier, M.D., M.P.H.
David L. Cutler, M.D.
Sarah DeMichele, M.D.
William R. Dubin, M.D.
Michael A. Fauman, M.D., Ph.D.
Joel Feiner, M.D.
Paul Jay Fink, M.D.
Peter Forster, M.D.
K.W.M. Fulford, D.Phil., F.R.C.P., F.R.C.Psych.
Paulette Marie Gillig, M.D., Ph.D.
Leslie H. Gise, M.D.
Sir David Goldberg, M.D.
Lawrence S. Gross, M.D.
Douglas G. Jacobs, M.D.
Douglas A. Kalunian, M.D.
Elisabeth J.S. Kunkel, M.D.
Ira Lesser, M.D.
James W. Lomax, M.D.
Henry Mallard, M.D.
David Mallott, M.D.
Marlin R. Mattson, M.D.
Peter McGeorge, M.D. M.B.Ch.B., F.R.A.N.Z.C.P.
Hunter L. McQuistion, M.D.
Jeffrey L. Metzner, M.D.
Kenneth Minkoff, M.D.
Mark Munetz, M.D.

Marvin Nierenberg, M.D.
Ann E. Norwood, M.D.
Lewis A. Opler, M.D., Ph.D.
John Peteet, M.D.
Herbert S. Peyser, M.D.
Harold Alan Pincus, M.D.
Henry Pinsker, M.D.
Brian Robertson, M.D.
Barbara R. Rosenfeld, M.D.
Barry W. Rovner, M.D.
M. David Rudd, Ph.D., A.B.P.P.
John Z. Sadler, M.D.
Warren Seides, M.D.
Michael Serby, M.D.
Joel J. Silverman, M.D.
Robert Stern, M.D., Ph.D.
Nada Stotland, M.D., M.P.H.
Jeffrey Stovall, M.D.
Paula T. Trzepacz, M.D.
Mitchell G. Weiss, M.D., Ph.D.
Cindy Wigg, M.D.
Bonnie Zima, M.D., M.P.H.
Mark Zimmerman, M.D.
Sidney Zisook, M.D.

Academy of Psychosomatic Medicine
American Academy of Addiction Psychiatry
American Academy of Clinical Psychiatrists
American Academy of Family Physicians
American Association for Emergency Psychiatry
American Association of Directors of Psychiatric Residency Training
American Association of Suicidology
American Group Psychotherapy Association
Association for Academic Psychiatry
Association for Behavioral and Cognitive Therapies
Group for the Advancement of Psychiatry
National Institute of Mental Health
Royal College of Psychiatrists
World Federation for Mental Health

REFERENCES

The following coding system is used to indicate the nature of the supporting evidence in the summary recommendations and references:

[A] *Double-blind, randomized clinical trial.* A study of an intervention in which subjects are prospectively followed over time; there are treatment and control groups; subjects are randomly assigned to the two groups; both the subjects and the investigators are blind to the assignments.

[A–] *Randomized clinical trial.* Same as above but not double-blind.

[B] *Clinical trial.* A prospective study in which an intervention is made and the results of that intervention are tracked longitudinally; study does not meet standards for a randomized clinical trial.

[C] *Cohort or longitudinal study.* A study in which subjects are prospectively followed over time without any specific intervention.

[D] *Control study.* A study in which a group of patients and a group of control subjects are identified in the present and information about them is pursued retrospectively or backward in time.

[E] *Review with secondary data analysis.* A structured analytic review of existing data, e.g., a meta-analysis or a decision analysis.
[F] *Review.* A qualitative review and discussion of previously published literature without a quantitative synthesis of the data.
[G] *Other.* Textbooks, expert opinion, case reports, and other reports not included above.

1. Othmer E, Othmer SC: The Clinical Interview Using DSM-IV-TR, vol 1: Fundamentals. Washington, DC, American Psychiatric Publishing, 2002 [G]
2. Shea SC: Psychiatric Interviewing, the Art of Understanding: A Practical Guide for Psychiatrists, Psychologists, Counselors, Social Workers, Nurses, and Other Mental Health Professionals, 2nd ed. Philadelphia, WB Saunders, 1998 [G]
3. Carlat DJ: The Psychiatric Interview: A Practical Guide. Philadelphia, Lippincott Williams & Wilkins, 1999 [G]
4. Pridmore S: Psychiatric Interview: A Guide to History Taking and the Mental State Examination. New York, Taylor & Francis, 2000 [G]
5. Hales RE, Yudofsky SC: The American Psychiatric Publishing Textbook of Clinical Psychiatry, 4th ed. Washington, DC, American Psychiatric Publishing, 2005 [G]
6. Sadock BJ, Sadock VA (eds): Kaplan and Sadock's Comprehensive Textbook of Psychiatry, 8th ed, vol 1 and 2. Philadelphia, Lippincott Williams & Wilkins, 2005 [G]
7. Institute of Medicine: Crossing the Quality Chasm: A New Health System for the 21st Century. Washington, DC, National Academy Press, 2001 [G]
8. Margulies A, Havens LL: The initial encounter: what to do first? Am J Psychiatry 1981; 138:421–428 [F]
9. Morrison J: The First Interview: Revised for DSM-IV, revised ed. New York, Guilford, 1994 [G]
10. American Psychiatric Association: The Principles of Medical Ethics With Annotations Especially Applicable to Psychiatry. Washington, DC, American Psychiatric Association, 2001 [G]
11. American Psychiatric Association: Practice guideline for the assessment and treatment of patients with suicidal behaviors. Am J Psychiatry 2003; 160(Nov suppl) [G]
12. Currier GW, Allen MH, Serper MR, Trenton AJ, Copersino ML: Medical, psychiatric, and cognitive assessment in the psychiatric emergency service, in Emergency Psychiatry. Edited by Allen MH. Washington, DC, American Psychiatric Publishing, 2002, pp 35–74 [G]
13. Slaby AE, Dubin WR, Baron DA: Other psychiatric emergencies, in Kaplan and Sadock's Comprehensive Textbook of Psychiatry, 8th ed. Edited by Sadock BJ, Sadock VA. Philadelphia, Lippincott Williams & Wilkins, 2005, pp 2453–2471 [G]
14. Hillard R, Zitek B: Emergency Psychiatry. New York, McGraw-Hill Medical, 2004 [G]
15. Petit JR: Handbook of Emergency Psychiatry. Philadelphia, Lippincott Williams & Wilkins, 2004 [G]
16. Reeves RR, Pendarvis EJ, Kimble R: Unrecognized medical emergencies admitted to psychiatric units. Am J Emerg Med 2000; 18:390–393 [G]
17. White AJ, Barraclough B: Thyroid disease and mental illness: a study of thyroid disease in psychiatric admissions. J Psychosom Res 1988; 32:99–106 [G]
18. Allen MH, Currier GW: Medical assessment in the psychiatric emergency service. New Dir Ment Health Serv 1999; 82:21–28 [G]
19. Williams ER, Shepherd SM: Medical clearance of psychiatric patients. Emerg Med Clin North Am 2000; 18:185–198 [F]
20. Schiller MJ, Shumway M, Batki SL: Utility of routine drug screening in a psychiatric emergency setting. Psychiatr Serv 2000; 51:474–478 [G]
21. Perrone J, De Roos F, Jayaraman S, Hollander JE: Drug screening versus history in detection of substance use in ED psychiatric patients. Am J Emerg Med 2001; 19:49–51 [G]
22. Olshaker JS, Browne B, Jerrard DA, Prendergast H, Stair TO: Medical clearance and screening of psychiatric patients in the emergency department. Acad Emerg Med 1997; 4:124–128 [G]

23. Korn CS, Currier GW, Henderson SO: "Medical clearance" of psychiatric patients without medical complaints in the Emergency Department. J Emerg Med 2000; 18:173–176 [G]
24. Kanich W, Brady WJ, Huff JS, Perron AD, Holstege C, Lindbeck G, Carter CT: Altered mental status: evaluation and etiology in the ED. Am J Emerg Med 2002; 20:613–617 [G]
25. Henneman PL, Mendoza R, Lewis RJ: Prospective evaluation of emergency department medical clearance. Ann Emerg Med 1994; 24:672–677 [G]
26. Gregory RJ, Nihalani ND, Rodriguez E: Medical screening in the emergency department for psychiatric admissions: a procedural analysis. Gen Hosp Psychiatry 2004; 26:405–410 [F]
27. Elie M, Rousseau F, Cole M, Primeau F, McCusker J, Bellavance F: Prevalence and detection of delirium in elderly emergency department patients. CMAJ 2000; 163:977–981 [G]
28. Weissberg MP: Emergency room medical clearance: an educational problem. Am J Psychiatry 1979; 136:787–790 [F]
29. Tintinalli JE, Peacock FW, Wright MA: Emergency medical evaluation of psychiatric patients. Ann Emerg Med 1994; 23:859–862 [G]
30. Riba M, Hale M: Medical clearance: fact or fiction in the hospital emergency room. Psychosomatics 1990; 31:400–404 [G]
31. Zun LS, Hernandez R, Thompson R, Downey L: Comparison of EPs' and psychiatrists' laboratory assessment of psychiatric patients. Am J Emerg Med 2004; 22:175–180 [G]
32. Broderick KB, Lerner EB, McCourt JD, Fraser E, Salerno K: Emergency physician practices and requirements regarding the medical screening examination of psychiatric patients. Acad Emerg Med 2002; 9:88–92 [G]
33. Hall RC, Gardner ER, Popkin MK, Lecann AF, Stickney SK: Unrecognized physical illness prompting psychiatric admission: a prospective study. Am J Psychiatry 1981; 138:629–635 [C]
34. Anfinson TJ, Stoudemire A: Laboratory and neuroendocrine assessment in medical-psychiatric patients, in Psychiatric Care of the Medical Patient, 2nd ed. Edited by Stoudemire A, Fogel BS, Greenberg DB. New York, Oxford University Press, 2000, pp 119–148 [F]
35. Meyers J, Stein S: The psychiatric interview in the emergency department. Emerg Med Clin North Am 2000; 18:173–183 [G]
36. Garrick TR, Stotland NL: How to write a psychiatric consultation. Am J Psychiatry 1982; 139:849–855 [G]
37. Karasu TB, Plutchik R, Conte H, Siegel B, Steinmuller R, Rosenbaum M: What do physicians want from a psychiatric consultation service? Compr Psychiatry 1977; 18:73–81 [C]
38. Group for the Advancement of Psychiatry: The Mental Health Professional and the Legal System: Report 131. New York, Brunner/Mazel, 1991 [F]
39. Gutheil TG, Appelbaum PS: Clinical Handbook of Psychiatry and the Law, 3rd ed. Baltimore, Lippincott Williams & Wilkins, 2000 [G]
40. Sederer LI: Brief hospitalization, in American Psychiatric Press Review of Psychiatry, vol 11. Edited by Tasman A, Riba MB. Washington, DC, American Psychiatric Press, 1992, pp 518–534 [G]
41. Sederer LI, Rothschild AJ (eds): Acute Care Psychiatry: Diagnosis and Treatment. Philadelphia, Lippincott Williams & Wilkins, 1997 [G]
42. George L, Durbin J, Sheldon T, Goering P: Patient and contextual factors related to the decision to hospitalize patients from emergency psychiatric services. Psychiatr Serv 2002; 53:1586–1591 [G]
43. Rolland JS: Families, Illness, and Disability: An Integrative Treatment Model. New York, Basic Books, 1994 [G]
44. Redelmeier DA, Schull MJ, Hux JE, Tu JV, Ferris LE: Problems for clinical judgement, 1: eliciting an insightful history of present illness. CMAJ 2001; 164:647–651 [F]

45. Bronheim HE, Fulop G, Kunkel EJ, Muskin PR, Schindler BA, Yates WR, Shaw R, Steiner H, Stern TA, Stoudemire A (Academy of Psychosomatic Medicine): The Academy of Psychosomatic Medicine practice guidelines for psychiatric consultation in the general medical setting. Psychosomatics 1998; 39(suppl 4):S8–S30 [G]
46. Posternak MA, Zimmerman M: How accurate are patients in reporting their antidepressant treatment history? J Affect Disord 2003; 75:115–124 [G]
47. Greenfield SF, Hennessy G: Assessment of the patient, in Textbook of Substance Abuse Treatment. Edited by Galanter M, Kleber HD. Washington, DC, American Psychiatric Publishing, 2004, pp 101–119 [G]
48. Center for Substance Abuse Treatment: Assessment and Treatment of Patients With Coexisting Mental Illness and Alcohol and Other Drug Abuse. Improvement Protocol Series #42 DHHS Publication (SMA) 05-3922. Rockville, Md, Substance Abuse and Mental Health Services Administration, Center for Substance Abuse Treatment, 2005. http://www.ncbi.nlm.nih.gov/books/bv.fcgi?rid=hstat5.chapter.74370 [G]
49. American Psychiatric Association: Practice guideline for the treatment of patients with substance use disorders (second edition). Am J Psychiatry (in press) [G]
50. Yates WR, Gleason O: Hepatitis C and depression. Depress Anxiety 1998; 7:188–193 [G]
51. Redelmeier DA, Tu JV, Schull MJ, Ferris LE, Hux JE: Problems for clinical judgement, 2: obtaining a reliable past medical history. CMAJ 2001; 164:809–813 [F]
52. Loewenstein RJ: An office mental status examination for complex chronic dissociative symptoms and multiple personality disorder. Psychiatr Clin North Am 1991; 14:567–604 [G]
53. Herman JL: Trauma and Recovery. New York, Basic Books, 1992 [G]
54. Group for the Advancement of Psychiatry: A Guide to the Assessment of Sexual Function. Washington, DC, American Psychiatric Press, 2001. http://www.groupadpsych.org/pdf%20files/Gapbook%20April%202001.pdf [G]
55. Ursano RJ, Bell C, Eth S, et al: Practice guideline for the treatment of patients with acute stress disorder and posttraumatic stress disorder. Am J Psychiatry 2004; 161(11 suppl):3–31 [G]
56. Rey JM, Stewart GW, Plapp JM, Bashir MR, Richards IN: Validity of axis V of DSM-III and other measures of adaptive functioning. Acta Psychiatr Scand 1988; 77:535–542 [C]
57. Sohlberg S: There's more in a number than you think: new validity data for the Global Assessment Scale. Psychol Rep 1989; 64:455–461 [F]
58. Harder DW, Strauss JS, Greenwald DF, Kokes RF, Ritzler BA, Gift TE: Predictors of outcome among adult psychiatric first admissions. J Clin Psychol 1992; 46:119–128 [C]
59. Galanter M: Spirituality and the Healthy Mind: Science, Therapy and the Need for Personal Meaning. New York, Oxford University Press, 2005 [G]
60. Scheiber S, Kramer T, Adamowski S (eds): Core Competencies for Psychiatric Practice: What Clinicians Need to Know. A Report of the American Board of Psychiatry and Neurology, Inc. Washington, DC, American Psychiatric Publishing, 2003 [G]
61. Politi BJ, Arena VC, Schwerha J, Sussman N: Occupational medical history taking: how are today's physicians doing? a cross-sectional investigation of the frequency of occupational history taking by physicians in a major US teaching center. J Occup Environ Med 2004; 46:550–555 [G]
62. MacDonald-Wilson K, Rogers ES, Anthony WA: Unique issues in assessing work function among individuals with psychiatric disabilities. J Occup Rehabil 2001; 11:217–232 [F]
63. Anthony WA, Rogers ES, Cohen M, Davies RR: Relationships between psychiatric symptomatology, work skills, and future vocational performance. Psychiatr Serv 1995; 46:353–358 [B]
64. Mueser KT, Becker DR, Torrey WC, Xie H, Bond GR, Drake RE, Dain BJ: Work and nonvocational domains of functioning in persons with severe mental illness: a longitudinal analysis. J Nerv Ment Dis 1997; 185:419–426 [B]

65. Metzner JL: An introduction to correctional psychiatry, part II. J Am Acad Psychiatry Law 1997; 25:571–579 [G]
66. Metzner JL, Buck JB: Psychiatric disability determinations and personal injury litigation, in Principles in Practice of Forensic Psychiatry. Edited by Rosner R. London, Arnold, 2003, pp 260–272 [G]
67. Bennett R: The Practical Guide to the Genetic Family History. New York, Wiley-Liss, 1999 [G]
68. American Medical Association: Family Medical History Pocket Information Card, 2004. http://www.ama-assn.org/ama1/pub/upload/mm/464/family_insert02.pdf [G]
69. American Society of Human Genetics: To Draw Your Family Tree, 2005. http://www.ashg.org/genetics/ashg/educ/007a.shtml [G]
70. March of Dimes: Genetics and Your Practice, 2005. http://www.marchofdimes.com/gyponline/index.bm2 [G]
71. Trzepacz PJ, Baker RW: The Psychiatric Mental Status Examination. New York, Oxford University Press, 1993 [G]
72. Reeves RR, Bullen JA: A standardized form for DSM-IV review of symptoms and mental status examination for students and residents. J Am Osteopath Assoc 1995; 95:381–387 [G]
73. Serby M: Psychiatric resident conceptualizations of mood and affect within the mental status examination. Am J Psychiatry 2003; 160:1527–1529 [G]
74. Tardiff K: The current state of psychiatry in the treatment of violent patients. Arch Gen Psychiatry 1992; 49:493–499 [G]
75. Hughes DH: Suicide and violence assessment in psychiatry. Gen Hosp Psychiatry 1996; 18:416–421 [F]
76. Shea SC: The chronological assessment of suicide events: a practical interviewing strategy for the elicitation of suicidal ideation. J Clin Psychiatry 1998; 59(suppl 20):58–72 [F]
77. Twemlow SW: Interviewing violent patients. Bull Menninger Clin 2001; 65:503–521 [F]
78. Tardiff K: Concise Guide to Assessment and Management of Violent Patients, 2nd ed. Washington, DC, American Psychiatric Press, 1996 [G]
79. Chiles JA, Strosahl KD: Clinical Manual for Assessment and Treatment of Suicidal Patients. Washington, DC, American Psychiatric Publishing, 2005 [G]
80. Prochaska J, DiClemente C: The Transtheoretical Approach: Crossing Traditional Boundaries of Therapy. Homewood, IL, Dow Jones-Irwin, 1984 [G]
81. Prochaska J, DiClemente C: Stages of Change in the Modification of Problem Behaviors. Newbury Park, CA, Sage, 1992 [G]
82. Prochaska JO, Velicer WF: The transtheoretical model of health behavior change. Am J Health Promot 1997; 12:38–48 [F]
83. Littell JH, Girvin H: Stages of change: a critique. Behav Modif 2002; 26:223–273 [E]
84. Miller WR, Rollnick S, Conforti K: Motivational Interviewing: Preparing People for Change, 2nd ed. New York, Guilford, 2002 [G]
85. Finnell DS: Use of the Transtheoretical model for individuals with co-occurring disorders. Community Ment Health J 2003; 39:3–15 [F]
86. Rogers ES, Martin R, Anthony W, Massaro J, Danley K, Crean T, Penk W: Assessing readiness for change among persons with severe mental illness. Community Ment Health J 2001; 37:97–112 [G]
87. Cox A, Hopkinson K, Rutter M: Psychiatric interviewing techniques, II: naturalistic study: eliciting factual information. Br J Psychiatry 1981; 138:283–291 [C]
88. Hopkinson K, Cox A, Rutter M: Psychiatric interviewing techniques, III: naturalistic study: eliciting feelings. Br J Psychiatry 1981; 138:406–415 [C]
89. Cox A, Rutter M, Holbrook D: Psychiatric interviewing techniques, V: experimental study: eliciting factual information. Br J Psychiatry 1981; 139:29–37 [B]
90. Cox A, Holbrook D, Rutter M: Psychiatric interviewing techniques, VI: experimental study: eliciting feelings. Br J Psychiatry 1981; 139:144–152 [B]

91. Cox A, Rutter M, Holbrook D: Psychiatric interviewing techniques: a second experimental study: eliciting feelings. Br J Psychiatry 1988; 152:64–72 [G]
92. Cruz M, Pincus HA: Research on the influence that communication in psychiatric encounters has on treatment. Psychiatr Serv 2002; 53:1253–1265 [E]
93. Maier W, Philipp M, Buller R: The value of structured clinical interviews. Arch Gen Psychiatry 1988; 45:963–964 [C]
94. Robins LN: Diagnostic grammar and assessment: translating criteria into questions. Psychol Med 1989; 19:57–68 [F]
95. Watson CG, Juba MP, Manifold V, Kucala T, Anderson PE: The PTSD interview: rationale, description, reliability, and concurrent validity of a DSM-III-based technique. J Clin Psychol 1991; 47:179–188 [C]
96. First MB (ed): Standardized Evaluation in Clinical Practice (Review of Psychiatry Series, vol 23; Oldham JM and Riba MB, series editors). Washington, DC, American Psychiatric Publishing, 2003 [G]
97. Kashner TM, Rush AJ, Suris A, Biggs MM, Gajewski VL, Hooker DJ, Shoaf T, Altshuler KZ: Impact of structured clinical interviews on physicians' practices in community mental health settings. Psychiatr Serv 2003; 54:712–718 [A–]
98. Miller PR, Dasher R, Collins R, Griffiths P, Brown F: Inpatient diagnostic assessments, 1: accuracy of structured vs unstructured interviews. Psychiatry Res 2001; 105:255–264 [G]
99. Steiner JL, Tebes JK, Sledge WH, Walker ML: A comparison of the structured clinical interview for DSM-III-R and clinical diagnoses. J Nerv Ment Dis 1995; 183:365–369 [G]
100. Ramirez BM, Bostic JQ, Davies D, Rush AJ, Witte B, Hendrickse W, Barnett V: Methods to improve diagnostic accuracy in a community mental health setting. Am J Psychiatry 2000; 157:1599–1605 [G]
101. Shear MK, Greeno C, Kang J, Ludewig D, Frank E, Swartz HA, Hanekamp M: Diagnosis of nonpsychotic patients in community clinics. Am J Psychiatry 2000; 157:581–587 [G]
102. Zimmerman M, Mattia JI: Psychiatric diagnosis in clinical practice: is comorbidity being missed? Compr Psychiatry 1999; 40:182–191 [G]
103. Pinderhughes E: Understanding Race, Ethnicity and Power. New York, Free Press, 1988 [G]
104. American Psychiatric Association: Position statement on bias-related incidents (official actions). Am J Psychiatry 1993; 150:686 [G]
105. American Psychiatric Association: Guidelines regarding possible conflict between psychiatrists' religious commitment and psychiatric practice. Am J Psychiatry 1990; 147:542 [G]
106. US Department of Health and Human Services Office of Minority Health: National standards on culturally and linguistically appropriate services (CLAS) in health care. Federal Register 2000; 65:80865–80879 [G]
107. US Congress: Americans With Disabilities Act of 1990. 42 USC 12101–12213, 1990 [G]
108. Westermeyer JJ: Cross-cultural psychiatric assessment, in Culture, Ethnicity, and Mental Illness. Edited by Gaw AC. Washington, DC, American Psychiatric Press, 1993, pp 125–144 [F]
109. Tribe R, Raval H: Working With Interpreters in Mental Health. London, Brunner-Routledge, 2002 [G]
110. Tribe R, Morrissey J: Using interpreters when working in mental health. Int J Psychol 2004; 35:380 [G]
111. Mailloux SL: Ethics and interpreters: are you practicing ethically? J Psychol Practice 2004; 10:37–44 [G]
112. Fochtmann LJ: Psychiatric assessment and management, in Emergency Toxicology. Edited by Viccellio P, Bania T. Philadelphia, Lippincott-Raven, 1998, pp 41–59 [G]
113. Brasic JR, Fogelman D: Clinician safety. Psychiatr Clin North Am 1999; 22:923–940 [F]
114. Khadivi AN, Patel RC, Atkinson AR, Levine JM: Association between seclusion and restraint and patient-related violence. Psychiatr Serv 2004; 55:1311–1312 [B]

115. Dubin WR, Lion JR (eds): American Psychiatric Association Task Force Report 33: Clinician Safety. Washington, DC, American Psychiatric Association, 1993 [G]
116. Dubin WR: Clinician safety, in Medical Management of the Violent Patient. Edited by Tardiff K. New York, Marcel Dekker, 1999, pp 219–236 [G]
117. American Psychiatric Association, American Psychiatric Nurses Association, National Association of Psychiatric Health Systems: Learning From Each Other: Success Stories and Ideas for Reducing Restraint/Seclusion in Behavioral Health. Arlington, Va, American Psychiatric Association, 2003. http://www.psych.org/psych_pract/treatg/pg/learningfrom eachother.cfm [G]
118. American Psychiatric Association: Handbook of Psychiatric Measures. Washington, DC, American Psychiatric Press, 2000 [G]
119. Escobar JI, Burnam A, Karno M, Forsythe A, Landsverk J, Golding JM: Use of the Mini-Mental State Examination (MMSE) in a community population of mixed ethnicity: cultural and linguistic artifacts. J Nerv Ment Dis 1986; 174:607–614 [C]
120. Lopez S, Nunez JA: Cultural factors considered in selected diagnostic criteria and interview schedules. J Abnorm Psychol 1987; 96:270–272 [F]
121. Flaherty JA, Gaviria FM, Pathak D, Mitchell T, Wintrob R, Richman JA, Birz S: Developing instruments for cross-cultural psychiatric research. J Nerv Ment Dis 1988; 176:257–263 [F]
122. Roberts RE, Rhoades HM, Vernon SW: Using the CES-D scale to screen for depression and anxiety: effects of language and ethnic status. Psychiatry Res 1990; 31:69–83 [C]
123. Sandoval J, Geisinger KF, Frisby C: Test Interpretation and Diversity: Achieving Equity in Assessment. Washington, DC, American Psychological Association, 1999 [G]
124. Samuda RJ: Psychological Testing of American Minorities: Issues and Consequences, 2nd ed. Thousand Oaks, Calif, Sage, 1998 [G]
125. Suzuki LA, Ponterotto JG, Meller PJ: The New Handbook of Multicultural Assessment: Clinical, Psychological, and Educational Applications, 2nd ed. San Francisco, Jossey-Bass, 2000 [G]
126. Kovess V, Sylla O, Fournier L, Flavigny V: Why discrepancies exist between structured diagnostic interviews and clinicians' diagnoses. Soc Psychiatry Psychiatr Epidemiol 1992; 27:185–191 [C]
127. Harrington R, Hill J, Rutter M, John K, Fudge H, Zoccolillo M, Weissman M: The assessment of lifetime psychopathology: a comparison of two interviewing styles. Psychol Med 1988; 18:487–493 [C]
128. North CS, Pollio DE, Thompson SJ, Ricci DA, Smith EM, Spitznagel EL: A comparison of clinical and structured interview diagnoses in a homeless mental health clinic. Community Ment Health J 1997; 33:531–543 [G]
129. Blacker D: Psychiatric rating scales, in Kaplan and Sadock's Comprehensive Textbook of Psychiatry, 8th ed. Edited by Sadock BJ, Sadock VA. Philadelphia, Lippincott Williams & Wilkins, 2005, pp 929–955 [G]
130. Applegate WB, Blass JP, Williams TF: Instruments for the functional assessment of older patients. N Engl J Med 1990; 322:1207–1214 [F]
131. Katz S: Assessing self-maintenance: activities of daily living, mobility, and instrumental activities of daily living. J Am Geriatr Soc 1983; 31:721–727 [F]
132. American Psychiatric Association: Position statement on the role of psychiatrists in assessing driving ability (official actions). Am J Psychiatry 1995; 152:819 [G]
133. Anfinson TJ, Kathol RG: Screening laboratory evaluation in psychiatric patients: a review. Gen Hosp Psychiatry 1992; 14:248–257 [G]
134. White AJ, Barraclough B: Benefits and problems of routine laboratory investigations in adult psychiatric admissions. Br J Psychiatry 1989; 155:65–72 [F]
135. Bostwick JM, Philbrick KL: The use of electroencephalography in psychiatry of the medically ill. Psychiatr Clin North Am 2002; 25:17–25 [F]

136. Gomez-Gil E, Trilla A, Corbella B, Fernandez-Egea E, Luburich P, de Pablo J, Ferrer RJ, Valdes M: Lack of clinical relevance of routine chest radiography in acute psychiatric admissions. Gen Hosp Psychiatry 2002; 24:110–113 [G]
137. Knutsen E, DuRand C: Previously unrecognized physical illnesses in psychiatric patients. Hosp Community Psychiatry 1991; 42:182–186 [G]
138. Koran LM, Sheline Y, Imai K, Kelsey TG, Freedland KE, Mathews J, Moore M: Medical disorders among patients admitted to a public-sector psychiatric inpatient unit. Psychiatr Serv 2002; 53:1623–1625 [G]
139. Lyketsos CG, Dunn G, Kaminsky MJ, Breakey WR: Medical comorbidity in psychiatric inpatients: relation to clinical outcomes and hospital length of stay. Psychosomatics 2002; 43:24–30 [G]
140. Ryan R, Sunada K: Medical evaluation of persons with mental retardation referred for psychiatric assessment. Gen Hosp Psychiatry 1997; 19:274–280 [G]
141. Sheline Y, Kehr C: Cost and utility of routine admission laboratory testing for psychiatric inpatients. Gen Hosp Psychiatry 1990; 12:329–334 [G]
142. Warner MD, Boutros NN, Peabody CA: Usefulness of screening EEGs in a psychiatric inpatient population. J Clin Psychiatry 1990; 51:363–364 [G]
143. Yudofsky SC, Kim HF (eds): Neuropsychiatric Assessment (Review of Psychiatry Series, vol 23; Oldham JM and Riba MB, series editors). Washington, DC, American Psychiatric Publishing, 2004 [G]
144. Pomeroy C, Mitchell JE, Roerig J, Crow S: Medical Complications of Psychiatric Illness. Washington, DC, American Psychiatric Publishing, 2002 [G]
145. American Psychiatric Association: Practice guideline for the treatment of patients with bipolar disorder (revision). Am J Psychiatry 2002; 159(April suppl) [G]
146. American Psychiatric Association: The Practice of Electroconvulsive Therapy. Recommendations for Treatment, Training, and Privileging: A Task Force Report of the American Psychiatric Association, 2nd ed. Washington, DC, American Psychiatric Press, 2001 [G]
147. Meyer GJ, Finn SE, Eyde LD, Kay GG, Moreland KL, Dies RR, Eisman EJ, Kubiszyn TW, Reed GM: Psychological testing and psychological assessment: a review of evidence and issues. Am Psychol 2001; 56:128–165 [F]
148. Ercoli LM, Siddarth P, Dunkin JJ, Bramen J, Small GW: MMSE items predict cognitive decline in persons with genetic risk for Alzheimer's disease. J Geriatr Psychiatry Neurol 2003; 16:67–73 [C]
149. Green MF, Kern RS, Braff DL, Mintz J: Neurocognitive deficits and functional outcome in schizophrenia: are we measuring the "right stuff"? Schizophr Bull 2000; 26:119–136 [E]
150. Phillips WA, Silverstein SM: Convergence of biological and psychological perspectives on cognitive coordination in schizophrenia. Behav Brain Sci 2003; 26:65–82 [G]
151. Ragland JD: Profiles of neuropsychologic function in schizophrenia. Curr Psychiatry Rep 2003; 5:299–302 [G]
152. Harrow M, Green KE, Sands JR, Jobe TH, Goldberg JF, Kaplan KJ, Martin EM: Thought disorder in schizophrenia and mania: impaired context. Schizophr Bull 2000; 26:879–891 [G]
153. Rubinsztein JS, Michael A, Paykel ES, Sahakian BJ: Cognitive impairment in remission in bipolar affective disorder. Psychol Med 2000; 30:1025–1036 [D]
154. Quraishi S, Frangou S: Neuropsychology of bipolar disorder: a review. J Affect Disord 2002; 72:209–226 [F]
155. Donaldson S, Goldstein LH, Landau S, Raymont V, Frangou S: The Maudsley Bipolar Disorder Project: the effect of medication, family history, and duration of illness on IQ and memory in bipolar I disorder. J Clin Psychiatry 2003; 64:86–93 [C]
156. Martinez-Aran A, Vieta E, Colom F, Reinares M, Benabarre A, Torrent C, Goikolea JM, Corbella B, Sanchez-Moreno J, Salamero M: Neuropsychological performance in depressed and euthymic bipolar patients. Neuropsychobiology 2002; 46(suppl 1):16–21 [G]

157. Nebes RD, Pollock BG, Houck PR, Butters MA, Mulsant BH, Zmuda MD, Reynolds CF III: Persistence of cognitive impairment in geriatric patients following antidepressant treatment: a randomized, double-blind clinical trial with nortriptyline and paroxetine. J Psychiatr Res 2003; 37:99–108 [A]
158. Alexopoulos GS: Role of executive function in late-life depression. J Clin Psychiatry 2003; 64(suppl 14):18–23 [G]
159. Shenal BV, Harrison DW, Demaree HA: The neuropsychology of depression: a literature review and preliminary model. Neuropsychol Rev 2003; 13:33–42 [F]
160. Wilson RS, Mendes De Leon CF, Bennett DA, Bienias JL, Evans DA: Depressive symptoms and cognitive decline in a community population of older persons. J Neurol Neurosurg Psychiatry 2004; 75:126–129 [G]
161. Gilotty L, Kenworthy L, Sirian L, Black DO, Wagner AE: Adaptive skills and executive function in autism spectrum disorders. Neuropsychol Dev Cogn Sect C Child Neuropsychol 2002; 8:241–248 [G]
162. Tager-Flusberg H, Joseph RM: Identifying neurocognitive phenotypes in autism. Philos Trans R Soc Lond B Biol Sci 2003; 358:303–314 [G]
163. Kaiser S, Unger J, Kiefer M, Markela J, Mundt C, Weisbrod M: Executive control deficit in depression: event-related potentials in a Go/No-go task. Psychiatry Res 2003; 122:169–184 [G]
164. Green MF, Nuechterlein KH: Should schizophrenia be treated as a neurocognitive disorder? Schizophr Bull 1999; 25:309–319 [G]
165. Schiffer RB, Klein RF, Sider RC: The Medical Evaluation of Psychiatric Patients. New York, Plenum, 1988 [G]
166. Talbot-Stern JK, Green T, Royle TJ: Psychiatric manifestations of systemic illness. Emerg Med Clin North Am 2000; 18:199–209 [F]
167. Nurcombe B, Fitzhenry-Coor I: How do psychiatrists think? clinical reasoning in the psychiatric interview: a research and education project. Aust N Z J Psychiatry 1982; 16:13–24 [F]
168. IGDA Workgroup WPA: IGDA, 8: idiographic (personalised) diagnostic formulation. Br J Psychiatry Suppl 2003; 45:S55–S57 [G]
169. Summers RF: The psychodynamic formulation updated. Am J Psychother 2003; 57:39–51 [G]
170. Bergner RM: Characteristics of optimal clinical case formulations: the linchpin concept. Am J Psychother 1998; 52:287–300 [G]
171. Pies RW: Clinical Manual of Psychiatric Diagnosis and Treatment: A Biopsychosocial Approach. Washington, DC, American Psychiatric Press, 1994 [G]
172. Weerasekera P: Formulation: a multiperspective model. Can J Psychiatry 1993; 38:351–358 [G]
173. McDougall GM, Reade B: Teaching biopsychosocial integration and formulation. Can J Psychiatry 1993; 38:359–362 [G]
174. Cleghorn JM, Bellissimo A, Will D: Teaching some principles of individual psychodynamics through an introductory guide to formulations. Can J Psychiatry 1983; 28:162–172 [G]
175. Ross CA, Leichner P, Matas M, Anderson D: A method of teaching and evaluating psychiatric case formulation. Acad Psychiatry 1990; 14:99–105 [G]
176. Perry S, Cooper AM, Michels R: The psychodynamic formulation: its purpose, structure, and clinical application. Am J Psychiatry 1987; 144:543–550 [G]
177. Sadock BJ: Psychiatric report, medical record and medical error, in Kaplan and Sadock's Comprehensive Textbook of Psychiatry, 8th ed. Edited by Sadock BJ, Sadock VA. Philadelphia, Lippincott Williams & Wilkins, 2005, pp 834–847 [G]
178. Engel GL: The need for a new medical model: a challenge for biomedicine. Science 1977; 196:129–136 [G]

179. Eells TD, Kendjelic EM, Lucas CP: What's in a case formulation? development and use of a content coding manual. J Psychother Pract Res 1998; 7:144–153 [G]
180. IGDA Workgroup WPA: IGDA, 4: evaluation of symptoms and mental state. Br J Psychiatry Suppl 2003; 45:S46–S47 [G]
181. Lu F, Lim R, Mezzich J: Issues in the assessment and diagnosis of culturally diverse individuals, in American Psychiatric Press Review of Psychiatry, vol 14. Edited by Oldham JO, Riba M. Washington, DC, American Psychiatric Press, 1995, pp 477–510 [G]
182. Group for the Advancement of Psychiatry: Cultural Assessment in Clinical Psychiatry. Washington, DC, American Psychiatric Publishing, 2002 [G]
183. Koskoff H: The Culture of Emotions (video recording). Boston, Fanlight Productions, 2002 [G]
184. Lim R: Cultural Psychiatry for Clinicians. Baltimore, Johns Hopkins University Press (in press) [G]
185. Hays P: Addressing Cultural Complexities in Practice: A Framework for Clinicians and Counselors. Washington, DC, American Psychological Association, 2001 [G]
186. Weinreich P, Saunderson W: Analyzing Identity: Cross-Cultural, Societal, and Clinical Contexts. New York, Routledge, 2003 [G]
187. Tervalon M, Murray-Garcia J: Cultural humility versus cultural competence: a critical distinction in defining physician training outcomes in multicultural education. J Health Care Poor Underserved 1998; 9:117–125 [G]
188. American Psychiatric Association: Diagnostic and Statistical Manual of Mental Disorders, 4th Edition, Text Revision. Washington, DC, American Psychiatric Association, 2000 [G]
189. Phillips KA, First MB, Pincus HA (eds): Advancing DSM Dilemmas in Psychiatric Diagnosis. Washington, DC, American Psychiatric Publishing, 2003 [G]
190. McHugh PR, Slavney PR: The Perspectives of Psychiatry, 2nd ed. Baltimore, Johns Hopkins University Press, 1998 [G]
191. Adams N, Grieder DM: Treatment Planning for Person-Centered Care: The Road to Mental Health and Addiction Recovery. Burlington, Mass, Elsevier, 2005 [G]
192. Grisso T, Appelbaum PS: Assessing Competence to Consent to Treatment: A Guide for Physicians and Other Health Professionals. New York, Oxford University Press, 1998 [G]
193. Maio JE: HIPAA and the special status of psychotherapy notes. Lippincotts Case Manag 2003; 8:24–29 [G]
194. American Psychiatric Association: Psychotherapy notes provision of the Health Insurance Portability and Accountability Act (HIPAA) privacy rule: a resource document. Washington, DC, American Psychiatric Association, 2001 [G]
195. Appelbaum PS: Privacy in psychiatric treatment: threats and responses. Am J Psychiatry 2002; 159:1809–1818 [G]
196. US Public Health Service: Confidentiality of Alcohol and Drug Abuse Patient Records. Code of Federal Regulations, Title 42, Chapter I, Part 2, 2000. http://www.access.gpo.gov/nara/cfr/waisidx_00/42cfr2_00.html [G]
197. Substance Abuse and Mental Health Services Administration: The Confidentiality of Alcohol and Drug Abuse Patient Records Regulation and the HIPAA Privacy Rule: Implications for Alcohol and Substance Abuse Programs, 2004. http://www.hipaa.samhsa.gov/Part2Applicability.htm [G]
198. Gutheil TG: Paranoia and progress notes: a guide to forensically informed psychiatric recordkeeping. Hosp Community Psychiatry 1980; 31:479–482 [G]
199. American Psychiatric Association: Minimum necessary guidelines for third-party payers for psychiatric treatment: a position statement. Washington, DC, American Psychiatric Association, 2002 [G]
200. American Psychiatric Association: Documentation of psychotherapy by psychiatrists: resource document. Washington, DC, American Psychiatric Association, 2002 [G]

201. McCormick JJ, Currier GW: Emergency medicine and mental health law. Top Emerg Med 1999; 21:28–37 [G]
202. Karlawish J, James B: Ethical issues in geriatric medicine: informed consent, surrogate decision making, and advanced care planning, in Principles of Geriatric Medicine and Gerontology, 5th ed. Edited by Hazzard WR, Glass JP, Halter JB, Ouslander JG, Tinetti M. New York, McGraw-Hill, 2003, pp 353–360 [G]
203. Srebnik DS, Rutherford LT, Peto T, Russo J, Zick E, Jaffe C, Holtzheimer P: The content and clinical utility of psychiatric advance directives. Psychiatr Serv 2005; 56:592–598 [G]
204. Simon RI: The law and psychiatry, in The American Psychiatric Publishing Textbook of Clinical Psychiatry, 4th ed. Edited by Hales RE, Yudofsky SC. Washington, DC, American Psychiatric Publishing, 2003, pp 1585–1628 [G]
205. Lamb HR, Weinberger LE: Persons with severe mental illness in jails and prisons: a review. Psychiatr Serv 1998; 49:483–492 [F]
206. National Institute of Corrections: Provision of Mental Health Care in Prisons. Washington, DC, US Department of Justice, 2001 [G]
207. National Commission on Correctional Health Care: Correctional Mental Health Care: Standards and Guidelines for Delivering Services. Chicago, National Commission on Correctional Health Care, 1999 [G]
208. Jones G, Connelly M: Mentally Ill Offenders and Mental Health Care Issues: An Overview of the Research. College Park, Md, Maryland State Commission on Criminal Sentencing Policy, 2002. http://www.msccsp.org/publications/mental.html [G]
209. Metzner JL: An introduction to correctional psychiatry, I. J Am Acad Psychiatry Law 1997; 25:375–381 [F]
210. Hayes LM: Prison Suicide: An Overview and Guide to Prevention. Washington, DC, US Department of Justice, National Institute of Corrections, 1995 [G]
211. Federal Bureau of Prisons: Federal Bureau of Prisons Clinical Practice Guidelines for Psychiatric Evaluations. Federal Bureau of Prisons, 2002. http://www.us.oup.com/us/pdf/pdr/psychEval.pdf [G]
212. American Psychiatric Association: Psychiatric Services in Jails and Prisons, 2nd ed. Washington, DC, American Psychiatric Association, 2000 [G]
213. Metzner JL, Miller RD, Kleinsasser D: Mental health screening and evaluation within prisons. Bull Am Acad Psychiatry Law 1994; 22:451–457 [F]
214. Bell CC: Correctional psychiatry, in Kaplan and Sadock's Comprehensive Textbook of Psychiatry, 8th ed. Edited by Sadock BJ, Sadock VA. Philadelphia, Lippincott Williams & Wilkins, 2005, pp 4002–4012 [G]
215. McKee GR: Lethal vs nonlethal suicide attempts in jail. Psychol Rep 1998; 82:611–614 [G]
216. Marcus P, Alcabes P: Characteristics of suicides by inmates in an urban jail. Hosp Community Psychiatry 1993; 44:256–261 [C]
217. Hayes LM, Kajden B: And Darkness Closes In: A National Study of Jail Suicides: Final Report to the National Institute of Corrections. Washington, DC, National Center on Institutions and Alternatives, 1981 [E]
218. Hayes LM: National study of jail suicides: seven years later. Psychiatr Q 1989; 60:7–29 [F]
219. Bonner RL: Isolation, seclusion, and psychosocial vulnerability as risk factors for suicide behind bars, in Assessment and Prediction of Suicide. Edited by Maris RW, Berman AL, Maltsberger JT, Yufit RI. New York, Guilford, 1992, pp 398–419 [F]
220. McQuistion HL, Felix A, Susser ES: Serving homeless people with mental illness, in Psychiatry, 2nd ed. Edited by Tasman A, Lieberman J, Kay J. London, Wiley, 2003, pp 2314–2321 [G]
221. Rush KS, Bowman LG, Eidman SL, Toole LM, Mortenson BP: Assessing psychopathology in individuals with developmental disabilities. Behav Modif 2004; 28:621–637 [F]

222. King BH, DeAntonio C, McCracken JT, Forness SR, Ackerland V: Psychiatric consultation in severe and profound mental retardation. Am J Psychiatry 1994; 151:1802–1808 [G]
223. Ferrell RB, Wolinsky EJ, Kauffman CI, Flashman LA, McAllister TW: Neuropsychiatric syndromes in adults with intellectual disability: issues in assessment and treatment. Curr Psychiatry Rep 2004; 6:380–390 [F]
224. Finlay WM, Lyons E: Methodological issues in interviewing and using self-report questionnaires with people with mental retardation. Psychol Assess 2001; 13:319–335 [F]
225. Ross E, Oliver C: The assessment of mood in adults who have severe or profound mental retardation. Clin Psychol Rev 2003; 23:225–245 [F]
226. Desrochers MN, Hile MG, Williams-Moseley TL: Survey of functional assessment procedures used with individuals who display mental retardation and severe problem behaviors. Am J Ment Retard 1997; 101:535–546 [G]
227. Beange H, McElduff A, Baker W: Medical disorders of adults with mental retardation: a population study. Am J Ment Retard 1995; 99:595–604 [G]
228. Kupfer DJ, First MB, Regier DA (eds): A Research Agenda for DSM-V. Washington, DC, American Psychiatric Association, 2002 [G]
229. McLean M, Armstrong D: Eliciting patients' concerns: a randomised controlled trial of different approaches by the doctor. Br J Gen Pract 2004; 54:663–666 [A–]
230. Brewer DD, Garrett SB: Evaluation of interviewing techniques to enhance recall of sexual and drug injection partners. Sex Transm Dis 2001; 28:666–677 [A–]
231. Swenson SL, Buell S, Zettler P, White M, Ruston DC, Lo B: Patient-centered communication: do patients really prefer it? J Gen Intern Med 2004; 19:1069–1079 [G]
232. O'Keefe M, Roberton D, Sawyer M, Baghurst P: Medical student interviewing: a randomized trial of patient-centeredness and clinical competence. Fam Pract 2003; 20:213–219 [G]
233. Stewart M, Brown JB, Donner A, McWhinney IR, Oates J, Weston WW, Jordan J: The impact of patient-centered care on outcomes. J Fam Pract 2000; 49:796–804 [G]
234. Dowsett SM, Saul JL, Butow PN, Dunn SM, Boyer MJ, Findlow R, Dunsmore J: Communication styles in the cancer consultation: preferences for a patient-centered approach. Psychooncology 2000; 9:147–156 [A–]
235. Williams N, Ogden J: The impact of matching the patient's vocabulary: a randomized control trial. Fam Pract 2004; 21:630–635 [A–]
236. Razavi D, Delvaux N, Marchal S, Durieux JF, Farvacques C, Dubus L, Hogenraad R: Does training increase the use of more emotionally laden words by nurses when talking with cancer patients? a randomised study. Br J Cancer 2002; 87:1–7 [A–]
237. Wells KB, Sherbourne C, Schoenbaum M, Duan N, Meredith L, Unutzer J, Miranda J, Carney MF, Rubenstein LV: Impact of disseminating quality improvement programs for depression in managed primary care: a randomized controlled trial. JAMA 2000; 283:212–220 [B]
238. Chinman M, Young AS, Schell T, Hassell J, Mintz J: Computer-assisted self-assessment in persons with severe mental illness. J Clin Psychiatry 2004; 65:1343–1351 [A–]
239. Newman JC, Des J, Turner CF, Gribble J, Cooley P, Paone D: The differential effects of face-to-face and computer interview modes. Am J Public Health 2002; 92:294–297 [G]
240. Solomon GL, Dechter M: Are patients pleased with computer use in the examination room? J Fam Pract 1995; 41:241–244 [A–]
241. Garrison GM, Bernard ME, Rasmussen NH: Twenty-first-century health care: the effect of computer use by physicians on patient satisfaction at a family medicine clinic. Fam Med 2002; 34:362–368 [G]
242. Main DS, Quintela J, Araya-Guerra R, Holcomb S, Pace WD: Exploring patient reactions to pen-tablet computers: a report from CaReNet. Ann Fam Med 2004; 2:421–424 [G]
243. Rudd MD, Rajab MH: Specificity of the Beck Depression Inventory and the confounding role of comorbid disorders in a clinical sample. Cognit Ther Res 1995; 19:51–68 [G]

244. Rocchi A, Pellegrini S, Siciliano G, Murri L: Causative and susceptibility genes for Alzheimer's disease: a review. Brain Res Bull 2003; 61:1–24 [F]
245. Egan MF, Goldberg TE, Kolachana BS, Callicott JH, Mazzanti CM, Straub RE, Goldman D, Weinberger DR: Effect of COMT Val108/158Met genotype on frontal lobe function and risk for schizophrenia. Proc Natl Acad Sci U S A 2001; 98:6917–6922 [G]
246. Goldberg TE, Egan MF, Gscheidle T, Coppola R, Weickert T, Kolachana BS, Goldman D, Weinberger DR: Executive subprocesses in working memory: relationship to catechol-*O*-methyltransferase Val158Met genotype and schizophrenia. Arch Gen Psychiatry 2003; 60:889–896 [G]
247. Harrison PJ, Owen MJ: Genes for schizophrenia? recent findings and their pathophysiological implications. Lancet 2003; 361:417–419 [G]
248. Ressler KJ, Nemeroff CB: Role of serotonergic and noradrenergic systems in the pathophysiology of depression and anxiety disorders. Depress Anxiety 2000; 12(suppl 1):2–19 [G]
249. Hariri AR, Weinberger DR: Imaging genomics. Br Med Bull 2003; 65:259–270 [G]
250. Caspi A, Sugden K, Moffitt TE, Taylor A, Craig IW, Harrington H, McClay J, Mill J, Martin J, Braithwaite A, Poulton R: Influence of life stress on depression: moderation by a polymorphism in the 5-HTT gene. Science 2003; 301:386–389 [C]
251. Bookheimer SY, Strojwas MH, Cohen MS, Saunders AM, Pericak-Vance MA, Mazziotta JC, Small GW: Patterns of brain activation in people at risk for Alzheimer's disease. N Engl J Med 2000; 343:450–456 [D]
252. Moffitt TE, Caspi A, Rutter M: Strategy for investigating interactions between measured genes and measured environments. Arch Gen Psychiatry 2005; 62:473–481 [G]
253. Killiany RJ, Gomez-Isla T, Moss M, Kikinis R, Sandor T, Jolesz F, Tanzi R, Jones K, Hyman BT, Albert MS: Use of structural magnetic resonance imaging to predict who will get Alzheimer's disease. Ann Neurol 2000; 47:430–439 [C]
254. Killiany RJ, Hyman BT, Gomez-Isla T, Moss MB, Kikinis R, Jolesz F, Tanzi R, Jones K, Albert MS: MRI measures of entorhinal cortex vs hippocampus in preclinical AD. Neurology 2002; 58:1188–1196 [G]
255. Kaye JA, Swihart T, Howieson D, Dame A, Moore MM, Karnos T, Camicioli R, Ball M, Oken B, Sexton G: Volume loss of the hippocampus and temporal lobe in healthy elderly persons destined to develop dementia. Neurology 1997; 48:1297–1304 [C]
256. Xu Y, Jack CR Jr, O'Brien PC, Kokmen E, Smith GE, Ivnik RJ, Boeve BF, Tangalos RG, Petersen RC: Usefulness of MRI measures of entorhinal cortex versus hippocampus in AD. Neurology 2000; 54:1760–1767 [D]
257. Jagust WJ, Budinger TF, Reed BR: The diagnosis of dementia with single photon emission computed tomography. Arch Neurol 1987; 44:258–262 [G]
258. DeKosky ST, Shih WJ, Schmitt FA, Coupal J, Kirkpatrick C: Assessing utility of single photon emission computed tomography (SPECT) scan in Alzheimer disease: correlation with cognitive severity. Alzheimer Dis Assoc Disord 1990; 4:14–23 [G]
259. Holman BL, Tumeh SS: Single-photon emission computed tomography (SPECT): applications and potential. JAMA 1990; 263:561–564 [G]
260. Silverman DH, Gambhir SS, Huang HW, Schwimmer J, Kim S, Small GW, Chodosh J, Czernin J, Phelps ME: Evaluating early dementia with and without assessment of regional cerebral metabolism by PET: a comparison of predicted costs and benefits. J Nucl Med 2002; 43:253–266 [G]
261. Herholz K, Salmon E, Perani D, Baron JC, Holthoff V, Frolich L, Schonknecht P, Ito K, Mielke R, Kalbe E, Zundorf G, Delbeuck X, Pelati O, Anchisi D, Fazio F, Kerrouche N, Desgranges B, Eustache F, Beuthien-Baumann B, Menzel C, Schroder J, Kato T, Arahata Y, Henze M, Heiss WD: Discrimination between Alzheimer dementia and controls by automated analysis of multicenter FDG PET. Neuroimage 2002; 17:302–316 [D]

262. Gill SS, Rochon PA, Guttman M, Laupacis A: The value of positron emission tomography in the clinical evaluation of dementia. J Am Geriatr Soc 2003; 51:258–264 [F]
263. Kulasingam SL, Samsa GP, Zarin DA, Rutschmann OT, Patwardhan MB, McCrory DC, Schmechel DE, Matchar DB: When should functional neuroimaging techniques be used in the diagnosis and management of Alzheimer's dementia? a decision analysis. Value Health 2003; 6:542–550 [E]
264. Silverman DH, Small GW, Chang CY, Lu CS, Kung De Aburto MA, Chen W, Czernin J, Rapoport SI, Pietrini P, Alexander GE, Schapiro MB, Jagust WJ, Hoffman JM, Welsh-Bohmer KA, Alavi A, Clark CM, Salmon E, de Leon MJ, Mielke R, Cummings JL, Kowell AP, Gambhir SS, Hoh CK, Phelps ME: Positron emission tomography in evaluation of dementia: regional brain metabolism and long-term outcome. JAMA 2001; 286:2120–2127 [C]
265. Hoffman JM, Hanson MW, Welsh KA, Earl N, Paine S, Delong D, Coleman RE: Interpretation variability of 18FDG-positron emission tomography studies in dementia. Invest Radiol 1996; 31:316–322 [G]
266. Drevets WC, Videen TO, Price JL, Preskorn SH, Carmichael ST, Raichle ME: A functional anatomical study of unipolar depression. J Neurosci 1992; 12:3628–3641 [G]
267. Coffey CE, Wilkinson WE, Weiner RD, Parashos IA, Djang WT, Webb MC, Figiel GS, Spritzer CE: Quantitative cerebral anatomy in depression: a controlled magnetic resonance imaging study. Arch Gen Psychiatry 1993; 50:7–16 [D]
268. Steffens DC, Krishnan KR: Structural neuroimaging and mood disorders: recent findings, implications for classification, and future directions. Biol Psychiatry 1998; 43:705–712 [F]
269. Drevets WC: Functional anatomical abnormalities in limbic and prefrontal cortical structures in major depression. Prog Brain Res 2000; 126:413–431 [G]
270. Bearden CE, Hoffman KM, Cannon TD: The neuropsychology and neuroanatomy of bipolar affective disorder: a critical review. Bipolar Disord 2001; 3:106–150 [F]
271. Kumar A, Gupta RC, Albert TM, Alger J, Wyckoff N, Hwang S: Biophysical changes in normal-appearing white matter and subcortical nuclei in late-life major depression detected using magnetization transfer. Psychiatry Res 2004; 130:131–140 [G]
272. Glahn DC, Ragland JD, Abramoff A, Barrett J, Laird AR, Bearden CE, Velligan DI: Beyond hypofrontality: a quantitative meta-analysis of functional neuroimaging studies of working memory in schizophrenia. Hum Brain Mapp 2005; 25:60–69 [E]
273. Meyer-Lindenberg AS, Olsen RK, Kohn PD, Brown T, Egan MF, Weinberger DR, Berman KF: Regionally specific disturbance of dorsolateral prefrontal-hippocampal functional connectivity in schizophrenia. Arch Gen Psychiatry 2005; 62:379–386 [D]
274. Szeszko PR, Ardekani BA, Ashtari M, Kumra S, Robinson DG, Sevy S, Gunduz-Bruce H, Malhotra AK, Kane JM, Bilder RM, Lim KO: White matter abnormalities in first-episode schizophrenia or schizoaffective disorder: a diffusion tensor imaging study. Am J Psychiatry 2005; 162:602–605 [D]
275. MacDonald AW III, Carter CS, Kerns JG, Ursu S, Barch DM, Holmes AJ, Stenger VA, Cohen JD: Specificity of prefrontal dysfunction and context processing deficits to schizophrenia in never-medicated patients with first-episode psychosis. Am J Psychiatry 2005; 162:475–484 [D]
276. Hill K, Mann L, Laws KR, Stephenson CM, Nimmo-Smith I, McKenna PJ: Hypofrontality in schizophrenia: a meta-analysis of functional imaging studies. Acta Psychiatr Scand 2004; 110:243–256 [E]
277. Davidson LL, Heinrichs RW: Quantification of frontal and temporal lobe brain-imaging findings in schizophrenia: a meta-analysis. Psychiatry Res 2003; 122:69–87 [E]
278. Konick LC, Friedman L: Meta-analysis of thalamic size in schizophrenia. Biol Psychiatry 2001; 49:28–38 [E]

279. Zakzanis KK, Poulin P, Hansen KT, Jolic D: Searching the schizophrenic brain for temporal lobe deficits: a systematic review and meta-analysis. Psychol Med 2000; 30:491–504 [E]
280. Wright IC, Rabe-Hesketh S, Woodruff PW, David AS, Murray RM, Bullmore ET: Meta-analysis of regional brain volumes in schizophrenia. Am J Psychiatry 2000; 157:16–25 [E]
281. Riffkin J, Yucel M, Maruff P, Wood SJ, Soulsby B, Olver J, Kyrios M, Velakoulis D, Pantelis C: A manual and automated MRI study of anterior cingulate and orbito-frontal cortices, and caudate nucleus in obsessive-compulsive disorder: comparison with healthy controls and patients with schizophrenia. Psychiatry Res 2005; 138:99–113 [D]
282. van den Heuvel OA, Veltman DJ, Groenewegen HJ, Cath DC, van Balkom AJ, van Hartskamp J, Barkhof F, van Dyck R: Frontal-striatal dysfunction during planning in obsessive-compulsive disorder. Arch Gen Psychiatry 2005; 62:301–309 [D]
283. Pujol J, Soriano-Mas C, Alonso P, Cardoner N, Menchon JM, Deus J, Vallejo J: Mapping structural brain alterations in obsessive-compulsive disorder. Arch Gen Psychiatry 2004; 61:720–730 [D]
284. Kitayama N, Vaccarino V, Kutner M, Weiss P, Bremner JD: Magnetic resonance imaging (MRI) measurement of hippocampal volume in posttraumatic stress disorder: a meta-analysis. J Affect Disord 2005; 88:79–86 [E]
285. Mathew SJ, Mao X, Coplan JD, Smith EL, Sackeim HA, Gorman JM, Shungu DC: Dorsolateral prefrontal cortical pathology in generalized anxiety disorder: a proton magnetic resonance spectroscopic imaging study. Am J Psychiatry 2004; 161:1119–1121 [D]
286. Bremner JD, Vythilingam M, Vermetten E, Southwick SM, McGlashan T, Nazeer A, Khan S, Vaccarino LV, Soufer R, Garg PK, Ng CK, Staib LH, Duncan JS, Charney DS: MRI and PET study of deficits in hippocampal structure and function in women with childhood sexual abuse and posttraumatic stress disorder. Am J Psychiatry 2003; 160:924–932 [D]
287. Massana G, Serra-Grabulosa JM, Salgado-Pineda P, Gasto C, Junque C, Massana J, Mercader JM, Gomez B, Tobena A, Salamero M: Amygdalar atrophy in panic disorder patients detected by volumetric magnetic resonance imaging. Neuroimage 2003; 19:80–90 [D]
288. Massana G, Serra-Grabulosa JM, Salgado-Pineda P, Gasto C, Junque C, Massana J, Mercader JM: Parahippocampal gray matter density in panic disorder: a voxel-based morphometric study. Am J Psychiatry 2003; 160:566–568 [D]
289. Morey RA, Inan S, Mitchell TV, Perkins DO, Lieberman JA, Belger A: Imaging frontostriatal function in ultra-high-risk, early, and chronic schizophrenia during executive processing. Arch Gen Psychiatry 2005; 62:254–262 [D]
290. Woods BT, Ward KE, Johnson EH: Meta-analysis of the time-course of brain volume reduction in schizophrenia: implications for pathogenesis and early treatment. Schizophr Res 2005; 73:221–228 [E]
291. Strasser HC, Lilyestrom J, Ashby ER, Honeycutt NA, Schretlen DJ, Pulver AE, Hopkins RO, Depaulo JR, Potash JB, Schweizer B, Yates KO, Kurian E, Barta PE, Pearlson GD: Hippocampal and ventricular volumes in psychotic and nonpsychotic bipolar patients compared with schizophrenia patients and community control subjects: a pilot study. Biol Psychiatry 2005; 57:633–639 [D]
292. Saxena S, Brody AL, Maidment KM, Smith EC, Zohrabi N, Katz E, Baker SK, Baxter LR Jr: Cerebral glucose metabolism in obsessive-compulsive hoarding. Am J Psychiatry 2004; 161:1038–1048 [D]
293. Kennedy SH, Evans KR, Houle S, Vaccarino FJ: PET analysis of antidepressant effects of paroxetine (abstract #47). Continuing Medical Education Syllabus and Scientific Proceedings of the 151st Annual Meeting of the American Psychiatric Association. Toronto, May 30–June 4, 1998 [G]
294. Sackeim HA, Prohovnik I, Moeller JR, Brown RP, Apter S, Prudic J, Devanand DP, Mukherjee S: Regional cerebral blood flow in mood disorders, I: comparison of major depressives and normal controls at rest. Arch Gen Psychiatry 1990; 47:60–70 [D]

295. Sackeim HA, Prohovnik I: Brain imaging studies of depressive disorders, in The Biology of Depressive Disorders, Part A: A Systems Perspective. Edited by Mann JJ, Kupfer DJ. New York, Plenum, 1993, pp 205–258 [G]
296. Nobler MS, Roose SP, Prohovnik I, Moeller JR, Louie J, Van Heertum RL, Sackeim HA: Regional cerebral blood flow in mood disorders, V: effects of antidepressant medication in late-life depression. Am J Geriatr Psychiatry 2000; 8:289–296 [G]
297. Figiel GS, Krishnan KR, Doraiswamy PM, Rao VP, Nemeroff CB, Boyko OB: Subcortical hyperintensities on brain magnetic resonance imaging: a comparison between late age onset and early onset elderly depressed subjects. Neurobiol Aging 1991; 12:245–247 [G]
298. Hickie I, Scott E, Mitchell P, Wilhelm K, Austin MP, Bennett B: Subcortical hyperintensities on magnetic resonance imaging: clinical correlates and prognostic significance in patients with severe depression. Biol Psychiatry 1995; 37:151–160 [G]
299. Saxena S, Brody AL, Ho ML, Zohrabi N, Maidment KM, Baxter LR Jr: Differential brain metabolic predictors of response to paroxetine in obsessive-compulsive disorder versus major depression. Am J Psychiatry 2003; 160:522–532 [G]
300. Drevets WC, Bogers W, Raichle ME: Functional anatomical correlates of antidepressant drug treatment assessed using PET measures of regional glucose metabolism. Eur Neuropsychopharmacol 2002; 12:527–544 [G]
301. Phan KL, Wager T, Taylor SF, Liberzon I: Functional neuroanatomy of emotion: a meta-analysis of emotion activation studies in PET and fMRI. Neuroimage 2002; 16:331–348 [E]
302. Carey PD, Warwick J, Niehaus DJ, van der Linden G, van Heerden BB, Harvey BH, Seedat S, Stein DJ: Single photon emission computed tomography (SPECT) of anxiety disorders before and after treatment with citalopram. BMC Psychiatry 2004; 4:30 [G]

GUIDELINE WATCH: PRACTICE GUIDELINE FOR THE TREATMENT OF PATIENTS WITH DELIRIUM

Ian A. Cook, M.D.

Since the 1999 publication of the APA's *Practice Guideline for the Treatment of Patients With Delirium* (1), advances in the clinical neurosciences and other areas have contributed to the understanding of delirium and have expanded options for its management. This guideline watch summarizes important elements of the incremental progress in this area.

DETECTION

The 1999 guideline noted that the presence of delirium is frequently undetected by clinicians until psychiatric consultation is obtained, often triggered by dangerous behaviors. In the years since 1999, many papers providing easily remembered strategies for clinical detection and management of delirium have been published, not only in the psychiatric literature but also in journals that focus on critical care, pain management, oncology, medical-surgical nursing, substance abuse, and geriatric medicine. Despite this broadening literature base, it has been noted that many cases of delirium continue to be missed (2). Reasons for this underrecognition are varied but may include the absence of routine, systematic screening (3). Improved attention to and recognition of delirium should be motivated by its clinical importance (e.g., association with elevated mortality [4]).

One step toward improved detection may be the use of instruments that have demonstrated sensitivity to the presence of delirium. Examples include the Delirium Rating Scale—Revised–98 (5, 6), including a version for use with children (7); the Delirium Observation Screening Scale (8); and the Confusion Assessment Method for the Intensive Care Unit (9–11). Instruments have variable concordance with the diagnostic criteria detailed in DSM-IV, and each instrument may be better suited to particular clinical contexts.

The American Psychiatric Association (APA) practice guidelines are developed by expert work groups using an explicit methodology that includes rigorous review of available evidence, broad peer review of iterative drafts, and formal approval by the APA Assembly and Board of Trustees. APA practice guidelines are intended to assist psychiatrists in clinical decision making. They are not intended to be a standard of care. The ultimate judgment regarding a particular clinical procedure or treatment plan must be made by the psychiatrist in light of the clinical data presented by the patient and the diagnostic and treatment options available. Guideline watches summarize significant developments in practice since publication of an APA practice guideline. Watches may be authored and reviewed by experts associated with the original guideline development effort and are approved for publication by APA's Executive Committee on Practice Guidelines. Thus, watches represent opinion of the authors and approval of the Executive Committee but not policy of the APA. This guideline watch was published in August 2004. Suggested citation: Cook IA: *Guideline Watch: Practice Guideline for the Treatment of Patients With Delirium.* Arlington, VA: American Psychiatric Association, 2004. Available online at http://www.psych.org/psych_pract/treatg/pg/prac_guide.cfm.

NEUROPATHOPHYSIOLOGIC MODELS

The etiologic heterogeneity of delirium is a persistent theme in the more recent literature (10, 12–15). The role of the anticholinergic properties of a variety of medications continues to be noted (16, 17). In a patient population with a mixture of putative causes of delirium, regional cerebral perfusion was consistently reported to show significant reductions during periods of delirium in comparison with blood flow patterns after recovery (18). The possibility of a final common pathway, involving acetylcholine and dopamine, has been advanced (15, 19, 20). The feature of sleep/wake cycle disruption in delirium has led others to speculate about the possible role of melatonin (21, 22). Although more research could prove illuminating, there are practical challenges to performing controlled clinical investigations with delirious persons, thoughtfully summarized by Meagher (23). Despite these challenges, there is pressing need for more research in this area.

MANAGEMENT

Management of patients with delirium continues to focus on ensuring safety from behavioral disturbances while simultaneously assessing for a probable etiology and definitive treatment. Safety can best be addressed by combining environmental, behavioral, and pharmacologic means. In addition to the alterations in the hospital environment noted in the 1999 guideline, low-tech but potentially labor-intensive changes in nurse–patient interactions, as well as flexibility within hospital systems to individualize processes of care, may be able to reduce the impact of delirium (24). Behavioral programs can be highly effective but appear to be critically dependent on adherence to the details of the program (25).

Current pharmacological interventions expand the options reported in the 1999 guideline. Data supporting the use of first-generation antipsychotic medications (12) have been joined by case reports, case series, and a limited number of open-label trials supporting the use of second-generation antipsychotic medications (26) such as olanzapine (27–29), risperidone (30–32), ziprasidone (33), and quetiapine (34–38). The prophylactic use of haloperidol has been examined in hip surgery patients in a prospective, double-blind, placebo-controlled trial (39), and although the incidence of delirium was not significantly altered by the intervention, there were significant differences in important secondary measures (duration of delirium, length of stay, Delirium Rating Scale scores) in this prevention trial. Given the dearth of research data, there is a clear need for prospective, randomized, controlled efficacy trials of second-generation antipsychotic medications for the management of delirium. Cholinesterase inhibitors also have shown success in managing delirium in some case reports, but usually for reversing drug-induced delirium, both for donepezil (40–43) and rivastigmine (44). The avoidance of benzodiazepines except for particular indications (e.g., alcohol or γ-hydroxybutyric acid [GHA] withdrawal delirium, delirium related to seizures) continues to be a recommendation (12). In addition, if patients in critical care settings are already receiving high doses of parenteral lorazepam, the clinician will want to be alert for toxicity (e.g., renal dysfunction, hyperosmolar metabolic acidosis) associated with lorazepam's propylene glycol vehicle (45–47).

REFERENCES

1. American Psychiatric Association: Practice guideline for the treatment of patients with delirium. Am J Psychiatry 1999; 156(5 suppl):1–20
2. Laurila JV, Pitkala KH, Strandberg TE, Tilvis RS: Detection and documentation of dementia and delirium in acute geriatric wards. Gen Hosp Psychiatry 2004; 26:31–35

3. Ely EW, Stephens RK, Jackson JC, Thomason JW, Truman B, Gordon S, Dittus RS, Bernard GR: Current opinions regarding the importance, diagnosis, and management of delirium in the intensive care unit: a survey of 912 healthcare professionals. Crit Care Med 2004; 32:106–112
4. McCusker J, Cole M, Abrahamowicz M, Primeau F, Belzile E: Delirium predicts 12-month mortality. Arch Intern Med 2002; 162:457–463
5. Trzepacz PT: The Delirium Rating Scale: its use in consultation-liaison research. Psychosomatics 1999; 40:193–204
6. Trzepacz PT, Mittal D, Torres R, Kanary K, Norton J, Jimerson N: Validation of the Delirium Rating Scale—Revised–98: comparison with the Delirium Rating Scale and the Cognitive Test for Delirium. J Neuropsychiatry Clin Neurosci 2001; 13:229–242
7. Turkel SB, Braslow K, Tavare CJ, Trzepacz PT: The Delirium Rating Scale in children and adolescents. Psychosomatics 2003; 44:126–129
8. Schuurmans MJ, Shortridge-Baggett LM, Duursma SA: The Delirium Observation Screening Scale: a screening instrument for delirium. Res Theory Nurs Pract 2003; 17:31–50
9. Inouye SK, van Dyck CH, Alessi CA, Balkin S, Siegal AP, Horwitz RI: Clarifying confusion: the Confusion Assessment Method. A new method for detection of delirium. Ann Intern Med 1990; 113:941–948
10. Ely EW, Margolin R, Francis J, May L, Truman B, Dittus R, Speroff T, Gautam S, Bernard GR, Inouye SK: Evaluation of delirium in critically ill patients: validation of the Confusion Assessment Method for the Intensive Care Unit (CAM-ICU). Crit Care Med 2001; 29:1370–1379
11. Laurila JV, Pitkala KH, Strandberg TE, Tilvis RS: Confusion Assessment Method in the diagnostics of delirium among aged hospital patients: would it serve better in screening than as a diagnostic instrument? Int J Geriatr Psychiatry 2002; 17:1112–1119
12. Meagher DJ: Delirium: optimising management. BMJ 2001; 322:144–149
13. Packard RC: Delirium. Neurologist 2001; 7:327–340
14. Cole MG: Delirium in elderly patients. Am J Geriatr Psychiatry 2004; 12:7–21
15. Trzepacz PT, Meagher DJ: Delirium, in The American Psychiatric Publishing Textbook of Psychosomatic Medicine. Edited by Levenson JL. Washington, DC, American Psychiatric Publishing, 2005, pp 91–130
16. Tune LE: Anticholinergic effects of medication in elderly patients. J Clin Psychiatry 2001; 62(suppl 21):11–14
17. Mulsant BH, Pollock BG, Kirshner M, Shen C, Dodge H, Ganguli M: Serum anticholinergic activity in a community-based sample of older adults: relationship with cognitive performance. Arch Gen Psychiatry 2003; 60:198–203
18. Yokota H, Ogawa S, Kurokawa A, Yamamoto Y: Regional cerebral blood flow in delirium patients. Psychiatry Clin Neurosci 2003; 57:337–339
19. Trzepacz PT: Update on the neuropathogenesis of delirium. Dement Geriatr Cogn Disord 1999; 10:330–334
20. Trzepacz PT: Is there a final common neural pathway in delirium? Focus on acetylcholine and dopamine. Semin Clin Neuropsychiatry 2000; 5:132–148
21. Hanania M, Kitain E: Melatonin for treatment and prevention of postoperative delirium. Anesth Analg 2002; 94:338–339
22. Balan S, Leibovitz A, Zila SO, Ruth M, Chana W, Yassica B, Rahel B, Richard G, Neumann E, Blagman B, Habot B: The relation between the clinical subtypes of delirium and the urinary level of 6-SMT. J Neuropsychiatry Clin Neurosci 2003; 15:363–366
23. Meagher DJ: Reply to "Optimising Management of Delirium." BMJ 2001; 322:1602
24. Flaherty JH, Tariq SH, Raghavan S, Bakshi S, Moinuddin A, Morley JE: A model for managing delirious older inpatients. J Am Geriatr Soc 2003; 51:1031–1035

25. Inouye SK, Bogardus ST Jr, Williams CS, Leo-Summers L, Agostini JV: The role of adherence on the effectiveness of nonpharmacologic interventions: evidence from the delirium prevention trial. Arch Intern Med 2003; 163:958–964
26. Schwartz TL, Masand PS: The role of atypical antipsychotics in the treatment of delirium. Psychosomatics 2002; 43:171–174
27. Passik SD, Cooper M: Complicated delirium in a cancer patient successfully treated with olanzapine. J Pain Symptom Manage 1999; 17:219–223
28. Kim KS, Pae CU, Chae JH, Bahk WM, Jun T: An open pilot trial of olanzapine for delirium in the Korean population. Psychiatry Clin Neurosci 2001; 55:515–519
29. Breitbart W, Tremblay A, Gibson C: An open trial of olanzapine for the treatment of delirium in hospitalized cancer patients. Psychosomatics 2002; 43:175–182
30. Sipahimalani A, Sime RM, Masand PS: Treatment of delirium with risperidone. Int J Geriatr Psychopharmacol 1997; 1:24–26
31. Furmaga KM, DeLeon OA, Sinha SB, Jobe TH, Gaviria M: Psychosis in medical conditions: response to risperidone. Gen Hosp Psychiatry 1997; 19:223–228
32. Horikawa N, Yamazaki T, Miyamoto K, Kurosawa A, Oiso H, Matsumoto F, Nishimura K, Karasawa K, Takamatsu K: Treatment for delirium with risperidone: results of a prospective open trial with 10 patients. Gen Hosp Psychiatry 2003; 25:289–292
33. Leso L, Schwartz TL: Ziprasidone treatment of delirium. Psychosomatics 2002; 43:61–62
34. Schwartz TL, Masand PS: Treatment of delirium with quetiapine. Prim Care Companion J Clin Psychiatry 2000; 2:10–12
35. Torres R, Mittal D, Kennedy R: Use of quetiapine in delirium: case reports. Psychosomatics 2001; 42:347–349
36. Sasaki Y, Matsuyama T, Inoue S, Sunami T, Inoue T, Denda K, Koyama T: A prospective, open-label, flexible-dose study of quetiapine in the treatment of delirium. J Clin Psychiatry 2003; 64:1316–1321
37. Al Samarrai S, Dunn J, Newmark T, Gupta S: Quetiapine for treatment-resistant delirium. Psychosomatics 2003; 44:350–351
38. Kim KY, Bader GM, Kotlyar V, Gropper D: Treatment of delirium in older adults with quetiapine. J Geriatr Psychiatry Neurol 2003; 16:29–31
39. Kalisvaart KJ, de Jonghe J, Bogaards MJ, Burger BJ, van Gool PA, Egberts TC, Eikelenboom P: A placebo-controlled study of haloperidol prophylaxis for post-operative delirium in elderly hip-surgery patients. J Am Geriatr Soc 2003; 51(suppl 4):239–255
40. Wengel SP, Roccaforte WH, Burke WJ: Donepezil improves symptoms of delirium in dementia: implications for future research. J Geriatr Psychiatry Neurol 1998; 11:159–161
41. Wengel SP, Burke WJ, Roccaforte WH: Donepezil for postoperative delirium associated with Alzheimer's disease. J Am Geriatr Soc 1999; 47:379–380
42. Burt T: Donepezil and related cholinesterase inhibitors as mood and behavioral controlling agents. Curr Psychiatry Rep 2000; 2:473–478
43. Gleason OC: Donepezil for postoperative delirium. Psychosomatics 2003; 44:437–438
44. Dautzenberg PL, Wouters CJ, Oudejans I, Samson MM: Rivastigmine in prevention of delirium in a 65 year old man with Parkinson's disease. Int J Geriatr Psychiatry 2003; 18:555–556
45. Yaucher NE, Fish JT, Smith HW, Wells JA: Propylene glycol–associated renal toxicity from lorazepam infusion. Pharmacotherapy 2003; 23:1094–1099
46. Mullins ME, Barnes BJ: Hyperosmolar metabolic acidosis and intravenous lorazepam. N Engl J Med 2002; 347:857–858
47. Reynolds HN, Teiken P, Regan ME, Habashi NM, Cottingham C, McCunn M, Scalea TM: Hyperlactatemia, increased osmolar gap, and renal dysfunction during continuous lorazepam infusion. Crit Care Med 2000; 28:1631–1634

PRACTICE GUIDELINE FOR THE Treatment of Patients With Delirium

WORK GROUP ON DELIRIUM

Paula Trzepacz, M.D., Chair
William Breitbart, M.D.
John Franklin, M.D.
James Levenson, M.D.
D. Richard Martini, M.D.
Philip Wang, M.D., Dr.P.H. (Consultant)

Originally published in May 1999. A guideline watch, summarizing significant developments in the scientific literature since publication of this guideline, may be available in the Psychiatric Practice section of the APA web site at www.psych.org.

CONTENTS

Introduction 69

Development Process 70

I. Summary of Recommendations 71
  A. Coding System 71
  B. General Considerations 71

II. Disease Definition, Epidemiology, and Natural History 72
  A. Definition and Clinical Features 72
  B. Associated Features 74
  C. Differential Diagnosis 74
  D. Prevalence and Course 74
  E. Causes 75
  F. Use of Formal Measures 77

III. Treatment Principles and Alternatives 79
  A. Psychiatric Management 79
  B. Environmental and Supportive Interventions 82
  C. Somatic Interventions 84

IV. Formulation and Implementation of a Treatment Plan 89
  A. Psychiatric Management 89
  B. Choice of Specific Environmental and Supportive Interventions 90
  C. Choice of Somatic Intervention 90
  D. Issues of Competency and Consent 91

V. Clinical Features Influencing Treatment 92
  A. Comorbid Psychiatric Disorders 92
  B. Comorbid General Medical Conditions 92
  C. Advanced Age 92

VI. Reviewers and Reviewing Organizations 93

VII. References 94

INTRODUCTION

This practice guideline seeks to summarize data regarding the care of patients with delirium. It begins at the point where the psychiatrist has diagnosed a patient as suffering from delirium according to the DSM-IV criteria for the disorder. The purpose of this guideline is to assist the psychiatrist in caring for a patient with delirium.

Psychiatrists care for patients with delirium in many different settings and serve a variety of functions. In many cases, a psychiatrist will serve as a consultant to the attending physician and will not have primary responsibility for the patient. This guideline reviews the treatment that patients with delirium may need. The psychiatrist should either provide or advocate for the appropriate treatments. In addition, many patients have comorbid conditions that cannot be described completely with one DSM diagnostic category. Therefore, the psychiatrist caring for patients with delirium should consider, but not be limited to, the treatments recommended in this practice guideline.

To share feedback on this or other published APA practice guidelines, a form is available at http://www.psych.org/psych_pract/pg/reviewform.cfm.

DEVELOPMENT PROCESS

This practice guideline was developed under the auspices of the Steering Committee on Practice Guidelines. The process is detailed in the Appendix to this volume. Key features of the process include the following:

- a comprehensive literature review (description follows) and development of evidence tables;
- initial drafting by a work group that included psychiatrists with clinical and research expertise in delirium;
- the production of multiple drafts with widespread review, in which 12 organizations and over 83 individuals submitted comments (see Section VI);
- approval by the APA Assembly and Board of Trustees; and
- planned revisions at 3- to 5-year intervals.

A computerized search of the relevant literature from MEDLINE, PsycINFO, and EMBASE was conducted.

The first literature search was conducted by searching MEDLINE, using PubMed, for the period 1966 to April 1996 and used the keywords "organic mental disorders," "psychotic," "delirium," "delusions," "acute organic brain syndrome," "alcohol amnestic disorder," "psychoses," "substance-induced," and "intensive care psychosis" with "haloperidol," "droperidol," "antipsychotic agents," "physostigmine," "tacrine," "cholinergic agents," "benzodiazepines," "thiamine," "folic acid," "vitamin b 12," "vitamins," "morphine," "paralysis," "electroconvulsive therapy," "risperidone," and "neuroleptic malignant syndrome." A total of 954 citations were found.

A second search in MEDLINE was completed for the period 1995 to 1998 and used the key words "delirium," "dementia," "amnestic," "cognitive disorders," and "delusions" with "haloperidol," "droperidol," "antipsychotic agents," "physostigmine," "tacrine," "cholinergic agents," "benzodiazepines," "vitamins," "morphine," "paralysis," "electroconvulsive therapy," "risperidone," and "neuroleptic malignant syndrome." A total of 1,386 citations were found.

The literature search conducted by using PsycINFO covered the period 1967 to November 1998 and used the key words "delirium" and "treatment & prevention" with "psychosocial," "behavioral," "restraint," "seclusion," "isolation," "structure," "support," "sensory deprivation," "orient," "reorient," and "delirium tremens." A total of 337 citations were found.

An additional literature search was conducted by using EMBASE for the period 1985 to November 1998 and used the key word "delirium" with "vitamins," "morphine," "paralysis," "electroconvulsive therapy," and "neuroleptic malignant syndrome." A total of 156 citations were found.

I. SUMMARY OF RECOMMENDATIONS

The following executive summary is intended to provide an overview of the organization and scope of recommendations in this practice guideline. The treatment of patients with delirium requires the consideration of many factors and cannot be adequately reviewed in a brief summary. The reader is encouraged to consult the relevant portions of the guideline when specific treatment recommendations are sought. This summary is not intended to stand on its own.

A. CODING SYSTEM

Each recommendation is identified as falling into one of three categories of endorsement, indicated by a bracketed Roman numeral following the statement. The three categories represent varying levels of clinical confidence regarding the recommendations:

[I] Recommended with substantial clinical confidence.
[II] Recommended with moderate clinical confidence.
[III] May be recommended on the basis of individual circumstances.

B. GENERAL CONSIDERATIONS

Delirium is primarily a disturbance of consciousness, attention, cognition, and perception but can also affect sleep, psychomotor activity, and emotions. It is a common psychiatric illness among medically compromised patients and may be a harbinger of significant morbidity and mortality. The treatment of patients with delirium begins with an essential array of psychiatric management tasks designed to provide immediate interventions for urgent general medical conditions, identify and treat the etiology of the delirium, ensure safety, and improve the patient's functioning. Environmental and supportive interventions are also generally offered to all patients with delirium and are designed to reduce factors that may exacerbate delirium, to reorient patients, and to provide them with support. Somatic interventions largely consist of pharmacologic treatment with high-potency antipsychotic medications. Other somatic interventions may be of help in particular cases of delirium due to specific etiologies or with particular clinical features.

1. Psychiatric management

Psychiatric management is an essential feature of treatment for delirium and should be implemented for all patients with delirium [I]. The specific tasks that constitute psychiatric management include the following: coordinating the care of the patient with other clinicians; identifying the underlying cause(s) of the delirium; initiating immediate interventions for urgent general medical conditions; providing treatments that address the underlying etiology of the delirium; assessing and ensuring the safety of the patient and others; assessing the patient's psychiatric status and monitoring it on an ongoing basis; assessing individual and family psychological and social characteristics; establishing and maintaining a supportive therapeutic stance with the patient, the family, and other clinicians; educating the patient, family, and other clinicians regarding the illness; and providing postdelirium management to support the patient and family and providing education regarding risk factors for future episodes.

2. Environmental and supportive interventions

These interventions are generally recommended for all patients with delirium [I]. Environmental interventions are designed to reduce or eliminate environmental factors that exacerbate delirium.

They include providing an optimal level of environmental stimulation, reducing sensory impairments, making environments more familiar, and providing environmental cues that facilitate orientation. Cognitive-emotional supportive measures include providing patients with reorientation, reassurance, and information concerning delirium that may reduce fear or demoralization. In addition to providing such supportive interventions themselves, it may be helpful for psychiatrists to inform nursing staff, general medical physicians, and family members of their importance.

3. Somatic interventions

The choice of somatic interventions for delirium will depend on the specific features of a patient's clinical condition, the underlying etiology of the delirium, and any associated comorbid conditions [I]. Antipsychotic medications are often the pharmacologic treatment of choice [I]. Haloperidol is most frequently used because it has few anticholinergic side effects, few active metabolites, and a relatively small likelihood of causing sedation and hypotension. Haloperidol may be administered orally, intramuscularly, or intravenously and may cause fewer extrapyramidal symptoms when administered intravenously. Haloperidol can be initiated in the range of 1–2 mg every 2–4 hours as needed (0.25–0.50 mg every 4 hours as needed for elderly patients), with titration to higher doses for patients who continue to be agitated. For patients who require multiple bolus doses of antipsychotic medications, continuous intravenous infusions of antipsychotic medication may be useful (e.g., haloperidol bolus, 10 mg i.v., followed by continuous intravenous infusion of 5–10 mg/hour; lower doses may be required for elderly patients). For patients who require a more rapid onset of action, droperidol, either alone or followed by haloperidol, can be considered. Recently some physicians have used the newer antipsychotic medications (risperidone, olanzapine, and quetiapine) in the treatment of patients with delirium. Patients receiving antipsychotic medications for delirium should have their ECGs monitored [I]. A QTc interval greater than 450 msec or more than 25% over baseline may warrant a cardiology consultation and reduction or discontinuation of the antipsychotic medication.

Benzodiazepine treatment as a monotherapy is generally reserved for delirium caused by withdrawal of alcohol or sedative-hypnotics [I]. Patients with delirium who can tolerate only lower doses of antipsychotic medications may benefit from the combination of a benzodiazepine and antipsychotic medication [III].

Other somatic interventions may be considered for patients with delirium who have particular clinical conditions or specific underlying etiologies. Cholinergics such as physostigmine may be useful in delirium known to be caused specifically by anticholinergic medications [II]. Paralysis, sedation, and mechanical ventilation may be required for agitated patients with delirium and hypercatabolic conditions [III]. Palliative treatment with opiates may be needed by patients with delirium for whom pain is an aggravating factor [III]. Multivitamin replacement should be given to patients with delirium for whom there is the possibility of B vitamin deficiencies (e.g., those who are alcoholic or malnourished) [II].

II. DISEASE DEFINITION, EPIDEMIOLOGY, AND NATURAL HISTORY

A. DEFINITION AND CLINICAL FEATURES

The essential features of delirium include disturbances of consciousness, attention, cognition, and perception. The disturbance develops over a short period of time (usually hours to days) and tends to fluctuate during the course of the day. Following are the DSM-IV criteria for delirium (1):

A. Disturbance of consciousness (i.e., reduced clarity of awareness of the environment) with reduced ability to focus, sustain, or shift attention.
B. A change in cognition (such as memory deficit, disorientation, language disturbance) or the development of a perceptual disturbance that is not better accounted for by a preexisting, established, or evolving dementia.
C. The disturbance develops over a short period of time (usually hours to days) and tends to fluctuate during the course of the day.

According to DSM-IV, delirium frequently represents a sudden and significant decline from a previous level of functioning and cannot be better accounted for by a preexisting or evolving dementia. There is usually evidence from the history, physical examination, or laboratory tests that the delirium is a direct physiological consequence of a general medical condition, substance intoxication or withdrawal, use of a medication, toxin exposure, or a combination of these factors. The disorders included in the DSM-IV delirium section have a common symptom presentation of a disturbance in consciousness and cognition but are differentiated by etiology:

1. Delirium due to a general medical condition.
2. Substance-induced delirium.
3. Delirium due to multiple etiologies.
4. Delirium not otherwise specified.

The disturbance in consciousness or arousal can be manifested by a reduced clarity or awareness of the environment that does not reach the level of stupor or coma. In addition, the ability to focus, sustain, or shift attention is frequently impaired and may result in the patient's being easily distracted.

There is also an accompanying decline in other areas of cognition. Cognitive deficits can include memory and visuoconstructional impairment, disorientation, or language disturbance. Memory impairment is most commonly evident in recent memory. Disorientation is usually manifested as disorientation to time (e.g., thinking it is morning in the middle of the night) or place (e.g., thinking one is at home rather than in the hospital). Disorientation to other persons occurs commonly, but disorientation to self is rare. It may be difficult for the clinician to fully assess cognitive function because the patient is inattentive and incoherent. Obtaining information from the medical chart, medical staff, and other informants, particularly family members, is often helpful in these circumstances.

Dysarthria is a frequent speech and language disturbance, and dysnomia (i.e., impaired ability to name objects), dysgraphia (i.e., impaired ability to write), or even frank aphasia may be observed.

Perceptual disturbances may include misinterpretations, illusions, or hallucinations. For example, the patient may see the nurse mixing intravenous solutions and conclude the nurse is trying to poison him or her (misinterpretation); the folds of the bedclothes may appear to be animate objects (illusion); or the patient may see a group of people around the bed when no one is actually there (hallucination). Although visual misperceptions and hallucinations are most common in delirium, auditory, tactile, gustatory, and olfactory misperceptions or hallucinations can also occur. Misperceptions range from simple and uniform to highly complex. A patient with delirium may have a delusional conviction of the reality of a hallucination and exhibit emotional and behavioral responses consistent with the hallucination's content.

B. ASSOCIATED FEATURES

Other commonly associated features of delirium include disturbances of sleep, psychomotor activity, and emotion. Disturbances in the sleep-wake cycle observed in delirium include daytime sleepiness, nighttime agitation, and disturbances in sleep continuity. In some cases, complete reversal of the night-day sleep-wake cycle or fragmentation of the circadian sleep-wake pattern can occur.

Delirium is often accompanied by disturbed psychomotor activity. Lipowski (2, 3) clinically described two subtypes of delirium based on psychomotor activity and arousal levels. These delirium subtypes included the "hyperactive" (or agitated, hyperalert) subtype and the "hypoactive" (lethargic, hypoalert) subtype. Others have included a "mixed" delirium subtype with alternating features of both. Ross et al. (4) suggested that the hyperactive form is more often characterized by hallucinations, delusions, agitation, and disorientation, while the hypoactive form is characterized by confusion and sedation and is less often accompanied by hallucinations, delusions, or illusions. Comparable levels of cognitive impairment have been observed with both motor subtypes.

The delirious individual may also exhibit emotional disturbances, such as anxiety, fear, depression, irritability, anger, euphoria, and apathy. There may be affective lability, with rapid and unpredictable shifts from one emotional state to another.

Depending on the etiology, delirium can be associated with a number of nonspecific neurological abnormalities, such as tremor, myoclonus, asterixis, and reflex or muscle tone changes. For example, nystagmus and ataxia may accompany delirium due to medication intoxications; cerebellar signs, myoclonus, and generalized hyperreflexia may be seen with lithium intoxication; cranial nerve palsies may occur with Wernicke's encephalopathy; and asterixis may be observed with renal or hepatic insufficiency. The background rhythm seen on EEG is typically abnormal, usually showing generalized slowing. However, in alcohol or sedative-hypnotic withdrawal, the EEG usually shows fast activity. In addition, laboratory findings that are characteristic of associated or etiological general medical conditions (or intoxication or withdrawal states) may be seen.

C. DIFFERENTIAL DIAGNOSIS

The differential diagnosis of patients with features of delirium is discussed in the delirium section of DSM-IV. The most common issue in differential diagnosis is whether the patient has dementia rather than delirium, has delirium alone, or has a delirium superimposed on a preexisting dementia. Cognitive disturbances, such as memory impairment, are common to both delirium and dementia; however, the patient with dementia usually is alert and does not have the disturbance of consciousness or arousal that is characteristic of delirium. The temporal onset of cognitive deficit symptoms and the temporal course and reversibility of cognitive impairments are helpful in distinguishing between delirium and dementia. The severity of delirium symptoms characteristically fluctuates during a 24-hour period, while dementia symptoms generally do not. Information from medical records, other caregivers, and family members may be helpful in determining whether a dementia was present before the onset of a delirium.

D. PREVALENCE AND COURSE

The prevalence of delirium in the hospitalized medically ill ranges from 10% to 30%. In the hospitalized elderly, the delirium prevalence ranges from 10% to 40% (2). As many as 25% of hospitalized cancer patients (5) and 30%–40% of hospitalized AIDS patients (6) develop delirium. As many as 51% of postoperative patients develop delirium (7), and up to 80% of patients with terminal illnesses develop delirium near death (8). Patients who have just had surgery, particularly cardiotomy, hip surgery, or a transplant, and patients with burns, dialysis, or central nervous system lesions are at increased risk for delirium.

Some patients manifest subclinical delirium or prodromal symptoms such as restlessness, anxiety, irritability, distractibility, or sleep disturbance in the days before the onset of overt delirium. Prodromal symptoms may progress to full-blown delirium over 1–3 days. The duration of symptoms of delirium has been reported to range from less than 1 week to more than 2 months (9–14). Typically the symptoms of delirium resolve within 10–12 days; however, up to 15% of patients with delirium have symptoms that persist for up to 30 days and beyond (10). Elderly patients with delirium may be more likely to have a prolonged course, with symptom durations frequently exceeding 1 month (11, 12).

While the majority of patients recover fully, delirium may progress to stupor, coma, seizures, or death, particularly if untreated. Full recovery is less likely in the elderly, with estimated rates of full recovery by the time of discharge varying from 4% to 40% (9, 15). Persistent cognitive deficits are also quite common in elderly patients recovering from delirium, although such deficits may be due to preexisting dementia that was not fully appreciated (9). Similarly, in a study of delirium in AIDS patients Fernandez et al. (16) found that only 27% had complete recovery of cognitive function, possibly because of underlying AIDS dementia.

Delirium in the medically ill is associated with significant morbidity. Medically ill patients, particularly the elderly, have a significantly increased risk of developing complications, such as pneumonia and decubitus ulcers, resulting in longer hospital stays (17, 18). In postoperative patients, delirium is a harbinger of limited recovery and poor long-term outcome. Patients who develop delirium, particularly after orthopedic surgery, are at increased risk for postoperative complications, longer postoperative recuperation periods, longer hospital stays, and long-term disability (19, 20). Seizures may occur in delirium, particularly among patients with alcohol or sedative-hypnotic withdrawal, cocaine intoxication, head trauma, hypoglycemia, strokes, or extensive burns (21).

Delirium in the medically ill is also associated with an increased mortality rate (22, 23). Elderly patients who develop delirium during a hospitalization have been estimated to have a 22%–76% chance of dying during that hospitalization (22, 24). Patients who develop delirium during a hospitalization also have a very high rate of death during the months following discharge. Several studies suggest that up to 25% of patients with delirium die within 6 months and that their mortality rate in the 3 months after diagnosis is 14 times as high as the mortality rate for patients with affective disorders (25, 26).

E. CAUSES

The disorders included in the delirium section of DSM-IV have a common symptom presentation but are differentiated according to presumed etiology (see Table 1 for a list of common etiologies).

1. Due to a general medical condition

In determining that delirium is due to a general medical condition, the clinician must first establish the presence of a general medical condition and then establish that the delirium is etiologically related. A careful and comprehensive assessment is necessary to make this judgment. A temporal association between the onset, exacerbation, or remission of the general medical condition and that of the delirium is a helpful guide. Evidence from the literature that suggests the condition in question can be directly associated with the development of delirium is also useful. Delirium can be associated with many different general medical conditions, each of which has characteristic physical examination and laboratory findings. When these are present they may help confirm the relationship between delirium and the general medical condition. General medical conditions commonly causing delirium are shown in Table 1.

TABLE 1. Underlying Conditions Commonly Associated With Delirium

Type	Disorder
Central nervous system disorder	Head trauma Seizures Postictal state Vascular disease (e.g., hypertensive encephalopathy) Degenerative disease
Metabolic disorder	Renal failure (e.g., uremia) Hepatic failure Anemia Hypoxia Hypoglycemia Thiamine deficiency Endocrinopathy Fluid or electrolyte imbalance Acid-base imbalance
Cardiopulmonary disorder	Myocardial infarction Congestive heart failure Cardiac arrhythmia Shock Respiratory failure
Systemic illness	Substance intoxication or withdrawal Infection Neoplasm Severe trauma Sensory deprivation Temperature dysregulation Postoperative state

2. Due to substance use or withdrawal

Delirium is frequently due to substance use or withdrawal (27). Substances with the potential to cause delirium include both agents that are not usually regarded as having psychoactive properties and those with established psychoactive properties. Delirium that occurs during substance intoxication may arise within minutes to hours after ingestion of high doses of drugs such as cocaine or hallucinogens; other drugs, such as alcohol, barbiturates, or meperidine, may cause delirium after intoxication is sustained for several days. During substance intoxication, the potential for additional agents with anticholinergic activity to cause delirium is increased. Usually the delirium resolves as the intoxication ends or within hours to days thereafter. Delirium associated with substance withdrawal develops as fluid and tissue concentrations of the substance decrease after reduction of sustained, high-dose use of certain substances. Substance-withdrawal delirium can also occur after the reduction of lower doses in patients having poor clearance, experiencing drug interactions, or taking combinations of drugs. The duration of the delirium usually varies with the half-life of the substance involved. Longer-acting substances usually are associated with less severe but more protracted withdrawal and may not have an onset of withdrawal symptoms for days or weeks after use of the substance is discontinued. Substance-withdrawal delirium may continue for only a few hours or may persist for as long as 2–4 weeks.

Table 2 lists substances associated with delirium, including substances of abuse, prescription medications, and toxins.

3. Due to multiple etiologies

Delirium, particularly in the critically ill and in elderly hospitalized patients, often has multiple etiologies (25). Francis and Kapoor (28) found that while 56% of elderly patients with delirium

TABLE 2. Substances That Can Cause Delirium Through Intoxication or Withdrawal

Category	Substance
Drugs of abuse	Alcohol
	Amphetamines
	Cannabis
	Cocaine
	Hallucinogens
	Inhalants
	Opioids
	Phencyclidine
	Sedatives
	Hypnotics
	Other
Medications	Anesthetics
	Analgesics
	Antiasthmatic agents
	Anticonvulsants
	Antihistamines
	Antihypertensive and cardiovascular medications
	Antimicrobials
	Antiparkinsonian medications
	Corticosteroids
	Gastrointestinal medications
	Muscle relaxants
	Immunosuppressive agents
	Lithium and psychotropic medications with anticholinergic properties
Toxins	Anticholinesterase
	Organophosphate insecticides
	Carbon monoxide
	Carbon dioxide
	Volatile substances, such as fuel or organic solvents

had a single definite or probable etiology for delirium, the remaining 44% had an average of 2.8 etiologies per patient.

4. Due to unspecified etiology

Occasionally, no clear etiology is immediately apparent. Often, unrecognized medication use or substance abuse is the cause of an intoxication or withdrawal delirium, and sometimes a rare cause of delirium, such as disseminated intravascular coagulation, is eventually revealed. There has been some controversy as to whether particular settings can themselves cause delirium (e.g., there has been speculation that the intensive care environment can cause "intensive care unit psychosis"). Koponen et al. (11) found a clear organic etiology in 87% of patients with delirium, and they found relatively little evidence that delirium was caused primarily by environmental factors.

F. USE OF FORMAL MEASURES

Although standard psychiatric, general medical, and neurological histories and examinations are usually sufficient to diagnose and evaluate the severity of delirium, they can be supplemented by assessments using formal instruments. A large number of delirium assessment methods have been designed, some intended for clinical evaluations and others for research. Detailed reviews of the psychometric properties of instruments, as well as suggestions for choosing among instruments for particular clinical evaluations or research purposes, are available (29–31). Four types of instruments are briefly mentioned in the following sections: tests that screen for delirium symptoms, delirium diagnostic instruments, delirium symptom severity ratings, and some experimental laboratory tests.

1. Screening instruments

Several tools have been developed to screen for delirium symptoms among patients, and most have been designed to be administered by nursing staff. These may aid in the recognition of delirium, especially in nursing homes, where physician visits are less frequent. The number of delirium symptoms covered, the specificity of items for delirium, and the complexity of administration all vary. Screening instruments include the Clinical Assessment of Confusion–A (CAC-A) (32), the Confusion Rating Scale (CRS) (33), the MCV Nursing Delirium Rating Scale (MCV-NDRS) (34), and the NEECHAM Confusion Scale (35).

2. Diagnostic instruments

Investigators have designed a variety of instruments to make a formal diagnosis of delirium. These instruments consist of operationalized delirium criteria from a variety of diagnostic systems, often in the form of a checklist incorporating information from patient observation and the medical record (e.g., DSM-III-R, DSM-IV, ICD-9, and ICD-10). The rate of delirium diagnosis obtained by using these diagnostic instruments varies according to both the diagnostic system that was used and the particular way in which the authors chose to operationalize the criteria. One structured diagnostic interview schedule, the Delirium Symptom Interview (DSI), can be administered by lay interviewers and used in epidemiological studies (36). Other delirium diagnostic instruments include the Confusion Assessment Method (CAM) (37), Delirium Scale (Dscale) (38), Global Accessibility Rating Scale (GARS) (39), Organic Brain Syndrome Scale (OBS) (40), and Saskatoon Delirium Checklist (SDC) (41).

3. Delirium symptom severity rating scales

Several instruments have been developed to rate the severity of delirium symptoms. Ratings are generally based both on behavioral symptoms and on confusion and cognitive impairment. Rating the severity of delirium over time may be useful for monitoring the effect of an intervention or plotting the course of a delirium over time. These scales have also been used to make the diagnosis of delirium by considering patients with scores above a specified cutoff to have the diagnosis. Such rating scales include the Delirium Rating Scale (DRS) (42) and the Memorial Delirium Assessment Scale (MDAS) (43).

4. Laboratory tests

Several laboratory evaluations have been investigated for possible use in evaluating delirium. With the exception of the EEG, these tests are experimental and currently appropriate only for research purposes. For several decades, investigators have observed EEG changes in patients with delirium (44). EEG changes consist mainly of generalized slowing, although low-voltage fast activity is seen in some types of delirium, such as delirium tremens (45). The presence of EEG abnormalities has fairly good sensitivity for delirium (in one study, the sensitivity was found to be 75%), but their absence does not rule out the diagnosis; thus, the EEG is no substitute for careful clinical observation. Among the experimental laboratory tests that have been investigated for use in delirium, those that appear to show some promise include brain imaging (46, 47) and measures of serum anticholinergic activity (48).

III. TREATMENT PRINCIPLES AND ALTERNATIVES

Several therapeutic modes are employed in the treatment of delirium and are discussed in this section. First, the cornerstone of treatment, psychiatric management, is defined and its components are described. Treatment of the delirium itself involves a set of environmental and supportive interventions and specific pharmacologic treatments. Environmental manipulations are generally designed to help reorient the patient and modulate the degree of stimulation. Supportive measures are designed to provide patient, family, and friends with both reassurance and education regarding the nature, temporal course, and sequelae of delirium.

A. PSYCHIATRIC MANAGEMENT

Psychiatric management involves an array of tasks that the psychiatrist should seek to ensure are performed for all patients with delirium. A psychologically informed understanding of the patient and the family may facilitate these tasks. These tasks are designed to facilitate the identification and treatment of the underlying cause(s) of delirium, improve the patient's level of functioning, and ensure the safety and comfort of patients and others. In many cases, the psychiatrist will be part of, or a consultant to, a multidisciplinary team and should encourage the administration of the full range of needed treatments.

1. Coordinate with other physicians caring for the patient

Delirium frequently heralds a medical emergency, and patients are usually managed in an acute-care hospital setting. For some patients with milder symptoms, once the etiology of delirium has been identified and general medical management has begun, psychiatric and general medical management can take place in an alternative setting (e.g., skilled nursing facility, home, hospice). The psychiatrist is commonly asked to consult when a patient develops delirium on a general medical or surgical unit in the hospital; however, delirium may also present as an emergency in either the psychiatric outpatient or inpatient setting.

The appropriate treatment of delirium involves interventions to search for and correct underlying causes, as well as relieve current symptoms. Joint and coordinated management of the patient with delirium by the psychiatrist and internist, neurologist, or other primary care or specialty physicians will frequently help ensure appropriate comprehensive evaluation and care.

2. Identify the etiology

An essential principle in the psychiatric management of delirium is the identification and correction of the etiologic factors. Careful review of the patient's medical history and interview of family members or others close to the patient may provide some direction. Appropriate laboratory and radiological investigations such as those listed in Table 3 may be necessary to determine the underlying cause(s) of delirium. The choice of specific tests to be undertaken will depend on the results of the clinical evaluation.

3. Initiate interventions for acute conditions

A patient with delirium may have life-threatening general medical conditions that demand therapeutic intervention even before a specific or definitive etiology is determined. In addition to ensuring that diagnostic tests essential to identifying the cause of delirium are ordered, when acting as a consultant, the psychiatrist should raise the level of awareness of the general medical staff concerning the potential morbidity and mortality associated with delirium. Increased observation and monitoring of the patient's general medical condition should include frequent monitoring of vital signs, fluid intake and output, and levels of oxygenation. A patient's medications should be carefully reviewed; nonessential medications should be discontinued, and doses of needed medications should be kept as low as possible.

TABLE 3. Assessment of the Patient With Delirium

Domain	Measure
Physical status	History Physical and neurological examinations Review of vital signs and anesthesia record if postoperative Review of general medical records Careful review of medications and correlation with behavioral changes
Mental status	Interview Cognitive tests (e.g., clock face, digit span, Trailmaking tests)
Basic laboratory tests—consider for all patients with delirium	Blood chemistries: electrolytes, glucose, calcium, albumin, blood urea nitrogen (BUN), creatinine, SGOT, SGPT, bilirubin, alkaline phosphatase, magnesium, PO_4 Complete blood count (CBC) Electrocardiogram Chest X-ray Measurement of arterial blood gases or oxygen saturation Urinalysis
Additional laboratory tests—ordered as indicated by clinical condition	Urine culture and sensitivity (C&S) Urine drug screen Blood tests (e.g., venereal disease research laboratory [VDRL], heavy metal screen, B_{12} and folate levels, lupus erythematosus [LE] prep, antinuclear antibody [ANA], urinary porphyrins, ammonia, human immunodeficiency virus [HIV]) Blood cultures Measurement of serum levels of medications (e.g., digoxin, theophylline, phenobarbital, cyclosporine) Lumbar puncture Brain computerized tomography (CT) or magnetic resonance imaging (MRI) Electroencephalogram (EEG)

Source. From guidelines by Trzepacz and Wise (49).

4. Provide other disorder-specific treatment

The goal of diagnosis is to discover reversible causes of delirium and prevent complications through prompt treatment of these specific disorders. One must give a high priority to identifying and treating such disorders as hypoglycemia, hypoxia or anoxia, hyperthermia, hypertension, thiamine deficiency, withdrawal states, and anticholinergic-induced or other substance-induced delirium. Examples of specific reversible causes of delirium and treatments for these disorders appear in Table 4.

5. Monitor and ensure safety

Behavioral disturbances, cognitive deficits, and other manifestations of delirium may endanger patients or others. Psychiatrists must assess the suicidality and violence potential of patients and implement or advocate interventions to minimize these risks (e.g., remove dangerous items, increase surveillance and supervision, and institute pharmacotherapy). Suicidal behaviors are often inadvertent in delirium and occur in the context of cognitive impairment and/or in response to hallucinations or delusions. Additional assessments of a patient's risk for falls, wandering, inadvertent self-harm, etc., should also be made with appropriate measures taken to ensure safety.

TABLE 4. Examples of Reversible Causes of Delirium and Their Treatments

Condition	Treatment
Hypoglycemia or delirium of unknown etiology where hypoglycemia is suspected	Tests of blood and urine for diagnosis Thiamine hydrochloride, 100 mg i.v. (before glucose) 50% glucose solution, 50 ml i.v.
Hypoxia or anoxia (e.g., due to pneumonia, obstructive or restrictive pulmonary disease, cardiac disease, hypotension, severe anemia, or carbon monoxide poisoning)	Immediate oxygen
Hyperthermia (e.g., temperature above 40.5°C or 105°F)	Rapid cooling
Severe hypertension (e.g., blood pressure of 260/150 mm Hg) with papilledema	Prompt antihypertensive treatment
Alcohol or sedative withdrawal	Appropriate pharmacologic intervention Thiamine, intravenous glucose, magnesium, phosphate, and other B vitamins, including folate
Wernicke's encephalopathy	Thiamine hydrochloride, 100 mg i.v., followed by thiamine daily, either intravenously or orally
Anticholinergic delirium	Withdrawal of offending agent In severe cases, physostigmine should be considered unless contraindicated

Whenever possible, means other than restraints, such as sitters, should be used to prevent the delirious patient from harming himself or herself, others, or the physical environment. Restraints themselves can increase agitation or carry risks for injuries and should be considered only when other means of control are not effective or appropriate (50). A patient who is restrained should be seen as frequently as is necessary to monitor changes in the patient's condition (51). The justification for initiating restraints and continuing use of restraints should be documented in the patient's medical record. Additional rules may apply in some jurisdictions, and the psychiatrist should become familiar with applicable regulations and institutional policies (52).

6. Assess and monitor psychiatric status

The psychiatrist must periodically assess the patient's delirium symptoms, mental status, and other psychiatric symptoms. The symptoms and behavioral manifestations of delirium can fluctuate rapidly, and regular monitoring will allow for the adjustment of treatment strategies.

Important behavioral issues that must be addressed include depression, suicidal ideation or behavior, hallucinations, delusions, aggressive behavior, agitation, anxiety, disinhibition, affective lability, cognitive deficits, and sleep disturbances. It is helpful to record serial assessments of mental status and symptoms over time, as these may indicate the effectiveness of interventions and new or worsening medical conditions. A structured or semistructured instrument, such as those described in Section II.F, may aid in the systematic completion of this task.

7. Assess individual and family psychological and social characteristics

Knowledge of the patient's and the family's psychodynamic issues, personality variables, and sociocultural environment may aid in dealing effectively with specific anxieties and reaction patterns on the part of both the patient and the family. This understanding may be based on prior acquaintance with the patient, current interviews or interaction with the patient or family, and/or history from the family.

8. Establish and maintain alliances

It is important for the psychiatrist who is treating the patient with delirium to establish and maintain a supportive therapeutic stance. Understanding the underlying affect, concerns, and premorbid personality of the patient is frequently helpful in maintaining a supportive alliance. A solid alliance with the family is also desirable, as family members are a critical source of potential support for patients and information on patients who may be unable to give reliable histories. Establishing strong alliances with the multiple clinicians and caregivers frequently involved in the care of delirious medically ill patients is also crucial.

9. Educate patient and family regarding the illness

Educating patients and families regarding delirium, its etiology, and its course is an important role for psychiatrists involved in the care of patients with delirium. Patients may vary in their ability to appreciate their condition; however, providing reassurance that delirium is usually temporary and that the symptoms are part of a medical condition may be extremely beneficial to both patients and their families. Specific educational and supportive interventions are discussed in more detail in the following paragraphs.

Nursing staff make frequent observations of patients over time, which places them in an excellent position to detect the onset and monitor the course of delirium. Education of nursing staff on each shift regarding the clinical features and course of delirium can be an important task for psychiatrists.

Because of the behavioral problems accompanying delirium, there may be a tendency for some general medical physicians to overlook underlying general medical problems contributing to a patient's delirium and to consider the problem to be entirely in the realm of the psychiatrist. In such instances, providing education to other physicians regarding the underlying physiological etiologies of delirium may be an important task for the psychiatrist.

10. Provide postdelirium management

Following recovery, patients' memory for the experience and events of the delirium is variable. Some patients gradually or abruptly lose all apparent recall of the delirious experience, while others have vivid, frightening recollections. Explanations regarding delirium, its etiology, and its course should be reiterated. Supportive interventions that are a standard part of psychiatric management following a traumatic experience should be used for those with distressing postdelirium symptoms. Following recovery, all patients who have experienced delirium should be educated about the apparent cause of their delirium (when this could be identified) so that the patient, family, and subsequent physicians can be made aware of risk factors that may lead to delirium in the future. Psychotherapy focused on working through the experience of the delirium may, at times, be necessary to resolve anxiety, guilt, anger, depression, or other emotional states. These states may be compounded by the patient's preexisting psychological, social, or cultural characteristics.

B. ENVIRONMENTAL AND SUPPORTIVE INTERVENTIONS

1. Environmental interventions

Management of delirium includes a specific array of interventions by nursing, psychological, general medical, and psychiatric staff that can be broadly categorized as environmental interventions. The general goals are to reduce environmental factors that exacerbate delirium, confusion, and misperception while providing familiarity and an optimal level of environmental stimulation. While there is no empirical evidence that the environment by itself causes delirium, certain environmental conditions may exacerbate delirium.

"Timelessness" in hospital intensive care units (ICUs) (i.e., a similar environment regardless of the time of day) appears to contribute to disorganization of sleep-wake cycles, which in turn aggravates fatigue and confusion. Some ICUs have introduced windows, while others change the lighting to cue night versus day. The ICU can be a very noisy environment, with beeps, alarms, pumps, respirators, overhead paging, resuscitation efforts, etc. The confused patient with delirium may become overstimulated by too much noise, and efforts should be made to reduce this whenever possible. On the other hand, understimulation from the environment may leave the patient with delirium undistracted from his or her own internal disorganized perceptions and thoughts; too quiet an environment may exacerbate delirium. It is important to provide a regular amount of modest stimulation (vocal, visual, tactile) to the patient with delirium.

Delirium can also be aggravated by sensory impairments, including visual impairment (53) and auditory impairment (54). By restoring a patient's glasses or hearing aid, one may substantially reduce the manifestations of delirium. Ensuring that there is an analog clock and a calendar that the patient can see will further facilitate orientation. Steps that render the environment more familiar and less alien, such as bringing in family photographs or favorite objects from home (e.g., stuffed animals) or actually having family members there when possible, are also helpful. Especially in a room that may be dark at night, night-lights can help reduce anxiety.

There is some empirical evidence that these environmental interventions can reduce the severity of delirium and improve outcomes (55–58). While there are no large, rigorous, randomized controlled trials, these environmental interventions are widely endorsed because of clinical experience and the lack of adverse effects. Although the value of environmental interventions is widely recognized, they remain substantially underutilized (59).

2. Structure and support for the patient

Nursing, psychological, general medical, and psychiatric staff and family members can also provide cognitive-emotional support designed to strengthen any retained adaptive cognitive functioning that the patient possesses. The goal of these interventions is to reduce anxiety and the unfamiliar while providing understanding and support.

Central to providing cognitive and emotional support are efforts to deal with disorientation. All who come in contact with the patient should provide reorientation, which entails reminding the patient in an unpressured manner of where he or she is, the date and time, and what is happening to him or her.

The patient's emotional reaction to symptoms of delirium can itself be a significant aggravating factor. The patient should be told that the symptoms are temporary and reversible and do not reflect a persistent psychiatric disorder. Similarly, the perception of cognitive deficits may lead patients to conclude that they have suffered brain damage. Unless the delirium is thought to be due to a major stroke or injury or to another event that may cause permanent brain injury, all who have contact with the patient should reassure her or him that these deficits are common and reversible symptoms associated with the particular illness, surgery, or other treatment.

There have been no large clinical trials examining the efficacy of cognitive and emotional support in delirium. However, as with environmental interventions, increased use of these currently underutilized supportive measures has been encouraged on the basis of clinical experience, common sense, and lack of adverse effects (59).

3. Support and education for the family

Educating patients' friends and family about delirium is extremely helpful since they may have the same worries as the patient (e.g., the patient has a permanent psychiatric illness or is brain damaged) and become frightened and demoralized instead of being hopeful and encouraging the patient (60).

It may be useful to recommend that family and friends spend time in the patient's room and bring familiar objects from home to help orient the patient and help him or her feel secure.

C. SOMATIC INTERVENTIONS

The primary treatment of the symptoms of delirium is largely pharmacologic. The high-potency antipsychotic medication haloperidol is most frequently employed, although other pharmacologic and somatic interventions have been used in particular instances. Recently, there has been increased use of risperidone (61, 62). The available studies of the efficacy and other outcomes from use of these treatments for patients with delirium are reviewed in this section.

Several important points should be considered when evaluating the evidence for specific somatic interventions. While haloperidol has been the most studied pharmacologic treatment, few studies have used a standardized definition of delirium (e.g., based on DSM-IV criteria). In addition, few investigations have used reliable and valid delirium symptom rating measures to assess symptom severity before and after intervention.

For somatic treatments other than haloperidol, there have been no large, prospective trials or studies including a control group. Information regarding the efficacy of these treatments comes mainly from small case series or case reports; interpretation of the results from many of these case presentations is also made difficult by the use of nonstandardized definitions of delirium or informal measures of delirium symptom severity.

1. Antipsychotics

a) Goals and efficacy

Antipsychotics have been the medication of choice in the treatment of delirium. Evidence for their efficacy has come from numerous case reports and uncontrolled trials (63, 64). A series of controlled trials also showed that antipsychotic medications can be used to treat agitation and psychotic symptoms in medically ill and geriatric patient populations (65–69). However, most of these trials were not conducted with patients who had clearly or consistently defined delirium; in some studies, agitation and disorientation were the sole criteria and symptom assessments ranged from questionnaires to simple identification without symptom descriptions.

A randomized, double-blind, comparison trial by Breitbart et al. (70) identified delirium by using standardized clinical measures, and it demonstrated the clinical superiority of antipsychotic medications over benzodiazepines in delirium treatment. The Delirium Rating Scale, Mini-Mental State examination, and DSM-III-R were used to make the diagnosis in 244 hospitalized AIDS patients. The subjects were randomly assigned to one of three medications: chlorpromazine, haloperidol, and lorazepam. There were statistically significant decreases in scores on the Delirium Rating Scale after 2 days in the haloperidol and chlorpromazine groups but not in the lorazepam group (the mean decreases in scores were 8.0, 8.5, and 1.0, respectively). The improvement in delirium symptoms observed among those treated with antipsychotic medications occurred quickly, usually before the initiation of interventions directed at the medical etiologies of the delirium.

Droperidol, a butyrophenone with a rapid onset of action and relatively short half-life that is more sedating than haloperidol, has also been found to be an effective treatment for hospitalized patients with agitation, although not necessarily delirium (71). Results of two double-blind clinical trials comparing droperidol to haloperidol suggest that a more rapid response may be obtained with droperidol. Resnick and Burton (72) reported that 30 minutes after intramuscular injections, 81% of patients initially treated with 5 mg of haloperidol required a second injection, compared to only 36% of patients initially given 5 mg of droperidol. Thomas and colleagues (69), comparing 5 mg i.m. of droperidol to 5 mg i.m. of haloperidol, found significantly decreased combativeness among the droperidol treatment group after 10, 15, and 30 minutes. There has been very little study of the newer antipsychotic medications (risperidone, olanzapine, and quetiapine) in the treatment of delirium. Although there have been several case reports of use of risperidone for patients with delirium (61, 62, 73, 74), there have been no published clinical trials of any of the new antipsychotic medications for patients with delirium.

b) Side effects

Phenothiazines can be associated with sedation, anticholinergic effects, and α-adrenergic blocking effects that can cause hypotension; each of these side effects may complicate delirium. Butyrophenones, particularly haloperidol and droperidol, are considered the safest and most effective antipsychotics for delirium. Haloperidol, a high-potency dopamine-blocking agent with few or no anticholinergic side effects, minimal cardiovascular side effects, and no active metabolites, has generally been considered the antipsychotic medication of first choice in the treatment of delirium. High-potency antipsychotic medications also cause less sedation than the phenothiazines and therefore are less likely to exacerbate delirium. Although droperidol may have the advantages of a more rapid onset of action and a shorter half-life than haloperidol, droperidol is associated with greater sedation and hypotensive effects (75).

The use of antipsychotic medications can be associated with neurological side effects, including the development of extrapyramidal side effects, tardive dyskinesia, and neuroleptic malignant syndrome. However, there is some evidence to suggest that extrapyramidal side effects may be less severe when antipsychotic medications are administered intravenously (76). One case series involved 10 consecutive general medical inpatients receiving doses of oral or intravenous haloperidol at approximately 10 mg/day. Four patients were given intravenous medication, and six were given oral doses. Although delirium was not identified as the reason for treatment, five patients met diagnostic criteria by description. There was no significant difference in the incidence of akathisia, but the group receiving intravenous medication experienced less severe extrapyramidal symptoms. Neither method of administration resulted in acute dystonic reactions or changes in blood pressure or pulse rate (76).

Haloperidol used in the treatment of delirium has been found in some instances to lengthen the QT interval, which can lead to torsades de pointes, a form of polymorphic ventricular tachycardia that can degenerate to ventricular fibrillation and sudden death. Estimates of the incidence of torsades de pointes among patients with delirium treated with intravenous haloperidol have ranged from four out of 1,100 patients (77) to eight out of 223 patients (78). Although development of this serious event has been associated with higher intravenous doses (>35 mg/day) of haloperidol, it is important to note that torsades de pointes has also been reported with low-dose intravenous haloperidol and oral haloperidol as well (78, 79). Droperidol has also been associated with lengthening of the QT interval, and it may also be associated with torsades de pointes and sudden death.

Other side effects of antipsychotic medication use can rarely include lowering of the seizure threshold, galactorrhea, elevations in liver enzyme levels, inhibition of leukopoiesis, neuroleptic malignant syndrome, and withdrawal movement disorders.

c) Implementation

Although different antipsychotic medications can be given orally, intramuscularly, or intravenously, in emergency situations or when there is lack of oral access, intravenous administration may be most effective. In addition, as described in the preceding section on side effects, there is some evidence that antipsychotic medications may cause less severe extrapyramidal side effects when administered intravenously (76). Intravenous administration of haloperidol has not yet received approval by the Food and Drug Administration (FDA).

There have been few studies to determine the optimal doses of antipsychotic medications in the treatment of delirium. On the basis of doses used in several studies, starting haloperidol in the range of 1–2 mg every 2–4 hours as needed has been suggested (80). Low doses, for example as low as 0.25–0.50 mg of haloperidol every 4 hours as needed, have been suggested for elderly patients (81). On the other hand, severely agitated patients may require titration to higher doses. Bolus intravenous haloperidol doses exceeding 50 mg with total daily doses up to 500 mg have been reported, and they were associated with minimal effects on heart rate, respiratory rate, blood pressure, and pulmonary artery pressure and minimal extrapyramidal side effects (82, 83).

Several studies (75, 84) have examined the use of continuous intravenous infusions of haloperidol or droperidol among agitated medically ill patients who have required multiple bolus intravenous injections of antipsychotic medications. The results indicate that this means of administration can be safe and may help avoid some of the complications associated with repeated bolus dosing (e.g., hypotension). The authors of one study (84) recommended continuous infusion of haloperidol for patients who required more than eight 10-mg haloperidol boluses in 24 hours or more than 10 mg/hour for more than 5 consecutive hours. They suggested initiating haloperidol with a bolus dose of 10 mg followed by continuous infusion at 5–10 mg/hour.

Because antipsychotic medications used in the treatment of delirium have occasionally been found to lengthen the QT interval, possibly leading to torsades de pointes, ventricular fibrillation, and sudden death, recommendations for medication management include a baseline ECG with special attention paid to the length of the QTc interval. A prolongation of the QTc interval to greater than 450 msec or to greater than 25% over that in previous ECGs may warrant telemetry, a cardiology consultation, and dose reduction or discontinuation (85, 86). It has also been recommended that serum levels of magnesium and potassium be monitored in critically ill patients, especially those whose baseline QTc interval is 440 msec or longer, those who are receiving other drugs that increase the QT interval, or those who have electrolyte disturbances (87).

2. Benzodiazepines

a) Goals and efficacy

Few controlled studies have evaluated the efficacy of benzodiazepines as a monotherapy (i.e., not in combination with other pharmacotherapies) for the treatment of delirium. The limited data that are available suggest that benzodiazepine monotherapy may be ineffective as a treatment for general cases of delirium caused by a variety of etiologies. For example, the comparison by Breitbart et al. (70), described in Section III.C.1, indicated that lorazepam, given alone, was less effective as a treatment for delirium than either haloperidol or chlorpromazine.

Although there appears to be little evidence to support the use of benzodiazepines alone for general cases of delirium, there may be certain types of delirium for which benzodiazepines have advantages and are preferable. For example, benzodiazepines are the treatment of choice for delirium related to alcohol or benzodiazepine withdrawal. Other specific clinical circumstances in which benzodiazepines may be useful include instances when there is a need for a medication that can raise the seizure threshold (unlike antipsychotics, which lower the seizure threshold) or when anticholinergic side effects or akathisia associated with antipsychotics would seriously exacerbate a patient's condition.

There have been several reports of the combination of antipsychotics and benzodiazepines for the treatment of delirium, and the results indicate that this combination may decrease medication side effects and potentially increase clinical effectiveness in special populations, for example severely ill cancer patients or AIDS patients. Results of several open studies using intravenous haloperidol along with intravenous lorazepam suggest that the combined treatment is more efficacious, with a shorter duration of the delirium and fewer extrapyramidal symptoms, than intravenous haloperidol alone (16, 63, 88). Most of these studies defined delirium according to DSM criteria but did not use standardized assessment tools.

b) Side effects

The adverse effects of benzodiazepines on mental status have received some attention. Marcantonio et al. (89) demonstrated an association between benzodiazepine use and postoperative delirium in a prospective study of psychoactive medications given to patients admitted for elective noncardiac procedures. Long-acting benzodiazepines in particular posed problems. Benzodiazepines have been associated with sedation, behavioral disinhibition, amnesia, ataxia, respiratory depression, physical dependence, rebound insomnia, withdrawal reactions, and delirium. Geriatric populations are at greater risk for the development of these complications; children and adolescents may also be at increased risk for disinhibition reactions, emotional lability, increased anxiety, hallucinations, aggression, insomnia, euphoria, and incoordination (16, 90, 91).

Benzodiazepines are generally contraindicated in delirium from hepatic encephalopathy due to accumulation of glutamine, which is related chemically to γ-aminobutyric acid (GABA). Benzodiazepines should also be avoided, or used with caution, in patients with respiratory insufficiency. For patients who have hepatic insufficiency or are taking other medications metabolized by the cytochrome P450 system, benzodiazepines that are predominantly metabolized by glucuronidation (lorazepam, oxazepam, and temazepam) should be used when a benzodiazepine is required.

c) Implementation

When benzodiazepines are used, relatively short-acting medications with no active metabolites (e.g., lorazepam) should be selected.

Few studies have investigated the optimal dose of benzodiazepines for the treatment of delirium. However, the dose must be carefully considered, given the possibility that benzodiazepines may exacerbate symptoms of delirium. In cases of delirium due specifically to alcohol or sedative-hypnotic withdrawal, higher doses of benzodiazepines and benzodiazepines with longer half-lives may be required.

In a report of a case series of 20 critically ill cancer patients for which benzodiazepines and antipsychotics were administered together, Adams et al. (63) suggested that treatment be started with 3 mg i.v. of haloperidol followed immediately by 0.5–1.0 mg i.v. of lorazepam. Additional doses and the frequency are then titrated to the patient's degree of improvement. For example, Adams et al. stated that if little or no improvement is observed within 20 minutes, an additional dose of 5 mg i.v. of haloperidol and 0.5–2.0 mg i.v. of lorazepam can be given. In some cases of severe agitation, the eventual doses of both medications have been quite large (e.g., daily doses of lorazepam between 20 and 30 mg and of haloperidol between 100 and 150 mg).

3. Cholinergics

a) Goals and efficacy

Anticholinergic mechanisms have been implicated in the pathogenesis of many medication-induced deliriums. In addition, anticholinergic mechanisms may be involved in delirium from hypoxia, hypoglycemia, thiamine deficiency, traumatic brain injury, and stroke (49). However, cholinergic medications have been used in a very limited fashion to treat delirium, almost exclusively in cases of delirium clearly caused by anticholinergic medications. Physostigmine, a centrally active cholinesterase inhibitor, has been used most often, with tacrine and donepezil receiving less attention.

In one prospective study (92), physostigmine reversed delirium among 30 patients in a postanesthesia recovery room, in whom either atropine or scopolamine had caused the delirium. In four single case reports of delirium diagnosed by clinical interviews, physostigmine reversed the delirium resulting from ranitidine (93), homatropine eyedrops (94), benztropine (95), and meperidine (96).

In a single case study (97), tacrine reversed delirium induced by anticholinergic medication. Newer cholinesterase inhibitors with fewer side effects than tacrine have not been studied for treatment of delirium.

b) Side effects

Many side effects of cholinesterase inhibitors are caused by cholinergic excess; such effects include bradycardia, nausea, vomiting, salivation, and increased gastrointestinal acid. Physostigmine can cause seizures, particularly if intravenous administration is too rapid (98). Tacrine has been associated with asymptomatic increases in liver enzyme levels. A threefold increase has been observed in approximately 30% of patients and is generally reversible with discontinuation of treatment; 5%–10% of patients develop more marked (e.g., tenfold) but still generally reversible increases in liver enzyme levels that warrant discontinuation of tacrine treatment (99).

c) Implementation

Physostigmine is usually administered parenterally. Doses that have been used in studies of delirium have included intravenous or intramuscular injections ranging from 0.16 to 2.00 mg and continuous intravenous infusions of 3 mg/hour (92–96).

In the single case study of tacrine used to reverse delirium induced by anticholinergic medication, 30 mg i.v. was used (97).

4. Vitamins

Certain vitamin deficiencies are commonly described as causing delirium. Consequently, one would expect such deliria to reverse at least to some extent with repletion of the deficient vitamin. Although this has not been subjected to rigorous trials, there are some case reports and case series supporting this effect. A malnourished hemodialysis patient with nicotinamide deficiency had a paranoid delirium that responded to parenteral nicotinamide, 500 mg/day (100). Bahr et al. (101) reported that of two chronic alcoholic patients with B vitamin deficiency, malnutrition, and central pontine myelinolysis, one improved quickly with intravenous vitamins. Thiamine deficiency delirium (DSM-III-R) was treated with vitamin B complex in six of 13 elderly medically ill patients, but only one patient had a dramatic response to treatment (102).

In one randomized controlled trial (103), 26 elderly patients undergoing orthopedic surgery received treatment with intravenous vitamins B and C preoperatively and postoperatively and were compared to 32 age-matched surgical control subjects who did not receive vitamins. There was no difference between the intervention and control groups in the incidence of postoperative confusion (39% versus 38%) or in the preoperative thiamine status as determined by serum assays.

In general, any patient with delirium who has a reason to be B vitamin deficient (e.g., alcoholic or malnourished) should be given multivitamin replacement.

5. Morphine and paralysis

Hypoxia, fatigue, and the metabolic consequences of overexertion all exacerbate delirium. Such hypercatabolic conditions are likely to accompany certain causes of agitated delirium (e.g., hyperdynamic heart failure, adult respiratory distress syndrome, hyperthyroid storm). For such patients and for any cases of agitated delirium unresponsive to other pharmacologic interventions, the patient may require a paralytic agent and mechanical ventilation. This improves oxygenation and reduces skeletal muscle exertion. The patient is usually heavily sedated. Morphine (or other opiate) is also an important palliative treatment in cases of delirium where pain is an aggravating factor (104). However, some opiates can exacerbate delirium, particularly through their metabolites, which possess anticholinergic activity (89). Among opiates, meperidine and fentanyl are particularly anticholinergic.

6. ECT

ECT has not been shown to be an effective treatment for general cases of delirium. Earlier case reports and case series had significant limitations: standardized diagnostic criteria and rating scales were not used; patients with schizophrenia, mania, postpartum psychosis, or psychotic depression were included and diagnosed with delirium because they had disorganized thinking and cognition; and few details concerning the manner in which ECT was performed were provided (105–111).

There is limited evidence for ECT as a treatment for particular cases of delirium due to specific etiologies. MEDLINE literature searches identified two case reports of ECT use for the delirium that is a component of neuroleptic malignant syndrome. In one study (112), the delirium symptoms improved in 24 of 29 patients with neuroleptic malignant syndrome who were treated with ECT. In the second study (113), 26 of 31 patients with neuroleptic malignant syndrome who were treated with ECT and hydration were described as having improved delirium symptoms. ECT has been studied in small samples of patients with delirium tremens. In one older study (109), 10 patients receiving ECT and conventional treatment had a shorter duration of delirium symptoms than 10 patients receiving conventional treatment alone (mean, 0.85 versus 2.8 days, respectively). In one case report (106), a patient with delirium tremens who had not responded to high-dose benzodiazepine treatment was described as recovering after ECT. In two case reports (114, 115), patients with protracted courses of delirium after traumatic brain injuries improved after receiving ECT. Because of the lack of compelling evidence, as well as the availability of alternative means of management, ECT is not presently used in the United States for treatment of delirium tremens.

In addition to the very limited evidence that ECT is an effective treatment for delirium, there may be considerable risks with ECT in medically unstable patients. For these reasons, ECT should be considered only rarely for patients with delirium due to specific etiologies such as neuroleptic malignant syndrome and should not be considered initially as a substitute for more conservative and conventional treatments. ECT itself may carry a risk of both postictal delirium (lasting minutes to hours) and interictal delirium (lasting days) after the procedure (116–120). Beyond that time period, ECT can also exacerbate cognitive deficits, such as memory impairment. Certain patient populations at higher risk for these adverse effects from ECT include patients with Parkinson's disease (particularly those taking carbidopa), Huntington's disease, or caudate or other basal ganglia strokes (119, 121–125).

IV. FORMULATION AND IMPLEMENTATION OF A TREATMENT PLAN

After the diagnosis of delirium is made (see Section II) a treatment plan is developed. The components of the treatment plan and factors that go into a psychiatrist's choice of treatment recommendations are discussed in this section. Although the treatment of delirium involves multiple modalities, certain components are essential and should be implemented with all patients. Other components of treatment may involve a choice between specific therapies, and this choice should be guided by a careful assessment of the patient's clinical condition, etiology, and comorbid conditions.

A. PSYCHIATRIC MANAGEMENT

Psychiatric management is the cornerstone of successful treatment for delirium and should be implemented for all patients with delirium. The goals of psychiatric management are similar for all patients with delirium and involve facilitating the identification and treatment of underlying etiologies, improving patient functioning and comfort, and ensuring the safety of patients and others. The specific elements (see Section III.A) include coordinating care with other clinicians; ensuring that the etiology is identified; ensuring that interventions for acute conditions are initiated; ensuring that disorder-specific treatments are provided; monitoring and ensuring safety; assessing and monitoring psychiatric status; establishing and maintaining supportive therapeutic alliances with patients, families, and other treaters; educating the patient and family regarding the illness; and postdelirium management.

B. CHOICE OF SPECIFIC ENVIRONMENTAL AND SUPPORTIVE INTERVENTIONS

One aspect of the management of delirium involves environmental interventions and cognitive-emotional support provided by nursing, general medical, and psychiatric treaters. The general goals of environmental interventions are to remove factors that exacerbate delirium while providing familiarity and an optimal level of environmental stimulation; the general goals of supportive management include reorientation, reassurance, and education concerning delirium. Specific examples of environmental and supportive interventions are given in Section III.B. These interventions are recommended for all patients with delirium, on the basis of some formal evidence but mainly because of the value observed through clinical experience and the absence of adverse effects.

C. CHOICE OF SOMATIC INTERVENTION

The specific features of a patient's clinical condition, the underlying cause(s) of the delirium, and associated conditions may be used by the psychiatrist to determine the choice of specific somatic therapy. Antipsychotic medications are the pharmacologic treatment of choice in most cases of delirium because of their efficacy in the treatment of psychotic symptoms. Haloperidol is most frequently used because of its short half-life, few or no anticholinergic side effects, no active metabolites, and lower likelihood of causing sedation. Haloperidol may be administered orally or intramuscularly, but it appears to cause fewer extrapyramidal side effects when administered intravenously. An optimal dose range for patients with delirium has not been determined. Initial doses of haloperidol in the range of 1–2 mg every 2–4 hours as needed have been used, and even lower starting doses (e.g., 0.25–0.50 mg every 4 hours as needed) are suggested for elderly patients. Titration to higher doses may be required for patients who continue to be agitated. Although total daily intravenous doses in the hundreds of milligrams have been given under closely monitored conditions, much lower doses usually suffice. Continuous intravenous infusions of antipsychotic medications can be used for patients who have required multiple bolus doses of antipsychotic medications. Initiating haloperidol with a bolus dose of 10 mg followed by continuous intravenous infusion of 5–10 mg/hour has been suggested. Droperidol, either alone or followed by haloperidol, can be considered for patients with delirium and acute agitation for whom a more rapid onset of action is required. The ECG should be monitored in patients receiving antipsychotic medications for delirium, and a QTc interval longer than 450 msec or more than 25% over baseline may warrant a cardiology consultation and consideration of discontinuation of the antipsychotic medication. The availability of new antipsychotic medications (risperidone, olanzapine, and quetiapine) with their different side effect profiles has led some physicians to use these agents for the treatment of delirium.

Benzodiazepines can exacerbate symptoms of delirium and, when used alone for general cases of delirium, have been shown to be ineffective. For these reasons, benzodiazepines as monotherapies are reserved for specific types of patients with delirium for which these medications may have particular advantages. For example, benzodiazepines are used most frequently to treat patients with delirium that has been caused by withdrawal of alcohol or benzodiazepines. When a benzodiazepine is used, medications such as lorazepam, which are relatively short-acting and have no active metabolites, are preferable. Combining a benzodiazepine with an antipsychotic medication can be considered for patients with delirium who can only tolerate lower doses of antipsychotic medications or who have prominent anxiety or agitation. Combined treatment can be started with 3 mg i.v. of haloperidol followed immediately by 0.5–1.0 mg i.v. of lorazepam and then adjusted according to the patient's degree of improvement.

Other somatic interventions have been suggested for patients with delirium who have particular clinical conditions or specific underlying etiologies; however, few data are available regarding the efficacy of these interventions in treating delirium. There is some suggestion that cholinergics such as physostigmine and tacrine may be useful in delirium caused by anticholinergic medications. Agitated patients with delirium with hypercatabolic conditions (e.g., hyperdynamic heart failure, adult respiratory distress syndrome, hyperthyroid storm) may require paralysis and mechanical ventilation. For patients with delirium in whom pain is an aggravating factor, palliative treatment with an opiate such as morphine is recommended. ECT may be a treatment consideration in a few cases of delirium due to a specific etiology such as neuroleptic malignant syndrome; any potential benefit of ECT should be weighed against the risks of ECT for patients who are often medically unstable. Any patient with delirium with a reason to be deficient in B vitamins (e.g., alcoholic or malnourished) should be given multivitamin replacement.

D. ISSUES OF COMPETENCY AND CONSENT

Decisions regarding the care of patients with delirium are often complex because of risks associated with treatments, and these decisions frequently have to be made quickly because of the seriousness of the underlying general medical conditions. Unfortunately, delirium intermittently affects consciousness, attention, and cognition and can impair a patient's decisional capacity (i.e., the ability to make decisions as determined by a clinician's evaluation) or competence (i.e., the ability to make decisions as determined by a court of law) (126, 127).

The presence or diagnosis of delirium does not in itself mean that a patient is incompetent or lacks capacity to give informed consent (128). Instead, a determination of decisional capacity or competence to give informed consent involves formal assessment of a patient's understanding about the proposed intervention (including the intervention's risks, benefits, and alternatives) and the consequences of the decisions to be made.

Decision-making guidelines have been suggested for patients with delirium who lack decisional capacity or competence to give informed consent (129). The urgency with which treatment is needed and the risks and benefits of treatments can be used by the treating physician to choose between several alternative courses of action. In medical emergencies requiring prompt intervention, the first alternative is to treat the patient with delirium without informed consent, under the common-law doctrine of implied consent (i.e., that treatment may be provided in medical emergencies without informed consent if it is appropriate treatment that a reasonable person would want). In nonemergency situations, the clinician should obtain input or consent from surrogates. Involving interested family members can be especially helpful for choosing among equally beneficial interventions that involve low or moderate risks. The opinion of a second clinician can be useful for making decisions involving more uncertainty or interventions associated with greater risks. Obtaining the consultation of a hospital's administrator, risk manager, or legal counsel may also provide a means for reassuring family members and the treatment team that reasonable decisions are being made. For decisions that involve significant risks or substantial disagreements involving family members, a court-appointed guardian can be sought if time permits. In more emergent cases, an urgent hearing with a judge may be required. All assessments of a patient's decisional capacity or competence and the reasons for a particular course of action should be documented in the patient's medical record.

V. CLINICAL FEATURES INFLUENCING TREATMENT

A. COMORBID PSYCHIATRIC DISORDERS

Delirium is often misdiagnosed as depression or dementia. These disorders can be diagnosed during a delirium only when the patient's history reveals symptoms that clearly existed before the delirium onset. When delirium is comorbid with other psychiatric disorders, the delirium should be treated first and the treatments for these other disorders, such as antidepressant or anxiolytic medications, should be minimized or not begun until the delirium is resolved. Medications for psychiatric disorders can both be the cause of delirium and exacerbate or contribute to delirium from other causes.

B. COMORBID GENERAL MEDICAL CONDITIONS

1. AIDS/HIV

Approximately 30%–40% of hospitalized AIDS patients develop delirium (6, 16, 70). Early reports concerning the increased sensitivity of AIDS patients to the extrapyramidal side effects of dopamine-blocking antipsychotic drugs have made clinicians cautious in using high doses of antipsychotics, such as haloperidol (130, 131). At lower doses, antipsychotics such as haloperidol and chlorpromazine have been demonstrated to be safe and effective with minimal extrapyramidal side effects (70).

2. Liver disease

The liver is the body's detoxifying organ for drugs and other molecules. Hepatic insufficiency significantly affects the metabolism of many medications. Most psychotropic medications undergo hepatic transformation. In addition, the liver produces albumin and other plasma proteins that transport bound medications in the bloodstream. When these protein levels decrease because of liver dysfunction, unbound medications can enter tissues at an accelerated rate—including crossing the blood-brain barrier—and can also be more available for catabolism or excretion. Thus, the former effect may alter therapeutic effects or cause side effects, while the latter may result in less therapeutic effect than expected at a given dose.

Haloperidol undergoes metabolism by the P450 2D6 enzyme system, which reduces it to reduced haloperidol. The latter is in equilibrium with the parent drug. In addition, glucuronidation is an important route of metabolism of haloperidol (132). This suggests that its pharmacokinetics in patients with liver insufficiency would be similar to those in other patients when used to treat delirium.

On the other hand, many benzodiazepines require oxidation by the liver. The exceptions are lorazepam, temazepam, and oxazepam, which require only glucuronidation. It is therefore preferred that benzodiazepines requiring only glucuronidation be used to treat delirium secondary to sedative-hypnotic or alcohol withdrawal in patients who have liver insufficiency. Of these, lorazepam is usually chosen because it is well absorbed when given orally, intramuscularly, or intravenously.

C. ADVANCED AGE

The elderly are particularly vulnerable to delirium due to changes in brain function, multiple general medical problems, polypharmacy, reduced hepatic metabolism of medications, multisensory declines, and brain disorders such as dementia. Conducting a careful medical evaluation that includes particular attention to a patient's level of oxygenation, possible occult infection (e.g., urinary tract infection), and the possible role of medications is an essential initial approach to the management of delirium in the elderly. Medications with anticholinergic effects are often the culprit; however, even medications not generally recognized as possessing anticholinergic effects (e.g., meperidine, digoxin, and ranitidine) can be responsible (133–135). Nursing home patients are at particular risk of delirium.

Low doses of antipsychotic medication usually suffice in treating delirium in elderly patients, for example, beginning with 0.5 mg haloperidol once or twice a day. The benefits of restraints may be greater for elderly patients than for younger patients because of the greater risk of falls and hip fractures in older populations; hip and other fractures often carry a grim prognosis for elderly patients, who may never return to independent functioning. On the other hand, the risks associated with restraints may be greater among the elderly, and other means to prevent falls should be considered if possible. When extrapyramidal side effects occur early in the treatment of delirium, Lewy body dementia should be considered in the differential diagnosis.

VI. REVIEWERS AND REVIEWING ORGANIZATIONS

Larry Altstiel, M.D.
Varda Peller Backus, M.D.
William T. Beecroft, M.D.
Jeffrey L. Berlant, M.D.
D. Peter Birkett, M.D.
Charles H. Blackinton, M.D.
Mel Blaustein, M.D.
Barton J. Blinder, M.D.
Harold E. Bronheim, M.D.
Thomas Markham Brown, M.D.
Stephanie Cavanaugh, M.D.
Christopher C. Colenda, M.D.
Dave M. Davis, M.D.
Horace A. DeFord, M.D.
Prakash Desai, M.D.
Joel E. Dimsdale, M.D.
Ann Maxwell Eward, Ph.D.
Laura J. Fochtmann, M.D.
David G. Folks, M.D.
Gilles L. Fraser, Pharm.D.
Richard K. Fuller, M.D.
Dolores Gallagher-Thompson
Larry Goldman, M.D.
Sheila Hafter Gray, M.D.
Robert M. Greenberg, M.D.
Jon E. Gudeman, M.D.
Edward Hanin, M.D.
Carla T. Herrerias, M.P.H.
Daniel W. Hicks, M.D.
John Hughes, M.D.
Keith Isenberg, M.D.
Sue C. Jacobs, Ph.D.
Sandra Jacobson, M.D.
Leslie Dotson Jaggers, Pharm.D.
Charles Kaelber, M.D.
Barbara Kamholz, M.D.
Gary Kaplan, M.D.
Fred Karlin, M.D.
Roger G. Kathol, M.D.
Sherry Katz-Bearnot, M.D.
David J. Knesper, M.D.
Bob G. Knight, Ph.D.
Ronald R. Koegler, M.D.
Sharon Levine, M.D.
Glenn Lippman, M.D.
Rex S. Lott, Pharm.D.
Velandy Manohar, M.D.
Peter J. Manos, M.D., Ph.D.
James R. McCartney, M.D.
Dinesh Mittel, M.D.
Kevin O'Connor, M.D.
Joseph F. O'Neill, M.D.
Edmond H. Pi, M.D.
Michael K. Popkin, M.D.
Peter V. Rabins, M.D.
Stephen R. Rapp, M.D.
Vaughn I. Rickert, Psy.D.
Jonathan Ritro, M.D.

Laura Roberts, M.D.
Stephen M. Saravay, M.D.
Marc A. Schuckit, M.D.
Ben Seltzer, M.D.
Todd Semla, Pharm.D.
David Servan-Schreiber, M.D., Ph.D.
Elisabeth J. Shakin Kunkel, M.D.
Winston W. Shen, M.D.
Edward Silberman, M.D.
Theodore A. Stern, M.D.
Janice Zalen Stiers
John Tanquary, M.D.
William R. Tatomer, M.D.
Larry E. Tripp, M.D.
Vera Trzepacz, M.D.
Gary J. Tucker, M.D.
Peter VanDyck, M.D.
John Wattis, M.D.
William Weddington, M.D.
Richard D. Weiner, M.D.
Joseph Westermeyer, M.D., M.P.H., Ph.D.
Donald Wexler, M.D.
Thomas N. Wise, M.D.
Linda Worley, M.D.
William Zurhellen, M.D.

Alabama Department of Mental Health and Mental Retardation
American Academy of Pediatrics
American College of Emergency Physicians
American Society of Health-System Pharmacists
Association for Academic Psychiatry
Association for the Advancement of Behavior Therapy
Association of Gay and Lesbian Psychiatrists
Group for the Advancement of Psychiatry
Michigan Psychiatric Society
National Institute on Alcohol Abuse and Alcoholism
Society of Adolescent Medicine
U.S. Department of Health and Human Services—HIV/AIDS Bureau

VII. REFERENCES

The following coding system is used to indicate the nature of the supporting evidence in the references:

[A] *Randomized clinical trial.* A study of an intervention in which subjects are prospectively followed over time; there are treatment and control groups; subjects are randomly assigned to the two groups; both the subjects and the investigators are blind to the assignments.

[B] *Clinical trial.* A prospective study in which an intervention is made and the results of that intervention are tracked longitudinally; study does not meet standards for a randomized clinical trial.

[C] *Cohort or longitudinal study.* A study in which subjects are prospectively followed over time without any specific intervention.

[D] *Case-control study.* A study in which a group of patients and a group of control subjects are identified in the present and information about them is pursued retrospectively or backward in time.

[E] *Review with secondary data analysis.* A structured analytic review of existing data (e.g., a meta-analysis or a decision analysis).

[F] *Review.* A qualitative review and discussion of previously published literature without a quantitative synthesis of the data.

[G] *Other.* Textbooks, expert opinion, case reports, and other reports not included above.

1. American Psychiatric Association: Diagnostic and Statistical Manual of Mental Disorders, 4th ed (DSM-IV). Washington, DC, APA, 1994 [F]
2. Lipowski ZJ: Delirium (acute confusional states). JAMA 1987; 258:1789–1792 [F]
3. Lipowski ZJ: Delirium: Acute Confusional States. New York, Oxford University Press, 1990 [G]
4. Ross CA, Peyser CE, Shapiro I: Delirium: phenomenologic and etiologic subtypes. Int Psychogeriatr 1991; 3:135–147 [F]
5. Stiefel F, Holland J: Delirium in cancer patients. Int Psychogeriatr 1991; 3:333–336 [F]
6. Perry S: Organic mental disorders caused by HIV: update on early diagnosis and treatment. Am J Psychiatry 1990; 147:696–710 [F]
7. Tune LE: Post-operative delirium. Int Psychogeriatr 1991; 3:325–332 [F]
8. Massie MJ, Holland J, Glass E: Delirium in terminally ill cancer patients. Am J Psychiatry 1983; 140:1048–1050 [C, G]
9. Rockwood K: The occurrence and duration of symptoms in elderly patients with delirium. J Gerontol 1993; 48:M162–M166 [C]
10. Sirois F: Delirium: 100 cases. Can J Psychiatry 1988; 33:375–378 [D]
11. Koponen H, Stenback U, Mattila E: Delirium among elderly persons admitted to a psychiatric hospital: clinical course during the acute stage and one-year follow-up. Acta Psychiatr Scand 1989; 79:579–585 [D]
12. Koizumi J, Shiraishi H, Suzuki T: Duration of delirium shortened by the correction of electrolyte imbalance. Jpn J Psychiatry Neurol 1988; 42:81–88 [D]
13. Rockwood K: Acute confusion in elderly medical patients. J Am Geriatr Soc 1989; 37:150–154 [C]
14. Manos PJ, Wu R: The duration of delirium in medical and postoperative patients referred for psychiatric consultation. Ann Clin Psychiatry 1997; 9:219–226 [C]
15. Levkoff SE, Evans DA, Liptzin B, Cleary PD, Lipsitz LA, Wetle TT, Reilly CH, Pilgrim DM, Schor J, Rowe J: Delirium: the occurrence and persistence of symptoms among elderly hospitalized patients. Arch Intern Med 1992; 152:334–340 [C]
16. Fernandez F, Levy JK, Mansell PWA: Management of delirium in terminally ill AIDS patients. Int J Psychiatry Med 1989; 19:165–172 [C]
17. Inouye S, Horowitz R, Tinetti M, Berkman L: Acute confusional states in the hospitalized elderly: incidence, risk factors and complications (abstract). Clin Res 1989; 37:524A [C]
18. Cole MG, Primeau FJ: Prognosis of delirium in elderly hospital patients. Can Med Assoc J 1993; 149:41–46 [E]
19. Rogers M, Liang M, Daltroy L: Delirium after elective orthopedic surgery: risk factors and natural history. Int J Psychiatry Med 1989; 19:109–121 [C]
20. Gustafson Y, Berggren D, Brannstrom B, Bucht G, Norberg A, Hansson LI, Winblad B: Acute confusional states in elderly patients treated for femoral neck fracture. J Am Geriatr Soc 1988; 36:525–530 [C]
21. Antoon AY, Volpe JJ, Crawford JD: Burn encephalopathy in children. Pediatrics 1972; 50:609–616 [C]
22. Rabins PV, Folstein MF: Delirium and dementia: diagnostic criteria and fatality rates. Br J Psychiatry 1982; 140:149–153 [C]
23. Varsamis J, Zuchowski T, Maini KK: Survival rates and causes of death in geriatric psychiatric patients: a six-year follow-up study. Can Psychiatr Assoc J 1972; 17:17–22 [C]
24. Cameron DJ, Thomas RI, Mulvihill M, Bronheim H: Delirium: a test of the Diagnostic and Statistical Manual III criteria on medical inpatients. J Am Geriatr Soc 1987; 35:1007–1010 [C]
25. Trzepacz P, Teague G, Lipowski Z: Delirium and other organic mental disorders in a general hospital. Gen Hosp Psychiatry 1985; 7:101–106 [G]
26. Weddington WW: The mortality of delirium: an under-appreciated problem? Psychosomatics 1982; 23:1232–1235 [E, F]

27. Inouye SK: The dilemma of delirium: clinical and research controversies regarding diagnosis and evaluation of delirium in hospitalized elderly medical patients. Am J Med 1994; 97:278–288 [F]
28. Francis J, Kapoor WN: Delirium in hospitalized elderly. J Gen Intern Med 1990; 5:65–79 [F]
29. Smith MJ, Breitbart WS, Platt MM: A critique of instruments and methods to detect, diagnose, and rate delirium. J Pain Symptom Manage 1995; 10:35–77 [F]
30. Trzepacz PT: A review of delirium assessment instruments. Gen Hosp Psychiatry 1994; 16:397–405 [F]
31. Levkoff S, Liptzin B, Cleary P, Reilly CH, Evans D: Review of research instruments and techniques used to detect delirium. Int Psychogeriatr 1991; 3:253–271 [F]
32. Vermeersch PE: The Clinical Assessment of Confusion—A. Appl Nurs Res 1990; 3:128–133 [D]
33. Williams MA, Ward SE, Campbell EB: Confusion: testing versus observation. J Gerontol Nurs 1988; 14:25–30 [D]
34. Rutherford L, Sessler C, Levenson JL, Hart R, Best A: Prospective evaluation of delirium and agitation in a medical intensive care unit (abstract). Crit Care Med 1991; 19:S81 [C]
35. Neelon V, Champagne MT, Carlson JR, Funk SG: The NEECHAM Confusion Scale: construction, validation, and clinical testing. Nurs Res 1996; 45:324–330 [C]
36. Albert MS, Levkoff SE, Reilly C, Liptzin B, Pilgrim D, Cleary PD, Evans D, Rowe JW: The Delirium Symptom Interview: an interview for the detection of delirium symptoms in hospitalized patients. J Geriatr Psychiatry Neurol 1992; 5:14–21 [C]
37. Inouye SK, van Dyck CH, Alessi CA, Balkin S, Siegal AP, Horwitz RI: Clarifying confusion: the confusion assessment method, a new method for the detection of delirium. Ann Intern Med 1990; 113:941–948 [C]
38. Lowy F, Engelsmann F, Lipowski Z: Study of cognitive functioning in a medical population. Compr Psychiatry 1973; 14:331–338 [C]
39. Anthony JC, LeResche LA, Von Korff MR, Niaz U, Folstein MF: Screening for delirium on a general medical ward: the tachistoscope and a global accessibility rating. Gen Hosp Psychiatry 1985; 7:36–42 [C]
40. Gustafsson I, Lindgren M, Westling B: The OBS Scale: a new rating scale for evaluation of confusional states and other organic brain syndromes (abstract). Presented at the II International Congress on Psychogeriatric Medicine, Umeå, Sweden, Aug 28–31, 1985, abstract 128 [G]
41. Miller PS, Richardson JS, Jyu CA, Lemay JS, Hiscock M, Keegan DL: Association of low serum anticholinergic levels and cognitive impairment in elderly presurgical patients. Am J Psychiatry 1988; 145:342–345 [A]
42. Trzepacz P, Baker R, Greenhouse J: A symptom rating scale for delirium. Psychiatry Res 1988; 23:89–97 [C]
43. Breitbart W, Rosenfeld B, Roth F, Smith MJ, Cohen K, Passik S: The Memorial Delirium Assessment Scale. J Pain Symptom Manage 1997; 13:128–137 [C]
44. Engel G, Romano J: Delirium, a syndrome of cerebral insufficiency. J Chronic Dis 1959; 9:260–277 [G]
45. Pro J, Wells C: The use of the electroencephalogram in the diagnosis of delirium. Dis Nerv Syst 1977; 38:804–808 [D]
46. Tsai L, Tsuang MT: The Mini-Mental State test and computerized tomography. Am J Psychiatry 1979; 136:436–439 [C]
47. Hemmingsen R, Vorstrup S, Clemmesen L, Holm S, Tfelt-Hansen P, Sørensen AS, Hansen C, Sommer W, Bolwig TG: Cerebral blood flow during delirium tremens and related clinical states studied with xenon-133 inhalation tomography. Am J Psychiatry 1988; 145:1384–1390 [C]
48. Golinger RC, Peet T, Tune LE: Association of elevated plasma anticholinergic activity with delirium in surgical patients. Am J Psychiatry 1987; 144:1218–1220 [C]

49. Trzepacz PT, Wise MG: Neuropsychiatric aspects of delirium, in American Psychiatric Press Textbook of Neuropsychiatry. Edited by Yudofsky SC, Hales RE. Washington, DC, American Psychiatric Press, 1997, pp 447–470 [G]
50. Inouye SK, Charpentier PA: Precipitating factors for delirium in hospitalized elderly persons: predictive model and interrelationships with baseline vulnerability. JAMA 1996; 275:852–857 [C]
51. American Psychiatric Association: Seclusion and Restraint: Psychiatric Uses. Washington, DC, APA, 1984, addendum 1992 [G]
52. Joint Commission on Accreditation of Healthcare Organizations: 1998 Accreditation Manual for Hospitals. Oak Brook Terrace, Ill, JCAHO, 1998 [G]
53. Inouye SK, Viscoli CM, Horwitz RI: A predictive model for delirium in hospitalized elderly medical patients based on admission characteristics. Ann Intern Med 1993; 119:474–481 [C]
54. Hashimoto H, Yamashiro M: Postoperative delirium and abnormal behaviour related with preoperative quality of life in elderly patients. Nippon Ronen Igakkai Zasshi 1994; 31:633–638 [C]
55. Lazarus HR, Hagens JH: Prevention of psychosis following open-heart surgery. Am J Psychiatry 1968; 124:1190–1195 [B]
56. Budd S, Brown W: Effect of a reorientation technique on postcardiotomy delirium. Nurs Res 1974; 23:341–348 [B]
57. Williams MA, Campbell EB, Raynor WJ, Mlynarczyk SM, Ward SE: Reducing acute confusional states in elderly patients with hip fractures. Res Nurs Health 1985; 8:329–337 [B]
58. Cole MG, Primeau FJ, Bailey RF, Bonnycastle MJ, Masciarelli F, Engelsmann F, Pepin MJ, Ducic D: Systematic intervention for elderly inpatients with delirium: a randomized trial. Can Med Assoc J 1994; 151:965–970 [A]
59. Meagher DJ, O'Hanlon D, O'Mahony E, Casey PR: The use of environmental strategies and psychotropic medication in the management of delirium. Br J Psychiatry 1996; 168:512–515 [C]
60. Allen JG, Lewis L, Blum S, Voorhees S, Jernigan S, Peebles MJ: Informing psychiatric patients and their families about neuropsychological assessment findings. Bull Menninger Clin 1986; 50:64–74 [G]
61. Sipahimalani A, Masand PS: Use of risperidone in delirium: case reports. Ann Clin Psychiatry 1997; 9:105–107 [G]
62. Ravona-Springer R, Dolberg OT, Hirschmann S, Grunhaus L: Delirium in elderly patients treated with risperidone: a report of three cases (letter). J Clin Psychopharmacol 1998; 18:171–172 [G]
63. Adams F, Fernandez F, Andersson BS: Emergency pharmacotherapy of delirium in the critically ill cancer patient. Psychosomatics 1986; 27(suppl 1):33–38 [F]
64. Muskin P, Mellman L, Kornfeld D: A "new" drug for treating agitation and psychosis in the general hospital: chlorpromazine. Gen Hosp Psychiatry 1986; 8:404–410 [D]
65. Rosen H: Double-blind comparison of haloperidol and thioridazine in geriatric patients. J Clin Psychiatry 1979; 40:17–20 [A]
66. Smith G, Taylor C, Linkous P: Haloperidol versus thioridazine for the treatment of psychogeriatric patients: a double-blind clinical trial. Psychosomatics 1974; 15:134–138 [A]
67. Tsuang MM, Lu LM, Stotsky BA, Cole JO: Haloperidol versus thioridazine for hospitalized psychogeriatric patients: double-blind study. J Am Geriatr Soc 1971; 19:593–600 [A]
68. Kirven LE, Montero EF: Comparison of thioridazine and diazepam in the control of nonpsychotic symptoms associated with senility: double-blind study. J Am Geriatr Soc 1973; 12:546–551 [A]
69. Thomas H, Schwartz E, Petrilli R: Droperidol versus haloperidol for chemical restraint of agitated and combative patients. Ann Emerg Med 1992; 21:407–413 [A]

70. Breitbart W, Marotta R, Platt MM, Weisman H, Derevenco M, Grau C, Corbera K, Raymond S, Lund S, Jacobsen P: A double-blind trial of haloperidol, chlorpromazine, and lorazepam in the treatment of delirium in hospitalized AIDS patients. Am J Psychiatry 1996; 153:231–237 [A]
71. van Leeuwen A, Molders J, Sterkmans P, Mielants P, Martens C, Toussaint C, Hovent A, Desseilles M, Koch H, Devroye A, Parent M: Droperidol in acutely agitated patients. J Nerv Ment Dis 1977; 164:280–283 [B]
72. Resnick M, Burton B: Droperidol vs haloperidol in the initial management of acutely agitated patients. J Clin Psychiatry 1984; 45:298–299 [A]
73. Chen B, Cardasis W: Delirium induced by lithium and risperidone combination (letter). Am J Psychiatry 1996; 153:1233–1234 [D]
74. Sipahimalani A, Sime RM, Masand PS: Treatment of delirium with risperidone. Int J Geriatric Psychopharmacology 1997; 1:24–26 [G]
75. Frye MA, Coudreaut MF, Hakeman SM, Shah BG, Strouse TB, Skotzko CE: Continuous droperidol infusion for management of agitated delirium in an intensive care unit. Psychosomatics 1995; 36:301–305 [G]
76. Menza MA, Murray GB, Holmes VF, Rafuls WA: Decreased extrapyramidal symptoms with intravenous haloperidol. J Clin Psychiatry 1987; 48:278–280 [B]
77. Wilt JL, Minnema AM, Johnson RF, Rosenblum AM: Torsade de pointes associated with the use of intravenous haloperidol. Ann Intern Med 1993; 119:391–394 [G]
78. Sharma ND, Rosman HS, Padhi D, Tisdale JE: Torsades de pointes associated with intravenous haloperidol in critically ill patients. Am J Cardiol 1998; 81:238–240 [G]
79. Jackson T, Ditmanson L, Phibbs B: Torsades de pointes and low-dose oral haloperidol. Arch Intern Med 1997; 157:2013–2015 [G]
80. Tesar GE, Murray GB, Cassem NH: Use of high-dose intravenous haloperidol in the treatment of agitated cardiac patients. J Clin Psychopharmacol 1985; 5:344–347 [G]
81. Liptzin B: Delirium, in Comprehensive Review of Geriatric Psychiatry, 2nd ed. Edited by Sadavoy J, Lazarus LW, Jarvik LF, Grossberg GT. Washington, DC, American Psychiatric Press, 1996, pp 479–495 [G]
82. Stern TA: The management of depression and anxiety following myocardial infarction. Mt Sinai J Med 1985; 52:623–633 [G]
83. Levenson JL: High-dose intravenous haloperidol for agitated delirium following lung transplantation. Psychosomatics 1995; 36:66–68 [G]
84. Riker RR, Fraser GL, Cox PM: Continuous infusion of haloperidol controls agitation in critically ill patients. Crit Care Med 1994; 22:433–439 [D]
85. Metzger E, Friedman R: Prolongation of the corrected QT and torsades de pointes cardiac arrhythmia associated with intravenous haloperidol in the medically ill. J Clin Psychopharmacol 1993; 13:128–132 [G]
86. Hunt N, Stern TA: The association between intravenous haloperidol and torsades de pointes: three cases and a literature review. Psychosomatics 1995; 36:541–549 [F, G]
87. Lawrence KR, Nasraway SA: Conduction disturbances associated with administration of butyrophenone antipsychotics in the critically ill: a review of the literature. Pharmacotherapy 1997; 17:531–537 [F]
88. Menza MA, Murray GB, Holmes VF: Controlled study of extrapyramidal reactions in the management of delirious medically ill patients: intravenous haloperidol versus intravenous haloperidol plus benzodiazepines. Heart Lung 1988; 17:238–241 [B]
89. Marcantonio ER, Goldman L, Mangione CM, Ludwig LE, Muraca B, Haslauer CM, Donaldson MC, Whittemore AD, Sugarbaker DJ, Poss R, Haas S, Cook EF, Orav EJ, Lee TH: A clinical prediction rule for delirium after elective noncardiac surgery. JAMA 1994; 271:134–139 [C]

90. Coffey B, Shader RI, Greenblatt DJ: Pharmacokinetics of benzodiazepines and psychostimulants in children. J Clin Psychopharmacol 1983; 3:217–225 [F]
91. Reiter S, Kutcher SP: Disinhibition and anger outbursts in adolescents treated with clonazepam (letter). J Clin Psychopharmacol 1991; 11:268 [G]
92. Greene LT: Physostigmine treatment of anticholinergic-drug depression in postoperative patients. Anesth Analg 1971; 50:222–226 [C]
93. Goff DC, Garber HJ, Jenike MA: Partial resolution of ranitidine-associated delirium with physostigmine: case report. J Clin Psychiatry 1985; 46:400–401 [G]
94. Delberghe X, Zegers de Beyl D: Repeated delirium from homatropine eyedrops. Clin Neurol Neurosurg 1987; 89:53–54 [G]
95. Stern TA: Continuous infusion of physostigmine in anticholinergic delirium: case report. J Clin Psychiatry 1983; 44:463–464 [G]
96. Eisendrath SJ, Goldman B, Douglas J, Dimatteo L, Van Dyke C: Meperidine-induced delirium. Am J Psychiatry 1987; 144:1062–1065 [D]
97. Mendelson G: Pheniramine aminosalicylate overdosage: reversal of delirium and choreiform movements with tacrine treatment. Arch Neurol 1977; 34:313 [G]
98. Physicians Desk Reference, 52nd ed. Montvale, NJ, Medical Economics Co, 1998 [G]
99. Watkins PB, Zimmerman HJ, Knapp MJ, Gracon SI, Lewis KW: Hepatoxic effects of tacrine administration in patients with Alzheimer's disease. JAMA 1994; 271:992–998 [A]
100. Waterlot Y, Sabot JP, Marchal M, Vanherweghem JL: Pellagra: unusual cause of paranoid delirium in dialysis. Nephrol Dial Transplant 1986; 1:204–205 [G]
101. Bahr M, Sommer N, Petersen D, Wietholter H, Dichgans J: Central pontine myelinolysis associated with low potassium levels in alcoholism. J Neurol 1990; 237:275–276 [G]
102. O'Keeffe ST, Tormey WP, Glasgow R, Lavan JN: Thiamine deficiency in hospitalized elderly patients. Gerontology 1994; 40:18–24 [G]
103. Day JJ, Bayer AJ, McMahon M, Pathy MS, Spragg BP, Rolands DC: Thiamine status, vitamin supplements and postoperative confusion. Age Ageing 1988; 17:29–34 [A]
104. Shapiro BA, Warren J, Egol AB, Greenbaum DM, Jacobi J, Nasraway SA, Schein RM, Spevetz A, Stone JR: Practice parameters for intravenous analgesia and sedation for adult patients in the intensive care unit: an executive summary. Society of Critical Care Medicine. Crit Care Med 1995; 23:1596–1600 [F]
105. Stromgren LS: ECT in acute delirium and related clinical states. Convuls Ther 1997; 13:10–17 [G]
106. Kramp P, Bolwig TG: Electroconvulsive therapy in acute delirious states. Compr Psychiatry 1981; 22:368–371 [G]
107. Krystal AD, Coffey CE: Neuropsychiatric considerations in the use of electroconvulsive therapy. J Neuropsychiatry Clin Neurosci 1997; 9:283–292 [G]
108. Fink M: Convulsive therapy in delusional disorders. Psychiatr Clin North Am 1995; 18:393–406 [F]
109. Dudley WHC, Williams JG: Electroconvulsive therapy in delirium tremens. Compr Psychiatry 1972; 13:357–360 [F]
110. Zwil AS, Pelchat RJ: ECT in the treatment of patients with neurological and somatic disease. Int J Psychiatry Med 1994; 24:1–29 [F]
111. Roberts AH: The value of ECT in delirium. Br J Psychiatry 1963; 109:653–655 [G]
112. Davis JM, Janicak PJ, Sakkar P, Gilmore C, Wang Z: Electroconvulsive therapy in the treatment of the neuroleptic malignant syndrome. Convuls Ther 1991; 7:111–120 [E]
113. Shefner WA, Shulman RB: Treatment choice in neuroleptic malignant syndrome. Convuls Ther 1998; 8:267–279 [F, G]
114. Silverman M: Organic stupor subsequent to severe head injury treated with ECT. Br J Psychiatry 1964; 110:648–650 [G]

115. Kant R, Bogyi A, Carasella N, Fishman E, Kane V, Coffey E: ECT as a therapeutic option in severe brain injury. Convuls Ther 1995; 11:45–50 [G]
116. Burke WJ, Rubin EH, Zorumski CP, Wetzel RD: The safety of ECT in geriatric psychiatry. J Am Geriatr Soc 1987; 35:516–521 [B]
117. Calev A, Gaudino EA, Squires NK, Zervas IM, Fink M: ECT and non-memory cognition: a review. Br J Clin Psychol 1995; 34:505–515 [F]
118. Devanand DP, Fitzsimons L, Prudic J, Sackeim HA: Subjective side effects during electroconvulsive therapy. Convuls Ther 1995; 11:232–240 [A]
119. Fink M: Post-ECT delirium. Convuls Ther 1993; 9:326–330 [F]
120. Nelson JP, Rosenberg DR: ECT treatment of demented elderly patients with major depression: a retrospective study of efficacy and safety. Convuls Ther 1991; 7:157–165 [D]
121. Martin M, Figiel G, Mattingly G, Zorumski CF, Jarvis MR: ECT-induced interictal delirium in patients with a history of a CVA. J Geriatr Psychiatry Neurol 1992; 5:149–155 [B]
122. Figiel GS, Coffey CE, Djang WT, Hoffman G Jr, Doraiswamy PM: Brain magnetic resonance imaging findings in ECT-induced delirium. J Neuropsychiatry Clin Neurosci 1990; 2:53–58 [G]
123. Figiel GS, Krishnan KR, Doraiswamy PM: Subcortical structural changes in ECT-induced delirium. J Geriatr Psychiatry Neurol 1990; 3:172–176 [G]
124. Figiel GS, Hassen MA, Zorumski C, Krishnan KR, Doraiswamy PM, Jarvis MR, Smith DS: ECT-induced delirium in depressed patients with Parkinson's disease. J Neuropsychiatry Clin Neurosci 1991; 3:405–411 [G]
125. Zervas IM, Fink M: ECT and delirium in Parkinson's disease (letter). Am J Psychiatry 1992; 149:1758 [G]
126. Parry JW: In defense of lawyers. Hosp Community Psychiatry 1988; 39:1108–1109 [G]
127. Grossberg GT, Zimny GH: Medical-legal issues, in Comprehensive Review of Geriatric Psychiatry, 2nd ed. Edited by Sadavoy J, Lazarus LW, Jarvik LF, Grossberg GT. Washington, DC, American Psychiatric Press, 1996, pp 1037–1049 [G]
128. Goldstein R: Non compos mentis: the psychiatrist's role in guardianship and conservatorship proceedings involving the elderly, in Geriatric Psychiatry and the Law. Edited by Rosner R, Schwartz HI. New York, Plenum, 1987, pp 269–278 [G]
129. Fogel B, Mills M, Landen J: Legal aspects of the treatment of delirium. Hosp Community Psychiatry 1986; 37:154–158 [F]
130. Breitbart W, Marotta RF, Call P: AIDS and neuroleptic malignant syndrome. Lancet 1988; 2:1488–1489 [D]
131. Hriso E, Kuhn T, Masdeu JC, Grundman M: Extrapyramidal symptoms due to dopamine-blocking agents in patients with AIDS encephalopathy. Am J Psychiatry 1991; 148:1558–1561 [D]
132. Someya T, Shibasaki M, Noguchi T, Takahashi S, Inaba T: Haloperidol metabolism in psychiatric patients: importance of glucuronidation and carbamyl reduction. J Clin Psychopharmacol 1992; 12:169–174 [B]
133. Tune L, Carr S, Hoag E, Cooper T: Anticholinergic effects of drugs commonly prescribed for the elderly: potential means for assessing risk of delirium. Am J Psychiatry 1992; 149:1393–1394 [G]
134. Tune L, Carr S, Cooper T: Association of anticholinergic activity of prescribed medications with postoperative delirium. J Neuropsychiatry Clin Neurosci 1993; 5:208–210 [C]
135. Tune LE, Damlouji NF, Holland A, Gardner TJ, Folstein MF, Coyle JT: Association of postoperative delirium with raised serum levels of anticholinergic drugs. Lancet 1981; 2:651–653 [C]

GUIDELINE WATCH: PRACTICE GUIDELINE FOR THE TREATMENT OF PATIENTS WITH ALZHEIMER'S DISEASE AND OTHER DEMENTIAS OF LATE LIFE

Peter V. Rabins, M.D., M.P.H.

Since the 1997 publication of the APA's *Practice Guideline for the Treatment of Patients With Alzheimer's Disease and Other Dementias of Late Life* (1), advances in treatment have been made. This guideline watch highlights those changes and indicates areas in which no changes have occurred.

SCREENING

No method for screening for dementia has been validated. The use of a screening instrument such as the Mini-Mental State Examination (MMSE) in patients older than age 75 is sometimes recommended to increase earlier detection, but data are lacking to support the efficacy or benefit of using the MMSE (2) or other instruments.

DIAGNOSIS

Preliminary evidence indicates that there may be a use for positron emission tomography (PET) and single photon emission computed tomography (SPECT) in the diagnosis of Alzheimer's disease (3–8). Studies using volumetric magnetic resonance imaging (MRI) to measure the size of key brain structures (e.g., hippocampus, amygdala, cingulate gyrus, ventricles, entorhinal cortex) have suggested that a smaller size of these structures in persons with only minor cognitive complaints can identify individuals who will have diagnosable Alzheimer's dementia within 3 years (9–12). No significant advances have been made in the use of biological markers for the diagnosis of dementia.

The American Psychiatric Association (APA) practice guidelines are developed by expert work groups using an explicit methodology that includes rigorous review of available evidence, broad peer review of iterative drafts, and formal approval by the APA Assembly and Board of Trustees. APA practice guidelines are intended to assist psychiatrists in clinical decision making. They are not intended to be a standard of care. The ultimate judgment regarding a particular clinical procedure or treatment plan must be made by the psychiatrist in light of the clinical data presented by the patient and the diagnostic and treatment options available. Guideline watches summarize significant developments in practice since publication of an APA practice guideline. Watches may be authored and reviewed by experts associated with the original guideline development effort and are approved for publication by APA's Executive Committee on Practice Guidelines. Thus, watches represent opinion of the authors and approval of the Executive Committee but not policy of the APA. This guideline watch was published in April 2006. Suggested citation: Rabins PV: *Guideline Watch: Practice Guideline for the Treatment of Patients With Alzheimer's Disease and Other Dementias of Late Life.* Washington, DC, American Psychiatric Association. Available online at http:// www.psych.org/ psych_pract/treatg/pg/prac_guide.cfm.

TREATMENT

Three cholinesterase inhibitor drugs—galantamine, rivastigmine, and donepezil—are now approved by the U.S. Food and Drug Administration (FDA) and are used for the treatment of Alzheimer's disease (13). Tacrine is rarely used because of hepatotoxicity. There is no convincing evidence that any one cholinesterase inhibitor has greater efficacy than another. Although each of these drugs has shown cognitive benefit over placebo, it remains unclear whether use of these drugs slows progression of the disease, delays nursing home placement, or alters mortality. Although these drugs are FDA approved for the treatment of Alzheimer's disease, there is some evidence that they are also beneficial in the treatment of dementia with Lewy bodies (14) and vascular dementia (15). A meta-analysis of 22 randomized trials of cholinesterase inhibitors found significant methodological weaknesses in the existing studies and modest evidence of benefit (16).

Memantine, an antagonist at NMDA-glutamatergic ion channels, has been shown to improve cognition in moderate to severe dementia, which is generally defined as having an MMSE score below 15 or a clinical dementia rating (CDR) of 2 or higher (17, 18). Therapeutic benefits are also observed when memantine is administered to patients already receiving a stable regimen of donepezil (18).

The only available study examining the efficacy of vitamin E supports the use of 2,000 IU daily in patients with moderately severe impairment for slowing disease progression (19), but vitamin E did not prevent development of dementia in individuals with mild cognitive impairment at 3 years (20).

The one study supporting use of ginkgo biloba as a treatment for dementia (21) has not been replicated (22).

Modest evidence is now available to support the benefits of exercise training to improve physical health and depression in patients with Alzheimer's disease (23).

New evidence provides moderate support for the efficacy of antidepressants, specifically sertraline, to treat major depression in patients with Alzheimer's disease (24). Although evidence does not exist for the treatment of major depression in dementia of other etiologies, extrapolation of these data to the treatment of major depression in all dementias may be warranted.

Further evidence suggests that neuroleptic medications offer modest benefit for concomitant psychosis and agitation in patients with Alzheimer's disease (13, 25). Although emerging data suggest that second-generation antipsychotic agents may offer some benefits in treating behavioral symptoms in dementia (26), these medications have also been associated with glucose dysregulation, hyperlipidemia, and weight gain (27). In addition, an increased risk of cerebrovascular adverse events, including stroke, was seen in clinical trials of risperidone and olanzapine in geriatric patients with dementia-related psychosis. Evidence does not support the use of trazodone or divalproex sodium for aggressive behaviors (28; P. Tariot, personal communication, 2004).

Although retrospective epidemiological studies have raised the possibility that specific interventions may decrease the likelihood of developing Alzheimer's disease (29, 30), efficacy has yet to be demonstrated in prospective trials.

REFERENCES

1. American Psychiatric Association: Practice guideline for the treatment of patients with Alzheimer's disease and other dementias of late life. Am J Psychiatry 1997; 154:1–39
2. White N, Scott A, Woods RT, Wenger GC, Keady JD, Devakumar M: The limited utility of the Mini-Mental State Examination in screening people over the age of 75 years for dementia in primary care. Br J Gen Pract 2002; 52:1002–1003

3. Herholz K, Salmon E, Perani D, Baron JC, Holthoff V, Frolich L, Schonknecht P, Ito K, Mielke R, Kalbe E, Zundorf G, Delbeuck X, Pelati O, Anchisi D, Fazio F, Kerrouche N, Desgranges B, Eustache F, Beuthien-Baumann B, Menzel C, Schroder J, Kato T, Arahata Y, Henze M, Heiss WD: Discrimination between Alzheimer dementia and controls by automated analysis of multicenter FDG PET. Neuroimage 2002; 17:302–316
4. Hoffman JM, Hanson MW, Welsh KA, Earl N, Paine S, Delong D, Coleman RE: Interpretation variability of 18FDG-positron emission tomography studies in dementia. Invest Radiol 1996; 31:316–322
5. Silverman DH, Gambhir SS, Huang HW, Schwimmer J, Kim S, Small GW, Chodosh J, Czernin J, Phelps ME: Evaluating early dementia with and without assessment of regional cerebral metabolism by PET: a comparison of predicted costs and benefits. J Nucl Med 2002; 43:253–266
6. Silverman DH, Small GW, Chang CY, Lu CS, Kung De Aburto MA, Chen W, Czernin J, Rapoport SI, Pietrini P, Alexander GE, Schapiro MB, Jagust WJ, Hoffman JM, Welsh-Bohmer KA, Alavi A, Clark CM, Salmon E, de Leon MJ, Mielke R, Cummings JL, Kowell AP, Gambhir SS, Hoh CK, Phelps ME: Positron emission tomography in evaluation of dementia: regional brain metabolism and long-term outcome. JAMA 2001; 286:2120–2127
7. Kulasingam SL, Samsa GP, Zarin DA, Rutschmann OT, Patwardhan MB, McCrory DC, Schmechel DE, Matchar DB: When should functional neuroimaging techniques be used in the diagnosis and management of Alzheimer's dementia? A decision analysis. Value Health 2003; 6:542–550
8. Gill SS, Rochon PA, Guttman M, Laupacis A: The value of positron emission tomography in the clinical evaluation of dementia. J Am Geriatr Soc 2003; 51:258–264
9. Killiany RJ, Gomez-Isla T, Moss M, Kikinis R, Sandor T, Jolesz F, Tanzi R, Jones K, Hyman BT, Albert MS: Use of structural magnetic resonance imaging to predict who will get Alzheimer's disease. Ann Neurol 2000; 47:430–439
10. Killiany RJ, Hyman BT, Gomez-Isla T, Moss MB, Kikinis R, Jolesz F, Tanzi R, Jones K, Albert MS: MRI measures of entorhinal cortex vs hippocampus in preclinical AD. Neurology 2002; 58:1188–1196
11. Kaye JA, Swihart T, Howieson D, Dame A, Moore MM, Karnos T, Camicioli R, Ball M, Oken B, Sexton G: Volume loss of the hippocampus and temporal lobe in healthy elderly persons destined to develop dementia. Neurology 1997; 48:1297–1304
12. Xu Y, Jack CR Jr, O'Brien PC, Kokmen E, Smith GE, Ivnik RJ, Boeve BF, Tangalos RG, Petersen RC: Usefulness of MRI measures of entorhinal cortex versus hippocampus in AD. Neurology 2000; 54:1760–1767
13. Lanctot KL, Best TS, Mittmann N, Liu BA, Oh PI, Einarson TR, Naranjo CA: Efficacy and safety of neuroleptics in behavioral disorders associated with dementia. J Clin Psychiatry 1998; 59:550–561
14. McKeith I, Del Ser T, Spano P, Emre M, Wesnes K, Anand R, Cicin-Sain A, Ferrara R, Spiegel R: Efficacy of rivastigmine in dementia with Lewy bodies: a randomised, double-blind, placebo-controlled international study. Lancet 2000; 356:2031–2036
15. Wilkinson D, Doody R, Helme R, Taubman K, Mintzer J, Kertesz A, Pratt RD: Donepezil in vascular dementia: a randomized, placebo-controlled study. Neurology 2003; 61:479–486
16. Kaduszkiewicz H, Zimmermann T, Beck-Bornholdt H-P, van den Bussche H: Cholinesterase inhibitors for patients with Alzheimer's disease: systematic review of randomised clinical trials. BMJ 2005; 331:321–327
17. Reisberg B, Doody R, Stoffler A, Schmitt F, Ferris S, Mobius HJ: Memantine in moderate-to-severe Alzheimer's disease. N Engl J Med 2003; 348:1333–1341
18. Tariot PN, Farlow MR, Grossberg GT, Graham SM, McDonald S, Gergel I: Memantine treatment in patients with moderate to severe Alzheimer disease already receiving donepezil: a randomized controlled trial. JAMA 2004; 291:317–324

19. Sano M, Ernesto C, Thomas RG, Klauber MR, Schafer K, Grundman M, Woodbury P, Growdon J, Cotman CW, Pfeiffer E, Schneider LS, Thal LJ: A controlled trial of selegiline, alpha-tocopherol, or both as treatment for Alzheimer's disease. The Alzheimer's Disease Cooperative Study. N Engl J Med 1997; 336:1216–1222
20. Petersen RC, Thomas RG, Grundman M, Bennett D, Doody R, Ferris S, Galasko D, Jin S, Kaye J, Levey A, Pfeiffer E, Sano M, van Dyck CH, Thal LJ: Vitamin E and donepezil for the treatment of mild cognitive impairment. N Engl J Med 2005; 352:2379–2388
21. Le Bars PL, Katz MM, Berman N, Itil TM, Freedman AM, Schatzberg AF: A placebo-controlled, double-blind, randomized trial of an extract of ginkgo biloba for dementia. North American EGb Study Group. JAMA 1997; 278:1327–1332
22. Solomon PR, Adams F, Silver A, Zimmer J, DeVeaux R: Ginkgo for memory enhancement: a randomized controlled trial. JAMA 2002; 288:835–840
23. Teri L, Gibbons LE, McCurry SM, Logsdon RG, Buchner DM, Barlow WE, Kukull WA, LaCroix AZ, McCormick W, Larson EB: Exercise plus behavioral management in patients with Alzheimer disease: a randomized controlled trial. JAMA 2003; 290:2015–2022
24. Lyketsos CG, DelCampo L, Steinberg M, Miles Q, Steele CD, Munro C, Baker AS, Sheppard JM, Frangakis C, Brandt J, Rabins PV: Treating depression in Alzheimer disease: efficacy and safety of sertraline therapy, and the benefits of depression reduction: the DIADS. Arch Gen Psychiatry 2003; 60:737–746
25. Katz IR, Jeste DV, Mintzer JE, Clyde C, Napolitano J, Brecher M: Comparison of risperidone and placebo for psychosis and behavioral disturbances associated with dementia: a randomized, double-blind trial. Risperidone Study Group. J Clin Psychiatry 1999; 60:107–115
26. Lee PE, Gill SS, Freedman M, Bronskill SE, Hillmer MP, Rochon PA: Atypical antipsychotic drugs in the treatment of behavioural and psychological symptoms of dementia: systematic review. BMJ 2004; 329:75
27. American Psychiatric Association: Practice guideline for the treatment of patients with schizophrenia, second edition. Am J Psychiatry 2004; 161(suppl):1–56
28. Teri L, Logsdon RG, Peskind E, Raskind M, Weiner MF, Tractenberg RE, Foster NL, Schneider LS, Sano M, Whitehouse P, Tariot P, Mellow AM, Auchus AP, Grundman M, Thomas RG, Schafer K, Thal LJ: Treatment of agitation in AD: a randomized, placebo-controlled clinical trial. Neurology 2000; 55:1271–1278
29. Etminan M, Gill S, Samii A: Effect of non-steroidal anti-inflammatory drugs on risk of Alzheimer's disease: systematic review and meta-analysis of observational studies. BMJ 2003; 327:128
30. Forette F, Seux ML, Staessen JA, Thijs L, Babarskiene MR, Babeanu S, Bossini A, Fagard R, Gil-Extremera B, Laks T, Kobalava Z, Sarti C, Tuomilehto J, Vanhanen H, Webster J, Yodfat Y, Birkenhager WH: The prevention of dementia with antihypertensive treatment: new evidence from the Systolic Hypertension in Europe (Syst-Eur) study. Arch Intern Med 2002; 162:2046–2052

PRACTICE GUIDELINE FOR THE Treatment of Patients With Alzheimer's Disease and Other Dementias of Late Life

WORK GROUP ON ALZHEIMER'S DISEASE AND RELATED DEMENTIAS

Peter Rabins, M.D., M.P.H., Chair
Walter Bland, M.D.
Lory Bright-Long, M.D.
Eugene Cohen, M.D.
Ira Katz, M.D.
Barry Rovner, M.D.
Lon Schneider, M.D.
Deborah Blacker, M.D., Sc.D. (Consultant)

Originally published in May 1997. A guideline watch, summarizing significant developments in the scientific literature since publication of this guideline, may be available in the Psychiatric Practice section of the APA web site at www.psych.org.

CONTENTS

Introduction 109

Development Process 110

I. Summary of Recommendations 111
- A. Coding System 111
- B. General Treatment Principles and Alternatives 111

II. Disease Definition, Natural History, and Epidemiology 115
- A. Definition of Dementia 116
- B. Associated Features 116
- C. Differential Diagnosis 116
- D. Prevalence and Course 117
- E. Staging of Dementia 117
- F. Specific Dementias 118

III. Treatment Principles and Alternatives 120
- A. Determining the Site of Treatment and Frequency of Visits 120
- B. Psychiatric Management; Psychotherapy and Other Psychosocial Treatments 121
- C. Specific Psychotherapies/Psychosocial Treatments 128
- D. Somatic Treatments 130

IV. Development of a Treatment Plan 147
- A. Mildly Impaired Patients 147
- B. Moderately Impaired Patients 148
- C. Severely and Profoundly Impaired Patients 148

V. Factors Modifying Treatment Decisions 149
- A. Comorbid Conditions 149
- B. Site-Specific Issues 150
- C. Demographic and Social Factors 153

VI. Research Directions 154

VII. Individuals and Organizations That Submitted Comments 155

VIII. References 156

INTRODUCTION

This guideline seeks to summarize data to inform the care of patients with dementia of the Alzheimer's type (referred to here as Alzheimer's disease) and other dementias associated with aging, including vascular dementia, Parkinson's disease, Lewy body disease, and Pick's and other frontal lobe dementias. The guideline does not purport to cover dementias associated with general medical conditions, such as human immunodeficiency virus (HIV) infection, Huntington's disease, head trauma, structural lesions, or endocrine and metabolic disturbances. However, while many of the research data on which the recommendations are based come from the study of Alzheimer's disease and to a lesser extent vascular dementia, many of the recommendations regarding the management of cognitive and functional changes and behavioral complications apply to dementia in general.

The guideline begins at the point where the psychiatrist has diagnosed a patient with a dementing disorder according to the criteria in DSM-IV (1) and has evaluated the patient for coexisting mental disorders, such as delirium, major depression, and substance use disorder. It also assumes that the psychiatrist, neurologist, or primary care physician has evaluated the patient for treatable factors that may be causing or exacerbating the dementia and for general medical or other conditions that may affect its treatment.

The purpose of this guideline is to assist the psychiatrist in caring for a demented patient. It should be noted that many patients have comorbid conditions that cannot be completely covered with one DSM diagnostic category. The guideline attempts to be inclusive and to cover the range of necessary treatments that might be used by a psychiatrist who provides or coordinates the overall care of the patient with dementia. The psychiatrist caring for a patient with dementia should consider, but not be limited to, the treatments recommended in this practice guideline. Psychiatrists care for patients with dementia in many different settings and serve a variety of functions. For some patients a psychiatrist will be the primary evaluator or treater, for some the psychiatrist will serve as a consultant to another physician regarding the care of psychiatric symptoms, and for other patients the psychiatrist will act as part of a multidisciplinary team.

Much of the emphasis of this practice guideline is on behavioral symptoms because most of the effective treatments available for dementing disorders are in this realm. The treatment of these symptoms is a role uniquely filled by a psychiatrist in the management of these disorders. Other key roles include administering treatments aimed at cognitive and functional deficits, which is expected to gain in importance over time as new treatments are developed, and providing support for family members and other caregivers, who will always remain critical to the care of patients with dementia.

To share feedback on this or other published APA practice guidelines, a form is available at http://www.psych.org/psych_pract/pg/reviewform.cfm.

DEVELOPMENT PROCESS

This practice guideline was developed under the auspices of the Steering Committee on Practice Guidelines. The process is detailed in the Appendix to this volume. Key features of the process include the following:

- initial drafting by a work group that included psychiatrists with clinical and research expertise in dementia;
- a comprehensive literature review (description follows);
- the production of multiple drafts with widespread review, in which 10 organizations and over 48 individuals submitted comments (see section VII);
- approval by the APA Assembly and Board of Trustees; and
- planned revisions at 3- to 5-year intervals.

The following computerized searches of relevant literature were conducted by using Excerpta Medica and MEDLINE for the period 1966 to 1994. The primary search was done in three parts: 1) medication treatment of dementia and complications (except depression), 2) nonmedication treatment of dementia and complications (except depression), and 3) treatment of depression in dementia.

In addition to this primary search, additional searches were performed where there did not appear to be adequate coverage, as follows. The key words used in Excerpta Medica searches for the period 1991–1995 were all terms indexed under "dementia," "alzheimer's," "hydergine," and "tacrine." These terms resulted in 376 citations. The key words used in MEDLINE searches were "chloral hydrate in treatment for dementia," "valproic acid in treatment for agitation," "lithium in treatment for agitation," "carbamazepine in treatment for agitation," and "beta blockers in treatment for agitation" for the period 1966–1995; "driving and dementia" for the period 1990–1995; and "MAO-inhibitors" with all terms indexed under "dementia" and "alzheimer's," all terms indexed under "dihydroergotoxine," all terms relevant for "tacrine," "NSAIDS in treatment of cognition disturbance," "estrogen in the treatment of cognition disorders," "chelation therapy in the treatment of cognition disorders," "day care—respite care—non-institutional treatment in dementia," and "zolpidem in the treatment of dementia or cognition" for the period 1991–1995.

I. SUMMARY OF RECOMMENDATIONS

The following executive summary is intended to provide an overview of the organization and scope of recommendations in this practice guideline. The treatment of patients with Alzheimer's disease and related dementias requires the consideration of many factors and cannot adequately be reviewed in a brief summary. The reader is encouraged to consult the relevant portions of the guideline when specific treatment recommendations are sought. This summary is not intended to stand by itself.

A. CODING SYSTEM

Each recommendation is identified as falling into one of these three categories of endorsement, indicated by a bracketed Roman numeral following the statement. The three categories represent varying levels of clinical confidence:

[I] Recommended with substantial clinical confidence.
[II] Recommended with moderate clinical confidence.
[III] May be recommended on the basis of individual circumstances.

B. GENERAL TREATMENT PRINCIPLES AND ALTERNATIVES

Patients with dementia display a broad range of cognitive impairments, behavioral symptoms, and mood changes. As a result, they require an individualized and multimodal treatment plan. Dementia is often progressive; thus, treatment must evolve with time in order to address newly emerging issues. At each stage the psychiatrist should be vigilant for symptoms likely to be present and should help the patient and family anticipate future symptoms and the care likely to be required [I].

1. Psychiatric management

The core of the treatment of demented patients is psychiatric management, which must be based on a solid alliance with the patient and family and thorough psychiatric, neurological, and general medical evaluations of the nature and cause of the cognitive deficits and associated noncognitive symptoms [I]. It is particularly critical to identify and treat general medical conditions that may be responsible for or contribute to the dementia or associated behavioral symptoms [I].

Ongoing assessment should include periodic monitoring of the development and evolution of cognitive and noncognitive psychiatric symptoms and their response to intervention [I]. In order to offer prompt treatment, assure safety, and provide timely advice to the patient and family, it is generally necessary to see patients in routine follow-up every 4–6 months [II]. More frequent visits (e.g., once or twice a week) may be required for patients with complex or potentially dangerous symptoms or during the administration of specific therapies [I]. Safety measures include evaluation of suicidality and the potential for violence; recommendations regarding adequate supervision, preventing falls, and limiting the hazards of wandering; vigilance regarding neglect or abuse; and restrictions on driving and use of other dangerous equipment [I]. Driving poses particular concern because of its public health impact. All patients and families should be informed that even mild dementia increases the risk of accidents [I]. Mildly impaired patients should be urged to stop driving or limit their driving to safer situations [II], and moderately and severely impaired patients should be advised not to drive [II]; in both cases, the advice should be given to the family as well as the patient [I]. Another critical aspect of psychiatric management is educating the patient and family about the illness, its treatment, and available sources of care and support (e.g., support groups, various types of respite care, nursing homes and other long-term care facilities, the Alzheimer's Association). It is also important to help patients and their families plan for financial and legal issues due to the patient's incapacity (e.g., power of attorney for medical and financial decisions, an up-to-date will, the cost of long-term care) [I].

2. Specific psychotherapies and other psychosocial treatments

In addition to the psychosocial interventions subsumed under psychiatric management, a number of specific interventions are appropriate for some patients with dementia. Few of these treatments have been subjected to double-blind, randomized evaluation, but some research, along with clinical practice, supports their effectiveness. Behavior-oriented treatments identify the antecedents and consequences of problem behaviors and institute changes in the environment that minimize precipitants and/or consequences. These approaches have not been subjected to randomized clinical trials but are supported by single-case studies and are in widespread clinical use [II]. Stimulation-oriented treatments, such as recreational activity, art therapy, and pet therapy, along with other formal and informal means of maximizing pleasurable activities for patients, have modest support from clinical trials for improving function and mood, and common sense supports their use as part of the humane care of patients with dementia [II]. Among the emotion-oriented treatments, supportive psychotherapy is used by some practitioners to address issues of loss in the early stages of dementia, reminiscence therapy has some modest research support for improvement of mood and behavior, while validation therapy and sensory integration have less research support; none of these modalities has been subjected to rigorous testing [III]. Cognition-oriented treatments, such as reality orientation, cognitive retraining, and skills training, are focused on specific cognitive deficits, are unlikely to be beneficial, and have been associated with frustration in some patients [III].

3. Special concerns regarding somatic treatments for elderly and demented patients

Psychoactive medications are effective in the management of some symptoms associated with dementia, but they must be used with caution [I]. Elderly individuals have decreased renal clearance and slowed hepatic metabolism of many medications, so lower starting doses, smaller increases in dose, and longer intervals between increments must be used [I]. General medical conditions and other medications may further alter the binding, metabolism, and excretion of many medications [I]. In addition, the elderly and patients with dementia are more sensitive to certain medication side effects, including anticholinergic effects, orthostasis, central nervous system (CNS) sedation, and parkinsonism [I]. For all of these reasons, medications should be used with considerable care, particularly when more than one agent is being used [I].

4. Treatment of cognitive symptoms

The available treatments for the cognitive symptoms of dementia are limited. Two cholinesterase inhibitors are available for Alzheimer's disease: tacrine and donepezil. Either may be offered to patients with mild to moderate Alzheimer's disease after a thorough discussion of its potential risks and benefits [I]. Tacrine has been shown to lead to modest improvements in cognition in a substantial minority of patients, but up to 30% of patients cannot tolerate the medication because of nausea and vomiting or substantial (but reversible) elevations in liver enzyme levels [I]. Donepezil has also been shown to lead to modest improvements in a substantial minority of patients, and it appears to have a similar propensity to cause nausea and vomiting [II]. Because donepezil does not share tacrine's risk for liver toxicity, and thus does not require frequent monitoring, it may prove preferable as a first-line treatment [III]. However, accumulated data from additional clinical trials and clinical practice will be necessary in order to establish a more complete picture of its efficacy and side effect profile.

Vitamin E may also be considered for patients with moderate Alzheimer's disease to prevent further decline [I] and might also be beneficial earlier or later in the course of the disease [III]. A single, large, well-conducted trial of vitamin E showed a significant delay in poor outcome over a 2-year period [I], and the agent appears to be very safe [I]. Thus, it might be considered alone or in combination with a cholinesterase inhibitor in the treatment of Alzheimer's disease [II]. Its role in the treatment of other dementing disorders is unknown.

Selegiline may also be considered for patients with moderate Alzheimer's disease to prevent further decline [II] and may possibly be beneficial earlier or later in the course of the disease [III]. A single, large, well-conducted trial showed a significant delay in poor outcome over a 2-year period [I]. However, selegiline is associated with orthostatic hypotension and a risk for medication interactions, so vitamin E, which appeared equally efficacious in a direct comparison, may be preferable [II]. However, because limited evidence suggests that selegiline may offer short-term improvement in dementia, it might be appropriate as an alternative to cholinesterase inhibitors in patients who are ineligible for, intolerant of, or unresponsive to these agents [III]. Because there was no evidence of an additive effect of vitamin E and selegiline, there is no empirical basis for using the two agents in combination [I]. The effect of selegiline in combination with cholinesterase inhibitors is unknown.

The mixture of ergoloid mesylates known by the trade name Hydergine cannot be recommended for the treatment of cognitive symptoms but may be offered to patients with vascular dementia and may be appropriately continued for patients who experience a benefit [III]. This agent has been assessed in a large number of studies with inconsistent findings, but there is a suggestion that it may have more benefit for patients with vascular dementia than those with degenerative dementias [III]. It has no significant side effects [I].

A variety of other agents have been suggested as possibly helpful in the treatment of cognitive symptoms, some of the most promising of which are under active study in clinical trials. Because these agents remain experimental, they are best taken in the context of a clinical trial. Such trials may be an appropriate option for some patients, since they offer the chance of clinical benefit while contributing to progress in treating dementia [III].

5. Treatment of psychosis and agitation

Psychosis and agitation are common in demented patients, often coexist, and may respond to similar therapies. In approaching any of these symptoms, it is critical to consider the safety of the patient and those around him or her [I]. The next step is a careful evaluation for a general medical, psychiatric, or psychosocial problem that may underlie the disturbance [I]. If attention to these issues does not resolve the problem and the symptoms do not cause undue distress to the patient or others, they are best treated with reassurance and distraction [I]. For agitation, some of the behavioral measures discussed in Section I.B.2 may be helpful as well [II]. If other measures are unsuccessful, these symptoms may be treated judiciously with one of the agents discussed in the following paragraphs [II]. The use of such agents must be evaluated and documented on an ongoing basis [I].

Antipsychotics are the only documented pharmacologic treatment for psychosis in dementia [I] and are the best documented for agitation [II]. While they have been shown to provide modest improvement in behavioral symptoms in general [I], some research evidence, along with considerable anecdotal evidence, suggests that this improvement is greater for psychosis than for other symptoms [II]. There is no evidence of a difference in efficacy among antipsychotic agents [II]. The efficacy of these agents beyond 8 weeks has limited research support, but there is considerable clinical experience with this practice [II]. Antipsychotics have a number of potentially severe side effects, including sedation and worsening of cognition, and thus must be used at the lowest effective dose: extremely low starting doses are recommended for this population [I]. High-potency agents are more likely to cause akathisia and parkinsonian symptoms; low-potency agents are more likely to cause sedation, confusion, delirium, postural hypotension, and peripheral anticholinergic effects [I]. All conventional antipsychotic agents are also associated with more serious complications, including tardive dyskinesia (for which the elderly, women, and individuals with dementia are at greater risk) and neuroleptic malignant syndrome. Risperidone appears to share the risks associated with high-potency agents, although it may be somewhat less likely to cause extrapyramidal reactions [III]. Clozapine is much less likely to be associated with extrapyramidal reactions, but it is associated with sedation, postural hypotension, and an elevated seizure risk and carries a risk of agranulocytosis, so it requires regular monitoring of blood counts [I]. The decision of which antipsychotic to use is based on the relationship between the side effect profile and the characteristics of a given patient [I]. It is expected that in the near future new agents that may alter decision making in this area will be released, but they have not yet been tested with geriatric or demented populations, so they cannot be recommended at this time.

Benzodiazepines are most useful for treating patients with prominent anxiety or for giving on an as-needed basis to patients who have infrequent episodes of agitation or to individuals who need to be sedated for a procedure such as a tooth extraction [II]. Benzodiazepines appear to perform better than placebo but not as well as antipsychotics in treating behavioral symptoms, although the data are of limited quality [II]. They can have many side effects, including sedation, worsening cognition, delirium, an increase in the risk of falls, and worsening of sleep-disordered breathing [I]. It may be preferable to use lorazepam and oxazepam, which have no active metabolites and are not metabolized in the liver [III].

The anticonvulsant agents carbamazepine and valproate, the sedating antidepressant trazodone, the atypical anxiolytic buspirone, and possibly selective serotonin reuptake inhibitors (SSRIs) are less well studied but may be appropriate for nonpsychotic patients with behavioral disorders, especially those with mild symptoms or sensitivity to antipsychotic medications. There is preliminary evidence to support their efficacy in the treatment of agitation [III]. Medroxyprogesterone and related hormones may have a role in the treatment of disinhibited sexual behavior in male patients with dementia [III]. Lithium and beta-blockers are not generally recommended: the few data supporting their use concern nondemented populations, and the potential side effects are serious [II].

6. Treatment of depression

Depression is common in patients with dementia. Patients with depression should be carefully evaluated for suicide potential [I]. Depressed mood may respond to improvements in the living situation or stimulation-oriented treatments [II], but patients with severe or persistent depressed mood with or without a full complement of neurovegetative signs should be treated with antidepressant medications [II]. Although formal evaluation of the efficacy of antidepressants for demented patients is limited, there is considerable clinical evidence supporting their use [II]. The choice among agents is based on the side effect profile and the characteristics of a given patient [I]. SSRIs are probably the first-line treatment, although one of the tricyclic antidepressants or newer agents, such as bupropion or venlafaxine, may be more appropriate for some patients [II]. Agents with significant anticholinergic effects (e.g., amitriptyline, imipramine) should be avoided [I]. Because of the elevated risk of dietary indiscretion in demented patients and the substantial risk of postural hypotension, monoamine oxidase inhibitors (MAOIs) are probably appropriate only for patients who have not responded to other treatments [II]. Although research data are limited, clinical experience suggests that electroconvulsive therapy (ECT) is effective in the treatment of patients who do not respond to other agents [II]. Twice- rather than thrice-weekly and unilateral rather than bilateral treatments may decrease the risk of delirium or memory loss associated with this modality [III].

Treatments for apathy are not well documented, but psychostimulants, bupropion, bromocriptine, and amantadine may be helpful [III]. Psychostimulants are also sometimes useful in the treatment of depression in patients with significant general medical illness [III].

7. Treatment of sleep disturbances

Sleep disturbances are common in patients with dementia. Pharmacologic intervention should be considered only when other interventions, including careful attention to sleep hygiene, have failed [I]. If a patient has a sleep disturbance and requires medication for another condition, an agent with sedating properties, given at bedtime, should be selected if possible [II]. If the sleep disturbance does not coexist with other problems, possibly effective agents include zolpidem and trazodone [II], but there are few data on the efficacy of specific agents for demented patients. Benzodiazepines and chloral hydrate are usually not recommended for other than brief use because of the risk of daytime sedation, tolerance, rebound insomnia, worsening cognition, disinhibition, and delirium [II]. Triazolam in particular is not recommended because of its association with amnesia [II]. Diphenhydramine is generally not recommended because of its anticholinergic properties [II].

8. Special issues for long-term care

Many patients with dementia eventually require placement in a nursing home or other long-term care facility, and approximately two-thirds of nursing home patients suffer from dementia. Facilities should be structured to meet the needs of patients with dementia, including those with behavioral problems [I], which are extremely common. Staff with knowledge and experience concerning dementia and the management of noncognitive symptoms appear to be important [II]. Special care units may offer a model of optimal care for patients with dementia, although there is no evidence that special care units achieve better outcomes than traditional units [III].

A particular concern is the use of physical restraints and antipsychotic medications. When used appropriately, antipsychotics can relieve symptoms and reduce distress for patients and can increase safety for patients, other residents, and staff [I]. However, overuse can lead to worsening of the dementia, oversedation, falls, and tardive dyskinesia. Thus, federal regulations and good clinical practice require careful consideration and documentation of the indications and available alternatives, both initially and over time [I]. A dose decrease or discontinuation should be considered periodically for all patients who receive antipsychotic medications [I]. A structured education program for staff may decrease the use of these medications in nursing homes [II]. Physical restraints should be used only for patients who pose an imminent risk of physical harm to themselves or others and only until more definitive treatment is provided or when other measures have been exhausted [I]. When restraints are used, the indications and alternatives should be carefully documented [I]. The need for restraints can be decreased by environmental changes that decrease the risk of falls or wandering and by careful assessment and treatment of possible causes of agitation [II].

II. DISEASE DEFINITION, NATURAL HISTORY, AND EPIDEMIOLOGY

Although there are many types of dementia, they have a number of features in common. This section contains a discussion of dementia in general and brief descriptions of some of its more common types.

A. DEFINITION OF DEMENTIA

The essential features of a dementia are multiple cognitive deficits that include memory impairment and at least one of the following: aphasia, apraxia, agnosia, or a disturbance in executive functioning (the ability to think abstractly and to plan, initiate, sequence, monitor, and stop complex behavior). The order of onset and relative prominence of the cognitive disturbances and associated symptoms vary with the specific type of dementia, as discussed in the following.

Memory impairment is generally a prominent early symptom. Individuals with dementia have difficulty learning new material and may lose valuables, such as wallets and keys, or forget food cooking on the stove. In more severe dementia, individuals also forget previously learned material, including the names of loved ones. Individuals with dementia may have difficulty with spatial tasks, such as navigating around the house or in the immediate neighborhood (where difficulties with memory are unlikely to play a role). Poor judgment and poor insight are common as well. Individuals may exhibit little or no awareness of memory loss or other cognitive abnormalities. They may make unrealistic assessments of their abilities and make plans that are not congruent with their deficits and prognosis (e.g., planning to start a new business). They may underestimate the risks involved in activities (e.g., driving).

In order to make a diagnosis of dementia, the cognitive deficits must be sufficiently severe to cause impairment in occupational or social functioning and must represent a decline from a previous level of functioning. The nature and degree of impairment are variable and often depend on the particular social setting of the individual. For example, mild cognitive impairment may significantly impair an individual's ability to perform a complex job but not a less demanding one.

B. ASSOCIATED FEATURES

Some individuals with dementia show disinhibited behavior, including making inappropriate jokes, neglecting personal hygiene, exhibiting undue familiarity with strangers, or disregarding conventional rules of social conduct. Occasionally, they may harm others by striking out. Suicidal behavior may occur, especially in mildly impaired individuals, who are more likely to have insight into their deficits and to be capable of formulating (and carrying out) a plan of action. Anxiety is fairly common, and some patients manifest "catastrophic reactions," overwhelming emotional responses to relatively minor stressors, such as changes in routine or environment. Depressed mood, with or without neurovegetative changes, is quite common, as are sleep disturbances independent of depression. Delusions can occur, especially those involving themes of persecution (e.g., the belief that misplaced possessions have been stolen). Misidentifications of familiar people as unfamiliar (or vice versa) frequently occur. Hallucinations can occur in all sensory modalities, but visual hallucinations are most common. Some patients exhibit a peak period of agitation (or other behavioral disturbances) during the evening hours, which is sometimes referred to as "sundowning."

Delirium is frequently superimposed on dementia because the underlying brain disease increases susceptibility to the effects of medications or concurrent general medical conditions. Individuals with dementia may also be especially vulnerable to psychosocial stressors (e.g., going to the hospital, bereavement), which may exacerbate their intellectual deficits and associated problems.

Dementia is sometimes accompanied by motor disturbances, which may include gait difficulties, slurred speech, and a variety of abnormal movements. Other neurological symptoms, such as myoclonus and seizures, may also occur.

C. DIFFERENTIAL DIAGNOSIS

The differential diagnosis of dementia is described in detail in DSM-IV (1) and is summarized only briefly here. Memory impairment occurs in both *delirium* and dementia. Delirium is also characterized by a reduced ability to maintain and shift attention appropriately, but the cognitive deficits tend to fluctuate, while those of dementia tend to be stable or progressive. An *amnestic disorder* is characterized by memory impairment without significant impairment in other cognitive domains. *Mental retardation* has an onset before age 18 and is characterized by significantly subaverage general intellectual functioning, which does not necessarily include memory impairment. *Schizophrenia* may be associated with multiple cognitive impairments and a decline in functioning, but the cognitive impairment tends to be less severe and occurs against a background of psychotic and behavioral symptoms meeting the established diagnostic criteria. Particularly in elderly persons, *major depressive disorder* may be associated with complaints of memory impairment, difficulty concentrating, and a reduction in intellectual abilities shown by history or mental status examination; this is sometimes referred to as *pseudodementia.* The two may sometimes be distinguished on the basis of an assessment of the course and onset of depressive and cognitive symptoms and by response to treatment of the depression. However, even when the onset of depressive symptoms precedes or coincides with the onset of cognitive symptoms and both resolve with antidepressant treatment, as many as one-half of patients go on to develop an irreversible dementia within 3 years (2). Dementia must be distinguished from *malingering* and *factitious disorder,* which generally manifest patterns of cognitive deficits that are inconsistent over time and are uncharacteristic of those typically seen in dementia. Dementia must also be distinguished from *age-related cognitive decline,* the mild decline in cognitive functioning that may occur with aging, which is nonprogressive and does not lead to functional impairment.

D. PREVALENCE AND COURSE

Exact estimates of the prevalence of dementia depend on the definition and specific threshold used, but it is clear that the prevalence increases dramatically with age. The syndrome affects approximately 5%–8% of individuals over age 65, 15%–20% of individuals over age 75, and 25%–50% of individuals over age 85. Alzheimer's disease is the most common dementia, accounting for 50%–75% of the total, with a greater proportion in the higher age ranges. Vascular dementia is probably next most common, but its prevalence is unknown. The remaining types of dementia account for a much smaller fraction of the total, although in the last few years it has been suggested that Lewy body disease may be more prevalent than previously realized (3).

The mode of onset and subsequent course of dementia depend on the underlying etiology. Classically, Alzheimer's disease has an insidious onset and gradual decline, while vascular dementia is characterized by a more acute onset and stepwise decline. However, since both disorders are common, the two frequently coexist, although only one diagnosis may be made during a person's life. Other dementias may be progressive, static, or remitting. The reversibility of a dementia is a function of the underlying pathology and of the availability and timely application of effective treatment.

E. STAGING OF DEMENTIA

Progressive dementias are generally staged according to the level of functional impairment, and the same categories may be used to describe the degree of severity of any dementia (4, 5). The ability to perform a specific function depends on baseline skills, deficits, and the social environment, so the severity of illness should be assessed in the context of past functioning in several domains. Individuals with *questionable* impairment show borderline functioning in several areas but definite impairment in none. Such individuals are not considered demented, but they should be evaluated over time: some may progress to a dementing disorder, some may return to normal functioning, and others may remain in a questionable state. Individuals with *mild* impairment are likely to have difficulties with balancing a checkbook, preparing a complex meal, or managing a difficult medication schedule. Those with *moderate* impairment also have difficulties with simpler food preparation, household cleanup, and yard work and may require assistance with some aspects of self-care (e.g., reminders to use the bathroom, help with fasteners or shaving). Those whose dementia is *severe* require considerable assistance with personal care, including feeding, grooming, and toileting. In *profound* dementia, the patients may become largely oblivious to their surroundings and are almost totally dependent on caregivers. In the *terminal* phase, patients are generally bed bound, require constant care, and may be susceptible to accidents and infectious diseases, which often prove fatal.

F. SPECIFIC DEMENTIAS

1. Dementia of the Alzheimer's type

Dementia of the Alzheimer's type, referred to here for brevity as Alzheimer's disease, is a dementia with an insidious onset and gradual progression. Various patterns of deficits are seen, but the disorder begins most commonly with deficits in recent memory, which are followed by aphasia, apraxia, and agnosia after several years. Deficits in executive function (e.g., performing tasks involving multiple steps, such as balancing a checkbook or preparing a meal) are also typically seen early in the course of the disease. Some individuals may show personality changes or increased irritability in the early stages. In the middle and later stages of the disease, psychotic symptoms are common. Patients also tend to develop incontinence and gait and motor disturbances, and eventually they become mute and bedridden. Seizures and myoclonus may also occur late in the disease.

The diagnosis of Alzheimer's disease should be made only when other etiologies for the dementia have been ruled out by careful history, physical and neurological examinations, and laboratory tests. A definitive diagnosis of Alzheimer's disease depends on microscopic examination of the brain (generally at autopsy), which reveals numerous characteristic senile plaques and neurofibrillary tangles widely distributed in the cerebral cortex. A clinical diagnosis of Alzheimer's disease conforms to the pathological diagnosis 70%–90% of the time.

Onset generally occurs in late life, most commonly in the 60s, 70s, and 80s and beyond, but in rare instances the disorder appears in the 40s and 50s. The incidence of Alzheimer's disease also increases with age, and it is estimated at 0.5% per year from age 65 to 69, 1% per year from age 70 to 74, 2% per year from age 75 to 79, 3% per year from 80 to 84, and 8% per year from age 85 onward (6). Progression is gradual but steadily downward, with an average duration from onset of symptoms to death of 8–10 years. Plateaus may occur, but progression generally resumes after 1 to several years.

DSM-IV subdivides Alzheimer's disease into the following subtypes, indicating the predominant feature of the current clinical presentation: With Delirium, With Delusions, With Depressed Mood (including but not limited to presentations that meet symptom criteria for a Major Depressive Episode), and Uncomplicated. In addition, the specifier "With Behavioral Disturbance" can also be used to indicate the presence of clinically significant difficulties, such as wandering or combativeness. DSM-IV further divides Alzheimer's disease arbitrarily into early onset, which is used if the symptoms of cognitive decline begin at or before age 65, and late onset, if they begin after age 65.

2. Vascular (multi-infarct) dementia

Vascular dementia is a dementia due to the effects of one or more strokes on cognitive function. Typically, it is characterized by an abrupt onset and stepwise course in the context of cerebrovascular disease documented by history, focal neurological signs and symptoms, and/or imaging studies. The pattern of cognitive deficits is often patchy, depending on which regions of the brain have been destroyed. Certain cognitive functions may be affected early, whereas others remain relatively unimpaired. Associated focal neurological signs and symptoms include extensor plantar response, pseudobulbar palsy, gait abnormalities, exaggeration of deep tendon reflexes, and weakness of an extremity. Structural imaging studies usually indicate multiple vascular lesions of the cerebral cortex and subcortical structures.

The onset of vascular dementia may occur any time in late life but becomes less common after age 75, while the incidence of Alzheimer's disease continues to rise. The relationship between Alzheimer's disease and vascular dementia is complex, in part because Alzheimer's disease and strokes are both common and frequently coexist (although generally only one diagnosis is recognized during a person's life), and because recent evidence suggests that small strokes may lead to increased clinical expression of Alzheimer's disease (7). The degree to which strokes alone are responsible for dementia is unclear. However, one study estimated that 8% of individuals over 60 who have a stroke develop dementia within the following year, compared to 1% of age-matched individuals without a history of stroke (8). Vascular dementia tends to progress in a stepwise fashion but can be static. Early treatment of hypertension and vascular disease may prevent further progression.

Like Alzheimer's disease, vascular dementia is subtyped in DSM-IV according to any prominent associated symptoms: With Delirium, With Delusions, With Depressed Mood, and Uncomplicated. The additional modifier "With Behavioral Disturbance" may also be used. No subtyping based on age of onset is used.

3. Dementia due to Parkinson's disease

Parkinson's disease is a slowly progressive neurological condition characterized by tremor, rigidity, bradykinesia, and postural instability; its onset is typically in middle to late life. In 20%–60% of the cases, it is accompanied by a dementia, which is particularly common late in the course. The dementia associated with Parkinson's disease has an insidious onset and slow progression and is characterized by cognitive and motor slowing, executive dysfunction, and impairment in memory retrieval. Parkinson's disease is important to psychiatrists because of the high prevalence of associated depression and the frequent occurrence of psychotic symptoms during pharmacologic treatment of the primary motor deficit.

4. Dementia due to Lewy body disease

Lewy body disease is a recently characterized disorder (9) that is clinically fairly similar to Alzheimer's disease but tends to have earlier and more prominent visual hallucinations and parkinsonian features and a somewhat more rapid evolution. Patients are notably sensitive to extrapyramidal effects of antipsychotic medications. Histopathologically, it is marked by the presence of Lewy inclusion bodies in the cerebral cortex. Recent studies suggest that Lewy body disease may account for many as 7%–26% of dementia cases, depending on the criteria used (3). The disorder is particularly likely to come to psychiatric attention because of the patients' prominent psychotic symptoms and sensitivity to antipsychotic medications.

5. Dementia due to Pick's disease and other frontal lobe dementias

Pick's disease and other frontal lobe dementias are characterized in their early stages by changes in personality, executive dysfunction, deterioration of social skills, emotional blunting, behavioral disinhibition, and prominent language abnormalities. Difficulties with memory, apraxia, and other features of dementia usually follow later in the course. Prominent primitive reflexes (snout, suck, grasp) may be present. As the dementia progresses, it may be accompanied by either apathy or extreme agitation. Individuals may develop such severe problems with language, attention, or behavior that it may be difficult to assess the degree of cognitive impairment. The diagnosis is difficult to make clinically, and it is especially difficult to distinguish from atypical Alzheimer's disease. In Pick's disease, structural brain imaging typically reveals prominent frontal and/or temporal atrophy, with relative sparing of the parietal and occipital lobes. The diagnosis of Pick's disease must be confirmed by the autopsy finding of characteristic Pick inclusion bodies. Other frontal lobe dementias tend to have more nonspecific histopathology. The disorder most commonly manifests itself in individuals between the ages of 50 and 60 years, although it can occur among older individuals. The course is progressive and tends to be more rapid than that of Alzheimer's disease. These disorders are fairly rare but are important for psychiatrists because they often present with psychiatric symptoms.

6. Other progressive dementing disorders

A number of other disorders can lead to progressive dementia. These include Huntington's disease—an autosomal dominant disorder that affects the basal ganglia and other subcortical structures and includes motor, behavioral, and cognitive symptoms—and Creutzfeldt-Jakob disease—a rapidly progressive spongiform encephalopathy associated with a slow virus or a prion (proteinaceous infectious particle).

7. Dementia due to other causes

In addition to the preceding categories, a number of general medical conditions can cause dementia. These conditions include structural lesions (primary or secondary brain tumor, subdural hematoma, slowly progressive or normal-pressure hydrocephalus), head trauma, endocrine conditions (hypothyroidism, hypercalcemia, hypoglycemia), nutritional conditions (deficiency of thiamine, niacin, or vitamin B_{12}), other infectious conditions (HIV, neurosyphilis, *Cryptococcus*), derangements of renal and hepatic function, neurological conditions (e.g., multiple sclerosis), effects of medications (e.g., benzodiazepines, beta-blockers, diphenhydramine), and the toxic effect of long-standing substance abuse, especially alcohol abuse. It is critical that psychiatrists caring for demented individuals be familiar with the general medical and neurological causes of dementia in order to assure that the diagnosis is accurate and, in particular, that potentially treatable conditions are not missed.

III. TREATMENT PRINCIPLES AND ALTERNATIVES

The treatment of Alzheimer's disease and related dementias is multimodal. It is guided by the stage of illness and is focused on the specific symptoms manifested by the patient. This discussion begins with psychiatric management, the cornerstone of the treatment of the demented patient, and then goes on to review specific treatments, first the broad range of psychosocial interventions used with dementia and then the pharmacologic options organized by target symptom.

A. DETERMINING THE SITE OF TREATMENT AND FREQUENCY OF VISITS

As for all patients, the site of treatment for an individual with dementia is determined by the need to provide safe and effective treatment in the least restrictive setting. Individuals with dementia may need to be admitted to an inpatient facility for the treatment of psychotic, affective, or behavioral symptoms. In addition, they may need to be admitted for treatment of comorbid general medical conditions or for psychiatric comorbidity. For patients who are very frail or who have significant medical illnesses, a geriatric psychiatry or medical psychiatric unit may be helpful when available. Indications for hospitalization include factors based on illness (e.g., threats of harm to self or others, violent or uncontrollable behavior) and those based on the intensity of services needed (e.g., the need for continuous skilled observation, ECT, or a medication or test that cannot be performed on an outpatient basis) (10, 11). The length of stay is similarly determined by the ability of the patient to safely receive the needed care in a less intensive setting.

Decisions regarding the need for placement in a long-term care facility often depend on the degree to which the patient's needs can be met in the home, by either relatives or other potential caregivers. The decision to remain at home should be reassessed regularly, with consideration of the patient's clinical status and the continued ability of the patient's caregivers to supervise the patient and manage the burden of care.

The necessary frequency of visits is determined by a number of factors, including the patient's clinical status and the likely rate of change, the current treatment plan and the need for any specific monitoring of treatment effects, and the reliability and skill of the patient's caregivers, particularly regarding the likelihood of their notifying the psychiatrist if a clinically important change occurs. In order to be able to offer prompt treatment, assure safety, and provide timely advice to the patient and family, it is generally, but not always, necessary to see patients in follow-up at least every 3 to 6 months. More frequent visits are likely to be required for patients with complex, distressing, or potentially dangerous symptoms or during the administration of specific therapies. For example, outpatients who present with or experience acute exacerbations of depressive or psychotic symptoms may need to be seen as frequently as once or twice a week.

B. PSYCHIATRIC MANAGEMENT; PSYCHOTHERAPY AND OTHER PSYCHOSOCIAL TREATMENTS

Successful management of patients with dementia requires a broad range of tasks, which are grouped under the term "psychiatric management." These tasks help to maximize the patient's level of function and to assure the safety and comfort of patients and their families in the context of living with a difficult disease. In some cases, psychiatrists perform all or most of these tasks themselves. In others, they are part of multidisciplinary teams. In either case, they must be aware of the full range of available treatments and take steps to assure that any necessary treatments are administered.

1. Establish and maintain an alliance with the patient and family

As with any psychiatric care, a solid alliance is critical to taking care of the demented patient. The care of a demented patient requires an alliance with the family and other caregivers, as well as the patient. Family members and other caregivers are a critical source of information, as the patient is frequently unable to give a reliable history, they are generally responsible for implementing and monitoring treatment plans, their own attitudes and behaviors have a profound effect on the patient, and they often need the treating psychiatrist's compassion and concern.

2. Perform a diagnostic evaluation and refer the patient for any needed general medical care

Patients with dementia need a thorough diagnostic evaluation. This serves to identify a diagnosis that may guide specific treatment decisions and to reveal any treatable psychiatric or general medical conditions (e.g., major depression, thyroid disease, B_{12} deficiency, tertiary syphilis, hydrocephalus, or structural brain lesion) that might be causing or exacerbating the dementia. The details of this evaluation are beyond the scope of this guideline: the reader is referred to the Consensus Conference on the Differential Diagnosis of Dementing Disorders of the National

Institute on Aging, National Institute of Neurological and Communication Disorders and Stroke, National Institute of Mental Health, and National Institutes of Health (12), the practice guideline on the diagnosis and evaluation of dementia of the American Academy of Neurology (13), and the Agency for Health Care Policy and Research's clinical practice guideline *Recognition and Initial Assessment of Alzheimer's Disease and Related Dementias* (14) for more-complete descriptions of the evaluation of patients with dementia. A brief summary follows.

The general principles of a complete psychiatric evaluation are outlined in the American Psychiatric Association's *Practice Guideline for Psychiatric Evaluation of Adults* (15; included in this volume). Evaluation of a patient with dementia frequently involves a number of physicians. The psychiatrist who has overall responsibility for the care of the patient oversees the evaluation, which should at a minimum include a clear history of the onset and progression of symptoms; a complete physical and neurological examination; a psychiatric examination, including a cognitive evaluation (e.g., the Mini-Mental State Exam) (16); a review of the patient's medications; and laboratory studies, i.e., complete blood count (CBC), blood chemistry battery (including glucose, electrolytes, calcium, and kidney and liver function tests), measurement of vitamin B_{12} level, syphilis serology, thyroid function tests, and determination of erythrocyte sedimentation rate. An assessment for past or current psychiatric illness, such as schizophrenia or major depression, that might mimic or exacerbate the dementia is also critical. For some patients, toxicology studies, HIV testing, a lumbar puncture, or an electroencephalogram may be indicated. If the history and neurological examination suggest a possible focal lesion, a structural imaging study, with computerized tomography (CT) or magnetic resonance imaging (MRI), should be obtained. Functional imaging techniques, such as positron emission tomography (PET) and single photon emission computed tomography (SPECT), have not yet shown clinical utility but are the focus of current study. Neuropsychological testing may be helpful in deciding whether a patient is actually demented or for more thoroughly characterizing an unusual symptom picture. It may also help identify strengths and weaknesses that might guide expectations for the patient and suggest interventions to improve overall function. Testing for the apolipoprotein E4 gene (*APOE4*), one form of a gene on chromosome 19 that is more common in individuals with Alzheimer's disease than in age-matched individuals without dementia, is not currently recommended for use in diagnosis because it is found in many undemented elderly and is not found in many patients with dementia (17, 18).

3. Assess and monitor psychiatric status

The psychiatrist must periodically assess the patient for the presence of noncognitive psychiatric symptoms and progression of cognitive symptoms.

Both cognitive and noncognitive symptoms of dementia tend to evolve over time, so regular monitoring allows adaptation of treatment strategies to current needs. For example, among the behavioral disturbances common in Alzheimer's disease, depression is more common early in the illness, while delusions and hallucinations are more common in the middle and later stages. Among the cognitive deficits, memory loss is a common early symptom, while language and spatial dysfunction tend to occur later.

Behavioral issues to be addressed include major depression and other depressive syndromes, suicidal ideation or behavior, hallucinations, delusions, agitation, aggressive behavior, disinhibition, anxiety, apathy, and sleep disturbances. Cognitive symptoms to address include memory, executive function, language, judgment, and spatial abilities. It is often helpful to track cognitive status with a simple examination such as the Mini-Mental State (16). A detailed assessment of functional status may also aid the clinician in documenting and tracking changes over time. These assessments of recent cognitive and functional status provide a baseline for assessing the effect of any intervention, and they improve the recognition and treatment of acute problems, such as delirium.

Whenever there is an acute worsening of cognition, functioning, behavior, or mood, the clinician should bear in mind that the elderly in general and demented patients in particular are at high risk for delirium associated with general medical problems, medications, and surgery. Newly developing or acutely worsening agitation in particular can be a sign of an occult general medical condition, untreated or undertreated pain, or physical or emotional discomfort. Thus, a thoughtful assessment of the patient's overall status and a general medical evaluation must precede any intervention with psychotropic medications or physical restraint except in an emergency.

Before undertaking an intervention, the psychiatrist should enlist the help of caregivers in carefully characterizing the target symptoms. Their nature, intensity, frequency, precipitants, and consequences should be reviewed and documented. This process is critical to monitoring the impact of any intervention and helps caregivers begin to achieve some mastery over the problem. It is also helpful if clinicians explicitly review their own, the patient's, and caregivers' expectations before embarking on any intervention.

4. Monitor safety and intervene when required

The psychiatrist treating demented patients must be vigilant regarding assessment of cognitive deficits or behavioral difficulties that might lead such patients to pose a danger to themselves or others. The psychiatrist should a) assess suicidality, b) assess violence potential, c) make recommendations regarding adequate supervision, d) make recommendations regarding the prevention of falls, and e) be vigilant regarding neglect or abuse. Other important safety issues in managing patients with dementia include interventions to decrease the hazards of wandering and recommendations concerning driving and other use of hazardous equipment, which will be discussed separately.

If suicidal ideation occurs in patients with Alzheimer's disease or others with dementia, it tends to be when the disease is mild—when depressive symptoms are common and insight is more likely to be preserved. It is a particular concern in patients who are clinically depressed but can occur in the absence of major depression. The elderly in general and elderly men in particular are at high risk for suicide, although the diagnosis of dementia confers no special risk. Interventions are similar to those for nondemented patients and may include, depending on the nature and intensity of the suicidal ideation or behavior and capacity and support system of the patient, psychotherapy; pharmacotherapy; removal of potentially dangerous items, such as medications, guns, or vehicles; increased supervision; and hospitalization.

Threats, combativeness, and physical violence are more likely to occur later in the illness and are often associated with frustration, misinterpretations, delusions, or hallucinations. These behaviors pose a particular problem for patients cared for at home, especially by frail spouses. If such behavior cannot be brought under control rapidly, hospitalization and/or nursing home placement must be considered.

The patient should be adequately supervised in the context of his or her cognitive abilities and the risk of dangerous activities. For instance, a patient with significant cognitive impairment may not be safe alone at home: he or she might improperly administer medications, be unable to cope with a household emergency, or use the stove, power tools, or other equipment in a dangerous manner.

Psychiatrists caring for demented patients should be aware that falls are a common and potentially serious problem for all elderly patients and especially those with dementia. They can lead to hip fracture, head trauma, and a variety of other injuries. In order to prevent falls, every effort should be made to minimize orthostatic hypotension. Medications associated with CNS sedation should also be kept to a minimum. If gait disturbances are present, canes, walkers, or other supports may be helpful if not contraindicated by the symptoms of the dementia. Patients at high risk for falling may need to be closely supervised while walking. The removal of loose rugs, low tables, and other obstacles can diminish risk. The use of lower beds, night-lights, and bedside commodes and/or frequent toileting may help prevent falls at night. Bed rails may also help prevent a patient from rolling out of bed but, for patients who tend to climb, may actually increase the risk of falls.

The psychiatrist should be vigilant regarding the possibility of elder abuse or neglect. Demented individuals are at particular risk for abuse because of their limited ability to protest and the added demands and emotional strain on caregivers, and those whose caregivers appear angry or frustrated may be at still higher risk. Any concern, especially one raised by the patient, must be thoroughly evaluated. However, corroborating evidence (e.g., from physical examination) should be sought in order to distinguish delusions, hallucinations, and misinterpretations from actual abuse. In most states, if neglect or abuse is suspected, the psychiatrist may be required to make a report to the appropriate local agency responsible for investigating elder abuse.

5. Intervene to decrease the hazards of wandering

Families should be advised that patients with dementia sometimes wander away from home and that wandering may be dangerous to patients who cannot find their way back or lack the judgment to recognize and deal with a dangerous situation. Since walking may be beneficial, both as stimulation and exercise, it should not be limited unnecessarily. A large, safe area for walking or an opportunity for supervised walks is ideal. When this cannot be made available to a patient who tends to wander, adequate supervision is important in order to prevent wandering into risky situations and to locate missing patients promptly. It may also be necessary to structure the environment to prevent unsupervised departures. At home, the addition of a more complex or less accessible door latch may be helpful. In institutional settings, electronic locks may be used or a high-risk patient may be fitted with an electronic Wanderguard, which triggers an alarm when the patient tries to leave. In addition, there is weak evidence that interventions such as floor grids, mirrors, and covers designed to disguise exits and doorknobs may decrease wandering (19–21), at least in institutional settings. If patients are prevented from leaving on their own, adequate supervision must be provided in order to assure egress in an emergency.

In addition, provision should be made for locating a patient should wandering occur. Such measures include sewing or pinning identifying information onto clothes, placing medical-alert bracelets on patients, and filing photographs with local police departments. Referrals to the Safe Return Program of the Alzheimer's Association (1-800-621-0379) or similar options provided by local police departments or other organizations are appropriate for many families.

6. Advise the patient and family concerning driving (and other activities that put other people at risk)

Most of the available evidence suggests that dementia, even when mild, impairs driving performance to some extent and that the risk of accidents increases with increasing severity of the dementia (22–28). The issue raises significant public health concerns, since extensive data document that individuals with dementia, even some with fairly serious impairment, continue to drive (29–33).

There is a strong consensus that demented patients with moderate impairment (e.g., those who cannot perform moderately complex tasks, such as preparing simple meals, household chores, yard work, or simple home repairs) pose an unacceptable risk and should not drive. Those with severe impairment are generally unable to drive and certainly should not do so. However, there is no consensus regarding the threshold level of dementia at which driving should be permanently curtailed (25, 34). Some clinicians argue that in mild dementia the benefits to the patient of continued independence and access to needed services outweigh the risk of an accident and that, while the risk is greater than for age-matched nondemented individuals, it is less than that for cognitively intact young drivers (e.g., under age 25). Others argue that no patient with dementia should drive because the risk of an accident is elevated even in mildly demented patients and that it is impossible to say at what point the risk becomes unacceptable. Many clinicians believe that the risk of driving is greater for patients with mild dementia whose deficits include substantial impairment in judgment, spatial function, or praxis, although research studies have been unable to confirm this (22, 26, 33). Increased risk may also be associated with concomitant motor deficits (e.g., due to stroke or a parkinsonian syndrome), sensory deficits (e.g., neglect, visual loss, deafness), general medical problems (e.g., symptomatic cardiac arrhythmia, syncope, seizures, poorly controlled diabetes), or the use of sedative-hypnotic or other sedating medications.

Psychiatrists should discuss the risks of driving with all demented patients and their families, and these discussions should be carefully documented. They should include an exploration of the patient's current driving patterns, transportation needs, and potential alternatives. The psychiatrist should ask the family about any history of getting lost or traffic accidents. For demented patients who continue to drive, the issue should be raised repeatedly and reassessed over time. This is especially true for patients with Alzheimer's disease or other progressive dementias. Eventually the point will be reached where the danger is undeniable, so patients and their families need to make plans for alternative modes of transportation. A social service referral may be helpful for some families to help with transportation arrangements and costs.

Patients with moderate to severe impairment should be strongly advised not to drive. This recommendation may also be appropriate for patients with mild dementia who have significant deficits in judgment, spatial function, or praxis or a history of at-fault traffic incidents. This advice should be communicated to family members, as well as to the patient, since the burden of the decision often falls on families. The psychiatrist can also lend moral authority and support to family members who wish to restrict driving but are reluctant to take responsibility for the decision (e.g., write on a prescription pad, "DO NOT DRIVE"). In addition, the psychiatrist can provide concrete advice regarding how best to accomplish this goal (e.g., confrontation regarding risks to grandchildren, discussion of the impact on insurance coverage and rates, removing the car from view, hiding the keys, removing ignition wires).

Patients with milder impairment should be urged to consider giving up driving. For those who are unwilling to do so, it may be helpful to advise them to consider the use of a spouse navigator and to begin limiting their driving to conditions likely to be less risky (e.g., familiar locations, modest speeds, good visibility, clear roads) (35). Mildly impaired patients who wish an independent assessment of their driving skills may be referred to an occupational therapist, rehabilitation center, driving school, or local department of motor vehicles, but the predictive value of these assessments for behind-the-wheel performance is not established.

Psychiatrists caring for demented patients should familiarize themselves with state regulations. In some states, disclosure is forbidden. In others, a diagnosis of dementia or Alzheimer's disease must be reported to the state department of motor vehicles, and the patient and family should be so informed. In most states, the physician may breach confidentiality to inform the state motor vehicle department of a patient who is judged to be a dangerous driver: on rare occasions this option is appropriate for patients with significant dementia who refuse to stop driving and whose families are unwilling or unable to stop them.

Although the data and recommendations just described refer to the operation of motor vehicles, similar principles apply to the operation of other equipment that puts the patient and others at risk. Thus, patients whose leisure or work activities involve firearms, heavy machinery, or other dangerous equipment or material may need to have these activities limited.

7. Educate the patient and family regarding the illness and available treatments

An important role of the psychiatrist caring for an individual with dementia is educating the patient and family regarding the illness and its natural history. Often the first step is to communicate the diagnosis of dementia or a specific dementing illness, such as Alzheimer's disease. Patients themselves vary in their awareness of and ability to discuss their diagnoses. Most mildly and some moderately impaired individuals are able to discuss the matter at some level, but the discussion must be adapted to the specific concerns and abilities of the patient; it may be helpful to seek the family's input regarding the nature and timing of any discussion with the patient (36). In most cases, the psychiatrist will have an explicit discussion with family members regarding the diagnosis, prognosis, and options for intervention, but this too must be adapted to the concerns and abilities of the patient and family. Recent work suggests that certain specific symptoms (e.g., psychosis, extrapyramidal symptoms) are predictive of more rapid decline, and thus may be used in tandem with other features to assess prognosis (37).

One critical part of educating the patient and family is help with the recognition of current symptoms and anticipation of future manifestations. This allows them to plan for the future and to recognize emergent symptoms that should be brought to medical attention. Family members and other caregivers may be particularly concerned about behavioral symptoms, which they often associate with a loss of dignity, social stigma, and an increased caregiving burden. It may be helpful to reassure patients and their families that these symptoms are part of the illness and are direct consequences of the damage to the brain. Moreover, they may be relieved to know that, while cognitive losses themselves may not be reversible much of the time, many symptoms, especially the more disruptive ones, can be alleviated or even eliminated with treatment, resulting in an overall increase in functional status and comfort.

It is also helpful to educate the family regarding basic principles of care. These include a) keeping requests and demands relatively simple and avoiding overly complex tasks that might lead to frustration; b) avoiding confrontation and deferring requests if the patient becomes angered; c) remaining calm, firm, and supportive if the patient becomes upset; d) being consistent and avoiding unnecessary change; e) providing frequent reminders, explanations, and orientation cues; f) recognizing declines in capacity and adjusting expectations appropriately; and g) bringing sudden declines in function and the emergence of new symptoms to professional attention. In addition, the psychiatrist can offer more specific behaviorally or psychodynamically informed suggestions for techniques that caregivers can use to avoid or deal with difficult behaviors.

Last, many patients and families are interested in understanding what is known regarding the pathophysiology and etiology of the disorder. The local chapter and national office of the Alzheimer's Association (1-800-621-0379) are often very helpful resources: they distribute a number of pamphlets written for patients, caregivers, and health professionals and operate hotlines staffed by well-informed volunteers. Many clinicians also recommend that families read articles or books written specifically for lay readers interested in understanding dementia and its care (e.g., *The Thirty-Six Hour Day: A Family Guide to Caring for Persons With Alzheimer's Disease, Related Dementing Illness, and Memory Loss in Later Life*) (38) or view informational videotapes that may be available from the local Alzheimer's Association chapter or public library.

One issue that comes up frequently is the etiology of dementia. The risk factors for vascular dementia and Alzheimer's disease are probably the best characterized. The principal risk factors for vascular dementia are the same as those for stroke: advanced age, hypertension, diabetes, and hyperlipidemia. Risk factors for Alzheimer's disease include increased age, female gender, head trauma, family history, and Down's syndrome. Apparent protective factors include education, use of nonsteroidal anti-inflammatory drugs (NSAIDs), estrogen replacement therapy, and possibly smoking. Aside from age, the best-studied risk factors are genetic. Abnormal genes on chromosomes 21, 14, and 1 appear to account for the vast majority of cases of the early-onset familial form of the illness (39–41), and one form of the apolipoprotein gene (*APOE4*) on chromosome 19 has been shown to carry an increased, but not definite, risk of Alzheimer's disease (42–44). Testing for *APOE4* has been suggested by some as a potential predictive test for Alzheimer's disease, but two independent expert panels (17, 18) strongly recommended against such testing because its predictive value is unknown, especially in the context of other risk factors for Alzheimer's disease and for mortality.

8. Advise the family regarding sources of care and support

Family members often feel overwhelmed by the combination of hard work and personal loss associated with caring for a demented individual. The caring attitude of the psychiatrist may provide a critical piece of support. This may include thoughtful inquiries about current needs and how they are being met; advice about available sources of help, both moral and practical; and more-extensive supportive psychotherapy. It also may include referrals to a variety of community resources.

A substantial literature, along with extensive practical experience, reinforces the value of support groups, especially those combining information with emotional support (45, 46). Support groups conforming to this general pattern are available in many localities through local chapters of the Alzheimer's Association and/or hospitals, community organizations, and religious groups. These groups may vary widely in their approaches, and caregivers may elect to try several before finding one that suits them. In addition to providing helpful information about the disease, how to care for it, and ways to decrease caregiver burden, these groups may enhance the quality of life of patients and spouses or other caregivers and may delay nursing home placement (46, 47). Other programs have been developed and may be appropriate for reducing the burden and relieving the stress and depression associated with long-term caregiving; these interventions include psychoeducational programs for coping with frustration or depression and workshops in stress management techniques (48, 49).

With or without such support, caregivers frequently become frustrated, overwhelmed, or clinically depressed. Psychiatrists caring for demented patients should be vigilant for these conditions in caregivers, which increase the risk of substandard care, neglect, or abuse of patients and are a sign that the caregivers themselves are in need of care. When caregivers are in significant distress, prompt treatment should be recommended; such treatment could be provided (according to the preference of psychiatrist, patient, and caregiver) by the patient's psychiatrist or through a referral.

As for the logistical aspects of care, many resources provide valuable help for those trying to care for demented individuals at home. Respite care allows the caregiver periods of relief from the responsibilities of caring for a demented individual. It provides essential physical and emotional support, serving the dual purposes of decreasing the burden of care and allowing caregivers to continue to work or fulfill other responsibilities. Respite care may last for hours to weeks and may be provided through companions, home health aides, visiting nurses, day care programs, and brief nursing home stays or other temporary overnight care. Depending on the local and individual circumstances, these types of care may be available from local senior services agencies, the local chapter of the Alzheimer's Association, religious groups, or other community organizations. Although there is little documentation of improvement in patient variables, these programs may lead to a delay in institutionalization (50–53). In addition, clinical experience suggests that, by decreasing caregiver burden, these programs may also improve the quality of life for patients and their families. Other resources that might be helpful include social service agencies, community-based social workers, home health agencies, cleaning services, Meals on Wheels, transportation programs, geriatric law specialists, and financial planners.

When families feel that they are no longer able to care for patients at home, they may need both logistical and emotional support in placing the patient in a long-term care facility (e.g., continuing care retirement community, group home, or nursing home). The psychiatrist can be a valuable resource in informing families about the available options and helping them evaluate and anticipate their needs in the context of their values, priorities, and other responsibilities. The question of placement in a long-term care facility should be raised well before it becomes an immediate necessity so that families who wish to pursue this option have time to select and apply for a suitable home, to plan for paying for long-term care, and to make needed emotional adjustments. A referral to a social service agency, private social worker, or the local chapter of the Alzheimer's Association may assist with this transition. Some social service agencies provide comprehensive home service assessment, which may help families recognize and address their needs.

9. Guide the family in financial and legal issues

Patients with dementia often lose their ability to make medical, legal, and financial decisions as the disorder progresses, and these functions must be taken over by others (54). In the case of a progressive dementing illness, such as Alzheimer's disease, if family members act while the patient is still able to participate, they can seek his or her guidance regarding long-term plans. In addition, documents such as durable powers of attorney for health care and for financial matters can help families avoid the difficulty and expense of petitioning the courts for guardianship or conservatorship should this become necessary later on in the illness. The specific rules vary from state to state, but the basic principles are the same.

Patients and family members should be advised about the opportunity to discuss preferences about medical treatment early in the course of the illness, while the patient is still able to make his or her wishes known. Issues that might be raised about care in the later stages of the illness include the use of feeding tubes, the care desired for infections and other potentially life-threatening medical conditions, and artificial life support. In most locales, medical decision making can be transferred to a trusted family member (or friend) in the form of a durable power of attorney for health care. For some patients, a living will or advance directive may also be appropriate, but which document is used and its specific features depend on the prevailing state law.

Patients may also pass authority for legal and financial decision making in the form of a durable power of attorney for financial matters. At a minimum, it is generally wise to include a trusted family member as a cosigner on any bank accounts so that payment of expenses can proceed smoothly even when the patient is no longer able to complete the task himself or herself. In some instances, it may be a good idea to warn families about the vulnerability of demented individuals to unscrupulous individuals seeking "charitable" contributions or selling inappropriate goods. If need be, the family can ask the patient to give up charge cards and checkbooks to prevent the loss of the patient's resources.

Patients and families should also be advised of the importance of financial planning early in the illness. This advice may include a frank discussion regarding the financing of home health care and/or institutional care. Unfortunately, once the patient is clearly demented it is too late to purchase long-term care insurance, but careful planning in the early stages may help to lessen the burden of nursing home care or home health services later in the disease.

Patients should also be advised to complete or update their wills while they are able to make and express decisions (55). A patient with more complex financial issues should be referred to an attorney or financial planner to establish any appropriate trusts, plan for transfer of assets, and so on.

C. SPECIFIC PSYCHOTHERAPIES/PSYCHOSOCIAL TREATMENTS

The psychiatric care of patients with dementia involves a broad range of psychosocial treatments for the patient and his or her family, as already described. In addition, some patients may benefit from more specific psychosocial interventions. These more specific psychosocial treatments for dementia can be divided into four broad groups: behavior oriented, emotion oriented, cognition oriented, and stimulation oriented.

Although few of these treatments have been subjected to rigorous double-blind, randomized, controlled trials, some are supported by research findings and practice. The studies were generally small, and many of the reports failed to fully characterize the intervention, the nature of the subjects' dementia or their baseline status, or the posttreatment outcome. Nonetheless, a review of the literature reveals modest efficacy of such treatments (although the limited available follow-up data suggest that the benefits of most do not persist beyond the duration of the interventions).

1. Goals

While these treatments differ in philosophy, focus, and methods, they have the broadly overlapping goals of improving quality of life and maximizing function in the context of existing deficits. Many have as an additional goal the improvement of cognitive skills, mood, or behavior. They are discussed together here because of their overlapping goals and apparent nonspecificity of action.

2. Types of psychotherapies/treatments and their efficacy

a) Behavior-oriented approaches

Although there are limited data from formal assessments of these treatments, there is widespread agreement that behavioral approaches (56, 57) can be effective in lessening or abolishing problem behaviors (e.g., aggression, screaming, incontinence) (58). The first step is a careful description of the behavior in question, including where it occurs, when it occurs, and how often it occurs. The next step is an assessment of the specific antecedents and consequences of each problem behavior, which will often suggest specific strategies for intervention. Activities that consistently precede the problem behavior may be acting as precipitants and should be avoided whenever possible. If the activity is a necessary one, such as bathing, it may be helpful to decrease its frequency or alter the environment so that the negative consequences are minimized (e.g., switch bath time to allow a home health aide to supervise, or change the location of baths to decrease the impact of aggressive outbursts on family members or other patients). When multistep activities, such as dressing and eating, precipitate problem behaviors, such as aggression, it often helps to simplify them or break them into parts (e.g., using clothing with Velcro closures, serving several simple snacks instead of a large meal). Whatever the intervention, it is critical to match the level of demand on the patient with his or her current capacities, avoiding both infantilization and frustration, and to modify the environment insofar as possible to compensate for deficits and capitalize on the patient's strengths.

b) Emotion-oriented approaches

These interventions include supportive psychotherapy (59), reminiscence therapy (reviewed by Burnside and Haight [60]), validation therapy (61, 62), sensory integration (63), and simulated presence therapy (64).

Reminiscence therapy, which aims to stimulate memory and mood in the context of the patient's life history, has been shown in three studies of "confused" elderly persons (65–67) to be associated with modest short-lived gains in mood, behavior, and cognition. In a single small study (68), the effects of validation therapy, which aims to restore self-worth and reduce stress by validating emotional ties to the past, on cognitive, functional, and mood measures were not significantly different from the effects of reality orientation or no intervention. Preliminary evidence from one small study (64) suggests that simulated presence therapy may be helpful in diminishing problem behaviors associated with social isolation. In another small study (63), sensory integration showed no difference from no intervention in effects on cognitive, behavioral, and functional measures. Supportive psychotherapy also falls under this rubric. It has received little or no formal assessment, but some clinicians find it useful in helping mildly impaired patients adjust to their illness.

c) Cognition-oriented approaches

These techniques include reality orientation (reviewed by Powell-Proctor and Miller [69]) and skills training (70). The aim of these treatments is to redress cognitive deficits, often in a classroom setting. In a number of studies of both institutionalized and noninstitutionalized patients, reality orientation has produced modest transient improvement in verbal orientation (65, 71–80). Some studies have also demonstrated slight transient improvement in other measures of cognition, function, behavior, and social interaction. Of note, there have been case reports of anger, frustration, and depression precipitated by reality orientation (81). There is also some evidence for transient benefit from cognitive remediation and from skills (or memory) training (70, 82–86) but there have been reports of frustration in patients and depression in caregivers associated with this type of intervention (47). The slight improvements observed with some of these treatments have not lasted beyond the treatment sessions and thus do not appear to warrant the risk of adverse effects.

d) Stimulation-oriented approaches

These treatments include activities or recreational therapies (e.g., crafts, games, pets) and art therapies (e.g., music, dance, art). They provide stimulation and enrichment and thus mobilize the patient's available cognitive resources. There is some evidence that, while they are in use, these interventions decrease behavioral problems and improve mood (79, 87, 88). Although the data supporting efficacy are limited either by small number of subjects (79, 87) or multiple interventions (87), there is anecdotal and commonsense support for their inclusion as part of the humane care of patients with dementia. Additional support for this approach comes from the work of Teri et al. (89, 90), who have developed a behavioral protocol for managing Alzheimer's disease that includes a number of interventions. The core of this protocol is identifying and increasing the number of pleasant activities, which has been shown in preliminary studies to improve the mood of patients and caregivers alike.

3. Side effects

Short-term adverse emotional consequences have been reported with psychosocial treatments. This is especially true of the cognitively oriented treatments, during which frustration, catastrophic reactions, agitation, and depression have been reported. Thus, treatment regimens must be tailored to the cognitive abilities and frustration tolerance of each patient.

4. Implementation

Behavioral interventions have strong support in clinical practice and deserve careful trials with patients who have behavioral problems that are difficult to manage. Many stimulation treatments provide the kind of environmental stimulation that is recognized as part of the humane care of patients, and thus such treatments are often included in the care of patients with dementia. Beyond this, the choice of therapy is generally based on patient characteristics and preference, availability, and cost. For instance, some approaches are available only in institutional settings, such as nursing homes or day care centers, while others can be used at home. In many cases, several modalities will be selected at the same time. Because these treatments generally do not provide lasting effects, those that can be offered regularly may be the most practical and beneficial. These treatments are generally delivered daily or weekly.

Rates of short-term response to emotion-oriented treatments are consistent with modest efficacy on a wide variety of outcome measures, and thus these treatments may be helpful for some patients. Cognition-oriented treatments are not supported by efficacy data and also have the potential to produce adverse effects.

D. SOMATIC TREATMENTS

The sections that follow describe medications (and for depression, ECT) used for the purpose of treating the cognitive and functional losses associated with dementia; psychosis, anxiety, and agitation; depression and apathy; and sleep disturbances. Although the sections are organized by these target symptoms, many medications have broader impact in actual practice.

1. Special considerations for elderly and demented populations

Certain principles underlie the pharmacologic treatment of elderly and demented patients. They will be discussed in more detail in the APA practice guideline for geriatric psychiatry (in preparation) and can be summarized as follows. First, it must be remembered that elderly individuals may have decreased renal clearance and slowed hepatic metabolism, so lower starting doses, smaller increases in dose, and longer intervals between increments must be used (this practice is sometimes referred to as "start low and go slow"). Because elderly individuals are more likely to have a variety of general medical problems and take multiple medications, one must be alert to general medical conditions and medication interactions that may further alter the serum binding, metabolism, and excretion of the medication. In addition, certain medication side effects pose particular problems for elderly and demented patients, so medications with these effects must be used especially judiciously. Anticholinergic side effects may be more burdensome in the elderly owing to coexisting cardiovascular disease, prostate or bladder disease, or other general medical conditions. Especially in demented elderly persons, these medications may also lead to worsening cognitive impairment, confusion, or even delirium (91). Elderly individuals have decreased vascular tone, are more likely to be taking other medications that cause orthostasis, and, especially if they are demented, are also more prone to falls and associated injuries. Medications associated with CNS sedation may worsen cognition, increase the risk of falls, and put patients with sleep apnea at risk of additional respiratory depression. Last, the elderly, especially those with Alzheimer's or Parkinson's disease, are especially susceptible to extrapyramidal side effects.

For all these reasons, medications should be used with considerable care. The use of multiple agents (sometimes referred to as "polypharmacy") should be avoided if possible. However, as elderly demented individuals frequently manifest multiple behavioral symptoms that do not respond to psychosocial interventions, and multiple general medical problems as well, some patients benefit from the use of several medications at once.

2. Treatments for cognitive and functional losses

a) Goals

There are a number of psychoactive medications that are used for the purposes of restoring cognitive abilities, preventing further decline, and increasing functional status in patients with dementia. These include cholinesterase inhibitors (tacrine and donepezil); α-tocopherol (vitamin E); selegiline (L-deprenyl), approved for Parkinson's disease but studied and used in demented populations; and ergoloid mesylates (Hydergine), which are approved for nonspecific cognitive decline. In addition, a number of other medications have been proposed for the treatment of cognitive decline, including NSAIDs, estrogen supplementation, melatonin, botanical agents (e.g., ginkgo biloba), and chelating agents. Many additional agents are currently being tested; for patients who have access to academic medical centers, participation in clinical trials is another option. Interventions for specific medical conditions, such as blood pressure control and use of aspirin to prevent further strokes, and prescription of L-dopa as a general treatment of Parkinson's disease, are beyond the purview of this guideline.

b) Cholinesterase inhibitors

In 1993 tacrine became the first agent approved specifically for the treatment of cognitive symptoms in Alzheimer's disease. Tacrine is a reversible cholinesterase inhibitor and is thought to work by increasing the availability of intrasynaptic acetylcholine in the brains of Alzheimer's disease patients. The medication may also have other actions. Donepezil, another reversible cholinesterase inhibitor, is now available for treatment of Alzheimer's disease. Additional agents that increase cholinergic function are in development.

(1) Efficacy

The efficacy of tacrine in mild to moderate Alzheimer's disease has been extensively studied. At least five double-blind, placebo-controlled trials with parallel group comparisons including a total of over 2,000 patients have been reported (92–96). Overall, these clinical trials consistently demonstrated differences between tacrine and placebo: approximately 30%–40% of patients taking tacrine who were able to complete the trials showed modest improvements in cognitive and functional measures over study periods ranging from 6 to 30 weeks, compared to up to 10% of those taking placebo. Modest improvement in these studies corresponds to maintaining or improving function by an amount typically lost over 6 months in untreated groups of similar Alzheimer's disease patients. Response appeared to be related to dose, at least in the largest clinical trial (94), in which patients who could tolerate 120–160 mg/day were more likely to respond. Only approximately 60% of the patients overall completed the tacrine trials even at moderate doses; 30% of subjects were dropped from these trials prior to completion because of elevation in hepatic transaminases, as specified in the protocols (i.e., more than three times the upper limit of normal, a lower threshold than the current prescribing guidelines, described in the section on implementation), and another 10% had to leave because of other adverse effects, mainly cholinergic effects (e.g., nausea and vomiting). The benefits and adverse effects of administration beyond 30 weeks are unknown. However, one observational study suggests that continued use of tacrine at doses above 120 mg/day was associated with delay in nursing home placement compared with patients who used daily doses below 120 mg (97). Anecdotal reports suggest that individuals who respond to the medication and then stop taking it may have a significant decline. The effects of tacrine on individuals with more severe or very mild Alzheimer's disease or with other dementing illnesses have not been assessed.

The efficacy of donepezil has been reported in three trials (98; Aricept package insert). A 12-week double-blind, randomized parallel group trial (99) included 160 patients with mild to moderate Alzheimer's disease randomized to receive placebo or 1, 3, or 5 mg/day of donepezil. Modest improvements in neuropsychological test results and clinicians' impressions were reported for higher doses. In another 12-week double-blind, parallel group trial (Aricept package insert), approximately 450 patients were randomized to receive placebo, 5 mg/day, or 10 mg/day of donepezil (after 5 mg/day for 1 week). A third trial (Aricept package insert), this one for 24 weeks, involved 473 patients similarly randomized to placebo, 5 mg, or 10 mg. In both of the latter two trials, the treatment groups showed modest improvement in neuropsychological test performance, clinician's impression of change, and Mini-Mental State examination scores with a trend for a somewhat greater response for the 10-mg dose during the course of the trial. Consistent with observations of tacrine, patients discontinued from donepezil after 12 or 24 weeks of treatment returned to the cognitive level of the placebo-treated patients within 3–6 weeks. In long-term observations over 2 years, patients continued on doses of 5 mg or greater of donepezil overall maintained their performance at or above baseline for an average of 40 weeks and deteriorated less when compared to a historical comparison group (100).

(2) Side effects and toxicity

As would be expected with cholinesterase inhibitors, side effects associated with cholinergic excess, particularly nausea and vomiting, are common, but tend to be mild to moderate for both agents. Observed rates are on the order of 10%–20% of patients. Additional cholinergic side effects include bradycardia, which can be dangerous in individuals with cardiac conduction problems, and increased gastrointestinal acid, a particular concern in those with a history of ulcer and those taking NSAIDs. However, these effects appear to occur infrequently with these agents. In general, cholinergic effects tend to wane within 2–4 days, so if patients can tolerate unpleasant effects in the early days of treatment, they may be more comfortable later on.

A unique property of tacrine is direct medication-induced hepatocellular injury. Approximately 30% of patients develop significant (e.g., three times the upper limit of normal) but reversible and asymptomatic elevations in liver enzyme levels, and for 5%–10% of patients the medication must be stopped owing to more marked elevations (e.g., 10 times the upper limit of normal). However, perhaps 80% of patients who initially develop elevations in liver enzyme levels can be successfully rechallenged with more-gradual increases in dose, as described in the following section. The hepatotoxicity is more common in women and tends to occur about 6–8 weeks into treatment. It has thus far proved to be reversible with discontinuation of the medication (101). No additional toxicities with donepezil have been reported, but the experience with this agent is limited.

(3) Implementation

Given the evidence for modest improvement in some patients and the lack of established alternatives, it is appropriate to consider a trial of one of these agents for mildly or moderately impaired patients with Alzheimer's disease for whom the medication is not contraindicated (e.g., in the case of tacrine, because of liver disease). Patients and their families should be apprised of the limited potential benefits and potential costs (including, in the case of tacrine, risk of hepatotoxicity) (102). Although the currently available data do not allow a direct comparison, they suggest similar degrees of efficacy for the two medications. However, donepezil has the advantage of greater ease of use because it can be given once instead of four times per day and does not require regular liver function tests. Thus, donepezil may prove preferable as a first-line treatment. However, accumulated data from clinical practice with typical Alzheimer's disease patients, along with the outcome of additional clinical trials, will be critical in developing a more complete picture of donepezil's efficacy and adverse effects. Because the efficacy of these two agents is modest, it is also appropriate to discuss alternative options, including vitamin E or possibly selegiline, psychosocial interventions, participation in a trial of an experimental treatment (if available locally), or no treatment.

For tacrine, the starting dose is currently 10 mg q.i.d. The dose may be increased by 10 mg q.i.d. (40 mg/day) every 6 weeks up to a maximum dose of 40 mg q.i.d. The highest tolerated dose (up to 160 mg/day) should be administered, since cognitive improvement is more likely to occur at higher doses. If there is no improvement in clinical status after 3–6 months, most clinicians would stop the medication.

Because of hepatotoxicity, the patient's baseline level of alanine aminotransferase (ALT) should be measured before tacrine treatment is begun; patients with elevations should not receive the medication. Once the medication is begun, ALT should be measured every 2 weeks for approximately 3 months after each dose increase, and once the dose has been stable for 3 months, ALT may be measured every 3 months. If the ALT level is three to five times the upper limit of normal, the dose should be decreased to the prior dose. A later repeat trial at the higher dose can often be accomplished without a significant increase in ALT. If it is five to 10 times the upper limit of normal, the medication should be temporarily discontinued, with a rechallenge considered after the ALT level returns to baseline. A later repeat trial can sometimes be accomplished without a significant increase in ALT. If the ALT level is more than 10 times the upper limit of normal, the medication should be discontinued. These recommendations are currently under review and may change in the near future. In addition, a trial of sustained-release tacrine is underway, so the frequency of administration may change and four-times-per-day dosing may no longer be necessary.

For donepezil, the currently recommended starting dose is 5 mg/day. After 1 week, the dose may be increased to 10 mg/day. The higher dose should be used if tolerated, as it is associated with greater efficacy; however, it has a greater tendency to cause cholinergic side effects. It should be noted that dosing and other aspects of administration may evolve as clinical experience with this medication accumulates.

c) Vitamin E

There has been considerable interest in vitamin E (α-tocopherol) as a treatment for Alzheimer's disease and other dementias because of its antioxidant properties. Vitamin E has been shown to slow nerve cell damage and death in animal models and cell culture (including damage associated with amyloid deposition, and thus possibly relevant to the development and progression of Alzheimer's disease) (103–106).

(1) Efficacy

A single clinical trial has been conducted concerning vitamin E in Alzheimer's disease (106). This placebo-controlled, double-blind, multicenter trial included 341 moderately impaired patients randomized to receive either 1000 IU b.i.d. of vitamin E alone, 5 mg b.i.d. of selegiline alone, both, or placebo, and found that vitamin E alone and selegiline alone were equivalently helpful in delaying the advent of a poor outcome (defined as death, institutionalization, or significant functional decline). Combined treatment performed somewhat worse than either agent alone, but the difference was not statistically significant. The benefit observed among individuals treated with vitamin E or selegiline alone was equivalent to approximately 7 months delay in reaching any of the endpoints designated as a poor functional outcome. It should be noted that there was no evidence of *improvement* in function compared to baseline, but only of *decreased rates of functional decline* on active treatment compared to on placebo. Despite the evidence for a better *functional* outcome in the treatment groups compared to the placebo group, all groups showed similar rates of *cognitive* decline during the 2-year study period. There are no data concerning the role of vitamin E in Alzheimer's disease with mild or severe impairment, or in other dementing illnesses. There are also no data concerning the effect of vitamin E in combination with medications other than selegiline.

(2) Side effects and toxicity

Vitamin E has been widely used clinically, has been observed in many clinical trials for other indications, and is considered to have low toxicity. Doses between 200 and 3000 IU/day have been shown to be safe and well-tolerated in many studies (107). At high doses, it has sometimes been noted to worsen blood coagulation defects in patients with vitamin K deficiency (107).

In the trial described above (106), the vitamin E group showed an elevated rate of falls and syncope compared to placebo, but the difference was not statistically significant and did not lead to attrition from the study. Vitamin E has not been associated with this effect in trials for other indications (107).

(3) Implementation

On the basis of these data, vitamin E may be used in moderately impaired patients with Alzheimer's disease in order to delay the progression of disease. Vitamin E has not been studied in Alzheimer's disease with mild or severe impairment, but, given its lack of toxicity (and possible other health benefits), some physicians might consider the medication for patients at these stages of disease as well. Vitamin E has not been studied in combination with cholinesterase inhibitors, and there is no clinical experience with this combination. However, given vitamin E's lack of medication interactions, it might be considered for use in combination with a cholinesterase inhibitor. Available evidence suggests that there is no benefit to giving vitamin E in combination with selegiline, since the combination treatment performed no better than either agent alone in the large clinical trial described above (106).

The efficacy data reported here are for a fairly high dose of 2000 IU/day. There are no data concerning other doses. Because of the association of vitamin E and worsening of coagulation defects in patients with vitamin K deficiency, vitamin E should be limited to conventional doses (200–800 IU/day) in this population.

d) Selegiline

Selegiline (also known as L-deprenyl) is a selective MAO-B inhibitor licensed in the United States for the treatment of Parkinson's disease. It is approved as a dementia medication in some European countries and is used by some clinicians in the United States for this indication. It has been suggested that selegiline may act as an antioxidant or neuroprotective agent and slow the progression of Alzheimer's disease, although, because of its effects on catecholamine metabolism, it could also act in a variety of other ways (106).

(1) Efficacy

Selegiline has been studied in six double-blind, randomized clinical trials involving over 500 patients with dementia followed over periods ranging from 1 month to 2 years (106, 108–115). The largest and most methodologically rigorous of these trials was the comparison of selegiline and vitamin E to placebo, described in Section III.D.2.c.1, in which selegiline appeared similar to vitamin E and both were superior to placebo in delaying poor outcome, and combined treatment appeared similar but somewhat worse than either agent alone.

The remaining five double-blind, randomized trials (108–115) were generally smaller, briefer (1–3 months), and had methodologic limitations. Nonetheless, all but one (110, 111) showed statistically significant or nearly significant improvements in a variety of measures across multiple domains, both cognitive and noncognitive. In addition there were five small, within-subject crossover studies of similar durations that supported a beneficial effect of selegiline (116–120).

(2) Side effects and toxicity

Selegiline's principal side effect is orthostatic hypotension, which has been reported to interfere with some patients' tolerance of the medication. However, this may be more common in patients with Parkinson's disease, since it was not observed in the large Alzheimer's disease trial reported above (106). The investigators reported that the agent was well tolerated, and, although a somewhat higher rate of falls and syncope were reported with selegiline than with placebo, the differences were not statistically significant and did not lead to dropout from the study.

Beyond these effects, selegiline is reported to be quite activating, which is helpful for some patients but may lead to anxiety and/or irritability in others (118). The 5- to 10-mg/day dose used in the treatment of dementia is relatively selective for MAO-B and does not fully inhibit MAO-A, so a tyramine-free diet and avoidance of sympathomimetic agents are not required. However, patients and caregivers should be warned about the symptoms of hypertensive crisis and the critical nature of the 10-mg dose ceiling. More critical, adverse effects of medication interactions, including changes in mental status, seizures, and even death have been observed with meperidine, SSRIs, and tricyclic antidepressants, although there are also reports of patients who have tolerated these combinations. Selegiline is generally considered contraindicated for patients who are taking any of these agents.

(3) Implementation

The recent large study confirms the efficacy of selegiline in delaying the progression of Alzheimer's disease with moderate impairment. However, in the same study, vitamin E, which is generally less expensive and has a more favorable side effect profile and less potential for medication interactions, had approximately equal efficacy, and thus might appear preferable to selegiline. On the other hand, there is also modest support for cognitive and functional improvement with selegiline, rather than simply the prevention of functional decline, so a trial of selegiline might be considered, especially for those patients who cannot take cholinesterase inhibitors. There are limited data concerning the role of selegiline at other stages of Alzheimer's disease, but it is possible that it would offer a benefit to either milder or more severely impaired patients. Last, if the side effects and medication interactions do not pose a problem, selegiline may be continued in patients whose families report a benefit. The standard dose of selegiline for dementia is 5–10 mg/day. In the largest trial (106), which was reported above, 10 mg was used.

e) Ergoloid mesylates

(1) Efficacy

A mixture of ergoloid mesylates, known by the trade name Hydergine, is currently marketed for the treatment of nonspecific cognitive impairment. It has been available for at least 40 years and has been studied in at least 150 clinical trials. Of these, seven were double-blind, placebo-controlled, randomized trials with a parallel group design involving a total of 297 patients with diagnoses consistent with Alzheimer's disease (84, 121–126). A recent meta-analysis (116) suggested that there might have been improvements in some neuropsychological and behavioral measures, but the overall effect sizes were not statistically significant. There was a general impression that any improvement observed was in behavioral rather than cognitive measures. In seven trials involving a total of 140 patients with vascular dementia (123, 125, 127–131), there was somewhat more compelling evidence of modest improvement on neuropsychological and behavioral measures.

(2) Side effects and toxicity

Ergoloid mesylates occasionally cause mild nausea or gastrointestinal distress, but no significant side effects or toxicity have emerged during long-term use. However, the medication is contraindicated for patients with psychosis.

(3) Implementation

The questionable efficacy of ergoloid mesylates suggested by extensive study argues against routine use of this medication in the treatment of dementia. However, under some circumstances it may be appropriate to offer a trial of this agent for vascular dementia. For Alzheimer's disease, a trial of a cholinesterase inhibitor, vitamin E, or selegiline is probably preferable, and for some patients participation in a clinical trial at an academic medical center may also be preferable. However, when these options are inappropriate or unsuccessful, a trial of ergoloid mesylates may be appropriate for patients with a strong interest in pharmacologic therapy. In addition, use of the medication may be safely continued for patients whose families report a benefit. The manufacturer's recommended dose is 3 mg/day, but studies using 4 or more (up to 9) mg/day were more likely to show significant improvements in patient outcomes.

f) Other agents

A number of additional medications marketed for other indications have been proposed for the treatment of dementia on the basis of epidemiologic data or pilot studies, but they cannot be recommended for use at this time. Aspirin and other NSAIDs have been proposed because of epidemiologic data suggesting that they protect against the development of the disease (132–135) and because of hypotheses regarding the involvement of inflammatory mechanisms (136). In a single small treatment trial for patients with Alzheimer's disease, patients receiving indomethacin, 100–150 mg/day, experienced less decline over 6 months than did a matched control group (134). Patients using or considering these agents for other indications (e.g., arthritis treatment) might consider this preliminary evidence when weighing the risks and benefits of nonsteroidal therapy.

Estrogen replacement therapy, which is known to affect cognitive function (137), has been shown to be beneficial in the treatment of dementia in at least two case series (138, 139), and it has been associated with later onset and/or decreased risk of cognitive decline in at least two observational studies of postmenopausal women (140, 141). A clinical trial of estrogen in the treatment of postmenopausal women with Alzheimer's disease is in progress. In the meantime, postmenopausal women weighing the risks and benefits of estrogen replacement might consider this preliminary evidence (142).

There is also interest in the hormone melatonin and in botanical agents, such as ginkgo biloba, which are available without a prescription. Because some of these agents are quite popular, psychiatrists should routinely inquire about their use and should advise patients and their families that these agents are marketed with limited quality control and have not been subjected to efficacy evaluations.

The chelating agent desferrioxamine has also been studied as a possible treatment for Alzheimer's disease on the basis of hypotheses regarding heavy metals in the pathogenesis of the disease. In one small single-blind trial, there was some evidence of a decrease in cognitive decline over 2 years (143). Study of another chelating agent has failed to confirm this finding (144). Because chelating agents are quite toxic and support for them is so weak, they cannot be recommended for the treatment of dementia.

3. Treatments for psychosis and agitation

a) Goals

Use of such treatments is intended to decrease psychotic symptoms (including paranoia, delusions, and hallucinations) and associated or independent agitation, screaming, combativeness, or violence and thereby increase the comfort and safety of patients and their families and caregivers. Although DSM-IV defines one subtype of Alzheimer's disease (and other dementias) on the basis of delusions and another subtype by behavioral disturbances, this section covers both, along with hallucinations, paranoia, and suspiciousness. This section also briefly addresses the treatment of anxiety in demented individuals.

In the consideration of an intervention, it is critical to be specific in describing target symptoms, both to select the optimal treatment and to monitor the effect of that treatment (145–147). However, the treatments used for this broad group of symptoms overlap to a considerable extent, so they are discussed together here.

b) General principles

Interventions for psychosis should be guided by the patient's level of distress and the risk to the patient or caregivers. If there is little distress or danger, reassurance and distraction are often all that is required. If the patient is distressed or if accompanying agitation, combativeness, or violent behavior puts the patient or others in danger, psychopharmacologic treatment is indicated. The principles for anxiety are similar, although it is less commonly associated with dangerous behavior.

"Agitation" is an umbrella term that can refer to a range of behavioral disturbances, including aggression, combativeness, hyperactivity, and disinhibition. The first priority in treating such conditions is a careful medical evaluation. Agitation can result from an occult general medical problem, untreated or undertreated pain, depression, sleep loss, or delirium. The agitation will often resolve with treatment of the underlying condition. The next step is an assessment of the patient's overall situation: agitation can also result from physical discomfort, such as hunger, constipation, or sleep deprivation; an interpersonal issue, such as a change in living situation or a new caregiver or roommate; or an emotional difficulty, such as frustration, boredom, or loneliness. Attending to unmet needs, providing reassurance, or redirecting activities may resolve the problem. If the agitation occurs repeatedly, it is often helpful to institute the behavioral measures discussed in Section III.C.2.a. If these measures are unsuccessful, then pharmacologic treatment should be considered, especially if the agitation puts the patient or others in danger.

If the psychosis and/or agitation is deemed dangerous to the patient and caregiver, the psychiatrist must undertake the measures necessary to assure safety, in addition to pharmacologic intervention. Such additional measures may include hospitalization, one-on-one care, or physical restraint.

Whatever agent is used in the treatment of behavioral disturbances, its continued use must be evaluated and justified on an ongoing basis. As a dementing illness evolves, psychosis and agitation may wax and wane or may change in character; more or less of a medication, a change in medications, or no medication at all may be indicated in response to these changes.

c) Antipsychotics

(1) Efficacy

Antipsychotic medications have been extensively studied in the treatment of psychosis and agitation in demented individuals. For example, a 1990 review (148) identified seven double-blind, placebo-controlled, randomized parallel group clinical trials including 252 patients studied over 3–8 weeks (149–155). Despite some methodologic flaws, notably small numbers of subjects and a lack of diagnostic specificity, taken together these studies constitute solid evidence for a modest improvement in behavioral symptoms with antipsychotic treatment. A meta-analysis of these seven trials (148), using clinician assessment of improvement in a variety of behavioral symptoms as the primary outcome, showed improvement in 59% of the subjects taking antipsychotics and 41% of those taking placebo. The studies varied widely in dose, ranging from 66 to 267 mg/day in chlorpromazine equivalents, and efficacy for behavioral symptoms was not correlated with standardized dose. Adverse effects were common, but specific rates are not available. Dropout rates were also high, whether associated with side effects or poor efficacy. Of note, one study suggested that antipsychotic agents are most effective specifically for psychotic symptoms (149). The available studies comparing antipsychotics to one another are of limited power but suggest no difference in efficacy (147, 148). Of note, there are limited data on the efficacy of antipsychotic medications for demented individuals beyond 8 weeks of follow-up, although extensive clinical experience suggests that they are helpful for longer periods of time.

Newer agents, such as risperidone and clozapine, have not been studied for demented populations in well-controlled trials. However, risperidone was effective in several case series of geriatric patients, including those with dementia (156), and also has support from some geriatric clinicians, who report that it is effective against agitation and psychosis in geriatric patients even at very low doses (i.e., 0.5–2.0 mg/day), which may limit extrapyramidal side effects. Clozapine has been found to be useful in controlling psychotic symptoms in Parkinson's disease (157) and Lewy body disease (158) and may also be useful for patients with Alzheimer's disease who are sensitive to the extrapyramidal effects of conventional antipsychotic agents (159). Olanzapine was released in 1996, and sertindole and quetiapine are due to be released in the near future. Early data suggest that their efficacy is similar to that of conventional antipsychotic agents, but they have not yet been tested in geriatric or demented populations.

(2) Side effects and toxicity

Antipsychotic agents have a broad range of common side effects that tend to vary with medication potency, although any effect can be seen with any agent. High-potency agents (e.g., haloperidol, fluphenazine) are most strongly associated with akathisia (which can worsen the target behaviors) and parkinsonian symptoms. Low-potency agents (e.g., thioridazine, chlorpromazine) are associated with sedation (which can lead to worsening cognition or falls), confusion, delirium, postural hypotension (which can also lead to falls), and a variety of peripheral anticholinergic effects (e.g., dry mouth, constipation). Risperidone shares many features with high-potency antipsychotic agents, although some clinicians feel that it has a somewhat lower risk of extrapyramidal effects, especially if low doses (0.5–2.0 mg/day) are used. Unfortunately, there are few data from direct comparisons of risperidone and conventional antipsychotics using equivalent doses, especially for elderly patients. Clozapine is less commonly associated with extrapyramidal side effects but is associated with sedation, postural hypotension, and an elevated risk of seizures. Early trials of the newer agents—olanzapine, sertindole, and quetiapine—suggest that they carry little or no risk of extrapyramidal effects for general psychiatric patients, but additional research and clinical experience will be necessary to characterize their performance for elderly and demented patients in general practice.

All of these side effects can be minimized by using the lowest effective dose. This principle is particularly important in order to minimize sedation and akathisia, both of which can actually worsen target behaviors and may thus make antipsychotics less effective (160). It may also be helpful to select an agent with the side effect profile most suited to a given patient. Anticholinergic agents may be effective in the treatment of parkinsonian side effects, but the high risk of associated cognitive decline, delirium, and other anticholinergic effects suggests that they should be used only with extreme caution for elderly and demented patients.

In addition to these common side effects, antipsychotic agents are associated with a risk of more serious complications that must be considered in weighing the risks and benefits of antipsychotic treatment. The first is tardive dyskinesia, which is more likely with increasing dose and duration of treatment and occurs more commonly in women, demented individuals, and the elderly in general. The risk may be as high as 30% for elderly patients with significant exposure (161–163). The second additional possible complication is neuroleptic malignant syndrome, which is rare but potentially lethal. Both of these complications have been reported with risperidone, although they may occur at lower frequencies. Clozapine appears less likely to be associated with these two complications, although they have been described with clozapine treatment. Clozapine has a significant risk of agranulocytosis, which is more common in the elderly than in younger patients (159), and regular monitoring of blood counts is required. Olanzapine, sertindole, and quetiapine have not been associated with these complications, although additional research data and practice experience will be needed to identify and characterize their effects on demented and geriatric patients in general practice.

(3) Implementation

Antipsychotics are the only pharmacologic treatment available for psychotic symptoms in dementia. They are also the most commonly used and best-studied pharmacologic treatment for agitation, and there is considerable evidence for their efficacy. However, there are a number of nonpharmacologic interventions that can be used before a trial of an antipsychotic or other medication is begun, as already outlined. Use of nonpharmacologic treatments is particularly critical given the large number and potential severity of side effects and more serious complications associated with antipsychotic medications.

There are no efficacy data to guide the choice among antipsychotic agents. Instead, the choice is based on the side effect profile. Some clinicians recommend agents that fall between the extremes of side effect profiles (e.g., perphenazine), but there are no data to support the contention that these agents have fewer adverse effects. It generally makes sense to select an agent whose most typical side effects are least likely to cause problems for a given patient (for instance, a higher-potency agent [e.g., haloperidol] might be selected if the patient is likely to be sensitive to anticholinergic effects, or a lower-potency agent [e.g., thioridazine] might be chosen if the patient has parkinsonian symptoms) or might actually be beneficial (e.g., a more sedating medication, given at bedtime, for a patient with difficulty falling asleep). Some clinicians believe that risperidone also poses a lower risk of extrapyramidal symptoms when used at doses of 2 mg/day or lower (164), but others disagree (165). Clozapine may be a good choice for individuals with Parkinson's disease (157) or Lewy body disease (158) and possibly for others who cannot tolerate extrapyramidal side effects (156). Olanzapine and the two novel agents due to be released soon (sertindole and quetiapine) may prove to be good choices for geriatric and demented patients, especially those who are sensitive to extrapyramidal side effects, but insufficient data are available to recommend them at this time.

Antipsychotics are most commonly administered in the evening, so that maximum blood levels occur when they will help foster sleep and treat behavioral problems that peak in the evening hours (sometimes called "sundowning"). Most of these medications have long half-lives, so once-a-day dosing is generally sufficient. However, morning doses or twice-a-day doses may be helpful for patients with different symptom patterns.

On the whole, antipsychotic agents are given as standing doses rather than as needed, although as-needed doses may be appropriate for symptoms that occur infrequently. Oral administration is generally preferred, although an intramuscular injection may sometimes be used in an emergency or when a patient is unable to take medications by mouth (e.g., for a surgical procedure). Very low doses of depot antipsychotic medications (e.g., 1.25–3.75 mg/month of fluphenazine decanoate) were shown in a small open study to be effective in managing chronic behavioral problems in this population (166).

Low starting doses are recommended (e.g., 0.5 mg/day of haloperidol, 10–25 mg/day of thioridazine, 2 mg/day of perphenazine, 1 mg/day of thiothixene, 0.5–1.0 mg/day of risperidone, 1–2 mg/day of trifluoperazine, 12.5 mg/day of clozapine). The dose can be increased on the basis of the response of the target symptom(s). The usual maximum doses of these agents for demented elderly patients are 2–5 mg/day of haloperidol, 50–100 mg/day of thioridazine, 16–24 mg/day of perphenazine, 10–15 mg/day of thiothixene, 4–6 mg/day of risperidone, 10–15 mg/day of trifluoperazine, and 75–100 mg/day of clozapine. Most patients with dementia do best with doses below these maxima, but younger and less frail individuals may tolerate and respond to somewhat higher doses.

Given their side effects and potential toxicity, the risks and benefits of antipsychotic agents must be reassessed on an ongoing basis. The lowest effective dose should be sought, and emergent side effects should first be treated by dose reduction. The routine prescribing of anticholinergic agents is to be avoided. In addition, periodic attempts (e.g., every several months) to reduce or withdraw antipsychotic medications should be considered for all patients in the context of the probability of a relapse and the dangerousness of the target behavior(s).

d) Benzodiazepines

(1) Efficacy

The use of benzodiazepines in the treatment of behavioral symptoms in dementia has been studied in at least seven randomized clinical trials. Five studies including a total of 825 patients compared benzodiazepines to antipsychotics (167–171), and two studies compared benzodiazepines to placebo (172, 173). These studies are limited by poorly specified diagnosis, a mixture of target symptoms, limited outcome measures, and, in most cases, high doses of long-acting agents. Nonetheless, they show fairly consistently that benzodiazepines perform better than placebo but not as well as antipsychotics in reducing behavior problems. However, it is somewhat difficult to extrapolate these results, most of which are based on substantial doses of long-acting agents (e.g., 12 mg/day of diazepam), to the lower doses or the shorter-acting agents more commonly used today. There are no data concerning the efficacy of benzodiazepines after 8 weeks or whether one benzodiazepine is more effective than another.

(2) Side effects and toxicity

The most commonly reported side effects are sedation, ataxia, amnesia, confusion (even delirium), and paradoxical anxiety. These can lead to worsening cognition and behavior and can also contribute to the risk of falls (174). They also carry a risk of respiratory suppression in patients with sleep-related breathing disorders. Because all of these effects are dose related, the minimum effective dose should be used. Agents with long half-lives and long-lived metabolites can take weeks to reach steady-state levels, especially in elderly patients, so these agents must be used with particular caution. There is some evidence that elderly patients taking long-acting benzodiazepines are more likely to fall, and to suffer hip fractures, than those taking short-acting agents (175), although it is possible that the total dose, and not the duration of action, is the culprit (176). Clinical experience suggests that, like alcohol, benzodiazepines may lead to disinhibition, although there are few data to support this. The risk of medication dependence (and withdrawal, if the medication is stopped abruptly) is also a concern for some patients.

(3) Implementation

Although benzodiazepines may have a higher likelihood of side effects and a lower likelihood of benefit than antipsychotics, they can be useful in treating agitation in some patients with dementia, particularly those in whom anxiety is prominent. They may be particularly useful on an as-needed basis for patients who have only rare episodes of agitation or those who need to be sedated for a particular procedure, such as a tooth extraction. However, given the risk of disinhibition (and thus worsening of the target behaviors), oversedation, falls (and associated injuries), and delirium, their use should be kept to a minimum.

Among the benzodiazepines, many clinicians favor agents such as oxazepam and lorazepam that do not require oxidative metabolism in the liver and have no active metabolites. Temazepam shares these characteristics but is more problematic because of its long half-life. Lorazepam may be given on an as-needed basis in doses from 0.5 to 1.0 mg every 4–6 hours. Standing doses of 0.5–1.0 mg may be given from one to four times per day. Oxazepam is absorbed more slowly, so it is less useful on an as-needed basis. Standing doses of 7.5–15.0 mg may be given one to four times per day. Some clinicians prefer long-acting agents, such as clonazepam (starting at 0.5 mg/day with increases up to 2 mg/day) (177). However, such agents must be used with caution: dose increases must be made very gradually, as the medication can continue to accumulate over a substantial period, and vigilance concerning the increased risk of falls must be exercised. If benzodiazepines are used for an extended period (e.g., a month), they should be tapered rather than stopped abruptly owing to the risk of withdrawal.

e) Anticonvulsants

(1) Efficacy

Use of carbamazepine has support from several case series (178), a small open trial (179), a double-blind, nonrandomized trial (180), and one randomized trial (181) in which it was associated with nonsignificant decreases in behavioral measures.

Several favorable case reports and open trials have been reported for the anticonvulsant valproate (182, 183).

(2) Side effects and toxicity

The principal side effects of carbamazepine include ataxia, sedation, and confusion, which are particular concerns for elderly and demented patients. In addition, in rare instances carbamazepine can lead to bone marrow suppression or hyponatremia.

Valproate's principal side effects are gastrointestinal disturbances and ataxia. In addition, in rare instances it can lead to bone marrow suppression or hepatic toxicity.

(3) Implementation

Given the sparse data on these agents, they cannot be recommended with confidence for the treatment of agitation in demented patients. Nonetheless, a therapeutic trial of one of these agents (especially carbamazepine, for which the data are somewhat stronger at this point) may be appropriate for some nonpsychotic patients, especially those who are mildly agitated or are sensitive or unresponsive to antipsychotics. Given the potential toxicity of these anticonvulsant agents, it is particularly critical to identify and monitor target symptoms and to stop administering the medication if no improvement is observed.

Carbamazepine may be given in two to four doses per day, started at a dose of 100 mg/day, and increased gradually as warranted by behavioral response and side effects or until blood levels reach 8–12 ng/ml. Valproate is given in two or three doses per day and should be started at 125–250 mg/day, with gradual increases based on behavioral response and side effects or until blood levels reach 50–60 ng/ml (or, for rare patients in this population, 100 ng/ml).

Many clinicians recommend monitoring CBC and electrolyte levels in patients taking carbamazepine and monitoring CBC and liver function values in patients taking valproate, owing to the possibility of bone marrow suppression, hyponatremia, and liver toxicity. However, this practice is not uniform. For details concerning the assessment and monitoring necessary during use of these agents, along with their side effects and potential toxicities, the reader is referred to the American Psychiatric Association's *Practice Guideline for the Treatment of Patients With Bipolar Disorder* (184; included in this volume). However, a particularly cautious approach is warranted when treating elderly and demented patients, who may be more vulnerable to adverse effects, particularly CNS effects, and yet less likely to be able to report warning symptoms.

f) Other agents

A number of other agents have been proposed for the treatment of agitation in patients with dementia (reviewed in references 148, 185, and 186). Efficacy data for these agents generally come from case reports or small open trials, often of mixed populations.

Data on trazodone have been provided by a few favorable case reports and case series (187–189), one small open trial (190), and one small double-blind, randomized clinical trial (191). Postural hypotension, sedation, and dry mouth are the principal side effects. Trazodone is generally given before bed but can be given in two or three divided doses per day. It can be started at 25–50 mg/day and gradually increased up to a maximum dose of 150–250 mg/day. Preliminary data suggest that SSRIs may also be useful in the treatment of agitation (190, 192, 193).

There have been at least two case reports (194, 195) and one open trial (196) concerning buspirone as a treatment for agitation or anxiety in elderly patients with dementia. Buspirone is generally well tolerated by elderly individuals but is sometimes associated with nausea, headache, dizziness, light-headedness, and fatigue. It is not associated with psychomotor impairment or tolerance and dependence. It is given in up to four doses per day and can be started at 5 mg/day and increased up to a total daily dose of 60 mg. There have been case reports of serotonin syndrome when buspirone is combined with SSRIs, so it should be used with SSRIs or other serotonergic agents only with cautious monitoring.

Given the limited efficacy data, none of these less-well-studied agents can be recommended with any confidence for the treatment of agitation and psychosis in patients with dementia. Nonetheless, a therapeutic trial of trazodone, buspirone, or perhaps an SSRI may be appropriate for some nonpsychotic patients, especially those with relatively mild symptoms or those who are intolerant of or unresponsive to antipsychotics.

When male patients display intrusive disinhibited sexual behavior, a particular problem in patients with frontal lobe dementias, medroxyprogesterone and related hormonal agents are sometimes recommended (197–199), but only case series support this recommendation at present.

Lithium carbonate has also been suggested because of its occasional utility for mentally retarded patients, but support for it is quite limited and side effects (including a considerable risk of delirium) are common (148).

Beta-blockers, notably propranolol, metoprolol, and pindolol, have also been reported to be helpful for some agitated patients with dementia (200). However, most of the patients included in the case reports had unusual illnesses. In addition, large doses (e.g., 200–300 mg/day of propranolol) were used, and such doses create a considerable risk of bradycardia, hypotension, and delirium for elderly patients.

4. Treatments for depression

a) Goals

Somatic treatments for depression in demented patients are used to improve mood, functional status, and quality of life. Even patients with depressed mood who do not meet the diagnostic criteria for major depression should be considered for treatment. This is in keeping with the subtypes of Alzheimer's disease and other dementias included in DSM-IV, which are diagnosed when a patient with dementia has a depressed mood *with* or *without* the full depressive syndrome. However, patients should be carefully evaluated for neurovegetative signs, suicidal ideation, and other indicators of major depression, since these may indicate a need for safety measures (e.g., hospitalization for suicidality) or more vigorous and aggressive therapies (such as higher medication doses, multiple medication trials, or ECT).

One goal of treating depression in dementia is to improve cognitive symptoms. Sometimes cognitive deficits partially or even fully resolve with successful treatment of the depression. Individuals whose cognitive symptoms recover fully with treatment of the depression are considered not to have been demented (this condition is sometimes referred to as "pseudodementia"); however, as many as one-half of such persons develop dementia within 5 years (2). Thus, caution is urged in ruling out an underlying early dementia in patients with both mood and cognitive impairment.

A related goal in the treatment of patients with dementia is diminishing apathy, which is common in Alzheimer's disease and many other dementing illnesses, especially those affecting the frontal lobes, and may occur even in the absence of depression. The treatments for apathy overlap those for depression, so they are reviewed here as well.

Before any treatment is instituted, patients should be evaluated for general medical problems (e.g., hypo- or hyperthyroidism, electrolyte imbalance), substance abuse, and medications (e.g., beta-blockers, corticosteroids, benzodiazepines) that may be causing or contributing to the depression. Correctable general medical problems should be addressed, and potentially offending medications should be discontinued (with appropriate substitutions as necessary).

b) Antidepressants

(1) Efficacy

The evidence for the efficacy of antidepressants for demented patients is limited. There have been five small placebo-controlled studies (192, 193, 201–203) and an additional two studies using a within-subject design (204, 205). These studies are limited by small number of subjects, mixed and poorly characterized dementia syndromes, mixed and poorly characterized depressive symptoms (defined variously by mood alone, by diagnosis, or by symptom severity threshold), lack of randomization, and the use of uncommon agents (including many not available in the United States). However, the available evidence suggests that depressive symptoms (including depressed mood alone and with neurovegetative changes) in dementia are responsive to antidepressant therapy. Cognitive symptoms beyond the impairment induced by the depression do not appear to respond to antidepressant treatment. Indeed, one imipramine trial suggested that antidepressant treatment might exert a *negative* effect on cognition, but this observation might have been due to the medication's anticholinergic properties (201).

Although the data from the best-designed trials concern unusual agents, they document that depression in patients with dementia is responsive to treatment. This, along with extensive clinical experience in using more-typical antidepressants for this population (206), suggests that the more substantial efficacy literature concerning pharmacologic treatment of depression may be cautiously applied to patients with dementia. The reader is referred to the *Practice Guideline for the Treatment of Patients With Major Depressive Disorder* (207; included in this volume) for a summary of this literature.

The literature concerning the treatment of apathy is much sparser. There is minimal evidence that dopaminergic agents, such as psychostimulants (*d*-amphetamine, methylphenidate), amantadine, bromocriptine, and bupropion, are helpful in the treatment of severe apathy, but promising case reports suggest that efficacy studies are warranted (208). Psychostimulants have also received some support for the treatment of depression in elderly individuals with severe general medical disorders (209–211).

(2) Side effects and toxicity

The reader is referred to the practice guideline on major depression (207, included in this volume) for a more detailed discussion of the side effects of antidepressant agents and to the forthcoming practice guideline on geriatric psychiatry for a discussion of the particular issues for the elderly. These effects, divided by medication class, are summarized briefly here.

SSRIs, including fluoxetine, paroxetine, and sertraline, tend to have a more favorable side effect profile than do cyclic agents. However, any SSRI can produce nausea and vomiting, agitation and akathisia, parkinsonian side effects, sexual dysfunction, and weight loss, although some of these effects are more common with one agent than another. In addition, physicians prescribing SSRIs should be aware of the many possible medication interactions.

The structurally unique agent bupropion is associated with a risk of seizures, especially at high doses. Venlafaxine is associated with elevations in blood pressure, which sometimes diminish over time.

Cyclic antidepressants generally have significant cardiovascular effects, including orthostatic hypotension and delays in cardiac conduction. Their effects on conduction make these agents dangerous in overdose, so they should be used only for patients who are adequately supervised to guard against accidental or purposeful overdose. Most cyclic antidepressants have anticholinergic properties to some degree, including blurred vision, tachycardia, dry mouth, urinary retention, constipation, sedation, impaired cognition, and delirium. These effects are most marked for amitriptyline and imipramine and least so for nortriptyline and desipramine, but there is considerable variation from patient to patient. Trazodone has minimal cardiac conduction or anticholinergic effects but is associated with postural hypotension, sedation, and a risk of priapism. Nefazodone is most commonly associated with sedation.

MAOIs, including tranylcypromine and phenelzine, can lead to postural hypotension, a particular concern with the elderly because of the risk of falls. In addition, they have complex medication interactions (sympathomimetic agents, narcotics, especially meperidine, and serotonergic agents must be avoided) and require dietary modifications (tyramine-containing foods, such as cheeses, preserved meat, and red wine, must be avoided), which may make them potentially dangerous for poorly supervised individuals with dementia.

Psychostimulants (*d*-amphetamine, methylphenidate) are associated with tachycardia, restlessness, agitation, sleep disturbances, and appetite suppression. Bromocriptine is associated with psychosis, confusion, and dyskinesias. Amantadine is sometimes associated with anticholinergic effects, including delirium.

(3) Implementation

There are no efficacy data on which to base the selection of one antidepressant over another. Thus, the choice of an antidepressant is generally based on the side effect profile and the general medical and psychiatric status of each patient. For example, if sedation is desired, trazodone or perhaps nortriptyline may be selected. If activation is desired, fluoxetine, bupropion, or desipramine may be selected. If the patient has urinary outflow obstruction, even agents with modest anticholinergic effects should be avoided. If the patient has a prolonged QT interval or A-V block, fascicular block, or significant coronary artery disease, cyclic antidepressants should be avoided if possible. These and other implementation issues are discussed in greater detail in the practice guidelines on depression and on geriatric psychiatry and are only briefly summarized here.

Many clinicians choose SSRIs as the initial treatment because of their better side effect profiles. Once-a-day dosing is appropriate. Fluoxetine should be started at 5–10 mg/day and increased at several-week intervals to a maximum of 40–60 mg/day. Paroxetine has the same dosing, but the dose can be increased every 1–2 weeks because of its shorter half-life. Sertraline may be started at 25 mg/day and increased at 1- to 2-week intervals up to a maximum dose of 150–200 mg/day.

Some clinicians favor bupropion. However, it appears to decrease the seizure threshold, so it should not be the first choice for individuals with a high risk of seizures. It is started at 37.5 mg b.i.d. and increased every 5 to 7 days as tolerated up to a maximum of 350–450 mg/day in divided doses. No more than 150 mg should be given within any 4-hour period because of the risk of seizures. Venlafaxine should be avoided for individuals with hypertension if good alternatives are available; if it is used, careful monitoring of blood pressure and adjustment of antihypertensive medication are required. It is started at 18.75–37.50 mg b.i.d. and may be increased at approximately weekly intervals up to a maximum dose of 300–375 mg/day. If elevations in blood pressure occur and do not diminish over time and venlafaxine is effective in treating depression in an individual who has not responded to trials of other agents, the medication may be continued and the hypertension may be treated.

Among the tricyclic and heterocyclic agents, theoretical reasoning and clinical experience suggest avoiding agents with prominent anticholinergic activity (e.g., amitriptyline, imipramine). Among the remaining agents, sample dosing strategies are given here for nortriptyline, desipramine, and trazodone. Nortriptyline may be started at 10–25 mg/day, with increases at 5- to 7-day intervals up to a maximum daily dose of 100–150 mg. Dosing is guided by clinical response and side effects. Blood levels, which should not exceed 100–150 ng/ml, may also be helpful. For desipramine, the starting dose is 25–50 mg/day, with increases at 5- to 7-day intervals up to a maximum daily dose of 200 mg. Blood levels should not exceed 150–250 ng/ml. For trazodone, the starting dose is 25–50 mg/day, with increases at 5- to 7-day intervals up to a maximum daily dose of 300–400 mg.

Because of their side effects and the extra monitoring required, MAOIs should be considered only for individuals who are unresponsive to or unable to take other agents. The MAOIs tranylcypromine and phenelzine may be used at starting doses of 10 mg/day and 15 mg/day, respectively, with monitoring of orthostatic blood pressure, and increased at weekly intervals to maximum doses of 40 and 60 mg/day (in divided doses), respectively. Patients and caregivers must be advised in detail about dietary and medication restrictions. They should also be educated about the symptoms of hypertensive crisis and advised to seek medical attention immediately if these symptoms arise. It is important to inform caregivers that dietary supervision is necessary, since demented patients are unlikely to remember dietary restrictions on their own.

Stimulants are sometimes used in the treatment of apathy or of depression in individuals with serious general medical illness. Dextroamphetamine and methylphenidate are started at 2.5–5.0 mg in the morning. They can be increased by 2.5 mg every 2 or 3 days to a maximum of 30–40 mg/day. As they are controlled substances, adequate steps to avoid abuse should be taken. Amantadine is sometimes used in the treatment of apathy as well. It may be started at 100 mg/day and increased to a maximum of 200 mg/day. Bromocriptine may be started at 1.25 mg b.i.d. and gradually increased; few patients tolerate more than 2.50 mg b.i.d.

Most patients with dementia will not tolerate the higher maxima given for antidepressant agents, but younger and less frail individuals may tolerate and respond to somewhat higher doses. When a rapid response is not critical, a still more gradual increase may increase the likelihood that a therapeutic dose will be tolerated.

c) Electroconvulsive therapy

There is no substantial literature on the efficacy of ECT in the treatment of depression in dementia. However, considerable clinical experience suggests that ECT may be beneficial for patients with severe major depression who are ineligible for, cannot tolerate, or do not respond to other agents (212). Dementia increases the likelihood of delirium and of memory loss following ECT, but these effects are generally of short duration: delirium tends to resolve within days and memory loss within weeks. Twice-weekly rather than thrice-weekly and unilateral rather than bilateral ECT may decrease the risk of cognitive side effects after ECT.

5. Treatments for sleep disturbance

a) Goals

Treatment of sleep disturbance in dementia is aimed at decreasing the frequency and severity of insomnia, interrupted sleep, and nocturnal confusion in patients with dementia. The goals are to increase patient comfort and to decrease the disruption to families and caregivers. Sleep disorder is common in dementia (213, 214) and is not always so disruptive that the risk of medication side effects is outweighed by the need for a pharmacologic trial. Thus, the psychiatrist assessing a patient for a sleep disorder should first consider whether treatment is needed and then whether appropriate sleep hygiene—including regular sleep and waking times, limited daytime sleeping, avoidance of fluid intake in the evening, calming bedtime rituals, and adequate daytime physical and mental activities (215)—has been tried. If the patient lives in a setting that can provide adequate supervision without undue disruption to others, permitting daytime sleep and nocturnal awakening may provide an alternative to pharmacologic intervention. Pharmacologic treatment should be instituted only after other measures have been unsuccessful. In addition, the clinician should consider whether the sleep disorder could be due to an underlying condition. It is particularly important to be aware of sleep apnea (216), which is relatively common in elderly individuals and contraindicates the use of benzodiazepines or other agents that suppress respiratory drive.

b) Efficacy

There are no available reports of studies that have assessed the efficacy of pharmacologic treatment for sleep disturbances specifically in individuals with dementia or that have compared pharmacologic to nonpharmacologic therapies. However, there are some data concerning use of various agents for mixed elderly populations. Reports of two small studies of chloral hydrate use with the elderly (217, 218) are available. Piccione et al. (217) found chloral hydrate to be better than placebo but not as good as triazolam in the short-term treatment of insomnia in elderly individuals. Linnoila et al. (218) found chloral hydrate to be superior to both tryptophan and placebo in the treatment of sleep disturbances in elderly psychiatric patients. Zolpidem was studied in 119 elderly psychiatric inpatients (219), of whom 50% suffered from dementia. In a double-blind, randomized parallel group clinical trial, zolpidem was superior to placebo on multiple sleep outcomes. A dose of 10 mg appeared to be superior to 20 mg: it was equally effective in promoting sleep and lacked the daytime sleepiness and ataxia sometimes observed at the higher dose. The impact of benzodiazepines and antipsychotics on sleep has not been studied systematically in demented elderly patients. Clinical experience suggests that low-dose antipsychotics (e.g., haloperidol, 0.5–1.0 mg) can be helpful in managing sleep problems in patients with dementia. Clinical experience with benzodiazepines is less favorable, although short- to medium-acting agents at low to moderate doses (e.g., lorazepam, 0.5–1.0 mg; oxazepam, 7.5–15.0 mg) are sometimes helpful for short-term disturbances (e.g., after a change in caregivers).

In addition to pharmacologic agents, there is preliminary evidence from three small open trials for elderly subjects with dementia (220–222) that early morning or evening bright light therapy may improve sleep (and possibly behavior as well). Others have reported preliminary evidence that the hormone melatonin may also be beneficial in the treatment of sleep disturbances in elderly individuals (223, 224), but the agent has not yet been subjected to controlled trials with demented individuals. In addition, it should be noted that such agents lack the quality controls of pharmaceutical agents.

c) Implementation

Given the sparse efficacy data, the choice of pharmacologic agents is generally guided by the presence of other symptoms. For instance, if the patient has psychotic symptoms and sleep disturbance, antipsychotics will generally be given at bedtime, and a relatively sedating antipsychotic (e.g., thioridazine, mesoridazine) may be chosen if not otherwise contraindicated. If the patient is depressed and has a sleep disturbance, an antidepressant with sedative properties (e.g., trazodone, nortriptyline) will be given at bedtime. When anxiety is prominent, a benzodiazepine (e.g., lorazepam) may be selected.

When sleep disturbances occur without other psychiatric symptoms beyond the dementia itself, there is little to guide the choice among agents. Some clinicians prefer trazodone at 25–100 mg h.s. for sleep disturbances. Some prefer zolpidem, 5–10 mg h.s. Benzodiazepines (e.g., lorazepam, 0.5–1.0 mg; oxazepam, 7.5–15.0 mg) and chloral hydrate (250–500 mg) may be used but are generally not recommended for other than short-term sleep problems because of the possibility of tolerance, daytime sleepiness, rebound insomnia, worsening cognition, disinhibition, and even delirium. Triazolam in particular is not recommended for individuals with dementia because of its association with amnesia. Diphenhydramine, which is found in most over-the-counter sleep preparations, is used by some clinicians, but its anticholinergic properties make it suboptimal for the treatment of demented patients.

IV. DEVELOPMENT OF A TREATMENT PLAN

When choosing specific treatments for a demented patient, one begins from the assessment of symptoms. A multimodal approach is often used, combining, for instance, a behavioral and a psychopharmacologic intervention as available and appropriate. When multiple agents or approaches are being used and problems persist (or new problems develop), it is advisable, if possible, to make one change at a time so that the effect of each change can be assessed; this is particularly critical when unusual treatments are being tried. Whatever interventions are implemented, their continuing utility must be periodically reevaluated.

The treatment of dementia varies through the course of the illness, as symptoms evolve over time. Although many symptoms can and do occur throughout the illness, certain symptoms are typical of the various stages, as outlined in Section II.E. At each stage of the illness, the psychiatrist should be vigilant for cognitive and noncognitive symptoms likely to be present and should help the patient and family anticipate future symptoms. The family may also benefit from a reminder to plan for the care likely to be necessary at later stages.

A. MILDLY IMPAIRED PATIENTS

At the early stages of a dementing illness, patients and their families are often dealing with recognition of the illness and associated limitations, and they may appreciate suggestions for how to cope with these limitations (e.g., making lists, using a calendar). It may be helpful to identify specific impairments and highlight remaining abilities. Families and patients may also suffer from a sense of loss and from a perceived stigma associated with the illness. Mildly impaired patients should also be advised about the risk of driving. Although there is no consensus on this issue, a review of the data coupled with a concern for the safety of the patient and others suggest that patients with mild impairment should be urged to stop driving or to limit their driving to familiar routes and less challenging situations (e.g., good road conditions, low speeds, spouse or other navigator in the car). At this stage of the illness, the patient should also be advised to draw up a power of attorney for medical and financial decision making, an advance directive, and/or a living will. Patients may also wish to revise their wills and to make the necessary financial arrangements to plan for long-term care. Caregivers should be made aware of the availability of support groups and social agencies.

Patients with Alzheimer's disease seen in the early stages may be offered a trial of tacrine or donepezil for cognitive impairment. Although available data are limited to moderately impaired patients, it is possible that vitamin E might also delay progression of Alzheimer's disease in patients with mild impairment. Thus, physicians might consider vitamin E alone or possibly in combination with a cholinesterase inhibitor at this stage. Selegiline, which also delayed progression in moderately impaired patients, might also be considered, although vitamin E may be preferable because of its more favorable side effect profile and lack of drug interactions. Mildly impaired patients might also be interested in referrals to local research centers for participation in clinical trials of experimental agents for the treatment of Alzheimer's disease. Additional information regarding such trials may be obtained from the local or national chapter of the Alzheimer's Association or from the National Institute on Aging.

Mildly impaired patients also deserve a careful evaluation for depressed mood or major depression, which suggests the need for pharmacologic intervention, as reviewed in Section III.D.4.b. Patients with moderate to severe major depression who do not respond to or cannot tolerate antidepressant medications should be considered for ECT. Particularly—but not only—if they are depressed, mildly impaired patients should also be carefully assessed for suicidality.

B. MODERATELY IMPAIRED PATIENTS

As patients become more impaired, they are likely to require more supervision to remain safe. Families should be advised regarding the possibility of accidents due to forgetfulness (e.g., fires while cooking), of difficulties coping with household emergencies, and of the possibility of wandering. Family members should be advised to determine whether the patient is handling finances appropriately and to consider taking over the paying of bills and other responsibilities. At this stage of the disease, patients should be strongly urged not to drive, and families should be urged to undertake measures (such as taking away the car keys) to prevent patients from driving.

As patients' dependency increases, caregivers may begin to feel more burdened. A referral for some form of respite care (e.g., home health aid, day care, or brief nursing home stay) may be helpful. At this stage, families should begin to consider and plan for additional support at home or possible transfer to a long-term care facility.

Treatment for cognitive symptoms should also be considered at this stage. For patients with Alzheimer's disease, currently available data suggest that a trial of tacrine or donepezil is the intervention most likely to lead to improvement in cognitive function. In addition, vitamin E or selegiline, which have been shown to delay progression in Alzheimer's disease patients with moderate impairment, may be offered to patients at this stage. Vitamin E appears preferable because of its low toxicity and lack of drug interactions. It may be appropriate to offer vitamin E in combination with a cholinesterase inhibitor.

Delusions and hallucinations often develop in moderately impaired patients. The patient and family may be troubled and fearful about these symptoms, and it may be helpful to reassure them that the symptoms are part of the illness and are often treatable. If these symptoms cause no distress to the patient and are unaccompanied by agitation or combativeness, they are probably best treated with reassurance and distraction. If they do cause distress or are associated with behavior that may place the patient or others at risk, they should be treated with low doses of antipsychotic medications. If a patient is agitated or combative in the absence of psychosis, treatment with an antipsychotic medication has the most support in the literature, but carbamazepine, valproate, trazodone, buspirone, or possibly an SSRI may be used in a careful therapeutic trial. If behavioral symptoms are time limited, a benzodiazepine may also prove useful. Depression often remains part of the picture at this stage and should be treated vigorously.

C. SEVERELY AND PROFOUNDLY IMPAIRED PATIENTS

At this stage of the illness, patients are severely incapacitated and are almost completely dependent on others for help with basic functions, such as dressing, bathing, and feeding. Families are often struggling with a combined sense of burden and loss and may benefit from a frank exploration of these feelings and any associated resentment or feelings of guilt. They may also need encouragement to get additional help at home or to consider nursing home placement.

There are no data available to guide decisions about the use of cognition-enhancing medications for the severely impaired: use of these medications may be continued, or a medication-free trial may be used to assess whether the medication is still providing a benefit.

Similarly, there are no data available about whether vitamin E or selegiline retards the progression at this stage, and, for patients who reach this stage of illness already taking one of these agents, even a medication-free interval may not clarify the picture, since the expected benefit is slower progression rather than frank improvement.

Depression is somewhat less likely to be present at this stage but should be treated vigorously if it is. Psychotic symptoms and agitation are often present and should be treated pharmacologically if they cause distress to the patient or significant danger or disruption to caregivers.

At this stage, it is important to ensure adequate nursing care, including measures to prevent bedsores and contractures. The psychiatrist should help the family prepare for the patient's death. Ideally, discussions about feeding tube placement, treatment of infection, and cardiopulmonary resuscitation and intubation will have taken place when the patient could also participate, but in any case it is important to raise these issues with the family before a decision about one of these options becomes urgent.

Hospice care is an underused resource for patients with end-stage dementia (225). It provides physical support for the patient (with an emphasis on attentive nursing care rather than medical intervention) and emotional support for the family during the last months of life. In most settings, a physician must certify that the patient is within 6 months of death; the use of a formal rating scale (226) may help in this determination.

V. FACTORS MODIFYING TREATMENT DECISIONS

A. COMORBID CONDITIONS

1. General medical conditions

The likelihood of chronic general medical illnesses and the likelihood of dementia both increase with age, so the two commonly coexist. The assessment and treatment of general medical comorbidity are complicated by memory impairment and aphasia, both of which interfere with the patient's ability to provide a reliable description of symptoms. Resistance to physical examination, laboratory testing, and radiologic procedures can also complicate assessment. The involvement of family members and other caregivers in gathering a history and completing an evaluation is essential.

2. Delirium

Dementia predisposes to the development of delirium (227, 228), especially in the presence of general medical and neurological illnesses. In addition, medications needed to treat comorbid general medical disorders can lead to further cognitive impairment or to delirium, even when doses are appropriate and blood levels are in the nontoxic range. Compounds with anticholinergic effects (e.g., tricyclic antidepressants, low-potency antipsychotics, diphenhydramine, disopyramide phosphate) or histamine-2 activity (cimetidine, ranitidine) are particularly likely to cause delirium, but many classes of medications can do so (229). Of particular relevance to psychiatrists, delirium has been associated with virtually all psychotropic medications, including lithium, other mood stabilizers, tricyclic antidepressants, SSRIs, and benzodiazepines. Avoidance of unnecessary medications, use of the lowest effective dose, vigilant monitoring aimed at early recognition, a thorough search for causes, and prompt treatment may diminish the prevalence and morbidity of delirium.

3. Parkinson's disease

Cognitive impairment coexisting with Parkinson's disease requires a broad treatment approach. First, mild cognitive impairment may be partially ameliorated by dopaminergic agents prescribed for the treatment of motor symptoms, so both cognitive and motor symptoms should be carefully monitored, especially after any intervention. Second, the use of dopaminergic agents predisposes to the development of visual hallucinations and other psychotic phenomena, especially in patients with coexisting dementia, so these agents must be used with particular care, and the minimal dose needed to control the motor symptoms should be used. In addition, these patients, like other elderly and demented patients, are vulnerable to delirium due to medications and concomitant general medical conditions, so the development of these symptoms deserves a thorough evaluation. Third, if psychotic symptoms result in distress or dangerousness, the judicious use of an antipsychotic agent is indicated. Some clinicians prefer the use of low-potency antipsychotic agents (e.g., thioridazine). Others now favor clozapine, but it has received limited study (157). Fourth, the patient must be carefully assessed and treated for depression, which is common in Parkinson's disease and may exacerbate or even be misinterpreted as dementia.

4. Stroke

For patients with dementia and a history of stroke, whether or not the strokes are responsible for or contribute to the dementia, it is critical to conduct a careful evaluation to determine the etiology of the strokes (e.g., atrial fibrillation, valvular disease) and to make any needed referrals for further evaluation and treatment. Beyond this, good control of blood pressure, and perhaps low-dose aspirin, may help to prevent further strokes. In addition, a trial of Hydergine, which appears to be possibly effective in dementia due to vascular disease, may be appropriate. Some clinicians favor pentoxifylline, alleged to improve cognition after stroke by increasing cerebral blood flow (230–232), but this treatment has limited support.

B. SITE-SPECIFIC ISSUES

The care of patients with dementia should be adapted not only to the patient's symptoms and associated general medical problems but also to his or her environment. Certain issues arise frequently in particular care settings.

1. Home

Of the 3–4.5 million Americans with dementia in the United States, only about 1 million reside in nursing homes, leaving over 2 million individuals with dementia who reside at home (233). Psychosocial problems include the need for family care providers to work at jobs outside the home during the day and the adverse emotional impact on caregivers and children or grandchildren. Particularly difficult behavior problems for patients with dementia living at home include poor sleep, wandering, accusations directed toward caregivers, threatening or combative behavior, and reluctance to accept help; all of these are potentially solvable. Interventions with the family that focus on the specific behavior problem and, where appropriate, carefully monitored pharmacologic treatment of behavioral symptoms can be helpful. In addition, the use of home health aides, day care, and respite care may provide stimulation for patients and needed relief for caregivers. The psychological stress on families from Alzheimer's disease appears to be more complex than simply the burden of caring for a disabled family member (234). It has been estimated that 30% of spousal caregivers experience a depressive disorder while providing care for a husband or wife with Alzheimer's disease (235). The prevalence of depressive disorders among adult children caring for a parent with Alzheimer's disease ranges from 22% among those with no prior history of affective disorder to 37% among those with a prior history of depression (235).

2. Day care

Ideally, day care provides a protected environment and appropriate stimulation to patients during the day and gives caregivers a needed break to attend to other responsibilities. Some centers specialize in the care of individuals with dementia and may thus offer more appropriate activities and supervision. Anecdotal reports and practice support the benefit to patients of scheduled activities. However, behavioral symptoms can be precipitated by overstimulation as well as understimulation, so activities must be selected with care and participation should be adjusted according to each patient's response. Of note, problems can arise when patients with different levels of severity are expected to participate together in the same activities.

3. Long-term care

A high proportion of patients with dementia eventually require placement in nursing homes or other long-term care facilities (e.g., assisted living, group home) because of the progression of the illness, the emergence of behavioral problems, the development of intercurrent illness, or the loss of social support. Approximately two-thirds of the residents of long-term care facilities suffer from dementia (233, 236), and as many as 90% of them have behavioral symptoms. Thus, these facilities should be tailored to meet the needs of patients with dementia and to adequately address behavioral symptoms (88, 237).

Research data on the optimum care of individuals with dementia in nursing homes are sparse. One important element is staff who are committed to working with demented patients and knowledgeable about dementia and the management of its noncognitive symptoms. Structured activity programs can improve both behavior and mood (88). Other factors valued in nursing homes include privacy, adequate stimulation, maximization of autonomy, and adaptation to change with the progression of the disease (see references 238, 239). Use of design features such as particular colors for walls, doors, and door frames is widely touted but lacks scientific support.

In recent years special care units have been specifically developed for persons with Alzheimer's disease or other dementing disorders. There are few data to demonstrate that these units are more effective than traditional nursing home units (237), and clinical experience suggests that they vary a great deal in quality. However, the better ones may offer a model for the optimal care of demented patients in any nursing home setting.

A particular concern regarding nursing homes is the use of physical restraints and antipsychotic medications. The Omnibus Budget Reconciliation Act of 1987 (OBRA) regulates the use of physical restraints and many psychotropic medications in nursing homes. Psychiatrists practicing in nursing homes must be familiar with these regulations, which can generally be obtained from the nursing home administrator, local public library, or regional office of the Health Care Financing Administration.

Antipsychotic medications are used in nursing homes, as elsewhere, for the treatment of behavioral and psychotic symptoms. When used appropriately, these medications can be effective in reducing patient distress and increasing safety for the demented patient, other residents, and staff. Overuse, on the other hand, can lead to worsening cognition, oversedation, falls, and numerous other complications and can place patients at risk of tardive dyskinesia. Thus, the OBRA regulations and good clinical practice require careful documentation of the indications for antipsychotic medication treatment and available alternatives and outcomes. In the context of these regulations, a clinical strategy of carefully considering which patients may be appropriate for withdrawal of antipsychotic medications and being prepared to maintain use of the medications in some cases and reinstate them in others, as deemed clinically necessary, may be optimal (240). Of note, a structured education program for nursing and medical staff has been shown to decrease antipsychotic usage in the nursing home setting without adverse outcomes (240). Ongoing use of antipsychotic medication requires regular reassessment of medication response, monitoring for adverse effects, and thorough documentation. Tardive dyskinesia, for which older age, female gender, and brain injury are risk factors, deserves particular attention.

Physical restraints (e.g., Posey restraints, geri-chairs) are sometimes used to treat agitation or combativeness that puts the patient, other residents, or staff at risk. Use of restraints is fairly common in nursing homes (241). However, regulations and humane care support keeping the use of restraints to a minimum, and there is even a suggestion that restraints may increase the risk of falls and contribute to cognitive decline (242, 243).

Although few studies are available to guide the appropriate use of restraints in nursing homes, clinical experience suggests that restraint use can be decreased by environmental changes that reduce the risk of falls or wandering and by careful assessment and treatment of possible causes of agitation. Chest or wrist restraints are appropriately used during a wait for more-definitive treatment for patients who pose an imminent risk of physical harm to themselves or others (e.g., during evaluation of a delirium or during an acute-care hospitalization for an intercurrent illness). For long-term care facilities, geri-chairs may have a place in the care of patients at extreme risk of falling. In any case, regular use of restraints is not recommended unless alternatives have been exhausted. When they are used, they require periodic reassessment and careful documentation.

Documentation of the need for temporary use of restraints should discuss the other measures that were tried and failed to bring the behavior under control. Such measures include a) routine assessment to identify risk factors for falls that would, if addressed, obviate the need for restraints; b) bed and chair monitors that alert nursing staff when patients may be climbing out of bed or leaving a chair; and c) prompted voiding schedules through the day and night in order to decrease the urge for unsupervised trips to the bathroom.

4. Inpatient general medical or surgical services

Patients with dementia on general medical and surgical services are at particular risk for three problems, all of which can lead to aggressive behavior, wandering, climbing over bed rails, removal of intravenous lines, and resistance to needed medical procedures. First, cognitive impairment makes demented individuals vulnerable to behavioral problems owing to fear, lack of comprehension, and lack of memory of what they have been told. No data are available to guide treatment recommendations, but general practice supports having family members or aides stay with the patient as one preventive approach. Frequent reorientation and explanation of hospital procedures and plans, adequate light, and avoidance of overstimulation may also be useful. Second, persons with dementia are at high risk for delirium (227, 228). Prevention of delirium by judicious use of any necessary medications and elimination of any unnecessary ones, attention to fluid and electrolyte status, and prompt treatment of infectious diseases can also diminish morbidity. Occasionally, psychopharmacologic treatment, generally with a high-potency antipsychotic such as haloperidol, is necessary. Third, patients with dementia may have difficulty understanding and communicating pain, hunger, and other troublesome states. For this reason, the development of irritability and/or agitation should prompt a thorough evaluation to identify an occult medical problem or a possible source of discomfort. A significant part of the psychiatrist's role in this setting is educating other physicians and hospital staff regarding the diagnosis and management of dementia and its behavioral manifestations.

5. General psychiatric inpatient units

Individuals with dementia may be admitted to psychiatric units for the treatment of psychotic, affective, or behavioral symptoms. For patients who are very frail or who have significant general medical illnesses, a geriatric psychiatry or medical psychiatric unit may be helpful when available. Indications for hospitalization include those based on severity of illness (e.g., threats of harm to self or others, violent or uncontrollable behavior) and those based on the intensity of services (e.g., need for continuous skilled observation, need for ECT or a medication or test that cannot be performed on an outpatient basis) (10, 11).

A thorough search for psychosocial, general medical, or noncognitive psychiatric difficulties that may be leading to the disturbance will often reveal a treatable problem. If it is reasonably safe, patients should be encouraged to walk freely. Both nonpharmacologic and pharmacologic interventions can be tried more readily and aggressively on inpatient units than in outpatient settings.

C. DEMOGRAPHIC AND SOCIAL FACTORS

1. Age

Because most dementias occur in the elderly, age is the major psychosocial factor affecting treatment. Individuals with dementia occurring in middle age (e.g., early-onset Alzheimer's disease) are likely to have particular difficulty coping with the diagnosis and its impact on their lives. In addition, they may require assistance with problems not generally seen with older patients, such as relinquishing work responsibilities (particularly if their jobs are such that their dementia may put others at risk), obtaining disability benefits, and arranging care for minor children. On the other hand, extremely old patients may be frail and have multiple other general medical problems that lead to more difficult diagnosis and treatment and much greater disability for a given level of dementia.

2. Gender

Another critical area affecting treatment is gender. Dementia, particularly Alzheimer's disease, is more common in women, partly because of greater longevity but possibly also because of other risk factors not yet identified. In addition, because of their greater life expectancy (and tendency to marry men older than themselves), women with dementia are more likely to have an adult child rather than a spouse as caregiver. Unlike an elderly spouse caregiver, who is more likely to be retired, adult child caregivers (most often daughters or daughters-in-law) are more likely to have jobs outside the home and/or to be raising children. These additional responsibilities of caregivers may contribute to earlier institutionalization for elderly women with dementia.

3. Other demographic factors

Perhaps the most critical demographic factor affecting the care of patients with dementia is social support. The availability of a spouse, adult child, or other loved one with the physical and emotional ability to supervise and care for the patient and communicate with treating physicians is critical in both the quality of life and need for institutionalization. In addition, a network of friends, neighbors, and community may play a key role in supporting the patient and primary caregivers.

Another factor is resource availability, which varies widely by geographic region and socioeconomic status. These issues need to be considered for all treatment decisions, but they have a particular impact on decisions about long-term care. A referral to the local chapter of the Alzheimer's Association or a social worker or other individual knowledgeable about local resources, treatment centers, and Medicaid laws can be important in helping families find local treatment options that fit their needs and their budget.

Ethnic background also has an impact on caregiving style, symptom presentation, and acceptance of behavioral disorder. This needs to be taken into account in assessment and treatment planning.

4. Family history

When there are other cases of Alzheimer's disease in the family of a patient with the disease, families may be particularly concerned about the risk to other family members. Such concern is warranted, as first-degree relatives of Alzheimer's disease patients have a risk for the disease that is two to four times that for the general population, and four genes associated with Alzheimer's disease have been identified (see Section III.B.7). Families with multiple cases of early-onset (before age 60 or 65) Alzheimer's disease may carry one of the known genes on chromosome 21, 14, or 1 (39–41). Even so, there are currently no associated genetic tests for the disease because it is not possible to screen for the specific mutations, which are often found in only a single family. However, it may be appropriate to refer such families to genetic counselors to help family members further characterize their risk and ensure that they receive up-to-date information on genetic testing and related issues. Late-onset Alzheimer's disease can also run in families, but the only identified gene associated with this pattern is *APOE4*, which also confers increased risk in early-onset and nonfamilial disease (42–44). Because *APOE4* is not found in many demented individuals and is found in many nondemented elderly individuals, it too is not considered appropriate for predictive testing for the illness (17, 18). However, information on the genetics of both early- and late-onset Alzheimer's disease is evolving rapidly, so it may be appropriate to refer interested families to a local academic medical center or to the national information number (1-800-621-0379) of the Alzheimer's Association for up-to-date information.

VI. RESEARCH DIRECTIONS

A review of currently available treatments suggests a number of areas for further study. Several of these are in the realm of evaluation and assessment. The first is better detection and evaluation of dementia, especially in the prodromal and early stages, when treatment that slows progression would be more likely to be beneficial. Another is earlier and more accurate detection of noncognitive problems, so as to facilitate optimal intervention. The next is better assessment of dangerous symptoms, especially impaired driving ability. The last is the development of a consensus on clinically meaningful outcome measures, including neuropsychological testing, functional assessment, and "hard" end points, such as institutionalization and mortality.

In the realm of pharmacologic treatments, there is a critical need for medications with greater ability to improve cognition or at least halt the progression of dementia. Promising leads being actively studied for patients with Alzheimer's disease include additional cholinergic agents, further work on vitamin E (especially for mildly impaired patients) and other antioxidants, NSAIDs, and estrogen supplementation. In addition, medication development needs to go beyond these areas to identify and test new cognition-enhancing medications based on the pathophysiological picture of dementia emerging from neuroscience and molecular genetics. For example, pharmacologic agents that prevent or slow down amyloid deposition or remove precipitated amyloid might function as preventive or reversing therapies for Alzheimer's disease. As the understanding of other dementing disorders advances, targeted therapies must be developed and tested for these illnesses as well. Efforts to prevent stroke and to decrease its destructive effect on brain tissue are particularly important avenues for dementia prevention.

Another arena is the optimal pharmacologic treatment of noncognitive symptoms, including psychosis, agitation, depression, and sleep disturbance. Many current recommendations are extrapolated from small uncontrolled studies of agents no longer in common use and/or at doses well above those used in current practice. There is a critical need for randomized, controlled studies of up-to-date treatments for psychosis, agitation, depression, and sleep disturbance in dementia.

Further research into nonpharmacologic interventions, such as behavioral and environmental modification, is also needed. One aspect of dementia care that deserves further study is the rehabilitation model, which focuses on identifying and maximizing remaining abilities as a way to maximize function. Further research into this and other strategies may help to identify specific aspects of these therapies that benefit persons with dementia or specific types of dementia. Similarly, research is needed to better characterize the aspects of nursing homes and other environments most likely to improve patient outcomes.

In the health services arena, managed care organizations are beginning to enroll large numbers of elderly individuals. It will be critical to study the impact of this major shift in payment for health services on the care of individuals with dementia so that any needed changes in policy can be made in a timely fashion.

Research is also needed to identify which patients will benefit from alternative forms of living environments and supplemental caregiving. The identification of sites that are more comfortable, less costly, and equally safe and effective for the care of individuals with moderate to severe dementia would have enormous benefits for patients, their families, and society.

VII. INDIVIDUALS AND ORGANIZATIONS THAT SUBMITTED COMMENTS

Marilyn Albert, Ph.D.
Leonard Berg, M.D.
Charles H. Blackington, M.D., P.A.
Dan G. Blazer, M.D., Ph.D.
Carlos A. Cabán, M.D.
Jeffrey L. Cummings, M.D.
Kenneth L. Davis, M.D.
D.P. Devanand, M.D.
Leah Dickstein, M.D.
George Dyck, M.D.
David V. Espino, M.D.
Laura Fochtmann, M.D.
William E. Falk, M.D.
Sanford Finkel, M.D.
Lois T. Flaherty, M.D.
Dolores Gallagher-Thompson, Ph.D.
Larry S. Goldman, M.D.
Marion Z. Goldstein, M.D.
Kevin Gray, M.D.
Sheila Hafter Gray, M.D.
William M. Greenberg, M.D.
George Grossberg, M.D.
Edward Hanin, M.D.
Hugh C. Hendrie, M.D.
Claudia Kawas, M.D.
Lawrence Y. Kline, M.D.
Ronald R. Koegler, M.D.
Rosalie J. Landy
Constantine G. Lyketsos, M.D., M.H.S.
Ronald L. Martin, M.D.
Richard Mayeux, M.D.
James R. McCarthy, M.D.
Jerome A. Motto, M.D.
Douglas E. Moul, M.D., M.P.H.
Germaine Odenheimer, M.D.
Roger Peele, M.D.
Elaine R. Peskind, M.D.
Charles Portney, M.D.
Sadie Robertson
Robert Roca, M.D.
Pedro Ruiz, M.D.
Steven C. Samuels, M.D.

Mary Sano, Ph.D.
Paul M. Schyve, M.D.
Nada Stotland, M.D.
Alan Stoudemire, M.D.
Pierre Tariot, M.D.
William R. Tatomer, M.D.
Joseph A. Troncale, M.D.
Lawrence Tune, M.D.
George Warren, M.D.
Myron F. Weiner, M.D.
Donald Wexler, M.D.
Rhonda Whitson, R.R.A.

American Academy of Family Physicians
American Academy of Neurology
American Association of General Hospital Psychiatrists
American Association for Geriatric Psychiatry
American Medical Association
American Psychoanalytic Association
American Society for Adolescent Psychiatry
Joint Commission on Accreditation of Healthcare Organizations
National Institute of Mental Health
Royal Australian and New Zealand College of Psychiatrists

VIII. REFERENCES

The following coding system is used to indicate the nature of the supporting evidence in the summary recommendations and references:

[A] *Randomized clinical trial.* A study of an intervention in which subjects are prospectively followed over time; there are treatment and control groups; subjects are randomly assigned to the two groups; both the subjects and the investigators are blind to the assignments.

[B] *Clinical trial.* A prospective study in which an intervention is made and the results of that intervention are tracked longitudinally; study does not meet standards for a randomized clinical trial.

[C] *Cohort or longitudinal study.* A study in which subjects are prospectively followed over time without any specific intervention.

[D] *Case-control study.* A study in which a group of patients and a group of control subjects are identified in the present and information about them is pursued retrospectively or backward in time.

[E] *Review with secondary data analysis.* A structured analytic review of existing data (e.g., a meta-analysis or a decision analysis).

[F] *Review.* A qualitative review and discussion of previously published literature without a quantitative synthesis of the data.

[G] *Other.* Textbooks, expert opinion, case reports, and other reports not included above.

1. American Psychiatric Association: Diagnostic and Statistical Manual of Mental Disorders, 4th ed (DSM-IV). Washington, DC, APA, 1994 [G]
2. Alexopoulos G, Meyers BS, Young RC, Mattis S, Kakuma T: The course of geriatric depression with "reversible dementia": a controlled study. Am J Psychiatry 1993; 150:1693–1699 [C]
3. Shergill S, Mullan E, D'Ath P, Katona C: What is the clinical prevalence of Lewy body dementia? Int J Geriatr Psychiatry 1994; 9:907–912 [G]

4. Reisberg B, Ferris SH, de Leon MJ, Crook T: The Global Deterioration Scale for assessment of primary degenerative dementia. Am J Psychiatry 1982; 139:1136–1139 [G]
5. Hughes CP, Berg L, Danziger WL, Coben LA, Martin RL: A new clinical scale for the staging of dementia. Br J Psychiatry 1982; 140:566–572 [G]
6. Hebert LE, Scherr PA, Beckett LA, Albert MS, Pilgrim DM, Chown MJ, Funkenstein HH, Evans DA: Age-specific incidence of Alzheimer's disease in a community population. JAMA 1995; 273:1354–1359 [C]
7. Snowdon DA, Greiner LH, Mortimer JA, Riley KP, Greiner PA, Markesbery WR: Brain infarction and the clinical expression of Alzheimer disease. JAMA 1997; 277:813–817 [C]
8. Tatemichi TK, Paik M, Bagiella E, Desmond DW, Stern Y, Sano M, Hauser WA, Mayeux R: Risk of dementia after stroke in a hospitalized cohort: results of a longitudinal study. Neurology 1994; 44:1885–1891 [C]
9. McKeith IG, Fairbairn AF, Perry RH, Thompson P: The clinical diagnosis and misdiagnosis of senile dementia of Lewy body type (SDLT). Br J Psychiatry 1994; 165:324–332 [G]
10. Rabins P, Nicholson M: Acute psychiatric hospitalization for patients with irreversible dementia. Int J Geriatr Psychiatry 1991; 6:209–211 [G]
11. Zubenko GS, Rosen J, Sweet RA, Mulsant BH, Rifai AH: Impact of psychiatric hospitalization on behavioral complications of Alzheimer's disease. Am J Psychiatry 1992; 149:1484–1491 [B]
12. NIH Consensus Development Panel on the Differential Diagnosis of Dementing Diseases: Differential diagnosis of dementing diseases. JAMA 1987; 258:3411–3416 [G]
13. Okagaki JF, Alter M, Byrne TN, Daube JR, Franklin G, Frishberg BM, Goldstein ML, Greenberg MK, Lanska DJ, Mishra S, Odenheimer GL, Paulson G, Pearl RA, Rosenberg JH, Sila C, Stevens JC: Practice parameter for diagnosis and evaluation of dementia. Neurology 1994; 44:2203–2206 [G]
14. Recognition and Initial Assessment of Alzheimer's Disease and Related Dementias: Clinical Practice Guideline, vol 19. Washington, DC, US Department of Health and Human Services, Agency for Health Care Policy and Research, 1996 [G]
15. American Psychiatric Association: Practice Guideline for Psychiatric Evaluation of Adults. Am J Psychiatry 1995; 152(Nov suppl):63–80 [G]
16. Folstein MF, Folstein SE, McHugh PR: "Mini-Mental State": a practical method for grading the cognitive state of patients for the clinician. J Psychiatr Res 1975; 12:189–198 [G]
17. American College of Medical Genetics/American Society of Human Genetics Working Group on ApoE and Alzheimer's Disease: Statement on use of apolipoprotein E testing for Alzheimer's disease. JAMA 1995; 274:1627–1629 [G]
18. National Institute on Aging/Alzheimer's Association Working Group: Apolipoprotein E genotyping in Alzheimer's disease. Lancet 1996; 347:1091–1095 [G]
19. Hussian RA, Brown DC: Use of two-dimensional grid patterns to limit hazardous ambulation in demented patients. J Gerontol 1987; 42:558–560 [B]
20. Namazi KH, Rosner TT, Calkins MP: Visual barriers to prevent ambulatory Alzheimer's patients from exiting through an emergency door. Gerontologist 1989; 29:699–702 [B]
21. Mayer R, Darby SJ: Does a mirror deter wandering in demented older people? Int J Geriatr Psychiatry 1991; 6:607–609 [B]
22. Hunt L, Morris JC, Edwards D, Wilson BA: Driving performance in persons with mild senile dementia of the Alzheimer type. J Am Geriatr Soc 1993; 41:747–753 [B]
23. Friedland RP, Koss E, Kumar A, Gaine S, Metzler D, Haxby J, Moore A: Motor vehicle crashes in dementia of the Alzheimer type. Ann Neurol 1988; 24:782–786 [C]
24. Dubinsky RM, Williamson A, Gray CS, Glatt SL: Driving in Alzheimer's disease. J Am Geriatr Soc 1992; 40:1112–1116 [G]
25. Drachman DA, Swearer JM: Driving and Alzheimer's disease: the risk of crashes. Neurology 1993; 43:2448–2456 [D]

26. Fitten LJ, Perryman KM, Wilkinson CJ, Little RJ, Burns MM, Pachana N, Mervis JR, Malmgren R, Siembieda DW, Ganzell S: Alzheimer and vascular dementias and driving: a prospective road and laboratory study. JAMA 1995; 273:1360–1365 [C]
27. Tuokko H, Tallman K, Beatti BL, Cooper P, Weir J: An examination of driving records in a dementia clinic. J Gerontol 1995; 50:S173–S181 [G]
28. Trobe JD, Waller PF, Cook-Flannagan CA, Teshima SM, Bieliauskas LA: Crashes and violations among drivers with Alzheimer disease. Arch Neurol 1996; 53:411–416 [D]
29. Lucas-Blaustein MJ, Filipp L, Dungan C, Tune L: Driving in patients with dementia. J Am Geriatr Soc 1988; 36:1087–1091 [G]
30. Gilley DW, Wilson RS, Bennett DA, Stebbins GT, Bernard BA, Whalen ME, Fox JH: Cessation of driving and unsafe motor vehicle operation by dementia patients. Arch Intern Med 1991; 151:941–946 [G]
31. Carr D, Jackson T, Alquire P: Characteristics of an elderly driving population referred to a geriatric assessment center. J Am Geriatr Soc 1990; 38:1145–1150 [D]
32. O'Neill D, Neubauer K, Boyle M, Gerrard J, Surmon D, Wilcock GK: Dementia and driving. J R Soc Med 1992; 85:199–202 [G]
33. Odenheimer GL, Beaudet M, Jette AM, Albert MS, Grande L, Minaker KL: Performance-based driving evaluation of the elderly driver: safety, reliability, and validity. J Gerontol 1994; 49(4):M153–M159 [G]
34. Adler G, Rottunda SJ, Dysken MW: The driver with dementia: a review of the literature. Am J Geriatr Psychiatry 1996; 4:110–120 [F]
35. Shua-Haim JR, Gross JS: The co-pilot driver syndrome. J Am Geriatr Soc 1996; 44:815–817 [G]
36. Drickamer MA, Lachs MS: Should patients with Alzheimer's disease be told their diagnosis? N Engl J Med 1992; 326:947–951 [G]
37. Stern Y, Tang M-X, Albert MS, Brandt J, Jacobs DM, Bell K, Marder K, Sano M, Devanand D, Albert SM, Bylsma F, Tsai W-Y: Predicting time to nursing home care and death in individuals with Alzheimer disease. JAMA 1997; 277:806–812 [C]
38. Mace NL, Rabins PV: The Thirty-Six Hour Day: A Family Guide to Caring for Persons With Alzheimer's Disease, Related Dementing Illness, and Memory Loss in Later Life, 2nd revised ed. New York, Warner Books, 1992 [G]
39. Goate A, Chartier-Harlin MC, Mullan M, Brown J, Crawford F, Fidani L, Giuffra L, Haynes A, Irving N, James L, Mant R, Newton P, Rooke K, Roques P, Talbot C, Pericak-Vance M, Roses A, Williamson R, Rossor M, Owen M, Hardy J: Segregation of a missense mutation in the amyloid precursor protein gene with familial Alzheimer's disease. Nature 1991; 349:704–706 [G]
40. Sherrington R, Rogaev EI, Liang Y, Rogaeva EA, Levesque G, Ikeda M, Chi H, Lin C, Li G, Holman K, Tsuda T, Mar L, Foncin J-F, Bruni AC, Montesi MP, Sorbi S, Rainero I, Pinessi L, Nee L, Chumakov I, Po D, Brookes A, Sanseau P, Polinsky RJ, Wasco W, Da Silva HAR, Hai JL, Pericak-Vance MA, Tanzi RE, Roses AD, Fraser PE, Rommens JM, George-Hyslop PH: Cloning of a gene bearing missense mutations in early-onset familial Alzheimer's disease. Nature 1995; 375:754–760 [G]
41. Levy-Lahad E, Wasco W, Poorkaj P, Romano DM, Oshima J, Pettingell WH, Yu CE, Jondro PD, Schmidt SD, Wang K, Crowley AC, Fu YH, Guenette SY, Galas D, Nemens E, Wijsman EM, Bird TD, Schellenberg GD, Tanzi RE: Candidate gene for the chromosome 1 familial Alzheimer's disease locus. Science 1995; 269:973–977 [G]
42. Strittmatter WJ, Saunders AM, Schmechel D, Pericak-Vance M, Enghild J, Salvesen GS, Roses AD: Apolipoprotein E: high-avidity binding to β-amyloid and increased frequency of type 4 allele in late-onset familial Alzheimer's disease. Proc Natl Acad Sci USA 1993; 90:1977–1981 [G]

43. Saunders AM, Strittmatter WJ, Schmechel D, George-Hyslop PH, Pericak-Vance MA, Joo SH, Rosi BL, Gusella JF, Crapper-MacLachlan DR, Alberts MJ: Association of apolipoprotein E allele ε4 with late-onset familial and sporadic Alzheimer's disease. Neurology 1993; 43:1467–1472 [G]
44. Locke PA, Conneally PM, Tanzi RE, Gusella JF, Haines JL: Apolipoprotein E4 allele and Alzheimer disease: examination of allelic association and effect on age at onset in both early- and late-onset cases. Genet Epidemiol 1995; 12:83–92 [G]
45. Chiverton P, Caine ED: Education to assist spouses in coping with Alzheimer's disease. J Am Geriatr Soc 1989; 37:593–598 [C]
46. Mittelman MS, Ferris SH, Steinberg G, Shulman E, Mackell JA, Ambinder A, Cohen J: An intervention that delays institutionalization of Alzheimer's disease patients: treatment of spouse-caregivers. Gerontologist 1993; 33:730–740 [A]
47. Brodaty H, Peters KE: Cost effectiveness of a training program for dementia carers. Int Psychogeriatr 1991; 3:11–22 [G]
48. Lovett S, Gallagher D: Psychoeducational interventions for family caregivers: preliminary efficacy data. Behav Ther 1988; 19:321–330 [B]
49. Gallagher-Thompson D: Direct services and interventions for caregivers: a review and critique of extant programs and a look ahead to the future, in Family Caregiving: Agenda for the Future. Edited by Cantor MM. San Francisco, American Society on Aging, 1994, pp 102–122 [G]
50. Flint AJ: Effects of respite care on patients with dementia and their caregivers. Int J Psychogeriatr 1995; 7:505–517 [F]
51. Burdz M, Eaton W, Bond J: Effect of respite care on dementia and nondementia patients and their caregivers. Psychol Aging 1988; 3:38–42 [G]
52. Conlin MM, Caranasos GJ, Davidson RA: Reduction of caregiver stress by respite care: a pilot study. South Med J 1992; 85:1096–1100 [B]
53. Wimo A, Mattsson B, Adolfsson R, Eriksson T, Nelvig A: Dementia day care and its effects on symptoms and institutionalization—a controlled Swedish study. Scand J Prim Health Care 1993; 11:117–123 [B]
54. Overman W Jr, Stoudemire A: Guidelines for legal and financial counseling of Alzheimer's disease patients and their families. Am J Psychiatry 1988; 145:1495–1500 [G]
55. Spar JE, Garb AS: Assessing competency to make a will. Am J Psychiatry 1992; 149:169–174 [G]
56. Robinson A, Spencer W, White L: Understanding Difficult Behaviors. Lansing, Mich, Geriatric Education Center of Michigan, 1988 [G]
57. Mintzer JE, Lewis L, Pennypacker L, Simpson W, Bachman D, Wohlreich G, Meeks A, Hunt S, Sampson R: Behavioral intensive care unit (BICU): a new concept in the management of acute agitated behavior in elderly demented patients. Gerontologist 1993; 33:801–806 [G]
58. Burgio LD, Engel BT, Hawkins AM, McCormick KA, Scheve A, Jones LT: A staff management system for maintaining improvements in continence with elderly nursing home residents. J Appl Behav Anal 1990; 23:111–118 [G]
59. Group for the Advancement of Psychiatry Committee on Aging: The Psychiatric Treatment of Alzheimer's Disease: Report 125. New York, Brunner/Mazel, 1988 [G]
60. Burnside I, Haight B: Reminiscence and life review: therapeutic interventions for older people. Nurse Pract 1994; 19(4):55–61 [F]
61. Jones GM: Validation therapy: a companion to reality orientation. Can Nurse 1985; 81(3):20–23 [G]
62. Feil N: The Feil Method—How to Help Disoriented Old-Old. Cleveland, Edward Feil Productions, 1992 [G]

63. Robichaud L, Hebert R, Desrosiers J: Efficacy of a sensory integration program on behaviors of inpatients with dementia. Am J Occup Ther 1994; 48:355–360 [A]
64. Woods P, Ashley J: Simulated presence therapy: using selected memories to manage problem behaviors in Alzheimer's disease patients. Geriatr Nurs 1995; 16(1):9–14 [B]
65. Baines S, Saxby P, Ehlert K: Reality orientation and reminiscence therapy: a controlled cross-over study of elderly confused people. Br J Psychiatry 1987; 151:222–231 [A]
66. Kiernat JM: The use of life review activity with confused nursing home residents. Am J Occup Ther 1979; 33:306–310 [B]
67. Cook J: Reminiscing: how can it help confused nursing home residents? Social Casework 1984; 65:90–93 [G]
68. Scanland SG, Emershaw LE: Reality orientation and validation therapy: dementia, depression, and functional status. J Gerontol Nurs 1993; 19:7–11 [B]
69. Powell-Proctor L, Miller E: Reality orientation: a critical appraisal. Br J Psychiatry 1982; 140:457–463 [F]
70. Tappen RM: The effect of skill training on functional abilities of nursing home residents with dementia. Res Nurs Health 1994; 17:159–165 [B]
71. Hanley IG, McGuire RJ, Boyd WD: Reality orientation and dementia: a controlled trial of two approaches. Br J Psychiatry 1981; 138:10–14 [A]
72. Koh K, Ray R, Lee J, Nair A, Ho T, Ang P: Dementia in elderly patients: can the 3R mental stimulation programme improve mental status? Age Ageing 1994; 23:195–199 [B]
73. Johnson CH, McLaren SM, McPherson FM: The comparative effectiveness of three versions of "classroom" reality orientation. Age Ageing 1981; 10:33–35 [B]
74. Woods RT: Reality orientation and staff attention: a controlled study. Br J Psychiatry 1979; 134:502–507 [A]
75. Brook P, Degun G, Mather M: Reality orientation, a therapy for psychogeriatric patients: a controlled study. Br J Psychiatry 1975; 127:42–45 [B]
76. Greene JG, Timbury GC, Smith R: Reality orientation with elderly patients in the community: an empirical evaluation. Age Ageing 1983; 12:38–43 [B]
77. Reeve W, Ivison D: Use of environmental manipulation and classroom and modified informal reality orientation with institutionalized, confused elderly patients. Age Ageing 1985; 14:119–121 [B]
78. Williams R, Reeve W, Ivison D, Kavanagh D: Use of environmental manipulation and modified informal reality orientation with institutionalized, confused, elderly subjects: a replication. Age Ageing 1987; 16:315–318 [B]
79. Gerber GJ, Prince PN, Snider HG, Atchinson K, Dubois L, Kilgour JA: Group activity and cognitive improvement among patients with Alzheimer's disease. Hosp Community Psychiatry 1991; 42:843–845 [A]
80. Baldelli MV, Pirani A, Motta M, Abati E, Mariani E, Manzi V: Effects of reality orientation therapy on elderly patients in the community. Arch Gerontol Geriatr 1993; 7:211–218 [B]
81. Dietch JT, Hewett LJ, Jones S: Adverse effects of reality orientation. J Am Geriatr Soc 1989; 37:974–976 [B]
82. Beck C, Heacock P, Mercer S, Thatcher R, Sparkman C: The impact of cognitive skills remediation training on persons with Alzheimer's disease or mixed dementia. J Geriatr Psychiatry 1988; 21:73–88 [A]
83. Zarit SH, Zarit JM, Reever KE: Memory training for severe memory loss: effects on senile dementia patients and their families. Gerontologist 1982; 22:373–377 [A]
84. Yesavage JA, Westphal J, Rush L: Senile dementia: combined pharmacologic and psychologic treatment. J Am Geriatr Soc 1981; 29:164–171 [A]
85. McEvoy CL, Patterson RL: Behavioral treatment of deficit skills in dementia patients. Gerontologist 1986; 26:475–478 [B]

86. Abraham IL, Reel SJ: Cognitive nursing interventions with long-term care residents: effects on neurocognitive dimensions. Arch Psychiatr Nurs 1992; 6:356–365 [B]
87. Karlsson I, Brane G, Melin E, Nyth AI, Rybo E: Effects of environmental stimulation on biochemical and psychological variables in dementia. Acta Psychiatr Scand 1988; 77:207–213 [B]
88. Rovner BW, Steel CD, Shmuely Y, Folstein MF: A randomized trial of dementia care in nursing homes. J Am Geriatr Soc 1996; 44:7–13 [B]
89. Teri L: Behavioral treatment of depression in patients with dementia. Alzheimer Dis Assoc Disord 1994; 8(3):66–74 [B]
90. Teri L, Logsdon RG: Identifying pleasant activities for Alzheimer's disease patients: the Pleasant Events Schedule-AD. Gerontologist 1991; 31:124–127 [G]
91. Sunderland T, Weingartner H, Cohen RM, Tariot PN, Newhouse PA, Thompson KE, Lawlor BA, Mueller EA: Low-dose oral lorazepam administration in Alzheimer subjects and age-matched controls. Psychopharmacology (Berl) 1989; 99:129–133 [D]
92. Davis KL, Thal LJ, Gamzu ER, Davis CS, Woolson RF, Gracon SI, Drachman DA, Schneider LS, Whitehouse PJ, Hoover TM, Morris JC, Kawas CH, Knopman DS, Earl NL, Kumar V, Doody RS, Tacrine Collaborative Study Group: A double-blind, placebo-controlled multicenter study of tacrine for Alzheimer's disease. N Engl J Med 1992; 327:1253–1259 [A]
93. Farlow M, Gracon SI, Hershey LA, Lewis KW, Sadowsky CH, Dolan-Ureno J: A controlled trial of tacrine in Alzheimer's disease. JAMA 1992; 268:2523–2529 [A]
94. Knapp MJ, Knopman DS, Solomon PR, Pendlebury WW, Davis CS, Gracon SI: A 30-week randomized controlled trial of high-dose tacrine in patients with Alzheimer's disease. JAMA 1994; 271:985–991 [A]
95. Forette F, Hoover T, Gracon S, de Rotrou J, Hervy MP: A double-blind, placebo-controlled, enriched population study of tacrine in patients with Alzheimer's disease. Eur J Neurology 1995; 2:1–10 [A]
96. Foster NL, Petersen RC, Gracon SI, Lewis K, Tacrine 970-6 Study Group: An enriched-population, double-blind, placebo-controlled, crossover study of tacrine and lecithin in Alzheimer's disease. Dementia 1996; 7:260–266 [A]
97. Knopman D, Schneider L, Davis K, Talwalker S, Smith F, Hoover T, Gracon S: Long-term tacrine (Cognex) treatment: effects on nursing home placement and mortality. Neurology 1996; 47:166–177 [C]
98. Rogers SL, Doody R, Mohs R, Friedhoff LT: E2020 produces both clinical global and cognitive test improvement in patients with mild to moderately severe Alzheimer's disease: results of a 30-week phase III trial (abstract). Neurology 1996; 46:A217 [A]
99. Rogers SL, Friedhoff LT, Apter JT, Richter RW, Hartford JT, Walshe TM, Baumel B, Linden RD, Kinney FC, Doody RS, Borison RL, Ahem GL: The efficacy and safety of donepezil in patients with Alzheimer's disease: results of a US multicentre, randomized, double-blind, placebo-controlled trial. Dementia 1996; 7:293–303 [A]
100. Rogers SL, Friedhoff LT: Donepezil (E2020) produces long-term clinical improvement in Alzheimer's disease. Presented at the 4th International Nice/Springfield Symposium on Advances in Alzheimer Therapy, April 10–14, 1996 [A]
101. Watkins PB, Zimmerman HJ, Knapp MJ, Gracon SI, Lewis KW: Hepatotoxic effects of tacrine administration in patients with Alzheimer's disease. JAMA 1994; 271:992–998 [C]
102. Lyketsos CG, Corazzini K, Steele CD, Kraus MF: Guidelines for the use of tacrine in Alzheimer's disease: clinical application and effectiveness. J Neuropsychiatry Clin Neurosci 1996; 8:67–73 [F]
103. Halliwell B, Gutteridge JMC: Oxygen radicals in the nervous system. Trends Neurosci 1985; 8:22–26 [G]

104. Behl C, Davis J, Cole G, Shubert D: Vitamin E protects nerve cells from beta-amyloid protein toxicity. Biochem Biophys Res Commun 1992; 186:944–950 [G]
105. Sano M, Ernesto C, Klauber MR, Schafer K, Woodbury P, Thomas R, Grundman F, Growdon S, Thal LJ: Rationale and design of a multicenter study of selegiline and α-tocopherol in the treatment of Alzheimer disease using novel clinical outcomes. Alzheimer Dis Assoc Disord 1996; 10:132–140 [G]
106. Sano M, Ernesto C, Thomas RG, Klauber MR, Schafer K, Grundman M, Woodbury P, Growdon J, Cotman CW, Pfeiffer E, Schneider LS, Thal LJ: A two-year, double blind randomized multicenter trial of selegeline and α-tocopherol in the treatment of Alzheimer's disease. N Engl J Med (in press) [A]
107. Kappus H, Diplock AT: Tolerance and safety of vitamin E: a toxicological position report. Free Radic Biol Med 1992; 13:55–74 [G]
108. Tatton WG, Greenwood CE: Rescue of dying neurons: a new action for deprenyl in MPTP parkinsonism. J Neurosci Res 1991; 30:666–672 [G]
109. Mangoni A, Grassi MP, Frattola L, Piolti R, Bassi S, Motta A, Marcone A, Smirne S: Effects of a MAO-B inhibitor in the treatment of Alzheimer disease. Eur Neurol 1991; 31:100–107; correction 31:433 [A]
110. Burke WJ, Roccaforte WH, Wengel SP, Bayer BL, Ranno AE, Willcockson NK: L-deprenyl in the treatment of mild dementia of the Alzheimer type: results of a 15-month trial. J Am Geriatr Soc 1993; 41:1219–1225 [A]
111. Burke WJ, Ranno AE, Roccaforte WH, Wengel SP, Bayer BL, Willcockson NK: L-deprenyl in the treatment of mild dementia of the Alzheimer type: preliminary results. J Am Geriatr Soc 1993; 41:367–370 [A]
112. Agnoli A, Martucci N, Fabbrini G, Buckley AE, Fioravanti M: Monoamine oxidase and dementia: treatment with an inhibitor of MAO-B activity. Dementia 1990; 1:109–114 [A]
113. Filip V, Kolibas E, Ceskova E, Hronek J, Novotna D, Novotny V: Selegiline in mild SDAT: results of a multi-center, double-blind, placebo-controlled trial (abstract). Neuropsychopharmacol 1991 [A]
114. Loeb C, Albano C: Selegiline: a new approach to DAT treatment (abstract). Presented at the European Conference on Parkinson's Disease and Extrapyramidal Disorders, Rome, July 1990 [A]
115. Martucci N, Fabbrini G, Fioravanti M: Monoaminossidasi e demenza: trattamento con un inibitore dell'attivita MAO-B. Giornale di Neuropsicofarmacologia 1989; 11:265–269 [A]
116. Schneider LS, Olin JT: Overview of clinical trials of Hydergine in dementia. Arch Neurol 1994; 51:787–798 [E]
117. Tariot PN, Cohen RM, Sunderland T, Newhouse PA, Yount D, Mellow AM, Weingartner H, Mueller EA, Murphy DL: L-Deprenyl in Alzheimer's disease: preliminary evidence for behavioral change with monoamine oxidase B inhibition. Arch Gen Psychiatry 1987; 44:427–433 [A]
118. Piccinin GL, Finali G, Piccirilli M: Neuropsychological effects of L-deprenyl in Alzheimer's type dementia. Clin Neuropharmacol 1990; 13:147–163 [A]
119. Finali G, Piccirilli M, Oliani C, Piccinin GL: L-deprenyl therapy improves verbal memory in amnesic Alzheimer patients. Clin Neuropharmacol 1991; 14:523–536 [B]
120. Schneider LS, Olin JT, Pawluczyk S: A double-blind crossover pilot study of l-deprenyl (selegiline) combined with cholinesterase inhibitor in Alzheimer's disease. Am J Psychiatry 1993; 150:321–323 [A]
121. Thompson TL II, Filley CM, Mitchell WD, Culig KM, LoVerde M, Byyny RL: Lack of efficacy of hydergine in patients with Alzheimer's disease. N Engl J Med 1990; 323:445–448; correction 323:691 [A]
122. McDonald WM, Krishnan KR: Pharmacologic management of the symptoms of dementia. Am Fam Physician 1990; 42:123–132 [A]

123. Irfan S, Linder L: The effect of dihydrogenated ergot alkaloids in the treatment of geriatric patients suffering from senile mental deterioration, in XIth International Congress of Gerontology. Tokyo, SCIMED, 1978, p 142 [A]
124. Puxty J: Community screening for dementia and evaluation of treatment, in Proceedings of the Basel Symposium (CH). Edited by Carlsson A, Kanowski S, Allain H, Spiegel R. Pearl River, NY, Parthenon Publishing Group, 1989, p 211–230 [A]
125. Soni SD, Soni SS: Dihydrogenated alkaloids of ergotoxine in nonhospitalised elderly patients. Curr Med Res Opin 1975; 3:464–468 [A]
126. Thienhaus OJ, Wheeler BG, Simon S, Zemlan FP, Hartford JT: A controlled double-blind study of high-dose dihydroergotoxine mesylate (Hydergine) in mild dementia. J Am Geriatr Soc 1987; 35:219–223 [A]
127. Rao DB, Norris JR: A double-blind investigation of hydergine in the treatment of cerebrovascular insufficiency in the elderly. Johns Hopkins Med J 1972; 130:317–324 [B]
128. Winslow IE: Clinical evaluation of hydergine. Unpublished manuscript, 1972 [A]
129. Lazzari R, Passeri M, Chierichetti SM: Le mésylate de dihydroergotoxine dans le traitement de l'insuffisance cérébrale sénile. Le Presse Médicale 1983; 12:3179–3185 [A]
130. Martucci N, Manna V: EEG-pharmacological and neuropsychological study of dihydroergocristine mesylate in patients with chronic cerebrovascular disease. Advances in Therapy 1986; 3:210–223 [A]
131. Moglia A, Bono G, Sinforiani E, Alfonsi E, Zandrini C, Pistarini C, Arrigo A, Franch F: La diidroergotossina mesilato dell'insufficienza cerebrovasculare cronica: analisi spettrale dell'EEG e correlati neuropsicologici. Farmaco 1983; 38:97–102 [A]
132. Breitner JCS, Gau BA, Welsh KA, Plassman BL, McDonald WM, Helm MJ, Anthony JC: Inverse association of anti-inflammatory treatments and Alzheimer's disease: initial results of a co-twin control study. Neurology 1994; 44:227–232 [D]
133. McGeer PL, Rogers J: Anti-inflammatory agents as a therapeutic approach to Alzheimer's disease. Neurology 1992; 42:447–448 [G]
134. Rogers J, Kirby LC, Hempelman SR, Berry DL, McGeer PL, Kaszniak AW, Zalinski J, Cofield M, Mansukhani L, Willson P, Kogan F: Clinical trial of indomethacin in Alzheimer's disease. Neurology 1993; 43:1609–1611 [A]
135. Stewart WF, Kawas C, Corrada M, Metter EJ: Risk of Alzheimer's disease and duration of NSAID use. Neurology 1997; 48:626–632 [C]
136. Aisen PS, Davis KL: Inflammatory mechanisms in Alzheimer's disease: implications for therapy. Am J Psychiatry 1994; 151:1105–1113 [G]
137. Sherwin BB: Estrogenic effects on memory in women. Ann NY Acad Sci 1994; 743:213–230 [G]
138. Fillit H, Weinreb H, Cholst I, Luine V, McEwen B, Amador R, Zabriskie J: Observations in a preliminary open trial of estradiol therapy for senile dementia-Alzheimer's type. Psychoneuroendocrinology 1986; 11:337–345 [B]
139. Ohkura T, Isse K, Akazawa K, Hamamoto M, Yaoi Y, Hagino N: Long-term estrogen replacement therapy in female patients with dementia of the Alzheimer type: 7 case reports. Dementia 1995; 6(2):99–107 [G]
140. Henderson VW, Paganini-Hill A, Emanuel CK, Dunn ME, Buckwalter JG: Estrogen replacement therapy in older women: comparisons between Alzheimer's disease cases and nondemented control subjects. Arch Neurol 1994; 51:896–900 [D]
141. Tang MX, Jacobs D, Stern Y, Marder K, Schofield P, Gurland B, Andrews H, Mayeux R: Effect of oestrogen during menopause on risk and age at onset of Alzheimer's disease. Lancet 1996; 348:429–432 [C]
142. Burns A, Murphy D: Protection against Alzheimer's disease? Lancet 1996; 348:420–421 [G]

143. Crapper-McLachlan DR, Dalton AJ, Kruck TPA, Bell MY, Smith WL, Kalow W, Andrews DF: Intramuscular desferrioxamine in patients with Alzheimer's disease. Lancet 1991; 337:1304–1308; correction 337:1618 [B]
144. Cardelli MB, Russell M, Bagne CA, Pomara N: Chelation therapy: unproved modality in the treatment of Alzheimer-type dementia. J Am Geriatr Soc 1985; 33:548–551 [G]
145. Leibovici A, Tariot PN: Agitation associated with dementia: a systematic approach to treatment. Psychopharmacol Bull 1988; 24:49–53 [G]
146. Reisberg B, Borenstein J, Salob SP, Ferris SH, Franssen E, Georgotas A: Behavioral symptoms in Alzheimer's disease: phenomenology and treatment. J Clin Psychiatry 1987; 48(May suppl):9–15 [G]
147. Devanand DP, Sackeim HA, Brown RP, Mayeux R: Psychosis, behavioral disturbance, and the use of neuroleptics in dementia. Compr Psychiatry 1988; 29:387–401 [F]
148. Schneider LS, Pollack VE, Lyness SA: A metaanalysis of controlled trials of neuroleptic treatment in dementia. J Am Geriatr Soc 1990; 38:553–563 [E]
149. Rada RT, Kellner R: Thiothixene in the treatment of geriatric patients with chronic organic brain syndrome. J Am Geriatr Soc 1976; 24:105–107 [A]
150. Barnes R, Veith R, Okimoto J, Raskind M, Gumbrecht G: Efficacy of antipsychotic medications in behaviorally disturbed dementia patients. Am J Psychiatry 1982; 139:1170–1174 [A]
151. Sugarman AA, Williams BH, Adlerstein AM: Haloperidol in the psychiatric disorders of old age. Am J Psychiatry 1964; 120:1190–1192 [A]
152. Petrie WM, Ban TA, Berney S, Fujimori M, Guy W, Ragheb M, Wilson WH, Schaffer JD: Loxapine in psychogeriatrics: a placebo- and standard-controlled clinical investigation. J Clin Psychopharmacol 1982; 2:122–126 [A]
153. Hamilton LD, Bennett JL: The use of trifluoperazine in geriatric patients with chronic brain syndrome. J Am Geriatr Soc 1962; 10:140–147 [A]
154. Hamilton LD, Bennett JL: Acetophenazine for hyperactive geriatric patients. Geriatrics 1962; 17:596–601 [A]
155. Abse DW, Dahlstrom WG, Hill C: The value of chemotherapy in senile mental disturbance. JAMA 1960; 174:2036–2042 [A]
156. Madhusoodanan S, Brenner R, Araujo L, Abaza A: Efficacy of risperidone treatment for psychoses associated with schizophrenia, schizoaffective disorder, bipolar disorder, or senile dementia in 11 geriatric patients: a case series. J Clin Psychiatry 1995; 56:514–518 [G]
157. Friedman JH, Lannon MC: Clozapine in the treatment of psychosis in Parkinson's disease. Neurology 1989; 39:1219–1221 [G]
158. Chacko R, Hurley R, Jankovic J: Clozapine use in diffuse Lewy body disease. J Neuropsychiatry Clin Neurosci 1993; 5:206–208 [G]
159. Salzman C, Vaccaro B, Lieff J, Weiner A: Clozapine in older patients with psychosis and behavioral disturbances. Am J Geriatr Psychiatry 1995; 3:26–33 [G]
160. Devanand DP, Sackeim HA, Brown RP, Mayeux R: A pilot study of haloperidol treatment of psychosis and behavioral disturbance in Alzheimer's disease. Arch Neurol 1989; 46:854–857 [B]
161. Woerner MG, Alvir JMJ, Kane JM, Saltz BL, Lieberman JA: Neuroleptic treatment of elderly patients. Psychopharmacol Bull 1995; 31:333–337 [B]
162. Jeste DV, Caliguiri MP, Paulsen JS, Heaton RK, Lacro JP, Harris M, Bailey A, Fell RL, McAdams LA: Risk of tardive dyskinesia in older patients: a prospective longitudinal study of 266 outpatients. Arch Gen Psychiatry 1995; 52:756–765 [B]
163. Salzman C: Treatment of the elderly agitated patient. J Clin Psychiatry 1987; 48(May suppl):19–22 [G]
164. Allen RL, Walker Z, D'Ath PJ, Katona CLE: Risperidone for psychotic and behavioural symptoms in Lewy body dementia (letter). Lancet 1995; 346:185 [G]

165. McKeith IG, Ballard CG, Harrison RW: Neuroleptic sensitivity to risperidone in Lewy body dementia (letter). Lancet 1995; 346:699 [G]
166. Gottlieb G, McAllister T, Gur R: Depot neuroleptics in the treatment of behavioral disorders in patients with Alzheimer's disease. J Am Geriatr Soc 1988; 36:619–621 [G]
167. Kirven LE, Montero EF: Comparison of thioridazine and diazepam in the control of nonpsychotic symptoms associated with senility: double-blind study. J Am Geriatr Soc 1973; 21:546–551 [A]
168. Covington J: Alleviating agitation, apprehension and related symptoms in geriatric patients. South Med J 1975; 68:719–724 [G]
169. Stotsky B: Multicenter study comparing thioridazine with diazepam and placebo in elderly nonpsychotic patients with emotional and behavioral disorders. Clin Ther 1984; 6:546–559 [A]
170. Coccaro EF, Kramer E, Zemishlany Z, Thorne A, Rice CM III, Giordani B, Duvvi K, Patel BM, Torres J, Nora R, Neufeld R, Mohs RC, Davis KL: Pharmacologic treatment of noncognitive behavioral disturbances in elderly demented patients. Am J Psychiatry 1990; 147:1640–1645 [G]
171. Cevera AA: Psychoactive drug therapy in the senile patient: controlled comparison of thioridazine and diazepam. Psychiatry Digest 1974: pp 15–21 [A]
172. Beber CR: Management of behavior in the institutionalized aged. Dis Nerv Syst 1965; 26:591–595 [A]
173. Lemos GP, Clement MA, Nickels E: Effects of diazepam suspension in geriatric patients hospitalized for psychiatric illnesses. J Am Geriatr Soc 1965; 13:355–359 [A]
174. Salzman C: Clinical Geriatric Psychopharmacology, 2nd ed. Baltimore, Williams & Wilkins, 1992 [G]
175. Grad R: Benzodiazepines for insomnia in community-dwelling elderly: a review of benefit and risk. J Fam Pract 1995; 41:473–481 [F]
176. Herings RM, Stricker BH, de Boer A, Bakker A, Sturmans F: Benzodiazepines and the risk of falling leading to femur fractures: dosage more important than elimination half-life. Arch Intern Med 1995; 155:1801–1807 [D]
177. Ashton H: Guidelines for the rational use of benzodiazepines: when and what to use. Drugs 1994; 48:25–40 [G]
178. Gleason RP, Schneider LS: Carbamazepine treatment of agitation in Alzheimer's outpatients refractory to neuroleptics. J Clin Psychiatry 1990; 51:115–118 [G]
179. Lemke MR: Effect of carbamazepine on agitation in Alzheimer's inpatients refractory to neuroleptics. J Clin Psychiatry 1995; 56:354–357 [B]
180. Tariot PN, Erb R, Leibovici A, Podgorski CA, Cox C, Asnis J, Kolassa J, Irvine C: Carbamazepine treatment of agitation in nursing home patients with dementia: a preliminary study. J Am Geriatr Soc 1994; 42:1160–1166 [B]
181. Chambers CA, Bain J, Rosbottom R, Ballinger BR, McLaren S: Carbamazepine in senile dementia and overactivity: a placebo controlled double blind trial. IRCS Med Sci 1982; 10:505–506 [A]
182. Lott AD, McElroy SL, Keys MA: Valproate in the treatment of behavioral agitation in elderly patients with dementia. J Neuropsychiatry Clin Neurosci 1995; 7:314–319 [G]
183. Mellow AM, Solano-Lopez C, Davis S: Sodium valproate in the treatment of behavioral disturbance in dementia. J Geriatr Psychiatry Neurol 1993; 6:205–209 [G]
184. American Psychiatric Association: Practice Guideline for the Treatment of Patients With Bipolar Disorder (Revised). Am J Psychiatry 2002; 159(April suppl) [G]
185. Risse SC, Barnes R: Pharmacologic treatment of agitation associated with dementia. J Am Geriatr Soc 1986; 34:368–376 [A]
186. Kunik ME, Yudofsky SC, Silver JM, Hales RE: Pharmacologic approach to management of agitation associated with dementia. J Clin Psychiatry 1994; 55(Feb suppl):13–17 [G]

187. Simpson DM, Foster D: Improvement in organically disturbed behavior with trazodone treatment. J Clin Psychiatry 1986; 47:191–193 [G]
188. Nair NP, Ban TA, Hontela S, Clarke R: Trazodone in the treatment of organic brain syndromes, with special reference to psychogeriatrics. Curr Ther Res 1973; 15:769–775 [G]
189. Houlihan DJ, Mulsant BH, Sweet RA, Rifai AH, Pasternak R, Rosen J, Zubenko GS: A naturalistic study of trazodone in the treatment of behavioral complications of dementia. Am J Geriatr Psychiatry 1994; 2:78–85 [G]
190. Lebert F, Pasquier F, Petit H: Behavioral effects of trazodone in Alzheimer's disease. J Clin Psychiatry 1994; 55:536–538 [B]
191. Sultzer D, Gray KF, Gunay I, Berisford MA, Mahler ME: A double-blind comparison of trazodone and haloperidol for treatment of agitation in patients with dementia. Am J Geriatr Psychiatry 1997; 5:60–69 [A]
192. Nyth AL, Gottfries CG: The clinical efficacy of citalopram in treatment of emotional disturbances in dementia disorders: a Nordic multicentre study. Br J Psychiatry 1990; 157:894–901 [B]
193. Nyth AL, Gottfries CG, Lyby K, Smedegaard-Andersen L, Gylding-Sabroe J, Kristensen M, Refsum HE, Ofsti E, Eriksson S, Syversen S: A controlled multicenter clinical study of citalopram and placebo in elderly depressed patients with and without concomitant dementia. Acta Psychiatr Scand 1992; 86:138–145 [B]
194. Colenda CC III: Buspirone in treatment of agitated demented patient (letter). Lancet 1988; 1:1169; correction 1988; 2:754 [G]
195. Tiller JW, Dakis JA, Shaw JM: Short-term buspirone treatment in disinhibition with dementia (letter). Lancet 1988; 2:510 [G]
196. Sakauye KM, Camp CJ, Ford PA: Effects of buspirone on agitation associated with dementia. Am J Geriatr Psychiatry 1993; 1:82–84 [B]
197. Weiner MF, Denke M, Williams K, Guzman R: Intramuscular medroxyprogesterone acetate for sexual aggression in elderly men. Lancet 1992; 339:1121–1122 [G]
198. Kyomen H, Nobel K, Wet J: The use of estrogen to decrease aggressive physical behavior in elderly men with dementia. J Am Geriatr Soc 1991; 39:1110–1112 [G]
199. Rich SS, Ovsiew F: Leuprolide acetate for exhibitionism in Huntington's disease. Mov Disord 1994; 9:353–357 [G]
200. Weiler PG, Mungas D, Bernick C: Propranolol for the control of disruptive behavior in senile dementia. J Geriatr Psychiatry Neurol 1988; 1:226–230 [G]
201. Reifler BV, Teri L, Raskind M, Veith R, Barnes R, White E, McLean P: Double-blind trial of imipramine in Alzheimer's disease patients with and without depression. Am J Psychiatry 1989; 146:45–49 [A]
202. Passeri M, Cucinotta D, DeMello M, Biziere K: Comparison of minaprine and placebo in the treatment of Alzheimer's disease and multi-infarct dementia. Int J Geriatr Psychiatry 1987; 2:97–103 [B]
203. Fuchs A, Henke U, Erhart DH, Schell CH, Pramshohler B, Danninger B, Schautzer F: Video rating analysis of effect of maprotiline in patients with dementia and depression. Pharmacopsychiatry 1993; 26:37–41 [B]
204. Conti L, Fosca RE, Lazzerini F, Morey LC, Ban TA, Santini V, Modafferi A, Postiglione A: Glycosaminoglycan polysulfate (Ateroid) in old-age dementias: effects upon depressive symptomatology in geriatric patients. Prog Neuropsychopharmacol Biol Psychiatry 1989; 13:977–981 [B]
205. Passeri M, Cucinotta D, Abate G, Senin U, Ventura A, Badiale MS, Diana R, La Greca P, Le Grazie C: Oral 5′-methyltetrahydrofolic acid in senile organic mental disorders with depression: results of a double-blind multicenter study. Aging 1993; 5:63–71 [B]
206. NIH Consensus Development Panel on Depression in Late Life: Diagnosis and treatment of depression in late life. JAMA 1992; 268:1018–1024 [G]

207. American Psychiatric Association: Practice Guideline for the Treatment of Patients With Major Depressive Disorder (Revision). Am J Psychiatry 2000; 157(April suppl) [G]
208. Marin RS, Fogel BS, Hawkins J, Duffy J, Krupp B: Apathy: a treatable syndrome. Clin Neuroscience 1995; 7(1):23–30 [G]
209. Wallace AE, Kofoed LL, West AN: Double-blind, placebo-controlled trial of methylphenidate in older, depressed, medically ill patients. Am J Psychiatry 1995; 152:929–931 [A]
210. Pickett P, Masand P, Murray G: Psychostimulant treatment of geriatric depressive disorders secondary to medical illness. J Geriatr Psychiatry Neurol 1990; 3:146–151 [G]
211. Lazarus LW, Moberg PJ, Langsley PR, Lingam VR: Methylphenidate and nortriptyline in the treatment of poststroke depression: a retrospective comparison. Arch Phys Med Rehabil 1994; 75:403–406 [G]
212. Price TR, McAllister TW: Safety and efficacy of ECT in depressed patients with dementia: a review of clinical experience. Convulsive Ther 1989; 5:1–74 [G]
213. Aharon-Peretz J, Masiah A, Pillar T, Epstein R, Tzischinsky O, Lavie P: Sleep-wake cycles in multi-infarct dementia and dementia of the Alzheimer type. Neurology 1991; 41:1616–1619 [G]
214. Satlin A: Sleep disorders in dementia. Psychiatr Ann 1994; 24:186–190 [G]
215. Hoch CC, Reynolds CF III, Houck PR: Sleep patterns in Alzheimer, depressed, and healthy elderly. West J Nurs Res 1988; 10:239–256 [G]
216. Strollo P, Rogers R: Obstructive sleep apnea. N Engl J Med 1996; 334:99–104 [G]
217. Piccione P, Zorick F, Lutz T, Grissom T, Kramer M, Roth T: The efficacy of triazolam and chloral hydrate in geriatric insomniacs. J Int Med Res 1980; 8:361–367 [B]
218. Linnoila M, Viukari M, Numminen A, Auvinen J: Efficacy and side effects of chloral hydrate and tryptophan as sleeping aids in psychogeriatric patients. Int Pharmacopsychiatry 1980; 15:124–128 [B]
219. Shaw SH, Curson H, Coquelin JP: A double-blind, comparative study of zolpidem and placebo in the treatment of insomnia in elderly psychiatric in-patients. J Int Med Res 1992; 20:150–161; correction 20:494 [A]
220. Satlin A, Volicer L, Ross V, Herz L, Campbell S: Bright light treatment of behavioral and sleep disturbances in patients with Alzheimer's disease. Am J Psychiatry 1992; 149:1028–1032 [B]
221. Okawa M, Mishima K, Nanami T, Shimizu T, Iijima S, Hishikawa Y, Takahashi K: Vitamin B12 treatment for sleep-wake rhythm disorders. Sleep 1990; 13(1):15–23 [A]
222. Mishima K, Okawa M, Hishikawa Y, Hozumi S, Hori H, Takahashi K: Morning bright light therapy for sleep and behavior disorders in elderly patients with dementia. Acta Psychiatr Scand 1994; 89:1–7 [B]
223. Maurizi CP: The therapeutic potential for tryptophan and melatonin: possible roles in depression, sleep, Alzheimer's disease and abnormal aging. Med Hypotheses 1990; 31:233–242 [E]
224. Singer C, McArthur A, Hughes R, Sack R, Kaye J, Lewy A: High dose melatonin administration and sleep in the elderly. Sleep Res 1995; 24A:151 [G]
225. Volicer L, Volicer BJ, Hurley AC: Is hospice care appropriate for Alzheimer patients? Caring 1993; 12(11):50–55 [G]
226. Volicer L, Hurley AC, Lathi DC, Kowall NW: Measurement of severity in advanced Alzheimer's disease. J Gerontol 1994; 49(5):M223–M226 [G]
227. Levkoff SE, Evans DA, Liptzin B, Wetle T, Reilly C, Pilgrim D, Schor J, Rowe J: Delirium: the occurrence and persistence of symptoms among elderly hospitalized patients. Arch Intern Med 1992; 152:334–340 [G]
228. Erkinjuntti T, Wikstrom J, Palo J, Autio L: Dementia among medical inpatients. Arch Intern Med 1986; 146:1923–1926 [C]

229. Tune L, Carr S, Hoag E, Cooper T: Anticholinergic effects of drugs commonly prescribed for the elderly: potential means for assessing risk of delirium. Am J Psychiatry 1992; 149:1393–1394 [G]
230. Torigoe R, Hayashi T, Anegawa S, Harada K, Toda K, Maeda K, Katsuragi M: Effect of propentofylline and pentoxifylline on cerebral blood flow using ^{123}I-IMP SPECT in patients with cerebral arteriosclerosis. Clin Ther 1994; 16:65–73 [G]
231. Blume J, Ruhlmann KU, de la Haye R, Rettig K: Treatment of chronic cerebrovascular disease in elderly patients with pentoxifylline. J Med 1992; 23:417–432 [A]
232. Black RS, Barclay LL, Nolan KA, Thaler HT, Hardiman ST, Blass JP: Pentoxifylline in cerebrovascular dementia. J Am Geriatr Soc 1992; 40:237–244 [A]
233. Rovner BW, Kafonek S, Filipp L, Lucas MJ, Folstein MF: Prevalence of mental illness in a community nursing home. Am J Psychiatry 1986; 143:1446–1449 [G]
234. Boss P, Caron W, Horbal J, Mortimer J: Predictors of depression in caregivers of dementia patients: boundary ambiguity and mastery. Fam Process 1990; 29:245–254 [G]
235. Dura JR, Stukenberg KW, Kiecolt-Glaser JK: Chronic stress and depressive disorders in older adults. J Abnorm Psychol 1990; 99:284–290 [D]
236. Tariot PN, Podgorski CA, Blazina L, Leibovici A: Mental disorders in the nursing home: another perspective. Am J Psychiatry 1993; 150:1063–1069 [G]
237. Sloane PD, Barrick AL: Improving long-term care for persons with Alzheimer's disease (editorial). J Am Geriatr Soc 1996; 44:91–92 [G]
238. Lawton MP, Brody EM, Saperstein AR: A controlled study of respite service for caregivers of Alzheimer's patients. Gerontologist 1989; 29:8–16 [B]
239. Pynoos J, Regnier V: Improving residential environments for frail elderly: bridging the gap between theory and application, in The Concept and Measurement of Quality of Life in the Frail Elderly. Edited by Birren JE, Lubben JE, Rowe JC, Deutchman DE. San Diego, Academic Press, 1991, pp 91–119 [G]
240. Horwitz GJ, Tariot PN, Mead K, Cox C: Discontinuation of antipsychotics in nursing home patients with dementia. Am J Geriatr Psychiatry 1995; 3:290–299 [C]
241. Tinetti ME, Liu WL, Marottoli RA, Ginter SF: Mechanical restraint use among residents of skilled nursing facilities. JAMA 1991; 265:468–471 [G]
242. Burton LC, German PS, Rovner BW, Brant LJ: Physical restraint use and cognitive decline among nursing home residents. J Am Geriatr Soc 1992; 40:811–816 [C]
243. Capezuti E, Evans L, Strumpf N, Maislin G: Physical restraint use and falls in nursing home residents. J Am Geriatr Soc 1996; 44:627–633 [D]

GUIDELINE WATCH: PRACTICE GUIDELINE FOR THE TREATMENT OF PATIENTS WITH HIV/AIDS

Marshall Forstein, M.D.
Francine Cournos, M.D.
Antoine Douaihy, M.D.
Karl Goodkin, M.D., Ph.D.
Milton L. Wainberg, M.D.
Khakasa H. Wapenyi, M.D.

Since publication in 2000 of APA's *Practice Guideline for the Treatment of Patients With HIV/AIDS* (1), new evidence has become available that affects the psychiatric care of patients with human immunodeficiency virus (HIV) infection and acquired immune deficiency syndrome (AIDS). This guideline watch highlights this evidence for the following areas: epidemiology, antiretroviral medication regimens, HIV-associated cognitive-motor disorders, treatment of psychiatric disorders and conditions when comorbid with HIV infection, hepatitis C virus (HCV) and HIV coinfection, and metabolic syndrome and lipodystrophy.

EPIDEMIOLOGY

HIV infection remains a global pandemic. According to the Joint United Nations Programme on HIV/AIDS, as of December 2004 more than 39 million people in the world were estimated to be living with HIV/AIDS; 95% of these people lived in low- and middle-income countries (2). Globally, more than 20 million persons have died of AIDS since the disease was first identified in 1981. Worldwide, 14,000 people are newly infected with HIV every day (3). According to the U.S. Centers for Disease Control and Prevention, through 2003, the cumulative

The American Psychiatric Association (APA) practice guidelines are developed by expert work groups using an explicit methodology that includes rigorous review of available evidence, broad peer review of iterative drafts, and formal approval by the APA Assembly and Board of Trustees. APA practice guidelines are intended to assist psychiatrists in clinical decision making. They are not intended to be a standard of care. The ultimate judgment regarding a particular clinical procedure or treatment plan must be made by the psychiatrist in light of the clinical data presented by the patient and the diagnostic and treatment options available. Guideline watches summarize significant developments in practice since publication of an APA practice guideline. Watches may be authored and reviewed by experts associated with the original guideline development effort and are approved for publication by APA's Executive Committee on Practice Guidelines. Thus, watches represent opinion of the authors and approval of the Executive Committee but not policy of the APA. This guideline watch was published in April 2006. Suggested citation: Forstein M, Cournos F, Douaihy A, Goodkin K, Wainberg ML, Wapenyi KH: *Guideline Watch: Practice Guideline for the Treatment of Patients With HIV/ AIDS.* Arlington, VA: American Psychiatric Association, 2006. Available online at http://www.psych.org/psych_pract/treatg/pg/prac_ guide.cfm.

estimated number of diagnoses of AIDS in the United States was 929,985; the cumulative estimated number of deaths of persons with AIDS was 524,060; and an estimated 1,039,000 to 1,185,000 persons in the United States were living with HIV/AIDS, with 24%–27% unaware of their HIV infection (4). In the United States, prevention efforts have been successful at decreasing HIV incidence. New infections, however, remain stabilized at 40,000 per year, with people of color bearing a disproportionate burden of new infections, suggesting that new strategies must be developed for further reducing the spread of HIV.

In recent years, there has been a change in the epidemiology of AIDS in the United States. Initially the epidemic mostly affected men who had sex with men, intravenous drug users, pregnant women, women who were breast-feeding, and recipients of blood products. Data now show an increasing number of individuals infected through unprotected heterosexual intercourse. For men, the majority of infections continues to result from drug use and sex between men. Among women, however, heterosexual intercourse accounts for most HIV infections (4). Recent studies have provided increasing evidence that the main risk factor for women is undisclosed risk behavior of their male partners, especially sex with other men (5). Increasingly, it is important for psychiatrists to assess specific risk behaviors that facilitate HIV transmission rather than making assumptions about risk based on patients' sexual orientation, marital status, or other characteristics. Identifying drug-using and sexual behaviors is an ongoing component of psychiatric practice.

ANTIRETROVIRAL AGENTS

Recommended regimens

Since publication of the APA practice guideline in 2000, changes have occurred in the U.S. Department of Health and Human Services (DHHS) guidelines on antiretroviral therapy for the management of HIV infection (available online at http://aidsinfo.nih.gov). According to the DHHS guidelines, as of October 2005 there were 21 approved antiretroviral agents, belonging to four classes (6). A new class of antiretroviral medications, the fusion/entry inhibitors, is engineered to work by preventing the virus from fusing with a cell membrane and entering the cell, thus preventing infection of cells. Antiretroviral agents are prescribed in combination regimens that are also known as *combination antiretroviral therapy* (CART) (previously termed *highly active antiretroviral therapy* [HAART]) (6). The timing of CART initiation has been debated and may depend on assessment of viral load, CD4 count, and history of associated symptoms. There has been consensus to recommend the following as first-line regimens: 1) efavirenz + (lamivudine or emtricitabine) + (zidovudine or tenofovir) or 2) lopinavir + (lamivudine or emtricitabine) + zidovudine.

Notably, three nonnucleoside reverse transcriptase inhibitors (NNRTIs) (namely, delavirdine, efavirenz, and nevirapine) are currently marketed for use. The NNRTI-based regimens are commonly prescribed as initial therapy for treatment-naive patients. These regimens have the advantage of lower pill burden compared with most protease inhibitor–based regimens. Use of NNRTI-based regimens as initial therapy spares the protease inhibitors for later use, reducing or delaying patient exposure to some of the treatment-limiting adverse effects more commonly associated with the protease inhibitors. The major disadvantage of these regimens is their low genetic barrier for resistance. Only a single mutation need exist to confer resistance to these agents. Moreover, resistance often develops across the entire class. As a result, patients who do not respond to this initial regimen may lose the utility of other NNRTIs and/or may transmit NNRTI-resistant virus to others. Efavirenz is recommended, on the basis of safety data, as the preferred NNRTI in initial therapy. Exceptions are pregnant women (especially during the first trimester), women who are planning to conceive, and women who are not using effective and consistent contraception. For such patients, nevirapine is recommended as the alternative to efavirenz. Delavirdine has the least potent antiviral activity in this class and is not recommended for initial treatment.

Because of the association of the protease inhibitor class of antiretrovirals with the development of metabolic syndrome (see "Metabolic Syndrome and Lipodystrophy" below), regimens are structured to reserve this class of antiretrovirals for future use in case of treatment failure.

Many new medications to manage HIV infection are in development.

Adherence

In patients receiving antiretroviral treatment, lack of almost perfect adherence to daily regimens continues to be the greatest barrier to sustaining a clinically effective response. Within the community, lack of adherence can also lead to the development of HIV strains resistant to the available antiretrovirals. The prevalence of HIV isolates that demonstrate resistance to antiretroviral agents is increasing, and such isolates can develop despite stable low-level viremia (7). Resistance testing, genotypic or phenotypic, is indicated when patients experience virologic failure (failure to achieve or maintain virologic suppression below 400 HIV RNA copies/mL plasma at 24 weeks or 50 copies/mL plasma at 48 weeks or >400 copies/mL plasma after viral suppression [6, 8]).

Directly observed therapy (DOT), originally used to improve cure rates of tuberculosis in hard-to-reach populations, has been adapted for individuals receiving treatment for HIV to decrease long-term morbidity and mortality. In treatment-experienced HIV-infected substance-using patients, DOT has been successfully used to promote adherence. A study of 69 HIV-infected individuals enrolled in a community-based modified DOT program showed a median decrease of 2.7 log in HIV viral load (9). DOT also provides a way to offer psychosocial support as well as connections to addiction, psychiatric, and social services (10).

Adherence to antiretroviral therapy improves in depressed patients treated with antidepressants. Untreated depression has been associated with medication nonadherence (11).

Drug-drug interactions between new antiretroviral agents and psychotropic medications

Interactions between psychotropic and antiretroviral medications are common in the HIV-infected patient. Drug-drug interactions are too numerous to be listed here in full. Most medications used in the treatment of psychiatric disorders are metabolized by the cytochrome P450 (CYP) enzymes, especially the subgroups 3A4 and 2D6. Of the antiretrovirals, the protease inhibitors tend to pose the greatest risk for changes in drug levels that are significant in the HIV patient. Ritonavir is the most potent of the protease inhibitors, with the greatest impact on the inhibition of 3A4 and to a lesser extent 2D6. Enfuvirtide, the fusion inhibitor, is not an inhibitor of CYP enzymes and does not alter the metabolism of CYP 3A4, CYP 2D6, CYP 2C19, or CYP 2E1 substrates. Thus, it has no significant impact on blood levels of psychiatric medications or other antiretrovirals (12).

Efavirenz has been shown in vivo to induce CYP 3A4 (12). Other compounds that are substrates of CYP 3A4 may have decreased plasma concentrations when coadministered with efavirenz. In vitro studies have demonstrated that efavirenz inhibits 2C9, 2C19, and 3A4 isoenzymes in the range of observed efavirenz plasma concentrations (13). Coadministration of efavirenz with drugs primarily metabolized by these isoenzymes may result in altered plasma concentrations of the coadministered drug. Therefore, appropriate dose adjustments may be necessary for these drugs.

Drugs that induce CYP 3A4 activity (e.g., phenobarbital, rifampin, rifabutin) would be expected to increase the clearance of efavirenz, resulting in lowered plasma concentrations (http: / /www.rxlist.com/cgi/generic/efaviren_ad.htm).

Antiretrovirals that inhibit or induce the CYP enzymes may increase or decrease methadone levels, leading to acute withdrawal symptoms or excessive dosing in otherwise stabilized methadone maintenance patients, which may lead to unfounded assumptions about opioid relapse (14–16).

TABLE 1. Useful Web Sites for Information on Drug-Drug Interactions

http://hivinsite.ucsf.edu/InSite?page=md-rr-24
http://www.projectinform.org/fs/druginter.html
http://www.rxlist.com/cgi/generic2/ritonavirsol_ad.htm
http://www.atforum.com/SiteRoot/pages/addiction_resources/Drug_Interactions.pdf
http://www.aidsetc.org/pdf/p02-et/et-03-00/pharm2005.pdf

It is important for psychiatrists to remain in contact with other medical providers, maintain updated lists of all medications and substances of abuse, and frequently consult updated web-based information sites regarding potential drug-drug interactions (17). Web sites (Table 1) provide the most up-to-date information about specific drug-drug interactions.

Central nervous system (CNS) side effects

Efavirenz has been reported to produce side effects including sleep disturbances and a transient neurovestibular symptom complex (18–20). Such side effects are common but generally short-term.

One randomized, controlled study of 100 patients supported the addition of efavirenz rather than a second drug from other classes of antiretrovirals for improved quality of life, despite a greater incidence of side effects; the study authors recommended, however, that patients with prior histories of emotional disturbances be monitored carefully over the long term (21). A cross-sectional study of 828 patients determined that factors independently associated with discontinuation of efavirenz were female gender, unemployment, a steady sexual partner, and multiple episodes of depression (22). Another cross-sectional study of 60 patients on regimens that included efavirenz and 60 patients on regimens that included a protease inhibitor found that mild and clinically tolerable neuropsychiatric disorders could persist after 2 years in patients receiving efavirenz; quality of life and psychological status remained good in both study groups (23).

In a study conducted by the AIDS Clinical Trials Group (24), efavirenz was associated not only with having vivid dreams but also with being off balance, having the sensation of falling over, feeling that the room is spinning, being unsteady in walking, feeling lightheaded, and being drowsy. Neuropsychological performance improved with initiation of therapy in an efavirenz-treated group compared with an NRTI-treated control group. Nevertheless, small negative significant correlations between efavirenz levels and neuropsychological performance persisted over time (24). Efavirenz causes subjective symptoms during the first week of treatment that are most consistently described as a vestibular disorder. Overall, sleep quality was not impaired by efavirenz and was improved at week 4 compared with the control group. Transient increases in vivid dreams associated with efavirenz use resolved by week 4 of therapy. No differences in changes of depressed mood or anxiety were detected. Overall, efavirenz-associated toxicities resolved without treatment by week 4 (24).

HIV-ASSOCIATED COGNITIVE-MOTOR DISORDERS

Cognitive-motor disorders in patients with HIV infection are common and may be progressive (25, 26). However, the incidence of HIV-associated dementia in the CART era has been reduced by 50%, and a similar reduction has been reported for minor cognitive-motor disorder. It is not yet clear whether this benefit persists over the long-term course of illness and treatment or which regimens are most effective in sustaining cognitive function. In developed countries, it has been suggested that the prevalence of cognitive disorders has increased because of the increased longevity of the patient population overall. It can be concluded that these disorders continue to be a significant source of morbidity among patients (25, 27, 28).

In many HIV patients with neurocognitive impairment, the impairment probably remains undiagnosed. Patients with HIV-associated cognitive-motor disorder may benefit from early intervention with combination antiretroviral therapy, as well as adjuvant treatments for the pathophysiological factors in the CNS that contribute to neurocognitive impairment. Available antiretroviral agents suppress HIV replication but do not eradicate the virus. The brain can serve as an important reservoir for the virus, contributing to an increased likelihood that a cognitive-motor disorder may develop over time.

Some antiretroviral agents can cross the blood-brain barrier and therefore decrease viral load in the cerebrospinal fluid. Improvements in neurocognitive function, however, have been shown even with regimens not containing cerebrospinal fluid (CSF)–penetrating antiretrovirals. In a study of 31 patients who received new antiretroviral treatment, patients whose regimens included CSF-penetrating agents showed greater reduction in CSF viral load and improved neuropsychological function. Treatment-naive patients had greater improvement in neuropsychological function than treatment-experienced patients (29). Other studies have not shown benefit, and thus the question of whether adding CSF-penetrating agents is beneficial is still controversial. Other immunological factors (i.e., chemokines, cytokines, tumor necrosis factor) are also implicated in the development of neuropathological changes leading to neurocognitive symptoms. Other factors that contribute to progression of cognitive disorders include age, concurrent methamphetamine use, and hepatitis coinfection (29–32).

CHANGES IN CLASSIFYING NEUROCOGNITIVE IMPAIRMENT

A June 13, 2005, conference (sponsored by the National Institute of Mental Health and the National Institute of Neurological Disorders and Stroke) on CNS disorders associated with HIV in developed and resource-limited settings included a meeting on revising the American Academy of Neurology criteria for HIV-associated cognitive-motor disorders (33). This conference identified and defined the diagnostic criteria for HIV-associated dementia and minor cognitive-motor disorder and added a condition: asymptomatic neurocognitive impairment. The proposed new criteria, described below, are expected to be published in early 2006.

Asymptomatic neurocognitive impairment occurs without any associated decrement in functional status. The presence of asymptomatic neurocognitive impairment poses a risk for progression to a cognitive-motor disorder, now to be termed *neurocognitive disorder.*

Mild neurocognitive disorder, previously termed *HIV-associated minor cognitive-motor disorder,* will now require neurocognitive impairment at least one standard deviation below the mean (normed for specific populations) in at least two neurocognitive domains, one of which must be primarily cognitive. This change from the criteria for minor cognitive-motor disorder reflects prioritization of deficits observed in the neurocognitive sphere over those observed in the motor and behavioral spheres. The criteria for mild neurocognitive disorder are determined by specific neuropsychological tests. In addition, a systematic exclusion of confounding conditions (e.g., opportunistic CNS disease, systemic illness, psychiatric illness, substance use disorders, or medications with CNS effects) is recommended. Where neuropsychological testing is unavailable, the criteria may also be determined by using an alternative clinical method (such as the HIV Dementia Scale or the International HIV Dementia Scale). Functional impairment is a necessary finding for a diagnosis of neurocognitive disorders.

HIV-associated dementia, previously termed *AIDS dementia complex,* is defined (for persons with moderate or severe impairment) as impairment within at least two cognitive domains that is greater than or equal to two standard deviations below the mean, or impairment within at least one cognitive domain that is greater than or equal to one standard deviation below the mean and impairment within one other domain that is greater than or equal to 2.5 standard deviations below the norm. Like the criteria for mild neurocognitive disorder, these criteria reflect prioritization of deficits observed in the neurocognitive sphere over those observed in the motor and behavioral spheres. The criteria are determined by specific neuropsychological tests that sample each of the neuropsychological domains as well as by a more systematic assessment of functional status and exclusion of confounding conditions. HIV dementia is more subcortical than cortical, and therefore clinical symptoms tend to involve motor functions, memory, mood with flattening of emotional range, apathy, and coarsening of personality. The HIV Dementia Scale is more sensitive to subcortical deficits than the Folstein Mini-Mental State Examination, which is directed mostly at cortical deficits and may not detect impairment until very late in the course of HIV dementia. Other tests directed at assessing psychomotor speed and subcortical processing, such as the grooved pegboard or Trail Making Test Part B, may be clinically useful. In resource-limited settings, alternative clinical methods may determine the criteria, after careful ruling out of other processes in the CNS that might account for the changes in mental status scores.

DEPRESSION

It has been established that depressive disorders among people with HIV infection may approach nearly 50% and that depression is associated with accelerated HIV disease progression, nonadherence to antiretroviral treatment, and mortality (34–37). Major depression remains underdiagnosed and undertreated in persons with HIV, especially African Americans, but using screening instruments can enhance detection (38, 39). In a double-blind, randomized, controlled trial of 25 patients infected with HIV, treatment of depression had a beneficial influence on health-related quality of life (40).

Psychotherapeutic or psychopharmacological treatments shown to be effective in other populations are useful also in the HIV-infected patient with co-occurring psychiatric disorders. Guidelines for the treatment of the major psychiatric disorders are available from APA (41).

To date, no specific antidepressant has been shown to be preferable or not to work in HIV patients, provided attention is paid to drug-drug interactions and sides effects that are more likely in the medically ill population. There are small studies of specific antidepressants and other agents. Mirtazapine, sustained-release bupropion, and venlafaxine seem to be effective, have at least equivalent tolerability to tricyclics and selective serotonin reuptake inhibitors, and do not have significant drug-drug interactions. Further studies to investigate these medications in a placebo-controlled fashion are still lacking (42–44).

A recent review described selective serotonin reuptake inhibitors as being safe and effective for the treatment of depression in patients with HIV and having better tolerability than tricyclic antidepressants (45). There is one report of serotonin syndrome occurring when antidepressants are used with some antiretrovirals (46).

There is also emerging evidence for other agents. A small, uncontrolled, open-label pilot study showed encouraging results for the use of modafinil to treat depressive symptoms and fatigue in patients with HIV (47). A small randomized, placebo-controlled trial showed significant improvement in mood and energy of HIV-infected men treated with dextroamphetamine (48). A large randomized, controlled trial did not support use of testosterone as a first-line treatment for depressive disorders in HIV-positive men; however, it was suggested that with additional study, testosterone may be indicated as a useful option for medically ill men experiencing significant fatigue as well as depression (49).

Cognitive behavior therapy groups, educational programs, and stress management techniques have also been shown to improve depression in patients with HIV (50–52). Psychodynamic, cognitive behavior, and interpersonal therapies are also applicable to the HIV population. A study by Nemeroff et al. (53) reported that in depressed patients with a history of early psychological trauma, psychotherapy alone was superior to psychopharmacology alone. Despite the methodological difficulties in such research, several studies have demonstrated the effectiveness of psychodynamic psychotherapy in depression (54–56) and in other psychiatric disorders, including personality disorders, which often co-occur with HIV and depression (57–60).

BIPOLAR DISORDERS AND PSYCHOSIS

There is a strong association between psychosis and HIV-related mood disorders (61). A retrospective review of the charts of 15 patients infected with HIV and receiving antiretroviral therapy suggested that the mood stabilizer divalproex sodium is well tolerated and does not increase viral load (62). In fact, new studies suggest that valproic acid might over time help to eradicate HIV from latent cells (63–65). Psychiatrists should closely monitor hepatic function and serum levels of valproic acid in the HIV patient, given the number of hepatically metabolized medications most patients with HIV have to take.

A study of 46 patients with HIV syndrome and mental illness showed that bipolar disorder was associated with nonadherence to antiretroviral therapy (66). A study of 2,459 New Jersey Medicaid beneficiaries found that patients with schizophrenia were not significantly less persistent in their use of antiretroviral therapy than those without serious mental illness, but patients with severe affective disorders were less persistent (67).

Primary psychosis can occur in HIV-positive patients, as can secondary psychoses associated with infectious, systemic, and cerebral complications of HIV infection (68). Case reports of psychosis, with or without manic features, have been associated with the use of efavirenz and other antiretroviral regimens, corticosteroids, antivirals such as ganciclovir and interferon-α, antimicrobials such as sulfadiazine and dapsone, and buspirone (69–72). One case of reversible coma associated with the use of ritonavir with risperidone has been reported (73). Concerns have grown about the metabolic complications associated with the use of second-generation (atypical) antipsychotics (see "Metabolic Syndrome and Lipodystrophy" below), although they remain better tolerated than first-generation antipsychotics in patients with HIV/AIDS (74).

HEPATITIS C VIRUS AND HIV INFECTION

HCV infection has become more prevalent in the general population and in the HIV-infected population. Overall, approximately 30% of all HIV-positive patients are HCV positive (75, 76). A recent study found a high prevalence of HCV among crystal methamphetamine users (77). Current evidence suggests that in patients treated with combination antiretroviral therapy, HCV infection may not increase HIV replication, but HIV infection appears to increase HCV replication, leading to more patients with coinfection having symptoms and medical illness related to their HCV infection. Studies have also shown that although HCV infection does not significantly change viral load or CD4 parameters in HIV-infected individuals, the survival time of such individuals is shortened (78, 79). Laboratory evidence suggests that HIV may facilitate HCV replication in monocytes, explaining the extrahepatic consequences of HCV in coinfected individuals (80).

Significant rates of HCV are found in patients with psychiatric disorders because of the high lifetime rates of intravenous drug use in the population with severe mental illness (81, 82). Psychiatric disorders are also prevalent in HCV-infected patients, as shown in Figure 1.

HIV, HCV, and cognitive impairment

Studies suggest that HCV may be able to replicate in the brain, and HCV has been associated with cognitive impairment independently of hepatic compromise. HCV viral load can be measured in the blood and CSF. HCV can cause cognitive impairment in the absence of systemic illness, elevated liver enzymes, or liver failure, and there appears to be an additive effect of HCV

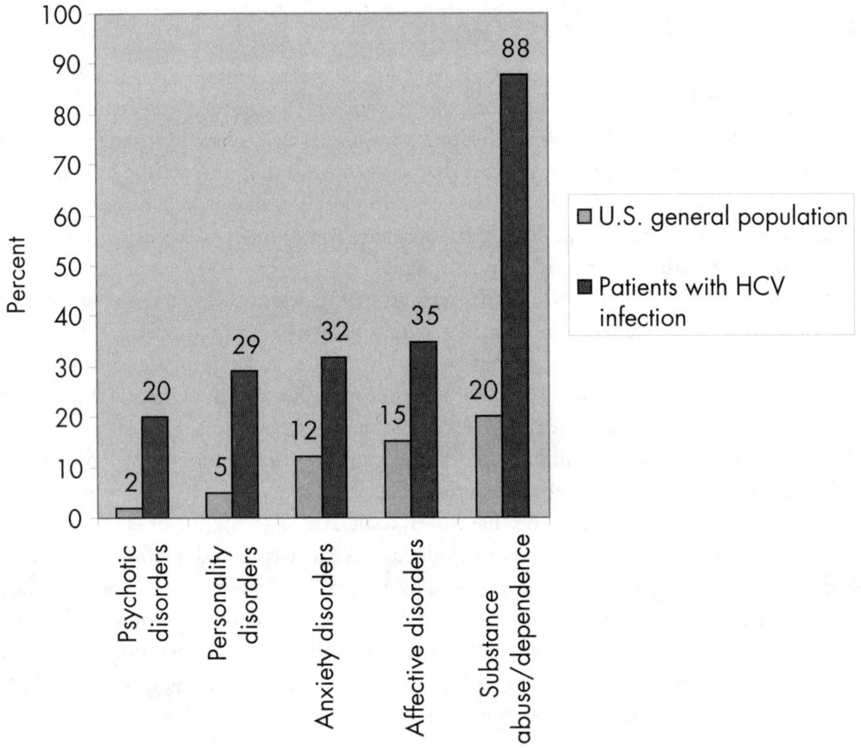

FIGURE 1. Prevalence of DSM-IV-TR Psychiatric Disorders in Patients With Hepatitis C, Compared With U.S. General Population.

Source. Reprinted with permission from Rifai and Rosenstein (83); data from Epidemiologic Catchment Area study (84, 85).

and HIV on cognitive dysfunction (86–88). Several studies have shown HCV infection to be a predictor of impairments in learning, abstraction, and motor skills in the HIV-negative population as well (77, 89, 90). In one study, 46% of HIV-positive/HCV-positive patients met criteria for HIV-associated dementia, as opposed to 10% of HIV-positive/HCV-negative patients; however, 45% of HIV-positive/HCV-negative patients met criteria for minor cognitive-motor disorder, as opposed to 23% of HIV-positive/HCV-positive patients (30). In advanced HCV disease, increasing ammonia levels can also lead to CNS impairment, usually reversible with appropriate treatment (77, 91).

Management of psychiatric consequences of HCV treatment

Psychiatrists are often asked to evaluate patients who have a current episode or history of mood disorders before the initiation of treatment for HCV. Depression is the most common side effect of interferon treatment with ribavirin for HCV infection. Current evidence of the value of antidepressant treatment in the non-HIV population suggests that antidepressant medication should be continued in those already being treated for depression and should be considered as prophylaxis in those with a prior history of depression (92, 93). A double-blind, randomized, controlled trial of 40 patients with malignant melanoma who received interferon treatment suggested that prophylactic treatment with paroxetine is an effective strategy for minimizing depression induced by interferon (94). A small open-label study suggested citalopram may be effective for depression in patients with HCV infection (95).

METABOLIC SYNDROME AND LIPODYSTROPHY

Since the 1990s, clinicians have observed changes in body morphology and metabolic parameters that appeared to be related to the combination antiretroviral treatment regimens that were prolonging and improving quality of life for people with HIV infection. Numerous factors contribute to body morphological changes, including antiretroviral therapy, HIV infection itself, and perhaps immune reconstitution occurring in the context of ongoing disease (96–100).

People with HIV present with body changes, including what is now called *lipoatrophy* and/or *lipohypertrophy* (also known together as the *lipodystrophy syndrome*). The associated profound metabolic abnormalities, such as hyperglycemia, hyperinsulinemia, hyperlipidemia, and hypertension, are now commonly referred to as the *metabolic syndrome.*

One of the reasons for the wide range of prevalence rates of metabolic syndrome reported in patients on protease inhibitor regimens (2%–84%) (96, 101–103) has been the lack of uniformity of definitions, criteria, and assessment methodology.

Risk factors for lipodystrophy include exposure to protease and nucleoside reverse transcriptase inhibitors, duration of use of a protease inhibitor or a nucleoside reverse transcriptase inhibitor, duration and severity of HIV disease, viral load, time since reversal of clinical progression of HIV infection, increasing age, female gender, and extreme changes in body mass index (104). Fat accumulation is correlated with female gender, low viral load, and high body mass index. Fat depletion is associated with low body mass index and the use of the nucleoside reverse transcriptase inhibitor stavudine (105).

A retrospective cohort study showed that 13% of 221 patients treated with protease inhibitor therapy for 5 years developed lipodystrophy, suggesting that the effect of antiretroviral medication may be an important contributor to the development of the syndrome (106).

Males are reported to be at greater risk of developing metabolic abnormalities, including hypertriglyceridemia, hypercholesterolemia, and hyperglycemia. Another study has suggested that mixed fat redistribution (concurrent fat wasting and fat accumulation) may be related to effective HIV suppression by combination antiretroviral therapy (107). The greatest risk factor identified thus far has been protease inhibitor use. Data from one study (96) showed that 64% of patients (74 of 116) receiving protease inhibitor therapy suffered from lipodystrophy, as opposed to only 3% of patients (1 of 32) who had never received protease inhibitor therapy.

Lipoatrophic changes are characterized by subcutaneous fat depletion in the face, arms, legs, and gluteal region. Muscles of the extremities may appear more pronounced, and veins may appear more prominent in fat-depleted regions. (The fat wasting observed in this syndrome is distinguished from other wasting conditions associated with HIV infection, including the AIDS wasting syndrome, malnutrition, cachexia, adrenal insufficiency, and severe chronic infections.) Lipohypertrophy is characterized by truncal obesity, dorsocervical fat accumulation (buffalo hump), and breast enlargement (108–112).

The lipodystrophy syndrome appears to increase risk in HIV-positive patients for cardiovascular and cerebrovascular disease (113). The hypercholesterolemia may predispose individuals to accelerated atherosclerosis and premature coronary artery disease (114–117). One retrospective study (118) of more than 1,300 patients demonstrated an increased frequency of myocardial infarction in HIV-infected patients receiving protease inhibitor therapy (119, 120).

Many HIV-infected patients may exhibit more than one risk factor for the development of coronary artery and cerebrovascular disease: hypertriglyceridemia, low high-density lipoprotein cholesterol, increased low-density lipoprotein cholesterol, elevated diastolic blood pressure, decreased tissue plasminogen activator levels, and increased plasminogen activator inhibitor–1 levels. The median time to the development of hypercholesterolemia may precede that of lipodystrophy by 3–6 months (121, 122).

It is important to consider a diagnosis of metabolic syndrome in patients receiving antiretroviral therapy who manifest insulin resistance, particularly if fat redistribution, dyslipidemia, or hyperglycemia is present. Second-generation antipsychotic medications, often prescribed for late-stage HIV-associated dementia, delirium, and psychotic disorders, can increase the risk of metabolic syndrome. Second-generation antipsychotics less associated with metabolic syndrome are ziprasidone and aripiprazole (123). Clozapine and olanzapine have been implicated in a greater risk for development of metabolic syndrome (123–126).

Currently, there are no medications or treatments approved by the U.S. Food and Drug Administration for metabolic syndrome, although the statin drugs are being used and specifically tested. There are controlled studies to suggest effective interventions to reverse the development of lipodystrophy syndrome; rosiglitazone (127) and pioglitazone are being used and specifically tested. However, use of psychiatric medications least likely to affect the metabolic parameters described above may reduce patients' risk for developing a metabolic syndrome.

The changes in body morphology may have significant psychological effects on people with HIV who are already living with a stigmatized illness. Development of lipodystrophy may contribute to nonadherence to antiretroviral medications or exacerbate mood and anxiety disorders. Psychiatrists can help patients with HIV whose treatments may adversely affect quality of life balance the competing wishes to sustain health and well-being.

ACKNOWLEDGMENT

The authors thank Kalonda Bradshaw, Natravis R. Cox, Darpun Dhawan, Leigh Ann Dooley, Lorraine E. Lothringer, Ana Elizabeth Miranda, Kristen C. Ochoa, Kathryn Suslov, Elizabeth Tien, and Arthur Jason Vaught for their contributions to this watch.

REFERENCES

1. American Psychiatric Association: Practice guideline for the treatment of patients with HIV/AIDS. Am J Psychiatry 2000; 157:1–62
2. UNAIDS: AIDS Epidemic Update: 2004. Geneva, Joint United Nations Programme on HIV/AIDS (UNAIDS), 2004. Also available: http://www.unaids.org/wad2004/report.html, 2004
3. UNAIDS: 2004 Report on the Global HIV/AIDS Epidemic: 4th Global Report. Geneva, Joint United Nations Programme on HIV/AIDS (UNAIDS), 2004. Also available: http://www.unaids.org/bangkok2004/report.html
4. Centers for Disease Control and Prevention: HIV/AIDS Surveillance Report, 2003 (vol 15). Atlanta, U.S. Department of Health and Human Services, Centers for Disease Control and Prevention, 2004. Also available: http://www.cdc.gov/hiv/stats/hasrlink.htm
5. McMahon JM, Tortu S, Pouget ER, Hamid R, Torres L: Increased sexual risk behaviour and high HIV sero-incidence among drug-using low-income women with primary heterosexual partners. Presented at the XV International AIDS Conference, Bangkok, Thailand, July 11–16, 2004. Abstract number TuOrD1220. Available at: http://www.iasociety.org/ejias/show.asp?abstract_id=2168225
6. Panel on Clinical Practice for the Treatment of HIV Infection: Guidelines for the Use of Antiretroviral Agents in HIV-1-Infected Adults and Adolescents. Washington, DC, U.S.

Department of Health and Human Services, 2005. Also available: http://aidsinfo.nih.gov/ContentFiles/AdultandAdolescentGL.pdf, 2005

7. Lafeuillade VA, Hittinger G, Chadapaud S, Poggi C: The HYDILE trial: a quadruple combination of nucleoside analog hydroxyurea and IL-2 as salvage therapy for HIV infection. Presented at the 9th Conference on Retroviruses and Opportunistic Infections, Seattle, WA, February 24–28, 2002. Abstract number 424-W. Available at: http:// www.retroconference.org/2002/Abstract/13005.htm
8. Gallant J: Choosing and using new antiretrovirals for multiclass-experienced HIV-infected patients. Symposium sponsored by University of Alabama School of Medicine and Clinical Care Options, Washington, DC, December 17, 2005. Available at: http://www.clinicaloptions.com/HIV/Treatment%20Updates/Choosing%20ARVs.aspx
9. Mitty JA, Macalino G, Taylor L, Harwell JI, Flanigan TP: Directly observed therapy (DOT) for individuals with HIV: successes and challenges. Med Gen Med 2005; 5(1):30
10. Flanigan TP, Taylor LE, Mitty JA: Use of community-based, directly observed therapy for HIV infection: lessons learned for treatment of hepatitis C virus infection. Clin Infect Dis 2005; 40(suppl 5):S346–S348
11. Yun LW, Maravi M, Kobayashi JS, Barton PL, Davidson AJ: Antidepressant treatment improves adherence to antiretroviral therapy among depressed HIV-infected patients. J Acquir Immune Defic Syndr 2005; 38:432–438
12. Wolbach-Lowes J, Jed SL, Johnson SC, Fletcher CV, Brown B: A Pharmacist's Guide to Antiretroviral Medications for HIV-Infected Adults and Adolescents. Denver, Mountain Plains AIDS Education and Training Center, University of Colorado at Denver and Health Sciences Center. Available at: http://www.aidsetc.org/pdf/p02-et/et-03-00/pharm2005.pdf
13. Hazen RJ, Harvey RJ, St Clair MH, Ferris RG, Freeman GA, Tidwell JH, Schaller LT, Cowan JR, Short SA, Romines KR, Chan JH, Boone LR: Anti-human immunodeficiency virus type 1 activity of the nonnucleoside reverse transcriptase inhibitor GW678248 in combination with other antiretrovirals against clinical isolate viruses and in vitro selection for resistance. Antimicrob Agents Chemother 2005; 49:4465–4473
14. Boffito M, Rossati A, Reynolds HE, Hoggard PG, Back DJ, Di Perri G: Undefined duration of opiate withdrawal induced by efavirenz in drug users with HIV infection and undergoing chronic methadone treatment. AIDS Res Hum Retroviruses 2002; 18:341–342
15. McCance-Katz EF, Rainey PM, Smith P, Morse G, Friedland G, Gourevitch M, Jatlow P: Drug interactions between opioids and antiretroviral medications: interaction between methadone, LAAM, and nelfinavir. Am J Addict 2004; 13:163–180
16. Stocker H, Kruse G, Kreckel P, Herzmann C, Arasteh K, Claus J, Jessen H, Cordes C, Hintsche B, Schlote F, Schneider L, Kurowski M: Nevirapine significantly reduces the levels of racemic methadone and (R)-methadone in human immunodeficiency virus-infected patients. Antimicrob Agents Chemother 2004; 48:4148–4153
17. Sandson NB, Armstrong SC, Cozza KL: An overview of psychotropic drug-drug interactions. Psychosomatics 2005; 46:464–494
18. Zaccarelli M, Soldani F, Liuzzi G, Sette P, Grisetti S, Trotta MP, Perno CF, Antinori A: CNS side effects as main risk factor for efavirenz failure and transient HIV-RNA elevation. Presented at the 9th Conference on Retroviruses and Opportunistic Infections, Seattle, Wash, February 24–28, 2002. Abstract number 720-T. Available at: http://www.retroconference.org/2002/Abstract/13744.htm
19. Welch KJ, Morse A: Association between efavirenz and selected psychiatric and neurological conditions. J Infect Dis 2002; 185:268–269
20. Marzolini C, Telenti A, Decosterd LA, Greub G, Biollaz J, Buclin T: Efavirenz plasma levels can predict treatment failure and central nervous system side effects in HIV-1-infected patients. AIDS 2001; 15:71–75

21. Fumaz CR, Tuldra A, Ferrer MJ, Paredes R, Bonjoch A, Jou T, Negredo E, Romeu J, Sirera G, Tural C, Clotet B: Quality of life, emotional status, and adherence of HIV-1-infected patients treated with efavirenz versus protease inhibitor-containing regimens. J Acquir Immune Defic Syndr 2002; 29:244–253
22. Spire B, Carrieri P, Garzot MA, L'henaff M, Obadia Y: Factors associated with efavirenz discontinuation in a large community-based sample of patients. AIDS Care 2004; 16:558–564
23. Fumaz CR, Munoz-Moreno JA, Molto J, Negredo E, Ferrer MJ, Sirera G, Perez-Alvarez N, Gomez G, Burger D, Clotet B: Long-term neuropsychiatric disorders on efavirenz-based approaches: quality of life, psychologic issues, and adherence. J Acquir Immune Defic Syndr 2005; 38:560–565
24. Clifford DB, Evans S, Yang Y, Acosta EP, Goodkin K, Tashima K, Simpson D, Dorfman D, Ribaudo H, Gulick RM: Impact of efavirenz on neuropsychological performance and symptoms in HIV-infected individuals. Ann Intern Med 2005; 143:714–721
25. Stern Y, McDermott MP, Albert S, Palumbo D, Selnes OA, McArthur J, Sacktor N, Schifitto G, Kieburtz K, Epstein L, Marder KS: Factors associated with incident human immunodeficiency virus-dementia. Arch Neurol 2001; 58:473–479
26. Maldonado J, Fernandez F: Neurobehavioral complications of HIV and AIDS, in Neuropsychiatry, 2nd ed. Edited by Fogel B, Schiffer R, Rao T, eds. Baltimore, Lippincott Williams & Wilkins, 2003, pp 1018–1033
27. Sacktor N, McDermott MP, Marder K, Schifitto G, Selnes OA, McArthur JC, Stern Y, Albert S, Palumbo D, Kieburtz K, De Marcaida JA, Cohen B, Epstein L: HIV-associated cognitive impairment before and after the advent of combination therapy. J Neurovirol 2002; 8:136–142
28. Starace F, Bartoli L, Aloisi MS, Antinori A, Narciso P, Ippolito G, Ravasio L, Moioli MC, Vangi D, Gennero L, Coronado OV, Giacometti A, Nappa S, Perulli ML, Montesarchio V, La Gala A, Ricci F, Cristiano L, De Marco M, Izzo C, Pezzotti P, D'Arminio MA: Cognitive and affective disorders associated to HIV infection in the HAART era: findings from the NeuroICONA study. Cognitive impairment and depression in HIV/AIDS. The NeuroICONA study. Acta Psychiatr Scand 2002; 106:20–26
29. Letendre SL, McCutchan JA, Childers ME, Woods SP, Lazzaretto D, Heaton RK, Grant I, Ellis RJ: Enhancing antiretroviral therapy for human immunodeficiency virus cognitive disorders. Ann Neurol 2004; 56:416–423
30. Ryan EL, Morgello S, Isaacs K, Naseer M, Gerits P: Neuropsychiatric impact of hepatitis C on advanced HIV. Neurology 2004; 62:957–962
31. Nukuna A, Gendelman HE, Limoges J, Rasmussen J, Poluektova L, Ghorpade A, Persidsky Y: Levels of human immunodeficiency virus type 1 (HIV-1) replication in macrophages determines the severity of murine HIV-1 encephalitis. J Neurovirol 2004; 10(suppl 1):82–90
32. Dou H, Kingsley JD, Mosley RL, Gelbard HA, Gendelman HE: Neuroprotective strategies for HIV-1 associated dementia. Neurotox Res 2004; 6:503–521
33. American Academy of Neurology: Nomenclature and research case definitions for neurologic manifestations of human immunodeficiency virus-type 1 (HIV-1) infection. Report of a Working Group of the American Academy of Neurology AIDS Task Force. Neurology 1991; 41:778–785
34. Bing EG, Burnam MA, Longshore D, Fleishman JA, Sherbourne CD, London AS, Turner BJ, Eggan F, Beckman R, Vitiello B, Morton SC, Orlando M, Bozzette SA, Ortiz-Barron L, Shapiro M: Psychiatric disorders and drug use among human immunodeficiency virus-infected adults in the United States. Arch Gen Psychiatry 2001; 58:721–728
35. Ammassari A, Antinori A, Aloisi MS, Trotta MP, Murri R, Bartoli L, Monforte AD, Wu AW, Starace F: Depressive symptoms, neurocognitive impairment, and adherence to highly active antiretroviral therapy among HIV-infected persons. Psychosomatics 2004; 45:394–402

36. Ickovics JR, Hamburger ME, Vlahov D, Schoenbaum EE, Schuman P, Boland RJ, Moore J: Mortality, CD4 cell count decline, and depressive symptoms among HIV-seropositive women: longitudinal analysis from the HIV Epidemiology Research Study. JAMA 2001; 285:1466–1474
37. Morrison MF, Petitto JM, Ten Have T, Gettes DR, Chiappini MS, Weber AL, Brinker-Spence P, Bauer RM, Douglas SD, Evans DL: Depressive and anxiety disorders in women with HIV infection. Am J Psychiatry 2002; 159:789–796
38. Asch SM, Kilbourne AM, Gifford AL, Burnam MA, Turner B, Shapiro MF, Bozzette SA: Underdiagnosis of depression in HIV: who are we missing? J Gen Intern Med 2003; 18:450–460
39. Kalichman SC, Rompa D, Cage M: Distinguishing between overlapping somatic symptoms of depression and HIV disease in people living with HIV-AIDS. J Nerv Ment Dis 2000; 188:662–670
40. Elliott AJ, Russo J, Roy-Byrne PP: The effect of changes in depression on health related quality of life (HRQoL) in HIV infection. Gen Hosp Psychiatry 2002; 24:43–47
41. American Psychiatric Association: American Psychiatric Association Practice Guidelines for the Treatment of Psychiatric Disorders: Compendium 2006. Arlington, Va, American Psychiatric Association, 2006
42. Klesmer J, Badescu R: Pharmacologic treatment of mood disorders in acquired immune deficiency syndrome (AIDS). Curr Psychiatry Rep 2002; 4:222–227
43. Currier MB, Molina G, Kato M: A prospective trial of sustained-release bupropion for depression in HIV-seropositive and AIDS patients. Psychosomatics 2003; 44:120–125
44. Elliott AJ, Roy-Byrne PP: Mirtazapine for depression in patients with human immunodeficiency virus. J Clin Psychopharmacol 2000; 20:265–267
45. Caballero J, Nahata MC: Use of selective serotonin-reuptake inhibitors in the treatment of depression in adults with HIV. Ann Pharmacother 2005; 39:141–145
46. DeSilva KE, Le Flore DB, Marston BJ, Rimland D: Serotonin syndrome in HIV-infected individuals receiving antiretroviral therapy and fluoxetine. AIDS 2001; 15:1281–1285
47. Rabkin JG, McElhiney MC, Rabkin R, Ferrando SJ: Modafinil treatment for fatigue in HIV+ patients: a pilot study. J Clin Psychiatry 2004; 65:1688–1695
48. Wagner GJ, Rabkin R: Effects of dextroamphetamine on depression and fatigue in men with HIV: a double-blind, placebo-controlled trial. J Clin Psychiatry 2000; 61:436–440
49. Rabkin JG, Wagner GJ, McElhiney MC, Rabkin R, Lin SH: Testosterone versus fluoxetine for depression and fatigue in HIV/AIDS: a placebo-controlled trial. J Clin Psychopharmacol 2004; 24:379–385
50. Blanch J, Rousaud A, Hautzinger M, Martinez E, Peri JM, Andres S, Cirera E, Gatell JM, Gasto C: Assessment of the efficacy of a cognitive-behavioural group psychotherapy programme for HIV-infected patients referred to a consultation-liaison psychiatry department. Psychother Psychosom 2002; 71:77–84
51. Weiss JL, Mulder CL, Antoni MH, de Vroome EM, Garssen B, Goodkin K: Effects of a supportive-expressive group intervention on long-term psychosocial adjustment in HIV-infected gay men. Psychother Psychosom 2003; 72:132–140
52. Antoni MH: Stress management and psychoneuroimmunology in HIV infection. CNS Spectr 2003; 8:40–51
53. Nemeroff CB, Heim CM, Thase ME, Klein DN, Rush AJ, Schatzberg AF, Ninan PT, McCullough JP Jr, Weiss PM, Dunner DL, Rothbaum BO, Kornstein S, Keitner G, Keller MB: Differential responses to psychotherapy versus pharmacotherapy in patients with chronic forms of major depression and childhood trauma. Proc Natl Acad Sci USA 2003; 100:14293–14296
54. Tyll MD, Goodkin K, Blaney TT, Baldewicz JD, Hunt, Asthana D: Theory-driven interventions in psychoneuroimmunology. CNS Spectr 2000; 5:25–32

55. Bond M, Perry JC: Long-term changes in defense styles with psychodynamic psychotherapy for depressive, anxiety, and personality disorders. Am J Psychiatry 2004; 161:1665–1671
56. Abbass A: Intensive short-term dynamic psychotherapy in a private psychiatric office: clinical and cost effectiveness. Am J Psychother 2002; 56:225–232
57. Leichsenring F, Leibing E: The effectiveness of psychodynamic therapy and cognitive behavior therapy in the treatment of personality disorders: a meta-analysis. Am J Psychiatry 2003; 160:1223–1232
58. Leichsenring F, Rabung S, Leibing E: The efficacy of short-term psychodynamic psychotherapy in specific psychiatric disorders: a meta-analysis. Arch Gen Psychiatry 2004; 61:1208–1216
59. Vinnars B, Barber JP, Noren K, Gallop R, Weinryb RM: Manualized supportive-expressive psychotherapy versus nonmanualized community-delivered psychodynamic therapy for patients with personality disorders: bridging efficacy and effectiveness. Am J Psychiatry 2005; 162:1933–1940
60. Svartberg M, Stiles TC, Seltzer MH: Randomized, controlled trial of the effectiveness of short-term dynamic psychotherapy and cognitive therapy for cluster C personality disorders. Am J Psychiatry 2004; 161:810–817
61. Uldall KK, Harris VL, Lalonde B: Outcomes associated with delirium in acutely hospitalized acquired immune deficiency syndrome patients. Compr Psychiatry 2000; 41:88–91
62. Maggi JD, Halman MH: The effect of divalproex sodium on viral load: a retrospective review of HIV-positive patients with manic syndromes. Can J Psychiatry 2001; 46:359–362
63. Lehrman G, Hogue IB, Palmer S, Jennings C, Spina CA, Wiegand A, Landay AL, Coombs RW, Richman DD, Mellors JW, Coffin JM, Bosch RJ, Margolis DM: Depletion of latent HIV-1 infection in vivo: a proof-of-concept study. Lancet 2005; 366:549–555
64. Routy JP: Valproic acid: a potential role in treating latent HIV infection. Lancet 2005; 366:523–524
65. Smith SM: Valproic acid and HIV-1 latency: beyond the sound bite. Retrovirology 2005; 2:56
66. Kemppainen JK, Levine R, Buffum M, Holzemer W, Finley P, Jensen P: Antiretroviral adherence in persons with HIV/AIDS and severe mental illness. J Nerv Ment Dis 2004; 192:395–404
67. Walkup JT, Sambamoorthi U, Crystal S: Use of newer antiretroviral treatments among HIV-infected Medicaid beneficiaries with serious mental illness. J Clin Psychiatry 2004; 65:1180–1189
68. Alciati A, Fusi A, D'Arminio MA, Coen M, Ferri A, Mellado C: New-onset delusions and hallucinations in patients infected with HIV. J Psychiatry Neurosci 2001; 26:229–234
69. Puzantian T, Lee J, Karasic D, et al: Psychiatric effects associated with efavirenz: a retrospective study. Presented at the 41st annual meeting of the Infectious Disease Society of America, Chicago, October 24–27, 2002. Abstract number 481
70. Foster R, Olajide D, Everall IP: Antiretroviral therapy-induced psychosis: case report and brief review of the literature. HIV Med 2003; 4:139–144
71. Wise ME, Mistry K, Reid S: Drug points: neuropsychiatric complications of nevirapine treatment. BMJ 2002; 324:879
72. Hoffman RG, Cohen MA, Alfonso CA, Weiss JJ, Jones S, Keller M, Condemarin JR, Chiu NM, Jacobson JM: Treatment of interferon-induced psychosis in patients with comorbid hepatitis C and HIV. Psychosomatics 2003; 44:417–420
73. Jover F, Cuadrado JM, Andreu L, Merino J: Reversible coma caused by risperidone-ritonavir interaction. Clin Neuropharmacol 2002; 25:251–253
74. Bagchi A, Sambamoorthi U, McSpiritt E, Yanos P, Walkup J, Crystal S: Use of antipsychotic medications among HIV-infected individuals with schizophrenia. Schizophr Res 2004; 71:435–444

75. Sulkowski MS, Thomas DL: Hepatitis C in the HIV-infected person. Ann Intern Med 2003; 138:197–207
76. Rockstroh JK, Mocroft A, Soriano V, Tural C, Losso MH, Horban A, Kirk O, Phillips A, Ledergerber B, Lundgren J: Influence of hepatitis C virus infection on HIV-1 disease progression and response to highly active antiretroviral therapy. J Infect Dis 2005; 192:992–1002
77. Cherner M, Letendre S, Heaton RK, Durelle J, Marquie-Beck J, Gragg B, Grant I: Hepatitis C augments cognitive deficits associated with HIV infection and methamphetamine. Neurology 2005; 64:1343–1347
78. Anderson KB, Guest JL, Rimland D: Hepatitis C virus coinfection increases mortality in HIV-infected patients in the highly active antiretroviral therapy era: data from the HIV Atlanta VA Cohort Study. Clin Infect Dis 2004; 39:1507–1513
79. Braitstein P, Yip B, Montessori V, Moore D, Montaner JS, Hogg RS: Effect of serostatus for hepatitis C virus on mortality among antiretrovirally naive HIV-positive patients. CMAJ 2005; 173:160–164
80. Laskus T, Radkowski M, Jablonska J, Kibler K, Wilkinson J, Adair D, Rakela J: Human immunodeficiency virus facilitates infection/replication of hepatitis C virus in native human macrophages. Blood 2004; 103:3854–3859
81. Carey MP, Carey KB, Kalichman SC: Risk for human immunodeficiency virus (HIV) infection among persons with severe mental illnesses. Clin Psychol Rev 1997; 17:271–291
82. Susser E, Miller M, Valencia E, Colson P, Roche B, Conover S: Injection drug use and risk of HIV transmission among homeless men with mental illness. Am J Psychiatry 1996; 153: 794–798
83. Rifai MA, Rosenstein DL: Hepatitis C and psychiatry. Focus 2005; 3:194–202
84. Regier DA, Narrow WE, Rae DS, Manderscheid RW, Locke BZ, Goodwin FK: The de facto US mental and addictive disorders service system: Epidemiologic Catchment Area prospective 1-year prevalence rates of disorders and services. Arch Gen Psychiatry 1993; 50:85–94
85. Norquist GS, Regier DA: The epidemiology of psychiatric disorders and the de facto mental health care system. Annu Rev Med 1996; 47:473–479
86. Hilsabeck RC, Perry W, Hassanein TI: Neuropsychological impairment in patients with chronic hepatitis C. Hepatology 2002; 35:440–446
87. Back-Madruga C, Fontana R, Bieliauskas L, et al: Predictors of cognitive impairment in chronic hepatitis C patients entering the HALT-C trial. J Int Neuropsychol Soc 2003; 9:245–246
88. Hilsabeck RC, Hassanein TI, Carlson MD, Ziegler EA, Perry W: Cognitive functioning and psychiatric symptomatology in patients with chronic hepatitis C. J Int Neuropsychol Soc (in press)
89. Kramer L, Bauer E, Funk G, Hofer H, Jessner W, Steindl-Munda P, Wrba F, Madl C, Gangl A, Ferenci P: Subclinical impairment of brain function in chronic hepatitis C infection. J Hepatol 2002; 37:349–354
90. Hilsabeck RC, Castellon SA, Hinkin CH: Neuropsychological aspects of coinfection with HIV and hepatitis C virus. Clin Infect Dis 2005; 41(suppl 1):S38–S44
91. Forton DM, Thomas HC, Taylor-Robinson SD: Central nervous system involvement in hepatitis C virus infection. Metab Brain Dis 2004; 19:383–391
92. Laguno M, Blanch J, Murillas J, Blanco JL, Leon A, Lonca M, Larrousse M, Biglia A, Martinez E, Garcia F, Miro JM, de Pablo J, Gatell JM, Mallolas J: Depressive symptoms after initiation of interferon therapy in human immunodeficiency virus-infected patients with chronic hepatitis C. Antivir Ther 2004; 9:905–909
93. Corcoran CP: Neuropsychiatric changes in HIV/hepatitis C coinfected patients undergoing interferon therapy. J Assoc Nurses AIDS Care 2003; 14(5 suppl):80S–86S
94. Musselman DL, Lawson DH, Gumnick JF, Manatunga AK, Penna S, Goodkin RS, Greiner K, Nemeroff CB, Miller AH: Paroxetine for the prevention of depression induced by high-dose interferon alfa. N Engl J Med 2001; 344:961–966

95. Gleason OC, Yates WR, Isbell MD, Philipsen MA: An open-label trial of citalopram for major depression in patients with hepatitis C. J Clin Psychiatry 2002; 63:194–198
96. Carr A, Samaras K, Burton S, Law M, Freund J, Chisholm DJ, Cooper DA: A syndrome of peripheral lipodystrophy, hyperlipidaemia and insulin resistance in patients receiving HIV protease inhibitors. AIDS 1998; 12:F51–F58
97. Henry K: Lipid abnormalities associated with use of protease inhibitors: prevalence, clinical sequelae and treatment, in Program of the 12th World AIDS Conference. Geneva, Marathon Multimedia, 1998. Abstract number 12319
98. Walli R, Herfort O, Michl GM, Demant T, Jager H, Dieterle C, Bogner JR, Landgraf R, Goebel FD: Treatment with protease inhibitors associated with peripheral insulin resistance and impaired oral glucose tolerance in HIV-1-infected patients. AIDS 1998; 12:F167–F173
99. Vigouroux C, Gharakhanian S, Salhi Y, Nguyen TH, Chevenne D, Capeau J, Rozenbaum W: Diabetes, insulin resistance and dyslipidaemia in lipodystrophic HIV-infected patients on highly active antiretroviral therapy (HAART). Diabetes Metab 1999; 25:225–232
100. Hadigan C, Miller K, Corcoran C, Anderson E, Basgoz N, Grinspoon S: Fasting hyperinsulinemia and changes in regional body composition in human immunodeficiency virus-infected women. J Clin Endocrinol Metab 1999; 84:1932–1937
101. Gervasoni C, Ridolfo AL, Trifiro G, Santambrogio S, Norbiato G, Musicco M, Clerici M, Galli M, Moroni M: Redistribution of body fat in HIV-infected women undergoing combined antiretroviral therapy. AIDS 1999; 13:465–471
102. Saint-Marc T, Partisani M, Poizot-Martin I, Bruno F, Rouviere O, Lang JM, Gastaut JA, Touraine JL: A syndrome of peripheral fat wasting (lipodystrophy) in patients receiving long-term nucleoside analogue therapy. AIDS 1999; 13:1659–1667
103. Carr A, Samaras K, Thorisdottir A, Kaufmann GR, Chisholm DJ, Cooper DA: Diagnosis, prediction, and natural course of HIV-1 protease-inhibitor-associated lipodystrophy, hyperlipidaemia, and diabetes mellitus: a cohort study. Lancet 1999; 353:2093–2099
104. Miller JE, Emery S, French M, Baker D, Cooper DA: The Australian prevalence survey of lipodystrophy. Presented at the 7th Conference on Retroviruses and Opportunistic Infections, San Francisco, January 30–February 4, 2000. Abstract number 201. Available at: http://www.retroconference.org/2000/Abstracts/201.htm
105. Galli M, Cozzi-Lepri A, Ridolfo AL, Gervasoni C, Ravasio L, Corsico L, Gianelli E, Vaccarezza M, Vullo V, Cargnel A, Minoli L, Coronado O, Giacometti A, Antinori A, Antonucci G, D'Arminio MA, Moroni M: Incidence of adipose tissue alterations in first-line antiretroviral therapy: the LipoICoNa Study. Arch Intern Med 2002; 162:2621–2628
106. Tsiodras S, Mantzoros C, Hammer S, Samore M: Effects of protease inhibitors on hyperglycemia, hyperlipidemia, and lipodystrophy: a 5-year cohort study. Arch Intern Med 2000; 160:2050–2056
107. Saint-Marc T, Partisani M, Poizot-Martin I, Rouviere O, Bruno F, Avellaneda R, Lang JM, Gastaut JA, Touraine JL: Fat distribution evaluated by computed tomography and metabolic abnormalities in patients undergoing antiretroviral therapy: preliminary results of the LIPOCO study. AIDS 2000; 14:37–49
108. Capeau J, Magre J, Lascols O, Caron M, Bereziat V, Vigouroux C, Bastard JP: Diseases of adipose tissue: genetic and acquired lipodystrophies. Biochem Soc Trans 2005; 33:1073–1077
109. Giordano N, Amendola A, Papakostas P, Cipolli F, Agate VM, Martini G, Figura N, Nuti R: Possible pathogenetic role of antiphospholipid antibodies in a clinical case of human immunodeficiency virus infection with peripheral polyneuropathy and arterial thrombosis. New Microbiol 2005; 28:261–263
110. Shaw AJ, McLean KA, Evans BA: Disorders of fat distribution in HIV infection. Int J STD AIDS 1998; 9:595–599
111. Kotler DP, Rosenbaum K, Wang J, Pierson RN: Studies of body composition and fat distribution in HIV-infected and control subjects. J Acquir Immune Defic Syndr Hum Retrovirol 1999; 20:228–237

112. Lo JC, Mulligan K, Tai VW, Algren H, Schambelan M: "Buffalo hump" in men with HIV-1 infection. Lancet 1998; 351:867–870
113. Maggi P, Serio G, Epifani G, Fiorentino G, Saracino A, Fico C, Perilli F, Lillo A, Ferraro S, Gargiulo M, Chirianni A, Angarano G, Regina G, Pastore G: Premature lesions of the carotid vessels in HIV-1-infected patients treated with protease inhibitors. AIDS 2000; 14:F123–F128
114. Henry K, Melroe H, Huebsch J, Hermundson J, Levine C, Swensen L, Daley J: Severe premature coronary artery disease with protease inhibitors. Lancet 1998; 351:1328
115. Flynn TE, Bricker LA: Myocardial infarction in HIV-infected men receiving protease inhibitors. Ann Intern Med 1999; 131:548
116. Mary-Krause M, Cotte L, Partisani M, Simon A, Costagliola D: Impact of treatment with protease inhibitor (PI) on myocardial infarction (MI) occurrence in HIV-infected men. Presented at the 8th Conference on Retroviruses and Opportunistic Infections, Chicago, February 4–8, 2001. Abstract number 657. Available at: http://www.retroconference.org/2001/Abstracts/Abstracts/Abstracts/657.htm
117. Klein D, Hurley L, Sorel M, Sidney S: Do protease inhibitors increase the risk for coronary heart disease among HIV positive patients-follow-up. Presented at the 8th Conference on Retroviruses and Opportunistic Infections, Chicago, February 4–8, 2001. Abstract number 655. Available at: http://www.retroconference.org/2001/Abstracts/Abstracts/Abstracts/655.htm
118. Juette A, Salzberger B, Franzen C, Roemer K, Diehl V, Faetkenheuer G: Increased morbidity from severe coronary heart disease in HIV-patients receiving protease inhibitors.Presented at the 6th Conference on Retroviruses and Opportunistic Infections, Chicago, January 31–February 4, 1999. Abstract number 656. Available at: http://www.retroconference.org/1999/Abstracts/656.htm
119. Cohen CJ: Ritonavir-boosted protease inhibitors, 2: cardiac implications of lipid alterations. AIDS Read. 2005; 15:528
120. Zareba KM, Miller TL, Lipshultz SE: Cardiovascular disease and toxicities related to HIV infection and its therapies. Expert Opin Drug Saf 2005; 4:1017–1025
121. Keruly J, Mehta S, Chaisson RE, Moore RD: Incidence of and factors associated with the development of hypercholesterolemia and hyperglycemia in HIV-infected patients using a protease inhibitor, in Program of the 38th Interscience Conference on Antimicrobial Agents and Chemotherapy, San Diego, September 24–27, 1998. Abstract number I-95
122. Mann M, Piazza-Hepp T, Koller E, Gibert C: Abnormal fat distribution in AIDS patients following protease inhibitor therapy: FDA summary. Presented at the 5th Conference on Retroviruses and Opportunistic Infections, Chicago, February 1–5, 1998. Abstract number 412. Available at: http://www.retroconference.org/1998/Abstracts/412.htm
123. Mackin P, Watkinson HM, Young AH: Prevalence of obesity, glucose homeostasis disorders and metabolic syndrome in psychiatric patients taking typical or atypical antipsychotic drugs: a cross-sectional study. Diabetologia 2005; 48:215–221
124. Newcomer JW, Nasrallah HA: A review of metabolic issues in atypical antipsychotic treatment. Advanced Studies in Medicine 2004; 4:S1045–S1058
125. Goff DC, Sullivan LM, McEvoy JP, Meyer JM, Nasrallah HA, Daumit GL, Lamberti S, D'Agostino RB, Stroup TS, Davis S, Lieberman JA: A comparison of ten-year cardiac risk estimates in schizophrenia patients from the CATIE study and matched controls. Schizophr Res 2005; 80:45–53
126. Lieberman JA, Stroup TS, McEvoy JP, Swartz MS, Rosenheck RA, Perkins DO, Keefe RS, Davis SM, Davis CE, Lebowitz BD, Severe J, Hsiao JK: Effectiveness of antipsychotic drugs in patients with chronic schizophrenia. N Engl J Med 2005; 353:1209–1223
127. van Wijk JP, de Koning EJ, Cabezas MC, op't Roodt J, Joven J, Rabelink TJ, Hoepelman AI: Comparison of rosiglitazone and metformin for treating HIV lipodystrophy: a randomized trial. Ann Intern Med 2005; 143:337–346

PRACTICE GUIDELINE FOR THE Treatment of Patients With HIV/AIDS

WORK GROUP ON HIV/AIDS

J. Stephen McDaniel, M.D., Chair

Larry Brown, M.D.
Francine Cournos, M.D.
Marshall Forstein, M.D.
Karl Goodkin, M.D., Ph.D.
Constantine Lyketsos, M.D., M.H.S.
Joyce Y. Chung, M.D. (Consultant)

Originally published in November 2000. A guideline watch, summarizing significant developments in the scientific literature since publication of this guideline, may be available in the Psychiatric Practice section of the APA web site at www.psych.org.

CONTENTS

Introduction 191

Development Process 192

Part A: Background Information and Treatment Recommendations for Patients With HIV/AIDS 193

I. Summary of Treatment Recommendations 193
- A. Coding System 193
- B. General Considerations 193

II. Disease Definition, Epidemiology, and Natural History 196
- A. Basic Facts About HIV Infection, AIDS, and Treatments 196
- B. Associated Features of Neuropsychiatric and Psychosocial Importance 204
- C. Prevalence of Comorbid Psychiatric Conditions 210

III. Formulation and Implementation of a Treatment Plan 211
- A. Individuals at High Risk for HIV Infection 211
- B. HIV-Infected Individuals 215

IV. Clinical and Environmental Features Influencing Treatment 223
- A. Sociodemographic Variables 223
- B. Clinical Features 226
- C. Special Treatment Situations 229

Part B: Review and Synthesis of Available Evidence 230

V. Data Regarding Prevention for Individuals at High Risk for HIV Infection 230
- A. HIV-Related Risk Assessment of Behavior 230
- B. HIV Antibody Testing 231
- C. Interventions to Reduce HIV Risk Behavior 231
- D. Reducing Maternal-Fetal Transmission 233
- E. Postexposure Prophylaxis 234
- F. Special Psychiatric Populations 234

VI. Data Regarding Psychiatric Treatments for Individuals With HIV Infection 235
A. Access to Services 236
B. Pharmacologic Treatment 237
C. Psychosocial Treatment 246
D. Legal and Ethical Issues 247
E. Adherence to Treatment 248
F. Specific Syndromes 250

Part C: Future Research Needs 261

Individuals and Organizations That Submitted Comments 265

References 266

INTRODUCTION

This practice guideline seeks to summarize data and specific forms of treatment regarding the care of patients with HIV/AIDS. The purpose of this guideline is to assist the psychiatrist in caring for a patient with HIV/AIDS.

Psychiatrists care for patients with HIV/AIDS in many different settings and serve a variety of functions. In many cases, a psychiatrist will serve as a consultant to the patient's primary care physician. This guideline reviews the treatment that patients with HIV/AIDS may need. The psychiatrist should either provide or advocate for the appropriate treatments.

To share feedback on this or other published APA practice guidelines, a form is available at http://www.psych.org/psych_pract/pg/reviewform.cfm.

DEVELOPMENT PROCESS

This document is a practical guide to the management of patients—primarily adults over the age of 18—with HIV/AIDS and represents a synthesis of current scientific knowledge and rational clinical practice. This guideline strives to be as free as possible of bias toward any theoretical approach to treatment.

This practice guideline was developed under the auspices of the Steering Committee on Practice Guidelines. The process is detailed in the Appendix to this volume. Key features of the process include the following:

- a comprehensive literature review (description follows) and development of evidence tables;
- initial drafting by a work group that included psychiatrists with clinical and research expertise in HIV/AIDS;
- the production of multiple drafts with widespread review, in which 14 organizations and over 60 individuals submitted significant comments;
- approval by the APA Assembly and Board of Trustees; and
- planned revisions at regular intervals.

A computerized search of the relevant literature from MEDLINE, PsycINFO, EMBASE, and AIDSLINE was conducted.

The first literature search was conducted by using MEDLINE for the period from 1966 to June 1998 and used the key words "acquired immunodeficiency syndrome," "HIV," "dementia," "mood disorders," "anxiety," "sleep," "depression mania," "substance use," and "adjustment disorders."

The literature search conducted by using PsycINFO covered the period from 1967 to March 1998 and used the key words "acquired immune deficiency syndrome," "adjustment disorders," "human immunodeficiency virus," "dementia," and "mood disorders."

The literature search conducted by using EMBASE covered the period from 1980 to 1998 and used the key words "acquired immune deficiency syndrome," "adjustment disorders," "human immunodeficiency virus," "manic depressive psychosis," "depression," and "mood disorders."

The literature search conducted by using AIDSLINE covered the period from 1980 to 1998 and used the key words "acquired immunodeficiency syndrome," "HIV," "adjustment disorders," "psychotherapy," "dementia," "treatment," "therapy," "therapeutic," and "mood disorders."

An additional literature search was conducted by using MEDLINE for the period from 1990 to 1999 and used the key words "correctional settings," "jail," "women," "minorities," and "suicide."

Additional, less formal, literature searches were conducted by APA staff and individual members of the work group on HIV/AIDS.

PART A:
BACKGROUND INFORMATION AND TREATMENT RECOMMENDATIONS FOR PATIENTS WITH HIV/AIDS

I. SUMMARY OF TREATMENT RECOMMENDATIONS

The following executive summary is intended to provide an overview of the organization and scope of recommendations in this practice guideline. Because psychiatric treatment of patients with HIV/AIDS requires the consideration of many factors, it cannot be adequately reviewed in a brief summary. The reader is encouraged to consult the relevant portions of the guideline when specific treatment recommendations are sought. This summary is not intended to stand on its own.

A. CODING SYSTEM

Each recommendation is identified as falling into one of three categories of endorsement, indicated by a bracketed Roman numeral following the statement. The three categories represent varying levels of clinical confidence regarding the recommendation:

[I] Recommended with substantial clinical confidence.
[II] Recommended with moderate clinical confidence.
[III] May be recommended on the basis of individual circumstances.

B. GENERAL CONSIDERATIONS

All psychiatrists need to have an adequate fund of knowledge about HIV/AIDS. Because scientific knowledge regarding virology, prevention, and interventions to treat HIV infection advances rapidly, this guideline attempts to summarize current knowledge and principles of treatment with the expectation that updated information will be needed. For this reason, several pertinent web site addresses have been included both in the text and in an appendix at the end of the guideline. The reader is encouraged to use the web sites to search for additional or more current information that will supplement the information provided in this guideline. Section II provides information about the following: the pathophysiology and virology of HIV, the epidemiology of HIV/AIDS, transmission of HIV, pathogenesis of HIV, assessment and staging of HIV disease, treatment for HIV infection, impact of HIV on the central nervous system, neuropsychiatric clinical syndromes, differential diagnosis of neuropsychiatric syndromes, pediatric HIV/AIDS syndromes, and prevalence of comorbid psychiatric conditions.

Section III serves as a guide for formulating and implementing a treatment plan, and its outline is mirrored in Sections V and VI, in which the data regarding prevention and treatment, respectively, are provided. Readers may find it useful to first read Section III and then refer to Sections V and VI for the scientific evidence on which the treatment recommendations have been made.

Because there are many clinical and environmental features that may influence treatment, Section IV provides additional information on sociodemographic variables such as race/ethnicity, sexual orientation, gender, age, economic factors, and setting (urban versus rural). Specific clinical topics of suicidality, bereavement, axis II disorders, and psychoneuroimmunology are also covered. Last, information about special treatment situations such as alternative/complementary treatments, institutional settings, and health care clinician issues is included.

1. Psychiatric management of individuals at high risk for HIV infection

Psychiatrists may encounter patients in the course of their clinical work who are at risk for acquiring HIV infection. Optimum management of patients at high risk for HIV infection uses a wide range of psychiatric skills such as comprehensive diagnostic evaluations, assessment of possible medical causes of new-onset symptoms, initiation of specific treatment interventions, and a keen understanding of psychodynamic issues [I]. Patients with substance use disorders, patients with severe mental illness, and victims of sexual abuse/crimes have specific risks for becoming infected with HIV [I]. Psychiatric management of individuals who, because of specific behaviors, are at risk for HIV infection involves obtaining a risk history, considering the need for HIV antibody testing, initiating risk reduction strategies, and initiating postexposure prophylaxis with antiretroviral medication when indicated. A psychiatrist will not be aware of a patient's risk for HIV infection unless risk behavior is accurately assessed [I]. Psychiatrists should be knowledgeable about which specific risk behaviors are more likely to result in HIV transmission [I]. Psychiatric units or individual practitioners who conduct HIV testing should be aware of their obligation to provide the necessary pre- and posttest counseling [I]. Because successful risk reduction requires more than knowledge of risk, ongoing discussions between patient and psychiatrist can help provide the motivating and skill-building factors that help ensure consistent changes in behavior [II].

Psychiatrists serve as primary clinicians of both medical and psychiatric care in some institutional settings. Thus, administrators of these facilities should formulate policies that support the full range of HIV prevention steps outlined in this guideline [I]. Postexposure prophylaxis is recommended for known occupational exposure, especially percutaneous or mucous membrane exposure, to blood or other body fluids [I]. The American College of Obstetricians and Gynecologists now recommends that an HIV antibody test be offered during annual exams to all women seeking preconception care, not just pregnant women [II].

2. Psychiatric management of HIV-infected individuals

Specific tasks that constitute the psychiatric management of patients with HIV/AIDS include the following: establishing and maintaining a therapeutic alliance; collaboration and coordination of care with other mental health and medical providers; diagnosing and treating all associated psychiatric disorders; facilitating adherence to the overall treatment plan; providing education about psychological, psychiatric, and neuropsychiatric disorders; providing risk reduction strategies to further minimize the spread of HIV; maximizing psychological and social/adaptive functioning; considering the role of religion/spirituality; preparing the patient for issues of disability, death, and dying; and advising significant others/family regarding sources of care and support.

The development of a psychiatric treatment plan for patients with HIV infection requires thoughtful and comprehensive consideration of the biopsychosocial context of the illness [I].

TABLE 2. Risk of HIV Transmission Associated With Various Sexual Activities

Risk Level	Sexual Activity
No risk	Dry kissing Body-to-body rubbing Massage Nipple stimulation Using unshared inserted sexual devices Being masturbated by partner without semen or vaginal fluids Erotic bathing and showering Contact with feces or urine on intact skin
Theoretical risk	Wet kissing Cunnilingus with barrier Anilingus Digital-anal and digital-vaginal intercourse, with or without glove Using shared but disinfected inserted sexual devices
Low risk	Sharing nondisinfected personal hygiene items (razors, toothbrushes) Cunnilingus without barrier during or outside menstruation Fellatio and ejaculation, with or without ingestion of semen Fellatio, with or without condom Penile-vaginal intercourse with condom Penile-anal intercourse with condom
High risk	Penile-vaginal intercourse without condom Penile-anal intercourse without condom Coitus interruptus (intercourse with withdrawal before ejaculation)

Source. From Counselling Guidelines for HIV Testing (6).

transmission has been documented in both directions. Penile-anal and penile-vaginal intercourse are considered the highest risk behaviors, with transmission more likely in the presence of other sexually transmitted diseases or genital lesions or during sexual activities that cause a rupture of tissue or bleeding (Table 2).

b) Injection drug use

Sharing the equipment used to prepare and inject drugs with an HIV-infected person is a very efficient means of transmitting HIV and essentially amounts to a direct inoculation of viral particles from one person to another. The risk of transmission is directly related to the concentration of virus present in the blood and the volume of blood exchanged. Injection drug use is the second most common risk factor for HIV infection, and injection drug users account for an increasing proportion of AIDS cases (24% in 1997). It has been estimated that there are more than 1.5 million injection drug users in the United States (7).

c) Blood transfusion

Blood transfusion with infected blood products remains a significant risk for acquiring HIV in some parts of the world. In the United States, donated blood has been screened for antibodies to HIV-1 since 1985 and for antibodies to HIV-2 since 1992. Therefore, the risk of transmission from a blood transfusion has become extraordinarily low—less than 0.001%. To further ensure that donated blood is not infected with HIV, since 1996 the American Red Cross has used the HIV antigen test. This test helps address the problem of false-negative HIV antibody tests in donors who may not have produced detectable antibodies after their initial infection. Before the use of lyophilized factor VIII, recurrent inoculation with pooled donated factor VIII was a major source of HIV transmission in hemophilia patients.

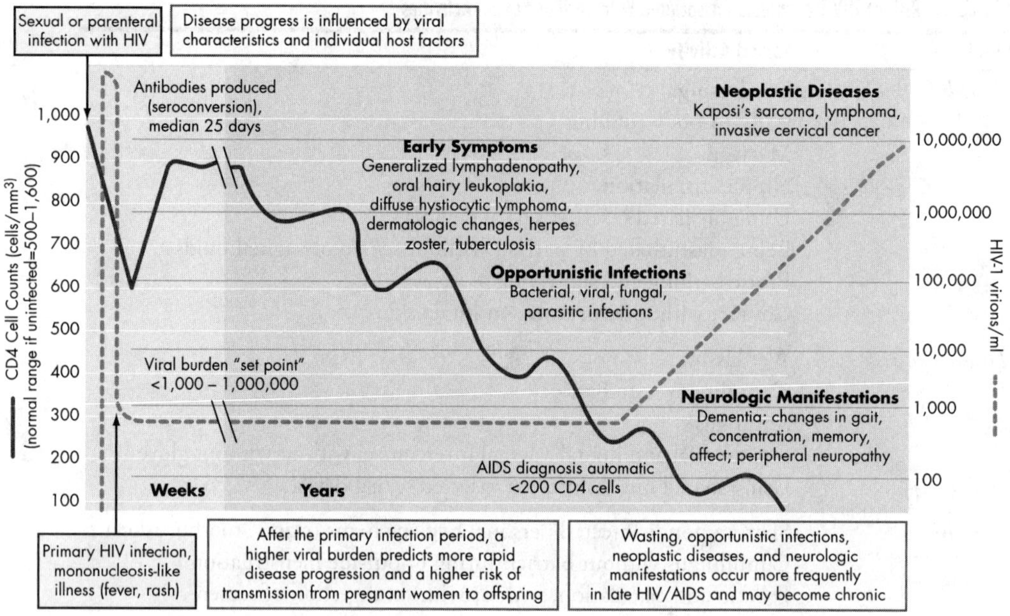

FIGURE 3. The Course of Untreated Adult HIV Infection.

Source. From the Southeast AIDS Training and Education Center, Emory University, Atlanta.

d) Perinatal

Infection from mother to infant can occur during gestation, delivery, or breast-feeding. Because breast milk contains significant numbers of lymphocytes that can lead to HIV transmission from mothers to newborns, it is recommended in the United States and other developed countries that HIV-infected mothers bottle-feed and not nurse their infants.

e) Cofactors for transmission

Cofactors can enhance but do not cause the transmission of HIV. *Physical* cofactors include the presence of sexually transmitted diseases (such as gonorrhea, syphilis, and chlamydia, which may cause genital lesions) or genital/mucous membrane bleeding during sexual activity. The use of mood or mind-altering substances may serve as a *behavioral* cofactor because they can lower sexual inhibitions, impair judgment, or increase impulsivity. Data are inconclusive regarding the effect of mind-altering substances on immunocompetence and HIV susceptibility or progression.

4. Pathogenesis of HIV

Three to 6 weeks after initial infection with HIV, there is a burst of viral replication, with wide dissemination of the virus throughout the body, particularly in lymphoid tissue and within the CNS. During this acute phase, approximately 50%–90% of people will experience a nonspecific "flu-like" syndrome of varying severity with fever, sore throat, rash, lymphadenopathy, and splenomegaly. Others do not have this seroconversion syndrome and may be unaware of their infection (8). As the host's immune system begins to recognize the pathogen and mounts a response to control the infection, plasma viral titers may drop 100-fold within 1 or 2 months of initial infection. When the host produces circulating antibodies against HIV, the host is said to "seroconvert," demonstrating a positive HIV antibody test. Although the immune system may

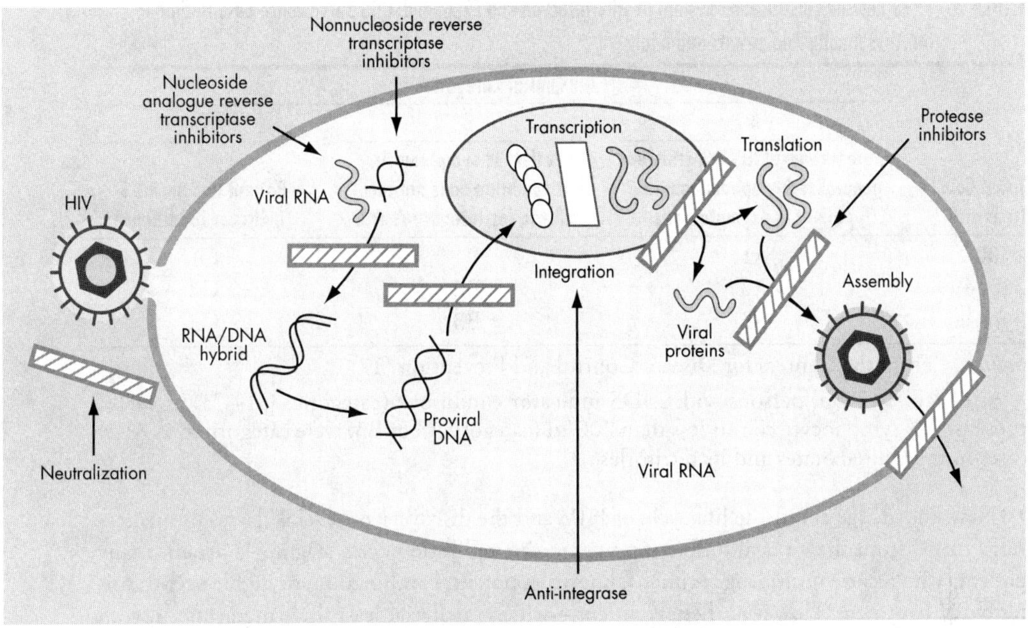

FIGURE 4. Antiviral Therapy Targets During the HIV Replication Cycle.
Source. Adapted from Paul (16).

appear to control the initial infection, chronic viral replication persists. There have been recent discoveries that "resting CD4 T cells" become infected rapidly after HIV transmission, and once HIV hides within resting T cells, antiretroviral therapy is unlikely to affect this sanctuary for HIV (9, 10).

The acute phase is followed by a clinically asymptomatic phase, during which the body has established a dynamic balance between the capacity of the virus to replicate and infect new CD4 cells and the capacity of the body to produce more CD4 cells. Even so, as many as 10 billion viral particles are produced daily, with a plasma virus half-life of about 6 hours. The asymptomatic phase may last for many years until symptoms arise that indicate that HIV infection is progressing. Progression to a symptomatic phase of illness may occur more rapidly in those with immune systems that are compromised before HIV infection and in infants with undeveloped immune systems. Other factors influencing disease progression include mutations of cell surface receptors and host factors such as HIV-specific cytotoxic lymphocyte response (Figure 3).

Viral load, a measurement of how many viral particles are present in a cubic millimeter of blood, is determined by several different assays that can detect as few as 20 viral particles per cubic millimeter of blood. Below that threshold, viral load is reported as "nondetectable." This does not mean that there is no HIV in the blood. Furthermore, this method does not measure the amount of HIV in lymphoid tissue, semen, or CNS. While some studies have shown a small correlation between serum viral load and lymphoid tissue and CSF viral load, in later stages of HIV infection, plasma and CSF viral load are largely uncorrelated (11, 12). Thus, the CNS can be seen as an independent "reservoir" of HIV replication. Current practice is to use serum viral load measurements, in combination with assays of immune cells such as CD4 counts and genotypic testing for viral resistance, to guide clinical decisions about the initiation of or changes in antiretroviral medication (13–15).

TABLE 3. 1993 Revised Classification System for HIV Infection and Expanded AIDS Surveillance Case Definition for AIDS Among Adolescents and Adults

	Clinical Categories		
	A	B	C
T Cell Count (cells/μl)	Acute (primary) HIV or persistent generalized lymphadenopathy; patient is asymptomatic	Patient is symptomatic, but condition does not meet criteria for category A or C	Patient has an AIDS indicator condition[a]
≥500	A1	B1	C1
200–499	A2	B2	C2
<200[a]	A3	B3	C3

Source. From the Centers for Disease Control and Prevention (17).

[a]As of Jan. 1, 1993, persons with AIDS indicator conditions (categories C1–C3) as well as those with T lymphocyte counts less than 200/μl (category A3 or B3) were categorized as AIDS cases in the United States and its territories.

New knowledge about the life cycle of HIV and the discovery of several classes of medications that disrupt the virus at different points in the replication cycle (Figure 4) benefit many patients who receive multidrug regimens, known as potent, combination, or highly active antiretroviral treatment. However, these regimens—which involve at least three medications, with short- and potential long-term side effects, taken multiple times per day for the life of the infected person—require strict adherence. The behavioral and psychological burden of early intervention is thus a mitigating factor against such an early and aggressive treatment approach. The rapid pace of changes to potent, combination, or highly active antiretroviral treatment guidelines adds to uncertainty about such interventions. Medications that can be taken less frequently are being developed to make the regimens more manageable.

5. Assessment and staging of HIV disease

HIV infection usually leads to clinical diseases that affect almost every organ system and present with a wide range of symptoms and syndromes. Accurate assessment and diagnosis of systemic as well as CNS impairment requires close medical and psychiatric management, with increasing vigilance as immune competence declines and the possibility of life-threatening disorders increases.

The CDC Revised Classification system for HIV infection and AIDS used CD4 counts and staging of illness (Table 3) to establish clinical categories for HIV disease. Generally, AIDS is defined by certain conditions marking advanced immunosuppression, such as a diagnosis of opportunistic infections (e.g., *Pneumocystis carinii* pneumonia) or other conditions (e.g., dementia or wasting). AIDS-defining criteria are listed in Table 4.

6. Treatment for HIV infection

Most of the world's HIV-infected population has little if any access to antimicrobial therapies for consequences of immune deficiency, let alone combination antiretroviral treatment. In the United States, revised standards of care for the treatment of HIV infection have improved treatment effectiveness, increased survival for patients, and potentially lessened development of viral resistance. Treatment is accomplished through numerous combinations of antiretroviral agents from four classes: nucleoside analogue reverse transcriptase inhibitors, nonnucleoside reverse transcriptase inhibitors, protease inhibitors, and the newest class, nucleotide analogues (Table 5). Guidelines for the use of antiretroviral agents in HIV-infected adults and adolescents are available from the HIV/AIDS Treatment Information Service (http://www.hivatis. org).

The current goal of antiretroviral therapy is to reduce viral load to undetectable levels and maintain such remission without interruption. Evidence suggests that the therapies suppress

TABLE 4. AIDS-Defining Conditions That Emerge With Advancing Immunosuppression

CD4 Cell Count (cells/mm^3)	Condition
200–500	Thrush Kaposi's sarcoma Tuberculosis reactivation Herpes zoster Herpes simplex Bacterial sinusitis/pneumonia
100–200	*Pneumocystis carinii* pneumonia
50–100	Systemic fungal infections Primary tuberculosis Cryptosporidiosis Cerebral toxoplasmosis Progressive multifocal leukoencephalopathy Peripheral neuropathy Cervical carcinoma
0–50	Cytomegalovirus disease Disseminated *Mycobacterium avium-intracellulare* complex Non-Hodgkin's lymphoma Central nervous system lymphoma HIV-associated dementia

replication but do not eradicate HIV from all parts of the body, particularly lymphoid tissue and the brain. Not all patients who initiate antiretroviral therapy respond. The lack of clinical response is likely explained by problems with adherence, suboptimal antiretroviral treatment potency, and genetic mutation of HIV strains (18). Many patients experience substantial side effects, and it is not uncommon for changes to be made in antiretroviral drug regimens because of such side effects. Adverse effects include lipodystrophy (fat redistribution syndromes), hyperlipidemia, nephrotoxicity, bone marrow suppression, neuropathy, and elevation of glucose to possibly diabetes mellitus–causing levels (19). Patients often experience nausea, diarrhea, sleep disturbances, and rashes. The cost of antiretroviral drugs alone is about $12,000 per year for a single individual, and the long-term health consequences of these agents are not known.

Adherence is of utmost concern with antiretroviral treatment because the regimens are so unforgiving; even minor deviations from the prescribed regimen can result in viral resistance and permanent loss of efficacy for existing medications. Studies of antiretroviral treatment continue to indicate that near-perfect adherence is needed to adequately repress viral replication. The potential implications of nonadherence are troubling, as evidenced by a study that found a primary viral resistance rate to antiretrovirals of 16.3% among a cohort of recently infected individuals (20). This study documented what was earlier considered a theoretical concern—namely that persons newly infected with HIV may carry viral strains already resistant to available antiretroviral agents, indicating transmission of resistant viral strains from persons who were taking nonsuppressive multiple drug therapy or who were nonadherent to treatment (21).

As the U.S. HIV epidemic spreads increasingly among disadvantaged persons with limited resources who may have multiple comorbid disorders, significantly more psychosocial stressors, and less access to ongoing primary or mental health care, these individuals are at risk of not receiving the recommended treatment for HIV infection. Services for HIV patients must balance medical interventions with the emotional, economic, and social supports required for good quality of life and prevention of further transmission.

TABLE 5. Antiretroviral Medications

Class	Drug Name
Nucleoside analogue reverse transcriptase inhibitors	Abacavir
	Didanosine[a]
	Lamivudine[b]
	Stavudine[c]
	Zalcitabine[d]
	Zidovudine[e]
	Lamivudine-zidovudine (combination)
Nonnucleoside reverse transcriptase inhibitors	Delavirdine
	Efavirenz
	Nevirapine
Protease inhibitors	Amprenavir
	Indinavir
	Lopinavir-ritonavir (combination)
	Nelfinavir
	Ritonavir
	Saquinavir
Nucleotide analogues	Adefovir

[a]Formerly called dideoxyinosine (ddI).
[b]Formerly called 3TC.
[c]Formerly called d4T.
[d]Formerly called 2′3′-dideoxycytidine (ddC).
[e]Formerly called azidothymidine (AZT).

B. ASSOCIATED FEATURES OF NEUROPSYCHIATRIC AND PSYCHOSOCIAL IMPORTANCE

1. Impact of HIV on the CNS

Clinical evidence for direct infection of the CNS by HIV emerged in the mid-1980s, when patients began to survive their presenting opportunistic infections but went on to develop neuropsychiatric syndromes that could not be attributed to CNS opportunistic infections or neoplasms. Additional evidence included signs of neurocognitive impairment in adults, loss or arrest of developmental milestones in children, ability to culture HIV from CSF, neuropathological lesions of the brain at autopsy, and abnormalities observed through brain imaging techniques, including cerebral atrophy.

HIV invades the CNS early in the course of infection, entering by way of macrophages, which along with microglial cells are largely responsible for HIV replication within the CNS. While HIV does not infect neurons in the CNS, it causes neuronal death by other mechanisms. It is hypothesized that HIV infection of microglial cells in the CNS causes the elaboration of neurotoxins that, in turn, cause neuronal damage (22, 23). Neuronal dysfunction usually takes place at a slow rate, and it is not clear whether the immune system plays a role in keeping HIV in the CNS under control (24). Some researchers believe that high systemic viral load may "drive" neurological disease (25), but there is converging evidence that the CNS compartment differs from that of the peripheral bloodstream, with independent viral evolution/mutation (leading to viral resistance) and different viral load decay kinetics (26, 27).

Major unanswered questions remain about the natural history of HIV in the CNS and whether current antiretroviral treatment regimens penetrate the blood-brain barrier sufficiently to reduce viral replication to the levels seen in the systemic circulation. Neuroprotective agents, immune modulators that increase macrophage activity within the CNS, and vaccines that boost immune response rather than prevent infection are all potential additional strategies to address neuropsychiatric syndromes.

2. Clinical syndromes

HIV infection can lead to neuropsychiatric syndromes that can occur at various stages of infection. Clinicians need to be aware of this possibility when evaluating new patients and observing changes in the patients whom they treat (28). Symptomatic HIV infection of the brain generally affects cognitive and motor functioning. Subtle neuropsychological impairment may be found in 22%–30% of otherwise asymptomatic patients with HIV infection (29, 30); these findings may or may not have functional significance. There is ample evidence for HIV causing the disorders HIV-associated dementia and HIV-associated minor cognitive motor disorder. HIV can affect other areas of the nervous system, causing syndromes such as painful sensory peripheral neuropathy or vacuolar myelopathy of the dorsolateral columns of the spinal cord. There are limited data in support of HIV infection of the CNS resulting in syndromes such as psychosis (31) or mania (32–34).

What separates HIV-associated dementia and HIV-associated minor cognitive motor disorder from the less severe cognitive changes seen in some HIV patients are the significance and duration of the functional deficits (Table 6, Table 7). HIV-associated minor cognitive motor disorder is a less severe disorder than HIV-associated dementia but does not necessarily progress to HIV-associated dementia (36). HIV-associated minor cognitive motor disorder is important to diagnose and treat, since it is thought to involve neuronal cell dysfunction rather than actual cell death, as seen in HIV-associated dementia. Both HIV-associated minor cognitive motor disorder and HIV-associated dementia are independent risk factors that decrease survival among patients with HIV infection (37, 38).

3. HIV-associated dementia

In contrast to Alzheimer's disease, which is a cortical dementia, HIV-associated dementia is classified as a subcortical dementia. HIV-associated dementia can produce different combinations of a clinical triad of progressive cognitive decline, motor dysfunction, and behavioral abnormalities. Symptoms commonly found in HIV-associated dementia include psychomotor slowing, decreased speed of information processing, impaired verbal memory and learning efficiency, and, later on, impairment in executive functioning. Behavioral manifestations vary throughout the range of HIV-related neurocognitive disorders, ranging from apathy to psychosis.

While the prevalence rate for HIV-associated dementia was estimated in the past to be 15%–20% of all AIDS patients (39), the incidence rate for HIV-associated dementia may be affected by the use of potent combination therapies. One report from the Multicenter AIDS Cohort Study (40) demonstrated declines of at least 50% in the incidence of HIV-associated dementia and CNS opportunistic complications (e.g., toxoplasmosis and primary CNS lymphoma) since the introduction of combination antiretroviral treatment in 1996. A second report has estimated that the incidence of HIV-associated dementia decreased from 21.1/1000 person-years in 1990–1992 to 14.7/1000 person-years in 1996–1997 (40). On the other hand, one group found that for patients who received combination antiretroviral treatment, the proportion of HIV-associated dementia as a percentage of all AIDS-defining illnesses rose from 4.4% to 6.5% between 1995 and 1997 (41). This shift in the rate of HIV-associated dementia is thought to reflect the decrease in rates of other AIDS-defining conditions, thereby leading to the relative rise in HIV-associated dementia cases.

TABLE 6. Definitional Criteria for HIV-Associated Dementia

Criterion	Description
1. Acquired abnormality in at least two of the following cognitive abilities (present for ≥1 month) Attention/concentration Speed of processing Abstraction/reasoning Visuospatial skills Memory learning Speech/language	Cognitive decline verified by history and mental status examination. When possible, history should be obtained from an informant and examination should be supplemented by neuropsychological testing. The cognitive dysfunction must cause impairment of work or in activities of daily living, with impairment not attributable solely to severe systemic illness.
2. At least one of the following:	
Acquired abnormality in motor function or performance	Abnormality verified by physical examination, neuropsychological tests, or both.
Decline in motivation or emotional control or change in social behavior	Change characterized by any of the following: apathy, inertia, irritability, emotional lability, or new-onset impaired judgment characterized by socially inappropriate behavior or disinhibition.
3. Absence of clouding of consciousness during a period long enough to establish the presence of criterion 1	
4. Exclusion of another etiology by history, physical, and psychiatric examination and appropriate laboratory and radiologic tests	Alternate possible etiologies include active central nervous system opportunistic infections or malignancy, psychiatric disorders (e.g., depressive disorders), active substance abuse, or acute or chronic substance withdrawal.

Source. From the American Academy of Neurology (35).

TABLE 7. Definitional Criteria for HIV-Associated Minor Cognitive Motor Disorder

Probable Diagnosis (must meet all four criteria)[a]

1. Acquired cognitive/motor/behavioral abnormalities, verified by both a reliable history and by neuropsychological tests
2. Mild impairment of work or activities of daily living
3. Does not meet criteria for HIV dementia or HIV myelopathy
4. No other etiology present

Source. From the American Academy of Neurology (35).
[a]A possible diagnosis of minor cognitive motor disorder can be given if criteria 1–3 are present and either 1) an alternative etiology is present and the cause of number 1 is not certain, or 2) the etiology of criterion 1 cannot be determined because of an incomplete evaluation.

4. Other psychiatric syndromes

Because HIV affects subcortical areas of the brain, it has been postulated that HIV may cause syndromes relating to mood and psychosis. New-onset psychosis and mania in HIV-infected patients tend to present at later stages of HIV disease and often occur in association with cognitive motor impairment. Lyketsos and colleagues (34) have described HIV-infected patients with so-called AIDS mania who present at advanced stages of HIV infection but generally have no family or personal history of mood disorder and have higher rates of comorbid dementia.

TABLE 8. Etiologies of Delirium in HIV/AIDS Patients

Intracranial	Extracranial
Seizures	Medications and other drugs (not exhaustive)
Infections	Amphotericin B
Cryptococcal meningitis	Acyclovir
Encephalitis due to HIV, herpes, cytomegalovirus	Ganciclovir
Progressive multifocal leukoencephalopathy	Ethambutol
Mass lesions	Trimethoprim/sulfamethoxazole
Lymphoma	Pentamidine
Toxoplasmosis	Foscarnet
	Ketoconazole
	Sedative/hypnotics
	Cycloserine
	Opiate analgesics
	Isoniazid
	Rifampin
	Zidovudine or didanosine
	Vincristine
	Dapsone
	Drug or alcohol withdrawal
	Infection/sepsis
	Endocrine dysfunction/metabolic abnormality
	Hypoglycemia due to pentamidine, protease inhibitors
	Hypoxia due to pneumonia
	Nonendocrine organ dysfunction
	Renal failure due to HIV nephropathy or medication toxicity
	Liver failure due to comorbid hepatitis and medication toxicity
	Nutritional deficiencies
	Wasting syndrome
	Failure to replace trace elements or vitamins in total parenteral nutrition

Source. Adapted from Bialer et al. (50).

They hypothesized that mania in this context is directly caused by HIV brain infection. Mijch and colleagues (32) conducted a prospective case-control study to test the hypothesis put forward by Lyketsos et al. In their study of 19 HIV patients with secondary mania, they found that treatment with zidovudine, which is known to penetrate the blood-brain barrier well, provided a protective effect against the development of mania. In addition, they found the incidence rate of HIV-associated dementia in the subjects with mania to be significantly greater than in HIV subjects without mania.

New-onset psychotic symptoms have been reported in HIV-positive individuals in the absence of medical/iatrogenic causes or concurrent substance abuse (42, 43). One case-control study systematically examined patients with HIV infection that predated the onset of psychosis (31). In this study, the psychotic subjects had significantly higher rates of past stimulant and sedative-hypnotic abuse and higher mortality at follow-up. While the study was limited by a sample size of 20, the authors postulated that direct effects of HIV infection on the brain could be one possible cause of new-onset psychosis in their subjects.

TABLE 9. Central Nervous System Manifestations of HIV-1 Infection

Type of Manifestation	Condition
Acute HIV-1 infection	Viral meningitis Encephalitis Ascending polyneuropathy
Opportunistic infections (late HIV-1 infection)	*Toxoplasma* cerebritis Cryptococcal meningitis Progressive multifocal leukoencephalopathy Neurosyphilis *Mycobacterium tuberculosis* meningitis Cytomegalovirus encephalitis Herpes simplex encephalitis
Neoplastic disease (late HIV-1 infection)	CNS lymphoma Kaposi's sarcoma
Other manifestations	HIV-associated dementia HIV-associated minor cognitive motor disorder

5. Differential diagnosis of neuropsychiatric syndromes

Differential diagnosis of an acute change in mental status includes but is not limited to delirium. Delirium occurs frequently in the medically ill and is more likely when a patient's illness is more severe. Estimates of rates of delirium in HIV patients range from 43% to greater than 65% in late-stage AIDS (44–46). Definition and management of the syndrome of delirium is well described in the APA *Practice Guideline for the Treatment of Patients With Delirium* (47; included in this volume). Identification of the delirious state and intervention to correct underlying causes reduces morbidity and mortality. In persons with HIV infection, the most common causes are iatrogenic and psychoactive-substance-induced toxicity, infection, neoplasms, and metabolic disturbances. Some antiretroviral medications can cause delirium (e.g., zidovudine at high doses [48] or efavirenz [49]) (Table 8).

The term "HIV encephalopathy" is occasionally used to refer to acute-onset cognitive deficits in adults, but its definition and usage vary. A wide range of conditions that primarily involve the CNS needs to be considered within the psychiatric differential diagnosis, since these conditions may present with psychiatric symptoms or cause psychiatric syndromes including psychosis (with or without an affective component) and mood episodes (mania, hypomania, depression) (51) (Table 9). The same concerns exist for medications commonly used to treat conditions associated with HIV infection (Table 10).

In adults and children with HIV infection, changes in mental status or the emergence of new psychiatric or cognitive disorders requires ruling out treatable and reversible causes; medical causes are of increasing concern if CD4 counts are low or viral load has begun to rise. Psychiatrists should consider adding assessments of basic immune function and viral load, CSF examination, and brain imaging studies to the standard medical workup of new- or acute-onset psychiatric syndromes for patients with or at high risk for HIV infection (Table 11).

6. Pediatric HIV/AIDS syndromes

To date, the proportion of children born with HIV who survive until the age of 9 is approximately 50%, but antiretroviral interventions will increase the number of infected youth who enter adolescence. HIV-related symptoms may develop at any age, but a prospective collaborative study found that only 10% of children were symptomatic before the onset of an AIDS-defining illness (53).

Certain clinical presentations characterized by lymphadenopathy, parotitis, skin diseases, and recurrent respiratory tract infections are associated with longer survival, while lymphoid

TABLE 10. Neuropsychiatric Side Effects of Selected Medications Used in HIV Disease

Drug	Target Illness	Side Effects
Acyclovir	Herpes encephalitis	Visual hallucinations, depersonalization, tearfulness, confusion, hyperesthesia, hyperacusis, thought insertion, insomnia
Amphotericin B	Cryptococcosis	Delirium, peripheral neuropathy, diplopia
β-Lactam antibiotics	Infections	Confusion, paranoia, hallucinations, mania, coma
Co-trimoxazole	*Pneumocystis carinii* pneumonia	Depression, loss of appetite, insomnia, apathy
Cycloserine	Tuberculosis	Psychosis, somnolence, depression, confusion, tremor, vertigo, paresis, seizure, dysarthria
Didanosine	HIV	Nervousness, anxiety, confusion, seizures, insomnia, peripheral neuropathy
Efavirenz	HIV	Nightmares, depression, confusion
Foscarnet	Cytomegalovirus	Paresthesias, seizures, headache, irritability, hallucinations, confusion
Interferon-α	Kaposi's sarcoma	Depression, weakness, headache, myalgias, confusion
Isoniazid	Tuberculosis	Depression, agitation, hallucinations, paranoia, impaired memory, anxiety
Lamivudine	HIV	Insomnia, mania
Methotrexate	Lymphoma	Encephalopathy (at high dose)
Pentamidine	*Pneumocystis carinii* pneumonia	Confusion, anxiety, lability, hallucinations
Procarbazine	Lymphoma	Mania, loss of appetite, insomnia, nightmares, confusion, malaise
Quinolones	Infection	Psychosis, delirium, seizures, anxiety, insomnia, depression
Stavudine	HIV	Headache, asthenia, malaise, confusion, depression, seizures, excitability, anxiety, mania, early morning awakening, insomnia
Sulfonamides	Infection	Psychosis, delirium, confusion, depression, hallucinations
Thiabendazole	Strongyloidiasis	Hallucinations, olfactory disturbance
Vinblastine	Kaposi's sarcoma	Depression, loss of appetite, headache
Vincristine	Kaposi's sarcoma	Hallucinations, headache, ataxia, sensory loss
Zalcitabine	HIV	Headaches, confusion, impaired concentration, somnolence, asthenia, depression, seizures, peripheral neuropathy
Zidovudine	HIV	Headache, malaise, asthenia, insomnia, unusually vivid dreams, restlessness, severe agitation, mania, auditory hallucinations, confusion

Source. Adapted from Grant and Atkinson (52).

interstitial pneumonitis and thrombocytopenia form an intermediate survival group. The worst prognosis is associated with bacterial infections, progressive neurological disease, anemia, and fevers (54).

HIV infection that occurs at the time of birth rather than early in gestation is thought to be associated with a better prognosis. While at any given time many HIV-infected children may not experience significant HIV-related medical morbidity, their overall health outcome may be compromised by the conditions of poverty.

TABLE 11. Evaluation of Altered Mental Status in Patients With HIV/AIDS

Physical/neurologic examination
- Focal deficits may indicate space-occupying lesion (e.g., CNS lymphoma, toxoplasmosis, progressive multifocal leukoencephalopathy)
- Sensory changes, which may indicate peripheral neuropathy
- Ataxia or changes in gait, which may indicate myelopathy

Laboratory analyses
- CBC with differential
- Serum chemistries
- Arterial blood gas in patients with pneumonia
- VDRL, fluorescent treponemal antibody
- B_{12}, folate

MRI, to rule out space-occupying lesion (progressive multifocal leukoencephalopathy)

Lumbar puncture, to rule out acute infection (e.g., cryptococcal meningitis, herpes, toxoplasmosis, syphilis)

Neuropsychological testing
- AIDS Dementia Rating Scale
- Finger Tapping Test
- Trail Making Test

Source. Adapted from Bialer et al. (50).

The impact of HIV on the developing nervous system of children is more significant than on the developed adult nervous system, and certain cognitive deficits may occur in some infected youth. The term "dementia" is not commonly used to describe cognitive deficits in children by pediatricians or child psychiatrists, who refer to this condition as either HIV-associated progressive encephalopathy or HIV encephalopathy. Nonetheless, "dementia due to HIV disease" in children is specifically mentioned in DSM-IV (p. 148).

HIV-associated progressive encephalopathy in children is characterized by a triad of symptoms: impaired brain growth, progressive motor dysfunction, and loss or plateau of developmental milestones (55). Progressive encephalopathy needs to be distinguished from mental retardation secondary to other causes, such as maternal drug addiction and prematurity, which can be determined only by longitudinal assessment. Despite the general fact that progressive encephalopathy is observed in the context of immunosuppression, markers of immunologic functioning (e.g., CD4 count) do not correlate with degree of neurocognitive impairment (54). The prevalence rate of progressive encephalopathy in a cohort of 128 HIV-infected children was 21% during a mean follow-up period of 24 months. Progressive encephalopathy was the first AIDS-defining condition in 67% of the group, and mean survival after diagnosis was 14 months (56).

Although many children with HIV are considered to be asymptomatic, numerous studies document at least some cognitive and language delays (57). In a sample of 36 HIV-infected children who were less than 10 years old, brain abnormalities detected by means of computerized tomography scans were significantly correlated with receptive and expressive language deficits, with expressive language more severely impaired than receptive language among those children with progressive encephalopathy (58). In addition, visual motor deficits are common and may be correlated with disease progression (59).

C. PREVALENCE OF COMORBID PSYCHIATRIC CONDITIONS

Since early in the HIV epidemic, researchers have studied the prevalence of psychiatric disorders in persons with HIV infection (60–63). Often these psychiatric disorders predated HIV infection or occurred during the course of living with the disease; they are not necessarily attributable to neuropathic effects of HIV. Psychiatric illness is generally related to poorer functioning and quality of life as well as increased use of HIV-related hospital services (64). A study conducted by researchers in California found that depression was associated with shorter survival times in men with HIV infection (65).

Prevalence rates of psychiatric disorders reported in published studies vary widely. In general, higher rates of psychiatric disorders are seen in later stages of HIV infection and are reported in studies that assess patients receiving care in HIV medical or psychiatric clinics rather than community-based samples (66). On one extreme, recent data from the national, multisite HIV/AIDS Mental Health Services Demonstration Program revealed high rates of depression (60%), dysthymic disorder (25%), and anxiety disorders (25%) among persons seeking HIV-related mental health services in the public sector (67). The study found high rates of comorbid substance use disorders, with nearly 50% of all patients also having a diagnosis of alcohol or drug dependence. These higher rates are most likely linked to characteristics of the population studied: HIV-positive individuals voluntarily seeking psychiatric care, a population that may be more reflective of patients receiving care from community mental health clinics. In contrast, prevalence studies in selected community-based samples have found much lower rates of psychiatric disorders, such as rates of major depressive disorder in the 4%–14% range (68–73).

III. FORMULATION AND IMPLEMENTATION OF A TREATMENT PLAN

A. INDIVIDUALS AT HIGH RISK FOR HIV INFECTION

HIV prevention strategies are an essential component of the comprehensive treatment of specific psychiatric populations and for other psychiatric patients who manifest high-risk sexual and drug use behavior. Some psychiatric patients, such as those confined to forensic units, in long-term hospitals, and locked nursing homes have almost no access to preventive strategies other than those provided and supported by staff. Administrators and institutions should formulate policies that support the full range of HIV prevention steps outlined in this section. Primary prevention strategies are those that seek to avert initial infection. Secondary and tertiary prevention strategies target infected individuals in order to prevent further transmission and reduce HIV-related medical complications, respectively.

1. Psychiatric management

Optimum management of patients at high risk for HIV infection involves a wide range of psychiatric skills: comprehensive diagnostic evaluations, assessment of possible medical causes of new-onset symptoms, initiation of specific treatment interventions, and a keen understanding of psychodynamic issues. In some institutional settings, psychiatrists serve as primary clinicians of both medical and psychiatric care. In such situations, psychiatrists should be mindful to include HIV risk assessment and prevention as part of patients' treatment plans.

a) Obtaining a risk history

A psychiatrist will not be aware of a patient's risk for HIV infection unless risk behavior is accurately assessed. Such an assessment should be considered in every psychiatric evaluation in order to identify individuals who are at high risk due to specific behaviors. Factors such as acute episodes of psychiatric illness, stressful or traumatic life events, and the developmental stage of the patient (e.g., initiation of sexual activity in adolescents) contribute to the need for ongoing appraisal of patient risk. Psychiatrists are particularly well-placed to assess HIV risk because

TABLE 12. Items for Clinicians to Cover When Conducting an Assessment of HIV Risk Behavior

Frequency of sexual intercourse (vaginal, anal, oral)
Number, gender, and known HIV risk of sex partners
Whether the patient has traded sex (for money, drugs, a place to stay, cigarettes)
Past and current symptoms of sexually transmitted infections
Use of condoms and other contraceptive methods
Use of drugs, particularly those that are injected or sniffed
Sharing of needles, syringes, or other injection equipment

Source. From McKinnon et al. (74).

they often follow patients for lengthy periods of time, which allows for multiple opportunities to assess behavior (74).

At times, the clinical state of the patient may preclude an accurate assessment, such as when the patient is acutely psychotic or intoxicated. In this situation, the risk history may need to be obtained either when the patient is able to provide valid answers or with the assistance of family or friends. Psychiatrists should be knowledgeable about which specific sexual behaviors are more likely to result in HIV transmission (Table 2). When conducting an assessment of risk behavior, psychiatrists should convey a nonjudgmental attitude.

When carrying out a risk assessment, it is important to clarify the vocabulary and cultural beliefs of the patient. For instance, it is not uncommon for patients and clinicians to use different terms to describe sexual or drug use behaviors, and slang terms change quickly. The National Institute on Drug Abuse has published a community drug alert that outlines common street drugs and their slang names, which is available at www.drugabuse.gov. Clinicians may be able to clarify risk behavior terms by first describing a risk behavior and then asking a patient what he or she would call that behavior (Table 12).

b) HIV antibody testing

Attitudes about HIV antibody testing have changed with the development of HIV treatment interventions and educational efforts. Formerly, patients were unwilling to learn their HIV status, since knowing could cause emotional distress, could engender possible discrimination, and did not lead to better clinical outcomes. Public policy now promotes earlier identification of HIV infection so that newly infected persons can be medically monitored and receive antiretroviral treatment as appropriate. Yet HIV testing still carries risks due to worries and fears associated with HIV/AIDS, as well as the possibility of physical assault by a partner or other relation after HIV diagnosis (75). Disclosure of HIV status to family, friends, or employers can be quite problematic for some patients.

Discussion of the pros and cons of a routine baseline HIV test are part of a comprehensive approach to HIV prevention in high-risk patients. Psychiatric units or individual practitioners who conduct HIV testing should be aware of their obligation to provide the necessary pre- and posttest counseling (76). Elements of pre- and posttest counseling include an explanation of the HIV test, including risks and benefits, confidentiality of the results, discussion of risk behavior and risk reduction strategies, and plans for dealing with a positive or negative test result. Federal guidelines for counseling have been established by the CDC (http://www.cdc.gov/hiv/pubs/hivctsrg.pdf).

Clinicians should remember that the timing of when to undergo HIV testing is a distinct clinical decision. For instance, it is generally not advisable to test a patient for HIV while he or she is confused or intoxicated with alcohol or drugs. In the event that a patient cannot give informed consent, the psychiatrist should be familiar with the local legal requirements regarding HIV testing and disclosure (77). Anonymous and confidential HIV testing is often provided by state public health agencies or community-based organizations; some patients prefer anonymity and may be more likely to agree to testing given this option. Many state health departments conduct "partner notification" or prevention counseling and referral services to identify and test past or present sexual partners or drug injection equipment-sharing partners of a newly reported HIV-seropositive person.

The American College of Obstetricians and Gynecologists now recommends that an HIV antibody test be offered during annual exams to all women seeking preconception care (not just pregnant women), which reflects the growing awareness that many women may not properly assess their personal risk for HIV infection (78). This recommendation goes beyond the previous recommendation that pregnant women undergo HIV antibody testing so that HIV-infected women can consider treatment with antiretroviral medication. For female patients who are at risk for HIV infection *and* for pregnancy, conducting a baseline pregnancy test along with a baseline HIV test is advised.

c) Risk reduction strategies

Risk reduction strategies include education of patients about behaviors that place them at risk for HIV infection, active discussions of changes in behavior, and treatment of problems that promote risky behavior. It is important to view undergoing an HIV antibody test as a "teachable moment," when counseling about risk for HIV can be tailored to the specific behavior of the patient and an individualized risk reduction plan can be developed.

Because successful risk reduction requires more than knowledge of risk, ongoing discussions between patient and psychiatrist can help provide the motivating and skill-building factors that help ensure consistent changes in behavior. Psychiatrists should consider unconscious motivations that may contribute to risk-taking behavior when developing risk reduction strategies. Some patients may need to be referred to community-based organizations or other clinicians who offer specific risk reduction programs (e.g., needle exchange programs or skills training groups). For some patients, risk reduction strategies can include extended counseling and case management, such as that modeled by the CDC (79).

When appropriate, psychiatrists should determine whether patients have access to condoms and the skills to use them (Table 13). Skills to discuss and negotiate safer sex with partners may need to be developed; psychotherapy can provide an opportunity to practice communication skills through role playing. Clinicians should be alert to feelings of powerlessness in sexual situations for patients with histories of sexual abuse and to the real possibility of violence for some if a sexual partner is threatened or angered.

Psychiatric conditions that could theoretically increase patient risk for engaging in high-risk behavior include impulse control disorders, untreated depression, hypersexuality associated with mania, psychotic disorders, mental disorders due to a general medical condition, binge alcohol or drug use, and personality disorders.

d) Postexposure prophylaxis

The premise underlying postexposure prophylaxis is that chemoprophylaxis during a window of opportunity may prevent initial cellular infection and local propagation of HIV, thus allowing the host immune defenses to eliminate the inoculum of virus (81). Currently, postexposure prophylaxis is recommended for known occupational exposure, especially percutaneous or mucous membrane exposure, to blood or other body fluids.

Psychiatrists who serve as administrators of mental health facilities should formulate policies and protocols for the expedient treatment of health care professionals or patients who have had such exposure. The protocol requires a rapid assessment of risk and, where risk is present, beginning a multiple drug regimen as soon as 1–2 hours after exposure and not later than 24–36 hours. It further requires 4 weeks of treatment with two or three antiretroviral agents that can have significant side effects.

TABLE 13. Condom Use

Condoms must be used consistently and correctly to provide maximum protection. Consistent use means using a new condom with each act of intercourse. Latex condoms and polyurethane condoms provide protection; lambskin condoms should not be used. Correct condom use includes all of the following steps.

- Check the expiration date.
- Use a new condom for each act of vaginal, anal, or oral intercourse.
- Put on the condom as soon as erection occurs and before any vaginal, anal, or oral contact with the penis.
- Apply lubricant to penis before and after putting the condom on. This will provide greater satisfaction for both the insertive and the receptive partners.
- Hold the tip of the condom and unroll it onto the erect penis, leaving space at the tip of the condom, yet ensuring that no air is trapped in the tip of the condom.
- Adequate lubrication is important to prevent condom breakage, but use only water-based lubricants, such as glycerine or lubricating jellies (which can be purchased at any pharmacy). Oil-based lubricants, such as petroleum jelly, cold cream, hand lotion, or baby oil, can weaken the condom.
- Withdraw from the partner immediately after ejaculation, holding the condom firmly to the base of the penis to keep it from slipping off.

Source. From the CDC National Center for HIV, STD and TB Prevention, Division of HIV/AIDS Prevention (80).

The CDC has issued guidelines for the use of antiretroviral medication following health care worker occupational exposure to HIV (82). There is a National Clinicians' Postexposure Hotline (888-448-4911) that can be accessed 24 hours a day for guidance in cases of possible or known exposure to HIV. A web site (www.ucsf.edu/hivcntr) offers a wealth of information to address this issue.

Data are being gathered to evaluate the use of postexposure prophylaxis in other exposure situations, but it is being increasingly offered for known or possible sexual exposure to HIV. Public health messages should emphasize that postexposure prophylaxis should be used only when primary prevention methods such as use of condoms or avoidance of high-risk behaviors have failed. Clinicians should counsel patients who receive postexposure prophylaxis to reduce their chance of future exposure (81).

2. Specific treatment situations

a) Patients with substance use disorders

The best way to prevent the spread of HIV through injection drug use is effective primary prevention of drug use. For people who are already injecting opioids, eliminating this behavior through adequately dosed substitution therapy, such as methadone or a long-acting form of methadone, L-α-acetylmethadol (LAAM), can serve an HIV prevention function.

Harm reduction policies have received more support in the last decade due to the spread of AIDS among injection drug users. The primary purpose of harm reduction is to decrease the negative consequences of drug use (83). As opposed to a policy of abstinence, harm reduction approaches realistically assume that some individuals will continue to use drugs. In this framework, a hierarchy of goals is established, with more immediate or attainable ones achieved on the way to risk-free use or possible abstinence. Risk reduction strategies such as methadone maintenance treatment, needle education and bleach distribution, safer sex education, legal clean needle purchase, and needle exchange programs are all examples of harm reduction strategies (84).

While injection drug use has a direct role in transmission of HIV, noninjection drugs and alcohol can play a potent role as cofactors of transmission because of their effects on behavior and cognition. The treatment success of substance use disorders varies, and the situation is further hampered because access to substance abuse services is often limited or is unwanted; relapses are common. Nonetheless, keeping substance use disorder intervention high on the list of treatment priorities is recommended for persons at risk for HIV infection.

One component of a comprehensive approach to HIV prevention among injection drug users is access to sterile syringes. The U.S. Public Health Service recommends that injection drug users who continue to inject use sterile syringes to prepare and inject drugs and obtain those syringes from a reliable source (e.g., a pharmacy). At the same time, a wide variety of laws and regulations restrict the ability of injection drug users to purchase and possess sterile syringes (7). Numerous national organizations, including the American Psychiatric Association (85), the American Medical Association, and the American Pharmaceutical Association, have recommended in policy statements and guidelines the removal of government restrictions on the availability of sterile syringes and have supported government-sponsored needle exchange programs. Cleaning drug injection equipment with bleach is an alternative that requires a multistep cleaning process that is impractical for many injection drug users (86).

b) Patients with severe mental illness

Rates of HIV infection among psychiatric inpatients averaged 7.8% in seroprevalence studies conducted in East Coast cities (87). Men and women were equally affected, with the highest rates occurring among patients who were under 40, were black or Latino, or used substances, especially injected drugs. Rates for other geographic areas in the United States were not available.

Despite not identifying themselves as gay, 10% of men with schizophrenia have reported same-sex sexual encounters (88). Public mental health systems should implement prevention policies and practices, educate both mental and medical health care clinicians about key treatment issues, and develop effective linkages between clinicians and systems of care (89, 90).

Severe mental illness may be associated with health risks due to poor access to health care or decreased capacity to care for oneself. Despite the challenges that chronically and severely mentally ill patients face, risk reduction programs tailored to their needs have been shown to reduce risk of HIV infection (91, 92).

c) Victims of sexual abuse/crimes

Psychiatrists frequently encounter child, adolescent, and adult psychiatric patients who have histories of being sexually abused, including when treating patients with posttraumatic stress disorder (PTSD), dissociative disorders, and borderline personality disorder. Victims of sexual crimes vary from those with long abuse histories to those with a single sexual assault. Sexual coercion often results in long-term emotional damage to those that have been assaulted and may be followed by PTSD or other psychiatric disorders. These emotional scars are associated with increased vulnerability to other HIV-risk situations.

A patient with a history of sexual abuse or trauma should be asked about specific behaviors that are associated with risk for HIV transmission. Patients with such a history may be reluctant to provide information initially. Psychiatrists should determine if a psychiatric disorder is present and whether treatment is indicated. In the case of sexual assault, psychiatrists should expediently gather enough information so that the decision about the appropriateness of postexposure prophylaxis can be made (93).

B. HIV-INFECTED INDIVIDUALS

1. Psychiatric management

The development of a psychiatric treatment plan for patients with HIV infection requires thoughtful and comprehensive consideration of the biopsychosocial context of the illness.

Treatment decisions must balance standard recommendations for psychiatric conditions against the medical stage of HIV illness and up-to-date information about available medical interventions targeted at the underlying HIV infection. At the same time, psychiatrists should be aware that emotional reactions and conflicts can interfere with a patient's ability to follow medical recommendations and thus have a profound effect on physical status. Psychiatrists should carefully consider possible medical causes of psychiatric symptoms and whether a medical workup is indicated to rule out a potentially life-threatening illness due to HIV or HIV-related illness. Organ malfunction, synergism of side effects of drugs, and drug-drug interactions are important factors to address in the management of patients.

a) Establish and maintain a therapeutic alliance

Establishing an alliance involves, in part, recognition of a patient's understanding of his or her stage of illness and an evaluation of how he or she is coping with it. The exploration of cultural/ethnic beliefs regarding psychiatric and HIV illnesses can also contribute to the formation of a solid alliance. Because of the potential for the patient to feel shame and stigma associated with HIV infection and the sensitive nature of discussing risk behavior, psychiatrists should be supportive and not judgmental to encourage trust.

Issues of confidentiality should be reviewed with the patient, and the patient should be asked to consider the psychiatrist's role in assisting with the process of disclosure of HIV status to appropriate persons (94). In establishing a therapeutic alliance, it is important to discuss with the patient whether he or she wants to extend the treatment relationship to include selected communication with the family or significant other(s). Lastly, given the importance of the therapeutic alliance and the emotional impact of issues related to HIV, the psychiatrist should be aware of transference and countertransference feelings as well as personal attitudes about HIV infection and how the patient acquired the virus.

b) Collaborate and coordinate care with other mental health and medical providers

Managing the health care needs of a patient with HIV infection can be challenging due to the complex nature of the illness. Psychiatrists must be aware that the illness changes over time and has many different clinical manifestations. In addition, because information about HIV-related treatment is constantly evolving, psychiatrists may feel that their fund of knowledge about the most current interventions, such as antiretroviral medications, is inadequate. To keep up to date and to provide good clinical care, it is essential to collaborate with other physicians in infectious disease, primary care, and other disciplines.

Discussions of drug-drug interactions and the close monitoring and workup of unexplained somatic or psychiatric symptoms are examples of how psychiatrists and primary care physicians can assist each other in providing high-quality comprehensive care. Patients should specify their agreement for the exchange of specific information between the psychiatrist and other clinicians in a written release of information. It is often appropriate to use a multidisciplinary team approach when managing a patient with HIV, especially as the disease becomes more advanced. Access to both general medical and specialty care may need to be addressed.

c) Diagnose and treat all associated psychiatric disorders

A number of surveys of persons with HIV infection have shown an elevated premorbid rate of psychiatric disorders when compared to rates in the general population. In addition, psychiatric disorders can develop during any stage of HIV illness.

Psychiatric treatment of patients with HIV infection should include active monitoring of substance abuse, since it is often associated with risk behaviors that can lead to further transmission of HIV. Clinicians must not assume that patients who have relatively good immune functioning have no risk for CNS HIV disorders. Thorough evaluation and accurate diagnosis are key to selecting the appropriate intervention, whether it is risk reduction counseling, neuropsychological testing, or the use of psychotropic and antiretroviral medications.

There are no data to suggest that the psychotherapeutic management of patients with HIV infection should be different from that of other patients. Many clinicians use a variety of approaches (e.g., both time-limited and longer-term individual and group psychotherapy) and psychotherapeutic models (e.g., cognitive behavior, supportive, interpersonal, or psychodynamic/psychoanalytic).

d) Facilitate adherence to overall treatment plan

Adherence to a treatment regimen is profoundly important for patients with HIV infection. Research has demonstrated that less than 95% adherence to antiretroviral medications results in the development of viral resistance (95). Translated into actual practice, if medication doses are taken twice a day, a patient cannot miss more than one dose every 10 days.

Because comorbid psychiatric disorders, such as substance abuse or depression, have been shown to adversely affect patients' compliance with a complicated treatment regimen, psychiatrists and patients should actively discuss adherence to both psychotropic and HIV medications (96). Psychoeducational approaches are especially useful, since they reinforce the importance of adherence, support appropriate help-seeking, and identify barriers to adherence. Some patients who are unable to modify their behavior after educational approaches may be helped by intensive psychodynamic psychotherapy. If indicated, outreach efforts with public health nurses and services can be used to provide adherence assistance.

e) Provide education about psychological, psychiatric, and neuropsychiatric disorders

Mental health problems can occur at any stage of HIV illness (e.g., around the time of serologic testing) (97), or they could be precipitated by the onset of somatic symptoms. Preexisting psychiatric disorders or personality traits may be exacerbated by the onset of HIV illness. Patients may seek mental health services on their own, but it is not uncommon for other clinicians to request psychiatric consultation for patients who are in crisis or who have psychiatric symptoms.

It is often the psychiatrist's role to educate other clinicians and patients about the neuropsychiatric complications of HIV infection and to initiate and encourage treatment of current or emergent psychiatric disorders. When seeing a patient in consultation, it is important to gather history about cognitive or motor symptoms and conduct a mental status screening examination to determine whether neurocognitive deficits are present (see Section III.B.2.a on screening exams).

f) Provide risk reduction strategies to further minimize the spread of HIV

Psychiatrists are obligated to assess the risk for HIV transmission from their HIV-infected patients to others and to provide risk reduction counseling. This task should be a long-term treatment priority, since many HIV-infected individuals continue risk behaviors. Risk assessment should be repeated when there are changes in the patient's clinical status or social situation, such as the onset of binge drug or alcohol use or new sexual relationships. Psychotherapy may help some individuals who are unaware of motivations that promote ongoing risk behavior. When a psychiatrist cannot provide the specific risk reduction intervention that is indicated for a patient, he or she should refer patients to resources such as HIV/AIDS service organizations and support the intervention when initiated.

g) Maximize psychological and social/adaptive functioning

Biomedical interventions have stemmed the progression of HIV illness so that its course has increasingly resembled that of other chronic medical illnesses. Therefore, maximizing psychosocial functioning is relevant to the long-term social and economic impact of HIV infection. Psychiatrists can enhance a patient's functioning by helping him or her cope with the illness. Psychiatrists should ask about and be aware of a patient's use of alternative or complementary treatments, including herbal remedies.

Assessment of social supports, utilization of appropriate community-based services, and resolution of financial and occupational concerns are all potential fruitful domains of inquiry. Many patients find support groups for persons with HIV infection helpful in coping with their illness, whereas others may prefer individual, couples, or family therapy.

h) Role of religion/spirituality

Inquiry about the spiritual beliefs and religious faith of a person with HIV infection should be a regular part of a psychiatric assessment and treatment planning, since they can be an important source of support for many with HIV/AIDS. Facing a serious illness often serves as a catalyst for a search for meaning and a renewal of spiritual beliefs and practices. A person's religious history includes not only current beliefs and practices but also religious traditions of one's family of origin and ethnic culture.

Religious congregations have had different, sometimes negative, responses to the spiritual needs of members with HIV/AIDS that often correspond to the core beliefs of the faith communities (98). Many ethnic minorities find the religious community or body of the church to be the network that most effectively addresses their need for support in crises.

The concept of spirituality goes beyond religious considerations to encompass multidimensional and existential perspectives that are important in maintaining well-being for many persons with HIV infection. It is not uncommon for persons with HIV/AIDS to seek alternative modes of spiritual expression, such as meditation. An assessment of the spiritual needs of a patient involves questions around the person's concept of God, sources of strength and hope, significance of practices and rituals, and perceived relationship between spiritual beliefs and health status (99). Information gathered may help caregivers assist patients to better cope with their illness at all stages but particularly as a patient nears death.

i) Prepare for issues of disability, death, and dying

As HIV illness advances, a psychiatrist may be asked to help evaluate the need for reasonable work or school accommodations or the ability to return to work in line with the Americans With Disabilities Act. Patients with minor children may need assistance with disclosure of illness and the establishment of a custody plan in the event of parental death from AIDS. Psychotherapy may be very helpful in reducing the emotional distress and turmoil activated by approaching death.

The fundamental right of a patient with advancing HIV illness to make treatment decisions can be supported when issues relating to disability, death, and dying are discussed by the appropriate parties in a timely and ongoing fashion. Discussions about preferences for care should be initiated by physicians, since it has been reported that only 36% of patients with AIDS had spoken with their physician about their preferred treatment (100). It is recommended that patients with HIV infection draw up a living will to guide end-of-life decisions in addition to a durable power of attorney. Copies of these documents should be placed in a patient's medical charts and in the files of their primary and specialty physicians.

j) Advice to significant others/family regarding sources of care and support

The HIV patient's significant others—partner, family, and friends—are often collaborative partners in care and support who often shoulder a significant share of the clinical day-to-day care of an acutely or terminally ill patient with AIDS. They also are a rich source of collateral information about the clinical status of the patient. The psychiatrist needs to take care that the patient has given consent before speaking directly with family and significant others.

Intimate involvement with the patient and his or her illness can lead to mental health difficulties for the significant others as well. Referral to support groups for significant others affected by HIV may be helpful, as can encouragement to participate in HIV/AIDS advocacy organizations. Both can provide emotional validation and a degree of respite for a significant

TABLE 14. Screening Examinations for HIV-Associated Cognitive Motor Dysfunction

Instrument	Administration	Comments
Mental Alteration Test (102)	Clinician administered	Timed test; verbal version of the Trail Making Test; alternates between numbers and letters
HIV Dementia Scale (103)	Clinician administered	Five sections cover memory registration, attention, psychomotor speed, memory recall, and construction
Executive Interview Test (104)	Clinician administered	A 10-minute, 25-item bedside test of executive function, including snout reflex, word fluency, echopraxia, go/no-go task

other. Some significant others and family members may be best served by referral for psychiatric evaluation and treatment, including individual or family therapy.

2. Diagnosis and treatment of disorders requiring specific psychiatric intervention

a) Dementia and the spectrum of cognitive disorders

Cognitive complaints are not uncommon among psychiatric patients in general, but the evaluation of such complaints in a patient with HIV infection requires a comprehensive psychiatric assessment, formulation of a differential diagnosis, and possible medical workup. Symptoms of early cognitive changes due to HIV can be subtle and can differ from symptoms associated with cortical dementia such as Alzheimer's. For example, HIV-associated dementia, due to its subcortical localization, more commonly presents with psychomotor slowing rather than deficits in language or visual recognition. Psychiatrists need to be aware of these differences in clinical phenomenology in order to identify HIV-associated dementia at early stages.

The widely used Mini-Mental State (101) is not sensitive in picking up early HIV-associated cognitive motor symptoms. Alternative screening examinations have been proposed that identify symptoms more likely to be present with subcortical dementia (102–105). Psychiatrists should become familiar with the available screening examinations for cognitive motor impairment that are more specific for subcortical symptoms (Table 14). It has been found that patient self-assessment of cognitive status is not reliable (106). Therefore, psychiatrists should administer a baseline screening examination on every patient with HIV infection and plan to readminister the test on a regular basis as part of the treatment plan. If there is evidence of early cognitive impairment, formal neuropsychological testing is useful to more comprehensively document cognitive dysfunction as well as areas of relative cognitive strength.

Once cognitive deficits are identified, the psychiatrist should work in collaboration with infectious disease specialists, neurologists, or primary care clinicians to develop a plan for further workup. A magnetic resonance imaging scan often reveals no abnormality in patients with early dementia, so this technique is not useful in providing specific confirmation of HIV-associated dementia. The overall immunological status of the patient should be assessed if not already known.

Pharmacologic treatment of HIV-associated dementia consists of intervening with potent antiretroviral therapy that targets the underlying HIV infection with consideration of whether the agents adequately penetrate the CNS. For comorbid conditions such as depression, psychiatrists should consider prescribing antidepressant medications as they would for other medically ill patients. Last, for management of symptoms associated with HIV-associated dementia (e.g., agitation or fatigue), medications such as antipsychotic or stimulant agents, respectively, should be considered.

Psychotherapy may be helpful for patients with mild to moderate dementia in order to help them understand, mourn, and adapt to this new impairment of functioning. Both medications and psychotherapy can thus improve the quality of life both for persons with HIV-related cognitive disorders and their significant others while also improving overall clinical outcomes.

b) Delirium

The evaluation of the cause of delirium in an HIV-infected patient requires the psychiatrist to be alert to multiple possible etiologic factors and be knowledgeable about specific diseases that are associated with HIV infection. Examples are hypoxemia due to *Pneumocystis carinii* pneumonia, uremia due to HIV nephropathy, or elevated ammonia levels due to cirrhosis. One of the most important factors is the multiple medications that HIV patients typically take, which often cause delirium or contribute to delirious states because of drug-drug interactions. Problems arising from such toxicity are often reversible. Patients with AIDS who reside in either nursing homes or assisted living facilities or who have been hospitalized and who develop delirium have been shown to have significantly shorter survival than AIDS patients without delirium (107, 108). HIV-associated delirium may present with symptoms that resemble classic mania or drug intoxication, thereby bringing patients to the attention of a psychiatrist for evaluation. Delirium in the context of HIV infection should be evaluated like delirium with other medical conditions (47). A psychiatrist should advocate for a complete medical/neurological evaluation for patients with HIV infection who present with an acute onset of psychiatric symptoms with no previous psychiatric history. A complete workup should include a toxicology screen, thorough neurological examination, laboratory evaluation, and brain imaging studies. A comprehensive assessment for infectious processes should be conducted and may entail lumbar puncture.

Management of delirium in the context of HIV infection includes judicious use of antipsychotic medications for symptoms of agitation or perceptual abnormalities such as hallucinations. Many clinicians use the newer, atypical antipsychotic agents due to their lower side effect profile.

c) Mood disorders

The management of disturbances in mood such as depression or mania for patients with HIV infection is similar to that for other patients with medical comorbidity. Fatigue and insomnia, frequent complaints in otherwise asymptomatic patients, are likely related to psychological disturbances such as major depressive disorder (109). In addition, the overall medical status of the patient should be assessed to take into account possible effects of concurrent illness or side effects of medications such as efavirenz. Psychiatrists should know all medications that a patient is taking. Choice of an antidepressant or mood-stabilizing agent may be influenced by the antiretroviral regimen in place, and doses may need to be adjusted if drug-drug interactions are likely. Psychotherapy should be recommended when indicated.

Manic syndromes are difficult to treat in HIV-infected patients for several reasons. First, mania may result from HIV infection (secondary mania) (33), AIDS-associated brain infections, neoplasms, or treatment with medications like steroids. In addition, manic syndromes can be related to comorbid substance use disorders, and case reports have documented manic symptoms induced by the antiretroviral agents didanosine and zidovudine (110, 111). Patients who experience their first manic episode later in the course of their HIV disease are less likely to have personal or family histories of mood disorders and are more likely to have dementia or neurocognitive slowing (34). Although the prevalence and incidence of mania associated with HIV are not well described, treatment studies suggest that traditional antimanic agents are effective and tolerated.

d) Substance use disorders

In the United States, substance use disorders are prevalent in the population of persons with or at risk for HIV infection, and treatment is a high priority. Because drug- and alcohol-dependent

HIV-infected patients form a large reservoir for HIV in the United States, and because behavior that risks transmission of HIV is often associated with concomitant substance use, psychiatrists should be aware that by treating substance abuse, they may well be preventing HIV infection (112). Unfortunately, the number of injection drug users in the United States outnumbers the available treatment slots.

Treatment with methadone or LAAM (113) can be an important treatment component for persons with opiate dependence. Since the quality of such programs varies, psychiatrists should help identify the best program for their patients. Factors that often indicate higher quality include the use of higher doses of methadone or LAAM and a close working relationship with primary medical clinicians and associated psychosocial services. It should be noted that doses of methadone may need to be increased or decreased in accordance with the use of specific antiretroviral agents that can have an impact on the metabolism of methadone.

Psychiatrists may be primary providers of care in a variety of clinical settings for HIV-infected patients who also have a substance use disorder. Psychiatrists should either provide treatment for their patients with comorbid substance abuse or collaborate with high-quality substance abuse programs. Substance use disorders themselves are often associated with comorbid psychiatric disorders such as anxiety, depression, and psychotic symptoms. Treatment of these comorbid conditions can help stabilize patients who are attempting to achieve sobriety or abstinence.

e) Anxiety disorders

Many problems involving anxiety symptoms can arise in relationship to HIV illness. An example of a clinical anxiety problem *without* HIV infection is AIDS phobia. For persons infected with HIV, there are numerous points at various stages of the illness when anxiety about the future, physical symptoms, or clinical decisions can become overwhelming. Psychotherapeutic approaches to situational anxiety can help patients work through intense affects and provide a structure within which sound decisions can be made.

Anxiety disorders can precede HIV infection or arise as its consequence. Treatment of anxiety disorders among HIV-infected patients has not been well studied; thus, psychiatrists should apply standard pharmacologic treatments for anxiety disorders with caution. For instance, many benzodiazepines are contraindicated when patients are taking protease inhibitors, particularly ritonavir, since predicted pharmacokinetics suggest blood levels of these psychotropic agents will be greatly elevated. Thus, benzodiazepines should be given as a short-term intervention in most instances. Psychiatrists may need to adjust medication doses and consider medical setbacks when treating patients with prominent anxiety symptoms. Psychotherapy may be effective in managing anxiety while reducing the need for medications. PTSD is a possible outcome of sexual assault or abuse and may be a focus of clinical treatment for some patients with HIV infection.

f) Psychotic disorders

Psychotic symptoms in the context of HIV infection, particularly at advanced stages of illness, do not necessarily indicate a primary psychotic disorder, such as schizophrenia, but may arise from causes ranging from opportunistic infections, mania, HIV-associated dementia, or delirium. Evaluation of new-onset psychosis requires a careful medical/neurological workup.

There is no literature to suggest that the use of antipsychotic medication needs to be modified for HIV-infected patients who have good immune functioning and are not taking antiretroviral medication. For patients taking antiretroviral medications, it is important to be aware of drug-drug interactions and overlapping toxicities. In particular, the use of clozapine is problematic with both ritonavir and zidovudine, the former because ritonavir may elevate blood levels of clozapine, the latter because clozapine and zidovudine can each cause significant bone marrow suppression.

In late-stage HIV infection, atypical antipsychotic medications are the first-line treatment because standard neuroleptic medications have been associated with very severe and difficult-to-treat extrapyramidal side effects. Also, in late-stage HIV illness, the lowest effective dose of any atypical antipsychotic medication should be given, since lower doses are sufficient to achieve efficacy and necessary to help prevent side effects.

g) Adjustment disorders

These disorders are interspersed among other diagnostic categories and are differentiated on the basis of onset after an identifiable stressor. Adjustment disorders are associated with significant emotional or behavioral symptoms. Although they may arise from stressful life events such as testing HIV-antibody positive, they may indicate a subsyndromal state that will evolve into a severe psychiatric disorder if left untreated. Various forms of psychotherapy may be indicated to prevent progression to a more severe psychiatric disturbance.

h) Sleep disorders

Sleep complaints are common in HIV patients in psychiatric treatment. Sleep disturbances may arise from a psychiatric disorder such as depression or stem from complications of HIV infection. For instance, because pain is a frequent accompaniment of HIV-related illness and is often treatable, clinicians should intervene to alleviate pain that causes sleep disturbance. The antiretroviral medication efavirenz is associated with a high incidence of vivid dreams and nightmares.

i) Disorders of infancy, childhood, and adolescence

The presenting psychiatric problems of HIV illness in children depend upon factors such as the age and developmental stage of the child, HIV clinical stage, psychosocial situation, and individual vulnerabilities for psychiatric disorders. Although there are few studies in this area, psychiatric disorders are common among infected youth, with rates of about 30% for mood disorders and 25% for attention deficit hyperactivity disorder (114, 115). As mood and anxiety disorders are more likely to be overlooked by caregivers than disorders with prominent behavioral manifestations (externalizing disorders), extra vigilance is required by the psychiatrist.

Just as the standard of care for HIV intervention has changed for adults, so have the treatments for children infected with HIV. Children have increased survival rates and slower progression to AIDS with the use of antiretroviral medications.

Psychiatrists, especially child and adolescent psychiatrists, need to help support children who survive to adolescence to negotiate this complex developmental stage. Psychotherapy may be of particular help for adolescents who are dealing with issues of developing sexuality. For some adolescents, sexuality may be a reminder of their infection. For others, sexual risk behavior may be a reenactment of parental behaviors, a method of mastering their trauma, or a response to their anger concerning their ill health. Substance abuse is frequent (33% in one study) and is likely to involve multiple drug use (116). The issues of risk behavior and autonomy have implications for HIV prevention, adherence to treatment, and effective coping with chronic illness. The family's understanding and capacity to respond in a supportive manner are essential—these adaptations will not only help the child or adolescent cope with the attendant biopsychosocial adversity, they may also influence morbidity and mortality. The importance of family dynamics for children and adolescents with chronic illness and handicapping conditions has long been recognized (117, 118).

j) HIV-associated syndromes with psychiatric implications

In the case of somatic syndromes that exist at the interface of medical and psychiatric disorders, psychiatrists can serve to integrate treatment approaches and promote interdisciplinary and interspecialty dialogue. Symptoms such as fatigue, weight loss, pain, and sexual dysfunction can be associated with HIV illness as well as psychiatric disorders. It is useful to avoid all-or-nothing, mind or body, approaches when evaluating such nonspecific symptoms. Good communication between psychiatrists and other physicians leads to better treatment decisions. Principles of palliative care apply when a patient is terminally ill and desires treatment that focuses on comfort and symptom relief.

Wasting syndrome generally occurs in patients with more advanced HIV illness and can be related to a number of physiologic disturbances, such as progressive HIV disease, hypogonadism, and gastrointestinal malabsorption. Loss of lean body mass is a strong predictor of increased mortality due to AIDS (119). Wasting is defined as loss of >10% of ideal body weight.

Fatigue is a common, often chronic symptom in HIV disease, frequently associated with depressed mood and physical disability, particularly among patients with more advanced HIV infection or AIDS (120–122).

Patients report pain at all stages of HIV illness, but complaints tend to be more frequent and more intense at advanced stages of systemic illness (123, 124). Common painful symptoms stem from headaches, herpetic lesions, peripheral neuropathy, back pain, throat pain, arthralgias, and muscle and abdominal pain (125).

Sexual dysfunction has been reported to occur in both men and women with HIV infection. In men, hypogonadism can be treated with testosterone replacement (126). As a rule, testosterone more effectively treats diminished libido than erectile dysfunction.

IV. CLINICAL AND ENVIRONMENTAL FEATURES INFLUENCING TREATMENT

A. SOCIODEMOGRAPHIC VARIABLES

1. Race/ethnicity

AIDS and HIV infection disproportionately affect both the African American and Hispanic populations in the United States. In 1998, African Americans accounted for 45% of AIDS cases reported that year while constituting only 12% of the total U.S. population. The same year, the rate of reported AIDS cases for Hispanics in the United States was 20%, although Hispanics constituted only 13% of the general population (Figure 5). In 1998, African Americans overtook whites as the group with the largest number of persons living with AIDS. The rates have been relatively constant in the Asian/Pacific Islander and American Indian/Alaska Native groups: about 1% of cases (Figure 6).

The statistics are even more skewed when classified according to both race *and* gender. For those cases of AIDS reported through 1998, 77% of all women with AIDS were black or Hispanic; 81% of all children with AIDS were black or Hispanic (127).

Three interrelated issues seem to account for the high rates of HIV/AIDS in minority communities: 1) inequities in the general health status in economically disadvantaged minorities, 2) problems controlling substance abuse in minority communities, and 3) the role of substance abuse in the spread of HIV sexually and perinatally.

HIV prevention efforts must be tailored for specific ethnic/cultural groups so that their effectiveness can be enhanced. This point is highlighted by the high levels of stigma associated with gay or bisexual activity in the African American and Hispanic communities. The impact of religious beliefs (Pentecostal, Catholic) in these communities may also affect HIV prevention efforts due to negative views of homosexuality.

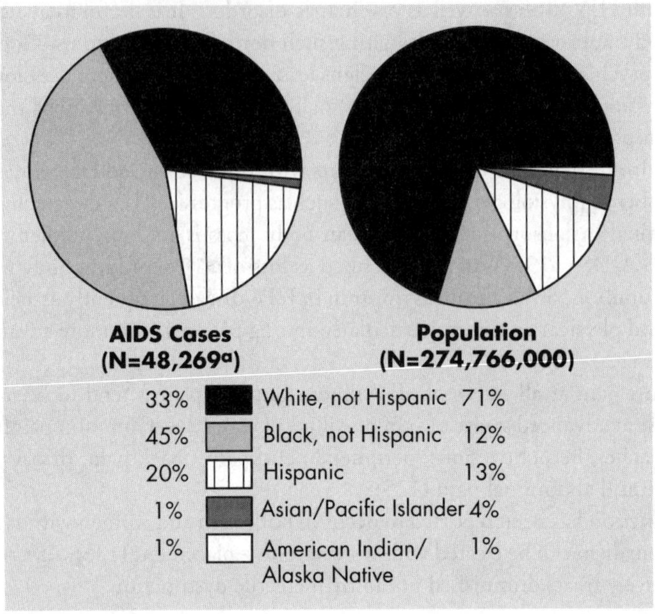

FIGURE 5. U.S. AIDS Cases Reported in 1998 and Estimated 1998 U.S. Population, by Race/Ethnicity (3).

[a]Includes 242 persons with unknown race/ethnicity.

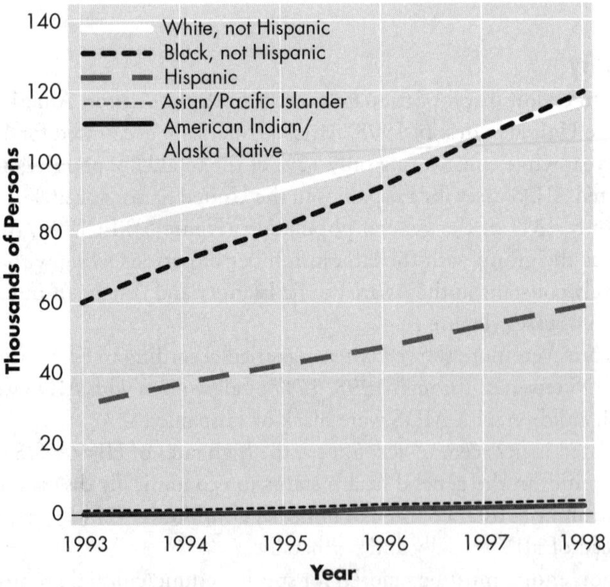

FIGURE 6. Estimated Number of Persons Living With AIDS in the United States, 1993–1998, by Race/Ethnicity (3).

Hispanics in the United States constitute a diverse group of cultures and countries of origin. Surveys have found that exposure to HIV varies in different Hispanic subgroups. For example, injection drug use is more prevalent among Hispanics from Puerto Rico, whereas the more common risk behavior for Hispanics who originate from Mexico, Cuba, and South and Central America is unsafe sex among men who have sex with men (128).

2. Sexual orientation

Throughout most of the earlier years of the HIV/AIDS epidemic, men who had sex with men were disproportionately affected. Although this group still constitutes the population with the highest AIDS incidence (37% of new AIDS cases in 1998), through massive prevention interventions, rates for men who have sex with men have declined, whereas other exposure categories are increasing annually. For example, in 1998, 12% of new AIDS cases were linked to heterosexual transmission (127).

Evidence from HIV prevalence studies and risk behavior surveys supports the need to continue HIV prevention efforts among each generation of gay and bisexual men. There are cohort differences in attitudes, behavior, and perceived risk in younger and older gay and bisexual men. In one study of six urban counties, 5%–8% of adolescents and young men between the ages of 15 and 22 who were having sex with men were already infected with HIV (3).

Bisexual women have been reported to have significantly more sexually transmitted diseases and HIV risk than heterosexual women (129), and women who have sex with women constitute a group with a combination of risks for HIV infection. In general, female-to-female transmission is thought to be uncommon, although theoretically possible. The CDC writes that "of the 347 (out of 2,220) women who were reported to have had sex only with women, 98% also had another risk—injection drug use in most cases" (130). Women who have sex with women do need to know that exposure to mucous membranes, such as the vagina or mouth, or to vaginal secretions or menstrual blood could transmit HIV, especially if the concentration of the virus is high (early or late-stage HIV infection).

3. Gender

The percentage of women with both HIV infection and AIDS has been steadily rising over the past decade. AIDS cases among women and adolescent girls rose 364% between 1991 and 1997. Trends in HIV diagnoses showed a 3% decrease in men but a 3% increase in women between 1995 and 1996. Heterosexual contact is the leading risk category for women (38%), with 29% of cases in women resulting from personal injection drug use (127).

The exposure category "other/not identified" represents 32% of AIDS cases in women (127). It is typical for more recently reported cases to be classified as "other/not identified," but after medical record review and investigation, most cases are eventually attributed to one of the defined exposure categories.

African American and Hispanic women are disproportionately affected, with AIDS rates 17 and 6 times higher, respectively, than for Caucasian women. Despite the difficult socioeconomic conditions many minority women live in, a recent survey of health concerns among low-income women found that AIDS was ranked as the most important concern (131).

There are issues that are unique to women and HIV/AIDS. Male-to-female transmission is estimated to be eight times more likely than female-to-male transmission (132). Sex differences in HIV measurements such as viral load, side effects of antiretroviral medications, and access to quality health care have all been documented (133). These biological differences make recommendations for antiretroviral therapies more uncertain for women. In addition, most clinical trials of interventions to treat HIV infection have enrolled male subjects. Women, particularly HIV-positive women, have psychological, psychosocial, reproductive, and gynecological concerns that differ from men (134, 135).

4. Age

AIDS has always had the greatest impact on Americans ages 25–44. For example, in 1996, almost 75% of persons with AIDS were between the ages of 25 and 44; 21% were over age 44, and less than 4% were between the ages of 13 and 24. More recent data have shown that one in four new infections in the United States occurs in people younger than 22 years of age (127).

Because of the impact associated with new medical therapies, many people's lives have significantly lengthened, which has led to older generations of persons living with HIV/AIDS. For instance, currently one out of 10 AIDS patients in the United States is over 50 years old; in Florida, one out of every six AIDS patients is older than 50 (136).

The age of diagnosis for 11% of AIDS cases is 50 years or older, and the age of diagnosis for 3% of AIDS cases is 60 years or older (127). However, there remains a common misperception that HIV is not a risk for older people. Many HIV-related symptoms mimic the effects of aging, so clinicians may be slow to diagnose HIV infection in older people and fail to question their older patients about risk behaviors (137). This is troublesome given research findings that document that adults over the age of 50 are up to one-sixth as likely to use condoms as people in their 20s (138). A particular diagnostic challenge for mental health clinicians treating HIV-infected older persons involves neurological symptoms, for which the differential diagnosis of cognitive impairment should be broadened to include dementias seen in older age.

5. Economic factors

According to data from the first national multisite HIV/AIDS Mental Health Services Demonstration Program, of nearly 2,000 persons with HIV/AIDS seeking mental health services, a majority were socially and economically disadvantaged (i.e., marginally employed, poor, relying on public assistance, or under- or uninsured) (139). Almost half of the 2,000 patients treated in this program lacked medical insurance, and for all patients median monthly income was only $575. Other sources of economic information yield seroprevalence data that suggest higher rates of HIV infection among the poor. For example, among Job Corps participants (who are primarily economically disadvantaged youth), HIV seroprevalence rates are twice that of youth seen at adolescent clinics and eight times higher than rates for similar age youth who apply for military service (140).

6. Urban versus rural

Although HIV has historically disproportionately affected urban areas, rural populations are increasingly at risk. Although more drug-related risk behaviors are reported by residents of large metropolitan areas, high-risk sexual behaviors have not been found to differ significantly among urban and rural residents (141). However, one recent study found rural low-income women less likely to use condoms than their urban counterparts (142). When compared to urban dwellers living with HIV/AIDS, rural inhabitants report significantly lower life satisfaction, lower perceptions of social support from family and friends, reduced access to medical and mental health care, elevated levels of loneliness, more community stigma, heightened personal fear that their HIV status might be disclosed by others, and more maladaptive coping strategies (143).

B. CLINICAL FEATURES

1. Suicidality

Suicide, attempted suicide, and suicidal ideation are complex clinical issues that may arise during the course of psychiatric care for HIV patients (144). Studies in the 1980s, before antiretroviral treatments, reported rates of completed suicide in HIV-positive men as high as 66 times that of the general population (145–147). However, more recent data show suicide rates only modestly elevated and comparable to those in other medically ill populations (148), although perhaps most elevated among men who have sex with men (149). A study among U.S. military service applicants found suicide rates for both HIV-positive and HIV-negative individuals that were only marginally more elevated than those in the U.S. general population (150).

A number of risk factors for suicide in HIV patients have been described. They include psychiatric morbidity such as substance abuse (151, 152), antisocial personality disorder (153), family psychiatric history and family history of attempted suicide (154), and major depressive disorder. Numerous psychosocial factors have also been identified, such as a history of multiple HIV-related losses, lack of social support, loss of employment or insurance coverage, painful and disfiguring physical deterioration, exhaustion of financial resources, and reliance on public assistance (155, 156).

Recent evidence has shown that patients with greater levels of "fighting spirit," a specific pattern of adjustment to life-threatening illnesses, tend to have lower levels of suicidal ideation. Evaluation of suicide risk and other violent acts is an integral part of a comprehensive evaluation for HIV/AIDS patients. Psychiatric treatments that promote greater adaptation to living with HIV infection may lower the risk of suicide for many patients (154).

2. Bereavement

There are unique features to bereavement in the context of HIV/AIDS. Deaths from AIDS often disproportionately affect specific segments of the U.S. population. For example, it is not uncommon for a member of the gay community to have lost multiple persons to AIDS. At the same time, a bereaved individual may himself or herself be infected with HIV. Reports have suggested increases in high-risk sexual behavior and suicidal ideation in partners of individuals who have died of AIDS (157, 158). Bereavement is often compounded by the fact that many people die from AIDS at a young age, out of synchrony with the normal developmental sequence (159, 160).

Growing numbers of children will lose one or both parents to HIV. Psychiatrists need to explore the capacity of families to communicate about HIV and the children's understanding of their parent's illness. Disclosure is difficult for many parents who worry about revealing stigmatized behaviors or overwhelming a child with information (161). Permanency planning is an essential step in communication and collaboration with social agencies. For many children, bereavement is complicated by the psychosocial problems that existed before HIV that are then compounded by disintegration of the immediate family. Problem behaviors in adolescents who anticipate losing one or both parents to AIDS have been described (162). Family-based, multidisciplinary team approaches may be effective in providing access to care and needed follow-up services.

Researchers have studied the relationship of AIDS bereavement and psychological or medical variables but have not necessarily found that greater numbers of AIDS losses are associated with a higher rate of depressive symptoms or depressive disorders (163) or that distress increases in a dose-response relationship to the number of losses (164). One investigation reported changes in measures of immune function relevant to HIV disease in bereaved HIV-positive men that suggested patterns consistent with disease progression (165). Bereavement has been associated with decreased lymphocyte proliferation (164, 166) and decreased natural killer cell function (167, 168).

Group therapy is often recommended for AIDS-related bereavement (169). Group participants include partners, friends, family, and caregivers of persons who have died of AIDS. A randomized, controlled trial of support group interventions for bereaved HIV-positive and HIV-negative men demonstrated significant improvement in grief symptoms for the treatment group compared to control subjects (170).

3. Axis II disorders

Several studies have reported that patients with HIV infection have a prevalence of personality disorders in the range of 19%–37%, which is higher than rates found in comparable patients who are not infected (171). Personality disorders categorized (per DSM) within cluster B, such as borderline and histrionic personality disorder, are the most common (172). These data are supported by clinical reports from settings that provide care for large numbers of HIV-infected patients (173). The findings are not surprising given the association between personality disorders—especially those disorders in which "impulsivity" is prominent—and risk factors for HIV infection such as high-risk drug use and sexual behaviors. Personality disorders among those infected with HIV are associated with a higher rate of depression, maladaptive coping, and other psychiatric symptoms (174, 175) as well as with a higher rate of injection drug use (176). In fact, one study has documented that among their sample of HIV-positive and "at risk" HIV-negative gay men, persons with personality disorders were at significant risk of onset of future axis I disorders and serious functional impairment, regardless of a past history of axis I disorders (177).

No studies have assessed the efficacy of specific treatments for personality disorders among individuals infected with HIV. There is no evidence against the use of standard psychiatric treatments for personality disorders, tailored to the individual patient. Some clinicians use an approach that includes limit setting, especially limits on the inappropriate use of medical resources and medications. Other strategies for complex cases emphasize the development and maintenance of a doctor-patient relationship, treatment of comorbid conditions such as depression and substance abuse, and supportive or cognitive psychotherapy techniques (173).

4. Psychoneuroimmunology

The relationship of behavior and psychopathology to immune measures has been the focus of ongoing research over recent years. With regard to HIV infection, the findings are mixed. On the one hand, a number of studies have found that stressful life event burden is associated with decreased CD4 cell count (178–180), decreased cytotoxic T lymphocyte count (181), clinical HIV disease progression (182, 183), and physical symptom burden (168). In contrast, the relationship of variables such as stressful life events and depressed mood levels with markers of immunological progression has not been supported by other studies (184, 185).

There appears to be an increase in the frequency and severity of depression around the time of the onset of AIDS that persists throughout the time of severe immunodeficiency (66). Whether depressed mood levels in general are associated with decreases in immune function is not clear, since one study has shown such an association (186), whereas another has not (187). The disparity across studies attempting to elicit such natural history relationships may be due to methodological differences related to the extent to which other factors, including immunological measures and clinical disease progression, had been controlled (179).

Interventions such as cognitive behavior stress management, coping skills enhancement training, massage therapy, existential therapy, bereavement support groups, and antidepressant medication have all been evaluated with regard to their effect on immune measures (188–190). The findings are mixed, with some interventions showing modest improvements of specific immune measures, whereas others did not result in positive changes. Most interventions are safe, including those that involved the antidepressants fluoxetine and imipramine (190). At this time, these types of interventions should be regarded as investigational in terms of their immunological and health effects. However, psychotherapeutic and psychopharmacologic interventions are indicated for their alleviation of distress and enhancement of functional status.

A caveat regarding the use of such interventions is that many patients hold beliefs that may lead to inappropriate expectations of the potential for immunological and clinical health effects. Patients who do not observe these effects may come to blame themselves (and their behavior) for the lack of such immunological and clinical effects and for disease progression. This could actually result in increased distress. Hence, patients must be carefully prepared for understanding the context in which behavioral interventions are being offered and which outcomes should be considered primary (psychological and functional) and which might be considered secondary and investigational (immunological and clinical health). On the other hand, clinicians should not discourage use of adjunctive techniques that can potentially add to the effect of current medical management by expanding the comprehensiveness of care.

C. SPECIAL TREATMENT SITUATIONS

1. Alternative and complementary treatment

Alternative and complementary medicine is an important part of the health care sought by many Americans. Surveys of the U.S. public in both 1990 and 1997 demonstrated that over one-third of Americans used at least one unconventional treatment in the past year, with rates rising from 34% to 42% between 1990 and 1997. It is estimated that the number of visits to nontraditional care clinicians exceeds total visits to all U.S. primary care physicians and represents $27.0 billion in annual out-of-pocket expenditures (191, 192). More than 60% of patients who use complementary/alternative treatments do not disclose the treatments to their doctors. Depression is one of the most common conditions for which patients seek alternative/complementary therapies.

Surveys specific to the HIV-infected population report similar findings, with between 30% and 68% of respondents reporting use of some form of complementary/alternative treatment (193–196). Patients with HIV/AIDS use complementary and alternative medicine to improve general health or quality of life, prevent progression of HIV disease, treat specific symptoms, or counter side effects that result from biomedical treatments (197, 198).

According to data from the first 1,016 participants of the Alternative Medical Care Outcomes in AIDS Study, the 10 most frequently used activities are aerobic exercise (64%), prayer (56%), massage (54%), needle acupuncture (48%), meditation (46%), support groups (42%), visualization and imagery (34%), breathing exercises (33%), spiritual activities (33%), and other exercise (33%) (199). Other nontraditional treatments include nutritional, vitamin, or herbal supplements and medicinal use of marijuana and anabolic steroids. Only one research study to date has examined complementary therapy in the context of HIV infection. A multisite project is currently being conducted in cooperation with the Office of Alternative Medicine, National Institutes of Health, to evaluate these treatments (200).

2. Institutional settings

Institutions that house, treat, or incarcerate have a responsibility to address issues of HIV education, prevention, and clinical services for persons served in these settings. Seroprevalence studies in institutional settings identify the scale of HIV infection and help inform policies for the institution. For example, concerns about HIV infection among institutionalized mentally retarded persons have been somewhat allayed by studies that found either no cases of HIV infection (201) or low rates (0.16%) (202). These institutions nonetheless need to maintain universal blood and body fluid precautions as well as develop prevention programs tailored to their patient population.

Some of the highest rates of HIV infection are found among jails and prisons due to the high frequency of drug-related sentences and high-risk behaviors that occur within the institutions. Prevalence rates among male inmates have been recorded between 6% and 8.5% (203, 204); one study of incarcerated women in New York found an 18.8% rate of HIV infection (205).

Despite the alarmingly high rates of HIV infection among prisoners in the United States, administrative and institutional barriers, such as not allowing the distribution of condoms, undermine prevention interventions. Collaboration between institutional staff and clinicians or researchers of HIV prevention efforts may lead to effective interventions for inmates and their partners (206). Psychiatrists working in correctional facilities may need to advocate for patients who may not receive antiretroviral medications in a timely manner due to lockdowns, solitary confinement, or other factors. Recommendations for handling HIV-related issues in psychiatric institutions can be found in policy and position statements issued by the APA Office on AIDS (www.psych.org/aids; click on "Policy Statements").

3. Health care clinician issues

HIV creates unique demands on clinicians. Stresses that are associated with the care of HIV-infected patients include fear of contagion, the emotional impact of dying patients, stigma associated with AIDS, anxiety concerning sexual and drug risk behavior, a constantly changing knowledge base, and often inadequate treatment resources (207). Health care workers have numerous reactions to these stresses. Clinicians have reported, for example, greater anxiety, more interference with nonwork activities, and symptoms similar to PTSD when treating AIDS patients as compared to non-AIDS patients (208, 209).

Despite the stresses and demands, most clinical staff members feel positively about their work, and only a small minority experience job burnout. The frequently cited rewards of working with HIV-infected patients include a sense of personal helpfulness, increased professional mastery, altruism, and admiration for patients' courage (210). In order to support employees, most multidisciplinary programs address issues that are likely to cause stress, such as death and dying, the management of sexuality, and fear of contagion. Interventions to address these issues range from weekly informal team meetings to leader-based staff support groups (211, 212).

Workshops that allow caregivers an opportunity to express grief, explore frustrations, and share resources may be helpful (213). Progress in HIV therapeutics requires frequent educational updates. Appropriate resolution of staff conflict and disagreement is useful in the HIV care setting, as it is in other settings that deal with chronic medical illness. One study, for example, found that HIV health care workers who perceived colleagues as significantly stressful were nearly 50% more likely to experience job burnout (214). Thus, a well-functioning HIV team may help buffer the stresses of providing care, and psychiatrists can be effective by assisting those teams.

PART B:
REVIEW AND SYNTHESIS OF AVAILABLE EVIDENCE

V. DATA REGARDING PREVENTION FOR INDIVIDUALS AT HIGH RISK FOR HIV INFECTION

A. HIV-RELATED RISK ASSESSMENT OF BEHAVIOR

In a national survey of 417 practicing psychiatrists conducted in 1997 by APA, the physicians reported that over 9% of patients they treat are at risk for HIV infection (215); the rate was derived from questions about psychiatrists' knowledge of patient risk behavior. This estimate is probably conservative, since many psychiatrists do not conduct a detailed HIV risk assessment. Nonetheless, the survey data support other findings that psychiatric patients report higher rates of HIV risk behavior than the general population (141) and underscore the important role that psychiatrists play in preventing HIV infection.

Studies of primary care clinicians who conduct HIV risk assessments among patients who express concern about HIV risk found that in 73% of the encounters, the physicians did not elicit enough information to adequately characterize patients' HIV risk status (216).

B. HIV ANTIBODY TESTING

It is estimated that only two-thirds of all HIV-infected people in the United States know their serological status. Hence, many do not know until they are diagnosed with AIDS. The CDC recommends routine voluntary HIV antibody testing of patients who are admitted to hospitals that have HIV seroprevalence rates of >1% among admitted patients.

A multistate evaluation found that *anonymous* HIV testing was associated with earlier HIV testing and HIV-related medical care when compared to those who were tested *confidentially* (217). Concerns about HIV test confidentiality led to a study of testing trends in six states that initiated name-based reporting of HIV test results. The researchers did not find significant declines in the total number of HIV tests performed at counseling and testing sites other than those expected from trends present before name-based reporting (218). Moreover, Osmond and colleagues (219) surveyed nearly 2,000 HIV-seropositive patients diagnosed during 1995–1996 in five states with name-based HIV surveillance (and three without) and reported that keeping records of people infected with HIV by name does not help or hinder treatment.

Home collection testing for HIV provides a method for testing among individuals who may not otherwise seek HIV testing through publicly funded sites or medical providers. A review of data collected by test manufacturers in the first year of availability (1996–1997) reported that of 174,316 tests performed, 0.9% were positive. Most users of home collection tests were white men aged 25–34 years; HIV prevalence was highest among nonwhites, men who had sex with men (particularly bisexual men), and injection drug users. Nearly 60% of those who submitted samples and 49% of those who tested positive had never had a previous HIV test (220).

C. INTERVENTIONS TO REDUCE HIV RISK BEHAVIOR

A wealth of literature addresses the issue of how to intervene to reduce HIV risk behavior at both the individual and community level. While this section will focus primarily on data concerning interventions at the individual level, macro-level changes in structure or policy can lead to powerful community-level support of specific behavior changes (221). The AIDS Community Demonstration Project is a good example of a community-level intervention. Community volunteers and "small" media were able to influence community norms about the use of condoms and disinfection of drug injection equipment by using bleach (222). Other examples of societal-level policies that influence the effectiveness of individual-level HIV risk behavior interventions are 1) laws that prohibit same-sex marriage, which hinder the establishment of long-term monogamous relationships for men who have sex with men (223), and 2) insufficient substance abuse treatment capacity, which decreases the opportunity for an injection drug user to receive treatment.

Sexual behavior is the target of most prevention efforts worldwide, but because of the diversity of sexual behavior and the influences of economics, culture, and environment, interventions to stem HIV necessarily vary as well (224). Because of the sheer size of the prevention literature and the many specific populations that have been targeted, these guidelines will not provide more detailed information about subgroups based on gender, ethnicity, or age. A publication from the CDC entitled "Compendium of HIV Prevention Interventions with Evidence of Effectiveness" provides a useful synopsis of the research in this area (225).

1. Counseling strategies

The HIV counseling and testing model has been widely used in studies that intend to promote behavior change in persons at risk for HIV infection. Yet, two large reviews of HIV counseling and testing studies (226, 227) found that HIV counseling and testing interventions do not consistently lead to risk reduction or promote help-seeking behavior in most populations studied. Both analyses found that serodiscordant heterosexual couples demonstrated the most change in risk behavior. A recent meta-analysis of the effect of HIV counseling and testing interventions found that they were more effective in secondary prevention for HIV-positive persons than as a primary prevention strategy (228).

The most widely used counseling models acknowledge that knowledge about HIV transmission and prevention is necessary but not sufficient for behavior change (229–231). More effective interventions rely on skills training and take into account individual psychosocial and cognitive strategies (232). Essential to effective counseling is helping patients perceive themselves as at risk for HIV infection, addressing motivation to reduce risk, and ensuring that patients have the skills and resources to implement risk reduction strategies. Changing peer norms with the help of peer leaders and matching the background characteristics (e.g., race, ethnicity, sexual orientation) of the leader to the targeted population often help increase intervention effectiveness.

The largest randomized, controlled HIV behavioral intervention study conducted in the United States found that even among persons served in public health settings, a small-group, seven-session risk reduction intervention cut reported high-risk sexual behaviors in half and more than doubled reported regular use of condoms (from 23% to at least 60%) (233). HIV prevention interventions have proven useful for psychiatric populations, including injection drug users and people with severe mental illness, and have been shown to be effective even when conducted in busy public clinics (234, 235).

2. Specific strategies for injection drug users

The principles for preventing the spread of HIV among active drug injectors are similar to those used to modify unsafe sexual behavior. Ethnographic research has clarified how injected drugs are purchased, dissolved, filtered, transferred into syringes, and injected, and how sharing practices at each step in the process contribute to the potential spread of HIV (236). Successful interventions focus on knowledge, motivation, and behavioral skills that are tailored to realistic strategies for changing sharing practices. These programs have also engaged members of the injection drug use community as prevention leaders.

An international study found that injection drug users are capable of changing their risk behavior and providing accurate reports of their behavior. Further, these behavioral changes are associated with lower rates of HIV infection (237). A review of the research literature on HIV prevention outreach efforts concluded that most such programs have led to changes in drug-related and sex-related risk behaviors in injection drug users (238). Specific reductions in drug injection, sharing of injection equipment, and crack use and increases in needle disinfection, condom use, and entry into drug treatment were seen with such programs.

The most controversial component of HIV transmission prevention in the injection drug use population has been the use of needle and syringe exchange programs that make sterile equipment available to drug injectors. These programs have met strong political opposition in many countries, including the United States, and assessment of their effectiveness has been fraught with methodological difficulties. There are unsubstantiated concerns that exchange programs may attract subjects who engage in the riskiest practices and that the number of needles or syringes in circulation may not be sufficient to ensure single-time use (239). Recent U.S. and international data make a strong argument for the benefits of needle exchange programs on reducing HIV transmission as well as other parenterally transmissible infections such as hepatitis B and C (240, 241). Nonetheless, since federal funds to date have been prohibited for use in needle exchange programs, they have had limited impact on lowering HIV transmission in the United States. Needle exchange programs that do exist are often small and cannot meet local demand.

D. REDUCING MATERNAL-FETAL TRANSMISSION

Before interventions with antiretroviral treatment were instituted, between 1,000 and 2,000 infants were born each year in the United States with HIV infection (242). Since recommendations were made for routine counseling and voluntary HIV testing of pregnant women, and for subsequent treatment with zidovudine for those who prove seropositive, the CDC has recorded dramatic decreases in perinatal transmission. From 1992 to 1997, cases of perinatal AIDS declined 67%, including an 80% decline in AIDS cases among infants and a 66% decline among children between the ages of 1 and 5 (243). It has been shown that elective cesarean delivery may further decrease the risk for fetal infection (244).

The protocol of administering zidovudine to a pregnant woman in the last two trimesters, followed by intravenous zidovudine during delivery, then 6 weeks of zidovudine treatment for newborns was found to reduce the incidence of HIV transmission from mother to child from 22.6% to 7.6%—a 66% reduction (245, 246). While the mechanism by which zidovudine reduces perinatal transmission is not known, research has shown that a risk factor for perinatal transmission is the amount of HIV in the pregnant woman's blood (247, 248). At the same time, the effect of zidovudine's lowering maternal HIV viral load does not fully explain the efficacy of zidovudine in reducing transmission. Another important component of protection may be preexposure prophylaxis of the fetus or infant to antiretroviral drugs. Because it has been shown to be metabolized into its active triphosphate form within the placenta, zidovudine may have distinct superiority in efficacy compared to other nucleoside analogues such as didanosine and zalcitabine (249).

There have been other studies of interventions to reduce perinatal transmission, such as short-course antenatal/intrapartum zidovudine in non-breast-feeding Thai women (250) or the combined agent lamivudine/zidovudine during gestation, intrapartum, and postpartum in African women (251). Both interventions were associated with reductions in perinatal transmission by approximately 50% (even though the group given lamivudine/zidovudine breast-fed). In the situation when the diagnosis of HIV infection is not made until near the end of gestation or during labor, treatment with the combined agent lamivudine/zidovudine or nevirapine in the intrapartum/postpartum period has been shown to be effective in reducing transmission (251, 252).

There are limited data on the effect of combination antiretroviral therapies on pregnancy outcome. A retrospective Swiss study reported that 80% of women experienced side effects to the drugs, which included reverse transcriptase inhibitors and protease inhibitors, and further, found a possible association with preterm birth (253).

Women who face decisions regarding the use of antiretroviral medications during pregnancy must consider the effects of treatment on their own health as well as on fetal or child health. These decisions are complex, since the standard of care has moved to multiple antiretroviral drugs, and yet the long-term consequences of exposure to such drugs by the infant are not known. In general, the three-stage zidovudine regimen (prenatal, intrapartum, and postpartum) alone or in combination with other antiretroviral agents should be discussed and offered to all HIV-infected pregnant women.

Antiretroviral protocols to prevent perinatal transmission are burdensome for patients and practitioners, and adherence is again a crucial factor in treatment effectiveness. A 1995 study found that only 15% of HIV-positive mothers and their newborns received the full zidovudine treatment regimen (252). This same study found that 26% of pregnant women with HIV infection did not receive any prenatal care. Coordination of care by providers of medical, mental health, drug abuse, and social services may be required for the successful implementation of antiretroviral treatment during pregnancy.

E. POSTEXPOSURE PROPHYLAXIS

While universal infection control precautions have become the standard of care in the U.S. health care system, as of June 1998, 54 health care workers had documented HIV infection through occupational exposure. Of the 54, 46 had percutaneous (puncture/cut injury) exposure, five had mucocutaneous (mucous membrane or skin) exposure, two had both percutaneous and mucocutaneous exposure, and one had an unknown exposure (82). The estimated risk of HIV infection in health care workers with percutaneous HIV exposure is approximately 0.3% (254).

Postexposure prophylaxis with antiretroviral agents has been shown to be safe and effective (82). The postexposure prophylaxis protocol outlines specific steps in assessing risk. First, the type of exposure—including type of material, contact surface type, volume, and severity of exposure—is determined. Next, the HIV status of the exposure source is assessed on the basis of factors such as probable viral titer (based on clinical HIV status of exposure source) and whether actual HIV status is known (it may be unknown). The exact postexposure prophylaxis recommendation—whether to intervene at all, use two agents (zidovudine and lamivudine), or use three (both of the above plus either indinavir or nelfinavir)—is based on these assessments. If done properly, postexposure prophylaxis can reduce the risk for occupational transmission of HIV infection in health care workers with known exposure, such as a needle stick injury involving blood or other body fluids, by 80% (255).

F. SPECIAL PSYCHIATRIC POPULATIONS

1. Patients with substance use disorders

HIV is spread both by sharing injection drug use equipment (most frequently practiced by opiate, cocaine, or methamphetamine users) and by engaging in unsafe sexual practices that are associated with substance use disorders. Documented sexual risk behaviors among those with substance use disorders include having multiple partners in the context of buying or selling sex for drugs or money to buy drugs; unprotected sex with injection drug users; and difficulty employing safer sex practices while intoxicated. These sexual encounters can also increase the risk of transmission of other sexually transmitted diseases that are cofactors for HIV transmission. Unfortunately, sexual risk behaviors are more resistant to change than drug-use risk behaviors in drug users (256).

Comorbidity of substance use disorders with other psychiatric disorders deserves mention. A study that used data from the 1992 National Survey of Veterans examined whether substance abuse or other mental disorders serve as risk factors for HIV infection. The investigators found that the combination of substance abuse and PTSD increased the rate of HIV infection by almost 12 times over that of those without either disorder (257).

Drug use disorders are associated with high rates of incarceration for drug-related crimes. Jails and prisons, in turn, bring people with elevated rates of HIV infection together in a confined space, increasing the chance that a sexual or injection drug use partner encountered in these settings will be infected with the virus (258, 259). Institutionalization in all-male settings also increases the likelihood of sex between men.

There are geographic differences in seroprevalence rates of HIV in injection drug use populations, with the highest rates in the United States occurring in the Northeast, on the East

Coast, and in Puerto Rico (3). Holding the risk behavior constant, the likelihood of acquiring HIV increases with its penetration into a given geographic area by increasing the chance that sexual and drug injection partners will be infected. Because substance use disorders are associated with decreased occupational functioning or disability, many of these individuals become impoverished and often cluster in urban neighborhoods that are endemic for HIV.

2. Patients with severe mental illness

The severely and persistently mentally ill population is at risk for HIV infection due to factors analogous to those of patients with substance use disorders. There are high rates of substance use disorders among those with severe mental illness, and both populations share similar tendencies to reside in institutions or poor urban neighborhoods where cases of HIV infection are concentrated. Chronically mentally ill adults have been documented to have misunderstandings about AIDS transmission, to have histories of treatment for sexually transmitted diseases, and to report behaviors such as "survival sex" (in exchange for shelter, food, or money) (260). When compared to the general population, people with severe mental illness have higher rates of same-sex sexual activity and intimate contact with multiple partners (261). One study found an association of positive symptoms of psychosis and the diagnosis of schizophrenia with specific high-risk sexual behaviors (74).

Randomized, controlled trials of relatively brief AIDS prevention programs for the chronically mentally ill led to significant improvements in rates of unprotected intercourse and condom use (262) and knowledge about AIDS (263) in the intervention groups. It is not known whether such improvements persist beyond the short follow-up period.

3. Victims of sexual abuse/crimes

A history of sexual abuse is highly prevalent among both women and men living with or at risk for HIV infection. One report of 408 mostly economically disadvantaged women (at least 18 years old) found a lifetime prevalence of sexual abuse of 43%; over one-half of the cases occurred during adulthood (264). A cohort of 327 homosexual or bisexual men had a 35.5% rate of childhood sexual abuse. Men with a history of childhood sexual abuse reported more lifetime male partners and a higher likelihood of unprotected receptive anal intercourse in the past 6 months (265). Women with a history of childhood sexual abuse have been found to have more sexual partners, heightened sexual activity, and more negative expectations of condom use (266). For example, a study of women in low-income housing developments found that those with a history of sexual coercion were likely to perceive that requesting a partner to use a condom would create a potentially violent situation (267).

In children, the occurrence of sexually transmitted diseases can be the first indication of sexual abuse. Although perinatal transmission of HIV accounts for the vast majority of HIV cases in children, HIV transmission has been reported to occur through childhood sexual abuse (268). Efforts to encourage active risk reduction in high-risk populations through AIDS education have found that adolescents who have been sexually abused are significantly less likely to use condoms and have much greater communication difficulties than their peers (269).

VI. DATA REGARDING PSYCHIATRIC TREATMENTS FOR INDIVIDUALS WITH HIV INFECTION

Psychiatric treatments for individuals with HIV infection follow the same principles as for any patient with a psychiatric diagnosis, but there are special considerations. As with other patients with comorbid medical and psychiatric illnesses, it is essential to help patients cope with HIV illness and, when appropriate, with death and dying. There is also an ongoing need to determine whether new psychiatric symptoms have a medical basis that requires intervention. Examples of unique treatment issues with HIV patients include but are not limited to the following:

- working with the patient on disclosure of HIV status;
- assessing dangerousness from the perspective of HIV transmission and intervening to reduce that risk;
- helping families with dependent children arrange permanency planning;
- treating HIV-infected children who have developmental delays resulting from prenatal drug exposure or from HIV infection;
- negotiating disability status and, for some patients, a return to work;
- bereavement/loss; and
- treatment adherence.

A. ACCESS TO SERVICES

Most patients are asymptomatic for many years after becoming infected. But once symptomatic with more advanced HIV disease, they may become high users of medical care, including mental health services (270). They may need frequent assessment and treatment visits, undergo many medical tests, require hospitalization, and take multiple medications (often as many as 10–15 different medications at different times of day). Many patients receive medical care from an HIV primary care or infectious disease clinic or from an infectious disease specialist in the community. A recent study reported better medical outcomes for patients with HIV infection who receive care from physicians with more experience treating HIV diseases (271).

The Ryan White CARE (Comprehensive AIDS Resources Emergency) Act was enacted in 1990 to help states, communities, and families provide care for people with HIV/AIDS who lack adequate health insurance or other resources. Since its inception, CARE Act grants have totaled $6.4 billion and have served approximately 500,000 individuals with HIV/AIDS annually. Administered by the Health Resources and Services Administration of the U.S. Department of Health and Human Services, CARE Act grants were reauthorized in 1996 and comprise several programs. Title I grants provide funds to cities for low-income or under- or uninsured persons to cover the cost of health care and medications, as well as support services like counseling and home and hospice care. Title II grants are for the 50 states, the District of Columbia, Puerto Rico, and U.S. territories to improve the quality, accessibility, and organization of both health care and support for patients with HIV/AIDS. Title III grants are given to public or nonprofit entities that provide comprehensive primary health care services for persons with AIDS or at-risk populations. Title IV grants fund efforts to coordinate HIV services and access to research for children, youth, women, and families. An additional component of the CARE program includes training for health care professionals, grants for innovative service delivery models for special populations, and dental services.

Despite CARE Act funding, lack of access to care remains a problem that affects morbidity and mortality for certain groups. One study documented that among urban patients who receive medical care, there are no differences in HIV disease progression or survival associated with sex, race, injection drug use, or socioeconomic status. This suggests access to medical care is a main determinant of how quickly a patient develops AIDS (272). More recently, investigators from the HIV Cost and Services Utilization Study, a national population-based sample, found that African American, Hispanic, female, uninsured, and Medicaid-insured individuals all had inferior patterns of medical care (e.g., later initiation of antiretroviral medication) than did Caucasian and privately insured individuals (273).

Persons with HIV infection have higher rates of most psychiatric disorders than the general population. Psychiatric patients with common medical problems, especially those with severe mental illness, receive suboptimal medical care and suffer greater morbidity and mortality from medical illnesses than the general population. Studies are now under way to determine the access of patients with severe mental illness to HIV-related medical treatments; it can be assumed that these patients need help to access medical services.

Psychiatric disorders can be underdetected, misdiagnosed, undertreated, or treated improperly in primary care settings. For example, while a substantial majority of HIV-infected persons presenting for intake to an HIV primary care clinic suffered from depression, substance dependence, or another current psychiatric disorder, most cases were not detected by clinicians (66). Underscoring the importance of mental health care is the finding that ongoing high-risk sexual behavior is predicted by higher levels of depression and recreational drug use (274).

There are several patient barriers to meeting the mental health needs of HIV-infected persons. These barriers include adherence difficulties (e.g., missed appointments or inability to follow treatment recommendations); fear of additional stigmatization (the "double stigma" of HIV and a mental disorder); negative prior experiences with the mental health system; lack of funds for transportation, payment of care, or medications; unstable housing and frequent relocation; and the complex comorbid presentations of patients with HIV infection (e.g., depression complicated by concurrent substance dependence and a personality disorder). On the other hand, health care professionals should not assume that depression is "normal" in a person with HIV infection.

Some innovative HIV clinics integrate medical, mental health, and substance abuse treatment within their programs (275). These model programs increase the opportunities for prevention and treatment and may reach a more impaired population (276). One model uses an outpatient psychiatric consultation-liaison clinic that specializes in the treatment of HIV-infected patients. The clinic can be physically off-site from an HIV clinic but receives most of its referrals from that clinic. Other models include HIV programs within community mental health centers, programs located within residential substance abuse treatment facilities, free-standing community-based agencies, and referrals to private practitioners with expertise in treating HIV patients. All of these models appear to be effective (67).

B. PHARMACOLOGIC TREATMENT

In general, the use of psychotropic agents in HIV patients follows similar principles for using these medications in such populations as geriatric patients or those with comorbid medical illnesses. This is particularly true for patients with more advanced HIV disease and those on complex antiretroviral regimens who may be more sensitive to medication dosages and side effects and are at higher risk for drug-drug interactions (277). Because some standard medications used to treat HIV infection or HIV-related conditions can potently inhibit or induce the cytochrome P450 system, psychotropic medications that share metabolic pathways should be used judiciously; however, this concern should not preclude appropriate pharmacologic intervention.

General guidelines, particularly for patients with symptomatic HIV disease, include 1) using lower starting doses and slower titration, 2) providing the least complicated dosing schedules possible, 3) focusing on drug side effect profiles to avoid unnecessary adverse events (e.g., anticholinergic effects from tricyclic antidepressants, leukopenia from carbamazepine), and 4) maintaining awareness of drug metabolism/clearance pathways to minimize drug-drug interactions and possible end organ damage.

Published reports of adverse events and side effects can offer specific guidance for the use of some psychotropic agents in HIV-infected patients. However, clinicians must be cautioned that many studies that have examined psychotropic effectiveness in HIV patients were conducted on relatively asymptomatic patients, often did not include women or youth, and were conducted before the availability of combination antiretroviral therapy. Liver disease, in particular hepatitis C,

TABLE 15. Cytochrome P450 Inhibition Potency of Protease Inhibitors, by Isoenzyme System

Protease Inhibitor	Cytochrome P450 Isoenzyme Inhibited
Ritonavir	3A4, 2C9, 2D6
Indinavir	3A4
Nelfinavir	3A4, 2C19, 2D6
Saquinavir	3A4, 2C9

is becoming increasingly important as a comorbid condition. Thus, routine liver function testing is necessary when prescribing psychotropic medications for patients with HIV infection.

Combination therapy with multiple medication classes constitutes the standard of care for successful treatment of HIV infection. Although limited clinical information is available concerning drug-drug interactions involving psychotropic and antiretroviral medications, effective psychotropic medication management in the setting of HIV requires attention to possible interactions.

Potential drug-drug interactions in the setting of antiretroviral therapy include the effects of antiretroviral agents on psychotropic medications and vice versa. Protease inhibitors and nonnucleoside reverse transcriptase inhibitors are metabolized by the cytochrome P450 system and may inhibit or induce multiple isoenzymes. For example, the protease inhibitor ritonavir inhibits the cytochrome P450 isoenzymes 3A, 2D6, and 2C9/19; thus, most psychotropic medications may be affected when concomitantly used with ritonavir. Other protease inhibitors tend to only inhibit the cytochrome P450 isoenzyme 3A, thus limiting possible drug-drug interactions to psychotropic medications metabolized via this pathway (e.g., some benzodiazepines, citalopram, and nefazodone).

The nonnucleoside reverse transcriptase inhibitors also require careful attention. For example, nevirapine and efavirenz are metabolized via the cytochrome P450 isoenzymes 3A and 2B6 and induce cytochrome P450 activity, which could result in decreased psychotropic concentrations at standard doses (278). Delavirdine, another nonnucleoside reverse transcriptase inhibitor, inhibits the cytochrome P450 isoenzyme 3A and reduces hepatic clearance of psychotropic agents primarily metabolized by this pathway (279). The protease inhibitors and nonnucleoside reverse transcriptase inhibitors are among the most problematic of the antiretrovirals when coadministered with psychotropic medication. Table 15 indicates the relative rank order of inhibition potency of the currently available protease inhibitors.

For combination antiretroviral therapy that includes protease inhibitors and nonnucleoside reverse transcriptase inhibitors, an overarching concern in terms of coadministration with psychotropic agents is not only the possibility of plasma levels of psychotropic medications outside the targeted therapeutic concentration range but also the possible reduction of antiretroviral levels to the point of risking their effectiveness. While most interactions *inhibit* the cytochrome P450 system, some clinically important drug interactions also *induce* this system with medications used to treat co-occurring medical conditions in HIV disease (e.g., glucocorticoids, rifampin, phenytoin). Table 16 provides an overview of psychotropic agents and HIV therapies, routes of metabolic inhibition and induction, and potential clinical concerns.

Although the aforementioned risks for drug-drug interactions may seem substantial, to date, clinical data have not revealed severe side effects among most patients receiving antiretrovirals in conjunction with psychotropic medications (50). A few reports have documented the inhibitory effects of protease inhibitors. For example, when coadministered with ritonavir, desipramine levels have been shown to increase 145% in vitro (280) and to increase to some extent when coadministered with other protease inhibitors (281). In a clinical setting, coadministration of saquinavir and midazolam has caused prolonged sedation (282). These in vitro and in vivo data should lead to careful monitoring for potentially problematic or dangerous side effects in patients taking antiretrovirals.

TABLE 16. HIV-Related Medications and Psychotropic Agents Involving the Cytochrome P450 System

Cytochrome P450 Isoenzyme	Common HIV-Related Medications That Inhibit Isoenzyme	Psychotropic Medications Primarily Metabolized by Isoenzyme	Possible Clinical Implications of Isoenzyme Inhibition	Common HIV-Related Medications That Induce Isoenzyme	Possible Clinical Implications of Isoenzyme Induction
3A4	Protease inhibitors (especially ritonavir) Delavirdine Clarithromycin Erythromycin Itraconazole Ketoconazole Macrolide antibiotics	Benzodiazepines Buspirone Citalopram Carbamazepine Nefazodone Trazodone	Increased plasma levels and increased side effects; for benzodiazepines, sedation and decreased respiratory drive	Nevirapine Efavirenz Glucocorticoids Rifampin Rifabutin	Decreased plasma levels of psychotropic medications and decreased effectiveness
2D6	Protease inhibitors (especially ritonavir and nelfinavir)	Mirtazapine Fluoxetine Paroxetine Sertraline Fluvoxamine Tricyclic antidepressants Venlafaxine Neuroleptics, typical and atypical	Increased plasma levels and increased side effects; for tricyclic antidepressants, potential increased risk for cardiac conduction delay	None	

Drugs of abuse can also cause drug-drug interactions. MDMA, an amphetamine derivative also known as "ecstasy" that is primarily metabolized via the cytochrome P450 isoenzyme 2D6, reportedly led to a lethal overdose when taken by a patient being treated with ritonavir (283). Other drugs of abuse, particularly those metabolized via the cytochrome P450 isoenzymes 2D6 or 3A (e.g., amphetamines, ketamine, heroin, cocaine, and γ-hydroxybutyrate) may lead to toxic events when taken by patients being treated with protease inhibitors.

Although some drug-drug interactions may be only theoretical, it is prudent for clinicians to explain these concerns during the informed consent process of psychotropic prescribing. Because of the extent of comorbid substance abuse among some HIV patients, a general warning of the possible interactions of combining antiretroviral agents, psychotropic medications, and recreational drugs is often indicated. Web sites are available to clinicians and patients that address antiretroviral drug interactions and may be useful educational and reference tools (www.aegis.com; www.drug-interactions.com; and www.dml.georgetown.edu/depts/pharmacology/davetab.html).

Psychiatrists should remember that HIV patients who have been clinically stable on regimens of maintenance psychotropic medications and who later initiate combination antiretroviral therapies may require adjustments or changes in their psychotropic regimen. The rational choice of psychotropic medications must also include critical considerations of adherence. Generally, it is important to minimize the number of drug doses and to tie dosing to times of the day with natural cues (e.g., meals, work schedule, bedtime). Outlined here are unique factors to consider in administering specific psychotropic agents to HIV patients, particularly those patients simultaneously receiving antiretroviral therapies.

1. Antidepressant agents

The prevalence of mood disorders in HIV patients is higher than general population rates; evidence from effectiveness studies and clinical trials indicates that antidepressants are generally well tolerated by HIV patients, even those with symptomatic HIV infection or AIDS (284–290). Thus, antidepressants are commonly prescribed to HIV patients for the treatment of depression as well as for other HIV-related conditions, such as chronic pain (e.g., peripheral neuropathy) (291). However, clinicians must be cautioned that two factors may limit the generalizability of some antidepressant studies. First, many studies of antidepressants in HIV patients were conducted before the availability of combination antiretroviral therapy and thus did not take into account possible pharmacokinetic complications (292). Second, a minority of published psychopharmacology studies has included patients with advanced stages of HIV infection or AIDS. There is, to date, no evidence to suggest adverse effects of antidepressants on the immune system (293).

a) SSRIs

Several studies have indicated that tricyclic antidepressants are less well tolerated than SSRIs (287, 294), leading some to recommend SSRIs over tricyclic antidepressants (277). One study found that despite efficacy for treating depression, fluvoxamine was poorly tolerated by HIV patients (295). Because similar metabolic pathways, particularly the cytochrome P450 isoenzyme 2D6, are utilized by SSRIs and ritonavir, the psychiatrist should maintain communication with other clinicians treating the patient. Although SSRIs are generally well tolerated across a broad range of blood levels, the untoward outcome of serotonin syndrome may be possible in some cases in which the cytochrome P450 isoenzyme 2D6 is inhibited (296). While the SSRIs themselves inhibit this isoenzyme, the potency of their inhibition is less than that of ritonavir. However, the potential impact of SSRI-related inhibition of the cytochrome P450 isoenzyme 2D6 should be remembered when coadministering SSRIs with other agents that are substrates of the cytochrome P450 2D6 isoenzyme.

b) Tricyclic antidepressants

While tricyclic antidepressants are metabolized by other cytochromes, they rely principally on the cytochrome P450 isoenzyme 2D6 for clearance. Therefore if tricyclic antidepressants are coadministered with ritonavir, monitoring of ECG results and tricyclic antidepressant plasma levels is recommended because of the possibility of increased tricyclic antidepressant plasma levels from cytochrome P450 inhibition and associated tricyclic antidepressant side effects (e.g., delayed cardiac conduction, anticholinergic effects, orthostasis).

c) Other antidepressants

Nefazodone and the protease inhibitors are both potent inhibitors of the cytochrome P450 isoenzyme 3A, and their combination may be problematic. Nefazodone administration may theoretically decrease the metabolism of some protease inhibitors, leading to increased protease inhibitor plasma levels and increased side effects. However, one study that examined the efficacy of nefazodone in HIV patients found that only one of 15 patients had a clinically significant drug interaction that was related to coadministration with ritonavir (288). Of general concern is the coadministration of nefazodone or protease inhibitors with the antipsychotic pimozide, which can cause cardiac arrhythmias at increased plasma levels (296). Other potentially dangerous interactions with inhibitors of the cytochrome P450 isoenzyme 3A include the coadministration of most benzodiazepines (respiratory depression), clozapine (seizures), ergot alkaloids (sustained systemic vasoconstriction), and sildenafil (priapism).

Venlafaxine has been reported to decrease the concentration of indinavir significantly even though a lack of such interaction was predicted based on each drug's pharmacokinetic parameters. At this time, venlafaxine should be avoided in those patients receiving indinavir, since decreases in concentration of protease inhibitors can affect treatment efficacy and increase the chances for viral resistance to develop (297).

Previously it was thought that bupropion was eliminated via the cytochrome P450 isoenzyme 2D6. However, recent data have shown that it is actually cleared via the 2B6 isoenzyme. Therefore, bupropion has been removed from the list of drugs contraindicated with ritonavir, and this is reflected in the revised product monograph.

No adverse events have been reported with the agents citalopram and mirtazapine. Citalopram has minimal inhibitory actions on the cytochrome system and may be particularly useful for patients taking multiple medications where drug-drug interactions are an ongoing concern. Mirtazapine, because of its sedating profile, may be particularly useful for depressed patients with insomnia. It may also be helpful for patients with poor appetite because of its tendency to increase appetite and also helpful for patients who may be prone to sexual dysfunction with other antidepressant agents.

2. Antipsychotic medications

Generally, the use of antipsychotic medication among patients with advanced HIV infection is associated with an increased incidence of extrapyramidal side effects. High-potency standard neuroleptics (haloperidol is the most commonly used in published reports) can be associated with severe dystonia, rigidity, akathisia, and parkinsonism (31, 298–301). Low-potency standard neuroleptics can also result in severe extrapyramidal side effects but overall appear to be less problematic than high-potency neuroleptics (302–305).

A study that contrasts with the perspective that standard neuroleptics are associated with severe extrapyramidal side effects in advanced HIV infection was conducted in hospitalized patients with AIDS who were randomly assigned pharmacologic treatment for delirium; 13 received chlorpromazine, and 11 received haloperidol (46). The study stated that "no clinically significant medication-related side effects were noted." However, patients were treated with very low doses of neuroleptic (i.e., average maintenance doses were 36 mg/day for chlorpromazine and 1.4 mg/day for haloperidol). The study is consistent with the rest of the literature in stressing the importance of treating patients with advanced HIV infection with the lowest possible effective dose when using a typical neuroleptic.

Neuroleptic malignant syndrome has been noted with standard neuroleptics in five reports. In one case, neuroleptic malignant syndrome occurred within 24 hours; in the four other cases, neuroleptic malignant syndrome occurred within days of initiating treatment (300, 306–309). All patients recovered with usual management. Onset of tardive dyskinesia has been reported within a period as short as 6 weeks or within months (31, 310, 311). Confusion has also been reported with standard neuroleptics (312).

Most patients with extrapyramidal side effects respond to typical treatments, but one case report of a patient with parkinsonian side effects noted a slow response (299). Another patient had no response to multiple antiparkinsonian agents (313). Scurlock et al. (298) reported an AIDS patient who developed a grand mal seizure while taking chlorpromazine, and Jones et al. (314) reported a grand mal seizure in one man with symptomatic HIV infection who was taking amitriptyline and chlorpromazine.

Atypical antipsychotic agents appear to be better tolerated with fewer serious side effects, as evidenced by two case series of 30 combined patients who received risperidone (310, 315), one report of four patients who received remoxipride (298), and another of four patients who received molindone (312). Some of these patients had previously experienced severe side effects while taking typical neuroleptics. All were able to tolerate the atypical agents, and most but not all patients had a good therapeutic response. The most common side effects seen with risperidone were drowsiness and drooling (315). Extensive clinical experience suggests that olanzapine is also well tolerated for the treatment of psychosis, delirium, and behavioral disturbances among HIV patients.

It is of interest that movement disorders, including dystonia and parkinsonism, have been reported in advanced HIV infection without exposure to neuroleptics (316, 317). In the one case report of irreversible extrapyramidal side effects in a man with HIV-associated dementia following exposure to standard neuroleptics, an autopsy revealed numerous microscopic changes, including neuronal loss in the basal ganglia (313). It may be that damage to the basal ganglia is a factor that increases the susceptibility of HIV patients to extrapyramidal side effects after neuroleptic administration (318). A similar pattern of extrapyramidal side effect susceptibility in concert with neuronal damage has been described in the elderly (311, 319).

For all antipsychotic agents, the possibility of drug-drug interactions must be considered for those patients also taking antiretroviral medication. Antipsychotic dosage adjustments may be required to minimize side effects such as extrapyramidal side effects. Because of the rare dose-related side effect of agranulocytosis among patients taking clozapine, this particular agent should be monitored closely if given to any HIV patient (320). Likewise, clinicians should monitor for risk of seizures if clozapine is administered with ritonavir, since ritonavir inhibits the cytochrome P450 isoenzyme 2D6, clozapine's primary metabolic pathway. Pimozide should also be used cautiously in combination with any inhibitor of the cytochrome P450 isoenzyme 3A because of risk of fatal arrhythmias at elevated doses. Depot antipsychotic medication should be avoided in advanced HIV disease.

3. Psychostimulants

Psychostimulants, such as methylphenidate and dextroamphetamine, are frequently used in HIV patients with neurocognitive impairment, fatigue, and, to a lesser extent, in some patients with depression (321, 322). These drugs are generally safe and well tolerated with no drug-drug interactions reported to date among HIV patients. The possibility of dopamine agonism inducing psychosis should be considered in vulnerable patients, such as those with a history of HIV-related CNS complications or a history of psychosis. Psychostimulants should be avoided or used judiciously among patients with a past or current history of amphetamine abuse.

4. Mood stabilizers

a) Valproate

Use of valproate in patients with bipolar disorder is not uncommon, particularly among HIV patients who develop mania secondary to HIV-related complications or psychoactive substance use. Concerns have been raised about the potential for valproate to possibly accelerate disease progression in HIV-positive patients. This concern is based on the fact that valproate has been shown in vitro to lower glutathione levels, which leads to activation of HIV replication (323). However, a retrospective review by Maggi and Halman (324) of 11 patients with HIV infection who were also treated with valproate found no evidence of increased viral load in those receiving adequate antiretroviral therapy.

The metabolic pathways of valproate are not fully delineated, but this agent has been associated with hepatotoxicity. There is a case report of valproic acid–induced hepatotoxicity when valproate was used together with ritonavir and nevirapine (325). Valproate inhibits glucuronyl transferase. Zidovudine uses glucuronyl transferase as its primary pathway of metabolic clearance. Therefore, increased plasma levels of zidovudine and associated side effects could result when the two agents are combined.

Generally, divalproex sodium is better tolerated than valproic acid, since it produces fewer gastrointestinal side effects and can be dosed less frequently (two or three times a day rather than four), particularly among HIV patients who may have preexisting gastrointestinal illness. Increased side effects may be caused by increased concentrations of free valproate in HIV patients because of factors such as the reduction of plasma protein levels, the increased percentage of free drug due to chronic illness, or drug-drug interactions that may decrease protein binding of valproate (326).

b) Lithium carbonate

Lithium is commonly used in HIV patients with primary bipolar disorder. Because it does not require hepatic metabolism, it is a rational choice for many patients taking antiretroviral agents who require extensive hepatic metabolism. Lithium should be used with great caution in patients who develop HIV-related nephropathy, a generally irreversible complication that can lead to decreased lithium clearance and possible lithium toxicity. When given at doses necessary to maintain serum lithium concentrations between 0.5 and 1.5 meq/liter, lithium has been associated with signs of toxicity in some HIV patients, even among patients without renal disease (327). Thus, clinical experience suggests that lithium is best avoided in patients with probable AIDS mania or advanced HIV disease due to risk of toxicity.

c) Carbamazepine

Although not absolutely contraindicated, carbamazepine is used less commonly in HIV patients because of its potential to cause bone marrow complications (e.g., leukopenia or aplastic anemia). This risk should be avoided in immunocompromised patients. Carbamazepine, like other anticonvulsants, phenobarbital, and phenytoin, is known to induce activity of the cytochrome P450 isoenzyme 3A. This induction can accelerate antiretroviral drug metabolism and possibly cause decreased plasma levels and diminished efficacy. It is recommended that carbamazepine concentrations be closely monitored.

d) Newer anticonvulsants

Lamotrigine, gabapentin, and topiramate are newer anticonvulsants that have recently been used off-label to treat selected populations of patients with bipolar disorder, typically those with rapid cycling, mixed mood states, or bipolar depression. While no data currently support their use for mood disorders in HIV patients, gabapentin may offer some advantages over other anticonvulsants because it is neither protein bound nor metabolized by the liver. Gabapentin is thus less likely than other anticonvulsants to lead to drug-drug interactions. Gabapentin has been successfully used in HIV patients to treat peripheral neuropathy, which can be both a complication of HIV disease and a side effect of some antiretroviral agents.

5. Anxiolytic and sedative-hypnotic medications

a) Buspirone

Buspirone is commonly used and generally well tolerated in HIV patients as a treatment for generalized anxiety disorder (328). There are no reports of HIV-related drug-drug interactions with buspirone. However, one case report describes induction of manic psychosis following a single dose of buspirone in a patient with asymptomatic HIV illness (329).

b) Benzodiazepines

Benzodiazepines are commonly used in HIV patients and are best used for short periods to minimize the risk of tolerance or addiction and to maximize effectiveness. This class of drugs is generally best avoided in patients with alcoholism and those with a history of substance abuse. Benzodiazepines are metabolized primarily by the cytochrome P450 isoenzyme 3A; however, oxazepam, lorazepam, and temazepam are metabolized by direct conjugation via glucuronyl transferase, resulting in shorter elimination half-lives and less likelihood of metabolite accumulation and associated side effects.

When some benzodiazepines are coadministered with inhibitors of the cytochrome P450 isoenzyme 3A (such as protease inhibitors), one would expect a decrease in benzodiazepine clearance with increased sedation, potentially resulting in respiratory depression. Even saquinavir's relatively low-potency inhibition of the cytochrome P450 isoenzyme 3A has been shown to prolong the sedative effect of midazolam (282). Although one study that examined the chronic effect of ritonavir administration on alprazolam metabolism reported a 10%–15% decrease in expected alprazolam levels (330), a more recent study found that short-term, low-dose ritonavir administration significantly impaired alprazolam clearance (331). These studies call attention to the need for judicious use of alprazolam in combination with ritonavir.

An additional consideration when using benzodiazepines that are metabolized by glucuronidation (e.g., oxazepam, lorazepam, temazepam) involves ritonavir's inductive effect on glucuronyl transferase activity (332). The concentration of glucuronyl transferase substrates may be decreased when these agents are coadministered with ritonavir. Therefore in some cases, patients taking one of these three benzodiazepines may require higher doses for symptom control. Benzodiazepine-dependent patients may also require higher doses to avoid the onset of withdrawal (296).

6. Medications for HIV-related wasting

Some patients with wasting syndrome can be helped by medications that serve as appetite stimulants to combat loss of appetite and associated weight loss. Four agents currently have been approved by the Food and Drug Administration (FDA). Two of these agents, dronabinol and oxandrolone, are Schedule II controlled substances. Because these agents have unique psychiatric side effect profiles, they should be monitored closely among patients who receive psychiatric care.

Dronabinol is a cannabinoid indicated for HIV-associated anorexia and nausea. It is a major active metabolite in marijuana and, like marijuana, has complex effects on the CNS, including sympathomimetic activity. Oxandrolone is an anabolic steroid synthetically derived from testosterone that is used for weight gain and promotion of lean body mass (333–335). Its side effect profile is similar to that of other anabolic steroids, including mood effects. Another agent, megestrol acetate, is a synthetic derivative of progesterone that increases fat rather than muscle gain. It also lowers testosterone and may produce side effects (e.g., mood disturbances) similar to those associated with glucocorticoids. Somatotropin is an injectable form of recombinant human growth hormone indicated for the treatment of AIDS wasting and cachexia (336–340). It is an anabolic and anticatabolic treatment that combats the loss of lean body mass and is generally well tolerated by patients. The effects of somatotropin are often lost when it is discontinued.

These medications can be extremely beneficial for patients with significant anorexia, weight loss, and nausea. However, because they are usually used in more advanced stages of HIV disease, when patients are more medically frail and receiving multiple other medications, psychiatrists should actively monitor response, side effects, and drug interactions. Limited data do not indicate a high incidence of psychiatric side effects.

Thalidomide, a potent teratogen once marketed as a sedative and morning sickness agent in the 1950s and 1960s, is currently available on a restricted basis for HIV patients for the treatment of wasting syndrome (341, 342). The agent is FDA-approved as an immunomodulatory drug for the treatment of severe HIV-related oral ulcers. Prescribing physicians must register under a special restricted distribution program with the FDA. Primary psychiatric side effects include CNS depression; few data are available concerning drug-drug interactions, although thalidomide does not appear to be metabolized by the liver to any large extent.

7. Testosterone

A number of clinical trials have found testosterone to be effective in the treatment of a number of HIV-related symptoms (e.g., fatigue, wasting, impaired sexual functioning, and mild depression) often associated with more advanced HIV disease (126, 343, 344). Although typically used to treat hypogonadism in the general population, clinical response to testosterone in HIV patients is not correlated with serum testosterone levels at baseline. HIV-infected men with normal levels of testosterone respond as well as those with lower than normal levels (126). The most common psychiatric side effects of testosterone are changes in mood and irritability.

8. Opiate analgesics

Many HIV patients are treated with opiate analgesics for both acute pain syndromes, such as that associated with *Candida* esophagitis, as well as chronic pain conditions (e.g., neuropathic and myopathic pain syndromes). Chronic pain is also common in advanced HIV disease, particularly among cachectic patients with wasting syndrome. Because opioids are metabolized primarily via the cytochrome P450 isoenzymes 2D6 and 3A, they should be used cautiously in conjunction with antiretroviral agents that are likely to increase their plasma levels.

Some opioids, such as codeine and hydrocodone (as well as the nonopiate tramadol), must be converted into active metabolites to produce analgesic effects. This conversion can be blocked by cytochrome P450 inhibitors, which results in reduced pain control in addition to adverse reactions from the buildup of unmetabolized drug (345). Oxycodone and morphine, which are primarily glucuronyl transferase substrates, are alternatives for pain control. However, in the presence of a glucuronyl transferase inducer such as ritonavir, their analgesic effect can be diminished as well (296, 332). As HIV disease progresses, the provision of safe, effective pain control requires clear understanding of the above factors.

9. Drugs used in the treatment of substance use disorders

a) Opioid dependence

There is limited information available on the extent and clinical implications of drug interactions in HIV-positive patients with comorbid substance use disorders. However, several studies have been published. Methadone has been shown to significantly increase zidovudine levels, but zidovudine has not been shown to affect methadone levels (346–348). Interim results from a study of the interaction of zidovudine with LAAM, buprenorphine, or naltrexone indicate that LAAM does not affect zidovudine levels, whereas buprenorphine may decrease levels nonsignificantly (349). Another report indicates that abacavir, a newer nucleoside analogue reverse transcriptase inhibitor, increases methadone clearance, although the proposed mechanism remains unclear (350). Preclinical studies of the coadministration of protease inhibitors and methadone revealed that ritonavir causes a twofold increase in the area under the curve for methadone level and that indinavir causes a 30% increase, compared to no increase with saquinavir (351). One case report has indicated that nelfinavir may induce cytochrome P450 enzymes leading to decreased methadone levels (352). Nevirapine and efavirenz induce cytochrome P450 enzymes important to methadone metabolism and are reported to precipitate opiate withdrawal symptoms in methadone maintenance patients (278, 353). The consequences of undetected drug interactions among opioid-dependent patients are complicated and include nonadherence with treatment regimens, the potential development of resistant HIV strains, increased illicit drug abuse, drug toxicity, and loss of efficacy. In administering methadone to HIV patients taking protease inhibitors or nonnucleoside reverse transcriptase inhibitors, clinicians should adjust doses to compensate for cytochrome P450 enzyme effects.

b) Alcohol dependence

There is no clinical information regarding the use of disulfiram in patients with HIV infection. Psychiatrists should therefore follow general guidelines for the use of disulfiram cautiously. Naltrexone, an opioid antagonist, is indicated in the treatment of alcohol dependence and for the blockage of the effects of exogenously administered opioids. Because naltrexone can cause hepatocellular damage when given in excessive doses, it should be used cautiously in patients with liver disease. It should also be noted that naltrexone's opioid antagonism might block the clinical effects of some commonly used medications in HIV patients that contain opioids (e.g., antidiarrheal medications, cough and cold preparations).

10. Alternative/complementary agents

Patients with HIV infection may use a wide range of alternative/complementary agents for preventive and symptomatic treatment of HIV-related complications. Of particular interest to psychiatrists are those agents used to treat psychiatric symptoms. For example, patients may take *Hypericum perforatum* (St. John's wort) or the nutritional supplement *S*-adenosylmethionine (or SAM-e) to treat depression, kava kava for anxiety, melatonin or valerian root for insomnia, and ginkgo biloba for memory problems. One published report found that St. John's wort, which contains an inducer of the cytochrome P450 isoenzyme 3A, dramatically lowered levels of indinavir (and presumably other substrates of the cytochrome P450 isoenzyme 3A) (354). The FDA thus issued a public health advisory that concomitant use of St. John's wort with protease inhibitors and nonnucleoside reverse transcriptase inhibitors is not recommended. There are no data regarding other alternative/complementary agents at this time.

C. PSYCHOSOCIAL TREATMENT

Since the beginning of the AIDS epidemic, psychosocial support has emerged as a cornerstone of the comprehensive treatment for many persons infected and affected by HIV/AIDS. For many HIV patients, psychotherapy and psychosocial interventions have been invaluable in the search for meaning during the course of living with HIV (355). Psychotherapy can be an important intervention to address conditions that may interfere with a patient's acceptance of HIV illness or their ability to work cooperatively with their health care team. With the advent of new antiretroviral treatments, new psychotherapy themes have emerged, including changes in role definitions and life trajectory as well as treatment adherence challenges (356–358).

For patients who are socially disenfranchised, psychosocial treatments may consist of basic services that assist them in gaining access to food, shelter, transportation, and child care—essential elements of a care plan that diminish health care delivery barriers and promote mental health care utilization.

Generally, psychosocial treatments are those treatments, often offered in the community, that provide direct assistance along such parameters as social adjustment, social support, coping, and overall adjustment to HIV infection. Psychosocial interventions often occur in group formats, such as informal support groups, although more formal groups may tailor their membership (i.e., women, men, mothers, caregivers) or their mission (HIV risk reduction, treatment adherence) (359, 360). Other formats include peer counseling, a supportive intervention typically offered by HIV-positive consumers based in community AIDS service organizations.

Other psychosocial treatments have been developed that incorporate a service model (e.g., psychosocial rehabilitation programs for persons with HIV/AIDS, day treatment programs for HIV-positive persons with neurocognitive impairment) or a service theme (e.g., permanency planning for parents with advanced AIDS, HIV prevention, case management, disclosure of HIV status) (67, 79, 355, 361).

Researchers have described a wide range of psychological and psychosocial sequelae from HIV/AIDS (251). In their review of empirical findings, Kalichman and Sikkema (362) showed that psychological complications include distress, anger, guilt, bereavement, and the full spectrum of psychiatric disorders. Syndromes such as depression may appear, subside, and recur during the course of living with HIV/AIDS. Moreover, certain psychosocial conditions, such as increased social support and fewer incidents of HIV-related discrimination, have been shown to predict greater life satisfaction among HIV patients (143).

Psychosocial treatment of HIV-related complications will often involve referral of patients to community AIDS service organizations that specialize in the provision of psychosocial support. While many of the treatment issues are also themes that will emerge in psychotherapy (i.e., stigma, coping strategies, or disclosure of HIV status), support groups and other interventions provide a model for structuring social support over the course of living with HIV infection (362). Psychosocial services may take on added importance for patients living in rural regions, in which more community HIV-related stigma has been documented (143).

Psychosocial interventions have been shown to enhance adaptive coping strategies, social support, perceived sense of meaning and purpose, and self-esteem and also have been shown to lower anxiety and HIV risk behaviors among HIV-positive adults (359, 363–365). Because of the spectrum of social, psychological, and neuropsychiatric consequences of HIV/AIDS, psychiatric treatment should consider the relevance for a given individual of a wide variety of potential psychosocial interventions, spanning the spectrum from individual to family or group psychotherapy as well as psychodynamic/psychoanalytic, interpersonal, behavioral, or supportive approaches.

D. LEGAL AND ETHICAL ISSUES

Psychiatrists caring for HIV-infected patients can be faced with complex legal and ethical issues, some of which are unique to HIV infection. The AIDS Litigation Project conducted a national review of cases that involved individuals with HIV/AIDS in the federal and state courts in the United States between 1991 and 1997. The review identified important subsets of litigation, which included issues of "testing and reporting; privacy, the duty to warn, and the right to know; physician standards of care in prevention and treatment; and discrimination and access to health care" (366).

Most U.S. states have legal requirements surrounding HIV testing that require written informed consent and a minimum amount of pre- and posttest counseling—both to those who test positive and to those who test negative. Furthermore, many states are required to report positive HIV test results to public health agencies. Some states mandate that the report include the name of the individual who tested HIV positive. All states have mandatory name reporting when a patient is diagnosed with an AIDS-defining condition.

For those infected with HIV, confidentiality of HIV status is often paramount, especially for patients who are asymptomatic or who are concerned about possible discrimination by their employers or by insurance companies. Psychiatrists are typically attuned to confidentiality issues and regard patient-doctor confidentiality as fundamental to effective treatment. Yet, there are limits to confidentiality, such as when there is potential for others to be harmed, and these limitations should be discussed with patients when treatment is initiated.

For persons infected with HIV, particularly those recently diagnosed, their recent sexual partners and/or those with whom they share injection equipment should be informed of their potential exposure to HIV. These partners can benefit from HIV counseling and testing and knowing their HIV infection status. Many health departments offer services known either as "partner notification" or prevention counseling and referral services (367–369).

Another important issue involves the dangerousness of HIV patients. A patient with HIV infection is not a danger to others in the absence of imminent threats to harm others. In general, there are no legal requirements for physicians to inform partners of HIV-infected patients of their HIV status, especially if the patient agrees to notify their partner or if they are clearly practicing "safer sex." However, because HIV-infected patients are able to transmit the virus and potentially put others in danger of infection, psychiatrists who care for HIV patients have an ethical requirement to counsel their patients about modes of HIV transmission and promote safer behavior, such as the consistent use of condoms and/or the use of clean needles. Psychiatrists can offer to assist patients in notifying individuals at risk or help refer a patient to public health officials for partner notification, if necessary.

On the other hand, if a patient has not disclosed their HIV-positive status to a partner and continues high-risk behavior, psychiatrists may have a duty to warn identifiable sexual partners or other at-risk individuals. APA policy reads that, "If a patient refuses to change behavior that places others at risk for HIV infection or to inform individuals at ongoing risk, or if the psychiatrist has good reason to believe that the patient has failed to or is unable to cease such behaviors or to inform those at risk, it is ethically permissible for the psychiatrist to notify identifiable individuals at risk or to arrange for public health authorities to do so" (370). Psychiatrists need to be mindful that while it may be *ethically* permissible to notify, it may not be *legally* permissible, and therefore psychiatrists should obtain legal advice before breaching confidentiality.

For patients who are impulsive or psychotic, protective measures such as voluntary or involuntary psychiatric hospitalization are options for treatment of psychiatric disorders and protection of others. For antisocial individuals, hospitalization should not be used merely as a means of social control.

During the course of HIV illness, and especially after the onset of AIDS, patients may experience cognitive impairment or symptoms of dementia. Such disturbances may affect a patient's ability to give informed consent to accept or refuse treatment. When psychiatrists are asked to conduct competency evaluations for patients with HIV/AIDS, a comprehensive mental status examination that includes an evaluation of cognition is critical, followed—if indicated—by formal neuropsychological testing and assessment of specific treatment decision-making capacity.

The opposite of a patient's refusal of treatment is the refusal on the part of physicians to provide HIV treatment to psychiatric patients. Because antiretroviral therapies involve complex medication regimens and adherence to treatment is critical, physicians may be biased against prescribing these treatments to patients with a comorbid mental illness such as a substance use disorder. While refusal of treatment due to poor adherence is appropriate, refusal of treatment solely on the grounds of a mental illness is not. When the psychiatrist is a consultant who does not intervene directly in the care of the patient, he or she will need to work with the primary clinician to help ensure that appropriate psychiatric treatment is received (371).

E. ADHERENCE TO TREATMENT

Potent antiretroviral treatment has given hope to patients infected with HIV yet simultaneously has increased the complexities of managing HIV illness (372). For instance, the combination of three or more medications used in most antiretroviral treatment regimens makes adherence difficult. In addition, some medications must be taken with food, others without food; dosing is usually twice a day but sometimes can be more frequent. Side effects can be significant, requiring discontinuation or the initiation of a new combination of medications. Because antiretroviral treatment should begin as an aggressive broad attack on HIV replication, doses of the drugs are generally not titrated upward but rather are initiated at the full dose. Thus, patients may experience many initiation side effects.

Adherence to antiretroviral therapy regimens is critical, as evidenced by a study that measured adherence by using a microelectronic monitoring system (95). The authors found that 95% adherence to treatment was associated with complete viral suppression but that failure rates increased sharply with less than 95% adherence. Researchers have documented that patients who receive potent antiretroviral treatment but who are not enrolled in clinical trials show viral suppression rates one-half those of study patients, which suggests the real-world difficulty of maintaining strict adherence (373).

Adherence to any kind of medical treatment is a well-established problem. Overall adherence rates vary from 20% to 80% and average 50% (374). Psychiatrists should make every effort to treat and control psychiatric disorders that affect a patient's ability to maintain close adherence to an HIV treatment regimen. Each year, about 7% of patients with AIDS develop HIV-associated dementia (375). This condition can interfere with ability to follow and understand treatment regimens. In addition, researchers have found that depression can be a cause of nonadherence and that treatment of depression might thus improve medical outcomes (96). Strategies that have proven useful in improving adherence for both psychotropic and antiretroviral medication have been reported and are summarized below (376).

1. Institutional factors

How a health care system is structured will strongly influence whether clinicians and patients can collaborate and enhance adherence. One important element is a respectful and culturally sensitive environment. The availability and continuity of clinicians over time with 24-hour/day phone coverage to handle crises that might disrupt a regimen (severe side effects, loss of medication), as well as clinician caseloads that permit time for adequate discussion with patients, all promote adherence. Hospitals do not always dispense medications on the 8- or 12-hour schedules required for antiretroviral dosing. Last, social service mechanisms such as case management for handling financial and logistical barriers to obtaining and following the regimens provide crucial support.

2. Physician factors

When initiating antiretroviral treatment, it is essential for the physician to prepare the patient. Because the best chance at viral suppression occurs with the first regimen, it makes sense to wait until the patient is ready. For a psychiatrist, it is important to treat or recommend treatment for comorbid alcohol/substance use disorders, depression, psychotic illnesses, or personality disorders that are likely to interfere with adherence (377). At the same time, if the patient is motivated to begin antiretroviral treatment, this can be a good opportunity to introduce psychiatric or substance use treatment if indicated.

3. Clinical strategies

Multiple approaches to enhancing adherence are often needed (Table 17). For longer-term adherence, individual medication management, in which a staff member provides assessment and problem-solving support, may improve adherence (378).

TABLE 17. Interventions to Increase Patient Adherence to Antiretroviral Regimens

Prepare patients
Discuss use of medications before prescribing
Outline pros and cons of therapy
Acknowledge commitment required, consequences of noncompliance, and benefits of therapy
Provide written instructions
Inform patients of expectations, including side effects
Provide information on who patients should call if significant side effects occur
Schedule a follow-up appointment soon after initiating therapy
Review importance of therapy
Inform patients that they must continue to take all medications
Review the effects of stopping one medication
Outline procedure for obtaining refills
Recognize patient lifestyle and preferences
Twice-daily dosing benefits may outweigh initial side effects; ritonavir may be preferred
Consider whether patients prefer tolerability over convenience; nelfinavir or indinavir may be preferred
Discuss midday dosing
Recommend medication timers or calendar
Help patients plan for away-from-home dosing
Simplify regimens
If possible, prioritize or eliminate medications when patients are overwhelmed
Look for and address nonadherence
Consider regimens that minimize cross-resistance
Use regimens that leave options for future effective antiretroviral therapy
Inquire about adherence
Inquire about medication-taking behavior at each visit
Anticipate relapses in adherence, even after long-term use of medication

F. SPECIFIC SYNDROMES

There are numerous psychiatric difficulties that can occur in the context of HIV infection, yet studies of the treatment of HIV-related psychiatric disorders are limited. This section summarizes the existing scientific literature on the treatment of specific psychiatric disorders for patients with concurrent HIV/AIDS.

1. Dementia and the spectrum of cognitive disorders

Most research studies on the treatment of cognitive disorders associated with HIV infection have focused on HIV-associated dementia. Fewer studies have looked at the benefits of intervention at earlier stages of cognitive decline despite the possibilities for treating disorders, such as minor cognitive motor disorder, that involve neuronal cell dysfunction rather than cell death. Treatment of neuropsychological impairment without clinical disorder has been studied to some extent, and protection against neuropsychological impairment has been studied least.

Pharmacologic treatment strategies for cognitive disorders can be divided into four types: 1) antiretroviral therapies, 2) therapies aimed at immunological measures or inflammatory mediators, 3) therapies aimed at bolstering the response of the brain to the onslaught of the infection (e.g., neurotransmitter manipulation), and 4) nutritional therapies. Most controlled studies have investigated the efficacy of antiretroviral therapies, and while these studies have advanced our knowledge about interventions for cognitive disorders, several key factors must be kept in mind. First is the fact that most published studies to date report on the treatment strategy of administering a single antiretroviral agent. Their findings are therefore difficult to interpret in light of the multidrug regimens that are now the standard of care in developed countries. Second, the reports vary widely with regard to the study population, since some studies enrolled subjects on the basis of established criteria for HIV-associated dementia or minor cognitive motor disorder but other studies enrolled cognitively impaired subjects without specifying whether they also met criteria for a clinical disorder. Third, the range of HIV clinical severity also varied widely in study subjects.

Whether antiretroviral agents penetrate the blood-brain barrier sufficiently to adequately suppress viral replication is a key issue that requires further study (379, 380). We know that near-perfect adherence to antiretroviral therapy is required to maintain plasma viral load at undetectable levels. Even in the best-case scenario, if decreased plasma viral load is achieved and levels of antiretroviral agents in CSF or brain tissue are optimized, it is not yet known whether complete suppression of replication in the CNS can be achieved (381). Another theoretical concern is that if antiretroviral resistance develops in the CNS, it is possible that resistant HIV could then reseed the peripheral circulation. This mechanism could potentially lead to increased prevalence of neurocognitive disorders as well as systemic progression of HIV disease.

a) Zidovudine treatment of cognitive disorders or dysfunction

Two randomized, placebo-controlled clinical trials have provided evidence for the effectiveness of zidovudine in reducing neuropsychological impairment for patients with HIV infection. Sidtis and colleagues (382) treated a group of 40 homosexual men (early-stage dementia and mean CD4 cell counts of 500 cells/mm^3) with 1000 or 2000 mg/day of zidovudine or placebo. They found that both treatment groups demonstrated significant combined mean neuropsychological z score improvements when compared to the placebo group. In another randomized, placebo-controlled clinical trial, Schmitt and colleagues (383) used zidovudine to treat 281 subjects who did not necessarily have clear-cut signs of neuropsychological impairment or cognitive disorder but were stratified into two groups, AIDS or early asymptomatic HIV infection, on the basis of CD4 cell count. Significant improvements were found in attention, memory, visual-motor, and simple motor function at 4 months in both groups, which led to premature discontinuation of the study.

An open study of zidovudine in injection drug users found improvements in neuropsychological functioning on a number of subtests (384). Four case control studies retrospectively examined whether zidovudine treatment was associated with outcomes such as reduced leukoencephalopathy (385, 386), lower CSF β_2-microglobulin levels (which are related to neuropsychological improvement) (387), or improved neuropsychological measures (388). Three of the four studies found that the zidovudine-treated patients had significantly positive findings compared to untreated patients.

While the above studies support the efficacy of zidovudine, they do not resolve the issue of optimal dosage nor zidovudine resistance (380). Doses of up to 2000 mg/day of zidovudine were used in some of the above studies, which are often associated with significant toxicity, including neutropenia and anemia. A typical zidovudine dose used now is 500–600 mg/day, and many patients cannot tolerate even these reduced doses (375). Patients can develop resistance to zidovudine, especially if used alone, and because zidovudine-resistant strains can be transmitted from one person to another, some HIV experts have considered the need for testing for zidovudine resistance before choosing which agents to use in treatment (389).

b) Other antiretroviral treatments of cognitive disorders or dysfunction

Treatment studies of antiretroviral agents other than zidovudine are fewer but illuminating. De Ronchi and colleagues (390) conducted a clinical trial (N=88) that compared zidovudine to didanosine to refusal of therapy in both symptomatic and asymptomatic HIV patients. They found that for subjects who were *symptomatic* for HIV disease, both zidovudine and didanosine treatment resulted in better performance on all neuropsychological subtests. In general, *asymptomatic* subjects did not show significant differences in neuropsychological performance compared to the untreated group. The findings suggest differences in effectiveness based on HIV clinical status.

A more recent placebo-controlled study involved the use of abacavir, a nucleoside analogue reverse transcriptase inhibitor with good CSF penetration, in 99 subjects with moderate to severe HIV-associated dementia (391). This study did not demonstrate significant differences in neuropsychological scores between abacavir and placebo groups, but a major limiting factor in this study design was that abacavir alone was added to an already failing antiretroviral treatment regimen.

Of currently available antiretroviral agents, the CSF penetration of stavudine is relatively high (0.4 ratio with serum), but a recent study indicated that stavudine nevertheless penetrates brain tissue poorly (392). The individual protease inhibitors have not been well studied for effects on neurocognitive impairment, and all but indinavir (0.16 ratio with serum) penetrate the CSF poorly (393). Regarding the nonnucleoside reverse transcriptase inhibitors, nevirapine has been shown to have a 0.45 CSF-to-serum ratio and therefore may be a good candidate to include in future controlled studies of HIV-associated cognitive disorders (381).

Ferrando and colleagues (394) studied the effects of various combination antiretroviral therapy regimens on measures of cognitive motor function. They found that tests of attention, concentration, psychomotor speed, learning, and memory were significantly better in those subjects taking antiretroviral therapy than in those who were untreated. Furthermore, they found that those without neuropsychological impairment had lower mean viral load levels, which suggests that antiretroviral treatment benefits neuropsychological functioning through lowering viral load. A similar conclusion was offered by Sacktor et al. (40).

c) Antiretroviral treatments to prevent HIV-associated dementia

A few studies have examined the use of antiretroviral medications to prevent HIV-associated dementia. Moore and colleagues (395) conducted a study of 863 homosexual men treated with zidovudine who were evaluated every 2 months for 2 years or until death. Development of HIV-associated dementia continued with zidovudine treatment but was significantly correlated with low CD4 cell count. Montforte and colleagues (396) used didanosine in a study of 1,047 subjects (median CD4 cell count of 47 cells/mm^3 and mean prior zidovudine treatment of 19 months). Subjects were followed every 2 months to a clinical endpoint (AIDS-defining condition, severe adverse event, or death). They reported a very low incidence of HIV-associated dementia (11 subjects, or 1%), although no formal criteria for defining HIV-associated dementia were offered. One randomized clinical trial with 32 subjects that compared zidovudine treatment to placebo found no significant difference in rate of developing dementia by treatment assignment (397). HIV-associated dementia prevention requires further study, but it appears that treatment with antiretroviral medications may prevent the development of HIV-associated dementia and other cognitive motor disorders.

d) Interventions that affect inflammatory mediators

Although peptide T can be thought of as "antiretroviral," since it blocks the binding of envelope glycoprotein to CD4 receptors, it more likely exerts its effects through decrements in the deleterious effects of inflammatory mediators known as cytokines, such as tumor necrosis factor. A multisite, randomized, placebo-controlled clinical trial with intranasal peptide T was conducted on a sample of 215 patients with HIV-associated neurocognitive impairment, most of whom were taking a single antiretroviral agent or a two-drug combination regimen (398). The study found no statistically significant differences between treatment and placebo groups on global neuropsychological z scores. However, subgroup analyses showed that subjects with a CD4 count of 201–500 cells/mm^3 and subjects with at least moderate neuropsychological impairment at baseline improved significantly with peptide T compared with those given placebo ($p<0.05$). In addition, peptide T was well tolerated with no clinically significant toxic effects.

Studies of inflammatory mediators are indicated because researchers have postulated that HIV-related neuronal injury involves the activation of voltage-dependent calcium channels and *N*-methyl-D-aspartate (NMDA) receptor-operated channels (399). Therefore, studies are underway using memantine (an NMDA antagonist), inhibitors of tumor necrosis factor-α, thalidomide, pentoxifylline, and naloxone (an inhibitor of interferon-α). Mapou and colleagues (400) conducted a clinical trial with interferon-α-n3 in 20 asymptomatic subjects with HIV infection and reported significant improvements in neuropsychological performance in selected subtests. While interferon has been associated with neuropsychological side effects, including depression, Skillman et al. (401) reported that such side effects are minimal.

Nimodipine is a voltage-dependent calcium channel antagonist that has been postulated to prevent HIV-related neuronal injury. Two controlled studies of nimodipine, one in combination with zidovudine (402) and one with nimodipine alone (403), found no significant differences in overall neuropsychological performance.

e) Treatments involving neurotransmitter manipulation

Stimulant drugs have been used as palliative agents to help manage symptoms of fatigue, decreased concentration, or memory deficits among patients with HIV-associated dementia or minor cognitive motor disorder. With regard to the specific effect of stimulants on neurocognitive impairment, there has been one randomized, placebo-controlled clinical trial of a small sample of eight opioid-dependent patients maintained on a regimen of methadone (404). This 7-day crossover study with sustained-release methylphenidate (20–40 mg/day) resulted in nonsignificant neuropsychological z score improvements from baseline with methylphenidate but not placebo. Fernandez and colleagues (321) presented case reports of treating patients with HIV-related disease with methylphenidate (30–90 mg/day) or dextroamphetamine (30–60 mg/day). All patients improved significantly; however, there was no placebo control group and the sample size was small. Similar data from a small trial are offered by Holmes et al. (405).

Studies of dopaminergic agonists are supported by preliminary data in the form of case studies of carbidopa and L-dopa (303). The Dana Consortium conducted a randomized, placebo-controlled clinical trial of 36 subjects with HIV-associated cognitive motor impairment who were given L-deprenyl, a putative antiapoptotic agent, and found that deprenyl-treated subjects showed an improvement in neuropsychological test performance, specifically in verbal memory (406). Investigation of the dopaminergic agent pramipexole is currently under way.

Other neurotransmitters such as serotonin and 5-hydroxyindoleacetic acid have been found to be decreased in CSF as HIV disease progresses (407). It is possible that increasing CNS serotonin levels through administration of agents such as SSRIs may be useful in the treatment of cognitive motor impairment.

f) Nutritional therapies and HIV-associated cognitive disorders

Nutritional therapies need to be considered as potential interventions for the cognitive motor symptoms associated with HIV infection. A case report of a subject with apparent late-stage HIV-associated dementia and a low cobalamin (vitamin B_{12}) level due to decreased intrinsic factor secretion responded over 2 months to B_{12} replacement therapy with complete symptom resolution (408). Oxidative free radical scavengers such as vitamin E, the experimental antioxidant OPC-14117, and the trace mineral and antioxidant selenium may prove to be therapeutically useful.

2. Delirium

Antipsychotic medications have been the treatment of choice in treating delirious states that develop in patients with HIV infection, with most evidence arising from case reports or uncontrolled trials (409, 410). For patients with HIV infection, a prominent issue is the observed increased sensitivity to side effects (299, 300). This sensitivity applies to extrapyramidal side effects with higher-potency agents and also to cognitive side effects with lower-potency antipsychotics.

To date, only one randomized clinical trial has studied the treatment of delirium associated with HIV infection. Breitbart and colleagues (46) approached 244 hospitalized AIDS patients and monitored them for the development of delirium. Among the 30 subjects who went on to develop delirium, 310 episodes of delirium occurred that met both DSM-III-R and Delirium Rating Scale criteria (411). The 30 subjects were randomly assigned to receive haloperidol (N=11), chlorpromazine (N=13), or lorazepam (N=6). Because the six subjects taking lorazepam developed signs of toxicity (oversedation, disinhibition, ataxia, and increased confusion), this treatment was terminated prematurely. Both haloperidol and chlorpromazine treatment resulted in significantly reduced scores on the Delirium Rating Scale in the first 24 hours. The researchers did not report significant problems with extrapyramidal side effects in study patients, but mean daily doses were low.

Scattered case reports or series suggest that other antipsychotic agents may be useful for treating HIV-associated delirium. For instance, molindone (312), risperidone (315), and droperidol (412, 413) have been suggested as alternatives to the standard antipsychotic medication because of differences in side effect profile, onset of action, or potency.

3. Mood disorders

Disturbances of mood occur frequently in the context of HIV infection. Treatment studies are quite varied with regard to variables such as severity of mood disorder, methodology to categorize or diagnose mood disorders, outcome measures, and stage of HIV illness.

a) Acute treatment of depressive disorders—somatic treatments

Many studies, including randomized controlled trials, open-label trials, case series, and case reports, support the efficacy and safety of many antidepressants in the acute treatment of depressive disorders, including major depression, in a wide range of HIV-infected populations at all disease stages.

Wagner and colleagues (286) reported on a series of 6-week studies that used random assignment and placebo control to examine the efficacy of standard and alternative antidepressants for major depression in HIV-infected patients. The agents used at standard doses were fluoxetine, sertraline, imipramine, dextroamphetamine, and testosterone. Response rates to the different agents ranged from 70% to 93% and were significantly higher than placebo.

Similar findings were reported in a randomized, placebo-controlled clinical trial conducted by Elliot and colleagues (287) in 75 HIV patients (45% with AIDS) who had major depression. Both imipramine- and paroxetine-treated groups improved significantly compared to placebo at weeks 6, 8, and 12. The dropout rate due to side effects was higher for those receiving imipramine (48%) than it was for placebo (24%) or paroxetine (20%).

One randomized, placebo-controlled clinical trial (N=120) found that fluoxetine was an efficacious antidepressant agent among depressed HIV patients; the response rate for fluoxetine was 74% versus 47% for placebo (289). The same study reported significant differences between ethnic groups in terms of antidepressant efficacy; the response rates were 84% for white, 67% for Latino, and 50% for black subjects (414). Despite the effectiveness of fluoxetine in treating depression, because both placebo response and attrition were high, the researchers suggested that the addition of another medication in patients with serious medical illness who require multiple concomitant medications may be a significant barrier to the treatment of depression.

In a double-blind, placebo-controlled trial that compared desipramine to fluoxetine in 14 women with advanced HIV disease, both agents were linked to symptom improvement; however, for most of the women significant depressive symptoms remained after the 6-week trial

(294). These findings are consistent with those of an open-label fluoxetine trial that compared HIV-positive and HIV-negative depressed men, which found that improvement in the HIV-positive cohort was significantly delayed beyond the 8-week trial compared to the HIV-negative patients (415).

The randomized trials are supported by uncontrolled studies of depression in HIV populations and confirm the effectiveness of fluvoxamine (295) and fluoxetine (293, 416, 417) in HIV-infected *asymptomatic* patients and of paroxetine, sertraline, and fluoxetine in *symptomatic* HIV patients (285, 418). In an open trial in which HIV-positive depressed women were given either fluoxetine or sertraline, both drugs were found to be effective treatments (419). Another open-label study found nefazodone effective in the treatment of depressed HIV-positive patients (288). One open-label trial of 32 patients with advanced HIV disease found venlafaxine effective among depressed patients who also had minor cognitive motor disorder (420).

The use of psychostimulants for treatment of major depression in HIV-infected outpatients has been supported in smaller studies, including five case reports, one open-label trial, and one placebo-drug-placebo clinical trial (321, 322, 421, 422). These studies suggest that methylphenidate, up to 35 mg/day, or dextroamphetamine, up to 10 mg/day, can improve major depression.

An open trial of testosterone replacement for hypogonadal men found that of 34 study participants with major depressive disorder, 79% had significant improvement in mood (126). There is a case report of a patient with HIV infection and comorbid major depressive disorder whose depression resolved with treatment with the antiretroviral agent zidovudine (423). For patients with severe major depression who are delusional or have failed medication treatment, ECT has been found to be safe and effective (424).

b) Acute treatment of depressive disorders—psychotherapy

Several studies of psychotherapeutic treatment of depression in HIV patients have been conducted. In a randomized, controlled trial, Targ and colleagues (425) compared structured group therapy plus fluoxetine to structured group therapy with placebo in 20 asymptomatic homosexual men with major depression or adjustment disorder and Hamilton Depression Rating Scale scores ≥16. Both groups showed significant improvements in depression after 6 weeks of treatment, but there were no differences between treatment groups (425). In contrast, another randomized, placebo-controlled clinical trial that compared the efficacy and safety of fluoxetine plus group psychotherapy versus group psychotherapy alone in 47 depressed HIV-positive men for 7 weeks found that fluoxetine in addition to group therapy was more efficacious than group psychotherapy alone. Differences were particularly apparent for patients whose initial depressive episodes were rated as severe (Hamilton depression score ≥24) (290).

Markowitz and colleagues (426) conducted a randomized, placebo-controlled clinical trial that compared 16-week interventions with interpersonal psychotherapy, cognitive behavior therapy, supportive psychotherapy, and supportive psychotherapy plus imipramine in 101 HIV patients with depressive symptoms (Hamilton depression score ≥15). Patients randomly assigned to interpersonal psychotherapy and supportive psychotherapy plus imipramine had significantly greater symptom improvement than those receiving supportive psychotherapy alone or cognitive behavior therapy.

In an earlier study (427), the Markowitz group demonstrated the benefits of interpersonal psychotherapy in HIV-positive, asymptomatic outpatients in an open study of men and women with DSM-III-R major depression or dysthymia. Twenty (87%) out of 23 patients achieved a full remission after 6 weeks by clinical assessment; mean Hamilton depression scores at baseline and follow-up were 25 and 6.8, respectively. Levine et al. (428) reported that four outpatients with major depression remained euthymic for 9 months with structured group psychotherapy after acute remission was achieved with fluoxetine, 20–40 mg/day.

Other studies such as two retrospective chart reviews (284, 429) and a prospective effectiveness study (430) support the findings from controlled and uncontrolled treatment studies of major depression that treatment with a number of different antidepressant agents is effective and generally tolerated in HIV patients.

c) Treatment of other types of depression

Other studies have investigated the efficacy of treatment for other types of depression in HIV patients. These studies generally use screening instruments (e.g., the Center for Epidemiologic Studies Depression Scale [CES-D Scale]) rather than structured interviews or clinical evaluations to diagnose specific depressive disorders. All involved ambulatory patients who had no significant clinical manifestations of HIV disease. In a study of patients with depression (CES-D Scale score >16) but with unknown psychiatric diagnoses, investigators compared cognitive behavior therapy and brief supportive group therapy to a waiting list control condition. Outpatients (N=68) were randomly assigned to an 8-week intervention of cognitive behavior therapy, support group, or a control group. While both types of psychotherapy were superior to the control condition, neither led to significant reductions on the CES-D Scale into the nondepressed range (431).

Eller (432) conducted a randomized, placebo-controlled clinical trial of alternative therapies for depression and assigned 81 male and female outpatients with HIV infection to guided imagery, relaxation therapy, or usual care. The sample had a mean CES-D Scale score of 19. There were no significant declines in CES-D Scale scores during treatment in any of the three groups.

d) Treatment of mania/bipolar disorder

One chart review (433) and one case report (434) have addressed the treatment of manic syndromes in HIV-infected patients. The chart review study identified seven male outpatients with mania who did not improve with lithium or neuroleptic treatment due to toxicity. Three patients had been treated with valproic acid (750–1750 mg/day), two with clonazepam (2 mg/day), one with phenytoin, and one with carbamazepine. All seven patients experienced remission of their manic syndrome with the agent used (433). The case report described the effectiveness of valproic acid in the treatment of acute mania in a patient with AIDS complicated by dementia (434). There are no published studies of maintenance treatments for mania or bipolar disorders in HIV-infected populations.

4. Substance use disorders

Clinical consensus has established the necessity of treating substance use disorders in order to produce optimal psychiatric and medical outcomes for patients with HIV infection. Despite this knowledge, remarkably few studies have investigated psychiatric treatment of substance use disorders in HIV-infected patients. This section will review the literature of the treatment of substance use disorders and associated syndromes.

a) Entry into a treatment program

Entry into a treatment program is probably one of the more critical steps for the assessment and treatment of substance use disorders. Guydish and colleagues (435) described a consultation-education-triage model program that referred drug users with HIV infection to follow-up care for substance use disorders. Of the 86 patients referred over an 8-month period, 81% were referred for further care to a substance use program, with 58% actually contacting the referral resource. Eighty percent had AIDS or symptomatic HIV disease; 37% of patients were dependent on alcohol, 36% were dependent on amphetamines, and 26% were dependent on heroin, marijuana, or cocaine.

b) Methadone maintenance

The Program for AIDS Counseling and Education in San Francisco is considered a model program for inner-city, poor, opiate-dependent, mostly minority men (436, 437). The program provides medical assessment and care, psychiatric treatment, methadone treatment, counseling, detoxification, and tolerance management for opiate addicts. Outcomes for patients enrolled in the Program for AIDS Counseling and Education have been reported in two conference papers. In one report, 29 opioid-dependent HIV patients with a mean of 28 days of drug use in the past month reduced their use to a mean of 5.9 days of use per month after 3 months in the program (438). The other report focused on clinical events related to drug use before and after enrollment for 62 patients in the program (439). Clinical events included medical complications and lapses in compliance with treatment. At baseline, patients experienced 0.72 clinically significant medical complications per 100 patient years, whereas the rate decreased significantly to 0.16 during enrollment in the Program for AIDS Counseling and Education. There was also a reduction in preventable HIV clinical events from 0.21 per 100 patient years to 0.02 per 100 patient years after starting the program. The reports provide some evidence that both the medical care as well as substance use behaviors of HIV-infected opioid addicts can benefit from a multidisciplinary, structured intervention.

c) Pharmacologic treatment of substance use disorders

One study of HIV-infected patients investigated the effect of antidepressant medications on symptoms of drug dependency, such as drug craving and comorbid depression. Batki (440) conducted a controlled trial that compared fluoxetine to placebo in 37 patients with cocaine and opiate dependency who were on a regimen of methadone maintenance. Of this sample, 41% also had major depression. Participants treated with fluoxetine (20–40 mg/day) had lower median measures of cocaine metabolites in urine and fewer mean days of cocaine use per week (1.6) compared to those given placebo (2.6); the fluoxetine-treated patients also reported reduced cocaine craving. Those with major depression showed significant improvement after the 12-week treatment.

d) Overall outcomes of psychiatric treatment

Lyketsos and colleagues (430) conducted a 14-month prospective effectiveness study of clinical outcomes in HIV patients who were referred to psychiatric treatment. Within the cohort, 110 patients had current (N=66) or recent (N=44) substance use disorders; there were high rates of polysubstance dependence, with only a small proportion of patients who abused alcohol. The psychiatric treatment took place within a primary care clinic and included treatment for substance abuse and concurrent psychiatric disorders. Psychiatric intervention led to a decrease in the use of substances and better clinical condition.

5. Anxiety disorders

Anxiety disorders are prevalent in the population of persons who have or are at risk for HIV infection, but studies of specific treatments for anxiety disorders in HIV patients are lacking. The literature provides only one retrospective chart review and two case reports that address the management of anxiety disorders in HIV-positive patients. There are no treatment studies of PTSD among HIV-infected patients, although PTSD rates are high in some HIV-affected groups (441).

A chart review study found that buspirone was an effective anxiolytic in opioid-dependent, HIV-positive patients who were on a regimen of methadone maintenance and who also had a comorbid anxiety disorder. The study additionally showed a modest reduction of urine tests positive for substances of abuse, from 42% to 30% (328).

McDaniel and Johnson (442) found fluoxetine to be effective in the treatment of obsessive-compulsive disorder (OCD) in two HIV-positive patients. Both patients tolerated the fluoxetine with minimal side effects and responded with resolution of OCD symptoms within 6–8 weeks.

A male patient with advanced AIDS complicated by comorbid trichotillomania and major depression was reported to have responded well to sertraline at a maximum dose of 150 mg/day. The patient reported experiencing a 70%–80% decrease in hair pulling and a modest improvement in depressed mood, with minimal medication side effects (443).

6. Psychotic disorders

Nine literature citations, two of them clinical trials and the remainder case reports, present evidence concerning the efficacy of psychotropic medication for the management of psychosis in the presence of HIV infection. The nine reports contain fewer than 100 subjects, approximately 90% of them male, and most with symptomatic HIV infection, usually AIDS. Where stated, the majority did not have a history of psychosis before HIV infection, and, where stated, the majority had cognitive impairment.

Antipsychotic medications were effective in treating psychosis whether or not cognitive dysfunction or delirium was present. One large case history series found that patients with manic psychosis showed more improvement than patients with schizophreniform psychosis (315). The two clinical trials (31, 444) found that positive symptoms responded better than negative symptoms. Across studies the subjects, who largely had advanced HIV disease, required lower doses of antipsychotic medication, similar to the pattern seen in the elderly. Lower doses were also useful due to increased sensitivity to side effects. If a patient did not respond to or tolerate one antipsychotic, it was useful to try another from a different class (300, 301, 310, 312).

In case reports, the use of adjunctive medications, including antianxiety drugs, antidepressants, and mood stabilizers, was a common practice and often useful in individual cases, but there have been no controlled studies on the efficacy of these combinations. Two case reports, each of a single male subject with AIDS, found that catatonia responded rapidly to lorazepam (445, 446). No side effects were noted.

Maintenance medication was not always necessary to sustain remission of psychotic symptoms (42, 312). In some cases it was specifically noted that symptoms of psychosis diminished as severe late-stage medical illness progressed (42). While it has been hypothesized that there is a window of vulnerability to psychosis or mania occurring early in the course of HIV-associated dementia (447), no data support this theory, and most patients treated for psychosis have continued their maintainance medication regimens.

There are few data on the treatment of psychosis in early-stage HIV infection or among women nor is there information concerning potential modifications in the treatment of preexisting psychotic illness, which might be necessary in the presence of advancing HIV infection.

7. Adjustment disorders

Two open-label clinical trials have assessed the effectiveness of psychotropic medications in the management of adjustment disorders in HIV-positive patients. As part of a larger study that examined the effectiveness of paroxetine in the treatment of depression in the context of HIV infection, Grassi and colleagues (418) included five patients with a diagnosis of adjustment disorder with depressed mood. All five patients received paroxetine (20 mg/day) and showed significant recovery as measured by the Hamilton depression scale at the 6-week endpoint.

Five male patients with neurocognitive impairment as well as a diagnosis of adjustment disorder with depressed mood were treated as part of a larger study of the effectiveness of psychostimulants in patients with HIV-associated dementia. Four of the five patients who received methylphenidate had moderate to marked improvement in symptoms; the one patient with minimal response was switched to dextroamphetamine and subsequently had a moderate response (405).

8. Sleep disorders

Numerous reports have documented disrupted sleep and altered sleep architecture in HIV patients (29, 448, 449), including one study which linked fatigue and sleep disturbances to morbidity and disability in homosexual men (450). While the etiologies remain unclear, some investigators have documented growth hormone dysregulation associated with sleep pathology (451), and one study found obstructive sleep apnea due to adenotonsillar hypertrophy to be a primary cause of sleep disruption in a cohort of HIV patients with excessive daytime sleepiness (452).

The treatment of sleep disorders in HIV-positive persons has been examined in only one open-label clinical trial of flurazepam in 12 patients (453). All patients were given a one-time dose of flurazepam, 30 mg, to examine changes in the patients' electroencephalographic recordings during sleep. Flurazepam mainly affected non-REM parameters, such as reduction of times awake during the night and increases in stage two and effective sleep time. As this study did not address treatment with flurazepam beyond a one-time dose, actual treatment recommendations cannot be made.

9. Disorders of infancy, childhood, and adolescence

Since HIV infection in childhood is associated with developmental delays or loss of acquired skills, it is hoped that early treatment will promote normal development. Currently, it appears that antiretroviral drug therapy reduces morbidity in children, especially in those with HIV-associated neurocognitive impairment. Several studies have reported a significant increase in mental ability, as measured by the WISC-R, the McCarthy Scales of Children's Abilities, or the Bayley Scales of Infant Development, in over 450 children during 12- and 36-month trials with zidovudine (58, 246, 454, 455). None of the studies included a control group.

The safety of zidovudine for children is similar to that for adults, although up to 40% of children experience hematological side effects that require dose alterations (246). The one published study of 54 children that did not find a significant improvement in cognitive functioning with zidovudine treatment did find a significant decrease in CD4 levels over the treatment period. No data were provided on adherence to treatment or zidovudine resistance (456). Other antiretroviral agents, such as didanosine, have been studied, with a multisite project showing that combination zidovudine and didanosine therapy was superior to either used as monotherapy for most of the CNS outcomes evaluated (457). Although combination antiretroviral therapy with three agents is standard practice with adults, there is only one case report of its use with a child (458). Caregivers noted the positive impact of this regimen on an 8-year-old boy's neurocognitive development.

The effectiveness of the treatment of other mental and behavioral disorders associated with HIV infection in children and adolescents is largely unstudied. Case reports of single patients suggest that attention deficit disorders and depressive disorders in those with HIV infection may be treated by using regimens that are standard for those without HIV infection (459). As in the treatment of adults, children with HIV infection may be especially sensitive to some treatment side effects, such as insomnia or appetite suppression associated with psychostimulant use.

Pain frequently accompanies pediatric HIV and can involve multiple organ systems (460). Clinicians should be aware that the inadequate verbal skills of younger children or the fact that some children are from non-English-speaking families can lead to the underrecognition and undertreatment of pain (461).

10. HIV-associated syndromes with psychiatric implications

A number of HIV-associated clinical syndromes have psychiatric implications, such as wasting syndrome, fatigue, pain, and sexual dysfunction. Because there are overlapping symptoms with these conditions and psychiatric disorders, it is useful for psychiatrists to be aware of treatment studies for such syndromes so that overall clinical outcomes can be improved.

a) Wasting syndrome

Several studies have focused on the use of testosterone for treatment of wasting syndrome in both patients with low testosterone levels and patients with "clinical hypogonadism" (normal hormone levels). Grinspoon and colleagues (462) conducted a double-blind, placebo-controlled study of hypogonadal HIV-positive men with wasting syndrome that demonstrated the safety and efficacy of testosterone replacement therapy (300 mg i.m. every 3 weeks). The treatment resulted in a significant increase of lean body mass, overall quality of life, and self-perception of appearance in treated subjects. Similar findings have been reported by Rabkin and colleagues (126, 343, 463), who conducted several randomized, placebo-controlled trials as well as open trials of testosterone replacement in men with clinical hypogonadism that led to significant positive effects on mood and weight (lean body mass). Another study that used oxymetholone, a testosterone derivative, demonstrated weight gain in cachectic men with AIDS (464). A controlled study of hypogonadal *women* with HIV infection that used transdermal testosterone replacement also reported improvement in lean body mass and quality of life (465).

Wagner and colleagues (466) reported an additional improvement of measures on the Brief Symptom Inventory and nutritional status for patients who exercised in addition to receiving testosterone replacement. In a double-blind, randomized, placebo-controlled trial, researchers found that resistance exercise in addition to testosterone and the anabolic steroid oxandrolone substantially increased lean body mass (467). Two open-label studies have reported that oxandrolone, 20 mg/day, in HIV patients with wasting syndrome led to significant weight gain, in particular, increases in body cell mass (334, 335).

Several clinical trials have used the recombinant growth hormone somatotropin for treatment of HIV-related wasting (336, 340). A large multicenter, double-blind, placebo-controlled study that used growth hormone in patients with AIDS wasting reported significant improvement in overall quality of life and weight gain, with no negative effect on virological or immunological markers (339). Treatment was well tolerated.

Since tumor necrosis factor-α has been postulated to have a role in the pathogenesis of wasting syndrome, the effect of thalidomide, a selective inhibitor of tumor necrosis factor-α, has been studied in patients with AIDS wasting syndrome. Two reports (a mail survey of thalidomide users and a small randomized, placebo-controlled clinical trial) have supported the positive effects of thalidomide on weight gain, appetite, and quality of life (341, 342).

b) Fatigue

Breitbart and colleagues (468) conducted a randomized, placebo-controlled clinical trial that used two psychostimulant medications, methylphenidate and pemoline, in treating fatigue among HIV patients. They found that both treatments were superior to placebo, with a stronger effect in the methylphenidate group. In addition, they reported that improvement in fatigue was associated with improvement in depressive symptoms and psychological distress. In an open trial of depressed patients with CD4 counts below 200, dextroamphetamine administration led to improvement of fatigue in 95% of patients along with reduction in depression scores (322). Testosterone replacement with dehydroepiandrosterone (DHEA) in HIV-infected hypogonadal men has also been found to improve symptoms of fatigue (469).

c) Pain

Studies of the frequency and adequacy of treatment for pain among patients with AIDS find wide variations in the effectiveness of interventions to manage pain. A study by Breitbart et al. (123) found that 85% of HIV patients in their ambulatory sample treated at a cancer center received inadequate pain therapy. Yet a different study reported that only 20% of their sample of AIDS patients treated in the hospital, home care, or nursing facility did not receive effective pain control (470).

While agents such as tricyclic antidepressants and anticonvulsant medications are often used to manage chronic pain from peripheral neuropathy, published treatment studies for HIV-associated peripheral neuropathy have not supported their use. Two randomized, controlled trials have focused on HIV-associated peripheral neuropathy; both trials used the agent mexiletine, an antiarrhythmic drug with local anesthetic properties that had been used in the treatment of diabetic neuropathy (317, 471). Neither study found pain relief different from that of placebo. Furthermore, Kieburtz et al. (317) did not find that treatment with amitriptyline provided significant pain relief compared to placebo. Shlay and colleagues (472) conducted a randomized, controlled trial that compared acupuncture, amitriptyline, and placebo for pain due to HIV-related peripheral neuropathy and found that neither acupuncture nor amitriptyline was more effective than placebo.

d) Sexual dysfunction

Sexual dysfunction is experienced commonly by HIV patients, both men and women, particularly with HIV disease progression. While no treatment trials are currently published, a cautionary note regarding sildenafil is clinically important. Sildenafil should be used judiciously in patients with erectile dysfunction who are also taking protease inhibitors, since the primary route of sildenafil metabolism is via the cytochrome P450 isoenzyme 3A4. One death has been reported in a 47-year-old male taking ritonavir and saquinavir who was administered 25 mg of sildenafil (473). The manufacturer of sildenafil has recommended that patients receiving ritonavir should not take more than a single sildenafil dose of 25 mg in a 48-hour period.

PART C:
FUTURE RESEARCH NEEDS

Considerable progress has been made in understanding HIV, AIDS, and treatment for these conditions. However, further studies are needed regarding specific, effective treatments for patients, including women and children, with HIV/AIDS. Areas of specific concern include:

1. The impact of antiretroviral therapy on the incidence of CNS opportunistic diseases and neuropsychiatric disorders.
2. The specific etiology of HIV-associated dementia and minor cognitive motor disorder and effective interventions to prevent or ameliorate these conditions.
3. The clinical significance of drug-drug interactions of psychotropic agents and HIV-related medications.
4. Whether HIV is directly linked to the occurrence of psychosis, mania, depression, or other psychiatric disorders in persons with HIV infection.
5. Whether the CNS serves as a reservoir of HIV-resistant strains and the clinical implications if it does.
6. The effectiveness of psychiatric care in critical areas of treatment adherence, prevention of HIV infection, and psychosocial adaptation.
7. Information about the impact of HIV infection on development in children, with possible differences in clinical course due to whether infected in utero or perinatally or due to type of treatment received.
8. More effective interventions for HIV risk reduction in specific psychiatric populations, particularly for primary prevention of HIV infection.
9. The need for more data about the effectiveness of psychiatric treatments such as psychotherapy, pharmacotherapy, and psychosocial services for adults, adolescents, and children with HIV/AIDS.
10. Investigating possible gender differences in the problems associated with HIV/AIDS and treatment for these conditions.

APPENDIX 1. HIV/AIDS Electronic Resources

Resource	Organization	URL
General information	AIDS Action Committee (AAC)	www.aac.org
	AIDS Daily Summary	www.cdcnpin.org/news/start.htm
	AIDS Education Training Centers (AETC)	www.service.emory.edu/SEATEC/AETCdir.html#USA
	AIDS Virtual Library	www.planetq.com/aidsvl/index.html
	American Medical Association	www.ama-assn.org
	American Psychiatric Association	www.psych.org/aids
	Business and Labor Resource Service	www.brta-hta.org
	Centers for Disease Control and Prevention (CDC)	www.cdc.gov
	CDC National Prevention Information Network (CDCNAC)	www.cdcpin.org
	CDC National AIDS Funding Database	www.cdcnpin.org/db/public/fundmain.htm
	CMV Retinitis Education and Treatment Information	www.piv.org
	Food and Drug Administration (FDA)	www.fda.gov
	FDA/OASHI: HIV/AIDS	www.fda.gov/oashi/aids/hiv.gov
	FDA Medical Bulletin	www.fda.gov/medbull/contents.html
	Healthcare Communications Group	www.healthcg.com
	Healthfinder	www.healthfinder.gov
	HIVDent	www.hivdent.org
	Human Retroviruses and AIDS Sequence Database	hiv-web.ianl.gov
	Johns Hopkins AIDS Service	www.hopkins-aids.edu
	Infectious Diseases Society	www.idsociety.org
	Insights in HIV Disease Management	www.meniscius.com/hiv
	Medical Matrix	www.medmatrix.org/index.asp
	National Academy of Sciences	www.nas.edu
	National AIDS Treatment Advocacy Project (NATAP)	www.natap.org
	National Hemophilia Foundation (NHF)	www.infoahf.org
	National Institutes of Health (NIH)	www.nih.gov
	National Science Foundation	www.nsf.gov
	New York Online Access on Health	www.noah.cuny.edu/aids/aids.html
	Pharmaceutical Research Manufacturers Association of America (PhRMA)	www.phrma.org

APPENDIX 1. HIV/AIDS Electronic Resources *(continued)*

Resource	Organization	URL
General information *(continued)*	The Access Project	204.179.124.69/network/access/index.html
	The Body	www.thebody.com
	University of California HIV/AIDS Program	hivinsite.ucsf.edu
	USP Pharmacopeia Practitioners Reporting Network	usp.org/index
	Yahoo: Health Medicines HIV/AIDS	www.yahoo.com/Health/Medicine
	Webber's AIDS/HIV Law and Policy Resource	www.critpath.org/aidslaw
Alternative treatments	American Chiropractic Association	www.amerchiro.org/aca
	ATDN's Alternative Treatments	204.179.124.69/network/altx.html
	Bastyr University AIDS Research Center	www.bastyr.edu/research/busrc
	Herb Research Foundation	www.herbs.org
	Homeopathic Educational Services	www.homeopathic.com
	Institute for Traditional Medicine	www.europa.com/-itm
Clinical trials	Adult AIDS Clinical Trials Group (ACTG)	aactg.a-3.com/links.com
	AIDS Clinical Trial Information Services	www.actic.org
	AIDS Treatment Information Service	www.atis.org
	American Foundation for AIDS Research (amFAR)	www.amfar.org/td
	Canadian HIV Trials Network	www.hivnet.ubc.ca/ctn.html
	Pediatric AIDS Clinical Trials Group	pactg.s-3.com/links.htm
	The Body	www.thebody.com/treatclintri.html
	USA HIV Clinical Trials/Trial Search	hivinsite.ucsf.edu/tsearch
	Vanderbilt Vaccines	www.mc.vanderbilt.edu/adl/aids_project/vac
Harm reduction/ needle exchange	Center for AIDS Prevention Studies (UCSF)	www.caps.ucsf.edu/capsweb
	The Lindesmith Center	www.lindesmith.org
	The XCHANGE POINT	members.aol.com/xchangept/aids.html
	North American Syringe Exchange Network	www.nasen.org
	Safe Works AIDS Project	www.safeworks.org

APPENDIX 1. HIV/AIDS Electronic Resources *(continued)*

Resource	Organization	URL
Recreational drugs and anti-HIV drug information	National AIDS Manual	www.nam.org/uk/atu/atu51.trt
	Notes from the Underground	www.aidsinfonyc.org/pwahg/notes/38.html
	Positively AWARE	www.tpan.com/library/pa/mayjun97/p.32.htm
	The Toronto Hospital	www.tthhivclinic.com/recreation.htm
	POZ	www.thebody.com/poz/survival/6_98/warning.html
	CATIE (Community AIDS Treatment Information Exchange)	www.catie.ca
	University of California, San Francisco	Hivinsite.ucsf.edu/topics/substance_use/hiv_aids_medications_and_interventions_with_legal_and_illegal_drugs/
	Medscape	www.medscape.com/medscape/hiv/clinicalmgmt/can/drug/public/toccm.drug.html
	NO/AIDS Task Force	www.crescentcity.com/noaids
	Project Inform	www.projinf.org/fe/drugin.html
	San Francisco AIDS Foundation	www.afa.org/treatment/beta/b34/b34piint.html

INDIVIDUALS AND ORGANIZATIONS THAT SUBMITTED COMMENTS

J. Atkinson, M.D.
Steven Batki, M.D.
Christy L. Beaudin, Ph.D., L.C.S.W., C.P.H.Q.
Carl Bell, M.D.
Marcia Bennett, D.N.S.
Alan Berkman, M.D.
Philip A. Bialer, M.D.
Charles H. Blackinton, M.D., P.A.
Mel Blaustein, M.D.
Michael T. Brady, M.D.
William Breitbart, M.D.
Robert Broadbent, M.D.
Robert Paul Cabaj, M.D.
Susan Chuck, Pharm.D.
Norman A. Clemens, M.D.
Dave Davis, M.D.
Steven A. Epstein, M.D.
Abraham Feingold, Psy.D.
Steve Ferrando, M.D.
Jack Gorman, M.D.
William M. Greenberg, M.D.
Susan Haikalis, L.C.S.W.
Mark Halman, M.D.
Lawrence Hartmann, M.D.
Roman M. Hendrickson, M.D.
Al Herzog, M.D.
Dan Hicks, M.D.
Ewald Horwath, M.D.
Michael Hughes, M.D.
Jeffrey S. Janofsky, M.D.
T. Stephen Jones, M.D.
Nalini V. Juthani, M.D.
Cheryl Ann Kennedy, M.D.
Robert Kertzner, M.D.
Lawrence Y. Kline, M.D.
Joyce Kobayashi, M.D.
Ronald R. Koegler, M.D.
Thomas Kosten, M.D.
Zev Labins, M.D.
Debra E. Lyon, Ph.D.
John C. Markowitz, M.D.
Elinore F. McCance-Katz, M.D.
Karen McKinnon, M.A.
Philip R. Muskin, M.D.
Judith Rabkin, M.D.
David Rosmarin, M.D.
Peter Ross
Pedro Ruiz, M.D.
Larry Siegel, M.D.
Robert Stasko, M.D.
William R. Tatomer, M.D.
Joshua T. Thornhill IV, M.D.
Glenn J. Treisman, M.D.
Milton L. Wainberg, M.D.
Bert Warren, M.D.
Jonathan L. Worth, M.D.
Claire Zilber, M.D.

American Academy of Family Physicians
American Academy of Psychiatry and the Law
American Group Psychotherapy Association, Inc.
American Psychiatric Nurses Association
American Society of Addiction Medicine
American Society of Clinical Psychopharmacology, Inc.
APA Commission on Psychotherapy by Psychiatrists
Association for Academic Psychiatry
Association of Gay and Lesbian Psychiatrists
Black Psychiatrists of America
National Association of Social Workers
PacifiCare Behavioral Health
Royal Australian and New Zealand College of Psychiatrists
San Francisco AIDS Foundation

REFERENCES

The following coding system is used to indicate the nature of the supporting evidence in the references:

[A] *Randomized clinical trial.* A study of an intervention in which subjects are prospectively followed over time; there are treatment and control groups; subjects are randomly assigned to the two groups; both the subjects and the investigators are blind to the assignments.

[B] *Clinical trial.* A prospective study in which an intervention is made and the results of that intervention are tracked longitudinally; study does not meet standards for a randomized clinical trial.

[C] *Cohort or longitudinal study.* A study in which subjects are prospectively followed over time without any specific intervention.

[D] *Case-control study.* A study in which a group of patients and a group of control subjects are identified in the present and information about them is pursued retrospectively or backward in time.

[E] *Review with secondary data analysis.* A structured analytic review of existing data (e.g., a meta-analysis or a decision analysis).

[F] *Review.* A qualitative review and discussion of previously published literature without a quantitative synthesis of the data.

[G] *Other.* Textbooks, expert opinion, case reports, and other reports not included above.

1. Ho DD: Viral counts count in HIV infection. Science 1996; 272:1124–1125 [G]
2. National Center for Health Statistics: AIDS falls from top ten causes of death; teen births, infant mortality, homicide all decline (press release). Hyattsville, Md, US Department of Health and Human Services, Oct 7, 1998 [G]
3. Centers for Disease Control and Prevention: HIV/AIDS Surveillance Report 1999; 1(11) [G]
4. Steinbrook R: Caring for people with human immunodeficiency virus infection (editorial). N Engl J Med 1998; 339:1926–1928 [G]
5. Mitka M: Slowing decline in AIDS deaths prompts concern. JAMA 1999; 282:1216–1217 [G]
6. Counselling Guidelines for HIV Testing. Ottawa, Canadian Medical Association, 1995 [G]
7. Gostin LO, Lazzarini Z, Jones TS, Flaherty K: Prevention of HIV/AIDS and other blood-borne diseases among injection drug users: a national survey on the regulation of syringes and needles. JAMA 1997; 277:53–62 [D]
8. Kinloch-de Loes S, de Saussure P, Saurat JH, Stalder H, Hirschel B, Perrin LH: Symptomatic primary infection due to human immunodeficiency virus type 1: review of 31 cases. Clin Infect Dis 1993; 17:59–65 [D]
9. Zhang Z, Schuler T, Zupancic M, Wietgrefe S, Staskus KA, Reimann KA, Reinhart TA, Rogan M, Cavert W, Miller CJ, Veazey RS, Notermans D, Little S, Danner SA, Richman DD, Havlir D, Wong J, Jordan HL, Schacker TW, Racz P, Tenner-Racz K, Letvin NL, Wolinsky S, Haase AT: Sexual transmission and propagation of SIV and HIV in resting and activated CD4+ T cells. Science 1999; 286:1353–1357 [G]
10. Chun TW, Engel D, Berrey MM, Shea T, Corey L, Fauci AS: Early establishment of a pool of latently infected, resting CD4(+) T cells during primary HIV-1 infection. Proc Natl Acad Sci USA 1998; 95:8869–8873 [G]
11. Schrager LK, D'Souza MP: Cellular and anatomical reservoirs of HIV-1 in patients receiving potent antiretroviral combination therapy. JAMA 1998; 280:67–71 [F]

12. Hengge UR, Brockmeyer NH, Esser S, Maschke M, Goos M: HIV-1 RNA levels in cerebrospinal fluid and plasma correlate with AIDS dementia (letter). AIDS 1998; 12:818–820 [G]
13. Hirsch MS, Conway B, D'Aquila RT, Johnson VA, Brun-Vezinet F, Clotet B, Demeter LM, Hammer SM, Jacobsen DM, Kuritzkes DR, Loveday C, Mellors JW, Vella S, Richman DD (International AIDS Society—USA Panel): Antiretroviral drug resistance testing in adults with HIV infection: implications for clinical management. JAMA 1998; 279:1984–1991 [E]
14. Hughes MD, Johnson VA, Hirsch MS, Bremer JW, Elbeik T, Erice A, Kuritzkes DR, Scott WA, Spector SA, Basgoz N, Fischl MA, D'Aquila RT (ACTG 241 Protocol Virology Substudy Team): Monitoring plasma HIV-1 RNA levels in addition to CD4+ lymphocyte count improves assessment of antiretroviral therapeutic response. Ann Intern Med 1997; 126:929–938 [A]
15. O'Brien WA, Hartigan PM, Daar ES, Simberkoff MS, Hamilton JD (VA Cooperative Study Group on AIDS): Changes in plasma HIV RNA levels and CD4+ lymphocyte counts predict both response to antiretroviral therapy and therapeutic failure. Ann Intern Med 1997; 126:939–945 [A]
16. Paul WE (ed): Fundamental Immunology, 3rd ed. Philadelphia, Lippincott-Raven, 1994, p 1386 [G]
17. Centers for Disease Control and Prevention: 1993 revised classification system for HIV infection and expanded surveillance case definition for AIDS among adolescents and adults. MMWR Morb Mortal Wkly Rep 1992; 41(RR-17):1–19 [E]
18. Descamps D, Flandre P, Calvez V, Peytavin G, Meiffredy V, Collin G, Delaugerre C, Robert-Delmas S, Bazin B, Aboulker JP, Pialoux G, Raffi F, Brun-Vezinet F: Mechanisms of virologic failure in previously untreated HIV-infected patients from a trial of induction-maintenance therapy. JAMA 2000; 283:205–211 [G]
19. Deeks SG, Smith M, Holodniy M, Kahn JO: HIV-1 protease inhibitors: a review for clinicians. JAMA 1997; 277:145–153 [F]
20. Boden D, Hurley A, Zhang L, Cao Y, Guo Y, Jones E, Tsay J, Ip J, Farthing C, Limoli K, Parkin N, Markowitz M: HIV-1 drug resistance in newly infected individuals. JAMA 1999; 282:1135–1141 [D]
21. Pomerantz RJ: Primary HIV-1 resistance: a new phase in the epidemic? (editorial). JAMA 1999; 282:1177–1179 [G]
22. Swindells S, Zheng J, Gendelman HE: HIV-associated dementia: new insights into disease pathogenesis and therapeutic interventions. AIDS Patient Care STDS 1999; 3:153–163 [F]
23. Zink WE, Zheng J, Persidsky Y, Poluektova L, Gendelman HE: The neuropathogenesis of HIV-1 infection. FEMS Immunol Med Microbiol 1999; 26:233–241 [F]
24. Kolson DL, Lavi E, Gonzalez-Scarano F: The effects of human immunodeficiency virus in the central nervous system. Adv Virus Res 1998; 50:1–47 [F]
25. Childs EA, Lyles RH, Selnes OA, Chen B, Miller EN, Cohen BA, Becker JT, Mellors J, McArthur JC: Plasma viral load and CD4 lymphocytes predict HIV-associated dementia and sensory neuropathy. Neurology 1999; 52:607–613 [C]
26. Inkina N, Price RW, Barbour J, Bandrapalli N, Novakovic-Agopian T, Staprans S, Grant RM: HIV-1 compartmentalization and discordant virologic failure in CSF and plasma (abstract 297). Sixth Conference on Retroviruses and Opportunistic Infections 1999; p 124 [G]
27. Haas DW, Spearman P, Johnson B, Harris VL, Donlon R, Wilkinson GR, Clough LA, Grosso RA, Stevens MR: Discordant HIV-1 RNA decay in CSF versus plasma following initiation of antiretroviral therapy: a prospective ultra-intensive CSF sampling study (abstract 405), in Abstracts From the 6th Conference on Retroviruses and Opportunistic Infections. Alexandria, VA, Foundation for Retrovirology and Human Health, 1999 [C]

28. McDaniel JS, Campos PE, Purcell DW, Farber EW, Bondurant A, Donahoe JE, Chang BM: A national, randomized survey of HIV/AIDS attitudes and knowledge among psychiatrists-in-training. Academic Psychiatry 1998; 22:107–116 [G]
29. White JL, Darko DF, Brown SJ, Miller JC, Hayduk R, Kelly T, Mitler MM: Early central nervous system response to HIV infection: sleep distortion and cognitive-motor decrements. AIDS 1995; 9:1043–1050 [C]
30. Wilkie FL, Eisdorfer C, Morgan R, Loewenstein DA, Szapocznik J: Cognition in early human immunodeficiency virus infection. Arch Neurol 1990; 47:433–440 [G]
31. Sewell DD, Jeste DV, McAdams LA, Bailey A, Harris MJ, Atkinson JH, Chandler JL, McCutchan JA, Grant I (HNRC Group): Neuroleptic treatment of HIV-associated psychosis. Neuropsychopharmacology 1994; 10:223–229 [B]
32. Mijch AM, Judd FK, Lyketsos CG, Ellen S, Cockram A: Secondary mania in patients with HIV infection: are antiretrovirals protective? J Neuropsychiatry Clin Neurosci 1999; 11: 475–480 [G]
33. Ellen SR, Judd FK, Mijch AM, Cockram A: Secondary mania in patients with HIV infection. Aust NZ J Psychiatry 1999; 33:353–360 [G]
34. Lyketsos CG, Schwartz J, Fishman M, Treisman G: AIDS mania. J Neuropsychiatry Clin Neurosci 1997; 9:277–279 [D]
35. Nomenclature and research case definitions for neurologic manifestations of human immunodeficiency virus-type 1 (HIV-1) infection: report of a working group of the American Academy of Neurology AIDS Task Force. Neurology 1991; 41:778–785 [F]
36. Masliah E, Ge N, Mucke L: Pathogenesis of HIV-1 associated neurodegeneration. Crit Rev Neurobiol 1996; 10:57–67 [F]
37. Mayeux R, Stern Y, Tang M-X, Todak G, Marder K, Sano M, Richards M, Stein Z, Ehrhardt AA, Gorman JM: Mortality risks in gay men with human immunodeficiency virus infection and cognitive impairment. Neurology 1993; 43:176–182 [C]
38. Ellis RJ, Deutsch R, Heaton RK, Marcotte TD, McCutchan JA, Nelson JA, Abramson I, Thal LJ, Atkinson JH, Wallace MR, Grant I (San Diego HIV Neurobehavioral Research Center Group): Neurocognitive impairment is an independent risk factor for death in HIV infection. Arch Neurol 1997; 54:416–424 [G]
39. Simpson DM: Human immunodeficiency virus-associated dementia: review pf pathogenesis, prophylaxis, and treatment studies of zidovudine therapy. Clin Infect Dis 1999; 29: 19–34 [F]
40. Sacktor NC, Lyles RH, Skolasky RL, Anderson DE, McArthur JC, McFarlane G, Selnes OA, Becker JT, Cohen B, Wesch J, Miller EN: Combination antiretroviral therapy improves psychomotor speed performance in HIV-seropositive homosexual men: Multicenter AIDS Cohort Study (MACS). Neurology 1999; 52:1640–1647 [B]
41. Dore GJ, Correll PK, Li Y, Kaldor JM, Cooper DA, Brew BJ: Changes to AIDS dementia complex in the era of highly active antiretroviral therapy. AIDS 1999; 13:1249–1253 [G]
42. Halstead S, Riccio M, Harlow P, Oretti R, Thompson C: Psychosis associated with HIV infection. Br J Psychiatry 1988; 153:618–623 [G]
43. Harris M, Jeste D, Gleghorn A, Sewell D: New-onset psychosis in HIV-infected patients. J Clin Psychiatry 1991; 52:369–376 [E]
44. Goodkin K: Psychiatric disorders in HIV-spectrum illness. Tex Med 1988; 84(9):55–61 [F]
45. Maj M: Organic mental disorders in HIV-1 infection. AIDS 1990; 4:831–840 [G]
46. Breitbart W, Marotta R, Platt M, Weisman H, Derevenco M, Grau C, Corbera K, Raymond S, Lund S, Jacobson P: A double-blind trial of haloperidol, chlorpromazine, and lorazepam in the treatment of delirium in hospitalized AIDS patients. Am J Psychiatry 1996; 153: 231–237 [A]
47. American Psychiatric Association: Practice Guideline for the Treatment of Patients With Delirium. Am J Psychiatry 1999; 156(May suppl):1–20 [G]

48. McKegney FP, Aronson MK, Oot WL: Identifying depression in the old old. Psychodynamics 1988; 29:175–181 [G]
49. Product monograph: Sustiva™ (efavirenz). Wilmington, DE, Dupont Pharmaceuticals, 1999 [F]
50. Bialer PA, Wallack JJ, McDaniel JS: Human immunodeficiency virus and AIDS, in Psychiatric Care of the Medical Patient. Edited by Stoudemire A, Fogel BS, Greenberg DB. New York, Oxford University Press, 2000, pp 871–888 [G]
51. McDaniel JS, Purcell DW, Farber EW: Severe mental illness and HIV-related medical and neuropsychiatric sequelae. Clin Psychol Rev 1997; 17:311–325 [G]
52. Grant I, Atkinson JH Jr: Neuropsychiatric aspects of HIV infection and AIDS, in Kaplan and Sadock's Comprehensive Textbook of Psychiatry. Edited by Sadock BJ, Sadock VA. Philadelphia, Lippincott Williams & Wilkins, 1999, pp 308–336 [G]
53. European Collaborative Study: Natural history of vertically acquired human immunodeficiency virus-1 infection. Pediatrics 1994; 94:815–819 [F]
54. Pavlakis SG, Frank Y, Nocyze M, Porricolo M, Prohovnik I, Wiznia A: Acquired immunodeficiency syndrome and the developing nervous system. Adv Pediatr 1994; 41:427–451 [F]
55. Mintz M: Neurological and developmental problems in pediatric HIV infection. J Nutr 1996; 126 (suppl 10):2663S–2673S [F]
56. Cooper ER, Hanson C, Diaz C, Mendez H, Abboud R, Nugent R, Pitt J, Rich K, Rodriguez EM, Smeriglio V (Women and Infants Transmission Study Group): Encephalopathy and progression of human immunodeficiency virus disease in a cohort of children with perinatally acquired human immunodeficiency virus infection. J Pediatr 1998; 132:808–812 [C]
57. Bachanas PJ, Kullgren KA, Morris MK, Jones JS: Influence of family factors and illness parameters on HIV-infected children's cognitive, academic and psychological functioning. NIMH Conference on the Role of Families in Adapting to and Preventing HIV/AIDS. Washington, DC, July, 1998 [D]
58. Wolters P, Brouwers P, Moss H, Pizzo P: Adaptive behavior of children with symptomatic HIV infection before and after zidovudine therapy. J Pediatr Psychol 1994; 19:47–61 [B]
59. Frank EG, Foley GM, Kuchuk A: Cognitive functioning in school-age children with human immunodeficiency virus. Percept Mot Skills 1997; 85:267–272 [G]
60. Atkinson JH Jr, Grant I, Kennedy CJ, Richman DD, Spector SA, McCutchan JA: Prevalence of psychiatric disorders among men infected with human immunodeficiency virus: a controlled study. Arch Gen Psychiatry 1988; 45:859–864 [D]
61. Brown GR, Rundell JR, McManis SE, Kendall SN, Zachary R, Temoshok L: Prevalence of psychiatric disorders in early stages of HIV infection. Psychosom Med 1992; 54:588–601 [D]
62. Williams JB, Rabkin JG, Remien RH, Gorman JM, Ehrhardt AA: Multidisciplinary baseline assessment of homosexual men with and without human immunodeficiency virus infection, II: standardized clinical assessment of current and lifetime psychopathology. Arch Gen Psychiatry 1991; 48:124–130 [D]
63. McDaniel JS, Fowlie E, Summerville MB, Farber EW, Cohen-Cole SA: An assessment of rates of psychiatric morbidity and functioning in HIV disease. Gen Hosp Psychiatry 1995; 17:346–352 [D]
64. Uldall KK, Koutsky LA, Bradshaw DH, Krone M: Use of hospital services by AIDS patients with psychiatric illness. Gen Hosp Psychiatry 1998; 20:292–301 [D]
65. Mayne TJ, Vittinghoff E, Chesney MA, Barrett DC, Coates TJ: Depressive affect and survival among gay and bisexual men infected with HIV. Arch Intern Med 1996; 156:2233–2238 [D]
66. Lyketsos CG, Hutton H, Fishman M, Schwartz J, Treisman GJ: Psychiatric morbidity on entry to an HIV primary care clinic. AIDS 1996; 10:1033–1039 [G]

67. Acuff C, Archambeault J, Greenberg B: Mental Health Care for People Living With or Affected by HIV/AIDS: A Practical Guide (SAMHSA Monograph). www.mentalhealth.org/cmhs/HIVAIDS/mhcarehiv.htm [G]
68. Rabkin JG, Johnson J, Lin SH, Lipsitz JD, Remien RH, Williams JB, Gorman JM: Psychopathology in male and female HIV-positive and negative injecting drug users: longitudinal course over 3 years. AIDS 1997; 11:507–515 [G]
69. Rabkin JG, Ferrando SJ, Jacobsberg LB, Fishman B: Prevalence of axis I disorders in an AIDS cohort: a cross-sectional, controlled study. Compr Psychiatry 1997; 38:146–154 [D]
70. Rosenberger PH, Bornstein RA, Nasrallah HA, Para MF, Whitaker CC, Fass RJ, Rice RR Jr: Psychopathology in human immunodeficiency virus infection: lifetime and current assessment. Compr Psychiatry 1993; 34:150–158 [D]
71. Perry S, Jacobsberg LB, Fishman B, Frances A, Bobo J, Jacobsberg BK: Psychiatric diagnosis before serological testing for the human immunodeficiency virus. Am J Psychiatry 1990; 147:89–93 [G]
72. Perkins DO, Stern RA, Golden RN, Murphy C, Naftolowitz D, Evans DL: Mood disorders in HIV infection: prevalence and risk factors in a nonepicenter of the AIDS epidemic. Am J Psychiatry 1994; 151:233–236 [D]
73. Lipsitz JD, Williams JB, Rabkin JG, Remien RH, Bradbury M, el Sadr W, Goetz R, Sorrell S, Gorman JM: Psychopathology in male and female intravenous drug users with and without HIV infection. Am J Psychiatry 1994; 151:1662–1668 [D]
74. McKinnon K, Cournos F, Sugden R, Guido JR, Herman R: The relative contributions of psychiatric symptoms and AIDS knowledge to HIV risk behaviors among people with severe mental illness. J Clin Psychiatry 1996; 57:506–513 [D]
75. Zierler S, Cunningham WE, Andersen R, Shapiro MF, Nakazono T, Morton S, Crystal S, Stein M, Turner B, St Clair P, Bozette SA: Violence victimization after HIV infection in a US probability sample of adult patients in primary care. Am J Public Health 2000; 90:208–215 [G]
76. Kassler WJ, Wu AW: Addressing HIV infection in office practice: assessing risk, counseling, and testing. Prim Care 1992; 19:19–33 [F]
77. APA Commission on AIDS: Guidelines for HIV Antibody Testing. Washington, DC, APA, 1998 [G]
78. American College of Obstetricians and Gynecologists: OB-GYNS Revise Screening Recommendations; Expand Testing for Diabetes, HIV and Hepatitis C Advised (press release). Washington, DC, ACOG, Nov 30, 1999 [G]
79. Purcell DW, DeGroff AS, Wolitski RJ: HIV prevention case management: current practice and future directions. Health Soc Work 1998; 23:282–289 [E]
80. Division of HIV/AIDS Prevention: Condoms and Their Use in Preventing HIV Infection and Other STDs. Atlanta, CDC National Center for HIV, STD and TB Prevention, 1999 [G]
81. Katz MH, Gerberding JL: Postexposure treatment of people exposed to the human immunodeficiency virus through sexual contact or injection-drug use. N Engl J Med 1997; 336:1097–1100 [G]
82. Centers for Disease Control and Prevention: Public health service guidelines for the management of health-care worker exposures to HIV and recommendations for postexposure prophylaxis. MMWR Morb Mortal Wkly Rep 1998; 47:1–39 [G]
83. Riley D, Sawka E, Conley P, Hewitt D, Mitic W, Poulin C, Room R, Single E, Topp J: Harm reduction: concepts and practice: a policy discussion paper. Subst Use Misuse 1999; 34:9–24 [F]
84. Ferrando SJ: Substance abuse and HIV. Psychiatric Annals (in press) [F]
85. APA Commission on AIDS: Position statement on needle exchange programs. Washington, DC, APA, 1996 [G]

86. Des Jarlais D, Friedman P, Hagan H, Friedman SR: The protective effect of AIDS-related behavioral change among injection drug users: a cross-national study. Am J Public Health 1996; 86:1780–1785 [C]
87. Cournos F, McKinnon K: HIV seroprevalence among people with severe mental illness in the United States: a critical review. Clin Psychol Rev 1997; 17:259–269 [F]
88. Cournos F, Guido JR, Coomaraswamy S, Meyer-Bahlburg H, Sugden R, Horwath E: Sexual activity and risk of HIV infection among patients with schizophrenia. Am J Psychiatry 1994; 151:228–232 [G]
89. Sullivan G, Koegel P, Kanouse DE, Cournos F, McKinnon K, Young AS, Bean D: HIV and people with serious mental illness: the public sector's role in reducing HIV risk and improving care. Psychiatr Serv 1999; 50:648–652 [F]
90. Brown EJ, Jemmott LS: HIV among people with mental illness: contributing factors, prevention needs, barriers, and strategies. J Psychosoc Nurs Ment Health Serv 2000; 38:14–19 [G]
91. Weinhardt LS, Carey MP, Carey KB, Verdecias RN: Increasing assertiveness skills to reduce HIV risk among women living with a severe and persistent mental illness. J Consult Clin Psychol 1998; 66:680–684 [A]
92. Kelly JA: HIV risk reduction interventions for persons with severe mental illness. Clin Psychol Rev 1997; 17:293–309 [F]
93. Bamberger JD, Waldo CR, Gerberding JL, Katz MH: Postexposure prophylaxis for human immunodeficiency virus (HIV) infection following sexual assault. Am J Med 1999; 106: 323–326 [F]
94. APA Commission on AIDS: Position statement on confidentiality, disclosure, and protection of others. Am J Psychiatry 1993; 150:852 [G]
95. Paterson DL, Swindells S, Mohr J, Brester M, Vergis EN, Squier C, Wagener MM, Singh N: Adherence to protease inhibitor therapy and outcomes in patients with HIV infection. Ann Intern Med 2000; 133:21–30 [C]
96. Singh N, Squier C, Sivek C, Wagener M, Nguyen MH, Yu VL: Determinants of compliance with antiretroviral therapy in patients with human immunodeficiency virus: prospective assessment with implications for enhancing compliance. AIDS Care 1996; 8:261–269 [C]
97. Perry S, Jacobsberg L, Card CA, Ashman T, Frances A, Fishman B: Severity of psychiatric symptoms after HIV testing. Am J Psychiatry 1993;150:775–779 [C]
98. Somlai AM, Heckman TG, Kelly JA, Mulry GW, Multhauf KE: The response of religious congregations to the spiritual needs of people living with HIV/AIDS. J Pastoral Care 1997; 51:415–426 [G]
99. Stoll R: Guidelines for spiritual assessment. Am J Nursing 1979; 79:1574–1577 [G]
100. Mouton C, Teno JM, Mor V, Piette J: Communication of preferences for care among human immunodeficiency virus-infected patients: barriers to informed decisions? Arch Fam Med 1997; 6:342–347 [G]
101. Folstein MF, Folstein SE, McHugh PR: "Mini-Mental State": a practical method for grading the cognitive state of patients for the clinician. J Psychiatr Res 1975; 12:189–198 [G]
102. Jones BN, Teng EL, Folstein MF, Harrison KS: A new bedside test of cognition for patients with HIV infection. Ann Intern Med 1993; 119:1001–1004 [C]
103. Power C, Selnes OA, Grim JA, McArthur JC: HIV Dementia Scale: a rapid screening test. Acquir Immune Defic Syndr Hum Retrovirol 1995; 8:273–278 [G]
104. Royall DR, Mahurin RK, Gray KF: Bedside assessment of executive cognitive impairment: the Executive Interview. J Am Geriatr Soc 1992; 40:1221–1226 [G]
105. Berghuis JP, Uldall KK, Lalonde B: Validity of two scales in identifying HIV-associated dementia. J Acquir Immune Defic Syndr 1999; 12:134–140 [G]
106. van Gorp WG, Satz P, Hinkin C, Selnes O, Miller EN, McArthur J, Cohen B, Paz D: Metacognition in HIV-1 seropositive asymptomatic individuals: self-ratings versus objective neuropsychological performance. J Clin Exp Neuropsychol 1991; 13:812–819 [C]

107. Uldall KK, Harris VL, Lalonde B: Outcomes associated with delirium in acutely hospitalized acquired immune deficiency syndrome patients. Compr Psychiatry 2000; 41:88–91 [C]
108. Uldall KK, Ryan R, Berghuis JP, Harris VL: Association between delirium and death in AIDS patients. AIDS Patient Care STDS 2000; 14:95–100 [G]
109. Perkins DO, Leserman J, Stern RA, Baum SF, Liao D, Golden RN, Evans DL: Somatic symptoms and HIV infection: relationship to depressive symptoms and indicators of HIV disease. Am J Psychiatry 1995; 152:1776–1781 [C]
110. Brouillette MJ, Chouinard G, Lalonde R: Didanosine-induced mania in HIV infection (letter). Am J Psychiatry 1994; 151:1839–1840 [G]
111. Maxwell S, Scheftner WA, Kessler HA, Busch K: Manic syndrome associated with zidovudine treatment (letter). JAMA 1988; 259:3406–3407 [G]
112. Hoffman JA, Klein H, Clark DC, Boyd FT: The effect of entering drug treatment on involvement in HIV-related risk behaviors. Am J Drug Alcohol Abuse 1998; 24:259–284 [C]
113. American Psychiatric Association: Practice Guideline for Treatment of Patients With Substance Use Disorders: Alcohol, Cocaine, Opioids. Am J Psychiatry 1995; 152(Nov suppl):1–59 [G]
114. Pao M, Lyon M, D'Angelo LD, Schuman WB, Tipnis T, Mrazek DA: Psychiatric risk factors in HIV seropositive adolescents. Presented at the 1998 Annual Meeting of the American Academy of Child and Adolescent Psychiatry. Washington, DC, AACAP, 1998 [D]
115. Havens JF, Whitaker AH, Feldman JF, Ehrhardt AA: Psychiatric morbidity in school-age children with congenital human immunodeficiency virus infection: a pilot study. J Dev Behav Pediatr 1994; 15:S18–S25 [G]
116. Ramafedi G: The University of Minnesota Youth and AIDS Projects' Adolescent Early Intervention Program: a model to link HIV-seropositive youth with care. J Adolesc Health 1998; 23(2 suppl):115–121 [G]
117. Mattsson A: Long-term physical illness in childhood: a challenge to psychosocial adaptation. Pediatrics 1972; 50:801–811 [F]
118. Garrad SD, Richmond JB: Psychological aspects of the management of chronic diseases and handicapping conditions in childhood, in The Psychological Basis of Medical Practice. Edited by Lief HI, Lief VF, Lief NR. New York, Harper and Row, 1963, pp 370–403 [G]
119. Kotler D, Tierney AR, Wang J, Pierson RN: Magnitude of body cell mass depletion and the timing of death from wasting in AIDS. Am J Clin Nutr 1989; 50:44–47 [C]
120. Breitbart W, McDonald MV, Rosenfeld B, Monkman ND, Passik S: Fatigue in ambulatory AIDS patients. J Pain Symptom Manage 1998; 15:159–167 [C]
121. Ferrando S, Evans S, Goggin K, Sewell M, Fishman B, Rabkin J: Fatigue in HIV illness: relationship to depression, physical limitations, and disability. Psychosom Med 1998; 60: 759–764 [C]
122. Groopman JE: Fatigue in cancer and HIV/AIDS. Oncology (Huntingt) 1998; 12:335–344 [G]
123. Breitbart W, McDonald MV, Rosenfeld B, Passik SD, Hewitt D, Thaler H, Portenoy RK: Pain in ambulatory AIDS patients, 1: pain characteristics and medical correlates. Pain 1996; 68:315–321 [A]
124. Laschinger SJ, Fothergill-Bourbonnais F: The experience of pain in persons with HIV/ AIDS. J Assoc Nurses AIDS Care 1999; 10:59–67 [G]
125. Singer EJ, Zorilla C, Fahy-Chandon B, Chi S, Syndulko K, Tourtellotte WW: Painful symptoms reported by ambulatory HIV-infected men in a longitudinal study. Pain 1993; 54:15–19 [C]
126. Rabkin JG, Wagner GJ, Rabkin R: Testosterone therapy for human immunodeficiency virus–positive men with and without hypogonadism. J Clin Psychopharmacol 1999; 19: 19–27 [A]

127. Centers for Disease Control and Prevention: HIV/AIDS Surveillance Report 1998; 10(2): 1–43 [G]
128. HIV/AIDS among racial/ethnic minority men who have sex with men—United States. MMWR Morb Mortal Wkly Rep 2000; 1:4–11 [G]
129. Gonzales V, Washienko KM, Krone MR, Chapman LI, Arredondo EM, Huckeba HJ, Downer A: Sexual and drug-use risk factors for HIV and STDs: a comparison of women with and without bisexual experiences. Am J Public Health 1999; 89:1841–1846 [A]
130. CDC Division of HIV/AIDS Prevention: HIV/AIDS and US women who have sex with women (fact sheet). Atlanta, CDC National Center for HIV, STD and TB Prevention, 1999 [G]
131. Carey MP: HIV and AIDS relative to other health, social, and relationship concerns among low-income urban women: a brief report. J Womens Health Gend Based Med 1999; 8: 657–661 [C]
132. Padian NS, Shiboski SC, Glass SO, Vittinghoff E: Heterosexual transmission of human immunodeficiency virus (HIV) in northern California: results from a ten-year study. Am J Epidemiol 1997;146:350–357 [C]
133. Farzadegan H, Hoover DR, Astemborski J, Lyles CM, Margolick JB, Markham RB, Quinn TC, Vlahov D: Sex differences in HIV-1 viral load and progression to AIDS. Lancet 1998; 352:1510–1514 [C]
134. Chung J, Magraw M: A group approach to psychosocial issues faced by HIV-positive women. Hosp Community Psychiatry 1992; 43:891–894 [G]
135. Gray JJ: The difficulties of women living with HIV infection. J Psychosoc Nurs Ment Health Serv 1999; 37:39–43 [G]
136. Thomas P: Americas: AIDS on the Rise Among Over-50s. BBC News Online, June 11, 1999. http://news6.thdo.bbc.co.uk/hi/english/world/americas/newsid_366000/366702.stm [G]
137. Kasper SJ, Cavalieri TA: HIV-related medical issues in older people. Focus: A Guide to AIDS Research and Counseling 1999; 14:5–6 [G]
138. Stall R, Catania J: AIDS risk behaviors among late middle-aged and elderly Americans: the National AIDS Behavior Surveys. Arch Intern Med 1994; 154:57–63 [G]
139. Acuff C, Archambeault J, Greenberg B: Mental Health Care for People Living With or Affected by HIV/AIDS: A Practical Guide (SAMHSA Monograph). www.mentalhealth.org/cmhs/HIVAIDS/mhcarehiv.htm [G]
140. CDC Division of HIV/AIDS Prevention: National data on HIV prevalence among disadvantaged youth in the 1990s (fact sheet). Atlanta, CDC National Center for HIV, STD and TB Prevention, 1998 [G]
141. Anderson JE, Wilson RW, Barker P, Doll L, Jones TS, Holtgrave D: Prevalence of sexual and drug-related HIV risk behaviors in the US adult population: results of the 1996 National Household Survey on Drug Abuse. J Acquir Immune Defic Syndr Hum Retrovirol 1999: 21:148–156 [C]
142. Crosby RA, Yarber WL, Meyerson B. Prevention strategies other than male condoms employed by low-income women to prevent HIV infection. Public Health Nursing 2000; 17:53–60 [D]
143. Heckman TG, Somlai AM, Sikkema KJ, Kelly JA, Franzoi SL: Psychosocial predictors of life satisfaction among persons living with HIV infection and AIDS. J Assoc Nurses AIDS Care 1997; 8:21–30 [C]
144. Beckett A, Shenson D: Suicide risk in patients with human immune deficiency virus infection and acquired immune deficiency syndrome. Harv Rev Psychiatry 1993; 1:27–35 [F]
145. Marzuk P, Tierney H, Tardiff K, Gross E, Morgan E, Hsu M, Mann J: Increased risk of suicide in persons with AIDS. JAMA 1988; 259:1333–1337 [D]

146. Kizer KW, Green M, Perkins CI, Doebbert G, Hughes MJ: AIDS and suicide in California (letter). JAMA 1998; 260:1881 [D]
147. Cote T, Biggar R, Dannenberg A: Risk of suicide among persons with AIDS: a national assessment. JAMA 1992; 268:2066–2068 [D]
148. Marzuk PM, Tardiff K, Leon AC, Hirsch CS, Hartwell N, Potera L, Iqbal MI: HIV seroprevalence among suicide victims in New York City, 1991–1993. Am J Psychiatry 1997; 154:1720–1725 [D]
149. McDaniel JS, Purcell DW, D'Augelli AR: The relationship between sexual orientation and risk for suicide: research findings and future directions for research and prevention. Suicide Life Threat Behav 2001; 31(suppl):84–105 [F]
150. Dannenberg AI, McNeil JG, Brundage JF, Brookmeyer R: Suicide and HIV infection: mortality follow-up of 4,147 HIV-seropositive military service applicants. JAMA 1996; 276:1743–1746 [C]
151. van Haastrecht HJ, Mientjes GH, van den Hoek AJ, Coutinho RA: Death from suicide and overdose among drug injectors after disclosure of first HIV test result. AIDS 1994; 8: 1721–1725 [C]
152. Westermeyer J, Seppala M, Gasow S, Carlson G: AIDS-related illness and AIDS risk in male homo/bisexual substance abusers: case reports and clinical issues. Am J Drug Alcohol Abuse 1989; 15:443–461 [G]
153. Lester D: Sexual versus psychiatric predictors of suicide in men with AIDS-related illnesses. Am J Drug Alcohol Abuse 1992; 19:139–140 [D]
154. Kelly B, Raphael B, Judd F, Perdices M, Kernutt G, Burnett P, Dunne M, Burrows G: Suicidal ideation, suicide attempts, and HIV infection. Psychosomatics 1998; 39:405–415 [D]
155. Goldblum P, Moulton J: HIV disease and suicide, in Face to Face: A Guide to AIDS Counseling. Edited by Dilley JW, Pies C, Helquist M. Berkeley, Calif, Celestial Arts, 1989, pp 152–164 [G]
156. Houston-Vega M, Ward J: Suicide assessment and intervention with persons infected with HIV, in HIV and Community Mental Healthcare. Edited by Knox M, Sparks C. Baltimore, Johns Hopkins University Press, 1998, pp 178–194 [G]
157. Mayne TJ, Acree M, Chesney MA, Folkman S: HIV sexual risk behavior following bereavement in gay men. Health Psychol 1998; 17:403–411 [C]
158. Rosengard C, Folkman S: Suicidal ideation, bereavement, HIV serostatus and psychosocial variables in partners of men with AIDS. AIDS Care 1997; 9:373–384 [C]
159. Martin JL, Dean L: Effects of AIDS-related bereavement and HIV-related illness on psychological distress among gay men: a 7-year longitudinal study, 1985–1991. J Consult Clin Psychol 1993; 61:94–103 [C]
160. Sherr L, Hedge B, Steinhart K, Davey T, Petrack J: Unique patterns of bereavement in HIV: implications for counselling. Genitourin Med 1992; 68:378–381 [G]
161. Rotheram-Borus MJ, Draimin BH, Reid HM, Murphy DA: The impact of illness disclosure and custody plans on adolescents whose parents live with AIDS. AIDS 1997; 11:1159–1164 [G]
162. Rotheram-Borus MJ, Stein JA: Problem behavior of adolescents whose parents are living with AIDS. Am J Orthopsychiatry 1999; 69:228–239 [G]
163. Neugebauer R, Rabkin JG, Williams JB, Remien RH, Goetz R, Gorman JM: Bereavement reactions among homosexual men experiencing multiple losses in the AIDS epidemic. Am J Psychiatry 1992; 149:1374–1379 [D]
164. Goodkin K, Blaney N, Tuttle R, Nelson R, Baidewicz T, Kumar M, Fletcher M, Leeds B, Feaster D: Bereavement and HIV infection. Int Rev Psychiatry 1996; 8:201–216 [F]
165. Kemeny ME, Weiner H, Taylor SE, Schneider S, Visscher B, Fahey JL: Repeated bereavement, depressed mood, and immune parameters in HIV seropositive and seronegative gay men. Health Psychol 1994; 13:14–24 [D]

166. Bartrop RW, Luckhurst E, Lazarus L, Kiloh LG, Penny R: Depressed lymphocyte function after bereavement. Lancet 1977; 8016:834–836 [C]
167. Irwin M, Daniels M, Smith TL, Bloom E, Weiner H: Impaired natural killer cell activity during bereavement. Brain Behav Immun 1987; 1:98–104 [D]
168. Goodkin K, Feaster DJ, Tuttle R, Blaney NT, Kumar M, Baum MK, Shapshak P, Fletcher MA: Bereavement is associated with time-dependent decrements in cellular immune function in asymptomatic human immunodeficiency virus type 1-seropositive homosexual men. Clin Diagn Lab Immunol 1996; 3:109–118 [C]
169. Sikkema KJ, Kalichman SC, Kelly JA, Koob JJ: Group intervention to improve coping with AIDS-related bereavement: model development and an illustrative clinical example. AIDS Care 1995; 7:463–475 [G]
170. Goodkin K, Blaney NT, Feaster DJ, Baldewicz T, Burkhalter JE, Leeds B: A randomized controlled clinical trial of a bereavement support group intervention in human immunodeficiency virus type 1-seropositive and -seronegative homosexual men. Arch Gen Psychiatry 1999; 56:52–59 [A]
171. Golding M, Perkins DO: Personality disorder in HIV infection. Int Rev Psychiatry 1996; 8:253 [F]
172. Jacobsberg L, Frances A, Perry S: Axis II diagnoses among volunteers for HIV testing and counseling. Am J Psychiatry 1995; 152:1222–1224 [G]
173. Treisman GJ, Lyketsos CG, Fishman M, Hanson AL, Rosenblatt A, McHugh PR: Psychiatric care for patients with HIV infection: the varying perspectives. Psychosomatics 1993; 34:432–439 [F]
174. Perkins DO, Davidson EJ, Leserman J, Liao D, Evans DL: Personality disorder in patients infected with HIV: a controlled study with implications for clinical care. Am J Psychiatry 1993; 150:309–315 [C]
175. Johnson JG, Williams JB, Rabkin JG, Goetz RR, Remien RH: Axis I psychiatric symptoms associated with HIV infection and personality disorder. Am J Psychiatry 1995; 152:551–554 [C]
176. Brooner RK, Bigelow GE, Strain E, Schmidt CW: Intravenous drug abusers with antisocial personality disorder: increased HIV risk behavior. Drug Alcohol Depend 1990; 26:39–44 [G]
177. Johnson JG, Williams JB, Goetz RR, Rabkin JG, Remien RH, Lipsitz JD, Gorman JM: Personality disorders predict onset of axis I disorders and impaired functioning among homosexual men with and at risk of HIV infection. Arch Gen Psychiatry 1996; 53:350–357 [C]
178. Goodkin K, Fuchs I, Feaster D, Leeka J, Rishel DD: Life stressors and coping style are associated with immune measures in HIV-1 infection—a preliminary report. Int J Psychiatry Med 1992; 22:155–172 [G]
179. Goodkin K, Mulder CL, Blaney NT, Ironson G, Kumar M, Fletcher MA: Psychoneuroimmunology and human immunodeficiency virus type 1 infection revisited. Arch Gen Psychiatry 1994; 51:246–248 [G]
180. Kemeny ME, Weiner H, Duran R, Taylor SE, Visscher B, Fahey JL: Immune system changes after the death of a partner in HIV-positive gay men. Psychosom Med 1995; 57:547–554 [D]
181. Evans DL, Leserman J, Perkins DO, Stern RA, Murphy C, Tamul K, Liao D, van der Horst CM, Hall CD, Folds JD: Stress-associated reductions of cytotoxic T lymphocytes and natural killer cells in asymptomatic HIV infection. Am J Psychiatry 1995; 152:543–550 [C]
182. Leserman J, Petitto JM, Perkins DO, Folds JD, Golden RN, Evans DL: Severe stress, depressive symptoms, and changes in lymphocyte subsets in human immunodeficiency virus-infected men. A 2-year follow-up study. Arch Gen Psychiatry 1997; 54:279–285 [C]
183. Leserman J, Jackson ED, Petitto JM, Golden RN, Silva SG, Perkins DO, Cai J, Folds JD, Evans DL: Progression to AIDS: the effects of stress, depressive symptoms, and social support. Psychosom Med 1999; 61:397–406 [C]

184. Rabkin JG, Williams JB, Remien RH, Goetz R, Kertzner R, Gorman JM: Depression, distress, lymphocyte subsets, and human immunodeficiency virus symptoms on two occasions in HIV-positive homosexual men. Arch Gen Psychiatry 1991; 48:111–119 [C]
185. Perry S, Fishman B, Jacobsberg L: Stress and HIV infection. Am J Psychiatry 1992; 149: 416–417 [G]
186. Burack JH, Barrett DC, Stall RD, Chesney MA, Ekstrand ML, Coates TJ: Depressive symptoms and CD4 lymphocyte decline among HIV-infected men. JAMA 1993; 270: 2568–2573 [C]
187. Lyketsos CG, Hoover DR, Guccione M, Senterfitt W, Dew MA, Wesch J, VanRaden MJ, Treisman GJ, Morgenstern H: Depressive symptoms as predictors of medical outcomes in HIV infection: Multicenter AIDS Cohort Study. JAMA 1993; 270:2563–2567 [C]
188. Antoni MH, Baggett L, Ironson G, LaPerriere A, August S, Klimas N, Schneiderman N, Fletcher MA: Cognitive-behavioral stress management intervention buffers distress responses and immunologic changes following notification of HIV-1 seropositivity. J Consult Clin Psychol 1991; 59:906–915 [C]
189. Goodkin K, Feaster DJ, Asthana D, Blaney NT, Kumar M, Baldewicz T, Tuttle RS, Maher KJ, Baum MK, Shapshak P, Fletcher MA: A bereavement support group intervention is longitudinally associated with salutary effects on the CD4 cell count and number of physician visits. Clin Diagn Lab Immunol 1998; 5:382–391 [A]
190. Rabkin JG, Rabkin R, Harrison W, Wagner G: Effect of imipramine on mood and enumerative measures of immune status in depressed patients with HIV illness. Am J Psychiatry 1994; 151:516–523 [A]
191. Eisenberg DM, Kessler RC, Foster C, Norlock FE, Calkins DR, Delbanco TL: Unconventional medicine in the United States: prevalence, costs, and patterns of use. N Engl J Med 1993; 328:246–252 [G]
192. Eisenberg DM, Davis RB, Ettner SL, Appel S, Wilkey S, Van Rompay M, Kessler RC: Trends in alternative medicine use in the United States, 1990–1997: results of a follow-up national survey. JAMA 1998; 280:1569–1575 [G]
193. Fairfield KM, Eisenberg DM, Davis RB, Libman H, Phillips RS: Patterns of use, expenditures, and perceived efficacy of complementary and alternative therapies in HIV-infected patients. Arch Intern Med 1998; 158:2257–2264 [D]
194. Ostrow MJ, Cornelisse PG, Heath KV, Craib KJ, Schechter MT, O'Shaughnessy M, Montaner JS, Hogg RS: Determinants of complementary therapy use in HIV-infected individuals receiving antiretroviral or anti-opportunistic agents. J Acquir Immune Defic Syndr Hum Retrovirol 1997; 15:115–120 [G]
195. Singh N, Squier C, Sivek C, Nguyen M, Wagener M, Yu VL: Determinants of nontraditional therapy use in patients with HIV infection: a prospective study. Arch Intern Med 1996; 156:197–201 [C]
196. Anderson W, O'Connor B, MacGregor R, Schwartz J: Patient use and assessment of conventional and alternative therapies for HIV infection and AIDS. AIDS 1993; 7:561–565 [F]
197. Calabrese C, Wenner C, Reeves C, Turet P, Standish L: Treatment of human immunodeficiency virus-positive patients with complementary and alternative medicine: a survey of practitioners. J Altern Complement Med 1998; 4:281–287 [G]
198. Macintyre R, Holzemer W: Complementary and alternative medicine and HIV/AIDS, part II: selected literature review. J Assoc Nurses AIDS Care 1997; 8:25–38 [F]
199. Greene KB, Berger J, Reeves C, Moffat A, Standish LJ, Calabrese C: Most frequently used alternative and complementary therapies and activities by participants in the AMCOA Study. J Assoc Nurses AIDS Care 1999; 10:60–73 [E]
200. Standish L, Calabrese C, Reeves C, Polissar N, Bain S, O'Donnell T: A scientific plan for the evaluation of alternative medicine in the treatment of HIV/AIDS. Altern Ther Health Med 1997; 3:58–67 [G]

201. Pincus SH, Schoenbaum EE, Webber M: A seroprevalence survey for human immunodeficiency virus antibody in mentally retarded adults. NY State J Med 1990; 90:139–142 [G]
202. Lohiya GS: Human immunodeficiency virus type-1 antibody in 6,703 institutionalized mentally retarded clients: an unlinked serosurvey at seven California developmental centers. AIDS Res Hum Retroviruses 1993; 9:247–249 [G]
203. Altice FL, Mostashari F, Selwyn PA, Checko PJ, Singh R, Tanguay S, Blanchette EA: Predictors of HIV infection among newly sentenced male prisoners. J Acquir Immune Defic Syndr Hum Retrovirol 1998; 18:444–453 [C]
204. Behrendt C, Kendig N, Dambita C, Horman J, Lawlor J, Vlahov D: Voluntary testing for human immunodeficiency virus (HIV) in a prison population with a high prevalence of HIV. Am J Epidemiol 1994; 139:918–926 [E]
205. Smith PF, Mikl J, Truman BI, Lessner L, Lehman JS, Stevens RW, Lord EA, Broaddus RK, Morse DL: HIV infection among women entering the New York State correctional system. Am J Public Health Suppl 1991; 81:35–40 [G]
206. Grinstead OA, Zack B, Faigeles B: Collaborative research to prevent HIV among male prison inmates and their female partners. Health Educ Behav 1999; 26:225–238 [G]
207. Silverman DC: Psychosocial impact of HIV-related caregiving on health providers: a review and recommendations for the role of psychiatry. Am J Psychiatry 1993; 150:705–712 [F]
208. McDaniel JS, Farber EW, Summerville MB: Mental health care providers working with HIV: avoiding stress and burnout, in Textbook of Homosexuality and Mental Health. Edited by Cabaj RP, Stein TS. Washington, DC, American Psychiatric Press, 1996, pp 839–858 [G]
209. Catalan J, Burgess A, Pergami A, Hulme N, Gazzard B, Phillips R: The psychological impact on staff of caring for people with serious diseases—the case of HIV infection and oncology. J Psychosom Res 1996; 40:425–435 [D]
210. Barbour RS: The impact of working with people with HIV/AIDS: a review of the literature. Soc Sci Med 1994; 39:221–232 [F]
211. Frost JC: Support groups for medical caregivers of people with HIV diseases. Group 1994; 18:141–153 [G]
212. Wainberg ML: 52nd American Group Psychotherapy Association Annual Meeting, Atlanta 1995 [G]
213. Aruffo JE, Thompson R, McDaniel JS, Sacco J, Herman R, Kaplan M, Andriote J, Washington R, Eversole T: Training programs for staff, in AIDS and People With Severe Mental Illness: A Handbook for Mental Health Professionals. Edited by Cournos F, Bakalar N. New Haven, Conn, Yale University Press, 1996, pp 201–224 [G]
214. Brown LK, Stermock AC, Ford HH, Geary M: Emotional reactions of haemophilia health care providers. Haemophilia 1999; 5:127–131 [G]
215. Chung JY, Suarez AP, Zarin DA, Pincus HA: Psychiatric patients and HIV. Psychiatr Serv 1999; 50:487 [G]
216. Epstein RM, Morse DS, Frankel RM, Frarey L, Anderson K, Beckman HB: Awkward moments in patient-physician communication about HIV risk. Ann Intern Med 1998; 128: 435–442 [C]
217. Bindman AB, Osmond D, Hecht FM, Lehman JS, Vranizan K, Keane D, Reingold A (Multistate Evaluation of Surveillance of HIV [MESH] Study Group): Multistate evaluation of anonymous HIV testing and access to medical care. JAMA 1998; 16:1416–1420 [D]
218. Nakashima AK, Horsley R, Frey RL, Sweeney PA, Weber JT, Fleming PL: Effect of HIV reporting by name on use of HIV testing in publicly funded counseling and testing programs. JAMA 1998; 16:1421–1426 [G]
219. Osmond DH, Bindman AB, Vranizan K, Lehman JS, Hecht FM, Keane D, Reingold A (Multistate Evaluation of Surveillance for HIV Study Group): Name-based surveillance and public health interventions for persons with HIV infection. Ann Intern Med 1999; 131: 775–779 [G]

220. Branson BM: Home sample collection tests for HIV infection. JAMA 1998; 280:1699–1701 [G]
221. Coates TJ: Strategies for modifying sexual behavior for primary and secondary prevention of HIV disease. J Consult Clin Psychol 1990; 58:57–69 [F]
222. Guenther-Grey C, Noroian D, Fonseka J, Higgins D: Developing community networks to deliver HIV prevention interventions. Public Health Rep 1996; 111(suppl 1):41–49 [G]
223. Cabaj RP, Purcell DW (eds): On the Road to Same-Sex Marriage: A Supportive Guide to Psychological, Political, and Legal Issues. San Francisco, Jossey-Bass, 1998 [G]
224. Joint United Nations Programme on HIV/AIDS: Sexual Behavioural Change for HIV: Where Have Theories Taken Us? Geneva, UNAIDS, 1999 [F]
225. HIV/AIDS Prevention Research Synthesis Project: Compendium of HIV Prevention Interventions With Evidence of Effectiveness. Atlanta, CDC, 1999 [G]
226. Higgins DL, Galavotti C, O'Reilly KR, Schnell DJ, Moore M, Rugg DL, Johnson R: Evidence for the effects of HIV antibody counseling and testing on risk behaviors. JAMA 1991; 266:2419–2429 [F]
227. Wolitski RJ, MacGowan RJ, Higgins DL, Jorgensen CM: The effects of HIV counseling and testing on risk-related practices and help-seeking behavior. AIDS Educ Prev 1997; 9(3 suppl):52–67 [F]
228. Weinhardt LS, Carey MP, Johnson BT, Bickham NL: Effects of HIV counseling and testing on sexual risk behavior: a meta-analytic review of published research, 1985–1997. Am J Public Health 1999; 89:1397–1405 [E]
229. Prochaska JO, DiClemente CC: Stages of change in the modification of problem behaviors. Prog Behav Modif 1992; 28:183–218 [F]
230. Azjen I, Fishbeign M: Understanding Attitudes and Predicting Behavior. Englewood Cliffs, NJ, Prentice Hall, 1980 [G]
231. Fisher JD, Fisher WA: Changing AIDS-risk behavior. Psychol Bull 1992; 111:455–474 [G]
232. Kalichman SC, Hospers HJ: Efficacy of behavioral-skills enhancement HIV risk-reduction interventions in community settings. AIDS 1997; 11(suppl A):S191–S199 [F]
233. National Institute of Mental Health (NIMH) Multisite HIV Prevention Trial Group: The NIMH Multisite HIV Prevention Trial: reducing HIV sexual risk behavior. Science 1998; 280:1889–1894 [A]
234. Kamb ML, Fishbein M, Douglas JM Jr, Rhodes F, Rogers J, Bolan G, Zenilman J, Hoxworth T, Malotte CK, Iatesta M, Kent C, Lentz A, Graziano S, Byers RH, Peterman TA (Project RESPECT Study Group): Efficacy of risk-reduction counseling to prevent human immunodeficiency virus and sexually transmitted diseases: a randomized controlled trial. JAMA 1998; 280:1161–1167 [A]
235. Kelly JA, McAuliffe TL, Sikkema KJ, Murphy DA, Somlai AM, Mulry G, Miller JG, Stevenson LY, Fernandez MI: Reduction in risk behavior among adults with severe mental illness who learned to advocate for HIV prevention. Psychiatr Serv 1997; 48:1283–1288 [A]
236. Zule WA, Desmond DP: An ethnographic comparison of HIV risk behaviors among heroin and methamphetamine injectors. Am J Drug Alcohol Abuse 1999; 25:1–23 [D]
237. Des Jarlais D, Friedman SR: HIV epidemiology and interventions among injecting drug users. Int J STD AIDS 1996; 7(suppl 2):57–61 [F]
238. Coyle SL, Needle RH, Normand J: Outreach-based HIV prevention for injecting drug users: a review of published outcome data. Public Health Rep 1998; 113(suppl 1):19–30 [F]
239. Strathdee SA, Celentano DD, Shah N, Lyles C, Stambolis VA, Macalino G, Nelson K, Vlahov D: Needle-exchange attendance and health care utilization promote entry into detoxification. J Urban Health 1999; 76:448–460 [C]
240. Viahov D, Junge B: The role of needle exchange programs in HIV prevention. Public Health Rep 1998; 113(suppl 1):75–80 [F]

241. Hurley SF, Jolley DJ, Kaldor JM: Effectiveness of needle-exchange programmes for prevention of HIV infection. Lancet 1997; 349:1797–1800 [E]
242. CDC Division of HIV/AIDS Prevention: Status of Perinatal HIV Prevention: U.S. Declines Continue (fact sheet). Atlanta, CDC National Center for HIV, STD and TB Prevention, 1999 [G]
243. Lindegren ML, Byers RH Jr, Thomas P, Davis SF, Caldwell B, Rogers M, Gwinn M, Ward JW, Fleming PL: Trends in perinatal transmission of HIV/AIDS in the United States. JAMA 1999; 282:531–538 [G]
244. Riley LE, Greene MF: Elective cesarean delivery to reduce the transmission of HIV. N Engl J Med 1999; 340:1032–1033 [G]
245. Centers for Disease Control and Prevention: AIDS among children—United States, 1996. MMWR Morb Mortal Wkly Rep 1996; 45:1005–1010 [G]
246. Brady M, McGrath N, Brouwers P, Gelber R, Fowler M, Yogev R, Hutton N, Bryson YJ, Mitchell CD, Fikrig S, Borkowsky W, Jimenez E, McSherry G, Rubinstein A, Wilfert CM, McIntosh K, Elkins MM, Weintrub PS (Pediatric AIDS Clinical Trials Group 128): Randomized study of the tolerance and efficacy of high- versus low-dose zidovudine in human immunodeficiency virus–infected children with mild to moderate symptoms. J Infect Dis 1996; 173:1097–1106 [B]
247. Mofenson LM, Lambert JS, Stiehm ER, Bethel J, Meyer WA III, Whitehouse J, Moye J, Jr, Reichelderfer P, Harris DR, Fowler MG, Mathieson BJ, Nemo GJ (Pediatric AIDS Clinical Trials Group Study 185 Team): Risk factors for perinatal transmission of human immunodeficiency virus type 1 in women treated with zidovudine. N Engl J Med 1999; 341:385–393 [A]
248. Garcia PM, Kalish LA, Pitt J, Minkoff H, Quinn TC, Burchett SK, Kornegay J, Jackson B, Moye J, Hanson C, Zorrilla C, Lew JF (Women and Infants Transmission Study Group): Maternal levels of plasma human immunodeficiency virus type I RNA and the risk of perinatal transmission. N Engl J Med 1999; 341:394–402 [G]
249. Sandberg JA, Slikker W Jr: Developmental pharmacology and toxicology of anti-HIV therapeutic agents: dideonucleosides. FASEB J 1995; 9:1157–1163 [G]
250. Centers for Disease Control and Prevention: Administration of zidovudine during late pregnancy and delivery to prevent perinatal HIV transmission—Thailand, 1996–1998. MMWR Morb Mortal Wkly Rep 1998; 47:151–154 [G]
251. Leroy V, Dabis F: Reduction of mother-child transmission of HIV infection in Africa: from clinical research to public health programs. Med Trop (Mars) 1999; 59:456–464 [F]
252. Public Health Service Task Force recommendations for the use of antiretroviral drugs in pregnant women infected with HIV-1 for maternal health and for reducing perinatal HIV-1 transmission in the United States. MMWR Morb Mortal Wkly Rep 1998; 47(RR-2):1–30; corrections, 47(14):287, 47(15):315 [G]
253. Lorenzi P, Spicher VM, Laubereau B, Hirschel B, Kind C, Rudin C, Irion O, Kaiser L: Antiretroviral therapies in pregnancy: maternal, fetal and neonatal effects: Swiss HIV Cohort Study, the Swiss Collaborative HIV and Pregnancy Study, and the Swiss Neonatal HIV Study. AIDS 1998; 12:F241–F247 [C]
254. Bell DM: Occupational risk of human immunodeficiency virus infection in healthcare workers: an overview. Am J Med 1997; 102(suppl 5B):9–15 [F]
255. Cardo DM, Culver DH, Ciesielski CA, Srivastava PU, Marcus R, Abiteboul D, Heptonstall J, Ippolito G, Lot F, McKibben PS, Bell DM: A case-control study of HIV seroconversion in health care workers after percutaneous exposure. N Engl J Med 1997; 337:1485–1490 [D]
256. Kotranski L, Semaan S, Collier K, Lauby J, Halbert J, Feighan K: Effectiveness of an HIV risk reduction counseling intervention for out-of-treatment drug users. AIDS Educ Prev 1998; 10:19–33 [A]

257. Hoff RA, Beam-Goulet J, Rosenheck RA: Mental disorder as a risk factor for human immunodeficiency virus infection in a sample of veterans. J Nerv Ment Dis 1997; 185:556–560 [G]
258. Polonsky S, Kerr S, Harris B, Gaiter J, Fichtner RR, Kennedy MG: HIV prevention in prisons and jails: obstacles and opportunities. Public Health Rep 1994; 109:615–625 [G]
259. Inciardi JA: HIV risk reduction and service delivery strategies in criminal justice settings. J Subst Abuse Treat 1996; 13:421–428 [F]
260. Katz RC, Watts C, Santman J: AIDS knowledge and high risk behaviors in the chronic mentally ill. Community Ment Health J 1994; 4:395–402 [G]
261. Carey MP, Carey KB, Kalichman SC: Risk for human immunodeficiency virus (HIV) infection among persons with severe mental illnesses. Clin Psychol Rev 1997; 17:271–291 [F]
262. Kalichman SC, Sikkema KJ, Kelly JA, Bulto M: Use of a brief behavioral skills intervention to prevent HIV infection among chronic mentally ill adults. Psychiatr Serv 1995; 46:275–280 [G]
263. Katz RC, Westerman C, Beauchamp K, Clay C: Effects of AIDS counseling and risk reduction training on the chronic mentally ill. AIDS Educ Prev 1996; 8:457–463 [A]
264. Zierler S, Witbeck B, Mayer K: Sexual violence against women living with or at risk for HIV infection. Am J Prev Med 1996; 12:304–310 [C]
265. Lenderking WR, Wold C, Mayer KH, Goldstein R, Losina E, Seage GR III: Childhood sexual abuse among homosexual men: prevalence and association with unsafe sex. J Gen Intern Med 1997; 12:250–253 [G]
266. Thompson NJ, Potter JS, Sanderson CA, Maibach EW: The relationship of sexual abuse and HIV risk behaviors among heterosexual adult female STD patients. Child Abuse Negl 1997; 21:149–156 [G]
267. Kalichman SC, Williams EA, Cherry C, Belcher L, Nachimson D: Sexual coercion, domestic violence, and negotiating condom use among low-income African American women. J Womens Health 1998; 7:371–378 [G]
268. Lindegren ML, Hanson IC, Hammett TA, Beil J, Fleming PL, Ward JW: Sexual abuse of children: intersection with the HIV epidemic. Pediatrics 1998; 102:E46 [G]
269. Brown LK, Kessel SM, Lourie KJ, Ford HH, Lipsitt LP: Influence of sexual abuse on HIV-related attitudes and behaviors in adolescent psychiatric inpatients. J Am Acad Child Adolesc Psychiatry 1997; 36:316–322 [G]
270. Fleishman JA, Hsia DC, Hellinger FJ: Correlates of medical service utilization among people with HIV infection. Health Serv Res 1994; 29:527–548 [C]
271. AIDS mortality rates lower at sites with HIV experience. AIDS Alert, Nov 1999, p 129 [G]
272. Chaisson RE, Keruly JC, Moore RD: Race, sex, drug use, and progression of human immunodeficiency virus disease. N Engl J Med 1995; 333:751–756 [G]
273. Shapiro MF, Morton SC, McCaffrey DF, Senterfitt JW, Fleishman JA, Perlman JF, Athey LA, Keesey JW, Goldman DP, Berry SH, Bozzette SA: Variations in the care of HIV-infected adults in the United States: results from the HIV Cost and Services Utilization Study. JAMA 1999; 281:2305–2315 [C]
274. Kelly JA, Murphy DA, Bahr GR, Koob JJ, Morgan MG, Kalichman SC, Stevenson LY, Brasfield TL, Bernstein BM, St Lawrence JS: Factors associated with severity of depression and high-risk sexual behavior among persons diagnosed with human immunodeficiency virus (HIV) infection. Health Psychol 1993; 12:215–219 [D]
275. Friedmann PD, Alexander JA, Jin L, D'Aunno TA: On-site primary care and mental health services in outpatient drug abuse treatment units. J Behav Health Serv Res 1999; 26:80–94 [F]
276. Gomez MF, Klein DA, Sand S, Marconi M, O'Dowd MA: Delivering mental health care to HIV-positive individuals: a comparison of two models. Psychosomatics 1999; 40:321–324 [G]

277. Ayuso JL: Use of psychotropic drugs in patients with HIV infection. Drugs 1994; 47:599–610 [G]
278. Tashima K, Bose T, Gormley J, Sousa H, Flanigan TP: The potential impact of efavirenz on methadone maintenance (abstract). Conference on Retroviruses and Opportunistic Infections 1999; 6 [G]
279. Morse GD, Fischl MA, Shelton MJ, Cox SR, Driver M, DeRemer M, Freimuth WW: Single-dose pharmacokinetics of delavirdine mesylate and didanosine in patients with human immunodeficiency virus infection. Antimicrob Agents Chemother 1997; 41:169–174 [A]
280. Beertz R, Cao G, Cavanaugh JH, Hsu A, Granneman GR, Leonard JM: Effect of ritonavir on the pharmacokinetics of desipramine (abstract 1201), in Abstracts of the 11th International Conference on AIDS. Vancouver, BC, International AIDS Society, 1996 [G]
281. von Moltke LL, Greenblatt DJ, Duan SX, Daily JP, Harmatz JS, Shader RI: Inhibition of desipramine hydroxylation (Cytochrome P450-2D6) in vitro by quinidine and by viral protease inhibitors: relation to drug interactions in vivo. J Pharm Sci 1998; 87:1184–1189 [G]
282. Merry C, Mulcahy F, Barry M, Gibbons S, Back D: Saquinavir interaction with midazolam; pharmacokinetic considerations when prescribing protease inhibitors for patients with HIV disease (letter). AIDS 1997; 11:268–269 [G]
283. Henry JA, Hill IR: Fatal interaction between ritonavir and MDMA. Lancet 1998; 352: 1751–1752 [G]
284. Hintz S, Kuck J, Peterkin J, Volk D, Zisook S: Depression in the context of human immunodeficiency virus infection: implications for treatment. J Clin Psychiatry 1990; 51: 497–501 [G]
285. Ferrando S, Goldman J, Charness W: Selective serotonin reuptake inhibitor treatment of depression in symptomatic HIV infection and AIDS. Gen Hosp Psychiatry 1997; 19:89–97 [B]
286. Wagner G, Rabkin J, Rabkin R: A comparative analysis of standard and alternative antidepressants in the treatment of human immunodeficiency virus patients. Compr Psychiatry 1996; 37:402–408 [A]
287. Elliott AJ, Uldall KK, Bergam K, Russo J, Claypoole K, Roy-Byrne PP: Randomized, placebo-controlled trial of paroxetine versus imipramine in depressed HIV-positive outpatients. Am J Psychiatry 1998; 155:367–372 [A]
288. Elliott AJ, Russo J, Bergam K, Claypoole K, Uldall KK, Roy-Byrne PP: Antidepressant efficacy in HIV-seropositive outpatients with major depressive disorder: an open trial of nefazodone. J Clin Psychiatry 1999; 60:226–231 [B]
289. Rabkin JG, Wagner GJ, Rabkin R: Fluoxetine treatment for depression in patients with HIV and AIDS: a randomized, placebo-controlled trial. Am J Psychiatry 1999; 156:101–107 [A]
290. Zisook S, Peterkin J, Goggin KJ, Sledge P, Atkinson JH, Grant I (HIV Neurobehavioral Research Center Group): Treatment of major depression in HIV-seropositive men. J Clin Psychiatry 1998; 59:217–224 [A]
291. Cornblath DR, McArthur JC: Predominantly sensory neuropathy in patients with AIDS and AIDS-related complex. Neurology 1988; 38:794–796 [C]
292. Vitiello B, Stover ES: Psychopharmacology in HIV-positive patients: research perspectives. Psychopharmacol Bull 1996; 32:293–297 [G]
293. Rabkin J, Rabkin R, Wagner G: Effects of fluoxetine on mood and immune status in depressed patients with HIV illness. J Clin Psychiatry 1994; 55:92–97 [B]
294. Schwartz JA, McDaniel JS: Double-blind comparison of fluoxetine and desipramine in the treatment of depressed women with advanced HIV disease: a pilot study. Depress Anxiety 1999; 9:70–74 [A]

295. Grassi B: Notes on the use of fluvoxamine as treatment of depression in HIV-1 infected subjects. Pharmacopsychiatry 1995; 28:93–94 [B]
296. Gillenwater DR, McDaniel JS: Rational psychopharmacology in patients with HIV infection and AIDS. Psychiatr Annals (in press) [F]
297. Levin GM, Nelson LA, Devane CL, Preston SL, Carson SW, Eisele G: Venlafaxine and indinavir: results of a pharmacokinetic interaction study (abstract 661), in Abstracts of the 39th Interscience Conference on Antimicrobial Agents and Chemotherapy. Washington, DC, American Society for Microbiology, 1999 [G]
298. Scurlock HJ, Singh AN, Catalan J: Atypical antipsychotic drugs in the treatment of manic syndromes in patients with HIV-1 infection. J Psychopharmacol 1995; 9:151–154 [G]
299. Hriso E, Kuhn T, Masdeu JC, Grundman M: Extrapyramidal symptoms due to dopamine-blocking agents in patients with AIDS encephalopathy. Am J Psychiatry 1991; 148:1558–1561 [D]
300. Breitbart W, Marotta RF, Call P: AIDS and neuroleptic malignant syndrome. Lancet 1988; 2:1488–1489 [G]
301. Maccario M, Scharre DW: HIV and acute onset of psychosis (letter). Lancet 1987; 2:342 [G]
302. Edelstein H, Knight RT: Severe parkinsonism in two AIDS patients taking prochlorperazine (letter). Lancet 1987; 2:341–342 [G]
303. Kieburtz K, Epstein L, Gelbard H, Greenamyre J: Excitotoxicity and dopaminergic dysfunction in the acquired immunodeficiency syndrome dementia complex. Arch Neurol 1991; 48:1281–1284 [G]
304. Swenson JR, Erman M, Labelle J, Dimsdale JE: Extrapyramidal reactions: neuropsychiatric mimics in patients with AIDS. Gen Hosp Psychiatry 1989; 11:248–253 [G]
305. Hollander H, Golden J, Mendelson T, Cortland D: Extrapyramidal symptoms in AIDS patients given low-dose metoclopramide or chlorpromazine (letter). Lancet 1985; 2:1186 [G]
306. Vogel-Scibilia S, Mulsant BH, Keshavan MS: HIV infection presenting as psychosis: a critique. Acta Psychiatr Scand 1988; 78:652–656 [G]
307. Rosebush P, Stewart T: A prospective analysis of 24 episodes of neuroleptic malignant syndrome. Am J Psychiatry 1989; 146:717–725 [B]
308. Gabel R, Barnard N, Norko M, O'Connell R: AIDS presenting as mania. Compr Psychiatry 1986; 27:251–254 [G]
309. Ferrando S, Eisendrath S: Adverse neuropsychiatric effects of dopamine antagonist medications: misdiagnosis in the medical setting. Psychosomatics 1991; 32:426–432 [C]
310. Belzie LR: Risperidone for AIDS-associated dementia—a case series. AIDS Patient Care and STDs 1996; 10:246–249 [G]
311. Shedlack KJ, Soldato-Couture C, Swanson CL Jr: Rapidly progressive tardive dyskinesia in AIDS (letter). Biol Psychiatry 1994; 35:147–148 [G]
312. Fernandez F, Joel L: The use of molindone in the treatment of psychotic and delirious patients infected with the human immunodeficiency virus: case reports. Gen Hosp Psychiatry 1993; 15:31–35 [G]
313. Factor S, Podskalny G, Barron K: Persistent neuroleptic-induced rigidity and dystonia in AIDS dementia complex: a clinico-pathological case report. J Neurol Sci 1994; 127:114–120 [G]
314. Jones GH, Kelly CL, Davies JA: HIV and onset of schizophrenia (letter). Lancet 1987; 1:982 [G]
315. Singh A, Goiledge H, Catalan J: Treatment of HIV-related psychotic disorders with risperidone: a series of 21 cases. J Psychosom Res 1997; 42:489–493 [G]
316. Nath A, Jankovic J, Pettigrew LC: Movement disorders and AIDS. Neurology 1987; 37:37–41 [G]

317. Kieburtz K, Simpson D, Yiannoutsos C, Max MB, Hall CD, Ellis RJ, Marra CM, McKendall R, Singer E, Dal Pan GJ, Clifford DB, Tucker T, Cohen B (AIDS Clinical Trial Group 242 Protocol Team): A randomized trial of amitriptyline and mexiletine for painful neuropathy in HIV infection. Neurology 1998; 51:1682–1688 [A]
318. Janssen RS (American Academy of Neurology Workgroup on the Nomenclature for HIV-Associated Cognitive Disorders): Nomenclature and research case definitions for neurologic manifestations of human immunodeficiency virus-type 1 (HIV-1) infection. Neurology 1991; 41:778–785 [A]
319. Wilson JA, Smith RG: Relation between elderly and AIDS patients with drug-induced Parkinson's disease (letter). Lancet 1987; 2:686 [G]
320. Lera G, Zirulnik J: Pilot study with clozapine in patients with HIV-associated psychosis and drug-induced parkinsonism. Mov Disord 1999; 14:128–131 [B]
321. Fernandez F, Levy JK, Galizzi H: Response of HIV-related depression to psychostimulants: case reports. Hosp Community Psychiatry 1988; 39:628–631 [G]
322. Wagner GJ, Rabkin JG, Rabkin R: Dextroamphetamine as a treatment for depression and low energy in AIDS patients: a pilot study. J Psychosom Res 1997; 42:407–411 [B]
323. Hardy MA, Nardacci D: Does valproate pose a threat to human immunodeficiency virus-infected patients? (letter). J Clin Psychopharmacol 1999; 19:189–190 [G]
324. Maggi JD, Halman MH: The effect of divalproex sodium on viral load: a retrospective review of HIV-positive patients with manic syndromes. Can J Psychiatry 2001; 46:359–362 [F]
325. Cozza KL, Swanton EJ, Humphreys CW: Hepatotoxicity with combination of valproic acid, ritonavir, and nevirapine: a case report. Psychosomatics 2000; 41:452–453 [G]
326. Jefferson JW: Possible risks associated with valproate treatment of AIDS-related mania. J Clin Psychiatry 1998; 59:317 [G]
327. Parenti DM, Simon GL, Scheib RG, Meyer WA III, Sztein MB, Paxton H, DiGioia RA, Schulof RS: Effect of lithium carbonate in HIV-infected patients with immune dysfunction. J Acquir Immune Defic Syndr 1988; 1:119–124 [C]
328. Batki SL: Buspirone in drug users with AIDS or AIDS-related complex. J Clin Psychopharmacol 1990; 10(June suppl):111S–115S [G]
329. Trachman SB: Buspirone-induced psychosis in a human immunodeficiency virus-infected man. Psychosomatics 1992; 33:332–335 [G]
330. Frye R: Effect of ritonavir on the pharmacokinetics and pharmacodynamics of alprazolam (abstract). Interscience Conference on Antimicrobial Agents and Chemotherapy 1997 [G]
331. Greenblatt DJ, von Moltke LL, Harmatz JS, Durol AL, Daily JP, Graf JA, Mertzanis P, Hoffman JL, Shader RI: Alprazolam-ritonavir interaction: implications for product labeling. Clin Pharmacol Ther 2000; 67:335–341[A]
332. Chuck SK, Rodvold KA, von Moltke LL, Greenblatt DJ, Shader RI: Pharmacokinetics of protease inhibitors and drug interactions with psychoactive drugs, in Psychological and Public Health Implications of New HIV Therapies. Edited by Ostrow D, Kalichman SC. New York, Plenum, 1998, pp 33–60 [G]
333. Fisher A, Abbatiola M: The effects of oxandrolone on body weight and composition in patients with HIV-associated weight loss (abstract 42351). International Conference on AIDS 1998; 12:844 [G]
334. Fisher AE, Abbatiola MM: Effects of oxandrolone on body weight and composition in patients with HIV-associated weight loss (abstract 477). Conference on Retroviruses and Opportunistic Infections 1998; 5:169 [G]
335. Poles MA, Meller JA, Lin A, Weiss WR, Gocke M, Dietrict DT: Oxandrolone as a treatment for AIDS-related weight loss and wasting (abstract 695). Conference on Retroviruses and Opportunistic Infections 1997; 4:193 [G]

336. Tai VW, Mulligan K, Culp J, Schambelan M: The effects of chronic growth hormone therapy on dietary intake in patients with HIV-associated weight loss (abstract MoB 1388). International Conference on AIDS 1996; 11(1):122 [A]
337. Luna-Castanos G, Osornio L, Gomez DM, Neigo L: Growth hormone in the treatment of weight loss AIDS-related (abstract MoB 1387). International Conference on AIDS 1996; 11(1):122 [G]
338. Gomez CWH, Feregrino-Goyos M, Alvarado-Diez R, Eid-Lidt G, Conde-Mercado JM, Fuentes-Del-Toro S, Mireles MP, Mora-Rodriquez G: Short and long time treatment with growth hormone in AIDS wasting syndrome increase in quality of life and nutritional status (abstract MoB 1386). International Conference on AIDS 1996; 11(1):122 [G]
339. Berger DS, LaMarca A, Landy H, Kaufman RS, Breitmeyer J: A phase III study of recombinant human growth hormone (mammalian cell-derived) in patients with AIDS wasting. International Conference on AIDS 1996; 11:B422 [G]
340. Koster F, Nightingale S, Gesundheit N, Waters D, Bukar J, Qualls C, Danska J, Watson D, Jackson L, Hardy K: A randomized, double-blind, placebo-controlled phase II trial of growth hormone and insulin-like growth factor I for AIDS wasting. Program and Abstracts of the Interscience Conference on Antimicrobial Agents and Chemotherapy 1994; 56 [A]
341. Sharp M, Getty J, Chambers S, Sekeres G: Thalidomide associated weight gain in HIV-1 positive clients (abstract WeB 180). International Conference on AIDS 1996; 20:112 [G]
342. Reyes-Teran G, Sierra-Madero JG, Martinez del Cerro V, Arroyo-Figueroa H, Pasquetti A, Calva JJ, Ruiz-Palacios GM: Effects of thalidomide on HIV-associated wasting syndrome: a randomized, double-blind, placebo controlled clinical trial. AIDS 1996; 10:1501–1507 [A]
343. Rabkin JG, Rabkin R, Wagner G: Testosterone replacement therapy in HIV illness. Gen Hosp Psychiatry 1995; 17:37–42 [B]
344. Confrancesco J, Whalen JJ, Dobs AS: Testosterone replacement options for HIV-infected men. J Acquir Immune Defic Syndr Hum Retrovirol 1997; 16:254–265 [F]
345. Chang GWM, Kam PCA: The physiologic and pharmacological roles of cytochrome P450 enzymes. Anaesthesia 1999; 54:42–50 [G]
346. Schwartz EL, Brechbuhl AB, Kahl P, Miller MA, Selwyn P, Friedland GH: Pharmacokinetic interactions of zidovudine and methadone in intravenous drug-using patients with HIV infection. J Acquir Immune Defic Syndr 1992; 5:619–626 [B]
347. Borg L, Kreek M: Clinical problems associated with interactions between methadone pharmacotherapy and medications used in the treatment of HIV-1 positive and AIDS patients. Current Opinion in Psychiatry 1995; 8:199–202 [F]
348. McCance-Katz EF, Rainey PM, Jatlow P, Friedland G (AIDS Clinical Trials Group 262): Methadone effects on zidovudine disposition. J Acquir Immune Defic Syndr Hum Retrovirol 1998; 18:435–443 [A]
349. Rainey P, McCance-Katz EF, Jatlow P, Kosten TR, Friedland G: Opioid effects on zidovudine disposition. NIDA Res Monogr (in press) [G]
350. Sellers E: The pharmacokinetics (PK) of abacavir (ABC) and methadone (M) following coadministration: CNAAL 01 2 (abstract 663). Program and Abstracts From the 39th Interscience Conference on Antimicrobial Agents and Chemotherapy, 1999 [G]
351. Guibert A, Furlan V, Martino J, Taburet AM: In vitro effect of HIV protease inhibitors on methadone metabolism (abstract A-58). Program and Abstracts From the 37th Interscience Conference of Antimicrobial Agents and Chemotherapy, 1997 [G]
352. McCance-Katz EF, Farber S, Selwyn PA, O'Connor A: Decrease in methadone levels with nelfinavir mesylate (letter). Am J Psychiatry 2000; 157:481 [G]
353. Altice FL, Friedland GH, Cooney EL: Nevirapine induced opiate withdrawal among injection drug users with HIV infection receiving methadone. AIDS 1999; 13:957–962 [D]
354. Piscitelli SC, Burstein AH, Chaitt D, Alfaro RM, Falloon J: Indinavir concentrations and St John's wort. Lancet 2000; 355:547–548 [G]

355. Winiarski MG: AIDS-Related Psychotherapy. New York, Pergamon Press, 1991 [G]
356. Farber EW, Schwartz JAJ, Shaper PE, Moonen DJ, McDaniel JS: Resilience factors associated with adaptation to HIV disease. Psychosomatics 2000; 41:140–146 [G]
357. Farber EW, McDaniel JS: Assessment and psychotherapy practice implications of new combination antiviral therapies in HIV disease. Professional Psychology: Research and Practice 1999; 30:173–179 [G]
358. Selwyn PA, Arnold R: From fate to tragedy: the changing meanings of life, death, and AIDS. Ann Intern Med 1998; 129:899–902 [G]
359. Robins AG, Dew MA, Davidson S, Penkower L, Becker JT, Kingsley L: Psychosocial factors associated with risky sexual behavior among HIV-seropositive gay men. AIDS Educ Prev 1994; 6:483–492 [G]
360. Aversa SL, Kimberlin C: Psychosocial aspects of antiretroviral medication use among HIV patients. Patient Educ Couns 1996; 29:207–219 [G]
361. Mason HR, Simoni JM, Marks G, Johnson CJ, Richardson JL: Missed opportunities? disclosure of HIV and support seeking among HIV positive African-American and European-American men. AIDS and Behavior 1996; 1:155 [C]
362. Kalichman S, Sikkema K: Psychological sequelae of HIV infection and AIDS: review of empirical findings. Clin Psychol Rev 1994; 14:611–632 [F]
363. Linn JG, Lewis FM, Cain VA, Kimbrough GA: HIV-illness, social support, sense of coherence, and psychosocial well-being in a sample of help-seeking adults. AIDS Educ Prev 1993; 5:254–262 [C]
364. Hall VP: The relationship between social support and health in gay men with HIV/AIDS: an integrative review. J Assoc Nurses AIDS Care 1999; 10:74–86 [E]
365. Leserman J, Perkins DO, Evans DL: Coping with the threat of AIDS: the role of social support. Am J Psychiatry 1992; 149:1514–1520 [C]
366. Gostin LO, Webber DW: HIV infection and AIDS in the public health and health care systems: the role of law and litigation. JAMA 1998; 279:1108–1113 [G]
367. Levy JA, Fox SE: The outreach-assisted model of partner notification with IDUS. Public Health Rep 1998; 113(suppl 1):160–169 [A]
368. West GR, Stark KA: Partner notification for HIV prevention: a critical reexamination. AIDS Educ Prev 1997; 9:68–78 [F]
369. Fenton KA, Peterman TA: HIV partner notification—taking a new look (editorial). AIDS 1997; 11:1535–1546 [G]
370. APA Commission on AIDS: AIDS policy: position statement on confidentiality, disclosure, and protection of others. Am J Psychiatry 1993; 150:852 [G]
371. Bronheim HE, Fulop G, Kunkel EJ, Muskin PR, Schindler BA, Yates WR, Shaw R, Steiner H, Stern TA, Stoudemire A: The Academy of Psychosomatic Medicine practice guidelines for psychiatric consultation in the general medical setting. Psychosomatics 1998; 39:S8–S30 [G]
372. Kalichman SC, Ramachandran B, Ostrow D: Protease inhibitors and the new AIDS combination therapies: implication for psychological services. Professional Psychol Res Practice 1998; 29:349–356 [G]
373. Lucas GM, Chaisson RE, Moore RD: Highly active antiretroviral therapy in a large urban clinic: risk factors for virologic failure and adverse drug reactions. Ann Intern Med 1999; 131:81–87 [D]
374. Wainberg ML, Cournos F: Adherence to treatment. New Dir Ment Health Serv Fall 2000; (87):85–93 [G]
375. McArthur JC GI: HIV Neurocognitive disorders, in The Neurology of AIDS. Edited by Gendelman HE, Lipton SA, Epstein L, Swindells S. New York, Chapman & Hall, 1996, pp 499–523 [F]
376. Ickovics JR, Meisler AW: Adherence in AIDS clinical trials: a framework for clinical research and clinical care. J Clin Epidemiol 1997; 50:385–391 [G]

377. Wall TL, Sorensen JL, Batki SL, Delucchi KL, London JA, Chesney MA: Adherence to zidovudine (AZT) among HIV-infected methadone patients: a pilot study of supervised therapy and dispensing compared to usual care. Drug Alcohol Depend 1995; 37:261–269 [B]
378. Sorensen JL, Mascovich A, Wall TL, DePhilippis D, Batki SL, Chesney M: Medication adherence strategies for drug abusers with HIV/AIDS. AIDS Care 1998; 10:297–312 [G]
379. Foudraine NA, Hoetelmans RM, Lange JM, de Wolf F, van Benthem BH, Maas JJ, Keet IP, Portegies P: Cerebrospinal-fluid HIV-1 RNA and drug concentrations after treatment with lamivudine plus zidovudine or stavudine. Lancet 1998; 351:1547–1551 [A]
380. Gulevich SJ, McCutchan JA, Thal LJ, Kirson D, Durand D, Wallace M, Mehta P, Heyes MP, Grant I: Effect of antiretroviral therapy on the cerebrospinal fluid of patients seropositive for the human immunodeficiency virus. J Acquir Immune Defic Syndr 1993; 6:1002–1007; correction, 1994; 7:994 [B]
381. Goodkin K, Wilkie FL, Concha M, Asthana D, Shapshak P, Douyon R, Fujimura RK, LoPiccolo C: Subtle neuropsychological impairment and minor cognitive-motor disorder in HIV-1 infection: neuroradiological, neurophysiological, neuroimmunological, and virological correlates. Neuroimaging Clin N Am 1997; 7:561–579 [F]
382. Sidtis JJ, Gatsonis C, Price RW, Singer EJ, Collier AC, Richman DD, Hirsch MS, Schaerf FW, Fischl MA, Kieburtz K: Zidovudine treatment of the AIDS dementia complex: results of a placebo-controlled trial. Ann Neurol 1993; 33:343–349 [A]
383. Schmitt FA, Bigley JW, McKinnis R, Logue PE, Evans RW, Drucker JL: Neuropsychological outcome of zidovudine (AZT) treatment of patients with AIDS and AIDS-related complex. N Engl J Med 1988; 319:1573–1578 [A]
384. Azzini M, Nanni S, Astori MR, Brunetto A, Massobrio L: Evaluation of neuropsychiatric parameters in HIV positive subjects treated with zidovudine. Acta Neurol (Napoli) 1990; 12:36–39 [G]
385. Vago L, Castagna A, Lazzarin A, Trabattoni G, Cinque P, Costanzi G: Reduced frequency of HIV-induced brain lesions in AIDS patients treated with zidovudine. J Acquir Immune Defic Syndr 1993; 6:42–45 [D]
386. Bell JE, Donaldson YK, Lowrie S, McKenzie CA, Elton RA, Chiswick A, Brettle RP, Ironside JW, Simmonds P: Influence of risk group and zidovudine therapy on the development of HIV encephalitis and cognitive impairment in AIDS patients. AIDS 1996; 10: 493–499 [B]
387. Brew BJ, Bhalla RB, Paul M, Sidtis JJ, Keilp JJ, Sadler AE, Gallardo H, McArthur JC, Schwartz MK, Price RW: Cerebrospinal fluid beta 2-microglobulin in patients with AIDS dementia complex: an expanded series including response to zidovudine treatment. AIDS 1992; 6:461–465 [C]
388. Gorman JM, Mayeux R, Stern Y, Williams JB, Rabkin J, Goetz RR, Ehrhardt AA: The effect of zidovudine on neuropsychiatric measures in HIV-infected men. Am J Psychiatry 1993; 150:505–507 [B]
389. Yerly S, Kaiser L, Race E, Bru JP, Clavel F, Perrin L: Transmission of antiretroviral-drug-resistant HIV-1 variants. Lancet 1999; 354:729–733 [G]
390. De Ronchi D, Lazzari C, Rucci P, Cangialosi A, Volterra V: Neurocognitive effects of zidovudine and 2',3'-dideoxyinosine during the treatment of asymptomatic and symptomatic HIV-1 seropositive patients: comparison with non-treated patients. Human Psychopharmacology 1996; 11:415–420 [G]
391. Brew BJ, Brown SJ, Catalan J: Safety and efficacy of abacavir (ABC, 1592) in AIDS dementia complex (study CNAB 3001). Abstracts of the 12th International Conference on AIDS. Geneva, International AIDS Society, 1998, p 559 [B]
392. Thomas SA, Segal MB: The transport of the anti-HIV drug, 2′,3′-didehydro-3′-deoxythymidine (D4T), across the blood-brain and blood–cerebrospinal fluid barriers. Br J Pharmacol 1998; 125:49–54 [G]

393. Stahle L, Martin C, Svensson JO, Sonnerborg A: Indinavir in cerebrospinal fluid of HIV-1-infected patients (letter). Lancet 1997; 350:1823 [G]
394. Ferrando S, van Gorp W, McElhiney M, Gogin K, Sewell M, Rabkin J: Highly active antiretroviral treatment in HIV infection: benefits for neuropsychological function. AIDS 1998; 12:F65–F70 [B]
395. Moore RD, Keruly J, Richman DD, Creagh-Kirk T, Chaisson RE: Natural history of advanced HIV disease in patients treated with zidovudine. AIDS 1992; 6:671–677 [B]
396. Montforte A, Musicco M, Galli M: Italian multicenter study of didanosine: compassionate use in advanced HIV infection. Eur J Microb Infect Dis 1997; 16:135–142 [G]
397. Day JJ, Grant I, Atkinson JH, Brysk LT, McCutchan JA, Hesselink JR, Heaton RK, Weinrich JD, Spector SA, Richman DD: Incidence of AIDS dementia in a two-year follow-up of AIDS and ARC patients on an initial phase II AZT placebo-controlled study: San Diego cohort. J Neuropsychiatry Clin Neurosci 1992; 4:15–20 [A]
398. Heseltine PN, Goodkin K, Atkinson JH, Vitiello B, Rochon J, Heaton RK, Eaton EM, Wilkie FL, Sobel E, Brown SJ, Feaster D, Schneider L, Goldschmidts WL, Stover ES: Randomized double-blind placebo-controlled trial of peptide T for HIV-associated cognitive impairment. Arch Neurol 1998; 55:41–51 [A]
399. Lipton SA: HIV-related neuronal injury: potential therapeutic intervention with calcium channel antagonists and NMDA antagonists. Mol Neurobiol 1994; 8:181–196 [F]
400. Mapou RL, Law WA, Wagner K, Malone JL, Skillman DR: Neuropsychological effects of interferon alfa-n3 treatment in asymptomatic human immunodeficiency virus-1-infected individuals. J Neuropsychiatry Clin Neurosci 1996; 8:74–81 [B]
401. Skillman DR, Malone JL, Decker CF, Wagner KF, Mapou RL, Liao MJ, Testa D, Meltzer MS: Phase I trial of interferon alfa-n3 in early-stage human immunodeficiency virus type 1 disease: evidence for drug safety, tolerance, and antiviral activity. J Infect Dis 1996; 173: 1107–1114 [B]
402. Galgani S, Balestra P, Narciso P, Tozzi V, Sette P, Pau F, Visco G: Nimodipine plus zidovudine versus zidovudine alone in the treatment of HIV-1-associated cognitive deficits (letter). AIDS 1997; 11:1520–1521 [G]
403. Navia BA, Dafni U, Simpson D, Tucker T, Singer E, McArthur JC, Yiannoutsos C, Zaborski L, Lipton SA: A phase I/II trial of nimodipine for HIV-related neurologic complications. Neurology 1998; 51:221–228 [A]
404. van Dyck CH, McMahon TJ, Rosen MI, O'Malley SS, O'Connor PG, Lin CH, Pearsall HR, Woods SW, Kosten TR: Sustained-release methylphenidate for cognitive impairment in HIV-1-infected drug abusers: a pilot study. J Neuropsychiatry Clin Neurosci 1997; 9:29–36 [A]
405. Holmes VF, Fernandez F, Levy JK: Psychostimulant response in AIDS-related complex patients. J Clin Psychiatry 1989; 50:5–8 [B]
406. Dana Consortium on the Therapy of HIV Dementia and Related Cognitive Disorders: A randomized, double-blind, placebo-controlled trial of deprenyl and thioctic acid in human immunodeficiency virus-associated cognitive impairment. Neurology 1998; 50:645–651 [A]
407. Gisslen M, Larsson M, Norkrans G, Fuchs D, Wachter H, Hagberg L: Tryptophan concentrations increase in cerebrospinal fluid and blood after zidovudine treatment in patients with HIV type 1 infection. AIDS Res Hum Retroviruses 1994; 10:947–951 [B]
408. Herzlich BC, Schiano TD: Reversal of apparent AIDS dementia complex following treatment with vitamin B12. J Intern Med 1993; 233:495–497 [G]
409. Adams F, Fernandez F, Andersson BS: Emergency pharmacotherapy in the critically ill cancer patient. Psychosomatics 1986; 27(Jan suppl):33–38 [G]
410. Muskin PR, Mellman LA, Kornfeld DS: A "new" drug for treating agitation and psychosis in the general hospital: chlorpromazine. Gen Hosp Psychiatry 1986; 8:404–410 [G]
411. Trzepacz PT, Baker RW, Greenhouse J: A symptom rating scale for delirium. Psychiatry Res 1988; 23:89–97 [G]

412. Resnick M, Burton BT: Droperidol vs haloperidol in the initial management of acutely agitated patients. J Clin Psychiatry 1984; 45:298–299 [A]
413. Thomas H Jr, Schwartz E, Petrilli R: Droperidol versus haloperidol for chemical restraint of agitated and combative patients. Ann Emerg Med 1992; 21:407–413 [A]
414. Wagner G, Maguen S, Rabkin J: Ethnic differences in response to fluoxetine in a controlled trial with depressed HIV-positive patients. Psychiatr Serv 1998; 49:239–240 [A]
415. Cazzulio CL, Bessone E, Bertrando P, Pedrazzoli L, Cusini M: Treatment of depression in HIV-infected patients. J Psychiatry Neurosci 1998; 23:293–297 [B]
416. Levine S, Anderson D, Bystritsky A, Baron D: A report of eight HIV-seropositive patients with major depression responding to fluoxetine. J Acquir Immune Defic Syndr 1990; 3: 1074–1077 [B]
417. Gottlieb JF: book review, A Lazare (ed): Outpatient Psychiatry: Diagnosis and Treatment, 2nd ed. Am J Psychiatry 1991; 148:805–806 [G]
418. Grassi B, Gambini O, Garghentini G, Lazzarin A, Scarone S: Efficacy of paroxetine for the treatment of depression in the context of HIV infection. Pharmacopsychiatry 1997; 30:70–71 [B]
419. Ferrando SJ, Rabkin JG, de Moore GM, Rabkin R: Antidepressant treatment of depression in HIV-seropositive women. J Clin Psychiatry 1999; 60:741–756 [B]
420. Fernandez F, Levy J: Efficacy of venlafaxine in HIV-depressive disorders. Psychosomatics 1997; 38:173–174 [B]
421. White J, Christensen J, Clifford M: Methylphenidate as a treatment for depression in acquired immunodeficiency syndrome: an n-of-1 trial. J Clin Psychiatry 1992; 53:153–156 [A]
422. Walling V, Pfefferbaum B: The use of methylphenidate in a depressed adolescent with AIDS. J Dev Behav Pediatr 1990; 11:195–197 [G]
423. Perkins D, Evans DL: HIV-related major depression: response to zidovudine treatment. Psychosomatics 1991; 32:451–454 [G]
424. Schaerf F, Miller RR, Lipsey JR, McPherson RW: ECT for major depression in four patients infected with human immunodeficiency. Am J Psychiatry 1989; 146:782–784 [G]
425. Targ E, Karasic D, Diefenbach P, Anderson D, Bystritsky A, Fawzy F: Structured group therapy and fluoxetine to treat depression in HIV-positive persons. Psychosomatics 1994; 35:132–137 [A]
426. Markowitz JC, Kocsis JH, Fishman B, Spielman LA, Jacobsberg LB, Frances AJ, Klerman GL, Perry SW: Treatment of depressive symptoms in human immunodeficiency virus–positive patients. Arch Gen Psychiatry 1998; 55:452–457 [A]
427. Markowitz JC, Klerman GL, Perry SW: Interpersonal psychotherapy of depressed HIV-positive outpatients. Hosp Community Psychiatry 1992; 43:885–890 [B]
428. Levine S, Bystritsky A, Baron D, Jones L: Group psychotherapy for HIV-seropositive patients with major depression. Am J Psychother 1991; 45:413–424 [B]
429. Treisman G: HIV, AIDS, and the Brain, vol 72. New York, Raven Press, 1994 [G]
430. Lyketsos C, Fishman M, Hutton H, Cox T, Hobbs S, Spoler C, Hunt W, Driscoll J, Treisman G: The effectiveness of psychiatric treatment for HIV-infected patients. Psychosomatics 1997: 38:423–432 [B]
431. Kelly JA, Murphy DA, Bahr GR, Kalichman SC, Morgan MG, Stevenson LY, Koob JJ, Brasfield TL, Bernstein BM: Outcome of cognitive-behavioral and support group brief therapies for depressed, HIV-infected persons. Am J Psychiatry 1993; 150:1679–1686 [A]
432. Eller L: Effects of two cognitive-behavioral interventions on immunity and symptoms in persons with HIV. Ann Behav Med 1995; 17:339–348 [B]
433. Halman MH, Worth JL, Sanders KM, Renshaw PF, Murray GB: Anticonvulsant use in the treatment of manic syndromes in patients with HIV-1 infection. J Neuropsychiatry Clin Neurosci 1993; 5:430–434 [D]
434. RachBeisel JA, Weintraub E: Valproic acid treatment of AIDS-related mania (letter). J Clin Psychiatry 1997; 58:406–407 [G]

435. Guydish J, Temoshok L, Dilley J, Rinaldi J: Evaluation of a hospital based substance abuse intervention and referral service for HIV affected patients. Gen Hosp Psychiatry 1990; 12:1–7 [B]
436. Sorensen J, Batki S, Good P, Wilkinson K: Methadone maintenance program for AIDS-affected opiate addicts. J Subst Abuse Treat 1989; 6:87–94 [G]
437. Ferrando SJ, Batki SL: HIV-infected intravenous drug users in methadone maintenance treatment: clinical problems and their management. J Psychoactive Drugs 1991; 23:217–224 [G]
438. Batki SL: Abstract. International Conference on AIDS 1995 [B]
439. Antela A, Casado JL, Gonzalez MJ, Perez P, Perez-Elias MJ, Montilla P, Buzon L: Influence of a methadone maintenance programme on the improved outcome of a cohort of injecting drug users with advanced HIV disease (letter). AIDS 1997; 11:1405–1406 [G]
440. Batki SL: Abstract. International Conference on AIDS 1993 [A]
441. McDaniel JS, Blalock A: Diagnosis and management of HIV-related mood and anxiety disorders. New Directions in Psychiatric Services (in press) [F]
442. McDaniel J, Johnson K: Obsessive-compulsive disorder in HIV disease: response to fluoxetine. Psychosomatics 1995; 36:147–150 [G]
443. Rahman M, Gregory R: Trichotillomania associated with HIV infection in response to sertraline. Psychosomatics 1995; 36:417–418 [G]
444. Perretta P, Nisita C, Zaccagnini E, Scasso A, Nuccorini A, Santa M, Cassano G: Diagnosis and clinical use of bromperidol in HIV-related psychoses in a sample of seropositive patients with brain damage. Int Clin Psychopharmacol 1992; 7:95–99 [B]
445. Scamvougeras A, Rosebush PI: AIDS-related psychosis with catatonia responding to low-dose lorazepam. J Clin Psychiatry 1992; 53:414–415 [G]
446. Snyder S, Prenzlauer S, Maruyama N, Rose DN: Catatonia in a patient with AIDS-related dementia (letter). J Clin Psychiatry 1992; 53:414 [G]
447. El-Mallakh R: AIDS dementia-related psychosis: is there a window of vulnerability? AIDS Care 1992; 4:381–387 [F]
448. Norman SE, Chediak AD, Kiel M, Cohn MA: Sleep disturbances in HIV-infected homosexual men. AIDS 1990; 4:775–781 [C]
449. Norman SE, Chediak AD, Freeman C, Kiel M, Mendez A, Duncan R, Simoneau J, Nolan B: Sleep disturbances in men with asymptomatic human immunodeficiency (HIV) infection. Sleep 1992; 15:150–155 [C]
450. Darko DF, McCutchan JA, Kripke DF, Gillin JC, Golshan S: Fatigue, sleep disturbance, disability, and indices of progression of HIV infection. Am J Psychiatry 1992; 149:514–520 [C]
451. Darko DF, Mitler MM, Miller JC: Growth hormone, fatigue, poor sleep, and disability in HIV infection. Neuroendocrinology 1998; 67:317–324 [C]
452. Epstein LJ, Strollo PJ Jr, Donegan RB, Delmar J, Hendrix C, Westbrook PR: Obstructive sleep apnea in patients with human immunodeficiency virus (HIV) disease. Sleep 1995; 18:368–376 [C]
453. Hansen M, Kubicki S, Henkes H, Terstegge G, Scholz, Weiss R: The effects of flurazepam on sleep in AIDS patients. New Trends in Clinical Neuropharmacology 1989; 3:134–135 [B]
454. Pizzo PA, Eddy J, Falloon J, Balis FM, Murphy RF, Moss H, Wolters P, Brouwers P, Jarosinski P, Rubin M: Effect of continuous intravenous infusion of zidovudine (AZT) in children with symptomatic HIV infection. N Engl J Med 1988; 319:889–896 [B]
455. Brouwers P, Moss H, Wolters P, Eddy J, Balis F, Poplack D, Pizzo P: Effect of continuous-infusion zidovudine therapy on neuropsychologic functioning in children with symptomatic human immunodeficiency virus infection. J Pediatr 117:980–985 [B]
456. Nozyce M, Hoberman M, Arpadi S, Wiznia A, Lambert G, Dobroszycki J, Chang CJ, St Louis Y: A 12-month study of the effects of oral zidovudine on neurodevelopmental functioning in a cohort of vertically HIV-infected inner-city children. AIDS 1994; 8:635–639 [B]

457. Raskino C, Pearson DA, Baker CJ, Lifschitz MH, O'Donnell K, Mintz M, Nozyce M, Bruwors P, McKinney RE, Jimenez E, England JA (Pediatric AIDS Clinical Trials Group 152 Study Team): Neurologic, neurocognitive, and brain growth outcomes in human immunodeficiency virus-infected children receiving different nucleoside antiretroviral regimens. Pediatrics 1999; 104(3):e32 [A]
458. Tepper VJ, Farley JJ, Rothman MI, Houck DL, Davis KF, Collins-Jones TL, Wachtel RC: Neurodevelopmental/neuroradiologic recovery of a child infected with HIV after treatment with combination antiretroviral therapy using the HIV-specific protease inhibitor ritonavir. Pediatrics 1998; 101:e7 [G]
459. Cesena M, Lee D, Cebollero A, Steingard R: Case study: behavioral symptoms of pediatric HIV-1 encephalopathy successfully treated with clonidine. J Am Acad Child Adolesc Psychiatry 1995; 34:302–306 [G]
460. Anand A, Carmosino L, Glatt A: Management of recalcitrant pain in a pediatric acquired immunodeficiency syndrome patient. Pediatr Infect Dis J 1993; 12:159–160 [G]
461. Hirschfeld S, Moss H, Dragisic K, Smith W, Pizzo PA: Pain in pediatric human immunodeficiency virus infection: incidence and characteristics in a single-institution pilot study. Pediatrics 1996; 98:449–452 [G]
462. Grinspoon S, Corcoran C, Askari H, Schoenfeld D, Wolf L, Burrows B, Walsh M, Hayden D, Parlman K, Anderson E, Basgoz N, Klibanski A: Effects of androgen administration in men with the AIDS wasting syndrome: a randomized, double-blind, placebo-controlled trial. Ann Intern Med 1998; 129:18–26 [A]
463. Rabkin JG, Rabkin R, Wagner GJ: Testosterone treatment of clinical hypogonadism in patients with HIV/AIDS. Int J STD AIDS 1997; 8:537–545 [F]
464. Hengge UR, Baumann M, Maleba R, Brockmeyer NH, Goos M: Oxymetholone promotes weight gain in patients with advanced human immunodeficiency virus (HIV-1) infection. Br J Nutr 1996; 75:129–138 [A]
465. Miller K, Corcoran C, Armstrong C, Caramelli K, Anderson E, Cotton D, Basgoz N, Hirschhorn L, Tuomala R, Schoenfeld D, Daugherty C, Mazer N, Grinspoon S: Transdermal testosterone administration in women with acquired immunodeficiency syndrome wasting: a pilot study. J Clin Endocrinol Metab 1998; 83:2717–2725 [B]
466. Wagner G, Rabkin J, Rabkin R: Exercise as a mediator of psychological and nutritional effects of testosterone therapy in HIV+ men. Med Sci Sports Exerc 1998; 30:811–817 [B]
467. Strawford A, Barbieri T, Van Loan M, Parks E, Catlin D, Barton N, Neese R, Christiansen M, King J, Hellerstein MK: Resistance exercise and supraphysiologic androgen therapy in eugonadal men with HIV-related weight loss: a randomized controlled trial. JAMA 1999; 281:1282–1290 [A]
468. Breitbart WS, Rosenfeld B, Kaim M, Funesti-Esch J: Psychostimulants for fatigue in the HIV+ patient: preliminary findings of a placebo-controlled trial of methylphenidate vs pemoline. Psychosomatics 1999; 40:160–161 [A]
469. Rabkin JG, Ferrando SJ, Wagner GJ, Rabkin R: DHEA treatment for HIV+ patients: effects on mood, androgenic and anabolic parameters. Psychoneuroendocrinology 2000; 25:53–68 [B]
470. Holzemer WL, Henry SB, Reilly CA: Assessing and managing pain in AIDS care: the patient perspective. J Assoc Nurses AIDS Care 1998; 9:22–30 [G]
471. Kemper CA, Kent G, Burton S, Deresinski SC: Mexiletine for HIV-infected patients with painful peripheral neuropathy: a double-blind, placebo-controlled, crossover treatment trial. J Acquir Immune Defic Syndr Hum Retrovirol 1998; 19:367–372 [A]
472. Shlay JC, Chaloner K, Max MB, Flaws B, Reichelderfer P, Wentworth D, Hillman S, Brizz B, Cohn DL: Acupuncture and amitriptyline for pain due to HIV-related peripheral neuropathy: a randomized controlled trial: Terry Beirn Community Programs for Clinical Research on AIDS. JAMA 1998; 280:1590–1595 [A]
473. Hall MC, Ahmad S: Interaction between sildenafil and HIV-1 combination therapy (letter). Lancet 1999; 353:2071–2072 [G]

PRACTICE GUIDELINE FOR THE
Treatment of Patients With Substance Use Disorders
Second Edition

WORK GROUP ON SUBSTANCE USE DISORDERS

Herbert D. Kleber, M.D., Chair

Roger D. Weiss, M.D., Vice-Chair

Raymond F. Anton Jr., M.D.
Tony P. George, M.D.
Shelly F. Greenfield, M.D., M.P.H.
Thomas R. Kosten, M.D.
Charles P. O'Brien, M.D., Ph.D.
Bruce J. Rounsaville, M.D.
Eric C. Strain, M.D.
Douglas M. Ziedonis, M.D.
Grace Hennessy, M.D. (Consultant)
Hilary Smith Connery, M.D., Ph.D. (Consultant)

This practice guideline was approved in December 2005 and published in August 2006. A guideline watch, summarizing significant developments in the scientific literature since publication of this guideline, may be available in the Psychiatric Practice section of the APA web site at www.psych.org.

CONTENTS

Guide to Using This Practice Guideline 295

Development Process 296

Part A: Treatment Recommendations for Patients With Substance Use Disorders 297

I. Executive Summary of Recommendations 297
- A. Coding System 297
- B. General Treatment Principles 297
- C. Nicotine Use Disorders: Treatment Principles and Alternatives 300
- D. Alcohol Use Disorders: Treatment Principles and Alternatives 301
- E. Marijuana Use Disorders: Treatment Principles and Alternatives 301
- F. Cocaine Use Disorders: Treatment Principles and Alternatives 301
- G. Opioid Use Disorders: Treatment Principles and Alternatives 302

II. General Treatment Principles 303
- A. Goals of Treatment 304
- B. Assessment 306
- C. Treatment Settings 310
- D. Psychiatric Management 316
- E. Somatic Treatments 321
- F. Psychosocial Treatments 324
- G. Clinical Features Influencing Treatment 333
- H. Legal and Confidentiality Issues 358

III. Treatment of Nicotine Dependence 359
- A. Overview 359
- B. Assessment 360
- C. Treatment Settings 362
- D. General Approach to Treatment 362
- E. Somatic Treatments 368
- F. Psychosocial Treatments 370
- G. Treatment of Smokers on Smoke-Free Wards 371
- H. Clinical Features Influencing Treatment 373

IV. Treatment of Alcohol-Related Disorders 377
- A. Overview 377
- B. Treatment Settings 378
- C. Somatic Treatments 379
- D. Psychosocial Treatments 385
- E. Clinical Features Influencing Treatment 388

V. Treatment of Marijuana-Related Disorders ... 391
A. Overview ... 391
B. Treatment Setting ... 391
C. Somatic Treatments ... 392
D. Psychosocial Treatments ... 392
E. Pregnancy ... 392

VI. Treatment of Cocaine-Related Disorders ... 393
A. Overview ... 393
B. Treatment Settings ... 393
C. Somatic Treatments ... 394
D. Psychosocial Treatments ... 396
E. Clinical Features Influencing Treatment ... 397

VII. Treatment of Opioid-Related Disorders ... 399
A. Overview ... 399
B. Treatment Settings ... 400
C. Somatic Treatments ... 401
D. Psychosocial Treatments ... 408
E. Clinical Features Influencing Treatment ... 409

Part B: Background Information and Review of Available Evidence ... 412

VIII. Disease Definition, Natural History and Course, and Epidemiology ... 412
A. Disease Definition and Diagnostic Features ... 412
B. Natural History and Course ... 414
C. Epidemiology ... 416

IX. Review and Synthesis of Available Evidence ... 421
A. Nicotine Dependence ... 421
B. Alcohol-Related Disorders ... 435
C. Marijuana-Related Disorders ... 446
D. Cocaine-Related Disorders ... 447
E. Opioid-Related Disorders ... 452

Part C: Future Research Needs ... 466

Individuals and Organizations That Submitted Comments ... 468

References ... 469

GUIDE TO USING THIS PRACTICE GUIDELINE

The *Practice Guideline for the Treatment of Patients With Substance Use Disorders,* 2nd Edition, consists of three parts (A, B, and C) and many sections, not all of which will be equally useful for all readers. The following guide is designed to help readers find the sections that will be most useful to them.

Part A, "Treatment Recommendations for Patients With Substance Use Disorders," is published as a supplement to the *American Journal of Psychiatry* and contains general and specific treatment recommendations. Section I summarizes the key recommendations of the guideline and codes each recommendation according to the degree of clinical confidence with which the recommendation is made. Section II, "General Treatment Principles," provides a general discussion of the formulation and implementation of a treatment plan as it applies to the individual patient. Section II.G, "Clinical Features Influencing Treatment," discusses a range of clinical considerations that could alter the general recommendations discussed in Section I. Sections III, IV, V, VI, and VII provide specific recommendations for the treatment of patients with nicotine-, alcohol-, marijuana-, cocaine-, and opioid-related disorders, respectively.

Part B, "Background Information and Review of Available Evidence," and Part C, "Future Research Needs," are not included in the *American Journal of Psychiatry* supplement but are provided with Part A in the complete guideline, which is available in print format from American Psychiatric Publishing, Inc. (http://www.appi.org) and online through the American Psychiatric Association (http://www.psych.org). Part B provides an overview of substance use disorders, including general information on their natural history, course, and epidemiology. It also provides a structured review and synthesis of the evidence that underlies the recommendations made in Part A. Part C draws from the previous sections and summarizes areas for which more research data are needed to guide clinical decisions.

To share feedback on this or other published APA practice guidelines, a form is available at http://www.psych.org/psych_pract/pg/reviewform.cfm.

DEVELOPMENT PROCESS

This practice guideline was developed under the auspices of the Steering Committee on Practice Guidelines. The development process is detailed in "APA Guideline Development Process," which is available from the APA Department of Quality Improvement and Psychiatric Services. The key features of this process with regard to this document include the following:

- A comprehensive literature review to identify all relevant randomized clinical trials as well as less rigorously designed clinical trials and case series when evidence from randomized trials was unavailable
- The development of evidence tables that summarized the key features of each identified study, including funding source, study design, sample sizes, subject characteristics, treatment characteristics, and treatment outcomes
- Initial drafting of the guideline by a work group that included psychiatrists with clinical and research expertise in substance use disorders
- The production of multiple revised drafts with widespread review (23 organizations and 70 individuals submitted significant comments)
- Approval by the APA Assembly and Board of Trustees
- Planned revisions at regular intervals

Relevant updates to the literature were identified through a MEDLINE literature search for articles published since the initial guideline edition, published in 1995. Thus MEDLINE was searched, using PubMed, between 1995 and 2002 using the keywords "substance use disorder OR substance use disorders OR substance use OR substance withdrawal OR substance intoxication OR substance abuse OR substance dependence OR alcohol abuse OR alcohol dependence OR cocaine abuse OR cocaine dependence OR cocaine use OR marijuana use OR marijuana abuse OR marijuana dependence OR opiate abuse OR opiate dependence OR opiate use OR opioid abuse OR opioid dependence OR opioid use OR heroin abuse OR heroin dependence OR heroin use OR cigarette OR cigarettes OR smoking OR tobacco OR tobacco use OR tobacco use disorder OR tobacco use cessation OR smoking cessation." This search yielded 89,231 references, of which 4,373 were controlled clinical trials; randomized, controlled trials; or meta-analyses; 4,101 of the 4,373 references were studies in humans, were written in the English language, and had abstracts. Evidence tables were developed for these results. Later in the development process, a second MEDLINE literature search, using PubMed, on the same keywords for the period 2003 to February 2005 yielded an additional 25,003 references, of which 1,114 were controlled clinical trials; randomized, controlled trials; or meta-analyses; 1,063 of these 1,114 references were studies in humans, were written in the English language, and had abstracts. Additional, less formal literature searches were conducted by APA staff and individual members of the Work Group on Substance Use Disorders. The Cochrane databases were also searched for relevant meta-analyses.

The summary of treatment recommendations is keyed according to the level of confidence with which each recommendation is made (indicated by a bracketed Roman numeral). In addition, each reference is followed by a bracketed letter that indicates the nature of the supporting evidence.

PART A

TREATMENT RECOMMENDATIONS FOR PATIENTS WITH SUBSTANCE USE DISORDERS

I. EXECUTIVE SUMMARY

A. CODING SYSTEM

Each recommendation is identified as meriting one of three categories of endorsement, based on the level of clinical confidence regarding the recommendation, as indicated by a bracketed Roman numeral after the statement. The three categories are as follows:

[I] Recommended with substantial clinical confidence.
[II] Recommended with moderate clinical confidence.
[III] May be recommended on the basis of individual circumstances.

B. GENERAL TREATMENT PRINCIPLES

Individuals with substance use disorders are heterogeneous with regard to a number of clinically important features and domains of functioning. Consequently, a multimodal approach to treatment is typically required. Care of individuals with substance use disorders includes conducting a complete assessment, treating intoxication and withdrawal syndromes when necessary, addressing co-occurring psychiatric and general medical conditions, and developing and implementing an overall treatment plan. The goals of treatment include the achievement of abstinence or reduction in the use and effects of substances, reduction in the frequency and severity of relapse to substance use, and improvement in psychological and social functioning.

1. Assessment

A comprehensive psychiatric evaluation is essential to guide the treatment of a patient with a substance use disorder [I]. The assessment includes 1) a detailed history of the patient's past and present substance use and the effects of substance use on the patient's cognitive, psychological, behavioral, and physiological functioning; 2) a general medical and psychiatric history and examination; 3) a history of psychiatric treatments and outcomes; 4) a family and social history; 5) screening of blood, breath, or urine for substance used; 6) other laboratory tests to help confirm the presence or absence of conditions that frequently co-occur with substance use disorders; and 7) with the patient's permission, contacting a significant other for additional information.

2. Psychiatric management

Psychiatric management is the foundation of treatment for patients with substance use disorders [I]. Psychiatric management has the following specific objectives: motivating the patient to change, establishing and maintaining a therapeutic alliance with the patient, assessing the patient's safety and clinical status, managing the patient's intoxication and withdrawal states, developing and facilitating the patient's adherence to a treatment plan, preventing the patient's relapse, educating the patient about substance use disorders, and reducing the morbidity and sequelae of substance use disorders. Psychiatric management is generally combined with specific treatments carried out in a collaborative manner with professionals of various disciplines at a variety of sites, including community-based agencies, clinics, hospitals, detoxification programs, and residential treatment facilities. Many patients benefit from involvement in self-help group meetings, and such involvement can be encouraged as part of psychiatric management.

3. Specific treatments

The specific pharmacological and psychosocial treatments reviewed below are generally applied in the context of programs that combine a number of different treatment modalities.

a) Pharmacological treatments

Pharmacological treatments are beneficial for selected patients with specific substance use disorders [I]. The categories of pharmacological treatments are 1) medications to treat intoxication and withdrawal states, 2) medications to decrease the reinforcing effects of abused substances, 3) agonist maintenance therapies, 4) antagonist therapies, 5) abstinence-promoting and relapse prevention therapies, and 6) medications to treat comorbid psychiatric conditions.

b) Psychosocial treatments

Psychosocial treatments are essential components of a comprehensive treatment program [I]. Evidence-based psychosocial treatments include cognitive-behavioral therapies (CBTs, e.g., relapse prevention, social skills training), motivational enhancement therapy (MET), behavioral therapies (e.g., community reinforcement, contingency management), 12-step facilitation (TSF), psychodynamic therapy/interpersonal therapy (IPT), self-help manuals, behavioral self-control, brief interventions, case management, and group, marital, and family therapies. There is evidence to support the efficacy of integrated treatment for patients with a co-occurring substance use and psychiatric disorder; such treatment includes blending psychosocial therapies used to treat specific substance use disorders with psychosocial treatment approaches for other psychiatric diagnoses (e.g., CBT for depression).

4. Formulation and implementation of a treatment plan

The goals of treatment and the specific therapies chosen to achieve these goals may vary among patients and even for the same patient at different phases of an illness [I]. Because many substance use disorders are chronic, patients usually require long-term treatment, although the intensity and specific components of treatment may vary over time [I]. The treatment plan includes the following components: 1) psychiatric management; 2) a strategy for achieving abstinence or reducing the effects or use of substances of abuse; 3) efforts to enhance ongoing adherence with the treatment program, prevent relapse, and improve functioning; and 4) additional treatments necessary for patients with a co-occurring mental illness or general medical condition.

The duration of treatment should be tailored to the individual patient's needs and may vary from a few months to several years [I]. It is important to intensify the monitoring for substance use during periods when the patient is at a high risk of relapsing, including during the early stages of treatment, times of transition to less intensive levels of care, and the first year after active treatment has ceased [I].

5. Treatment settings

Treatment settings vary with regard to the availability of specific treatment modalities, the degree of restricted access to substances that are likely to be abused, the availability of general medical and psychiatric care, and the overall milieu and treatment philosophy.

Patients should be treated in the least restrictive setting that is likely to be safe and effective [I]. Commonly available treatment settings include hospitals, residential treatment facilities, partial hospitalization programs, and outpatient programs. Decisions regarding the site of care should be based on the patient's ability to cooperate with and benefit from the treatment offered, refrain from illicit use of substances, and avoid high-risk behaviors as well as the patient's need for structure and support or particular treatments that may be available only in certain settings [I]. Patients move from one level of care to another based on these factors and an assessment of their ability to safely benefit from a different level of care [I].

Hospitalization is appropriate for patients who 1) have a substance overdose who cannot be safely treated in an outpatient or emergency department setting; 2) are at risk for severe or medically complicated withdrawal syndromes (e.g., history of delirium tremens, documented history of very heavy alcohol use and high tolerance); 3) have co-occurring general medical conditions that make ambulatory detoxification unsafe; 4) have a documented history of not engaging in or benefiting from treatment in a less intensive setting (e.g., residential, outpatient); 5) have a level of psychiatric comorbidity that would markedly impair their ability to participate in, adhere to, or benefit from treatment or have a co-occurring disorder that by itself would require hospital-level care (e.g., depression with suicidal thoughts, acute psychosis); 6) manifest substance use or other behaviors that constitute an acute danger to themselves or others; or 7) have not responded to or were unable to adhere to less intensive treatment efforts and have a substance use disorder(s) that endangers others or poses an ongoing threat to their physical and mental health [I].

Residential treatment is indicated for patients who do not meet the clinical criteria for hospitalization but whose lives and social interactions have come to focus predominantly on substance use, who lack sufficient social and vocational skills, and who lack substance-free social supports to maintain abstinence in an outpatient setting [II]. Residential treatment of ≥3 months is associated with better long-term outcomes in such patients [II]. For patients with an opioid use disorder, therapeutic communities have been found effective [II].

Partial hospitalization should be considered for patients who require intensive care but have a reasonable probability of refraining from illicit use of substances outside a restricted setting [II]. Partial hospitalization settings are frequently used for patients leaving hospitals or residential settings who remain at high risk for relapse. These include patients who are thought to lack sufficient motivation to continue in treatment, have severe psychiatric comorbidity and/or a history of relapse to substance use in the immediate posthospitalization or postresidential period, and are returning to a high-risk environment and have limited psychosocial supports for abstaining from substance use. Partial hospitalization programs are also indicated for patients who are doing poorly despite intensive outpatient treatment [II].

Outpatient treatment of substance use disorders is appropriate for patients whose clinical condition or environmental circumstances do not require a more intensive level of care [I]. As in other treatment settings, a comprehensive approach is optimal, using, where indicated, a variety of psychotherapeutic and pharmacological interventions along with behavioral monitoring [I]. Most treatment for patients with alcohol dependence or abuse can be successfully conducted outside the hospital (e.g., in outpatient or partial hospitalization settings) [II], although patients with alcohol withdrawal must be detoxified in a setting that provides frequent clinical assessment and any necessary treatments [I]. For many patients with a cocaine use disorder, clinical and research experience suggests the effectiveness of intensive outpatient treatment in which a variety of treatment modalities are simultaneously used and in which the focus is the maintenance of abstinence [II]. The treatment of patients with nicotine dependence or a marijuana use disorder occurs on an outpatient basis unless patients are hospitalized for other reasons [I].

6. Clinical features influencing treatment

In planning and implementing treatment, a clinician should consider several variables with regard to patients: comorbid psychiatric and general medical conditions, gender-related factors, age, social milieu and living environment, cultural factors, gay/lesbian/bisexual/transgender issues, and family characteristics [I]. Given the high prevalence of comorbidity of substance use disorders and other psychiatric disorders, the diagnostic distinction between substance use symptoms and those of other disorders should receive particular attention, and specific treatment of comorbid disorders should be provided [I]. In addition to pharmacotherapies specific to a patient's substance use disorder, various psychotherapies may also be indicated when a patient has a co-occurring psychiatric disorder, psychosocial stressors, or other life circumstances that exacerbate the substance use disorder or interfere with treatment [I]. A patient's cessation of substance use may also be associated with changes in his or her psychiatric symptoms or the metabolism of medications (e.g., altered antipsychotic metabolism via cytochrome P450 1A2 with smoking cessation) that will necessitate adjustment of psychotropic medication doses [I].

In women of childbearing age, the possibility of pregnancy needs to be considered [I]. Each of the substances discussed in this practice guideline has the potential to affect the fetus, and psychosocial treatment to encourage substance abstinence during pregnancy is recommended [I]. With some substances, concomitant agonist treatment may be preferable to continued substance use. In pregnant smokers, treatment with nicotine replacement therapy (NRT) may be helpful [II]. For pregnant women with an opioid use disorder, treatment with methadone [I] or buprenorphine [II] can be a useful adjunct to psychosocial treatment.

C. NICOTINE USE DISORDERS: TREATMENT PRINCIPLES AND ALTERNATIVES

1. Pharmacological treatments

Pharmacological treatment is recommended for individuals who wish to stop smoking and have not achieved cessation without pharmacological agents or who prefer to use such agents [I]. There are six medications approved by the U.S. Food and Drug Administration (FDA) for nicotine dependence, including five NRTs (patch, gum, spray, lozenge, and inhaler) and bupropion. These are all first-line agents that are equally effective in alleviating withdrawal symptoms and reducing smoking. Any of these could be used based on patient preference, the route of administration, and the side-effect profile [I]. Significant adverse events to NRTs, including dependence, are rare. Although combined psychosocial and medication treatment produces the best outcomes in treating nicotine use disorders, these medications are effective even when no psychosocial treatment is provided [I]. Using a combination of these first-line treatments may also improve outcome [II]. Nortriptyline and clonidine have utility as second-line agents but appear to have more side effects [II]. Other medications and acupuncture have not been proven to be effective.

2. Psychosocial treatments

Psychosocial treatments are also effective for the treatment of nicotine dependence and include CBTs [I], behavioral therapies [I], brief interventions [II], and MET [II] provided in individual [I], group [I], or telephone [I] formats or via self-help materials [III] and Internet-based formats [III]. The efficacy of treatment is related to the amount of psychosocial treatment received. The 12-step programs, hypnosis, and inpatient therapy have not been proven effective.

D. ALCOHOL USE DISORDERS: TREATMENT PRINCIPLES AND ALTERNATIVES

1. Management of intoxication and withdrawal

The acutely intoxicated patient should be monitored and maintained in a safe environment [II]. Symptoms of alcohol withdrawal typically begin within 4–12 hours after cessation or reduction of alcohol use, peak in intensity during the second day of abstinence, and generally resolve within 4–5 days. Serious complications include seizures, hallucinations, and delirium.

The treatment of patients in moderate to severe withdrawal includes efforts to reduce central nervous system (CNS) irritability and restore physiological homeostasis [I] and generally requires the use of thiamine and fluids [I], benzodiazepines [I], and, in some patients, other medications such as anticonvulsants, clonidine, or antipsychotic agents [II]. Once clinical stability is achieved, the tapering of benzodiazepines and other medications should be carried out as necessary, and the patient should be observed for the reemergence of withdrawal symptoms and the emergence of signs and symptoms suggestive of co-occurring psychiatric disorders [I].

2. Pharmacological treatments

Specific pharmacotherapies for alcohol-dependent patients have well-established efficacy and moderate effectiveness. Naltrexone may attenuate some of the reinforcing effects of alcohol [I], although data on its long-term efficacy are limited. The use of long-acting, injectable naltrexone may promote adherence, but published research is limited and FDA approval is pending. Acamprosate, a γ-aminobutyric acid (GABA) analog that may decrease alcohol craving in abstinent individuals, may also be an effective adjunctive medication in motivated patients who are concomitantly receiving psychosocial treatment [I]. Disulfiram is an effective adjunct to a comprehensive treatment program for reliable, motivated patients whose drinking may be triggered by events that suddenly increase alcohol craving [II].

3. Psychosocial treatments

Psychosocial treatments found effective for some patients with an alcohol use disorder include MET [I], CBT [I], behavioral therapies [I], TSF [I], marital and family therapies [I], group therapies [II], and psychodynamic therapy/IPT [III]. Recommending that patients participate in self-help groups, such as Alcoholics Anonymous (AA), is often helpful [I].

E. MARIJUANA USE DISORDERS: TREATMENT PRINCIPLES AND ALTERNATIVES

Studies of treatment for marijuana use disorders are limited. No specific pharmacotherapies for marijuana withdrawal or dependence can be recommended [I]. In terms of psychosocial therapies, an intensive relapse prevention approach that combines motivational interventions with the development of coping skills may be effective for the treatment of marijuana dependence [III], but further study of these approaches is necessary.

F. COCAINE USE DISORDERS: TREATMENT PRINCIPLES AND ALTERNATIVES

1. Management of intoxication and withdrawal

Cocaine intoxication is usually self-limited and typically requires only supportive care [II]. However, hypertension, tachycardia, seizures, and persecutory delusions can occur with cocaine intoxication and may require specific treatment [II]. Acutely agitated patients may benefit from sedation with benzodiazepines [III].

2. Pharmacological treatments

Pharmacological treatment is not ordinarily indicated as an initial treatment for patients with cocaine dependence. In addition, no pharmacotherapies have FDA indications for the treatment of cocaine dependence. However, for individuals who fail to respond to psychosocial treatment alone, some medications (topiramate, disulfiram, or modafinil) may be promising when integrated into psychosocial treatments.

3. Psychosocial treatments

For many patients with a cocaine use disorder, psychosocial treatments focusing on abstinence are effective [I]. In particular, CBTs [I], behavioral therapies [I], and 12-step-oriented individual drug counseling [I] can be useful, although efficacy of these therapies varies across subgroups of patients. Recommending regular participation in a self-help group may improve the outcome for selected patients with a cocaine use disorder [III].

G. OPIOID USE DISORDERS: TREATMENT PRINCIPLES AND ALTERNATIVES

1. Management of intoxication and withdrawal

Acute opioid intoxication of a mild to moderate degree usually does not require specific treatment [II]. However, severe opioid overdose, marked by respiratory depression, may be fatal and requires treatment in an emergency department or inpatient setting [I]. Naloxone will reverse respiratory depression and other manifestations of opioid overdose [I].

The treatment of opioid withdrawal is directed at safely ameliorating acute symptoms and facilitating the patient's entry into a long-term treatment program for opioid use disorders [I]. Strategies found to be effective include substitution of methadone or buprenorphine for the opioid followed by gradual tapering [I]; abrupt discontinuation of opioids, with the use of clonidine to suppress withdrawal symptoms [II]; and clonidine-naltrexone detoxification [II]. It is essential that the treating physician assess the patient for the presence of other substances, particularly alcohol, benzodiazepines, or other anxiolytic or sedative agents, because the concurrent use of or withdrawal from other substances can complicate the treatment of opioid withdrawal [I]. Anesthesia-assisted rapid opioid detoxification (AROD) is not recommended because of lack of proven efficacy and adverse risk-benefit ratios.

2. Pharmacological treatments

Maintenance treatment with methadone or buprenorphine is appropriate for patients with a prolonged history (>1 year) of opioid dependence [I]. The goals of treatment are to achieve a stable maintenance dose of opioid agonist and facilitate engagement in a comprehensive program of rehabilitation [I]. Maintenance treatment with naltrexone is an alternative strategy [I], although the utility of this strategy is often limited by lack of patient adherence and low treatment retention.

3. Psychosocial treatments

Psychosocial treatments are effective components of a comprehensive treatment plan for patients with an opioid use disorder [II]. Behavioral therapies (e.g., contingency management) [II], CBTs [II], psychodynamic psychotherapy [III], and group and family therapies [III] have been found to be effective for some patients with an opioid use disorder. Recommending regular participation in self-help groups may also be useful [III].

II. GENERAL TREATMENT PRINCIPLES

Although many of the principles presented in this section apply to all substances reviewed in this guideline (i.e., nicotine, alcohol, marijuana, cocaine, and opioids), not all principles are applicable to the treatment of every substance use disorder. This is particularly true for nicotine dependence treatment, as nicotine dependence rarely causes the behavioral or social harm seen with other substance dependencies.

Individuals with substance use disorders are heterogeneous with regard to a number of clinically important features:

- The number and type of substances used
- The individual's genetic vulnerability for developing a substance use disorder(s)
- The severity of the disorder, the rapidity with which it develops, and the degree of associated functional impairment(s)
- The individual's awareness of the substance use disorder as a problem
- The individual's readiness for change and motivation to enter into treatment for the purpose of change
- The associated general medical and psychiatric conditions (either co-occurring or induced by substance use)
- The individual's strengths (protective and resiliency factors) and vulnerabilities
- The social, environmental, and cultural context in which the individual lives and will be treated

It is clinically helpful when assessing patients to use a spectrum that includes *use, misuse, abuse,* and *dependence.* The latter two terms represent formal diagnostic categories. Use of a substance may or may not be clinically significant. If use of a substance is thought to be potentially clinically significant but does not meet diagnostic criteria for abuse or dependence, it may be characterized as "misuse," although this is not a formal diagnostic category. Even when functional impairment is absent or limited, substance misuse can be an early indicator of an individual's vulnerability to developing a chronic substance use disorder. Brief early interventions can effectively reduce this progression (1–3), although follow-up reinforcement appears necessary for sustained utility. Most individuals presenting or referred for treatment of a substance use disorder, however, have been unable to stop using substances on their own. They often exhibit functional impairments across many categories (e.g., health, social and family, occupational, financial, legal) and have a history of chronic or relapsing episodes of problematic substance use. This practice guideline refers primarily to the care of such individuals.

As with treatment models for chronic diseases, treatment for individuals with substance use disorders occurs in temporal phases that include initial assessment, acute intervention, and long-term intervention and/or maintenance, with frequent reassessment during episodic flares in substance use (4). During the assessment phase, the specific variables associated with an individual's substance use are evaluated (e.g., genetic vulnerability, environmental influences, behavioral patterns of use, positive and negative consequences of use, associated conditions that trigger or otherwise interact with use, risk of withdrawal). In addition, the level of risk for morbidity or mortality associated with substance use is determined. Immediate intervention to provide safety to the patient in a medically monitored environment is recommended for individuals who present with high-risk intoxication or withdrawal states or altered mental states (e.g., psychosis, suicidality, agitation) that are associated with a risk of danger to self or others. After the patient is stabilized, the patient's immediate needs regarding safety and stability should be addressed to prepare the patient to enter into comprehensive, long-term treatment of the substance use disorder and its associated conditions. Such acute interventions may be focused on goals such as preserving health, achieving financial security, and finding stable housing. It is recommended that individuals in the patient's family or social network be included in the treatment process so they may learn about the disorder, help monitor the patient's progress, and assist in the patient's maintaining existing relationships or repairing troubled ones (5).

Depending on the clinical circumstances and an individual's readiness for change (6), treatment strategies may emphasize providing motivational enhancement, teaching risk-reduction behaviors and skills, helping the patient achieve abstinence and learn relapse prevention skills, or combining substitution agonist therapies (e.g., methadone or buprenorphine for opioid-dependent individuals, NRTs for tobacco-dependent individuals) with therapy to help the patient acquire relapse prevention skills. In addition, individuals with substance use disorders often require multimodal treatment to address associated conditions that have contributed to or resulted from the substance use disorder. Specific pharmacological and psychosocial treatments for patients with a substance use disorder are reviewed separately in this guideline; however, in practice they are often implemented together, as combined treatments lead to better treatment retention and outcomes (7).

A. GOALS OF TREATMENT

The evidence to date suggests that substance-dependent individuals who achieve sustained abstinence from the abused substance have the best long-term outcomes (8, 9). Psychiatrists will, however, frequently encounter individuals who wish to reduce their substance use to a "controlled" level (i.e., use without apparent functional consequences). Although some of these individuals, particularly those with less severe problems, may be helped to reach a stable level of use (e.g., "controlled" drinking) that does not cause morbidity (10), a goal of "controlled" substance use is unrealistic for most individuals presenting with a substance use disorder. Furthermore, setting "controlled" use as a primary goal of treatment may initially dissuade individuals from working toward abstinence. However, treatment may be initially facilitated by the clinician's accepting the patient's goal for moderation while sharing with the patient any reservations the clinician may have about the likelihood of success. If the clinician believes that any level of substance use for the individual carries a risk of acute or chronic negative consequences, he or she should share with the patient this concern and the belief that long-term abstinence would be the best course of action. In certain circumstances it may be reasonable, however, for an individual to begin treatment by setting a short-term goal of reducing or containing dangerous substance use as a first step toward achieving the longer-term goal of sustained abstinence (11).

The goals for treating a substance use disorder begin with engaging the patient in treatment and may ultimately progress to the patient's achieving and maintaining complete abstinence from all problematic substances. Along this treatment spectrum or timeline, an individual and his or her physician may develop immediate goals involving risk reduction, such as reducing the frequency and quantity of substances taken, abstaining from some (but not all) substances according to assessment of risk (e.g., abstaining from injected heroin without abstaining from cannabis use), or limiting substance use to lower-risk situations (e.g., continuing to drink at home but avoiding drinking in other environments or driving while drinking). The guiding elements of treatment planning consist of ongoing efforts to reduce the patient's substance use and prevent a return to previously dangerous patterns of use. It is essential to complement this approach with parallel setting of goals to repair an individual's functional decline and develop new pathways for safe, sober pleasures. These issues are outlined below.

1. Treatment retention and substance use reduction or abstinence as initial goals of treatment

The ideal outcome for most individuals with substance use disorders is total cessation of substance use. Nonetheless, many individuals are either unable or unmotivated to reach this goal, particularly in the early phases of treatment and/or after a relapse to substance use. Such individuals can still be helped to minimize the direct and indirect negative effects of ongoing substance use. The interventions discussed in this practice guideline may result in substantial reductions in the general medical, psychiatric, interpersonal, familial/parental, occupational, or other difficulties commonly associated with substance abuse or dependence. For example, reductions in the amount or frequency of substance use, substitution of a less risky substance, and reduction of high-risk behaviors associated with substance use may be achievable goals when abstinence is initially unobtainable (12, 13). Engaging an individual to participate and remain in treatment that may eventually lead to further reductions in substance use and its associated morbidity is a critical early goal of treatment planning and is often enhanced by motivational interviewing techniques (14).

2. Reduction in the frequency and severity of substance use episodes

Reduction in the frequency and severity of substance use episodes is a primary goal of long-term treatment (15). The individual is educated about common types of substance use triggers, such as environmental cues, stress, and exposure to a priming substance (16, 17). The individual is then helped to develop skills to prevent substance use; these skills include identifying and avoiding high-risk situations as well as developing alternative responses to situations in which substance use may occur. Individuals are at a greater risk of using substances when any of the following are present: 1) craving or urges to use a substance due to acute or protracted withdrawal states and/or classically conditioned responses to cues associated with substance use (18–20); 2) easy access to substances; 3) social facilitation of substance use (e.g., holiday parties, association with other substance users); 4) negative affective states; 5) negative life events, or any significant, even positively viewed, life event if the event carries with it a significant increase in responsibility (e.g., marriage, the birth of a child, beginning school or a new job, work promotion); 6) physical discomfort; 7) unstructured time or boredom; or 8) nonadherence to prescribed treatment. Many clinicians do not recognize that individuals with substance use disorders have a chronic condition and may have future episodes of substance use. Therefore, the clinician may become discouraged when an individual doing well in treatment over an extended period of time resumes substance use. A useful clinical strategy is to explicitly anticipate the reality of future substance use and plan a strategy for recovery in the event of substance use relapse; such a strategy helps both the patient and the clinician optimally manage and contain the negative consequences resulting from a return to substance use.

3. Improvement in psychological, social, and adaptive functioning

Substance use disorders are associated with impairments in psychological development and social adjustment, family and social relations, school and work performance, financial status, health, and personal independence (e.g., as a result of legal charges associated with substance use, suspension of the individual's driver's license after being convicted of driving under the influence of an intoxicating substance) (21). For optimal outcome, the treatment of a substance use disorder may also include strategies that target repair of damages or losses that resulted from the individual's substance use; aid in developing effective interpersonal, vocational, and proactive coping skills; and enhance familial and interpersonal relations that will support an abstinent lifestyle. It is particularly important to provide comprehensive treatments when individuals have co-occurring psychiatric or general medical conditions that significantly influence relapse risk (e.g., chronic pain, depression, anxiety, impaired cognition, and impulse control disorders) (22–24).

TABLE 1. DSM-IV-TR Criteria for Substance Abuse

A. A maladaptive pattern of substance use leading to clinically significant impairment or distress, as manifested by one (or more) of the following, occurring within a 12-month period:

1) recurrent substance use resulting in a failure to fulfill major role obligations at work, school, or home (e.g., repeated absences or poor work performance related to substance use; substance-related absences, suspensions, or expulsions from school; neglect of children or household)
2) recurrent substance use in situations in which it is physically hazardous (e.g., driving an automobile or operating a machine when impaired by substance use)
3) recurrent substance-related legal problems (e.g., arrests for substance-related disorderly conduct)
4) continued substance use despite having persistent or recurrent social or interpersonal problems caused or exacerbated by the effects of the substance (e.g., arguments with spouse about consequences of intoxication, physical fights)

B. The symptoms have never met the criteria for substance dependence for this class of substance.

B. ASSESSMENT

The term "substance use disorder" encompasses a number of different substances and disorders (i.e., abuse, dependence, intoxication, withdrawal, and psychiatric syndromes and disorders that result from substance use). Substance abuse and substance dependence are two disorders that are frequently encountered, and their criteria are applicable across substances. The criteria for these disorders are presented in Tables 1 and 2. However, it is beyond the scope of this practice guideline to describe all the substance use disorders, and the reader is referred to DSM-IV-TR for a full description.

A clinician's approach to assessing a substance use disorder will differ depending on the context in which an individual presents for treatment. An individual who recognizes the presence of a substance use disorder may present willingly for treatment and be amenable to a thorough assessment (as outlined below). However, many individuals will not be similarly motivated, and retaining them in treatment may require adapting the assessment process to their level of insight and motivational state. For example, individuals with benzodiazepine dependence will often present for treatment of an anxiety disorder but have no motivation to reduce their benzodiazepine use. Likewise, individuals with bipolar disorder will often present with a co-occurring substance use disorder but may not identify or recognize substance use as problematic (e.g., the use of alcohol at night to facilitate sleep onset). In such cases, educational efforts to help the individual recognize the substance use disorder as a problem may be helpful. This may involve extending the assessment phase over time rather than attempting to acquire all the patient's information at once so that the clinician can tailor the intervention to the patient's particular stage of change (25).

In an alternative scenario, an individual may be coerced into an assessment by frustrated family members or drug treatment diversion programs within the justice system. Such individuals may be resentful of the assessment process and have no motivation for changing their behavior other than the stipulations of family or the court system. Under these conditions, the clinician must attempt to establish an alliance with the individual in order to be viewed as a valuable source of information and aid rather than as a punitive extension of the referring sources. Retaining the individual in treatment will also take precedence over treating the disorder but may not always be possible. A full assessment of the individual's substance use disorder(s) may need to be gathered in pieces over time, with details being added to the initial picture when the individual is more comfortable sharing information pertinent to the pattern of his or her substance use and more motivated to contemplate change.

TABLE 2. DSM-IV-TR Criteria for Substance Dependence

A maladaptive pattern of substance use, leading to clinically significant impairment or distress, as manifested by three (or more) of the following, occurring at any time in the same 12-month period:

1) tolerance, as defined by either of the following:
   a) a need for markedly increased amounts of the substance to achieve intoxication or desired effect
   b) markedly diminished effect with continued use of the same amount of the substance
2) withdrawal, as manifested by either of the following:
   a) the characteristic withdrawal syndrome for the substance
   b) the same (or a closely related) substance is taken to relieve or avoid withdrawal symptoms
3) the substance is often taken in larger amounts or over a longer period than was intended
4) there is a persistent desire or unsuccessful efforts to cut down or control substance use
5) a great deal of time is spent in activities necessary to obtain the substance (e.g., visiting multiple doctors or driving long distances), use the substance (e.g., chain-smoking), or recover from its effects
6) important social, occupational, or recreational activities are given up or reduced because of substance use
7) the substance use is continued despite knowledge of having a persistent or recurrent physical or psychological problem that is likely to have been caused or exacerbated by the substance (e.g., current cocaine use despite recognition of cocaine-induced depression, or continued drinking despite recognition that an ulcer was made worse by alcohol consumption)

The diagnosis should specify "With Physiological Dependence" (either item 1 or 2 is present) or "Without Physiological Dependence" (neither item 1 nor 2 is present).

All individuals undergoing a psychiatric evaluation should be screened for a substance use disorder, regardless of their age, presentation, or referral source. Several empirically validated screening tools are available that do not require extensive training or time to use during an initial assessment. Commonly used screens include the four-item CAGE screen for alcohol abuse (Have you ever felt the need to **C**ut down on drinking, been **A**nnoyed by others' criticism of your drinking, felt **G**uilty about drinking, needed an **E**ye-opener drink first thing in the morning?) (26), the 10-item Alcohol Use Disorders Identification Test (27), and the Drug Abuse Screening Test, a 20-item self-report assessment that screens for commonly abused substances other than alcohol (28). If screening instruments or other assessment questions reveal that an individual has ever used substances, it is important to obtain a history of current and past substance use, including the frequency of substance use and the quantity of the substance used per using episode. The clinician should also inquire about the individual's current caffeine and nicotine use, past cigarette use in pack-years (defined as the number of packs per day multiplied by the number of years of smoking), and, for current smokers, the time from waking in the morning to their first cigarette.

It is also important for the assessing clinician to inquire about specific substance misuse if an individual's work is associated with increased risk because of occupational demands, privileged access to controlled substances, or a desire to enhance performance. For example, firefighters, police, and emergency personnel have a high prevalence of alcohol dependence related to job stress (29). Misuse of prescription substances or anesthetics is common among health care or veterinary medicine personnel; when compared with other physicians who misuse substances, anesthesiologists have been shown to be more likely to misuse opioids (30). Synthesis and misuse of controlled substances have also been observed in medicinal chemists. Anabolic steroid hormone precursors may be misused by athletes, and stimulant drugs may be misused by commercial truck drivers attempting to stay awake longer or by models and actors wanting to lose weight. Cocaine use appears to be a hazard among staff in restaurants and the entertainment industry. The clinician will also want to ask about other situations in an individual's history that may put him or her at higher risk for substance misuse, such as a history of trauma, psychiatric disorders, or chronic medical conditions.

In evaluating an individual with a suspected or confirmed substance use disorder, a comprehensive psychiatric evaluation is essential. Information should be sought from the individual and, with the individual's consent, available family members and peers, current and past health professionals, employers, and others as appropriate. The goals of the assessment are to establish a multiaxial DSM-IV-TR diagnosis, including identification of current and past substance use disorders as well as other comorbid psychiatric and physical disorders, and to identify other factors that are important to developing a treatment plan. Specific elements of the assessment may include the following:

1. A systematic inquiry into the mode of onset, quantity, frequency, and duration of substance use; the escalation of use over time; the motivation for use; the specific circumstances of the individual's substance use (e.g., where, with whom, how much, by what route of administration); the desired effect of the substance used; the most recent dose of each substance used; the time elapsed since the most recent use; the degree of associated intoxication; the severity of associated withdrawal syndromes; and the subjective effects of all substances used, including substances other than the individual's "drug of choice." As the psychiatrist elicits the individual's substance use history, he or she should also determine if the individual meets DSM-IV-TR criteria for abuse or dependence (see Tables 1 and 2) for each substance used. Because many patients entering treatment for a specific substance use disorder are using more than one substance, assessment should routinely include questions about the use of multiple substances, including which substances are used in combination, in what order, and for what effect. Use of over-the-counter and prescription medications should also be ascertained. If prescription medications are being used, it is important to learn if the medication has been prescribed for the individual or for someone else.
2. A history of any prior treatment for a substance use disorder, including the characteristics of the treatment such as setting; context (e.g., voluntary or involuntary); modalities used; duration and, if applicable, dose of treatment; adherence to treatment; and short-term (3-month), intermediate (1-year), and longer-term outcomes as measured by subsequent substance use, level of social and occupational functioning achieved, and other outcome variables. Previous efforts to control or stop substance use outside of a formal treatment setting should also be discussed. For individuals who had previous treatment or periods of abstinence, additional history may include the duration of abstinence, the factors that promoted or helped sustain abstinence, the impact of abstinence on psychiatric functioning, the circumstances surrounding relapse (e.g., whether the relapse was related to withdrawal symptoms, exacerbation of a psychiatric disorder, or psychosocial stressors), the individual's attitude toward prior treatment, nontreatment experiences, and expectations about future treatments.
3. A comprehensive general medical and psychiatric history, including mental status and physical examination, to ascertain the presence or absence of co-occurring psychiatric or general medical disorders as well as signs and symptoms of intoxication or withdrawal. Psychological or neuropsychological testing may also be indicated for some individuals (e.g., to assess an individual's level of cognitive impairment). When a clinician is attempting to ascertain an individual's current medication use, he or she should specifically ask about prescribed and nonprescribed medications, including vitamins and herbal products.

4. Qualitative and quantitative blood and urine screening for substances of abuse and laboratory tests for abnormalities that may accompany acute or chronic substance use. These tests may also be used during treatment to monitor for potential relapse. For some substances, such as alcohol and nicotine, breath tests may also be useful.
5. Screening for infectious and other diseases often found in substance-dependent individuals (e.g., human immunodeficiency virus [HIV], tuberculosis, hepatitis). Such individuals, particularly those with evidence of compromised immune function, are at high risk for these diseases.
6. A complete family and social history, including information on familial substance use or other psychiatric disorders; social factors contributing to the development or perpetuation of the substance use disorder (e.g., social facilitation of substance use); financial or legal problems; social supports, including peer relationships; school or vocational adjustment; and other functional impairments. When obtaining the family and social history, the psychiatrist may also wish to ask for permission to speak to family members, friends, or other significant people in the individual's life who may be able to provide important information regarding the individual's substance use disorder. In evaluating the impact of the individual's current living environment on his or her ability to adhere to treatment and refrain from substance use, it is important to determine whether and how household members and friends have supported or interfered with prior attempts at abstinence. The substance use status of others in the household and close friends (e.g., never used substances, former substance user, current substance user) should also be considered. If others in the household are currently using substances, their willingness to quit at the same time as the individual or to refrain from substance use in the presence of the individual should be assessed.
7. Individual preferences, motivations, and barriers for treatment. Individuals vary in their treatment preferences regarding pharmacotherapy, group therapy, individual therapy, and self-help treatments. Working with the individual's preferences is likely to lead to better treatment adherence and outcomes (31). For individuals who have a co-occurring psychiatric disorder, exacerbation of psychiatric symptoms can be an additional barrier (31, 32).

When a clinician is assessing a new patient and establishing a diagnosis, it is often difficult to distinguish between psychiatric symptoms resulting from substance use and those from a co-occurring psychiatric disorder. Anxiety, depression, mania, and psychosis are all commonly induced by various substances and can be observed with chronic use as well as during specific substance-induced states, including intoxication and withdrawal. Evaluation of psychiatric symptoms in substance-using individuals can be enhanced with repeated, longitudinal psychiatric assessments. As part of the initial assessment, it may also be useful to draw a timeline of all substances used and all psychiatric symptoms and/or disorders and to include in this timeline all prior treatments. This timeline approach can help determine the chronology of symptom development (i.e., whether the signs and symptoms predate or follow the onset of repetitive substance use), the presence or absence of symptoms during extended substance-free periods (e.g., 3 months or more), and the impact of each disorder on the presentation, clinical course, and outcome of the other(s).

The probability that an individual with a substance use disorder has a co-occurring psychiatric disorder and not a substance-induced psychiatric disorder is increased if at least one first-degree relative has a documented history of a similar disorder, the individual's symptoms are not typically observed in conjunction with the use of a particular substance, there is a clear history that psychiatric symptoms preceded the onset of the substance use disorder, or the symptoms were evident during extended substance-free periods. Such a distinction is relevant when a clinician must decide whether to treat the psychiatric symptoms with medications and determine how long to maintain a medication once it is started. For example, individuals with certain substance-induced psychotic symptoms, such as paranoia resulting from the use of stimulants or phencyclidine (PCP), may benefit from the short-term use of an antipsychotic medication. Conversely, symptoms of depression and anxiety coexisting with a substance use disorder may initially be addressed in psychosocial treatment but may require medication management if they do not improve over time.

C. TREATMENT SETTINGS

Individuals with substance use disorders may receive care in a variety of settings. Treatment settings vary according to the availability of resources (e.g., the presence or absence of medical monitoring, the specialization of services and therapy provided, the availability of psychiatric consultation), the freedom allowed the individual (e.g., locked versus open unit), the intensity of treatment duration/participation, and the milieu philosophy driving the primary interventions (e.g., medical model, educational, 12-step, peer support, faith based). Because treatment best occurs in a system that encourages cessation of all harmful substance use (33), consideration should be given to making treatment sites smoke free (33, 34). Although most studies indicate that smoking cessation does not increase alcohol relapse and may aid recovery in substance-dependent patients (35–37), one study found that smoking cessation worsened drinking outcomes in a group of alcohol-dependent patients (38).

1. Factors affecting choice of treatment setting

Individuals should be treated in the least restrictive setting that is likely to prove safe and effective. Decisions regarding the site of care should be based on the individual's 1) capacity and willingness to cooperate with treatment; 2) ability for self-care; 3) social environment (which may be supportive or high risk); 4) need for structure, support, and supervision to remain safe and abstinent; 5) need for specific treatments for co-occurring general medical or psychiatric conditions; 6) need for particular treatments or an intensity of treatment that may be available only in certain settings; and 7) preference for a particular treatment setting. In addition, the choice of setting should be guided by the particular substance(s) used, the medical risks associated with use of the substance(s), the accessibility of appropriate levels of care, and the stated goals of the individual's treatment plan (as described in Sections III through VII and as determined by the individual's clinical status).

Patients should be moved from one level of care to another on the basis of these factors; the decision to move to a less intensive level of care should consider these factors plus the clinician's assessment of a patient's readiness and ability to benefit from the less restrictive setting. To appropriately match patients and treatment settings, many clinicians, health insurers, hospitals, and treatment agencies use the American Society of Addiction Medicine (ASAM) patient placement criteria (39). These criteria provide an algorithm for placement that represents expert consensus and that is updated as additional evidence becomes available on treatment outcomes and levels of care.

Studies comparing the short-term, intermediate, and long-term benefits of treatment in various settings (i.e., inpatient, residential, partial hospitalization, outpatient) have a variety of methodological problems, including heterogeneity of individual populations, high dropout rates, lack of controlled trials, inappropriate comparison of outcomes after time-limited treatment interventions, and reliance on individual self-reports uncorroborated by data from collateral sources (40). Stated treatment goals, program features, and outcome measures vary across studies (41). A common finding among different treatments available for substance use disorders is that retention in treatment improves outcomes (42–45).

2. Commonly available treatment settings and services

Settings and services used in the treatment of substance use disorders may be considered as points along a continuum of care from most to least intensive. The specific factors leading to the choice of a particular setting for an individual patient are described below. The choice of a treatment setting may also be influenced by availability, given that communities differ in the variety of treatment services they offer and certain specialized treatment settings (e.g., dual-diagnosis partial hospitalization care) may not be widely available. For individuals with primary nicotine dependence or marijuana use disorders, treatment occurs in outpatient settings; information presented about other treatment settings may not be applicable to these populations.

a) Hospitals

The range of services available in hospital-based programs typically includes emergency detoxification and stabilization during withdrawal; assessment and treatment of general medical and psychiatric conditions; group, individual, and family therapies; psychoeducation; motivational counseling; and social service facilitation of follow-up care in available community services (46, 47). Psychiatric hospitals may offer dual-diagnosis inpatient units that specialize in the stabilization of co-occurring psychiatric and substance use disorders. For patients admitted to hospital-level care for other reasons (general medical or psychiatric), smoking cessation programs may also be available.

Hospital-based treatment settings may be secure (i.e., locked) or may permit individuals and visitors to come and go in a monitored but generally less restrictive fashion. Secure hospital settings should be considered for individuals with co-occurring psychiatric conditions whose clinical state would ordinarily require such a unit (e.g., actively suicidal individuals). Individuals with poor impulse control and judgment who in the presence of an "open door" are likely to leave the program or obtain or receive drugs on the unit are also candidates for a secure unit. In some states, individuals can reside on a secure unit in "conditional voluntary" status, which requires written notice and a time delay (e.g., 3 days) before the patient's request for discharge is approved or another disposition (e.g., commitment) is implemented. Such restrictions can provide a useful period of delay in which poorly motivated individuals can reconsider their wish to leave a program prematurely.

The available data do not support the notion that hospitalization per se has specific benefits over other treatment settings beyond the ability to address treatment objectives that require a medically monitored environment (48, 49). There is consensus (e.g., ASAM patient placement criteria) that individuals in one or more of the following categories may require hospital-level care:

1. Individuals with drug overdoses who cannot be safely treated in an outpatient or emergency department setting (e.g., individuals with severe respiratory depression, individuals in a coma)
2. Individuals in withdrawal who are at risk for a severe or complicated withdrawal syndrome (e.g., individuals dependent on multiple substances, individuals with a history of delirium tremens) or cannot receive the necessary medical assessment, monitoring, and treatment in a less intensive setting
3. Individuals with acute or chronic general medical conditions that make detoxification in a residential or ambulatory setting unsafe (e.g., individuals with severe cardiac disease)
4. Individuals with a documented history of not engaging in or benefiting from treatment in a less intensive setting (e.g., residential, outpatient)
5. Individuals with marked psychiatric comorbidity who are an acute danger to themselves or others (e.g., individuals who have depression with suicidal thoughts, acute psychosis)
6. Individuals manifesting substance use or other behaviors who are an acute danger to themselves or others
7. Individuals who have not responded to less intensive treatment efforts and whose substance use disorder(s) poses an ongoing threat to their physical and mental health

In general, the duration of hospital-based treatment should be dictated by the individual's current need to receive treatment in a restrictive setting and his or her capacity to access, safely participate in, and benefit from treatment in a less restrictive setting.

b) Partial hospitalization programs and intensive outpatient programs

Partial hospitalization and intensive outpatient programs can provide an intensive, structured treatment experience for individuals with substance use disorders who require more services than those generally available in traditional outpatient settings. Although the terms "partial hospitalization," "day treatment," and "intensive outpatient" programs may be used nearly interchangeably in different parts of the country, the ASAM patient placement criteria (39) define structured programming in partial hospitalization programs as 20 hours per week and in intensive outpatient programs as 9 hours per week. Partial hospitalization programs provide ancillary medical and psychiatric services, whereas intensive outpatient programs may be more variable in the accessibility of these services. Some patients enter these programs directly from the community. Alternatively, these programs are sometimes used as "step-down" programs for individuals leaving hospital or residential settings who are at a high risk of relapsing because of problems with motivation, the presence of frequent cravings or urges to use a substance, poor social supports, immediate environmental cues for relapse and/or availability of substances, and co-occurring medical and/or psychiatric disorders. The goal of such a "step-down" approach is to stabilize patients by retaining them in treatment and providing more extended intensive outpatient monitoring of relapse potential and co-occurring disorders. Partial hospitalization and intensive outpatient programs may also be used as a brief "step-up" in treatment for an outpatient who has had a relapse but who does not require medical detoxification or who has entered into a high-risk period for relapse because of life circumstances or recurrence of a co-occurring medical and/or psychiatric symptom (e.g., depressed mood, increased pain).

The treatment components of partial hospitalization programs may include some combination of individual and group therapy, vocational and educational counseling, family meetings, medically supervised use of adjunctive medications (e.g., opioid antagonists, antidepressants), random urine screening for substances of abuse, and treatment for any co-occurring psychiatric disorders. Intensive outpatient programs use individual therapy, group therapy, family therapy, and urine toxicology but vary in the amount of other therapeutic components used (50). An advantage of intensive outpatient programs is the availability of evening programs that accommodate day-shift employees. The availability of weekend programs varies for both partial hospitalization and intensive outpatient programs. Both kinds of programs aim to prepare the individual for transition to less intensive outpatient services and increased self-reliance through the practice and mastery of relapse prevention skills and the active use of self-help programs.

Limited data are available for the efficacy of partial hospitalization and intensive outpatient programs. Randomized, controlled trials have demonstrated that some individuals who would ordinarily be referred for residential- or hospital-level care do just as well in partial hospitalization care (51, 52). One study (53) comparing a more time-intensive day hospital program to an intensive outpatient program that was actually less time intensive found no differences in outcome for cocaine-dependent individuals, and another study comparing intensive with traditional outpatient treatment of the same population found no differences in outcome (54).

c) Residential treatment

Residential treatment is indicated primarily for individuals who do not meet clinical criteria for hospitalization but whose lives and social interactions have come to focus exclusively on substance use and who currently lack sufficient motivation and/or substance-free social supports to remain abstinent in an ambulatory setting. For these individuals, residential facilities provide a safe and substance-free environment in which residents learn individual and group living skills for preventing relapse. As in the case of hospital-based programs, residential treatment programs frequently provide psychosocial, occupational, and family assessment; psychoeducation; an introduction to self-help groups; and referral for social or vocational rehabilitative services where necessary (55). Many residential programs provide their own individual, group, and vocational counseling programs but rely on affiliated partial hospitalization or outpatient programs to supply the psychosocial and psychopharmacological treatment components of their programs. Residential treatment settings should have access to general medical and psychiatric care that is required to meet individual needs.

The duration of residential treatment should be dictated by the length of time necessary for the patient to meet specific criteria that would predict his or her successful transition to a less structured, less restrictive treatment setting (e.g., outpatient care). These criteria may include a demonstrated motivation to continue in outpatient treatment, the ability to remain abstinent even in situations where substances are potentially available, the availability of a living situation and associated support system conducive to remaining substance free (e.g., family, substance-free peers), sufficient stabilization of any co-occurring general medical or psychiatric disorder so that the patient is considered suitable for outpatient aftercare, and the availability of adequate follow-up care.

In some areas, particularly urban centers, residential treatment programs specifically designed for adolescents, pregnant or postpartum women, or women with young children are available (56, 57).

d) Therapeutic communities

Individuals with opioid, cocaine, or multiple substance use disorders may benefit from referral to a long-term residential therapeutic community. These programs are generally reserved for individuals with a low likelihood of benefiting from outpatient treatment, such as individuals who have a history of multiple treatment failures or whose profound impairment in social relational skills or ability to attain and sustain employment impede adherence to outpatient treatment (58). Rather than viewing substance abuse as an illness (as defined by the disease concept), therapeutic community theory views it as a deviant behavior; that is, it is seen as a symptom of pathological development in personality structure, social relating, and educational and economic skills (reviewed by De Leon in reference 59). The therapeutic community milieu provides individual, social, and vocational rehabilitation through the community method of social learning. It is a highly structured, substance-free community setting in which the primary interventions are behavioral modeling, supportive peer confrontation, contingency management, community recreation, and work therapy designed to facilitate adherence to social norms and substance-free lifestyles (44).

Therapeutic communities are characteristically organized along strict hierarchies, with newcomers being assigned to the most menial social status and work tasks. Residents achieve higher status and take on increasing responsibility as they demonstrate that they can remain substance free and conform to community rules. Supportive confrontation, individually and in groups, is a primary intervention used to break through denial about the role of substance use in one's life, identify maladaptive behaviors and coping styles that lead to interpersonal conflict and vocational failure, suggest alternative ways of handling disturbing affects, and encourage the development of attitudes and beliefs that are incompatible with continued substance use.

Data regarding the effectiveness of traditional long-term (2-year commitment) therapeutic communities are limited by the fact that only 15%–25% of individuals admitted voluntarily complete a program, with maximum attrition occurring in the first 3 months (60, 61). Retention rates differ with program sites (62), and retention lengths predict outcomes on abstinence and lack of criminal recidivism indexes, with 2-year postcompletion success rates at 90% for graduates, 50% for dropouts completing >1 year, and 25% for dropouts completing <1 year (44, 63).

Cost-containment concerns and increasing knowledge of dual-diagnosis needs have led to modifications of the traditional therapeutic community model. Shorter-term programs (e.g., 3–12 months) and nonresidential programs are offered for those with fewer social and vocational impairments. The expanded availability of social services has allowed improved treatment of special populations (e.g., dual-diagnosis, HIV-positive, single-parent, adolescent) in the therapeutic community setting, and some methadone maintenance programs are provided in this setting.

Potential voluntary applicants to a residential therapeutic community setting should have some understanding of the severity of their substance use disorder and a readiness to change their lifestyle; they should also have a willingness to conform to the structure of the therapeutic community and to temporarily sever ties with family and friends while they assimilate into the community environment. An individual's violation of community rules or shirking of work responsibilities is disclosed to all community members and may be grounds for discharge.

Therapeutic community settings have provided some of the better studied and more successful programs for treating incarcerated substance abusers (64). This has influenced the development of standardized staff training curricula (65).

e) Community residential facilities

Community residential facilities are commonly known as "halfway houses" or "sober houses," with the former typically offering more structure and supervision. They provide an outpatient substance-free housing environment as a transitional setting for individuals in recovery who are not yet able to manage independent housing without a significant risk for relapse. Some studies have shown that for patients with multiple service needs (e.g., vocational, housing, transportation), the provision of stable housing in the form of long-term community residential facilities leads to significantly improved substance use outcomes (66–68). This benefit has been demonstrated for adult substance users of both sexes. Community residential facilities show more variability in substance use outcomes for youth and adolescents (69); this may be related to inadequate matching of services to individual needs.

f) Aftercare

Aftercare occurs after an intense treatment intervention (e.g., hospital or partial hospitalization program) and generally includes outpatient care, involvement in self-help approaches, or both. The clinician should consider the possibility that cognitive impairment may be present in recently detoxified patients when determining their next level of care. Research on aftercare has examined different treatment models, including eclectic, medically oriented, motivational, 12-step, cognitive-behavioral, group, and marital strategies (see Section II.F). Given the chronic, relapsing nature of many types of substance use disorders, especially those requiring hospitalization, it is expected that aftercare will be recommended with few exceptions. In fact, if addiction is reconceptualized along the lines of a chronic rather than an acute disease model, as recommended by McLellan et al. (4), the distinction between a "treatment episode" and "aftercare" should be removed and the different modalities of care (e.g., inpatient, outpatient) be reconsidered as part of a continuous, long-term treatment plan.

g) Outpatient settings

Outpatient treatment settings include but are not limited to mental health clinics, integrated dual-diagnosis programs, private practice settings, primary care clinics, and substance abuse treatment centers, including opioid treatment programs. For individuals with primary nicotine dependence or a marijuana use disorder, treatment is always provided in an outpatient setting. For individuals with other substance use disorders, outpatient treatment is appropriate when clinical conditions or environmental and social circumstances do not require a more intensive level of care.

As in other treatment settings, the optimal outpatient approach is a comprehensive one that includes a variety of psychotherapeutic and pharmacological interventions along with behavioral monitoring, where indicated. The evidence base for empirically supported outpatient treatments is larger for alcohol, nicotine, and opioid dependence treatments than for other substance dependence treatments (70–74). In addition to medication therapies (see Section II.E), outpatient treatments with strong evidence of effectiveness include CBTs (e.g., relapse prevention, social skills training), MET, behavioral therapies (e.g., community reinforcement, contingency management), TSF, psychodynamic therapies/IPT, self-help manuals, behavioral self-control, brief interventions, case management, and group, marital, and family therapies (see Section II.F).

Many specific outpatient treatments have been designed to enhance an individual's participation in treatment and sense of self-efficacy regarding the reduction or cessation of problematic substance use. As in the case of residential and partial hospitalization programs, high rates of attrition can be problematic in outpatient settings, particularly in the early phase (i.e., the first 6 months). Because intermediate and long-term outcomes are highly correlated with retention in treatment, individuals should be strongly encouraged to remain in treatment (42, 43, 45). Clinicians should also encourage and attempt to integrate into treatment a patient's participation in self-help programs where appropriate (see Section II.F.9) (75).

h) Case management

Case management, by definition, exists as an adjunctive treatment. The goals of case management interventions are to provide advocacy and coordination of care and social services and to improve patient adherence to prescribed treatment and follow-up care (76). Case management initially provides psychoeducation about the patient's diagnosis and treatment as well as assessment and stabilization of basic necessities required for the individual to actively participate in treatment (e.g., housing, utilities, income, health insurance, transportation). Beyond this, case managers aid individuals in maintaining stability and understanding and adhering to prescribed treatment. The variability in case management models has complicated research on the effectiveness of this approach (77, 78). Nevertheless, studies show that case management interventions are effective for individuals with an alcohol use disorder (79) or co-occurring psychiatric and substance use disorders (80) and for adolescents with substance use disorders (81).

i) Legally mandated treatment

Treatment of substance use disorders may be legally mandated under a variety of circumstances, including substance-related criminal offenses such as driving under the influence of alcohol or drugs. Drug court programs recognize the effectiveness of diverting offenders with lesser drug-related convictions from correctional facilities into court-mandated community programs for the treatment of substance use disorders (82). Standard procedures for drug court programs include 1) assessment of individual substance use treatment needs, 2) appropriate referral for treatment after arrest, 3) periodic monitoring of adherence to treatment through the use of clinician report and mandatory drug testing, 4) reduction in the severity of charges contingent on successful utilization of programs for the treatment of substance use disorders, and 5) aftercare planning for maintaining sobriety in the community. For offenses related to driving under the influence of alcohol or drugs, state and community sanctions include incarceration, license suspension, driver's education, and community service requirements. Some evidence indicates that more severe sanctions lead to less recidivism for intoxicated drivers with high blood alcohol content readings (83).

Despite the high frequency at which substance use disorders and criminal behaviors co-occur, it has been estimated that only 1%–20% of substance abusers receive adequate treatment while incarcerated (84). The most studied effective treatment programs for incarcerated individuals are therapeutic communities (see Section II.C.2.d) (64).

j) Employee assistance programs

Employee assistance programs (EAPs) provide an employment-based treatment setting and referral platform for employees with substance use disorders. EAPs differ according to workplace size and location. A critical difference for substance use treatment received through an EAP versus through an alternate community outpatient setting is the definition of successful intervention outcome. Whereas most community settings define successful outcome as a reduction of substance use and related medical and social problems, an EAP defines and measures success primarily through job performance. This reflects the employer's need to serve and retain an employee while simultaneously protecting the workplace from inadequate job performance and attributable losses (85). EAPs are cost-effective in the short term (86, 87), but posttreatment follow-up rates are poor (88).

D. PSYCHIATRIC MANAGEMENT

Successful treatment of substance use disorders may involve the use of multiple specific treatments, the choice of which may vary for any one individual over time, and may involve clinicians from a variety of backgrounds. Psychiatric management entails the ongoing process of choosing from among various treatments, monitoring patients' clinical status, and coordinating different treatment components. The frequency, intensity, and focus of psychiatric management must be tailored to meet each patient's needs, and the type of management is likely to vary over time, depending on the patient's clinical status.

1. Motivating change

In recent years, there has been a great deal of research and clinical emphasis on the clinician's role in motivating patients with substance use disorders to change their behaviors. Motivational interviewing techniques (49) were developed specifically for the treatment of patients with a substance use disorder. These involve the use of an empathic, nonjudgmental, and supportive approach to examining the patient's ambivalence about changing addictive behaviors. Understanding the patient's stage of readiness to change (precontemplation, contemplation, preparation, action, or maintenance stage) (25) allows the clinician to determine what motivational strategies are most appropriate for the patient at that time. One of the goals of motivational interviewing is to elicit the patient's reasons for change and assist the patient in moving through the subsequent stages of change (89).

Other techniques involved in motivating change include A-FRAMES (see Section II.F.10) and METs. Manuals describing these techniques are available (49, 90).

2. Establishing and maintaining a therapeutic framework and alliance

An essential feature of psychiatric management of patients with a substance use disorder is the establishment and maintenance of a therapeutic alliance wherein the psychiatrist empathically obtains the necessary diagnostic and treatment-related information, gains the confidence of the patient and perhaps significant others, and is available in times of crisis. The frequency and duration of treatment contacts should be sufficient to engage the patient and, where appropriate, significant others in a sustained effort to participate in all relevant treatment modalities and, where appropriate, self-help groups. Within the context of this alliance, the primary goal of treatment is to help the patient learn, practice, and internalize changes in attitudes and behaviors that are conducive to relapse prevention (91, 92). The strength of the therapeutic alliance has been found to be a significant predictor of psychotherapy outcome (93). For example, several studies of individuals with substance use disorders have found that a stronger patient-clinician alliance predicts less substance use and better psychological functioning by the patient (94–96), although one of these studies found no association between therapeutic alliance strength and treatment retention for patients enrolled in a methadone maintenance program (96). Despite the finding of this one study, the chronic and relapsing nature of substance use disorders highlights the importance of establishing a therapeutic relationship so that patients will return for additional treatment, if necessary (33, 97–99). Ackerman and Hilsenroth (100) reviewed therapist attributes and strategies that facilitate a positive therapeutic alliance for all patient populations. They found that being flexible, honest, respectful, confident, warm, and open all contributed to the development of a positive therapeutic alliance. The most effective strategies for developing such an alliance included exploration, reflection, highlighting past therapy successes, providing accurate interpretation, facilitating the expression of affect, and attending to the patient's experience.

A review of the literature on effective characteristics of therapists concluded that the characteristic most associated with patient retention and reduced substance use is strong interpersonal skills (101). Safran and Muran (102) reviewed techniques for repairing ruptures in the therapeutic alliance, such as clarifying misunderstandings, helping patients learn that they can express their needs in an individuated fashion and assert themselves without destroying the therapeutic relationship, and changing the tasks and goals to be more relevant to the patient's current needs. Limit setting has an important role in treatment of substance use disorders and may be particularly important for individuals with co-occurring personality disorders (103, 104).

3. Assessing safety and clinical status

The psychiatric assessment establishes a diagnosis and provides a baseline determination of a patient's clinical status. Ongoing evaluation of the patient's safety is also critical, as the patient's clinical status may change over time. It is particularly important to assess patients for suicidal or homicidal thoughts or other dangerous behavior—such as driving while under the influence of substances, domestic violence, or child abuse or neglect—that may need to be addressed through a change in the treatment plan or care setting.

Because relapse to substance use is common and inconsistently reported by patients (particularly when use is met with negative consequences or a judgmental response), breath, blood, saliva, and urine testing are helpful in the early detection of relapse. These tests are often initially conducted on a frequent and random schedule, as many substances and their metabolites may be detected for only a few days after use. Random urine screening for recent (i.e., within the last 1–3 days) substance use may be supplemented by nonrandom testing when recent substance use is suspected.

Methods of urine screening vary as to levels of sensitivity, specificity, and cost. The psychiatrist should be familiar with the applicability and sensitivity of the available analytic methods and collection procedures used in local laboratories, and he or she should specify the suspected type of substance used when requesting testing. Direct supervision of a patient's voiding or the use of other procedures (e.g., temperature-sensitive cups) will help to increase the validity and reliability of the test results.

The decision to test a patient's breath, blood, or urine depends on the type of substance use suspected, the substance's duration of action, the sensitivity of the test used, and the clinical setting in which care is being rendered. For example, blood testing is useful for assessing very recent substance use because it reflects current blood levels, and breath testing is useful for detecting alcohol intoxication and generally gives results comparable to those from blood tests. However, breath testing for alcohol is frequently preferred because the results are immediate and it is a noninvasive and low-cost procedure. Breath testing can also detect carbon monoxide, an indicator of smoking, as recent as a few hours before the test (105).

Urine testing is useful for detecting substance use over the preceding 5-day period for common substances of abuse (cocaine, opiates, cannabis, amphetamines, benzodiazepines, and PCP); however, certain opioids (buprenorphine, oxycodone, hydrocodone, and fentanyl) cannot be detected with routine methods and require special assays. Alcohol can be detected for up to 24 hours in urine, whereas ethyl glucuronide (EtG), a minor metabolite of alcohol, can be detected in the urine for 2–3 days after alcohol ingestion (106–108). Because EtG is produced by in vivo metabolism of alcohol prior to excretion in urine, the assay for EtG is highly sensitive and specific and is sometimes used in monitoring programs. Finally, there is some evidence that certain state markers can be used to detect recent alcohol use (e.g., elevation of carbohydrate-deficient transferrin, mean corpuscular volume, or γ-glutamyl transpeptidase).

Results from some studies have indicated that more intensive monitoring of substance use may increase recovery rates from a substance use disorder, as has been demonstrated with physicians and pilots (109–111). Ongoing assessment of the substance use disorder and psychiatric status is also necessary to ensure that the patient is receiving the appropriate treatment(s) and to monitor the patient's response to treatment (i.e., to determine the optimal dose of a medication, evaluate its efficacy, and detect treatment-emergent side effects). Co-occurring psychiatric disorders may complicate the treatment of the substance use disorder (111) and require the addition of specific treatments (e.g., an antidepressant medication for a patient with co-occurring major depressive disorder). An ongoing longitudinal assessment of the patient may be critical to the accurate diagnosis of a co-occurring condition (see Section II.B).

4. Managing intoxication

In general, acutely intoxicated patients require a safe, monitored environment in which they can receive decreased exposure to external stimulation, as well as reassurance, reorientation, and reality testing. Clinical assessment involves ascertaining which substances have been used; the route of administration, dose, and time since the last dose; whether the level of intoxication is waxing or waning; and other diagnostic information, as has been already described. Management of acute intoxication may also be directed toward hastening the removal of substances from the body, which may be accomplished through gastric lavage (in the case of substances that have been recently ingested) or techniques that increase the excretion rate of substances or their active metabolites. Medications that antagonize the actions of the abused substances may be used to reverse their effect. Examples include the administration of naloxone to patients who have overdosed with heroin or other opioids or flumazenil to patients who have overdosed with benzodiazepines.

Many patients use multiple substances simultaneously to enhance, ameliorate, or otherwise modify the degree or nature of their intoxication or to relieve withdrawal symptoms. Intoxication with alcohol and cocaine, the use of heroin and cocaine ("speedball"), and the combined use of alcohol, marijuana, and/or benzodiazepines by opioid-dependent patients are particularly frequent. When intoxication with multiple substances is present, the effects of each substance need to be taken into consideration in managing the patient. More information on the management of alcohol, cocaine, and opioid intoxication can be found in the specific section for each substance (Sections IV.C.1, VI.C.1, and VII.C.2, respectively).

5. Managing withdrawal

Not all individuals who are intoxicated or using substances will develop withdrawal symptoms. Withdrawal syndromes usually occur in physically dependent individuals who discontinue or reduce their substance use after a period of heavy and regular use. Patients using multiple substances (including alcohol and nicotine) are at risk for withdrawal from each substance. Factors that predict the severity of a withdrawal syndrome include 1) type of substance used, 2) time elapsed since last use, 3) metabolic rates of the substance, 4) dissociation rates of the substance from receptor sites, 5) synergistic effects or drug-drug interactions from the concomitant use of other prescribed or nonprescribed medications, 6) the presence or absence of concurrent general medical or psychiatric disorders, and 7) past withdrawal experiences (especially for alcohol). More information on the management of withdrawal from alcohol, cocaine, and opioids can be found in the specific section for each substance (Sections IV.C.2, VI.C.2, and VII.C.3, respectively).

6. Reducing the morbidity and sequelae of substance use disorders

The clinician should engage the patient and, when appropriate, significant others in developing a comprehensive treatment plan to address problems in biological, psychological, and social functioning. Coordination with a patient's primary care physician may also be important in the medical management of patients with substance use disorders (112).

Substance use disorders are commonly associated with substance-related medical morbidity. Although an individual patient's presentation may warrant specific screening and intervention, a number of baseline screening tests are frequently recommended based on epidemiological studies documenting the high risk for co-occurring medical disorders. For example, electrolyte panels and complete blood counts may be considered for those with severe substance dependence of any type because of the high correlation of substance dependence with poor nutritional status. For women of childbearing age, testing for pregnancy is an important part of medical screening. Tuberculin skin testing may be appropriate because of substance users' increased risk for tuberculosis exposure and to address public health concerns. Blood pressure monitoring may be advisable for substance users because of associated hypertension (e.g., with alcohol, nicotine, and stimulants) and hypotension (e.g., dehydration associated with poor self-care) risks. For individuals with specific substance use disorders, additional laboratory and other screening tests may be considered. These include the following:

- *Alcohol use.* Hepatic panel to screen for liver toxicity and functioning; complete blood count to determine mean corpuscular volume, which can be increased with hepatic toxicity, thiamine, folate, and vitamin B_{12} deficiency, as well as the direct effects of alcohol on hematopoiesis; stool sampling for occult blood reflecting gastritis, peptic ulcerative disease, or esophageal varices; mental status examination to detect cognitive functioning deficits
- *Nicotine dependence.* Examination of lymph nodes, mouth, and throat to assess for occult cancer and pulmonary disease; auscultation of chest and lungs; chest X-ray; pulmonary function testing, if warranted; electrocardiogram because of increased risk for cardiovascular disease; urine or blood cotinine level
- *Injection drug use.* Blood testing for blood-borne and sexually transmitted diseases, such as HIV, hepatitis B and C virus, and syphilis; skin examination for cellulitis; complete blood count to detect occult infection; genital examination and sampling for chlamydia, gonococcal disease, and human papilloma virus

Even if not initially caused by substance use, co-occurring medical disorders may be exacerbated by substance use, such as respiratory disease worsened by nicotine use; cardiovascular disease worsened by cocaine, alcohol, or nicotine use; hepatic disease aggravated by alcohol abuse; and seizure disorder exacerbated by withdrawal from alcohol, benzodiazepines, or other sedatives. In addition, individuals with substance use disorders frequently neglect preventive health care and follow-up medical care (113). All substance use disorders can be a cause for nonadherence to prescribed medications. Delayed dosing, missed dosing, or overuse of prescribed medications may occur during intoxication and withdrawal states. To finance substance use, individuals may sell prescribed medications (e.g., opiate analgesics) or avoid filling prescriptions to save insurance copayments. "Downward drift" and homelessness among substance-dependent individuals also often curtails their access to medical and dental care.

Individuals with a co-occurring psychiatric disorder are particularly vulnerable to the self-neglect and morbidity associated with substance use, possibly resulting in exacerbation of depression and suicidal thinking, worsening of psychosis, destabilization of bipolar disorder, and increased impulsivity leading to high-risk behaviors. Nonadherence to prescribed medication occurs frequently in those with a substance use disorder and further exacerbates these sequelae. Such individuals are best served by being referred to an integrated psychiatric and substance use disorder treatment program (114). Psychiatrists are often the only medical contacts for patients with co-occurring psychiatric and substance use disorders and therefore are important resources for the facilitation of appropriate medical screening, referral for medical care, and follow-up with medical care (115).

7. Facilitating adherence to a treatment plan and preventing relapse

Because individuals with substance use disorders are often ambivalent about giving up their substance use, it can be useful to monitor their attitudes about participating in treatment and adhering to specific recommendations. These patients often deny or minimize the negative consequences attributable to their substance use; this tendency is often erroneously interpreted by clinicians and significant others as evidence of dishonesty. Even patients entering treatment with high motivation to achieve abstinence will struggle with the reemergence of craving for a substance or preoccupation with thoughts about attaining or using a substance. Moreover, social influences (e.g., substance-using family or friends), economic influences (e.g., unemployment), medical conditions (e.g., chronic pain, fatigue), and psychological influences (e.g., hopelessness, despair) may make an individual more vulnerable to a relapse episode even when he or she adheres to prescribed treatment. For these reasons, it can be helpful for clinicians and patients to anticipate the possibility that the patient may return to substance use and to agree on a corrective plan of action should this occur. If the patient is willing, it can be helpful to involve significant others in preventing the patient's relapse and prepare significant others to manage relapses should they occur.

Supporting patients in their efforts to reduce or abstain from substance use positively reinforces their progress. Overt recognition of patient efforts and successes helps to motivate patients to remain in treatment despite setbacks. Clinicians can optimize patient engagement and retention in treatment through the use of motivational enhancement strategies (49, 116) and by encouraging patients to actively partake in self-help strategies. Monitoring programs, such as EAPs and impaired-physician programs (86, 111, 117), can sometimes help patients adhere to treatment.

Early in treatment a clinician may educate patients about cue-, stress-, and substance-induced relapse triggers (17, 118). Patients benefit from being educated in a supportive manner about relapse risk situations, thoughts, or emotions; they must learn to recognize these as triggers for relapse and learn to manage unavoidable triggers without resorting to substance-using behaviors. Participation in AA or similar self-help group meetings can also support patients' sobriety and help them avoid relapse. Many other strategies can also help prevent relapse. Social skills training is targeted at improving individual responsibility within family relationships, work-related interactions, and social relationships. During the early recovery phase, it can be helpful to encourage patients to seek new experiences and roles consistent with a substance-free existence (e.g., greater involvement in vocational, social, or religious activities) and to discourage them from instituting major life changes that might increase the risk of relapse. Facilitating treatment of co-occurring psychiatric and medical conditions that significantly interact with substance relapse is a long-term intervention for maintaining sobriety (119–121).

Therapeutic strategies to prevent relapse have been well studied and include teaching individuals to anticipate and avoid substance-related cues (e.g., assessing individual capacity to avoid relapse in the presence of substance-using peers), training individuals how to monitor their affective or cognitive states associated with increased craving and substance use, behavioral contingency contracting, training individuals in cue extinction and relaxation therapies to reduce the potency of substance-related stimuli and modulate craving intensity, and supporting patients in the development of coping skills and lifestyle changes that support sobriety (122, 123). Behavioral techniques that enhance the availability and perceived value of social reinforcement as an alternative to substance use or reward for remaining abstinent have also been used (124).

If relapse does occur, individuals should be praised for even limited success and encouraged to continue in or resume treatment. Clinicians may help patients analyze relapses as well as periods of sobriety from a functional and behavioral standpoint and use what is learned to adjust the treatment plan to fit the individual's present needs. For chronically relapsing substance users, medication therapies may be necessary adjuncts to treatment.

8. Providing education about substance use disorders and their treatment

Patients with substance use disorders should receive education and feedback about their disorder, prognosis, and treatment. Clinicians are responsible for educating patients and their significant others about the etiology and nature of substance use, the benefits of abstinence, the risk of switching addictions (e.g., to other substances, to addictive behaviors such as compulsive gambling), the identification of relapse triggers, the availability of treatment options, and the role of family and friends in aiding or impeding recovery. When appropriate, psychiatrists may provide education about the effects of alcohol and other substances on the brain, the positive changes that occur with abstinence, substance-related medical problems (e.g., hepatitis C virus), and the effects of smoking, alcohol, and other substances on fetal development. Education on reducing behavioral harm may include advice about the use of sterile needles, procedures for safer sex, contraceptive options, and the availability of treatment services for drug-exposed newborns. Patients may also be directed to other educational resources. For example, public health services for the treatment of nicotine dependence are offered free of charge and are available by telephone (e.g., the "telephone quitlines" for individual states sponsored by the Centers for Disease Control and Prevention [CDC], available at http://www.cdc.gov/tobacco/quitlines.htm), on the Internet (e.g., the CDC's Tobacco Information and Prevention Source, available at http://www.cdc.gov/tobacco/), and by mail. As in all clinical settings, patient education is best delivered with due consideration to the individual's educational background and cultural setting.

9. Facilitating access to services and coordinating resources among mental health, general medical, and other service systems

In all aspects of patient management, the psychiatrist may work collaboratively with members of other professional disciplines, community-based agencies, treatment programs, and lay organizations to coordinate and integrate the patient's care and address the patient's social, vocational, educational, and rehabilitative needs. This is particularly important for patients lacking resources or the capacity for self-care because of a psychiatric or medical disorder. Case management services are aimed at such coordination of care (125).

In treating an individual with significant comorbidities or treatment-resistant disorders (e.g., chronic pain syndromes, personality disorders, cognitive impairment, chronic suicidality), it may be important for the treating clinician to consult with colleagues and experts in specialty care. In some cases, it may be necessary to place patients in a highly supervised setting to protect them and society from their dangerous behaviors associated with substance use.

E. SOMATIC TREATMENTS

Medication therapies for substance use disorders are effective adjuncts to behavioral therapies and self-help groups; the settings for medication therapies include hospitals, partial hospitalization and intensive outpatient programs, and a variety of outpatient settings including primary care clinics, mental health clinics, substance use disorder treatment facilities, and private practice offices.

The types of accepted and effective medication strategies used in the treatment of specific substance use disorders are discussed in greater detail in later sections of this practice guideline. The following sections describe the general principles of these main categories of medication interventions: 1) medications to treat intoxication states, 2) medications to treat withdrawal syndromes,

3) agonist maintenance therapies, 4) antagonist therapies, 5) abstinence-promoting and relapse prevention therapies, and 6) medications to treat co-occurring psychiatric conditions.

1. Medications to treat intoxication states

Most clinicians treating patients with substance use disorders do not direct medical treatment of life-threatening intoxication states, because this role belongs to trained emergency physicians. However, clinicians who treat patients with substance use disorders should be able to recognize potentially dangerous intoxication states so they can make a rapid referral to emergency services. This section briefly describes potentially dangerous states of substance intoxication and emergency medication therapies.

In general, there are two types of medication interventions for acute intoxication and overdose: the administration of specific antagonists (e.g., naloxone for acute opioid overdose, flumazenil for acute benzodiazepine overdose complicated by ingestion of multiple substances) and therapies that stabilize the physical effects of substance overdose (e.g., anticholinergics, adrenergic pressor agents, anti-arrhythmics, anticonvulsants). Other adjunctive supportive treatments for overdose include establishing an adequate airway, decreasing the risk of aspiration (e.g., positioning the patient on his or her side, use of a cuffed endotracheal tube), and, if indicated, providing ventilatory support and hemodialysis. Hemodialysis or lavage therapies may also be used to enhance elimination of ingested substances.

The syndrome of acute opioid overdose is recognizable by respiratory depression, extreme miosis, and stupor or coma (126). Pulmonary edema may also be observed. Naloxone is a competitive antagonist at all three types of opiate receptors (mu, kappa, and sigma) and has no intrinsic agonist activity (127). It is clinically indicated to rapidly reverse a known or suspected opioid overdose (126, 128). Because of its poor bioavailability from significant hepatic first-pass effects, naloxone is typically administered intravenously, but it may also be given intramuscularly, subcutaneously, or endotracheally if intravenous access is unattainable (126). The dosing of naloxone varies depending on whether the patient is known to be opioid dependent as well as on the extent of respiratory depression. For example, in patients with CNS but not respiratory depression, an initial dose of 0.05–0.4 mg i.v. is recommended. The lower dose is used for opioid-dependent individuals, who will show withdrawal symptoms within minutes of being given the medication (129). For any person who presents with significant respiratory depression, the initial suggested dose is 2.0 mg i.v., regardless of the individual's drug use history; a beneficial response should occur within 2 minutes. Repeated doses can be administered every 3 minutes until respiratory or CNS depression is completely reversed or until a maximum dose of 10 mg i.v. has been given (128). If no response is observed after administration of the 10 mg of naloxone, the diagnosis of opioid overdose should be reconsidered. Because naloxone is rapidly absorbed by the brain and then quickly redistributed and eliminated from the body, its activity in the brain is short-lived (126, 130). Thus, further monitoring and infusion of additional naloxone are needed to continue antagonizing the effects of severe opioid overdose, particularly if longer-acting opioids have been ingested (128, 131). Monitoring for opioid withdrawal symptoms is also indicated because patients may experience significant distress that can last for several hours after reversal of an opioid overdose with an antagonist (129).

Acute sedative-hypnotic overdose is recognizable by slurred speech, loss of coordination, and confusion and, in a severe overdose, stupor, respiratory depression, and coma. Flumazenil is a potent benzodiazepine-specific antagonist that competes at central synaptic GABA receptor sites in a dose-dependent manner (132). In addition, it may antagonize the sedative effects of other compounds that act through GABA receptors, such as zolpidem, zaleplon, and eszopiclone (133). However, it does not antagonize benzodiazepine effects at peripheral GABAergic (e.g., renal, cardiac) receptor sites (134). Like naloxone, flumazenil has poor bioavailability and a brief duration of activity and is administered by repeated boluses or through continuous intravenous infusion. Although it can be used as a low-dose (2 mg i.v.) diagnostic probe for suspected benzodiazepine overdose or in the reversal of benzodiazepines given for diagnostic or therapeutic procedures, flumazenil must be carefully administered to benzodiazepine-dependent patients and patients who have ingested mixed substances to avoid the production of withdrawal seizures (135). Flumazenil can also affect cerebral hemodynamics and is not recommended for situations in which intracranial pressure may already be increased (e.g., in the case of a head injury) (135). For these reasons, as well as cost, flumazenil is not recommended for uncomplicated benzodiazepine overdose that can be successfully managed by supportive ventilation therapies.

2. Medications to treat withdrawal syndromes

Patients who develop tolerance to a particular substance also develop cross-tolerance to other substances in the same pharmacological class. Physicians can take advantage of cross-tolerance in the treatment of withdrawal states by replacing the abused substance with a medication that is in the same pharmacological class. Examples of this include the use of methadone or buprenorphine in the treatment of opioid withdrawal, benzodiazepines in the treatment of alcohol and sedative-hypnotic withdrawal, and NRTs in the treatment of nicotine dependence (136–141).

Other medications are used to ameliorate indirect withdrawal-related symptoms. For example, clonidine is an α_2-adrenergic agonist that is useful in treating opioid withdrawal symptoms as well as anxiety syndromes (129, 142). Nonspecific symptoms of withdrawal such as headache and stomach upset may also require treatment using medications such as acetaminophen and histamine$_2$-receptor antagonists, respectively.

3. Agonist maintenance therapies

Opioid agonist maintenance therapy may be the primary tool available to engage an opioid-dependent individual in treatment because it relieves unpleasant withdrawal syndromes and craving associated with abstinence. The central and subjective effects of agonist therapies render these agents more acceptable to opioid-dependent patients than antagonist therapies, and adherence with treatment with agonist therapies is greater than with antagonist therapies.

Opioid agonist maintenance therapies (described further below) include methadone, a long-acting potent agonist at the mu opiate receptor sites (126), and buprenorphine, a potent long-acting compound that acts as a partial opioid agonist at mu receptor sites (126) and that is prescribed alone or with naloxone (in a combination tablet). An additional opioid agonist therapy, L-α-acetylmethadol (LAAM), has an extended duration of action and high intrinsic activity at the mu opiate receptor, but it has been withdrawn from the U.S. market by its manufacturer because of the risk of cardiac arrhythmia.

4. Antagonist therapies

Antagonist therapies are used to block or otherwise counteract the physiological and/or subjective reinforcing effects of substances. The narcotic antagonist naltrexone blocks the subjective and physiological effects of subsequently administered opioid drugs (e.g., heroin) (143, 144) without tolerance developing to its antagonist effect (145) (see Sections VII.C.1.c and IX.E.1.b). Compared with naloxone, naltrexone has good oral bioavailability (126) and a relatively long half-life; it is also available in a long-acting injectable preparation that may improve treatment adherence.

Mecamylamine, a nicotine antagonist, has also been studied, but its effectiveness remains unclear (146, 147).

5. Abstinence-promoting and relapse prevention therapies

For promoting abstinence and preventing relapse in patients with substance use disorders, certain medications may be useful. Examples of such medications are disulfiram, naltrexone, and acamprosate for alcohol use disorders and bupropion for nicotine dependence.

The ingestion of alcohol after disulfiram, an inhibitor of the enzyme aldehyde dehydrogenase, has been taken results in the accumulation of toxic levels of acetaldehyde accompanied by a host of unpleasant, potentially dangerous but rarely lethal signs and symptoms (148–151). The purpose of disulfiram is not to make the patient ill but to prevent the patient from drinking impulsively because he or she knows the symptoms that will result from drinking while taking disulfiram (see Sections IV.C.3.b and IX.B.3.b).

Naltrexone, described above as an antagonist therapy for the treatment of opiate dependence, is also effective in reducing alcohol craving and preventing alcohol-induced relapse (152–154), presumably because of the effect of mu opiate receptor antagonism in blocking the centrally mediated reinforcing effects of alcohol (155) (see Sections IV.C.3.a and IX.B.3.a).

Acamprosate (calcium bis-acetyl homotaurine) is a small, flexible molecule that resembles GABA and decreases glutamatergic neurotransmission, perhaps by acting as an *N*-methyl-D-aspartate antagonist (151, 156). It has been proposed that this medication helps sustain abstinence in detoxified alcohol-dependent individuals by reducing neuronal hyperexcitability during early recovery (156, 157) (see Sections IV.C.3.c and IX.B.3.c).

Treatment of nicotine dependence with the sustained-release formulation of the antidepressant bupropion has been associated with reductions in nicotine craving and smoking urges (158–160). The mechanism of action for bupropion in the treatment of nicotine dependence is unclear but is likely related to blockade of dopamine and norepinephrine reuptake (161) as well as antagonism of high-affinity nicotinic acetylcholine receptors (162) (see Sections III.E.2 and IX.A.1.b).

6. Medications to treat co-occurring psychiatric conditions

The treatment of co-occurring psychiatric disorders may or may not improve treatment outcome for the substance use disorder, but if treatment of the co-occurring psychiatric disorder does not occur, it is less likely that the treatment of substance use disorder will be successful. The high prevalence of co-occurring psychiatric disorders in substance-dependent patients implies that many such patients will require specific pharmacotherapy for a co-occurring disorder. Examples include the use of mood stabilizers for substance-dependent patients with bipolar disorder, antipsychotics for patients with psychotic disorders, and antidepressants for patients with major depressive disorder (see also Section II.G.2.d).

Clinically significant issues for substance-dependent patients receiving pharmacotherapy for co-occurring psychiatric disorders include 1) synergy of prescribed medications and effects of the abused substance (e.g., benzodiazepines and alcohol), 2) drug-drug interactions that affect the efficacy of psychiatric treatment (e.g., antipsychotics and smoked tobacco), 3) nonadherence to treatment because of intoxication and withdrawal states as well as drug-seeking behaviors, and 4) intentional or unintentional overdose. Certain medications used to treat co-occurring psychiatric disorders may themselves be abused. For example, patients with a co-occurring anxiety disorder may abuse benzodiazepines, patients with attention deficit hyperactivity disorder (ADHD) may abuse prescribed stimulants, and patients with a co-occurring psychotic disorder who are treated with anticholinergics for antipsychotic adverse side effects may abuse the anticholinergic adjunct. Substance-dependent patients may also misuse prescribed medications in an attempt to ameliorate withdrawal syndromes, enhance the effect of other substances of abuse, or accelerate the action of the prescribed medication. Whenever possible, medications with low abuse potential and relative safety in overdose should be selected for the treatment of patients with a co-occurring substance use disorder.

F. PSYCHOSOCIAL TREATMENTS

Some type of psychosocial intervention is usually available in specialized substance use disorder treatment programs. These approaches are the mainstay of treatment for users of certain classes of substances (e.g., cocaine) for which there are no pharmacological treatments with established efficacy. The major psychotherapeutic treatments that have been studied in patients with substance use disorders are cognitive-behavioral, behavioral, psychodynamic/interpersonal, and recovery-oriented therapies. A growing body of efficacy data from controlled clinical trials suggests that psychotherapy is superior to control conditions as a treatment for patients with a substance use disorder. However, no particular type of psychotherapy has been found to be consistently superior when compared with other active psychotherapies for treating substance use disorders. Even comparatively brief psychotherapies appear to have durable effects among patients with a substance use disorder (123).

After a discussion of the role of psychotherapy in substance abuse treatment and the relation between psychotherapy and pharmacotherapy, this section reviews the major psychosocial treatment approaches, the principles underlying their use, and their application in the treatment of patients with substance use disorders.

1. Role of psychosocial treatments

Psychosocial treatments for substance use disorders attempt to counteract compulsive substance use by bringing about changes in patients' behaviors, thought processes, affect regulation, and social functioning. Although the techniques and theories of therapeutic action vary widely across the different approaches reviewed below, they all address one or more of a set of common tasks: 1) enhancing motivation to stop or reduce substance use, 2) teaching coping skills, 3) changing reinforcement contingencies, 4) fostering management of painful affects, and 5) enhancing social supports and interpersonal functioning (163). A central challenge for clinicians treating individuals with substance use disorders is that the core symptom, compulsive substance use, at least initially results in euphoria or relief of dysphoria, with the aversive and painful effects of substance use occurring some time after the rewarding effects. This contrasts with the course of most other psychiatric disorders (e.g., mood or anxiety disorders), in which the primary symptoms are painful or aversive. In addition, substance use has come to serve an important function in the individual's life by the time treatment is sought. Sustained recovery from a substance use disorder entails both relinquishing a valued element of life and developing different behaviors, thought patterns, and relationships that serve the functions previously met by substance use (164).

Psychosocial treatments are often essential for many aspects of this recovery process: Sustained motivation is required to forgo the rewards of substance use, tolerate the discomforts of early and protracted withdrawal symptoms, and gather the energy to avoid relapse despite episodes of craving that can occur throughout a lifetime. Coping skills are required to manage and avoid situations that place the individual at high risk for relapse. Alternative sources of reward or symptom relief must be sought and used to fill the place of substance use. Dysphoric affects, such as anger, sadness, or anxiety, must be managed in ways that do not involve continued substance use. Social relationships that are supportive of recovery need to be developed or repaired.

Patients with substance use disorders vary widely in their need for attention to each of these aspects of recovery, and brief treatment or self-help methods may be sufficient for the recovery of highly motivated patients with good interpersonal functioning and social support. However, none of these processes can be assumed to occur simply as a result of detoxification or with the administration of medications. It is essential that these psychosocial aspects of recovery be evaluated during treatment planning to determine the need for behavioral treatments.

2. Relation of psychosocial treatments to pharmacotherapy for substance use disorders

Research has demonstrated that the utility of pharmacotherapies for substance use disorders may be limited unless they are delivered with adjunctive psychotherapy. For example, naltrexone maintenance for opioid dependence is plagued by high rates of premature dropout (165,

166) that can be lessened by concurrent behavioral or family therapy (167). Without adjunctive psychotherapy, the utility of disulfiram may be limited, in part because of low rates of medication adherence (150); however, its effectiveness can be enhanced when it is delivered in the context of a contract with a family member or significant other (168). Methadone maintenance for opioid dependence is the most successful pharmacological treatment of a substance use disorder, with substantial evidence of its impact on treatment retention and associated reductions in opioid use and illegal activity (169). However, cross-program effectiveness varies widely in relation to the quality and amount of ancillary psychosocial services delivered (169). Moreover, McLellan et al. (170) have shown that methadone maintenance alone yields acceptable results for only a small fraction of patients and that outcome is enhanced in proportion to the intensity of concomitant psychosocial services. More recently, a meta-analysis confirmed that a combination of psychosocial treatment and methadone maintenance produced greater reductions in heroin use by opioid-dependent individuals than methadone maintenance alone (171). Similar results have been found with nicotine replacement treatments: rates of sustained abstinence are increased two- to fourfold when they are combined with behavioral therapies (172, 173).

These findings suggest that even the most efficacious pharmacotherapies for substance use disorders have limitations that need to be addressed with psychosocial interventions. First, medications frequently affect only part of the substance dependence syndrome while leaving other aspects untouched. For example, methadone is highly effective in relieving withdrawal symptoms and minimizing the impact of continued opioid use, but by itself it has limited impact on counteracting social impairments resulting from protracted substance use prior to a patient's entering treatment (169). Also, most medications have variable or partial effects on the target symptom. Second, side effects or delayed effects of medications may limit acceptability and adherence. Third, medications typically target only one class of substances, whereas abuse of multiple substances is the norm in treatment populations (174). Fourth, gains made while taking the medication tend to diminish when the treatment is discontinued, whereas vulnerability to relapse is lifelong. Psychosocial strategies for countering these limitations and enhancing effectiveness of pharmacotherapies include 1) increasing a patient's motivation to stop substance use by taking the prescribed medication, 2) providing guidance to the patient on using the medication and managing its side effects, 3) maintaining the patient's motivation to continue the medication after an initial period of abstinence is achieved, 4) providing the patient with a supportive therapeutic relationship aimed at preventing premature termination, and 5) helping the patient develop skills to adjust to a life without substance use.

The importance of psychosocial treatments is reinforced by the recognition that there are only a handful of effective pharmacotherapies for substance use disorders and that, for the most part, these therapies are limited to the treatment of opioid, alcohol, and nicotine dependence (175). Effective pharmacotherapies for dependence on cocaine and other stimulants, marijuana, hallucinogens, and sedative-hypnotics have yet to be developed. For individuals who abuse these latter substances, psychosocial therapies remain the principal treatments.

Although the foregoing discussion has emphasized the need for psychotherapy to enhance the effectiveness of pharmacotherapy, this section would not be complete without considering the role of pharmacotherapy in enhancing the efficacy of psychotherapy. These two treatments have different mechanisms of action and targeted effects that can counteract the weaknesses of either treatment alone. Psychotherapies effect change by psychological means in the psychosocial aspects of substance abuse, such as motivation, coping skills, dysfunctional thoughts, or social relationships. The weaknesses of these treatments include a limited effect on the physiological aspects of substance abuse or withdrawal. Also, the impact of behavioral treatments tends to be delayed, requiring practice, repeated sessions, and a "working through" process. In contrast, the relative strength of pharmacological treatments is their rapid action in reducing immediate or protracted withdrawal symptoms, craving, and the rewarding effects of continued substance use. In effect, pharmacotherapies for substance use disorders reduce the patients' immediate access to and preoccupation with the abused substance, freeing the patient to address other concerns such as long-term goals or interpersonal relationships. When medications are used in conjunction with psychotherapy, the dropout rate from therapy is reduced because the patient's urges to use and relapse to substance use are alleviated by the effects of the medication. In addition, a longer duration of abstinence can further enhance the efficacy of psychotherapy by preventing substance-related effects on attention and mental acuity, thereby maximizing the patient's ability for learning new behaviors in therapy.

Because of the complementary actions of psychotherapies and pharmacotherapies, combined treatment has a number of potential advantages. As is reviewed later, research evidence on combined treatment is sparse but generally supportive. Although factors such as patient acceptance can limit the use of combined approaches, it is important to note that for the treatment of substance use disorders, no studies have shown that combined treatments are less effective than either psychotherapy or pharmacotherapy alone.

3. Cognitive-behavioral therapies

CBTs for the treatment of substance use disorders are based on social learning theories regarding the acquisition and maintenance of the disorder (176). These therapies target two processes conceptualized as underlying substance abuse: 1) dysfunctional thoughts, such as the belief that the use of substances is completely uncontrollable, and 2) maladaptive behaviors, such as acceptance of offers to use drugs. Early versions of this approach (177, 178) were derived from cognitive therapy for depression and anxiety by Beck and Emery (179) and placed primary emphasis on identifying and modifying dysfunctional thinking patterns. Other adaptations of this approach have broadened the focus of therapy to help the patient master an individualized set of coping strategies as an effective alternative to substance use (176, 180). Typical cognitive strategies include fostering the patient's resolve to stop using substances by exploring positive and negative consequences of continued use, recognizing seemingly irrelevant decisions that could culminate in high-risk situations, and identifying and confronting thoughts about substance use. Behavioral strategies are based on a functional analysis of substance use (i.e, understanding substance use in relation to its antecedents and consequences) and include the development of strategies for coping with craving, preparing for emergencies, and coping with relapse to substance use.

Social skills training, an element of CBT, recognizes that alcohol and drug dependence commonly results in the interruption of normal developmental acquisition of social skills as well as the deterioration of previously learned social skills because of the interference of drug-seeking and drug-using behaviors. Social skills training targets an individual's capacity for 1) effective and meaningful communication, 2) listening, 3) being able to imagine someone else's feelings and thoughts to inform one's own behavioral interactions, 4) being able to monitor and modify one's own nonverbal communications, 5) being able to adapt to circumstances to maintain relationships, and 6) being assertive (181). This strategy has been successfully used as an adjunct to a more comprehensive treatment plan and can be delivered in a wide variety of outpatient treatment settings. It may be particularly useful in certain dually diagnosed populations, such as patients with schizophrenia (182) and adolescents at risk for beginning substance abuse (183).

Relapse prevention is a treatment approach in which CBT techniques are used to help patients develop greater self-control to avoid relapse (184, 185). Specific relapse prevention strategies include discussing the patient's ambivalence about the substance use disorder, identifying emotional and environmental triggers of craving and substance use, developing and reviewing specific coping strategies to deal with internal or external stressors, exploring the decision chain leading to reinitiation of substance use, learning from brief episodes of relapse (slips) about triggers leading to relapse, and developing effective techniques for early intervention (184, 186). In more recent clinical trials (43, 187), techniques drawn from cognitive therapy and relapse prevention have been combined with the aims of initiating abstinence and preventing relapse.

4. Motivational enhancement therapy

MET is the longer-term follow-up to an initial brief intervention strategy. It continues the use of motivational interviewing and moves a patient closer to a readiness to change substance use behaviors (reviewed in DiClemente et al. [6] and Miller and Rollnick [49]). It combines techniques from cognitive, client-centered, systems, and social-psychological persuasion approaches and may be provided by trained clinicians in substance abuse facilities, mental health clinics, and private practice offices. MET is characterized by an empathic approach in which the therapist helps to motivate the patient by asking about the pros and cons of specific behaviors, exploring the patient's goals and associated ambivalence about reaching those goals, and listening reflectively to the patient's responses. This treatment modality is effective even for patients who are not highly motivated to change, which gives it a practical advantage over other therapies for substance use disorders in many settings.

5. Behavioral therapies

Behavioral therapies are based on basic principles of learning theory (188), which deals with the role of externally applied positive or negative contingencies on learning or unlearning of behaviors that can range from simple autonomic reactions such as salivation to complex behavioral routines such as purchasing drugs. When these theories are applied to substance use disorders, the target behavior is habitual excessive substance use, which is altered through systematic environmental manipulations that vary widely depending on the specific substance use behavior. These theories differ from those underlying CBTs by not recognizing cognition as a domain independent of behavior.

The shared goals of behavioral therapies are to interrupt the sequence of substance use in response to internal or external cues and substitute behaviors that take the place of or are incompatible with substance use. There are two broad classes of learning theory-based treatments: 1) those that are based on classical conditioning and focus more on antecedent stimuli such as cue exposure therapy (189) and 2) those that are based on operant conditioning and focus more on consequences such as community reinforcement therapy (190). Representative behavioral approaches are briefly described here.

a) Contingency management

Contingency management therapy involves introducing rewards for therapeutically desired behaviors (e.g., attending therapy sessions, providing substance-negative urine samples) and/or aversive consequences for undesirable behaviors (e.g., failure to adhere to clinic rules) (191–193). As an adjunctive treatment, contingency management has been used with a variety of substances of abuse, including cocaine (193–196), opiates (197–200), and marijuana (201). Incentives to be offered, behaviors to be reinforced, and the reinforcement schedule vary widely by substance and also depend on the role of contingency management within the larger treatment plan (188). Although most studies have centered on abstinence from substance use, contingency management procedures are potentially applicable to a wide range of target behaviors and problems, including treatment retention, adherence to treatment (e.g., retroviral therapies for individuals with HIV), and reinforcement of other treatment goals such as employment seeking (202) or work attendance (203). Contingency management is effective when desired behaviors are rewarded with vouchers that can be exchanged for mutually agreed-on items such as movie tickets. Other reinforcers (e.g., free housing, direct compensation) can be substituted for vouchers. The use of large but low-probability reinforcers (e.g., earning the chance to draw from a bowl and win prizes of varying magnitudes ranging from $1 to more than $100) is also effective (204, 205) and may reduce the total costs of contingency management approaches (206).

Contingency contracting is a subtype of contingency management based on the use of predetermined positive or negative consequences to reward abstinence or punish, and thus deter, drug-related behaviors. Negative consequences of substance use may include notification of courts, employers, or family members. The effectiveness of this approach depends heavily on the concurrent use of frequent, random, supervised urine screening for substance use. When negative contingencies are based on the anticipated response of others (e.g., spouses, employers), the treating physician should obtain the patient's written informed consent to contact these individuals at the time the contract is initiated (207).

b) Community reinforcement

The community reinforcement approach (CRA) is based on the theory that environmental reinforcers for substance use perpetuate substance use disorders and that, at the same time, patients with substance use disorders lack positive environmental reinforcers for sober activities and pleasures (208). CRA aims to provide individuals with substance use disorders with natural alternative reinforcers by rewarding their involvement in the family and social community; thus, family members or peers play a role in reinforcing behaviors that demonstrate or facilitate abstinence (190). In CRA, emphasis is placed on improving environmental contingencies for activities of a sober lifestyle to make that type of lifestyle preferable to a substance-dependent lifestyle. In addition to individual behavioral treatment and contingency management, the multifaceted CRA treatment package typically includes conjoint marital therapy, training in finding a job, counseling on substance-free social and recreational activities, and a substance-free social club. CRA is often applied with contingency management incentives (e.g., vouchers for recreation or food) that are used to reward evidence of sober behavior (209, 210). CRA has been shown to be effective in treating alcohol dependence, with adjunctive disulfiram treatment increasing its effectiveness (211). CRA can be clinic or office based, but it is largely practiced in residential or partial hospitalization programs, therapeutic communities, and community residential facilities.

c) Cue exposure and relaxation training

Cue exposure treatment involves exposing a patient to cues that induce craving while preventing actual substance use and, therefore, the experience of substance-related reinforcement (212). Cue exposure can also be paired with relaxation techniques and drug-refusal training to facilitate the extinction of classically conditioned craving (213, 214). As an alternative, relaxation training has been used alone to provide a nonsubstance response to counteract dysphoric affects or anxiety.

d) Aversion therapy

Aversion therapy involves coupling substance use with an unpleasant experience such as mild electric shock, pharmacologically induced vomiting, or exaggerated effects of the substance. This treatment seeks to eliminate substance use behaviors by pairing them with punishment.

6. Psychodynamic and interpersonal therapies

Psychodynamic psychotherapies vary but generally attribute symptom formation and personality characteristics to traumas and deficits during an individual's development that result in unconscious psychological conflict, faulty learning, and distortions of intrapsychic structures as well as internal object relations (215) and that have a profound effect on interpersonal relationships. These developmental events and their sequelae are inextricably interconnected to the individual's underlying neurobiology (as determined by genetic and other influences), which can in turn be altered by life experience, including learning, psychological events, and psychotherapy (216). Systematic testing of the efficacy of psychodynamic treatments for substance use disorders has occurred only with supportive-expressive therapy (217), a comparatively brief psychodynamically oriented treatment based on the use of interpretation and a supportive therapeutic relationship to modify negative views of the self and others. Two trials have supported the efficacy of supportive-expressive therapy for methadone-maintained, opioid-dependent patients (177, 218). However, an additional randomized trial found that combined individual and group drug counseling was superior to a combination of individual support-expressive therapy and group drug counseling in treating patients with cocaine dependence (219).

IPT for substance use disorders is based on the concept that dysfunctional social relationships either cause or prevent recovery from a substance use disorder (220). By discovering the relation between interpersonal problems and substance use, the patient can move toward making changes aimed at building a social network that is supportive of recovery. Clinical study of IPT for substance use disorders has been limited.

7. Group therapy

Group therapy is viewed as an integral and valuable part of the treatment regimen for many patients with a substance use disorder. Many different types of therapies have been used in a group format with this population, including CBT, IPT, and behavioral marital, modified psychodynamic, interactive, rational emotive, Gestalt, and psychodrama therapies (221–225).

Group therapies permit efficient use of therapist time (226). In addition, aspects of group therapy may make this modality more effective than individual treatment for individuals with a substance use disorder. For example, given the social stigma attached to having lost control of substance use, the presence of other group members who acknowledge having a similar problem can provide comfort. In addition, other group members who are further along in their recovery can act as models, illustrating that attempts to stop substance use are not futile. These more experienced group members can offer a wide variety of coping strategies that go beyond the repertoire known even by the most skilled individual therapist. Furthermore, group members frequently can act as "buddies" who offer continued support outside of group sessions in a way that most professional therapists do not.

Finally, the public nature of group therapy provides a powerful incentive to individuals to avoid relapse. The ability to publicly declare the number of days sober coupled with the fear of having to publicly admit to relapse is a strong force that helps group members fight a disorder that is characterized by a breakdown of internalized control mechanisms. Individuals with substance use disorders have been characterized as having poorly functioning internal self-control mechanisms (227, 228), and the group process can provide a robust source of external control. Moreover, because the group is composed of individuals recovering from substance use disorders, members may be better at detecting each other's concealed substance use or early relapse signals than would an individual therapist who may not have personal experience with a substance use disorder.

Although clinical trials of group therapy for substance use disorders are comparatively rare, the available data suggest that the efficacy of group treatment is comparable with that of individual therapies (229, 230). No compelling empirical evidence is available to document the advantages or disadvantages of choosing group or individual treatment for substance use disorders. Because many patients have experience with group or individual therapy, patient preferences should be considered when choosing between the two types of treatment delivery or when developing a combined treatment program.

8. Family therapies

Dysfunctional families, characterized by impaired communication among family members and an inability of family members to set appropriate limits or maintain standards of behavior, are associated with poor short- and long-term treatment outcome for patients with substance use disorders (231). Family therapy may be delivered in a formal, ongoing therapeutic relationship or through periodic contact. Goals of family therapy include obtaining information about the patient's current attitudes toward substance use, treatment adherence, social and vocational adjustment, level of contact with substance-using peers, and degree of abstinence, as well as encouraging family support for abstinence, maintaining marital and family relationships, and improving treatment adherence and long-term outcome (232–235). They may also include behavioral contracting to maintain treatment (e.g., contracting with a partner for disulfiram treatment) or increasing positive incentives associated with sober family activities. Even the brief involvement of family members in the treatment program can enhance treatment engagement and retention.

Controlled studies have shown positive outcomes of involving non-alcohol-abusing family members in the treatment of an alcohol-abusing individual (236). More recent studies have demonstrated the effectiveness of family involvement in substance use disorder treatment for both women and men (237, 238), including patients on methadone maintenance (170). Family therapy, often in combination with other approaches, has also been studied extensively and has shown good evidence for efficacy in adolescents (239–242).

Different theoretical orientations of family therapy include structural, strategic, psychodynamic, systems, and behavioral approaches. Family interventions include those focused on the nuclear family; on the patient and his or her spouse or partner; on concurrent treatment for patients, spouses or partners, and siblings; on multifamily groups; and on social networks (120, 243, 244). Of the many types of family therapy used to treat substance use disorders, the preponderance of clinical trial evidence has been obtained for the behavioral and strategic approaches (245). The support for behavioral couples treatment is particularly strong (246).

Family intervention is indicated in circumstances in which a patient's abstinence upsets a previously well-established but maladaptive style of family interaction (233, 247) and in which other family members need help adjusting to a new set of individual and family goals, attitudes, and behaviors. Family therapy that addresses interpersonal and family interactions leading to conflict or enabling behaviors can reduce the risk of relapse for patients with high levels of family involvement. A major role for family and couples intervention is to enlist concerned significant others to foster treatment seeking and retention in family members who are unmotivated to change substance abuse behaviors. As reviewed by Miller et al. (248), most attention has been paid to behavioral coping strategies, 12-step approaches, and confrontational interventions (249), all of which are associated with high rates of treatment entry for patients who receive the intervention. However, in helping family members engage their significant others in treatment, concerned significant others and identified patients are more likely to follow through and show better results with less confrontational approaches, including CRA and community reinforcement and family training (250), than with more traditional interventions (248). Couples and family therapy are also useful for promoting psychological differentiation of family members, providing a forum for the exchange of information and ideas about the treatment plan, developing behavioral management contracts and ground rules for continued family support, and reinforcing behaviors that help prevent relapse and enhance the prospects for recovery. There is also some evidence that these approaches can improve the psychosocial functioning and decrease the likelihood of substance use in children living with a parent abusing alcohol or other substances (251, 252).

9. Self-help groups and 12-step-oriented approaches

The most widely available self-help groups (also called *mutual help groups*) are based on the 12-step approach, originally embodied in AA (253, 254), which emphasizes the concept of substance dependence as an incurable, progressive disease that has physical, emotional, and spiritual components. The 12-step programs firmly endorse the need for abstinence and consider themselves lifelong programs of recovery, even though initial success is attained one day at a time. The importance of recognizing and relying on a "higher power" or a power greater than the individual is a central element of these programs. Also key are the 12 steps of recovery, which focus first on surrender and acceptance of one's disease, second on a personal inventory, third on making amends and personal change, and finally on bringing the message to others. In addition, 12-step groups help members with relapse prevention by providing role models, social support, social strategies for maintaining a sober lifestyle, and opportunities for structured and unstructured substance-free social events and interactions. Members of self-help groups can attend meetings on a self-determined or prescribed schedule, which, if necessary, could be every day or even more than once a day. Periods associated with high risk for relapse (e.g., weekends, holidays, evenings) are particularly appropriate for attendance. A sponsor who is compatible with the patient can provide important guidance and support during the recovery process, particularly when the patient is facing periods of emotional distress and increased craving. The straightforward advice and encouragement about avoiding relapse from a recovering sponsor as well as his or her personalized support are important features of 12-step groups. For clinicians who are treating patients who report involvement in self-help groups, it is useful to ask if they are attending meetings, if they have obtained a sponsor, and if they are attending other activities associated with the self-help group (e.g., self-help group–sponsored social gatherings, retreats).

Another significant advantage to 12-step groups is their broad availability. AA is a worldwide organization with an estimated 2.2 million members in 150 countries (255), and 12-step groups have expanded to include treatment of nearly every type of substance use (Cocaine Anonymous, Marijuana Anonymous, Methadone Anonymous, Narcotics Anonymous, Nicotine Anonymous, "Crystal Meth" Anonymous). Self-help groups based on the 12-step model are also available for family members and friends (e.g., Al-Anon, Alateen, Nar-Anon) and provide group support and education about the disorder, with the goal of reducing maladaptive enabling behavior in family and friends.

In general, active participation in self-help groups has been correlated with better outcomes (256). AA has been effective for both men and women and appears to be particularly useful for those with more severe alcohol dependence (257–259). Other recent research has suggested that 12-step groups may also benefit patients dependent on substances such as cocaine (256). For patients concurrently receiving professional substance abuse treatment, there is growing empirical evidence that improved treatment outcomes are associated with participation in self-help groups (260–266). Furthermore, several studies (43, 219, 265, 267) support the efficacy of professional treatment, including TSF therapy (268) and individual drug counseling (269), that enhances a patient's motivation to participate in 12-step programs. These findings have important clinical implications, given that these approaches are similar to the dominant model applied in most community treatment programs (270). Thus, for many patients, even those who may still be actively using substances, referral to a 12-step program can be helpful at all stages in the treatment process.

An individual's refusal to participate in a self-help group is not synonymous with his or her resistance to treatment in general. Despite their many potential benefits, self-help groups are not useful for all patients. Some individuals' apparent resistance to self-help group participation can be addressed by individualizing the choice of a group to the patient's needs. For example, young people generally do better in groups that include age-appropriate peers in addition to some older recovering members. Patients who require psychotropic medications for co-occurring psychiatric disorders should be directed to groups in which this activity is recognized and supported as useful treatment rather than as another form of substance abuse. The spiritual tenets of traditional 12-step programs can be a deterrent to participation for individuals who do not embrace these ideas. Although not widely available, alternative self-help groups such as Women for Sobriety (271), Secular Organizations for Sobriety (272), and Self-Management and Recovery Training (273) have been developed to address this problem and may be an option for some patients.

10. Brief therapies

The efficacy of brief interventions has been studied mostly in connection with alcohol use disorders. The interventions were initially designed to facilitate the treatment of alcohol abuse or dependence in a setting other than a substance abuse treatment facility (e.g., primary care clinic, mental health clinic, EAP) (274, 275). More recent evidence suggests that brief interventions are also effective with other substance use disorders, including cannabis (276), opioid (277), and nicotine (278) dependence and in special populations such as adolescents (279), patients with co-occurring psychiatric and substance use disorders (280), and patients in the military (281).

The A-FRAMES model is the core structure of a brief intervention: Assessment, providing objective Feedback, emphasizing that Responsibility for change belongs to the patient, giving clear Advice about the benefits of change, providing a Menu of options for treatment to facilitate change, using Empathic listening, and emphasizing and encouraging Self-efficacy with the patient (49). Despite the short time required to implement a brief intervention, treatment facilities that do not specialize in substance abuse treatment often experience difficulties in using this strategy, including inadequate time available during face-to-face encounters and clinicians' negative attitudes toward substance use (282, 283).

11. Self-guided therapies

Self-help therapies guided by written, programmed, or Internet-based instruction have been shown to be effective for heavy users of legal substances (i.e., alcohol, nicotine) who do not meet criteria for a substance use disorder. The target population for such approaches typically includes students or general medical patients rather than individuals who are seeking treatment for a substance use disorder.

Self-help manuals and behavioral self-control training teach patients how to 1) set goals for substance reduction or cessation, 2) monitor progress toward achievement of these goals, 3) reward oneself for progress, 4) learn new coping skills that will facilitate substance reduction or abstinence, and 5) perform functional analysis of behaviors associated with substance use (284). These therapies are available as manual-guided self-help programs, manual-guided therapies with a clinician, and computer-guided programs (285, 286). They are therefore available for home use as well as office- and clinic-based use.

Although these approaches are sometimes helpful for those at high risk for developing a substance use disorder or substance-related medical consequences, such minimal therapies may not be sufficient for treatment-seeking patients who already have a substance use disorder.

12. Hypnosis

The use of hypnotherapy for substance use disorders has been most studied as an aid in the cessation of cigarette smoking, with its usual goal being to implant unconscious suggestions that will deter use of a substance, such as "smoking will be unpleasant." Despite the widespread use of hypnosis in this context, there is little scientific validation to support its effectiveness in the treatment of nicotine dependence (287).

G. CLINICAL FEATURES INFLUENCING TREATMENT

1. Use of multiple substances

Many patients entering treatment for a specific substance use disorder abuse more than one substance, and co-occurring nicotine dependence is particularly common. For some patients, there is a "drug of choice," with other substances serving as a substitute when the primary substance is unavailable. Others routinely use multiple substances simultaneously. An individual's concurrent use of two or more substances may be motivated by his or her wish to modify the effects of the primary drug of choice or to prevent or relieve withdrawal symptoms. In addition, many patients use multiple substances because of their availability. Frequent drug combinations include 1) cocaine and alcohol; 2) cocaine and heroin; 3) heroin and benzodiazepines; 4) alcohol, cocaine, and benzodiazepines; 5) nicotine and any other drug; 6) multiple "club drugs" (e.g., 3,4-methylenedioxymethamphetamine [MDMA], γ-hydroxybutyrate [GHB], ketamine); 7) "club drugs" with prescription medications (e.g., MDMA with sildenafil and/or fluoxetine); and 8) opioids, stimulants, sedatives, steroids, and other substances. The severity of abuse of each substance and the motivation to stop using each substance may vary widely in individuals who abuse multiple substances.

The treatment of patients using multiple substances may be complicated by 1) simultaneous intoxication or withdrawal from two or more drugs, 2) varying time frames for experiencing withdrawal symptoms, 3) the need to detoxify the patient from more than one drug, and 4) potential interactions between an abused substance and medications used to treat a comorbid substance use disorder (e.g., inadvertent precipitation of opioid withdrawal in patients treated with naltrexone for alcohol dependence).

Although the presence of multiple substance use disorders is the norm, there is limited research to guide clinicians on adapting the usual evidence-based clinical interventions to the treatment of individuals using more than one substance, including medication and psychosocial treatments. The best recommendation is for the clinician to do a comprehensive assessment of the patient and integrate the evidence-based treatment approaches, including pharmacological and psychosocial treatments, for each specific substance use disorder (288).

2. Psychiatric factors

The presence of a substance use disorder will have an impact on psychiatric issues, such as the risk of suicide or other self-injurious behaviors and the risk of aggressive behaviors, including homicide. In addition, the presence of co-occurring psychiatric symptoms or disorders affects the patient's treatment adherence as well as the onset, course, and prognosis of the substance use disorder (170, 288–292). These factors need to be taken into consideration when arriving at a treatment plan for an individual patient.

a) Risk of suicide

The frequency of suicide attempts and death by suicide is substantially higher among patients with a substance use disorder than in the general population. A systematic review of retrospective and prospective cohort studies of substance use disorders and suicide (293) demonstrated that individuals with alcohol use disorder, opioid dependence, or mixed drug use have a substantially greater likelihood of suicide compared with the general population, with a 9.8-, 13.5-, and 16.9-fold elevated risk, respectively. This review reported insufficient evidence to compare the suicide risk among patients with other drug use disorders (e.g., cocaine dependence). In terms of lifetime suicide mortality, a review of 83 studies demonstrated a lifetime suicide risk of 7% in individuals with an alcohol use disorder, which is comparable to that of individuals with a mood disorder (6%) or schizophrenia (4%) (294). These rates vary by country and may be slightly lower in the United States (295). In addition, significant rates of substance use disorders are found in psychological autopsy studies of individuals who have died by suicide (296–300), with a recent or impending interpersonal loss being a frequent apparent precipitant (301).

Rates of suicidal ideation and suicidal behaviors, including suicide attempts, are also increased in individuals with a substance use disorder. For example, in a recent prospective study, treatment-seeking individuals with alcohol dependence were found to have attempted suicide seven times more frequently than age-matched, non-alcohol-dependent comparison subjects during the 5-year follow-up period after the initial evaluation (302). The alcohol-dependent individuals who attempted suicide (4.5%) were more likely than the other individuals to have made prior attempts; other related factors were earlier onset of the substance disorder, more severe substance dependence, dependence on multiple substances, more panic symptoms, being separated or divorced, having had prior treatment, and having been diagnosed with a substance-induced psychiatric disorder (302). In addition, significant high rates of substance use disorders are seen among individuals who have attempted suicide (296, 303–305).

The risk of suicidal behaviors and death by suicide is further increased for individuals with a substance use disorder in the context of certain co-occurring psychiatric disorders, such as major depressive disorder, bipolar disorder, and cluster B personality disorders. The presence of major depressive disorder substantially increases impulsive suicidal behaviors and suicide risk (298, 303, 306–308). A recent review of the literature on co-occurring alcohol use disorders and major depressive disorder demonstrated that this comorbidity increases the risk of suicidal ideation, suicidal behaviors, and death by suicide (309). Among patients diagnosed with major depressive disorder and bipolar disorder, cigarette smoking has also been found to be an independent predictor of future suicidal behavior (310).

Prospective studies of patients with co-occurring bipolar and substance use disorders consistently report greater frequency of lifetime suicide attempts and suicidal ideation compared with bipolar disorder patients with no co-occurring substance use disorder (311–313). Bipolar patients with co-occurring anxiety symptoms or cluster B personality disorder features and a substance use disorder may be at the greatest risk for suicidal behaviors (314, 315).

Patients with co-occurring cluster B personality and substance use disorders also have a greater risk of suicidal ideation and death by suicide (316, 317). This population is also at greater risk for accidental death by injection drug overdose (318).

Despite this clear evidence for an increased risk of suicidal behaviors in individuals with a substance use disorder, few controlled studies are available to assist in guiding the treatment of such patients (319). As in the care of any patient with a psychiatric disorder, suicide risk should be assessed regularly and in a systematic manner. Assessment of suicide risk includes determining the presence or absence of current suicidal thoughts, intent, and plan; a history of suicide attempts (e.g., lethality of method, circumstances); a family history of suicide; a history of aggression (e.g., weapon use, circumstances); the intensity of current depressive and other mood symptoms; the current treatment regimen and response; recent life stressors (e.g., marital separation, job loss); substance use patterns; psychotic symptoms; and current living situation (e.g., social supports, availability of weapon). In substance-using individuals, suicidal ideation and suicide attempts may occur in the context of a major depressive episode or result from substance-induced sadness or dysphoria combined with increased impulsivity and poor judgment. However, individuals with a substance use disorder can also be at risk for suicide even in the apparent absence of depression. In terms of treatment implications, care should be used when prescribing potentially toxic medications to a suicidal patient. For additional recommendations on the assessment and treatment of suicidal patients with substance use disorders, the reader is referred to APA's *Practice Guideline for the Assessment and Treatment of Patients With Suicidal Behaviors* (301).

b) Risk of aggressive behaviors, including homicide

Substance use disorders are associated with an increased risk for aggressive behaviors toward others, including physical assault, sexual aggression, domestic violence, child abuse, and homicide (320–322). Substance intoxication and withdrawal states may be associated with anxiety, irritability, agitation, impaired impulse control, disinhibition, decreased pain sensitivity, and impaired reality testing; these effects are hypothesized to account for the increased aggressive behaviors associated with substance use. In particular, intoxication with substances such as alcohol, cocaine, methamphetamine, PCP, anabolic steroids, and hallucinogens may be associated with aggression (138, 323–327), whereas withdrawal from substances such as alcohol, opioids, sedative-hypnotics, and cannabis can lead to withdrawal syndromes associated with a risk of aggressive behaviors (138, 320, 328). Intoxication with marijuana or hallucinogens may inadvertently lead individuals to perform aggressive acts because of a faulty perception of reality coupled with high levels of anxiety and paranoia (329–331). Substance use disorders are also indirectly associated with aggressive behaviors engaged in to obtain illicit or expensive substances. Although it is important to assess for and be aware of the potential for aggressive behaviors in individuals with a substance use disorder, it is also important to assess for substance use disorders in all individuals who present with a history of agitation or aggression. Because family and partners may be affected by substance-related domestic violence, systematic screening and referral for domestic violence treatment interventions may effectively reduce domestic violence. Some treatments such as abstinent partner therapy (e.g., coping skills training [332]) and couples therapy (e.g., behavioral couples therapy [333]) have been shown to reduce alcohol-related domestic violence in randomized, controlled trials.

c) Sleep disturbances

Individuals with substance use disorders frequently report sleep disturbances, particularly after being detoxified. For some patients, managing sleep disturbances will be an important component of the treatment plan. Indeed, some studies have demonstrated that among detoxified alcohol-dependent individuals, insomnia is a strong predictor of relapse (334–336). Despite the recognition that sleep disturbances are a problem among individuals with substance use disorders, only a handful of studies have examined the treatment of sleep disturbances in these individuals, and these studies have focused only on individuals with alcohol dependence. For example, one small double-blind study found that trazodone was superior to placebo in improving sleep in alcohol-dependent individuals with insomnia (337). In an open-label study comparing trazodone and gabapentin for the treatment of insomnia in alcohol-dependent individuals, both medications were found to improve insomnia, but the gabapentin group showed greater improvements than the trazodone group (338). Given the open-label nature of this study, more research is needed to determine if gabapentin is an effective treatment for sleep disturbances related to alcohol dependence. In addition, more research is needed to determine if trazodone and gabapentin, as well as other sedating psychotropic medications, can effectively treat sleep disturbances not only in individuals with alcohol dependence but also in those with other substance use disorders.

In addition to the studies of pharmacological agents, there has been one randomized, controlled study that showed that CBT strategies helped improve sleep disturbances in alcohol-dependent individuals in recovery (339). As with the pharmacological treatments for sleep disturbances, more research is needed to determine if these strategies will help improve insomnia in individuals with other substance use disorders as well.

d) Co-occurring psychiatric and substance use disorders

(1) General principles

Co-occurring psychiatric and substance use disorders are common in all treatment settings (e.g., centers for the treatment of substance use disorders, mental health clinics, primary care settings, emergency departments) and in the general community. In fact, only a few differences (e.g., higher prevalence of schizophrenia and primary psychotic disorders in mental health care settings, more severe patterns of substance use in substance use treatment settings) are observable between patients with co-occurring psychiatric disorders receiving treatment in substance abuse treatment centers and patients with co-occurring substance use disorders receiving treatment in mental health treatment centers (340). In community population samples studied in the National Comorbidity Survey (341), individuals with alcohol dependence had high rates of clinically significant depression during their lifetime (men: 24% depression and 11% dysthymia; women: 49% depression and 21% dysthymia). Individuals with bipolar disorder had high rates of alcohol (61%) and other substance (41%) dependence (342). Treatment-seeking individuals have even higher rates of co-occurring disorders (343–345). For example, Penick et al. (346) studied a U.S. Department of Veterans Affairs (VA) hospital outpatient population with alcohol dependence or abuse and found that 56% reported co-occurring psychiatric disorders. In substance use disorder treatment settings, depression, anxiety, and personality disorders frequently occur. However, posttraumatic stress disorder (PTSD), adult ADHD, learning disabilities, social anxiety disorder, eating disorders, and pathological gambling are also common and are often underrecognized and undertreated (121, 288).

Individuals with nicotine dependence are more likely to have co-occurring psychiatric disorders than the general U.S. population (347). Furthermore, in mental health and substance use disorder treatment settings, nicotine dependence continues to be the most common co-occurring substance use disorder, with approximately 60%–95% of patients being nicotine dependent, although this varies by the type of psychiatric disorder and the treatment setting (348). One analysis of nicotine use as reported in the National Comorbidity Survey found that individuals with psychiatric disorders were about twice as likely to smoke as the general population and that about 44% of the cigarettes smoked in the United States were smoked by individuals with a psychiatric disorder (349).

Use of multiple substances and co-occurring psychiatric and substance use disorders are now so common in treatment settings that these combinations should be expected. Thus, all patients with a substance use disorder should be carefully assessed for the presence of co-occurring psychiatric disorders, including additional substance use disorders. Conversely, patients with identified psychiatric disorders should be routinely assessed for the presence of a co-occurring substance use disorder (350, 351).

Treating individuals with co-occurring psychiatric and substance use disorders in traditional inpatient and outpatient programs is challenging. Patients' motivation to change may vary according to the type of substance(s) they use and the severity of their psychiatric issues, and this needs to be taken into consideration in treatment planning. Recent research and consensus opinions by experts in the field support the notion that the integration of substance abuse and mental health treatment strategies, including integrated systems, programs, and clinical treatment, improves patient outcome (80, 121, 352, 353). There is growing evidence that patients in psychiatric or substance abuse treatment settings have better outcomes if they receive integrated treatment for their coexisting psychiatric and substance use disorders (121, 288, 354–356). Integrated treatment usually requires incorporating and modifying traditional psychiatric and substance abuse treatment methods so that the co-occurring disorders receive simultaneous treatment.

a. Integrated treatment

Recent research and clinical experience (80, 288) has also shed light on the question of treatment timing (e.g., if co-occurring disorders should be treated together in an integrated manner or in what circumstances one problem should be addressed before another). In general, the length of the observation period for a psychiatric or substance use disorder will be determined by balancing the following considerations: the degree of diagnostic certainty, the severity of the patient's condition, and the anticipated benefits and risks of the proposed treatment (288, 353).

The integrated treatment of co-occurring psychiatric and substance use disorders can include psychosocial and/or pharmacological interventions. Initial treatment efforts should include engaging the patient in treatment and assessing and managing the most severe symptoms of both types of disorders. This may include addressing symptoms of intoxication or withdrawal. Sometimes severe psychiatric symptoms (e.g., psychosis, suicidal ideation) can be managed while a patient is intoxicated or experiencing withdrawal; such patients may require immediate treatment in an emergency department or an inpatient psychiatric unit. Once a patient's acute psychiatric symptoms and intoxication or withdrawal states have been stabilized, the patient can be evaluated for treatment in an ongoing rehabilitative treatment program. When patients are being treated in a substance abuse treatment setting, their psychiatric symptoms should be monitored and addressed clinically through psychiatric medications, when appropriate, as well as through integrated psychosocial strategies (e.g., teaching patients mood management as part of relapse prevention therapy) and integrated treatment approaches for psychiatric disorders and substance use disorders (357).

In a psychiatric treatment setting, it would be incorrect to assume that successful treatment of a psychiatric disorder will resolve the substance use disorder. The substance use disorder will require specific treatment even when it arises in the context of another psychiatric disorder, a situation that is quite common and that presents an opportunity for the prevention of a secondary disorder (358).

Certain psychosocial and pharmacological treatments have been studied for specific combinations of psychiatric and substance use disorders (e.g., major depression and alcohol dependence, schizophrenia and cocaine dependence) (288, 353); the literature about these treatments is presented in the specific substance use disorder sections of this practice guideline. The reader is also advised to review other APA practice guidelines for the treatment of patients with specific psychiatric disorders for additional information.

b. Pharmacological management of psychiatric disorders

In most patients, the same medications are recommended for the treatment of a specific psychiatric disorder whether that disorder co-occurs with a substance use disorder or not. Clinical issues such as medication tolerability, safety, and abuse potential are important considerations in choosing a medication and will influence traditional psychopharmacological treatment algorithms. There is no evidence to suggest that the duration of pharmacotherapy for a psychiatric disorder in conjunction with a co-occurring substance use disorder would differ from that needed to treat the psychiatric condition alone, and there are no data to suggest that decisions about continuation and maintenance treatment should differ (288). An important clinical question in treating a co-occurring psychiatric disorder in a substance use disorder treatment setting is whether the prescribing clinician should initiate psychiatric medications during the acute treatment of the substance use disorder. For some psychiatric disorders (especially depression, generalized anxiety disorder [GAD], social anxiety disorder, and PTSD), there have been widely differing opinions about the amount of time a patient should be abstinent from a substance before a definitive diagnosis of a co-occurring psychiatric disorder versus a substance-induced psychiatric disorder can be made. If there is little overlap between the symptoms observed and the expected abstinence syndrome (such as bulimia nervosa in an opioid-dependent patient), then the psychiatric diagnosis can be immediately established. In circumstances when prominent mood or anxiety symptoms could be equally attributable to early abstinence or an independent co-occurring psychiatric disorder, a clinician may consider whether similar symptoms occurred before the substance use or during previous abstinence periods or whether the individual's family history suggests a vulnerability to a co-occurring mood or anxiety disorder. A common recommendation is to consider the severity of an individual's functional impairment when deciding whether or not to initiate pharmacotherapy, continue ongoing monitoring of symptoms, and initiate psychosocial treatment strategies for the management of anxiety and depression (288).

Medication nonadherence is common among individuals with co-occurring psychiatric and substance use disorders (359, 360). Nonadherence can be due to many factors, including cognitive impairment, the patient's fear of the interaction between prescribed medication and substances being abused, fear that the prescribed medication is itself harmful, change in motivation, and lack of support. Some patients attending 12-step meetings may feel pressure from some group members not to take psychiatric medications because they are "mood altering"; however, AA does support the appropriate use of needed medications (361, 362). AA brochures and other resources do state a reasonable concern about individuals' avoiding psychotropic medications with an abuse potential (e.g., sedative-hypnotics, anxiolytics, stimulants). When such medications are necessary, a clinician should prescribe them with caution and closely monitor their use (e.g., dispense in limited quantities, track prescription refills, monitor ongoing medical necessity for and the patient's response to the medication).

c. Medications to treat substance use disorders

Medications for treating substance use disorders, such as those for managing acute withdrawal and protracted withdrawal symptoms or reducing craving, have not been well studied in dually diagnosed populations but should be considered for these patients. The presence of a co-occurring mental illness may influence a clinician's decision to prescribe disulfiram for alcohol-dependent patients if, for example, the clinician is concerned about a patient's capacity to adhere to prescribing instructions due to acute psychiatric symptoms. However, a 12-week multicenter, randomized, controlled trial of disulfiram in patients with co-occurring alcohol dependence and psychiatric illness demonstrated the safety and effectiveness of this medication with this population (363). This same study also substantiated the safety and efficacy of naltrexone use in this population. However, no further benefit was achieved in this study by combining disulfiram and naltrexone.

d. Integrated psychosocial treatments

Psychosocial treatment is very important in the treatment of a substance use disorder both with and without a co-occurring psychiatric disorder. Integrated psychotherapy approaches represent some of the most recent advances in psychosocial treatments, and several have been developed for specific subtypes of co-occurring disorders. A common feature of these integrated therapies is their blending of traditional evidence-based psychotherapies with traditional evidence-based substance use disorder therapies such as MET, relapse prevention therapy/CBT, and TSF therapy. Examples of psychiatric disorders for which integrated treatments have been developed include PTSD (364–368), bipolar disorder (369), schizophrenia (80, 360, 370–372), and personality disorders (373, 374). The efficacy of these integrated psychotherapies is being actively investigated in individual as well as in family and group modalities (375–377).

(2) Treatment in the presence of specific co-occurring psychiatric disorders

a. Schizophrenia

A review of the literature examining nicotine dependence among individuals with schizophrenia demonstrated prevalence rates of 68%–88% among outpatients and 81%–88% among inpatients (378), suggesting that substance use vulnerability alone cannot account for the high smoking rates among patients with schizophrenia. Patterns of nicotine use among patients with schizophrenia are more severe than in patients with other psychiatric diagnoses (379), and these usage patterns are associated with increased morbidity and mortality due to tobacco-related medical diseases such as cancer and cardiovascular and respiratory diseases (359, 380–383). Apart from nicotine dependence, about 40%–60% of individuals with schizophrenia will have another co-occurring substance use disorder during their lifetime (353, 384, 385). Substance-abusing individuals with schizophrenia are more likely to be male, young, and less educated and have better social skills than those not abusing substances, but they have less peer support and poorer treatment outcomes in traditional substance abuse treatment settings because of the stress associated with the confrontational treatment approaches sometimes used in these programs (353, 386). Because substance abuse treatment staff typically have limited training in managing psychosis and because mental health clinicians are trained and able to provide both medications and psychosocial treatment for schizophrenia, this population most commonly receives integrated treatment for the co-occurring disorders within the mental health system.

Effective integrated treatment programs have used one clinical team to provide long-term, comprehensive care (i.e., medication and psychosocial treatment interventions) for both psychotic and substance use disorders (80, 353). Treatment is provided in the patient's natural environment, is matched to the patient's motivational state, provides comprehensive community services (e.g., stable housing, financial assistance through entitlements, vocational rehabilitation), and is not limited in duration (80, 387). Integrated treatment often begins by stabilizing a patient's psychotic symptoms, which may require psychiatric hospitalization. Integrated treatment programs can then initiate substance abuse treatment when the patient is sufficiently stable to participate in the psychosocial treatments for the psychiatric and substance use disorders. Thus, the acute stabilization phase may initially emphasize appropriate antipsychotic and psychosocial treatments that help stabilize the illnesses (353, 371).

1) Pharmacotherapy

Existing studies and reports from expert consensus meetings on co-occurring disorders support the same first-line agents recommended in APA's *Practice Guideline for the Treatment of Patients With Schizophrenia* (388) for individuals with co-occurring schizophrenia and substance use disorders (80, 288). With the possible exception of clozapine for patients with treatment-resistant symptoms, antipsychotics generally have similar efficacy in treating the positive symptoms of schizophrenia (389), although there is emerging evidence and an ongoing debate regarding whether second-generation antipsychotics may have superior efficacy in treating global psychopathology and cognitive, negative, and mood symptoms (388). Various smaller studies have found better outcomes with clozapine (390–398), risperidone (394, 399–402), and olanzapine (403, 404) than with first-generation antipsychotics for patients with co-occurring schizophrenia and substance use disorders. However, most of these studies were retrospective, nonrandomized, or uncontrolled pilot studies. Furthermore, no evidence to date suggests that any one second-generation antipsychotic is more efficacious than another in this population, and no trials have been reported that compare these agents in the same clinical study. Some have thought that clozapine should be considered as a first-line agent in patients with schizophrenia co-occurring with a substance use disorder because of the number of studies supporting its use (394) and its ability to reduce the risk of suicidal behaviors (405). In addition, clozapine may have beneficial effects in decreasing smoking (406–408). However, most experts have continued to recommend clozapine as a second-line agent (288) because of the need for regular monitoring of the patient's white blood count to detect granulocytopenia or impending agranulocytosis, as well as other concerns about clozapine's side-effect profile (i.e., increased seizure risk and sedation). Because significant nonadherence to clozapine necessitates the retitration of the medication dose and because blood monitoring is an essential part of clozapine treatment, clozapine is generally used in more motivated patients and in well-integrated treatment programs.

In choosing an antipsychotic medication, a clinician should assess patient preferences and vulnerabilities regarding side effects, interactions with abused substances, and other safety considerations. It should be noted that individuals with schizophrenia who abuse alcohol and cocaine may have an increased risk for seizures or liver toxicity and may have cardiac abnormalities as a result of their substance use. Medications that may induce QT prolongation should be used with caution, with electrocardiographic monitoring as needed. Because most antipsychotic medications are hepatically metabolized and can lower seizure threshold to some degree, these factors should also be taken into consideration when choosing among antipsychotic medications. Patients with schizophrenia may also experience increased somnolence and orthostatic hypotension if they abuse alcohol or other sedating drugs while taking antipsychotic medications. Tobacco smoking substantially lowers blood levels of clozapine, olanzapine, and numerous first-generation antipsychotics (e.g., haloperidol, fluphenazine, chlorpromazine, thioridazine) by increasing cytochrome P450 (CYP) 1A2 enzyme hepatic metabolism, a moderate effect that may necessitate an increase in the medication dose. The metabolism of other second-generation antipsychotics is not significantly affected by changes in smoking status.

Another clinically important issue in this population is addressing poor adherence with both pharmacological and psychosocial interventions. The use of long-acting, injectable antipsychotic medications can help increase medication adherence. A long-acting, injectable form of the second-generation antipsychotic risperidone is available as are long-acting decanoate preparations of first-generation antipsychotics (i.e., haloperidol, fluphenazine); there have been no direct comparisons of these long-acting first- and second-generation antipsychotic agents in this population.

In general, medications targeting specific substance use disorders can be safely prescribed for patients with co-occurring schizophrenia and substance use disorders (288). However, careful assessment is indicated before initiating treatment with disulfiram. Given the cognitive difficulties associated with schizophrenia, disulfiram should be reserved for use in individuals whose judgment and memory are adequate and for whom impulsivity is not a significant concern. In addition, there may be some further concern about using high-dose disulfiram in this population because carbon disulfide, a metabolite of disulfiram, inhibits dopamine β-hydroxylase, increases dopamine levels, and could potentially worsen psychosis (409, 410). Specific studies also support the use of naltrexone for alcohol dependence and methadone for opioid dependence in this population (411–413). The treatment of nicotine dependence with NRTs (i.e., nicotine patch, gum, spray, inhaler, or lozenge) and bupropion has helped improve treatment outcomes for tobacco smokers with schizophrenia (414, 415). There is a theoretical concern that bupropion may increase psychotic symptoms; however, this concern has not been borne out in studies to date (414). There are improved outcomes with combining NRT and bupropion with psychosocial treatments that are specific to nicotine dependence (348, 416).

2) Psychosocial treatments

Integrated psychosocial treatments for individuals with co-occurring schizophrenia and substance use disorders most commonly occur in mental health settings and include unique psychotherapy approaches as well as modified treatment programs and systems (352). One key aspect of integrated treatment is that patients do better when clinicians are able to maintain an optimistic, empathic, and helpful approach (417). Integrated programs often provide comprehensive services, including active outreach and case management in the community setting, in an effort to better engage and retain patients and help them transition between different levels of care (370, 417). Model integrated treatment programs have been described and evaluated in the literature (417), including assertive community treatment teams and integrated stage-based motivational models; these models tend to emphasize a recovery-oriented perspective while combining medications, MET, relapse prevention therapy, social skills training, and specific dual recovery therapy approaches (80, 371, 386, 418, 419). Other helpful components to integrated treatment programs include contingency management and money management (360, 372). Money management helps patients prevent relapse, given that many receive Social Security disability or Supplemental Security Income payments and are most vulnerable to substance use and relapse soon after receiving these funds (372).

b. Depressive disorders

Major depressive and substance use disorders commonly co-occur in clinical populations and in the community (341, 343, 344, 420). Studies have demonstrated that individuals diagnosed with major depressive disorder have high lifetime co-occurrence rates of alcohol abuse (men 9% and women 30%) and alcohol dependence (men 24% and women 48.5%) (421). Among individuals with major depressive disorder, approximately 25% have a co-occurring substance use disorder (422). A large prospective, longitudinal study has demonstrated that alcohol and drug use disorders during adolescence predict later development of major depressive disorder in young adults (423).

Mood disturbance is one of the most common symptoms reported by individuals in substance use disorder treatment programs. In addition to the high rate of co-occurring major depressive and substance use disorders, patients in substance use disorder treatment settings frequently experience substance-induced mood disorders in which signs and symptoms of depression are related to acute substance intoxication or to acute or protracted withdrawal from substances; these symptoms remit with maintained abstinence (424). Because it is often difficult for a clinician to discern whether a cluster of symptoms is due to co-occurring major depressive disorder, substance intoxication, substance withdrawal, substance-induced mood disorder, or some combination thereof, guidelines have been established for diagnosing and treating mood symptoms in the context of a substance use disorder (425). When possible, it is advisable to delay antidepressant pharmacotherapy by 1–4 weeks, depending on the nature and severity of the mood symptoms, to allow the clinician to identify substance-induced mood symptoms that may remit without medication intervention.

In general, treatment of depressive symptoms of moderate to severe intensity should begin concurrently or soon after initiating treatment of the co-occurring substance use disorder, particularly if there is evidence of prior mood episodes. In individuals without prior episodes of depression or a family history of mood disorders, it may be appropriate to delay the treatment of mild to moderate depressive symptoms for the purpose of diagnostic clarification. Clinicians are advised to monitor symptoms, assess and reassess for suicidal ideation, provide education, encourage abstinence from substances, and observe changes in mental status during the substance-free period while actively considering whether antidepressant intervention is indicated (288, 426–429).

1) Pharmacotherapy

Existing studies and expert consensus support the use of first-line agents recommended in APA's *Practice Guideline for the Treatment of Patients With Major Depressive Disorder* (430) and substance use disorder medications for detoxification, protracted withdrawal, and agonist maintenance treatment (288). Randomized, controlled trials supporting the efficacy of antidepressant pharmacotherapies for co-occurring major depressive disorder and specific substance use disorders exist for alcohol dependence, opioid dependence, cocaine use disorders, and nicotine dependence.

A meta-analysis of 14 well-designed placebo-controlled trials of antidepressant medication for co-occurring major depression and alcohol, opioid, or cocaine dependence (425) showed an overall beneficial effect of medication on mood outcome, similar in magnitude to the effect size observed in clinical trials involving depressed patients without substance problems. Studies showing the largest effects of medication on mood outcome also showed significant beneficial effects of medication on self-report measures of substance use, although rates of abstinence were low. The results across studies were inconsistent, with eight positive and six negative studies. The positive studies, those demonstrating a beneficial effect of antidepressant medication, had low placebo response rates and were more likely to have required at least a week of abstinence prior to diagnosing depression and starting medication. The evidence for medication effectiveness was more consistent among studies of patients with alcohol dependence than among studies of patients with drug dependence, in agreement with the conclusion of another recent meta-analysis (430a).

Of the selective serotonin reuptake inhibitors (SSRIs), fluoxetine (431) and sertraline (432–434) have been studied in the treatment of co-occurring major depressive disorder and alcohol dependence, and evidence is also available for the use of nefazodone (435, 436) and the tricyclic antidepressants (TCAs) imipramine (428, 437) and desipramine (438). These agents, however, have not been compared with each other nor has there been an adequate number of studies of other SSRIs to make recommendations for specific antidepressants as first-line agents in this population. A review of the literature indicates that antidepressant treatment is more effective in ameliorating mood symptoms than in improving drinking outcomes for this dually diagnosed population (439). Given the reported risks of hepatotoxicity and death with nefazodone use (440), this medication is not generally recommended unless other therapies have failed.

The evidence base for antidepressant pharmacotherapy in co-occurring opioid dependence and major depressive disorder is inconsistent and well studied only in methadone-maintained populations. Results of randomized, placebo-controlled trials of TCA treatment are mixed, with some showing no differences between antidepressant treatment and placebo (441–443) and others showing superior efficacy of TCAs compared with placebo (444–447). Evidence for SSRI efficacy in the same population is weaker (448), and many studies have failed to demonstrate beneficial effects of SSRIs on mood symptoms (413, 449, 450). Nevertheless, the relative safety of SSRIs as compared with TCAs in this population continues to influence the choice of SSRIs as first-line agents for patients with co-occurring opioid use disorder and major depressive disorder. Although the duration of antidepressant treatment in these studies was not >3 months, there are no available data to suggest that the duration of an antidepressant trial should be different than that used for treating major depressive disorder without a substance use disorder.

Treating mood symptoms in individuals with co-occurring cocaine use and major depressive disorders is complicated by the frequent occurrence of depressive symptoms during acute withdrawal from cocaine. Some randomized, controlled trials support the use of antidepressant intervention in these individuals (451, 452); this population also appears to have a more favorable mood response to TCAs than to SSRIs (453).

Nicotine dependence commonly co-occurs with major depressive disorder. In large well-designed, placebo-controlled trials, the antidepressant medications bupropion (158, 454) and nortriptyline (455, 456) have been found to improve smoking cessation rates and to prevent relapse after successful quit attempts. Smokers with a current major depression were excluded from these studies. The beneficial effects of both nortriptyline (456) and bupropion (454, 1587) have been shown not to depend on a past history of major depression—that is, the medications are equally effective for smokers with and without past depression. An analysis of mediators of treatment effect (456) suggested nortriptyline improves smoking cessation by reducing postquit dysphoria, with the effect, again, independent of past history of major depression. Serious depression sometimes emerges after a patient has successfully quit smoking (457, 457a, 763), suggesting the importance of monitoring mood during quit attempts. Studies are needed of the treatment of smokers with current depressive disorders. However, in such patients, most clinicians will prioritize stabilization of the depressive episode and then subsequently address treatment of nicotine dependence during the maintenance phase of depression treatment (348). Sustained-release bupropion for treating nicotine dependence may be safely added to other antidepressants (e.g., SSRIs, which do not alter smoking cessation rates) being used to treat major depressive disorder (458). NRTs are also recommended as a first-line option in treating nicotine dependence in depressed smokers. In addition, integrating standard tobacco dependence–related psychosocial treatment into ongoing psychosocial treatment for depression improves both tobacco dependence and depression outcomes among smokers with recurrent depression and heavy smoking (459).

Many patients with co-occurring major depressive and substance use disorders will report experiencing insomnia or anxiety symptoms. Such symptoms are optimally addressed using behavioral strategies (e.g., stress reduction, relaxation skills, adherence to sleep hygiene) and/or pharmacological interventions with medications that do not have a potential for abuse (e.g., buspirone) before medications with abuse potential (e.g., benzodiazepines, nonbenzodiazepine hypnotics such as zolpidem) are considered. Although not specifically studied in co-occurring major depressive and substance use disorders, the antidepressant trazodone may represent an additional option (see Section II.G.2.c).

In the context of continued substance use, inadequate symptom improvement should not lead the clinician to conclude that a medication regimen is a therapeutic failure. Patients with persistent depression and substance use may benefit from more frequent outpatient visits or referral to a higher level of care (e.g., intensive outpatient, partial or residential hospitalization, inpatient treatment).

2) Psychosocial treatments

Integrated psychosocial therapies have been developed, and their efficacy is being tested in controlled trials for patients with co-occurring major depressive disorder and substance use disorders (456, 460, 461). These psychotherapy approaches combine traditional therapies for substance use disorders (e.g., MET, TSF, relapse prevention therapies, CBT, contingency management) with traditional therapies for depression (e.g., cognitive therapy, behavioral therapy, IPT, and brief psychodynamic therapy) (357, 462). These approaches commonly try to help patients identify and manage triggers for substance use, understand and manage feelings, deal with grief and anger, change thoughts and beliefs that worsen mood, improve relationships, and change behaviors and lifestyles (463).

c. Bipolar disorder

Individuals with bipolar disorder are at high risk for a co-occurring substance use disorder; community lifetime prevalence rates of co-occurrence are ≥50% (341, 420). Substance use disorders influence bipolar disorder by worsening each episode as well as worsening the overall course of the disorder by causing more mixed episodes, earlier onset, more frequent episodes, and slower symptom remission (464).

Few medication studies have been conducted with co-occurring bipolar and specific substance use disorders; however, the existing research (464–468) and expert consensus (469, 470) support use of the first-line agents recommended in APA's *Practice Guideline for the Treatment of Patients With Bipolar Disorder* (471) and the use of adjunctive medications that target specific substance use disorders. The few medication studies examining co-occurring bipolar and substance use disorders support the use of valproate (or valproic acid or divalproex) as a mood stabilizer because it shows some evidence of efficacy and appears to help overall treatment adherence (472). In addition, some evidence suggests that patients with these co-occurring disorders are more likely to respond to valproate or a combination of valproate plus lithium than to lithium alone (465–468, 472, 473). The relative lack of efficacy with lithium may be due to an increase in side effects or the difficulty that patients with co-occurring bipolar and substance use disorders have in achieving stable lithium blood levels. The use of carbamazepine in this population is supported by a few studies with positive outcomes (474). There is only one small pilot study to date evaluating the role of second-generation antipsychotics in patients with co-occurring substance use and bipolar disorders (475). Therefore, treatment recommendations follow those presented in APA's *Practice Guideline for the Treatment of Patients With Bipolar Disorder* (471), with first-line pharmacological treatment for more severe manic or mixed episodes with lithium or valproate plus an antipsychotic. For less ill patients, monotherapy with lithium, valproate, or an antipsychotic may be sufficient. Second-generation antipsychotics are generally preferred over first-generation antipsychotics because they appear less likely to cause tardive dyskinesia and extrapyramidal side effects; however, the possibility of weight gain, diabetes, and hyperlipidemia with these agents requires consideration. Second-generation antipsychotic agents with an FDA indication for use in treating acute manic or mixed episodes in bipolar disorder include olanzapine, risperidone, ziprasidone, and aripiprazole. Quetiapine has an FDA indication for the treatment of acute episodes of mania. In the acute setting of a manic episode, a benzodiazepine may be helpful. However, the general concern about using a medication with high abuse potential must be considered; therefore, caution should be exercised in using benzodiazepines beyond the time period of the acute manic episode. For mixed episodes, valproate may be somewhat more efficacious and thus may be preferred over lithium (465–468). Pharmacological alternatives to lithium and valproate include carbamazepine or oxcarbazepine. The possibility of pregnancy should be considered when prescribing valproate or carbamazepine for women of childbearing age, particularly given the increased risk of neural tube defects if the fetus is exposed to these medications in utero.

Because there are no specific studies of the treatment of bipolar depression in substance-abusing individuals, medication strategies should follow the recommendations for managing bipolar depression described in APA's *Practice Guideline for the Treatment of Patients With Bipolar Disorder* (471). The guideline recommends the initiation of lithium or lamotrigine as a first-line pharmacological treatment. Lamotrigine should be used cautiously in individuals with co-occurring bipolar and substance use disorders because active substance users may be unreliable in reporting rashes; gradual titration of lamotrigine is needed and may be problematic in individuals who may be inclined to take excess medication doses, and drug-drug interactions may alter lamotrigine levels and increase the risk of rash (476). Antidepressant monotherapy is not recommended due to concerns about precipitating a mixed or manic episode or contributing to the development of rapid cycling. As an alternative, especially for more severely impaired patients, some clinicians will initiate simultaneous treatment with lithium and an antidepressant. Also, IPT and CBT may help treat symptoms of bipolar depression when they are added to pharmacotherapy.

Integrated psychosocial treatments for bipolar and substance use disorders have been developed and demonstrated to be effective by Weiss et al. (369). The group therapy–based treatment approach in this study integrated cognitive-behavioral approaches that were effective in treating both disorders. The approach has been described in a clinical treatment manual for clinicians that includes educational, motivational, and coping strategies to enhance medication adherence and self-efficacy with cues and triggers for drug use (369).

Although nicotine dependence is common among individuals with bipolar disorder, there have been no reports on treating nicotine dependence in this population (348). Recommendations for treating co-occurring bipolar disorder and nicotine dependence are to integrate the standard somatic and psychosocial treatments for nicotine dependence (see Section III) into the context of the maintenance phase of treating bipolar disorder.

d. Anxiety disorders

Symptoms of anxiety and anxiety disorders commonly co-occur with substance use disorders (341). Based on a sample of individuals between ages 15 and 54 years, lifetime rates of anxiety disorders (including GAD, panic disorder, specific phobia, social phobia, obsessive-compulsive disorder, PTSD, and acute stress disorder) in the community are estimated to be about 19% in men and 31% in women (341). About 50% of individuals with a substance use disorder have an anxiety disorder (341, 420), with different rates for different anxiety disorders. For example, about 4.5% of patients with a substance use disorder have panic disorder, and 16% of panic disorder patients have a co-occurring substance use disorder (341). Despite the high prevalence rates, anxiety disorders are frequently underdiagnosed in substance abuse treatment settings (477). Because many substances cause state-dependent anxiety symptoms (i.e., during intoxication, acute withdrawal, or protracted withdrawal), the assessment of anxiety disorders in substance-using populations is challenging and requires careful assessment. The clinician should ask about symptoms that relate to specific anxiety disorders and use similar considerations during the assessment process to those recommended for depression symptoms and substance use disorders. Although nicotine dependence is also common among individuals with anxiety disorders, there are almost no treatment studies for this population, and treatment should follow the standard somatic and psychosocial treatment recommendations for nicotine dependence (see Section III).

Integrated treatment for co-occurring anxiety and substance use disorders may include medications and psychosocial treatments from both substance abuse and psychiatric treatment perspectives. Specific medications and CBTs for specific anxiety disorders have been developed and can be combined with the usual treatments for substance use disorders. Providing education about the anxiety and substance use disorders and the effects the disorders have on each other is also important.

The recommended medications for treating panic disorder with a co-occurring substance use disorder are SSRIs plus integrated psychosocial treatment (288, 478). If several SSRIs are tried and found to be ineffective, then a TCA may be considered; however, TCAs may be of concern when using them in the context of co-occurring substance use disorders because of the risk of cardiac toxicity and seizures and the potential for overdose in a suicide attempt. Although benzodiazepines are usually considered a first-line treatment for panic disorder in patients without an active substance use disorder, the risk of benzodiazepine abuse is a significant concern and precludes this class of medications from being first-line agents in treating panic disorder in the context of a coexisting substance use disorder. In rare cases, physicians have treated severe panic symptoms by using benzodiazepines on a time-limited basis, selecting patients without a history of misusing benzodiazepines but who have a family history of panic disorder, and fully informing the patient and sometimes the family of the risks of taking benzodiazepines. Physicians may also limit prescriptions, supervise medication administration, monitor medication adherence with pill counts, and request that patients come for more frequent office visits while patients are taking benzodiazepines. Two double-blind, placebo-controlled studies have demonstrated the efficacy of buspirone in patients with alcohol dependence and anxiety (479, 480).

Pharmacotherapy for social anxiety disorder in the context of co-occurring substance use disorder may include beta-blockers or SSRIs along with integrated psychosocial treatment. In a recent study in which simultaneous treatment of social anxiety disorder and co-occurring alcohol dependence was compared with treatment of alcohol dependence alone, both treatment conditions improved alcohol-related outcomes and social anxiety; however, treatment focused on alcohol only was associated with better alcohol use outcomes (481). Although more studies of concurrent treatments for social anxiety and substance use disorders are needed, these findings suggest that combination treatment of social anxiety and alcohol use disorders may not be effective for all patients.

The treatment of obsessive-compulsive disorder in the context of a co-occurring substance use disorder uses pharmacotherapy with SSRIs and integrated psychosocial treatment. TCAs, including clomipramine, may be of concern for use in patients with co-occurring substance use disorders because of the risk of seizures and the potential for overdose in a suicide attempt. Second-generation antipsychotics may be an option for some individuals (288).

GAD commonly co-occurs with other psychiatric and substance use disorders. CBT approaches can be particularly helpful for symptoms of preoccupation/rumination and exaggerated perceptions of danger. First-line agents for this population include buspirone and SSRIs. Although benzodiazepines may be used chronically in GAD patients with no substance use disorder, their use should be limited or applied in only the previously described circumstances in patients with a substance use disorder because of their abuse potential (288).

PTSD is common among individuals with a substance use disorder (about 20%), with women having about twice the rate of co-occurring PTSD as men (482); however, clinicians are advised not to overlook the possibility of PTSD in male patients, because in the general community, rates of PTSD are higher for men than for women (483). Rates of PTSD appear to be high in substance use disorder treatment settings, with one study reporting that 40% of 95 substance-abusing/dependent inpatients met criteria for current PTSD (484). Women with PTSD and a substance use disorder often experienced childhood physical and/or sexual abuse, whereas men typically experienced combat or were victims of crime (483). PTSD symptoms are a common trigger of substance use, and patients may perceive the substances as a way of coping with overwhelming emotional pain (485–488). Indeed, one study showed that individuals with PTSD and either cocaine or alcohol dependence experienced increased craving when exposed to both trauma and drug cues (489). As patients with co-occurring PTSD and a substance use disorder participate in treatment and become able to maintain continued abstinence, they may feel overwhelmed by a flood of memories and unprocessed feelings about the past traumas that have been masked by substance use (490). Simply because patients have become abstinent from substances does not mean that symptoms of PTSD have resolved, and these will need to be addressed in treatment (491, 492). Patients may carry a great burden of shame and guilt, as both PTSD and substance abuse may be associated with keeping secrets and denial. These individuals are sometimes perceived as "crazy," "lazy," or "bad" by others and by themselves, and these issues are similarly important to anticipate in psychotherapy (490).

Specific integrated psychotherapies for PTSD co-occurring with a substance use disorder have been developed and evaluated (365, 368, 490). These approaches have similar components in that they educate the patient about both disorders and how the two problems interact to worsen the course of either disorder alone. Treatment focuses on stabilizing the substance use disorder and developing coping skills to manage the PTSD symptoms and trauma memories as they occur during the early phase of abstinence as well as after prolonged periods of abstinence (490). Seeking Safety (490), an empirically tested group treatment for patients with PTSD and a coexisting substance use disorder, and integrated treatment approaches that combine the 12-step treatment model from substance use disorder treatment with traditional psychotherapeutic approaches to PTSD have been developed to treat this patient population (493, 494). One study of 107 women were randomly assigned to receive Seeking Safety treatment, a manual-guided relapse prevention therapy, or standard community treatment found that women receiving Seeking Safety or relapse prevention therapy had significant reductions in substance use, PTSD, and psychiatric symptoms over the 3-month treatment period, whereas the symptoms of women who received standard community treatment worsened (364); furthermore, the Seeking Safety and relapse prevention groups maintained the greater improvements in substance use and PTSD symptoms at the 6- and 9-month follow-ups. Outcomes did not differ between the Seeking Safety and relapse prevention groups.

Many integrated treatment approaches discourage having the patient describe or explore traumatic memories as might be done in exposure therapy. Only a few pilot studies have been published that evaluate trauma exploration therapies (e.g., exposure therapy) in substance-abusing patients (365, 368). In those few studies, positive results were generally reported. One recently published effectiveness trial of integrated exposure-based therapy for PTSD and psychosocial treatment of substance use disorders reported feasibility and clinical effectiveness within an inner-city mental health treatment setting serving dually diagnosed patients (366). Future research is needed to define which patients may benefit from this type of treatment. Other psychosocial treatments used to treat PTSD are being considered for adaptation to patients with PTSD and a co-occurring substance use disorder; these include mourning therapy (495), eye movement desensitization and reprocessing (496), and the counting method (497).

Medication recommendations for treating PTSD in the context of a co-occurring substance use disorder follow the general recommendations from APA's *Practice Guideline for the Treatment of Patients With Acute Stress Disorder and Posttraumatic Stress Disorder* (498). The SSRIs are considered first-line medication treatment for PTSD. Given the abuse potential of benzodiazepines, prescribing them to patients for the treatment of PTSD presents a risk for substance relapse and/or the development of a new substance use disorder.

e. Attention deficit hyperactivity disorder

Substance use disorders are common in adolescents and adults with ADHD, with about 33% of adult ADHD patients having a history of an alcohol use disorder and about 20% having a drug use disorder; even higher prevalence rates (50%–60%) of co-occurring nicotine dependence have been reported (341, 499). Among patients with alcohol, cocaine, or opioid dependence, 17%–50% have co-occurring ADHD (499). Establishing a diagnosis of ADHD can be complicated in the context of ongoing substance use, because attention problems are often caused by the acute and prolonged effects of specific substances of abuse, and these attention problems will often improve with prolonged abstinence. On the other hand, delaying adequate treatment of co-occurring ADHD may compromise a patient's capacity to fully participate in treatment for a substance use disorder (500, 501). Therefore, it is recommended that treating physicians attempt to gather evidence supporting a co-occurring ADHD diagnosis (e.g., childhood ADHD, evidence of symptoms during prolonged abstinence from substance use) during early assessment and treatment planning. Clinicians are also advised to assess patients with co-occurring ADHD and a substance use disorder for other commonly co-occurring psychiatric disorders (e.g., learning disorders, mood and anxiety disorders, conduct disorder/antisocial personality disorder) (499).

The occurrence of childhood ADHD contributes independently of other psychiatric disorders to the risk of developing an early-onset substance use disorder (502, 503). Early interventions for childhood ADHD (psychosocial and/or pharmacotherapy) may help to prevent new-onset substance use disorders in this population in adulthood.

Even though stimulants are commonly recommended for the treatment of childhood ADHD, concerns that childhood use of prescribed stimulants may predispose an individual to a future substance use disorder are unsubstantiated (504). In fact, a recent meta-analysis of the literature indicated that childhood stimulant therapy lowers the risk of developing a concurrent alcohol or drug use disorder during adolescence and adulthood (505, 506).

Stimulant pharmacotherapy is effective for adolescent and adult ADHD (507) and may be effective for patients with a co-occurring substance use disorder (508–510); however, clinicians must carefully assess symptom improvement with stimulant treatment against the risk for misuse or diversion of prescribed stimulants. Prescription monitoring (e.g., limited dispensing, medication logs) and the use of long-acting stimulant preparations and standardized clinical symptom assessments (511, 512) are recommended. When there is concern about the safety of stimulant treatment in patients with ADHD and a substance use disorder, alternative ADHD pharmacotherapies without an abuse potential may be considered, such as atomoxetine, bupropion, and desipramine (513).

ADHD symptoms often interfere with a patient's adherence to substance use treatment, and therefore integrated psychosocial and pharmacotherapy treatment is recommended for patients with ADHD and a substance use disorder (501, 514). Although integrated psychosocial interventions for this population are recommended, research to support their use is limited. Expert consensus recommends providing patients with education about both disorders, encouraging their active participation in support groups, and modifying psychosocial treatments to facilitate learning (e.g., using brief structured sessions with written handouts) (288, 499).

f. Eating disorders

Epidemiological studies indicate an association between bulimia nervosa and substance use disorders, but not between anorexia nervosa and substance use disorders (515). Bulimia nervosa is more common among individuals with a substance use disorder than in the general population (515). Inpatient substance abuse treatment studies report that about 15% of women and 1% of men have an eating disorder; this group is more likely to abuse stimulants and less likely to use opioids than individuals without an eating disorder (515). In clinical samples, substance use disorders have been found to be common among patients with bulimia (about 23%) (516) and less frequent among those with anorexia nervosa (about 15%) (515). The types of agents abused by individuals with an eating disorder include diet pills, stimulants, laxatives, diuretics, emetics, and many other substances (515, 517). With chronic use, tolerance to the effects of and withdrawal from these medications can occur. Tobacco use and dependence are also common among individuals with bulimia and anorexia nervosa and may be linked with attempts to lose weight. Individuals with co-occurring bulimia and substance use disorders are more likely to be younger when they seek treatment for their bulimia nervosa and have an earlier onset of problem drinking compared with those individuals with bulimia nervosa only (516).

Integrated treatment may occur within psychiatric or substance use disorder treatment programs, and can combine traditional psychosocial treatments for substance use disorders with treatments for bulimia, including relapse prevention or CBT strategies (e.g., identifying automatic thoughts, thought restructuring, identifying cues and triggers for bingeing/purging and substance use). Substance abuse treatment programs may need to add nutritional consultation and education for these patients, help them set goals for an acceptable weight range, and observe them at and between meals for bingeing and/or purging behaviors (515, 518). The 12-

step recovery–oriented community groups for both disorders (such as AA and Overeaters Anonymous) can provide additional structure and support.

Medication strategies to treat bulimia or anorexia nervosa should follow the recommendations in APA's *Practice Guideline for the Treatment of Patients With Eating Disorders* (518). There are no controlled medication trials to guide treatment of bulimia nervosa co-occurring with a substance use disorder. Naltrexone may be worth considering for patients with co-occurring alcohol dependence and bulimia nervosa, given its clinical utility in bulimic patients (519, 520) and its established use with alcohol use disorders (see Sections IV.C.3.a and IX.B.3.a).

g. Personality disorders

Personality disorders and substance use disorders commonly co-occur, with an estimated 50%–60% of individuals with a substance use disorder having a co-occurring personality disorder (463, 521). Prevalence rates of borderline personality disorder (BPD) are approximately 30%–50% across inpatient, outpatient, and community samples of individuals with a substance use disorder (522). Antisocial personality disorder (ASPD) has a lifetime prevalence of 60% among injection drug users (523, 524), although there are recognized problems with the accuracy of an ASPD diagnosis in patients with a co-occurring substance use disorder due in part to drug-associated criminal behavior (525) and overlap with BPD (318). Establishing a personality disorder diagnosis in the context of a substance use disorder can be difficult and may be best done after a patient has achieved a prolonged period of abstinence from substance use. Because patients with a substance use disorder and BPD or ASPD have higher-risk behaviors and a higher suicide risk (303, 318, 526) as well as poorer treatment outcomes (527–532), improved instruments for assessing a co-occurring personality disorder in this context would help to identify high-risk patients who may require more intensive treatments.

Integrated treatments for this population initially focus on helping the therapist manage countertransference issues, develop a therapeutic alliance, and integrate existing behavioral therapy approaches for personality disorders into the substance use disorder treatment. Specific integrated psychosocial therapies that combine traditional substance use disorder treatment with the treatment of a personality disorder have been developed to address these co-occurring disorders (373, 374, 463). Although dialectical behavioral therapy has been shown to be effective for treating BPD with or without a co-occurring substance use disorder, it is not always effective in improving substance use outcomes (533), and there remains a need for improved integrated therapies for this high-risk population.

There have been few medication studies for co-occurring personality and substance use disorders. Medication recommendations in the APA's *Practice Guideline for the Treatment of Patients With Borderline Personality Disorder* (534) may be used to guide treatment. In some cases, medications for personality disorders are used episodically to treat specific symptoms. Benzodiazepines should be used with caution in patients with co-occurring personality and substance use disorders due to the risk of benzodiazepine abuse (535) and overdose and suicide attempts (536).

h. Pathological gambling

Individuals with a substance use disorder are vulnerable to other non-substance-related compulsive behaviors such as pathological gambling and compulsive sexual behaviors. Only pathological gambling is recognized as a DSM-IV-TR disorder. Individuals with a substance use disorder have about a four- to fivefold higher rate of pathological gambling when compared with the general population, and studies suggest that about 15% of substance abusers meet criteria for pathological gambling (537–539). The National Epidemiologic Survey on Alcohol and Related Conditions, a large nationally representative community study, reported that among adults with a lifetime history of pathological gambling, 73% have had a co-occurring alcohol use disorder, 38% have had a co-occurring drug use disorder, and 60% have had co-occurring nicotine dependence (540). It is likely that pathological gambling, though common, is underdiagnosed, because substance abuse or psychiatric treatment settings do not always screen for it (541). Individuals with pathological gambling and a substance use disorder are also at increased risk for engaging in unsafe sexual behaviors and having mood or anxiety problems, ADHD, ASPD, or legal problems (537, 539, 542, 543).

Integrated treatment programs rarely include pathological gambling treatment and generally do not provide Gamblers Anonymous meetings on-site (542, 544). However, integrated treatment could readily incorporate behavioral therapies for pathological gambling that are similar to traditional substance use disorder treatment, such as gambling relapse prevention strategies, social skills training, problem solving, and cognitive restructuring (544).

Medications that appear to help reduce the desire to gamble and gambling behaviors have not been examined in individuals with a co-occurring substance use disorder. Medications studied in pathological gambling alone include fluvoxamine (545–547) and naltrexone (548, 549). A large, multicenter, randomized, controlled trial of paroxetine plus psychosocial treatment failed to demonstrate a significant difference from placebo (550), and an open-label, flexible-dose study of sertraline also failed to demonstrate superiority to placebo (551). Lithium and valproate may be effective in the treatment of pathological gambling for those with bipolar disorder (552, 553). In general, medication trials for pathological gambling show a high early placebo rate; longer-duration studies may be needed to confirm the positive effects of medication.

3. Comorbid general medical disorders

Concurrent general medical conditions frequently complicate the treatment of substance use disorders. A full description of the medical problems associated with substance use disorders is beyond the scope of this practice guideline and has been provided elsewhere (554, 555).

Substance use causes a variety of health problems (Table 3), which vary depending on the substance used and its route of administration. These medical problems may be further complicated by the use of multiple substances and nutritional deficiencies that may accompany ongoing substance use. Many substance use disorder patients with a co-occurring medical disorder do not seek or receive adequate general medical care for a variety of reasons, including the chaotic and disorganized lifestyles often associated with substance abuse and these patients' lack of access to health care. Physicians may be reluctant to adequately treat the pain of individuals who have a painful medical condition but also a current or past substance use disorder (556). Thus, the substance abuse treatment encounter may be the first opportunity to address the general medical care needs of these patients.

At present, the medical risks associated with marijuana use are not well understood. Because it is likely that marijuana contains many of the same carcinogens as cigarettes, it is possible that lung cancer may occur in marijuana smokers, although there is no evidence to support this (557).

Substance use–related conditions such as hepatitis and tuberculosis and associated events such as motor vehicle accidents, falls, suicide, and homicide contribute to an increased risk of death and disability in the substance-using population. Tobacco-related medical disorders are a greater cause of mortality than alcohol-related medical disorders among individuals dependent on alcohol or other nonnicotine substances (558). This finding highlights the importance of assessing substance-abusing patients for tobacco use and recommending psychosocial and/or pharmacological intervention that will help them quit. Among individuals who inject drugs, infectious diseases are the most common cause of general medical comorbidity. Approximately 30%-40% of inner-city intravenous drug users test positive for HIV (559, 560), and depending on the treatment setting, as many as 30%–75% of substance use disorder treatment patients have been diagnosed with hepatitis C. Indeed, intravenous drug use accounts for 60% of new cases of hepatitis C and 25% of new HIV infections per year (561). Regardless of treatment setting, the adoption of universal precautions against body contamination by infectious agents is a necessary part of protecting staff and patients against the spread of HIV (562).

TABLE 3. Medical Disorders Associated With Specific Substances

Substance	Medical Disorders
Alcohol	*Gastrointestinal:* esophagitis, Mallory-Weiss tear, gastritis, peptic ulcer disease, fatty liver, alcohol-induced hepatitis, cirrhosis, acute or chronic pancreatitis *Cardiovascular:* hypertension, cardiomyopathy, coronary artery disease *Neurological:* Wernicke's encephalopathy, alcohol-related dementia, cerebellar degeneration, peripheral neuropathy, stroke, seizures *Hematological:* thrombocytopenia, anemia *Neoplastic:* cancers of the esophagus, liver, and pancreas *Other:* sexual dysfunction, sleep disorders, vitamin B deficiency, peripheral myopathy
Nicotine	*Cardiovascular:* coronary artery disease, vascular disease *Respiratory:* chronic obstructive pulmonary disease *Neoplastic:* cancers of the mouth, esophagus, and lung
Cocaine	*Cardiovascular:* ischemic heart disease, cardiac arrhythmias, cardiomyopathy, aortic dissection, myocardial infarction *Respiratory:* spontaneous pneumothorax, pneumomediastinum, bronchitis, pneumonitis and bronchospasm (when smoked) *Neurological:* seizures, stroke *Other:* sinusitis, nasal irritation, septal bleeding and perforation (with intranasal use), HIV and hepatitis (with intravenous use), weight loss and malnutrition
Opioids (when used intravenously)	*Gastrointestinal:* acute and chronic viral hepatitis *Cardiovascular:* endocarditis *Respiratory:* tuberculosis (which may be treatment resistant) *Neurological:* meningitis *Other:* cellulitis, abscesses, osteomyelitis, HIV

The risks of contracting sexually transmitted diseases commonly differ between the sexes. Among individuals with severe psychiatric disorders, men with hepatitis C have increased lifetime rates of drug-related risk behaviors (e.g., needle use, needle sharing, crack cocaine use), whereas women have higher lifetime rates of sexual risk behaviors (e.g., unprotected sex in exchange for drugs, money, or gifts; unprotected vaginal or anal sex) (563). All substance-using patients should be counseled about safe sex practices and taught specific interpersonal skills (e.g., assertiveness, negotiation) for discussing and requiring the use of safe sex practices with their partners. Gender-specific group treatments using educational/skills building approaches have been developed and are being studied (e.g., in the National Institute on Drug Abuse [NIDA] Clinical Trials Network studies to reduce HIV-related and sexually transmitted disease–related risk behaviors in patients in substance abuse treatment). Needle exchange programs and effective treatment of the substance use disorder and HIV or hepatitis C also reduce the spread of HIV and hepatitis C infection (561, 564).

When treating HIV-seropositive, opioid-dependent individuals with antiretrovirals and methadone, the physician needs to be aware of the clinically significant interactions between these two medications that can decrease the efficacy of antiviral medications and/or require methadone dose adjustments (565). It is recommended that individuals with hepatitis C receiving treatment with interferon be assessed for lifetime or current major depressive disorder because of the frequent development and/or exacerbation of depressive symptoms during treatment with interferon (566). All patients receiving interferon should be monitored for the development of depression, and consideration should be given to initiating antidepressants and counseling. Guidelines for the psychiatric treatment of patients with HIV or AIDS are available in the APA's *Practice Guideline for the Treatment of Patients With HIV/AIDS* (567).

The rise of treatment-resistant tuberculosis among patients with a substance use disorder suggests the need to consider periodic tuberculosis screening for patients and staff who treat these patients, along with efforts to reduce the spread of tuberculosis in treatment environments. Supervised on-site chemoprophylaxis or treatment for tuberculosis within substance abuse treatment programs is also strongly recommended (568, 569).

4. Pregnancy

The treatment of substance use disorders is crucial in the pregnant woman because ongoing substance use during pregnancy has the following multiple implications for both the mother and the developing fetus:

1. *The health of the pregnant woman.* Pregnant women with a substance use disorder are at high risk for sexually transmitted diseases (e.g., HIV infection), hepatitis, anemia, tuberculosis, hypertension, and preeclampsia (570, 571). In addition, the presence of a substance use disorder may affect a woman's ability to maintain a healthy lifestyle, including proper nutrition and prenatal care.
2. *The course of the pregnancy.* Women with certain substance use disorders may be at greater-than-average risk for spontaneous abortions, preeclampsia, abruptio placentae, and early and prolonged labor (572–574), in addition to complications of other general medical conditions that may be attributable to the substance use (e.g., hypertension in cocaine users) (575).
3. *Fetal development.* Some abused substances, including nicotine, opioids, cocaine, and alcohol, are known to pass through the placenta and directly affect fetal metabolism and development (576–578). This may happen at any stage of development but is particularly likely during the third trimester, when maternal fetal blood flow and rates of placental transport are increased. Fetal concentrations of abused substances average 50%–100% of maternal blood levels and may be higher than maternal blood levels (579). The circulation of active metabolites is another source of fetal exposure to potentially toxic substances. The fetus may be at higher-than-average risk for birth defects, cardiovascular problems, impaired growth and development, prematurity, low birth weight, and stillbirth (573, 580–585). After delivery, the neonate may experience withdrawal from the substance, which may be difficult to recognize, particularly if the pediatrician is unaware of the mother's substance use disorder.
4. *Child development.* Some substances (e.g., alcohol) are associated with long-term negative effects on physical and cognitive development, as is seen in fetal alcohol spectrum disorders (586–588).
5. *Parenting behavior.* In addition to ongoing treatment for the disorder itself, mothers with a substance use disorder are frequently in need of education and training in parenting skills, social services, nutritional counseling, assistance in obtaining health and welfare entitlements, and other interventions aimed at reducing the likelihood of child abuse or neglect (589, 590). This is particularly true of women with co-occurring substance use and psychiatric disorders.

Goals for the treatment of pregnant, substance-using women include 1) providing appropriate treatment for the substance use disorder (e.g., methadone maintenance for opioid dependence and abstinence from other substances, including alcohol, cocaine, marijuana, and nicotine), 2) treating co-occurring medical or psychiatric disorders, 3) monitoring the safety of patient behaviors during pregnancy as well as during the postpartum period, 4) facilitating competent parenting behaviors, and 5) motivating the patient to remain abstinent after childbirth.

The optimal therapeutic approach is nonpunitive and maintains patient confidentiality. Education and counseling to help women make an informed decision about continuing or terminating a pregnancy should be provided. Women likely to return to a substance-abusing milieu should be counseled about long-term treatment options available in the community.

5. Gender-related factors

Information on the natural history, clinical presentation, physiology, and treatment of substance use disorders in women is limited. Although women are estimated to comprise 34% of all individuals with a substance use disorder other than nicotine dependence in the United States (591), psychosocial and financial barriers (e.g., lack of child care, lack of health insurance) prevent many women from seeking treatment (592). Another explanation for women's low utilization of substance use disorder treatment services may be women's perception of greater social stigma associated with their substance abuse (593–595). Once in treatment, women have been found to have a higher prevalence than men of primary co-occurring mood and anxiety disorders that require psychiatric care (593, 596). Many women with a substance use disorder have a history of physical and/or sexual abuse (both as children and as adults), which may also influence treatment planning, participation, and outcomes (597, 598). Female patients, particularly single mothers, may have more family responsibilities and may require more help with family-related problems. There is some evidence that tailoring the goals of treatment to meet the needs of women improves treatment outcomes for substance-using women (599, 600).

In terms of nicotine dependence, there is some evidence to suggest that women may smoke less for nicotine reinforcement and more for nonnicotine factors such as other sensory effects of smoke inhalation, conditioned responses to smoke stimuli, and secondary social reinforcement (601). It has also been suggested that women have more difficulties with smoking cessation than men, although recent studies have suggested that cessation rates are similar between the two sexes. There is some evidence that NRT is less effective in female smokers, but the evidence for this is not strong; any initial failures with NRT could be followed by nonnicotine therapies such as bupropion and clonidine (602). Two recent studies showed that women have improved rates of smoking cessation when treated with naltrexone in combination with either smoking cessation therapy alone (603) or NRT and psychosocial therapy (604). Naltrexone as an adjunctive treatment to NRT and/or smoking cessation therapy may also be a treatment option for women who have had initial failures with NRT, although more research is needed to support this. Factors that may lead to poorer outcomes in women include depressive symptoms, negative affect, and reduced social supports. Women also frequently cite the fear of weight gain or actual weight gain after smoking cessation as a reason for relapsing to smoking. Therefore, smoking cessation therapies for women should emphasize weight-management strategies.

Women may also experience more adverse physical outcomes from tobacco use. Women may be more sensitive to secondhand smoke than men (605), and studies indicate that women smokers are at increased risk for lung cancer of all histological types, even after controlling for the number of cigarettes smoked (606). Estrogen effects on carcinogenesis in the lung may account for this difference in women.

The prevalence of smokeless tobacco use in young men over the last several years has dramatically increased (607). This is particularly alarming given the high rates of oral cancer associated with smokeless tobacco use. Smokeless tobacco use should be taken into consideration in addition to cigarette, cigar, and pipe use during the assessment and treatment planning processes.

With regard to alcohol use, female-to-male ratios for alcohol abuse are highest in the younger age groups, suggesting more alcohol use among young women and a closure of the original gap in usage rates between the sexes (596, 608). Of notable concern is the poorer prognosis for medical sequelae of alcohol abuse and dependence in women. Alcohol-dependent women consume less alcohol than men yet progress to late stages of alcohol-related illness more rapidly

(609) and have a shorter time course to the initial development of alcohol-related medical morbidity than do men. Prevalence rates of alcohol-related cirrhosis of the liver and cardiomyopathy in women are twice that in men with alcohol abuse or dependence. Breast cancer and mortality are increased in women consuming more than two standard unit drinks per day (610). Alcohol-abusing women are also at higher risk for death when compared with same-sex, sober control populations (reviewed in Greenfield and O'Leary [611]).

One study of individuals with a substance use disorder in three outpatient treatment settings (methadone maintenance clinic, intensive outpatient program for cocaine dependence, and general outpatient substance abuse treatment clinic) showed that women with a substance use disorder reported significantly more cardiovascular, mood, nose/throat, CNS, skin, and gastrointestinal symptoms related to substance use than did men (612). This occurred despite the lack of differences between men and women in this sample in their preference for cocaine, alcohol, or opioid drugs. Women frequently initiate cocaine and opioid use in the context of a substance-using partner and tend to initiate use at a younger age than men (593, 613).

6. Age

a) Children and adolescents

An in-depth review of the evaluation and treatment of substance use disorders in children and adolescents is beyond the scope of this practice guideline. However, because an adult psychiatrist may be called on to evaluate children or adolescents with a substance use disorder, some general information and treatment principles are reviewed here. For more detailed information, the reader is referred to the American Academy of Child and Adolescent Psychiatry's *Practice Parameter for the Assessment and Treatment of Children and Adolescents With Substance Use Disorders* (614) and the Substance Abuse and Mental Health Services Administration (SAMHSA) recommendations for screening and assessing adolescents for substance use disorders (615–617).

Alcohol and other psychoactive substance use, abuse, and dependence in children and adolescents continue to present a serious public health problem in the United States. Alcohol and other substance use are among the leading causes of morbidity and mortality from motor vehicle accidents, suicidal behavior, violence, drowning, and unprotected sexual activity in this population (618).

Regional studies reveal that 7%-10% of adolescents are in need of treatment for substance use disorders (619). Children and adolescents are generally more likely to have abuse rather than dependence disorders and are less likely to appreciate the need for entering and remaining in treatment. Abuse is not necessarily a prodrome to dependence, and it may be developmentally limited in many adolescents. In addition, Pollock and Martin (620) demonstrated the importance of a new nosological entry in youth diagnoses entitled "orphan diagnoses" that includes subthreshold symptomatology of alcohol dependence (i.e., one or two symptoms only) but no abuse symptoms. A 3-year follow-up study demonstrated that this entity has a unique trajectory dissimilar to that of abuse and dependence.

Assessment and treatment of children and adolescents with a substance use disorder must take into account their psychosocial developmental levels and the possible role of their substance use disorder in impeding the successful attainment of developmental milestones, including a sense of autonomy, the ability to form interpersonal relationships, and general integration into society. The assessment should be multidimensional and address problems in several life domains, including psychiatric comorbidity, school or employment performance, family functioning, peer social relationships, legal status, and recreational activities (621).

Children reared in family environments in which other family members abuse or are dependent on alcohol or other substances are at higher risk for physical and sexual abuse, particularly when family members exhibit antisocial behaviors; these children may exhibit psychological and behavioral sequelae (including substance abuse) as a result (622, 623).

Most adolescents with substance use disorders also have one or more co-occurring psychiatric disorders, most often conduct disorder and/or major depression, although ADHD, anxiety disorders (including social phobia and PTSD), bipolar disorder, eating disorders, learning disabilities, and other axis II disorders are also common (624–626). Many adolescents with substance use disorders also have preexisting and concurrent impulsive, oppositional, self-injurious, and suicidal symptoms or syndromes (627). Treatment should also address these problems, with treatment of the substance use disorder(s) and coexisting psychiatric symptoms occurring simultaneously.

In general, the range of treatment modalities used with adults can be used with adolescents as well. These modalities include brief interventions, motivational enhancement strategies, cognitive-behavioral approaches, psychodynamic/interpersonal approaches (individual, group, and family), self-help groups (628), and medications when needed (629). Most adolescents are treated in outpatient settings, and treatment is often delivered in a group therapy format. Although research data establishing the efficacy of specific treatment modalities for adolescent substance use disorders are sparse, program outcomes for adolescents appear to be enhanced by the availability of treatment that is developmentally appropriate and peer oriented and includes educational, vocational, and recreational services. Corrective experiences in family interaction should be part of the treatment plan (628). Family therapy also appears to have benefit (241, 242, 630). Residential facilities are very effective in reducing substance use, but gains are lost when aftercare is not well coordinated (56).

The prevention of substance use and abuse is considered the primary intervention for schools and clinicians (631–633). At-risk children and adolescents include those with a substance-abusing parent and those living under deprived conditions (i.e., neglect and/or abuse). Educational programs describe the negative consequences of substance use and teach drug refusal and harm-reduction behavioral strategies. Life skills training is a substance use prevention curriculum (634) that focuses on teaching youths the skills necessary to avoid social pressures to experiment with smoking, drinking, and drug use. In addition to showing efficacy in white middle-class youth (634, 635), the effects of the life skills training approach has also been demonstrated to be beneficial in African American and Hispanic youth (636). Masterman and Kelly (637) noted that the empirical literature suggests that universal prevention programs may delay the onset of drinking among low-risk baseline abstainers (i.e., individuals who are not drinking at the baseline assessment and who would be predicted to be at low risk of developing an alcohol use disorder on the basis of multiple risk factors); however, not enough studies support the utility of such programs for at-risk adolescents. Furthermore, they argue that motivational interviewing within a harm-reduction framework is well suited to adolescents.

Interventions aimed at preventing smoking are similarly crucial, given that smoking rates among adolescents continue to rise, despite reductions in other age groups (638). Smoking in adolescents is often a marker of psychiatric problems such as another substance use disorder or depression. In adolescents who smoke, the motivation to quit is often low; many of these adolescents are nicotine dependent and will have difficulties stopping smoking without behavioral and pharmacological support. There have been relatively few studies of smoking cessation in adolescent smokers, and success rates with interventions such as brief motivational enhancement, nicotine patch, and bupropion appear to be very low, at approximately 20% by the end of treatment (639–641).

Two common assumptions concerning adolescent substance use that are unfounded should be mentioned. Supporting the findings of a recent meta-analysis (506), a 16-year prospective, controlled trial showed that the use of stimulant medication (e.g., methylphenidate) in adolescence to treat ADHD does not lead to increased substance use in adulthood (642). Furthermore, contrary to the common perception, cannabis withdrawal is highly prevalent in adolescents (643).

b) Elderly individuals

Substance use disorders in elderly individuals are often undiagnosed and undertreated (644, 645). Abuse of and dependence on prescribed medications, particularly benzodiazepines, sedative-hypnotic medications, and opioids, can contribute to excessive confusion and sedation in elderly patients, poor adherence with prescribed treatment regimens, and inadvertent overdose, particularly when these drugs are combined with alcohol (646–648). In addition, alcohol use disorders, whether an extension of a long-standing disorder or of later onset, are a major problem among elderly individuals, particularly those living alone (649–651). Alcohol-related cognitive impairment, co-occurring depressive disorder, dementia, poststroke syndromes, and other conditions are also common among elderly individuals and may impair their ability to obtain or adhere to treatment for a substance use disorder or other general medical or psychiatric disorder (652).

Although rates of smoking decline with age (by 15%–20%), elderly patients who do smoke should be encouraged to quit. Even in older smokers, smoking cessation can lead to health improvements, including improved quality and length of life. There are few published studies of smoking cessation in the elderly; however, clinical experience suggests that the use of NRT is a safe and effective option. However, caution should be used when prescribing bupropion to elderly individuals because of its potential hypertensive effects (653, 654). This agent should be considered as a second-line agent, as controlled studies have not been conducted in this population.

There is a paucity of empirical data on the treatment of substance use disorders in the elderly population; it is generally accepted that empirically supported treatments of adult substance use disorders can be effectively applied to the treatment of elderly patients. Some modifications, such as slowing the pace of therapy, placing follow-up outreach calls, and providing patients with written information, improve the effectiveness of some therapies. In a recent study of 250 elderly men screened for substance abuse from a VA outpatient population, predictors of patient engagement in substance abuse treatment included severity of substance use, co-occurrence of depression, healthy cognitive status, and higher educational achievement (655). A large multisite study (PRISM-E) has also shown that primary care patients screening positive for a substance use disorder prefer to be treated within the medical system, with integrated psychiatric and substance abuse services, rather than to have facilitated referral to outside treatment (31).

Studies of individuals with alcohol use disorders also suggest that the needs of older adults may be different from those of younger patients. Kofoed et al. (656) reported that VA patients age 54 years or older who received specialized services for elderly patients as part of a treatment program were four times more likely to complete the program and remained in treatment longer than those who received conventional services, although posttreatment relapse rates were comparable in the two groups.

7. Racial, ethnic, and cultural factors

Current research suggests poorer prognoses for ethnic and racial minorities in conventional treatment programs, although this may be accounted for by socioeconomic group differences (657–659). Although there is a paucity of research on the efficacy of culturally specific programming, treatment services that are culturally sensitive and address the special concerns of ethnic minority groups may improve acceptance of, adherence to, and, ultimately, the outcome of treatment. The training of staff to be sensitive to and incorporate culture-specific beliefs about healing and recovery should be part of a comprehensive treatment program that serves different minority and ethnic groups (660). For example, Native Americans and Alaskans may have a greater acceptance of treatment that incorporates the use of the Medicine Wheel (661, 662). Still, clinical judgment in determining what cultural-based modifications to treatment are appropriate is advised, because some ethnic groups have large heterogeneity (e.g., Latino/Latina [663]); specialized cultural approaches (664) can be considered with a patient to determine whether or not the approach would be perceived as useful.

In terms of nicotine dependence, African Americans and Hispanics appear to be less likely to initiate smoking, tend to smoke in lower amounts, and have increased cotinine levels (due to slower metabolism of nicotine). When compared with whites, they appear less likely to become dependent but have less success in smoking cessation efforts (665–668). Recent studies suggest that the nicotine patch (669) and bupropion (670) are safe and effective treatments for African American smokers, but further study is needed.

8. Gay/lesbian/bisexual/transgender issues

Controversies in the literature exist about whether or not substance use rates are elevated in homosexual and bisexual populations. For example, earlier reports that lesbians are at higher risk than heterosexual women for alcohol-related disorders (671) have not been consistently replicated (672). Nonetheless, multiple studies do indicate increased rates of drug use among gay and bisexual sexually active men and lesbian women as compared with exclusively heterosexual men and women, with a prominence of cannabis and nicotine dependence for both homosexual men and lesbian women (673–675). In one undergraduate college student population, a higher incidence of drug use and smoking was found among gay and bisexual men and lesbian women as compared with heterosexual men and women (676). Among older gay, lesbian, and bisexual populations (ages 60–91 years), the incidence of alcohol abuse is greater for men than for women (677). Methodological issues of population sampling may confound interpretation of these findings. For example, in one community with a high concentration of gay and bisexual men, few differences were observed in drug use patterns among gay, bisexual, and heterosexual men (678). Furthermore, demographic variables other than sexual orientation influence the presence of substance abuse (679).

Because of concerns about increased risk and prevalence of substance use disorders in gay, lesbian, and bisexual populations, substance use disorder treatment programs frequently inquire about an individual's sexual orientation and whether or not the individual believes that his or her sexual orientation contributes in any way to the substance use. Special therapeutic strategies have been developed that target known regional associations between sexual orientation and substance abuse, such as a Los Angeles program for the treatment of male methamphetamine abusers who have sex with other men (680, 681). The rationale for this program was the discovery that this population has a high rate of HIV transmission. A similar concern over the higher prevalence of smoking among adolescent and adult gay, lesbian, and bisexual individuals has triggered the development of prevention and cessation programs for these populations (682, 683). SAMHSA published a statement in 2001 concerning the need to address substance abuse issues among gay, lesbian, bisexual, and transgender populations (684).

9. Family characteristics

Substance use disorders exact an enormous toll on family members. High levels of interpersonal conflict, domestic violence, inadequate parenting, child abuse and neglect, separation and divorce, financial and legal difficulties, and substance-related general medical problems (e.g., AIDS, tuberculosis), if present, can add to the family burden. In addition, children reared in family environments in which other family members abuse or are dependent on alcohol or other substances are also at increased risk of physical or sexual abuse (685).

Families who have one or more members with a substance use disorder often display a multigenerational pattern of transmission of both a substance use disorder and other frequently associated psychiatric disorders (e.g., ASPD, pathological gambling) (686, 687). The impact of maternal substance use on fetal development and childhood cognitive and emotional adjustment, coupled with the influence of genetically inherited risk factors (e.g., high genetic loading for alcoholism in the male population) and negative role models, plays a role in the development of substance use disorders across generational lines (688).

The substantial burden that having one or more members with a substance use disorder imposes on families and the impact of family interactions in perpetuating or ameliorating these problems affect the initiation of, perpetuation of, and patient's recovery from the substance use disorder; the patient's motivation and ability to adhere to treatment; and the patient's clinical course and outcome. These relationships, combined with the high prevalence of substance use disorders, co-occurring general medical and psychiatric disorders, psychosocial disability, and family burden make family screening and interventions extremely important (232, 236, 689, 690).

10. Social milieu and living environment

The patient's overall social milieu has an important impact on the development of and recovery from a substance use disorder. The social milieu shapes attitudes about the appropriate context for substance use (e.g., the difference between social drinking on family occasions and recreational drinking to achieve intoxication). Role models among one's family or peers influence the social and psychological context for substance use, the choice of substance, and the degree of control exerted over substance-using behaviors.

Once a pattern of dependence or abuse has developed, an individual's motivation and ability to adhere to treatment are influenced by the degree of support within his or her immediate peer group and social environment. Poor outcome is predicted by continued involvement with substance-using peer groups or family members as well as by residence in an environment in which substances are readily available. Addressing these issues is an important component of any treatment plan. Patients with high levels of psychosocial and environmental stressors need correspondingly high levels of community-based support or, in some cases, temporary relief from these stressors through treatment in a residential setting until the patient is able to develop specific relapse prevention strategies that can be applied in a community setting. Sexually active individuals should be educated about the prevalence and prevention of HIV infection and other sexually transmitted diseases (691).

Socioeconomic status may also play a role in the initiation and cessation of substance use. For example, smokers with lower education level, wages, and socioeconomic status are more likely to initiate smoking and less likely to quit; this may be due to less support for attempts to quit and less access to smoking cessation services. (692, 693).

H. LEGAL AND CONFIDENTIALITY ISSUES

1. Effect of legal pressure on treatment participation and outcome

Many patients with substance use disorders seek treatment in response to pressure from family members, employers, legal authorities, or other sources. Although being internally motivated for treatment is often regarded as a good prognostic sign, outcome studies of patients in therapeutic communities have shown that individuals who enter treatment under legal compulsion (e.g., as a condition of probation, to avoid incarceration) stay longer and do as well as comparable patients who enter treatment voluntarily (694, 695). The use of the opiate antagonist naltrexone has produced higher rates of adherence to court-mandated treatment by patients and physicians or other professionals who are at risk of losing their professional licenses should they fail to comply. Similar findings have been reported for professionals being treated for substance use disorders by means of contingency contracting approaches in which the contingency for nonadherence with treatment is being reported to a professional board of registration (696).

2. Confidentiality and reporting of treatment information

To protect patients' privacy and encourage their entry into treatment, federal law and regulations mandate strict confidentiality for information about patients being treated for substance use disorders (i.e., 42 U.S.C. Sections 290 dd-3 and ee-3; 42 C.F.R. Part 2). Disclosure of information from treatment records is prohibited unless the patient has given written consent, the disclosure is in response to a medical emergency, or there is a court order authorizing disclosure. Other times when patient confidentiality may be attenuated include disclosure needed to protect or warn third parties of potential harm by the patient, disclosure in response to a crime committed at the treatment program or against program staff, reporting of suspected child abuse or neglect, or, depending on the requirements of the local jurisdiction, reporting of suspected abuse of elderly individuals. Consequently, psychiatrists should be familiar with local and state reporting laws concerning the possible abuse and neglect of children, other dependents, or elderly individuals who may be at risk in the families of substance users.

Federal law generally does not make specific reference to the confidentiality of information pertaining to the HIV/AIDS status of a patient in substance abuse treatment, but there are many different state laws restricting disclosure of such status. The federal Health Insurance Portability and Accountability Act of 1996 has been particularly prominent in protecting the privacy of patients with a psychiatric disorder (697). Psychiatric disorders commonly co-occur with substance use disorders, and these patients are "doubly protected" by law.

3. Legal requirements for pharmacotherapy with opioids

Federal and state regulations govern the use of methadone, LAAM, and buprenorphine, the three opioids approved by the FDA for the treatment of opioid dependence. Programs that use these agents to treat opioid-dependent patients are registered with and accredited by the Center for Substance Abuse Treatment. The center holds opioid agonist treatment programs to a variety of accreditation standards that regulate issues such as admissions, record keeping, and the frequency of drug testing. In addition, individual states may also impose stricter licensing criteria for these programs.

In an effort to expand access beyond the highly regulated opioid agonist treatment programs, Congress passed the Drug Addiction Treatment Act of 2000, which allows "qualified physicians" in office-based practices to prescribe FDA-approved schedule III, IV, and V medications for the detoxification and maintenance of opioid dependence. Currently, sublingual buprenorphine and sublingual buprenorphine/naloxone are the only agents approved by the FDA for this purpose. Most physicians qualify by completing 8 hours of formal training and obtaining a special U.S. Drug Enforcement Agency number ("x" number). To obtain this number, physicians must have the capacity to refer patients for appropriate counseling and other ancillary services. Once qualified, physicians may treat patients in an individual or group practice with sublingual buprenorphine or sublingual buprenorphine/naloxone. As with all opioid agonist therapies, strict documentation of informed consent, qualification of the patient as being dependent on opioids with a history of relapse or medical risk, ongoing monitoring of efficacy, and evidence of abstinence or substance use through urine toxicology testing are required for safe prescribing. Physicians should also document the protection of children from accidental access to medication.

III. TREATMENT OF NICOTINE DEPENDENCE

A. OVERVIEW

Smoking is common among individuals with other substance use and psychiatric disorders (698, 699). Although most psychiatrists do not offer comprehensive nicotine dependence

TABLE 4. Fagerström Test for Nicotine Dependence

Questions	Answers	Points
1. How many cigarettes a day do you smoke?	≤10	0
	11–20	1
	21–30	2
	≥31	3
2. Do you smoke more in the morning than during the day?	No	0
	Yes	1
3. How soon after you wake up do you smoke your first cigarette?	>60 min	0
	31–60 min	1
	6–30 min	2
	≤5 min	3
4. Which cigarette would you hate most to give up?	Not first	0
	First of day	1
5. Do you find it difficult to refrain from smoking in places where it is forbidden, for example, in church, at the library, in the cinema, etc.?	No	0
	Yes	1
6. Do you smoke if you are so ill that you are in bed most of the day?	No	0
	Yes	1

Source. Heatherton et al. (709). More information about the test is available in APA's *Handbook of Psychiatric Measures* (711).

treatment, the multiple negative health effects of tobacco use make it important for clinicians to identify tobacco smokers and smokeless tobacco users, provide motivational interventions to encourage patients to quit tobacco use, and be familiar with medications and psychosocial interventions that are effective in treating nicotine dependence. Although there have been several recent controlled studies of smoking cessation treatments among psychiatric patients (414, 700–705), most of these studies have been of limited sample size and primarily involved cohorts of patients with schizophrenia. Thus, much of what is recommended in this section is similar to other recommendations for psychiatric patients who smoke (173, 414, 698, 705) as well as being consistent with guidelines from the U.S. Public Health Service (706) for the treatment of smokers who do not have a current psychiatric disorder. It is also important to note that the treatment of nicotine dependence differs from that of other drug dependencies in the following ways: 1) treatment commonly uses pharmacotherapies (e.g., NRT, bupropion), with varying levels of behavioral treatment given to those willing to receive it; 2) a specific "quit date" when all tobacco use is to cease is set; 3) a nicotine-dependent individual generally does not experience substantial social/occupational dysfunction due to tobacco use; 4) there is less of a need for family involvement in such treatment; and 5) effective over-the-counter medication treatments are available for treating this dependence.

B. ASSESSMENT

In addition to the general aspects of assessment outlined in Section II.B, the patient's current level of tobacco use (e.g., number of cigarettes per day) and degree of nicotine dependence also need to be determined, because highly nicotine-dependent individuals are more likely to need more intensive therapy, especially pharmacotherapy. The Fagerström Test for Nicotine Dependence (Table 4) is widely used in treatment studies and has proven reliability and validity (707–710).

A score of <3 on this scale indicates that an individual has very low or no nicotine dependence, whereas a score of ≥6 suggests that an individual is highly dependent on nicotine (708). This scale can also predict which smokers are likely to quit smoking and which may benefit from high-dose NRT (described in Section III.E.1). Nicotine dependence in smokeless tobacco users is common, and attempts have been made to measure dependence levels in this group as well (712).

Several other markers of nicotine dependence have been proposed, such as number of cigarettes per day, time to first cigarette (an item on the Fagerström test), cotinine levels, degree of withdrawal on last attempt, and number of unsuccessful attempts to quit. However, with the possible exception of time to first cigarette (713), these markers have yet to be shown to have significant treatment utility. DSM criteria for substance dependence (Table 2) also appear to be reliable and have prospective validity in diagnosing nicotine dependence (714).

As indicators of use, nicotine and cotinine levels can be measured in blood, saliva, and urine (105). Nicotine levels can reflect tobacco use over the last few hours, whereas the level of cotinine, a metabolite of nicotine, is sensitive to tobacco use in the last 7 days and offers a better measure of total daily nicotine exposure (105). It has been proposed that the measurement of cotinine levels be used to help guide nicotine replacement, but the utility of this strategy has not been well tested (173). An individual's carbon monoxide level is usually measured by breath and reflects smoking only over the last few hours (105). It has been suggested that the measurement of carbon monoxide is a means of motivating a patient to cease tobacco use or reinforcing abstinence (715), but the efficacy of this is unclear. The major benefit to using carbon monoxide levels as a marker is that it is easily measured and can be used to verify cessation of tobacco use when patients are using an NRT (105). Because smokers in nontreatment (or minimal treatment) settings are usually truthful about their smoking status and the number of cigarettes smoked per day (716), the described measures are not necessary for evaluating smoking cessation, although they show promise as helpful assessments.

Because 70% of smokers make more than one attempt to stop smoking (602), it is important and useful to inquire about and assess patient perceptions about prior attempts and past treatment adequacy. In addition to determining the patient's reasons for previous attempts to quit tobacco use and the amount of time he or she remained abstinent, it is important to assess the perceived cause of relapse. For example, was the relapse due to uncontrolled withdrawal symptoms, environmental stressors, alcohol use, negative or positive mood, psychiatric instability, or being around other smokers or tobacco users? Were there factors (e.g., fatigue, life disappointments, family or other social stressors) that undermined abstinence? What did the patient learn from prior failures? Past efforts to quit may also influence a patient's readiness and motivation to try quitting again. Thus, it is also important to understand the changes that a patient thinks need to occur before he or she can make another attempt to quit tobacco use, his or her fears about quitting, and the barriers to another attempt to quit.

For patients who have returned to tobacco use despite past efforts at treatment, a first consideration is the adequacy of prior treatment. For example: What was the duration of therapy? How many sessions of behavioral therapy were attended? What was the quality of the behavioral treatment in the last attempt to quit? What were the doses of gum or patch used? What was the level of adherence with the psychosocial or somatic therapy? It is also helpful to determine the patient's satisfaction with prior treatments. For example, did he or she believe that treatment was helpful? Did treatment experiences change his or her expectations of future treatment or its outcome?

The assessment of psychiatric patients in terms of cessation of tobacco use focuses on a number of other key points:

1. Is the patient motivated to quit using tobacco in the next month?
2. Are there any psychiatric reasons for concern about whether this is the best time for cessation? Is the patient about to undergo a new therapy? Is the patient presently in crisis? Is there a problem that is so pressing that time is better spent on this problem than on cessation of tobacco use?

3. What is the likelihood that cessation would worsen the non-nicotine-related psychiatric disorder?
4. Are there any signs or symptoms of other undiagnosed psychiatric or substance use disorders that might interfere with efforts to quit tobacco use?
5. What is the patient's ability to mobilize coping skills to deal with cessation?
6. What is the tobacco use status (e.g., never smoked, former smoker, current smoker) of others in the patient's household and among the patient's close friends?
7. What are the patient's treatment preferences and the basis for these preferences?

A discussion of the impact of these factors on the approach to treatment can be found in Section III.D, below.

C. TREATMENT SETTINGS

With the exception of patients hospitalized for other reasons, treatment of nicotine dependence occurs on an outpatient basis. However, an inpatient model for smoking cessation has been described (717) and appears to produce high cessation rates, especially given the level of nicotine dependence among smokers who enroll. There are no controlled trials that substantiate this at the current time.

Regardless of the specific setting, treatment best occurs in a system that encourages cessation (33). This may be especially important to achieve on psychiatric inpatient units, as discussed below in Section III.G. The psychiatrist should also consider maintaining a smoke-free work site (33, 34).

D. GENERAL APPROACH TO TREATMENT

As with treating other substance use disorders, the general goals in treating nicotine dependence include motivating and engaging an individual in treatment to reduce or preferably cease using tobacco. However, the general approach to treatment of nicotine dependence will depend on a number of factors, including the patient's psychiatric status, level of nicotine dependence, past treatment and efforts at quitting tobacco use, and current motivation for reducing or quitting tobacco use. This section discusses the general approach to nicotine dependence treatment; specific aspects of the pharmacotherapy and psychosocial treatments of nicotine dependence are discussed in Sections III.E and III.F, respectively.

Meta-analyses have found that the general techniques described below increase rates of quitting by a factor of 1.5–2.0 (718–721). Descriptive reviews of the skills and techniques critical to smoking interventions have also been published (33, 172, 722–728).

Research shows that 98% of tobacco use involves cigarettes, and most of the studies of treatments for nicotine dependence and smoking cessation have been in cigarette smokers (602). The available evidence suggests that other forms of tobacco use (e.g., pipe, cigars, smokeless tobacco) are becoming increasingly common (692). Although studies of treatment interventions are limited, pipe and cigar use are associated with higher rates of nicotine dependence because of their higher nicotine content. Thus, these other forms of nicotine use should also be taken into consideration in the assessment and treatment planning process.

1. Establishing and maintaining a therapeutic framework and alliance

Nicotine dependence is a chronic relapsing disorder; most smokers require five to seven attempts before they finally quit for good (729). Many patients do not realize that several attempts are often needed to stop smoking, and they will need to be remotivated to attempt to quit after a previous failure (33). Because of this, it is important to establish a therapeutic relationship so that the patient will accept treatment for subsequent attempts to quit, if necessary (33).

Clinician advice for individuals attempting to quit tobacco use is best given in a nonjudgmental, empathic, and supportive manner (32, 33). No studies have been conducted to test whether confrontational interventions applied in treating other substance use disorders are useful with nicotine dependence. In patients with a present or past psychiatric disorder, it is important to convey the message that simply having a psychiatric disorder is not a reason not to make a quit attempt (725, 730).

2. Increasing readiness and motivation for smoking cessation

A patient's current motivation will determine what strategies should be used to enhance and support his or her readiness and attempts to quit smoking. Because many psychiatric patients are ambivalent about stopping smoking or are not ready to attempt to quit (731–733), nicotine dependence treatment will most often consist of enhancing their motivation and dealing with anticipated barriers to cessation (33).

Brief advice from a physician (using protocols similar to those recommended by the National Cancer Institute) to stop smoking typically doubles quit rates, from approximately 5% to 10% (718–721, 734, 735). Advice from nonphysicians is also effective (718, 721), and advice from multiple sources is more effective (718, 721). Thus, clear direct advice from the psychiatrist and other psychiatric personnel (e.g., nurses, social workers) to stop smoking is an essential initial therapeutic step that may increase patient readiness and motivation to try other therapies as needed.

Stages-of-change approaches and motivational enhancement models (32, 736) may help formalize interventions to enhance a patient's motivation. Such interventions will generally include providing information and feedback on the risks of smoking and reasons for quitting that are specific to the individual patient. The most common reasons for trying to stop smoking are to improve health and respond to social pressure (737). Revisiting the issue of smoking cessation at periodic intervals, especially with the occurrence of smoking-related medical conditions (e.g., bronchitis) or other special situations (e.g., pregnancy, living with a child with asthma), can sometimes motivate smokers to consider quitting (737–740). Documenting smoking status (as well as concurrent alcohol or other drug use) in the medical record may help facilitate such a follow-up.

3. Overcoming barriers to smoking cessation

Patients who smoke may express negative feelings or fears related to quitting that may serve as a barrier to their smoking cessation. The most common concerns are fear of weight gain, fear of withdrawal, and fear of failure (737). Women frequently cite the fear of weight gain or actual weight gain after quitting smoking as negative reinforcers contributing to smoking relapse. The exacerbation of psychiatric symptoms is likely to be an additional barrier for psychiatric patients (32). There is little evidence that smoking cessation can exacerbate psychiatric symptoms in patients diagnosed with schizophrenia or major depression whose symptoms are stabilized. However, any patient fears about withdrawal symptoms or a worsening of psychiatric problems may be dealt with by problem-solving approaches, increased monitoring by the clinician, behavioral therapy, or treatment with NRT, bupropion, or both.

Patients who smoke may also be uninformed and demoralized about their inability to change or may be defensive and resistant to change. Thus, it may be helpful for a clinician to clarify and legitimize patients' feelings, explore the reasons for their smoking, and offer expressions of support and respect. If feelings of demoralization are uncovered, they can be addressed by informing the patient that even smokers who are very committed to quitting may make several attempts to quit before they finally succeed. Patients who become chronically ambivalent about quitting may benefit from encouragement to take small steps toward their goal of quitting, such as reducing the number of cigarettes they smoke or trying to quit for just 24 hours.

The psychiatrist supports self-efficacy by identifying and praising past behavioral change and encouraging the use of strategies that were effective in the past.

Smoking by others in the household and close friends may also present a barrier to treatment. Whether and how others in the household and friends have supported or undermined a patient's prior attempts to quit should be evaluated. Conversely, social support is a major predictor of cessation (741). If others in the household are current smokers, it is useful to determine their willingness to quit at the same time as the patient or not to smoke in front of the patient.

4. Eliciting patient preferences about treatment

Patients' treatment preferences and the reasons for those preferences should be elicited and considered when developing a treatment plan. For example, some patients may prefer to stop smoking on a certain date or may have strong likes or dislikes about pharmacotherapy, group therapy, or individual therapy. These factors will be important in setting a specific quit date as well as enhancing the patient's adherence to the treatment plan.

5. Determining timing of smoking cessation

When and how cessation advice is best delivered must be determined by the patient's status; for example, smoking cessation is not likely to be successful when the patient is in crisis. The best time for cessation would appear to be when the patient is psychiatrically stable, there are no recent or planned changes in medications, and no urgent problems take precedence (730). On the other hand, admission to a smoke-free inpatient unit or integrating smoking cessation into other lifestyle changes that are a part of ongoing psychiatric treatment (e.g., during cessation of alcohol use) can sometimes motivate a patient to quit smoking. More immediate cessation is indicated if the patient has recently been diagnosed with a smoking-related medical disorder; individuals with such disorders generally have high success rates for quitting (737, 740). Whenever a smoking quit date is postponed, it is helpful to list smoking cessation as a goal on the master psychiatric treatment plan so that it can be addressed at a later time.

6. Determining whether smoking cessation will be abrupt versus gradual

Most patients attempt and most clinicians recommend abrupt cessation of smoking rather than gradual reduction (742). Previous thinking has held that gradual reduction is less successful because patients appear to have difficulty achieving further reductions once they have cut down smoking to 5–10 cigarettes per day (173). On the other hand, most of the scientific data available suggest no difference in the outcomes of abrupt versus gradual cessation (173, 718, 719, 743); thus, patient preference to follow a gradual reduction strategy should be respected. A gradual approach may also be considered if the patient is historically uninterested or unable to quit smoking, as a significant and sustained reduction in smoking might still be achievable. Whether reductions in smoking are related to decreasing risk for smoking-related medical illnesses has not been clearly established (744, 745).

7. Setting a quit date

Once the above factors have been addressed and the patient agrees to stop smoking, a specific quit date is set and a concrete discussion of cessation procedures occurs. In addition, the psychiatrist may give the patient written materials that provide suggestions for succeeding in quitting. Even if a gradual approach to smoking cessation is chosen, patients should generally be advised to set a date by which they will completely stop smoking and that they should not use NRT until they have stopped smoking. Because many patients relapse within the first few days of smoking cessation (746), it is important for the psychiatrist or the psychiatrist's staff to call or see the patient in the first 1–3 days after the quit date.

If the patient is not ready to make a commitment to a quit date, the psychiatrist should plan to readdress smoking at a later date, encourage the patient to reconsider, and offer to help if the patient changes his or her mind. In addition, the psychiatrist may give the patient written materials that are intended to motivate the patient to make a quit attempt or that give tips on how to successfully quit.

8. Developing a plan of psychosocial and pharmacological treatment

a) Initial approaches

In the general population, most smokers quit on their own or with minimal treatment (747); for those who are unable to stop with minimal intervention, many algorithms and guidelines recommend a stepped-care approach, with minimal intervention early on and more intensive intervention later in the course of treatment (140, 172, 748–750). At the same time, most smokers who quit on their own require several attempts before they succeed (750); thus any success later in the algorithm cannot be attributed to the specific treatment being given at that point. Just as important, early cessation of smoking can prevent much of the devastating consequences of smoking (751); thus, delaying delivery of a treatment known to be effective could allow a serious, irreversible consequence of smoking (e.g., acute myocardial infarction, lung cancer) to develop. Consequently, the availability of effective treatments for smoking cessation as well as the rarity of significant adverse effects of those treatments suggests that pharmacotherapy be offered to all patients who wish to stop smoking. Combining psychosocial and medication treatment generally produces the best outcomes; however, medications are effective even when no psychosocial treatment is provided.

b) Monitoring clinical status

After the first follow-up 1–3 days after the quit date (see Section III.D.7), additional follow-ups may be scheduled, depending on the patient's perceived need, history of cessation, and psychiatric history. Follow-up visits may also be needed to assess a medication blood level that might increase with cessation. Follow-up visits may also be needed to monitor side effects or plan tapering of antismoking medications.

At follow-up, the psychiatrist assesses whether the patient has smoked and, if so, the number of cigarettes smoked per day; the severity of the patient's withdrawal symptoms; the onset of any psychiatric symptoms; the patient's use of alcohol or other drugs; how the patient dealt with situations in which he or she felt a strong urge to smoke; medication side effects; and other relevant issues and then tailors treatment accordingly (33). Most but not all studies suggest that brief follow-ups (including telephone calls) increase quit rates (720, 721, 752–754).

(1) Identifying symptoms of withdrawal

Nicotine withdrawal symptoms typically begin a few hours after the patient has ceased smoking and include dysphoric or depressed mood; insomnia; irritability, frustration or anger; anxiety; difficulty concentrating; restlessness; decreased heart rate; and increased appetite or weight gain. Although most symptoms peak 24–48 hours after cessation, they last an average of 4 weeks, with hunger and craving for tobacco lasting 6 months or more in some individuals (755). The duration of nicotine withdrawal symptoms may be a more important determinant of smoking relapse than the severity of the symptoms (756). Smoking cessation can cause physiological problems such as slowing of electroencephalographic activity in the awake and sleep state, decreases in cortisol and catecholamine levels, and a decline in the patient's metabolic rate (757). The mean heart rate decline is about 8 bpm, and the mean weight gain is 2–3 kg (757).

Nicotine withdrawal can occur in association with all forms of tobacco use (cigarettes, chewing tobacco, snuff, pipes, cigars) as well as with NRTs (755, 757). The ability of these products to induce or maintain dependence and withdrawal increases with the rapidity of the absorption of nicotine, the nicotine dose, and the availability of the product (758). Consequently, although symptom severity varies among patients (757), withdrawal is usually most severe with cigarette abstinence compared with abstinence from other forms of tobacco and nicotine medications (755, 757, 759).

(2) Identifying exacerbations of psychiatric symptoms

Patients with current or past psychiatric symptoms or disorders need particularly close monitoring in the first 14 days after smoking cessation because nicotine withdrawal symptoms such as anxiety, depression, increased rapid eye movement sleep, insomnia, irritability, restlessness, and weight gain can mimic, disguise, or aggravate the symptoms of other psychiatric disorders or side effects of medications. For example, when an alcohol-dependent individual who is also nicotine dependent is admitted to a smoke-free ward for alcohol detoxification, his or her anxiety, depression, difficulty concentrating, insomnia, irritability, and restlessness could be due to or aggravated by nicotine withdrawal. Although more studies support concurrent attempts to quit smoking and drinking, there is one study that suggests that relapse to alcohol is more likely with concurrent smoking cessation (38). There have been several prospective studies (760, 761) that have examined whether smoking cessation can exacerbate depressive (762–766) or psychotic (414, 702, 703, 767) symptoms in patients with major depression and schizophrenia, respectively; most of the available evidence suggests that this risk is low when patients' psychiatric symptoms are stabilized prior to the cessation attempt.

A patient's psychiatric status should also be monitored because blood levels of some psychiatric medications (e.g., those metabolized by the CYP 1A2 microsomal system, including clozapine, fluphenazine, haloperidol, oxazepam, desmethyldiazepam, clomipramine, nortriptyline, imipramine, desipramine, doxepin, and propranolol) may increase substantially within 3–6 weeks when patients taking such medications stop smoking, and these increases could worsen side effects or cause toxicity (414, 698, 760, 768, 769). This effect appears to be due not to nicotine but rather to the effects of benzopyrenes (tobacco carcinogens) and related compounds on the P450 system.

9. Providing education and enhancing adherence

Many patients do not realize their smoking may be a form of nicotine dependence (770). Key points to convey to patients include the following: 1) most smokers try to quit multiple times before they finally succeed, but with persistence, half of all smokers quit; 2) most smokers fail early on, but if the smoker is able to remain abstinent for 3 months, relapse is unlikely; 3) nicotine withdrawal can be relieved with NRT; 4) true withdrawal symptoms generally last 4 weeks or longer and may include dysphoric or depressed mood, insomnia, irritability, frustration or anger, anxiety, difficulty concentrating, restlessness, decreased heart rate, increased appetite, or weight gain (33).

To support a patient's adherence to treatment, it is important to deal with the patient's concerns about weight gain. Even though the health benefits of stopping smoking clearly outweigh the health risks of weight gain (771), fear of weight gain is common and is a major deterrent to smoking cessation, especially in women (772, 773). On average, smokers weigh 2–3 kg less than individuals who have never smoked, and when smokers stop smoking, they gain weight until they are similar in weight to those who have never smoked (771). Most smokers gain weight over the first few months after quitting smoking, but many later lose much or all of this weight. Women who are already trying to decrease their weight gain the most (773). However, smoking cessation-related weight gain does not cause a relapse to smoking (755). In fact, a concentrated effort to control weight gain by dieting during abstinence increases, not decreases, the chances of a relapse to smoking (774, 775). This may be because attempting to quit smoking and dieting at the same time is just too difficult. Clinicians can recommend that patients increase their physical activity and learn healthy eating strategies rather than diet or convince patients to tolerate a moderate amount of weight gain over the first 3 months after smoking cessation and work on losing weight later (775). Nicotine gum, but not the nicotine patch, appears to delay weight gain and could be used to delay attempts to control weight until a relapse to smoking is less likely (776).

Alcohol use is a risk factor in most studies for relapsing to smoking (777); thus, it is recommended that patients who are attempting to quit smoking either diminish their alcohol intake or abstain from alcohol. Caffeine use typically does not change with smoking cessation (755), and it is unclear whether caffeine use is a risk factor for relapse (769). Smoking increases the metabolism of caffeine, and smoking cessation increases caffeine levels by 50%–60% (778). Because many of the symptoms of caffeine intoxication and nicotine withdrawal overlap (e.g., anxiety, insomnia, restlessness), reducing caffeine intake after smoking cessation might be helpful; however, the one study to test this hypothesis found caffeine does not increase the severity of tobacco withdrawal (778). In addition, abruptly stopping caffeine could induce a withdrawal syndrome of its own (779). In summary, with this contradictory evidence, patient preferences on whether to change caffeine intake should be respected.

Because smoking even one cigarette during a cessation attempt often portends a full-blown relapse (780), reports of any slips should prompt immediate planning around changes in behavioral therapy (e.g., discuss ways to avoid or cope with the situation that led to the slip) or changes in pharmacotherapy (e.g., increased dose, change in medication). If the patient has fully relapsed, the psychiatrist should praise the patient for even limited success. The patient and psychiatrist should then discuss what was learned with this quit attempt and when the patient would like to think about trying again. Most patients who relapse continue to be interested in stopping smoking; thus, the psychiatrist should discuss setting a time to reconsider another cessation attempt.

10. Determining approaches for patients who do not respond to initial treatment

When a patient does not respond to a trial of a known effective formal therapy (e.g., behavioral therapy, NRT, bupropion, a combination of these therapies), it is first important to determine if the treatment was adequately or inadequately implemented. If inadequately implemented, the therapy may be repeated with changes to ensure the fidelity to therapeutic steps, treatment adherence, and adequacy of treatment dose and duration.

If the treatment was both appropriate and adequately implemented, rescreening the patient for other co-occurring disorders is indicated, as other unrecognized substance use or psychiatric disorders can interfere with smoking cessation (698, 760, 781). The psychiatrist should also attempt to determine whether the relapse was related to withdrawal symptoms or other causes. If the patient has not previously been treated with NRT and the prior relapse appeared to be caused by withdrawal symptomatology, NRT is appropriate. If the patient has been adequately treated with NRT, the psychiatrist may consider bupropion and/or a different formulation or dose of NRT. If these approaches are also ineffective, the use of clonidine or nortriptyline could be considered.

Other NRT delivery systems can also be considered. Although its side effects can limit its acceptability to some patients, nicotine nasal spray produces a more bolus-like effect that might better relieve withdrawal symptoms and craving (782), especially in heavy smokers who report that they relapsed to smoking both for withdrawal relief and for the positive effects of nicotine and tobacco (e.g., liking, satisfaction). A nicotine inhaler has the added advantage of replicating the hand-to-mouth motor acts associated with smoking, which may further support its utility. A strategy of initially using nicotine nasal spray and then switching to a nicotine patch or concomitantly using nicotine nasal spray and patch has been proposed and received some empirical support from controlled studies (782a, 782b, 1563). The combination of a patch with a faster-acting NRT such as gum, lozenge, spray, or inhaler may have some rationale, as the patch provides a steady level of nicotine for withdrawal relief and the faster delivery systems address the positive aspects of smoking (satisfaction and liking).

If the patient has relapsed because of a stressful life event and has not previously been treated with behavioral therapy, this type of therapy should be considered. If the patient has already had behavioral therapy, two choices are available: 1) more intensive behavioral therapy or 2) behavioral therapy within a different content or format (e.g., group therapy, individual therapy, combined individual and group therapy, involvement of family members). Whether these treatments are effective for those who have not responded to prior behavioral therapy has not been studied. Sometimes it is difficult to distinguish withdrawal versus nonwithdrawal causes of relapse. Under such circumstances, the patient may be a candidate for combined pharmacological and behavioral therapy (783, 784).

The results of three small controlled studies of acupuncture are promising (785–787), but due to methodological limitations, they do not justify the use of acupuncture for treating nicotine dependence either alone or in combination with other treatments. Furthermore, a meta-analysis of 22 controlled studies suggests acupuncture lacks efficacy in promoting smoking cessation (788).

When the treating psychiatrist does not have the knowledge necessary to implement the treatments outlined herein, or if the strategies are administered and the patient is not able to quit smoking, the psychiatrist should consider referring the patient to someone who specializes in treating nicotine dependence.

E. SOMATIC TREATMENTS

1. Nicotine replacement therapies

NRTs can be used as a first-line treatment approach for any individual who wishes to stop smoking. At present, there are five FDA-approved forms of NRT: patch, gum, lozenge, nasal spray, and inhaler. Because all are effective in alleviating withdrawal symptoms (789) and reducing smoking (790) in men and in women (791, 792), the choice of a specific NRT typically depends on patient preference and the NRT's route of administration and side effect profile (793). It is unclear what adjustments to NRTs are needed for pipe and cigar users; probably these therapies should be implemented according to the patient's nicotine dependence level as measured by the Fagerström Test (794). Using a combination of NRTs (790) or combining NRT with bupropion (795) or psychosocial therapies (790) may improve outcome.

The optimal duration of NRT is debatable (693). Although some individuals appear to require long-term use of NRT (e.g., ≥6 months), almost all eventually stop using such agents, and the development of dependence on these agents is rare (796, 797). Thus, patient preference should be the major determinant for the duration of an NRT.

Of the NRTs, many individuals find it easier to adhere to nicotine patch therapy. Typically, nicotine patch therapy will begin with a high-dose patch (21 or 22 mg); however, patients who smoke <15 cigarettes per day are candidates for starting with an intermediate-dose patch (e.g., 11 or 14 mg) or for using another form of NRT (798). Whether the 24- or 16-hour patch is better is debatable (71, 798). The 24-hour patch may better relieve morning craving but appears to cause insomnia in some patients (799, 800). Other common side effects are skin irritation (which can be diminished by rotating patch placement sites), nausea, and vivid dreams; however, patients usually develop tolerance to these side effects (790, 801). The recommended duration of nicotine patch therapy is 6–12 weeks, with a tapering of the patch dose over that period; longer durations of patch therapy have not been found to be more effective (790).

When nicotine gum or lozenges are used, scheduled dosing (e.g., one 2-mg lozenge or piece of gum every hour) rather than ad libitum dosing is often best. The 4-mg dose is recommended for heavy smokers (>25 cigarettes/day) or more nicotine-dependent smokers (790, 802, 803). The dose of nicotine replacement can be tapered over 6–12 weeks by decreasing the gum or lozenge dose (i.e., from 4 to 2 mg) and/or increasing the time between doses. Patients also benefit from receiving instructions about proper use of these NRTs. With nicotine gum, patients should be instructed to chew one piece of gum very slowly until a slight tingling or distinctive taste is noted, at which time the gum should be placed ("parked") between the cheek and gum until the taste or tingling is almost gone. This process is then repeated over about 30 minutes for each piece of gum. Nicotine lozenges should be sucked on rather than bitten or chewed. Typical side effects of lozenges are minor but include nausea, heartburn, and mild throat or mouth irritation; side effects of the gum are jaw soreness or difficulty chewing (802, 804). In addition, the lozenge contains phenylalanine and should not be used by individuals with a history of phenylketonuria. With both the lozenge and the gum, it is important to avoid beverages other than water immediately before or during NRT use because associated pH changes can blunt nicotine absorption (804a).

Nicotine nasal spray and vapor inhaler systems provide faster delivery of nicotine than gum or lozenges, but still deliver nicotine more slowly and with lower peak nicotine levels than cigarettes. Nicotine nasal sprays produce droplets that average 1 mg per administration, and patients administer the spray to each nostril every 1–2 hours. Nicotine vapor inhalers are cartridges of nicotine that are placed inside hollow cigarette-like plastic rods and produce a nicotine vapor (0.013 mg/puff) when smokers puff on them (805, 806). The recommended dose is 6–16 cartridges daily, with the inhaler being used ad libitum for about 12 weeks. Short-term side effects from nicotine nasal spray include nasal and throat irritation, rhinitis, sneezing, coughing, and watering eyes in up to 75% of users (807–809), and nicotine inhaler use is most often associated with throat irritation or coughing in up to 50% of users (806, 810). When compared with other forms of NRTs, the nasal spray and inhaler may have somewhat higher rates of continued use for periods >6 months (782, 796, 811).

2. Bupropion

The antidepressant agent bupropion in the sustained-release formulation is a first-line pharmacological treatment for nicotine-dependent smokers who want to quit smoking. Bupropion appears to have comparable tolerability and effectiveness to NRTs (158–160, 795, 812) and is equally beneficial in men and women (813). The target dosage for individuals with nicotine dependence is 300 mg/day. The medication is initiated at 150 mg/day 7 days prior to the target quit date; after 3–4 days, dosing is increased to 300 mg/day (150 mg b.i.d.). Bupropion can also be used in combination with an NRT, although the evidence is mixed on the extent to which this improves outcomes (795).

The primary side effects associated with bupropion are headache, jitteriness, insomnia, and gastrointestinal symptoms (795). Caution is needed when prescribing bupropion to individuals with a history of seizures of any etiology, as seizures have also been observed with bupropion treatment. The use of bupropion, especially the short-acting preparation, is also discouraged in patients with a past, and particularly a current, diagnosis of an eating disorder (i.e., anorexia nervosa or bulimia nervosa) because of higher rates of seizures observed in initial studies of the medication (161). In other individuals, the rate of de novo seizures is low (<0.5%), and such seizures are predominantly observed when daily dosing exceeds 450 mg/day (795).

3. Other agents

There is also support for the use of nortriptyline and clonidine as treatments for nicotine dependence; however, given the number of other available treatments for which results are well validated, these should be viewed as second-line therapies. Nortriptyline may be particularly promising as a second-line nonnicotine pharmacotherapy, and its efficacy does not appear to depend on the presence of co-occurring depressive symptoms or major depressive disorder (795, 814). However, the side effects of nortriptyline are more prominent than those of NRTs or bupropion, and nortriptyline is also toxic in overdose amounts (455, 815–817). Clonidine may also have some merit as a second-line agent (818), but its side effects may limit its use (819). Acupuncture (788) and other agents (e.g., naltrexone, mecamylamine, buspirone, monoamine oxidase inhibitors [MAOIs], SSRI antidepressants) (603, 795, 820–823) have also been studied, but their efficacy for smoking cessation has not been established.

F. PSYCHOSOCIAL TREATMENTS

There is extensive evidence of the efficacy of psychosocial therapies for treating individuals with nicotine dependence, whether delivered in a group (824) or individual (825) format. These therapies are typically provided as a multimodal package of several specific treatments and aim to provide patients with the skills to quit smoking and avoid smoking in high-risk situations. Behavioral coping skills may include removing oneself from the situation, substituting other behaviors (e.g., walking, exercising), or using skills to manage triggers (e.g., assertiveness, refusal skills, time management). Cognitive coping skills may include identifying maladaptive thoughts, challenging them, and substituting more effective thought patterns to prevent a slip from becoming a relapse (e.g., not viewing the slip as a catastrophe). The 6-month quit rates for behavioral therapies in general are typically 20%–25%, or about twofold greater than quit rates with control conditions (824–828). A review of behavioral therapy studies also suggests that 1) more intensive behavioral therapies can produce better treatment outcomes versus low-intensity interventions (701, 703), and 2) behavioral therapies can augment smoking cessation outcomes with pharmacotherapies, including all NRTs and bupropion (414, 701, 703, 704).

1. Social support

Social support appears to be of benefit in encouraging an individual to quit smoking, whether it is measured according to the degree of support provided by a spouse or partner (829) or is provided in the form of a specific intervention (e.g., buddy system) (718, 826, 828, 830–833). Thus, social support is recommended as a treatment for smoking cessation.

2. Brief therapies

Brief therapies, such as behavioral supportive cessation counseling, may lead to enhanced rates of treatment retention or smoking cessation (639, 826, 828, 834–837). Such therapies can often be implemented successfully and economically in a broad range of health care settings. These therapies often incorporate elements of MET and encourage the patient to examine the reasons for and against quitting smoking. When brief interventions are used, patients are likely to have a greater number of quit attempts and a greater likelihood of success in smoking cessation (825, 826, 828).

3. Behavioral therapies

Behavioral therapies are recommended as a first-line treatment for smoking cessation, with a large database of over 100 controlled prospective studies on multimodal behavioral therapy supporting this recommendation (720, 734, 735, 826, 838). In most reviews and meta-analyses, 6-month quit rates with behavioral therapy are double those observed in control groups (824, 826, 828) and similar to long-term outcomes obtained with NRTs and bupropion. Specific types of behavioral therapy that have also been studied include contingency management, cue exposure, and "rapid smoking" aversion therapy; however, none of these are sufficiently well studied to support their use clinically.

4. Cognitive-behavioral therapies

Several controlled studies suggest that CBTs are effective for smoking cessation (700, 839, 840) and are possibly effective for smokers with comorbid depressive symptoms, major depression, and alcohol and other substance use disorders (456, 459, 841–844). CBT may also help in addressing weight concerns associated with smoking cessation (840). However, the long-term effectiveness of CBT in this population has not been established.

5. Self-guided therapies

Self-help materials are designed to increase patients' motivation to quit smoking and teach them smoking cessation skills. In most (845–853) but not all (854, 855) studies, approaches such as community support groups, telephone counseling, written manuals, videos, and computer-generated, tailored self-help materials have shown promise in increasing smoking cessation rates. The use of multiple modes of therapy (e.g., written materials plus phone contact) (718, 720, 721, 856–859) and tailoring materials to the specific needs and concerns of each patient improves the effectiveness of self-help methods (736, 851, 860).

6. Other therapies

A number of other psychosocial therapies have been evaluated in a small number of clinical trials, with the results showing variable success. For example, some evidence suggests that exercise programs may help prevent a relapse to smoking in women (861, 862), whereas other studies do not (863, 864). However, based on the other health benefits of exercise, increased activity is encouraged in smokers attempting to quit or those who have recently quit smoking. There is also some support for the effectiveness of stimulus control techniques in reducing smoking urges, such as discarding cigarettes; removing ashtrays, lighters, and matches; avoiding smokers; and avoiding situations associated with smoking (718). However, these strategies are probably best used within the context of multicomponent therapies. Little evidence is available that would support the use of physiological feedback (i.e., giving immediate positive feedback on the benefits of smoking cessation such as decreasing carbon monoxide levels), gradual cessation (i.e., "nicotine fading"), or relaxation techniques (718). In addition, there is an insufficient number of studies of adequate research design regarding the use of 12-step programs, hypnosis, biofeedback, family therapy, IPT, or psychodynamic therapies for treating nicotine dependence, although clinical consensus suggests that such therapies may be useful in some patients.

G. TREATMENT OF SMOKERS ON SMOKE-FREE WARDS

This section focuses on the treatment of psychiatric patients on smoke-free wards, a common issue confronted by psychiatrists. The principles described also apply to smokers on general medical wards seen in consultation and to smokers in smoke-free nonmedical settings, such as residential care settings. Controlled studies of treating nicotine withdrawal symptoms on psychiatric inpatient wards have not been published; thus, the recommendations below are based on treating withdrawal in outpatient settings (755, 757).

An inpatient stay may be an opportune time for initiating treatment for nicotine dependence because of the intensity of exposure to medical staff, diagnosis of medical conditions, and removal from usual smoking cues. It may therefore be helpful to include smoking cessation on the master treatment plan whenever relevant. As in other settings, smokers should be assessed for their readiness and motivation for change (32). Those considering quitting should be asked about their interest in using the temporary abstinence of the smoke-free unit as a beginning step toward permanently stopping smoking. In addition to the aspects of assessment discussed above in Section III.B, it may also be helpful to elicit from the patient any history of withdrawal symptoms in prior hospitalizations, withdrawal during prior voluntary quit attempts, or significant fear of withdrawal. An important but often neglected issue is the incorporation of NRTs and smoking cessation-related advice and aftercare into treatment plans on patient discharge (865).

1. System issues

Although many inpatient units have been concerned about implementing smoke-free units, most have found it less difficult than anticipated (34, 866, 867). Most (34, 866, 868–870) but not all (871) reports before and after the institution of smoke-free units indicate no increases in aggression, disruption, discharges against medical advice, use of medications or restraints, or admission refusals. However, a recent retrospective study on a smoke-free unit suggested that smokers may be more likely to be irritable or agitated than nonsmokers and that smokers who are not prescribed an NRT were more likely to be discharged against medical advice than other patients (865). Giving special off-ward privileges to allow patients to smoke or labeling off-ward passes as "smoking breaks" implicitly condones smoking (34, 866). In addition, there are risks in allowing some patients to have smoking breaks, such as patients with suicidal ideation or those with a history of eloping or exhibiting other problematic behavior on passes. Policies that provide breaks for smokers and nonsmokers on the same schedule may be preferable to policies that provide smokers with extra passes. Other recommendations for implementing a smoke-free unit are discussed in reviews (34, 866).

2. Patient education

Patients need to be educated about the rationale for a smoke-free unit; that is, that its purpose is not to force patients to stop smoking but to prevent secondhand smoke exposure to other patients and be consistent with the institution's goal to encourage healthy behaviors (34, 866). Patients should also be educated about the goal of smoking cessation treatment: to reduce withdrawal symptoms and, if patients are interested, to help them begin a cessation attempt (see Section III.D.9). Many patients are unaware of the valid symptoms of nicotine withdrawal and their time course; thus education about these can be helpful (34, 866).

3. Monitoring of symptoms

Although true for all individuals who stop smoking, it is particularly important to monitor patients in smoke-free inpatient settings for changes in psychiatric symptoms. Smoking cessation can worsen anxiety, insomnia, concentration, and weight gain, thereby confounding assessment and treatment of the patient's other psychiatric disorders (865). For example, because many alcohol-dependent patients smoke, it may not be clear whether their irritability, anxiety, insomnia, restlessness, difficulty concentrating, and depression are due to alcohol or nicotine withdrawal during alcohol detoxification on a smoke-free ward. Although nicotine withdrawal symptoms are thought to be milder than alcohol withdrawal symptoms, there is substantial person-to-person variability so that some alcohol-dependent smokers have nicotine withdrawal symptoms that are more severe than their alcohol withdrawal symptoms (872). When patients with schizophrenia are hospitalized and given higher doses of medications to treat acute psychosis, any increases in restlessness could be due to nicotine withdrawal rather than to neuroleptic-induced akathisia. Further confounding the source of the increased symptoms is the fact that smoking cessation can cause dramatic increases in blood levels of some medications (e.g., those metabolized by the CYP 1A2 microsomal system) (760, 873). In particular, clozapine levels can increase by up to 40% with smoking cessation (874).

4. Treatment of withdrawal symptoms

For some individuals, nicotine withdrawal during hospitalization is often not as severe as anticipated because of the absence of smoking cues, the distraction of the primary psychiatric problem, and the effects of medications. However, a recent retrospective study suggests there are clear benefits of providing NRTs to smokers on smoke-free inpatient psychiatric units (865), findings that are consistent with recommendations of the U.S. Agency for Healthcare Research and Quality's *A Clinical Practice Guideline for Treating Tobacco Use and Dependence*

(826) and with a meta-analysis of studies in nonpsychiatric inpatients (875). Thus, given the low risk of NRTs, prophylactic treatment with an NRT is suggested for all psychiatric inpatients who smoke. The advantages of nicotine gum in this context include the patient's ability to self-titrate the nicotine dose and stop using the gum immediately before intermittent smoking (e.g., during passes). In addition, many patients find that only a few pieces of gum per day are sufficient to prevent withdrawal symptoms (34, 866). The nicotine patch has the advantage of improved adherence and providing stable nicotine replacement. This may be especially advantageous in patients for whom a clinician is trying to differentiate nicotine withdrawal symptoms from psychiatric symptoms (873). For highly nicotine-dependent individuals, the use of more than one form of NRT (e.g., nicotine patch plus gum) may be helpful (865). A frequent question about prescribing NRT to patients on smoke-free units relates to those individuals who do not wish to stop smoking entirely and may use NRTs and cigarettes concurrently. However, such use of NRTs appears to be unlikely to produce significant adverse effects (865, 876–881). Bupropion can also be used in inpatient settings given its fixed dosing, easy monitoring, and efficacy in reducing signs and symptoms of the withdrawal syndrome (158).

Although the existing evidence does not show direct effects of psychosocial treatments on withdrawal symptoms, clinical experience suggests several strategies that may be useful for individuals in inpatient settings. Relaxation tapes can be used to alleviate anxiety. Anger can be averted by temporarily avoiding interactions; insomnia can be decreased by improving sleep hygiene; weight gain can be combated by increasing activity; and distraction and activities aimed at keeping busy can be used to get through craving episodes. Support groups for those going smoke free and support from family and significant others for going smoke free can be helpful as well.

H. CLINICAL FEATURES INFLUENCING TREATMENT

1. Use of multiple substances

There is strong evidence that rates of smoking are much higher in patients with a substance use disorder than in the general population (347). For example, in the National Epidemiologic Survey on Alcohol and Related Conditions, the 12-month prevalence of nicotine dependence is 34.5% among individuals with any alcohol use disorder and 52.4% among individuals with any drug use disorder (347). Conversely, among subjects with nicotine dependence, the 12-month prevalence of an alcohol use disorder is 22.8% and that of a drug use disorder is 8.2%, rates that are 4.4- and 8.1-fold higher, respectively, those observed in non-nicotine-dependent individuals (347). A similar association between nicotine dependence and other substance use disorders has been observed in data from the National Comorbidity Study (349). In addition, the presence of alcohol or illicit drug use may be a negative predictor of smoking cessation treatment outcomes (698, 872). Although substance use and smoking are often concurrent and conditioned effects may be one important factor in determining the high rates of comorbidity and treatment failure, rates of smoking cessation among these individuals can still be substantial (349). In addition, many individuals with a substance use disorder express an interest in smoking cessation. In patients who do not express a current interest in quitting, motivational interventions should be used.

There is conflicting evidence about whether concurrent smoking cessation can increase, decrease, or affect at all the risk of relapse to alcohol (38), and it is also unclear whether cessation should be attempted concurrently or after initial abstinence from other substances. For these reasons, this decision may be guided by patient preference. In addition, there are few studies of pharmacotherapies in individuals with substance use disorders (705), but there is some evidence for the utility of NRT and behavioral approaches. The use of alcohol treatment-related pharmacotherapies such as disulfiram or naltrexone might be considered in alcohol-dependent smokers, but there are no empirical studies to suggest the efficacy of these therapies in smoking cessation. In any case, such smoking cessation treatment should be made available in substance use disorder treatment programs.

2. Treatment in the presence of specific co-occurring psychiatric disorders

In the presence of a co-occurring psychiatric disorder, smoking cessation may be more difficult (349, 698, 760, 882). Psychiatric patients appear to have more withdrawal symptomatology when they stop smoking (414, 703, 767), probably as a function of their higher levels of nicotine dependence and smoking consumption. Cessation rates with NRTs (702, 703, 883) appear promising in patients with serious psychiatric disorders. Nicotine nasal spray and vapor inhaler systems provide faster delivery of nicotine, which may increase the rewarding effects of their use. However, no specific studies on these systems have been published in psychiatric patients, and the degree of difficulty of using these delivery systems and their side effects may limit their utility in this population (758, 884). Although many psychiatric patients smoke large numbers of cigarettes and inhale cigarette smoke deeply (885), using higher-than-normal doses of nicotine for heavier smokers has not been consistently shown to be more effective (790, 886). However, supplementation of the nicotine patch with ad libitum use of nicotine gum, lozenges, or inhaler appears helpful (887, 888). NRTs may also be considered as a way to reduce smoking even when patients do not have smoking cessation as a goal.

Initial psychosocial interventions for psychiatric patients may need to include higher intensities of behavioral therapy, because briefer psychosocial treatments are often unsuccessful (414, 702–704). There has been little study of behavioral therapies for smoking cessation in chronic psychiatric patients, although preliminary studies provide modest evidence that higher-intensity therapies may improve outcomes (701, 703). These studies have typically lacked a treatment as usual or minimal intervention controls, necessitating more controlled studies to establish the efficacy of these treatments. Combining higher-intensity behavioral treatments with an NRT or bupropion should be considered and has shown some modest success rates in preliminary studies (414, 701, 703, 704). In addition, psychiatric patients, including those who abuse or are dependent on substances, are more likely to benefit from behavioral therapy because of their high incidence of psychosocial problems, poor coping skills, and often, history of benefit from such therapy (730). When deciding between individual or group therapy, it is important to consider patient preference, as many psychiatric patients have experience with one or both kinds of psychotherapy. For some patients, both individual and group therapy may be indicated; for example, a specific problem that undermines cessation (e.g., a problem with assertiveness) might be addressed by individual therapy, whereas smoking cessation in general might be addressed in group therapy. Patients with low levels of coping skills or supports might also benefit from both individual and group behavioral therapy.

a) Schizophrenia

Rates of smoking in patients with schizophrenia are much higher (58%–88%) than in the general population (349, 889). The motivation to address smoking is often poor in these patients (882, 890), and thus motivational interventions as initial treatments are strongly suggested (891). In addition, the very low quit rates observed for these patients (349) suggest that more intense interventions are needed. Several controlled trials (414, 701–704) using combinations of higher-intensity behavioral support and pharmacotherapies (NRTs or bupropion) have shown modest short-term cessation rates, whereas one open-label trial of bupropion and supportive group therapy showed a decreased consumption of cigarettes in patients with schizophrenia (415). Concurrent alcohol and drug abuse in individuals with schizophrenia is high and can complicate cessation efforts; most studies have attempted cessation in patients whose drug use is in recovery and whose psychiatric symptoms are stable. Regular monitoring of antipsychotic side effects and plasma concentrations may be needed because smoking cessation may increase levels of antipsychotic medications that are metabolized via the CYP 1A2 system (e.g., clozapine, olanzapine, fluphenazine, haloperidol) (see Section III.D.8.b.2). There is some evidence that in smokers with schizophrenia, the use of second-generation antipsychotic agents can either reduce smoking (e.g., clozapine) in those not wanting to quit (407) or facilitate cessation in those attempting to quit with the nicotine patch (703) or bupropion (414), but further studies of this effect are needed in larger samples.

b) Depressive disorders

Individuals with major depressive or dysthymic disorder also have high rates of smoking, with 12-month prevalence rates of about 30% (347). Similarly, about 17% of nicotine-dependent individuals have a 12-month prevalence of major depressive disorder (347), and 40% of smokers seeking treatment have a history of depression (760, 781). Current (765, 892, 893) and perhaps past (894) depression appears to be a negative predictor of treatment outcome during smoking cessation. Although pharmacotherapies for smoking cessation have not been carefully tested in patients with current (458) or past (456) major depression, antidepressants such as bupropion (158) or nortriptyline (456) should be strongly considered. In general, SSRIs do not appear to be efficacious in promoting smoking cessation (602, 795). Behavioral therapies such as CBT should also be considered for depressed smokers (456, 459, 893, 895), as these individuals are likely to fail with more minimal interventions. After a patient has quit smoking, his or her plasma levels of some antidepressants (e.g., TCAs) that are metabolized by CYP 1A2 may increase, necessitating close monitoring of levels and antidepressant side effects.

c) Other psychiatric disorders

Smoking rates in patients with a bipolar or anxiety disorder (e.g., PTSD, panic disorder), ADHD, or another substance use disorder (e.g., marijuana, opioids, cocaine) are also higher than in the general population, but there has been little study of factors associated with these patients' interest in quitting smoking or the efficacy of smoking cessation interventions with these patients (698, 699).

3. Comorbid general medical disorders

a) General issues

Nicotine dependence is the most frequent substance use disorder in all medical settings. In 2001, an estimated 46.2 million adults in the United States smoked cigarettes (896). A 2004 report of the U.S. Surgeon General (897) concluded that there is sufficient evidence to infer a causal relation between smoking and many medical conditions, including cancer and cardiovascular and respiratory diseases. Despite improved public awareness of its dangers, tobacco use continues to be the leading preventable cause of disease and death in the United States, leading to approximately 440,000 deaths per year (898). Because the duration of smoking is a substantial contributor to the associated harms from inhalation of tar and carbon monoxide, early intervention is important if smoking-related morbidity and mortality are to be prevented.

It is not surprising that smokers with psychiatric disorders have an increased risk for nicotine-related medical disorders because individuals with a psychiatric and/or a substance use disorder are two to three times more likely to be dependent on nicotine than the general population (347) and smokers with psychiatric disorders consume nearly half of all the cigarettes consumed in the United States (349). In addition, many of these individuals are obese, consume harmful levels of alcohol and salt, and do not exercise or undergo cholesterol screenings (899). As well as having increased medical comorbidity, smokers on psychiatric or other medications that are metabolized through CYP 1A2 will require higher medication doses compared with nonsmokers (414, 698, 760, 768, 769).

Environmental tobacco smoke (secondhand smoke) also contributes to increased morbidity and mortality and has been classified by the U.S. Environmental Protection Agency as a known cause of lung cancer in humans (group A carcinogen). Secondhand smoke is estimated by the agency to cause approximately 3,000 lung cancer deaths in nonsmokers each year (900). Given the high proportion of individuals with psychiatric disorders who smoke, those who reside or attend treatment programs with large numbers of other smokers may be at increased risk from environmental tobacco smoke.

b) Issues related to specific physical disorders

Cardiovascular disease, lung cancer, and chronic obstructive pulmonary disease are the most common causes of morbidity and mortality among smokers, making it important to screen smokers for the signs and symptoms of these conditions (751, 901). Among smokeless tobacco, cigar, and pipe users, mouth and upper airway cancers are the most common causes of tobacco-induced mortality, and users of these forms of tobacco should be screened for the presence of these diseases (751, 901).

With smoking-related physical disorders, the duration of smoking abstinence is directly related to decreases in risk within 5 years of cessation (902–906). Smoking cessation also leads to an improved quality of life. Because medical hospitalization, cancer diagnosis, impending surgery, or exacerbation of cardiorespiratory symptoms may motivate individuals to consider smoking cessation, treatment for nicotine dependence is particularly important at these junctures. Screening for other substance use is also indicated, as smokers with pulmonary problems may be highly dependent and have a comorbid alcohol use disorder.

In general, the treatments for nicotine dependence that are recommended for use in the general population are effective in patients with co-occurring general medical conditions. NRTs decrease acute symptoms of nicotine withdrawal and increase smoking cessation rates (839, 907–912) without appearing to have any increased risk of adverse outcomes (836, 876, 913–916). Bupropion also appears to be safe as well as effective in individuals with cardiovascular (917) and pulmonary disease (918). Behavioral interventions improve smoking cessation rates when administered alone (875, 919, 920), as a package of several behavioral interventions (836, 875, 920, 921), or in combination with an NRT (908, 911, 912); they appear particularly useful when delivered in more intensive formats (855, 875, 920) or in conjunction with a program of smoking cessation aftercare (836, 875, 920, 921).

4. Pregnancy

Pregnant women who smoke pose an immediate and considerable challenge, given the risks of smoking to the fetus (574, 922–928). Screening patients for their smoking status during pregnancy is essential, and biochemical measures may be more accurate than self-report measures in identifying those in need of intervention (929). The primary risk of smoking during pregnancy appears to be low-birth-weight infants. If a woman quits smoking by her third trimester, the risk of giving birth to a low-birth-weight infant is no greater than the risk to a nonsmoker (930–935).

There is good evidence that physician counseling about smoking during pregnancy is effective (936, 937). In addition, behavioral interventions may be preferred by many women (938, 939); thus, these interventions should be considered first-line treatments for pregnant smokers (939).

The evidence is mixed on the ability of NRTs to augment rates of smoking cessation in pregnant women compared with behavioral interventions alone (940, 941). Although there appears to be no increased risk for NRTs in pregnancy (930, 938), this has not been well studied. Nevertheless, the consensus suggests that any increase in risk that might occur with NRTs is likely to be less than the risk of ongoing smoking (942, 943). Intermittent forms of NRTs may be preferred over the nicotine patch as the former minimize nicotine exposure to the fetus (930). Although there are no reports on the teratogenicity of bupropion, the decision to treat a pregnant woman with bupropion should include consideration of the potential benefits and risks to the woman and the fetus.

Regardless of the form of treatment used to augment smoking cessation in pregnant women, postpartum relapse rates are high (738, 929, 944, 945), suggesting a need for additional efforts at relapse prevention.

IV. TREATMENT OF ALCOHOL-RELATED DISORDERS

A. OVERVIEW

The focus of this section is on the treatment of patients with alcohol dependence or abuse. However, treatment of these disorders may be complicated by episodes of intoxication and withdrawal, the treatment of which is discussed in Sections IV.C.1 and IV.C.2. Alcohol use disorders are common. In the National Epidemiologic Survey on Alcohol and Related Conditions, the 12-month prevalences were 4.65% for alcohol abuse and 3.61% for alcohol dependence (23), with corresponding 12-month prevalences in the National Comorbidity Study of 3.1% and 1.3%, respectively (946), and prevalences of lifetime disorder that were about five times the 12-month prevalences (947).

The course of alcohol use disorders is variable and frequently characterized by periods of remission and relapse. The first episode of alcohol intoxication is likely to occur in the midteens, and the age at onset of alcohol dependence peaks at ages 18–25 years (947, 948). The first evidence of withdrawal, if it occurs, is not likely to appear until many other aspects of dependence have developed. Although some individuals with alcohol dependence achieve long-term sobriety without active treatment, others need treatment to stop the cycles of remission and relapse (949).

The relation of alcohol dependence to alcohol abuse is also variable. In one study (950), only 30% of male subjects with alcohol abuse at baseline met criteria for alcohol dependence 4 years later; the other 70% either continued to meet criteria for alcohol abuse or saw their alcohol problems remit entirely.

The long-term goals of treatment for patients with an alcohol use disorder are identical to those for patients with any type of substance use disorder and include abstinence (or reduction in use and effects), relapse prevention, and rehabilitation. There is some controversy in the literature, however, regarding the possible benefits of striving for a reduction in alcohol intake, as opposed to total abstinence, for those who are unlikely to achieve the latter. A comprehensive review of the issue (951) concluded that a lower severity of pretreatment alcohol dependence and an individual's belief that he or she could control his or her drinking were associated with the individual's achieving controlled drinking after treatment. Interventions aimed at achieving moderate drinking have also been used with patients in the early stages of alcohol abuse (952, 953). Controlled drinking may be an acceptable outcome of treatment for a select group of patients when it is accompanied by substantial improvements in morbidity and psychosocial functioning. However, abstinence is the optimal goal that achieves the best long-term overall functioning (9).

Numerous studies (43, 954, 955) have documented positive outcomes among individuals who receive treatment for alcohol dependence; approximately 70% of all such patients manifest a reduction in the number of drinking days and improved health status within 6 months (43).

The majority of patients who are treated for an alcohol use disorder have at least one relapse episode during the first year after treatment. However, there is considerable evidence to show that most individuals with an alcohol use disorder drink less frequently and consume less alcohol after receiving treatment compared with before treatment (956–959). For example, patients typically report drinking heavily on 75% of the days during a 3-month period before treatment, whereas during posttreatment follow-ups, they report being abstinent on 70%–90% of the days and engage in heavy drinking on 5%–10% of the days (231).

Treatment has also been shown to bring about improvements in family functioning, marital satisfaction, and psychiatric impairments (43, 290, 960–963). Although improvements after treatment for alcohol dependence are at least in part attributable to nontreatment factors such as patient motivation (964), it is generally accepted that treatment does make a difference, at least in the short run.

B. TREATMENT SETTINGS

The choice of treatment setting for an alcohol-dependent individual will be determined by the results of the initial medical and psychiatric evaluation (see also Section II.C). In addition, the optimal treatment setting and subsequent treatment outcome are likely to vary depending on the characteristics of the individual patient (965, 966).

Patients with alcohol withdrawal must be detoxified in a setting that provides for frequent clinical assessment and the provision of any necessary treatments (967). Some outpatient settings can accommodate these requirements and may be appropriate for patients deemed to be at low risk for a complicated withdrawal syndrome, with medical detoxification being accomplished using the medications described below (see Section IV.C.3). Postdetoxification treatment can also be successfully conducted outside of the hospital (e.g., in outpatient, day hospital, or partial hospitalization settings) for most patients with alcohol dependence or abuse (51, 956, 967). Intensive outpatient care involving frequent visits or conducted in a day hospital is generally preferable for the early phase of treatment. It is usually preferred that a significant other be available for travel to and from the treatment site, medication monitoring, symptom evaluation, support for abstinence, and communication with a responsible health care professional on behalf of the alcoholic patient. Relapse prevention medications should always be considered after detoxification. Currently available medications are naltrexone, disulfiram, and acamprosate (see Sections IV.C.3.a–c).

Patients who are unlikely to benefit from less intensive and less restrictive alternatives may need to be hospitalized at times during their treatment. In particular, those who have a history of withdrawal seizures or delirium tremens, whose documented history of very heavy alcohol use and high tolerance places them at risk for a complicated withdrawal syndrome, who are concurrently abusing other substances, who have a severe comorbid general medical or psychiatric disorder, or who repeatedly fail to cooperate with or benefit from outpatient detoxification are more likely to require a residential or hospital setting that can safely provide the necessary care. Patients in severe withdrawal (i.e., delirium tremens) always require treatment in a hospital setting. Patients who fail to achieve abstinence or who relapse frequently should also be given a trial of inpatient care. Under some circumstances, psychiatrically or socially unstable individuals may similarly benefit from the stabilization provided by a residential treatment setting.

Inpatient care should include medical detoxification and a program of rehabilitation. Although many inpatient and residential treatment programs have been traditionally organized around a treatment length of 28 days, empirical studies have not yet identified a specific optimal length of stay for the treatment of patients with an alcohol use disorder. Moreover, 28 days is a brief period in the natural history of a chronic disease.

Regardless of whether treatment for an alcohol use disorder begins in an inpatient or outpatient setting, the pivotal factor in successful treatment is engaging the patient in long-term outpatient relapse prevention with a duration measured in years rather than days. Patients should also be encouraged to participate in 12-step or other self-help group programs during outpatient rehabilitation.

C. SOMATIC TREATMENTS

1. Treating intoxication states

In general, the acutely intoxicated patient requires reassurance and maintenance in a safe and monitored environment in which efforts are made to decrease external stimulation and provide orientation and reality testing. Adequate hydration and nutrition are also essential. Clinical assessment should follow the general guidelines described in Section II.B, giving particular emphasis to the patient's general medical and mental status, substance use history, and any associated social problems. Patients presenting with signs of intoxication should also be assessed for the possibility of recent use of other substances that could complicate their clinical course. Patients with a history of prolonged or heavy drinking or a history of withdrawal symptoms are at particular risk for medically complicated withdrawal syndromes and may require hospitalization.

2. Treating withdrawal syndromes

The treatment of alcohol withdrawal has two major goals: 1) help the patient achieve detoxification in a manner that is as safe and comfortable as possible and 2) enhance the patient's motivation for abstinence and recovery (968). According to DSM-IV-TR, the syndrome of mild to moderate alcohol withdrawal generally occurs within the first several hours after the cessation or reduction of heavy, prolonged ingestion of alcohol. It includes signs and symptoms such as gastrointestinal distress, anxiety, irritability, elevated blood pressure, tachycardia, and autonomic hyperactivity.

The syndrome of severe alcohol withdrawal, including delirium tremens, occurs especially within the first several days after cessation or reduction of heavy, prolonged ingestion of alcohol; the syndrome includes signs and symptoms such as clouding of consciousness, difficulty in sustaining attention, disorientation, generalized tonic-clonic seizures (grand mal) seizures, respiratory alkalosis, and fever (969–971). As described in DSM-IV-TR and elsewhere (972, 973), <5% of individuals with alcohol withdrawal develop severe symptoms and <3% develop grand mal seizures. In the past, the mortality rate for patients experiencing alcohol withdrawal delirium was as high as 20%; currently, it is closer to 1% because of improved diagnosis and medical treatment (972). The presence of a co-occurring medical disorder may also increase the likelihood of a complicated withdrawal syndrome (974–976). Because mounting evidence suggests that repeated episodes of alcohol withdrawal may lead to a worsening of future withdrawal episodes (a phenomenon known as the alcohol withdrawal kindling or sensitization effect), individuals with multiple previous withdrawals may require more aggressive treatment (977). To aid in identifying individuals at risk for severe alcohol withdrawal, a number of standardized instruments have been developed that assess and qualify the severity of withdrawal symptoms, with perhaps the most widely used being the Clinical Institute Withdrawal Assessment for Alcohol Scale, Revised (978, 979).

For approximately 67% of the patients with mild to moderate withdrawal symptoms, generalized support, reassurance, and frequent monitoring are sufficient treatment (980), although the effectiveness of supportive treatment for these patients relative to pharmacotherapy is not well established (981, 982). In one case-control study (981), 74% of hospitalized alcohol-dependent patients without a serious comorbid general medical problem responded to supportive treatment for alcohol withdrawal. Consensus does suggest that thiamine be given routinely to all patients receiving treatment for a moderate to severe alcohol use disorder to treat or prevent common neurological sequelae of chronic alcohol use (983–986). In addition, patients in more severe withdrawal and those who develop hallucinations require pharmacological treatment.

The criteria for an ideal pharmacological agent to treat alcohol withdrawal include effectiveness in relieving symptoms and preventing seizures and delirium; a benign side effect profile, including safety in overdose; limited interactions with other medications; tolerability by those with comorbid medical conditions; tolerability by outpatients who may have cognitive impairment; and the ability to suppress drinking during and after alcohol withdrawal (987). Because no single agent or class of agents meets all of these criteria, a pharmacotherapeutic agent needs to be chosen according to the needs of the individual patient.

There are numerous reviews of the pharmacological treatment of moderate to severe withdrawal (987–993). The pharmacotherapy is directed toward reducing CNS irritability and restoring physiological homeostasis. This often requires the use of fluids, benzodiazepines, and, in selected cases, other medications (138, 987, 992, 994), as described below. In particular, benzodiazepines effectively reduce withdrawal severity and the incidence of seizures and delirium (991, 992). Carbamazepine, beta-blockers, and clonidine also diminish the severity of alcohol withdrawal symptoms but have not been proven to prevent delirium or seizures, which suggests that beta-blockers, clonidine, carbamazepine, and neuroleptics can be used adjunctively but not as monotherapy (992). In fact, there is some suggestion that protracted withdrawal symptoms and the relapse rate that occurs after successful detoxification may depend in part on what type of agent (benzodiazepine or anticonvulsant) is used during the acute detoxification period (977).

Additional factors need to be taken into consideration when choosing a medication in an outpatient detoxification setting. It is clear that benzodiazepines can cause sedation and, if used with alcohol, can be especially dangerous. Use of an anticonvulsant agent such as carbamazepine may be considered. Anticonvulsants, clonidine, and beta-blockers do not have the abuse potential of benzodiazepines and are not likely to be diverted for other uses. These factors may be particularly important in the outpatient detoxification of a person who abuses multiple substances.

a) Benzodiazepines

The use of benzodiazepines to control withdrawal symptoms takes advantage of the cross-tolerance between alcohol and this class of medication (972). A substantial body of evidence, including several meta-analyses (991, 992, 995), supports the use of benzodiazepines in the treatment of alcohol withdrawal.

The literature is less clear about specific benzodiazepines or a specific protocol for detoxification with benzodiazepines. Some authors suggest a single oral loading dose of 200–400 mg chlordiazepoxide or 20–40 mg diazepam, or as needed, may be used (996, 997). Orally administered chlordiazepoxide (50 mg every 2–4 hours), diazepam (10 mg every 2–4 hours), oxazepam (60 mg q2h), and lorazepam (1 mg q2h) are commonly used (982, 998). Another approach is to take the total dose necessary to suppress CNS irritability and autonomic hyperactivity in the first 24 hours (i.e., the stabilization dose) and give it in four divided doses the following day, after which the dose can usually be tapered over 3–5 days, with monitoring for reemergence of symptoms (999). For most patients, the equivalent of 600 mg/day of chlordiazepoxide is the maximum dosage, and many patients require less; a few, however, may require substantially more (1000). Patients in severe withdrawal and those with a history of withdrawal-related symptoms may require up to 10 days of treatment before benzodiazepines can be completely withdrawn. Benzodiazepine administration should be discontinued once detoxification is completed. Multiple randomized, controlled trials demonstrate the use of less medication as well as shorter duration of treatment in symptom-triggered detoxification protocols (998, 1001–1003).

For patients who have severe hepatic disease, are elderly, or have delirium, dementia, or another cognitive disorder, short-acting benzodiazepines such as oxazepam or lorazepam (1004) are preferred by some clinicians and appear to be efficacious (1005). Oxazepam and lorazepam do not require multistep biotransformation; they are metabolized by phase II enzymes (glucuronidation) that are not as affected by alcohol-related hepatitis. Glucuronidation is preserved even in severe liver disease and cirrhosis (1006, 1007), making these medications safer choices for such patients. Lorazepam also has the advantage of being able to be administered parenterally. However, because of their brief half-lives, the short-acting benzodiazepines need to be given more frequently (1008–1011).

b) Adrenergic agonists and antagonists

Beta-adrenergic antagonists (e.g., propranolol, 10 mg p.o. q6h) have been used to reduce signs of autonomic nervous system hyperactivity (e.g., tremor, tachycardia, elevated blood pressure, diaphoresis) and, at higher doses, arrhythmias (1012–1014). Atenolol has been used for a similar purpose, usually in combination with benzodiazepines (1015), thus allowing the use of lower doses of benzodiazepines and thereby reducing the sedation and cognitive impairment often associated with benzodiazepine use. Clonidine, an α-adrenergic agonist (0.5 mg p.o. b.i.d. or t.i.d.) has been shown to reduce tremor, heart rate, and blood pressure (1016, 1017). However, the use of beta-blockers or clonidine alone for the treatment of alcohol withdrawal is not recommended because of their lack of efficacy in preventing seizures (992).

c) Anticonvulsants

The use of anticonvulsants as a treatment for acute alcohol withdrawal has been investigated in several studies (977, 994, 1018–1020) and considered in two meta-analyses (991, 992) and a review (987). Anticonvulsants and benzodiazepines appear to have comparable efficacy in preventing seizures during alcohol withdrawal (995); however, the prophylactic use of anticonvulsants such as phenytoin is not generally recommended (1005, 1021–1023) except in individuals with a co-occurring seizure disorder who have stopped their anticonvulsant medications while drinking (1024). Other withdrawal symptoms may also be diminished by anticonvulsants (992, 994, 1018, 1020), particularly in patients with mild to moderate withdrawal, although the evidence for this is mixed (987) and sample sizes of studies considering this usage have generally been small, making meta-analysis problematic (1025). Carbamazepine (600–800 mg/day for the first 48 hours; then tapered by 200 mg/day) has also been demonstrated to be effective in preventing withdrawal-related seizures, although its tendency to lower white blood cell counts in some patients may pose an added risk of infection (1026–1030). Although the evidence for the use of oxcarbazepine is sparse, this medication may be useful as an alternative to carbamazepine (1031). Divalproex sodium at a dosage of 500 mg t.i.d. (994) and intramuscular magnesium sulfate (1032) have also been used for preventing withdrawal seizures. Barbiturates (e.g., pentobarbital, phenobarbital, secobarbital) may be useful in reducing withdrawal symptoms in patients whose symptoms are refractory to benzodiazepines (1033). However, more recent reviews indicate that well-controlled studies of phenobarbital are rare and do not recommend phenobarbital for routine treatment of alcohol withdrawal (987).

d) Antipsychotic agents

For patients manifesting delirium, delusions, or hallucinations, antipsychotic agents, particularly haloperidol (0.5–2.0 mg i.m. q2h, as needed) are recommended. Because antipsychotic agents are not effective for treating the underlying withdrawal state (992), they should be used as an adjunct to benzodiazepines. Most patients will require <10 mg of haloperidol every 24 hours, although some patients may require considerably more.

e) Intravenous ethanol

Although some hospitals maintain oral and intravenous ethanol in their formularies to treat alcohol withdrawal syndromes, there is no clear evidence for the effectiveness of ethanol in this application. Given the published evidence of intravenous or oral benzodiazepine treatment for minor and major abstinence syndromes and the lack of any controlled trials comparing the use of intravenous benzodiazepines such as chlordiazepoxide with intravenous ethanol, the use of intravenous ethanol is not supported by the current published data (1034, 1035).

3. Medications to treat alcohol abuse and dependence

a) Naltrexone

Naltrexone, an opiate receptor antagonist, is thought to act by preventing the opiate receptor-mediated euphoric and rewarding effects of alcohol, diminishing the rewarding aspects of alcohol-induced dopamine release, and blunting the subsequent craving for alcohol. Naltrexone is one of the most widely studied medications for the treatment of alcohol dependence. Meta-analyses have found it to be more effective than placebo in promoting abstinence, reducing heavy drinking days, and decreasing rates of relapse (152–154, 1036). Depending on the study and outcome measure used, naltrexone is associated with small to moderate benefits (e.g., with effect sizes of 0.1–0.5 and/or relative risk decreases of 10%–14%). In addition, individual responsiveness to naltrexone varies, with some evidence that a family history of alcoholism and high levels of craving may predict better naltrexone response.

Some single-site and small multisite trials from several countries have shown therapeutic benefits of oral naltrexone (187, 954, 1037–1041), whereas other larger multisite studies have not (1042, 1043). Long-acting injectable naltrexone also appears to be efficacious (1044). In a number of these studies, the type and amount of concomitant psychosocial interventions may confound the interpretation of the study findings (1042, 1043). Several studies have indicated that naltrexone works best when combined with a relapse prevention approach, such as coping skills or CBT (187, 1038, 1039, 1041). Conversely, when more severely dependent subjects have been studied without concomitant relapse prevention interventions, the efficacy of naltrexone has been less robust (1045) or nonexistent (1043).

With the initiation of naltrexone therapy, patients taking opioids may experience withdrawal symptoms; therefore, before starting naltrexone, patients should be opioid free for at least 5 days after the last dose of a short-acting opioid such as heroin or 7 days after the last dose of a longer-acting opioid such as methadone (see Section VII.C.1.c). A urine toxicology screen for opiate medication may be indicated before naltrexone therapy is initiated. In non-opioid-abusing patients, the 50-mg dose of naltrexone used in most studies has been associated with mild and transient side effects, including CNS-related symptoms (headache, fatigue, dysphoria) and gastrointestinal problems (nausea, vomiting, abdominal pain). Similar side effects are reported with the long-acting injectable naltrexone and are more prominent in doses of 380 vs. 190 mg i.m. per month (1044). In addition, injection site pain was noted in about 10% of patients (1044).

Although significant hepatotoxicity has been reported with naltrexone, this side effect is rare at the usual doses. Moreover, liver function may improve in naltrexone-treated patients as a result of decreased drinking (1046). Hepatotoxicity may be more likely in morbidly obese individuals or at doses higher than those normally used in clinical treatment (>100 mg/day). Hepatoxicity resulting from an interaction between nonsteroidal anti-inflammatory drugs (NSAIDs) and high-dose naltrexone has also been described (1047); clinicians should use high doses of naltrexone cautiously and warn patients accordingly. In addition, because naltrexone is an opioid antagonist, it would be inappropriate for patients requiring opioid analgesics. The naltrexone-treated patient should carry a card explaining these issues and provide it to health care personnel in an emergency.

b) Disulfiram

Treatment with the aversive agent disulfiram (usually 250 mg/day, range 125–500 mg/day) is aimed at motivating abstinent alcoholic individuals to resist alcohol consumption. When aldehyde dehydrogenase is inhibited by disulfiram (151), alcohol consumption causes toxic levels of acetaldehyde to accumulate, which in turn is associated with a host of unpleasant and potentially dangerous signs and symptoms, including a sensation of heat in the face and neck, headache, flushing, nausea, vomiting, hypotension, and anxiety (148–150). Chest pain, seizures, liver dysfunction, respiratory depression, cardiac arrhythmias, myocardial infarction, and death have also been reported. The purpose of disulfiram is not to make the patient ill but to prevent a patient from drinking impulsively because he or she knows that illness will result from drinking while he or she is taking disulfiram. However, disulfiram is only effective to the degree that an alcohol-using individual adheres to taking it as prescribed. Methods to improve adherence include behavioral contracting between an alcohol-dependent individual and his or her spouse and other forms of monitored administration with set contingencies.

Controlled trials have not demonstrated any advantage of disulfiram over placebo in achieving total abstinence, delaying relapse, or improving employment status or social stability (1048, 1049), and a meta-analysis showed only some diminution in drinking with disulfiram (1036). However, a large VA multisite cooperative study did find that patients receiving 250 mg of disulfiram reported significantly fewer drinking days than those who either received no disulfiram or 1 mg of disulfiram (150). Moreover, some clinicians believe that this medication, when combined with other therapeutic interventions, has some benefit for selected individuals who remain employed and socially stable (150, 1048, 1050–1052). Patients who are intelligent, motivated, and not impulsive and whose drinking is often triggered by unanticipated internal or external cues that increase alcohol craving are the best candidates for disulfiram treatment. Treatment effectiveness is enhanced when adherence is encouraged through frequent behavioral monitoring (e.g., breath tests), group support for remaining abstinent (e.g., group therapy, AA) (1053), contingency contracting, or, where feasible, supervised administration of disulfiram (1054, 1055).

Disulfiram should never be used without the patient's knowledge and consent; understanding and explaining disulfiram's toxic or potentially lethal effects to patients is a prerequisite for its use (1056–1058). Patients taking disulfiram must be advised to avoid all forms of ethanol (including, for example, that found in some cough syrups). Disulfiram requires hepatic metabolism to convert it into an active medication. A metabolite of disulfiram is an inhibitor of CYP 450 3A4 (1059) and can interfere with the metabolism of a variety of psychotropic and other medications that are substrates for CYP 450 3A4. In addition to its aversive effects after the ingestion of alcohol, disulfiram can cause a variety of adverse effects that are rare but potentially severe, including neuropathies and hepatotoxicity. Thus, it should be used cautiously in patients with moderate to severe hepatic dysfunction, peripheral neuropathies, renal failure, and cardiac disease (1048). A patient who is impulsive, has poor judgment, or has a severe co-occurring psychiatric disorder (e.g., schizophrenia, bipolar disorder) that makes him or her unreliable or self-destructive (149, 1060) may also be a poor candidate for disulfiram treatment. Moreover, disulfiram is eliminated from the body slowly. Ingesting alcohol even 1–2 weeks after the last dose of disulfiram could cause an alcohol-disulfiram reaction (1061).

c) Acamprosate

In 2004 the FDA approved a new medication, acamprosate, for the treatment of alcohol dependence. The approval was based primarily on data derived from studies done in Europe (reviewed in 1062, 1063). Although the neuropharmacological action of acamprosate is not completely known, researchers do know that it is an amino acid derivative of taurine that is thought to work at brain glutamate receptor sites and stabilize glutamatergic function (155). As such, it has been hypothesized that it might normalize an aberrant glutamate system present during early abstinence that may be the basis of protracted withdrawal and early abstinence craving (1064).

Studies in Europe have evaluated patients who have generally started on the medication while in a hospitalized setting and who were abstinent for at least 7–10 days before taking the medication; the results of those studies showed that an increased number of patients maintain abstinence. Those who relapsed had more abstinent time before their first drinking day and also more overall abstinent days during a year or more of treatment (1062, 1063, 1065, 1066). In contrast, a multisite trial completed in the United States did not find acamprosate to be effective in a primary intent-to-treat analysis but did find that when subjects' motivation to maintain abstinence and adhere to medication treatment was taken into account, acamprosate was more effective than placebo in increasing the number of abstinent days (1067). The U.S. trial included outpatients who had a varied number of abstinent days prior to medication initiation, but, in general, the overall pretreatment abstinent time was much shorter than that in the European trials. Also, subjects in the U.S. trial received a standardized medical management type of counseling, whereas the European studies generally used varied traditional psychosocial alcohol treatment approaches focusing on the maintenance of abstinence. It would appear that, although not specifically studied, a number of days (perhaps 7 or more) of abstinence prior to starting acamprosate might be needed for acamprosate to be most effective.

There is also some evidence that acamprosate and naltrexone can be given together, but the benefit of doing so has not been clearly established (954, 1068). The COMBINE Study, a multisite trial supported by the National Institute on Alcohol Abuse and Alcoholism is in the process of further assessing the efficacy of acamprosate alone and in combination with naltrexone with and without a specialist-delivered behavioral intervention (1069, 1070). Acamprosate has also been studied in combination with disulfiram and has shown an apparent improvement in efficacy (1071).

At a dosage of two 333-mg pills t.i.d. (total dose of 1,998 mg), which is an approved dose in the United States, acamprosate is well tolerated, with generally self-limited and symptomatically treated diarrhea being the main adverse effect. Because acamprosate is excreted by the kidneys and not metabolized by the liver, caution must be taken with patients who have renal impairment (1072). However, liver disease should not affect its metabolism or blood level concentrations. Acamprosate has minimal if any negative interaction with alcohol so that it is expected to be generally safe in active or relapsed drinkers.

d) Medications acting on the serotonin system

SSRIs have been used in the treatment of alcoholism to directly affect alcohol consumption, with the goal of reducing drinking or promoting abstinence. SSRIs also may reduce psychiatric symptoms or syndromes (e.g., anxiety, depression) that might influence drinking behavior.

In addition to evidence that serotonin modulates the behavioral effects of alcohol (479, 1073–1075), several randomized, double-blind, placebo-controlled human studies with nondepressed heavy drinkers found that SSRIs reduce short-term alcohol consumption by 15%–20% (1076, 1077). However, subsequent studies in patients diagnosed with alcohol dependence have been less consistent (1078–1080) and suggest that SSRIs may worsen drinking behaviors in some individuals. The use of SSRIs in the treatment of alcohol dependence is similar to their use in other disorders (430), although gastrointestinal side effects may be more prominent in alcohol users.

TCAs also have nonselective effects on serotonin reuptake and have been used to treat depression associated with alcohol use disorders with equivocal results (138). However, two studies showed improved mood and reduced alcohol consumption in open (428) and double-blind, placebo-controlled trials (1081) with desipramine. Subsequent randomized, double-blind, controlled trials with desipramine (438) and imipramine (437), as well as a recent meta-analysis (425), concluded that TCAs may offer modest benefits in treating patients with alcohol use disorders and depression but not those with alcohol use disorders in the absence of depression.

Based on animal studies (1082, 1083) and early clinical laboratory findings (1084), the selective serotonin-3 receptor antagonist ondansetron was thought to have effects on alcohol reward and thereby reduce alcohol consumption and promote abstinence. Although patients with early-onset alcoholism and lower levels of drinking showed some benefit with low-dose ondansetron (1085, 1086), other patient subgroups did not demonstrate a response. Replication studies have yet to be conducted, and ondansetron is not approved by the FDA for alcoholism treatment. (Dosing, side effects, and implementation of treatment with ondansetron are discussed in greater detail in Section IX.B.3.d.)

e) Lithium

The use of lithium to treat patients with an alcohol use disorder not comorbid with bipolar disorder was supported by some early anecdotal reports and by a small double-blind, placebo-controlled study (1087). However, a large VA collaborative study (1088) showed no benefits of lithium over placebo for patients with or without depressive symptoms. A more recent meta-analysis also showed no efficacy for lithium in treating alcohol use disorders (1036). Consequently, lithium is not recommended as a primary treatment in patients who do not have co-occurring bipolar disorder.

D. PSYCHOSOCIAL TREATMENTS

A variety of psychosocial treatments have been used in the treatment of alcohol use disorders (1089), and the efficacy of specific psychotherapies for these disorders has been reviewed by a number of authors (79, 956, 1090, 1091). The sections that follow provide an overview of the use of CBT, behavioral therapies, psychodynamic therapies, IPT, self-help groups, brief interventions, marital and family therapy, and aftercare in the treatment of alcohol use disorders.

1. Cognitive-behavioral therapies

CBT and relapse prevention therapies aimed at improving self-control and social skills have been consistently found to reduce drinking (79, 1090, 1092–1094); such cognitive-behavioral therapies, as well as MET and TSF, are therefore recommended for use in individuals with an alcohol use disorder. Cognitive-behavioral stress management interventions and behavioral self-control training (consisting of cognitive and behavioral strategies, including self-monitoring, goal setting, rewards for goal attainment, functional analysis of drinking situations, and the learning of alternative coping skills) produced better outcomes than control treatments in about half of the studies (79, 1090, 1095–1097). Better outcomes during follow-up also seem to occur in individuals who show increased coping responses or "self-efficacy" at the end of treatment (184, 1098–1100) and in those who use problem solving or mastery rather than relying on avoidance of high-risk situations as a coping strategy (43, 265, 959, 1101). In contrast, cognitive therapy interventions that are focused on identifying and modifying maladaptive thoughts but that do not include a behavioral component are not as effective.

In group settings, CBT approaches are similarly effective, although treatment benefits may vary with patient characteristics (1102–1104). Finally, most studies show efficacy for social skills training, which focuses on learning skills for forming and maintaining interpersonal relationships, being assertive, and refusing alcohol (79).

MET and motivational interviewing are typically brief therapies that last one to four sessions and are aimed at maximizing the patient's intrinsic desire to change or enhancing a patient's adherence to more intensive or extended treatment. Motivational approaches have been found to be efficacious in most studies (reviewed by Dunn et al. [1105] and Miller and Wilbourne [79]), including the findings from Project MATCH (43, 90, 265, 1106) in which four

MET sessions given as a stand-alone treatment either initially or as part of posthospitalization care were comparable to 12 sessions of CBT or TSF, with benefits of treatment persisting through 3 years of follow-up.

2. Behavioral therapies

Individual behavioral therapy, particularly involving positive reinforcements for targeted behaviors, has been found to be effective for patients with an alcohol use disorder (191, 956, 1090) and is also a recommended treatment approach. Also effective are behavioral contracting (79) and the community reinforcement approach (190, 1107, 1108), which uses behavioral principles and usually includes conjoint therapy, training in job finding, counseling focused on alcohol-free social and recreational activities, monitoring of disulfiram use, and an alcohol-free social club. When compared with usual outpatient treatment or disulfiram plus a behavioral adherence program, community reinforcement led to significantly better patient outcomes (190, 1108). Community reinforcement also has documented effectiveness in combination with marital therapy (690). Compared with positive reward approaches, aversive therapies have been less successful (79). Relaxation training, although widely studied, has been ineffective in virtually all controlled trials (79).

3. Psychodynamic and interpersonal therapies

There are insufficient studies of adequate research design regarding the use of group or individual psychodynamically oriented psychotherapies for the treatment of individuals with an alcohol use disorder (79, 1090). It is difficult to draw conclusions in this area because of the paucity of well-controlled and designed studies, and the small extant literature is limited by poor research design and short duration of studies. However, there is some clinical consensus that such treatment is particularly helpful when other psychiatric disorders or interpersonal issues are present and when combined with other psychosocial or biological interventions. There are large numbers of patients in this type of treatment, and clinical consensus suggests the therapy is effective in at least some of these patients (956, 1090). In addition to addressing alcohol abuse or dependence, treatment goals often include stabilization of the patient's social and interpersonal life, disorganization of which may both accompany and perpetuate the alcohol use disorder.

4. Brief therapies

Brief interventions are generally delivered over one to three sessions and include an abbreviated assessment of drinking severity and related problems as well as the provision of motivational feedback and advice. Typically studied in general medical or school-based settings and in non-treatment-seeking heavy drinkers, brief therapies have been shown to be effective in reducing alcohol use and improving general health and social functioning (79, 275, 1109). In these subgroups of patients, the efficacy of brief therapies is often comparable with that of longer, more intense treatment; even very brief interventions (i.e., a few hours) may have some positive effect (1110, 1111).

5. Self-help groups and 12-step-oriented treatments

The effectiveness of AA, per se, has not been evaluated in randomized studies. However, other sources of information provide growing support for the utility of AA and 12-step-oriented treatments (259, 261, 956, 958, 959) as well as the efficacy of professional therapies such as TSF that are aimed at motivating patients to participate in AA (43, 219, 265, 267, 269). In addition, a large number of studies have documented that greater AA participation is associated with greater rates of abstinence from alcohol (1112) as well as with better drinking outcomes

(260–266, 289, 1113, 1114). Thus, most patients should be encouraged to attend at least several AA meetings to ascertain the appropriateness and utility of AA in helping them remain alcohol free. Individual patient needs and concerns should, however, be taken into consideration when making this recommendation.

As a spiritual but nonreligious program requiring belief in something beyond oneself (268), AA provides tools for its participants to maintain sobriety, including the 12 steps, group identification, and mutual help. More specifically, "AA is a fellowship of men and women who share their experience, strength and hope with each other that they may solve their common problem and help others to recover from alcoholism. The only requirement for membership is a desire to stop drinking" (253). Al-Anon (friends and family), Alateen (teenage children of alcoholic individuals), and Adult Children of Alcoholics (those who grew up in alcoholic or otherwise dysfunctional homes) help family members and friends of alcoholic individuals focus on the need to avoid enabling behaviors and care for oneself whether a loved one is drinking or not. Other mutual help programs include Women for Sobriety, Rational Recovery, Double Trouble (for patients with alcohol dependence comorbid with other psychiatric disorders), and Mentally Ill Chemical/Substance Abusers.

Patients may be more likely to benefit from AA groups composed of individuals with similar personal characteristics, such as age, sex, or cultural and occupational status. Evidence from small-scale trials on patient-to-program matching suggests that patients with a greater severity of drinking problems, an affective rather than cognitive focus, a concern about purpose and meaning in life, better interpersonal skills, and a high need for affiliation are good candidates for AA (254, 1115). In the landmark Project MATCH study (43), TSF-based aftercare was more effective than that using CBT for outpatients who did not show psychiatric symptoms and was of comparable efficacy for those with psychiatric symptoms. At 1-year follow-up, patients rated as high in seeking meaning of life fared better with TSF compared with MET and CBT, and patients with high social support for abstinence had better drinking outcomes at 1- and 3-year follow-up.

Although official AA policy encourages members to adhere to medical treatment, many individual members interpret the ethos of coping without the use of drugs to mean that recovering individuals should also forgo psychiatric medications (1116). Consequently, patients with a co-occurring psychiatric disorder requiring medication should be encouraged to attend dual-diagnosis AA groups or those in which regular attendees do not oppose medically prescribed psychotropic treatment.

6. Marital and family therapies

For patients who are married or living with family members, such relationships can be an important factor in the posttreatment environment (1090, 1117). Thus, it is not surprising that therapies aimed at enhancing marital or family relationships can be effective in the treatment of alcohol use disorders. In particular, behavioral marital therapy has demonstrated efficacy and cost-effectiveness (79, 225, 236, 238, 690, 961, 1118, 1119). Marital approaches for which there is significant support are Al-Anon facilitation and disulfiram contracting (168, 248); other approaches to marital therapy have shown lesser degrees of efficacy (79).

7. Self-guided therapies

Strong evidence is available to support the efficacy of self-monitoring of drinking patterns, guided by pamphlets provided by practitioners (79). Such approaches have typically been evaluated in general populations of primary care patients or with heavy drinkers who do not meet full criteria for alcohol dependence. Patients presenting to specialized substance use disorder treatment settings have generally experienced multiple failures at self-treatment and are poorer candidates for this approach.

8. Aftercare

A patient's involvement in aftercare after completing inpatient treatment for an alcohol use disorder is an important predictor of outcome (264, 1120, 1121). The lowest rates of relapse have been noted in those completing an aftercare program (1121, 1122), with some evidence that completion rates vary with therapists' efforts to maintain patients in the aftercare program (1122). Although the number of trials on specific aftercare approaches is limited, there is evidence for efficacy for TSF (43, 265), MET (43, 265), CBT administered alone (43, 265) or with coping skills training (223, 1102, 1103), a version of behavioral marital therapy that includes relapse prevention techniques (1118, 1119), insight-oriented interactional group therapy (223, 1102, 1103), and nurse visits delivered over a 12-month period (1123).

E. CLINICAL FEATURES INFLUENCING TREATMENT

The treatment implications of various clinical features are summarized in Section II.G. In addition to these considerations, specific sequelae and patterns of co-occurring disorders need to be considered for patients with an alcohol use disorder.

1. Co-occurring psychiatric disorders

Co-occurring psychiatric disorders are common among individuals with an alcohol use disorder. Integrated psychosocial treatments that combine traditional therapies for the psychiatric condition with therapies for the alcohol use disorder have been shown to be effective (376, 1124, 1125). In general, medications recommended to treat patients with an alcohol use disorder alone are also effective in patients with a co-occurring psychiatric disorder, and pharmacological treatment of the psychiatric disorder is similar to that recommended when the psychiatric disorder occurs independently of an alcohol use disorder. Some exceptions to these general principles are discussed below.

Given the propensity of individuals with alcohol and other substance use disorders to misuse prescribed medications, the treating clinician should give preference to prescribing medications that have a low abuse potential. Patients with a high level of depression, impulsivity, or poor judgment or the potential for making a suicide attempt should receive medications with a low potential for lethality in overdose (e.g., SSRIs) (1126, 1127). Given the tendency of patients with co-occurring disorders to have poor medication adherence and an increased risk of overdose, medications should be dispensed in limited amounts, the number of refills should be limited, and random or frequent blood or urine toxicology screening should be used to determine use of both prescribed and nonprescribed medications.

Many patients with alcohol dependence present with signs and symptoms suggestive of major depression or an anxiety disorder. In many patients, however, these signs and symptoms are related to alcohol intoxication or withdrawal and remit in the first few weeks of abstinence (424). Consequently, many psychiatrists feel that patients should be observed over a 3- to 4-week substance-free period before a diagnosis of a co-occurring mood or anxiety disorder is made and a disorder-specific medication is prescribed. Others suggest that in selected cases, earlier initiation of treatment is warranted. For example, depressed patients with particularly severe symptoms, a history of major depression unrelated to periods of alcohol use, and/or a strong family history of mood disorders are more likely to have a co-occurring depression that should be treated soon after detoxification is completed (426–429).

Although studies of SSRIs in individuals with an alcohol use disorder who are not depressed have shown mixed benefit (see Section IV.C.3.d), studies of those who are depressed have shown a moderate positive effect on the patients' addiction and mood (431, 1128, 1129). TCAs may also be effective for alcohol-dependent patients with comorbid depression (425, 437, 438), although the risk of poor adherence, tricyclic-to-alcohol interactions, and overdose should be considered with such patients. In addition, tricyclic plasma levels may be lower than expected because of the alcohol-induced increase in liver microsomal oxidases (1130, 1131). MAOIs have been used to treat patients with atypical depression, but there is a high risk of poor adherence to dietary and medication restrictions (including those for alcohol) and subsequent adverse reactions (e.g., hypertension) in patients with alcohol use disorders (1132). Consequently, because SSRIs and other nontricyclic, non-MAOI antidepressants have fewer adverse effects and less risk of morbidity and mortality in overdose situations, they are preferred over tricyclic and MAOI antidepressants in the treatment of patients with a co-occurring alcohol use disorder and depression (1133).

Studies of antidepressant agents in individuals with an alcohol use disorder and co-occurring anxiety are limited (1134). Consensus would suggest that these medications can be used as recommended for patients with an anxiety disorder alone.

The use of benzodiazepines for alcohol-dependent patients with comorbid anxiety or panic disorder is more controversial, as benzodiazepines have a high abuse potential in these patients. For patients with generalized or performance anxiety, beta-blockers (e.g., propranolol) and buspirone are preferable to benzodiazepines because they have no cross-tolerance with ethanol or other CNS depressants and minimal abuse potential. Buspirone has also been reported to reduce alcohol consumption in patients with high levels of comorbid anxiety (479, 1135). In patients with otherwise treatment-resistant panic disorder, clonazepam or other long-acting benzodiazepines can be cautiously administered if the principles outlined in Section II.G.2.d.2.d. are observed.

For patients with comorbid bipolar and alcohol use disorders, lithium, valproate, or carbamazepine may be used. A recent double-blind, controlled study of patients with bipolar disorder and alcoholism who were being maintained with valproate showed promising results of this medication as an adjunct to treatment (472). However, when prescribing lithium, valproate, or carbamazepine, the clinician may need to closely monitor the patient for side effects. In particular, the low therapeutic index of lithium may lead to a greater risk of toxicity in individuals with an alcohol use disorder who are actively drinking, and hematological abnormalities may be more pronounced in alcohol-dependent individuals who are treated with valproate or carbamazepine.

In patients with schizophrenia, some data suggest that clozapine may be useful for treating the symptoms of both schizophrenia and a comorbid substance use disorder, including an alcohol use disorder (384, 391, 393, 398), a possibility that requires further study in double-blind, randomized, controlled trials.

2. Comorbid general medical disorders

Chronic high-dose alcohol use can affect several different organ systems, including the gastrointestinal tract, the cardiovascular system, and the central and peripheral nervous systems. Alcohol-induced gastrointestinal problems include gastritis, ulcers of the stomach or duodenum, esophageal varices, portal hypertension, and, in approximately 15% of heavy users, cirrhosis of the liver and pancreatitis (1136–1138). Alcohol-dependent individuals also experience higher-than-average rates of cancer of the esophagus, stomach, and other parts of the gastrointestinal tract (1139, 1140).

Common comorbid cardiovascular conditions include low-grade hypertension and increased levels of triglycerides and low-density lipoprotein cholesterol, which increase the risk of heart disease. Cardiomyopathy occurs primarily among very heavy drinkers (1141).

For men, endocrinological changes associated with chronic alcohol use include decreases in testosterone, loss of facial hair, breast enlargement, decreased libido, and impotence (1142); endocrinological changes for women include amenorrhea, luteal phase dysfunction, anovulation, early menopause, and hyperprolactinemia (1143). Blunting of the thyroid-stimulating hormone response to thyrotropin-releasing hormone, hypoglycemia, ketosis, and hyperuricemia have also been reported (1144, 1145).

Alcohol-induced peripheral myopathy with muscle weakness, atrophy, tenderness, and pain is accompanied by elevations in creatine phosphokinase levels and the presence of myoglobins in the urine (1146). Histological evidence of myopathy can be observed in a significant proportion of patients with an alcohol use disorder, even in the absence of symptoms (1147). When it is severe, alcohol-induced myopathy can involve rapidly progressive muscle wasting.

Many patients seeking treatment of alcohol dependence manifest cognitive abnormalities (1148–1150). Chronic, heavy drinkers can experience an alcoholic dementia with characteristic cognitive deficits that include impairment in short- and long-term memory, abstract thinking, judgment, and other higher cortical functions as well as personality change. Usually the memory deficits are less severe than in Korsakoff's syndrome (alcohol-induced persisting amnestic disorder) or Alzheimer's disease (1151). Neuropathological abnormalities in the frontal lobes, in the area surrounding the third ventricle or diffusely through the cortex, have been reported. More commonly, however, there is subtle cognitive dysfunction that hampers a patient's ability to comprehend or adhere to a treatment plan (1148, 1149, 1152, 1153). For such patients, family members or other responsible parties should be actively involved from the beginning of and throughout the course of treatment. Initial placement of the patient in a more structured (e.g., residential) treatment setting may also be indicated to assess the impact of cognitive problems on the patient's ability to adhere to short- and long-term treatment. In patients who remain abstinent, reversal of alcohol-induced cognitive disturbance is often observed over time (1154, 1155).

Other nervous system sequelae of chronic alcohol use, including peripheral neuropathies, degenerative changes in the cerebellum, Wernicke's encephalopathy, and Korsakoff's syndrome, are related to vitamin deficiencies, particularly deficiencies in thiamine and other B vitamins (1156). Peripheral neuropathy is common, occurring in up to 33% of hospitalized individuals with an alcohol use disorder, with an even greater proportion of alcohol users showing electrophysiological evidence of peripheral nerve damage (1157). Symptoms of alcoholic neuropathy typically include sensory loss, paresthesias, a burning sensation of the feet, numbness, cramps, weakness, calf pain, and ataxia. Ataxia in alcohol-dependent patients can also occur due to cerebellar dysfunction.

Wernicke's encephalopathy is characterized by ophthalmoplegia, ataxia, and confusion (972, 1158). Ocular abnormalities include nystagmus, eye muscle palsies, and pupillary abnormalities. The mortality rate for acute untreated Wernicke's encephalopathy is 15%–20% (1159, 1160); recovery is incomplete in 40% of cases. Most patients (approximately 80%) with Wernicke encephalopathy also develop Korsakoff's syndrome, characterized by anterograde and retrograde amnesia, disorientation, poor recall, and impairment of recent memory coupled with confabulation. Lesions in the mammillary bodies and thalamic nuclei may be the result of vitamin deficiencies or the direct toxic effects of alcohol. Recovery is variable and not possible to predict on the basis of brain imaging. In more than half of the patients, elements of Korsakoff's syndrome are permanent.

These neurological complications should be treated vigorously with B complex vitamins (e.g., thiamine, 50–100 mg/day i.m. or i.v.), usually after adequate fluids and glucose levels are maintained. Some patients may require treatment with B complex vitamins over a prolonged period, and improvements may continue to occur up to 1 year after treatment is begun (1161).

Alcoholic hallucinosis during or after cessation of prolonged alcohol use may respond to antipsychotic medication. Unlike the visual hallucinations that may occur during alcohol withdrawal, these are primarily auditory and occur in conjunction with a clear sensorium (1162).

3. Pregnancy

The general effects of substance use during pregnancy are described in Section II.G.4. Alcohol-related disorders may have specific adverse effects on the health of the pregnant woman, the course of the pregnancy, fetal and early child development, and parenting behavior. The most well-established effect of in utero alcohol exposure is fetal alcohol spectrum disorder (587, 1163 ,1164). Some children with this disorder will exhibit the characteristic features of fetal alcohol syndrome, including low birth weight, poor coordination, hypotonia, neonatal irritability, retarded growth and development, craniofacial abnormalities (including microcephaly), cardiovascular defects, mild to moderate retardation, childhood hyperactivity, and impaired school performance (586, 972, 1165, 1166). Others will not have the classically described features of fetal alcohol syndrome but will exhibit cognitive and behavioral effects of in utero alcohol exposure (587, 1163, 1164). Thus, the goals in treating pregnant women with an alcohol use disorder include eliminating the use of alcohol, treating any comorbid psychiatric or general medical disorders, guiding the patient safely through the pregnancy, facilitating appropriate parenting behavior, and motivating the patient to remain in treatment after delivery to minimize the risk of relapse.

V. TREATMENT OF MARIJUANA-RELATED DISORDERS

A. OVERVIEW

Marijuana (cannabis) is the most widely used illicit drug in the United States (1167) and in the world. Although marijuana's relative dependence potential is less than that of other substances of abuse, the large number of users will yield high population rates of marijuana dependence (1168). Furthermore, although the overall prevalence of marijuana use has remained stable over the past decade, the initial age at onset of marijuana use has been declining (1169) and the prevalence of marijuana abuse or dependence has increased significantly, perhaps due to an increased potency of available marijuana (1170).

Marijuana use is often considered benign, but it has been associated with a number of psychological, behavioral, and social problems. Marijuana use is common and can be problematic in individuals with other psychiatric disorders, including major mood, anxiety, and personality disorders (1171–1174). Cannabis use can precipitate initial episodes of psychosis in vulnerable individuals (1175) and is associated with an earlier age at first psychotic episode in male patients with schizophrenia, 6.9 years younger than in non-cannabis users (1176). Cannabis abuse or dependence is highly associated with increased risk of other substance dependence (1177).

Contrary to the popular belief among laypeople and professionals that treatment for cannabis dependence is usually neither needed nor sought, the demand for such treatment at substance use disorder programs doubled between 1992 and 1998 in the United States. The percentage of illicit drug abuse treatment admissions for marijuana (23%) approximated that for cocaine (27%) and heroin (23%) (1178). Despite this, the treatment of marijuana abuse and dependence is a comparatively understudied area to date.

B. TREATMENT SETTING

Treatment for marijuana-related disorders usually occurs in an outpatient setting, either individually or in groups. Inpatient treatment is most likely to occur if the individual is hospitalized for another psychiatric disorder, including another substance use disorder.

C. SOMATIC TREATMENTS

Somatic treatments for marijuana dependence have been studied infrequently, perhaps because of the belief held by many that marijuana is a benign substance whose use is easy to stop when desired. However, interest in treatment has grown as evidence from animal and clinical studies has suggested that a withdrawal syndrome occurs if chronic heavy use of cannabis or tetrahydrocannabinol is discontinued (1179–1181). The magnitude and severity of these symptoms appear substantial, and their onset and time course appear similar to those of other substance withdrawal syndromes. Common symptoms are primarily emotional and behavioral, although appetite change, weight loss, and physical discomfort are frequently reported. With our increased knowledge of the marijuana withdrawal syndrome has come a heightened awareness of the drug's role in hampering many individuals from ceasing marijuana use.

Although more attention is now being paid to treatments for marijuana withdrawal symptoms, there have been no successful controlled trials of pharmacotherapy to date. Human trials of medications to ameliorate symptoms of marijuana withdrawal have included bupropion (1182), divalproex (1183, 1184), naltrexone, and nefazodone (1185); all these trials have had negative results. No pharmacotherapy trials to prevent marijuana reinstatement after abstinence have been reported. Thus, no specific pharmacotherapies can be recommended at this time.

D. PSYCHOSOCIAL TREATMENTS

Treatment of cannabis-related disorders has primarily used psychotherapies (1178). Specific psychosocial approaches that have been studied in the treatment of marijuana dependence have included a brief motivational approach and a more intensive relapse prevention approach that combines motivational approaches with coping skills development. Compared with delayed treatment control conditions, both treatments decreased marijuana use (276, 1186–1188), and, in the more robust study, intensive treatment showed a greater impact through the 15-month follow-up period (276). Adding voucher-based incentives to coping skills and motivational enhancement may lead to further improvements in outcomes (201). Nonetheless, even after achieving at least 2 weeks of abstinence, rates of relapse among marijuana-dependent patients receiving behavioral/psychosocial treatment are high, reaching >67% by 6 months in one study (1189). A recent study of a manual-guided, group-based treatment for adolescents with mild to moderate substance abuse found that marijuana use (but not alcohol use) was significantly reduced at 6 months, with the reduction sustained at 12 months (1190). Thus, although there are few studies of psychosocial treatments for marijuana dependence, those that have been conducted show evidence of benefit, particularly with more intensive approaches. Given the lack of pharmacotherapies for marijuana dependence and its psychological, behavioral, and social consequences, psychosocial treatments such as motivational therapy and relapse prevention are recommended for those with marijuana dependence.

E. PREGNANCY

There is increasingly robust evidence that marijuana use during pregnancy is associated with a number of deleterious outcomes. Case-control data (1190a) obtained at 17–22 weeks of gestation suggest that marijuana exposure has negative effects on fetal growth as measured by foot length and body weight. Behavioral, cognitive, and academic difficulties have also been observed in longitudinal follow-up studies of individuals with prenatal exposure to marijuana. As with prenatal exposure to maternal smoking or alcohol use, maternal use of marijuana during pregnancy appears to be related to increased impulsivity (1190b, 1190c), inattention (1190c, 1190d), and externalizing behaviors during childhood (1190c). Learning and memory tasks

(1190b, 1190c) and other aspects of cognitive functioning, such as executive functioning or visual analysis and hypothesis testing (1190d), also seem to be negatively affected by prenatal marijuana exposure.

Data from the 10-year follow-up of mother-child pairs who participated in the Maternal Health Practices and Child Development Project indicated differences in the effects of maternal marijuana use depending on the trimester in which exposure occurred. For example, independent of prenatal alcohol exposure, first-trimester marijuana exposure was associated with deficits in reading and spelling scores and lower teacher ratings of performance, whereas second-trimester exposure was associated with impaired reading comprehension and school performance (1190e). In the same cohort, prenatal marijuana exposure in the first and third trimesters predicted significantly increased levels of depressive symptoms in offspring at 10-year follow-up (1190f). An additional longitudinal study found that prenatal exposure to marijuana was associated with increased likelihood of both cigarette smoking and marijuana use in 16- to 21-year-old adolescent offspring compared with adolescents whose mothers had not used marijuana during pregnancy (1190g).

These findings suggest that pregnant women should be asked about marijuana use and advised to abstain from marijuana use during pregnancy.

VI. TREATMENT OF COCAINE-RELATED DISORDERS

A. OVERVIEW

At the time of the 2003 National Survey on Drug Use and Health (1191), approximately 2.3 million individuals were currently using cocaine, with approximately 33% of that group smoking crack cocaine. In addition, 1.1 million people used cocaine for the first time during that year. Although this figure does not approach the peak of 1.6 million new users seen in 1980, it does represent a slight increase over the approximately 1 million new users in each of the previous 3 years.

In recent years, the abuse of methamphetamine has also become a significant public health problem, beginning primarily in Hawaii, the West Coast, and the southwestern United States and steadily moving eastward.

Although this section focuses on cocaine dependence, pharmacotherapy of amphetamine dependence is expected to be similar. Neither disorder has an FDA-approved pharmacotherapy, and very few clinical trials have been completed with amphetamine-dependent patients, with none of these studies showing different results than those described later for cocaine dependence (1192, 1193). A possibly significant difference between cocaine and amphetamine is cocaine's interaction with alcohol to form cocaethylene. This metabolite has cocaine-like effects and toxicity (1194–1196).

B. TREATMENT SETTINGS

Patients with a cocaine or other stimulant use disorder generally do not require treatment in an inpatient setting as withdrawal syndromes are not severe or medically complex. Several studies have indicated that most patients can be effectively treated for cocaine abuse in intensive outpatient programs (1197, 1198).

C. SOMATIC TREATMENTS

1. Treating intoxication

The treatment of acute cocaine intoxication has been the subject of relatively little systematic investigation. In general, because there is no specific antidote to cocaine, treatment is typically supportive and aimed at treating symptoms such as delusions or autonomic hyperactivity. Cocaine intoxication can produce hypertension, tachycardia, cardiac arrhythmias, coronary artery vasospasm, myocardial infarction, stroke, and seizures (1199). Although the beta-blocker labetalol has been cited as being helpful in reducing this cocaine toxicity, animal studies and some clinical experience suggest that the use of adrenergic blockers and dopaminergic antagonists should be carefully monitored when treating acute cocaine intoxication (1200–1202). Benzodiazepines are used for acute cocaine intoxication in patients who become extremely agitated and/or potentially dangerous (1203). Although antipsychotic medications have been reported to be effective in treating delusions associated with cocaine intoxication, most individuals recover spontaneously within hours (1204, 1205) and thus require no treatment (1206–1208). There is no evidence that anticonvulsants prevent stimulant-induced seizures, and they are not recommended for this purpose.

2. Treating withdrawal

The clinical features and duration of the cocaine abstinence syndrome are still somewhat controversial. Although anhedonia and cocaine craving are common (1204), craving can be difficult to define (1204, 1209), and the cessation of cocaine use does not always cause specific withdrawal symptoms. However, many people do experience a characteristic withdrawal syndrome within a few hours to several days after the acute cessation of, or reduction in, heavy and prolonged cocaine use. An early uncontrolled outpatient study (1204) characterized withdrawal as progressing from a "crash" associated with intense depression, fatigue, and at times suicidal ideation to dysphoria and sleep difficulties lasting 1–10 weeks. Results from more recent inpatient studies (1209, 1210) and one outpatient study (1211) have suggested that cessation of regular cocaine use is associated with relatively mild symptoms of depression, anxiety, anhedonia, sleep disturbance (insomnia or hypersomnia), increased appetite, and psychomotor retardation, which decrease steadily over several weeks.

Dopamine agonists, such as amantadine (200–400 mg/day), were initially thought to be effective in reducing symptoms of cocaine withdrawal, craving, and subsequent use (1212–1214), but two other studies (1209, 1215) failed to confirm this finding. Similarly, initial studies of bromocriptine yielded promising results in the treatment of cocaine withdrawal (1216, 1217). A subsequent randomized, double-blind, controlled trial (1214) found a higher rate of cocaine-negative urine samples but a higher dropout rate among patients given bromocriptine than among patients given amantadine. An uncontrolled inpatient study (1218) found no reduction of cocaine craving with bromocriptine, and a randomized, double-blind, controlled trial (1219) found no significant difference between bromocriptine and placebo in reducing cocaine use in outpatients. Finally, a large study of pergolide (1220) found no difference from placebo in either symptom reduction or continued cocaine use.

Propranolol has recently been shown to have promise in reducing cocaine withdrawal symptoms, although its efficacy as a pharmacotherapy for cocaine dependence in general appears to be limited to those with relatively severe withdrawal symptoms (1221). There may be a subgroup of patients who will respond to some form of pharmacotherapy with reduced craving and, subsequently, reduced use (see below); however, to date there are few research data to help the psychiatrist identify such patients.

3. Medications to treat cocaine dependence

For many patients, pharmacological treatment is not ordinarily indicated as an initial treatment of cocaine dependence because no medication has been found to have clear-cut efficacy (1222–1225). However, a number of studies have shown promising results with pharmacotherapeutic agents, and patients with more severe forms of cocaine dependence (e.g., those with more severe cocaine withdrawal symptoms) (1221, 1226) or patients who do not respond to psychosocial treatment may be candidates for a pharmacotherapy trial.

Studies of desipramine have yielded inconsistent findings, with some studies showing benefit of the medication (1227–1229) and others showing no response by patients (1215, 1230, 1231). An additional study that compared desipramine with placebo showed improvement with desipramine in the short term (6 weeks) but not at 12 weeks or 1 year (503). Interpretation of studies of desipramine may be confounded by differences in patient population, route of cocaine administration, and use of concomitant psychotherapies or other pharmacotherapies. Fluoxetine (1232, 1233) and bupropion (1234) have also shown some benefit in small studies but have demonstrated no superiority to placebo when evaluated in larger trials (413, 1235–1238).

The evidence for using dopamine agonists in treating cocaine dependence is also mixed. Of the dopamine agonist medications, amantadine is the best studied but has shown no overall benefit in most studies (1225, 1231, 1239). However, it may be useful for some patients, as it did demonstrate efficacy in one controlled trial (1240) and in another trial may have led subjects with more severe withdrawal symptoms to have a better response (1226). Inconclusive or negative findings have been seen with other dopamine agonists, including selegiline (1241; F. Vocci, personal communication), L-dopa/carbidopa (1242), and pergolide (1220, 1243). Although replacement therapies with methylphenidate or sustained-release amphetamine are associated with better patient retention and greater reduction in cocaine use than placebo, these studies need further replication (1244–1247).

In treating patients who are dually dependent on cocaine and opioids, the mixed opioid agonist-antagonist buprenorphine has shown some promise in open trials (1248, 1249) but not in large-scale double-blind studies (1250–1252). Again, responses may vary depending on factors such as buprenorphine dose, with doses of 12–16 mg/day being more effective (1253), or concomitant treatment (e.g., desipramine plus contingency management) (1228, 1229, 1254). Naltrexone has also been tested but has not been found to be useful for cocaine dependence (1255).

Although initial studies of the anticonvulsant carbamazepine showed some favorable results in the treatment of cocaine dependence (1256), subsequent double-blind, placebo-controlled studies failed to confirm this (1257–1261). More recent research, including one double-blind study (1262), has suggested some promise for another anticonvulsant, topiramate, for cocaine-dependent patients. The $GABA_B$ agonist baclofen has shown some success in treating cocaine dependence (1263), and a recent double-blind clinical trial of tiagabine, a GABA reuptake blocker, was superior to placebo for reducing cocaine use (1264). However, these findings require replication. Modafinil (400 mg/day) has recently shown some efficacy for reducing cocaine abuse in an 8-week controlled study and merits further investigation (1265). Two previous cocaine interaction studies also support the potential efficacy and safety of modafinil (1266, 1267).

4. Medications to change the subjective effects of cocaine

Attempts to find a medication that blocks or attenuates the subjective (e.g., euphorigenic) effects of cocaine have included trials of neuroleptics (1268, 1269) and mazindol (1270–1273), neither of which has been shown to be effective. Recent data with disulfiram suggest that this medication may increase the aversive effects of cocaine and reduce its use (1274–1277). Other recent work has suggested that a cocaine vaccine may induce the formation of sufficient antibodies to reduce cocaine use (1278).

5. Acupuncture

Acupuncture is a somatic treatment that has been frequently used in the treatment of patients with a substance use disorder. Two recent large randomized, controlled trials (1279, 1280) of auricular acupuncture, a type of acupuncture that is supposed to be helpful specifically for patients with a substance use disorder, found the treatment to be no more effective than relaxation techniques or the needle insertion/sham acupuncture control condition. Moreover, cocaine craving and physiological arousal were not differentially affected by auricular acupuncture compared with sham acupuncture (1281). Although many studies have reported positive results for the use of acupuncture in clinical settings (1279, 1282–1287), none have used randomized assignment or appropriate controls. Thus, evidence for the benefits of acupuncture is weak, and if acupuncture is used, it should be part of a biopsychosocial treatment approach.

D. PSYCHOSOCIAL TREATMENTS

1. Cognitive-behavioral therapies

For the treatment of cocaine dependence, CBT confers greater therapeutic benefits than less-intensive approaches that have been evaluated as control conditions (267, 1288). It is at least as effective as manual-guided disease-model approaches (267, 1289) and can be associated with further decreases in cocaine use even after subjects leave treatment (1192, 1275, 1290, 1291). Furthermore, CBT appears to be particularly effective with more severe cocaine users or those with a comorbid disorder (229, 452, 503, 1289, 1292, 1293).

2. Behavioral therapies

The effectiveness of contingency management as a treatment for cocaine dependence has been demonstrated by Higgins and colleagues (188, 191–194, 1294). In addition to their work, the benefits of contingency management procedures have been replicated in other settings and samples, including cocaine-dependent individuals receiving methadone maintenance (195, 196, 1295, 1296), substance-abusing homeless individuals (1297), freebase cocaine users (1298), and pregnant substance users (1299).

3. Psychodynamic and interpersonal therapies

No randomized clinical trials have been conducted for psychodynamically oriented treatments for cocaine abuse or dependence, although a case series of individual psychodynamically oriented psychotherapy (1300) and reports of psychodynamically oriented group psychotherapy (1301, 1302) have supported the efficacy of this approach. The clinical study of IPT has been limited to a single 12-week randomized trial in cocaine-dependent outpatients in whom CBT was found to be superior to IPT (1276). Supportive-expressive therapy has been studied as part of the NIDA Collaborative Cocaine Treatment Study, a multisite randomized trial of psychotherapeutic treatments for cocaine dependence, and was found to be less effective than individual plus group drug counseling in decreasing cocaine use (219).

4. Self-help groups and 12-step-oriented treatments

Although self-help groups have not been shown to be a sufficient alternative to professional treatment (1303), greater participation in AA, Cocaine Anonymous, or other 12-step self-help groups seems to predict less cocaine use at subsequent follow-up points (256, 1304).

Manual-guided, professionally delivered treatments are based on 12-step principles, and patients treated with these approaches are actively encouraged (but not required) to attend AA or Cocaine Anonymous meetings, become involved in traditional fellowship activities, and maintain journals of their self-help group attendance and participation. These therapies, including TSF (268) and individual drug counseling (219, 269, 1305), also have demonstrated efficacy in treatment of cocaine use disorders. For example, in alcoholic cocaine-dependent individuals, TSF was found to be significantly more effective than clinical management, was comparable with CBT in reducing cocaine use (267), and was associated with continuing reductions in cocaine use throughout the follow-up period. Furthermore, the attainment of significant periods of abstinence during treatment was associated with abstinence during follow-up, emphasizing that the inception of abstinence is an important goal of treatment (194, 1275).

The effectiveness of 12-step-oriented individual drug counseling (269) was demonstrated in the NIDA Collaborative Cocaine Treatment Study (219, 1305). Cocaine use was significantly reduced relative to baseline use after intensive treatment (36 individual and 24 group sessions over 24 weeks, for a total of 60 sessions) with group drug counseling alone; cognitive therapy (1306) plus group drug counseling; or supportive-expressive therapy, a psychodynamically oriented approach (217), plus group drug counseling. However, the greatest reductions in cocaine use were noted with 12-step-based individual drug counseling plus group drug counseling (219); 12-step-oriented standard group counseling also appears to be comparable in efficacy with relapse prevention aftercare (229).

E. CLINICAL FEATURES INFLUENCING TREATMENT

The treatment implications of various clinical features are summarized in Section II.G. In addition to these considerations, specific sequelae and patterns of co-occurring disorders need to be considered for patients with a cocaine use disorder.

1. Specific co-occurring psychiatric disorders

Co-occurring psychiatric and medical disorders are common among cocaine-dependent patients (1307). Several reports have addressed the treatment of patients with a psychiatric disorder who also have a cocaine-related disorder (1308–1315). Specific treatments that have been reported to be effective in certain populations of patients with cocaine abuse include lithium for patients with co-occurring bipolar disorder, desipramine for patients with co-occurring depression, and bromocriptine for patients with co-occurring ADHD (1223, 1310, 1311, 1316). In addition, the results of a randomized, double-blind, placebo-controlled trial (445) suggest that desipramine or amantadine treatment for depressed cocaine-abusing, methadone-maintained patients may reduce cocaine use. Several focused and reasonably well-controlled studies have shown that patients with schizophrenia who primarily abuse cocaine experience some decreases in craving with antipsychotic agents (401, 1317–1319). Given the evidence to date, however, these treatments alone cannot be expected to reduce cocaine use in these patients and must therefore be accompanied by appropriate psychosocial treatment for a cocaine use disorder (1309, 1310).

2. Comorbid general medical disorders

A range of general medical conditions are associated with cocaine use, depending on the route of administration of cocaine. Intranasal use may cause sinusitis, irritation and bleeding of the nasal mucosa, and nasal septum perforation. Smoking cocaine is associated with respiratory problems, such as coughing, bronchitis, bronchospasm, and pneumonitis, resulting from irritation and inflammation of the tissues lining the respiratory tract (1320, 1321). Barotrauma such as pneumothorax, pneumomediastinum, and pneumopericardium may occur as a result of coughing or a Valsalva-like maneuver that is performed to better absorb the drug (1322, 1323).

Puncture marks and "tracks," most commonly in the forearms, occur in individuals who inject cocaine. HIV infection is associated with cocaine dependence as a result of frequent injections, increased promiscuous sexual behavior, or both; other sexually transmitted diseases, hepatitis, tuberculosis, and other lung infections are also seen, as described in DSM-IV-TR (p. 247).

General medical conditions independent of the administration route of cocaine include weight loss and malnutrition from appetite suppression, myocardial infarction, and stroke (657, 1225, 1324). Seizures, palpitations, and arrhythmias have also been observed in cocaine-using individuals. Among individuals who sell cocaine, traumatic injuries from violent behavior are common, as described in DSM-IV-TR (p. 248).

3. Pregnancy

In addition to the general effects of substance use during pregnancy (Section II.G.4), cocaine-related disorders may have specific adverse effects on the health of the pregnant woman, the course of the pregnancy, fetal and early childhood development, and parenting behavior. Possible effects of cocaine use on the course of the pregnancy include irregularities in placental blood flow, abruptio placentae, and premature labor and delivery, as described in DSM-IV-TR (p. 248). Although earlier studies suggested that cocaine use during pregnancy results in adverse effects on fetal development (e.g., very low birth weight, congenital anomalies, urogenital system malformations, mild neurodysfunction, transient electroencephalographic abnormalities, cerebral infarction, seizures, vascular disruption syndrome, smaller head circumference) (1325–1328), more recent studies (583, 1329) have challenged the specific role of cocaine in adversely affecting the course of pregnancy. Behnke et al. (1329) assessed the offspring of a sample of 154 identified cocaine users and a matched group of 154 non-cocaine-using control subjects to compare perinatal outcomes. The cocaine-exposed infants were significantly more likely to be premature and have smaller birth weight, length, and head circumference but showed no other major or minor anomalies to a greater degree than non-cocaine-exposed infants. Addis et al. (583) conducted a meta-analysis of 33 studies of the potential teratogenicity of cocaine. They found that although all of the complications they examined (prematurity, abruptio placentae, low birth weight, prevalence of major malformations, premature rupture of membrane, and mean birth weight, head circumference, and length) demonstrated worse outcomes in infants who had been exposed to cocaine in utero than those who had not, only the risk for abruptio placentae and premature rupture of membrane remained statistically associated with cocaine use. Thus, although children of women who used cocaine during pregnancy did appear to have worse perinatal outcomes, this may have been due to other factors associated with cocaine or other substance use during pregnancy.

The possible effects on early childhood development that have been reported in cocaine-exposed newborns include hypertonicity, spasticity, convulsions, hyperreflexia, irritability, and inattention. However, the role of exposure to cocaine or other substances, poor maternal nutrition, birth prematurity, low infant birth weight, and neonatal withdrawal in the development of these signs and symptoms remains unclear (1330, 1331). Signs of CNS irritability usually disappear within the first year of life, as do any differences in head circumference or retardation in brain growth. Studies in cocaine-exposed children have revealed deficits in attention span at 7 months, and in utero exposure to amphetamines has been found to be associated with slightly lower IQs (albeit still in the normal range) in 4-year-old children (1332). A recent review of early child development after prenatal cocaine exposure (1333) systematically examined 36 studies on this subject and documented no independent effects of cocaine exposure on most measures of child development, although it did find that some reduction in attentiveness and emotional expressivity may occur. Thus, although no clear correlation between in utero cocaine exposure and subsequent intellectual or neurological development has been established, associated conditions, such as low birth weight, the complications of untreated (or undertreated) withdrawal, and congenital abnormalities may have adverse effects on offspring's cognitive and psychosocial development. In addition, as stated above, many children of women who used cocaine during pregnancy have other risk factors that may affect their development.

A clinician who is developing a treatment plan for a pregnant patient who is withdrawing from cocaine should take into account the risks and benefits to the mother and fetus in deciding about the use and choice of pharmacotherapies. When present, the concurrent use of other substances will also need to be addressed.

VII. TREATMENT OF OPIOID-RELATED DISORDERS

A. OVERVIEW

According to the 2003 National Survey on Drug Use and Health (1191), there were approximately 3.7 million lifetime users of heroin in 2003. Of these lifetime users, 314,000 individuals had used heroin in the previous year and 169,000 reported heroin dependence at some point in the previous year. This suggests that a high proportion (54%) of individuals who used heroin in the previous year were dependent on this opiate. These numbers are likely to be significant underestimates because of the difficulty in ascertaining community rates of heroin dependence; the Office of National Drug Control Policy estimates that 750,000 to 1,000,000 individuals are heroin dependent (1333a).

Heroin is not the only opiate that is abused; there has been a growing awareness of misuse or "nonmedical use" of prescription pain relievers (e.g., hydromorphone, morphine, oxycodone, codeine, propoxyphene). The 2003 survey found that there were approximately 31.2 million individuals who reported nonmedical use of prescription pain relievers in their lifetime, a rate markedly higher than the rate of lifetime heroin use. Approximately 11.7 million reported using opiates for nonmedical reasons in the previous year, and 943,000 individuals fulfilled criteria for opioid dependence that same year. Although a considerably lower proportion of individuals with past-year use were dependent on prescription opioid pain relievers compared with heroin (8% vs. 54%), it is important to note that over five times as many individuals are dependent on prescription opioid pain relievers than on heroin.

Given the number of individuals who are using and are dependent on opiates, it is not surprising that the most commonly studied substance-related conditions, and those for which treatments have been most extensively studied, are opioid dependence, opioid abuse, opioid intoxication, and opioid withdrawal. Treatment for opioid-related conditions can be highly effective. Interventions include pharmacological treatments with agents such as methadone, buprenorphine, and naltrexone and nonpharmacological services such as behavioral therapies and counseling. The treatment of opioid dependence, in particular, is one of the most extensively researched areas in the field of addictions, and the range of available treatments is more extensive than for most other substance use disorders.

Despite the number of effective treatments for opioid dependence and the scientific basis for their efficacy and safety, the availability of treatment programs for this and other illicit drug use is limited. Among the multiple factors that probably contribute to the limited availability of such treatment generally and opioid dependence treatment in particular are the social stigma associated with treatment facilities and their patient population, limited funding for treatment, and a history of variability in the quality of treatment supplied by clinicians and existing programs. In addition, social ambivalence about the nature of addictions and the medicalization of substance use disorder treatment may be significant contributing factors for the difficulty of expanding such treatment.

There are two general thoughts regarding the treatment goals for patients with an opioid use disorder: 1) there should be abstinence from all illicit opioid use or 2) there should be a substantial decrease in use but abstinence is not an absolute requirement. The logic of the latter is that decreased use of illicit substances will translate into lower rates of risky behavior and that this is a worthy goal of treatment. Although these two general goals may seem opposed, it may be helpful to conceptualize the latter as an acceptable intermediate stage toward the ultimate achievement of the first goal—abstinence.

Additional goals of treatment include addressing other substance use, psychosocial outcomes (e.g., impact of drug use on employment, reconciliation with family members), and psychiatric and somatic needs (e.g., treatment for comorbid affective disorders, management of chronic physical disorders). Treatment goals will vary depending on the circumstances of the particular patient, the specific opioid-related disorder for which the patient seeks treatment, the treatment setting, the resources available to the practitioner, and the resources available to the patient.

Defining specific goals that are applicable to all patients is unrealistic, but a few further general points regarding treatment goals are worth noting. For example, cessation or stabilization of substance use should be an early and primary treatment goal. It is probably premature to attempt to rectify many early psychiatric symptoms or psychosocial problems while a patient is actively using opioids. However, exceptions may be made in certain circumstances, such as with a patient who has a clear history of a psychiatric disorder that is independent of the substance use or a patient who is acutely suicidal. In particular, the patient who maintains that he or she needs pharmacological treatment for anxiety or depressive symptoms to control illicit opioid use is probably best initially managed with a focus on the substance use. Another general treatment goal may include educating patients about the possibility of relapses during treatment and the importance of making a plan to prevent further substance use if a relapse occurs. Finally, treatment expectations, such as the patient's behavior (e.g., tardiness, missed appointments, presenting while intoxicated) and the clinician's responsibilities (e.g., providing emergency contact information, providing other resources to optimize outcomes) are related to treatment goals and may be addressed through a discussion with the patient.

B. TREATMENT SETTINGS

In general, there are five settings or modalities in which most treatment of opioid-related disorders occurs: inpatient hospital settings, outpatient clinics and offices, opioid treatment programs, self-help programs, and therapeutic communities. The choice of treatment setting depends on the clinical characteristics and preferences of the patient, the patient's perceived treatment needs, and the available alternatives. As in the treatment of all patients, the least restrictive setting that is likely to facilitate safe and effective treatment is preferred.

There are some general guidelines and recommendations for treatment settings for opioid-related disorders. An opioid overdose, which in severe cases can be a life-threatening emergency, should be evaluated and initially managed in a supervised medical setting such as an emergency department or inpatient service. Treatment typically includes reversal of opioid effects with an opioid antagonist (e.g., naloxone). Opioid withdrawal may also be treated in an inpatient setting and can be effectively managed with pharmacological agents such as opioid agonist medications (e.g., methadone, buprenorphine) or nonopioid medications (e.g., clonidine). Although management of opioid withdrawal symptoms can be effectively achieved relatively quickly in an inpatient setting (i.e, within 7 days), long-term outcome for such withdrawal is generally poor, with high rates of relapse after discharge from the controlled setting. Continued treatment for the opioid use disorder after withdrawal is indicated in most cases. Inpatient opioid withdrawal without specific outpatient follow-up (e.g., drug-free treatment) is an inadequate intervention that has a low likelihood of long-term success.

The second possible setting is outpatient clinics and offices. This can include so-called drug-free programs (treatment programs that do not provide opioid agonist medications to the patient), group practices, and the individual practitioner's office. Drug-free programs can provide services to patients who have undergone an inpatient, medically supervised opioid withdrawal. Although these programs do not provide opioid agonists to patients, they may provide naltrexone for the treatment of opioid dependence. Group practices and the individual practitioner's office may provide buprenorphine or naltrexone for the treatment of opioid dependence. The Drug Addiction Treatment Act of 2000 allows physicians in the United States to prescribe schedule III, IV, and V medications that are approved for the treatment of opioid dependence from office-based settings, although there are stipulations on this practice. Currently, sublingual buprenorphine and sublingual buprenorphine plus naloxone are the only FDA-approved agents for this purpose. There also has been interest in developing office-based methadone treatment, which is generally not available in the United States except under certain circumstances in which a physician works with an opioid treatment program (1334).

Outpatient opioid treatment programs, a third treatment setting, are primarily methadone maintenance programs, although buprenorphine can also be provided in this setting. These operate under special federal and state regulations, and expansion of this modality has been difficult in many parts of the United States. However, when properly operated, these programs can be highly effective for patients who have been unable to maintain abstinence from illicit opioid use. Methadone maintenance is the most common form of pharmacological treatment for opioid dependence, with more than 240,000 individuals estimated to be receiving methadone treatment in the United States in 2004. Routine office-based pharmacological treatment with buprenorphine, and possibly methadone, in the future has considerable promise based on research studies and the growing clinical experience with this form of treatment in the United States. Experience from France (1334a) suggests these treatments can substantially reduce opioid-related mortality, but there is a risk of buprenorphine diversion to other uses and abuse in the outpatient setting.

Self-help programs such as Narcotics Anonymous are another form of treatment used by individuals with opioid abuse or dependence. Because anonymity is an integral part of these programs, it is difficult to know the extent of their utilization, outcomes achieved, or factors that predict a particular person's success in such programs. However, anecdotal reports from patients and the pervasive availability of the meetings suggest these programs serve a valuable function and are effective for many people who have used illicit opioids. Self-help groups can also be effective when used within the different treatment settings previously discussed (see Section II.F.8).

Therapeutic communities are yet another treatment setting for patients who abuse or are dependent on opiates (see Section II.C.2.d). Therapeutic communities can be an effective treatment for some patients with opioid dependence but have decreased in prominence over time. However, there is renewed interest and evidence of efficacy for therapeutic communities in special circumstances, such as with criminal justice populations.

C. SOMATIC TREATMENTS

1. Treating dependence and abuse

a) Full mu agonist therapy: methadone and LAAM

There are two approved full mu agonist opioid medications available for the treatment of patients with chronic and relapsing opioid dependence: methadone and LAAM, both schedule II medications. Methadone is the most thoroughly studied and widely used pharmacological treatment for opioid dependence (1335, 1336). It is orally active, can be dosed once per day, and at sufficient doses does suppress opioid withdrawal and block the effects of other opioids. LAAM is structurally related to methadone and shares many similar features (oral activity, withdrawal suppression, blockade effects) but has a longer duration of action, allowing dosing on a less than daily basis. Although it is still an FDA-approved medication, LAAM has been withdrawn from the United States market by its manufacturer because of an associated risk of cardiac arrhythmias (1337).

Each of these medications is available only through specially licensed opioid treatment programs. Oversight of these programs was recently shifted from the FDA to SAMHSA, and the programs are now accredited by an outside agency such as the Joint Commission on Accreditation of Healthcare Organizations. Many of the prior treatment regulations have been revised (including greater flexibility in take-home doses of medication).

The primary goals of opioid agonist maintenance treatment are to 1) achieve a stable maintenance dose that suppresses withdrawal, reduces opioid craving, blocks the effects of illicit opioids, and eventually stops illicit opioid use; and 2) facilitate patient engagement in a comprehensive program designed to prevent dependence or abuse of other substances and promote rehabilitation.

The choice of treatment for opioid dependence is based on patient preference, assessment of the patient's past response to treatment, the probability of the patient's achieving and maintaining abstinence for the different treatment modalities, and the physician's assessment of the short- and long-term effects of continued use of illicit opioids on the patient's life adjustment and overall health status. Because methadone maintenance may become a lifelong therapy, some physicians prefer to avoid it as a first-line treatment for opioid dependence in adolescents. In addition, the higher demand versus availability of opioid treatment programs can be an additional and significant factor influencing referral to this type of program.

Methadone maintenance treatment for opioid-dependent individuals has generally been shown to be effective in 1) decreasing illicit opioid use, 2) decreasing psychosocial and general medical morbidity associated with opioid dependence, 3) improving overall health status, 4) decreasing mortality, 5) decreasing criminal activity, and 6) improving social functioning (171, 1338–1340). Several studies also support the usefulness of methadone maintenance in reducing the spread of HIV infection among intravenous drug users (1341). It should be noted that methadone maintenance treatment involves a combination of methadone medication and nonpharmacological services. The latter can include individual and group counseling, urine testing, and behavioral treatments, with the purpose of addressing opioid and other substance use as well as the psychosocial problems associated with drug use. Further discussion of psychosocial treatments for opioid-related disorders is provided in Section VII.D.

One of the key issues in methadone maintenance is determining a dose sufficient to suppress the patient's opioid withdrawal and craving, as no single dose is optimal for all patients. Some may benefit from maintenance on lower doses such as ≤40 mg/day, whereas others may require >100 mg/day to achieve maximum benefit. Controlled studies of methadone dosing have not tested daily doses of >100 mg/day, although there are anecdotal reports of such use in the United States, and doses greater than 100 mg/day are used in several other countries (1342–1346). Although 40–60 mg/day of methadone (and sometimes less) is usually sufficient to block opioid withdrawal symptoms (1339), higher doses are usually needed during maintenance treatment to block craving for opiates and associated drug use. Higher doses of methadone are also generally needed for heroin addicts with axis I psychiatric comorbidity (1347, 1348). In general, higher doses are associated with better treatment retention and lower rates of illicit opioid use (1349–1352).

Maintenance on methadone is generally safe. Methadone undergoes hepatic metabolism by CYP 450 3A4 in conjunction with other P450 enzymes; its half-life is approximately 24 hours, so methadone can be administered once daily (1353). However, other concurrent medications and/or substances of abuse that a patient might be taking need to be considered because they may induce symptoms of withdrawal, toxicity, and even death by interfering with the metabolism of methadone (1354, 1355). The most common side effects of methadone are constipation, increased sweating, and sexual difficulties. Although early studies of methadone found the medication had no significant effect on cognition or performance measures (1356–1358), other studies have found evidence of some subtle but significant effects (1359, 1360). Finally, overdose with methadone or any mu agonist can produce respiratory depression and death. Methadone can be used as an analgesic, and there has been evidence of increased methadone-related deaths as the frequency of prescribing methadone for pain management has increased. Methadone can be diverted for abuse, as can other opiates that have agonist effects at the mu receptor (e.g., LAAM, buprenorphine).

b) Partial mu agonist therapy: buprenorphine

Buprenorphine is a mixed opioid agonist-antagonist with a pharmacological profile different from that of full mu agonists such as methadone. Buprenorphine produces a less than maximal or partial agonist effect at the mu receptor (its primary action with respect to the treatment of opioid dependence) and an antagonistic effect at the kappa receptor (126). These receptor interactions are thought to account for buprenorphine's unique profile of effects, which have clinical implications for treating opioid dependence.

Buprenorphine has been marketed worldwide as a parenteral analgesic for many years. Because it has poor oral but fair sublingual bioavailability, a sublingual buprenorphine tablet has been developed for the treatment of opioid dependence. Buprenorphine enters the bloodstream more slowly through the sublingual route than with parenteral administration and thus has less abuse potential compared with the parenterally delivered form. There are two forms of the sublingual tablet: a buprenorphine-only tablet and a combination tablet of buprenorphine and the opioid antagonist naloxone. Because naloxone has poor sublingual but good parenteral bioavailability (1361), it is hoped that the combination tablet may decrease the risk of buprenorphine diversion to other uses and parenteral abuse even further because naloxone used parenterally will precipitate opioid withdrawal in opioid-dependent patients. Both forms of buprenorphine tablets are schedule III medications in the United States.

Like methadone, buprenorphine can suppress opioid withdrawal and block the effects of other opioids. Clinical trials comparing daily sublingual buprenorphine (equivalent of 12–16 mg of the tablet form per day) to moderate doses of daily oral methadone (i.e., 50–60 mg/day) have generally shown comparable outcomes on treatment retention and decreased illicit opioid use (1251). However, higher doses of methadone (≥80 mg/day) appear to produce superior outcomes to daily buprenorphine (1250, 1251, 1336, 1362–1364). It is not known if comparable effects could be produced by increasing the dose of buprenorphine; current evidence suggests buprenorphine may be best suited for patients with mild to moderate levels of physical dependence. Nonpharmacological treatment in combination with buprenorphine can help to achieve abstinence. For example, a study by Galanter et al. (1365) demonstrated that psychosocial support (in this study, network therapy) tailored to promoting abstinence from illicit opioids during buprenorphine maintenance can improve clinical outcomes.

Buprenorphine has a long duration of action and can be dosed on a less than daily basis. When used in this way, the dose administered should be increased to compensate for the longer between-dose interval (for example, doubling the daily dose for a 48-hour interval and tripling the daily dose for a 72-hour interval). Between-dose intervals of 48–72 hours are generally well tolerated in most patients; some patients may tolerate even longer intervals, such as 96 hours (1366–1370).

In the United States, buprenorphine can be distributed not only in special clinics but also through clinicians' offices; access in this latter setting provides a means for expanding treatment capacity and mainstreaming the care of opioid dependence. Daily sublingual maintenance doses typically fall between 8 and 32 mg. The buprenorphine-naloxone combination tablet significantly reduces the risk the medicine will be diverted for other uses because naloxone will exert a potent opioid antagonist effect if the combination tablet is crushed and administered intravenously by an opioid-dependent person. Details on use of the medication (e.g., induction, withdrawal) are available through specific guidelines published by the Center for Substance Abuse Treatment and through courses sponsored by professional societies, including APA.

Buprenorphine is generally safe, and its side effects can be similar to those seen with full mu agonist opioids. However, in the context of abrupt cessation of opioid use, buprenorphine is associated with a comparatively mild withdrawal syndrome (126). Another notable difference from methadone is that overdose with buprenorphine generally does not produce significant respiratory depression (1371); this probably reflects buprenorphine's partial mu agonist effects. Nevertheless, there have been reports of fatalities when individuals overdose with a combination of buprenorphine and a benzodiazepine, typically when both are taken parenterally. These reports have come from France, where buprenorphine is used extensively for the outpatient treatment of opioid dependence and where prescribing benzodiazepines is also quite common. Finally, there is some evidence that buprenorphine may produce mild elevations in liver function tests, especially in individuals with a history of liver disease. This is more likely to occur if large amounts (greater-than-usual clinical doses) of buprenorphine are taken parenterally.

c) Opioid antagonist therapy: naltrexone

Naltrexone is an opioid antagonist that can be an alternative to maintenance on full or partial mu opioid agonists. By tightly binding to opioid receptors without producing a psychoactive effect, naltrexone blocks the pleasurable effects of the usual street doses of heroin and other opioids, thereby discouraging opioid use and diminishing conditioned craving. Naltrexone cannot be given to individuals while they are actively dependent on opioids because it can precipitate an immediate opioid withdrawal syndrome. Before starting naltrexone, patients must be completely withdrawn and abstinent for at least 5 days from a short-acting opioid such as heroin or 7 days from a longer-acting opioid such as methadone. A urine toxicology screen for opiate medication may be indicated before naltrexone therapy is initiated. The risk of relapse during the interval between opioid withdrawal and the initiation of naltrexone treatment is high; for this reason, rapid opioid withdrawal, using clonidine and naloxone, has been used to shorten the interval between withdrawal and initiation of naltrexone treatment. Repeated doses of naloxone, a short-acting opioid antagonist related to naltrexone, have also been used with clonidine to shorten opioid withdrawal.

After withdrawal and the appropriate period of abstinence, a test dose of 0.8 mg i.m. of naloxone can be used to determine that the individual is no longer dependent on opioids before naltrexone treatment is initiated. Naltrexone can be taken as a daily dose of 50 mg or, because of its long duration of action, three times per week with doses of 100 mg on Monday and Wednesday and 150 mg on Friday. Naltrexone is approved for the treatment of opioid dependence in the United States; it has no abuse potential and is not a scheduled substance.

Studies of naltrexone's efficacy are mixed. Although inpatient studies of naltrexone-treated, opioid-dependent individuals who were given the opportunity to self-administer opioids have shown that naltrexone is highly effective at attenuating opioid use (1372), outpatient clinical trials have failed to demonstrate a similar robust effect (1373). Patients often drop out of such studies shortly after completing opioid withdrawal and starting on naltrexone. This is probably related, in part, to the absence of a psychoactive effect with naltrexone. In certain populations of motivated patients (e.g., patients on federal probation), however, naltrexone can be useful and effective (1374, 1375).

The adverse effects of naltrexone may include dysphoria, anxiety, and gastrointestinal distress. As previously noted, naltrexone can precipitate withdrawal in actively opioid-dependent individuals. Naltrexone's label notes that there is a risk that liver function test values will increase for some patients, but a review of the evidence shows that these cases occurred only with higher daily doses of naltrexone (300 mg/day) or, in rare cases, in patients who were over age 40 years and on a dose of <300 mg/day (1376). Finally, after discontinuation of chronically administered naltrexone for the treatment of opioid dependence, there is an increased sensitivity to opioid effects and an increased risk that opioid overdose will lead to significant respiratory depression; this is likely related to the up-regulation of opioid receptors while a patient is being treated with naltrexone (1377).

2. Treating intoxication

The care of patients with an opioid use disorder is frequently complicated by episodes of relapse. Consequently, it is important in ongoing treatment to recognize and treat intoxication with opioids or other substances.

Mild to moderate opioid intoxication usually does not require treatment. An uncomplicated overdose with a short-acting opioid that has a relatively short half-life, such as heroin, may be treated in an emergency department, with release after a few hours. Overdose with longer-acting opioids such as methadone, however, requires closer inpatient observation for a minimum of 24–48 hours. In addition, severe opioid overdose, marked by respiratory depression, may be fatal and requires treatment in an emergency department or inpatient setting. Naloxone, an opioid antagonist, reverses respiratory and CNS depression as well as other manifestations of overdose. (Its use is described in detail in Section II.E.1.) A patient who deliberately takes an overdose as part of a suicide attempt requires thorough psychiatric evaluation typically in a hospital setting. For patients who do not require medical or psychiatric hospitalization, appropriate follow-up is a necessary part of discharge planning.

3. Treating withdrawal

An opioid-dependent individual may undergo opioid withdrawal rather than be maintained in methadone or buprenorphine treatment if, for example, the patient has a relatively short history of opioid abuse with a good prognosis for remaining abstinent without pharmacological maintenance, no maintenance treatment program is available locally, or the patient desires to not be restricted by the requirements of maintenance medication. Some patients successfully maintained on a medication such as methadone or buprenorphine will also want to undergo medically supervised withdrawal.

Criteria for withdrawing patients from long-term maintenance on methadone or buprenorphine include demonstrated progress toward a drug-free lifestyle, stability in personal and occupational adjustment, the absence of other substance use disorders, and successful treatment and remission of any co-occurring psychiatric disorders.

Precipitous discharge from maintenance programs and concurrent withdrawal of methadone are associated with a high rate of relapse to illicit opioid use, arrests, and death. Voluntary termination of methadone maintenance also carries a high risk of relapse, even for patients who have responded well to treatment. Patients who voluntarily discontinue maintenance treatment should receive supportive treatment during withdrawal as well as aftercare services to aid in maintaining abstinence. Patients who relapse repeatedly despite such support should be given the option of voluntary long-term maintenance on methadone or buprenorphine.

The goal of opioid tapering is to minimize acute withdrawal symptoms and help patients transition to long-term treatment for opioid dependence. The use of standard rating scales for withdrawal (e.g., Clinical Institute Narcotic Assessment) can help guide dosing in an objective and routine manner. Five pharmacological strategies are in general use: 1) methadone substitution, with gradual methadone tapering; 2) abrupt discontinuation of opioids, with use of clonidine to suppress withdrawal symptoms; 3) clonidine-naltrexone detoxification, where withdrawal symptoms are precipitated by naltrexone and then suppressed by clonidine; 4) buprenorphine substitution, followed by abrupt or gradual discontinuation of buprenorphine; and 5) use of other medications to treat the symptoms of opioid withdrawal.

a) Use of methadone for withdrawal

Methadone hydrochloride is highly effective in ameliorating the symptoms of opioid withdrawal. Although the use of opioids to detoxify or maintain opioid-dependent patients requires special licensing (see Section II.H.3), this regulation is waived for inpatients admitted primarily because of a life-threatening general medical or psychiatric condition who also require methadone to stabilize their opioid dependence during the inpatient stay.

Inpatient opioid withdrawal with methadone involves stabilizing a patient on a daily methadone dose that is determined by the patient's response based on objective withdrawal signs (1378, 1379). Once the stabilization dose is determined (usually 40–60 mg/day and sometimes less), methadone can be tapered, for example, by increments of 5 mg/day. In inpatient settings, detoxification from heroin or other short-acting opioids can usually be completed within 7 days, but a more gradual tapering will result in a smoother clinical course.

When compared with inpatient withdrawal, outpatient opioid withdrawal uses a higher initial dose of methadone and occurs over a longer period of time. The goal of using a higher initial dose of methadone is to help dependent individuals end illicit opioid use. Because studies have suggested that slow tapers are associated with better outcomes, methadone should be tapered gradually over a period of weeks. Many patients tolerate methadone reductions to 20–30 mg/day with little difficulty, but further dose reductions may lead to increasing withdrawal distress. Even with gradual reductions in the dose, such distress may be difficult for some patients to tolerate and may be accompanied by high dropout and relapse rates during this later phase of withdrawal.

b) Use of clonidine for withdrawal

Clonidine is a centrally acting α_2-adrenergic antihypertensive medication that effectively decreases the noradrenergic hyperactivity associated with opioid withdrawal. Clonidine is not approved for opioid withdrawal in the United States but has been extensively studied and used for this indication elsewhere. Clonidine reduces withdrawal symptoms such as nausea, vomiting, diarrhea, cramps, and sweating but, unlike methadone, does little to reduce other symptoms such as muscle aches, insomnia, distress, and drug craving (1380, 1381). As a nonopioid medication, clonidine has some advantages over methadone for withdrawal. For example, clonidine does not produce opioid-like tolerance or dependence or the postmethadone rebound in withdrawal symptoms (1382). In addition, patients completing a course of clonidine-assisted withdrawal can immediately be given an opioid antagonist (e.g., naltrexone) if indicated. The disadvantages of clonidine include its aforementioned inability to improve certain opioid withdrawal symptoms, associated hypotension that can be profound despite the use of low doses of this medication, and its possible sedative effects. Contraindications to the use of clonidine include acute or chronic cardiac disorders, renal or metabolic disease, and moderate to severe hypotension (1383).

On the first day of clonidine-aided detoxification, a clonidine dose of 0.1 mg three times daily (totaling 0.3 mg per 24 hours) is usually sufficient to suppress signs of opioid withdrawal; inpatients can generally receive higher doses to block withdrawal symptoms because of the availability of medical staff to monitor the patient for hypotension and sedation. The dose is adjusted until withdrawal symptoms are reduced. If the patient's blood pressure falls below 90/60 mm Hg, the next dose should be withheld, after which tapering can be resumed while the patient is monitored for signs of withdrawal. In the case of short-acting opioids such as heroin, clonidine-aided withdrawal usually takes 4–6 days. Other medications may be used along with clonidine to treat withdrawal symptoms.

In general, clonidine-assisted detoxification is easier to carry out and monitor in inpatient settings. Clonidine-induced sedation is also less of a problem for inpatients. However, when delivered by experienced staff, outpatient detoxification with clonidine is a reasonable approach (1384–1386). Outpatients should not be given more than a 3-day supply of clonidine for unsupervised use because treatment requires careful dose titration and clonidine overdoses can be life-threatening (1387, 1388).

Clonidine can be an effective alternative to methadone for treating opiate withdrawal; the completion rate for clonidine-treated outpatients is relatively low and roughly comparable to that of methadone withdrawal (1387, 1389).

c) Use of clonidine-naltrexone for rapid withdrawal

The combined use of clonidine and naltrexone for rapidly withdrawing patients from an opioid has been demonstrated to be safe and effective. Essentially, naltrexone-precipitated withdrawal is avoided by pretreating the patient with clonidine. This technique is most useful for opioid-dependent patients who are in transition to narcotic antagonist treatment. The limitations of this method include the need to monitor patients for 8 hours on the first day because of the potential severity of naltrexone-induced withdrawal and the need for careful blood pressure monitoring during the entire detoxification procedure. However, relapse rates with naltrexone maintenance are high.

A related technique is to withdraw a patient from an opioid while the patient is maintained under general anesthesia. This technique has been called ultra-rapid opioid detoxification and has included naltrexone maintenance after the acute withdrawal is completed. Although some small uncontrolled studies have reported good long-term outcomes with this method, it appears to be no more effective than methadone detoxification in achieving beneficial outcomes such as maintenance of abstinence (1390). In addition, complications associated with such rapid withdrawal procedures (e.g., general anesthesia) coupled with the lack of better long-term results suggest that the procedure should not be commonly used (1390).

d) Use of buprenorphine for withdrawal

Prior to buprenorphine's approval in the United States for the treatment of opioid dependence, there were reports of the efficacy and safety of its analgesic form when used for medically supervised opioid withdrawal. Clinicians used parenteral buprenorphine for relatively short opioid withdrawal (≤1 week), administered by injection or provided in the liquid (analgesic) form sublingually. Now with FDA approval of the sublingual form of this medication, the analgesic form for opioid withdrawal should no longer be used, and this nonapproved use of injectable buprenorphine is not recommended.

Studies of buprenorphine for opioid withdrawal have generally found that it has greater patient acceptability and is more effective than clonidine (1384, 1391–1393), with the two medications differing on measures of subjective symptoms of opioid withdrawal. Well-designed and executed studies comparing buprenorphine to methadone for the treatment of opioid withdrawal have not been published.

When buprenorphine is used for inpatient opioid withdrawal, patients can be stabilized on a relatively low dose of daily sublingual buprenorphine (e.g., 8 mg/day), with the goal of suppressing opioid withdrawal symptoms. Both tablet forms (with or without naloxone) can be used in an inpatient setting, as the risk of diversion and parenteral abuse is low. The dose can be decreased in increments of 2 mg/day over several days. Because buprenorphine has a long duration of action, minimal withdrawal symptoms are seen during the dose reduction. However, some clinicians report that withdrawal symptoms can appear several days after the last dose of buprenorphine, after a patient is discharged from an inpatient setting.

If buprenorphine is used for the outpatient treatment of opioid withdrawal, then procedures similar to those described earlier for methadone should be followed. But the tablet form combined with naloxone is preferred. For example, patients should be initially stabilized on a daily dose (probably 8–32 mg/day) of buprenorphine that suppresses opioid withdrawal and results in abstinence from illicit opioid use. Dose reductions should then occur gradually over a period of 10–14 days. Because buprenorphine tablets are not scored, the smallest dose increment reduction possible is 2 mg.

It should be emphasized that concurrent nonpharmacological treatments should be used to maximize the likelihood of maintaining abstinence throughout and after withdrawal. However, long-term outcomes associated with withdrawal are generally poorer than those seen with maintenance treatments (1394).

e) Use of other medications

Some clinicians and treatment programs have used medications targeting the symptoms of opioid withdrawal as the primary means for treating this condition. For example, sedative-hypnotics or anxiolytics are used to treat insomnia and/or anxiety, antiemetics are prescribed to treat nausea and vomiting, NSAIDs are provided for muscle cramps, and antispasmodics are used to treat gastrointestinal cramping. There are limited controlled data about the use of such medications for the treatment of opioid withdrawal. Some psychiatrists maintain that the abuse potential of sedative-hypnotics and anxiolytics is too great to be used with these patients and that these medications may also precipitate craving for opioids and relapse. Others feel that for carefully selected patients and with appropriate monitoring, the use of benzodiazepines over a relatively brief period (i.e., 1–2 weeks) may be helpful in ameliorating the often debilitating insomnia that can accompany opioid withdrawal (1395). Diphenhydramine, hydroxyzine, and sedating antidepressants (e.g., doxepin, amitriptyline, trazodone) have also been used for this purpose. It should be noted that these medications have also been abused, although much less often than benzodiazepines (129). Other medications such as NSAIDs and antispasmodics may be safely provided but appear to be less effective than mu agonist opioids for symptom relief.

D. PSYCHOSOCIAL TREATMENTS

When considering psychosocial treatments for treating opioid-related disorders, it is essential to note that all clinical trials of psychosocial interventions for opioid abusers have taken place in programs that also provide either opioid agonist maintenance (e.g., methadone) or treatment with opioid antagonists. Although some follow-up studies of naturalistic treatment have found equivalent efficacy for methadone maintenance and outpatient drug-free programs for heroin users (61, 1396–1398), early attempts at providing psychotherapy alone yielded unacceptably high attrition rates (1399).

1. Cognitive-behavioral therapies

In individuals who are receiving methadone maintenance, CBT is efficacious in reducing illicit substance use and achieving a wide range of other treatment goals. The benefits of CBT in combination with drug counseling are equivalent to those of drug counseling alone or drug counseling plus supportive-expressive psychotherapy in patients with low levels of psychiatric symptoms; however, in the presence of higher degrees of depression or other psychiatric symptoms, supportive-expressive therapy or CBT has been shown to be much more effective than drug counseling alone (177, 218, 531, 1400, 1401). CBT may also help reduce other target symptoms or behaviors (e.g., HIV risk behaviors) in opioid-using individuals (1402). Group-based relapse prevention therapy, when combined with self-help group participation, may also help recently detoxified patients reduce opioid use and criminal activities and decrease unemployment rates (1403).

2. Behavioral therapies

Contingency management approaches are beneficial in reducing the use of illicit substances in opioid-dependent individuals who are maintained on methadone (170, 195, 1295). Although other reinforcers or rewards (e.g., vouchers for movie tickets or sporting goods) may be provided to patients who demonstrate specified target behaviors (e.g., providing drug-free urine specimens, accomplishing specific treatment goals, attending treatment sessions), methadone take-home privileges are a commonly offered and effective incentive that is made contingent on reduced drug use (197–199, 202). Furthermore, contingency management, either alone or in conjunction with family therapies, can also be used to enhance adherence with unpopular treatments such as naltrexone and has been shown to result in diminutions in drug use among recently detoxified opioid-dependent individuals (165–167, 1404–1407).

3. Psychodynamic and interpersonal therapies

The utility of adding a psychodynamic therapy to a program of methadone maintenance has been investigated. The provision of supportive-expressive therapy, a specific approach to such treatment, may be particularly helpful for patients with high levels of other psychiatric symptoms (177, 218) (see Section VII.D.1). However, in terms of individual IPT, the potential benefits of treatment are unclear, as it is very difficult to engage opioid-dependent patients in such approaches. Psychodynamically oriented group therapy, modified for substance-dependent patients, appears to be effective in promoting abstinence when combined with behavioral monitoring and individual supportive psychotherapy (1301).

4. Family therapies

Family therapy has been demonstrated to enhance treatment adherence and facilitate implementation and monitoring of contingency contracts with opioid-dependent patients (1408, 1409). Family therapies are described in detail in Section II.F.8.

5. Self-help groups and 12-step-oriented treatments

Self-help groups, such as Narcotics Anonymous, are beneficial for some individuals in providing peer support for continued participation in treatment, avoiding substance-using peers and high-risk environments, confronting denial, and intervening early in patterns of thinking and behavior that often lead to relapse. Because of the emphasis on abstinence in the 12-step treatment philosophy, patients maintained on methadone or other opioid agonists may encounter disapproval for this type of pharmacotherapy at Narcotics Anonymous meetings.

E. CLINICAL FEATURES INFLUENCING TREATMENT

The treatment implications of various clinical features are summarized in Section II.G. In addition to these considerations, specific sequelae and patterns of co-occurring disorders need to be considered for patients with an opioid use disorder.

1. Use of multiple substances

Dependence on alcohol, cocaine, or other substances of abuse is a frequent problem for opioid-dependent patients. In one study, cocaine abuse was found to occur in about 60% of patients entering methadone programs (169). In studies of opioid-dependent patients in active treatment, rates of cocaine use as high as 40% or more have been reported (1410–1413). Similarly, heavy drinking is a problem for an estimated 15%–30% of methadone-maintained patients, and benzodiazepine abuse may be just as common in this population (1414, 1415). Comparable data regarding rates of co-occurring substance use disorders in patients treated in naltrexone programs are not generally available.

Other co-occurring substance use disorders require special attention because treatment directed at opioid dependence alone is unlikely to lead to the cessation of other substance use. Treatment is generally similar to that described for individual substances elsewhere in this practice guideline. Increased frequency of behavioral monitoring (e.g., daily breath or semiweekly urine toxicology testing), intensified counseling, contingency contracting, referral to specific self-help groups (e.g., AA), and specialized pharmacological treatments (e.g., disulfiram) have all been used with varying degrees of success. The results of two studies suggest that higher methadone doses coupled with intensive outpatient treatment may decrease cocaine use by methadone-maintained patients (1416).

Opioid-dependent patients who are also dependent on other substances, particularly CNS depressants, should be stabilized with methadone and then gradually withdrawn from the other substances. Efforts to abruptly eliminate all substances of abuse will not be successful with all patients. In such cases, the elimination of the drugs one at a time may be warranted.

The use of aversive contingencies, such as methadone dose reduction or even withdrawal, for continued abuse of cocaine (or sedatives or alcohol) for patients in methadone maintenance treatment is controversial. Some psychiatrists believe that requiring methadone withdrawal for persistent substance abuse causes many patients to cease or greatly limit use, whereas failure to enforce such limits implicitly gives patients license to continue use. Others believe that methadone withdrawal is never justified for patients abusing alcohol or other substances because of the proven efficacy of methadone in reducing intravenous heroin use, improving social and occupational functioning, and providing the opportunity to continue to motivate patients to reduce other substance use.

2. Psychiatric factors

The reduction of opioid use in patients with a preexisting co-occurring psychiatric disorder may precipitate the reemergence of previously controlled psychiatric symptoms (e.g., depression, mania, psychosis), which in turn may increase the risk of relapse to substance use (1417).

In prescribing medications for co-occurring non-substance-related psychiatric disorders, psychiatrists should be alert to the dangers of medications with a high abuse potential and to possible drug-drug interactions between opioids and other psychoactive substances (e.g., benzodiazepines) (442, 1378, 1400). For example, the use of MAOIs should be avoided because of their potential interaction with alcohol, cocaine and other stimulants, and opioids, including meperidine and dextromethorphan. In general, benzodiazepines with a rapid onset, such as diazepam and alprazolam, should also be avoided because of their abuse potential (1418). However, benzodiazepines with a slow onset and substantially lower abuse potential (e.g., oxazepam, clorazepate) can probably be used safely for selected patients to, for example, ameliorate insomnia (Section VII.C.3.e), provided that appropriate controls are applied (1419). With all other psychotropic medications, decisions about prescriptions should consider that patients may not take medications as prescribed; random blood or urine monitoring can sometimes help in determining adherence.

3. Comorbid general medical disorders

The injection of opioids may result in the sclerosing of veins, cellulitis, abscesses, or, more rarely, tetanus infection. Other life-threatening infections associated with opioid use by injection include bacterial endocarditis, hepatitis, and HIV infection. HIV infection rates have been reported to be as high as 60% among individuals dependent on heroin in some areas of the United States (see DSM-IV-TR, p. 275). Counseling on how to reduce HIV risk should be a routine part of treatment for intravenous opioid users (559).

Tuberculosis is a particularly serious problem among individuals who inject drugs, especially those dependent on heroin. Infection with the tubercle bacillus occurs in approximately 10% of these individuals. For non-HIV-infected patients who test positive for the purified protein derivative of tuberculin, the lifetime risk of developing active tuberculosis is approximately 10% and the 1-year risk is 7%–10% (1420). Guidelines regarding prophylactic treatment for patients with a positive skin test have been published (1421).

As described in DSM-IV-TR (p. 275), in addition to the presence of life-threatening infections, opioid dependence is associated with a death rate as high as 1.5%–2% per year from overdose, accidents, injuries, or other general medical complications.

4. Pregnancy

In addition to the general effects of substance use during pregnancy (Section II.G.4), opioid use disorders may have adverse effects on the health of the pregnant woman, the course of the pregnancy, fetal and early child development, and parenting behavior. In pregnant women these effects include 1) poor nourishment, with accompanying vitamin deficiencies or iron- and folic acid-deficiency anemias; 2) general medical complications from frequent use of contaminated needles (abscesses, ulcers, thrombophlebitis, bacterial endocarditis, hepatitis, urinary tract infections, and HIV infection); 3) sexually transmitted diseases (gonorrhea, chlamydia, syphilis, herpes); and 4) hypertension.

Possible effects of opioid use and the related lifestyle on the course of the pregnancy include preeclampsia (toxemia), miscarriage, premature rupture of membranes, and infections. Possible short- and long-term effects on the infant include low birth weight, prematurity, stillbirth, neonatal abstinence syndrome, and sudden infant death syndrome (1327, 1422, 1423). Approximately 50% of the infants born to women with opioid dependence are physiologically dependent on opioids and may experience a moderate to severe withdrawal syndrome requiring pharmacological intervention. However, when socioeconomic factors (e.g., family disruption, poverty) are controlled for, mild to moderate neonatal withdrawal does not appear to affect psychomotor or intellectual development (1423).

The goals of treatment for the pregnant opioid-using patient include ensuring physiological stabilization and avoidance of opioid withdrawal; preventing further substance abuse; improving maternal nutrition; encouraging participation in prenatal care and rehabilitation; reducing the risk of obstetrical complications, including low birth weight and neonatal withdrawal, which can be lethal if untreated; and arranging for appropriate postnatal care when necessary.

Pregnant patients who lack the motivation or psychosocial support to remain substance free should be considered for methadone maintenance regardless of their treatment history, as methadone maintenance improves infant outcomes relative to continued maternal heroin use (1424–1426). In a randomized comparison of enhanced and standard methadone maintenance for pregnant opioid-dependent women, Carroll et al. (1427) found that enhanced treatment—consisting of standard treatment (daily methadone medication, weekly group counseling, and thrice-weekly urine screening) plus weekly prenatal care by a nurse-midwife, weekly relapse prevention groups, positive contingency rewards for abstinence, and the provision of therapeutic child care during treatment visits—resulted in improved neonatal outcomes (longer gestations and higher birth weights) but did not affect maternal substance use. Contingency management approaches may also be implemented to enhance adherence (1299, 1428, 1429). Withdrawal from methadone is not recommended, except in cases where methadone treatment is logistically not possible. In cases where medical withdrawal is necessary, there are no data to suggest that withdrawal is worse during any one trimester.

Although the long history of methadone use in pregnant women makes this medication the preferred pharmacotherapeutic agent, a growing body of evidence suggests that buprenorphine may also be used. Jones et al. (1430), in a randomized, double-blind, double-dummy, flexible-dosing, parallel-group controlled trial, compared 4–24 mg/day sublingual buprenorphine to 20–100 mg/day oral methadone, with treatment starting in the second trimester of pregnancy. Although the study was limited by its small sample size, buprenorphine and methadone showed comparable outcomes in terms of neonatal abstinence syndrome. Data from uncontrolled observations in more than 300 neonates also suggest that buprenorphine may be useful in pregnant women, with rates of neonatal abstinence syndrome possibly less than those observed with methadone treatment during pregnancy (1431).

Data on other treatments for opioid withdrawal or dependence during pregnancy are sparse. In particular, data on the safety of clonidine in pregnant patients are not available. However, a narcotic antagonist should never be given to a pregnant substance-using patient because of the risk of spontaneous abortion, premature labor, or stillbirth.

PART B

BACKGROUND INFORMATION AND REVIEW OF AVAILABLE EVIDENCE

VIII. DISEASE DEFINITION, NATURAL HISTORY AND COURSE, AND EPIDEMIOLOGY

A. DISEASE DEFINITION AND DIAGNOSTIC FEATURES

As delineated in DSM-IV-TR, substance-related disorders are divided into two groups: substance use disorders, which include substance dependence and substance abuse, and substance-induced disorders, which include substance intoxication, substance withdrawal, substance-induced delirium, substance-induced persisting dementia, substance-induced persisting amnestic disorder, substance-induced psychotic disorder, substance-induced mood disorder, substance-induced anxiety disorder, substance-induced sexual dysfunction, and substance-induced sleep disorder. This section of the guideline focuses on the first group, substance use disorders.

1. DSM-IV-TR criteria for substance dependence and abuse

The DSM-IV-TR criteria for substance dependence, which are applicable to each of the substances described in this guideline, include cognitive, behavioral, and physiological signs and symptoms indicating ongoing substance use despite significant problems associated with such use. Usually this continuous use will result in tolerance, withdrawal, and a pattern of compulsive use. Table 2 lists the specific DSM-IV-TR criteria for substance dependence. Individuals who meet DSM-IV-TR criteria for substance abuse have not experienced signs or symptoms of withdrawal or tolerance or met the criteria for compulsive substance use required for a diagnosis of substance dependence. However, they have shown a maladaptive pattern of substance use that is associated with significant recurring adverse consequences. The specific DSM-IV-TR criteria for substance abuse are delineated in Table 1. With DSM-IV-TR criteria, patients may be classified as currently manifesting a pattern of abuse or dependence or as being in remission. Those in remission can be divided into six subtypes—full, early partial, sustained full, sustained partial, on agonist therapy, and in a controlled environment—on the basis of whether any of the criteria for abuse or dependence have been met and over what time frame. Patients receiving agonist therapy (e.g., methadone maintenance) or living in a controlled substance-free environment are also categorized as being in remission, with the corresponding diagnostic modifier used to denote the circumstances of remission.

DSM-IV-TR includes nicotine dependence and nicotine withdrawal as disorders. Nicotine abuse is not included because clinically significant psychosocial problems from tobacco use are rare unless dependence is also present (1432); nicotine intoxication is also not included because it is very rare.

2. Associated features of substance use disorders

a) Cross-sectional features

Patients presenting for treatment of a substance use disorder frequently manifest signs and symptoms of substance-induced intoxication or withdrawal. The clinical picture varies with the substance used, the dosage, the duration of action, the time elapsed since the last dose, the presence or absence of tolerance, and co-occurring psychiatric or general medical conditions. The expectations of the patient, his or her style of responding to states of intoxication or physical discomfort, and the setting in which intoxication or withdrawal is taking place also play a role.

Patients experiencing substance-induced intoxication generally manifest changes in mood, cognition, and/or behavior. Mood-related changes may range from euphoria to depression, with considerable lability in response to or independent of external events. Cognitive changes may include shortened attention span, impaired concentration, and disturbances of thinking (e.g., delusions) and/or perceptions (e.g., hallucinations). Behavioral changes may include wakefulness or somnolence and lethargy or hyperactivity. Impairment in social and occupational functioning is also common in intoxicated individuals.

Other cross-sectional diagnostic features commonly found in patients with a substance use disorder include those related to any co-occurring psychiatric or general medical disorders that may be present. Psychiatric disorders that are often found in such patients include conduct disorder (particularly the aggressive subtype) in children and adolescents (1433–1435), depression, bipolar disorder, schizophrenia, anxiety disorders, eating disorders, pathological gambling, antisocial personality disorder, and other personality disorders (470, 624, 1434, 1436–1444).

Examples of general medical problems that may be directly related to substance use include cardiac toxicity resulting from acute cocaine intoxication, respiratory depression and coma in severe opioid overdose, and hepatic cirrhosis after prolonged heavy drinking (559). General medical conditions frequently associated with opioid-dependent individuals who administer opioids by injection include subacute bacterial endocarditis, HIV infection, and hepatitis. Patients whose substance use disorder is accompanied by diminished self-care and/or high levels of risk-taking behavior are at increased risk of experiencing malnutrition, physical trauma, and HIV infection (1445, 1446).

b) Longitudinal features

Patients with substance use disorders frequently present with a long history of repeated episodes of intoxication and withdrawal, interspersed with attempts to cease use of the substance. In patients who meet DSM-IV-TR criteria for substance abuse, episodes of intoxication may be sporadic and brief and rarely require general medical or psychiatric intervention; however, patients who meet DSM-IV-TR criteria for substance dependence often experience repeated episodes of intoxication that may last for weeks or months, interrupted by voluntary or involuntary periods of self-managed or medically managed withdrawal. Partial or complete withdrawal from abused substances may be followed by variable periods of self-imposed or involuntary (e.g., during periods of incarceration) abstinence, often ending in relapse to substance use and, eventually, resumption of dependence.

In some patients, dependence on a single substance may lead to use of and ultimately dependence on another substance (e.g., the development of alcohol dependence in patients already dependent on opioids or cocaine) (1447, 1448). These patients may replace one form of substance dependence with another.

Although many individuals who abuse alcohol or illicit substances maintain their ability to function in interpersonal relationships and in the work setting, substance-dependent patients presenting for treatment often have profound psychological, social, general medical, legal, and financial problems. These may include disrupted interpersonal (particularly family) relationships, absenteeism, job loss, criminal behavior, poor academic or work performance, failure to develop adaptive coping skills, and a general constriction of normal life activities. Peer relationships often focus extensively on obtaining and using illicit substances or alcohol. The risk of accidents, violence, and suicide is significantly greater for these individuals than for the general population (1449, 1450).

B. NATURAL HISTORY AND COURSE

1. Nicotine dependence

About 33% of adults who smoke make a serious attempt to stop smoking each year (729). Over 90% of these attempts to quit are made without formal treatment (729). Among those who quit by their own efforts, 33% remain abstinent for only 2 days and 3%–5% remain abstinent for 1 year, after which little relapse occurs (746, 1451). Most smokers make several attempts to quit, and 50% of smokers eventually succeed in quitting (729). Smokers with a history of or current anxiety, depression, or schizophrenia are less likely to stop smoking (731, 760, 873, 1452). This could be due to several factors, including increased nicotine withdrawal or nicotine dependence, less social support, or fewer coping skills (760). Smokers who have current alcohol abuse or dependence are unlikely to stop smoking unless their alcohol-related problem resolves (1452). Whether alcohol or other substance abusers in recovery are less likely to stop smoking is unclear (1452).

About 50% of adults who attempt to stop smoking will meet DSM criteria for nicotine withdrawal (755). Smokers who have withdrawal-induced depression or severe craving are less likely to be successful in smoking cessation efforts (755, 760). In addition, fear of weight gain appears to be a major deterrent to cessation attempts, especially among women (771). The presence of cues for smoking is thought to be crucial in producing withdrawal; thus, withdrawal during inpatient stays on smoke-free units is often not as severe as expected (757).

2. Other substance use disorders

It is common for initial experiences with substance use to occur before puberty. At the earliest stages of use, experimenters or casual users who go on to develop a substance use disorder are generally indistinguishable from their peers with respect to the type and frequency of substance use. However, there is increasing evidence that individuals have differential vulnerability for the progression from use to abuse to addiction. This has led to a disease concept of addiction (4), including a neuronal basis for many of its clinical features (1453), the presence of genetic vulnerability (1454), and a characteristic chronic, relapsing course that resembles that of many medical disorders. However, because substance use disorders are frequently viewed as purely behavioral problems, many adolescents with these disorders are managed by their parents, school authorities, or the judicial system rather than being treated in specialized adolescent substance abuse treatment programs. The problem is further complicated by the lack of substance abuse treatment programs for adolescents, even in the private sector.

In adolescents, growing preoccupation with substance use, frequent episodes of intoxication, use of substances with greater dependence liability (e.g., opioids, cocaine), and a preference for routes of administration that result in quicker onset of the substance's effects (e.g., injection) and for more rapidly acting preparations (e.g., crack cocaine) presage the development of substance dependence. Although in most cases the onset of a substance use disorder occurs in the late teens and early 20s, some individuals begin abusing substances in mid- to late adulthood (948, 1455, 1456).

TABLE 5. Estimated Drug Use and Dependence Among 15- to 45-Year-Olds in the United States

	Estimated Cumulative[a] Occurrence of Extra-medical[b] Drug Use (%)	Estimated Cumulative Occurrence of Drug Dependence (%)	Estimated Proportion Becoming Dependent, Once Use Has Occurred (%)
Tobacco	75.6	24.1	31.9
Cocaine	16.2	2.7	16.7
Heroin	1.5	0.4	23.1
Alcohol	91.5	14.1	15.4
Cannabis	46.3	4.2	9.1

Source. Anthony et al. (1168).
[a]"Cumulative" to age at the time of assessment.
[b]"Extra-medical" refers to drug use outside the boundaries of what is prescribed.

Although the use of multiple substances often continues throughout adolescence, some individuals settle on a "drug of choice" early on. A preference for a particular substance is shaped by a variety of factors, including current fashion, availability, peer influences, and individual biological and psychological factors. Sex-specific differences in substance preference (e.g., heroin use in male users, sedative-hypnotic and benzodiazepine use in females) have diminished somewhat over the last two decades. Although substance abuse and dependence appear to aggregate in families, which would support a genetic influence (1457), some of this effect may be explained by the concurrent familial distribution of antisocial personality disorder, which may predispose individuals to the development of these disorders. On the other hand, genetic factors do affect the risk of developing alcohol dependence, particularly in male alcohol users with male biological relatives who are also alcohol dependent (1458–1459) and, to a lesser extent, in female users with a strong family history of the disorder (1460–1462).

Although there is considerable heterogeneity among patients with substance use disorders, the disease course is often chronic, lasting for years. Periods of sustained use are interrupted by periods of partial or complete remission. Although some individuals are able to achieve prolonged periods of abstinence without formal treatment, abstinence or periods of greatly reduced substance use are more likely to be sustained by patients who are able to maintain active participation in formalized treatment and/or self-help groups (e.g., AA) (43, 289, 1463–1465). Patients who experience a severe life crisis (e.g., loss of an important relationship, incarceration, serious general medical sequelae of substance use) are generally more motivated to seek treatment, but most still require external support to maintain their motivation to continue in treatment beyond the initial stages (e.g., detoxification).

During the first several years of treatment, most substance-dependent patients continue to relapse, although with decreasing frequency. Risk of relapse is higher in the first 12 months after the onset of a remission (8). Many patients experience several cycles of remission and relapse before they conclude that a return to "controlled" substance use is not possible for them. Regardless of the treatment site or the modalities used, the frequency, intensity, and duration of treatment participation are positively correlated with improved outcome (356).

In one sample of alcoholic individuals followed for 60 years, of those who remained abstinent for 2 years, almost 90% were still substance free at 10 years, and those who remained substance free for 10 years had a very high likelihood (i.e., >90%) of being substance free at 20 years (9, 1465–1467). Prolonged abstinence, accompanied by improvement in social and occupational functioning, is more apt to occur in those who have lower levels of premorbid psychopathology, demonstrate the ability to develop new relationships, and consistently make use of self-help groups (e.g., AA) (9, 1464, 1468).

C. EPIDEMIOLOGY

By any measure, substance use disorders constitute a major public health problem, costing the United States in excess of $400 billion annually, including the costs of treatment, related health problems, absenteeism, lost productivity, drug-related crime and incarceration, and education and prevention efforts (1469).

The motivation for using any psychoactive substance is, in part, related to the acute and chronic effects of these agents on mood, cognition, and behavior. In some individuals, the subjective changes (e.g., euphoria, tension relief) that accompany substance intoxication are experienced as highly pleasurable and lead to repetitive use. The proportion of users who eventually meet criteria for dependence varies according to substance (1168). Table 5 shows the percentage of adults who have used a particular substance and the risk of becoming dependent.

Thus, 31.9% of individuals who ever used tobacco developed dependence, and 16.7% of individuals who ever used cocaine developed dependence. This does not imply that nicotine pharmacology is twice as potent as cocaine. Indeed, laboratory studies (1470) show that cocaine has the most powerful reinforcing effects of any abused substance. In U.S. society, however, where nicotine is a widely available, legal drug with strong marketing to young people in movies and the media, the net effect is a high risk of dependence.

Given these significant rates of substance use disorders, it is not surprising that there is a considerable need for treatment of substance use disorders. For example, in the National Comorbidity Survey Replication (1471), about 67% of individuals with an alcohol or other substance use disorder did not receive even minimally adequate mental health specialty services, with even a lower portion receiving minimally adequate health care services. As another example, it was estimated that 2.3 million U.S. youth ages 12–17 years needed substance abuse treatment in 2004 (1472). Of these, 185,000 received treatment, leaving a gap of an estimated 2.1 million untreated adolescents nationwide. Although this gap is partly due to the failure of youths to recognize that they have a problem or their reluctance to disclose information to their parents and guardians, it is mostly attributable to the inadequacy of the health care system in addressing the needs of individuals who require treatment for a substance use disorder.

Substance use disorders are associated with a significant increase in morbidity and mortality, particularly among men. Each year non-nicotine-related substance dependence is, directly or indirectly, responsible for at least 40% of all hospital admissions and approximately 25% of all deaths (500,000 per year) (1448, 1473, 1474). The total economic cost of substance use disorders was estimated to be $414 billion for 1995 (1469). This estimate includes substance use disorder treatment and prevention costs as well as other health care costs, costs associated with reduced job productivity or lost earnings, and other costs to society such as crime- and social welfare-related expenses (1469).

A significant portion of new HIV infections occur among users of intravenous drugs or individuals who have had sexual contact with such individuals, with high-risk sexual behaviors among injecting drug users being the biggest predictor of HIV infection in men and women (1475, 1476).

Substance use disorders also exert a profound impact on those who come into contact with affected individuals. For example, an estimated 13.6% of individuals age 12 years or older drove under the influence of alcohol at least once over a 1-year period (1191), and approximately half of all highway fatalities involve a driver or pedestrian who is intoxicated (1477–1479). Similarly, more than half of all cases of domestic violence occur under the influence of alcohol or illicit substances (1476, 1479), and evidence from a broad range of studies suggests that alcohol may play a role in enhancing the possibility of domestic violence (1479). In addition, estimates based on urine testing in general populations suggest that 7.5%–15.0% of all pregnant women had been recently exposed to substances of abuse (excluding alcohol) at the time they first sought prenatal care (1480–1482). Although heavy use of alcohol was reported by <1% of pregnant women in the 2003 National Survey on Drug Use and Health (1191), 9.8% reported using alcohol and 4.1% reported binge drinking in the month before the survey.

Finally, substance use disorders are frequently associated with other forms of psychopathology. The lifetime prevalence of comorbid axis I psychiatric disorders in individuals with substance use disorders (including those with alcohol dependence or abuse) is 20%–90%, depending on the population screened and the rigor of the diagnostic criteria used, with treatment-seeking patients being at the higher end of the range (344, 426, 427, 1308, 1448, 1483–1486). Approximately 33% of hospitalized psychiatric patients manifest a co-occurring non-nicotine-related substance use disorder (10, 1487).

1. Nicotine dependence

Smoking has been labeled the most important preventable cause of death and disease (1488–1490). It is responsible for 20% of all deaths in the United States (over 400,000 deaths/year), and 45% of smokers will die of a tobacco-induced disorder (901, 1490). Cigarette smoking causes multiple physical problems, including lung, oral, and other cancers (1491–1494); cardiovascular disease (1495, 1496); respiratory infections (1497); chronic obstructive pulmonary disease (1498); gastrointestinal disorders (1499); and maternal/fetal complications (751, 901, 923). Secondhand smoke causes death in thousands of nonsmokers and morbidity in children and other relatives of smokers (1500–1502). Although only about 5% of tobacco use is via cigars, pipes, or smokeless tobacco (770, 1191), these have also been linked to oral cancers as well as to other medical problems (901). Most of the tobacco-induced disorders appear to be due to the carcinogens and carbon monoxide in tobacco smoke, although nicotine itself might also cause health problems (804, 1503, 1504). Smoking cessation can dramatically reduce the risk of heart disease and cancer and stop the decline in lung function in those with chronic obstructive lung disease (1489, 1502, 1505).

Nicotine, a potent alkaloid in tobacco leaves, is the substance that produces tobacco dependence. Tobacco dependence usually begins with a decision in adolescence to begin smoking, which has lifelong consequences. The beginning of tobacco dependence, as with other substance dependencies, is influenced mostly by nonpharmacological, learned, or conditioned factors. Peer influence, social setting, personality, and genetics are all important in determining who begins and who continues to smoke. Twin studies have found that the heritability of smoking is as great as, if not greater than, that for alcohol dependence (1506, 1507). Some of the heritability of smoking is shared with and some is independent of that for alcohol dependence (1508, 1509). Although smoking usually precedes the onset of most psychiatric disorders, other psychiatric factors that may also predict initiation of smoking include use and abuse of substances other than alcohol, attention deficit disorders, and mood symptoms (760).

The strength of nicotine dependence relates to the efficiency with which the smoked drug is delivered to the brain, a person's ability to precisely control the nicotine dose depending on the way the cigarette is smoked, the frequency of cigarette smoking, and the multiple cues for cigarette use as well as the many positive reinforcing effects of nicotine (758). However, the severity of nicotine dependence via cigarette smoking can be illustrated by the fact that only 33% of self-quitters remain abstinent for 2 days and fewer than 5% are ultimately successful on a given quit attempt (746, 1451). Despite the strength of nicotine dependence, tobacco use by adults has decreased in recent years. In contrast, levels of adolescent smoking have remained at about 6,000 more adolescents beginning to smoke each day (770, 1510, 1511). According to the 2003 National Survey on Drug Use and Health (1191), approximately 70 million Americans (or about 30% of those age 12 years or older) reported using a tobacco product in the previous month and smoking a mean of 13 cigarettes each day. About 60% of current smokers (corresponding to approximately 36 million individuals in the United States) met criteria for nicotine dependence. Young adults (ages 18–25 years) reported the highest rates of use, with approximately 40% having smoked a cigarette in the previous month. In a CDC report on adolescent tobacco use, 64% of respondents reported ever having smoked cigarettes, 28% reported having smoked on at least one day in the previous month, and 14% reported having smoked on at least 20 of the previous 30 days (1511). Of high school seniors who reported having smoked, 29% already reported symptoms that met criteria for nicotine dependence (1512). More than 50% of adolescents indicate that they experience withdrawal symptoms after an attempt to quit (1513). Male and female adolescents have comparable rates of smoking in contrast to the case in adults, in whom tobacco use is more frequent in men (1191).

The prevalences of tobacco use and nicotine dependence are significantly increased among individuals with another psychiatric disorder. For example, in the 2001–2002 National Epidemiologic Survey on Alcohol and Related Conditions (347), highly significant associations were found between nicotine dependence and specific axis I and II disorders. Furthermore, nicotine-dependent individuals with a co-occurring psychiatric disorder made up 7.1% of the population yet consumed 34.2% of all cigarettes smoked in the United States (347). Epidemiologic findings from Germany have shown similar increases in nicotine dependence among psychiatrically ill individuals (1514). (The clinical implications of these findings are reviewed in greater detail in Section III.H.2.)

2. Alcohol-related disorders

Alcohol, like tobacco, is a commonly used and widely available licit substance that significantly affects public health (1515). According to the 2004 National Survey on Drug Use and Health (1472), about 50% of respondents age 12 years or older reported having had at least one drink and >20% reported at least one episode of binge drinking (consuming five or more drinks on the same occasion) in the previous month. Heavy drinking, defined as consuming at least five drinks on the same occasion for at least 5 of the previous 30 days, was reported by 6.9% of the population over age 12 years in the United States (approximately 16 million people). Across age groups, rates of binge and heavy drinking increase through adolescence and young adulthood, peak at ages 21–25 years, and then gradually fall through the adult years. When compared with their non-college-attending peers, college students were more likely to report alcohol use, binge drinking, and heavy drinking. At later ages, however, those who had completed college were less likely to engage in binge or heavy drinking, although they were still more likely to report current alcohol use. With the exception of individuals ages 12–17 years, in whom equivalent proportions of current alcohol use are reported by both sexes, men are more likely to report drinking than women (62% vs. 46%). Although whites were most likely to report current alcohol use, rates of binge and heavy drinking were highest in American Indians/Alaskan Natives and Native Hawaiians or other Pacific Islanders. Binge and heavy drinking were lowest among Asians, with intermediate rates reported in blacks and Hispanics.

Demographic patterns in the 12-month prevalence of DSM diagnoses of alcohol abuse and dependence tend to parallel reported rates of binge and heavy drinking. For example, the 2001–2002 National Epidemiologic Survey on Alcohol and Related Conditions found a 12-month prevalence of alcohol abuse and dependence in the United States of 4.7% and 3.8%, respectively, with both abuse and dependence being more prevalent in whites, in male respondents, and in younger individuals (1516). In Europe, an epidemiological study in six countries using a different interviewing methodology (1517) found lower overall prevalences for alcohol use disorders (4.1 and 1.1 lifetime and 0.7 and 0.3 12-month prevalences for alcohol abuse and alcohol dependence, respectively). However, demographic patterns were similar to those in the United States, with an increased prevalence of alcohol abuse and dependence observed in men and in those ages 18–24 years and a progressive decline in prevalence with increasing age.

There is some evidence that the demographic patterns of alcohol use disorders may be changing in the United States. As compared with nationally representative data obtained in the 1991–1992 National Longitudinal Alcohol Epidemiologic Survey, data from the 2001–2002 National Epidemiologic Survey on Alcohol and Related Conditions showed an overall increase in the prevalence of alcohol abuse, whereas the 12-month prevalence of alcohol dependence declined (1516). However, rates of alcohol dependence rose among male, young black female, and Asian male respondents. In addition, disproportionate increases in alcohol abuse were observed among female respondents and black and Hispanic youth (1516).

Although a DSM-IV-TR diagnosis of alcohol dependence takes precedence over a DSM-IV-TR diagnosis of alcohol abuse, and signs of alcohol abuse are sometimes used as an initial screen before inquiring about dependence, not everyone with alcohol dependence also meets criteria for alcohol abuse. Hasin and Grant (1518) found that 33.7% of respondents in the 2001–2002 National Epidemiologic Survey on Alcohol and Related Conditions with current alcohol dependence did not meet criteria for alcohol abuse. This finding was seen to a lesser extent among respondents with lifetime diagnoses of dependence, of whom 13.9% did not meet criteria for abuse. In terms of lifetime as well as current rates of alcohol use disorders, the presence of alcohol dependence without alcohol abuse was particularly common among women and among nonwhite populations.

Given the significant number of physical disorders that have been causally associated with alcohol use (1515), it is not surprising that the prevalence of alcohol use disorders is particularly high among general hospital inpatients. For example, Smothers et al. (1519), in a study of individuals admitted to nonfederal U.S. acute care general hospitals, found a 7.4% overall prevalence of a current alcohol use disorder and an estimated prevalence of 24% in those who had consumed at least 12 alcoholic drinks in the preceding 12 months, with approximately equal rates in men and women.

Use of alcohol, particularly binge or heavy drinking, is associated with greater rates of using tobacco or other substances. For example, in the 2003 National Survey on Drug Use and Health (1191), approximately 60% of heavy drinkers reported having smoked cigarettes in the previous month as compared with approximately 20% of those who were neither drinkers nor binge drinkers; approximately 33% of heavy drinkers reported using an illicit substance in the previous month, a rate that was 10-fold greater than in those who did not use alcohol. The increased association of alcohol and tobacco use disorders has also been noted longitudinally in follow-up assessments of subjects from the St. Louis Epidemiologic Catchment Area study (1520).

Rates of other psychiatric disorders are similarly increased in individuals with an alcohol use disorder. For example, mirroring the findings of earlier studies (1521–1523) and epidemiological data from Europe (1524), the National Epidemiologic Survey on Alcohol and Related Conditions (23) found that individuals meeting DSM-IV criteria for alcohol abuse were somewhat more likely to have a 12-month diagnosis of a mood or anxiety disorder (odds ratios 1.3 and 1.1, respectively). Furthermore, those meeting criteria for alcohol dependence had substantial increases in risk for a mood or anxiety disorder (odds ratios of 4.1 and 2.6, respectively) (23) as well as an increased likelihood of meeting diagnostic criteria for a personality disorder (1525). Such high rates of co-occurring disorders have important implications for the assessment and treatment of individuals with an alcohol use disorder (see Section IV.E.1).

3. Marijuana-related disorders

Marijuana is the most widely used illicit drug in the United States (1167) and worldwide. In the United States, a variety of studies suggest that the age at initial marijuana use has been lowering (1169). In the 2001 National Household Survey on Drug Abuse, more than 75 million (>34%) of Americans age 12 years or older reported having tried marijuana at least once and almost 19 million reported using it in the previous year (1167). It is estimated that 9%–10% of those who try marijuana will meet criteria for marijuana dependence at some time in their lives, and lifetime prevalence rates of marijuana have been estimated at 4% of the population (1168), making it the highest dependence rate of any illicit drug. Thus, although marijuana's relative dependence potential of 9% is lower than that of nicotine (32%), heroin (23%), cocaine (17%), or alcohol (15%), the large number of users will yield a high dependence rate in the population (1168). Although the overall prevalence of marijuana use remained stable from 1992 to 2002, the prevalence of marijuana abuse or dependence increased significantly during that time, with the greatest increases found among young black men and women and young Hispanic men (1170). Because the frequency and quantity of marijuana use have not changed, the increase in marijuana use disorders may be related to an increased potency of available marijuana (1170). Such increases in the prevalence of marijuana abuse and dependence may carry an added public health burden, given the increasing epidemiological evidence for adverse health consequences of marijuana use (1526–1528). In addition, rates of other substance use disorders (1529) and rates or symptoms of other psychiatric disorders may be increased among long-term marijuana users (1173, 1530–1535).

4. Cocaine- and other stimulant-related disorders

Although the prevalence of cocaine use has declined since the peak of the cocaine epidemic in 1980 (1536–1539), the 2003 National Survey on Drug Use and Health (1191) estimated that 2.3 million individuals (1.0% of the United States population) were current cocaine users in the United States, with 604,000 (0.3%) of those having used crack during the same 30-day period. Among eighth, tenth, and twelfth graders, the 30-day prevalence of cocaine abuse increased by more than twofold between 1991 and 1998, but during the 1990s the annual prevalence of cocaine use among high school seniors declined to 1%–2% (1539).

It is more typical for initial cocaine use to occur after age 18 years (1191), and cocaine-related disorders are most commonly found in individuals ages 18–30 years, with greater rates in men than women. Smoking of cocaine is associated with a more rapid progression from use to abuse or dependence than is intranasal use (1540, 1541).

An additional 1.2 million individuals in the United States use stimulants other than cocaine for nonmedicinal purposes (1191). Of special interest to psychiatrists is that the nonprescription use of methylphenidate increased among high school seniors from an annual prevalence of 0.1% in 1992 to 2.8% in 1997 and then remained at that level through 2003 (1539). In addition, localized epidemics of amphetamine and methamphetamine abuse have developed, particularly in the western and midwestern United States and more recently spreading to eastern U.S. cities (1542).

5. Opioid-related disorders

The Office of National Drug Control Policy estimates that 750,000 to 1,000,000 individuals are heroin dependent (1333a). However, heroin users constitute a small proportion of individuals using opiates for nonmedical purposes. Although rates of opiate dependence were not reported in the 2003 National Survey on Drug Use and Health (1191) and are difficult to ascertain (1543), the survey estimated that 31.2 million individuals (4.7% of U.S. population) had used narcotic pain-relief medication for nonmedical purposes in the previous month, most commonly combination medicines containing narcotic analgesics and acetaminophen (Vicodin, Lortab, Lorcet, Percocet, or Tylox) or aspirin (Percodan) (1191). Furthermore, there were statistically significant increases in the current and lifetime prevalence of nonmedical pain reliever use between 2002 and 2003 (1191).

IX. REVIEW AND SYNTHESIS OF AVAILABLE EVIDENCE

A. NICOTINE DEPENDENCE

1. Somatic treatments

Pharmacotherapies for nicotine dependence can be divided into NRTs and nonnicotine medications. The following sections describe these therapies in terms of treatment goals, efficacy in smoking cessation, side effects, and implementation. For more information, the reader is referred to descriptive (602, 706, 750, 1544–1548) and meta-analytic (789, 790, 793, 795, 1549) reviews.

a) Nicotine replacement therapy

(1) Goals

The primary goal of NRT is to relieve withdrawal symptoms when patients stop smoking and thus allow them to focus on conditioning factors that typically trigger a relapse to smoking. After the acute withdrawal period, NRT is reduced gradually so that little withdrawal should occur. A secondary goal of NRT may be to reduce smoking, but this approach has not been well studied.

(2) Description of products

a. Nicotine transdermal patch

The nicotine transdermal patch takes advantage of the ready absorption of nicotine across the skin (799, 1550). It is available in four formulations: three 24-hour patches and one 16-hour patch for use while an individual is awake. Treatment initiation typically uses a 21- to 22-mg 24-hour patch or a 15-mg 16-hour patch. Patches are applied on the first morning of smoking cessation and then each morning thereafter. The nicotine is slowly absorbed so that on the first day venous nicotine levels peak 6–10 hours after administration. Thereafter, nicotine levels remain fairly steady, with a decline from peak to trough of 25%–40% with 24-hour patches (799). The 16-hour nicotine patches demonstrate similar nicotine pharmacokinetics after discontinuation of smoking. Nicotine levels obtained with the use of patches are typically half those obtained by smoking (799).

After 4–6 weeks, the nicotine patch dose is tapered to a middle dose (e.g., 14 mg/24 hours or 10 mg/16 hours) and then tapered again in 2–4 weeks to the lowest dose (7 mg/24 hours or 5 mg/16 hours). The recommended total duration of treatment is usually 6–12 weeks (71, 1550). Most, but not all, studies indicate abrupt discontinuation of the patch usually causes no significant withdrawal so that tapering may not be necessary (71). There are now two nicotine patches available over the counter: a 21-, 14-, and 7-mg strength patch (24-hour application) and a 22- and 11-mg strength patch (16-hour application). The 15-mg patch does not require tapering.

b. Nicotine gum

Nicotine ingested through the gastrointestinal tract is extensively metabolized on first pass through the liver (1551). In addition, nicotine is a gastrointestinal irritant that makes orally ingested nicotine an unpleasant treatment for patients who are already experiencing nicotine withdrawal. Nicotine gum (nicotine polacrilex) avoids this problem via buccal absorption

(1551). The gum, which is available as an over-the-counter medication, contains 2 or 4 mg of nicotine that can be released from a resin by chewing (886).

When compared with nicotine delivery via smoking, nicotine gum produces lower steady-state blood levels of nicotine and does not reach peak levels of nicotine absorption for >30 minutes (1551). Because cigarette nicotine is absorbed directly into the arterial circulation, arterial blood levels from smoking are 5–10 times higher than those from the 2- and 4-mg gum (1552). Venous nicotine levels from the 2- and 4-mg gum are about 33% and 67% of the steady-state (i.e., between cigarettes) levels of nicotine achieved by cigarette smoking, respectively (1551). Absorption of nicotine in the buccal mucosa and the resulting steady-state levels are further decreased by an acidic environment; thus, patients should not drink acidic beverages (e.g., coffee, soda, juice) immediately before, during, or after nicotine gum use (1552).

In terms of dosing, the original recommendation was to use one piece of 2-mg gum every 15–30 minutes as needed for craving. More recent work, however, suggests greater efficacy with scheduled dosing (e.g., 1 piece of 2-mg gum/hour) and 4-mg gum for highly nicotine-dependent smokers (724). Although the original recommended treatment duration was 3 months, many experts believe longer treatment is more effective. However, two trials of longer treatment durations produced contradictory results (801).

c. Nicotine lozenges

The nicotine lozenge contains nicotine bound to a polacrilex ion-exchange resin, similar to the nicotine gum. It is available in 2- and 4-mg dose formulations. Because it does not have to be chewed, the lozenge may be preferable for smokers with dental problems or for those who do not like to chew gum. Compared with an equal dose of nicotine gum, the lozenge delivers 25% more nicotine (802). It is recommended that the lozenge be used every 1–2 hours for the first 2–4 weeks of treatment, with the frequency of use reduced to every 2–4 hours in subsequent weeks.

d. Nicotine nasal spray

This type of NRT consists of a nicotine solution in a nasal spray bottle similar to those used with saline sprays and antihistamines (71, 809, 1553). Nasal sprays produce droplets that average 1 mg per administration (spray solutions are dispensed at 10 mg/ml); patients administer the spray to each nostril every 1–2 hours. This formulation produces a more rapid rise in and higher nicotine levels than the nicotine gum but less than that obtained with cigarettes. There is approximately a 30% replacement of plasma nicotine levels with nasal spray use (809). Peak nicotine levels occur within 10 minutes, and venous nicotine levels are about 67% of between-cigarette levels (782). Smokers are to use the product ad libitum up to 30 times/day for 12 weeks, including a tapering period.

e. Nicotine vapor inhalers

Nicotine vapor inhalers are cartridges of nicotine containing about 1 mg of nicotine each placed inside hollow cigarette-like plastic rods. The cartridges produce a nicotine vapor when warm air is passed through them (805, 806). Absorption from the inhaler is primarily buccal rather than respiratory (1554). Nicotine blood levels produced by the nicotine vapor inhaler are about 33% of between-cigarette levels (1555). Smokers are instructed to puff continuously on the inhaler (0.013 mg/puff) during the day, with a recommended dose of 6–16 cartridges daily. The inhaler is to be used ad libitum for about 12 weeks.

(3) Efficacy of nicotine replacement therapies

a. General issues

In general, the various NRTs have shown comparable efficacy in studies using the rigorous outcome measure of at least 6 months of abstinence from smoking (790, 793, 1556). Although specific rates of smoking cessation vary across studies, there is typically a twofold increase in rates of smoking abstinence with an NRT. Many studies have shown that NRTs decrease withdrawal symptoms such as anxiety, anger/irritability, depression, difficulty concentrating, and impatience in outpatient settings (602, 755); insomnia and weight gain, however, are not consistently decreased by all forms of NRT (801). For example, nicotine gum at 2 mg ad libitum appears less likely to reduce craving compared with the nicotine patch or nasal spray; however, this may be a dose-related issue, as the 4-mg gum does appear to better reduce craving (1557). Finally, higher doses of an NRT only marginally decrease withdrawal symptoms (801).

b. Nicotine transdermal patch

The overall efficacy of the nicotine transdermal patch for smoking cessation has been well documented. A 1994 meta-analysis of 17 randomized, placebo-controlled trials of the patch (71) documented abstinence rates of 27% vs. 13% at the end of treatment and 22% vs. 9% at 6-month follow-up for the nicotine and placebo patch, respectively. These effects of the nicotine transdermal patch were independent of patch type, treatment duration, tapering procedures, and behavioral therapy format or intensity, although it should be noted that behavioral treatment plus nicotine patch enhanced treatment outcomes compared with the patch alone. A recent meta-analysis of patch trials suggests an odds ratio of 1.81 (95% confidence interval [CI] = 1.63–2.02) for nicotine patch versus placebo patch treatment effects (790). Because the nicotine patch is available as an over-the-counter product, it is also noteworthy that randomized, double-blind, placebo-controlled studies (1549, 1558) as well as a meta-analysis (793) have demonstrated the efficacy of nicotine patch therapy in over-the-counter settings.

Several studies have addressed the issue of matching the patch dose to the patient's nicotine-dependence level, and there is modest evidence that higher patch doses are more helpful for more heavy and dependent smokers, at least with short-term outcomes. For example, Hughes et al. (1544) evaluated the effects of four doses of the patch (0, 21, 35, and 42 mg/day) for smoking cessation in 1,039 cigarette smokers using >30 cigarettes/day. In conjunction with weekly smoking cessation group therapy, patches were used daily for 6 weeks, after which the dose was tapered over an additional 10 weeks. At 12 weeks, there was a dose-dependent effect of nicotine patch therapy on smoking cessation rates, but it was less pronounced at 1-year follow-up. In an 8-week trial of 504 cigarette smokers using at least 15 cigarettes per day, Jorenby et al. (1559) compared two doses of the patch (44 and 22 mg/day) with three different intensities of counseling and found superior smoking cessation rates with the higher-dose patch only in combination with the minimal therapy condition and at the 4-week time point. Similar findings were reported by Killen et al. (1560) in their double-blind trial of 408 cigarette smokers who smoked >25 cigarettes per day. The subjects in that trial were randomized to receive either a high- (25-mg) or low- (15-mg) dose 16 hour/day patch for 6 weeks. Paoletti et al. (1561) stratified 297 cigarette smokers to a dose of patch based on low (≤250 ng/ml) or high (>250 ng/ml) baseline plasma cotinine levels and found comparable cessation rates for the 25- and 15-mg patches in individuals with high baseline plasma cotinine levels. Thus, further treatment studies are needed to determine if higher-dose patches are effective for heavier and more dependent smokers. In addition, evidence from one randomized, double-blind, placebo-controlled study suggests that nicotine patch therapy may improve smoking cessation outcomes even in individuals who had resumed smoking after previous nicotine patch treatment and were smoking at least 15 cigarettes per day (1562).

Other studies have assessed whether combining nicotine transdermal patch and other smoking cessation treatments results in improved outcomes. A randomized, double-blind, placebo-controlled trial by Bohadana et al. (1563) studied the efficacy of the nicotine inhaler in combination with a nicotine or placebo patch for up to 12 weeks in 400 nicotine-dependent subjects. The inhaler plus nicotine patch group had higher abstinence rates than the inhaler plus placebo patch group at 6 and 12 weeks but not at 6- or 12-month follow-up. These results suggest that the use of the nicotine patch can augment outcomes with the nicotine inhaler and these two NRTs can be safely combined. The combination of nicotine patch with behavioral therapy has been studied in several trials. One trial suggested a modest additional benefit of nicotine patch at 10 weeks when combined with CBT (1564), but no difference was found at 6- and 12-month follow-ups. Two other trials (1559, 1565) used other behavioral interventions (e.g., self-help pamphlets, self-help video-enhanced manual, physician motivational messages, brief follow-up nurse visits, weekly cessation counseling groups) and found no augmenting effects of behavioral treatments over the nicotine patch alone.

Some studies have also shown efficacy for nicotine patch treatment in a variety of patient subgroups and specialized contexts. For example, a large double-blind, randomized, placebo-controlled study by Ahluwalia et al. (669) specifically examined the usefulness of the nicotine patch in African Americans, an important subset of the smoking population for which there is an insufficient number of studies assessing the efficacy of standard smoking cessation pharmacotherapies. Greater smoking cessation rates were observed with active patch (21 mg/day) relative to placebo patch at the end of the 10-week trial, with a trend toward significance at 6-month follow-up.

Three randomized, placebo-controlled trials have examined the efficacy of the nicotine patch in outpatient or hospitalized medical patients with smoking-related cardiac and pulmonary diseases. These trials demonstrated short- but not longer-term (i.e., >6 month) improvements in smoking cessation rates (910, 916, 1566). The negative outcomes, including mortality, were no greater with nicotine patch treatment than with placebo patch.

There have also been three preliminary controlled studies of the nicotine patch in patients with a psychiatric or substance use disorder. There have been two open-label studies of the patch (21 mg/day for 6 weeks, followed by 14 and 7 mg/day for 2 weeks each) for patients with co-occurring schizophrenia and nicotine dependence that demonstrated short-term smoking cessation in about 33% of patients (702, 703). In the study by George et al. (703), treatment of subjects with second-generation as compared with first-generation antipsychotics led to enhanced smoking cessation outcomes. However, in both studies there was a significant return to smoking in patients with schizophrenia 6 months after patch discontinuation. Finally, a single small, randomized, controlled trial in alcohol-dependent smokers (705) showed no significant effect of nicotine patch therapy on smoking cessation rates. Nevertheless, the patch was well tolerated by patients in all three studies. It is clear that placebo-controlled trials to establish the relative efficacy of the patch in psychiatric and substance-using populations are needed, but it appears that the patch has utility in treating smokers with a co-occurring psychiatric disorder.

c. Nicotine gum

Several placebo-controlled trials have established the safety and efficacy of nicotine gum for smoking cessation (790), with a pooled odds ratio of 1.66 (95% CI = 1.52–1.81). There is some evidence from randomized, controlled trials supporting the use of 4-mg nicotine gum in more highly dependent cigarette smokers (803, 1557, 1567, 1568). This finding supports the idea of matching the nicotine gum dose to the smoker's dependence level. The efficacy of matching gum dose to the patient's smoking dependence level appears to be independent of the intensity of behavioral therapy support, although this needs further study.

To manage the heavy smoker with treatment-resistant dependence, the combination of nicotine gum with nicotine patch is often used clinically, and its efficacy is supported by some evidence. For example, in a randomized trial of 374 nicotine-dependent cigarette smokers, Kornitzer et al. (888) found that the combination of active nicotine gum (2 mg) and active nicotine patch (15 mg/day) was superior to active patch plus placebo gum and placebo gum plus placebo patch at the end of the 12-week trial (34.2% vs. 22.7% vs. 17.3%) as well as at 1-year follow-up (18.1% vs. 12.7% vs. 13.3%).

d. Nicotine lozenges

Nicotine lozenges have been less well studied but also appear to be efficacious in improving short- and long-term smoking cessation rates. In a 6-week double-blind, randomized, placebo-controlled, multicenter study of 2- and 4-mg nicotine lozenges compared with placebo gum (802), smokers with low nicotine dependence (first cigarette >30 minutes after waking) were assigned to the 2-mg lozenge or placebo and those with a high nicotine dependence (first cigarette <30 minutes after waking) were assigned to the 4-mg lozenge or placebo. Both doses of the lozenge significantly increased carbon monoxide-verified continuous abstinence rates, with significant reduction in nicotine craving and withdrawal. At the 4-mg dose, abstinence rates were more than doubled (48.7% vs. 20.8%; $p<0.001$), suggesting that the higher 4-mg lozenge may be more efficacious in more highly dependent smokers and that the lozenge dose can be matched with the dependence level. The efficacy of the lozenge compared with placebo was also demonstrated at 12-month follow-up.

e. Nicotine nasal spray

Nicotine nasal spray has been found to be a safe and effective aid for smoking cessation in two randomized, double-blind, placebo-controlled trials (809, 1569). Both trials provided treatment for 3–6 months. Active nasal spray led to a doubling of quit rates during active use, but the differences between the active and placebo treatment were reduced or absent with extended follow-up, suggesting the need for maintenance use of this agent. The results of a recent Cochrane meta-analysis (790) suggested that the odds ratio for nicotine nasal spray versus placebo is 2.35 (95% CI=1.63–3.38). To date, long-term studies of the spray as well as studies of the spray in combination with the patch, gum, or bupropion have not been published.

f. Nicotine inhalers

Two randomized, double-blind, placebo-controlled trials (1570, 1571) have demonstrated the superiority of nicotine vapor inhalers to placebo inhalers for smoking cessation in trials of 4–6 months' duration, with two- to threefold increases in quit rates (17%–26%), compared with placebo at the trial endpoints, but smaller between-group differences at follow-up periods ≥1 year. The results of the Cochrane meta-analysis (790) suggest that the odds ratio for nicotine inhaler versus placebo is 2.14 (95% CI=1.44–3.18). Although these data support the short-term efficacy of the inhaler in cigarette smokers, longer-term trials are needed.

(4) Side effects of nicotine replacement therapies

a. Nicotine patch

No significant medical problems with nicotine patches have been found (798, 801, 1550, 1551). The most common minor side effects are skin reactions (50%), insomnia and increased or vivid dreams (15% with 24-hour patches), and nausea (5%–10%) (798, 801, 1550). Tolerance to these side effects usually develops within a week. In addition, the rotation of patch sites can decrease skin irritation, and a 24-hour patch can be removed before bedtime or changed to a 16-hour patch to determine if nicotine replacement is contributing to insomnia. Although the results of an early study suggested that the concomitant use of cigarettes and nicotine patches caused myocardial infarction (800), later analyses and prospective empirical studies in smokers with active heart disease indicated that the use of nicotine patches is safe in cardiac patients (836, 916). Abrupt cessation of the nicotine patch does not appear to produce significant withdrawal symptoms, and long-term use of the patch has not been associated with any long-term medical or psychiatric sequelae (140, 602, 798). There appears to be little dependence liability associated with patch use, as only 2% of patch users continue to use this product for an extended period after a cessation trial (796).

b. Nicotine gum

Major side effects from nicotine gum are uncommon and rarely deter use (790, 793, 804); minor side effects are of mechanical (e.g., difficulty chewing, sore jaw) or local pharmacological (e.g., burning in mouth, throat irritation) origin. Tolerance develops to most side effects over the first week (804). Education about the proper use of the gum (e.g., do not chew too vigorously) also decreases the side effects (804). In earlier research, some disorders were listed as contraindications to the use of nicotine gum (e.g., cardiovascular disease, pregnancy, hypertension). However, because nicotine blood levels are much lower with nicotine gum than with cigarettes, these contraindications have been removed (804, 1551).

The only potential psychological side effect of nicotine gum is the continuance of nicotine dependence (758). Abrupt cessation of nicotine gum can produce withdrawal symptoms similar to but less intense than that from cigarettes (758), whereas gradual reduction in the use of nicotine gum usually produces very minor or no withdrawal symptoms (758, 1572). There are several lines of evidence indicating that most long-term use is not dependence. Instead, long-term use appears to represent patients' desire to extend the duration of therapy based on their fear that they will return to smoking if they stop using the nicotine gum. West et al. (796) conducted a study on the continued use of NRT 15 weeks after smoking cessation and found that only 7% of smokers continued to use the gum after a cessation attempt compared with 2% continuing the patch and 10% continuing the nasal spray or inhaler. By 2 years, all but 1%–2% of smokers had stopped gum use, and the amount of gum use at long-term follow-up was minimal (usually 12 mg/day) (797). The potential harmful effects of long-term use of nicotine gum have not been studied; however, it is unlikely there are any, given the absence of exposure to carcinogens or carbon monoxide and the much lower levels of nicotine obtained from nicotine gum than from cigarettes (804, 1551).

c. Nicotine lozenges

Mild throat and mouth irritation have been reported in preliminary trials (802). Side effects of the nicotine lozenge include heartburn, hiccups, and nausea (802). In addition, because the lozenge contains phenylalanine, it should not be used by individuals with a history of phenylketonuria.

d. Nicotine nasal spray

The major short-term side effects of nicotine nasal spray are nasal and throat irritation, rhinitis, sneezing, coughing, and watering eyes (807–809). One or more of these occur in >75% of patients, although long-term nasal problems from use of nicotine nasal spray do not usually occur (807). Whether abrupt cessation of the spray produces withdrawal has not been studied. Nicotine nasal spray may have some potential to induce dependence. Several patients who quit smoking with nicotine nasal spray in some studies continued to use it for long periods (782, 811). Indeed, one controlled study of nicotine nasal spray by West et al. (796) determined that continued use of the spray occurred in 10% of smokers, and the results of a human laboratory study (811) suggest that nicotine nasal spray has modest reinforcing effects. Thus, follow-up of smokers using nasal spray is recommended.

e. Nicotine inhaler

No serious medical side effects have been reported with nicotine inhalers (810). About 50% of subjects report throat irritation or coughing (806). The results of the controlled study by West et al. (796) suggest that about 10% of smokers quitting with a nicotine inhaler continue to use it for extended periods, and thus follow-up of inhaler users is recommended.

(5) Implementation

Nicotine-dependent smokers benefit equally from nicotine gum, patch, inhaler, or nasal spray (790, 793, 1573, 1574). Some have suggested that NRT be used only if the patient is enrolled in behavioral therapy; however, the data clearly show that NRT is effective in the absence of behavioral therapy (790) and that not all individuals are receptive to concomitant behavioral therapy. Although nicotine gum and patches are available over the counter, psychiatrists may still encourage appropriate use of the patch consistent with package instructions, provide adjunctive psychiatric management and, when appropriate, psychosocial and other pharmacological therapies. It has been suggested that a patient's precessation blood level of cotinine, a metabolite of nicotine with a half-life of about 20 hours, may be a useful benchmark to examine the percent of nicotine replaced by NRTs (1575), presumably because the level from nicotine replacement is higher; however, this area is controversial and requires further study (1576).

Although most smoking cessation treatment lasts 6–12 weeks, some authors (71, 140, 602, 1577) have advocated longer-term use of NRT and even a nicotine replacement program. However, the European multicenter CEASE trial compared high (25-mg) versus low (15-mg) patch doses and shorter (22 weeks) versus longer (8 weeks) periods of treatment and found that although higher doses of the nicotine patch led to better outcomes, extending patch treatment beyond 8–12 weeks did not increase cessation rates (1578). In addition, a meta-analysis of nicotine patches did not find that longer treatment was associated with higher quit rates (71). However, no data examining whether longer NRT treatment is associated with higher abstinence rates are available for nicotine nasal spray, inhaler, or lozenges.

b) Sustained-release bupropion

(1) Goals

Bupropion is a first-line pharmacological treatment for nicotine-dependent smokers who want to quit smoking. It is a phenylaminoketone that is an atypical antidepressant and is available in immediate-release, sustained-release (SR), and extended-release (XR) formulations. Bupropion's mechanism of action in the treatment of nicotine dependence likely involves blockade of dopamine and norepinephrine reuptake (161) as well as antagonism of high-affinity nicotinic acetylcholine receptors (162). The goals of bupropion therapy entail cessation of smoking behavior, reduction of nicotine craving and withdrawal symptoms, and prevention of cessation-induced weight gain.

(2) Efficacy

Since the pivotal study by Hurt et al. (158) established the efficacy and safety of bupropion SR for treatment of nicotine dependence, which led to its FDA approval in 1998, multiple studies have confirmed its utility (160, 795, 812, 1579, 1580, 1582). A recent meta-analysis showed that rates of smoking cessation are doubled by bupropion treatment (795).

The 7-week double-blind, placebo-controlled multicenter trial of Hurt et al. (158) assigned 615 subjects who smoked 15 cigarettes per day to placebo or to 100, 150, or 300 mg/day bupropion SR; all treatment conditions also included weekly individual smoking cessation counseling. The end-of-trial, 7-week prevalence cessation rates were 19.0%, 28.8%, 38.6%, and 44.2%, respectively. At 1-year follow-up, the cessation rates were 12.4%, 19.6%, 22.9%, and 23.1%, respectively. In addition, bupropion SR treatment reduced weight gain associated with smoking cessation in a dose-dependent manner and significantly reduced nicotine withdrawal symptoms at the 150 and 300 mg/day doses. In this study, the major side effects associated with bupropion SR compared with placebo were insomnia and dry mouth. In accordance with these results, the 300 mg/day dose (150 mg b.i.d.) was recommended as the target dose for bupropion therapy for smoking cessation, with an initial dose of 150 mg/day for 3–4 days.

Several recent studies have extended the use of bupropion for smoking cessation. Hays et al. (160) examined the effects of bupropion versus placebo on the prevention of smoking relapse in 784 cigarette smokers who achieved smoking abstinence after a 7-week open-label trial of bupropion (300 mg/day). Those subjects who were abstinent from smoking at the end of the open-label phase of the trial (58.8%) were then randomized to receive bupropion (300 mg/day) or placebo for an additional 45 weeks. At the end of the 52-week treatment period, significantly more smokers in the bupropion group were abstinent than in the placebo group (55.1% vs. 42.3%; $p<0.01$) but not at the 1-year postmedication follow-up assessment (41.6% vs. 40.0%). The number of days to smoking relapse was higher in the bupropion than in the placebo group (156 vs. 65; $p<0.05$), and weight gain was significantly less in the bupropion group at the end of the 52-week treatment and at 1-year follow-up.

Dale et al. (1580) randomly assigned 615 subjects who smoked at least 15 cigarettes/day to placebo or to 100, 150, or 300 mg/day bupropion SR in a double-blind fashion. At the end of the 7 weeks of active treatment, bupropion SR showed improved rates of smoking abstinence in a dose-dependent manner.

It is not clear whether bupropion is superior to NRT or whether the addition of NRT to bupropion improves overall cessation rates. In one study, the combination of bupropion with the nicotine patch was evaluated in a double-blind, placebo-controlled, randomized, multicenter trial (159). The 893 cigarette smokers in that study, who smoked at least 15 cigarettes/day, were randomized to one of four experimental groups: 1) placebo bupropion (0 mg/day) plus placebo patch; 2) bupropion (300 mg/day) plus placebo patch; 3) placebo bupropion plus nicotine patch (21 mg/day for 4 weeks, with 2 weeks of 14 mg/day and 2 weeks of 7 mg/day); or 4) bupropion plus nicotine patch. Bupropion was administered 1 week before the target quit date (day 15), at which time patch treatment was initiated for a total of 8 weeks. All subjects received weekly individual smoking cessation counseling. Cessation rates at the 1-year follow-up assessment were 15.6% for placebo, 16.4% for active patch alone, 30.3% for bupropion alone, and 35.5% for the combination of nicotine patch and bupropion. The bupropion plus nicotine patch and bupropion alone conditions were significantly better than the placebo and nicotine patch alone conditions, but the combination (35.5%) was not significantly better than bupropion alone (30.3%). Weight suppression after cessation was most robust in the combination therapy group. Side effects were consistent with the profiles of patch and bupropion, and the combination was well tolerated. However, a higher-than-expected rate of treatment-emergent hypertension (4%–5%) was noted with the combination of bupropion and nicotine patch (159). The patch alone treatment was significantly different from placebo at the end of the trial but not at the follow-up assessments.

Other studies have suggested the efficacy of bupropion SR for smoking cessation in African Americans (670) and for smokers who have not responded to initial bupropion therapy (1583), smokers with chronic obstructive pulmonary disease (918) or cardiovascular disease (917), and users of smokeless tobacco (1584, 1585).

Finally, studies have suggested the utility of bupropion SR for smoking cessation/reduction in psychiatric and substance-abusing smokers. Using a secondary analysis of the Hurt et al. (158) study, Hayford et al. (1586) found that bupropion SR was equally efficacious for smoking cessation in individuals with or without a history of major depression or alcoholism. Similarly, Cox et al. (454), in a multicenter, randomized, double-blind relapse prevention trial of bupropion (300 mg/day) with 784 smokers, found bupropion to be effective regardless of whether patients had a history of depression or not. Finally, Chengappa et al. (458) found good rates of response to an open-label trial of bupropion for smoking cessation in 25 smokers with remitted major depression who were receiving maintenance SSRI, with 8 of the 25 (32%) subjects stopping smoking at the end of the 9-week trial. These findings suggest that bupropion's actions on nicotine dependence are independent of its antidepressant effects.

Bupropion SR has also been evaluated in three trials of patients with schizophrenia and nicotine dependence, including an open-label trial of 300 mg/day (415) and placebo-controlled trials of 150 (704) and 300 (414) mg/day. Weiner et al. (415) conducted a 26-week open-label trial of bupropion SR (300 mg/day), with 14 weeks of initial group CBT in eight patients with schizophrenia and nicotine dependence. Although none of the patients quit smoking during the trial, they did decrease their cigarette use, as indicated by an overall reduction (about 40%) in expired carbon monoxide levels at the end of the trial compared with pretrial levels. Of the four patients who chose to continue bupropion treatment for an additional 12 weeks after the trial, one stopped smoking completely, two had further decreases in expired carbon monoxide levels, and one maintained the decrease attained during the trial. In additional, negative symptoms of schizophrenia were reduced by bupropion during the trial, but this finding was not significant.

In a 12-week double-blind, placebo-controlled trial, Evins and colleagues (704) added bupropion SR or placebo to concurrent CBT for 18 patients with schizophrenia and nicotine dependence. Compared with placebo, treatment with bupropion led to an approximately 40%–50% reduction in carbon monoxide levels by the end of the trial. In addition, one of the nine subjects in the bupropion group versus none of the nine subjects in the placebo group achieved smoking cessation by the end of the trial. Both the positive and negative symptoms of schizophrenia were found to be reduced by bupropion during the trial.

In the third study, George et al. (414) conducted a 10-week double-blind, placebo-controlled trial of bupropion SR (300 mg/day) in 32 nicotine-dependent smokers with schizophrenia or schizoaffective disorder. All subjects received weekly group therapy emphasizing motivational enhancement, relapse prevention, and social skills training. Trial endpoint cessation rates (confirmed by a carbon monoxide level <10 ppm) were 50% (8 of 16) in the bupropion group and 12.5% (2 of 16) in the placebo group ($p<0.05$). Positive symptoms of schizophrenia were not affected, but negative symptom scores were reduced by about 15% in the bupropion group. In addition, treatment with a second- versus a first-generation antipsychotic medication strongly predicted success in smoking cessation in patients with schizophrenia.

The results from these preliminary placebo-controlled trials of bupropion suggest that smoking reduction and cessation are possible in patients with schizophrenia, exacerbation of psychotic symptoms is unlikely, and negative symptoms of schizophrenia may be reduced. With endpoint cessation rates of 11%–50%, bupropion may be more effective at higher doses (300 vs. 150 mg/day) in this population.

(3) Side effects

The primary side effects reported with bupropion administration in cigarette smokers are headache, nausea and vomiting, insomnia, and activation, most of which occur during the first week of treatment, although insomnia can persist (158, 159, 795, 1587–1590). Seizures are of exceedingly low occurrence (<0.5%) at doses of ≤300 mg/day, but a history of seizures or a seizure disorder would suggest a need for caution in prescribing bupropion (795, 1590). In addition, the use of bupropion is not recommended in individuals with a past or particularly a current diagnosis of an eating disorder because one study found an increased risk of generalized tonic-clonic (grand mal) seizures in bupropion-treated patients with bulimia (1591). The risk of hypertension with bupropion is <1% in smokers but may be higher in combination with an NRT (159).

(4) Implementation of bupropion therapy

For the treatment of nicotine dependence, the target dose of bupropion is 300 mg/day, taken in two doses of 150 mg each. Bupropion is started 7 days before the target quit date at 150 mg/day and, after 4–5 days, the dose is increased to 150 mg b.i.d. Currently there are few data as to which subgroups of smokers may benefit most for treatment with bupropion, although smokers with depressive symptoms may benefit from the medication's antidepressant properties independent of its efficacy in treating nicotine dependence.

c) Nortriptyline

Nortriptyline is a TCA that has been shown to be superior to placebo for smoking cessation in randomized, double-blind, placebo-controlled trials (456, 795, 814, 815, 1592) and to have comparable efficacy to bupropion (795, 814, 1579). Some evidence suggests that its benefits persist for up to a year of treatment (895) and that its efficacy can be augmented by concomitant use of the nicotine patch (455); however, data on adding psychosocial therapies to nortriptyline treatment are mixed (456, 895, 1579).

Nortriptyline's mechanism of action in treating nicotine dependence is unclear, although the medication does block reuptake of norepinephrine and serotonin and may have indirect effects on dopamine (816). In addition, its mechanism in nicotine dependence may be distinct from its mechanism in treating depression, because its efficacy in smoking cessation is unrelated to the presence or absence of depressive symptoms or major depressive disorder (456, 795, 815, 816).

Side effects of nortriptyline are frequent (455, 815, 816) and include anticholinergic effects (e.g., dry mouth, blurred vision, constipation, tachycardia, and urinary hesitancy or retention), sedation, orthostatic hypotension, and cardiac conduction changes (817). The toxicity of nortriptyline in overdose amounts also needs to be taken into consideration when prescribing this medication. Nevertheless, nortriptyline appears to have some utility in smokers and can be recommended as a second-line agent after NRT and bupropion, although further study of this agent is necessary.

d) Clonidine

Clonidine is a presynaptic α_2-adrenergic agonist that dampens sympathetic activity originating at the locus coeruleus (602, 749, 1593). Because of its suggested efficacy for alcohol and opioid withdrawal, it was tried with nicotine withdrawal as well (749, 1593). Several clinical trials have used oral or transdermal clonidine in doses of 0.1–0.4 mg/day for 2–6 weeks with and without behavioral therapy; a meta-analysis of these trials suggested that clonidine is efficacious (818). In general, however, the effects of clonidine have not been as robust as the effects of NRTs or bupropion. The most common side effects of clonidine treatment are dry mouth, sedation, and constipation (818, 819, 1594). Postural hypotension, rebound hypertension, and depression are rare when clonidine is used for smoking cessation treatment (1594).

e) Other pharmacotherapies

A number of other pharmacotherapies for nicotine dependence have been studied, but there is insufficient evidence to support their use. Mecamylamine, an oral antihypertensive agent, is a noncompetitive ion channel blocker of high-affinity CNS and peripheral nicotinic receptors (820, 821, 1595) that decreases the positive subjective effects from cigarettes. In several small trials (820, 821), it was shown to result in an initial increase but a subsequent decrease in cigarette use. It has been postulated that naltrexone, the long-acting oral form of the short-acting intravenous opioid antagonist naloxone, would be useful in treating nicotine dependence because the performance-enhancing and other positive effects of nicotine may be opioid mediated (1596). Although one preliminary study showed benefits of naltrexone in combination with nicotine patch therapy (1597), naltrexone did not appear to decrease smoking in other studies (603, 822) and may even have increased smoking in some individuals (749, 1598). Buspirone, a 5-HT_{1A} receptor partial agonist anxiolytic agent, has been noted to improve short-term smoking cessation rates in a general population of smokers; it improved abstinence in high-anxiety smokers in one study (1599) but not in another (823, 1600). The alkaloid lobeline, which appears to have dopamine reuptake blockade and nicotinic receptor antagonist properties (1601), was evaluated in a 6-week, randomized, double-blind, placebo-controlled, multicenter trial but did not produce any differences in smoking cessation rates (1602). Thus, there is little evidence that these diverse pharmacotherapies are useful for smoking cessation.

In addition to bupropion and nortriptyline, other antidepressive agents have been studied in nicotine-dependent patients. The available evidence gives little support for the use of SSRIs to assist in smoking cessation, either alone (1603, 1604) or in combination with NRT (1605, 1606). Although possible benefits have been found for the monoamine oxidase A inhibitor moclobemide (1607) and the monoamine oxidase B inhibitor selegiline hydrochloride (1608) for smoking cessation, larger trials of these agents are warranted. At the present time there is no evidence that other antidepressants are efficacious in treating nicotine dependence (795).

f) Somatic treatments

Acupuncture is often proposed for use in nicotine dependence, with the rationale that it may release endorphins that assist in smoking cessation. The efficacy of auricular acupuncture has been supported by some (786) but not other (1609) studies. The results of two more recent controlled studies (785, 1610) suggest that active versus sham acupuncture can lead to short- and long-term reduction in cigarette smoking but not smoking cessation. In addition, a meta-analysis of multiple other smaller studies of acupuncture has found no evidence for acupuncture efficacy in smoking cessation (788). In accordance with these results, acupuncture cannot be recommended as a treatment for smoking cessation.

Other somatic treatments that have been proposed include black pepper extracts (1611), capsaicin (1612), denicotinized tobacco (1613–1615), cigarette flavorings (1616), regenerated (denicotinized) smoke (1617), and citric acid inhaler (1618, 1619), all of which decrease cigarette craving or withdrawal symptoms or provide a substitute for the satisfaction from cigarettes in laboratory tests. However, none of these modalities have been sufficiently studied to recommend their use.

Cigarette filters have also been used to help smokers gradually reduce the amount of nicotine inhalation; however, studies of the efficacy of filters are inconclusive (1620, 1621), and smokers may to some extent adjust the frequency or depth of inhalation to compensate for such changes (1620, 1621). Thus, there is insufficient evidence to recommend filters as a treatment at this time.

2. Psychosocial treatments

a) Goals

The goals of psychosocial therapies for nicotine dependence include 1) providing individuals with the necessary skills to initiate abstinence, 2) teaching skills to avoid relapse to tobacco use in high-risk situations, 3) supporting and extending the effects of proven pharmacotherapies for nicotine dependence, and 4) facilitating a transition toward eventual smoking abstinence in smokers who are unable to quit immediately.

b) Efficacy

Psychosocial therapies appear to be effective treatments for nicotine dependence either alone or in combination with pharmacotherapies. The descriptive (827, 1580, 1622) and meta-analytic (720, 824–826, 828) reviews of psychosocial interventions for smoking cessation provide more information on efficacy.

c) Side effects

The side effects of psychosocial therapies for smoking cessation are considered minimal. Some factors should be taken into account when more intensive psychosocial therapies are considered, including their length and intensity. For these reasons, the majority (about 95%) of smokers do not desire or tolerate psychosocial therapies beyond minimal interventions.

d) Implementation

Although pharmacotherapy (bupropion or NRT) is recommended for all patients, a stepped-care approach in implementing psychosocial treatments for smoking cessation in general medical populations is recommended; thus, in initial smoking cessation attempts, social support and brief interventions (e.g., brief counseling, telephone support) should be tried first (826). If they are ineffective, more intensive behavioral treatments can be considered because there is a strong association between the intensity (826) and duration (895) of tobacco dependence counseling and its effectiveness. This strategy of a stepped-care approach to psychosocial treatment is supported by the fact that most smokers will continue to seek treatment despite repeated unsuccessful attempts at abstaining from smoking (1623, 1624).

Both group and individual formats of psychosocial therapies have been used for smoking cessation (720, 721, 742); groups can increase social support and individual treatment can address the particular problems of the smoker. In terms of the format of interventions, it is not clear whether individual or group psychosocial treatments are superior to one another; this may depend on the subtype of smoker and/or the treatment setting. Although studies of matching therapies to particular types of smokers have been published (1625, 1626), at present there are insufficient data to recommend specific matching strategies. Thus, patient preference should be considered when recommending group or individual treatment or when choosing a specific psychosocial treatment approach.

Because nearly 67% of patients relapse in the first week after a smoking cessation attempt (698, 794), most treatment is timed to occur over the few weeks immediately before and after the quit date (742). The most common providers of psychosocial therapies for smoking cessation are self-help groups (e.g., Nicotine Anonymous), state health departments, community organizations (e.g., American Cancer Society, American Lung Association), wellness programs, clinics for the treatment of substance use disorders, or health educators and psychologists in health care organizations (172). However, some treatments may not be available or be available only intermittently to patients, be costly, and not be integrated into the health care system. Consequently, many of those motivated to quit smoking forgo psychosocial therapy (172).

e. Specific techniques

The specific psychosocial interventions that have been evaluated for the treatment of nicotine dependence are described below.

(1) Social support

A number of studies have demonstrated the effectiveness of social supports (e.g., buddy systems, partner support) as treatments for smoking cessation (718, 826, 830–833). In some research, social support has been provided as an active intervention, whereas in other studies the supportiveness of a spouse or partner has been assessed independently without a specific intervention occurring (829). Interventions to enhance the degree of support provided by a spouse or partner have not produced significant differences in support levels and, not surprisingly, have not influenced smoking cessation rates (1627). Nevertheless, the effect of social support as an active intervention is significant, and it is thus recommended as a treatment for smoking cessation.

(2) Brief therapies

Several studies in controlled settings have documented that smoking cessation rates can be augmented by minimal behavioral interventions such as community support groups (845) and telephone counseling (846, 847). MET, which is often a component of brief interventions, encourages the smoker to weigh the reasons for and against quitting, thereby facilitating a choice of whether to quit or not. Several studies have suggested that brief interventions may be effective in promoting confidence in smoking cessation and treatment retention, even when cessation rates do not seem to be significantly improved (639, 834, 1628). In addition, training programs for physicians in basic behavioral counseling to support cessation may lead to enhanced cessation rates simply because physicians are more likely to engage patients in a discussion about smoking cessation (835). Such brief interventions also seem to have efficacy in promoting smoking cessation in hospitalized medical patients (836, 837), although this was not true across all studies (855). Thus, there is good evidence to recommend brief interventions in smokers making initial attempts at cessation and without prior unsuccessful treatment (826, 828).

(3) Behavioral therapies

Behavioral therapy is based on the theory that learning processes operate in the development, maintenance, and cessation of smoking. There have been >100 controlled prospective studies verifying the efficacy of behavioral therapy (720, 734, 735, 838). Behavioral therapies are typically a multimodal package of several specific treatments. In most reviews and meta-analyses, 6-month quit rates with behavioral therapy packages have been 20%–25%, and groups treated with behavioral therapy typically have had a twofold increase in quit rates as compared with control groups (718–720, 734, 735, 824, 825, 838, 1620). These cessation rates with behavioral therapy are similar to long-term outcomes obtained with medications such as NRTs and bupropion. Given this large database of efficacy, multimodal behavioral therapy is a recommended first-line treatment.

Several specific types of behavioral therapies have also been studied, but none are recommended at the present time. With contingency management, which has some evidence for short-term efficacy, behaviors consistent with smoking cessation are reinforced by giving a reward (e.g., money, vouchers) when patients are abstinent and denying them the same rewards if they are not (1629). However, once the contingencies are removed, smoking tends to return quickly. Thus, contingency management approaches might be best indicated in settings where a finite period of smoking abstinence is needed (e.g., during pregnancy, before surgical procedures). In addition, these techniques are probably best combined with CBT strategies.

Cue exposure involves repeatedly exposing patients to real or imagined situations that evoke potent urges to smoke to extinguish the ability of these situations to evoke these urges (1630–1633). Controlled studies (718), however, do not support the efficacy of cue exposure.

In aversion therapy, patients are asked to engage in "rapid smoking," in which inhaling cigarette smoke every few seconds produces a state of mild nicotine intoxication accompanied by nausea, dizziness, tremors, and other symptoms that will negatively reinforce smoking behavior (693, 734, 735). This technique has shown efficacy in many controlled studies, and most reviews and meta-analyses have concluded that rapid smoking is efficacious; however, the available studies have had methodological problems (1634) and adherence to the technique is low (718, 719, 734, 735, 741, 742, 838).

(4) Cognitive-behavioral therapies

For smokers who have failed initial treatments, the use of more specialized and higher-intensity behavioral treatments such as CBT in combination with NRT or bupropion is recommended. In CBT, patients anticipate situations where they are likely to smoke (e.g., at a party, during an argument) and plan strategies to cope with these situations without smoking. Behavioral coping includes removing oneself from the situation, substituting other behaviors (e.g., walking, exercising), or using skills (e.g., assertiveness, refusal skills, time management) to manage triggers. Cognitive coping includes identifying maladaptive thoughts, challenging them, and substituting more effective thought patterns (e.g., reminding oneself of why it is important to stop smoking or that the urge will pass) or trying to prevent a slip from becoming a relapse (e.g., not viewing the slip as a catastrophe). Some degree of efficacy of CBT has been demonstrated in smokers with a history of depression, alcohol dependence, and substance abuse (456, 459,

841–844). CBT has also demonstrated some degree of efficacy in addressing weight concerns associated with smoking cessation (840). However, differences in study design and control groups make comparisons of the studies difficult.

(5) Self-guided therapies

The major goals of self-help materials and procedures are to increase a smoker's motivation to quit and to teach smoking cessation skills. Most self-help materials are behaviorally oriented, and written manuals are the most common form of self-help material, although computer and video versions have also been developed (856, 859). In controlled settings, computer-generated tailored self-help materials (848, 849, 852, 853) can augment smoking cessation rates in those who adhere to the self-help program. Whether self-help interventions used without additional contact or support increase smoking cessation is debatable (720, 734, 735, 742, 838, 851, 859, 1451). Self-help materials appear to be more effective in patients who are less nicotine dependent (860, 1635) and more motivated (859). The use of multiple modes of therapy (e.g., written materials plus phone contact) appears to enhance the effectiveness of self-help (721, 856, 859). Tailoring materials to the specific needs and concerns of each patient also appears helpful (736, 851, 860). Telephone counseling in response to smokers' calls to a hot line appears to increase cessation when added to other self-help interventions (856–858), and meta-analyses suggest a small positive effect for such combined support (718, 720).

(6) Other therapies

A number of other therapies have been studied in small samples or used in clinical settings. One well-controlled randomized study provided evidence that exercise may assist with the prevention of smoking relapse and weight gain related to cessation (1636); however, another did not (863). In fact, a recent meta-analysis found that only 1 out of 11 studies examining the effects of exercise for smoking cessation had positive results; most of these studies were of small sample size and insufficient design (864). Nonetheless, it is recommended that exercise and increased activity be encouraged in smokers attempting to quit or who have recently quit smoking. Biofeedback, 12-step programs, family therapy, and psychodynamic therapies for the treatment of nicotine dependence have been minimally studied, and scientific evidence for their use is limited. Nevertheless, there is clinical consensus that such therapies may be useful in some patients.

Stimulus control is probably best used in the context of multicomponent therapies. It involves initially removing or avoiding cues associated with smoking to reduce urges to smoke. These strategies include discarding cigarettes; removing ashtrays, lighters, and matches; avoiding smokers; and avoiding situations associated with smoking. There is some support for the effectiveness of these techniques alone (718), but they require further study.

Physiological feedback, which presumes that abstinence will be reinforced by giving smokers immediate positive feedback about the decline in carbon monoxide levels when they stop smoking (718), has also been assessed. Although the rationale behind physiological feedback seems logical, actual findings are weak.

Gradual cessation procedures require smokers to gradually reduce the nicotine yield of their cigarettes by 1) increasing the time between cigarettes, 2) switching to cigarette brands with a lower nicotine content, or 3) using graduated filters ("faders") to progressively reduce the delivery of nicotine from the same brand of cigarettes (743, 1637). However, evidence for the efficacy of these treatments in improving quit rates is mixed, and meta-analyses have not supported their efficacy (718, 719).

Relaxation techniques are often taught to smokers to help them manage relapse situations that are associated with anxiety. Although often used in multicomponent programs, relaxation itself has not been shown to increase smoking cessation in most studies (734, 735, 741, 742, 1620) or in a meta-analysis (718). There is also little scientific validation for the effectiveness of hypnotherapies for smoking cessation, despite the fact that they are commonly used by individuals who wish to stop smoking.

B. ALCOHOL-RELATED DISORDERS

1. Treatment settings

Studies of specific settings for the treatment of alcohol-related disorders have been relatively limited. Such studies may also be subject to selection bias in terms of the characteristics of patients willing to be randomized to different treatment settings (1638).

Most (52, 1639–1641) but not all (1303) studies that have randomly assigned patients to different levels of treatment have not found an advantage for inpatient care over less restrictive settings. However, for safety reasons, these studies have been required to exclude from randomization individuals who would ordinarily be considered to require inpatient treatment (1642). For example, the study by Hayashida et al. (48) randomly assigned alcohol-dependent patients coming to a VA hospital to inpatient or outpatient detoxification but excluded those who required hospitalization for medical reasons. However, those excluded were only 10% of the population applying to this clinic. Another study among male veterans (1643) showed that the mortality rates for individuals with an alcohol use disorder 3 years after discharge varied with the initial treatment setting. Veterans who completed inpatient rehabilitation had the lowest mortality rate, whereas those in the following groups had an increasingly high mortality rate, respectively: 1) those who had at least 6 days of inpatient treatment (but did not complete the program), 2) those who were admitted for brief detoxification lasting <5 days, and 3) those who received no specific treatment for their alcohol use disorder. This study provided preliminary evidence that more intensive treatment may lower the mortality associated with a chronic alcohol use disorder. However, patients in this study were not randomly assigned to treatment conditions, so it is possible that self-selection influenced the results.

Some evidence suggests that longer treatment stays and treatment completion may be associated with better outcomes (959, 1304). This probably reflects the fact that more motivated patients are more likely to stay in treatment and have better outcomes, because differences in outcome are not typically observed when patients are randomly assigned to shorter versus longer treatments (51, 956).

Other evidence suggests that the association between treatment setting and outcome may be a complex one that is influenced by the characteristics and treatment needs of the individual patient. Magura et al. (965) studied a cohort of 248 patients who were newly admitted to inpatient rehabilitation or intensive or regular outpatient care and determined whether they were naturalistically matched or mismatched to care according to ASAM patient placement criteria. At 3 months after intake, individuals who received regular outpatient care when intensive outpatient care would have been recommended as more appropriate had poorer drinking outcomes. In individuals who received residential as compared with intensive outpatient treatment, there also was a trend for a better outcome. Rychtarik et al. (966) also examined individual factors that might determine the appropriateness of a given treatment setting for an individual patient. They found that individuals with a high level of involvement with alcohol and lower cognitive abilities had better outcomes when treated in inpatient settings, whereas those with lower levels of alcohol involvement did better in outpatient settings.

2. Pharmacological treatments for withdrawal

Benzodiazepines are effective in treating alcohol withdrawal symptoms, particularly when compared with placebo in the prevention of withdrawal seizures (991, 992, 995). In preventing seizures, benzodiazepines appear comparable in efficacy to anticonvulsants, although the significant heterogeneity of relevant clinical trials makes comparisons difficult (995). Nevertheless, meta-analyses have consistently demonstrated the benefits of benzodiazepines in treating alcohol withdrawal. One meta-analysis (992) examined 134 studies, including 65 prospective controlled trials involving 42 different medications. This analysis concluded that benzodiazepines reduce withdrawal severity and the incidence of seizures and delirium (992). Another meta-analysis of 11 randomized, controlled trials found benzodiazepines to be superior to placebo, with no study demonstrating that any other class of agent, including beta-blockers, carbamazepine, and clonidine, was more beneficial than benzodiazepines (991). Most recently, Ntais et al. (995) analyzed 57 trials that included a total of 4,051 people and concluded that benzodiazepines are effective against alcohol withdrawal symptoms when compared with placebo.

Evidence from multiple randomized, controlled trials also supports the use of symptom-triggered therapy, with symptom-triggered detoxification protocols leading to less use of medication as well as shorter duration of treatment than fixed-dose protocols (998, 1001–1003). An additional clinical trial of outpatient detoxification using chlordiazepoxide prescribed according to a symptom-triggered detoxification protocol showed that, on average, patients received 167 mg of the medication over 2.7 days and 85% completed the protocol (1644); however, this study did not use a randomized, placebo-controlled design.

One randomized, double-blind, placebo-controlled study compared lorazepam with placebo for the prevention of recurrent seizures related to alcohol withdrawal (1005). This study found that treatment with intravenous lorazepam was associated with a significant reduction in the risk of recurrent seizures related to alcohol.

One meta-analysis (992) considered four randomized, controlled trials of carbamazepine and concluded that carbamazepine was superior to placebo and equal in efficacy to phenobarbital and oxazepam for patients with mild to moderate withdrawal. Another study compared the efficacy of carbamazepine and lorazepam for detoxification in patients with more than one previous detoxification for alcohol withdrawal compared with those with one or no previous alcohol withdrawals (977, 1019). The authors found that healthy middle-age male outpatients randomized to carbamazepine or lorazepam had comparable outcomes in terms of symptoms of alcohol withdrawal. However, carbamazepine was superior to lorazepam in preventing rebound withdrawal symptoms and reducing posttreatment drinking, especially among those with multiple past detoxifications (977).

With respect to the use of other anticonvulsants for detoxification, one recent review concluded that there is no current evidence that divalproex sodium is effective in treating alcohol withdrawal (987), but one study demonstrated that divalproex sodium used as adjunctive pharmacotherapy with oxazepam reduced the total amount of oxazepam needed for detoxification (994). There have been two other open-label trials of divalproex to treat alcohol withdrawal: one compared divalproex with lorazepam in 11 patients and concluded that divalproex ameliorated alcohol withdrawal symptoms and decreased the amount of lorazepam needed for detoxification (1020), and another found that valproate was as effective as phenobarbital in managing acute withdrawal (1018).

Studies of adrenergic agents have been quite small, limiting the generalizability of their conclusions. For example, one randomized, controlled trial of 37 male patients admitted for uncomplicated detoxification compared diazepam 10 mg p.o. with propranolol 20 mg p.o., repeating the medication dose every 4 hours for continued withdrawal symptoms (1645). The patients randomized to diazepam or propranolol showed improvements in blood pressure level, pulse rate, and withdrawal tremors. However, one subject in the propranolol group had a withdrawal seizure, whereas no subject randomized to diazepam manifested a withdrawal seizure or hallucinations. Another study compared intravenous diazepam, clonidine, and alprazolam treatment of alcohol withdrawal and found diazepam was more effective than clonidine and placebo for some measures of withdrawal (1646).

3. Pharmacological treatments for dependence and abuse

a) Naltrexone

(1) Goals

The goals of pharmacotherapy for alcohol dependence can be multifaceted. Medications may help maintain or improve abstinence, reduce heavy alcohol consumption, decrease relapse rates to heavy drinking, or more generically reduce craving, an intermediary step to the above clinical goals.

(2) Efficacy

It is thought that alcohol exerts its rewarding, euphoric, and subsequent craving effects, at least in part, by stimulating opiate receptors. Naltrexone, an opiate receptor antagonist, blocks this effect. Alternatively, opiate receptor antagonism may play a role in diminishing the rewarding aspects of alcohol-induced dopamine release. Naltrexone is one of the most widely studied medications for the treatment of alcohol dependence, with randomized, controlled clinical trials having been performed not only in the United States but also in many European countries and Australia. Most published studies have evaluated naltrexone against placebo for its ability to promote abstinence, reduce heavy drinking days, and decrease rates of relapse. Enough data from randomized, controlled trials have been published to allow for several meta-analyses (e.g., references 152, 153). These meta-analyses concluded that naltrexone was more efficacious than placebo across most of the drinking outcome variables referred to above.

This advantage of naltrexone is small to moderate, with effect sizes of 0.1–0.5 and/or relative risk decreases of 10%–14% depending on the drinking measure. It also appears from research studies and clinical experience that some patients respond to naltrexone and others do not. It has been suggested that a family history of alcoholism, genetic differences in opiate alleles (1647), and high levels of craving may be predictive of naltrexone response. However, when evaluating published studies on naltrexone, there are two significant issues to consider: patient adherence to treatment and the concomitant psychosocial intervention used.

The role of medication adherence was emphasized by Pettinati et al. (1648) in their reanalysis of data from several clinical trials completed at their site. In that review, they observed a marked difference in naltrexone response between patients who adhered to the medication regimen and those who did not. This finding has led others to evaluate the factors that predict adherence to naltrexone treatment among alcohol-dependent subjects (1513). These authors and others (1649) have suggested that high levels of side effects during the first several weeks of treatment reduces adherence and that higher craving levels at study entry, as well as a greater belief in naltrexone's efficacy, may predict better medication adherence. Day-to-day fluctuations in patient motivation to take naltrexone may be overcome through the use of a long-acting injectable form of the medication. This formulation has been designed to release a small amount of naltrexone in the first few days (1650) and has been shown to have good tolerability in a multisite study (24 sites with 624 subjects) without dose titration or initial oral naltrexone (1044).

Several studies (187, 1039) have indicated that naltrexone works best when combined with a relapse prevention (coping skills, CBT) approach. This observation is supported by other studies (1038, 1041). In general, when naltrexone was given to more severely alcohol-dependent subjects without a concomitant defined relapse prevention intervention, its efficacy was less robust (1045) or nonexistent (1043).

The FDA approved naltrexone for use in treating alcohol dependence in 1994 based on several small single-site studies (187, 1037). Although the results from a number of single-site and small multisite studies from several countries have supported the utility of naltrexone (954, 1038–1041) in intent-to-treat analyses, those from a few larger multisite studies have been negative (1042, 1043). In one multisite randomized, controlled trial (1043), 627 predominantly male alcohol-dependent veterans were treated for up to 52 weeks with 50 mg naltrexone or placebo. Participants also received TSF and other treatment "as usual." The results showed that compared with placebo, naltrexone had no effect on abstinence rates, number of days to relapse, percentage of drinking days, or number of drinks per drinking day. In this trial there were several differences compared with other naltrexone studies that had positive results; the most significant of these were 1) the subjects were older and more severely affected by alcohol, 2) the background psychosocial intervention (TSF) may have been more varied, 3) the dropout rate was slightly higher, and 4) there was more variability inherent in this multisite study when compared with single-site studies.

In a 12-week German multisite study (1042), 171 "detoxified" alcoholic subjects from seven centers were treated with 50 mg/day naltrexone and at least 1 hour a week of psychosocial intervention "as usual." There was no statistical difference between naltrexone and placebo on time to first heavy drinking episode, time to first drink, or overall alcohol consumption or craving. However, the naltrexone group had a statistically significant reduction in γ-glutamyl transpeptidase (a liver enzyme measured in blood that serves as a marker of heavy alcohol consumption) compared with placebo. These study results need to be interpreted cautiously, however, because 1) the average participant was abstinent for almost 20 days before starting naltrexone and the relapse rate overall was lower than that in most other studies, 2) the psychosocial treatment was not standardized, and 3) the dropout rate was relatively high (33%–38%).

(3) Side effects

Naltrexone's side effects have generally been moderate at the 50-mg dose used in most studies, and have included gastrointestinal problems (nausea, vomiting, abdominal pain) and CNS-related symptoms (headache, fatigue). The U.S. product label (as described in the *Physicians' Desk Reference*) warns that significant hepatoxicity may occur with naltrexone. This complication has been observed mostly in morbidly obese subjects receiving higher doses of naltrexone, whereas many clinical trials, including a safety study conducted for FDA review (1046), did not observe significant hepatoxicity. However, a more recent report (1047) describing an interaction between NSAIDs and high-dose naltrexone (>100 mg/day) that leads to hepatoxicity should be noted. Although the exact risk of this interaction is unknown, clinicians should use high doses of naltrexone cautiously and warn their patients of this potentially dangerous medication interaction.

(4) Implementation issues

To minimize any potential interaction of side effects caused by naltrexone and those normally occurring during alcohol withdrawal, a few days of alcohol abstinence should be achieved before naltrexone is initiated. In general, naltrexone is begun at 25 mg/day for a few days, followed by an increase in the dose to 50 mg/day, as tolerated. A gradual dose increase might reduce the gastrointestinal side effects that occasionally emerge early in treatment and generally moderate over time. Women might be more sensitive to the gastrointestinal effects of naltrexone and could be especially aided by a slower titration. At this time, there is no strong evidence that naltrexone doses of >50 mg/day are more efficacious, but some individual cases of greater efficacy at higher doses have been noted. Clearly explaining to patients the potential mild adverse effects of naltrexone and the tendency of these effects to improve over time and providing motivational enhancement to promote patient adherence to medication and alcohol reduction/abstinence may all lead to improved patient cooperation with medication and psychosocial treatments. Although it is not clear how specific psychosocial interventions interact with naltrexone, there is good evidence that relapse prevention therapies (e.g., CBT, coping skills) may allow naltrexone to have its maximal effect.

Because naltrexone is an opiate antagonist, individuals abusing opiates may experience opiate withdrawal when treatment is initiated, and those taking opiates for analgesic effects will find them ineffective during naltrexone treatment. Therefore, a complete medication history and urine toxicology screen for opiate medication may be indicated before naltrexone therapy is initiated. In addition, caution should be taken if acute opiate analgesia is required during the course of treatment. For example, higher doses of opiates may be required, in which case the signs of respiratory distress should be monitored and treated appropriately. The naltrexone-treated patient should carry a card explaining these issues and provide it to health care personnel in an emergency.

b) Disulfiram

(1) Goals

The goal of treatment with disulfiram is to enhance the motivation of abstinent alcoholic individuals to resist alcohol consumption. Pretreatment with disulfiram establishes the conditions in which the subsequent use of alcohol will result in a toxic and highly aversive reaction. In theory, this knowledge should improve the patient's cognitive control over any urge to drink.

(2) Efficacy

Disulfiram inhibits the activity of aldehyde dehydrogenase, the enzyme that metabolizes acetaldehyde, a major metabolite of alcohol. The usual therapeutic dose is 250 mg/day, although some patients achieve optimal benefit at either a higher or a lower dose (range 125–500 mg/day). In the presence of disulfiram, alcohol consumption results in the accumulation of toxic levels of acetaldehyde, which in turn produces a host of unpleasant signs and symptoms including a sensation of heat in the face and neck, headache, flushing, nausea, vomiting, hypotension, and anxiety. Chest pain, seizures, liver dysfunction, respiratory depression, cardiac arrhythmias, myocardial infarction, and death have also been reported.

Controlled trials have not demonstrated any advantage of disulfiram over placebo in achieving total abstinence, delaying relapse, or improving employment status or social stability (1048, 1049). However, some clinicians believe that this medication, when combined with other therapeutic interventions, has benefit for some individuals who remain employed and socially stable (150, 1048, 1050–1052). Treatment effectiveness is enhanced when adherence is encouraged through frequent behavioral monitoring (e.g., breath tests), group support for remaining abstinent (e.g., group therapy, AA) (1053), contingency contracting, or, where feasible, supervised administration of disulfiram. Patients who are intelligent, motivated, and not impulsive and whose drinking is often triggered by unanticipated internal or external cues that increase alcohol craving are the best candidates for disulfiram treatment. Poor candidates might include patients who are impulsive, have poor judgment, or have a co-occurring psychiatric disorder (e.g., schizophrenia) that is severe enough to make the patient unreliable or self-destructive (149, 1060). However, some patients with schizophrenia might be able to use disulfiram correctly while under active maintenance with antipsychotics (363).

(3) Side effects

Disulfiram can cause a variety of adverse effects; hepatotoxicity and neuropathies with use of this medication are rare but potentially severe. In patients with moderate to severe hepatic dysfunction, peripheral neuropathies, pregnancy, renal failure, or cardiac disease, disulfiram should be used cautiously and potential benefits and risks for the individual patient should be considered (1048). Because one of the metabolites of disulfiram inhibits dopamine beta-hydroxylase, resulting in increased levels of dopamine, there is a theoretical risk of augmenting psychotic symptoms (409, 410). Thus, patients with a psychotic disorder should be observed for evidence of a worsening psychosis if treated with disulfiram.

(4) Implementation issues

Understanding and explaining disulfiram's toxic or lethal effects to patients are a prerequisite for its use (1056–1058), so it should never be used without the patient's knowledge and consent. Patients taking disulfiram must be advised to avoid all forms of ethanol (including, for example, that found in cough syrup). In addition, disulfiram interferes with the metabolism of many medications, including TCAs, so that care must be taken to avoid toxicity (1651).

c) Acamprosate

(1) Goals

The goal of using a medication like acamprosate is to decrease the relapse rate to any drinking after an initial abstinence period has been achieved. It may work best in combination with a psychosocial intervention that promotes and facilitates abstinence.

(2) Efficacy

In 2004, the FDA approved acamprosate for the treatment of alcohol dependence, primarily based on data derived from European studies (reviewed in references 1062, 1063). Although the neuropharmacological action of acamprosate is not completely known, it is an amino acid derivative of taurine that is thought to work at brain glutamate receptor sites. In general, it is thought to stabilize glutamatergic function (155). As such, it has been hypothesized that it normalizes an aberrant glutamate system present during early abstinence that might be the basis of protracted withdrawal and craving during that period (1064).

European studies evaluating patients who generally started on acamprosate while in a hospitalized setting and were abstinent for at least 7–10 days have shown that with acamprosate treatment, there is an increase in the number of patients who maintain abstinence. Those who relapse have more abstinent time before their first drinking day and also more overall abstinent days during a year or more of treatment (1062, 1063). In contrast, a multisite trial completed in the United States did not find acamprosate to be effective in a primary intent-to-treat analysis, but it did find that when subjects' motivation to maintain abstinence and adhere to medication was taken into account, acamprosate was more effective than placebo in increasing the number of abstinent days (1067). The U.S. trial included outpatients who had a varied number of abstinent days before medication initiation, but, in general, overall pretreatment abstinent time was much shorter than that in the European trials. Also, in the U.S. trial, subjects received standardized medical management counseling, whereas in the European studies (1062, 1063) traditional psychosocial alcohol treatment approaches focusing on the maintenance of abstinence were generally used. It would appear that acamprosate is most effective in patients who have achieved a number of days (perhaps ≥7) of abstinence before starting the medication, although this theory has not been specifically studied.

(3) Side effects

Acamprosate at the FDA-approved dosage of two 333-mg pills three times each day (total dose 1998 mg) is well tolerated, with generally self-limiting and symptomatically treated diarrhea being the main adverse effect. Liver disease should not affect its metabolism or blood levels. Because acamprosate has minimal if any negative interaction with alcohol, it is expected to be generally safe in active or relapsed drinkers.

(4) Implementation issues

It is not clear if certain subgroups of alcohol-dependent individuals will benefit from acamprosate more than others. Data from European studies and a U.S. multisite trial suggest that some days of abstinence prior to initiation of acamprosate treatment might improve efficacy. In addition, a patient's strong motivation to maintain or achieve abstinence might also improve treatment response. Acamprosate can be started at a full dose immediately. It is generally taken three times per day to maintain blood levels and avoid unnecessary gastrointestinal problems. It should be well tolerated in individuals with compromised liver function because it is metabolized and excreted primarily through the kidneys. Individuals with renal impairment should be monitored carefully when taking the medication; depending on the severity of the impairment, acamprosate might need to be avoided.

Data suggest it is safe to take acamprosate with naltrexone or disulfiram, and there are no known significant medication interactions.

d) Medications acting on the serotonin system

(1) Goals

The use of SSRIs in the treatment of alcoholism may have two distinct goals: 1) reduce drinking or promote abstinence through these medications' effect on the serotonin system, which is hypothesized to directly effect alcohol consumption (see discussion below); and 2) treat psychiatric syndromes/symptoms in alcoholic patients through the well-documented antidepressant and antianxiety effects of these agents. To the extent that anxiety and depression underlie drinking behavior, SSRI amelioration of these symptoms should lead to reduced drinking, a reduction of relapse, and the maintenance of abstinence. The selective 5-HT_3 antagonist ondansetron is thought to have effects on alcohol reward and thereby reduce alcohol consumption and promote abstinence.

(2) Efficacy

There is considerable evidence that serotonin modulates the behavioral effects of alcohol (479, 1073–1075). SSRIs augment brain serotonergic function and have been shown to reduce alcohol consumption in animals. Medications in this class include fluoxetine, sertraline, paroxetine, and citalopram.

Several randomized, double-blind, placebo-controlled human studies with nondepressed heavy drinkers found SSRIs reduce alcohol consumption by 15%–20% in the short term (4–6 weeks) (1076, 1077). The results of these initial studies suggested that these medications could have an effect in reducing alcohol consumption. However, the results could not be easily generalized to the more severely impaired alcohol-dependent person. Indeed, results of trials using SSRIs to treat patients diagnosed with alcohol dependence have been less consistent (1078). A double-blind study comparing fluoxetine treatment with placebo in which both groups received CBT found no overall difference in drinking between groups (1079). However, further analysis showed that type B alcoholic individuals, characterized by early onset of drinking, heavier alcohol dependence, and greater co-occurring psychopathology, showed less favorable drinking outcomes in response to treatment with fluoxetine than with placebo. In contrast, the type A alcoholic individuals, characterized by later onset of drinking, less severity of dependence, and less psychopathology, did appear to benefit from fluoxetine. These findings were confirmed in a 14-week placebo-controlled trial of sertraline (200 mg/day) in alcohol-dependent patients stratified by subtype (1080). At this time, the treatment of nondepressed alcoholic patients with SSRIs remains controversial and may worsen drinking behaviors in some individuals.

Based on animal studies (1082, 1083) and early clinical laboratory findings (1084), the 5-HT_3 receptor antagonist ondansetron was thought to have promise as a therapeutic agent in alcohol dependence, which led to its clinical evaluation. In a placebo-controlled outpatient trial with 71 mildly alcohol-dependent male subjects, a low dose (0.25 mg b.i.d.) but not a high dose (2.0 mg b.i.d.) of ondansetron moderately reduced alcohol consumption (1085). Using relatively low doses of ondansetron (2–32 μg/kg per day), Johnson et al. (1086) conducted a 12-week placebo-controlled clinical trial in 271 alcohol-dependent patients who also received weekly CBT. Patients with early-onset alcoholism who received ondansetron showed significant reductions in drinking (especially in the 4 μg/kg b.i.d. group) compared with those who received placebo. Patients with late-onset alcoholism had higher levels of drinking across all groups but showed no significant differences between medication and placebo treatment. The efficacy of ondansetron in the treatment of alcohol dependence in patients with early-onset alcoholism has been documented in only this single-site placebo-controlled study (1086) and in an open-label study in which the same dose of ondansetron was used (1652). Replication studies have yet to be conducted, and ondansetron has not been approved by the FDA for alcoholism treatment.

(3) Side effects

SSRIs are generally well-tolerated medications and have many patient-years of use worldwide. They appear to have a good safety profile in heavy alcohol consumers. However, some side effects of these medications clearly overlap with alcohol-related effects. The most frequent side effects of SSRIs occur in the gastrointestinal tract (nausea, diarrhea), which is also affected by alcohol, both during withdrawal and during active drinking. SSRIs have effects on the CNS (activation/sedation and headache) that also may occur during alcohol withdrawal and active drinking. Perhaps the most difficult side effects to evaluate in the alcoholic patient are potential SSRI-induced changes in libido and sexual performance. These complaints may occur during changes in alcohol consumption under normal conditions, and the differential role of SSRIs may be particularly hard to evaluate.

Ondansetron may cause some gastrointestinal disturbances, headache, and fatigue. It has been generally well tolerated at the low doses used in alcoholism trials to date.

(4) Implementation issues

Because there is an overlap of signs and symptoms of alcohol withdrawal and SSRI side effects, a few days of abstinence from alcohol and monitoring of amelioration of alcohol withdrawal effects should occur before initiating an SSRI. A more gradual titration might minimize any interaction of alcohol-related and SSRI effects.

Awareness and documentation of individual differences in sleep at baseline, which may or may not be alcohol related (334), will assist the clinician in evaluating the potential SSRI effect on sleep during treatment. For example, many alcoholic individuals drink to be able to get to sleep, so if an SSRI is causing nocturnal activation, this may not only reduce its effectiveness for alcohol treatment but also may be a reason to avoid its use. If an SSRI causes sedation during the day, this effect may be augmented by alcohol if an individual relapses.

Because SSRI-related sexual complaints overlap with alcohol-related effects, a good medical and longitudinal history of these complaints is likely to be helpful. Documentation of these issues before initiating SSRI treatment should also assist the clinician in assessing these complaints should they arise during treatment.

If ondansetron is to be prescribed, the clinician and patient must be reminded that the doses used in the published clinical trials have been an order of magnitude lower than what is generally prescribed for the treatment of nausea. Ondansetron is currently available in pill form but at a higher dose strength than that found to be efficacious in early-onset alcoholic patients. It is also available in liquid form. In either case, care must be taken to provide the correct dosing.

4. Psychosocial treatments

a) Cognitive-behavioral and relapse prevention therapies

There is abundant evidence that CBT approaches aimed at improving a patient's self-control and social skills consistently lead to reduced drinking (79, 1090, 1092–1094). Subtypes of CBT strategies have been supported with generally positive but variable degrees of success. Cognitive therapy interventions that focus on identifying and modifying maladaptive thoughts but that do not include a behavioral component have not been as effective as cognitive-behavioral treatments (1090) and were found to be effective in only 4 out of 10 studies reviewed by Miller and Wilbourne (79).

Behavioral self-control training consists of cognitive and behavioral strategies, including self-monitoring, goal setting, rewards for goal attainment, functional analysis of drinking situations, and the learning of alternative coping skills (1095, 1096). Holder et al. (1090) and Hodgeson (1097) both found that cognitive-behavioral stress management interventions were effective in the majority of studies reviewed. Although some studies of behavioral self-control training have included controlled drinking as well as abstinence as a goal for treatment, behavioral self-control techniques should be used with the explicit long-term goal of abstinence.

General self-control strategies include goal setting, self-monitoring, functional analysis of drinking antecedents, and learning alternative coping skills. Miller and Wilbourne (79) found that self-control training produced better outcomes than control treatments in 17 of 35 studies.

In several studies, increases in coping responses or "self-efficacy" (1098) at the end of treatment predicted better drinking outcomes during follow-up (184, 1099, 1100). Individuals who report more frequent use of cognitive or behavioral strategies aimed at problem solving or mastery ("approach coping") typically have better drinking outcomes than those who rely on staying away from high-risk situations ("avoidant coping") (959, 1101).

Outcome studies have typically supported the efficacy of group behavioral and CBT treatments, including group marital therapy. The results of studies matching patients to treatment in which patients were randomly assigned to cognitive-behaviorally oriented treatment groups or interactional therapy groups suggest that patients with fewer antisocial personality features or with neurological impairment fare better in interactional therapy; those with higher levels of antisocial personality features and psychopathology fare better in CBT groups (1102, 1103). Litt et al. (1104), in a randomized, controlled study, also found a positive effect of matching patients to treatment strategy.

(1) Relapse prevention strategies

In a meta-analysis of relapse prevention therapies, Irvin et al. (1094) found an effect size of 0.27 for treatment of alcohol use derived from five studies.

(2) Motivational enhancement therapy

MET and motivational interviewing, brief treatments aimed at maximizing the patient's intrinsic desire to change, were found to be efficacious in 7 of 9 studies reviewed by Dunn et al. (1105) and 12 of 17 studies reviewed by Miller and Wilbourne (79). This type of treatment is typically brief, lasting 1–4 sessions, and has been frequently used to enhance adherence with more intensive or extensive subsequent treatments. The use of MET as a stand-alone treatment was most notably supported by Project MATCH (43), in which 4 sessions of MET yielded equivalent results to 12 sessions of CBT or 12 sessions of TSF as an initial treatment or care after hospitalization. Alcohol-dependent patients in all three treatments experienced substantial and enduring improvement in drinking outcomes (43, 265).

b) Behavioral therapies

Individual behavioral therapy has been found to be effective for patients with an alcohol use disorder (191, 956, 1090), particularly those treatments that emphasize positive reinforcements for targeted behaviors. Behavioral contracting was found to be effective in four of five studies reviewed by Miller and Wilbourne (79). In contrast, relaxation training, a behavioral treatment that has been widely studied, was found to be ineffective in 17 of 18 controlled trials (79).

(1) Community reinforcement

The most comprehensive behavioral approach to the treatment of patients with alcohol use disorders is the community reinforcement approach, which uses behavioral principles and usually includes conjoint therapy, training in finding a job, counseling focused on alcohol-free social and recreational activities, monitoring of disulfiram use, and an alcohol-free social club (1107).

Using random assignment to community reinforcement treatment or standard hospital treatments, Azrin (190) found that patients in the community reinforcement group drank less, spent fewer days away from home, worked more days, and were institutionalized less over a 24-month follow-up period. A second controlled study comparing 1) the community reinforcement approach, 2) disulfiram plus a behavioral adherence program, and 3) regular outpatient treatment showed that patients treated with community reinforcement did substantially better on all outcome measures than those in the other treatment conditions (190). A meta-analytic review conducted by O'Farrell and Fals-Stewart (690) documented a medium effect size for the community reinforcement approach combined with marital therapy.

(2) Aversion therapy

Compared with positive reward approaches, aversion therapies have been less successful. Only a small number of studies (12 of 28) have documented the efficacy for aversion therapy using nausea or electric shock (79).

c) Social skills training

Social skills training focuses on learning skills for forming and maintaining interpersonal relationships, being assertive, and refusing alcohol. Miller and Wilbourne (79) found social skills training to be effective in 17 out of 25 studies.

d) Psychodynamic and interpersonal therapies

Holder et al. (1090) concluded that there was little empirical evidence from controlled studies that insight-oriented psychotherapy or counseling is an effective treatment for an alcohol use disorder. Individual psychotherapy produced better outcomes than a control condition in 2 of 8 studies reviewed, and psychodynamically oriented group psychotherapy produced better outcomes in 2 of 11 studies. Empirical research on the efficacy of psychodynamic treatment for substance abuse is limited by the long-term nature of this approach and difficulties in developing representative training manuals. However, there is a large body of clinical literature documenting success in individual patients in uncontrolled conditions (1653). A more recent review found support for individual therapy in 11 of 18 trials reviewed, although the quality of the studies was noted to be generally poor (79).

e) Self-help groups and 12-step-oriented treatments

The effectiveness of AA, per se, has not been evaluated in randomized studies because of a host of ethical and practical problems associated with assigning patients to a group that does not attend AA (261). However, there is growing support for the utility of AA and 12-step-oriented treatments from a range of sources (reviewed by McCrady and Irvine [1115]). Several naturalistic studies have suggested that AA can be an important support for promoting an alcohol-free lifestyle in patients who are willing to attend (956, 958, 959). A large number of studies have documented that more AA participation is linked to better drinking outcomes (260–266, 289, 1113, 1114). For example, in an evaluation of 8,087 patients in 57 programs, Hoffman and Miller (1112) reported that those attending AA at 1-year follow-up were 50% more likely to be abstinent than those not attending AA.

Professional therapies based on AA have been also found to be effective (1115). Moos and colleagues (260, 262–264, 266), in a series evaluating outcome in alcoholic veterans treated in a 12-step or CBT-oriented program, documented overall better outcome for 12-step treatments and a strong association between AA involvement and improved outcome. The findings of Project MATCH were generally positive for TSF, an individual-based, professionally delivered psychotherapy aimed at motivating patients to adhere to AA principles. Compared with MET and CBT, main effects for drinking outcomes were comparable or modestly superior for TSF (43, 265), and selected significant matching effects favored TSF for patients who had low severity of psychiatric symptoms, rated high on seeking meaning of life, and had high social support for not drinking.

Regarding patient-program matching, evidence from small-scale trials has suggested that patients with more severe drinking problems, an affective rather than a cognitive focus, a concern about purpose and meaning in life, better interpersonal skills, and a high need for affiliation are good candidates for AA (1115, 1654). In the landmark study Project MATCH, aftercare patients who rated high in the seeking meaning category fared better with TSF compared with MET and CBT at 1-year follow-up. Also, TSF was more effective than CBT for outpatients who did not show psychiatric symptoms and comparably equivalent for those with symptoms. Patients with high social support for not drinking had better drinking outcomes over the 3-year posttreatment period if they were treated with TSF rather than MET (1- and 3-year reports) (43, 265).

f) Brief interventions

Brief interventions generally delivered over one to three sessions include an abbreviated assessment of drinking severity and related problems and the provision of motivational feedback and advice. Brief therapies have typically been studied in general medical settings or school-based settings and have focused on non-treatment-seeking heavy drinkers who do not meet criteria for alcohol abuse or dependence. In 22 of 31 controlled treatment trials reviewed by Miller and Wilbourne (79), brief interventions were found to be effective. Reviews by Babor (1109) and Bien et al. (275) concluded that brief interventions 1) are typically more effective (in terms of alcohol use, general health, or social functioning) than no intervention; 2) often have efficacy comparable with that of traditional, more intense, longer-term programs; and 3) increase the effectiveness of later treatment. Even interventions that are very brief (i.e., a few hours) may have some positive effect (1110). For example, Fleming et al. (1111) conducted a trial of a brief physician advice condition plus a general health booklet versus the general health booklet alone in 774 primary care patients who screened positive for an alcohol use problem. This sample comprised 4.4% of 17,795 general medical patients screened. At 12-month follow-up, two 15–20-minute sessions of physician advice yielded significantly greater improvements in the number of alcoholic drinks taken over 7 days, the 30-day rate of binge drinking, and the rate of excessive drinking. Further research is needed to determine which patients are optimally served by receiving a brief intervention.

g) Marital and family therapy

The state of the patient's relationship with family members or significant others can be a critical factor in the posttreatment environment for patients who are married, in a committed relationship, or living with family members (1090, 1117). A meta-analytic review by O'Farrell and Fals Stewart (690) found a moderate effect size in 16 controlled trials of behavioral marital therapy. Other marital approaches with significant support were Al-Anon facilitation and disulfiram contracting (168, 248). Similarly, Miller and Wilbourne's box score review (79) found five of eight high-quality studies favored the efficacy of behavioral marital therapy; in contrast, other approaches to marital therapy were found to be effective in only three of eight trials (79). A noteworthy series of trials by O'Farrell and colleagues (225, 236, 238, 690, 961, 1118, 1119) demonstrated not only the efficacy but also the cost-effectiveness of behavioral marital therapy for patients with an alcohol use disorder.

h) Aftercare

Walker et al. (1120) found that involvement in aftercare was a stronger predictor of outcome than length of hospitalization, neuropsychological functioning, or pretreatment drinking and social stability measures. Ouimette et al. (264) found that participation in both aftercare and 12-step groups was associated with better 12-month outcomes in a sample of hospitalized male veterans. McLatchie and Lomp (1121) randomly assigned patients to mandatory, voluntary, or no aftercare for a 12-week period and found that those who completed aftercare had the lowest relapse rate, with no difference between the mandatory and voluntary groups. Gilbert (1122) randomly assigned patients to one of three aftercare conditions that varied in the degree of the therapist's efforts to maintain the patient in aftercare over 30 appointments. Patients in the maximal effort group were the most likely to complete aftercare, and all who completed aftercare, regardless of their study group, had better outcomes than those who did not. Results from studies that did not include random assignment suggest that greater participation in aftercare is generally associated with fewer drinks on drinking days, but not with diminished frequency of drinking (1655). A controlled study by O'Farrell et al. (225, 1118, 1119) demonstrated that a version of behavioral marital therapy that included relapse prevention techniques (184) and was delivered as an aftercare intervention led to better drinking outcomes. In two separate trials, Kadden and colleagues (223, 1102, 1103) compared inpatient aftercare programs consisting of 1) CBT and coping skills training and 2) insight-oriented interactional group therapy and reported similar outcomes in the two groups. Patterson et al. (1123) found nurse visits delivered over 12 months yielded better abstinence rates than clinical-based review visits. In Project MATCH (43, 265), 12 weeks of individual aftercare treatment using MET, TSF, or CBT showed comparable positive drinking outcomes in a sample of 774 alcohol-dependent patients. Also, 1 of 10 hypothesized matching effects was significant, suggesting that TSF was superior to CBT and MET for patients rated high in the seeking meaning category.

C. MARIJUANA-RELATED DISORDERS

1. Somatic treatments

There have been no successful controlled trials to date of pharmacotherapy for marijuana dependence. Trials with negative results have studied bupropion (1182), divalproex (1183, 1184), naltrexone, and nefazodone (1185). The main active ingredient of cannabis, Δ-9-tetrahydrocannabinol, has been tried in a laboratory study with human research volunteers and found to reverse withdrawal-associated psychomotor performance impairment and weight loss (1184) and warrants further study. No pharmacotherapy trials to prevent marijuana reinstatement after abstinence have been reported.

2. Psychosocial treatments

Given the absence of effective pharmacotherapies for marijuana dependence, the treatment of marijuana-related psychiatric disorders has primarily focused on psychosocial approaches (1178). Controlled trials have used cognitive-behavioral relapse prevention group therapy, social support group treatment, contingency management therapies, motivational individualized assessment and intervention, and MET therapy. However, it is difficult to discuss comparative efficacy across trials because the trials differed methodologically (e.g., in the diagnostic criteria and control groups used, the length of treatment and follow-up, the use of urine toxicology screens to confirm marijuana abstinence, the way in which interventions were delivered). Study samples also differed in their size and ethnic diversity. In general, existing trials consistently support the efficacy of the active treatments being studied.

a) Cognitive-behavioral and relapse prevention therapies

A number of studies in individuals with marijuana-related problems have compared outcomes after motivational or CBT interventions (1178). Stephens et al. (1187) randomized 212 subjects to receive relapse prevention therapy or a social support discussion group intervention. Both treatment conditions were associated with significant reductions in marijuana use relative to baseline, although no significant group differences were found in abstinence rates, marijuana-related problems, or days of marijuana use. Subsequently, 291 subjects were randomized into a delayed-treatment control group, a two-session motivational treatment group, and an intensive (14-session) relapse prevention treatment group (1186). Although no significant differences were observed between the brief and the more intensive treatment, marijuana-related outcomes for the two active treatments were found to be better than those with the delayed-treatment control condition. More recently, a replication and extension of that study involving a multisite trial of 450 marijuana-dependent patients compared three approaches: 1) a delayed-treatment control, 2) a two-session motivational approach, and 3) a nine-session combined motivational and coping skills approach (276). The results suggested that both active treatments were associated with significantly greater reductions in marijuana use than the delayed-treatment control condition at 4- and 15-month follow-up. Moreover, the nine-session intervention was significantly more effective than the two-session intervention, and this effect was sustained to 15-month follow-up.

Copeland et al. (1188) also studied CBT interventions for cannabis dependence, randomly assigning 229 participants to a six-session CBT program, a single-session CBT intervention, or a delayed-treatment control group. Participants in the treatment groups were assisted in acquiring skills to promote cannabis cessation and maintain abstinence. At about 6-month follow-up, both treatment groups reported better outcomes (greater abstinence rates, fewer marijuana use–related problems, less concern about control over marijuana use) than the delayed-treatment control group.

b) Behavioral therapies

Budney et al. (201) applied contingency management to marijuana users. They randomized 60 subjects to receive 4 sessions of MET, 14 sessions of MET in combination with coping skills therapy, or 14 sessions of MET in combination with coping skills therapy and voucher incentives. Although no differences in abstinence rates were noted between individuals receiving 4 sessions of MET or 14 sessions of MET plus coping skills therapy by the end of treatment, greater rates and durations of abstinence were seen in the group receiving MET plus coping skills therapy and voucher incentives. Thus, adding voucher-based incentives to coping skills and MET appears to improve outcomes during treatment for marijuana dependence.

D. COCAINE-RELATED DISORDERS

1. Somatic treatments

a) Medications to treat cocaine dependence

More than 45 different medications have been studied in the search for an effective pharmacological treatment for cocaine dependence (1225). Although a number of studies have shown promising results with a variety of pharmacotherapeutic agents, no medication has been found to have clear-cut efficacy in the treatment of cocaine dependence (1222–1224). Most studies have been hampered by methodological problems, including lack of adequate controls and consistent outcome measures (e.g., urine tests rather than self-reports), failure to standardize the type and "dose" of the accompanying psychosocial interventions, lack of clarity about the importance of craving in the maintenance of cocaine dependence, the role of craving in the natural course of untreated cocaine abstinence syndrome, and lack of agreement as to the exact meaning of the term "craving" (1204, 1209).

(1) Antidepressants

Gawin et al. (1227) found desipramine to be more effective than lithium or placebo in reducing cocaine use by outpatients without a coexisting mood disorder. Other reports (1215, 1230, 1231) failed to confirm these positive findings, possibly because of differences in patient population and route of cocaine administration. A subsequent study of desipramine and placebo with and without psychotherapy showed improvement with desipramine compared with placebo in the short term (6 weeks) but not at 12 weeks or 1 year (503). In buprenorphine-treated patients, desipramine was better than placebo for cocaine use (1228), and in methadone-treated patients, contingency management with desipramine produced more cocaine abstinence than desipramine alone, contingency management alone, or no treatment (1229).

Fluoxetine (1232, 1233) and bupropion (1234) also showed some benefit in small studies but demonstrated no superiority to placebo when evaluated in larger trials (413, 1235–1238).

(2) Dopamine agonists

Dopamine agonists are another class of agents that have been used in the treatment of cocaine dependence. The evidence for amantadine's effectiveness is inconsistent in that efficacy was observed in one controlled trial (1240) but not in two others (1225, 1231). Another controlled trial with amantadine found no overall difference between individuals receiving amantadine and those receiving placebo (1239), although those with more severe withdrawal symptoms appeared to have a better response to amantadine (1226).

The selective MAOI selegiline showed safety and some promise in laboratory studies in humans during cocaine administration, but a recent large multisite study failed to show its superiority to placebo (1241; F. Vocci, personal communication). Evidence for the benefits of L-dopa/carbidopa is limited (1242). Pergolide has been studied in larger trials and shown to have no superiority over placebo (1220, 1243). Laboratory studies in humans have suggested that a dopamine D_1 agonist (ABT-431) might reduce cocaine craving, but no oral formulations are available for outpatient trials (1656, 1657). Finally, replacement therapies using methylphenidate or sustained-release amphetamine have been superior to placebo for patient retention and reduction in cocaine use, but these studies need further replication (1244, 1245, 1247, 1658, 1659).

(3) Opioid-related agents

The mixed opioid agonist-antagonist buprenorphine has shown some promise in open trials in the treatment of patients dependent on both cocaine and opioids (1248, 1249), although three large-scale double-blind, clinical trials comparing patients maintained on buprenorphine with those receiving methadone showed no decrease in cocaine use among the former group (1250–1252). Although work by Schottenfeld et al. (1253) suggests that higher doses of buprenorphine (12–16 mg/day) may be effective, larger-scale clinical trials have found this medication to be effective only in combination with desipramine or, particularly, contingency management (1228, 1229, 1254). Naltrexone has also been tested and shown to be not useful for cocaine dependence (1255).

(4) Other medications

Anticonvulsants and agonists for GABA have been studied with some promise. Initial studies of carbamazepine in the treatment of cocaine dependence yielded some favorable results (1256), but subsequent double-blind, placebo-controlled studies failed to establish the efficacy of this drug in cocaine-dependent patients (1257–1261). A pilot study of the anticonvulsant topiramate showed promise (1262). The $GABA_B$ agonist baclofen has shown some success in treatment (1263), and a recent double-blind clinical trial of tiagabine, a GABA-reuptake blocker, was superior to placebo for reducing cocaine use (1264). Finally, modafinil shows promise for reducing cocaine abuse (1265).

b) Medications to change the subjective effects of cocaine

Attempts to find a medication that blocks or attenuates the subjective (e.g., euphorigenic) effects of cocaine have included trials of neuroleptics (1268, 1269), mazindol (1270), disulfiram, and a cocaine vaccine. At doses that can be tolerated by patients, neuroleptics and mazindol have not been effective (1271–1273). However, recent data with disulfiram have suggested that it may increase the aversive effects of cocaine and reduce its use (1277, 1660). Animal studies have demonstrated that a cocaine vaccine may form sufficient antibodies to reduce cocaine use (1278).

c) Acupuncture

Although it is not a pharmacological treatment, acupuncture is a somatic treatment that has been frequently used in the treatment of patients with a substance use disorder. Two recent randomized, controlled trials, however, one with 412 subjects (1279) and one with 620 subjects (1280), compared auricular acupuncture (which is supposed to be specifically helpful for patients with a substance use disorder) with a needle insertion control condition (sham acupuncture); the latter study also had a relaxation control condition. In both studies, acupuncture was no more effective than the sham acupuncture control or the relaxation condition in reducing cocaine use. The results of these studies, therefore, do not support the use of auricular acupuncture as a sole treatment for cocaine dependence.

d) Pharmacological treatment in individuals with a co-occurring psychiatric disorder

Several focused and reasonably well-controlled studies have examined the use of second-generation antipsychotics as anticraving agents among individuals with schizophrenia who primarily abuse cocaine. A 6-week open-label study showed that compared with patients taking first-generation antipsychotics, those receiving risperidone showed a significant reduction in cue-elicited cocaine craving, relapse to substance use, and symptom severity (401). A double-blind, randomized trial of olanzapine versus haloperidol was conducted with 31 cocaine-dependent patients with schizophrenia (1661). At the study completion, patients treated with olanzapine showed significantly less cue-elicited craving on two of four craving dimensions and fewer relapses compared with those treated with haloperidol.

2. Psychosocial treatments

a) Cognitive-behavioral therapies

A number of randomized clinical trials among several diverse cocaine-dependent populations have demonstrated that 1) compared with other commonly used psychotherapies for cocaine dependence, CBT appears to be particularly more effective with more severe cocaine users or those with co-occurring disorders (229, 452, 503, 1289, 1292, 1293); 2) CBT is significantly more effective than less intensive approaches that have been evaluated as control conditions (267, 1288); and 3) CBT is as effective or more effective than manual-guided disease-model approaches (267, 1289). Moreover, CBT appears to have a particularly durable impact, with patients continuing to reduce their cocaine use even after they leave treatment (1275, 1290, 1291, 1662).

b) Behavioral therapies

(1) Contingency management

Perhaps the most exciting findings pertaining to the effectiveness of behavioral treatments for cocaine dependence have been the reports by Petry et al. (188) and Higgins et al. (191–194) on the use of behavioral incentives for abstinence. The strategy of Higgins's group has four organizing features that are grounded in principles of behavioral pharmacology: 1) drug use and abstinence must be swiftly and accurately detected, 2) abstinence is positively reinforced,

3) drug use results in loss of reinforcement, and 4) emphasis is placed on the development of reinforcers to compete with drug use (1294). In this approach, urine specimens are required three times a week to systematically detect all episodes of drug use. Abstinence, verified through drug-free urine screens, is reinforced through a voucher system in which patients receive points redeemable for items consistent with a drug-free lifestyle (e.g., movie tickets, sporting goods).

In a series of well-controlled clinical trials, Higgins's group has demonstrated high rates of acceptance, retention, and abstinence in patients receiving this approach, as compared with standard counseling oriented toward 12-step programs (191, 192). Rates of abstinence do not decline substantially when less valuable incentives are substituted for the voucher system (192). The value of the voucher system itself, as opposed to other program elements, in producing good outcomes was demonstrated by comparing the behavioral system with and without the vouchers (193). Although the strong effects of this treatment declined somewhat after the contingencies were terminated, the voucher system has been shown to have durable effects (194). Moreover, the efficacy of a variety of contingency management procedures (including vouchers, direct payments, and free housing) has been replicated in other settings and samples, including cocaine-dependent individuals within methadone maintenance (195, 1295), substance-abusing homeless individuals (1297), freebase cocaine users (1298), and pregnant drug users (1299).

These findings are of great importance because contingency management procedures are potentially applicable to a wide range of target behaviors and problems, including treatment retention and adherence with pharmacotherapy (e.g., retroviral therapies for individuals with HIV). For example, Iguchi et al. (202) showed that contingency management can be effective in reinforcing desired treatment goals (e.g., looking for a job) in addition to abstinence.

In a line of research attempting to reduce the costs of contingency management, Petry and colleagues (204, 205) demonstrated that a variable ratio schedule of reinforcement that provides access to large reinforcers but at lower probabilities is effective in retaining subjects in treatment and reducing substance use. Rather than earning vouchers, subjects earn the chance to draw from a bowl and win prizes of varying magnitudes. The prizes range from small $1 prizes (e.g., bus tokens, McDonald's coupons) to large $20 prizes (e.g., portable radios, watches, and phone cards) to jumbo $100 prizes (e.g., small televisions). This system is far less expensive than the standard voucher system because only a proportion of behaviors are reinforced with a prize. In a study of 42 alcohol-dependent veterans who were randomly assigned to standard treatment or standard treatment plus contingency management, 84% of the contingency management subjects were retained in treatment throughout an 8-week period compared with 22% of standard treatment subjects. By the end of the treatment period, 69% of those receiving contingency management had not experienced a relapse to alcohol use, but only 39% of those receiving standard treatment were abstinent (205); there were similar findings among cocaine abusers (204).

(2) Cue exposure treatment

Cue exposure therapy has also been used in the treatment of cocaine use disorders, with equivocal results (189).

c) Psychodynamic and interpersonal therapies

No randomized clinical trials have been conducted for psychodynamically oriented treatments for cocaine abuse or dependence. A case series of patients successfully treated with individual psychodynamically oriented psychotherapy was reported by Schiffer (1300), and there is a preliminary report revealing a high rate of retention with modified psychodynamically oriented group psychotherapy (1301). Spitz (1302) has also described the use of group therapy for this population.

d) Self-help groups and 12-step-oriented treatments

Several trials have evaluated manual-guided professionally delivered treatments, including TSF (268) and individual drug counseling (269), that enhance a patient's motivation to participate in 12-step programs. As part of these professional treatments, patients are actively encouraged (but not required) to attend Narcotics Anonymous or Cocaine Anonymous meetings, become involved in traditional fellowship activities, and maintain journals of their self-help group attendance and participation.

In a comparison of TSF, CBT, and clinical management (a supportive approach in which patients received comparable empathy, support, and other "common elements" of psychotherapy but none of the unique "active ingredients" of TSF or CBT) for alcoholic cocaine-dependent individuals, TSF was found to be significantly more effective than clinical management and was comparable with CBT in reducing cocaine use (267). In addition, results at 1-year follow-up suggested that gains from treatment were maintained for subjects who received TSF or CBT; these subjects reported continuing to reduce their cocaine use throughout the follow-up period compared with subjects who received clinical management. Moreover, there was a strong association between the attainment of significant periods of abstinence during treatment and abstinence during follow-up, which emphasizes that the inception of abstinence, even for comparatively brief periods, is an important goal of treatment (194, 1275).

The results of the NIDA Collaborative Cocaine Treatment Study, a multisite randomized trial of psychotherapeutic treatments for cocaine dependence (219, 1305), suggest the effectiveness of a similar approach: 12-step-oriented individual drug counseling (269). In that study, 487 cocaine-dependent participants in four sites were randomly assigned to one of four conditions: 1) cognitive therapy (1306) plus group drug counseling; 2) supportive-expressive therapy, a psychodynamically oriented approach (217) plus group drug counseling; 3) 12-step-based individual drug counseling plus group drug counseling; or 4) group drug counseling alone. The treatments offered were intensive (36 individual and 24 group sessions over 24 weeks, for a total of 60 sessions) (219). On the whole, outcomes were good, with all groups significantly reducing their cocaine use from baseline; however, the best outcomes were seen for subjects who received individual drug counseling.

McKay et al. (229) compared 12-step-oriented standard group counseling to relapse prevention aftercare in 98 cocaine-dependent patients. Rates of complete abstinence in the 6-month study period were higher in the standard group counseling group than in the relapse prevention group, whereas relapse prevention was more effective in limiting the extent of cocaine use in those who currently used cocaine. Overall effectiveness was judged to be equivalent for the two treatments.

The studies above evaluated professional treatments based on 12-step concepts and not participation in self-help groups, per se. The literature on participation in Cocaine Anonymous or other 12-step self-help groups is more limited than that for patients with an alcohol use disorder participating in AA. In one study of day hospital rehabilitation for patients with a cocaine use disorder (1304), greater participation in self-help programs 3 months after treatment predicted less cocaine use 6 months after treatment, even after pretreatment patient characteristics and degree of success in the day hospital program were controlled for in the study.

Self-help groups have not been shown to be a sufficient alternative to professional treatment. For example, a large randomized trial that directly compared referral to self-help with professional treatments found poorer outcomes, with high rates of treatment utilization for the patients referred to self-help compared with inpatient treatment (1303).

E. OPIOID-RELATED DISORDERS

1. Somatic treatments

a) Opioid agonist therapies

(1) Methadone

Methadone is the most thoroughly studied and widely used pharmacological treatment for opioid dependence. Studies of its efficacy and safety have focused on its use as a maintenance medication and a medication for the treatment of opioid withdrawal. This section will review studies of methadone's efficacy and safety for these two purposes.

a. Use of methadone as a maintenance agent

Studies of methadone's efficacy and safety fall into two general categories: controlled clinical trials and naturalistic/survey studies. When designed and conducted properly under controlled conditions that are related to but distinct from routine clinical practice, clinical trials provide evidence of methadone's efficacy. The scientific value inherent in the methods of such studies (e.g., double-blind dosing) is offset by the somewhat unusual experimental conditions of a clinical trial (e.g., intensive monitoring of participants). Naturalistic survey studies of methadone provide complementary evidence to clinical trials and typically report results for larger populations that have been treated in routine settings. There is little control for factors such as expectancy, but these studies do provide data that are more closely tied to real-world clinical settings.

1) Naturalistic/survey studies of methadone treatment

Examples of naturalistic/survey studies of methadone efficacy include the Drug Abuse Reporting Program (61), the Treatment Outcome Prospective Study (1399), the Drug Abuse Treatment Outcome Study (45, 73, 1663), and the Effectiveness of Methadone Maintenance Treatment Study (169). The first three of these survey studies assessed methadone treatment as one of several substance abuse treatment modalities. Participants in these projects were not randomized to a treatment modality, and services were given in routine clinic settings and were not delivered in a blinded fashion. Results from such studies generally showed that methadone is effective when post- and pretreatment functioning are compared and that better outcomes are associated with longer periods of treatment. However, the relative efficacy of different doses of methadone has generally not been addressed in such survey studies.

The Effectiveness of Methadone Maintenance Treatment Study (169) was somewhat different from these national survey studies, as it assessed methadone treatment in a relatively restricted geographic region—six clinics located on the East Coast (two each in New York, Philadelphia, and Baltimore). However, the study did provide intensive evaluation of a large number of patients treated specifically with methadone (versus a more heterogeneous population of patients in the other surveys). A total of 617 patients were initially assessed; of these, 126 were new methadone admissions, 346 were in treatment for <4.5 years, and 145 were in treatment for ≥4.5 years.

At the 1-year follow-up, the methadone dose was inversely related to self-reported heroin use in the 30 days prior to the interview. The study found that longer time in treatment was associated with decreased rates of intravenous drug use. For patients in treatment for 4 years, self-reported use declined from 81% at the time of admission to 29% after 4 years. Among patients who had been in treatment for ≥4.5 years, 92% reported no heroin use and 83% reported no cocaine use in the 30 days before the study assessment. Other factors besides methadone dose were also found to be related to treatment and outcome in this study, such as the level of involvement of the clinic director.

Other naturalistic studies of methadone treatment provide further evidence of methadone's efficacy, especially with regard to methadone dose. For example, one study of 652 methadone maintenance patients found that heroin use was greatest among those with daily methadone maintenance doses <70 mg/day and that, independent of dose, time in treatment was associated with less heroin use (1664). Similarly, a review of methadone dosing for 62 patients treated in an Australian clinic found that higher doses were associated with less heroin use (1665). This study also concluded that the relative odds of heroin use were reduced by 2% for every 1 mg increase in maintenance dose.

It is important to note that an inherent weakness to survey studies is that patients are not randomly assigned to the conditions being compared. There may be other patient or program characteristics besides methadone dose or time in treatment that may account for the differences seen in such studies. In addition, these studies often rely on patient self-reports of substance use, including retrospective assessments of past use that are then used to calculate changes over time. Expectancy effects may also play an important role in outcomes seen. Thus, although survey studies can be helpful and informative, these and other liabilities compromise the degree of certainty that can be assigned to their conclusions.

2) Clinical trials of methadone dose and treatment

Numerous clinical trials have tested methadone for the treatment of opioid dependence. In general, these studies have found that methadone medication is a safe and effective pharmacotherapy for the treatment of opioid dependence and that methadone combined with other services such as counseling, behavioral interventions, and urine monitoring can broaden the efficacy of this intervention to include a greater range of treatment outcomes such as increased prosocial behavior and decreased nonopioid substance use.

There have been two double-blind, placebo-controlled studies of methadone for the treatment of opioid dependence. The first was conducted in Hong Kong in the early 1970s and enrolled 100 male opioid-dependent patients who were initially hospitalized for 2 weeks and treated with 60 mg/day of methadone (1666). Participants were then randomly assigned to 1) the placebo condition, in which they underwent 1-mg dose reductions of methadone each day on an outpatient basis and then were maintained on placebo after 60 days, or 2) the maintenance condition, in which they could have outpatient dose adjustments with a maximum possible dose of 130 mg/day. For this latter group, the average dose was 97 mg/day (range 30–130 mg) after 1 year. Subjects were withdrawn from the study if they missed 6 consecutive weeks of treatment or had six consecutive opioid-positive urine samples. At the 32-week evaluation point, 10% of placebo-treated patients remained in treatment (most of the rest having been withdrawn because of urine evidence of persisting illicit opioid use) compared with 76% of maintenance patients.

The second placebo-controlled study of methadone treatment was conducted in the late 1980s in Baltimore, Maryland, and enrolled 247 opioid-dependent outpatient participants (1350, 1351). The study began by randomly assigning subjects to one of three fixed doses of oral methadone (0, 20, or 50 mg/day). Participants were required to attend the clinic daily for supervised dose ingestion and were discharged for missing 3 consecutive days of treatment. Primary outcomes were treatment retention and urine test results. At the end of the 20-week study, significant differences were found among the three groups for treatment retention (primarily between the 50- and 0-mg groups), with the 20-mg group generally doing better than the 0-mg group. In addition, there were significantly lower rates of opioid-positive urine test results for the 50-mg group compared with the other two groups. A variety of secondary outcome measures, such as self-reported illicit opioid use, also showed dose-related effects. In addition to the demonstrated dose-related efficacy of methadone, these study results also indicated that the 20-mg dose of methadone might keep some patients in treatment but was not as effective in decreasing illicit opioid use as the 50-mg dose. Study limitations included the use of fixed doses of methadone and the absence of a dose condition ≥50 mg/day.

Further controlled clinical trials of methadone have tested higher versus lower doses of methadone. For example, a 40-week multicenter VA outpatient study of LAAM for the treatment of 430 opioid-dependent males included two fixed methadone dose control conditions of 50 and 100 mg/day (1349). The induction procedure for the 288 methadone-treated subjects was relatively slow; subjects were started on 30 mg of methadone per day and received 10-mg dose increases once per week until the target dose was achieved. Induction, therefore, lasted 5 weeks longer for patients in the 100-mg versus the 50-mg methadone group. Urine samples were collected and tested once per week, and the results were summarized using a set of rules that weighted results based on when the sample was collected and how missing values were handled. Outcomes for the methadone-treated subjects showed higher opioid urine scores (poorer outcomes) for the 50-mg versus the 100-mg group. Although this study provided evidence of methadone's dose-related efficacy on illicit opioid use, its results are limited by its use of an all male population, a slow induction procedure, fixed doses, and a somewhat unusual method for summarizing urine test results.

Another outpatient study compared a moderate dose (40–50 mg/day; N=97) with a higher dose (80–100 mg/day; N=95) of methadone for the treatment of opioid dependence (1352). This 40-week double-blind, randomized trial used a flexible dosing procedure in which participants could receive dose increases based on evidence of continued illicit opioid use. Primary outcome measures were treatment retention, the results of twice-weekly urinalyses, and self-reported illicit opioid use. The results showed no significant difference in treatment retention for the two groups but found a significantly lower rate of opioid-positive urine samples for the higher-dose condition. Both groups had marked declines in self-reported illicit opioid use, with significantly less use by the high-dose versus the moderate-dose group. Although significant effects were found on some outcomes in this study, both doses produced clinically meaningful decreases in illicit opioid use. The lack of difference between the study groups for treatment retention suggests that there may be a plateau in the dose-related efficacy of methadone in maintaining patients in treatment but not in decreasing illicit opioid use for the doses tested. However, the schedule of twice-weekly urinalyses used in this study may have failed to capture all illicit opioid use occurring in the study population.

Other controlled trials of methadone treatment and methadone dosing have also been conducted (1250, 1251, 1667–1670). In general, these studies have shown that methadone has dose-related efficacy, although it is important to note that not all randomized double-blind methadone studies have shown such an effect. However, it is also important to note that no double-blind, randomized, controlled clinical trials have tested daily doses of methadone ≥100 mg/day. There have been single-blind and open studies of higher doses of methadone that were conducted primarily in the early years of methadone treatment (1671–1673), and reports from clinical practice in both the United States and other countries indicate higher doses of methadone are used by some clinicians (1342–1346). Currently, there is no research database that provides information about the relative efficacy and safety of higher doses (i.e., ≥100 mg/day) of methadone.

b. Use of methadone as a withdrawal (detoxification) agent

The number of studies examining methadone for treating opioid withdrawal is more limited than the number examining methadone in maintenance treatment of opioid dependence. Outcomes from methadone withdrawal are generally poor (1674–1676), especially when compared with the success associated with methadone maintenance treatment. These studies have examined the various parameters under which methadone tapering can occur in an effort to determine optimal withdrawal schedules.

An early double-blind, randomized, outpatient study of methadone withdrawal by Senay et al. (1677) used a four-group design: dose reductions of 10% per week for 10 weeks, reductions of 3% per week for 30 weeks, stable dosing with patients knowing their dose would not change, and double-blind stable dosing. The 127 study participants were in methadone maintenance treatment, with an average dose of 31 mg/day. They could request a 1-week dose halt or increase during their withdrawal. Results from the study showed the poorest outcomes occurred for patients in the rapid dose-reduction (10% per week) group as measured by taper interruptions, positive urine sample rates, and withdrawal symptom complaints. As a group, patients undergoing the rapid withdrawal essentially stabilized around an average of 10 mg/day of methadone due to their requests for dose halts and temporary dose increases. These results suggested that a more gradual methadone taper (3% per week) leads to better outcomes than a more rapid taper (10% per week), although methadone maintenance treatment is even more effective.

Another randomized clinical trial compared methadone withdrawal—120 days of methadone induction/stabilization followed by a 60-day withdrawal and then 8 months of nonmethadone treatment—to 14 months of maintenance treatment in 179 opioid-dependent patients (1678). The study was not conducted in a blinded fashion, and the withdrawal group had more nonpharmacological services available to them. Results from the study showed significantly better treatment retention for the maintenance group but similar rates of illicit opioid use for the two groups until month 5, when patients withdrawn ftom methadone began to have higher rates of illicit opioid use. These study results support the value of methadone for maintenance treatment compared with withdrawal from methadone, although certain qualifiers to the study should be noted: expectancy effects could contribute to the outcomes shown, the requirement that withdrawn patients attend more groups and counseling may have contributed to the high dropout rate, and the length of the withdrawal (60 days) may have been too quick, as suggested by the results from the Senay et al. study (1677) reviewed above.

Other studies of methadone withdrawal have been conducted but generally with smaller sample sizes or in atypical treatment settings (e.g., inpatient units) that make their results limited in their applicability to current treatment circumstances. For example, an inpatient study of a 10-day methadone withdrawal comparing a linear schedule of daily dose reductions (based on a fixed percentage of the starting dose) to an exponential schedule of daily dose reductions (based on a percentage of the previous day's dose) found no differences in the time course of withdrawal symptoms, peak symptom severity, and patient adherence (1679). Other studies (1675, 1677, 1680) examining whether or not informing patients about their methadone dose-reduction schedule influences treatment outcome have concluded that informed patients have better outcomes. There is some evidence that patients do not have better outcomes, however, if they, rather than clinicians, are allowed to control their methadone withdrawal schedule (1675, 1681). Finally, one study found that lower rates of illicit opioid use occurred when patients received voucher incentives for opioid-negative urine samples during methadone withdrawal, although it appears this intervention primarily delayed relapse to illicit opioid use (1682).

c. Safety and side effects of methadone

Like all mu agonist opioids, overdose with methadone can produce respiratory depression and death. When used under physician supervision, methadone is a safe medication with limited side effects. Constipation, sweating, sexual dysfunction, and sedation are the most commonly reported side effects. When patients first start on methadone, they may experience some side effects (e.g., sedation) to which they will develop a tolerance. The two most common side effects reported by patients, constipation and sweating, may persist despite chronic treatment on a stable dose. Small effects that are not clinically significant have been noted on some physiological measures assessed during chronic methadone dosing (e.g., heart rate, pupil diameter) (1359, 1683). Studies of chronic dosing with methadone have shown no evidence of organ damage, such as hepatotoxic effects (1684–1686). There have been case reports of high-dose methadone treatment associated with torsade de pointes and a prolonged corrected QT interval (1687–1689). Methadone-related increases in the corrected QT interval appear to be related to dose (1690–1692), and patients experiencing this problem often have had other risk factors for torsade de pointes.

Early studies of psychomotor and cognitive performance tasks in methadone-maintained patients showed no significant impairments (1356–1358), but more recent studies have shown significantly poorer performance on these tasks in methadone-maintained patients versus matched control subjects (1359, 1360). Whether such effects are due to the acute or chronic effects of methadone or to other factors associated with a long history of substance use is not entirely clear despite efforts in these more recent studies to carefully match patients.

(2) LAAM

LAAM is an opioid agonist medication that has effects similar to those of methadone but a longer duration of action. LAAM has demonstrated efficacy as a maintenance agent in large multisite, randomized, double-blind studies (1349, 1693); smaller randomized, double-blind studies (1667, 1694–1696); and nonblind clinical trials (1697–1705). It also appears to be effective as a withdrawal (detoxification) agent (1674, 1706). Clinical trials with LAAM reported typical opioid agonist side effects (1349, 1707) but no cases of deaths or other significant adverse events that seemed linked to LAAM use. However, later case reports of corrected QT interval (QTc) prolongation and torsade de pointes (1337) led to LAAM's withdrawal from the U.S. and European markets.

(3) Buprenorphine

Clinical studies of buprenorphine have used two different formulations: solution and tablets. Because of its poor oral bioavailability, most clinical trials of buprenorphine for the treatment of opioid dependence have used a sublingual, often alcohol-based, solution. A liquid sublingual form of buprenorphine, however, was felt to be an impractical long-term treatment option, and as the evidence for its efficacy and safety in the treatment of opioid dependence grew, a water-soluble sublingual tablet form of buprenorphine was developed. However, the tablet form of buprenorphine appears to have lower bioavailability compared with the alcohol-based solution form (1708–1710), suggesting dosing parameters from clinical trials should be interpreted with caution if the solution form of buprenorphine is used.

Because buprenorphine can be abused (1711–1716), it is possible for the sublingual tablet to be dissolved and used parenterally. In France, where buprenorphine is the primary medication used for the treatment of opioid dependence, there have been reports of abuse of buprenorphine tablets (1713, 1717–1719). For this reason, a formulation that combines buprenorphine with naloxone was developed for the U.S. market. Naloxone has poor sublingual bioavailability (1361), so use of this combination tablet sublingually would produce a predominant buprenorphine effect. However, if an opioid-dependent individual dissolved and injected the combination tablet, he or she would risk precipitating a withdrawal syndrome due to naloxone's good parenteral bioavailability. Studies of the combination buprenorphine-naloxone tablet have confirmed such differential effects to be a function of the route of administration (1720–1724). Although the combination tablet is the more commonly used form of this medication, many clinical trials have used a monotherapy tablet, and the monotherapy tablet is the primary form of sublingual buprenorphine used outside the United States. Under chronic dosing conditions, there may be slightly better bioavailability for the combination versus the monotherapy tablets (1710). However, for a given dose of buprenorphine, there is considerable between-subject variability in buprenorphine blood levels.

a. Use of buprenorphine on a daily basis as a maintenance agent

Numerous randomized, double-blind clinical trials have studied the efficacy and safety of sublingual buprenorphine for the outpatient treatment of opioid dependence. This section reviews the three representative studies that compared buprenorphine with placebo and then provides a more limited review of the many studies that compared buprenorphine with methadone.

The first study was a 16-week multisite double-blind, randomized outpatient clinical trial using four different doses of sublingual buprenorphine solution: 1, 4, 8, and 16 mg/day (1725). The primary goal was to compare the 8- and 1-mg doses, with the 1-mg dose serving as the placebo condition. The study enrolled 736 opioid-dependent patients (about 33% female); primary outcome measures were treatment retention, opioid urinalysis results, craving, and global ratings by staff and patients. Results from the study showed significantly better outcomes for the 8- versus the 1-mg groups on all the primary outcome measures. In general, there was no clear pattern of increased side effects or adverse events for the 8-mg group, with the exception of ratings of constipation (but multiple comparisons were made). Although not the primary purpose of the study, the outcomes also showed dose-related effects for buprenorphine, where 4 mg of buprenorphine was better than 1 mg, 8 mg was better than 4 mg, and 16 mg was better than 8 mg, although these differences were not always robust in their magnitude.

The second study was a double-blind, placebo-controlled study that used a somewhat novel clinical trial design that lasted only 2 weeks (1726). In this study, the 150 male and female participants were fast-tracked into treatment and randomly assigned to 0 (N=60), 2 (N=60), or 8 (N=30) mg/day of sublingual buprenorphine solution. Subjects were informed that they could receive placebo or one of two buprenorphine doses and that after 6 days, they could request to have a blind change to one of the other two conditions. Primary outcomes were the percentage of patients in each condition who remained on their original dose and the percentage of patients in each condition who requested a dose change. Other study outcomes such as opioid urine test results and self-reports of drug use were also provided. This study found that, regardless of dose, a significantly higher percentage of patients in the two active conditions remained on their doses compared with the placebo group. Similarly, a significantly higher percentage of patients in the placebo condition requested a dose change compared with the other two groups, but, once again, there was no significant difference between the two active buprenorphine groups. In an interesting finding, male subjects in the two active buprenorphine groups had a significantly lower rate of opioid-positive urine samples, but there was no difference across the three conditions for female subjects. This study provides an alternative demonstration of the efficacy of buprenorphine compared with placebo.

The third study was an office-based protocol that compared sublingual placebo tablets to active buprenorphine/naloxone (16 mg/4 mg) and buprenorphine alone (16 mg) tablets (1727). This multicenter study enrolled 326 opioid-dependent individuals, and study participation lasted 4 weeks for each volunteer. Subjects received supervised dose administration on weekdays and take-home doses of tablets on weekends. Urine samples were collected thrice weekly. Study enrollment was discontinued early because significant differences between the two active conditions and placebo were found on an interim analysis. For example, rates of opioid-negative urine samples were significantly higher for both active treatment groups compared with the placebo group. After the 4-week period, there was a further period of open-label treatment for purposes of safety assessment; the results from this phase showed that buprenorphine was safe and well tolerated. The results from this study provide further evidence of buprenorphine's efficacy compared with placebo, especially when the tablet form is studied (rather than the solution form used in the previous two studies described).

In addition to these three studies, two others have compared buprenorphine with placebo (1394, 1728). Like the studies previously described, these reports also showed that buprenorphine maintenance is superior to placebo treatment as measured by treatment retention, opioid urine test results, and mortality.

Numerous studies have compared buprenorphine's efficacy and, to a more limited extent, its safety to methadone. These studies have generally been randomized, double-blind, clinical trials conducted at a single site with fixed doses of sublingual buprenorphine solution and oral methadone (137, 1251, 1362, 1668, 1729). Variations on this basic methodological approach include studies that have compared methadone with buprenorphine tablets rather than solution (1730–1732), have used double-blind, flexible-dosing schedules rather than fixed doses of methadone and buprenorphine (74, 1363, 1364), or have compared thrice-weekly buprenorphine to daily methadone (74). Some of these studies had relatively small groups of subjects (1364, 1730), although other features of these studies may represent important methodological advances in this line of research.

In general, these studies comparing buprenorphine with methadone demonstrated that outcomes for the two medications can be very similar. An important qualification to this conclusion is that it is not always clear that the studies used comparable doses of the two medications. For example, a study comparing a very low fixed methadone dose with an average fixed buprenorphine dose could lead to the conclusion that buprenorphine is more effective than methadone, but such a study would be a comparison of dose efficacy rather than medication efficacy. When studies have used flexible doses, compared doses of methadone and buprenorphine that are thought to be approximately equivalent, or used more than one fixed dose of each medication for comparison, they have generally found similar outcomes on measures of treatment retention and rates of opioid-positive urine samples for buprenorphine and methadone. However, it appears that based on these studies, buprenorphine's maximal therapeutic effect occurs in the range of 8–16 mg/day of sublingual tablets, which is equivalent to outcomes seen with daily doses of about 50–60 mg of methadone.

b. Use of buprenorphine on a less than daily basis as a maintenance agent

Buprenorphine's long duration of action suggests that it may be effective on a less than daily basis. Clinical trials of intermittent buprenorphine dosing have typically stabilized patients on a daily dose and then switched them to a less than daily schedule where buprenorphine was administered on active dosing days and placebo was given on the other days. In some studies, buprenorphine doses were not increased (1733, 1734), whereas in other studies the dose was doubled (1367, 1735) on active dosing days. Although there is some evidence that significant withdrawal can occur if the daily dose is not increased when switching to intermittent dosing (1733), increasing the dose to compensate for the 48-hour interdose period generally provides adequate effects for patients and is preferred to daily dosing (1367).

There are several studies of intervals between active doses that are ≥48 hours. For example, a study where triple the daily buprenorphine maintenance dose was administered to patients every 72 hours found some mild increase in opioid agonist effects in the first 24 hours and some mild withdrawal at 72 hours, but neither effect was robust or clinically significant (1368). Similar results were reported in another study testing buprenorphine's effects over a 72-hour time interval (1366). A double-blind study examining a quadruple daily maintenance dose of buprenorphine given at up to 96-hour intervals (1369) did not find excessive opioid agonist effects 24 hours after the quadrupled dose and only mild withdrawal effects at 96 hours. A follow-up open report on double, triple, and quadruple buprenorphine doses for 48-, 72-, and 96-hour intervals, respectively, found similar tolerability of the 96-hour interval as well as a preference by patients for all intermittent, rather than daily, dosing schedules of buprenorphine (1368). These results suggest dosing with buprenorphine on every fourth day is clinically possible, with no significant adverse effects from the higher doses of buprenorphine and comparable efficacy with daily dosing. However, findings from studies that have tested even longer intervals between active buprenorphine doses suggest that 96 hours may be the upper limit of the interdose interval (1736, 1737). In these studies, significant but clinically mild opioid agonist effects were noted 24 hours after the quintuple or sextuple dose, with clinically mild withdrawal effects appearing after 96 hours. Studies have not tested if higher doses of buprenorphine, such as seven times a daily dose, might be effective and safe for shorter periods such as 5 days.

One of the largest controlled clinical trials of intermittent buprenorphine dosing was a double-blind, randomized study comparing thrice-weekly to daily buprenorphine dosing (1738). This study assigned 92 opioid-dependent outpatients to receive sublingual buprenorphine solution daily or sublingual buprenorphine solution on Tuesdays, Fridays, and Sundays and placebo on the other four days. The daily buprenorphine dose was 16 mg/70 kg, whereas buprenorphine dosing in the intermittent condition was 34 mg/70 kg on Friday and Sunday and 44 mg/70 kg on Tuesday. The 72-hour dosing interval was from Tuesday to Friday to avoid potential study confounders associated with the weekend. There were no differences in rates of opioid-positive urine tests, self-reports of illicit opioid use, treatment retention, and medication adherence between the two groups and no significant adverse events noted for either group. The results from this large controlled study suggest that intermittent buprenorphine can be as equally effective as daily buprenorphine.

Although the studies reviewed here have all used the solution form of buprenorphine, there have also been studies of intermittent dosing with buprenorphine tablets. One double-blind outpatient clinical trial compared daily dosing of 8-mg buprenorphine tablets to thrice-weekly dosing with 16-mg tablets on Mondays and Wednesdays, 24-mg tablets on Fridays, and placebo tablets on the four nonactive dosing days. The study found equivalent retention for the two groups but a higher rate of opioid-positive urine samples in the intermittent dosing group (1739). Using the buprenorphine/naloxone combination tablets, Another study showed that patients prefer thrice-weekly take-home doses of the medication to both daily and thrice-weekly medication visits at a clinic (1740). These two studies provide evidence of the practicality of using buprenorphine tablets on an intermittent basis.

c. Use of buprenorphine as a withdrawal (detoxification) agent

Controlled clinical trials and reports of buprenorphine for the treatment of opioid withdrawal have varied in several ways. Some withdrawal studies have compared buprenorphine with methadone (1741), whereas others have compared it with clonidine (1393, 1742, 1743). Different formulations of buprenorphine (1384, 1744) and rapid or prolonged withdrawals (1392, 1745, 1746) have also been used in these studies. There has been some interest in and research on using buprenorphine as a bridging agent to treatment with naltrexone (1745, 1747). Several reports of buprenorphine's use in opioid withdrawal are open studies describing clinicians' experience with buprenorphine (1384, 1748–1752). Although the outcomes noted in these reports are confounded by the lack of important features found in appropriately conducted clinical trials, they do provide important clinical evidence of buprenorphine's acceptability as a withdrawal medication.

An early double-blind, double-dummy, random-assignment, outpatient clinical trial compared fixed doses of sublingual buprenorphine solution with oral methadone in the treatment of opioid withdrawal (1741). A total of 45 heroin-dependent male subjects were stabilized on 30 mg of methadone or 2 mg of buprenorphine for 3 weeks, underwent a dose taper for 4 weeks and then received placebo for 6 weeks. A novel feature to this study's design was that subjects underwent a 6-mg hydromorphone challenge session during the second week of stabilization (to test the relative blockade efficacy of the two treatment medications). Results from the withdrawal assessments showed the two medications were quite similar on measures of treatment retention, drug use, and rating of withdrawal. However, results from the hydromorphone challenge sessions showed that methadone produced significantly greater blockade than buprenorphine. The results from this early buprenorphine withdrawal study demonstrate that similar outcomes can be achieved with these two medications, although the study used relatively low doses of both medications and the overall results showed poor outcomes for both groups.

An inpatient, randomized, double-blind clinical trial compared sublingual buprenorphine solution to oral clonidine in a relatively short opioid withdrawal procedure (1742). In this study of 25 opioid-dependent male and female patients, participants received 3 days of a fixed-dose schedule of buprenorphine or a 5-day fixed-dose schedule of clonidine. Because this was an inpatient study, reports of withdrawal symptoms were not confounded by illicit substance use. Overall, patients treated with buprenorphine were found to have less opioid withdrawal than those treated with clonidine, whereas there was more hypotension in patients treated with clonidine. This study demonstrated that sublingual buprenorphine was more effective than clonidine in the inpatient treatment of opioid withdrawal; other studies and reports comparing buprenorphine with clonidine have shown similar results (1384, 1391–1393).

A large double-blind, randomized, outpatient clinical trial compared withdrawal using buprenorphine with clonidine and clonidine plus naltrexone in an outpatient primary care clinic setting (1747). This study randomly assigned 162 opioid-dependent male and female patients to one of three conditions: sublingual buprenorphine for 3 days, followed by clonidine and naltrexone; 7 days of clonidine; or 7 days of clonidine plus naltrexone. Results from the study showed that treatment retention was not significantly different for the three groups. However, there were significantly less opioid withdrawal symptoms (both overall withdrawal and peak effects) for buprenorphine-treated patients compared with the other two groups. These study results give further evidence of the clinical value of buprenorphine compared with clonidine provided on an outpatient basis.

d. Safety and side effects of buprenorphine

Buprenorphine has been extensively tested in a variety of outpatient clinical trials, with no reports of significant adverse events from these studies. In addition, it has been used extensively in other countries, especially France, where it is estimated that there are over 70,000 buprenorphine-treated patients.

There is some evidence that buprenorphine may have effects on hepatic function. One report, based on a retrospective review of 120 patients treated with sublingual buprenorphine, suggested that buprenorphine is associated with elevated results on liver function tests for some patients with a history of hepatitis (1753). Although these elevations were relatively mild, there is also evidence that intravenous use of buprenorphine can produce marked increases in liver function test values (1754, 1755). One inpatient study of buprenorphine also found mild increases in liver transaminases over time, although the lack of a control group, the nonspecificity of these laboratory results, and the relatively mild effects seen make interpretation of such findings difficult (1756).

Systematic evaluations of buprenorphine's other side effects have been relatively scarce. One report by Lange et al. (1756) on safety and side effect measures collected during a 12-week inpatient study of buprenorphine induction as well as a study on daily versus alternate-day dosing (1733, 1757) found that no symptoms were rated as definitely related to buprenorphine; the only two symptoms rated as probably related to buprenorphine were drowsiness/sedation and, most frequently, constipation. Nausea/vomiting and headache, which occurred in the first 1–2 weeks of treatment, were rated as possibly related to buprenorphine. A second report that compared safety and side effect measures from a clinical trial comparing daily buprenorphine solution to daily oral methadone found that there were few significant differences in side effect reports from the two medications (1758). However, as was found in the Lange et al. (1756) study, ratings of constipation were higher for the buprenorphine versus the methadone group, although they were relatively low for both groups.

Available evidence varies with respect to mortality and serious adverse events such as respiratory depression associated with buprenorphine. Because of buprenorphine's unusual pharmacological profile, which includes a bell-shaped dose-response curve observed in preclinical studies (1759–1761), it has been thought that overdose with buprenorphine would have a low likelihood of producing significant respiratory depression. Indeed, there have been at least two case reports of buprenorphine overdose in which patients did not experience respiratory depression (1762, 1763). However, there have also been case reports from France of deaths associated with buprenorphine use, typically when buprenorphine was injected in combination with a benzodiazepine, most typically flunitrazepam, which is not available by prescription in the United States (1764, 1765). There is also preclinical evidence that the combination of buprenorphine and a benzodiazepine can cause respiratory depression (1766) and evidence that suggests the interaction of buprenorphine with flunitrazepam is due to pharmacodynamic rather than pharmacokinetic effects (1767). Finally, benzodiazepine abuse is not uncommon in opioid-dependent patients in the United States; in one outpatient clinical trial of buprenorphine-treated patients, 6.2% of the patients' urine samples were positive for benzodiazepines (1363). However, buprenorphine-related deaths in U.S. clinical trials were not found, suggesting that use of buprenorphine as prescribed, even when combined with illicit benzodiazepine use, is typically not associated with fatalities. However, more liberal availability of buprenorphine in the United States could lead to deaths as has been seen in France.

b) Opioid antagonist therapy: naltrexone

Naltrexone is the only opioid antagonist medication currently approved in the United States for the maintenance treatment of opioid dependence.

(1) Efficacy of naltrexone as a maintenance agent

Naltrexone's efficacy in the treatment of opioid dependence has been studied under two general experimental designs: the inpatient human laboratory and outpatient clinical trials.

a. Naltrexone's efficacy as demonstrated in human laboratory studies

Studies of naltrexone in the human laboratory setting have typically withdrawn opioid-dependent volunteers from opioids and then tested the acute effects of opioids while maintaining the subjects on naltrexone. Under such conditions, naltrexone has been shown to be effective in blocking the effects of acute opioid use (145, 1768–1772).

In one study, for example, 12 heroin-dependent inpatients were withdrawn from opiates and then maintained on 50 mg/day of naltrexone (N=3) or daily placebo (N=9) (1372). The subjects were then allowed to self-administer four doses of heroin each day over the next 10 days. At the end of the study, the placebo group self-administered significantly more doses of heroin than did the naltrexone group. The naltrexone group self-administered heroin six times over the 10 days, whereas every placebo-maintained subject took heroin at least twice per day and three of the nine took all available heroin over the 10-day period. Results such as these demonstrate that naltrexone can be highly effective in blocking the effects of short-acting opioids such as heroin.

b. Naltrexone's efficacy as demonstrated in clinical trials

There have been numerous reports on clinician experience with the use of naltrexone in the outpatient treatment of opioid dependence (1773–1779). Large, double-blind, placebo-controlled studies of naltrexone are more uncommon, partly because maintaining the blind in an outpatient study of naltrexone is virtually impossible. Participants can easily guess their condition assignment if they use opiates and feel or do not feel an effect.

One of the earliest and still one of the largest double-blind studies comparing naltrexone with placebo for the treatment of opioid dependence illustrates the difficulties in such clinical trials (1375). This multisite study enrolled 735 patients who were recently withdrawn from illicit opioids, maintained on but withdrawn from methadone prior to receiving the study medication, or withdrawn from opioids and participating in drug-free treatment. The attrition rate for this study was high, with 543 (74%) participants dropping out before receiving any study medication. Of the 192 who received medication, 170 (89%) dropped out before completing the 9-month study, with >50% dropping out in the first 2 months of the study. For participants who submitted at least five urine samples, there was no significant difference in rates of opioid-positive urine samples. However, an analysis of a subgroup of patients who had at least one opioid-positive urine sample, implying they would have experienced naltrexone's beneficial effect or placebo's lack of effect, found a significantly lower rate of opioid-positive urine samples in the naltrexone-treated (N=17) versus the placebo-treated (N=18) group. This study, which sought to test the overall acceptability and efficacy of naltrexone treatment, showed there could be some possible efficacy in a small group of patients and concluded that this group is most likely to be those who are already in drug-free counseling and who have a high level of motivation.

Voucher incentives have been shown to improve patient adherence with naltrexone treatment (1406, 1407), and improved adherence implies that there should be less illicit opioid use. In the study by Preston et al. (1406), for example, 58 naltrexone-treated patients were randomly assigned to a contingent group where voucher incentives were given for each naltrexone dose taken (N=19), a noncontingent group where voucher incentives were given unsystematically and independent of medication adherence (N=19), or a no-voucher group (N=20). Comparing illicit opioid use among the three groups was extremely difficult because the group receiving vouchers contingent on adherence had substantially greater rates of treatment completion and mean time remaining in treatment. Nevertheless, there was a tendency for the contingent group to have the lowest rate of opioid-positive urine samples. The study by Carroll et al. (1407) also found voucher incentives enhanced naltrexone adherence, which in turn was associated with less illicit opioid use.

The legal system can also provide an external motivation for adherence with naltrexone treatment. A random assignment study of 51 individuals on federal probation compared probation plus naltrexone and counseling with probation and counseling alone (1375). At the end of the 6-month study, no significant differences in treatment retention were found between the two groups, but the group that also received naltrexone had significantly lower rates of opioid-positive urine samples and reincarceration. Other studies of individuals with high levels of motivation to remain abstinent, such as business executives and physicians (1374), provide further evidence that this medication can be useful under the proper clinical circumstances.

(2) Safety and side effects of naltrexone

In general, naltrexone is a safe medication with few side effects. There has been concern that naltrexone can produce elevations in liver function tests, but these effects were observed in only four studies where patients were treated for atypical indications (e.g., obesity, dementia) with naltrexone doses higher than those used for the treatment of opioid dependence (e.g., up to 300 mg/day). These elevations in liver function tests occurred only with the 300 mg/day dose of naltrexone, were seen in only 1 out of 40 (2.5%) subjects under age 40 years compared with 18.5% of individuals older than age 40, and resolved with naltrexone discontinuation (1374). However, there is one letter reporting that the risk of increased liver function tests may occur if naltrexone is taken with NSAIDs (1047). Although the approved label for naltrexone cautions about its potential effects on liver function tests, the likelihood that these hepatic effects will occur in patients treated within the usual dose range (50–150 mg/day) and without preexisting liver disease is minimal.

c) Clonidine and other nonopioid medications used for the treatment of opioid withdrawal

Clonidine is an α_2-adrenergic agonist approved in the United States for the treatment of hypertension but not for the treatment of opioid withdrawal. Clonidine has been used as an aid in controlling opioid withdrawal symptoms; unlike methadone, LAAM, buprenorphine, and naltrexone, it is not used as a maintenance treatment agent.

A related medication is lofexidine, another α_2-adrenergic agonist approved for the treatment of opioid withdrawal in the United Kingdom but not currently available in the United

States. There is evidence that lofexidine can be as effective as clonidine in the treatment of opioid withdrawal and that it produces less hypotension than does clonidine (1780–1782). However, at least one controlled inpatient study did not show that lofexidine markedly attenuated opioid withdrawal symptoms that were produced by a naloxone challenge (1783), and another study found buprenorphine was more effective than lofexidine when used in the treatment of opioid withdrawal (1784). The remainder of this section focuses on clonidine; no further review of lofexidine is provided here.

(1) Use of clonidine as a withdrawal (detoxification) agent

Several early studies tested the efficacy of clonidine when used on an inpatient basis for the treatment of opioid withdrawal (1388, 1785–1787). For example, a study that sought to determine optimal clonidine dosing parameters used a 2-week inpatient design and enrolled 25 methadone-maintained male and female patients (1380). Subjects had a double-blind abrupt discontinuation of their methadone dose and then started receiving thrice-daily clonidine 24 or 48 hours later, with flexible dosing based on signs and symptoms of withdrawal. Clonidine was found to reduce opioid withdrawal symptoms (compared with patient perception of previous withdrawal attempts), although symptoms of anxiety, restlessness, insomnia, and muscle aches were not relieved completely.

Another inpatient study used a classic substitution design to test the efficacy of acute doses of clonidine to suppress spontaneous opioid withdrawal symptoms in 10 male patients maintained on daily subcutaneous doses of morphine (1383). In this study, clonidine was found to be more effective than morphine in suppressing opioid withdrawal signs, although it was less effective than morphine in attenuating subjective complaints of opioid withdrawal.

Finally, a double-blind study from Spain compared the inpatient use of clonidine to a relatively low dose of methadone for short-term (8- to 10-day) withdrawal from heroin (1382). There were initially 45 subjects in the study; most of those who left the study early were taking clonidine. For those who remained (N=30), clonidine and methadone were found to be equally effective on measures of withdrawal. In an interesting finding, it appears that there was actually less residual opioid withdrawal at the end of this inpatient study for the clonidine patients compared with the methadone patients. However, the relatively short period of treatment and the low dose of methadone may have contributed to the finding of comparable efficacy for the two medications among patients who remained in the study.

Clonidine has also been examined for its efficacy in the outpatient treatment of opioid withdrawal (1384–1386). For example, a double-blind outpatient study with 49 opioid-dependent male and female participants compared methadone and clonidine in the treatment of withdrawal (1381). Participants in the study had relatively low levels of physical dependence (20 mg of daily methadone). In the study, participants underwent a double-blind 20-day methadone withdrawal or a 15-day clonidine withdrawal. There was no difference in the two groups among those successfully completing the withdrawal, although the clonidine-treated subjects tended to have greater withdrawal symptoms and to drop out earlier compared with the methadone-treated patients.

(2) Safety and side effects of clonidine

The most significant side effect associated with the use of clonidine in the treatment of opioid withdrawal is hypotension; the lowering of blood pressure by clonidine can be clinically significant for some opioid-dependent patients. This effect has been noted in many of the clinical studies of clonidine (1380, 1382, 1383, 1392, 1742, 1787) and has led to the common recommendation that when clonidine is used for opioid withdrawal, the treating physician regularly check the patient's blood pressure and hold the dose if hypotensive effects are noted.

Other side effects noted with clonidine when used for the treatment of opioid withdrawal have included sedation and other sleep difficulties, dry mouth, and constipation. In some cases, it can be difficult to know if these more uncommon symptoms are side effects of clonidine or opioid withdrawal effects that are not fully treated by clonidine.

2. Psychosocial treatments

As noted previously, psychosocial treatments for opioid-related disorders have been studied only in programs that also provide maintenance treatment with either opioid agonists (e.g., methadone) or antagonists.

a) Cognitive-behavioral therapies

Woody et al. (177, 531, 1400, 1401) randomly assigned methadone maintenance patients to one of three groups: 1) drug counseling alone, 2) drug counseling plus supportive-expressive psychotherapy, or 3) drug counseling plus CBT. Outcomes were determined at 7 and 12 months. In patients with a moderate to high degree of depression or other psychiatric symptoms, drug counseling with supportive-expressive therapy or CBT was much more effective than drug counseling alone; for patients with low levels of psychiatric symptoms, all three treatment conditions were equally effective. These findings were essentially replicated in three community-based methadone maintenance clinics (218). O'Neill et al. (1402) evaluated a CBT intervention added to a methadone program for pregnant, injecting drug users at risk for HIV infection. CBT resulted in significantly greater reductions in HIV risk behaviors.

(1) Relapse prevention strategies

McAuliffe (1403) reported that when combined with participation in a self-help group, group relapse prevention based on a conditioning model of addiction was more effective than no treatment in reducing opioid use, unemployment, and criminal activities in recently detoxified patients.

b) Behavioral therapies

(1) Contingency management

In a study evaluating the intensity of behavioral treatments for methadone patients, McLellan et al. (170) determined whether the addition of contingency-based counseling, general medical care, and psychosocial services improved the efficacy of methadone maintenance treatment in a study of newly admitted opioid patients randomly assigned to three levels of care. Patients who received counseling and contingencies based on urine test results, in addition to methadone, had better drug use outcomes than those who received methadone only. Patients who in addition received on-site general medical and psychiatric care, employment services, and family therapy had the best outcomes of all three conditions. Methadone alone was an effective treatment for only a small percentage of patients.

Several studies have evaluated the use of contingency management in reducing the use of illicit drugs in opioid-dependent individuals who are maintained on methadone. In these studies, a reinforcer (reward) is provided to patients who demonstrate specified target behaviors such as providing drug-free urine specimens, accomplishing specific treatment goals, or attending treatment sessions. For example, offering methadone take-home privileges contingent on reduced drug use is an approach that capitalizes on an inexpensive reinforcer that is potentially available in all methadone maintenance programs. Stitzer and colleagues (197–199) have done extensive work in evaluating methadone take-home privileges as a reward for decreased illicit drug use. In a series of well-controlled trials, these researchers have demonstrated 1) the relative benefits of positive (e.g., rewarding desired behaviors such as abstinence) compared with negative (e.g., punishing undesired behaviors such as continued drug use through discharges or dose reductions) contingencies (197), 2) the attractiveness of take-home privileges over other incentives available within methadone maintenance clinics (198), and 3) the relative effectiveness of rewarding drug-free urine specimens compared with other target behaviors (202).

Silverman and colleagues (195, 1295), drawing on the compelling work of Higgins and colleagues (described below), evaluated in a series of studies the efficacy of a voucher-based contingency management system to address concurrent illicit drug use (typically cocaine) among methadone-maintained opioid-dependent individuals. In this approach, urine specimens were required three times a week to systematically detect all episodes of drug use. Abstinence, verified through urine screens, was reinforced through a voucher system in which patients received points redeemable for items consistent with a drug-free lifestyle that were intended to help the patient develop alternate reinforcers to drug use (e.g., movie tickets, sporting goods). Silverman and colleagues (195, 1295) demonstrated the efficacy of this approach in reducing illicit opioid and cocaine use.

Opioid antagonist treatment (naltrexone) offers many advantages over methadone maintenance, including the fact that it is nonaddicting and can be prescribed without concerns about diversion, has a benign side effect profile, and can be less costly in terms of demands on professional time and patient time than the daily or near-daily clinic visits required for methadone maintenance (165). Most important are the behavioral aspects of treatment, as unreinforced opiate use allows the extinction of the association between cues and drug use. Although naltrexone treatment is likely to be attractive only to a small number of opioid-dependent individuals (166), naltrexone's unique properties make it an important alternative to methadone maintenance and other agonist approaches.

However, despite its many advantages, naltrexone has not fulfilled its promise. Naltrexone treatment programs remain comparatively rare and underutilized as compared with methadone maintenance programs (165), largely because of problems with retention, particularly during the induction phase; an average of 40% of patients drop out during the first month of treatment and 60% drop out by 3 months (166). In the 1970s, several preliminary evaluations identified the promise of using behavioral interventions to address naltrexone's weaknesses, including providing incentives for adherence with naltrexone treatment (1404, 1405) and the addition of family therapy to naltrexone treatment (1788). However, the interventions were not widely adopted, adherence remained a major problem, and naltrexone treatment and research dropped off considerably until the past few years, when the need for alternatives to methadone maintenance stimulated a modest revival of interest in naltrexone.

Some of the most recent promising data about strategies to enhance retention and outcome in naltrexone treatment have come from investigations of contingency management approaches. Preston et al. (1406) found improved retention and naltrexone treatment adherence with an approach that provided vouchers for adherence as compared with standard naltrexone treatment that did not provide vouchers. Carroll and colleagues (167, 1407) found that reinforcement of naltrexone treatment adherence and drug-free urine specimens, alone or in combination with family involvement in treatment, improved retention rates and reduced drug use among recently detoxified opioid-dependent individuals.

(2) Cue exposure treatment

Cue exposure treatment has been demonstrated to be effective in reducing classically conditioned responses to substance-related cues in a small group of patients with opioid use disorders (189).

c) Psychodynamic and interpersonal therapies

The effectiveness of adding a psychodynamic therapy to a program of methadone maintenance has been investigated. Woody et al. (177, 218) found that supportive-expressive therapy was more effective than drug counseling alone for patients with high levels of other psychiatric symptoms. Rounsaville et al. (1789) attempted to compare the efficacy of a 6-month course of weekly individual IPT with a low-contact comparison condition for individuals in a full-service methadone maintenance program that included weekly group psychotherapy. Patients with opioid dependence who met the inclusion criteria (including the presence of an additional nonpsychotic psychiatric diagnosis) were randomly assigned to the two groups. However, only 5% of the eligible patients agreed to participate (compared with 60% in the Woody et al. study), and only about 50% completed the trial. The highly selective nature of the participants (i.e., 95% of eligible patients refused), the high attrition rate, and the lack of significant outcome differences between the two groups led to the conclusions that it is very difficult to engage opioid-dependent patients in individual IPT and that the potential benefit of such treatment is unclear for those who do participate.

Psychodynamically oriented group therapy modified for substance-dependent patients appears to be effective in promoting abstinence when combined with behavioral monitoring and individual supportive psychotherapy (1301).

Although some follow-up studies of naturalistic treatment have found equivalent efficacy for methadone maintenance and outpatient drug-free programs for heroin users (61, 1396–1398), early attempts at providing psychotherapy alone have yielded unacceptably high attrition rates (1399).

PART C

FUTURE RESEARCH NEEDS

Despite the significant amount already known about substance use disorders, our understanding of these disorders as well as the treatment of patients would be improved by research focusing on a number of areas. One broad area involves delineating the multiple factors that alter the development, manifestations, clinical course, and prognosis of substance use disorders. Such factors may include developmental, biological, cognitive, and sociocultural factors, as well as the impact of early experiences with substances of abuse and the effects of co-occurring psychiatric or general medical conditions. Given the significant numbers of individuals with a co-occurring psychiatric and substance use disorder, improved methods for diagnosis are needed, including approaches for defining the precise temporal and etiological relation between substance use and other forms of psychopathology. Enhanced approaches for identifying prescription opioid dependence would also be beneficial, particularly in individuals with underlying physical disorders that are associated with significant pain.

Research on the modifying factors and underlying causes of substance use disorders is inextricably linked to a need for studies of the gene or genes that influence the heritability of abuse and dependence on specific substances (e.g., alcohol, opioids) as well as the heritability of substance use disorders in general. Genetic factors may also augment risk for or exert protective influences on the development and manifestations of substance use disorders. In a similar vein, other research approaches, including epidemiological studies, can assist in identifying risk and protective factors that influence vulnerability to substance use disorders.

Another topic that requires further research relates to the acute and chronic effects of abused substances. This includes the effects of substances on a variety of organ systems as well as the pathogenesis of substance-induced fetal abnormalities after in utero exposure to substances of abuse. In the CNS, the acute effects of substances on brain morphology, biochemistry, and physiology may be revealed through brain imaging or other assessment techniques. The time course of recovery from these effects once a patient is free of substances also needs delineating.

Such studies may complement assessments of the biological, cognitive, and behavioral factors contributing to the development of prolonged abstinence syndromes in patients previously dependent on nicotine, alcohol, marijuana, cocaine, or opioids.

Virtually every aspect of substance use disorder treatment provides an opportunity for further study and improvements in clinical care. More information is needed about the selection of treatment settings according to the unique needs of the individual patient. The utility of a particular treatment setting for specific disorders may also be worthy of further study (e.g., inpatient approach to smoking cessation). Treatment programs may exhibit differential efficacies or cost-effectiveness depending on the site of treatment, the mix of specific treatment modalities used, the organizational and managerial aspects of the treatment program, and the specific population of patients being served (e.g., individuals using more than one substance or having a co-occurring psychiatric disorder, at-risk individuals receiving preventive services or early interventions).

In addition to learning about specific treatment settings, more information is needed on the specific treatments for intoxication and withdrawal. Even in the treatment of alcohol withdrawal, for which there is considerable evidence and consensus, questions remain about the most effective class(es) of agents, the most effective agent(s) within a particular class, the most effective dosing regimen(s), and the choice of specific agents for treating specific patient subgroups or specific symptoms of withdrawal. For all substance use disorders, research should delineate the intensity and staging of treatment (i.e., using different treatments in different settings at different phases of the disorder) and the interactive (i.e., additive, synergistic, or antagonistic) effects of various treatment modalities when applied concurrently or in sequence. Such studies of treatment modalities, including those in current use and those being developed, will need to examine short-, intermediate-, and long-term outcomes in specific patient populations. The impact of sociodemographic, psychiatric, and general medical characteristics and patient treatment preferences on treatment adherence and outcome are also relevant.

In terms of pharmacotherapeutic approaches to treatment, the development of new therapies might focus on effectively decreasing symptoms of withdrawal (e.g., use of delta-9 tetrahydrocannabinol in marijuana dependence, nonopioid agents for opioid dependence), reducing short- and long-term craving in active and abstinent substance users (e.g., mixed agonist/antagonists for opioid dependence, novel agents including vaccines for cocaine dependence), treating dependence (e.g., to marijuana, cocaine, prescription opioids), and reversing the physiological effects of chronic substance use on the functioning of the brain and other affected organs. For pregnant substance-abusing women, it will be important to develop new pharmacotherapies that do not affect the fetus. In terms of existing pharmacotherapies, additional studies are needed on using combinations of pharmacotherapies (e.g., use of multiple NRTs or NRT and bupropion for nicotine dependence) as well as on the effects of specific pharmacotherapies in treating patients with co-occurring psychiatric and substance use disorders. Additional studies may help guide the identification of patient populations that will benefit from specific treatments (e.g., characteristics of patients who would benefit from naltrexone versus acamprosate for the treatment of an alcohol use disorder). Other therapeutic options could be developed depending on the gene or genes involved in the etiology or treatment responsiveness of substance use disorders (e.g., gene therapy, pharmacogenetics approach to optimizing the choice of pharmacotherapy).

Equally essential is additional research on psychosocial therapies for substance use disorders. Effective psychosocial interventions for the treatment of marijuana dependence are particularly important given the limited options for addressing this problem at present. However, the study of a broad range of psychosocial therapies will enhance therapeutic options for each substance use disorder. For children, adolescents, and adults at risk for a substance use disorder, research is needed on the long-term efficacy of behavioral, psychosocial, and family-based interventions. Other specific subgroups of patients (e.g., those with prescription opioid dependence, those with a co-occurring psychiatric and substance use disorder, individuals with treatment-resistant disorders) may require modified approaches to treatment. For individuals with multiple disorders, integrated approaches to treatment are likely to be needed. Combinations of psychosocial and pharmacological therapies should be examined in terms of augmenting short-term, immediate, and long-term patient outcomes. With each of the psychosocial therapies, research should determine the impact of sociodemographic, psychiatric, and general medical characteristics and patient treatment preferences on treatment participation and outcome.

INDIVIDUALS AND ORGANIZATIONS THAT SUBMITTED COMMENTS

Maryann Amodeo, Ph.D., M.S.W.
James C. Anthony, Ph.D.
Corinne Axelrod, M.P.H., L.Ac., Dipl.Ac.
David Baron, M.S.Ed., D.O.
Sheila Blume, M.D.
Lisa Borg, M.D.
Kathleen T. Brady, M.D., Ph.D.
Michael Brody, M.D.
David W. Brook, M.D.
Kirk J. Brower, M.D., F.A.S.A.M.
Kenneth Carter, M.D., M.P.H.
Scott Coffey, Ph.D.
Mirean Coleman, M.S.W., L.I.C.S.W., C.T.
Wilson Compton, M.D., M.P.E.
George De Leon, Ph.D.
Andrea DiMartini, M.D., F.A.P.M.
Lance M. Dodes, M.D.
Chad D. Emrick, Ph.D.
Michael Farrell, M.B. B.Ch., M.R.C.P., M.R.C.Psych.
David A. Fiellin, M.D.
Loretta Finnegan, M.D.
Marc Fishman, M.D.
Philip J. Flores, Ph.D., A.B.P.P., C.G.P., F.A.G.P.A.
Marc Galanter, M.D.
David R. Gastfriend, M.D.
Eilish Gilvarry, F.R.C.Psych.
Leslie H. Gise, M.D.
Mark S. Gold, M.D.
David Gorelick, M.D., Ph.D.
John Grabowski, Ph.D.
Sanjay Gupta, M.D.
Larry Hammer, M.D.
Allen Harlor, M.D.
Tina Haynes, MT-BC
Alfred Herzog, M.D.
Susan Hoppenworth, L.M.H.C.
John R. Hughes, M.D.
Andy Jagoda, M.D., F.A.C.E.P.
Yifrah Kaminer, M.D., M.B.A.
Kyle M. Kampman, M.D.
Debra K. Katzman, M.D., F.S.A.M.
Janice Kauffman, R.N., M.P.H., C.A.S.
Patricia K. Kokotailo, M.D., M.P.H.
George F. Kolodner, M.D.
Martin Leamon, M.D.
Frances Levin, M.D.
Joseph G. Liberto, M.D.
Theresa E. Madden, D.D.S., Ph.D.
Peter A. Mansky, M.D.
Icro Maremmani, M.D.
G. Alan Marlatt, Ph.D.
Elinore F. McCance-Katz, M.D., Ph.D.
Michael R. McCoy, Ph.D.
Barbara S. McCrady, Ph.D.
Edward P. Monnelly, M.D.
William R. Morris, O.M.D., MS.Ed., L.Ac.
Edgar P. Nace, M.D.
Edward Nunes, M.D.
Herbert S. Peyser, M.D.
Jonathan I. Ritvo, M.D.
Brian Robertson, M.D.
Victor Schermer, M.A., L.P.C.
Jeffrey Selzer, M.D.
Ian Shaffer, M.D., M.M.M.
Tammy L.H. Sims, M.D., M.S.
Robert Stern, M.D., Ph.D.
Maxine Stitzer, Ph.D.
William R. Tatomer, M.D.
Joseph R. Volpicelli, M.D., Ph.D.
Robert Weinstock, M.D.

Academy of Psychosomatic Medicine
American Academy of Addiction Psychiatry
American Academy of Child and Adolescent Psychiatry
American Academy of Clinical Psychiatrists
American Academy of Pediatrics
American Academy of Psychiatry and the Law
American Association of Oriental Medicine
American Group Psychotherapy Association
American Mental Health Counselors Association
American Music Therapy Association
American Psychological Association
American Society of Addiction Medicine
Association for Academic Psychiatry
Association for Cognitive and Behavioral Therapies
Association for Medical Education and Research on Substance Abuse
Group for the Advancement of Psychiatry
Managed Health Network, Inc.
National Acupuncture and Oriental Medicine Alliance
National Association of Social Workers
Royal College of Psychiatrists
Society for Adolescent Medicine
Texas Society of Psychiatric Physicians
World Federation for Mental Health

REFERENCES

The following coding system is used to indicate the nature of the supporting evidence in the summary recommendations and references:

[A] *Double-blind, randomized clinical trial.* A study of an intervention in which subjects are prospectively followed over time; there are treatment and control groups; subjects are randomly assigned to the two groups; both the subjects and the investigators are blind to the assignments.

[A–] *Randomized clinical trial.* Same as above but not double-blind.

[B] *Clinical trial.* A prospective study in which an intervention is made and the results of that intervention are tracked longitudinally; study does not meet standards for a randomized clinical trial.

[C] *Cohort or longitudinal study.* A study in which subjects are prospectively followed over time without any specific intervention.

[D] *Case-control study.* A study in which a group of patients is identified in the present and information about them is pursued retrospectively or backward in time.

[E] *Review with secondary data analysis.* A structured analytic review of existing data, e.g., a meta-analysis or a decision analysis.

[F] *Review.* A qualitative review and discussion of previously published literature without a quantitative synthesis of the data.

[G] *Other.* Textbooks, expert opinion, case reports, and other reports not included above.

1. Wutzke SE, Conigrave KM, Saunders JB, Hall WD: The long-term effectiveness of brief interventions for unsafe alcohol consumption: a 10-year follow-up. Addiction 2002; 97:665–675 [A–]
2. Baker A, Boggs TG, Lewin TJ: Randomized controlled trial of brief cognitive-behavioural interventions among regular users of amphetamine. Addiction 2001; 96:1279–1287 [A–]
3. Bernstein J, Bernstein E, Tassiopoulos K, Heeren T, Levenson S, Hingson R: Brief motivational intervention at a clinic visit reduces cocaine and heroin use. Drug Alcohol Depend 2005; 77:49–59 [A]
4. McLellan AT, Lewis DC, O'Brien CP, Kleber HD: Drug dependence, a chronic medical illness: implications for treatment, insurance, and outcomes evaluation. JAMA 2000; 284:1689–1695 [G]
5. Weiss RD: Adherence to pharmacotherapy in patients with alcohol and opioid dependence. Addiction 2004; 99:1382–1392 [F]
6. DiClemente CC, Schlundt D, Gemmell L: Readiness and stages of change in addiction treatment. Am J Addict 2004; 13:103–119 [F]
7. Siqueland L, Crits-Christoph P: Current developments in psychosocial treatments of alcohol and substance abuse. Curr Psychiatry Rep 1999; 1:179–184 [G]
8. Vaillant GE: A long-term follow-up of male alcohol abuse. Arch Gen Psychiatry 1996; 53:243–249 [C]
9. Vaillant GE: A 60-year follow-up of alcoholic men. Addiction 2003; 98:1043–1051 [C]
10. Marlatt GA, Larimer ME, Baer JS, Quigley LA: Harm reduction for alcohol problems: moving beyond the controlled drinking controversy. Behav Res Ther 1993; 24:461–504 [F]
11. Marlatt GA, Witkiewitz K: Harm reduction approaches to alcohol use: health promotion, prevention, and treatment. Addict Behav 2002; 27:867–886 [F]
12. Miller WR, Page AC: Warm turkey: other routes to abstinence. J Subst Abuse Treat 1991; 8:227–232 [G]
13. Hodgins DC, Leigh G, Milne R, Gerrish R: Drinking goal selection in behavioral self-management treatment of chronic alcoholics. Addict Behav 1997; 22:247–255 [G]
14. Tatarsky A: Harm reduction psychotherapy: extending the reach of traditional substance use treatment. J Subst Abuse Treat 2003; 25:249–256 [G]
15. Marlatt GA, Donovan DM: Relapse Prevention: Maintenance Strategies in the Treatment of Addictive Behaviors, 2nd ed. New York, Guilford, 2005 [G]
16. Saladin ME, Drobes DJ, Coffey SF, Dansky BS, Brady KT, Kilpatrick DG: PTSD symptom severity as a predictor of cue-elicited drug craving in victims of violent crime. Addict Behav 2003; 28:1611–1629 [G]
17. Stewart J: Pathways to relapse: the neurobiology of drug- and stress-induced relapse to drug-taking. J Psychiatry Neurosci 2000; 25:125–136 [G]
18. Wikler A, Pescor FT: Classical conditioning of a morphine abstinence phenomenon, reinforcement of opioid-drinking behavior and "relapse" in morphine-addicted rats. Psychopharmacologia 1967; 10:255–284 [G]
19. Childress A, Ehrman R, Rohsenow DJ, Roberts LJ, O'Brien C: Classically conditioned actors in drug dependence, in Substance Abuse: A Comprehensive Textbook, 2nd ed. Edited by Lowenstein JH, Ruiz P, Millman RB. Baltimore, Md, Williams & Wilkins, 1992, pp 56–69 [F]
20. Wise RA: The neurobiology of craving: implications for the understanding and treatment of addiction. J Abnorm Psychol 1988; 97:118–132 [G]
21. McLellan AT, Alterman AI, Cacciola J, Metzger D, O'Brien CP: A new measure of substance abuse treatment: initial studies of the treatment services review. J Nerv Ment Dis 1992; 180:101–110 [G]

22. Geppert CM: To help and not to harm: ethical issues in the treatment of chronic pain in patients with substance use disorders. Adv Psychosom Med 2004; 25:151–171 [G]
23. Grant BF, Stinson FS, Dawson DA, Chou SP, Dufour MC, Compton W, Pickering RP, Kaplan K: Prevalence and co-occurrence of substance use disorders and independent mood and anxiety disorders: results from the National Epidemiologic Survey on Alcohol and Related Conditions. Arch Gen Psychiatry 2004; 61:807–816 [G]
24. Walker R, Hiller M, Staton M, Leukefeld CG: Head injury among drug abusers: an indicator of co-occurring problems. J Psychoactive Drugs 2003; 35:343–353 [D]
25. Prochaska JO, DiClemente CC, Norcross JC: In search of how people change: applications to addictive behaviors. Am Psychol 1992; 47:1102–1114 [G]
26. Mayfield D, McLeod G, Hall P: The CAGE questionnaire: validation of a new alcoholism screening instrument. Am J Psychiatry 1974; 131:1121–1123 [G]
27. Babor TF, de la Fuente JR, Saunders J, Grant M: AUDIT: The Alcohol Use Disorders Identification Test: Guidelines for Use in Primary Health Care. Geneva, World Health Organization, 1992 [G]
28. Skinner HA: The Drug Abuse Screening Test. Addict Behav 1982; 7:363–371 [G]
29. North CS, Tivis L, McMillen JC, Pfefferbaum B, Spitznagel EL, Cox J, Nixon S, Bunch KP, Smith EM: Psychiatric disorders in rescue workers after the Oklahoma City bombing. Am J Psychiatry 2002; 159:857–859 [G]
30. Paris RT, Canavan DI: Physician substance abuse impairment: anesthesiologists vs other specialties. J Addict Dis 1999; 18:1–7 [D]
31. Bartels SJ, Coakley EH, Zubritsky C, Ware JH, Miles KM, Arean PA, Chen H, Oslin DW, Llorente MD, Costantino G, Quijano L, McIntyre JS, Linkins KW, Oxman TE, Maxwell J, Levkoff SE: Improving access to geriatric mental health services: a randomized trial comparing treatment engagement with integrated versus enhanced referral care for depression, anxiety, and at-risk alcohol use. Am J Psychiatry 2004; 161:1455–1462 [A–]
32. Prochaska JO, Goldstein MG: Process of smoking cessation: implications for clinicians. Clin Chest Med 1991; 12:727–735 [F]
33. Glynn TJ, Manley MW: How to Help Your Patients Stop Smoking. Washington, DC, US Government Printing Office, 1989 [G]
34. Hurt RD, Eberman KM, Slade JD, Karan L: Treating nicotine addiction in patients with other addictive disorders, in Nicotine Addiction: Principles and Management. Edited by Orleans CT, Slade J. New York, Oxford University Press, 1993, pp 310–326 [F]
35. Sullivan MA, Covey LS: Current perspectives on smoking cessation among substance abusers. Curr Psychiatry Rep 2002; 4:388–396 [G]
36. Cooney JL, Cooney NL, Pilkey DT, Kranzler HR, Oncken CA: Effects of nicotine deprivation on urges to drink and smoke in alcoholic smokers. Addiction 2003; 98:913–921 [B]
37. Kohn CS, Tsoh JY, Weisner CM: Changes in smoking status among substance abusers: baseline characteristics and abstinence from alcohol and drugs at 12-month follow-up. Drug Alcohol Depend 2003; 69:61–71 [B]
38. Joseph AM, Willenbring ML, Nugent SM, Nelson DB: A randomized trial of concurrent versus delayed smoking intervention for patients in alcohol dependence treatment. J Stud Alcohol 2004; 65:681–691 [A–]
39. Mee-Lee D, Shulman GD, Fishman M, Gastfriend DR, Griffith JH (eds): ASAM Patient Placement Criteria for the Treatment of Substance-Related Disorders, 2nd ed., revised. Chevy Chase, Md, American Society of Addiction Medicine, 2001 [G]
40. Dennis ML, Perl HI, Huebner RB, McLellan AT: Twenty-five strategies for improving the design, implementation and analysis of health services research related to alcohol and other drug abuse treatment. Addiction 2000; 95(suppl 3):S281–S308 [G]

41. Apsler R, Harding WM: Cost-effectiveness analysis of drug abuse treatment: current status and recommendations for future research, in Drug Abuse Services Research Series, No. 1: Background Papers on Drug Abuse Financing and Services Approach. Rockville, Md, National Institute on Drug Abuse, 1991, pp 58–81 [E]
42. Gerstein DR: Outcome research: drug abuse, in The American Psychiatric Publishing Textbook of Substance Abuse Treatment, 3rd ed. Edited by Galanter M, Kleber HD. Washington, DC, American Psychiatric Publishing, 2004, pp 137–147 [G]
43. Project MATCH Research Group: Matching alcoholism treatments to client heterogeneity: Project MATCH posttreatment drinking outcomes. J Stud Alcohol 1997; 58:7–29 [A–]
44. De Leon G, Wexler HK, Jainchill N: The therapeutic community: success and improvement rates 5 years after treatment. Int J Addict 1982; 17:703–747 [C]
45. Hubbard RL, Craddock SG, Anderson J: Overview of 5-year follow-up outcomes in the Drug Abuse Treatment Outcome Studies (DATOS). J Subst Abuse Treat 2003; 25:125–134 [C]
46. Dackis CA, Gold MS: Psychiatric hospitals for treatment of dual diagnosis, in Substance Abuse: A Comprehensive Textbook, 2nd ed. Edited by Lowinson JH, Ruiz P, Millman RB. Baltimore, MD, Williams & Wilkins, 1992, pp 467–485 [F]
47. Weiss RD, Sharpe Potter J: Inpatient treatment, in The American Psychiatric Publishing Textbook of Substance Abuse Treatment, 3rd ed. Edited by Galanter M, Kleber HD. Washington, DC, American Psychiatric Publishing, 2004, pp 445–456 [G]
48. Hayashida M, Alterman AI, McLellan AT, O'Brien CP, Purtill JJ, Volpicelli JR, Raphaelson AH, Hall CP: Comparative effectiveness and costs of inpatient and outpatient detoxification of patients with mild-to-moderate alcohol withdrawal syndrome. N Engl J Med 1989; 320:358–365 [A–]
49. Miller WR, Rollnick S: Motivational Interviewing: Preparing People for Change, 2nd ed. New York, Guilford, 2002 [G]
50. McLellan AT, Hagan TA, Meyers K, Randall M, Durell J: "Intensive" outpatient substance abuse treatment: comparisons with "traditional" outpatient treatment. J Addict Dis 1997; 16:57–84 [G]
51. Longabaugh R: Longitudinal outcome studies, in Alcoholism: Origins and Outcome. Edited by Rose RM, Barrett JE. New York, Raven Press, 1987, pp 267–280 [F]
52. Fink EB, Longabaugh R, McCrady BM, Stout RL, Beattie M, Ruggieri-Authelet A, McNeil D: Effectiveness of alcoholism treatment in partial versus inpatient settings: twenty-four month outcomes. Addict Behav 1985; 10:235–248 [B]
53. Coviello DM, Alterman AI, Rutherford MJ, Cacciola JS, McKay JR, Zanis DA: The effectiveness of two intensities of psychosocial treatment for cocaine dependence. Drug Alcohol Depend 2001; 61:145–154 [A–]
54. Gottheil E, Weinstein SP, Sterling RC, Lundy A, Serota RD: A randomized controlled study of the effectiveness of intensive outpatient treatment for cocaine dependence. Psychiatr Serv 1998; 49:782–787 [A–]
55. Friedman AS, Glickman NW: Residential program characteristics for completion of treatment by adolescent drug abusers. J Nerv Ment Dis 1987; 175:419–424 [C]
56. Dasinger LK, Shane PA, Martinovich Z: Assessing the effectiveness of community-based substance abuse treatment for adolescents. J Psychoactive Drugs 2004; 36:27–33 [B]
57. French MT, McCollister KE, Cacciola J, Durell J, Stephens RL: Benefit-cost analysis of addiction treatment in Arkansas: specialty and standard residential programs for pregnant and parenting women. Subst Abus 2002; 23:31–51 [G]
58. McLellan AT, Childress AR, Griffith J, Woody GE: The psychiatrically severe drug abuse patient: methadone maintenance or therapeutic community? Am J Drug Alcohol Abuse 1984; 10:77–95 [C]

59. De Leon G: Therapeutic communities, in The American Psychiatric Publishing Textbook of Substance Abuse Treatment, 3rd ed. Edited by Galanter M, Kleber HD. Washington, DC, American Psychiatric Publishing, 2004, pp 485–501 [G]
60. De Leon G, Schwartz S: Therapeutic communities: what are the retention rates? Am J Drug Alcohol Abuse 1984; 10:267–284 [C]
61. Simpson DD, Sells S (eds): Opioid Addiction and Treatment: A 12-Year Follow-Up. Melbourne, Fla, Robert E. Krieger, 1990 [G]
62. Simpson DD, Joe GW, Brown BS: Treatment retention and follow-up outcomes in the Drug Abuse Treatment Outcome Study (DATOS). Psychol Addict Behav 1997; 11:294–307 [G]
63. De Leon G: The Therapeutic Community: Study of Effectiveness. Rockville, Md, National Institute on Drug Abuse, 1984 [C]
64. Wexler HK, Falkin GP, Lipton DS: Outcome evaluation of a prison therapeutic community for substance abuse treatment. Crim Justice Behav 1990; 17:71–90 [G]
65. Therapeutic Communities of America: Therapeutic Communities in Correctional Settings: The Prison-Based TC Standards Development Project. Final Report of Phase II. Washington, DC, White House Office of National Drug Control Policy, 1999 [G]
66. Friedmann PD, Hendrickson JC, Gerstein DR, Zhang Z: The effect of matching comprehensive services to patients' needs on drug use improvement in addiction treatment. Addiction 2004; 99:962–972 [G]
67. Lemke S, Moos RH: Treatment and outcomes of older patients with alcohol use disorders in community residential programs. J Stud Alcohol 2003; 64:219–226 [B]
68. Jason LA, Davis MI, Ferrari JR, Bishop PD: Oxford House: a review of research and implications for substance abuse recovery and community research. J Drug Educ 2001; 31:1–27 [G]
69. Weiner DA, Abraham ME, Lyons J: Clinical characteristics of youths with substance use problems and implications for residential treatment. Psychiatr Serv 2001; 52:793–799 [G]
70. Miller WR, Wilbourne PL, Hettema JE: What works? a summary of alcohol treatment outcome research, in Handbook of Alcoholism Treatment Approaches: Effective Alternatives, 3rd ed. Edited by Hester RK, Miller WR. Needham Heights, Mass, Allyn & Bacon, 2003, pp 13–63 [G]
71. Fiore MC, Smith SS, Jorenby DE, Baker TB: The effectiveness of the nicotine patch for smoking cessation: a meta-analysis. JAMA 1994; 271:1940–1947 [E]
72. US Department of Health and Human Services: Treating Tobacco Use and Dependence: A Clinical Practice Guideline. Rockville, Md, US Department of Health and Human Services, 2000 [G]
73. Hubbard RL, Craddock SG, Flynn PM, Anderson J, Etheridge RM: Overview of 1-year follow-up outcomes in the Drug Abuse Treatment Outcome Study (DATOS). Psychol Addict Behav 1997; 11:261–278 [C]
74. Johnson RE, Chutuape MA, Strain EC, Walsh SL, Stitzer ML, Bigelow GE: A comparison of levomethadyl acetate, buprenorphine, and methadone for opioid dependence. N Engl J Med 2000; 343:1290–1297 [A]
75. Kleber H, Slobetz F: Outpatient drug-free treatment, in Handbook on Drug Abuse. Edited by DuPont RL, Goldstein A, O'Donnell J. Rockville, Md, National Institute on Drug Abuse, 1979, pp 31–38 [G]
76. Center for Substance Abuse Treatment: Comprehensive Case Management for Substance Abuse Treatment Improvement Protocol (TIP) Series No. 27. DHHS Publication (SMA) 98-3222. Rockville, MD, US Department of Health and Human Services, 1998 [G]
77. McNeese-Smith DK: Case management within substance abuse treatment programs in Los Angeles County. Care Manag J 1999; 1:10–18 [G]

78. Graham K, Timney CB: Case management in addictions treatment. J Subst Abuse Treat 1990; 7:181–188 [G]
79. Miller WR, Wilbourne PL: Mesa Grande: a methodological analysis of clinical trials of treatments for alcohol use disorders. Addiction 2002; 97:265–277 [F]
80. Drake RE, Mercer-McFadden C, Mueser KT, McHugo GJ, Bond GR: Review of integrated mental health and substance abuse treatment for patients with dual disorders. Schizophr Bull 1998; 24:589–608 [F]
81. Godley MD, Godley SH, Dennis ML, Funk R, Passetti LL: Preliminary outcomes from the assertive continuing care experiment for adolescents discharged from residential treatment. J Subst Abuse Treat 2002; 23:21–32 [A–]
82. Belenko S: Research on drug courts: a critical review. National Drug Court Institute Review 1998; 1:1–42 [F]
83. McCartt AT, Northrup VS: Effects of enhanced sanctions for high-BAC DWI offenders on case dispositions and rates of recidivism. Traffic Inj Prev 2004; 5:270–277 [C]
84. Peters RH, May RI, Kearns WD: Drug treatment in jails: results of a nationwide survey. J Crim Justice 1997; 20:283–295 [G]
85. Roman PM, Blum TC: Effectiveness of workplace alcohol problem interventions. Am J Health Promot 1996; 11:112–128 [G]
86. Zarkin GA, Bray JW, Qi J: The effect of employee assistance programs use on healthcare utilization. Health Serv Res 2000; 35:77–100 [G]
87. French MT, Zarkin GA, Bray JW, Hartwell TD: Costs of employee assistance programs: findings from a national survey. Am J Health Promot 1997; 11:219–222. [G]
88. Blum TC, Roman PM: A description of clients using employee assistance programs. Alcohol Health Res World 1992; 16:120–128 [G]
89. US Department of Health and Human Services: Enhancing Motivation for Change in Substance Abuse Treatment: Treatment Improvement Protocol (TIP) Series No. 35. DHHS Publication (SMA) 99-3354. Rockville, Md, Substance Abuse and Mental Health Services Administration, 1999 [G]
90. Project MATCH Research Group: Project MATCH (Matching Alcoholism Treatment to Client Heterogeneity): rationale and methods for a multisite clinical trial matching patients to alcoholism treatment. Alcohol Clin Exp Res 1993; 17:1130–1145 [G]
91. Fleisch B: Approaches in the Treatment of Adolescents With Emotional and Substance Abuse Problems. Rockville, Md, US Department of Health and Human Services, 1991 [G]
92. Friedman AS, Bickel WK: Treatment Services for Adolescent Substance Abusers. DHHS Publication (ADM) 85-1342. Rockville, Md, National Institute on Drug Abuse, 2003 [G]
93. Horvath AO, Luborsky L: The role of the therapeutic alliance in psychotherapy. J Consult Clin Psychol 1993; 61:561–573 [G]
94. Luborsky L, McLellan AT, Woody GE, O'Brien CP, Auerbach A: Therapist success and its determinants. Arch Gen Psychiatry 1985; 42:602–611 [D]
95. Connors GJ, Carroll KM, DiClemente CC, Longabaugh R, Donovan DM: The therapeutic alliance and its relationship to alcoholism treatment participation and outcome. J Consult Clin Psychol 1997; 65:588–598 [B]
96. Belding MA, Iguchi MY, Morral AR, McLellan AT: Assessing the helping alliance and its impact in the treatment of opiate dependence. Drug Alcohol Depend 1997; 48:51–59 [B]
97. De Weert-Van Oene GH, Schippers GM, De Jong CA, Schrijvers GJ: Retention in substance dependence treatment: the relevance of in-treatment factors. J Subst Abuse Treat 2001; 20:253–261 [G]

98. Barber JP, Luborsky L, Gallop R, Crits-Christoph P, Frank A, Weiss RD, Thase ME, Connolly MB, Gladis M, Foltz C, Siqueland L: Therapeutic alliance as a predictor of outcome and retention in the National Institute on Drug Abuse Collaborative Cocaine Treatment Study. J Consult Clin Psychol 2001; 69:119–124 [G]
99. Raytek HS, McGrady BS, Epstein EE, Hirsch LS: Therapeutic alliance and the retention of couples in conjoint alcoholism treatment. Addict Behav 1999; 24:317–330 [G]
100. Ackerman SJ, Hilsenroth MJ: A review of therapist characteristics and techniques positively impacting the therapeutic alliance. Clin Psychol Rev 2003; 23:1–33 [F]
101. Najavits LM, Weiss RD: Variations in therapist effectiveness in the treatment of patients with substance use disorders: an empirical review. Addiction 1994; 89:679–688 [F]
102. Safran JD, Muran JC: Resolving therapeutic alliance ruptures: diversity and integration. J Clin Psychol 2000; 56:233–243 [G]
103. Seymour PM: Long-term treatment of an addictive personality. Bull Menninger Clin 2003; 67:328–346 [G]
104. Klein RH, Orleans JF, Soule CR: The axis II group: treating severely characterologically disturbed patients. Int J Group Psychother 1991; 41:97–115 [G]
105. Benowitz NL: The use of biologic fluid samples in assessing tobacco smoke consumption. NIDA Res Monogr 1983; 48:6–26 [F]
106. Wurst FM, Wiesbeck GA, Metzger JW, Weinmann W: On sensitivity, specificity, and the influence of various parameters on ethyl glucuronide levels in urine: results from the WHO/ISBRA study. Alcohol Clin Exp Res 2004; 28:1220–1228 [G]
107. Skipper GE, Weinmann W, Thierauf A, Schaefer P, Wiesbeck G, Allen JP, Miller M, Wurst FM: Ethyl glucuronide: a biomarker to identify alcohol use by health professionals recovering from substance use disorders. Alcohol Alcohol 2004; 39:445–449 [G]
108. Seidl S, Wurst FM, Alt A: Ethyl glucuronide: a biological marker for recent alcohol consumption. Addict Biol 2001; 6:205–212 [G]
109. Centrella M: Physician addiction and impairment, current thinking: a review. J Addict Dis 1994; 13:91–105 [G]
110. Pakull B: The Federal Aviation Administration's role in evaluation of pilots and others with alcoholism or drug addiction. Occup Med 2002; 17:221–226, iv [G]
111. Domino KB, Hornbein TF, Polissar NL, Renner G, Johnson J, Alberti S, Hankes L: Risk factors for relapse in health care professionals with substance use disorders. JAMA 2005; 293:1453–1460 [C]
112. Weisner C, Mertens J, Parthasarathy S, Moore C, Lu Y: Integrating primary medical care with addiction treatment: a randomized controlled trial. JAMA 2001; 286:1715–1723 [A–]
113. Hazelton LD, Sterns GL, Chisholm T: Decision-making capacity and alcohol abuse: clinical and ethical considerations in personal care choices. Gen Hosp Psychiatry 2003; 25:130–135 [G]
114. Granholm E, Anthenelli R, Monteiro R, Sevcik J, Stoler M: Brief integrated outpatient dual-diagnosis treatment reduces psychiatric hospitalizations. Am J Addict 2003; 12:306–313 [B]
115. Meyer JM: Treating the mind and body in schizophrenia: risks and prevention. CNS Spectr 2004; 9:25–33 [G]
116. Connors GJ, Walitzer KS, Dermen KH: Preparing clients for alcoholism treatment: effects on treatment participation and outcomes. J Consult Clin Psychol 2002; 70:1161–1169 [A–]
117. Chan KK, Neighbors C, Marlatt GA: Treating addictive behaviors in the employee assistance program: implications for brief interventions. Addict Behav 2004; 29:1883–1887 [G]

118. Lowman C, Allen J, Stout RL: Replication and extension of Marlatt's taxonomy of relapse precipitants: overview of procedures and results. The Relapse Research Group. Addiction 1996; 91(suppl):S51–S71 [G]
119. Khantzian EJ: The primary care therapist and patient needs in substance abuse treatment. Am J Drug Alcohol Abuse 1988; 14:159–167 [G]
120. Galanter M: Network therapy for addiction: a model for office practice. Am J Psychiatry 1993; 150:28–36 [G]
121. Substance Abuse and Mental Health Services Administration: Report to Congress on the Prevention and Treatment of Co-Occurring Substance Abuse Disorders and Mental Disorders. Washington, DC, US Department of Health and Human Services, 2002. http://alt.samhsa.gov/reports/congress2002/index.html [G]
122. Daley DC, Marlatt GA: Relapse prevention: cognitive and behavioral interventions, in Substance Abuse: A Comprehensive Textbook, 2nd ed. Edited by Lowinson JH, Ruiz P, Millman RB, Langrod JG. Baltimore, Md, Williams & Wilkins, 1992, pp 533–542 [F]
123. US Department of Health and Human Services: Brief Interventions and Brief Therapies for Substance Abuse: Treatment Improvement Protocol (TIP) Series No. 34. DHHS Publication (SMA) 99-3353. Rockville, Md, Substance Abuse and Mental Health Services Administration, 1999 [G]
124. Miller WR, Hester RK: The effectiveness of alcoholism treatment: what research reveals, in Treating Addictive Behaviors: Processes of Change. Edited by Miller WR, Heather N. New York, Plenum, 1986, pp 121–174 [F]
125. US Department of Health and Human Services: Comprehensive Case Management for Substance Abuse Treatment: Treatment Improvement Protocol (TIP) Series No. 27. DHHS Publication (SMA) 98-3222. Rockville, Md, Substance Abuse and Mental Health Services Administration, 1998 [G]
126. Gutstein HB, Akil H: Opioid analgesics, in Goodman and Gilman's The Pharmacological Basis of Therapeutics, 10th ed. Edited by Hardman JG, Limbird LE, Gilman AG. New York, McGraw-Hill, 2001, pp 569–620 [G]
127. Martin WR: Naloxone. Ann Intern Med 1976; 85:765–768 [G]
128. Doyon S: Opioids, in Emergency Medicine: A Comprehensive Study Guide, 6th ed. Edited by Tintinalli JE, Kelen GD, Stapczynski JS. New York, McGraw-Hill, 2004, pp 1071–1074 [G]
129. Collins ED, Kleber H: Opioids: detoxification, in The American Psychiatric Publishing Textbook of Substance Abuse Treatment, 3rd ed. Edited by Galanter M, Kleber HD. Washington, DC, American Psychiatric Publishing, 2004, pp 265–289 [G]
130. Berkowitz BA: The relationship of pharmacokinetics to pharmacological activity: morphine, methadone and naloxone. Clin Pharmacokinet 1976; 1:219–230 [F]
131. Watson WA, Steele MT, Muelleman RL, Rush MD: Opioid toxicity recurrence after an initial response to naloxone. J Toxicol Clin Toxicol 1998; 36:11–17 [D]
132. Hoffman EJ, Warren EW: Flumazenil: a benzodiazepine antagonist. Clin Pharm 1993; 12:641–656 [F]
133. Schears RM: Nonbenzodiazepine hypnosedatives, in Emergency Medicine: A Comprehensive Study Guide, 6th ed. Edited by Tintinalli JE, Kelen GD, Stapczynski JS. New York, McGraw-Hill, 2004, pp 1057–1064 [G]
134. Hunkeler W, Mohler H, Pieri L, Polc P, Bonetti EP, Cumin R, Schaffner R, Haefely W: Selective antagonists of benzodiazepines. Nature 1981; 290:514–516 [G]
135. Bosse GM: Benzodiazepines, in Emergency Medicine: A Comprehensive Study Guide, 6th ed. Edited by Tintinalli JE, Kelen GD, Stapczynski JS. New York, McGraw-Hill, 2004, pp 1055–1057 [G]
136. Gowing L, Farrell M, Bornemann R, Ali R: Substitution treatment of injecting opioid users for prevention of HIV infection. Cochrane Database Syst Rev 2004; CD004145 [E]

137. Jaffe JH: Drug addiction and drug abuse, in The Pharmacological Basis of Therapeutics, 7th ed. Edited by Gilman AG, Goodman LS, Rall TW, Murad F. New York, Macmillan, 1985, pp 532–581 [F]
138. Liskow BI, Goodwin DW: Pharmacological treatment of alcohol intoxication, withdrawal and dependence: a critical review. J Stud Alcohol 1987; 48:356–370 [F]
139. Jaffe JH: Drugs used in the treatment of alcoholism, in Diagnosis and Treatment of Alcoholism. Edited by Mendelson JH, Mello K. New York, McGraw-Hill, 1985, pp 355–389 [G]
140. Fiore MC, Hatsukami DK, Baker TB: Effective tobacco dependence treatment. JAMA 2002; 288:1768–1771 [G]
141. Mayo-Smith MF, Beecher LH, Fischer TL, Gorelick DA, Guillaume JL, Hill A, Jara G, Kasser C, Melbourne J: Management of alcohol withdrawal delirium: an evidence-based practice guideline. Arch Intern Med 2004; 164:1405–1412 [G]
142. Gowing L, Farrell M, Ali R, White J: $Alpha_2$ adrenergic agonists for the management of opioid withdrawal. Cochrane Database Syst Rev 2004; CD002024 [E]
143. Meyer RE, Mirin SM, Zackon F: Community outcome on narcotic antagonist, in The Heroin Stimulus: Implications for a Theory of Addiction. Edited by Meyer RE, Mirin SM. New York, Plenum, 1979, pp 215–230 [B]
144. Meyer RE, Mirin SM: A psychology of craving: implications of behavioral research, in Substance Abuse: Clinical Problems and Perspectives. Edited by Lowinson JH, Ruiz P. Baltimore, Md, Williams & Wilkins, 1991, pp 57–62 [G]
145. Kleber HD, Kosten TR, Gaspari J, Topazian M: Nontolerance to the opioid antagonism of naltrexone. Biol Psychiatry 1985; 20:66–72 [A]
146. Rose JE, Behm FM, Westman EC, Levin ED, Stein RM, Ripka GV: Mecamylamine combined with nicotine skin patch facilitates smoking cessation beyond nicotine patch treatment alone. Clin Pharmacol Ther 1994; 56:86–99 [G]
147. Rose JE, Behm FM, Westman EC: Nicotine-mecamylamine treatment for smoking cessation: the role of pre-cessation therapy. Exp Clin Psychopharmacol 1998; 6:331–343 [A]
148. Gragg DM: Drugs to decrease alcohol consumption (letter). N Engl J Med 1982; 306:747–748 [G]
149. Banys P: The clinical use of disulfiram (Antabuse): a review. J Psychoactive Drugs 1988; 20:243–261 [F]
150. Fuller RK, Branchey L, Brightwell DR, Derman RM, Emrick CD, Iber FL, James KE, Lacoursiere RB, Lee KK, Lowenstam I: Disulfiram treatment of alcoholism: a Veterans Administration cooperative study. JAMA 1986; 256:1449–1455 [A]
151. Fleming MF, Mihic SJ, Harris RA: Ethanol, in Goodman and Gilman's The Pharmacological Basis of Therapeutics, 10th ed. Edited by Hardman JG, Limbird LE, Gilman A.G. New York, McGraw-Hill, 2001, pp 429–446 [G]
152. Kranzler HR, Van Kirk J: Efficacy of naltrexone and acamprosate for alcoholism treatment: a meta-analysis. Alcohol Clin Exp Res 2001; 25:1335–1341 [E]
153. Streeton C, Whelan G: Naltrexone, a relapse prevention maintenance treatment of alcohol dependence: a meta-analysis of randomized controlled trials. Alcohol Alcohol 2001; 36:544–552 [E]
154. Srisurapanont M, Jarusuraisin N: Opioid antagonists for alcohol dependence. Cochrane Database Syst Rev 2005; CD001867 [E]
155. Littleton J, Zieglgansberger W: Pharmacological mechanisms of naltrexone and acamprosate in the prevention of relapse in alcohol dependence. Am J Addict 2003; 12(suppl 1): S3–S11 [G]
156. Acamprosate campral for alcoholism. Med Lett Drugs Ther 2005; 47:1–3 [F]

157. Spanagel R, Zieglgansberger W: Anti-craving compounds for ethanol: new pharmacological tools to study addictive processes. Trends Pharmacol Sci 1997; 18:54–59 [G]
158. Hurt RD, Sachs DP, Glover ED, Offord KP, Johnston JA, Dale LC, Khayrallah MA, Schroeder DR, Glover PN, Sullivan CR, Croghan IT, Sullivan PM: A comparison of sustained-release bupropion and placebo for smoking cessation. N Engl J Med 1997; 337:1195–1202 [A]
159. Jorenby DE, Leischow SJ, Nides MA, Rennard SI, Johnston JA, Hughes AR, Smith SS, Muramoto ML, Daughton DM, Doan K, Fiore MC, Baker TB: A controlled trial of sustained-release bupropion, a nicotine patch, or both for smoking cessation. N Engl J Med 1999; 340:685–691 [A]
160. Hays JT, Hurt RD, Rigotti NA, Niaura R, Gonzales D, Durcan MJ, Sachs DP, Wolter TD, Buist AS, Johnston JA, White JD: Sustained-release bupropion for pharmacologic relapse prevention after smoking cessation: a randomized, controlled trial. Ann Intern Med 2001; 135:423–433 [A]
161. Ascher JA, Cole JO, Colin JN, Feighner JP, Ferris RM, Fibiger HC, Golden RN, Martin P, Potter WZ, Richelson E: Bupropion: a review of its mechanism of antidepressant activity. J Clin Psychiatry 1995; 56:395–401 [F]
162. Slemmer JE, Martin BR, Damaj MI: Bupropion is a nicotinic antagonist. J Pharmacol Exp Ther 2000; 295:321–327 [G]
163. Rounsaville BJ, Carroll KM, Back S: Individual psychotherapy, in Substance Abuse: A Comprehensive Textbook, 4th ed. Edited by Lowinson JH, Ruiz P, Millman RB, Langrod, JG. Baltimore, Md, Lippincott, Williams & Wilkins, 2004, pp 653–670 [G]
164. Marlatt GA, Gordon GR: Determinants of relapse: implications for the maintenance of behavior change, in Behavioral Medicine: Changing Health Lifestyles. Edited by Davidson PO, Davidson SM. New York, Brunner/Mazel, 1980, pp 410–452 [G]
165. Rounsaville BJ: Can psychotherapy rescue naltrexone treatment of opioid addiction? in Integrating Behavior Therapies With Medication in the Treatment of Drug Dependence. NIDA Research Monograph 150. Edited by Onken LS, Blaine JD, Boren JJ. Rockville, Md, National Institute on Drug Abuse, 1995, pp 37–52 [F]
166. Greenstein R, Fudala PJ, O'Brien CP: Alternative pharmacotherapies for opiate addiction, in Substance Abuse: A Comprehensive Textbook, 3rd ed. Edited by Lowinson JH, Ruiz P, Millman RB, Langrod JG. New York, Williams & Wilkins, 1997, pp 415-424 [G]
167. Carroll KM, Sinha R, Nich C, Babuscio T, Rounsaville BJ: Contingency management to enhance naltrexone treatment of opioid dependence: a randomized clinical trial of reinforcement magnitude. Exp Clin Psychopharmacol 2002; 10:54–63 [A–]
168. Allen JP, Litten RZ: Techniques to enhance compliance with disulfiram. Alcohol Clin Exp Res 1992; 16:1035–1041 [F]
169. Ball JC, Ross A: The Effectiveness of Methadone Maintenance Treatment: Patients, Programs, Services, and Outcome. New York, Springer Verlag, 1991 [G]
170. McLellan AT, Arndt IO, Metzger DS, Woody GE, O'Brien CP: The effects of psychosocial services in substance abuse treatment. JAMA 1993; 269:1953–1959 [A–]
171. Amato L, Minozzi S, Davoli M, Vecchi S, Ferri M, Mayet S: Psychosocial combined with agonist maintenance treatments versus agonist maintenance treatments alone for treatment of opioid dependence. Cochrane Database Syst Rev 2004; CD004147 [E]
172. Hughes JR, Francis RJ: Behavioral support programs for smoking cessation. Mod Med 1994; 62:22–26 [F]
173. Hughes JR: Treatment of nicotine dependence: is more better? JAMA 1995; 274:1390–1391 [F]
174. Rounsaville BJ, Petry NM, Carroll KM: Single versus multiple drug focus in substance abuse clinical trials research. Drug Alcohol Depend 2003; 70:117–125 [G]

175. O'Brien CP: A range of research-based pharmacotherapies for addiction. Science 1997; 278:66–70 [G]
176. Carroll KM: A Cognitive-Behavioral Approach: Treating Cocaine Addiction. NIH Publication 98-4308. Rockville, Md, National Institute on Drug Abuse, 1998 [G]
177. Woody GE, Luborsky L, McLellan AT, O'Brien CP, Beck AT, Blaine J, Herman I, Hole A: Psychotherapy for opiate addicts: does it help? Arch Gen Psychiatry 1983; 40:639–645 [A–]
178. Wright FD, Beck AT, Newman CF, Liese BS: Cognitive therapy of substance abuse: theoretical rationale. NIDA Res Monogr 1993; 137:123–146 [F]
179. Beck AT, Emery GE: Anxiety Disorders and Phobias: A Cognitive Perspective. New York, Basic Books, 1985 [F]
180. Monti P, Abrams D, Kadden R, Cooney N: Treating Alcohol Dependence: A Coping Skills Training Guide. New York, Guilford, 1989 [G]
181. Monti PM: Coping and social skills training, in Handbook of Alcoholism Treatment Approaches: Effective Alternatives, 3rd ed. Edited by Hester RK, Miller WR. Needham Heights, Mass, Allyn & Bacon, 2003, pp 213–236 [G]
182. Shaner A, Eckman T, Roberts LJ, Fuller T: Feasibility of a skills training approach to reduce substance dependence among individuals with schizophrenia. Psychiatr Serv 2003; 54:1287–1289 [B]
183. Griffin KW, Botvin GJ, Nichols TR, Doyle MM: Effectiveness of a universal drug abuse prevention approach for youth at high risk for substance use initiation. Prev Med 2003; 36:1–7 [A–]
184. Marlatt GA, Gordon JR (eds): Relapse Prevention: Maintenance Strategies in the Treatment of Addictive Behaviors. New York, Guilford, 1985 [F]
185. Annis HM, Davis CS: Relapse prevention, in Handbook of Alcoholism Treatment Approaches. Edited by Hester RK, Miller WR. New York, Pergamon, 1989, pp 170–182 [F]
186. Annis HM: A relapse prevention model for treatment of alcoholics, in Treating Addictive Behaviors: Processes of Change. Edited by Miller WR, Heather N. New York, Plenum, 1986, pp 407–433 [F]
187. O''Malley SS, Jaffe AJ, Chang G, Schottenfeld RS, Meyer RE, Rounsaville B: Naltrexone and coping skills therapy for alcohol dependence: a controlled study. Arch Gen Psychiatry 1992; 49:881–887 [A–]
188. Petry NM: A comprehensive guide to the application of contingency management procedures in clinical settings. Drug Alcohol Depend 2000; 58:9–25 [G]
189. O'Brien CP, Childress AR, McLellan T, Ehrman R: Integrating systemic cue exposure with standard treatment in recovering drug dependent patients. Addict Behav 1990; 15:355–365 [G]
190. Azrin NH: Improvements in the community-reinforcement approach to alcoholism. Behav Res Ther 1976; 14:339–348 [G]
191. Higgins ST, Delaney DD, Budney AJ, Bickel WK, Hughes JR, Foerg F, Fenwick JW: A behavioral approach to achieving initial cocaine abstinence. Am J Psychiatry 1991; 148:1218–1224 [B]
192. Higgins ST, Budney AJ, Bickel WK, Hughes JR, Foerg F, Badger G: Achieving cocaine abstinence with a behavioral approach. Am J Psychiatry 1993; 150:763–769 [A–]
193. Higgins ST, Budney AJ, Bickel WK, Foerg FE, Donham R, Badger GJ: Incentives improve outcome in outpatient behavioral treatment of cocaine dependence. Arch Gen Psychiatry 1994; 51:568–576 [A–]
194. Higgins ST, Wong CJ, Badger GJ, Ogden DE, Dantona RL: Contingent reinforcement increases cocaine abstinence during outpatient treatment and 1 year of follow-up. J Consult Clin Psychol 2000; 68:64–72 [A–]

195. Silverman K, Higgins ST, Brooner RK, Montoya ID, Cone EJ, Schuster CR, Preston KL: Sustained cocaine abstinence in methadone maintenance patients through voucher-based reinforcement therapy. Arch Gen Psychiatry 1996; 53:409–415 [A–]
196. Silverman K, Robles E, Mudric T, Bigelow GE, Stitzer ML: A randomized trial of long-term reinforcement of cocaine abstinence in methadone-maintained patients who inject drugs. J Consult Clin Psychol 2004; 72:839–854 [A–]
197. Stitzer ML, Bickel WK, Bigelow GE, Liebson IA: Effect of methadone dose contingencies on urinalysis test results of polydrug-abusing methadone-maintenance patients. Drug Alcohol Depend 1986; 18:341–348 [A–]
198. Stitzer ML, Bigelow GE: Contingency management in a methadone maintenance program: availability of reinforcers. Int J Addict 1978; 13:737–746 [A–]
199. Stitzer ML, Iguchi MY, Felch LJ: Contingent take-home incentive: effects on drug use of methadone maintenance patients. J Consult Clin Psychol 1992; 60:927–934 [A–]
200. Silverman K, Wong CJ, Higgins ST, Brooner RK, Montoya ID, Contoreggi C, Umbricht-Schneiter A, Schuster CR, Preston KL: Increasing opiate abstinence through voucher-based reinforcement therapy. Drug Alcohol Depend 1996; 41:157–165 [B]
201. Budney AJ, Higgins ST, Radonovich KJ, Novy PL: Adding voucher-based incentives to coping skills and motivational enhancement improves outcomes during treatment for marijuana dependence. J Consult Clin Psychol 2000; 68:1051–1061 [A–]
202. Iguchi MY, Lamb RJ, Belding MA, Platt JJ, Husband SD, Morral AR: Contingent reinforcement of group participation versus abstinence in methadone maintenance program. Exp Clin Psychopharmacol 1996; 4:1–7 [A–]
203. Silverman K, Svikis D, Wong CJ, Hampton J, Stitzer ML, Bigelow GE: A reinforcement-based therapeutic workplace for the treatment of drug abuse: three-year abstinence outcomes. Exp Clin Psychopharmacol 2002; 10:228–240 [A–]
204. Petry NM, Martin B: Low-cost contingency management for treating cocaine- and opioid-abusing methadone patients. J Consult Clin Psychol 2002; 70:398–405 [A–]
205. Petry NM, Martin B, Cooney JL, Kranzler HR: Give them prizes, and they will come: contingency management for treatment of alcohol dependence. J Consult Clin Psychol 2000; 68:250–257 [G]
206. Petry NM, Tedford J, Austin M, Nich C, Carroll KM, Rounsaville BJ: Prize reinforcement contingency management for treating cocaine users: how low can we go, and with whom? Addiction 2004; 99:349–360 [A–]
207. Crowley TJ: Contingency contracting treatment of drug-abusing physicians, nurses, and dentists. NIDA Res Monogr 1984; 46:68–83 [B]
208. Meyers RJ, Smith JE: Clinical Guide to Alcohol Treatment: The Community Reinforcement Approach. New York, Guilford, 1995 [G]
209. Petry NM, Simcic F Jr: Recent advances in the dissemination of contingency management techniques: clinical and research perspectives. J Subst Abuse Treat 2002; 23:81–86 [G]
210. Higgins ST, Alessi SM, Dantona RL: Voucher-based incentives: a substance abuse treatment innovation. Addict Behav 2002; 27:887–910 [G]
211. Roozen HG, Boulogne JJ, van Tulder MW, van den Brink W, De Jong CA, Kerkhof AJ: A systematic review of the effectiveness of the community reinforcement approach in alcohol, cocaine and opioid addiction. Drug Alcohol Depend 2004; 74:1–13 [F]
212. Niaura RS, Rohsenow DJ, Binkoff JA, Monti PM, Pedraza M, Abrams DB: Relevance of cue reactivity to understanding alcohol and smoking relapse. J Abnorm Psychol 1988; 97:133–152 [F]
213. Klajner F, Hartman LM, Sobell MB: Treatment of substance abuse by relaxation training: a review of its rationale, efficacy and mechanisms. Addict Behav 1984; 9:41–55 [F]

214. Childress A, Ehrman R, McLellan A, O'Brien C: Update on behavioral treatments for substance abuse. NIDA Res Monogr 1988; 90:183–192 [G]
215. Gabbard G: Psychodynamic Psychotherapy in Clinical Practice, 4th ed. Washington, DC, American Psychiatric Publishing, 2005 [G]
216. Kandel ER: Biology and the future of psychoanalysis: a new intellectual framework for psychiatry revisited. Am J Psychiatry 1999; 156:505–524 [F]
217. Luborsky L: Principles of Psychoanalytic Psychotherapy: A Manual for Supportive-Expressive Treatment. New York, Basic Books, 1984 [F]
218. Woody GE, McLellan AT, Luborsky L, O'Brien CP: Psychotherapy in community methadone programs: a validation study. Am J Psychiatry 1995; 152:1302–1308 [A–]
219. Crits-Christoph P, Siqueland L, Blaine J, Frank A, Luborsky L, Onken LS, Muenz LR, Thase ME, Weiss RD, Gastfriend DR, Woody GE, Barber JP, Butler SF, Daley D, Salloum I, Bishop S, Najavits LM, Lis J, Mercer D, Griffin ML, Moras K, Beck AT: Psychosocial treatments for cocaine dependence: National Institute on Drug Abuse Collaborative Cocaine Treatment Study. Arch Gen Psychiatry 1999; 56:493–502 [A–]
220. Klerman GL, Weissman MM, Rounsaville BJ, Chevron E: The Theory and Practice of Interpersonal Psychotherapy for Depression. New York, Basic Books, 1984 [G]
221. Zimberg S, Wallace J, Blume SB: Practical Approaches to Alcoholism Psychotherapy. New York, Plenum, 1978 [G]
222. Brandsma JM, Pattison EM: The outcome of group psychotherapy for alcoholics: an empirical review. Am J Drug Alcohol Abuse 1985; 11:151–162 [F]
223. Kadden RM, Litt MD, Cooney NL, Kabela E, Getter H: Prospective matching of alcoholic clients to cognitive-behavioral or interactional group therapy. J Stud Alcohol 2001; 62:359–369 [B]
224. Wetzel H, Szegedi A, Scheurich A, Lorch B, Singer P, Schlafke D, Sittinger H, Wobrock T, Muller MJ, Anghelescu I, Hautzinger M: Combination treatment with nefazodone and cognitive-behavioral therapy for relapse prevention in alcohol-dependent men: a randomized controlled study. J Clin Psychiatry 2004; 65:1406–1413 [A]
225. O'Farrell TJ, Choquette KA, Cutter HS, Floyd FJ, Bayog R, Brown ED, Lowe J, Chan A, Deneault P: Cost-benefit and cost-effectiveness analyses of behavioral marital therapy as an addition to outpatient alcoholism treatment. J Subst Abuse 1996; 8:145–166 [A–]
226. Marques AC, Formigoni ML: Comparison of individual and group cognitive-behavioral therapy for alcohol and/or drug-dependent patients. Addiction 2001; 96:835–846 [A–]
227. Khantzian EJ: The self-medication hypothesis of addictive disorders: focus on heroin and cocaine dependence. Am J Psychiatry 1985; 142:1259–1264 [G]
228. Wurmser L: The Hidden Dimension: Psychopathology of Compulsive Drug Use. New York, Jason Aronson, 1979 [G]
229. McKay JR, Alterman AI, Cacciola JS, Rutherford MJ, O'Brien CP, Koppenhaver J: Group counseling versus individualized relapse prevention aftercare following intensive outpatient treatment for cocaine dependence: initial results. J Consult Clin Psychol 1997; 65:778–788 [A–]
230. Weiss RD, Jaffee WB, de Menil VP, Cogley CB: Group therapy for substance use disorders: what do we know? Harv Rev Psychiatry 2004; 12:339–350 [F]
231. McKay JR, Longabaugh R, Beattie MC, Maisto SA, Noel NE: The relationship of pretreatment family functioning to drinking behavior during follow-up by alcoholic patients. Am J Drug Alcohol Abuse 1992; 18:445–460 [C]
232. Steinglass P, Bennett L, Wolin S, Reiss D: The Alcoholic Family. New York, Basic Books, 1987 [F]
233. Stanton MD: Family treatment approaches of substance abuse: a review. Fam Process 1979; 18:251–280 [F]

234. McCrady BS, Epstein EE, Sell RD: Theoretical bases of family approaches to substance abuse treatment, in Treating Substance Abuse: Theory and Technique. Edited by Rotgers F, Morgenstern J, Walters ST. New York, Guilford, 2003, pp 112–139 [G]
235. Fals-Stewart W, O'Farrell TJ, Birchler GR: Family therapy techniques, in Treating Substance Abuse: Theory and Technique. Edited by Rotgers F, Morgenstern J, Walters ST. New York, Guilford Press, 2003, pp 140–165 [G]
236. O'Farrell TJ: Marital and family therapy in alcoholism treatment. J Subst Abuse Treat 1989; 6:23–29 [G]
237. Winters J, Fals-Stewart W, O'Farrell TJ, Birchler GR, Kelley ML: Behavioral couples therapy for female substance-abusing patients: effects on substance use and relationship adjustment. J Consult Clin Psychol 2002; 70:344–355 [A–]
238. Fals-Stewart W, Birchler GR, O'Farrell TJ: Behavioral couples therapy for male substance-abusing patients: effects on relationship adjustment and drug-using behavior. J Consult Clin Psychol 1996; 64:959–972 [A–]
239. Liddle HA, Rowe CL, Dakof GA, Ungaro RA, Henderson CE: Early intervention for adolescent substance abuse: pretreatment to posttreatment outcomes of a randomized clinical trial comparing multidimensional family therapy and peer group treatment. J Psychoactive Drugs 2004; 36:49–63 [A]
240. Latimer WW, Winters KC, D'Zurilla T, Nichols M: Integrated family and cognitive-behavioral therapy for adolescent substance abusers: a stage I efficacy study. Drug Alcohol Depend 2003; 71:303–317 [A–]
241. Santisteban DA, Coatsworth JD, Perez-Vidal A, Kurtines WM, Schwartz SJ, LaPerriere A, Szapocznik J: Efficacy of brief strategic family therapy in modifying Hispanic adolescent behavior problems and substance use. J Fam Psychol 2003; 17:121–133 [A–]
242. Waldron HB, Slesnick N, Brody JL, Turner CW, Peterson TR: Treatment outcomes for adolescent substance abuse at 4- and 7-month assessments. J Consult Clin Psychol 2001; 69:802–813 [A–]
243. Heath A, Atkinson B: Systematic treatment of substance abuse: a graduate course. J Marital Fam Ther 1988; 14:411–418 [G]
244. Stanton MD: Course-work and self-study in the family treatment of alcohol and drug abuse: expanding health and Atkinson's curriculum. J Marital Fam Ther 1988; 14:419–427 [B]
245. Stanton MD, Shadish WR: Outcome, attrition, and family-couples treatment for drug abuse: a meta-analysis and review of the controlled, comparative studies. Psychol Bull 1997; 122:170–191 [E]
246. O'Farrell TJ, Fals-Stewart W: Behavioral couples and family therapy for substance abusers. Curr Psychiatry Rep 2002; 4:371–376 [F]
247. Stanton MD, Thomas TC: Family Therapy of Drug Abuse and Addiction. New York, Guilford, 1982 [G]
248. Miller WE, Meyers RJ, Tonigan JS: Engaging the unmotivated in treatment for alcohol problems: a comparison of three strategies for intervention through family members. J Consult Clin Psychol 1999; 67:688–697 [A–]
249. Johnson VE: Intervention: How to Help Someone Who Doesn't Want Help. Center City, Minn, Hazelden Foundation, 1986 [G]
250. Meyers RJ, Smith JE, Lash DN: The Community Reinforcement Approach. Recent Dev Alcohol 2003; 16:183–195 [G]
251. Kelley ML, Fals-Stewart W: Couples- versus individual-based therapy for alcohol and drug abuse: effects on children's psychosocial functioning. J Consult Clin Psychol 2002; 70:417–427 [A–]

252. Catalano RF, Gainey RR, Fleming CB, Haggerty KP, Johnson NO: An experimental intervention with families of substance abusers: one-year follow-up of the Focus on Families Project. Addiction 1999; 94:241–254 [A–]
253. Alcoholics Anonymous: The Big Book. New York, Alcoholics Anonymous World Services, 1973 [G]
254. Emrick CD, Tonigan JS: Alcoholics Anonymous and other 12-step groups, in American Psychiatric Publishing Textbook of Substance Abuse Treatment, 3rd ed. Edited by Galanter M, Kleber HD. Washington, DC, American Psychiatric Publishing, 2004, pp 433–443 [G]
255. Alcoholics Anonymous: Estimates of AA Groups and Members as of January 1, 2002. New York, Alcoholics Anonymous World Services, 2002 [G]
256. Weiss RD, Griffin ML, Gallop RJ, Najavits LM, Frank A, Crits-Christoph P, Thase ME, Blaine J, Gastfriend DR, Daley D, Luborsky L: The effect of 12-step self-help group attendance and participation on drug use outcomes among cocaine-dependent patients. Drug Alcohol Depend 2005; 77:177–184 [A–]
257. Connors GJ, Tonigan JS, Miller WR: A longitudinal model of intake symptomatology, AA participation and outcome: retrospective study of the project MATCH outpatient and aftercare samples. J Stud Alcohol 2001; 62:817–825 [C]
258. Humphreys K, Moos RH, Cohen C: Social and community resources and long-term recovery from treated and untreated alcoholism. J Stud Alcohol 1997; 58:231–238 [C]
259. Humphreys K, Wing S, McCarty D, Chappel J, Gallant L, Haberle B, Horvath AT, Kaskutas LA, Kirk T, Kivlahan D, Laudet A, McCrady BS, McLellan AT, Morgenstern J, Townsend M, Weiss R: Self-help organizations for alcohol and drug problems: toward evidence-based practice and policy. J Subst Abuse Treat 2004; 26:151–158 [G]
260. Humphreys K, Huebsch PD, Finney JW, Moos RH: A comparative evaluation of substance abuse treatment, V: substance abuse treatment can enhance the effectiveness of self-help groups. Alcohol Clin Exp Res 1999; 23:558–563 [C]
261. McCrady BS: Recent research in twelve step programs, in Principles of Addiction Medicine. Edited by Graham AW, Schultz TK, Wilford BB. Chevy Chase, Md, American Society of Addiction Medicine, 1998, pp 707-718 [F]
262. Moos RH, Moos BS, Andrassy JM: Outcomes of four treatment approaches in community residential programs for patients with substance use disorders. Psychiatr Serv 1999; 50:1577–1583 [C]
263. Moos RH, Finney JW, Ouimette PC, Suchinsky RT: A comparative evaluation of substance abuse treatment, I: treatment orientation, amount of care, and 1-year outcomes. Alcohol Clin Exp Res 1999; 23:529–536 [C]
264. Ouimette PC, Moos RH, Finney JW: Influence of outpatient treatment and 12-step group involvement on one-year substance abuse treatment outcomes. J Stud Alcohol 1998; 59:513–522 [C]
265. Project MATCH Research Group: Matching alcoholism treatments to client heterogeneity: Project MATCH three-year drinking outcomes. Alcohol Clin Exp Res 1998; 22:1300–1311 [A–]
266. Timko C, Moos RH, Finney JW, Lesar MD: Long-term outcomes of alcohol use disorders: comparing untreated individuals with those in Alcoholics Anonymous and formal treatment. J Stud Alcohol 2000; 61:529–540 [B]
267. Carroll KM, Nich C, Ball SA, McCance E, Rounsaville BJ: Treatment of cocaine and alcohol dependence with psychotherapy and disulfiram. Addiction 1998; 93:713–727 [A]
268. Nowinski J, Baker S, Carroll KM: Twelve-Step Facilitation Therapy Manual: A Clinical Research Guide for Therapists Treating Individuals With Alcohol Abuse and Dependence. Rockville, Md, National Institute on Alcohol Abuse and Alcoholism, 1992 [G]

269. Mercer DE, Woody G: An Individual Drug Counseling Approach to Treat Cocaine Addiction: The Collaborative Cocaine Treatment Study Model. Rockville, Md, National Institute on Drug Abuse, 1999 [G]
270. Horgan CM, Levine HJ: The substance abuse treatment system: what does it look like and whom does it serve? preliminary findings from the Alcohol and Drug Services Study, in Bridging the Gap Between Practice and Research: Forging Partnerships With Community-Based Drug and Alcohol Treatment. Edited by Lamb S, Greenlick MR, McCarty D. Washington, DC, National Academies Press, 1999, pp 186–197 [G]
271. Kaskutas LA: Pathways to self-help among Women for Sobriety. Am J Drug Alcohol Abuse 1996; 22:259–280 [G]
272. Connors GJ, Dermen KH: Characteristics of participants in Secular Organizations for Sobriety (SOS). Am J Drug Alcohol Abuse 1996; 22:281–295 [G]
273. Ellis A, Volten E: When AA Doesn't Work for You: Rational Steps to Quitting Alcohol. Fort Lee, NJ, Barricade Books, 1992 [G]
274. Edwards G, Orford J, Egert S, Guthrie S, Hawker A, Hensman C, Mitcheson M, Oppenheimer E, Taylor C: Alcoholism: a controlled trial of "treatment" and "advice." J Stud Alcohol 1977; 38:1004–1031 [B]
275. Bien TH, Miller WR, Tonigan JS: Brief interventions for alcohol problems: a review. Addiction 1993; 88:315–335 [F]
276. Marijuana Treatment Project Research Group: Brief treatments for cannabis dependence: findings from a randomized multisite trial. J Consult Clin Psychol 2004; 72:455–466 [A–]
277. Saunders B, Wilkinson C, Phillips M: The impact of a brief motivational intervention with opiate users attending a methadone programme. Addiction 1995; 90:415–424 [A–]
278. Fiore MC, Kenford SL, Jorenby DE, Wetter DW, Smith SS, Baker TB: Two studies of the clinical effectiveness of the nicotine patch with different counseling treatments. Chest 1994; 105:524–533 [A]
279. Tevyaw TO, Monti PM: Motivational enhancement and other brief interventions for adolescent substance abuse: foundations, applications and evaluations. Addiction 2004; 99(suppl 2):63–75 [G]
280. Baker A, Lewin T, Reichler H, Clancy R, Carr V, Garrett R, Sly K, Devir H, Terry M: Evaluation of a motivational interview for substance use within psychiatric in-patient services. Addiction 2002; 97:1329–1337 [A–]
281. Storer RM: A simple cost-benefit analysis of brief interventions on substance abuse at Naval Medical Center Portsmouth. Mil Med 2003; 168:765–768 [G]
282. Barry KL, Blow FC, Willenbring ML, McCormick R, Brockmann LM, Visnic S: Use of alcohol screening and brief interventions in primary care settings: implementation and barriers. Subst Abus 2004; 25:27–36 [G]
283. Anderson P, Kaner E, Wutzke S, Funk M, Heather N, Wensing M, Grol R, Gual A, Pas L: Attitudes and managing alcohol problems in general practice: an interaction analysis based on findings from a WHO collaborative study. Alcohol Alcohol 2004; 39:351–356 [G]
284. Miller WR, Leckman AL, Delaney HD, Tinkcom M: Long-term follow-up of behavioral self-control training. J Stud Alcohol 1992; 53:249–261 [C]
285. Hester RK: Behavioral self-control training, in Handbook of Alcoholism Treatment Approaches: Effective Alternatives, 3rd ed. Edited by Hester RK, Miller WR. Needham Heights, Mass, Allyn & Bacon, 2003, pp 152–187 [G]
286. Bock B, Graham A, Sciamanna C, Krishnamoorthy J, Whiteley J, Carmona-Barros R, Niaura R, Abrams D: Smoking cessation treatment on the Internet: content, quality, and usability. Nicotine Tob Res 2004; 6:207–219 [G]

287. Abbot NC, Stead LF, White AR, Barnes J, Ernst E: Hypnotherapy for smoking cessation. Cochrane Database Syst Rev 2000; CD001008 [E]
288. Center for Substance Abuse Treatment: Substance Abuse Treatment for Persons With Co-occurring Disorders: Treatment Improvement Protocol (TIP) Series No. 42. DHHS Publication (SMA) 05-3922. Rockville, Md, Substance Abuse and Mental Health Services Administration, 2005 [G]
289. Vaillant GE: The Natural History of Alcoholism: Causes, Patterns, and Paths to Recovery. Cambridge, Mass, Harvard University Press, 1983 [E]
290. McLellan AT, Woody GE, Luborsky L, O'Brien CP, Druley KA: Increased effectiveness of substance abuse treatment: a prospective study of patient-treatment "matching." J Nerv Ment Dis 1983; 171:597–605 [C]
291. McLellan AT, Luborsky L, O'Brien CP, Barr HL, Evans F: Alcohol and drug abuse treatment in three different populations: is there improvement and is it predictable? Am J Drug Alcohol Abuse 1986; 12:101–120 [B]
292. McLellan AT: "Psychiatric severity" as a predictor of outcome from substance abuse treatment, in Psychopathology and Addictive Disorders. Edited by Meyer RE. New York, Guilford, 1986, pp 97–139 [G]
293. Wilcox HC, Conner KR, Caine ED: Association of alcohol and drug use disorders and completed suicide: an empirical review of cohort studies. Drug Alcohol Depend 2004; 76(suppl):S11–S19 [E]
294. Inskip HM, Harris EC, Barraclough B: Lifetime risk of suicide for affective disorder, alcoholism and schizophrenia. Br J Psychiatry 1998; 172:35–37 [F]
295. Murphy GE, Wetzel RD: The lifetime risk of suicide in alcoholism. Arch Gen Psychiatry 1990; 47:383–392 [F]
296. Cherpitel CJ, Borges GL, Wilcox HC: Acute alcohol use and suicidal behavior: a review of the literature. Alcohol Clin Exp Res 2004; 28:18S–28S [F]
297. Conner KR, Beautrais AL, Conwell Y: Moderators of the relationship between alcohol dependence and suicide and medically serious suicide attempts: analyses of Canterbury Suicide Project data. Alcohol Clin Exp Res 2003; 27:1156–1161 [D]
298. Conwell Y, Duberstein PR, Cox C, Herrmann JH, Forbes NT, Caine ED: Relationships of age and axis I diagnoses in victims of completed suicide: a psychological autopsy study. Am J Psychiatry 1996; 153:1001–1008 [G]
299. Rich CL, Young D, Fowler RC: San Diego suicide study, I: young versus old subjects. Arch Gen Psychiatry 1986; 43:577–582 [G]
300. Arsenault-Lapierre G, Kim C, Turecki G: Psychiatric diagnoses in 3275 suicides: a meta-analysis. BMC Psychiatry 2004; 4:37 [E]
301. American Psychiatric Association: Practice guideline for the assessment and treatment of patients with suicidal behaviors. Am J Psychiatry 2003; 160:1–60 [G]
302. Preuss UW, Schuckit MA, Smith TL, Danko GP, Bucholz KK, Hesselbrock MN, Hesselbrock V, Kramer JR: Predictors and correlates of suicide attempts over 5 years in 1,237 alcohol-dependent men and women. Am J Psychiatry 2003; 160:56–63 [C]
303. Beautrais AL, Joyce PR, Mulder RT, Fergusson DM, Deavoll BJ, Nightingale SK: Prevalence and comorbidity of mental disorders in persons making serious suicide attempts: a case-control study. Am J Psychiatry 1996; 153:1009–1014 [D]
304. Beautrais AL, Joyce PR, Mulder RT: Cannabis abuse and serious suicide attempts. Addiction 1999; 94:1155–1164 [D]
305. Suominen K, Henriksson M, Suokas J, Isometsa E, Ostamo A, Lonnqvist J: Mental disorders and comorbidity in attempted suicide. Acta Psychiatr Scand 1996; 94:234–240 [G]
306. Cornelius JR, Thase ME, Salloum IM, Cornelius MD, Black A, Mann JJ: Cocaine use associated with increased suicidal behavior in depressed alcoholics. Addict Behav 1998; 23:119–121 [G]

307. Cornelius JR, Salloum IM, Day NL, Thase ME, Mann JJ: Patterns of suicidality and alcohol use in alcoholics with major depression. Alcohol Clin Exp Res 1996; 20:1451–1455 [G]
308. Tondo L, Baldessarini RJ, Hennen J, Minnai GP, Salis P, Scamonatti L, Masia M, Ghiani C, Mannu P: Suicide attempts in major affective disorder patients with comorbid substance use disorders. J Clin Psychiatry 1999; 60(suppl 2):63–69 [G]
309. Sullivan LE, Fiellin DA, O'Connor PG: The prevalence and impact of alcohol problems in major depression: a systematic review. Am J Med 2005; 118:330–341 [F]
310. Oquendo MA, Galfalvy H, Russo S, Ellis SP, Grunebaum MF, Burke A, Mann JJ: Prospective study of clinical predictors of suicidal acts after a major depressive episode in patients with major depressive disorder or bipolar disorder. Am J Psychiatry 2004; 161:1433–1441 [C]
311. Weiss RD, Ostacher MJ, Otto MW, Calabrese JR, Fossey M, Wisniewski SR, Bowden CL, Nierenberg AA, Pollack MH, Salloum IM, Simon NM, Thase ME, Sachs GS: Does recovery from substance use disorder matter in patients with bipolar disorder? J Clin Psychiatry 2005; 66:730–735 [C]
312. Goldberg JF, Garno JL, Portera L, Leon AC, Kocsis JH, Whiteside JE: Correlates of suicidal ideation in dysphoric mania. J Affect Disord 1999; 56:75–81 [D]
313. Feinman JA, Dunner DL: The effect of alcohol and substance abuse on the course of bipolar affective disorder. J Affect Disord 1996; 37:43–49 [C]
314. Garno JL, Goldberg JF, Ramirez PM, Ritzler BA: Bipolar disorder with comorbid cluster B personality disorder features: impact on suicidality. J Clin Psychiatry 2005; 66:339–345 [G]
315. Simon NM, Otto MW, Wisniewski SR, Fossey M, Sagduyu K, Frank E, Sachs GS, Nierenberg AA, Thase ME, Pollack MH: Anxiety disorder comorbidity in bipolar disorder patients: data from the first 500 participants in the Systematic Treatment Enhancement Program for Bipolar Disorder (STEP-BD). Am J Psychiatry 2004; 161:2222–2229 [G]
316. Kim CD, Seguin M, Therrien N, Riopel G, Chawky N, Lesage AD, Turecki G: Familial aggregation of suicidal behavior: a family study of male suicide completers from the general population. Am J Psychiatry 2005; 162:1017–1019 [D]
317. Stone MH: The Fate of Borderline Patients: Successful Outcome and Psychiatric Practice. New York, Guilford, 1990 [G]
318. Darke S, Williamson A, Ross J, Teesson M, Lynskey M: Borderline personality disorder, antisocial personality disorder and risk-taking among heroin users: findings from the Australian Treatment Outcome Study (ATOS). Drug Alcohol Depend 2004; 74:77–83 [G]
319. Cornelius JR, Salloum IM, Lynch K, Clark DB, Mann JJ: Treating the substance-abusing suicidal patient. Ann N Y Acad Sci 2001; 932:78–90 [F]
320. Hoaken PN, Stewart SH: Drugs of abuse and the elicitation of human aggressive behavior. Addict Behav 2003; 28:1533–1554 [F]
321. Budde RD: Cocaine abuse and violent death. Am J Drug Alcohol Abuse 1989; 15:375–382 [D]
322. Langevin R, Paitich D, Orchard B, Handy L, Russon A: The role of alcohol, drugs, suicide attempts and situational strains in homicide committed by offenders seen for psychiatric assessment: a controlled study. Acta Psychiatr Scand 1982; 66:229–242 [D]
323. Trenton AJ, Currier GW: Behavioural manifestations of anabolic steroid use. CNS Drugs 2005; 19:571–595 [G]
324. Cohen JB, Dickow A, Horner K, Zweben JE, Balabis J, Vandersloot D, Reiber C: Abuse and violence history of men and women in treatment for methamphetamine dependence. Am J Addict 2003; 12:377–385 [C]

325. Chermack ST, Blow FC: Violence among individuals in substance abuse treatment: the role of alcohol and cocaine consumption. Drug Alcohol Depend 2002; 66:29–37 [D]
326. Luisada PV: The phencyclidine psychosis: phenomenology and treatment. NIDA Res Monogr 1978; Aug:241–253 [F]
327. Brecher M, Wang BW, Wong H, Morgan JP: Phencyclidine and violence: clinical and legal issues. J Clin Psychopharmacol 1988; 8:397–401 [F]
328. Kouri EM, Pope HG Jr, Lukas SE: Changes in aggressive behavior during withdrawal from long-term marijuana use. Psychopharmacology (Berl) 1999; 143:302–308 [B]
329. Melges FT, Tinklenberg JR, Hollister LE, Gillespie HK: Temporal disintegration and depersonalization during marihuana intoxication. Arch Gen Psychiatry 1970; 23:204–210 [G]
330. Bowers MB Jr: Acute psychosis induced by psychotomimetic drug abuse, I: clinical findings. Arch Gen Psychiatry 1972; 27:437–440 [G]
331. Bowers MB Jr: Acute psychosis induced by psychotomimetic drug abuse, II: neurochemical findings. Arch Gen Psychiatry 1972; 27:440–442 [G]
332. Rychtarik RG, McGillicuddy NB: Coping skills training and 12-step facilitation for women whose partner has alcoholism: effects on depression, the partner's drinking, and partner physical violence. J Consult Clin Psychol 2005; 73:249–261 [A–]
333. Fals-Stewart W, Kashdan TB, O'Farrell TJ, Birchler GR: Behavioral couples therapy for drug-abusing patients: effects on partner violence. J Subst Abuse Treat 2002; 22:87–96 [A–]
334. Brower KJ, Aldrich MS, Robinson EA, Zucker RA, Greden JF: Insomnia, self-medication, and relapse to alcoholism. Am J Psychiatry 2001; 158:399–404 [G]
335. Brower KJ, Aldrich MS, Hall JM: Polysomnographic and subjective sleep predictors of alcoholic relapse. Alcohol Clin Exp Res 1998; 22:1864–1871 [D]
336. Drummond SP, Gillin JC, Smith TL, DeModena A: The sleep of abstinent pure primary alcoholic patients: natural course and relationship to relapse. Alcohol Clin Exp Res 1998; 22:1796–1802 [G]
337. Le Bon O, Murphy JR, Staner L, Hoffmann G, Kormoss N, Kentos M, Dupont P, Lion K, Pelc I, Verbanck P: Double-blind, placebo-controlled study of the efficacy of trazodone in alcohol post-withdrawal syndrome: polysomnographic and clinical evaluations. J Clin Psychopharmacol 2003; 23:377–383 [A]
338. Karam-Hage M, Brower KJ: Open pilot study of gabapentin versus trazodone to treat insomnia in alcoholic outpatients. Psychiatry Clin Neurosci 2003; 57:542–544 [B]
339. Currie SR, Clark S, Hodgins DC, el Guebaly N: Randomized controlled trial of brief cognitive-behavioural interventions for insomnia in recovering alcoholics. Addiction 2004; 99:1121–1132 [A–]
340. Havassy BE, Alvidrez J, Owen KK: Comparisons of patients with comorbid psychiatric and substance use disorders: implications for treatment and service delivery. Am J Psychiatry 2004; 161:139–145 [D]
341. Kessler RC, Nelson CB, McGonagle KA, Liu J, Swartz M, Blazer DG: Comorbidity of DSM-III-R major depressive disorder in the general population: results from the US National Comorbidity Survey. Br J Psychiatry 1996; 30(Jun suppl):17–30 [G]
342. Kessler RC, Nelson CB, McGonagle KA, Edlund MJ, Frank RG, Leaf PJ: The epidemiology of co-occurring addictive and mental disorders: implications for prevention and service utilization. Am J Orthopsychiatry 1996; 66:17–31 [G]
343. McLellan AT, Druley KA: Non-random relation between drugs of abuse and psychiatric diagnosis. J Psychiatr Res 1977; 13:179–184 [G]
344. Ross HE, Glaser FB, Germanson T: The prevalence of psychiatric disorders in patients with alcohol and other drug problems. Arch Gen Psychiatry 1988; 45:1023–1031 [G]
345. Hien D, Zimberg S, Weisman S, First M, Ackerman S: Dual diagnosis subtypes in urban substance abuse and mental health clinics. Psychiatr Serv 1997; 48:1058–1063 [G]

346. Penick EC, Powell BJ, Liskow BI, Jackson JO, Nickel EJ: The stability of coexisting psychiatric syndromes in alcoholic men after one year. J Stud Alcohol 1988; 49:395–405 [C]
347. Grant BF, Hasin DS, Chou SP, Stinson FS, Dawson DA: Nicotine dependence and psychiatric disorders in the United States: results from the National Epidemiologic Survey on Alcohol and Related Conditions. Arch Gen Psychiatry 2004; 61:1107–1115 [G]
348. Ziedonis DM, Williams JM: Addressing tobacco in mental health and addictions settings. Psychiatr Ann 2003; 22:425–426 [G]
349. Lasser K, Boyd JW, Woolhandler S, Himmelstein DU, McCormick D, Bor DH: Smoking and mental illness: a population-based prevalence study. JAMA 2000; 284:2606–2610 [G]
350. RachBeisel J, Scott J, Dixon L: Co-occurring severe mental illness and substance use disorders: a review of recent research. Psychiatr Serv 1999; 50:1427–1434 [F]
351. Tarter RE: Evaluation and treatment of adolescent substance abuse: a decision tree method. Am J Drug Alcohol Abuse 1990; 16:1–46 [G]
352. Ziedonis D: Integrated treatment of co-occurring mental illness and addiction: clinical intervention, program, and system perspectives. CNS Spectr 2004; 9:892–904, 925 [F]
353. Center for Substance Abuse Treatment: Assessment and Treatment of Patients With Coexisting Mental Illness and Alcohol and Other Drug Abuse: Treatment Improvement Protocol (TIP) Series No. 9. DHHS Publication (SMA) 95-3061. Rockville, Md, Substance Abuse and Mental Health Services Administration, 1994 [G]
354. Brunette MF, Mueser KT, Drake RE: A review of research on residential programs for people with severe mental illness and co-occurring substance use disorders. Drug Alcohol Rev 2004; 23:471–481 [F]
355. Rounsaville BJ, Dolinsky ZS, Babor TF, Meyer RE: Psychopathology as a predictor of treatment outcome in alcoholics. Arch Gen Psychiatry 1987; 44:505–513 [C]
356. McLellan AT, Luborsky L, Woody GE, O'Brien CP, Druley KA: Predicting response to alcohol and drug abuse treatments: role of psychiatric severity. Arch Gen Psychiatry 1983; 40:620–625 [C]
357. Ziedonis DM, Krejci J: Dual recovery therapy: blending psychotherapies for depression and addiction, in Integrated Treatment for Mood and Substance Disorders. Edited by Westermeyer JJ, Weiss RD, Ziedonis DM. Baltimore, Md, Johns Hopkins University Press, 2003, pp 90–121 [G]
358. Jaffe JH, Ciraulo DA: Alcoholism and depression, in Psychopathology as a Predictor of Treatment Outcome in Alcoholics. Edited by Meyer RE. New York, Guilford, 1986, pp 90–121 [F]
359. Dixon L, Postrado L, Delahanty J, Fischer PJ, Lehman A: The association of medical comorbidity in schizophrenia with poor physical and mental health. J Nerv Ment Dis 1999; 187:496–502 [G]
360. Bellack AS, DiClemente CC: Treating substance abuse among patients with schizophrenia. Psychiatr Serv 1999; 50:75–80 [B]
361. Alcoholics Anonymous: The AA Member: Medications and Other Drugs. New York, Author, 1984 [G]
362. Chappel JN: Effective use of Alcoholics Anonymous and Narcotics Anonymous in treating patients. Psychiatric Ann 1992; 22:409–418 [G]
363. Petrakis IL, Poling J, Levinson C, Nich C, Carroll K, Rounsaville B: Naltrexone and disulfiram in patients with alcohol dependence and comorbid psychiatric disorders. Biol Psychiatry 2005; 57:1128–1137 [A–]
364. Hien DA, Cohen LR, Miele GM, Litt LC, Capstick C: Promising treatments for women with comorbid PTSD and substance use disorders. Am J Psychiatry 2004; 161:1426–1432 [A–]

365. Brady KT, Dansky BS, Back SE, Foa EB, Carroll KM: Exposure therapy in the treatment of PTSD among cocaine-dependent individuals: preliminary findings. J Subst Abuse Treat 2001; 21:47–54 [B]
366. Coffey SF, Schumacher JA, Brimo ML, Brady KT: Exposure therapy for substance abusers with PTSD: translating research to practice. Behav Modif 2005; 29:10–38 [G]
367. Najavits LM, Weiss RD, Shaw SR, Muenz LR: "Seeking Safety": outcome of a new cognitive-behavioral psychotherapy for women with posttraumatic stress disorder and substance dependence. J Trauma Stress 1998; 11:437–456 [B]
368. Triffleman E, Carroll K, Kellogg S: Substance dependence posttraumatic stress disorder therapy: an integrated cognitive-behavioral approach. J Subst Abuse Treat 1999; 17:3–14 [G]
369. Weiss RD, Griffin ML, Greenfield SF, Najavits LM, Wyner D, Soto JA, Hennen JA: Group therapy for patients with bipolar disorder and substance dependence: results of a pilot study. J Clin Psychiatry 2000; 61:361–367 [B]
370. Carey KB: Substance use reduction in the context of outpatient psychiatric treatment: a collaborative, motivational, harm reduction approach. Community Ment Health J 1996; 32:291–306 [G]
371. Ziedonis DM, Stern R: Dual recovery therapy for schizophrenia and substance abuse. Psychiatr Ann 2001; 31:255–264 [G]
372. Shaner A, Roberts LJ, Eckman TA, Tucker DE, Tsuang JW, Wilkins JN, Mintz J: Monetary reinforcement of abstinence from cocaine among mentally ill patients with cocaine dependence. Psychiatr Serv 1997; 48:807–810 [C]
373. Ball SA: Manualized treatment for substance abusers with personality disorders: dual focus schema therapy. Addict Behav 1998; 23:883–891 [G]
374. Linehan MM, Schmidt H III, Dimeff LA, Craft JC, Kanter J, Comtois KA: Dialectical behavior therapy for patients with borderline personality disorder and drug-dependence. Am J Addict 1999; 8:279–292 [A–]
375. James W, Preston NJ, Koh G, Spencer C, Kisely SR, Castle DJ: A group intervention which assists patients with dual diagnosis reduce their drug use: a randomized controlled trial. Psychol Med 2004; 34:983–990 [A–]
376. Barrowclough C, Haddock G, Tarrier N, Lewis SW, Moring J, O'Brien R, Schofield N, McGovern J: Randomized controlled trial of motivational interviewing, cognitive behavior therapy, and family intervention for patients with comorbid schizophrenia and substance use disorders. Am J Psychiatry 2001; 158:1706–1713 [A–]
377. Haddock G, Barrowclough C, Tarrier N, Moring J, O'Brien R, Schofield N, Quinn J, Palmer S, Davies L, Lowens I, McGovern J, Lewis S: Cognitive-behavioural therapy and motivational intervention for schizophrenia and substance misuse: 18-month outcomes of a randomised controlled trial. Br J Psychiatry 2003; 183:418–426 [A–]
378. de Leon J: Smoking and vulnerability for schizophrenia. Schizophr Bull 1996; 22:405–409 [G]
379. Tidey JW, Rohsenow DJ, Kaplan GB, Swift RM: Cigarette smoking topography in smokers with schizophrenia and matched non-psychiatric controls. Drug Alcohol Depend 2005; 80:259–265 [D]
380. Curkendall SM, Mo J, Glasser DB, Rose SM, Jones JK: Cardiovascular disease in patients with schizophrenia in Saskatchewan, Canada. J Clin Psychiatry 2004; 65:715–720 [D]
381. Brown S, Inskip H, Barraclough B: Causes of the excess mortality of schizophrenia. Br J Psychiatry 2000; 177:212–217 [C]
382. Dalack GW, Healy DJ, Meador-Woodruff JH: Nicotine dependence in schizophrenia: clinical phenomena and laboratory findings. Am J Psychiatry 1998; 155:1490–1501 [F]

383. Stroup TS, Gilmore JH, Jarskog LF: Management of medical illness in persons with schizophrenia. Psychiatr Ann 2000; 30:35–40 [G]
384. Buckley PF: Substance abuse in schizophrenia: a review. J Clin Psychiatry 1998; 59(suppl 3):26–30 [F]
385. Drake RE, Rosenberg SD, Mueser KT: Assessing substance use disorder in persons with severe mental illness. New Dir Ment Health Serv; 1996; 30:3–17 [G]
386. Minkoff K: An integrated treatment model for dual diagnosis of psychosis and addiction. Hosp Community Psychiatry 1989; 40:1031–1036 [G]
387. Mueser KT, Drake RE, Noordsy DL: Integrated mental health and substance abuse treatment for severe psychiatric disorders. Journal of Practical Psychiatry and Behavioral Health 1998; 4:129–139 [G]
388. American Psychiatric Association: Practice guideline for the treatment of patients with schizophrenia, 2nd ed. Am J Psychiatry 2004; 161:1–56 [G]
389. Lieberman JA, Stroup TS, McEvoy JP, Swartz MS, Rosenheck RA, Perkins DO, Keefe RS, Davis SM, Davis CE, Lebowitz BD, Severe J, Hsiao JK: Effectiveness of antipsychotic drugs in patients with chronic schizophrenia. N Engl J Med 2005; 353:1209–1223 [A]
390. Albanese MJ, Khantzian EJ, Murphy SL, Green AI: Decreased substance use in chronically psychotic patients treated with clozapine. Am J Psychiatry 1994; 151:780–781 [G]
391. Buckley P, Thompson PA, Way L, Meltzer HY: Substance abuse and clozapine treatment. J Clin Psychiatry 1994; 55(suppl B):114–116 [B]
392. Buckley PF: Novel antipsychotic medications and the treatment of comorbid substance abuse in schizophrenia. J Subst Abuse Treat 1998; 15:113–116 [G]
393. Drake RE, Xie H, McHugo GJ, Green AI: The effects of clozapine on alcohol and drug use disorders among patients with schizophrenia. Schizophr Bull 2000; 26:441–449 [B]
394. Green AI, Burgess ES, Dawson R, Zimmet SV, Strous RD: Alcohol and cannabis use in schizophrenia: effects of clozapine vs risperidone. Schizophr Res 2003; 60:81–85 [D]
395. Lee ML, Dickson RA, Campbell M, Oliphant J, Gretton H, Dalby JT: Clozapine and substance abuse in patients with schizophrenia. Can J Psychiatry 1998; 43:855–856 [B]
396. Marcus P, Snyder R: Reduction of comorbid substance abuse with clozapine. Am J Psychiatry 1995; 152:959 [G]
397. Tsuang JW, Eckman TE, Shaner A, Marder SR: Clozapine for substance-abusing schizophrenic patients. Am J Psychiatry 1999; 156:1119–1120 [D]
398. Zimmet SV, Strous RD, Burgess ES, Kohnstamm S, Green AI: Effects of clozapine on substance use in patients with schizophrenia and schizoaffective disorder: a retrospective survey. J Clin Psychopharmacol 2000; 20:94–98 [D]
399. Albanese MJ: Safety and efficacy of risperidone in substance abusers with psychosis. Am J Addict 2001; 10:190–191 [B]
400. Kosten TR, Brady KT, George TP, McCance-Katz EF, Stine SM, Weiss RD: Risperidone for substance dependent psychotic patients. CPDD Scientific Meeting Abstracts, Jun 2003 [D]
401. Smelson DA, Losonczy MF, Davis CW, Kaune M, Williams J, Ziedonis D: Risperidone decreases craving and relapses in individuals with schizophrenia and cocaine dependence. Can J Psychiatry 2002; 47:671–675 [B]
402. Tsuang JW, Eckman T, Marder S, Tucker D: Can risperidone reduce cocaine use in substance abusing schizophrenic patients? J Clin Psychopharmacol 2002; 22:629–630 [G]

403. Conley RR, Kelly DL, Gale EA: Olanzapine response in treatment-refractory schizophrenic patients with a history of substance abuse. Schizophr Res 1998; 33:95–101 [B]
404. Littrell KH, Petty RG, Hilligoss NM, Peabody CD, Johnson CG: Olanzapine treatment for patients with schizophrenia and substance abuse. J Subst Abuse Treat 2001; 21:217–221 [B]
405. Meltzer HY, Alphs L, Green AI, Altamura AC, Anand R, Bertoldi A, Bourgeois M, Chouinard G, Islam MZ, Kane J, Krishnan R, Lindenmayer JP, Potkin S: Clozapine treatment for suicidality in schizophrenia: International Suicide Prevention Trial (InterSePT). Arch Gen Psychiatry 2003; 60:82–91 [A–]
406. Procyshyn RM, Ihsan N, Thompson D: A comparison of smoking behaviours between patients treated with clozapine and depot neuroleptics. Int Clin Psychopharmacol 2001; 16:291–294 [G]
407. George TP, Sernyak MJ, Ziedonis DM, Woods SW: Effects of clozapine on smoking in chronic schizophrenic outpatients. J Clin Psychiatry 1995; 56:344–346 [G]
408. McEvoy J, Freudenreich O, McGee M, VanderZwaag C, Levin E, Rose J: Clozapine decreases smoking in patients with chronic schizophrenia. Biol Psychiatry 1995; 37:550–552 [A–]
409. Bourdelat-Parks BN, Anderson GM, Donaldson ZR, Weiss JM, Bonsall RW, Emery MS, Liles LC, Weinshenker D: Effects of dopamine beta-hydroxylase genotype and disulfiram inhibition on catecholamine homeostasis in mice. Psychopharmacology (Berl) 2005; 183:72–80 [A]
410. Gorelick DA, Gardner EL, Xi ZX: Agents in development for the management of cocaine abuse. Drugs 2004; 64:1547–1573 [F]
411. Maxwell S, Shinderman MS: Use of naltrexone in the treatment of alcohol use disorders in patients with concomitant major mental illness. J Addict Dis 2000; 19:61–69 [G]
412. Batki S, Dimmock J, Cornell M, Wade M, Carey K, Maisto S: Naltrexone treatment of alcohol dependence in schizophrenia: relationship of alcohol use to psychosis severity and antipsychotic medication. Poster presented at the 13th annual meeting of the American Academy of Addiction Psychiatry, Las Vegas, December 12–15, 2002 [B]
413. Petrakis I, Carroll KM, Nich C, Gordon L, Kosten T, Rounsaville B: Fluoxetine treatment of depressive disorders in methadone-maintained opioid addicts. Drug Alcohol Depend 1998; 50:221–226 [A]
414. George TP, Vessicchio JC, Termine A, Bregartner TA, Feingold A, Rounsaville BJ, Kosten TR: A placebo controlled trial of bupropion for smoking cessation in schizophrenia. Biol Psychiatry 2002; 52:53–61 [A]
415. Weiner E, Ball MP, Summerfelt A, Gold J, Buchanan RW: Effects of sustained-release bupropion and supportive group therapy on cigarette consumption in patients with schizophrenia. Am J Psychiatry 2001; 158:635–637 [B]
416. Addington J: Group treatment for smoking cessation among persons with schizophrenia. Psychiatr Serv 1998; 49:925–928 [F]
417. Drake RE, Mueser KT: Psychosocial approaches to dual diagnosis. Schizophr Bull 2000; 26:105–118 [G]
418. Ziedonis D, Fisher W: Motivation-based assessment and treatment of substance abuse in patients with schizophrenia, in Hatherleigh Guide to Treating Substance Abuse, Part 2. New York, Hatherleigh Press, 1996, pp 270–287 [G]
419. Hellerstein DJ, Meehan B: Outpatient group therapy for schizophrenic substance abusers. Am J Psychiatry 1987; 144:1337–1339 [B]
420. Regier DA, Farmer ME, Rae DS, Locke BZ, Keith SJ, Judd LL, Goodwin FK: Comorbidity of mental disorders with alcohol and other drug abuse: results from the Epidemiologic Catchment Area (ECA) study. JAMA 1990; 264:2511–2518 [G]

421. Kessler RC, Crum RM, Warner LA, Nelson CB, Schulenberg J, Anthony JC: Lifetime co-occurrence of DSM-III-R alcohol abuse and dependence with other psychiatric disorders in the National Comorbidity Survey. Arch Gen Psychiatry 1997; 54:313–321 [G]
422. Kessler RC, Berglund P, Demler O, Jin R, Koretz D, Merikangas KR, Rush AJ, Walters EE, Wang PS: The epidemiology of major depressive disorder: results from the National Comorbidity Survey Replication (NCS-R). JAMA 2003; 289:3095–3105 [G]
423. Brook DW, Brook JS, Zhang C, Cohen P, Whiteman M: Drug use and the risk of major depressive disorder, alcohol dependence, and substance use disorders. Arch Gen Psychiatry 2002; 59:1039–1044 [C]
424. Linnoila MI: Anxiety and alcoholism. J Clin Psychiatry 1989; 50(suppl):26–29 [G]
425. Nunes EV, Levin FR: Treatment of depression in patients with alcohol or other drug dependence: a meta-analysis. JAMA 2004; 291:1887–1896 [E]
426. Mirin SM, Weiss RD: Substance abuse and mental illness, in Clinical Textbook of Addictive Disorders. Edited by Frances RJ, Miller SI. New York, Guilford, 1991, pp 271–298 [G]
427. Mirin SM, Weiss RD, Griffin ML, Michael JL: Psychopathology in drug abusers and their families. Compr Psychiatry 1991; 32:36–51 [D]
428. Nunes EV, McGrath PJ, Quitkin FM, Stewart JP, Harrison W, Tricamo E, Ocepek-Welikson K: Imipramine treatment of alcoholism with comorbid depression. Am J Psychiatry 1993; 150:963–965 [B]
429. Nunes EV, Quitkin FM, Brady R, Stewart JW: Imipramine treatment of methadone maintenance patients with affective disorder and illicit drug use. Am J Psychiatry 1991; 148:667–669 [B]
430. American Psychiatric Association: Practice guideline for the treatment of patients with major depressive disorder (revision). Am J Psychiatry 2000; 157(suppl):1–45 [G]
430a. Torrens M, Fonseca F, Mateu G, Farre M: Efficacy of antidepressants in substance use disorders with and without comorbid depression: a systematic review and meta-analysis. Drug Alcohol Depend 2005; 78:1–22 [E]
431. Cornelius JR, Salloum IM, Ehler JG, Jarrett PJ, Cornelius MD, Perel JM, Thase ME, Black A: Fluoxetine in depressed alcoholics: a double-blind, placebo-controlled trial. Arch Gen Psychiatry 1997; 54:700–705 [A]
432. Moak DH, Anton RF, Latham PK, Voronin KE, Waid RL, Durazo-Arvizu R: Sertraline and cognitive behavioral therapy for depressed alcoholics: results of a placebo-controlled trial. J Clin Psychopharmacol 2003; 23:553–562 [A]
433. Pettinati HM, Volpicelli JR, Luck G, Kranzler HR, Rukstalis MR, Cnaan A: Double-blind clinical trial of sertraline treatment for alcohol dependence. J Clin Psychopharmacol 2001; 21:143–153 [A]
434. Roy A: Placebo-controlled study of sertraline in depressed recently abstinent alcoholics. Biol Psychiatry 1998; 44:633–637 [A]
435. Hernandez-Avila CA, Modesto-Lowe V, Feinn R, Kranzler HR: Nefazodone treatment of comorbid alcohol dependence and major depression. Alcohol Clin Exp Res 2004; 28:433–440 [A]
436. Roy-Byrne PP, Pages KP, Russo JE, Jaffe C, Blume AW, Kingsley E, Cowley DS, Ries RK: Nefazodone treatment of major depression in alcohol-dependent patients: a double-blind, placebo-controlled trial. J Clin Psychopharmacol 2000; 20:129–136 [A]
437. McGrath PJ, Nunes EV, Stewart JW, Goldman D, Agosti V, Ocepek-Welikson K, Quitkin FM: Imipramine treatment of alcoholics with primary depression: a placebo-controlled clinical trial. Arch Gen Psychiatry 1996; 53:232–240 [A–]
438. Mason BJ, Kocsis JH, Ritvo EC, Cutler RB: A double-blind, placebo-controlled trial of desipramine for primary alcohol dependence stratified on the presence or absence of major depression. JAMA 1996; 275:761–767 [A]

439. Pettinati HM: Antidepressant treatment of co-occurring depression and alcohol dependence. Biol Psychiatry 2004; 56:785–792 [F]
440. Stewart DE: Hepatic adverse reactions associated with nefazodone. Can J Psychiatry 2002; 47:375–377 [G]
441. Nunes E, Quitkin F, Brady R, Post-Koenig T: Antidepressant treatment in methadone maintenance patients. J Addict Dis 1994; 13:13–24 [F]
442. Kleber HD, Weissman MM, Rounsaville BJ, Wilber CH, Prusoff BA, Riordan CE: Imipramine as treatment for depression in addicts. Arch Gen Psychiatry 1983; 40:649–653 [A]
443. Woody GE, O'Brien CP, McLellan AT, Marcovici M, Evans BD: The use of antidepressants with methadone in depressed maintenance patients. Ann N Y Acad Sci 1982; 398:120–127 [F]
444. Nunes EV, Quitkin FM, Donovan SJ, Deliyannides D, Ocepek-Welikson K, Koenig T, Brady R, McGrath PJ, Woody G: Imipramine treatment of opiate-dependent patients with depressive disorders: a placebo-controlled trial. Arch Gen Psychiatry 1998; 55:153–160 [A]
445. Ziedonis DM, Kosten TR: Depression as a prognostic factor for pharmacological treatment of cocaine dependence. Psychopharmacol Bull 1991; 27:337–343 [A]
446. Titievsky J, Seco G, Barranco M, Kyle EM: Doxepin as adjunctive therapy for depressed methadone maintenance patients: a double-blind study. J Clin Psychiatry 1982; 43:454–456 [A]
447. Woody GE, O'Brien CP, Rickels K: Depression and anxiety in heroin addicts: a placebo-controlled study of doxepin in combination with methadone. Am J Psychiatry 1975; 132:447–450 [A]
448. Stein MD, Solomon DA, Herman DS, Anthony JL, Ramsey SE, Anderson BJ, Miller IW: Pharmacotherapy plus psychotherapy for treatment of depression in active injection drug users. Arch Gen Psychiatry 2004; 61:152–159 [A–]
449. Carpenter KM, Brooks AC, Vosburg SK, Nunes EV: The effect of sertraline and environmental context on treating depression and illicit substance use among methadone maintained opiate dependent patients: a controlled clinical trial. Drug Alcohol Depend 2004; 74:123–134 [A]
450. Dean AJ, Bell J, Mascord DJ, Parker G, Christie MJ: A randomised, controlled trial of fluoxetine in methadone maintenance patients with depressive symptoms. J Affect Disord 2002; 72:85–90 [A–]
451. Nunes EV, McGrath PJ, Quitkin FM, Ocepek-Welikson K, Stewart JW, Koenig T, Wager S, Klein DF: Imipramine treatment of cocaine abuse: possible boundaries of efficacy. Drug Alcohol Depend 1995; 39:185–195 [A]
452. Carroll KM, Nich C, Rounsaville BJ: Differential symptom reduction in depressed cocaine abusers treated with psychotherapy and pharmacotherapy. J Nerv Ment Dis 1995; 183:251–259 [A–]
453. Rounsaville BJ: Treatment of cocaine dependence and depression. Biol Psychiatry 2004; 56:803–809 [G]
454. Cox LS, Patten CA, Niaura RS, Decker PA, Rigotti N, Sachs DP, Buist AS, Hurt RD: Efficacy of bupropion for relapse prevention in smokers with and without a past history of major depression. J Gen Intern Med 2004; 19:828–834 [A–]
455. Prochazka AV, Kick S, Steinbrunn C, Miyoshi T, Fryer GE: A randomized trial of nortriptyline combined with transdermal nicotine for smoking cessation. Arch Intern Med 2004; 164:2229–2233 [A]
456. Hall SM, Reus VI, Munoz RF, Sees KL, Humfleet G, Hartz DT, Frederick S, Triffleman E: Nortriptyline and cognitive-behavioral therapy in the treatment of cigarette smoking. Arch Gen Psychiatry 1998; 55:683–690 [A–]

457. Patten CA, Rummans TA, Croghan IT, Hurt RD, Hays JT: Development of depression during placebo-controlled trials of bupropion for smoking cessation: case reports. J Clin Psychiatry 1999; 60:436–441 [G]

457a. Glassman AH, Covey LS, Stetner F, Rivelli S: Smoking cessation and the course of major depression: a follow-up study. Lancet 2001; 357:1929–1932 [C]

458. Chengappa KN, Kambhampati RK, Perkins K, Nigam R, Anderson T, Brar JS, Vemulapalli HK, Atzert R, Key P, Kang JS, Levine J: Bupropion sustained release as a smoking cessation treatment in remitted depressed patients maintained on treatment with selective serotonin reuptake inhibitor antidepressants. J Clin Psychiatry 2001; 62:503–508 [B]

459. Brown RA, Kahler CW, Niaura R, Abrams DB, Sales SD, Ramsey SE, Goldstein MG, Burgess ES, Miller IW: Cognitive-behavioral treatment for depression in smoking cessation. J Consult Clin Psychol 2001; 69:471–480 [A–]

460. Carroll KM: Behavioral therapies for co-occurring substance use and mood disorders. Biol Psychiatry 2004; 56:778–784 [F]

461. Brown RA, Evans DM, Miller IW, Burgess ES, Mueller TI: Cognitive-behavioral treatment for depression in alcoholism. J Consult Clin Psychol 1997; 65:715–726 [A–]

462. Daley DC, Salloum IM, Thase ME: Integrated treatment using a recovery-oriented approach, in Integrated Treatment for Mood and Substance Use Disorders. Edited by Westermeyer JJ, Weiss RD, Ziedonis DM. Baltimore, Md, Johns Hopkins University Press, 2003, pp 68–89 [G]

463. Daley D, Moss H: Dual Disorders: Counseling Clients With Chemical Dependency and Mental Illness. Center City, Minn, Hazelden, 2002 [G]

464. Salloum IM, Thase ME: Impact of substance abuse on the course and treatment of bipolar disorder. Bipolar Disord 2000; 2:269–280 [F]

465. Geller B, Cooper TB, Sun K, Zimerman B, Frazier J, Williams M, Heath J: Double-blind and placebo-controlled study of lithium for adolescent bipolar disorders with secondary substance dependency. J Am Acad Child Adolesc Psychiatry 1998; 37:171–178 [A]

466. Brady KT, Sonne SC, Anton R, Ballenger JC: Valproate in the treatment of acute bipolar affective episodes complicated by substance abuse: a pilot study. J Clin Psychiatry 1995; 56:118–121 [B]

467. Bowden CL: Clinical correlates of therapeutic response in bipolar disorder. J Affect Disord 2001; 67:257–265 [G]

468. Weiss RD, Greenfield SF, Najavits LM, Soto JA, Wyner D, Tohen M, Griffin ML: Medication compliance among patients with bipolar disorder and substance use disorder. J Clin Psychiatry 1998; 59:172–174 [G]

469. Kosten TR, Kosten TA: New medication strategies for comorbid substance use and bipolar affective disorders. Biol Psychiatry 2004; 56:771–777 [F]

470. Levin FR, Hennessy G: Bipolar disorder and substance abuse. Biol Psychiatry 2004; 56:738–748 [F]

471. American Psychiatric Association: Practice guideline for the treatment of patients with bipolar disorder (revision). Am J Psychiatry 2002; 159(suppl):1–50 [G]

472. Salloum IM, Cornelius JR, Daley DC, Kirisci L, Himmelhoch JM, Thase ME: Efficacy of valproate maintenance in patients with bipolar disorder and alcoholism: a double-blind placebo-controlled study. Arch Gen Psychiatry 2005; 62:37–45 [A]

473. Le Fauve CE, Litten RZ, Randall CL, Moak DH, Salloum IM, Green AI: Pharmacological treatment of alcohol abuse/dependence with psychiatric comorbidity. Alcohol Clin Exp Res 2004; 28:302–312 [G]

474. Brady KT, Myrick H, Henderson S, Coffey SF: The use of divalproex in alcohol relapse prevention: a pilot study. Drug Alcohol Depend 2002; 67:323–330 [A]

475. Brown ES, Nejtek VA, Perantie DC, Bobadilla L: Quetiapine in bipolar disorder and cocaine dependence. Bipolar Disord 2002; 4:406–411 [B]

476. Huang CW, Tsai JJ, Lai ML: Lamotrigine-related skin rashes in adults. Kaohsiung J Med Sci 2002; 18:566–572 [D]

477. Romach MK, Doumani S: Alcoholism and anxiety disorders, in Dual Diagnosis and Treatment: Substance Abuse & Comorbid Medical & Psychiatric Disorders: Medical Psychiatry, vol 8. Edited by Kranzler HR, Rounsaville BJ. New York, Marcel Dekker, 1998, pp 137–175 [G]

478. American Psychiatric Association: Practice guideline for the treatment of patients with panic disorder. Am J Psychiatry 1998; 155(suppl):1–34 [G]

479. Kranzler HR, Burleson JA, Del Boca FK, Babor TF, Korner P, Brown J, Bohn MJ: Buspirone treatment of anxious alcoholics: a placebo-controlled trial. Arch Gen Psychiatry 1994; 51:720–731 [A]

480. Tollefson GD, Montague-Clouse J, Tollefson SL: Treatment of comorbid generalized anxiety in a recently detoxified alcoholic population with a selective serotonergic drug (buspirone). J Clin Psychopharmacol 1992; 12:19–26 [A]

481. Randall CL, Thomas S, Thevos AK: Concurrent alcoholism and social anxiety disorder: a first step toward developing effective treatments. Alcohol Clin Exp Res 2001; 25:210–220 [A–]

482. Leskin GA, Sheikh JL: Lifetime trauma history and panic disorder: findings from the National Comorbidity Survey. J Anxiety Disord 2001; 16:599–603 [E]

483. Kessler RC, Sonnega A, Bromet E, Hughes M, Nelson CB: Posttraumatic stress disorder in the National Comorbidity Survey. Arch Gen Psychiatry 1995; 52:1048–1060 [G]

484. Dansky BS, Roitzsch JC, Brady KT, Saladin ME: Posttraumatic stress disorder and substance abuse: use of research in a clinical setting. J Trauma Stress 1997; 10:141–148 [G]

485. Chilcoat HD, Breslau N: Posttraumatic stress disorder and drug disorders: testing causal pathways. Arch Gen Psychiatry 1998; 55:913–917 [C]

486. Cottler LB, Compton WM III, Mager D, Spitznagel EL, Janca A: Posttraumatic stress disorder among substance users from the general population. Am J Psychiatry 1992; 149:664–670 [G]

487. Grice DE, Brady KT, Dustan LR, Malcolm R, Kilpatrick DG: Sexual and physical assault history and posttraumatic stress disorder in substance-dependent individuals. Am J Addict 1995; 4:297–305 [D]

488. Najavits LM, Runkel R, Neuner C, Frank AF, Thase ME, Crits-Christoph P, Blaine J: Rates and symptoms of PTSD among cocaine-dependent patients. J Stud Alcohol 2003; 64:601–606 [G]

489. Coffey SF, Saladin ME, Drobes DJ, Brady KT, Dansky BS, Kilpatrick DG: Trauma and substance cue reactivity in individuals with comorbid posttraumatic stress disorder and cocaine or alcohol dependence. Drug Alcohol Depend 2002; 65:115–127 [C]

490. Najavits LM: Clinicians' views on treating posttraumatic stress disorder and substance use disorder. J Subst Abuse Treat 2002; 22:79–85 [G]

491. Brady KT: Comorbid posttraumatic stress disorder and substance use disorders. Psychiatric Ann 2001; 31:313–319 [G]

492. Kofoed L, Friedman MJ, Peck R: Alcoholism and drug abuse in patients with PTSD. Psychiatr Q 1993; 64:151–171 [G]

493. Evans K, Sullivan JM: Treating Addicted Survivors of Trauma. New York, Guilford, 1995 [G]

494. Trotter C: Stages of recovery and relapse prevention for the chemically dependent adult sexual trauma survivor, in Adult Survivors of Sexual Abuse: Treatment Innovations. Edited by Hunter M. Thousand Oaks, Calif, Sage, 1995, pp 98–135 [G]

495. Herman JL: Complex PTSD: a syndrome in survivors of prolonged and repeated trauma. J Trauma Stress 1992; 5:377–391 [G]
496. Shapiro F: Eye movement desensitization: a new treatment for post-traumatic stress disorder. J Behav Ther Exp Psychiatry 1989; 20:211–217 [G]
497. Ochberg FM: The counting method for ameliorating traumatic memories. J Trauma Stress 1996; 9:873–880 [G]
498. American Psychiatric Association: Practice guideline for the treatment of patients with acute stress disorder and posttraumatic stress disorder. Am J Psychiatry 2004; 161(suppl):3–31 [G]
499. Waid LR, Johnson DE, Anton RF: Attention-deficit hyperactivity disorder and substance abuse, in Dual Diagnosis and Treatment: Substance Abuse & Comorbid Medical & Psychiatric Disorders. Medical Psychiatry, vol 8. Edited by Kranzler HR, Rounsaville BJ. New York, Marcel Dekker, 1998, pp 393–425 [G]
500. Wilens TE: Attention-deficit/hyperactivity disorder and the substance use disorders: the nature of the relationship, subtypes at risk, and treatment issues. Psychiatr Clin North Am 2004; 27:283–301 [F]
501. Levin FR, Evans SM, Kleber HD: Practical guidelines for the treatment of substance abusers with adult attention-deficit hyperactivity disorder. Psychiatr Serv 1999; 50:1001–1003 [F]
502. Wilens TE, Biederman J, Mick E, Faraone SV, Spencer T: Attention deficit hyperactivity disorder (ADHD) is associated with early onset substance use disorders. J Nerv Ment Dis 1997; 185:475–482 [F]
503. Carroll KM, Rounsaville BJ, Gordon LT, Nich C, Jatlow P, Bisighini RM, Gawin FH: Psychotherapy and pharmacotherapy for ambulatory cocaine abusers. Arch Gen Psychiatry 1994; 51:177–187 [B]
504. Barkley RA, Fischer M, Smallish L, Fletcher K: Does the treatment of attention-deficit/hyperactivity disorder with stimulants contribute to drug use/abuse? a 13-year prospective study. Pediatrics 2003; 111:97–109 [C]
505. Wilens TE, Faraone SV, Biederman J, Gunawardene S: Does stimulant therapy of attention-deficit/hyperactivity disorder beget later substance abuse? a meta-analytic review of the literature. Pediatrics 2003; 111:179–185 [E]
506. Faraone SV, Wilens T: Does stimulant treatment lead to substance use disorders? J Clin Psychiatry 2003; 64(suppl 11):9–13 [E]
507. Wilens TE: Drug therapy for adults with attention-deficit hyperactivity disorder. Drugs 2003; 63:2395–2411 [F]
508. Riggs PD, Hall SK, Mikulich-Gilbertson SK, Lohman M, Kayser A: A randomized controlled trial of pemoline for attention-deficit/hyperactivity disorder in substance-abusing adolescents. J Am Acad Child Adolesc Psychiatry 2004; 43:420–429 [A]
509. Schubiner H, Saules KK, Arfken CL, Johanson CE, Schuster CR, Lockhart N, Edwards A, Donlin J, Pihlgren E: Double-blind placebo-controlled trial of methylphenidate in the treatment of adult ADHD patients with comorbid cocaine dependence. Exp Clin Psychopharmacol 2002; 10:286–294 [A]
510. Levin FR, Evans SM, McDowell DM, Kleber HD: Methylphenidate treatment for cocaine abusers with adult attention-deficit/hyperactivity disorder: a pilot study. J Clin Psychiatry 1998; 59:300–305 [B]
511. Murphy KR, Adler LA: Assessing attention-deficit/hyperactivity disorder in adults: focus on rating scales. J Clin Psychiatry 2004; 65(suppl 3):12–17 [G]
512. Collett BR, Ohan JL, Myers KM: Ten-year review of rating scales, V: scales assessing attention-deficit/hyperactivity disorder. J Am Acad Child Adolesc Psychiatry 2003; 42:1015–1037 [F]

513. Wilens TE: Impact of ADHD and its treatment on substance abuse in adults. J Clin Psychiatry 2004; 65(suppl 3):38–45 [G]
514. Sullivan M, Rudnik-Levin F: Attention deficit/hyperactivity disorder and substance abuse: diagnostic and therapeutic considerations. Ann N Y Acad Sci 2001; 931:251–270 [G]
515. Bulik CM, Sullivan PF: Comorbidity of eating disorders and substance-related disorders, in Dual Diagnosis and Treatment: Substance Abuse & Comorbid Medical & Psychiatric Disorders: Medical Psychiatry, vol 8. Edited by Kranzler HR, Rounsaville BJ. New York, Marcel Dekker, 1998, pp 365–392 [G]
516. Holderness CC, Brooks-Gunn J, Warren MP: Co-morbidity of eating disorders and substance abuse review of the literature. Int J Eat Disord 1994; 16:1–34 [F]
517. Bulik CM: Abuse of drugs associated with eating disorders. J Subst Abuse 1992; 4:69–90 [G]
518. American Psychiatric Association: Practice guideline for the treatment of patients with eating disorders, 3rd ed. Am J Psychiatry (in press) [G]
519. Marrazzi MA, Bacon JP, Kinzie J, Luby ED: Naltrexone use in the treatment of anorexia nervosa and bulimia nervosa. Int Clin Psychopharmacol 1995; 10:163–172 [A]
520. Marrazzi MA, Kinzie J, Luby ED: A detailed longitudinal analysis on the use of naltrexone in the treatment of bulimia. Int Clin Psychopharmacol 1995; 10:173–176 [C]
521. Nace EP: Substance abuse and personality disorder. J Chem Depend Treat 1990; 3:183–198 [G]
522. Trull TJ, Sher KJ, Minks-Brown C, Durbin J, Burr R: Borderline personality disorder and substance use disorders: a review and integration. Clin Psychol Rev 2000; 20:235–253 [F]
523. Darke S, Hall W, Swift W: Prevalence, symptoms and correlates of antisocial personality disorder among methadone maintenance clients. Drug Alcohol Depend 1994; 34:253–257 [G]
524. Darke S, Kaye S, Finlay-Jones R: Antisocial personality disorder, psychopathy and injecting heroin use. Drug Alcohol Depend 1998; 52:63–69 [G]
525. Gerstley LJ, Alterman AI, McLellan AT, Woody GE: Antisocial personality disorder in patients with substance abuse disorders: a problematic diagnosis? Am J Psychiatry 1990; 147:173–178 [F]
526. Brooner RK, Bigelow GE, Strain E, Schmidt CW: Intravenous drug abusers with antisocial personality disorder: increased HIV risk behavior. Drug Alcohol Depend 1990; 26:39–44 [C]
527. Zanarini MC, Frankenburg FR, Hennen J, Reich DB, Silk KR: Axis I comorbidity in patients with borderline personality disorder: 6-year follow-up and prediction of time to remission. Am J Psychiatry 2004; 161:2108–2114 [D]
528. Ross S, Dermatis H, Levounis P, Galanter M: A comparison between dually diagnosed inpatients with and without axis II comorbidity and the relationship to treatment outcome. Am J Drug Alcohol Abuse 2003; 29:263–279 [G]
529. Cacciola JS, Alterman AI, Rutherford MJ, McKay JR, Mulvaney FD: The relationship of psychiatric comorbidity to treatment outcomes in methadone maintained patients. Drug Alcohol Depend 2001; 61:271–280 [C]
530. Gill K, Nolimal D, Crowley TJ: Antisocial personality disorder, HIV risk behavior and retention in methadone maintenance therapy. Drug Alcohol Depend 1992; 30:247–252 [D]
531. Woody GE, McLellan AT, Luborsky L, O'Brien CP: Sociopathy and psychotherapy outcome. Arch Gen Psychiatry 1985; 42:1081–1086 [A–]

532. Rounsaville BJ, Kosten TR, Weissman MM, Kleber HD: Prognostic significance of psychopathology in treated opiate addicts: a 2.5-year follow-up study. Arch Gen Psychiatry 1986; 43:739–745 [C]
533. Linehan MM, Dimeff LA, Reynolds SK, Comtois KA, Welch SS, Heagerty P, Kivlahan DR: Dialectical behavior therapy versus comprehensive validation therapy plus 12-step for the treatment of opioid dependent women meeting criteria for borderline personality disorder. Drug Alcohol Depend 2002; 67:13–26 [A–]
534. American Psychiatric Association: Practice guideline for the treatment of patients with borderline personality disorder. Am J Psychiatry 2001; 158(suppl):1–52 [G]
535. Busto UE, Romach MK, Sellers EM: Multiple drug use and psychiatric comorbidity in patients admitted to the hospital with severe benzodiazepine dependence. J Clin Psychopharmacol 1996; 16:51–57 [G]
536. Lekka NP, Paschalis C, Beratis S: Suicide attempts in high-dose benzodiazepine users. Compr Psychiatry 2002; 43:438–442 [D]
537. Crockford DN, el Guebaly N: Psychiatric comorbidity in pathological gambling: a critical review. Can J Psychiatry 1998; 43:43–50 [F]
538. Lesieur HR, Blume SB, Zoppa RM: Alcoholism, drug abuse, and gambling. Alcohol Clin Exp Res 1986; 10:33–38 [G]
539. McCormick RA: Disinhibition and negative affectivity in substance abusers with and without a gambling problem. Addict Behav 1993; 18:331–336 [G]
540. Petry NM, Stinson FS, Grant BF: Comorbidity of DSM-IV pathological gambling and other psychiatric disorders: results from the National Epidemiologic Survey on Alcohol and Related Conditions. J Clin Psychiatry 2005; 66:564–574 [G]
541. Lesieur HR, Blume SB: The South Oaks Gambling Screen (SOGS): a new instrument for the identification of pathological gamblers. Am J Psychiatry 1987; 144:1184–1188 [G]
542. Langenbucher J, Bavly L, Labouvie E, Sanjuan PM, Martin CS: Clinical features of pathological gambling in an addictions treatment cohort. Psychol Addict Behav 2001; 15:77–79 [D]
543. Petry NM: Psychiatric symptoms in problem gambling and non-problem gambling substance abusers. Am J Addict 2000; 9:163–171 [D]
544. Sharpe L: Cognitive-behavioural treatment of problem gambling, in International Handbook of Cognitive and Behavioural Treatments for Psychological Disorders. Edited by Caballo VE. Oxford, UK, Elsevier Science, 1998, pp 393–416 [G]
545. Hollander E, DeCaria CM, Finkell JN, Begaz T, Wong CM, Cartwright C: A randomized double-blind fluvoxamine/placebo crossover trial in pathologic gambling. Biol Psychiatry 2000; 47:813–817 [A]
546. Hollander E, DeCaria CM, Mari E, Wong CM, Mosovich S, Grossman R, Begaz T: Short-term single-blind fluvoxamine treatment of pathological gambling. Am J Psychiatry 1998; 155:1781–1783 [B]
547. Blanco C, Petkova E, Ibanez A, Saiz-Ruiz J: A pilot placebo-controlled study of fluvoxamine for pathological gambling. Ann Clin Psychiatry 2002; 14:9–15 [A]
548. Kim SW, Grant JE, Adson DE, Shin YC: Double-blind naltrexone and placebo comparison study in the treatment of pathological gambling. Biol Psychiatry 2001; 49:914–921 [A]
549. Hollander E, Buchalter AJ, DeCaria CM: Pathological gambling. Psychiatr Clin North Am 2000; 23:629–642 [G]
550. Grant JE, Kim SW, Potenza MN, Blanco C, Ibanez A, Stevens L, Hektner JM, Zaninelli R: Paroxetine treatment of pathological gambling: a multi-centre randomized controlled trial. Int Clin Psychopharmacol 2003; 18:243–249 [A]

551. Saiz-Ruiz J, Blanco C, Ibanez A, Masramon X, Gomez MM, Madrigal M, Diez T: Sertraline treatment of pathological gambling: a pilot study. J Clin Psychiatry 2005; 66:28–33 [B]
552. Hollander E, Pallanti S, Allen A, Sood E, Baldini RN: Does sustained-release lithium reduce impulsive gambling and affective instability versus placebo in pathological gamblers with bipolar spectrum disorders? Am J Psychiatry 2005; 162:137–145 [A]
553. Pallanti S, Quercioli L, Sood E, Hollander E: Lithium and valproate treatment of pathological gambling: a randomized single-blind study. J Clin Psychiatry 2002; 63:559–564 [A–]
554. Wadland WC, Ferenchick GS: Medical comorbidity in addictive disorders. Psychiatr Clin North Am 2004; 27:675–687 [F]
555. Sullivan LE, O'Connor PG: Medical disorders in substance abuse patients, in Dual Diagnosis and Psychiatric Treatment: Substance Abuse and Comorbid Disorders, 2nd ed. Edited by Kranzler HR, Tinsley JA, Rounsaville BJ. New York, Marcel Dekker, 2004, pp 515–554 [G]
556. American Academy of Pain Medicine, American Pain Society: The use of opioids for the treatment of chronic pain: a consensus statement from the American Academy of Pain Medicine and the American Pain Society. Glenview, Ill, AAPM, 1997. http://www.ampainsoc.org/advocacy/opioids.htm [G]
557. Hall W: The health risks of cannabis. Aust Fam Physician 1995; 24:1237–1240 [G]
558. Hurt RD, Offord KP, Croghan IT, Gomez-Dahl L, Kottke TE, Morse RM, Melton LJ III: Mortality following inpatient addictions treatment: role of tobacco use in a community-based cohort. JAMA 1996; 275:1097–1103 [C]
559. Batki SL, Sorensen JL, Faltz B, Madover S: Psychiatric aspects of treatment of iv drug abusers with AIDS. Hosp Community Psychiatry 1988; 39:439–441 [G]
560. Bridge TP, Mirsky AF, Goodwin FK (eds): Psychological, Neuropsychiatric, and Substance Abuse Aspects of AIDS: Advances in Biochemical Psychopharmacology. New York, Raven, 1988 [G]
561. Sullivan LE, Fiellin DA: Hepatitis C and HIV infections: implications for clinical care in injection drug users. Am J Addict 2004; 13:1–20 [F]
562. Sorensen JL, Costantini MF, London JA: Coping with AIDS: strategies for patients and staff in drug abuse treatment programs. J Psychoactive Drugs 1989; 21:435–440 [G]
563. Butterfield MI, Bosworth HB, Meador KG, Stechuchak KM, Essock SM, Osher FC, Goodman LA, Swanson JW, Bastian LA, Horner RD: Gender differences in hepatitis C infection and risks among persons with severe mental illness. Psychiatr Serv 2003; 54:848–853 [G]
564. Ball JC, Lange WR, Myers CP, Friedman SR: Reducing the risk of AIDS through methadone maintenance treatment. J Health Soc Behav 1988; 29:214–226 [C]
565. Gourevitch MN, Friedland GH: Interactions between methadone and medications used to treat HIV infection: a review. Mt Sinai J Med 2000; 67:429–436 [F]
566. NIH Consensus Statement on Management of Hepatitis C, 2002. NIH Consens State Sci Statements 2002; 19:1–46 [G]
567. American Psychiatric Association: Practice guideline for the treatment of patients with HIV/AIDS. Am J Psychiatry 2000; 157(suppl):1–62 [G]
568. Novick DM, Haverkos HW, Teller DW: The medically ill substance abuser, in Substance Abuse: A Comprehensive Textbook, 3rd ed. Edited by Lowenstein JH, Ruiz P, Millman RB, Langrod JG. Baltimore, Md, Williams & Wilkins, 1997, pp 534–550 [G]
569. Centers for Disease Control: Tuberculosis and human immunodeficiency virus infection: recommendations of the Advisory Committee for the Elimination of Tuberculosis (ACET). MMWR Morb Mortal Wkly Rep 1989; 38:236–238, 243–250 [G]

570. Bauer CR, Shankaran S, Bada HS, Lester B, Wright LL, Krause-Steinrauf H, Smeriglio VL, Finnegan LP, Maza PL, Verter J: The Maternal Lifestyle Study: drug exposure during pregnancy and short-term maternal outcomes. Am J Obstet Gynecol 2002; 186:487–495 [C]
571. Bolnick JM, Rayburn WF: Substance use disorders in women: special considerations during pregnancy. Obstet Gynecol Clin North Am 2003; 30:545–558, vii [F]
572. Faiz AS, Ananth CV: Etiology and risk factors for placenta previa: an overview and meta-analysis of observational studies. J Matern Fetal Neonatal Med 2003; 13:175–190 [E]
573. Kennare R, Heard A, Chan A: Substance use during pregnancy: risk factors and obstetric and perinatal outcomes in South Australia. Aust NZ J Obstet Gynaecol 2005; 45:220–225 [C]
574. Ananth CV, Savitz DA, Luther ER: Maternal cigarette smoking as a risk factor for placental abruption, placenta previa, and uterine bleeding in pregnancy. Am J Epidemiol 1996; 144:881–889 [C]
575. Woods JR: Maternal and transplacental effects of cocaine. Ann N Y Acad Sci 1998; 846:1–11 [F]
576. Szeto HH: Maternal-fetal pharmacokinetics and fetal dose-response relationships. Ann N Y Acad Sci 1989; 562:42–55 [F]
577. Thadani PV, Strauss JF III, Dey SK, Anderson VM, Audus KL, Coats KS, Cross JC, Erlebacher A, Ganapathy V, Linzer DI, Miller RK, Novak DA, Rapaka RS, Sadovsky Y, Salafia CM, Soares M, Unadkat J: National Institute on Drug Abuse conference report on placental proteins, drug transport, and fetal development. Am J Obstet Gynecol 2004; 191:1858–1862 [G]
578. Schenker S, Yang Y, Johnson RF, Downing JW, Schenken RS, Henderson GI, King TS: The transfer of cocaine and its metabolites across the term human placenta. Clin Pharmacol Ther 1993; 53:329–339 [G]
579. Dattel BJ: Substance abuse in pregnancy. Semin Perinatol 1990; 14:179–187 [F]
580. Fried PA: Postnatal consequences of maternal marijuana use. NIDA Res Monogr 1985; 59:61–72 [F]
581. Little RE, Asker RL, Sampson PD, Renwick JH: Fetal growth and moderate drinking in early pregnancy. Am J Epidemiol 1986; 123:270–278 [C]
582. Handler A, Kistin N, Davis F, Ferre C: Cocaine use during pregnancy: perinatal outcomes. Am J Epidemiol 1991; 133:818–825 [D]
583. Addis A, Moretti ME, Ahmed SF, Einarson TR, Koren G: Fetal effects of cocaine: an updated meta-analysis. Reprod Toxicol 2001; 15:341–369 [E]
584. Wolfe EL, Davis T, Guydish J, Delucchi KL: Mortality risk associated with perinatal drug and alcohol use in California. J Perinatol 2005; 25:93–100 [D]
585. Armstrong MA, Gonzales OV, Lieberman L, Carpenter DM, Pantoja PM, Escobar GJ: Perinatal substance abuse intervention in obstetric clinics decreases adverse neonatal outcomes. J Perinatol 2003; 23:3–9 [D]
586. Prenatal exposure to alcohol. Alcohol Res Health 2000; 24:32–41 [F]
587. Chudley AE, Conry J, Cook JL, Loock C, Rosales T, LeBlanc N: Fetal alcohol spectrum disorder: Canadian guidelines for diagnosis. CMAJ 2005; 172:S1–S21 [F]
588. Jacobson SW, Jacobson JL, Sokol RJ, Chiodo LM, Corobana R: Maternal age, alcohol abuse history, and quality of parenting as moderators of the effects of prenatal alcohol exposure on 7.5-year intellectual function. Alcohol Clin Exp Res 2004; 28:1732–1745 [C]
589. Suchman N, Mayes L, Conti J, Slade A, Rounsaville B: Rethinking parenting interventions for drug-dependent mothers: from behavior management to fostering emotional bonds. J Subst Abuse Treat 2004; 27:179–185 [F]

590. Dawe S, Harnett PH, Staiger P, Dadds MR: Parent training skills and methadone maintenance: clinical opportunities and challenges. Drug Alcohol Depend 2000; 60:1–11 [F]
591. Finnegan LP, Kendall SR: Maternal and neonatal effects of alcohol and drugs, in Substance Abuse: A Comprehensive Textbook, 2nd ed. Edited by Lowenstein JH, Ruiz P, Millman RB. Baltimore, Md, Williams & Wilkins, 1992, pp 628–656 [G]
592. Blume SB, Zilberman ML: Addiction in women, in The American Psychiatric Publishing Textbook of Substance Abuse Treatment, 3rd ed. Edited by Galanter M, Kleber HD. Washington, DC, American Psychiatric Publishing, 2004, 539–546 [G]
593. Griffin ML, Weiss RD, Mirin SM, Lange U: A comparison of male and female cocaine abusers. Arch Gen Psychiatry 1989; 46:122–126 [G]
594. Blume SB: Sexuality and stigma: the alcoholic woman. Alcohol Health Res World 1991; 15:139–146 [G]
595. Roberts LW, Dunn LB: Ethical considerations in caring for women with substance use disorders. Obstet Gynecol Clin North Am 2003; 30:559–582 [F]
596. Stein MD, Cyr MG: Women and substance abuse. Med Clin North Am 1997; 81:979–998 [F]
597. Winfield I, George LK, Swartz M, Blazer DG: Sexual assault and psychiatric disorders among a community sample of women. Am J Psychiatry 1990; 147:335–341 [E]
598. Canterbury RJ: Alcohol and other substance abuse, in Women's Mental Health: A Comprehensive Textbook. Edited by Kornstein SG, Clayton AH. New York, Guilford, 2002, pp 222–243 [G]
599. Ladwig GB, Andersen MD: Substance abuse in women: relationship between chemical dependency of women and past reports of physical and/or sexual abuse. Int J Addict 1989; 24:739–754 [G]
600. Stevens S, Arbiter N, Glider P: Women residents: expanding their role to increase treatment effectiveness in substance abuse programs. Int J Addict 1989; 24:425–434 [G]
601. Perkins KA: Sex differences in nicotine versus nonnicotine reinforcement as determinants of tobacco smoking. Exp Clin Psychopharmacol 1996; 4:166–177 [F]
602. George TP, O'Malley SS: Current pharmacological treatments for nicotine dependence. Trends Pharmacol Sci 2004; 25:42–48 [F]
603. Covey LS, Glassman AH, Stetner F: Naltrexone effects on short-term and long-term smoking cessation. J Addict Dis 1999; 18:31–40 [A]
604. Byars JA, Frost-Pineda K, Jacobs WS, Gold MS: Naltrexone augments the effects of nicotine replacement therapy in female smokers. J Addict Dis 2005; 24:49–60 [A]
605. Bolego C, Poli A, Paoletti R: Smoking and gender. Cardiovasc Res 2002; 53:568–576 [F]
606. Gasperino J, Rom WN: Gender and lung cancer. Clin Lung Cancer 2004; 5:353–359 [F]
607. Ebbert JO, Carr AB, Dale LC: Smokeless tobacco: an emerging addiction. Med Clin North Am 2004; 88:1593–1605 [G]
608. Substance Abuse and Mental Health Services Administration: Results from the 2002 National Survey on Drug Use and Health: National Findings. NHSDA Series H-22. DHHS Publication (SMA) 03–3836. Rockville, Md, Substance Abuse and Mental Health Services Administration, 2003 [G]
609. Piazza NJ, Vrbka JL, Yeager RD: Telescoping of alcoholism in women alcoholics. Int J Addict 1989; 24:19–28 [G]
610. Bradley KA, Badrinath S, Bush K, Boyd-Wickizer J, Anawalt B: Medical risks for women who drink alcohol. J Gen Intern Med 1998; 13:627–639 [F]
611. Greenfield SF, O'Leary G: Sex differences in substance use disorders, in Psychiatric Illness in Women: Emerging Treatments and Research. Edited by Lewis-Hall F, Williams

TS, Panetta JA, Herrera JM. Washington, DC, American Psychiatric Publishing, 2002, pp 467–534 [G]

612. Patkar AA, Sterling RC, Gottheil E, Weinstein SP: A comparison of medical symptoms reported by cocaine-, opiate-, and alcohol-dependent patients. Subst Abus 1999; 20:227–235 [G]

613. Hser YI, Anglin MD, McGlothlin W: Sex differences in addict careers, 1: initiation of use. Am J Drug Alcohol Abuse 1987; 13:33–57 [D]

614. American Academy of Child and Adolescent Psychiatry: Practice parameter for the assessment and treatment of children and adolescents with substance use disorders. J Am Acad Child Adolesc Psychiatry 2005; 44:609–621 [G]

615. Center for Substance Abuse Treatment: Screening and Assessing Adolescents for Substance Use Disorders. Treatment Improvement Protocol (TIP) Series No. 31. DHHS Publication (SMA) 99-3282. Rockville, Md, Substance Abuse and Mental Health Services Administration, 1999 [G]

616. Wagner EF, Waldron HB: Innovations in Adolescent Substance Abuse Interventions. New York, Elsevier, 2001 [G]

617. Liddle H, Rowe C: Adolescent Substance Abuse Treatment Research Update: a NIDA monograph. Bethesda, Md, National Institute on Drug Abuse, 2005 [G]

618. American Academy of Pediatrics Committee on Substance Abuse: Tobacco, alcohol, and other drugs: the role of the pediatrician in prevention and management of substance abuse. Pediatrics 1998; 101:125–128 [G]

619. Kaminer Y, Tarter RE: Adolescent substance abuse, in The American Psychiatric Publishing Textbook of Substance Abuse Treatment, 3rd ed. Edited by Galanter M, Kleber HD. Washington, DC, American Psychiatric Publishing, 2004, pp 505–517 [G]

620. Pollock NK, Martin CS: Diagnostic orphans: adolescents with alcohol symptoms who do not qualify for DSM-IV abuse or dependence diagnoses. Am J Psychiatry 1999; 156:897–901 [C]

621. Kaminer Y, Bukstein O, Tarter RE: The Teen-Addiction Severity Index: rationale and reliability. Int J Addict 1991; 26:219–226 [G]

622. Reilly D: Family factors in the etiology and treatment of youthful drug abuse. Fam Ther 1976; 2:149–171 [G]

623. Stanton MD, Landau-Stanton J: Therapy with families of adolescent substance abusers, in Treatment Choices for Alcoholism and Substance Abuse. Edited by Milkman HB, Sederer LI. Lexington, Mass, Lexington Books, 1990, pp 329–339 [G]

624. Bukstein OG, Brent DA, Kaminer Y: Comorbidity of substance abuse and other psychiatric disorders in adolescents. Am J Psychiatry 1989; 146:1131–1141 [G]

625. Grilo CM, Becker DF, Walker ML, Levy KN, Edell WS, McGlashan TH: Psychiatric comorbidity in adolescent inpatients with substance use disorders. J Am Acad Child Adolesc Psychiatry 1995; 34:1085–1091 [D]

626. Riggs PD, Baker S, Mikulich SK, Young SE, Crowley TJ: Depression in substance-dependent delinquents. J Am Acad Child Adolesc Psychiatry 1995; 34:764–771 [G]

627. Goldston DB: Conceptual issues in understanding the relationship between suicidal behavior and substance use during adolescence. Drug Alcohol Depend 2004; 76(suppl): S79–S91 [G]

628. Catalano RF, Hawkins JD, Wells EA, Miller J, Brewer D: Evaluation of the effectiveness of adolescent drug abuse treatment, assessment of risks for relapse, and promising approaches for relapse prevention. Int J Addict 1991; 25:1085–1140 [F]

629. Bukstein OG, Kithas J: Adolescent substance use disorders, in Child Adolescent Psychopharmacology. Edited by Rosenberg D, Davanzo P, Gershon S. New York, Marcel Dekker, 2002, pp 675–710 [G]

630. Coatsworth JD, Santisteban DA, McBride CK, Szapocznik J: Brief strategic family therapy versus community control: engagement, retention, and an exploration of the moderating role of adolescent symptom severity. Fam Process 2001; 40:313–332 [A–]
631. Faggiano F, Vigna-Taglianti FD, Versino E, Zambon A, Borraccino A, Lemma P: School-based prevention for illicit drug use. Cochrane Database Syst Rev 2005; CD003020 [E]
632. Skara S, Sussman S: A review of 25 long-term adolescent tobacco and other drug use prevention program evaluations. Prev Med 2003; 37:451–474 [E]
633. Backinger CL, Fagan P, Matthews E, Grana R: Adolescent and young adult tobacco prevention and cessation: current status and future directions. Tob Control 2003; 12(suppl 4):IV46–IV53 [E]
634. Botvin GJ, Baker E, Dusenbury L, Botvin EM, Diaz T: Long-term follow-up results of a randomized drug abuse prevention trial in a white middle-class population. JAMA 1995; 273:1106–1112 [A–]
635. Botvin GJ, Griffin KW, Diaz T, Scheier LM, Williams C, Epstein JA: Preventing illicit drug use in adolescents: long-term follow-up data from a randomized control trial of a school population. Addict Behav 2000; 25:769–774 [A–]
636. Botvin GJ, Griffin KW: Life skills training: theory, methods, and effectiveness of a drug abuse prevention approach, in Innovations in Adolescent Substance Abuse Interventions. Edited by Wagner EF, Waldron HB. Oxford, UK, Elsevier Science, 2001, pp 31–50 [G]
637. Masterman PW, Kelly AB: Reaching adolescents who drink harmfully: fitting intervention to developmental reality. J Subst Abuse Treat 2003; 24:347–355 [G]
638. Garrison MM, Christakis DA, Ebel BE, Wiehe SE, Rivara FP: Smoking cessation interventions for adolescents: a systematic review. Am J Prev Med 2003; 25:363–367 [F]
639. Colby SM, Monti PM, Barnett NP, Rohsenow DJ, Weissman K, Spirito A, Woolard RH, Lewander WJ: Brief motivational interviewing in a hospital setting for adolescent smoking: a preliminary study. J Consult Clin Psychol 1998; 66:574–578 [B]
640. Hurt RD, Croghan GA, Beede SD, Wolter TD, Croghan IT, Patten CA: Nicotine patch therapy in 101 adolescent smokers: efficacy, withdrawal symptom relief, and carbon monoxide and plasma cotinine levels. Arch Pediatr Adolesc Med 2000; 154:31–37 [A–]
641. Backinger CL, Leischow SJ: Advancing the science of adolescent tobacco use cessation. Am J Health Behav 2001; 25:183–190 [F]
642. Mannuzza S, Klein RG, Moulton JL III: Does stimulant treatment place children at risk for adult substance abuse? a controlled, prospective follow-up study. J Child Adolesc Psychopharmacol 2003; 13:273–282 [A–]
643. Vandrey R, Budney AJ, Kamon JL, Stanger C: Cannabis withdrawal in adolescent treatment seekers. Drug Alcohol Depend 2005; 78:205–210 [G]
644. Widlitz M, Marin DB: Substance abuse in older adults: an overview. Geriatrics 2002; 57:29–34 [F]
645. Menninger JA: Assessment and treatment of alcoholism and substance-related disorders in the elderly. Bull Menninger Clin 2002; 66:166–183 [F]
646. Atkinson JH, Schuckit MA: Geriatric alcohol and drug misuse and abuse. Advances in Substance Abuse 1983; 3:195–237 [G]
647. Foy A, O'Connell D, Henry D, Kelly J, Cocking S, Halliday J: Benzodiazepine use as a cause of cognitive impairment in elderly hospital inpatients. J Gerontol A Biol Sci Med Sci 1995; 50:M99–M106 [C]
648. Moore AR, O'Keeffe ST: Drug-induced cognitive impairment in the elderly. Drugs Aging 1999; 15:15–28 [F]

649. Atkinson RM (ed): Alcohol and Drug Abuse in Old Age. Washington, DC, American Psychiatric Press, 1984 [G]
650. Breslow RA, Faden VB, Smothers B: Alcohol consumption by elderly Americans. J Stud Alcohol 2003; 64:884–892 [G]
651. Oslin DW: Alcohol use in late life: disability and comorbidity. J Geriatr Psychiatry Neurol 2000; 13:134–140 [F]
652. Abrams RC, Alexopoulos GS: Geriatric addictions, in Clinical Textbook of Addictive Disorders, 2nd ed. Edited by Frances RJ, Miller SI. New York, Guilford, 1998, pp 374–396 [G]
653. Hays JT, Ebbert JO: Bupropion sustained release for treatment of tobacco dependence. Mayo Clin Proc 2003; 78:1020–1024 [G]
654. Roose SP, Dalack GW, Glassman AH, Woodring S, Walsh BT, Giardina EG: Cardiovascular effects of bupropion in depressed patients with heart disease. Am J Psychiatry 1991; 148:512–516 [B]
655. Satre DD, Knight BG, Dickson-Fuhrmann E, Jarvik LF: Substance abuse treatment initiation among older adults in the GET SMART program: effects of depression and cognitive status. Aging Ment Health 2004; 8:346–354 [G]
656. Kofoed LL, Tolson RL, Atkinson RM, Toth RL, Turner JA: Treatment compliance of older alcoholics: an elder-specific approach is superior to "mainstreaming." J Stud Alcohol 1987; 48:47–51 [B]
657. National Institute on Alcohol Abuse and Alcoholism: Alcohol and minorities, in Alcohol Alert, No. 23 (23 PH 347). Washington, DC, National Academies Press, 1994. http://pubs.niaaa.nih.gov/publications/aa23.htm. Update in January 2002 (No. 55): http://pubs.niaaa.nig.gov/publications/aa55.htm [G]
658. Institute of Medicine: The treatment of special populations: overview and definitions, in Broadening the Base of Treatment for Alcohol Problems. Washington, DC, National Academies Press, 1990, pp 344–355 [G]
659. Dolan MP, Roberts WR, Penk WE, Robinowitz R, Atkins HG: Personality differences among black, white, and Hispanic-American male heroin addicts on MMPI content scales. J Clin Psychol 1983; 39:807–813 [G]
660. Cabaj RP: Substance abuse in the gay and lesbian community, in Substance Abuse: A Comprehensive Textbook. 2nd ed. Edited by Lowinson JH, Ruiz P, Millman RB. Baltimore, Md, Williams & Wilkins, 1992, pp 852–860 [G]
661. Gray N, Nye PS: American Indian and Alaska Native substance abuse: co-morbidity and cultural issues. Am Indian Alsk Native Ment Health Res 2001; 10:67–84 [G]
662. Noe T, Fleming C, Manson S: Healthy nations: reducing substance abuse in American Indian and Alaska Native communities. J Psychoactive Drugs 2003; 35:15–25 [G]
663. Alvarez J, Olson BD, Jason LA, Davis MI, Ferrari JR: Heterogeneity among Latinas and Latinos entering substance abuse treatment: findings from a national database. J Subst Abuse Treat 2004; 26:277–284 [G]
664. Gloria AM, Peregoy JJ: Counseling Latino alcohol and other substance users/abusers: cultural considerations for counselors. J Subst Abuse Treat 1996; 13:119–126 [G]
665. Kandel DB, Kiros GE, Schaffran C, Hu MC: Racial/ethnic differences in cigarette smoking initiation and progression to daily smoking: a multilevel analysis. Am J Public Health 2004; 94:128–135 [G]
666. Royce JM, Hymowitz N, Corbett K, Hartwell TD, Orlandi MA: Smoking cessation factors among African Americans and whites. COMMIT Research Group. Am J Public Health 1993; 83:220–226 [C]
667. Benowitz NL: Smoking cessation trials targeted to racial and economic minority groups. JAMA 2002; 288:497–499 [G]

668. Kabat GC, Morabia A, Wynder EL: Comparison of smoking habits of blacks and whites in a case-control study. Am J Public Health 1991; 81:1483–1486 [D]
669. Ahluwalia JS, McNagny SE, Clark WS: Smoking cessation among inner-city African Americans using the nicotine transdermal patch. J Gen Intern Med 1998; 13:1–8 [A]
670. Ahluwalia JS, Harris KJ, Catley D, Okuyemi KS, Mayo MS: Sustained-release bupropion for smoking cessation in African Americans: a randomized controlled trial. JAMA 2002; 288:468–474 [A]
671. Cochran SD, Keenan C, Schober C, Mays VM: Estimates of alcohol use and clinical treatment needs among homosexually active men and women in the US population. J Consult Clin Psychol 2000; 68:1062–1071 [D]
672. Hughes TL: Lesbians' drinking patterns: beyond the data. Subst Use Misuse 2003; 38:1739–1758 [F]
673. Cochran SD, Ackerman D, Mays VM, Ross MW: Prevalence of non-medical drug use and dependence among homosexually active men and women in the US population. Addiction 2004; 99:989–998 [D]
674. Jordan KM: Substance abuse among gay, lesbian, bisexual, transgender, and questioning adolescents. School Psych Rev 2000; 29:201–206 [G]
675. Skinner WF, Otis MD: Drug and alcohol use among lesbian and gay people in a southern US sample: epidemiological, comparative, and methodological findings from the Trilogy Project. J Homosex 1996; 30:59–92 [C]
676. McCabe SE, Boyd C, Hughes TL, d'Arcy H: Sexual identity and substance use among undergraduate students. Subst Abuse 2003; 24:77–91 [G]
677. D'Augelli AR, Grossman AH, Hershberger SL, O'Connell TS: Aspects of mental health among older lesbian, gay, and bisexual adults. Aging Ment Health 2001; 5:149–158 [G]
678. Stall R, Wiley J: A comparison of alcohol and drug use patterns of homosexual and heterosexual men: the San Francisco Men's Health Study. Drug Alcohol Depend 1988; 22:63–73 [G]
679. Stall R, Paul JP, Greenwood G, Pollack LM, Bein E, Crosby GM, Mills TC, Binson D, Coates TJ, Catania JA: Alcohol use, drug use and alcohol-related problems among men who have sex with men: the Urban Men's Health Study. Addiction 2001; 96:1589–1601 [G]
680. AIDS Alert: Behavioral intervention for meth-using MSM: researchers want to spread word. AIDS Alert 2002; 17:143–144 [G]
681. Frosch D, Shoptaw S, Huber A, Rawson RA, Ling W: Sexual HIV risk among gay and bisexual male methamphetamine abusers. J Subst Abuse Treat 1996; 13:483–486 [G]
682. Tang H, Greenwood GL, Cowling DW, Lloyd JC, Roeseler AG, Bal DG: Cigarette smoking among lesbians, gays, and bisexuals: how serious a problem? (United States). Cancer Causes Control 2004; 15:797–803 [G]
683. Ryan H, Wortley PM, Easton A, Pederson L, Greenwood G: Smoking among lesbians, gays, and bisexuals: a review of the literature. Am J Prev Med 2001; 21:142–149 [F]
684. Craft EM, Mulvey KP: Addressing lesbian, gay, bisexual, and transgender issues from the inside: one federal agency's approach. Am J Public Health 2001; 91:889–891 [G]
685. Liles RE, Childs D: Similarities in family dynamics of incest and alcohol abuse. Alcohol Health Res World 1986; Fall:66–69 [G]
686. Kosten TR, Rounsaville BJ, Kleber HD: Parental alcoholism in opioid addicts. J Nerv Ment Dis 1985; 173:461–469 [D]
687. Lessov CN, Swan GE, Ring HZ, Khroyan TV, Lerman C: Genetics and drug use as a complex phenotype. Subst Use Misuse 2004; 39:1515–1569 [F]

688. Barnard M, McKeganey N: The impact of parental problem drug use on children: what is the problem and what can be done to help? Addiction 2004; 99:552–559 [F]
689. Werner MJ, Joffe A, Graham AV: Screening, early identification, and office-based intervention with children and youth living in substance-abusing families. Pediatrics 1999; 103:1099–1112 [F]
690. O'Farrell TJ, Fals-Stewart W: Family-involved alcoholism treatment: an update. Recent Dev Alcohol 2001; 15:329–356 [E]
691. Strathdee SA, Sherman SG: The role of sexual transmission of HIV infection among injection and non-injection drug users. J Urban Health 2003; 80(suppl 3):7–14 [F]
692. Giovino GA: Epidemiology of tobacco use in the United States. Oncogene 2002; 21:7326–7340 [G]
693. Hughes JR: The future of smoking cessation therapy in the United States. Addiction 1996; 91:1797–1802 [G]
694. Leukefeld CG, Tims FM: Compulsory treatment for drug abuse. Int J Addict 1990; 25:621–640 [G]
695. Beane EA, Beck JC: Court based civil commitment of alcoholics and substance abusers. Bull Am Acad Psychiatry Law 1991; 19:359–366 [G]
696. Anker AL, Crowley TJ: Use of contingency contracts in specialty clinics for cocaine abuse. NIDA Res Monogr 1981; 41:452–459 [B]
697. Brendel RW, Bryan E: HIPAA for psychiatrists. Harv Rev Psychiatry 2004; 12:177–183 [G]
698. Kalman D, Morrisette SB, George TP: Co-morbidity of smoking in patients with psychiatric and substance use disorders. Am J Addict 2005; 14:106–123 [F]
699. Ziedonis DM, Williams JM: Management of smoking in people with psychiatric disorders. Curr Opin Psychiatry 2003; 16:305–315 [G]
700. Hall SM, Munoz RF, Reus VI: Cognitive-behavioral intervention increases abstinence rates for depressive-history smokers. J Consult Clin Psychol 1994; 62:141–146 [A–]
701. Ziedonis DM, George TP: Schizophrenia and nicotine use: report of a pilot smoking cessation program and review of neurobiological and clinical issues. Schizophr Bull 1997; 23:247–254 [B]
702. Addington J, el Guebaly N, Campbell W, Hodgins DC, Addington D: Smoking cessation treatment for patients with schizophrenia. Am J Psychiatry 1998; 155:974–976 [B]
703. George TP, Ziedonis DM, Feingold A, Pepper WT, Satterburg CA, Winkel J, Rounsaville BJ, Kosten TR: Nicotine transdermal patch and atypical antipsychotic medications for smoking cessation in schizophrenia. Am J Psychiatry 2000; 157:1835–1842 [A–]
704. Evins AE, Mays VK, Rigotti NA, Tisdale T, Cather C, Goff DC: A pilot trial of bupropion added to cognitive behavioral therapy for smoking cessation in schizophrenia. Nicotine Tob Res 2001; 3:397–403 [A]
705. Kalman D, Hayes K, Colby SM, Eaton CA, Rohsenow DJ, Monti PM: Concurrent versus delayed smoking cessation treatment for persons in early alcohol recovery: a pilot study. J Subst Abuse Treat 2001; 20:233–238 [A–]
706. Anderson JE, Jorenby DE, Scott WJ, Fiore MC: Treating tobacco use and dependence: an evidence-based clinical practice guideline for tobacco cessation. Chest 2002; 121:932–941 [F]
707. Fagerström KO, Schneider NG: Measuring nicotine dependence: a review of the Fagerström Tolerance Questionnaire. J Behav Med 1989; 12:159–182 [F]
708. Storr CL, Reboussin BA, Anthony JC: The Fagerström Test for Nicotine Dependence: a comparison of standard scoring and latent class analysis approaches. Drug Alcohol Depend 2005; 80:241–250 [G]

709. Heatherton TF, Kozlowski LT, Frecker RC, Fagerström KO: The Fagerström Test for Nicotine Dependence: a revision of the Fagerström Tolerance Questionnaire. Br J Addict 1991; 86:1119–1127 [G]
710. Pomerleau CS, Carton SM, Lutzke ML, Flessland KA, Pomerleau OF: Reliability of the Fagerström Tolerance Questionnaire and the Fagerström Test for Nicotine Dependence. Addict Behav 1994; 19:33–39 [G]
711. American Psychiatric Association: Handbook of Psychiatric Measures. Washington, DC, American Psychiatric Press, 2000 [G]
712. Boyle RG, Jensen J, Hatsukami DK, Severson HH: Measuring dependence in smokeless tobacco users. Addict Behav 1995; 20:443–450 [G]
713. Pomerleau CS, Majchrzak MJ, Pomerleau OF: Nicotine dependence and the Fagerström Tolerance Questionnaire: a brief review. J Subst Abuse 1989; 1:471–477 [F]
714. Woody GE, Cottler LB, Cacciola J: Severity of dependence: data from the DSM-IV field trials. Addiction 1993; 88:1573–1579 [G]
715. Lerman C, Orleans CT, Engstrom PF: Biological markers in smoking cessation treatment. Semin Oncol 1993; 20:359–367 [F]
716. Velicer WF, Prochaska JO, Rossi JS, Snow MG: Assessing outcome in smoking cessation studies. Psychol Bull 1992; 111:23–41 [F]
717. Hurt RD, Dale LC, Offord KP, Bruce BK, McClain FL, Eberman KM: Inpatient treatment of severe nicotine dependence. Mayo Clin Proc 1992; 67:823–828 [B]
718. US Department of Health and Human Services: Clinical Practice Guideline No. 18: Smoking Cessation, AHCPR Publication 96-0692. Washington, DC, US Government Printing Office, 1996 [G]
719. Law M, Tang JL: An analysis of the effectiveness of interventions intended to help people stop smoking. Arch Intern Med 1995; 155:1933–1941 [E]
720. Baille A, Mattick RP, Hall W, Webster P: Meta-analytic review of the efficacy of smoking cessation interventions. Drug Alcohol Rev 1994; 13:157–170 [E]
721. Kottke TE, Battista RN, DeFriese GH, Brekke ML: Attributes of successful smoking cessation interventions in medical practice: a meta-analysis of 39 controlled trials. JAMA 1988; 259:2883–2889 [E]
722. Fiore MC: Trends in cigarette smoking in the United States: the epidemiology of tobacco use. Med Clin North Am 1992; 76:289–303 [G]
723. Abrams D: Treatment issues: towards a stepped-care model. Tob Control 1993; 2(suppl): S17–S37 [F]
724. Sachs DP: Advances in smoking cessation treatment. Current Pulmonology 1991; 12:139–198 [F]
725. Goldstein MG, Niaura R, Abrams DB: Pharmacological and behavioral treatment of nicotine dependence: nicotine as a drug of abuse, in Medical Psychiatric Practice, vol 1. Edited by Stoudemire A, Fogel BS. Washington, DC, American Psychiatric Press, 1991, pp 541–596 [F]
726. Sachs DPL, Leischow SJ: Pharmacological approaches to smoking cessation. Clin Chest Med 1991; 12:9–10 [F]
727. Orleans CT, Slade J (eds): Nicotine Addiction: Principles and Management. New York, Oxford University Press, 1993 [F]
728. Mattick RP, Baillie A: An Outline for Approaches to Smoking Cessation: Quality Assurance Project. Australian Government Publishing Service, 1992 [G]
729. Centers for Disease Control and Prevention: National trends in smoking cessation, in The Health Benefits of Smoking Cessation: A Report of the Surgeon General. DHHS Publication (CDC) YO-K-116. Washington, DC, US Government Printing Office, 1990, pp 579–616 [F]
730. Hughes JR, Frances RJ: How to help psychiatric patients stop smoking. Psychiatr Serv 1995; 46:435–436 [G]

731. Ziedonis DM, Kosten TR, Glazer WM, Frances RJ: Nicotine dependence and schizophrenia. Hosp Community Psychiatry 1994; 45:204–206 [F]
732. Hall RG, Duhamel M, McClanahan R, Miles G, Nason C, Rosen S, Schiller P, Tao-Yonenaga L, Hall SM: Level of functioning, severity of illness, and smoking status among chronic psychiatric patients. J Nerv Ment Dis 1995; 183:468–471 [G]
733. Addington J, el Guebaly N, Addington D, Hodgins D: Readiness to stop smoking in schizophrenia. Can J Psychiatry 1997; 42:49–52 [G]
734. Schwartz JL: Methods of smoking cessation. Med Clin North Am 1992; 76:451–476 [E]
735. Schwartz JL: Review and Evaluation of Smoking Cessation Methods: The United States and Canada 1978–1985. NIH Publication 87-2940. Washington, DC, US Department of Health and Human Services, 1987 [E]
736. Prochaska JO, DiClemente CC, Velicer WF, Rossi JS: Standardized, individualized, interactive, and personalized self-help programs for smoking cessation. Health Psychol 1993; 12:399–405 [A]
737. Orleans CT: Treating nicotine dependence in medical settings: a stepped-care model, in Nicotine Addiction: Principles and Management. Edited by Orleans CT, Slade J. New York, Oxford University Press, 1993, pp 145–161 [G]
738. Pbert L, Ockene JK, Zapka J, Ma Y, Goins KV, Oncken C, Stoddard AM: A community health center smoking-cessation intervention for pregnant and postpartum women. Am J Prev Med 2004; 26:377–385 [G]
739. Borrelli B, McQuaid EL, Becker B, Hammond K, Papandonatos G, Fritz G, Abrams D: Motivating parents of kids with asthma to quit smoking: the PAQS project. Health Educ Res 2002; 17:659–669 [G]
740. Gritz ER, Kristeller J, Burns DM: Treating nicotine addiction in high-risk groups and patients with medical co-morbidity, in Nicotine Addiction: Principles and Management. Edited by Orleans CT, Slade J. New York, Oxford University Press, 1993, pp 279–309 [F]
741. US Department of Health and Human Services: Treatment of tobacco dependence, in The Health Consequences of Smoking: Nicotine Addiction. A Report of the Surgeon General. Washington, DC, US Government Printing Office, 1988, pp 459-560 [F]
742. Lando H: Formal quit smoking treatments, in Nicotine Addiction: Principles and Management. Edited by Orleans CT, Slade J. New York, Oxford University Press, 1993, pp 221–244 [F]
743. Cinciripini PM, Lapitsky L, Seay S, Wallfisch A, Kitchens K, Van Vunakis H: The effects of smoking schedules on cessation outcome: can we improve on common methods of gradual and abrupt nicotine withdrawal? J Consult Clin Psychol 1995; 63:388–399 [A]
744. Hatsukami DK, Henningfield JE, Kotlyar M: Harm reduction approaches to reducing tobacco-related mortality. Annu Rev Public Health 2004; 25:377–395 [F]
745. Hughes JR: Harm-reduction approaches to smoking: the need for data. Am J Prev Med 1998; 15:78–79 [G]
746. Hughes JR, Gulliver SB, Fenwick JW, Valliere WA, Cruser K, Pepper S, Shea P, Solomon LJ, Flynn BS: Smoking cessation among self-quitters. Health Psychol 1992; 11:331–334 [C]
747. Fiore MC, Novotny TE, Pierce JP, Giovino GA, Hatziandreu EJ, Newcomb PA, Surawicz TS, Davis RM: Methods used to quit smoking in the United States: do cessation programs help? JAMA 1990; 263:2760–2765 [G]
748. Cox JL: Algorithms for nicotine withdrawal therapy. Health Values 1993; 17:41–50 [G]
749. Hughes JR: Non-nicotine pharmacotherapies for smoking cessation. Journal of Drug Development 1994; 6:197–203 [F]

750. Rigotti NA: Clinical practice: treatment of tobacco use and dependence. N Engl J Med 2002; 346:506–512 [A–]
751. MacKenzie TD, Bartecchi CE, Schrier RW: The human costs of tobacco use, part 2. N Engl J Med 1994; 330:975–980 [F]
752. Lando HA, Rolnick S, Klevan D, Roski J, Cherney L, Lauger G: Telephone support as an adjunct to transdermal nicotine in smoking cessation. Am J Public Health 1997; 87:1670–1674 [A–]
753. Mermelstein R, Hedeker D, Wong SC: Extended telephone counseling for smoking cessation: does content matter? J Consult Clin Psychol 2003; 71:565–574 [A–]
754. Zhu SH, Stretch V, Balabanis M, Rosbrook B, Sadler G, Pierce JP: Telephone counseling for smoking cessation: effects of single-session and multiple-session interventions. J Consult Clin Psychol 1996; 64:202–211 [A–]
755. Hughes JR, Hatsukami DK: The nicotine withdrawal syndrome: a brief review and update. International Journal of Smoking Cessation 1992; 1:21–26 [F]
756. Piasecki TM, Niaura R, Shadel WG, Abrams D, Goldstein M, Fiore MC, Baker TB: Smoking withdrawal dynamics in unaided quitters. J Abnorm Psychol 2000; 109:74–86 [G]
757. Hughes JR, Higgins ST, Hatsukami DK: Effects of abstinence from tobacco: a critical review, in Research Advances in Alcohol and Drug Problems, vol. 10. Edited by Kozlowski LT, Annis HM, Cappell HD, Glaser FB, Goodstadt MS, Israel Y, Kalant H, Sellers EM, Vingilis ER. New York, Plenum, 1990, pp 317–398 [F]
758. Hughes JR: Dependence potential and abuse liability of nicotine replacement therapies. Biomed Pharmacother 1989; 43:11–17 [F]
759. Hatsukami D, Huber M, Callies A, Skoog K: Physical dependence on nicotine gum: effect of duration of use. Psychopharmacology (Berl) 1993; 111:449–456 [A]
760. Glassman AH: Cigarette smoking: implications for psychiatric illness. Am J Psychiatry 1993; 150:546–553 [F]
761. Glassman AH, Covey LS, Dalack GW, Stetner F, Rivelli SK, Fleiss J, Cooper TB: Smoking cessation, clonidine, and vulnerability to nicotine among dependent smokers. Clin Pharmacol Ther 1993; 54:670–679 [A]
762. Glassman AH, Helzer JE, Covey LS, Cottler LB, Stetner F, Tipp JE, Johnson J: Smoking, smoking cessation, and major depression. JAMA 1990; 264:1546–1549 [F]
763. Covey LS, Glassman AH, Stetner F: Major depression following smoking cessation. Am J Psychiatry 1997; 154:263–265 [B]
764. Tsoh JY, Humfleet GL, Munoz RF, Reus VI, Hartz DT, Hall SM: Development of major depression after treatment for smoking cessation. Am J Psychiatry 2000; 157:368–374 [C]
765. Niaura R, Britt DM, Shadel WG, Goldstein M, Abrams D, Brown R: Symptoms of depression and survival experience among three samples of smokers trying to quit. Psychol Addict Behav 2001; 15:13–17 [C]
766. Thorsteinsson HS, Gillin JC, Patten CA, Golshan S, Sutton LD, Drummond S, Clark CP, Kelsoe J, Rapaport M: The effects of transdermal nicotine therapy for smoking cessation on depressive symptoms in patients with major depression. Neuropsychopharmacology 2001; 24:350–358 [A]
767. Dalack GW, Becks L, Hill E, Pomerleau OF, Meador-Woodruff JH: Nicotine withdrawal and psychiatric symptoms in cigarette smokers with schizophrenia. Neuropsychopharmacology 1999; 21:195–202 [A]
768. Meyer JM: Individual changes in clozapine levels after smoking cessation: results and a predictive model. J Clin Psychopharmacol 2001; 21:569–574 [G]
769. Hughes JR, Oliveto AH: Coffee and alcohol intake as predictors of smoking cessation and tobacco withdrawal. J Subst Abuse 1993; 5:305–310 [C]

770. Giovino GA, Henningfield JE, Tomar SL, Escobedo LG, Slade J: Epidemiology of tobacco use and dependence. Epidemiol Rev 1995; 17:48–65 [F]
771. Klesges RC, Meyers AW, Klesges LM, La Vasque ME: Smoking, body weight, and their effects on smoking behavior: a comprehensive review of the literature. Psychol Bull 1989; 106:204–230 [F]
772. French SA, Jeffery RW: Weight concerns and smoking: a literature review. Ann Behav Med 1995; 17:234–244 [F]
773. Gritz ER, Klesges RC, Meyers AW: The smoking and body weight relationship: implications for intervention and post-cessation weight control. Ann Behav Med 1989; 11:144–153 [F]
774. Hall SM, Tunstall CD, Vila KL, Duffy J: Weight gain prevention and smoking cessation: cautionary findings. Am J Public Health 1992; 82:799–803 [A]
775. Pirie PL, McBride CM, Hellerstedt W, Jeffery RW, Hatsukami D, Allen S, Lando H: Smoking cessation in women concerned about weight. Am J Public Health 1992; 82:1238–1243 [A]
776. Perkins K: Issues in the prevention of weight gain after smoking cessation. Ann Behav Med 1994; 16:46–52 [F]
777. Shiffman SM: Relapse following smoking cessation: a situational analysis. J Consult Clin Psychol 1982; 50:71–86 [C]
778. Oliveto AH, Hughes JR, Terry SY, Bickel WK, Higgins ST, Pepper SL, Fenwick JW: Effects of caffeine on tobacco withdrawal. Clin Pharmacol Ther 1991; 50:157–164 [A]
779. Hughes JR: Caffeine withdrawal, dependence, and abuse, in DSM-IV Sourcebook. Edited by Widiger TA, Frances AJ, Pincus HA, First MB, Ross R, Davis W. Washington, DC, American Psychiatric Association, 1994, pp 129–134 [F]
780. Kenford SL, Fiore MC, Jorenby DE, Smith SS, Wetter D, Baker TB: Predicting smoking cessation: who will quit with and without the nicotine patch. JAMA 1994; 271: 589–594 [C]
781. Hall SM, Munoz RF, Reus VI, Sees KL: Nicotine, negative affect, and depression. J Consult Clin Psychol 1993; 61:761–767 [F]
782. Sutherland G, Russell MA, Stapleton J, Feyerabend C, Ferno O: Nasal nicotine spray: a rapid nicotine delivery system. Psychopharmacology (Berl) 1992; 108:512–518 [G]
782a. Croghan GA, Sloan JA, Croghan IT, Novotny P, Hurt RD, DeKrey WL, Mailliard JA, Ebbert LP, Swan DK, Walsh DJ, Wiesenfeld M, Levitt R, Stella P, Johnson PA, Tschetter LK, Loprinzi C: Comparison of nicotine patch alone versus nicotine nasal spray alone versus a combination for treating smokers: a minimal intervention, randomized multicenter trial in a nonspecialized setting. Nicotine Tob Res 2003; 5:181–187 [A–]
782b. Blondal T, Gudmundsson LJ, Olafsdottir I, Gustavsson G, Westin A: Nicotine nasal spray with nicotine patch for smoking cessation: randomised trial with six year follow up. BMJ 1999; 318(7179):285–288 [A]
783. Hughes JR: Combined psychological and nicotine gum treatment for smoking: a critical review. J Subst Abuse 1991; 3:337–350 [E]
784. Hughes JR: Combining behavioral therapy and pharmacotherapy for smoking cessation: an update, in Integrating Behavior Therapies With Medication in the Treatment of Drug Dependence. NIDA Research Monograph 150. Edited by Onken LS, Blaine JD, Boren JJ. Rockville, Md, National Institute on Drug Abuse, 1995, pp 92–109 [E]
785. He D, Medbo JI, Hostmark AT: Effect of acupuncture on smoking cessation or reduction: an 8-month and 5-year follow-up study. Prev Med 2001; 33:364–372 [A–]
786. Waite NR, Clough JB: A single-blind, placebo-controlled trial of a simple acupuncture treatment in the cessation of smoking. Br J Gen Pract 1998; 48:1487–1490 [A]

787. Ausfeld-Hafter B, Marti F, Hoffmann S: [Smoking cessation with ear acupuncture: descriptive study on patients after a smoking cessation treatment with ear acupuncture]. Forsch Komplementarmed Klass Naturheilkd 2004; 11:8–13 (German) [B]
788. White AR, Rampes H, Ernst E: Acupuncture for smoking cessation. Cochrane Database Syst Rev 2002; CD000009 [E]
789. West R, Shiffman S: Effect of oral nicotine dosing forms on cigarette withdrawal symptoms and craving: a systematic review. Psychopharmacology (Berl) 2001; 155:115–122 [E]
790. Silagy C, Lancaster T, Stead L, Mant D, Fowler G: Nicotine replacement therapy for smoking cessation. Cochrane Database Syst Rev 2004; CD000146 [E]
791. Munafo M, Bradburn M, Bowes L, David S: Are there sex differences in transdermal nicotine replacement therapy patch efficacy? a meta-analysis. Nicotine Tob Res 2004; 6:769–776 [E]
792. Cepeda-Benito A, Reynoso JT, Erath S: Meta-analysis of the efficacy of nicotine replacement therapy for smoking cessation: differences between men and women. J Consult Clin Psychol 2004; 72:712–722 [E]
793. Hughes JR, Shiffman S, Callas P, Zhang J: A meta-analysis of the efficacy of over-the-counter nicotine replacement. Tob Control 2003; 12:21–27 [E]
794. Hughes JR: An algorithm for smoking cessation. Arch Fam Med 1994; 3:280–285 [G]
795. Hughes J, Stead L, Lancaster T: Antidepressants for smoking cessation. Cochrane Database Syst Rev 2004; CD000031 [E]
796. West R, Hajek P, Foulds J, Nilsson F, May S, Meadows A: A comparison of the abuse liability and dependence potential of nicotine patch, gum, spray and inhaler. Psychopharmacology (Berl) 2000; 149:198–202 [G]
797. Shiffman S, Hughes JR, Pillitteri JL, Burton SL: Persistent use of nicotine replacement therapy: an analysis of actual purchase patterns in a population based sample. Tob Control 2003; 12:310–316 [C]
798. Fiore MC, Jorenby DE, Baker TB, Kenford SL: Tobacco dependence and the nicotine patch: clinical guidelines for effective use. JAMA 1992; 268:2687–2694 [F]
799. Palmer KJ, Buckley MM, Faulds D: Transdermal nicotine: a review of its pharmacodynamic and pharmacokinetic properties, and therapeutic efficacy as an aid to smoking cessation. Drugs 1992; 44:498–529 [F]
800. Hughes JR: Pharmacotherapy for smoking cessation: unvalidated assumptions, anomalies, and suggestions for future research. J Consult Clin Psychol 1993; 61:751–760 [E]
801. Hughes JR, Novy P, Hatsukami DK, Jensen J, Callas PW: Efficacy of nicotine patch in smokers with a history of alcoholism. Alcohol Clin Exp Res 2003; 27:946–954 [A]
802. Shiffman S, Dresler CM, Hajek P, Gilburt SJ, Targett DA, Strahs KR: Efficacy of a nicotine lozenge for smoking cessation. Arch Intern Med 2002; 162:1267–1276 [A]
803. Garvey AJ, Kinnunen T, Nordstrom BL, Utman CH, Doherty K, Rosner B, Vokonas PS: Effects of nicotine gum dose by level of nicotine dependence. Nicotine Tob Res 2000; 2:53–63 [A]
804. Hughes JR: Risk-benefit assessment of nicotine preparations in smoking cessation. Drug Saf 1993; 8:49–56 [F]
804a. Henningfield JE, Radzius A, Cooper TM, Clayton RR: Drinking coffee and carbonated beverages blocks absorption of nicotine from nicotine polacrilex gum. JAMA 1990; 264:1560–1564 [G]
805. Rose JE, Behm F: Refined cigarette smoke as a method for reducing nicotine intake. Pharmacol Biochem Behav 1987; 28:305–310 [A]
806. Tonnesen P, Norregaard J, Mikkelsen K, Jorgensen S, Nilsson F: A double-blind trial of a nicotine inhaler for smoking cessation. JAMA 1993; 269:1268–1271 [A]

807. Sutherland G, Stapleton JA, Russell MA, Jarvis MJ, Hajek P, Belcher M, Feyerabend C: Randomised controlled trial of nasal nicotine spray in smoking cessation. Lancet 1992; 340:324–329 [A]
808. Hjalmarson A, Franzon M, Westin A, Wiklund O: Effect of nicotine nasal spray on smoking cessation: a randomized, placebo-controlled, double-blind study. Arch Intern Med 1994; 154:2567–2572 [A]
809. Schneider NG, Olmstead R, Mody FV, Doan K, Franzon M, Jarvik ME, Steinberg C: Efficacy of a nicotine nasal spray in smoking cessation: a placebo-controlled, double-blind trial. Addiction 1995; 90:1671–1682 [A]
810. Leischow SJ: Nicotine vaporiser: review of results, in Future Directions in Nicotine Replacement Therapy. Chester, UK, Adis, 1994, pp 99–103 [F]
811. Perkins KA, Grobe JE, Caggiula A, Wilson AS, Stiller RL: Acute reinforcing effects of low-dose nicotine nasal spray in humans. Pharmacol Biochem Behav 1997; 56:235–241 [G]
812. Richmond R, Zwar N: Review of bupropion for smoking cessation. Drug Alcohol Rev 2003; 22:203–220 [F]
813. Scharf D, Shiffman S: Are there gender differences in smoking cessation, with and without bupropion? pooled- and meta-analyses of clinical trials of bupropion SR. Addiction 2004; 99:1462–1469 [E]
814. Wagena EJ, Knipschild P, Zeegers MP: Should nortriptyline be used as a first-line aid to help smokers quit? results from a systematic review and meta-analysis. Addiction 2005; 100:317–326 [E]
815. Prochazka AV, Weaver MJ, Keller RT, Fryer GE, Licari PA, Lofaso D: A randomized trial of nortriptyline for smoking cessation. Arch Intern Med 1998; 158:2035–2039 [A]
816. Hughes JR, Stead LF, Lancaster T: Nortriptyline for smoking cessation: a review. Nicotine Tob Res 2005; 7:491–499 [E]
817. Baldessarini RJ: Drug therapy of depression and anxiety disorders, in Goodman and Gilman's The Pharmacological Basis of Therapeutics, 11th ed. Edited by Brunton LL, Lazo JS, Parker KL. New York, McGraw-Hill, 2006, pp 429–459 [G]
818. Gourlay SG, Stead LF, Benowitz NL: Clonidine for smoking cessation. Cochrane Database Syst Rev 2004; CD000058 [E]
819. Westfall TC, Westfall DP: Adrenergic agonists and antagonists, in Goodman and Gilman's The Pharmacological Basis of Therapeutics, 11th ed. Edited by Brunton LL, Lazo JS, Parker KL. New York, McGraw-Hill, 2006, pp 237–315 [G]
820. Stolerman IP, Goldfarb T, Fink R, Jarvik ME: Influencing cigarette smoking with nicotine antagonists. Psychopharmacologia 1973; 28:247–259 [F]
821. Clarke PB: Nicotinic receptor blockade therapy and smoking cessation. Br J Addict 1991; 86:501–505 [F]
822. Wong GY, Wolter TD, Croghan GA, Croghan IT, Offord KP, Hurt RD: A randomized trial of naltrexone for smoking cessation. Addiction 1999; 94:1227–1237 [A–]
823. Hughes JR, Stead LF, Lancaster T: Anxiolytics for smoking cessation. Cochrane Database Syst Rev 2000; CD002849 [E]
824. Stead LF, Lancaster T: Group behaviour therapy programmes for smoking cessation. Cochrane Database Syst Rev 2005; CD001007 [E]
825. Lancaster T, Stead LF: Individual behavioural counselling for smoking cessation. Cochrane Database Syst Rev 2005; CD001292 [E]
826. The Tobacco Use and Dependence Clinical Practice Guideline Panel, Staff, and Consortium Representatives: A clinical practice guideline for treating tobacco use and dependence: a US Public Health Service report. JAMA 2000; 283:3244–3254 [G]
827. Fiore MC: US public health service clinical practice guideline: treating tobacco use and dependence. Respir Care 2000; 45:1200–1262 [E]

828. Miller M, Wood L: Effectiveness of smoking cessation interventions: review of evidence and implications for best practice in Australian health care settings. Aust N Z J Public Health 2003; 27:300–309 [E]
829. Roski J, Schmid LA, Lando HA: Long-term associations of helpful and harmful spousal behaviors with smoking cessation. Addict Behav 1996; 21:173–185 [C]
830. May S, West R: Do social support interventions ("buddy systems") aid smoking cessation? a review. Tob Control 2000; 9:415–422 [F]
831. Murray RP, Johnston JJ, Dolce JJ, Lee WW, O'Hara P: Social support for smoking cessation and abstinence: the Lung Health Study. Lung Health Study Research Group. Addict Behav 1995; 20:159–170 [B]
832. Gruder CL, Mermelstein RJ, Kirkendol S, Hedeker D, Wong SC, Schreckengost J, Warnecke RB, Burzette R, Miller TQ: Effects of social support and relapse prevention training as adjuncts to a televised smoking-cessation intervention. J Consult Clin Psychol 1993; 61:113–120 [A–]
833. West R, Edwards M, Hajek P: Randomized controlled trial of a "buddy" system to improve success at giving up smoking in general practice. Addiction 1998; 93:1007–1011 [A–]
834. Stotts AL, DeLaune KA, Schmitz JM, Grabowski J: Impact of a motivational intervention on mechanisms of change in low-income pregnant smokers. Addict Behav 2004; 29:1649–1657 [B]
835. Cornuz J, Humair JP, Seematter L, Stoianov R, van Melle G, Stalder H, Pecoud A: Efficacy of resident training in smoking cessation: a randomized, controlled trial of a program based on application of behavioral theory and practice with standardized patients. Ann Intern Med 2002; 136:429–437 [A–]
836. Rigotti NA, Arnsten JH, McKool KM, Wood-Reid KM, Pasternak RC, Singer DE: Efficacy of a smoking cessation program for hospital patients. Arch Intern Med 1997; 157:2653–2660 [A–]
837. Dornelas EA, Sampson RA, Gray JF, Waters D, Thompson PD: A randomized controlled trial of smoking cessation counseling after myocardial infarction. Prev Med 2000; 30:261–268 [A–]
838. Viswesvaran C, Schmidt FL: A meta-analytic comparison of the effectiveness of smoking cessation methods. J Appl Psychol 1992; 77:554–561 [E]
839. Simon JA, Carmody TP, Hudes ES, Snyder E, Murray J: Intensive smoking cessation counseling versus minimal counseling among hospitalized smokers treated with transdermal nicotine replacement: a randomized trial. Am J Med 2003; 114:555–562 [A–]
840. Perkins KA, Marcus MD, Levine MD, D'Amico D, Miller A, Broge M, Ashcom J, Shiffman S: Cognitive-behavioral therapy to reduce weight concerns improves smoking cessation outcome in weight-concerned women. J Consult Clin Psychol 2001; 69:604–613 [A–]
841. Patten CA, Martin JE, Myers MG, Calfas KJ, Williams CD: Effectiveness of cognitive-behavioral therapy for smokers with histories of alcohol dependence and depression. J Stud Alcohol 1998; 59:327–335 [A]
842. Garcia MP, Becona E: Evaluation of the amount of therapist contact in a smoking cessation program. Span J Psychol 2000; 3:28–36 [B]
843. Alterman AI, Gariti P, Mulvaney F: Short- and long-term smoking cessation for three levels of intensity of behavioral treatment. Psychol Addict Behav 2001; 15:261–264 [A–]
844. Burling TA, Burling AS, Latini D: A controlled smoking cessation trial for substance-dependent inpatients. J Consult Clin Psychol 2001; 69:295–304 [A–]
845. Bakkevig O, Steine S, von Hafenbradl K, Laerum E: Smoking cessation: a comparative, randomised study between management in general practice and the behavioural programme SmokEnders. Scand J Prim Health Care 2000; 18:247–251 [A–]

846. Curry SJ, McBride C, Grothaus LC, Louie D, Wagner EH: A randomized trial of self-help materials, personalized feedback, and telephone counseling with nonvolunteer smokers. J Consult Clin Psychol 1995; 63:1005–1014 [A–]
847. Borland R, Segan CJ, Livingston PM, Owen N: The effectiveness of callback counselling for smoking cessation: a randomized trial. Addiction 2001; 96:881–889 [A–]
848. Dijkstra A, De Vries H, Roijackers J: Targeting smokers with low readiness to change with tailored and nontailored self-help materials. Prev Med 1999; 28:203–211 [A–]
849. Etter JF, Perneger TV: Effectiveness of a computer-tailored smoking cessation program: a randomized trial. Arch Intern Med 2001; 161:2596–2601 [A–]
850. Strecher VJ, Shiffman S, West R: Randomized controlled trial of a web-based computer-tailored smoking cessation program as a supplement to nicotine patch therapy. Addiction 2005; 100:682–688 [A–]
851. Lancaster T, Stead LF: Self-help interventions for smoking cessation. Cochrane Database Syst Rev 2002; CD001118 [E]
852. Shiffman S, Paty JA, Rohay JM, Di Marino ME, Gitchell J: The efficacy of computer-tailored smoking cessation material as a supplement to nicotine polacrilex gum therapy. Arch Intern Med 2000; 160:1675–1681 [A–]
853. Shiffman S, Paty JA, Rohay JM, Di Marino ME, Gitchell JG: The efficacy of computer-tailored smoking cessation material as a supplement to nicotine patch therapy. Drug Alcohol Depend 2001; 64:35–46 [A–]
854. Reid RD, Pipe A, Dafoe WA: Is telephone counselling a useful addition to physician advice and nicotine replacement therapy in helping patients to stop smoking? a randomized controlled trial. CMAJ 1999; 160:1577–1581 [A–]
855. Hajek P, Taylor TZ, Mills P: Brief intervention during hospital admission to help patients to give up smoking after myocardial infarction and bypass surgery: randomised controlled trial. BMJ 2002; 324:87–89 [A–]
856. Gould RA, Clum GA: A meta-analysis of self-help treatment approaches. Clin Psychol Rev 1993; 13:169–186 [E]
857. Lichtenstein E, Glasgow RE, Lando HA, Ossip-Klein DJ, Boles SM: Telephone counseling for smoking cessation: rationales and meta-analytic review of evidence. Health Educ Res 1996; 11:243–257 [F]
858. Orleans CT, Schoenbach VJ, Wagner EH, Quade D, Salmon MA, Pearson DC, Fiedler J, Porter CQ, Kaplan BH: Self-help quit smoking interventions: effects of self-help materials, social support instructions, and telephone counseling. J Consult Clin Psychol 1991; 59:439–448 [A]
859. Curry SJ: Self-help interventions for smoking cessation. J Consult Clin Psychol 1993; 61:790–803 [F]
860. Strecher VJ, Kreuter M, Den Boer DJ, Kobrin S, Hospers HJ, Skinner CS: The effects of computer-tailored smoking cessation messages in family practice settings. J Fam Pract 1994; 39:262–270 [A]
861. Marcus BH, Albrecht AE, Niaura RS, Abrams DB, Thompson PD: Usefulness of physical exercise for maintaining smoking cessation in women. Am J Cardiol 1991; 68:406–407 [A]
862. Marcus BH, Albrecht AE, Niaura RS, Taylor ER, Simkin LR, Feder SI, Abrams DB, Thompson PD: Exercise enhances the maintenance of smoking cessation in women. Addict Behav 1995; 20:87–92 [A]
863. Ussher M, West R, McEwen A, Taylor A, Steptoe A: Efficacy of exercise counselling as an aid for smoking cessation: a randomized controlled trial. Addiction 2003; 98:523–532 [A–]
864. Ussher M: Exercise interventions for smoking cessation. Cochrane Database Syst Rev 2005; CD002295 [E]

865. Prochaska JJ, Gill P, Hall SM: Treatment of tobacco use in an inpatient psychiatric setting. Psychiatr Serv 2004; 55:1265–1270 [G]
866. Resnick MP: Treating nicotine addiction in patients with psychiatric co-morbidity, in Nicotine Addiction: Principles and Management. Edited by Orleans CT, Slade J. New York, Oxford University Press, 1993, pp 327–336 [F]
867. el Guebaly N, Cathcart J, Currie S, Brown D, Gloster S: Public health and therapeutic aspects of smoking bans in mental health and addiction settings. Psychiatr Serv 2002; 53:1617–1622 [F]
868. Haller E, McNiel DE, Binder RL: Impact of a smoking ban on a locked psychiatric unit. J Clin Psychiatry 1996; 57:329–332 [G]
869. Taylor NE, Rosenthal RN, Chabus B, Levine S, Hoffman AS, Reynolds J, Santos L, Willets I, Friedman P: The feasibility of smoking bans on psychiatric units. Gen Hosp Psychiatry 1993; 15:36–40 [G]
870. Thorward SR, Birnbaum S: Effects of a smoking ban on a general hospital psychiatric unit. Gen Hosp Psychiatry 1989; 11:63–67 [G]
871. Greeman M, McClellan TA: Negative effects of a smoking ban on an inpatient psychiatry service. Hosp Community Psychiatry 1991; 42:408–412 [G]
872. Hughes JR: Smoking and alcoholism, in Behavioral Approaches to Addiction. Edited by Cox J, Hatsukami DK. New York, Cahners Healthcare Communications, 1994, pp 1–3 [G]
873. Hughes JR: Possible effects of smoke-free inpatient units on psychiatric diagnosis and treatment. J Clin Psychiatry 1993; 54:109–114 [F]
874. Haring C, Barnas C, Saria A, Humpel C, Fleischhacker WW: Dose-related plasma levels of clozapine. J Clin Psychopharmacol 1989; 9:71–72 [G]
875. Rigotti NA, Munafo MR, Murphy MF, Stead LF: Interventions for smoking cessation in hospitalised patients. Cochrane Database Syst Rev 2003; CD001837 [E]
876. Working Group for the Study of Transdermal Nicotine in Patients with Coronary Artery Disease: Nicotine replacement therapy for patients with coronary artery disease. Arch Intern Med 1994; 154:989–995 [A]
877. Fagerström KO, Hughes JR: Nicotine concentrations with concurrent use of cigarettes and nicotine replacement: a review. Nicotine Tob Res 2002; 4(suppl 2):S73–S79 [F]
878. Stahl MM, Wohlfart B, Pahlm O: Tolerability of concurrent use of nicotine gum and smoking in healthy volunteers. Nicotine Tob Res 2001; 3:157–165 [A–]
879. Hughes JR, Pillitteri JL, Callas PW, Callahan R, Kenny M: Misuse of and dependence on over-the-counter nicotine gum in a volunteer sample. Nicotine Tob Res 2004; 6:79–84 [G]
880. Benowitz NL, Zevin S, Jacob P III: Suppression of nicotine intake during ad libitum cigarette smoking by high-dose transdermal nicotine. J Pharmacol Exp Ther 1998; 287: 958–962 [G]
881. Shiffman S, Hughes JR, Di Marino ME, Sweeney CT: Patterns of over-the-counter nicotine gum use: persistent use and concurrent smoking. Addiction 2003; 98:1747–1753 [G]
882. McChargue DE, Gulliver SB, Hitsman B: "Would" smokers with schizophrenia benefit from a more flexible approach to smoking treatment?" Addiction 2001; 97:785–793 [E]
883. Hall SM, Munoz RF, Reus VI, Sees KL, Duncan C, Humfleet GL, Hartz DT: Mood management and nicotine gum in smoking treatment: a therapeutic contact and placebo-controlled study. J Consult Clin Psychol 1996; 64:1003–1009 [A]
884. Williams JM, Ziedonis DM, Foulds J: A case series of nicotine nasal spray in the treatment of tobacco dependence among patients with schizophrenia. Psychiatr Serv 2004; 55:1064–1066 [B]

885. Olincy A, Young DA, Freedman R: Increased levels of the nicotine metabolite cotinine in schizophrenic smokers compared to other smokers. Biol Psychiatry 1997; 42:1–5 [G]
886. Hughes JR, Goldstein MG, Hurt RD, Shiffman S: Recent advances in the pharmacotherapy of smoking. JAMA 1999; 281:72–76 [F]
887. Fagerström K: Combined use of nicotine replacement products. Health Values 1994; 18:15–20 [F]
888. Kornitzer M, Boutsen M, Dramaix M, Thijs J, Gustavsson G: Combined use of nicotine patch and gum in smoking cessation: a placebo-controlled clinical trial. Prev Med 1995; 24:41–47 [A]
889. George TP, Vessicchio JC: Nicotine addiction and schizophrenia. Psychiatric Times 2001; 18:39–42 [G]
890. George TP, Vessicchio JC: Treating tobacco addiction in schizophrenia: where do we go from here? Addiction 2002; 97:795–796 [G]
891. Steinberg ML, Ziedonis DM, Krejci JA, Brandon TH: Motivational interviewing with personalized feedback: a brief intervention for motivating smokers with schizophrenia to seek treatment for tobacco dependence. J Consult Clin Psychol 2004; 72:723–728 [A–]
892. Covey LS, Sullivan MA, Johnston JA, Glassman AH, Robinson MD, Adams DP: Advances in non-nicotine pharmacotherapy for smoking cessation. Drugs 2000; 59:17–31 [E]
893. Haas AL, Munoz RF, Humfleet GL, Reus VI, Hall SM: Influences of mood, depression history, and treatment modality on outcomes in smoking cessation. J Consult Clin Psychol 2004; 72:563–570 [A–]
894. Hitsman B, Borrelli B, McChargue DE, Spring B, Niaura R: History of depression and smoking cessation outcome: a meta-analysis. J Consult Clin Psychol 2003; 71:657–663 [E]
895. Hall SM, Humfleet GL, Reus VI, Munoz RF, Cullen J: Extended nortriptyline and psychological treatment for cigarette smoking. Am J Psychiatry 2004; 161:2100–2107 [A–]
896. Centers for Disease Control and Prevention: Cigarette smoking among adults: United States, 2001. MMWR Morb Mortal Wkly Rep 2003; 52:953–956 [G]
897. Centers for Disease Control and Prevention, National Center for Chronic Disease Prevention and Health Promotion, Office on Smoking and Health: The Health Consequences of Smoking: A Report of the Surgeon General. Washington, DC, US Government Printing Office, 2004 [G]
898. Centers for Disease Control and Prevention: Annual smoking-attributable mortality, years of potential life lost, and economic costs: United States, 1995–1999. MMWR Morb Mortal Wkly Rep 2002; 51:300–303 [G]
899. Marder SR, Essock SM, Miller AL, Buchanan RW, Casey DE, Davis JM, Kane JM, Lieberman JA, Schooler NR, Covell N, Stroup S, Weissman EM, Wirshing DA, Hall CS, Pogach L, Pi-Sunyer X, Bigger JT Jr, Friedman A, Kleinberg D, Yevich SJ, Davis B, Shon S: Physical health monitoring of patients with schizophrenia. Am J Psychiatry 2004; 161:1334–1349 [G]
900. US Department of Health and Human Services: Report on Carcinogens, 9th ed. Public Health Service, National Toxicology Program, 2000 [G]
901. Peto R, Lopez AD, Boreham J, Thun M, Heath C Jr: Mortality from tobacco in developed countries: indirect estimation from national vital statistics. Lancet 1992; 339: 1268–1278 [G]
902. Anthonisen NR, Skeans MA, Wise RA, Manfreda J, Kanner RE, Connett JE: The effects of a smoking cessation intervention on 14.5-year mortality: a randomized clinical trial. Ann Intern Med 2005; 142:233–239 [C]

903. Critchley J, Capewell S: Smoking cessation for the secondary prevention of coronary heart disease. Cochrane Database Syst Rev 2004; CD003041 [E]
904. Scanlon PD, Connett JE, Waller LA, Altose MD, Bailey WC, Buist AS: Smoking cessation and lung function in mild-to-moderate chronic obstructive pulmonary disease: the Lung Health Study. Am J Respir Crit Care Med 2000; 161:381–390 [A–]
905. Kanner RE, Connett JE, Williams DE, Buist AS: Effects of randomized assignment to a smoking cessation intervention and changes in smoking habits on respiratory symptoms in smokers with early chronic obstructive pulmonary disease: the Lung Health Study. Am J Med 1999; 106:410–416 [A–]
906. Peters RW, Brooks MM, Todd L, Liebson PR, Wilhelmsen L: Smoking cessation and arrhythmic death: the CAST experience. The Cardiac Arrhythmia Suppression Trial (CAST) Investigators. J Am Coll Cardiol 1995; 26:1287–1292 [C]
907. van der Meer RM, Wagena EJ, Ostelo RW, Jacobs JE, van Schayck CP: Smoking cessation for chronic obstructive pulmonary disease. Cochrane Database Syst Rev 2003; CD002999 [E]
908. Wagena EJ, van der Meer RM, Ostelo RJ, Jacobs JE, van Schayck CP: The efficacy of smoking cessation strategies in people with chronic obstructive pulmonary disease: results from a systematic review. Respir Med 2004; 98:805–815 [E]
909. Wennike P, Danielsson T, Landfeldt B, Westin A, Tonnesen P: Smoking reduction promotes smoking cessation: results from a double blind, randomized, placebo-controlled trial of nicotine gum with 2-year follow-up. Addiction 2003; 98:1395–1402 [A]
910. Lewis SF, Piasecki TM, Fiore MC, Anderson JE, Baker TB: Transdermal nicotine replacement for hospitalized patients: a randomized clinical trial. Prev Med 1998; 27:296–303 [A–]
911. Wolfenden L, Campbell E, Walsh R, Wiggers J: Smoking cessation interventions for in-patients: a selective review with recommendations for hospital-based health professionals. Drug Alcohol Rev 2003; 22:437–452 [F]
912. Molyneux A, Lewis S, Leivers U, Anderton A, Antoniak M, Brackenridge A, Nilsson F, McNeill A, West R, Moxham J, Britton J: Clinical trial comparing nicotine replacement therapy (NRT) plus brief counselling, brief counselling alone, and minimal intervention on smoking cessation in hospital inpatients. Thorax 2003; 58:484–488 [A–]
913. Tzivoni D, Keren A, Meyler S, Khoury Z, Lerer T, Brunel P: Cardiovascular safety of transdermal nicotine patches in patients with coronary artery disease who try to quit smoking. Cardiovasc Drugs Ther 1998; 12:239–244 [A]
914. Murray RP, Bailey WC, Daniels K, Bjornson WM, Kurnow K, Connett JE, Nides MA, Kiley JP: Safety of nicotine polacrilex gum used by 3,094 participants in the Lung Health Study. Lung Health Study Research Group. Chest 1996; 109:438–445 [C]
915. Benowitz NL, Gourlay SG: Cardiovascular toxicity of nicotine: implications for nicotine replacement therapy. J Am Coll Cardiol 1997; 29:1422–1431 [F]
916. Joseph AM, Norman SM, Ferry LH, Prochazka AV, Westman EC, Steele BG, Sherman SE, Cleveland M, Antonnucio DO, Hartman N, McGovern PG: The safety of transdermal nicotine as an aid to smoking cessation in patients with cardiac disease. N Engl J Med 1996; 335:1792–1798 [A]
917. Tonstad S, Farsang C, Klaene G, Lewis K, Manolis A, Perruchoud AP, Silagy C, van Spiegel PI, Astbury C, Hider A, Sweet R: Bupropion SR for smoking cessation in smokers with cardiovascular disease: a multicentre, randomised study. Eur Heart J 2003; 24:946–955 [A]
918. Tashkin D, Kanner R, Bailey W, Buist S, Anderson P, Nides M, Gonzales D, Dozier G, Patel MK, Jamerson B: Smoking cessation in patients with chronic obstructive pulmonary disease: a double-blind, placebo-controlled, randomised trial. Lancet 2001; 357: 1571–1575 [A]

919. Quist-Paulsen P, Gallefoss F: Randomised controlled trial of smoking cessation intervention after admission for coronary heart disease. BMJ 2003; 327:1254–1257 [A–]
920. Munafo M, Rigotti N, Lancaster T, Stead L, Murphy M: Interventions for smoking cessation in hospitalised patients: a systematic review. Thorax 2001; 56:656–663 [E]
921. Miller NH, Smith PM, DeBusk RF, Sobel DS, Taylor CB: Smoking cessation in hospitalized patients: results of a randomized trial. Arch Intern Med 1997; 157:409–415 [A–]
922. Benowitz N, Dempsey D: Pharmacotherapy for smoking cessation during pregnancy. Nicotine Tob Res 2004; 6(suppl 2):S189–S202 [F]
923. Cnattingius S: The epidemiology of smoking during pregnancy: smoking prevalence, maternal characteristics, and pregnancy outcomes. Nicotine Tob Res 2004; 6(suppl 2): S125–S140 [F]
924. DiFranza JR, Aligne CA, Weitzman M: Prenatal and postnatal environmental tobacco smoke exposure and children's health. Pediatrics 2004; 113:1007–1015 [F]
925. Little J, Cardy A, Munger RG: Tobacco smoking and oral clefts: a meta-analysis. Bull World Health Organ 2004; 82:213–218 [E]
926. Windsor R: Smoking cessation or reduction in pregnancy treatment methods: a meta-evaluation of the impact of dissemination. Am J Med Sci 2003; 326:216–222 [F]
927. Shah NR, Bracken MB: A systematic review and meta-analysis of prospective studies on the association between maternal cigarette smoking and preterm delivery. Am J Obstet Gynecol 2000; 182:465–472 [E]
928. Hofhuis W, de Jongste JC, Merkus PJ: Adverse health effects of prenatal and postnatal tobacco smoke exposure on children. Arch Dis Child 2003; 88:1086–1090 [F]
929. Mullen PD: How can more smoking suspension during pregnancy become lifelong abstinence? lessons learned about predictors, interventions, and gaps in our accumulated knowledge. Nicotine Tob Res 2004; 6(suppl 2):S217–S238 [F]
930. Dempsey DA, Benowitz NL: Risks and benefits of nicotine to aid smoking cessation in pregnancy. Drug Saf 2001; 24:277–322 [A]
931. Tuthill DP, Stewart JH, Coles EC, Andrews J, Cartlidge PH: Maternal cigarette smoking and pregnancy outcome. Paediatr Perinat Epidemiol 1999; 13:245–253 [D]
932. MacArthur C, Knox EG, Lancashire RJ: Effects at age nine of maternal smoking in pregnancy: experimental and observational findings. BJOG 2001; 108:67–73 [A–]
933. Cope GF, Nayyar P, Holder R: Feedback from a point-of-care test for nicotine intake to reduce smoking during pregnancy. Ann Clin Biochem 2003; 40:674–679 [A]
934. England LJ, Kendrick JS, Wilson HG, Merritt RK, Gargiullo PM, Zahniser SC: Effects of smoking reduction during pregnancy on the birth weight of term infants. Am J Epidemiol 2001; 154:694–701 [C]
935. Li CQ, Windsor RA, Perkins L, Goldenberg RL, Lowe JB: The impact on infant birth weight and gestational age of cotinine-validated smoking reduction during pregnancy. JAMA 1993; 269:1519–1524 [A–]
936. Lumley J, Oliver SS, Chamberlain C, Oakley L: Interventions for promoting smoking cessation during pregnancy. Cochrane Database Syst Rev 2004; CD001055 [E]
937. Windsor RA, Woodby LL, Miller TM, Hardin JM, Crawford MA, DiClemente CC: Effectiveness of Agency for Health Care Policy and Research clinical practice guideline and patient education methods for pregnant smokers in Medicaid maternity care. Am J Obstet Gynecol 2000; 182:68–75 [A–]
938. Oncken CA, Kranzler HR: Pharmacotherapies to enhance smoking cessation during pregnancy. Drug Alcohol Rev 2003; 22:191–202 [G]
939. Melvin C, Gaffney C: Treating nicotine use and dependence of pregnant and parenting smokers: an update. Nicotine Tob Res 2004; 6(suppl 2):S107–S124 [F]

940. Hegaard HK, Kjaergaard H, Moller LF, Wachmann H, Ottesen B: Multimodal intervention raises smoking cessation rate during pregnancy. Acta Obstet Gynecol Scand 2003; 82:813–819 [A–]
941. Wisborg K, Henriksen TB, Jespersen LB, Secher NJ: Nicotine patches for pregnant smokers: a randomized controlled study. Obstet Gynecol 2000; 96:967–971 [A]
942. Herbert R, Coleman T, Britton J: UK general practitioners' beliefs, attitudes, and reported prescribing of nicotine replacement therapy in pregnancy. Nicotine Tob Res 2005; 7:541–546 [G]
943. Oncken CA, Pbert L, Ockene JK, Zapka J, Stoddard A: Nicotine replacement prescription practices of obstetric and pediatric clinicians. Obstet Gynecol 2000; 96:261–265 [G]
944. Ratner PA, Johnson JL, Bottorff JL, Dahinten S, Hall W: Twelve-month follow-up of a smoking relapse prevention intervention for postpartum women. Addict Behav 2000; 25:81–92 [A–]
945. Mullen PD, Richardson MA, Quinn VP, Ershoff DH: Postpartum return to smoking: who is at risk and when. Am J Health Promot 1997; 11:323–330 [C]
946. Kessler RC, Chiu WT, Demler O, Merikangas KR, Walters EE: Prevalence, severity, and comorbidity of 12-month DSM-IV disorders in the National Comorbidity Survey Replication. Arch Gen Psychiatry 2005; 62:617–627 [G]
947. Kessler RC, Berglund P, Demler O, Jin R, Merikangas KR, Walters EE: Lifetime prevalence and age-of-onset distributions of DSM-IV disorders in the National Comorbidity Survey Replication. Arch Gen Psychiatry 2005; 62:593–602 [G]
948. Li TK, Hewitt BG, Grant BF: Alcohol use disorders and mood disorders: a National Institute on Alcohol Abuse and Alcoholism perspective. Biol Psychiatry 2004; 56:718–720 [G]
949. Sobell LC, Cunningham JA, Sobell MB: Recovery from alcohol problems with and without treatment: prevalence in two population surveys. Am J Public Health 1996; 86:966–972 [G]
950. Hasin DS, Grant B, Endicott J: The natural history of alcohol abuse: implications for definitions of alcohol use disorders. Am J Psychiatry 1990; 147:1537–1541 [C]
951. Rosenberg H: Prediction of controlled drinking by alcoholics and problem drinkers. Psychol Bull 1993; 113:129–139 [F]
952. Baer JS, Marlatt GA, Kivlahan DR, Fromme K, Larimer ME, Williams E: An experimental test of three methods of alcohol risk reduction with young adults. J Consult Clin Psychol 1992; 60:974–979 [A–]
953. Kivlahan DR, Marlatt GA, Fromme K, Coppel DB, Williams E: Secondary prevention with college drinkers: evaluation of an alcohol skills training program. J Consult Clin Psychol 1990; 58:805–810 [A–]
954. Kiefer F, Jahn H, Tarnaske T, Helwig H, Briken P, Holzbach R, Kampf P, Stracke R, Baehr M, Naber D, Wiedemann K: Comparing and combining naltrexone and acamprosate in relapse prevention of alcoholism: a double-blind, placebo-controlled study. Arch Gen Psychiatry 2003; 60:92–99 [A]
955. Balldin J, Berglund M, Borg S, Mansson M, Bendtsen P, Franck J, Gustafsson L, Halldin J, Nilsson LH, Stolt G, Willander A: A 6-month controlled naltrexone study: combined effect with cognitive behavioral therapy in outpatient treatment of alcohol dependence. Alcohol Clin Exp Res 2003; 27:1142–1149 [A]
956. Miller WR, Hester RK: Inpatient alcoholism treatment: who benefits? Am Psychol 1986; 41:794–805 [G]
957. National Institute of Medicine: Patient-treatment matching and outcome improvement in alcohol rehabilitation, in Prevention and Treatment of Alcohol Problems: Research Opportunities. Washington, DC, National Academies Press, 1990, pp 231–246 [G]

958. McKay JR, Murphy R, Longabaugh R: The effectiveness of alcoholism treatment: evidence from outcome studies, in Psychiatric Treatment: Advances in Outcome Research. Edited by Mirin SM, Gossett JT, Grob MC. Washington, DC, American Psychiatric Press, 1991, pp 143–158 [F]
959. Moos RH, Finney JW, Cronkite RC: Alcoholism Treatment: Context, Process, and Outcome. New York, Oxford University Press, 1990 [F]
960. McCrady BS, Noel NE, Abrams DB, Stout RL, Nelson HF, Hay WM: Comparative effectiveness of three types of spouse involvement in outpatient behavioral alcoholism treatment. J Stud Alcohol 1986; 47:459–467 [B]
961. O'Farrell TJ, Cutter HS, Floyd FJ: Evaluating behavioral marital therapy for male alcoholics: effects on marital adjustment and communication from before to after treatment. Behavior Therapy 1985; 16:147–167 [A]
962. Maisto SA, McKay JR, O'Farrell TJ: Twelve-month abstinence from alcohol and long-term drinking and marital outcomes in men with severe alcohol problems. J Stud Alcohol 1998; 59:591–598 [C]
963. O'Farrell TJ, Murphy CM, Stephan SH, Fals-Stewart W, Murphy M: Partner violence before and after couples-based alcoholism treatment for male alcoholic patients: the role of treatment involvement and abstinence. J Consult Clin Psychol 2004; 72:202–217 [B]
964. Miller WR: Motivation for treatment: a review with special emphasis on alcoholism. Psychol Bull 1985; 98:84–107 [F]
965. Magura S, Staines G, Kosanke N, Rosenblum A, Foote J, DeLuca A, Bali P: Predictive validity of the ASAM Patient Placement Criteria for naturalistically matched vs mismatched alcoholism patients. Am J Addict 2003; 12:386–397 [C]
966. Rychtarik RG, Connors GJ, Whitney RB, McGillicuddy NB, Fitterling JM, Wirtz PW: Treatment settings for persons with alcoholism: evidence for matching clients to inpatient versus outpatient care. J Consult Clin Psychol 2000; 68:277–289 [A–]
967. Fiellin DA, Reid MC, O'Connor PG: Outpatient management of patients with alcohol problems. Ann Intern Med 2000; 133:815–827 [G]
968. Gallant D: Alcohol, in The American Psychiatric Press Textbook of Substance Abuse Treatment, 2nd ed. Edited by Galanter M, Kleber H. Washington, DC, American Psychiatric Press, 1999, pp 151–164 [G]
969. DeBellis R, Smith BS, Choi S, Malloy M: Management of delirium tremens. J Intensive Care Med 2005; 20:164–173 [F]
970. Trevisan LA, Boutros N, Petrakis IL, Krystal JH: Complications of alcohol withdrawal: pathophysiological insights. Alcohol Health Res World 1998; 22:61–66 [F]
971. Erwin WE, Williams DB, Speir WA: Delirium tremens. South Med J 1998; 91:425–432 [F]
972. Ciraulo DA, Shader RI: Clinical Manual of Chemical Dependence. Washington, DC, American Psychiatric Press, 1991 [F]
973. Shaw GK, Waller S, Latham CJ, Dunn G, Thomson AD: The detoxification experience of alcoholic in-patients and predictors of outcome. Alcohol Alcohol 1998; 33:291–303 [G]
974. Ferguson JA, Suelzer CJ, Eckert GJ, Zhou XH, Dittus RS: Risk factors for delirium tremens development. J Gen Intern Med 1996; 11:410–414 [G]
975. Schuckit MA, Tipp JE, Reich T, Hesselbrock VM, Bucholz KK: The histories of withdrawal convulsions and delirium tremens in 1,648 alcohol dependent subjects. Addiction 1995; 90:1335–1347 [D]
976. Feuerlein W, Kufner H, Flohrschutz T: Mortality in alcoholic patients given inpatient treatment. Addiction 1994; 89:841–849 [G]
977. Malcolm R, Myrick H, Roberts J, Wang W, Anton RF, Ballenger JC: The effects of carbamazepine and lorazepam on single versus multiple previous alcohol withdrawals in an outpatient randomized trial. J Gen Intern Med 2002; 17:349–355 [A]

978. Sullivan JT, Sykora K, Schneiderman J, Naranjo CA, Sellers EM: Assessment of alcohol withdrawal: the revised Clinical Institute Withdrawal Assessment for Alcohol Scale (CIWA-Ar). Br J Addict 1989; 84:1353–1357 [G]
979. Kraemer KL, Mayo-Smith MF, Calkins DR: Independent clinical correlates of severe alcohol withdrawal. Subst Abuse 2003; 24:197–209 [G]
980. Whitfield CL, Thompson G, Lamb A, Spencer V, Pfeifer M, Browning-Ferrando M: Detoxification of 1,024 alcoholic patients without psychoactive drugs. JAMA 1978; 239:1409–1410 [G]
981. Shaw JM, Kolesar GS, Sellers EM, Kaplan HL, Sandor P: Development of optimal treatment tactics for alcohol withdrawal, I: assessment and effectiveness of supportive care. J Clin Psychopharmacol 1981; 1:382–387 [C]
982. Naranjo CA, Sellers EM, Chater K, Iversen P, Roach C, Sykora K: Nonpharmacologic intervention in acute alcohol withdrawal. Clin Pharmacol Ther 1983; 34:214–219 [A]
983. Tallaksen CM, Bohmer T, Bell H: Blood and serum thiamin and thiamin phosphate esters concentrations in patients with alcohol dependence syndrome before and after thiamin treatment. Alcohol Clin Exp Res 1992; 16:320–325 [B]
984. Bond NW, Homewood J: Wernicke's encephalopathy and Korsakoff's psychosis: to fortify or not to fortify? Neurotoxicol Teratol 1991; 13:353–355 [G]
985. Blass JP, Gibson GE: Abnormality of a thiamine-requiring enzyme in patients with Wernicke-Korsakoff syndrome. N Engl J Med 1977; 297:1367–1370 [G]
986. Day E, Bentham P, Callaghan R, Kuruvilla T, George S: Thiamine for Wernicke-Korsakoff syndrome in people at risk from alcohol abuse. Cochrane Database Syst Rev 2004; CD004033 [E]
987. Malcolm R, Myrick H, Brady KT, Ballenger JC: Update on anticonvulsants for the treatment of alcohol withdrawal. Am J Addict 2001; 10(suppl):16–23 [G]
988. Femino J, Lewis DC: Clinical Pharmacology and Therapeutics of the Alcohol Withdrawal Syndrome: Monograph 272. Rockville, Md, National Institute on Alcohol Abuse and Alcoholism, 1982 [F]
989. Rosenbloom A: Emerging treatment options in the alcohol withdrawal syndrome. J Clin Psychiatry 1988; 49(suppl):28–32 [G]
990. Victor M: Treatment of alcohol intoxication and the withdrawal syndrome: a critical analysis of the use of drugs and other forms of therapy. Psychosom Med 1966; 28:636–650 [G]
991. Holbrook AM, Crowther R, Lotter A, Cheng C, King D: Meta-analysis of benzodiazepine use in the treatment of acute alcohol withdrawal. CMAJ 1999; 160:649–655 [E]
992. Mayo-Smith MF: Pharmacological management of alcohol withdrawal: a meta-analysis and evidence-based practice guideline. American Society of Addiction Medicine Working Group on Pharmacological Management of Alcohol Withdrawal. JAMA 1997; 278:144–151 [E]
993. Gatch MB, Lal H: Pharmacological treatment of alcoholism. Prog Neuropsychopharmacol Biol Psychiatry 1998; 22:917–944 [G]
994. Reoux JP, Saxon AJ, Malte CA, Baer JS, Sloan KL: Divalproex sodium in alcohol withdrawal: a randomized double-blind placebo-controlled clinical trial. Alcohol Clin Exp Res 2001; 25:1324–1329 [A]
995. Ntais C, Pakos E, Kyzas P, Ioannidis J: Benzodiazepines for alcohol withdrawal. Cochrane Database Syst Rev 2005; CD005063 [E]
996. Naranjo CA, Sellers EM: Clinical assessment and pharmacotherapy of the alcohol withdrawal syndrome. Recent Dev Alcohol 1986; 4:265–281 [G]
997. Schaffer A, Naranjo CA: Recommended drug treatment strategies for the alcoholic patient. Drugs 1998; 56:571–585 [G]

998. Saitz R, Mayo-Smith MF, Roberts MS, Redmond HA, Bernard DR, Calkins DR: Individualized treatment for alcohol withdrawal: a randomized double-blind controlled trial. JAMA 1994; 272:519–523 [A]
999. Bradley KA: Management of alcoholism in the primary care setting. West J Med 1992; 156:273–277 [G]
1000. Woo E, Greenblatt DJ: Massive benzodiazepine requirements during acute alcohol withdrawal. Am J Psychiatry 1979; 136:821–823 [G]
1001. Manikant S, Tripathi BM, Chavan BS: Loading dose diazepam therapy for alcohol withdrawal state. Indian J Med Res 1993; 98:170–173 [A–]
1002. Daeppen JB, Gache P, Landry U, Sekera E, Schweizer V, Gloor S, Yersin B: Symptom-triggered vs fixed-schedule doses of benzodiazepine for alcohol withdrawal: a randomized treatment trial. Arch Intern Med 2002; 162:1117–1121 [A–]
1003. Spies CD, Otter HE, Huske B, Sinha P, Neumann T, Rettig J, Lenzenhuber E, Kox WJ, Sellers EM: Alcohol withdrawal severity is decreased by symptom-orientated adjusted bolus therapy in the ICU. Intensive Care Med 2003; 29:2230–2238 [A]
1004. Bird RD, Makela EH: Alcohol withdrawal: what is the benzodiazepine of choice? Ann Pharmacother 1994; 28:67–71 [F]
1005. D'Onofrio G, Rathlev NK, Ulrich AS, Fish SS, Freedland ES: Lorazepam for the prevention of recurrent seizures related to alcohol. N Engl J Med 1999; 340:915–919 [A]
1006. Pacifici GM, Viani A, Franchi M, Santerini S, Temellini A, Giuliani L, Carrai M: Conjugation pathways in liver disease. Br J Clin Pharmacol 1990; 30:427–435 [G]
1007. Huet PM, Villeneuve JP: Determinants of drug disposition in patients with cirrhosis. Hepatology 1983; 3:913–918 [G]
1008. Sellers EM, Naranjo CA: New strategies for the treatment of alcohol withdrawal. Psychopharmacol Bull 1986; 22:88–92 [F]
1009. Seppala T, Aranko K, Mattila MJ, Shrotriya RC: Effects of alcohol on buspirone and lorazepam actions. Clin Pharmacol Ther 1982; 32:201–207 [G]
1010. Gessner PK: Treatment of the alcohol withdrawal syndrome. Substance Abuse 1979; 1:2–5 [G]
1011. Gessner PK: Drug therapy of the alcohol withdrawal syndrome, in The Biochemistry and Pharmacology of Ethanol. Edited by Majchrowicz E, Noble E. New York, Plenum, 1979, pp 375–434 [G]
1012. Gross GA: The use of propranolol as a method to manage acute alcohol detoxification. J Am Osteopath Assoc 1982; 82:206–207 [G]
1013. Zilm DH, Sellers EM, MacLeod SM, Degani N: Propranolol effect on tremor in alcoholic withdrawal (letter). Ann Intern Med 1975; 83:234–236 [G]
1014. Sellers EM, Zilm DH, MacLeod SM: Chlordiazepoxide and propranolol treatment of alcoholic withdrawal (abstract). Clin Res 1975; 23:610A [A]
1015. Kraus ML, Gottlieb LD, Horwitz RI, Anscher M: Randomized clinical trial of atenolol in patients with alcohol withdrawal. N Engl J Med 1985; 313:905–909 [A]
1016. Robinson BJ, Robinson GM, Maling TJ, Johnson RH: Is clonidine useful in the treatment of alcohol withdrawal? Alcohol Clin Exp Res 1989; 13:95–98 [A]
1017. Wilkins AJ, Jenkins WJ, Steiner JA: Efficacy of clonidine in treatment of alcohol withdrawal state. Psychopharmacology (Berl) 1983; 81:78–80 [A]
1018. Rosenthal RN, Perkel C, Singh P, Anand O, Miner CR: A pilot open randomized trial of valproate and phenobarbital in the treatment of acute alcohol withdrawal. Am J Addict 1998; 7:189–197 [A–]
1019. Malcolm R, Roberts JS, Wang W, Myrick H, Anton RF: Multiple previous detoxifications are associated with less responsive treatment and heavier drinking during an index outpatient detoxification. Alcohol 2000; 22:159–164 [D]

1020. Myrick H, Brady KT, Malcolm R: Divalproex in the treatment of alcohol withdrawal. Am J Drug Alcohol Abuse 2000; 26:155–160 [B]
1021. Rothstein E: Prevention of alcohol withdrawal seizures: the roles of diphenylhydantoin and chlordiazepoxide. Am J Psychiatry 1973; 130:1381–1382 [G]
1022. Sampliner R, Iber FL: Diphenylhydantoin control of alcohol withdrawal seizures: results of a controlled study. JAMA 1974; 230:1430–1432 [A–]
1023. Rathlev NK, D'Onofrio G, Fish SS, Harrison PM, Bernstein E, Hossack RW, Pickens L: The lack of efficacy of phenytoin in the prevention of recurrent alcohol-related seizures. Ann Emerg Med 1994; 23:513–518 [A]
1024. Shaw GK: Alcohol dependence and withdrawal. Br Med Bull 1982; 38:99–102 [G]
1025. Polycarpou A, Papanikolaou P, Ioannidis J, Contopoulos-Ioannidis D: Anticonvulsants for alcohol withdrawal. Cochrane Database Syst Rev 2005; CD005064 [E]
1026. Wilbur R, Kulik FA: Anticonvulsant drugs in alcohol withdrawal: use of phenytoin, primidone, carbamazepine, valproic acid, and the sedative anticonvulsants. Am J Hosp Pharm 1981; 38:1138–1143 [F]
1027. Poutanen P: Experience with carbamazepine in the treatment of withdrawal symptoms in alcohol abusers. Br J Addict Alcohol Other Drugs 1979; 74:201–204 [B]
1028. Malcolm R, Ballenger JC, Sturgis ET, Anton R: Double-blind controlled trial comparing carbamazepine to oxazepam treatment of alcohol withdrawal. Am J Psychiatry 1989; 146:617–621 [A]
1029. Chu NS: Carbamazepine: prevention of alcohol withdrawal seizures. Neurology 1979; 29:1397–1401 [B]
1030. Post RM, Ballenger JC, Putnam FW, Bunney WE Jr: Carbamazepine in alcohol withdrawal syndromes: relationship to the kindling model. J Clin Psychopharmacol 1983; 3:204–205 [G]
1031. Schik G, Wedegaertner FR, Liersch J, Hoy L, Emrich HM, Schneider U: Oxcarbazepine versus carbamazepine in the treatment of alcohol withdrawal. Addict Biol 2005; 10:283–288 [A–]
1032. Wilson A, Vulcano B: A double-blind, placebo-controlled trial of magnesium sulfate in the ethanol withdrawal syndrome. Alcohol Clin Exp Res 1984; 8:542–545 [A]
1033. Smith DE: Use of psychotropic drugs in alcoholism treatment: a summary. Addictions Alert 1989; 2:47–48 [F]
1034. Blondell RD, Dodds HN, Blondell MN, Looney SW, Smoger SH, Sexton LK, Wieland LS, Swift RM: Ethanol in formularies of US teaching hospitals. JAMA 2003; 289:552 [G]
1035. Smoger SH, Looney SW, Blondell RD, Wieland LS, Sexton L, Rhodes SB, Swift RM: Hospital Use of Ethanol Survey (HUES): preliminary results. J Addict Dis 2002; 21:65–73 [G]
1036. Garbutt JC, West SL, Carey TS, Lohr KN, Crews FT: Pharmacological treatment of alcohol dependence: a review of the evidence. JAMA 1999; 281:1318–1325 [E]
1037. Volpicelli JR, Alterman AI, Hayashida M, O'Brien CP: Naltrexone in the treatment of alcohol dependence. Arch Gen Psychiatry 1992; 49:876–880 [A]
1038. Anton RF, Moak DH, Waid LR, Latham PK, Malcolm RJ, Dias JK: Naltrexone and cognitive behavioral therapy for the treatment of outpatient alcoholics: results of a placebo-controlled trial. Am J Psychiatry 1999; 156:1758–1764 [A–]
1039. Heinala P, Alho H, Kiianmaa K, Lonnqvist J, Kuoppasalmi K, Sinclair JD: Targeted use of naltrexone without prior detoxification in the treatment of alcohol dependence: a factorial double-blind, placebo-controlled trial. J Clin Psychopharmacol 2001; 21:287–292 [A]
1040. Latt NC, Jurd S, Houseman J, Wutzke SE: Naltrexone in alcohol dependence: a randomised controlled trial of effectiveness in a standard clinical setting. Med J Aust 2002; 176:530–534 [A]

1041. Morris PL, Hopwood M, Whelan G, Gardiner J, Drummond E: Naltrexone for alcohol dependence: a randomized controlled trial. Addiction 2001; 96:1565–1573 [A]
1042. Gastpar M, Bonnet U, Boning J, Mann K, Schmidt LG, Soyka M, Wetterling T, Kielstein V, Labriola D, Croop R: Lack of efficacy of naltrexone in the prevention of alcohol relapse: results from a German multicenter study. J Clin Psychopharmacol 2002; 22:592–598 [A]
1043. Krystal JH, Cramer JA, Krol WF, Kirk GF, Rosenheck RA: Naltrexone in the treatment of alcohol dependence. N Engl J Med 2001; 345:1734–1739 [A]
1044. Garbutt JC, Kranzler HR, O'Malley SS, Gastfriend DR, Pettinati HM, Silverman BL, Loewy JW, Ehrich EW: Efficacy and tolerability of long-acting injectable naltrexone for alcohol dependence: a randomized controlled trial. JAMA 2005; 293:1617–1625 [A]
1045. Chick J, Anton R, Checinski K, Croop R, Drummond DC, Farmer R, Labriola D, Marshall J, Moncrieff J, Morgan MY, Peters T, Ritson B: A multicentre, randomized, double-blind, placebo-controlled trial of naltrexone in the treatment of alcohol dependence or abuse. Alcohol Alcohol 2000; 35:587–593 [A]
1046. Croop RS, Faulkner EB, Labriola DF: The safety profile of naltrexone in the treatment of alcoholism: results from a multicenter usage study. The Naltrexone Usage Study Group. Arch Gen Psychiatry 1997; 54:1130–1135 [B]
1047. Kim SW, Grant JE, Adson DE, Remmel RP: A preliminary report on possible naltrexone and nonsteroidal analgesic interactions. J Clin Psychopharmacol 2001; 21:632–634 [D]
1048. Arana GW, Hyman SE: Handbook of Psychiatric Drug Therapy, 2nd ed. Boston, Little, Brown, 1991 [G]
1049. Fuller RK, Roth HP: Disulfiram for the treatment of alcoholism: an evaluation in 128 men. Ann Intern Med 1979; 90:901–904 [A]
1050. Lister RG, Nutt DJ: Alcohol antagonists: the continuing quest. Alcohol Clin Exp Res 1988; 12:566–569 [G]
1051. Peachey JE: Clinical uses of the alcohol-sensitizing drugs, in Pharmacological Treatments for Alcoholism. Edited by Little EG. New York, Croom Helm, 1984, pp 531–557 [G]
1052. Peachey JE, Brien JF, Loomis CW, Rogers BJ: A study of the calcium carbimide-ethanol interaction in man: symptom responses. Alcohol Clin Exp Res 1980; 4:322–329 [G]
1053. Keso L, Salaspuro M: Inpatient treatment of employed alcoholics: a randomized clinical trial on Hazelden-type and traditional treatment. Alcohol Clin Exp Res 1990; 14:584–589 [A–]
1054. Martin B, Clapp L, Bialkowski D, Bridgeford D, Amponsah A, Lyons L, Beresford TP: Compliance to supervised disulfiram therapy: a comparison of voluntary and court-ordered patients. Am J Addict 2003; 12:137–143 [B]
1055. O'Farrell TJ, Allen JP, Litten RZ: Disulfiram (antabuse) contracts in treatment of alcoholism. NIDA Res Monogr 1995; 150:65–91 [F]
1056. Fox R: Disulfiram: alcohol side effects. JAMA 1968; 204:271–272 [G]
1057. Marchner J: The pharmacology of alcohol-sensitizing drugs, in Pharmacological Treatments for Alcoholism. Edited by Edwards G, Littleton J. New York, Methuen, 1984 [G]
1058. Peachey JE: A review of the clinical use of disulfiram and calcium carbimide in alcoholism treatment. J Clin Psychopharmacol 1981; 1:368–375 [F]
1059. Madan A, Parkinson A, Faiman MD: Identification of the human P-450 enzymes responsible for the sulfoxidation and thiono-oxidation of diethyldithiocarbamate methyl ester: role of P-450 enzymes in disulfiram bioactivation. Alcohol Clin Exp Res 1998; 22:1212–1219 [G]
1060. Gerrein JR, Rosenberg CM, Manohar V: Disulfiram maintenance in outpatient treatment of alcoholism. Arch Gen Psychiatry 1973; 28:798–802 [A–]

1061. Physicians Medical Economics: Physicians' Desk Reference. Montvale, NJ, Thomson Healthcare, 2005 [G]
1062. Mann K, Lehert P, Morgan MY: The efficacy of acamprosate in the maintenance of abstinence in alcohol-dependent individuals: results of a meta-analysis. Alcohol Clin Exp Res 2004; 28:51–63 [E]
1063. Mason BJ: Treatment of alcohol-dependent outpatients with acamprosate: a clinical review. J Clin Psychiatry 2001; 62(suppl 20):42–48 [F]
1064. Littleton J: Acamprosate in alcohol dependence: how does it work? Addiction 1995; 90:1179–1188 [G]
1065. Verheul R, Lehert P, Geerlings PJ, Koeter MW, van den Brink W: Predictors of acamprosate efficacy: results from a pooled analysis of seven European trials including 1485 alcohol-dependent patients. Psychopharmacology (Berl) 2005; 178:167–173 [E]
1066. Bouza C, Angeles M, Munoz A, Amate JM: Efficacy and safety of naltrexone and acamprosate in the treatment of alcohol dependence: a systematic review. Addiction 2004; 99:811–828 [E]
1067. Mason BJ: Analysis of USA Multicenter Trial Results, 2002. http://www.fda.gov/ohrms/dockets/ac/02/Slides/3857S1_05_Lipha%20-%20Mason/ [G]
1068. Kiefer F, Wiedemann K: Combined therapy: what does acamprosate and naltrexone combination tell us? Alcohol Alcohol 2004; 39:542–547 [F]
1069. COMBINE Study Research Group: Testing combined pharmacotherapies and behavioral interventions in alcohol dependence: rationale and methods. Alcohol Clin Exp Res 2003; 27:1107–1122 [A–]
1070. COMBINE Study Research Group: Testing combined pharmacotherapies and behavioral interventions for alcohol dependence (the COMBINE study): a pilot feasibility study. Alcohol Clin Exp Res 2003; 27:1123–1131 [A]
1071. Besson J, Aeby F, Kasas A, Lehert P, Potgieter A: Combined efficacy of acamprosate and disulfiram in the treatment of alcoholism: a controlled study. Alcohol Clin Exp Res 1998; 22:573–579 [A–]
1072. Saivin S, Hulot T, Chabac S, Potgieter A, Durbin P, Houin G: Clinical pharmacokinetics of acamprosate. Clin Pharmacokinet 1998; 35:331–345 [F]
1073. Kranzler HR, Anton RF: Implications of recent neuropsychopharmacologic research for understanding the etiology and development of alcoholism. J Consult Clin Psychol 1994; 62:1116–1126 [F]
1074. LeMarquand D, Pihl RO, Benkelfat C: Serotonin and alcohol intake, abuse, and dependence: findings of animal studies. Biol Psychiatry 1994; 36:395–421 [F]
1075. Linnoila M, Eckardt M, Durcan M, Lister R, Martin P: Interactions of serotonin with ethanol: clinical and animal studies. Psychopharmacol Bull 1987; 23:452–457 [G]
1076. Naranjo CA, Poulos CX, Bremner KE, Lanctot KL: Fluoxetine attenuates alcohol intake and desire to drink. Int Clin Psychopharmacol 1994; 9:163–172 [A–]
1077. Naranjo CA, Sellers EM, Roach CA, Woodley DV, Sanchez-Craig M, Sykora K: Zimelidine-induced variations in alcohol intake by nondepressed heavy drinkers. Clin Pharmacol Ther 1984; 35:374–381 [A]
1078. Pettinati HM, Oslin D, Decker K: Role of serotonin and serotonin-selective pharmacotherapy in alcohol dependence. CNS Spectr 2000; 5:33–46 [G]
1079. Kranzler HR, Burleson JA, Korner P, Del Boca FK, Bohn MJ, Brown J, Liebowitz N: Placebo-controlled trial of fluoxetine as an adjunct to relapse prevention in alcoholics. Am J Psychiatry 1995; 152:391–397 [A–]
1080. Pettinati HM, Volpicelli JR, Kranzler HR, Luck G, Rukstalis MR, Cnaan A: Sertraline treatment for alcohol dependence: interactive effects of medication and alcoholic subtype. Alcohol Clin Exp Res 2000; 24:1041–1049 [B]

1081. Mason BJ, Kocsis JH: Desipramine treatment of alcoholism. Psychopharmacol Bull 1991; 27:155–161 [A]
1082. Hodge CW, Samson HH, Lewis RS, Erickson HL: Specific decreases in ethanol- but not water-reinforced responding produced by the 5-HT3 antagonist ICS 205–930. Alcohol 1993; 10:191–196 [G]
1083. Rodd-Henricks ZA, McKinzie DL, Edmundson VE, Murphy JM, McBride WJ, Lumeng L, Li TK: Serotonin-3 receptor antagonists reduce alcohol intake during acquisition and maintenance but not following a period of alcohol deprivation in alcohol preferring (P) rats. Alcohol Clin Exp Res 1999; 23:49A [G]
1084. Johnson BA, Cowen PJ: Alcohol-induced reinforcement: dopamine and 5-HT3 receptor interactions in animals and humans. Drug Dev Res 1993; 30:153–169 [G]
1085. Sellers EM, Toneatto T, Romach MK, Somer GR, Sobell LC, Sobell MB: Clinical efficacy of the 5-HT3 antagonist ondansetron in alcohol abuse and dependence. Alcohol Clin Exp Res 1994; 18:879–885 [A]
1086. Johnson BA, Roache JD, Javors MA, DiClemente CC, Cloninger CR, Prihoda TJ, Bordnick PS, Ait-Daoud N, Hensler J: Ondansetron for reduction of drinking among biologically predisposed alcoholic patients: a randomized controlled trial. JAMA 2000; 284:963–971 [A]
1087. Fawcett J, Clark DC, Aagesen CA, Pisani VD, Tilkin JM, Sellers D, McGuire M, Gibbons RD: A double-blind, placebo-controlled trial of lithium carbonate therapy for alcoholism. Arch Gen Psychiatry 1987; 44:248–256 [A]
1088. Dorus W, Ostrow DG, Anton R, Cushman P, Collins JF, Schaefer M, Charles HL, Desai P, Hayashida M, Malkerneker U: Lithium treatment of depressed and nondepressed alcoholics. JAMA 1989; 262:1646–1652 [A]
1089. Silber A: Rationale for the technique of psychotherapy with alcoholics. Int J Psychoanal Psychother 1974; 3:28–47 [G]
1090. Holder HD, Longabaugh R, Miller WR, Rubonis AV: The cost effectiveness of treatment for alcoholism: a first approximation. J Stud Alcohol 1991; 52:517–540 [E]
1091. McKay JR, Maisto SA: An overview and critique of advances in the treatment of alcohol use disorders. Drugs Soc 1993; 8:1–29 [F]
1092. Chaney EF: Social skills training, in Handbook of Alcoholism Treatment Approaches. Edited by Hester RK, Miller WR. New York, Pergamon, 1989, pp 206–221 [F]
1093. Monti PM, Abrams DB, Binkoff JA, Zwick WR, Liepman MR, Nirenberg TD, Rohsenow DJ: Communication skills training, communication skills training with family and cognitive behavioral mood management training for alcoholics. J Stud Alcohol 1990; 51:263–270 [B]
1094. Irvin JE, Bowers CA, Dunn ME, Wang MC: Efficacy of relapse prevention: a meta-analytic review. J Consult Clin Psychol 1999; 67:563–570 [E]
1095. Miller WR, Munoz RF: How to Control Your Drinking, revised ed. Albuquerque, University of New Mexico Press, 1982 [F]
1096. Sanchez-Craig M: Therapist's Manual for Secondary Prevention of Alcohol Problems: Procedures for Teaching Moderate Drinking and Abstinence. Toronto, Addiction Research Foundation, 1984 [F]
1097. Hodgson R: Treatment of alcohol problems. Addiction 1994; 89:1529–1534 [G]
1098. Bandura A: Self-efficacy: toward a unifying theory of behavioral change. Psychol Rev 1977; 84:191–215 [G]
1099. McKay JR, Maisto SA, O'Farrell TJ: End-of-treatment self-efficacy, aftercare, and drinking outcomes of alcoholic men. Alcohol Clin Exp Res 1993; 17:1078–1083 [A–]
1100. Burling TA, Reilly PM, Moltzen JO, Ziff DC: Self-efficacy and relapse among inpatient drug and alcohol abusers: a predictor of outcome. J Stud Alcohol 1989; 50:354–360 [C]

1101. Edwards G, Brown D, Duckitt A, Oppenheimer E, Sheehan M, Taylor C: Outcome of alcoholism: the structure of patient attributions as to what causes change. Br J Addict 1987; 82:533–545 [G]
1102. Cooney NL, Kadden RM, Litt MD, Getter H: Matching alcoholics to coping skills or interactional therapies: two-year follow-up results. J Consult Clin Psychol 1991; 59:598–601 [B]
1103. Kadden RM, Cooney NL, Getter H, Litt MD: Matching alcoholics to coping skills or interactional therapies: posttreatment results. J Consult Clin Psychol 1989; 57:698–704 [A–]
1104. Litt MD, Babor TF, DelBoca FK, Kadden RM, Cooney NL: Types of alcoholics, II: application of an empirically derived typology to treatment matching. Arch Gen Psychiatry 1992; 49:609–614 [A–]
1105. Dunn C, Deroo L, Rivara FP: The use of brief interventions adapted from motivational interviewing across behavioral domains: a systematic review. Addiction 2001; 96:1725–1742 [E]
1106. Project MATCH Research Group: Matching alcoholism treatments to client heterogeneity: treatment main effects and matching effects on drinking during treatment. J Stud Alcohol 1998; 59:631–639 [A–]
1107. Hunt GM, Azrin NH: A community-reinforcement approach to alcoholism. Behav Res Ther 1973; 11:91–104 [G]
1108. Smith JE, Meyers RJ, Delaney HD: The community reinforcement approach with homeless alcohol-dependent individuals. J Consult Clin Psychol 1998; 66:541–548 [A–]
1109. Babor TF: Avoiding the Horrible and Beastly Sin of Drunkenness: Does Dissuasion Make a Difference? Storrs, Conn, University of Connecticut School of Medicine, 1992 [G]
1110. Anderson P, Scott E: The effect of general practitioners' advice to heavy drinking men. Br J Addict 1992; 87:891–900 [A–]
1111. Fleming MF, Manwell LB, Barry KL, Adams W, Stauffacher EA: Brief physician advice for alcohol problems in older adults: a randomized community-based trial. J Fam Pract 1999; 48:378–384 [A–]
1112. Hoffman NG, Miller NS: Treatment outcomes for abstinence-based programs. Psychiatr Ann 1992; 22:402–408 [F]
1113. Cross GM, Morgan CW, Mooney AJ III, Martin CA, Rafter JA: Alcoholism treatment: a ten-year follow-up study. Alcohol Clin Exp Res 1990; 14:169–173 [C]
1114. Gilbert FS: Development of a "Steps Questionnaire." J Stud Alcohol 1991; 52:353–360 [G]
1115. McCrady BS, Irvine S: Self-help groups, in Handbook of Alcoholism Treatment Approaches. Edited by Hester RK, Miller WR. New York, Pergamon, 1989, pp 153–169 [G]
1116. Rychtarik RG, Connors GJ, Dermen KH, Stasiewicz PR: Alcoholics Anonymous and the use of medications to prevent relapse: an anonymous survey of member attitudes. J Stud Alcohol 2000; 61:134–138 [G]
1117. Moos RH, Moos BS: The process of recovery from alcoholism, III: comparing functioning in families of alcoholics and matched control families. J Stud Alcohol 1984; 45:111–118 [D]
1118. O'Farrell TJ, Choquette KA, Cutter HS: Couples relapse prevention sessions after behavioral marital therapy for male alcoholics: outcomes during the three years after starting treatment. J Stud Alcohol 1998; 59:357–370 [A–]
1119. O'Farrell TJ, Choquette KA, Cutter HS, Brown ED, McCourt WF: Behavioral marital therapy with and without additional couples relapse prevention sessions for alcoholics and their wives. J Stud Alcohol 1993; 54:652–666 [A–]

1120. Walker RD, Donovan DM, Kivlahan DR, O'Leary MR: Length of stay, neuropsychological performance, and aftercare: influences on alcohol treatment outcome. J Consult Clin Psychol 1983; 51:900–911 [C]
1121. McLatchie BH, Lomp KG: An experimental investigation of the influence of aftercare on alcoholic relapse. Br J Addict 1988; 83:1045–1054 [A–]
1122. Gilbert FS: The effect of type of aftercare follow-up on treatment outcome among alcoholics. J Stud Alcohol 1988; 49:149–159 [C]
1123. Patterson DG, Macpherson J, Brady NM: Community psychiatric nurse aftercare for alcoholics: a five-year follow-up study. Addiction 1997; 92:459–468 [B]
1124. Herman SE, Frank KA, Mowbray CT, Ribisl KM, Davidson WS, Boots Miller B, Jordan L, Greenfield AL, Loveland D, Luke DA: Longitudinal effects of integrated treatment on alcohol use for persons with serious mental illness and substance use disorders. J Behav Health Serv Res 2000; 27:286–302 [A–]
1125. Drake RE, Mueser KT, Brunette MF, McHugo GJ: A review of treatments for people with severe mental illnesses and co-occurring substance use disorders. Psychiatr Rehabil J 2004; 27:360–374 [F]
1126. Robins E: The Final Months: A Study of the Lives of 134 Persons Who Committed Suicide. New York, Oxford University Press, 1981 [D]
1127. Berglund M: Suicide in alcoholism: a prospective study of 88 suicides, I: the multidimensional diagnosis at first admission. Arch Gen Psychiatry 1984; 41:888–891 [C]
1128. Cornelius JR, Salloum IM, Haskett RF, Daley DC, Cornelius MD, Thase ME, Perel JM: Fluoxetine versus placebo in depressed alcoholics: a 1-year follow-up study. Addict Behav 2000; 25:307–310 [B]
1129. Naranjo CA, Bremner KE, Bazoon M, Turksen IB: Using fuzzy logic to predict response to citalopram in alcohol dependence. Clin Pharmacol Ther 1997; 62:209–224 [G]
1130. Ciraulo DA, Jaffe JH: Tricyclic antidepressants in the treatment of depression associated with alcoholism. J Clin Psychopharmacol 1981; 1:146–150 [F]
1131. Ciraulo DA, Barnhill JG, Jaffe JH: Clinical pharmacokinetics of imipramine and desipramine in alcoholics and normal volunteers. Clin Pharmacol Ther 1988; 43:509–518 [G]
1132. Schottenfeld RS, O'Malley SS, Smith L, Rounsaville BJ, Jaffe JH: Limitation and potential hazards of MAOIs for the treatment of depressive symptoms in abstinent alcoholics. Am J Drug Alcohol Abuse 1989; 15:339–344 [G]
1133. Cornelius JR, Salloum IM, Cornelius MD, Perel JM, Thase ME, Ehler JG, Mann JJ: Fluoxetine trial in suicidal depressed alcoholics. Psychopharmacol Bull 1993; 29:195–199 [B]
1134. Randall CL, Johnson MR, Thevos AK, Sonne SC, Thomas SE, Willard SL, Brady KT, Davidson JR: Paroxetine for social anxiety and alcohol use in dual-diagnosed patients. Depress Anxiety 2001; 14:255–262 [A–]
1135. Bruno F: Buspirone in the treatment of alcoholic patients. Psychopathology 1989; 22(suppl 1):49–59 [A]
1136. Hanck C, Whitcomb DC: Alcoholic pancreatitis. Gastroenterol Clin North Am 2004; 33:751–765 [F]
1137. Teyssen S, Singer MV: Alcohol-related diseases of the oesophagus and stomach. Best Pract Res Clin Gastroenterol 2003; 17:557–573 [F]
1138. Lieber CS: Hepatic and other medical disorders of alcoholism: from pathogenesis to treatment. J Stud Alcohol 1998; 59:9–25 [F]
1139. Cho E, Smith-Warner SA, Ritz J, van den Brandt PA, Colditz GA, Folsom AR, Freudenheim JL, Giovannucci E, Goldbohm RA, Graham S, Holmberg L, Kim DH, Malila N, Miller AB, Pietinen P, Rohan TE, Sellers TA, Speizer FE, Willett WC, Wolk

A, Hunter DJ: Alcohol intake and colorectal cancer: a pooled analysis of 8 cohort studies. Ann Intern Med 2004; 140:603–613 [E]

1140. Riedel F, Goessler U, Hormann K: Alcohol-related diseases of the mouth and throat. Best Pract Res Clin Gastroenterol 2003; 17:543–555 [F]

1141. Spies CD, Sander M, Stangl K, Fernandez-Sola J, Preedy VR, Rubin E, Andreasson S, Hanna EZ, Kox WJ: Effects of alcohol on the heart. Curr Opin Crit Care 2001; 7:337–343 [F]

1142. Van Thiel DH, Gavaler JS: Endocrine effects of chronic alcohol abuse: hypothalamic-pituitary-gonadal axis, in Alcohol and the Brain: Chronic Effects. Edited by Tarter RE, Van Thiel DH. New York, Plenum, 1985, pp 69–79 [G]

1143. Mendelson JH, Babor TF, Mello NK, Pratt H: Alcoholism and prevalence of medical and psychiatric disorders. J Stud Alcohol 1986; 47:361–366 [G]

1144. Korsten MA, Lieber CS: Medical complications of alcoholism, in The Diagnosis and Treatment of Alcoholism. Edited by Mendelson JH, Mello NK. New York, McGraw-Hill, 1985, pp 21–64 [G]

1145. Hermann D, Heinz A, Mann K: Dysregulation of the hypothalamic-pituitary-thyroid axis in alcoholism. Addiction 2002; 97:1369–1381 [F]

1146. Sacanella E, Fernandez-Sola J, Cofan M, Nicolas JM, Estruch R, Antunez E, Urbano-Marquez A: Chronic alcoholic myopathy: diagnostic clues and relationship with other ethanol-related diseases. QJM 1995; 88:811–817 [G]

1147. Urbano-Marquez A, Estruch R, Fernandez-Sola J, Nicolas JM, Pare JC, Rubin E: The greater risk of alcoholic cardiomyopathy and myopathy in women compared with men. JAMA 1995; 274:149–154 [G]

1148. Bates ME, Bowden SC, Barry D: Neurocognitive impairment associated with alcohol use disorders: implications for treatment. Exp Clin Psychopharmacol 2002; 10:193–212 [F]

1149. Parsons OA: Neurocognitive deficits in alcoholics and social drinkers: a continuum? Alcohol Clin Exp Res 1998; 22:954–961 [F]

1150. Oscar-Berman M, Marinkovic K: Alcoholism and the brain: an overview. Alcohol Res Health 2003; 27:125–133 [F]

1151. Williams CM, Skinner AE: The cognitive effects of alcohol abuse: a controlled study. Br J Addict 1990; 85:911–917 [D]

1152. Moselhy HF, Georgiou G, Kahn A: Frontal lobe changes in alcoholism: a review of the literature. Alcohol Alcohol 2001; 36:357–368 [F]

1153. Gorenstein EE: Cognitive-perceptual deficit in an alcoholism spectrum disorder. J Stud Alcohol 1987; 48:310–318 [G]

1154. Bowden SC: Separating cognitive impairment in neurologically asymptomatic alcoholism from Wernicke-Korsakoff syndrome: is the neuropsychological distinction justified? Psychol Bull 1990; 107:355–366 [G]

1155. Allen DN, Goldstein G, Seaton BE: Cognitive rehabilitation of chronic alcohol abusers. Neuropsychol Rev 1997; 7:21–39 [F]

1156. Rindi G: Alcohol and thiamine of the brain. Alcohol Alcohol 1989; 24:493–495 [G]

1157. Goetz CG: Textbook of Clinical Neurology, 2nd ed. Philadelphia, WB Saunders, 2003 [G]

1158. Turner S, Daniels L, Greer S: Wernicke's encephalopathy in an 18-year-old woman. Br J Psychiatry 1989; 154:261–262 [G]

1159. Naidoo DP, Bramdev A, Cooper K: Wernicke''s encephalopathy and alcohol-related disease. Postgrad Med J 1991; 67:978–981 [G]

1160. McNamara ME, Campbell JJ, Recupero PR: Wernicke-Korsakoff syndrome. J Neuropsychiatry Clin Neurosci 1991; 3:232 [G]

1161. Martin PR, Eckardt MJ, Linnoila M: Treatment of chronic organic mental disorders associated with alcoholism. Recent Dev Alcohol 1989; 7:329–350 [G]

1162. Saravay SM, Pardes H: Auditory elementary hallucinations in alcohol withdrawal psychosis. Arch Gen Psychiatry 1967; 16:652–658 [G]
1163. Riley EP, McGee CL: Fetal alcohol spectrum disorders: an overview with emphasis on changes in brain and behavior. Exp Biol Med (Maywood) 2005; 230:357–365 [F]
1164. Meschke LL, Holl JA, Messelt S: Assessing the risk of fetal alcohol syndrome: understanding substance use among pregnant women. Neurotoxicol Teratol 2003; 25:667–674 [F]
1165. Lemoine P, Harroussea H, Borteyru JP: Les enfants de parents alcoholiques: anomalies observées à propos de 127 cas. Ouest Med 1968; 25:477–482 [C]
1166. Clarren SK, Smith DW: The fetal alcohol syndrome. N Engl J Med 1978; 298:1063–1067 [G]
1167. Substance Abuse and Mental Health Services Administration: Results From the 2001 National Household Survey on Drug Abuse, vol 1: Summary of National Findings. NHSDA Series H-17. DHHS Publication (SMA) 02-3758. Rockville, Md, Office of Applied Studies, 2002 [G]
1168. Anthony JC, Warner LA, Kessler RC: Comparative epidemiology of dependence on tobacco, alcohol, controlled substances and inhalants: basic findings from the National Comorbidity Survey. Exp Clin Psychopharmacol 1994; 2:244–268 [G]
1169. Johnston LD, O'Malley PM, Bachman JG: Monitoring the Future National Survey Results on Drug Use, 1975–2002. Bethesda, Md, National Institute on Drug Abuse, 2003 [G]
1170. Compton WM, Grant BF, Colliver JD, Glantz MD, Stinson FS: Prevalence of marijuana use disorders in the United States: 1991–1992 and 2001–2002. JAMA 2004; 291:2114–2121 [E]
1171. Brook JS, Cohen P, Brook DW: Longitudinal study of co-occurring psychiatric disorders and substance use. J Am Acad Child Adolesc Psychiatry 1998; 37:322–330 [C]
1172. Tims FM, Dennis ML, Hamilton N, Buchan J, Diamond G, Funk R, Brantley LB: Characteristics and problems of 600 adolescent cannabis abusers in outpatient treatment. Addiction 2002; 97(suppl 1):46–57 [G]
1173. Agosti V, Nunes E, Levin F: Rates of psychiatric comorbidity among US residents with lifetime cannabis dependence. Am J Drug Alcohol Abuse 2002; 28:643–652 [G]
1174. Aharonovich E, Liu X, Samet S, Nunes E, Waxman R, Hasin D: Postdischarge cannabis use and its relationship to cocaine, alcohol, and heroin use: a prospective study. Am J Psychiatry 2005; 162:1507–1514 [G]
1175. Arseneault L, Cannon M, Witton J, Murray RM: Causal association between cannabis and psychosis: examination of the evidence. Br J Psychiatry 2004; 184:110–117 [F]
1176. Veen ND, Selten JP, van der Tweel I, Feller WG, Hoek HW, Kahn RS: Cannabis use and age at onset of schizophrenia. Am J Psychiatry 2004; 161:501–506 [D]
1177. Degenhardt L, Hall W, Lynskey M: The relationship between cannabis use and other substance use in the general population. Drug Alcohol Depend 2001; 64:319–327 [G]
1178. McRae AL, Budney AJ, Brady KT: Treatment of marijuana dependence: a review of the literature. J Subst Abuse Treat 2003; 24:369–376 [F]
1179. Budney AJ, Hughes JR, Moore BA, Vandrey R: Review of the validity and significance of cannabis withdrawal syndrome. Am J Psychiatry 2004; 161:1967–1977 [F]
1180. Haney M, Ward AS, Comer SD, Foltin RW, Fischman MW: Abstinence symptoms following oral THC administration to humans. Psychopharmacology (Berl) 1999; 141:385–394 [A]
1181. Haney M, Ward AS, Comer SD, Foltin RW, Fischman MW: Abstinence symptoms following smoked marijuana in humans. Psychopharmacology (Berl) 1999; 141:395–404 [A–]

1182. Haney M, Ward AS, Comer SD, Hart CL, Foltin RW, Fischman MW: Bupropion SR worsens mood during marijuana withdrawal in humans. Psychopharmacology (Berl) 2001; 155:171–179 [A]
1183. Levin FR, McDowell D, Evans SM, Nunes E, Akerele E, Donovan S, Vosburg SK: Pharmacotherapy for marijuana dependence: a double-blind, placebo-controlled pilot study of divalproex sodium. Am J Addict 2004; 13:21–32 [A]
1184. Haney M, Hart CL, Vosburg SK, Nasser J, Bennett A, Zubaran C, Foltin RW: Marijuana withdrawal in humans: effects of oral THC or divalproex. Neuropsychopharmacology 2004; 29:158–170 [A]
1185. Haney M, Hart CL, Ward AS, Foltin RW: Nefazodone decreases anxiety during marijuana withdrawal in humans. Psychopharmacology (Berl) 2003; 165:157–165 [A]
1186. Stephens RS, Roffman RA, Curtin L: Comparison of extended versus brief treatments for marijuana use. J Consult Clin Psychol 2000; 68:898–908 [A–]
1187. Stephens RS, Roffman RA, Simpson EE: Treating adult marijuana dependence: a test of the relapse prevention model. J Consult Clin Psychol 1994; 62:92–99 [A–]
1188. Copeland J, Swift W, Roffman R, Stephens R: A randomized controlled trial of brief cognitive-behavioral interventions for cannabis use disorder. J Subst Abuse Treat 2001; 21:55–64 [A–]
1189. Moore BA, Budney AJ: Relapse in outpatient treatment for marijuana dependence. J Subst Abuse Treat 2003; 25:85–89 [C]
1190. Battjes RJ, Gordon MS, O'Grady KE, Kinlock TW, Katz EC, Sears EA: Evaluation of a group-based substance abuse treatment program for adolescents. J Subst Abuse Treat 2004; 27:123–134 [B]
1190a. Hurd YL, Wang X, Anderson V, Beck O, Minkoff H, Dow-Edwards D: Marijuana impairs growth in mid-gestation fetuses. Neurotoxicol Teratol 2005; 27:221–229 [D]
1190b. Richardson GA, Ryan C, Willford J, Day NL: Prenatal alcohol and marijuana exposure: effects on neuropsychological outcomes at 10 years. Neurotoxicol Teratol 2002; 24: 309–320 [C]
1190c. Huizink AC, Mulder EJ: Maternal smoking, drinking or cannabis use during pregnancy and neurobehavioral and cognitive functioning in human offspring. Neurosci Biobehav Rev (in press) [F]
1190d. Fried PA, Smith AM: A literature review of the consequences of prenatal marihuana exposure: an emerging theme of a deficiency in aspects of executive function. Neurotoxicol Teratol 2001; 23:1–11 [F]
1190e. Goldschmidt L, Richardson GA, Cornelius MD, Day NL: Prenatal marijuana and alcohol exposure and academic achievement at age 10. Neurotoxicol Teratol 2004; 26:521–532 [C]
1190f. Gray KA, Day NL, Leech S, Richardson GA: Prenatal marijuana exposure: effect on child depressive symptoms at ten years of age. Neurotoxicol Teratol 2005; 27:439–448 [C]
1190g. Porath AJ, Fried PA: Effects of prenatal cigarette and marijuana exposure on drug use among offspring. Neurotoxicol Teratol 2005; 27:267–277 [C]
1191. Substance Abuse and Mental Health Services Administration: Results from the 2003 National Survey on Drug Use and Health: National Findings. NSDUH Series H-25. DHHS Publication (SMA) 04-3964. Rockville, Md, Substance Abuse and Mental Health Services Administration, Office of Applied Studies, 2004. https://nsduhweb.rti.org [G]
1192. Rawson RA, Huber A, Brethen P, Obert J, Gulati V, Shoptaw S, Ling W: Status of methamphetamine users 2–5 years after outpatient treatment. J Addict Dis 2002; 21:107–119 [D]

1193. Srisurapanont M, Jarusuraisin N, Kittirattanapaiboon P: Treatment for amphetamine dependence and abuse. Cochrane Database Syst Rev 2001; 4:CD003022 [E]
1194. McCance EF, Price LH, Kosten TR, Jatlow PI: Cocaethylene: pharmacology, physiology and behavioral effects in humans. J Pharmacol Exp Ther 1995; 274:215–223 [A]
1195. Jatlow P, McCance EF, Bradberry CW, Elsworth JD, Taylor JR, Roth RH: Alcohol plus cocaine: the whole is more than the sum of its parts. Ther Drug Monit 1996; 18:460–464 [G]
1196. McCance-Katz EF, Kosten TR, Jatlow P: Concurrent use of cocaine and alcohol is more potent and potentially more toxic than use of either alone: a multiple-dose study. Biol Psychiatry 1998; 44:250–259 [A]
1197. McKay JR, McLellan AT, Alterman AI: An evaluation of the Cleveland criteria for inpatient treatment of substance abuse. Am J Psychiatry 1992; 149:1212–1218 [D]
1198. Alterman AI, O'Brien CP, McLellan AT, August DS, Snider EC, Droba M, Cornish JW, Hall CP, Raphaelson AH, Schrade FX: Effectiveness and costs of inpatient versus day hospital cocaine rehabilitation. J Nerv Ment Dis 1994; 182:157–163 [A]
1199. Perrone J, Hoffman RS: Cocaine, amphetamines, caffeine, and nicotine, in Emergency Medicine: A Comprehensive Study Guide, 6th ed. Edited by Tintinalli JE, Kelen GD, Stapczynski JS. New York, McGraw-Hill, 2004, pp 1075–1079 [G]
1200. Jin C, McCance-Katz EF: Substance abuse: cocaine use disorders, in Psychiatry, 2nd ed. Edited by Tasman A, Kay J, Lieberman JA. Chichester, UK, John Wiley & Sons, 2003, pp 1010–1036 [G]
1201. Leikin JB: Cocaine and beta-adrenergic blockers: a remarriage after a decade-long divorce? Crit Care Med 1999; 27:688–689 [G]
1202. Zimmerman JL: Poisonings and overdoses in the intensive care unit: general and specific management issues. Crit Care Med 2003; 31:2794–2801 [F]
1203. Goldfrank LR, Hoffman RS: The cardiovascular effects of cocaine. Ann Emerg Med 1991; 20:165–175 [F]
1204. Gawin FH, Kleber HD: Abstinence symptomatology and psychiatric diagnosis in cocaine abusers: clinical observations. Arch Gen Psychiatry 1986; 43:107–113 [B]
1205. Satel SL, Price LH, Palumbo JM, McDougle CJ, Krystal JH, Gawin F, Charney DS, Heninger GR, Kleber HD: Clinical phenomenology and neurobiology of cocaine abstinence: a prospective inpatient study. Am J Psychiatry 1991; 148:1712–1716 [C]
1206. Chen CK, Lin SK, Sham PC, Ball D, Loh EW, Hsiao CC, Chiang YL, Ree SC, Lee CH, Murray RM: Pre-morbid characteristics and co-morbidity of methamphetamine users with and without psychosis. Psychol Med 2003; 33:1407–1414 [D]
1207. Ujike H, Harano M, Inada T, Yamada M, Komiyama T, Sekine Y, Sora I, Iyo M, Katsu T, Nomura A, Nakata K, Ozaki N: Nine- or fewer repeat alleles in VNTR polymorphism of the dopamine transporter gene is a strong risk factor for prolonged methamphetamine psychosis. Pharmacogenomics J 2003; 3:242–247 [D]
1208. Yui K, Goto K, Ikemoto S: The role of noradrenergic and dopaminergic hyperactivity in the development of spontaneous recurrence of methamphetamine psychosis and susceptibility to episode recurrence. Ann N Y Acad Sci 2004; 1025:296–306 [G]
1209. Weddington WW, Brown BS, Haertzen CA, Cone EJ, Dax EM, Herning RI, Michaelson BS: Changes in mood, craving, and sleep during short-term abstinence reported by male cocaine addicts: a controlled, residential study. Arch Gen Psychiatry 1990; 47: 861–868 [C]
1210. Satel SL, Southwick SM, Gawin FH: Clinical features of cocaine-induced paranoia. Am J Psychiatry 1991; 148:495–498 [C]
1211. Coffey SF, Dansky BS, Carrigan MH, Brady KT: Acute and protracted cocaine abstinence in an outpatient population: a prospective study of mood, sleep and withdrawal symptoms. Drug Alcohol Depend 2000; 59:277–286 [C]

1212. Cornish JW, Alterman AA, Maany I, Droba M, O'Brien CP: Amantadine and carbamazepine treatment of cocaine abuse, in CME Syllabus and Scientific Proceedings in Summary Form, 145th Annual Meeting of the American Psychiatric Association. Washington, DC, American Psychiatric Association, 1992, p 131 [A]
1213. Handelsman L, Chordia PL, Escovar IL, Marion IJ, Lowinson JH: Amantadine for treatment of cocaine dependence in methadone-maintained patients. Am J Psychiatry 1988; 145:533 [C]
1214. Tennant FS Jr, Sagherian AA: Double-blind comparison of amantadine and bromocriptine for ambulatory withdrawal from cocaine dependence. Arch Intern Med 1987; 147:109–112 [A]
1215. Kosten TR, Morgan CM, Falcione J, Schottenfeld RS: Pharmacotherapy for cocaine-abusing methadone-maintained patients using amantadine or desipramine. Arch Gen Psychiatry 1992; 49:894–898 [A]
1216. Dackis CA, Gold MS: Bromocriptine as treatment of cocaine abuse. Lancet 1985; 1:1151–1152 [A–]
1217. Giannini AJ, Baumgartel P, DiMarzio LR: Bromocriptine therapy in cocaine withdrawal. J Clin Pharmacol 1987; 27:267–270 [A]
1218. Teller DW, Devenyi P: Bromocriptine in cocaine withdrawal: does it work? Int J Addict 1988; 23:1197–1205 [C]
1219. Moscovitz H, Brookoff D, Nelson L: A randomized trial of bromocriptine for cocaine users presenting to the emergency department. J Gen Intern Med 1993; 8:1–4 [A]
1220. Malcolm R, Kajdasz DK, Herron J, Anton RF, Brady KT: A double-blind, placebo-controlled outpatient trial of pergolide for cocaine dependence. Drug Alcohol Depend 2000; 60:161–168 [A]
1221. Kampman KM, Volpicelli JR, Mulvaney F, Alterman AI, Cornish J, Gariti P, Cnaan A, Poole S, Muller E, Acosta T, Luce D, O'Brien C: Effectiveness of propranolol for cocaine dependence treatment may depend on cocaine withdrawal symptom severity. Drug Alcohol Depend 2001; 63:69–78 [A]
1222. Kosten TR: Pharmacotherapeutic interventions for cocaine abuse: matching patients to treatments. J Nerv Ment Dis 1989; 177:379–389 [G]
1223. Gorelick DA: Overview of pharmacologic treatment approaches for alcohol and other drug addiction: intoxication, withdrawal, and relapse prevention. Psychiatr Clin North Am 1993; 16:141–156 [G]
1224. Kosten TR, McCance-Katz E: New pharmacotherapies, in American Psychiatric Press Review of Psychiatry, vol 14. Edited by Oldham J, Riba MB. Washington, DC, American Psychiatric Press, 1995, pp 105–126 [G]
1225. Kosten TR: Pathophysiology and treatment of cocaine dependence, in Neuropsychopharmacology: The Fifth Generation of Progress. Edited by Davis KL, Charney DS, Coyle JT, Nemeroff C. Baltimore, Md, Lippincott, Williams & Wilkins, 2002, pp 1461–1475 [G]
1226. Kampman KM, Volpicelli JR, Alterman AI, Cornish J, O'Brien CP: Amantadine in the treatment of cocaine-dependent patients with severe withdrawal symptoms. Am J Psychiatry 2000; 157:2052–2054 [A]
1227. Gawin FH, Kleber HD, Byck R, Rounsaville BJ, Kosten TR, Jatlow PI, Morgan C: Desipramine facilitation of initial cocaine abstinence. Arch Gen Psychiatry 1989; 46:117–121 [A]
1228. Oliveto AH, Feingold A, Schottenfeld R, Jatlow P, Kosten TR: Desipramine in opioid-dependent cocaine abusers maintained on buprenorphine vs methadone. Arch Gen Psychiatry 1999; 56:812–820 [A]

1229. Kosten TR, Poling J, Oliveto A: Effects of reducing contingency management values on heroin and cocaine use for buprenorphine and desipramine treated patients. Addiction 2003; 98:665–671 [A]
1230. Arndt I, Dorozynsky L, Woody G, McLellan AT, O'Brien CP: Desipramine treatment of cocaine abuse in methadone maintenance patients. NIDA Res Monogr 1989; 95:322–323 [A]
1231. Weddington WW Jr, Brown BS, Haertzen CA, Hess JM, Mahaffey JR, Kolar AF, Jaffe JH: Comparison of amantadine and desipramine combined with psychotherapy for treatment of cocaine dependence. Am J Drug Alcohol Abuse 1991; 17:137–152 [A]
1232. Pollack MH, Rosenbaum JF: Fluoxetine treatment of cocaine abuse in heroin addicts. J Clin Psychiatry 1991; 52:31–33 [E]
1233. Batki SL, Manfredi LB, Jacob P III, Jones RT: Fluoxetine for cocaine dependence in methadone maintenance: quantitative plasma and urine cocaine/benzoylecgonine concentrations. J Clin Psychopharmacol 1993; 13:243–250 [B]
1234. Margolin A, Kosten T, Petrakis I, Avants SK, Kosten T: An open pilot study of bupropion and psychotherapy for the treatment of cocaine abuse in methadone-maintained patients. NIDA Res Monogr 1991; 105:367–368 [B]
1235. Covi L, Hess JM, Kreiter NA, Haertzen CA: Three models for the analysis of a fluoxetine placebo controlled treatment in cocaine abuse, in Problems of Drug Dependence: Proceedings of the 55th Annual Scientific Meeting of the College on Problems of Drug Dependence, vol II. NIH Publication 94-3749. Edited by Harris L-S. Rockville, Md, US Department of Health and Human Services, 1994, p 138 [F]
1236. Montoya ID, Preston K, Cone E, Rothman R, Gorelick DA: Safety and efficacy of bupropion in combination with bromocriptine for treatment of cocaine dependence. Neuropsychopharmacology 1994; 10:129S [A]
1237. Montoya I, Preston KL, Cone EJ, Rothman R, Gorelick DA: Combination of bupropion and bromocriptine for treatment of cocaine dependence (abstract). CPDD Scientific Meeting Abstracts, 1994 [B]
1238. Margolin A, Kosten TR, Avants SK, Wilkins J, Ling W, Beckson M, Arndt IO, Cornish J, Ascher JA, Li SH: A multicenter trial of bupropion for cocaine dependence in methadone-maintained patients. Drug Alcohol Depend 1995; 40:125–131 [A]
1239. Kampman K, Volpicelli JR, Alterman A, Cornish J, Weinrieb R, Epperson L, Sparkman T, O'Brien CP: Amantadine in the early treatment of cocaine dependence: a double-blind, placebo-controlled trial. Drug Alcohol Depend 1996; 41:25–33 [A]
1240. Alterman AI, Droba M, Antelo RE, Cornish JW, Sweeney KK, Parikh GA, O'Brien CP: Amantadine may facilitate detoxification of cocaine addicts. Drug Alcohol Depend 1992; 31:19–29 [A]
1241. Bartzokis G, Beckson M, Newton T, Mandelkern M, Mintz J, Foster JA, Ling W, Bridge TP: Selegiline effects on cocaine-induced changes in medial temporal lobe metabolism and subjective ratings of euphoria. Neuropsychopharmacology 1999; 20:582–590 [B]
1242. Wolfsohn R, Angrist B: A pilot trial of levodopa/carbidopa in early cocaine abstinence. J Clin Psychopharmacol 1990; 10:440–442 [C]
1243. Malcolm R, Hutto BR, Phillips JD, Ballenger JC: Pergolide mesylate treatment of cocaine withdrawal. J Clin Psychiatry 1991; 52:39–40 [C]
1244. Grabowski J, Rhoades H, Schmitz J, Stotts A, Daruzska LA, Creson D, Moeller FG: Dextroamphetamine for cocaine-dependence treatment: a double-blind randomized clinical trial. J Clin Psychopharmacol 2001; 21:522–526 [A]
1245. Grabowski J, Roache JD, Schmitz JM, Rhoades H, Creson D, Korszun A: Replacement medication for cocaine dependence: methylphenidate. J Clin Psychopharmacol 1997; 17:485–488 [A]

1246. Grabowski J, Rhoades H, Stotts A, Cowan K, Kopecky C, Dougherty A, Moeller FG, Hassan S, Schmitz J: Agonist-like or antagonist-like treatment for cocaine dependence with methadone for heroin dependence: two double-blind randomized clinical trials. Neuropsychopharmacology 2004; 29:969–981 [A]
1247. Shearer J, Wodak A, van Beek I, Mattick RP, Lewis J: Pilot randomized double blind placebo-controlled study of dexamphetamine for cocaine dependence. Addiction 2003; 98:1137–1141 [A]
1248. Kosten TR, Kleber HD, Morgan C: Treatment of cocaine abuse with buprenorphine. Biol Psychiatry 1989; 26:170–172 [C]
1249. Gastfriend DR, Mendelson JH, Mello NK, Teoh SK: Preliminary results of an open trial of buprenorphine in the outpatient treatment of combined heroin and cocaine dependence, in Problems of Drug Dependence: Proceedings of the 53rd Annual Scientific Meeting of the Committee on Problems of Drug Dependence, 1992, p 461 [B]
1250. Johnson RE, Jaffe JH, Fudala PJ: A controlled trial of buprenorphine treatment for opioid dependence. JAMA 1992; 267:2750–2755 [A]
1251. Schottenfeld RS, Pakes JR, Oliveto A, Ziedonis D, Kosten TR: Buprenorphine vs methadone maintenance treatment for concurrent opioid dependence and cocaine abuse. Arch Gen Psychiatry 1997; 54:713–720 [A]
1252. Strain EC, Stitzer ML, Liebson IA, Bigelow GE: Buprenorphine versus methadone in the treatment of opioid-dependent cocaine users. Psychopharmacology (Berl) 1994; 116:401–406 [A]
1253. Schottenfeld RS, Pakes J, Ziedonis D, Kosten TR: Buprenorphine: dose-related effects on cocaine and opioid use in cocaine-abusing opioid-dependent humans. Biol Psychiatry 1993; 34:66–74 [B]
1254. Kosten T, Oliveto A, Feingold A, Poling J, Sevarino K, McCance-Katz E, Stine S, Gonzalez G, Gonsai K: Desipramine and contingency management for cocaine and opiate dependence in buprenorphine maintained patients. Drug Alcohol Depend 2003; 70:315–325 [A]
1255. Hersh D, Van Kirk JR, Kranzler HR: Naltrexone treatment of comorbid alcohol and cocaine use disorders. Psychopharmacology (Berl) 1998; 139:44–52 [A]
1256. Halikas JA, Crosby RD, Carlson GA, Crea F, Graves NM, Bowers LD: Cocaine reduction in unmotivated crack users using carbamazepine versus placebo in a short-term, double-blind crossover design. Clin Pharmacol Ther 1991; 50:81–95 [A]
1257. Cornish JW, Alterman AA, Maany I, Droba M, O'Brien CP: Amantadine and carbamazepine treatment for cocaine abuse, in CME Syllabus and Scientific Proceedings in Summary Form, 145th Annual Meeting of the American Psychiatric Association. Washington, DC, American Psychiatric Association, 1992, p 131 [A]
1258. Montoya ID, Levin FR, Fudala P, Gorelick DA: A double-blind comparison of carbamazepine and placebo treatment of cocaine dependence. NIDA Res Monogr 1994; 141:435 [A]
1259. Cornish JW, Maany I, Fudala PJ, Neal S, Poole SA, Volpicelli P, O'Brien CP: Carbamazepine treatment for cocaine dependence. Drug Alcohol Depend 1995; 38:221–227 [A]
1260. Kranzler HR, Bauer LO, Hersh D, Klinghoffer V: Carbamazepine treatment of cocaine dependence: a placebo-controlled trial. Drug Alcohol Depend 1995; 38:203–211 [A]
1261. Montoya ID, Levin FR, Fudala PJ, Gorelick DA: Double-blind comparison of carbamazepine and placebo for treatment of cocaine dependence. Drug Alcohol Depend 1995; 38:213–219 [A]

1262. Kampman KM, Pettinati H, Lynch KG, Dackis C, Sparkman T, Weigley C, O'Brien CP: A pilot trial of topiramate for the treatment of cocaine dependence. Drug Alcohol Depend 2004; 75:233–240 [A]
1263. Ling W, Shoptaw S, Majewska D: Baclofen as a cocaine anti-craving medication: a preliminary clinical study. Neuropsychopharmacology 1998; 18:403–404 [B]
1264. Gonzalez G, Sevarino K, Sofuoglu M, Poling J, Oliveto A, Gonsai K, George TP, Kosten TR: Tiagabine increases cocaine-free urines in cocaine-dependent methadone-treated patients: results of a randomized pilot study. Addiction 2003; 98:1625–1632 [A]
1265. Dackis CA, Kampman KM, Lynch KG, Pettinati HM, O'Brien CP: A double-blind, placebo-controlled trial of modafinil for cocaine dependence. Neuropsychopharmacology 2005; 30:205–211 [A]
1266. Dackis CA, Lynch KG, Yu E, Samaha FF, Kampman KM, Cornish JW, Rowan A, Poole S, White L, O'Brien CP: Modafinil and cocaine: a double-blind, placebo-controlled drug interaction study. Drug Alcohol Depend 2003; 70:29–37 [A]
1267. Donovan JL, DeVane CL, Malcolm RJ, Mojsiak J, Chiang CN, Elkashef A, Taylor RM: Modafinil influences the pharmacokinetics of intravenous cocaine in healthy cocaine-dependent volunteers. Clin Pharmacokinet 2005; 44:753–765 [B]
1268. Gawin FH, Allen D, Humblestone B: Outpatient treatment of "crack" cocaine smoking with flupenthixol decanoate: a preliminary report. Arch Gen Psychiatry 1989; 46:322–325 [B]
1269. Gawin FH: Neuroleptic reduction of cocaine-induced paranoia but not euphoria? Psychopharmacology (Berl) 1986; 90:142–143 [G]
1270. Margolin A, Azants SK, Kosten TR, Nichou C: A double-blind study of mazindol for the treatment of cocaine abuse in newly abstinent cocaine abusing methadone-maintained patients: a preliminary report. NIDA Res Monogr 1994; 141:446 [A]
1271. Stine SM, Krystal JH, Kosten TR, Charney DS: Mazindol treatment for cocaine dependence. Drug Alcohol Depend 1995; 39:245–252 [A]
1272. Margolin A, Avants SK, Malison RT, Kosten TR: High- and low-dose mazindol for cocaine dependence in methadone-maintained patients: a preliminary evaluation. Subst Abuse 1997; 18:125–131 [A–]
1273. Margolin A, Avants SK, Kosten TR: Mazindol for relapse prevention to cocaine abuse in methadone-maintained patients. Am J Drug Alcohol Abuse 1995; 21:469–481 [A]
1274. Petrakis IL, Carroll KM, Nich C, Gordon LT, McCance-Katz EF, Frankforter T, Rounsaville BJ: Disulfiram treatment for cocaine dependence in methadone-maintained opioid addicts. Addiction 2000; 95:219–228 [A]
1275. Carroll KM, Nich C, Ball SA, McCance E, Frankforter TL, Rounsaville BJ: One-year follow-up of disulfiram and psychotherapy for cocaine-alcohol users: sustained effects of treatment. Addiction 2000; 95:1335–1349 [A–]
1276. Carroll KM, Fenton LR, Ball SA, Nich C, Frankforter TL, Shi J, Rounsaville BJ: Efficacy of disulfiram and cognitive behavior therapy in cocaine-dependent outpatients: a randomized placebo-controlled trial. Arch Gen Psychiatry 2004; 61:264–272 [A–]
1277. George TP, Chawarski MC, Pakes J, Carroll KM, Kosten TR, Schottenfeld RS: Disulfiram versus placebo for cocaine dependence in buprenorphine-maintained subjects: a preliminary trial. Biol Psychiatry 2000; 47:1080–1086 [A]
1278. Kosten TR, Rosen M, Bond J, Settles M, Roberts JS, Shields J, Jack L, Fox B: Human therapeutic cocaine vaccine: safety and immunogenicity. Vaccine 2002; 20:1196–1204 [A]
1279. Bullock ML, Kiresuk TJ, Pheley AM, Culliton PD, Lenz SK: Auricular acupuncture in the treatment of cocaine abuse: a study of efficacy and dosing. J Subst Abuse Treat 1999; 16:31–38 [A–]

1280. Margolin A, Kleber HD, Avants SK, Konefal J, Gawin F, Stark E, Sorensen J, Midkiff E, Wells E, Jackson TR, Bullock M, Culliton PD, Boles S, Vaughan R: Acupuncture for the treatment of cocaine addiction: a randomized controlled trial. JAMA 2002; 287:55–63 [A–]
1281. Killeen TK, Haight B, Brady K, Herman J, Michel Y, Stuart G, Young S: The effect of auricular acupuncture on psychophysiological measures of cocaine craving. Issues Ment Health Nurs 2002; 23:445–459 [A]
1282. Gurevich MI, Duckworth D, Imhof JE, Katz JL: Is auricular acupuncture beneficial in the inpatient treatment of substance-abusing patients? a pilot study. J Subst Abuse Treat 1996; 13:165–171 [B]
1283. Konefal J, Duncan R, Clemence C: The impact of the addition of an acupuncture treatment program to an existing metro-Dade County outpatient substance abuse treatment facility. J Addict Dis 1994; 13:71–99 [A–]
1284. Richard AJ, Montoya ID, Nelson R, Spence RT: Effectiveness of adjunct therapies in crack cocaine treatment. J Subst Abuse Treat 1995; 12:401–413 [B]
1285. Russell LC, Sharp B, Gilbertson B: Acupuncture for addicted patients with chronic histories of arrest: a pilot study of the Consortium Treatment Center. J Subst Abuse Treat 2000; 19:199–205 [B]
1286. Shwartz M, Saitz R, Mulvey K, Brannigan P: The value of acupuncture detoxification programs in a substance abuse treatment system. J Subst Abuse Treat 1999; 17:305–312 [D]
1287. Smith MO, Kahn I: An acupuncture programme for the treatment of drug-addicted persons. Bull Narc 1988; 40:35–41 [G]
1288. Monti PM, Rohsenow DJ, Michalec E, Martin RA, Abrams DB: Brief coping skills treatment for cocaine abuse: substance use outcomes at three months. Addiction 1997; 92:1717–1728 [A–]
1289. Maude-Griffin PM, Hohenstein JM, Humfleet GL, Reilly PM, Tusel DJ, Hall SM: Superior efficacy of cognitive-behavioral therapy for urban crack cocaine abusers: main and matching effects. J Consult Clin Psychol 1998; 66:832–837 [A–]
1290. Carroll KM, Rounsaville BJ, Nich C, Gordon LT, Wirtz PW, Gawin F: One-year follow-up of psychotherapy and pharmacotherapy for cocaine dependence: delayed emergence of psychotherapy effects. Arch Gen Psychiatry 1994; 51:989–997 [A]
1291. McKay JR, Alterman AI, Cacciola JS, O'Brien CP, Koppenhaver JM, Shepard DS: Continuing care for cocaine dependence: comprehensive 2-year outcomes. J Consult Clin Psychol 1999; 67:420–427 [A–]
1292. Carroll KM, Rounsaville BJ, Gawin FH: A comparative trial of psychotherapies for ambulatory cocaine abusers: relapse prevention and interpersonal psychotherapy. Am J Drug Alcohol Abuse 1991; 17:229–247 [A–]
1293. Rosenblum A, Magura S, Palij M, Foote J, Handelsman L, Stimmel B: Enhanced treatment outcomes for cocaine-using methadone patients. Drug Alcohol Depend 1999; 54:207–218 [A–]
1294. Budney AJ, Higgins ST: A Community Reinforcement Plus Vouchers Approach: Treating Cocaine Addiction. Rockville, Md, National Institute on Drug Abuse, 1998 [G]
1295. Silverman K, Wong CJ, Umbricht-Schneiter A, Montoya ID, Schuster CR, Preston KL: Broad beneficial effects of cocaine abstinence reinforcement among methadone patients. J Consult Clin Psychol 1998; 66:811–824 [A–]
1296. Schottenfeld RS, Chawarski MC, Pakes JR, Pantalon MV, Carroll KM, Kosten TR: Methadone versus buprenorphine with contingency management or performance feedback for cocaine and opioid dependence. Am J Psychiatry 2005; 162:340–349 [A]

1297. Milby JB, Schumacher JE, Raczynski JM, Caldwell E, Engle M, Michael M, Carr J: Sufficient conditions for effective treatment of substance abusing homeless persons. Drug Alcohol Depend 1996; 43:39–47 [G]
1298. Kirby KC, Marlowe DB, Festinger DS, Lamb RJ, Platt JJ: Schedule of voucher delivery influences initiation of cocaine abstinence. J Consult Clin Psychol 1998; 66:761–767 [B]
1299. Svikis DS, Lee JH, Haug NA, Stitzer ML: Attendance incentives for outpatient treatment: effects in methadone- and nonmethadone-maintained pregnant drug dependent women. Drug Alcohol Depend 1997; 48:33–41 [A–]
1300. Schiffer F: Psychotherapy of nine successfully treated cocaine abusers: techniques and dynamics. J Subst Abuse Treat 1988; 5:131–137 [G]
1301. Khantzian EJ, Halliday KS, McAuliffe WE: Addiction and the Vulnerable Self: Modified Dynamic Group Therapy for Substance Abusers. New York, Guilford, 1990 [F]
1302. Spitz HI: Cocaine abuse: therapeutic group approaches, in Cocaine Abuse: New Directions in Treatment and Research. Edited by Spitz HI, Rosecan JS. New York, Brunner/Mazel, 1987, pp 156–201 [G]
1303. Walsh DC, Hingson RW, Merrigan DM, Levenson SM, Cupples LA, Heeren T, Coffman GA, Becker CA, Barker TA, Hamilton SK: A randomized trial of treatment options for alcohol-abusing workers. N Engl J Med 1991; 325:775–782 [A–]
1304. McKay JR, Alterman AI, McLellan AT, Snider EC: Treatment goals, continuity of care, and outcome in a day hospital substance abuse rehabilitation program. Am J Psychiatry 1994; 151:254–259 [B]
1305. Crits-Christoph P, Siqueland L, McCalmont E, Weiss RD, Gastfriend DR, Frank A, Moras K, Barber JP, Blaine J, Thase ME: Impact of psychosocial treatments on associated problems of cocaine-dependent patients. J Consult Clin Psychol 2001; 69:825–830 [A–]
1306. Beck AT, Wright FD, Newman CF, Liese BS: Cognitive Therapy of Substance Abuse. New York, Guilford, 1993 [G]
1307. Kranzler H, Rounsaville B: Dual Diagnosis: Substance Abuse and Comorbid Medical and Psychiatric Disorders. New York, Marcel Dekker, 1998 [G]
1308. Weiss RD, Mirin SM, Griffin ML, Michael JL: Psychopathology in cocaine abusers: changing trends. J Nerv Ment Dis 1988; 176:719–725 [D]
1309. Rounsaville BJ, Anton SF, Carroll K, Budde D, Prusoff BA, Gawin F: Psychiatric diagnoses of treatment-seeking cocaine abusers. Arch Gen Psychiatry 1991; 48:43–51 [G]
1310. Nunes EV, McGrath PJ, Wager S, Quitkin FM: Lithium treatment for cocaine abusers with bipolar spectrum disorders. Am J Psychiatry 1990; 147:655–657 [B]
1311. Cocores JA, Patel MD, Gold MS, Pottash AC: Cocaine abuse, attention deficit disorder, and bipolar disorder. J Nerv Ment Dis 1987; 175:431–432 [G]
1312. Gawin FH, Kleber HD: Cocaine abuse treatment: open pilot trial with desipramine and lithium carbonate. Arch Gen Psychiatry 1984; 41:903–909 [B]
1313. Weiss RD, Pope HG Jr, Mirin SM: Treatment of chronic cocaine abuse and attention deficit disorder, residual type, with magnesium pemoline. Drug Alcohol Depend 1985; 15:69–72 [E]
1314. Khantzian EJ: An extreme case of cocaine dependence and marked improvement with methylphenidate treatment. Am J Psychiatry 1983; 140:784–785 [G]
1315. Giannini AJ, Malone DA, Giannini MC, Price WA, Loiselle RH: Treatment of depression in chronic cocaine and phencyclidine abuse with desipramine. J Clin Pharmacol 1986; 26:211–214 [C]
1316. Arndt IO, McLellan AT, Dorozynsky L, Woody GE, O'Brien CP: Desipramine treatment for cocaine dependence: role of antisocial personality disorder. J Nerv Ment Dis 1994; 182:151–156 [A]

1317. Buckley P, Thompson P, Way L, Meltzer HY: Substance abuse among patients with treatment-resistant schizophrenia: characteristics and implications for clozapine therapy. Am J Psychiatry 1994; 151:385–389 [B]

1318. Green AI, Tohen MF, Hamer RM, Strakowski SM, Lieberman JA, Glick I, Clark WS: First episode schizophrenia-related psychosis and substance use disorders: acute response to olanzapine and haloperidol. Schizophr Res 2004; 66:125–135 [A]

1319. Sayers SL, Campbell EC, Kondrich J, Mann SC, Cornish J, O'Brien C, Caroff SN: Cocaine abuse in schizophrenic patients treated with olanzapine versus haloperidol. J Nerv Ment Dis 2005; 193:379–386 [A–]

1320. Osborn HH, Tang M, Bradley K, Duncan BR: New-onset bronchospasm or recrudescence of asthma associated with cocaine abuse. Acad Emerg Med 1997; 4:689–692 [D]

1321. O'Donnell AE, Mappin FG, Sebo TJ, Tazelaar H: Interstitial pneumonitis associated with "crack" cocaine abuse. Chest 1991; 100:1155–1157 [G]

1322. Shesser R, Davis C, Edelstein S: Pneumomediastinum and pneumothorax after inhaling alkaloidal cocaine. Ann Emerg Med 1981; 10:213–215 [G]

1323. Leitman BS, Greengart A, Wasser HJ: Pneumomediastinum and pneumopericardium after cocaine abuse. AJR Am J Roentgenol 1988; 151:614 [G]

1324. Levine SR, Brust JC, Futrell N, Brass LM, Blake D, Fayad P, Schultz LR, Millikan CH, Ho KL, Welch KM: A comparative study of the cerebrovascular complications of cocaine: alkaloidal versus hydrochloride: a review. Neurology 1991; 41:1173–1177 [F]

1325. Centers for Disease Control: Urogenital anomalies in the offspring of women using cocaine during early pregnancy: Atlanta, 1968–1980. MMWR Morb Mortal Wkly Rep 1989; 38:536, 541–542 [D]

1326. Chasnoff IJ, Burns WJ, Schnoll SH, Burns KA: Cocaine use in pregnancy. N Engl J Med 1985; 313:666–669 [F]

1327. Ward SL, Bautista DB, Chan L, Derry M, Lisbin A, Durfee MJ, Mills KS, Keens TG: Sudden infant death syndrome in infants of substance-abusing mothers. J Pediatr 1990; 117:876–881 [D]

1328. Fulroth R, Phillips B, Durand DJ: Perinatal outcome of infants exposed to cocaine and/or heroin in utero. Am J Dis Child 1989; 143:905–910 [C]

1329. Behnke M, Eyler FD, Garvan CW, Wobie K: The search for congenital malformations in newborns with fetal cocaine exposure. Pediatrics 2001; 107:E74 [C]

1330. Schneider JW, Chasnoff IJ: Cocaine abuse during pregnancy: its effects on infant motor development: a clinical perspective. Topics in Acute Care and Trauma Rehabilitation 1987; 2:59–69 [F]

1331. Neuspiel DR, Hamel SC, Hochberg E, Greene J, Campbell D: Maternal cocaine use and infant behavior. Neurotoxicol Teratol 1991; 13:229–233 [C]

1332. Delaney-Black V, Roumell N, Shankaran S, Bedard M: Maternal cocaine use and infant outcomes (abstract). Pediatr Res 1990; 25:242A [G]

1333. Frank DA, Augustyn M, Knight WG, Pell T, Zuckerman B: Growth, development, and behavior in early childhood following prenatal cocaine exposure: a systematic review. JAMA 2001; 285:1613–1625 [E]

1333a. Office of National Drug Control Policy: Drug Policy Information Clearinghouse Fact Sheet: Heroin. Rockville, Md, Drug Policy Information Clearinghouse, June 2003. http://www.whitehousedrugpolicy.gov/publications/factsht/heroin/index.html. [G]

1334. Kreek MJ, Vocci FJ: History and current status of opioid maintenance treatments: blending conference session. J Subst Abuse Treat 2002; 23:93–105 [G]

1334a. Auriacombe M, Fatseas M, Dubernet J, Daulouede JP, Tignol J: French field experience with buprenorphine. Am J Addict 2004; 13(suppl 1):S17–S28 [G]

1335. Jansson LM, Velez M, Harrow C: Methadone maintenance and lactation: a review of the literature and current management guidelines. J Hum Lact 2004; 20:62–71 [F]
1336. Mattick RP, Kimber J, Breen C, Davoli M: Buprenorphine maintenance versus placebo or methadone maintenance for opioid dependence. Cochrane Database Syst Rev 2004; CD002207 [E]
1337. Deamer RL, Wilson DR, Clark DS, Prichard JG: Torsades de pointes associated with high dose levomethadyl acetate (ORLAAM). J Addict Dis 2001; 20:7–14 [G]
1338. Mattick RP, Breen C, Kimber J, Davoli M: Methadone maintenance therapy versus no opioid replacement therapy for opioid dependence. Cochrane Database Syst Rev 2003; CD002209 [E]
1339. Farre M, Mas A, Torrens M, Moreno V, Cami J: Retention rate and illicit opioid use during methadone maintenance interventions: a meta-analysis. Drug Alcohol Depend 2002; 65:283–290 [E]
1340. Prendergast ML, Podus D, Chang E: Program factors and treatment outcomes in drug dependence treatment: an examination using meta-analysis. Subst Use Misuse 2000; 35:1931–1965 [E]
1341. Prendergast ML, Urada D, Podus D: Meta-analysis of HIV risk-reduction interventions within drug abuse treatment programs. J Consult Clin Psychol 2001; 69:389–405 [E]
1342. Uchtenhagen A: Swiss Methadone Report: Narcotic Substitution in the Treatment of Heroin Addicts in Switzerland. Zurich, Swiss Federal Office of Public Health, 1996 [G]
1343. Farrell M: A Review of the Legislation, Regulation and Delivery of Methadone in 12 Member States of the European Union: Final Report. Luxembourg, Office for Official Publications of the European Communities, 1996 [G]
1344. Byrne A: Methadone awareness (column comment). Patient Advocacy Newsletter 1998; 3 [G]
1345. Byrne A: Methadone in the Treatment of Narcotic Addiction. New South Wales, Australia, Tosca Press, 1995 [G]
1346. Shinderman M: Antidepressants and MMT methadone awareness (column). Patient Advocacy Newsletter 1997; 2 [G]
1347. Maremmani I, Zolesi O, Aglietti M, Marini G, Tagliamonte A, Shinderman M, Maxwell S: Methadone dose and retention during treatment of heroin addicts with axis I psychiatric comorbidity. J Addict Dis 2000; 19:29–41 [B]
1348. Maremmani I, Canoniero S, Pacini M: Methadone dose and retention in treatment of heroin addicts with bipolar I disorder comorbidity: preliminary results. Heroin Addiction and Related Clinical Problems 2000; 2:39–46 [B]
1349. Ling W, Charuvastra C, Kaim SC, Klett CJ: Methadyl acetate and methadone as maintenance treatments for heroin addicts: a Veterans Administration cooperative study. Arch Gen Psychiatry 1976; 33:709–720 [A]
1350. Strain EC, Stitzer ML, Liebson IA, Bigelow GE: Dose-response effects of methadone in the treatment of opioid dependence. Ann Intern Med 1993; 119:23–27 [A]
1351. Strain EC, Stitzer ML, Liebson IA, Bigelow GE: Methadone dose and treatment outcome. Drug Alcohol Depend 1993; 33:105–117 [A]
1352. Strain EC, Bigelow GE, Liebson IA, Stitzer ML: Moderate- vs high-dose methadone in the treatment of opioid dependence: a randomized trial. JAMA 1999; 281:1000–1005 [A]
1353. Iribarne C, Dreano Y, Bardou LG, Menez JF, Berthou F: Interaction of methadone with substrates of human hepatic cytochrome P450 3A4. Toxicology 1997; 117:13–23 [G]
1354. Langrod J, Lowinson J, Ruiz P: Methadone treatment and physical complaints: a clinical analysis. Int J Addict 1981; 16:947–952 [B]

1355. Corkery JM, Schifano F, Ghodse AH, Oyefeso A: The effects of methadone and its role in fatalities. Hum Psychopharmacol 2004; 19:565–576 [G]
1356. Gordon NB: Psychomotor and intellectual performance under methadone maintenance. Committee on Problems of Drug Dependence, Minutes of the 29th Meeting. Lexington, Ky, National Academy of Sciences, National Research Council, 1967 [G]
1357. Gordon NB: Reaction-times of methadone treated ex-heroin addicts. Psychopharmacologia 1970; 16:337–344 [G]
1358. Gritz ER, Shiffman SM, Jarvik ME, Haber J, Dymond AM, Coger R, Charuvastra V, Schlesinger J: Physiological and psychological effects of methadone in man. Arch Gen Psychiatry 1975; 32:237–242 [G]
1359. Darke S, Sims J, McDonald S, Wickes W: Cognitive impairment among methadone maintenance patients. Addiction 2000; 95:687–695 [D]
1360. Mintzer MZ, Stitzer ML: Cognitive impairment in methadone maintenance patients. Drug Alcohol Depend 2002; 67:41–51 [G]
1361. Preston KL, Bigelow GE, Liebson IA: Effects of sublingually given naloxone in opioid-dependent human volunteers. Drug Alcohol Depend 1990; 25:27–34 [B]
1362. Ling W, Wesson DR, Charuvastra C, Klett CJ: A controlled trial comparing buprenorphine and methadone maintenance in opioid dependence. Arch Gen Psychiatry 1996; 53:401–407 [A]
1363. Strain EC, Stitzer ML, Liebson IA, Bigelow GE: Comparison of buprenorphine and methadone in the treatment of opioid dependence. Am J Psychiatry 1994; 151:1025–1030 [A]
1364. Petitjean S, Stohler R, Deglon JJ, Livoti S, Waldvogel D, Uehlinger C, Ladewig D: Double-blind randomized trial of buprenorphine and methadone in opiate dependence. Drug Alcohol Depend 2001; 62:97–104 [A]
1365. Galanter M, Dermatis H, Glickman L, Maslansky R, Sellers MB, Neumann E, Rahman-Dujarric C: Network therapy: decreased secondary opioid use during buprenorphine maintenance. J Subst Abuse Treat 2004; 26:313–318 [A–]
1366. Eissenberg T, Johnson RE, Bigelow GE, Walsh SL, Liebson IA, Strain EC, Stitzer ML: Controlled opioid withdrawal evaluation during 72 h dose omission in buprenorphine-maintained patients. Drug Alcohol Depend 1997; 45:81–91 [A]
1367. Amass L, Bickel WK, Crean JP, Blake J, Higgins ST: Alternate-day buprenorphine dosing is preferred to daily dosing by opioid-dependent humans. Psychopharmacology (Berl) 1998; 136:217–225 [B]
1368. Bickel WK, Amass L, Crean JP, Badger GJ: Buprenorphine dosing every 1, 2, or 3 days in opioid-dependent patients. Psychopharmacology (Berl) 1999; 146:111–118 [A]
1369. Petry NM, Bickel WK, Badger GJ: A comparison of four buprenorphine dosing regimens in the treatment of opioid dependence. Clin Pharmacol Ther 1999; 66:306–314 [A]
1370. Petry NM, Bickel WK, Badger GJ: A comparison of four buprenorphine dosing regimens using open-dosing procedures: is twice-weekly dosing possible? Addiction 2000; 95:1069–1077 [B]
1371. Davids E, Gastpar M: Buprenorphine in the treatment of opioid dependence. Eur Neuropsychopharmacol 2004; 14:209–216 [F]
1372. Mello NK, Mendelson JH, Kuehnle JC, Sellers MS: Operant analysis of human heroin self-administration and the effects of naltrexone. J Pharmacol Exp Ther 1981; 216:45–54 [A]
1373. Hollister LE: Clinical evaluation of naltrexone treatment of opiate-dependent individuals: report of the National Research Council on Clinical Evaluation of Narcotic Antagonists. Arch Gen Psychiatry 1978; 35:335–340 [G]
1374. Washton AM, Gold MS, Pottash AC: Successful use of naltrexone in addicted physicians and business executives. Adv Alcohol Subst Abuse 1984; 4:89–96 [B]

1375. Cornish JW, Metzger D, Woody GE, Wilson D, McLellan AT, Vandergrift B, O'Brien CP: Naltrexone pharmacotherapy for opioid dependent federal probationers. J Subst Abuse Treat 1997; 14:529–534 [A–]

1376. Pfohl DN, Allen JI, Atkinson RL, Knopman DS, Malcolm RJ, Mitchell JE, Morley JE: Naltrexone hydrochloride (Trexan): a review of serum transaminase elevations at high dosage. NIDA Res Monogr 1986; 67:66–72 [F]

1377. Zukin RS, Sugarman JR, Fitz-Syage ML, Gardner EL, Zukin SR, Gintzler AR: Naltrexone-induced opiate receptor supersensitivity. Brain Res 1982; 245:285–292 [G]

1378. Kleber HD: Treatment of drug dependence: what works. Int Rev Psychiatry 1989; 1:81–100 [F]

1379. Kleber HD: Detoxification from narcotics, in Substance Abuse: Clinical Problems and Perspectives. Edited by Lowinson J, Ruiz P. Baltimore, Md, Williams & Wilkins, 1981, pp 317–338 [F]

1380. Charney DS, Sternberg DE, Kleber HD, Heninger GR, Redmond DE Jr: The clinical use of clonidine in abrupt withdrawal from methadone: effects on blood pressure and specific signs and symptoms. Arch Gen Psychiatry 1981; 38:1273–1277 [B]

1381. Kleber HD, Riordan CE, Rounsaville B, Kosten T, Charney D, Gaspari J, Hogan I, O'Connor C: Clonidine in outpatient detoxification from methadone maintenance. Arch Gen Psychiatry 1985; 42:391–394 [A]

1382. Cami J, de Torres S, San L, Sole A, Guerra D, Ugena B: Efficacy of clonidine and of methadone in the rapid detoxification of patients dependent on heroin. Clin Pharmacol Ther 1985; 38:336–341 [A]

1383. Jasinski DR, Johnson RE, Kocher TR: Clonidine in morphine withdrawal: differential effects on signs and symptoms. Arch Gen Psychiatry 1985; 42:1063–1066 [A]

1384. Fingerhood MI, Thompson MR, Jasinski DR: A comparison of clonidine and buprenorphine in the outpatient treatment of opiate withdrawal. Subst Abus 2001; 22:193–199 [A–]

1385. Spencer L, Gregory M: Clonidine transdermal patches for use in outpatient opiate withdrawal. J Subst Abuse Treat 1989; 6:113–117 [B]

1386. Washton AM, Resnick RB: Clonidine for opiate detoxification: outpatient clinical trials. Am J Psychiatry 1980; 137:1121–1122 [B]

1387. Kleber HD, Topazian M, Gaspari J, Riordan CE, Kosten T: Clonidine and naltrexone in the outpatient treatment of heroin withdrawal. Am J Drug Alcohol Abuse 1987; 13:1–17 [B]

1388. Gold MS, Pottash AC, Sweeney DR, Kleber HD: Opiate withdrawal using clonidine: a safe, effective, and rapid nonopiate treatment. JAMA 1980; 243:343–346 [B]

1389. Vining E, Kosten TR, Kleber HD: Clinical utility of rapid clonidine-naltrexone detoxification for opioid abusers. Br J Addict 1988; 83:567–575 [B]

1390. Collins ED, Kleber HD, Whittington RA, Heitler NE: Anesthesia-assisted vs buprenorphine- or clonidine-assisted heroin detoxification and naltrexone induction: a randomized trial. JAMA 2005; 294:903–913 [A]

1391. Janiri L, Mannelli P, Persico AM, Serretti A, Tempesta E: Opiate detoxification of methadone maintenance patients using lefetamine, clonidine and buprenorphine. Drug Alcohol Depend 1994; 36:139–145 [A]

1392. Nigam AK, Ray R, Tripathi BM: Buprenorphine in opiate withdrawal: a comparison with clonidine. J Subst Abuse Treat 1993; 10:391–394 [A–]

1393. Oreskovich MR, Saxon AJ, Ellis ML, Malte CA, Reoux JP, Knox PC: A double-blind, double-dummy, randomized, prospective pilot study of the partial mu opiate agonist, buprenorphine, for acute detoxification from heroin. Drug Alcohol Depend 2005; 77:71–79 [A]

1394. Kakko J, Svanborg KD, Kreek MJ, Heilig M: 1-year retention and social function after buprenorphine-assisted relapse prevention treatment for heroin dependence in Sweden: a randomised, placebo-controlled trial. Lancet 2003; 361:662–668 [A–]
1395. O'Connor PG, Waugh ME, Schottenfeld RS, Diakogiannis IA, Rounsaville BJ: Ambulatory opiate detoxification and primary care: a role for the primary care physician. J Gen Intern Med 1992; 7:532–534 [B]
1396. Simpson DD, Savage LJ, Lloyd MR: Follow-up evaluation of treatment of drug abuse during 1969 to 1972. Arch Gen Psychiatry 1979; 36:772–780 [C]
1397. Simpson DD, Joe GW, Bracy SA: Six-year follow-up of opioid addicts after admission to treatment. Arch Gen Psychiatry 1982; 39:1318–1323 [C]
1398. Hubbard RL, Marsden ME, Rachal JV: Drug Abuse Treatment: A National Study of Effectiveness. Chapel Hill, University of North Carolina Press, 1989 [C]
1399. Nyswander M, Winick C, Berstein A, Brill I, Kauger G: The treatment of drug addicts as voluntary outpatients: a progress report. Am J Orthopsychiatry 1958; 28:714–727 [G]
1400. Woody GE, McLellan AT, O'Brien CP: Treatment of behavioral and psychiatric problems associated with opiate dependence. NIDA Res Monogr 1984; 46:23–35 [G]
1401. Woody GE, McLellan AT, Luborsky L, O'Brien CP: Twelve-month follow-up of psychotherapy for opiate dependence. Am J Psychiatry 1987; 144:590–596 [A–]
1402. O'Neill K, Baker A, Cooke M, Collins E, Heather N, Wodak A: Evaluation of a cognitive-behavioural intervention for pregnant injecting drug users at risk of HIV infection. Addiction 1996; 91:1115–1125 [A–]
1403. McAuliffe WE: A randomized controlled trial of recovery training and self-help for opioid addicts in New England and Hong Kong. J Psychoactive Drugs 1990; 22:197–209 [A–]
1404. Grabowski J, O'Brien CP, Greenstein R, Ternes J, Long M, Steinberg-Donato S: Effects of contingent payment on compliance with a naltrexone regimen. Am J Drug Alcohol Abuse 1979; 6:355–365 [A–]
1405. Meyer RE, Mirin SM, Altman JL, McNamee HB: A behavioral paradigm for the evaluation of narcotic antagonists. Arch Gen Psychiatry 1976; 33:371–377 [G]
1406. Preston KL, Silverman K, Umbricht A, DeJesus A, Montoya ID, Schuster CR: Improvement in naltrexone treatment compliance with contingency management. Drug Alcohol Depend 1999; 54:127–135 [A–]
1407. Carroll KM, Ball SA, Nich C, O'Connor PG, Eagan DA, Frankforter TL, Triffleman EG, Shi J, Rounsaville BJ: Targeting behavioral therapies to enhance naltrexone treatment of opioid dependence: efficacy of contingency management and significant other involvement. Arch Gen Psychiatry 2001; 58:755–761 [A–]
1408. Fals-Stewart W, O'Farrell TJ, Birchler GR: Behavioral couples therapy for male methadone maintenance patients: effects on drug-using behavior and relationship adjustment. Behavior Therapy 2001; 32:391–411 [A–]
1409. Fals-Stewart W, O'Farrell TJ: Behavioral family counseling and naltrexone for male opioid-dependent patients. J Consult Clin Psychol 2003; 71:432–442 [A–]
1410. Kosten TR, Schumann B, Wright D, Carney MK, Gawin FH: A preliminary study of desipramine in the treatment of cocaine abuse in methadone maintenance patients. J Clin Psychiatry 1987; 48:442–444 [B]
1411. Kosten TR, Gawin FH, Rounsaville BJ, Kleber HD: Cocaine abuse among opioid addicts: demographic and diagnostic factors in treatment. Am J Drug Alcohol Abuse 1986; 12:1–16 [G]
1412. Kosten TR, Rounsaville BJ, Kleber HD: A 2.5-year follow-up of cocaine use among treated opioid addicts: have our treatments helped? Arch Gen Psychiatry 1987; 44:281–284 [C]

1413. Condelli WS, Fairbank JA, Dennis ML, Rachal JV: Cocaine use by clients in methadone programs: significance, scope, and behavioral interventions. J Subst Abuse Treat 1991; 8:203–212 [F]
1414. Anglin MD, Almog IJ, Fisher DG, Peters KR: Alcohol use by heroin addicts: evidence for an inverse relationship; a study of methadone maintenance and drug-free treatment samples. Am J Drug Alcohol Abuse 1989; 15:191–207 [G]
1415. Stimmel B, Cohen M, Sturiano V, Hanbury R, Korts D, Jackson G: Is treatment for alcoholism effective in persons on methadone maintenance? Am J Psychiatry 1983; 140:862–866 [A–]
1416. Stine SM, Freeman M, Burns B, Charney DS, Kosten TR: Effects of methadone dose on cocaine abuse in a methadone program. Am J Addict 1992; 1:294–303 [B]
1417. Schottenfeld RS, Kleber HD: Methadone maintenance, in Comprehensive Textbook of Psychiatry, 6th ed. Edited by Kaplan HI, Sadock BJ. Baltimore, Williams & Wilkins, 1995, pp 2031–2038 [F]
1418. Sellers EM, Ciraulo DA, DuPont RL, Griffiths RR, Kosten TR, Romach MK, Woody GE: Alprazolam and benzodiazepine dependence. J Clin Psychiatry 1993; 54(suppl): 64–75 [G]
1419. Griffiths RR, McLeod DR, Bigelow GE, Liebson IA, Roache JD, Nowowieski P: Comparison of diazepam and oxazepam: preference, liking and extent of abuse. J Pharmacol Exp Ther 1984; 229:501–508 [G]
1420. American Thoracic Society: Diagnostic standards and classification of tuberculosis. Am Rev Respir Dis 1990; 142:725–735; correction, 142:1470 [G]
1421. Dooley SW Jr, Castro KG, Hutton MD, Mullan RJ, Polder JA, Snider DE Jr: Guidelines for preventing the transmission of tuberculosis in health-care settings, with special focus on HIV-related issues. MMWR Recomm Rep 1990; 39:1–29 [G]
1422. Kaltenbach KK, Nathanson L, Finnegan LP: Temperament characteristics of infants born to drug dependent women (abstract). Pediatr Res 1989; 25:15A [D]
1423. Suffet F, Brotman R: A comprehensive care program for pregnant addicts: obstetrical, neonatal, and child development outcomes. Int J Addict 1984; 19:199–219 [B]
1424. Hulse GK, Milne E, English DR, Holman CD: The relationship between maternal use of heroin and methadone and infant birth weight. Addiction 1997; 92:1571–1579 [E]
1425. Hulse GK, Milne E, English DR, Holman CD: Assessing the relationship between maternal opiate use and neonatal mortality. Addiction 1998; 93:1033–1042 [E]
1426. Kandall SR, Doberczak TM, Jantunen M, Stein J: The methadone-maintained pregnancy. Clin Perinatol 1999; 26:173–183 [F]
1427. Carroll KM, Chang G, Behr H, Clinton B, Kosten TR: Improving treatment outcome in pregnant, methadone-maintained women. Am J Addict 1995; 4:56–59 [B]
1428. Jones HE, Haug N, Silverman K, Stitzer M, Svikis D: The effectiveness of incentives in enhancing treatment attendance and drug abstinence in methadone-maintained pregnant women. Drug Alcohol Depend 2001; 61:297–306 [A–]
1429. Jones HE, Haug NA, Stitzer ML, Svikis DS: Improving treatment outcomes for pregnant drug-dependent women using low-magnitude voucher incentives. Addict Behav 2000; 25:263–267 [A–]
1430. Jones HE, Johnson RE, Jasinski DR, O'Grady KE, Chisholm CA, Choo RE, Crocetti M, Dudas R, Harrow C, Huestis MA, Jansson LM, Lantz M, Lester BM, Milio L: Buprenorphine versus methadone in the treatment of pregnant opioid-dependent patients: effects on the neonatal abstinence syndrome. Drug Alcohol Depend 2005; 79:1–10 [A]
1431. Johnson RE, Jones HE, Fischer G: Use of buprenorphine in pregnancy: patient management and effects on the neonate. Drug Alcohol Depend 2003; 70:S87–S101 [F]
1432. Hughes JR, Higgins ST, Bickel WK: Nicotine withdrawal versus other drug withdrawal syndromes: similarities and dissimilarities. Addiction 1994; 89:1461–1470 [F]

1433. Elliott DS, Huizinga D, Menard S: Multiple Problem Youth: Delinquency, Substance Use and Mental Health. New York, Springer-Verlag, 1989 [F]
1434. Burke KC, Burke JD Jr, Regier DA, Rae DS: Age at onset of selected mental disorders in five community populations. Arch Gen Psychiatry 1990; 47:511–518 [G]
1435. Deykin EY, Levy JC, Wells V: Adolescent depression, alcohol and drug abuse. Am J Public Health 1987; 77:178–182 [G]
1436. Mirin SM, Weiss RD, Michael J, Griffin ML: Psychopathology in substance abusers: diagnosis and treatment. Am J Drug Alcohol Abuse 1988; 14:139–157 [F]
1437. O'Brien CP, Charney DS, Lewis L, Cornish JW, Post RM, Woody GE, Zubieta JK, Anthony JC, Blaine JD, Bowden CL, Calabrese JR, Carroll K, Kosten T, Rounsaville B, Childress AR, Oslin DW, Pettinati HM, Davis MA, Demartino R, Drake RE, Fleming MF, Fricks L, Glassman AH, Levin FR, Nunes EV, Johnson RL, Jordan C, Kessler RC, Laden SK, Regier DA, Renner JA Jr, Ries RK, Sklar-Blake T, Weisner C: Priority actions to improve the care of persons with co-occurring substance abuse and other mental disorders: a call to action. Biol Psychiatry 2004; 56:703–713 [G]
1438. Treffert DA: Marijuana use in schizophrenia: a clear hazard. Am J Psychiatry 1978; 135:1213–1215 [G]
1439. Alterman AI, Erdlen DL, Laporte DJ, Erdlen FR: Effects of illicit drug use in an inpatient psychiatric population. Addict Behav 1982; 7:231–242 [G]
1440. Inman DJ, Bascue LO, Skoloda T: Identification of borderline personality disorders among substance abuse inpatients. J Subst Abuse Treat 1985; 2:229–232 [B]
1441. Hesselbrock MN, Meyer RE, Keener JJ: Psychopathology in hospitalized alcoholics. Arch Gen Psychiatry 1985; 42:1050–1055 [G]
1442. Lesieur HR, Blume SB: Pathological gambling, eating disorders, and the psychoactive substance use disorders. J Addict Dis 1993; 12:89–102 [G]
1443. Volkow ND: The reality of comorbidity: depression and drug abuse. Biol Psychiatry 2004; 56:714–717 [G]
1444. Gonzales JJ, Insel TR: The conundrum of co-occurring mental and substance use disorders: opportunities for research. Biol Psychiatry 2004; 56:723–725 [G]
1445. Trocki KF, Leigh BC: Alcohol consumption and unsafe sex: a comparison of heterosexuals and homosexual men. J Acquir Immune Defic Syndr 1991; 4:981–986 [G]
1446. Woody GE, Metzger D, Navaline H, McLellan T, O'Brien CP: Psychiatric symptoms, risky behavior, and HIV infection. NIDA Res Monogr 1997; 172:156–170 [G]
1447. Ausubel DP: Methadone maintenance treatment: the other side of the coin. Int J Addict 1983; 18:851–862 [G]
1448. Kessler RC: The epidemiology of dual diagnosis. Biol Psychiatry 2004; 56:730–737 [F]
1449. Donovan JE, Jessor R: Structure of problem behavior in adolescence and young adulthood. J Consult Clin Psychol 1985; 53:890–904 [G]
1450. Comtois KA, Russo JE, Roy-Byrne P, Ries RK: Clinicians' assessments of bipolar disorder and substance abuse as predictors of suicidal behavior in acutely hospitalized psychiatric inpatients. Biol Psychiatry 2004; 56:757–763 [D]
1451. Cohen S, Lichtenstein E, Prochaska JO, Rossi JS, Gritz ER, Carr CR, Orleans CT, Schoenbach VJ, Biener L, Abrams D: Debunking myths about self-quitting: evidence from 10 prospective studies of persons who attempt to quit smoking by themselves. Am Psychol 1989; 44:1355–1365 [A]
1452. Hughes JR: Clinical implications of the association between smoking and alcoholism, in Alcohol and Tobacco: From Basic Science to Policy: NIAAA Research Monograph 30. NIH Publication 95-3931. Edited by Fertig JB, Allen JP. Washington, DC, US Government Printing Office, 1995, pp 171–185 [F]
1453. Dackis CA, Miller NS: Neurobiological effects determine treatment options for alcohol, cocaine, and heroin addiction. Psychiatr Ann 2003; 33:585–592 [F]

1454. Vanyukov MM, Tarter RE: Genetic studies of substance abuse. Drug Alcohol Depend 2000; 59:101–123 [G]
1455. Substance Abuse and Mental Health Services Administration: Results from the 1992 National Household Survey on Drug Abuse: Main Findings 1992. DHHS Publication (SMA) 94-3012. Rockville, Md, Office of Applied Studies, 1995 [D]
1456. Allan CA, Cooke DJ: Stressful life events and alcohol misuse in women: a critical review. J Stud Alcohol 1985; 46:147–152 [F]
1457. Merikangas KR, Stolar M, Stevens DE, Goulet J, Preisig MA, Fenton B, Zhang H, O'Malley SS, Rounsaville BJ: Familial transmission of substance use disorders. Arch Gen Psychiatry 1998; 55:973–979 [D]
1458. Cloninger CR, Bohman M, Sigvardsson S: Inheritance of alcohol abuse: cross-fostering analysis of adopted men. Arch Gen Psychiatry 1981; 38:861–868 [G]
1459. Cloninger CR: Neurogenetic adaptive mechanisms in alcoholism. Science 1987; 236:410–416 [G]
1460. Wilhelmsen KC, Schuckit M, Smith TL, Lee JV, Segall SK, Feiler HS, Kalmijn J: The search for genes related to a low-level response to alcohol determined by alcohol challenges. Alcohol Clin Exp Res 2003; 27:1041–1047 [G]
1461. Bohman M, Sigvardsson S, Cloninger CR: Maternal inheritance of alcohol abuse: cross-fostering analysis of adopted women. Arch Gen Psychiatry 1981; 38:965–969 [G]
1462. Kendler KS, Heath AC, Neale MC, Kessler RC, Eaves LJ: Alcoholism and major depression in women: a twin study of the causes of comorbidity. Arch Gen Psychiatry 1993; 50:690–698 [D]
1463. Nurco DN, Stephenson PE, Hanlon TE: Aftercare/relapse prevention and the self-help movement. Int J Addict 1990; 25:1179–1200 [G]
1464. Vaillant GE, Milofsky ES: Natural history of male alcoholism, IV: paths to recovery. Arch Gen Psychiatry 1982; 39:127–133 [C]
1465. Vaillant GE: What can long-term follow-up teach us about relapse and prevention of relapse in addiction? Br J Addict 1988; 83:1147–1157 [G]
1466. Vaillant GE: A 20-year follow-up of New York narcotic addicts. Arch Gen Psychiatry 1973; 29:237–241 [C]
1467. Brecht ML, Anglin MD, Woodward JA, Bonett DG: Conditional factors of maturing out: personal resources and preaddiction sociopathy. Int J Addict 1987; 22:55–69 [C]
1468. Schuckit MA: Prediction of outcome among alcoholics. Drug Abuse and Alcoholism Newsletter, 1988; 27(4) [F]
1469. The Robert Wood Johnson Foundation: Substance Abuse: The Nation's Number One Health Problem, 2nd ed. Princeton, NJ, 2001. http://www.rwjf.org/files/publications/other/SubstanceAbuseChartbook.pdf [G]
1470. Risner ME, Goldberg SR, Prada JA, Cone EJ: Effects of nicotine, cocaine and some of their metabolites on schedule-controlled responding by beagle dogs and squirrel monkeys. J Pharmacol Exp Ther 1985; 234:113–119 [G]
1471. Wang PS, Lane M, Olfson M, Pincus HA, Wells KB, Kessler RC: Twelve-month use of mental health services in the United States: results from the National Comorbidity Survey Replication. Arch Gen Psychiatry 2005; 62:629–640 [G]
1472. Substance Abuse and Mental Health Services Administration: Results From the 2004 National Survey on Drug Use and Health: National Findings. DHHS Publication (SMA) 05-4062. Rockville, Md, Office of Applied Studies, 2005 [G]
1473. Annual Medical Examiner Data 1990: Data from the Drug Abuse Warning Network (DAWN) Statistical Series: Series 1, No. 10-B. DHHS Publication (ADM) 91–1840. Rockville, Md, US Department of Health and Human Services, National Institute on Drug Abuse, 1991 [G]

1474. Centers for Disease Control: Alcohol-related mortality and years of potential life lost: United States, 1987. MMWR Morb Mortal Wkly Rep 1990; 39:173–177 [D]
1475. Semaan S, Des Jarlais DC, Sogolow E, Johnson WD, Hedges LV, Ramirez G, Flores SA, Norman L, Sweat MD, Needle R: A meta-analysis of the effect of HIV prevention interventions on the sex behaviors of drug users in the United States. J Acquir Immune Defic Syndr 2002; 30(suppl 1):S73–S93 [E]
1476. Strathdee SA, Galai N, Safaiean M, Celentano DD, Vlahov D, Johnson L, Nelson KE: Sex differences in risk factors for HIV seroconversion among injection drug users: a 10-year perspective. Arch Intern Med 2001; 161:1281–1288 [C]
1477. The Robert Wood Johnson Foundation: Substance Abuse: The Nation's Number One Health Problem: Key Indicators for Policy. Princeton, NJ, 1993 [G]
1478. Hingson R, Winter M: Epidemiology and consequences of drinking and driving. Alcohol Res Health 2003; 27:63–78 [F]
1479. Leonard KE: Alcohol and intimate partner violence: when can we say that heavy drinking is a contributing cause of violence? Addiction 2005; 100:422–425 [G]
1480. National Institute on Drug Abuse: National Pregnancy and Health Survey: Drug Use Among Women Delivering Livebirths. NIH Publication 96-3819. Rockville, Md, National Institutes of Health, 1996 [G]
1481. Centers for Disease Control: Current trends: statewide prevalence of illegal drug use by pregnant women: Rhode Island. MMWR Morb Mortal Wkly Rep 1990; 39:225–227 [D]
1482. Chasnoff IJ, Landress HJ, Barrett ME: The prevalence of illicit-drug or alcohol use during pregnancy and discrepancies in mandatory reporting in Pinellas County, Florida. N Engl J Med 1990; 322:1202–1206 [D]
1483. Kessler RC, McGonagle KA, Zhao S, Nelson CB, Hughes M, Eshleman S, Wittchen HU, Kendler KS: Lifetime and 12-month prevalence of DSM-III-R psychiatric disorders in the United States: results from the National Comorbidity Survey. Arch Gen Psychiatry 1994; 51:8–19 [G]
1484. Mirin SM, Weiss RD: Psychiatric comorbidity in drug and alcohol addiction, in Comprehensive Handbook of Drug and Alcohol Addiction. Edited by Miller NS. New York, Marcel Dekker, 1991, pp 641–661 [G]
1485. Mirin SM, Weiss RD, Greenfield S: Psychoactive substance use disorders, in the Practitioner's Guide to Psychoactive Drugs, 3rd ed. Edited by Gelenberg A, Bassuk E, Schoonover S. New York, Plenum, 1991, pp 243–316 [F]
1486. Weiss RD, Griffin ML, Mirin SM: Diagnosing major depression in cocaine abusers: the use of depression rating scales. Psychiatry Res 1989; 28:335–343 [G]
1487. Crowley TJ, Chesluk D, Dilts S, Hart R: Drug and alcohol abuse among psychiatric admissions: a multidrug clinical-toxicologic study. Arch Gen Psychiatry 1974; 30:13–20 [G]
1488. Centers for Disease Control: The Health Benefits of Smoking Cessation: A Report of the Surgeon General. DHHS Publication (CDC) 90-8416. Washington, DC, US Government Printing Office, 1990 [F]
1489. Public Health Service: Smoking and Health: A Report of the Surgeon General: DHEW Publication (PHS) 79-50066. Washington, DC, US Government Printing Office, 1979 [F]
1490. Lerman C, Patterson F, Berrettini W: Treating tobacco dependence: state of the science and new directions. J Clin Oncol 2005; 23:311–323 [G]
1491. Bilello KS, Murin S, Matthay RA: Epidemiology, etiology, and prevention of lung cancer. Clin Chest Med 2002; 23:1–25 [F]

1492. Whitrow MJ, Smith BJ, Pilotto LS, Pisaniello D, Nitschke M: Environmental exposure to carcinogens causing lung cancer: epidemiological evidence from the medical literature. Respirology 2003; 8:513–521 [E]
1493. Crew KD, Neugut AI: Epidemiology of upper gastrointestinal malignancies. Semin Oncol 2004; 31:450–464 [F]
1494. Ghadirian P, Lynch HT, Krewski D: Epidemiology of pancreatic cancer: an overview. Cancer Detect Prev 2003; 27:87–93 [F]
1495. Yusuf S, Hawken S, Ounpuu S, Dans T, Avezum A, Lanas F, McQueen M, Budaj A, Pais P, Varigos J, Lisheng L: Effect of potentially modifiable risk factors associated with myocardial infarction in 52 countries (the INTERHEART study): case-control study. Lancet 2004; 364:937–952 [G]
1496. Mamun AA, Peeters A, Barendregt J, Willekens F, Nusselder W, Bonneux L: Smoking decreases the duration of life lived with and without cardiovascular disease: a life course analysis of the Framingham Heart Study. Eur Heart J 2004; 25:409–415 [G]
1497. Arcavi L, Benowitz NL: Cigarette smoking and infection. Arch Intern Med 2004; 164:2206–2216 [F]
1498. Kamholz SL: Pulmonary and cardiovascular consequences of smoking. Med Clin North Am 2004; 88:1415–1430, ix–x [F]
1499. Kulig M, Nocon M, Vieth M, Leodolter A, Jaspersen D, Labenz J, Meyer-Sabellek W, Stolte M, Lind T, Malfertheiner P, Willich SN: Risk factors of gastroesophageal reflux disease: methodology and first epidemiological results of the ProGERD study. J Clin Epidemiol 2004; 57:580–589 [G]
1500. Centers for Disease Control: The Health Consequences of Involuntary Smoking: A Report of the Surgeon General. Washington, DC, US Government Printing Office, 1986 [F]
1501. Office of Health and Environmental Assessment: Respiratory Health Effects of Passive Smoking: Lung Cancer and Other Disorders. Publication EPA/600/6-90/006F. Washington, DC, US Government Printing Office, 1992 [F]
1502. Anthenelli RM: Recent advances in the treatment of tobacco dependence. Clinical Neuroscience Research (in press) [F]
1503. Benowitz NL: Toxicity of nicotine: implications with regard to nicotine replacement therapy. Prog Clin Biol Res 1988; 261:187–217 [F]
1504. Brownson RC, Figgs LW, Caisley LE: Epidemiology of environmental tobacco smoke exposure. Oncogene 2002; 21:7341–7348 [F]
1505. Fagerström K: The epidemiology of smoking: health consequences and benefits of cessation. Drugs 2002; 62(suppl 2):1–9 [F]
1506. Hughes JR: Genetics of smoking: a brief review. Behavior Therapy 1986; 17:335–345 [F]
1507. Heath AC, Madden PAF: Genetic influences on smoking behavior, in Behavior Genetic Approaches in Behavioral Medicine: Perspectives on Individual Differences. Edited by Turner JR, Cardon LR, Hewitt JK. New York, Plenum, 1995, pp 45–66 [F]
1508. Swan GE, Carmelli D, Rosenman RH, Fabsitz RR, Christian JC: Smoking and alcohol consumption in adult male twins: genetic heritability and shared environmental influences. J Subst Abuse 1990; 2:39–50 [B]
1509. O"Brien C, Anthony JC, Carroll K, Childress AR, Dackis C, Diamond G, Hornik R, Johnston LD, Jones R, Koob GF, Kosten T, Lerman C, McLellan AT, Moss H, Pettinati H, Spoth R: Substance use disorders, in Treating and Preventing Adolescent Mental Health Disorders: What We Know and What We Don't Know: A Research Agenda for Improving the Mental Health of Our Youth. Edited by Evans DL, Foa EB, Gur RE, Hendin H, O'Brien CP, Seligman MEP, Walsh BT. New York, Oxford University Press, 2005, pp 335–389 [G]

1510. Bauman A, Phongsavan P: Epidemiology of substance use in adolescence: prevalence, trends and policy implications. Drug Alcohol Depend 1999; 55:187–207 [G]
1511. Centers for Disease Control and Prevention: Youth tobacco surveillance: United States, 1998–1999. MMWR CDC Surveill Summ 2000; 49:1–94 [G]
1512. Stanton WR: DSM-III-R tobacco dependence and quitting during late adolescence. Addict Behav 1995; 20:595–603 [G]
1513. Rohsenow DJ, Colby SM, Monti PM, Swift RM, Martin RA, Mueller TI, Gordon A, Eaton CA: Predictors of compliance with naltrexone among alcoholics. Alcohol Clin Exp Res 2000; 24:1542–1549 [A]
1514. John U, Meyer C, Rumpf HJ, Hapke U: Smoking, nicotine dependence and psychiatric comorbidity: a population-based study including smoking cessation after three years. Drug Alcohol Depend 2004; 76:287–295 [G]
1515. Room R, Babor T, Rehm J: Alcohol and public health. Lancet 2005; 365:519–530 [F]
1516. Grant BF, Dawson DA, Stinson FS, Chou SP, Dufour MC, Pickering RP: The 12-month prevalence and trends in DSM-IV alcohol abuse and dependence: United States, 1991–1992 and 2001–2002. Drug Alcohol Depend 2004; 74:223–234 [G]
1517. Alonso J, Angermeyer MC, Bernert S, Bruffaerts R, Brugha TS, Bryson H, Girolamo G, Graaf R, Demyttenaere K, Gasquet I, Haro JM, Katz SJ, Kessler RC, Kovess V, Lepine JP, Ormel J, Polidori G, Russo LJ, Vilagut G, Almansa J, Arbabzadeh-Bouchez S, Autonell J, Bernal M, Buist-Bouwman MA, Codony M, Domingo-Salvany A, Ferrer M, Joo SS, Martinez-Alonso M, Matschinger H, Mazzi F, Morgan Z, Morosini P, Palacin C, Romera B, Taub N, Vollebergh WA: Prevalence of mental disorders in Europe: results from the European Study of the Epidemiology of Mental Disorders (ESEMeD) project. Acta Psychiatr Scand Suppl 2004; (420):21–27 [G]
1518. Hasin DS, Grant BF: The co-occurrence of DSM-IV alcohol abuse in DSM-IV alcohol dependence: results of the National Epidemiologic Survey on Alcohol and Related Conditions on heterogeneity that differ by population subgroup. Arch Gen Psychiatry 2004; 61:891–896 [G]
1519. Smothers BA, Yahr HT, Sinclair MD: Prevalence of current DSM-IV alcohol use disorders in short-stay, general hospital admissions, United States, 1994. Arch Intern Med 2003; 163:713–719 [G]
1520. Jackson KM, Sher KJ, Wood PK, Bucholz KK: Alcohol and tobacco use disorders in a general population: short-term and long-term associations from the St. Louis Epidemiologic Catchment Area study. Drug Alcohol Depend 2003; 71:239–253 [G]
1521. Berglund M, Ojehagen A: The influence of alcohol drinking and alcohol use disorders on psychiatric disorders and suicidal behavior. Alcohol Clin Exp Res 1998; 22:333S–345S [F]
1522. Schuckit MA, Hesselbrock V: Alcohol dependence and anxiety disorders: what is the relationship? Am J Psychiatry 1994; 151:1723–1734 [G]
1523. Swendsen JD, Merikangas KR, Canino GJ, Kessler RC, Rubio-Stipec M, Angst J: The comorbidity of alcoholism with anxiety and depressive disorders in four geographic communities. Compr Psychiatry 1998; 39:176–184 [G]
1524. Farrell M, Howes S, Bebbington P, Brugha T, Jenkins R, Lewis G, Marsden J, Taylor C, Meltzer H: Nicotine, alcohol and drug dependence, and psychiatric comorbidity: results of a national household survey. Int Rev Psychiatry 2003; 15:50–56 [G]
1525. Grant BF, Stinson FS, Dawson DA, Chou SP, Ruan WJ, Pickering RP: Co-occurrence of 12-month alcohol and drug use disorders and personality disorders in the United States: results from the National Epidemiologic Survey on Alcohol and Related Conditions. Arch Gen Psychiatry 2004; 61:361–368 [G]
1526. Gerberich SG, Sidney S, Braun BL, Tekawa IS, Tolan KK, Quesenberry CP: Marijuana use and injury events resulting in hospitalization. Ann Epidemiol 2003; 13:230–237 [D]

1527. Tashkin DP, Baldwin GC, Sarafian T, Dubinett S, Roth MD: Respiratory and immunologic consequences of marijuana smoking. J Clin Pharmacol 2002; 42:71S–81S [F]
1528. Kalant H: Adverse effects of cannabis on health: an update of the literature since 1996. Prog Neuropsychopharmacol Biol Psychiatry 2004; 28:849–863 [F]
1529. Agrawal A, Neale MC, Prescott CA, Kendler KS: A twin study of early cannabis use and subsequent use and abuse/dependence of other illicit drugs. Psychol Med 2004; 34:1227–1237 [G]
1530. Chen CY, Wagner FA, Anthony JC: Marijuana use and the risk of major depressive episode: epidemiological evidence from the United States National Comorbidity Survey. Soc Psychiatry Psychiatr Epidemiol 2002; 37:199–206 [G]
1531. Lynskey MT, Glowinski AL, Todorov AA, Bucholz KK, Madden PA, Nelson EC, Statham DJ, Martin NG, Heath AC: Major depressive disorder, suicidal ideation, and suicide attempt in twins discordant for cannabis dependence and early-onset cannabis use. Arch Gen Psychiatry 2004; 61:1026–1032 [G]
1532. Fergusson DM, Horwood LJ, Swain-Campbell NR: Cannabis dependence and psychotic symptoms in young people. Psychol Med 2003; 33:15–21 [C]
1533. Zammit S, Allebeck P, Andreasson S, Lundberg I, Lewis G: Self reported cannabis use as a risk factor for schizophrenia in Swedish conscripts of 1969: historical cohort study. BMJ 2002; 325:1199 [C]
1534. Patton GC, Coffey C, Carlin JB, Degenhardt L, Lynskey M, Hall W: Cannabis use and mental health in young people: cohort study. BMJ 2002; 325:1195–1198 [C]
1535. van Os J, Bak M, Hanssen M, Bijl RV, de Graaf R, Verdoux H: Cannabis use and psychosis: a longitudinal population-based study. Am J Epidemiol 2002; 156:319–327 [C]
1536. Johnston LD, O'Malley PM, Bachman JG: National Survey Results on Drug Use From the Monitoring the Future Study, 1975–1997, vol I: Secondary school students. NIH Publication 98-4345. Rockville, Md, National Institute on Drug Abuse, 1998 [G]
1537. Substance Abuse and Mental Health Services Administration: Preliminary Results From the 1997 National Household Survey on Drug Abuse. Rockville, Md, Substance Abuse and Mental Health Services Administration, 1998. http://www.oas.samhsa.gov/nhsda/nhsda97/httoc.htm [G]
1538. Abelson HI, Miller JD: A decade of trends in cocaine use in the household population. NIDA Res Monogr 1985; 61:35–49 [F]
1539. Johnston LD, O'Malley PM, Bachman JG, Schulenberg JE: Monitoring the Future: National Survey Results on Drug Use, 1975–2003, vol I: Secondary school students. NIH Publication 04-5507. Bethesda, Md, National Institute on Drug Abuse, 2004 [G]
1540. Gorelick DA: Progression of dependence in male cocaine addicts. Am J Drug Alcohol Abuse 1992; 18:13–19 [C]
1541. O'Brien MS, Anthony JC: Risk of becoming cocaine dependent: epidemiological estimates for the United States, 2000–2001. Neuropsychopharmacology 2005; 30:1006-1018; correction, 30:1588 [G]
1542. Anglin MD, Burke C, Perrochet B, Stamper E, Dawud-Noursi S: History of the methamphetamine problem. J Psychoactive Drugs 2000; 32:137–141 [F]
1543. De Angelis D, Hickman M, Yang S: Estimating long-term trends in the incidence and prevalence of opiate use/injecting drug use and the number of former users: back-calculation methods and opiate overdose deaths. Am J Epidemiol 2004; 160:994–1004 [G]
1544. Hughes JR, Lesmes GR, Hatsukami DK, Richmond RL, Lichtenstein E, Jorenby DE, Broughton JO, Fortmann SP, Leischow SJ, McKenna JP, Rennard SI, Wadland WC, Heatley SA: Are higher doses of nicotine replacement more effective for smoking cessation? Nicotine Tob Res 1999; 1:169–174 [A]

1545. Talwar A, Jain M, Vijayan VK: Pharmacotherapy of tobacco dependence. Med Clin North Am 2004; 88:1517–1534 [F]
1546. Patkar AA, Vergare MJ, Batra V, Weinstein SP, Leone FT: Tobacco smoking: current concepts in etiology and treatment. Psychiatry 2003; 66:183–199 [F]
1547. Sutherland G: Current approaches to the management of smoking cessation. Drugs 2002; 62(suppl 2):53–61 [F]
1548. Karnath B: Smoking cessation. Am J Med 2002; 112:399–405 [F]
1549. Hays JT, Croghan IT, Schroeder DR, Offord KP, Hurt RD, Wolter TD, Nides MA, Davidson M: Over-the-counter nicotine patch therapy for smoking cessation: results from randomized, double-blind, placebo-controlled, and open label trials. Am J Public Health 1999; 89:1701–1707 [A]
1550. Silagy C, Mant D, Fowler G, Lodge M: Meta-analysis on efficacy of nicotine replacement therapies in smoking cessation. Lancet 1994; 343:139–142 [E]
1551. Benowitz NL: Drug therapy: pharmacologic aspects of cigarette smoking and nicotine addition. N Engl J Med 1988; 319:1318–1330 [F]
1552. Henningfield JE, Stapleton JM, Benowitz NL, Grayson RF, London ED: Higher levels of nicotine in arterial than in venous blood after cigarette smoking. Drug Alcohol Depend 1993; 33:23–29 [G]
1553. Perkins KA, Grobe JE, Stiller RL, Fonte C, Goettler JE: Nasal spray nicotine replacement suppresses cigarette smoking desire and behavior. Clin Pharmacol Ther 1992; 52:627–634 [A]
1554. Russell MA, Jarvis MJ, Sutherland G, Feyerabend C: Nicotine replacement in smoking cessation: absorption of nicotine vapor from smoke-free cigarettes. JAMA 1987; 257:3262–3265 [G]
1555. Sutherland G, Russell MA, Stapleton JA, Feyerabend C: Glycerol particle cigarettes: a less harmful option for chronic smokers. Thorax 1993; 48:385–387 [A]
1556. Fiore MC: Treatment options for smoking in the '90s. J Clin Pharmacol 1994; 34:195–199 [G]
1557. Sachs DP: Effectiveness of the 4-mg dose of nicotine polacrilex for the initial treatment of high-dependent smokers. Arch Intern Med 1995; 155:1973–1980 [A]
1558. Davidson M, Epstein M, Burt R, Schaefer C, Whitworth G, McDonald A: Efficacy and safety of an over-the-counter transdermal nicotine patch as an aid for smoking cessation. Arch Fam Med 1998; 7:569–574 [A]
1559. Jorenby DE, Smith SS, Fiore MC, Hurt RD, Offord KP, Croghan IT, Hays JT, Lewis SF, Baker TB: Varying nicotine patch dose and type of smoking cessation counseling. JAMA 1995; 274:1347–1352 [A]
1560. Killen JD, Fortmann SP, Davis L, Strausberg L, Varady A: Do heavy smokers benefit from higher dose nicotine patch therapy? Exp Clin Psychopharmacol 1999; 7:226–233 [A]
1561. Paoletti P, Fornai E, Maggiorelli F, Puntoni R, Viegi G, Carrozzi L, Corlando A, Gustavsson G, Sawe U, Giuntini C: Importance of baseline cotinine plasma values in smoking cessation: results from a double-blind study with nicotine patch. Eur Respir J 1996; 9:643–651 [A]
1562. Gourlay SG, Forbes A, Marriner T, Pethica D, McNeil JJ: Double blind trial of repeated treatment with transdermal nicotine for relapsed smokers. BMJ 1995; 311:363–366 [A]
1563. Bohadana A, Nilsson F, Rasmussen T, Martinet Y: Nicotine inhaler and nicotine patch as a combination therapy for smoking cessation: a randomized, double-blind, placebo-controlled trial. Arch Intern Med 2000; 160:3128–3134 [A]
1564. Cinciripini PM, Cinciripini LG, Wallfisch A, Haque W, Van Vunakis H: Behavior therapy and the transdermal nicotine patch: effects on cessation outcome, affect, and coping. J Consult Clin Psychol 1996; 64:314–323 [B]

1565. Killen JD, Fortmann SP, Davis L, Varady A: Nicotine patch and self-help video for cigarette smoking cessation. J Consult Clin Psychol 1997; 65:663–672 [A]
1566. Campbell IA, Prescott RJ, Tjeder-Burton SM: Transdermal nicotine plus support in patients attending hospital with smoking-related diseases: a placebo-controlled study. Respir Med 1996; 90:47–51 [A]
1567. Herrera N, Franco R, Herrera L, Partidas A, Rolando R, Fagerström KO: Nicotine gum, 2 and 4 mg, for nicotine dependence: a double-blind placebo-controlled trial within a behavior modification support program. Chest 1995; 108:447–451 [A]
1568. Glover ED, Sachs DPL, Stitzer ML, Rennard SI, Wadland WC, Pomerleau OF, Nowak RT, Daughton DM, Glover PN, Hughes JR, Gross J: Smoking cessation in highly dependent smokers with 4 mg nicotine polacrilex. Am J Health Behav 1996; 20:319–332 [A]
1569. Blondal T, Franzon M, Westin A: A double-blind randomized trial of nicotine nasal spray as an aid in smoking cessation. Eur Respir J 1997; 10:1585–1590 [A]
1570. Schneider NG, Olmstead R, Nilsson F, Mody FV, Franzon M, Doan K: Efficacy of a nicotine inhaler in smoking cessation: a double-blind, placebo-controlled trial. Addiction 1996; 91:1293–1306 [A]
1571. Bolliger CT, Zellweger JP, Danielsson T, van Biljon X, Robidou A, Westin A, Perruchoud AP, Sawe U: Smoking reduction with oral nicotine inhalers: double blind, randomised clinical trial of efficacy and safety. BMJ 2000; 321:329–333 [A]
1572. Hurt RD, Offord KP, Lauger GG, Marusic Z, Fagerström KO, Enright PL, Scanlon PD: Cessation of long-term nicotine gum use: a prospective, randomized trial. Addiction 1995; 90:407–413 [A]
1573. Hajek P, West R, Foulds J, Nilsson F, Burrows S, Meadow A: Randomized comparative trial of nicotine polacrilex, a transdermal patch, nasal spray, and an inhaler. Arch Intern Med 1999; 159:2033–2038 [B]
1574. West R, Hajek P, Nilsson F, Foulds J, May S, Meadows A: Individual differences in preferences for and responses to four nicotine replacement products. Psychopharmacology (Berl) 2001; 153:225–230 [G]
1575. Hurt RD, Dale LC, Fredrickson PA, Caldwell CC, Lee GA, Offord KP, Lauger GG, Marusic Z, Neese LW, Lundberg TG: Nicotine patch therapy for smoking cessation combined with physician advice and nurse follow-up: one-year outcome and percentage of nicotine replacement. JAMA 1994; 271:595–600 [A]
1576. Benowitz NL, Jacob P III, Ahijevich K, Jarvis MJ, Hall S, LeHouzec J, Lichenstein E, Henningfield J, Tsoh J, Hurt RD, Velicer W: Biochemical verification of tobacco use and cessation: report from the SRNT Subcommittee on Biochemical Verification. Nicotine Tob Res 2002; 4:149–159 [G]
1577. Hughes JR, Glasser M: Transdermal nicotine for smoking cessation. Health Values 1993; 17:24–31 [F]
1578. Tonnesen P, Paoletti P, Gustavsson G, Russell MA, Saracci R, Gulsvik A, Rijcken B, Sawe U: Higher dosage nicotine patches increase one-year smoking cessation rates: results from the European CEASE trial. Collaborative European Anti-Smoking Evaluation. European Respiratory Society. Eur Respir J 1999; 13:238–246 [A]
1579. Hall SM, Humfleet GL, Reus VI, Munoz RF, Hartz DT, Maude-Griffin R: Psychological intervention and antidepressant treatment in smoking cessation. Arch Gen Psychiatry 2002; 59:930–936 [A–]
1580. Dale LC, Glover ED, Sachs DP, Schroeder DR, Offord KP, Croghan IT, Hurt RD: Bupropion for smoking cessation: predictors of successful outcome. Chest 2001; 119:1357–1364 [A]
1581. Reference not used.

1582. Jorenby D: Clinical efficacy of bupropion in the management of smoking cessation. Drugs 2002; 62(suppl)2:25–35 [F]
1583. Gonzales DH, Nides MA, Ferry LH, Kustra RP, Jamerson BD, Segall N, Herrero LA, Krishen A, Sweeney A, Buaron K, Metz A: Bupropion SR as an aid to smoking cessation in smokers treated previously with bupropion: a randomized placebo-controlled study. Clin Pharmacol Ther 2001; 69:438–444 [A]
1584. Glover ED, Glover PN, Sullivan CR, Cerullo CL, Hobbs G: A comparison of sustained-release bupropion and placebo for smokeless tobacco cessation. Am J Health Behav 2002; 26:386–393 [A]
1585. Dale LC, Ebbert JO, Schroeder DR, Croghan IT, Rasmussen DF, Trautman JA, Cox LS, Hurt RD: Bupropion for the treatment of nicotine dependence in spit tobacco users: a pilot study. Nicotine Tob Res 2002; 4:267–274 [A–]
1586. Hayford KE, Patten CA, Rummans TA, Schroeder DR, Offord KP, Croghan IT, Glover ED, Sachs DP, Hurt RD: Efficacy of bupropion for smoking cessation in smokers with a former history of major depression or alcoholism. Br J Psychiatry 1999; 174:173–178 [B]
1587. Dalsgareth OJ, Hansen NC, Soes-Petersen U, Evald T, Hoegholm A, Barber J, Vestbo J: A multicenter, randomized, double-blind, placebo-controlled, 6-month trial of bupropion hydrochloride sustained-release tablets as an aid to smoking cessation in hospital employees. Nicotine Tob Res 2004; 6:55–61 [A]
1588. Swan GE, McAfee T, Curry SJ, Jack LM, Javitz H, Dacey S, Bergman K: Effectiveness of bupropion sustained release for smoking cessation in a health care setting: a randomized trial. Arch Intern Med 2003; 163:2337–2344 [A–]
1589. Johnston JA, Fiedler-Kelly J, Glover ED, Sachs DP, Grasela TH, DeVeaugh-Geiss J: Relationship between drug exposure and the efficacy and safety of bupropion sustained release for smoking cessation. Nicotine Tob Res 2001; 3:131–140 [A]
1590. Aubin HJ: Tolerability and safety of sustained-release bupropion in the management of smoking cessation. Drugs 2002; 62(suppl 2):45–52 [F]
1591. Horne RL, Ferguson JM, Pope HG Jr, Hudson JI, Lineberry CG, Ascher J, Cato A: Treatment of bulimia with bupropion: a multicenter controlled trial. J Clin Psychiatry 1988; 49:262–266 [A]
1592. da Costa CL, Younes RN, Lourenco MT: Stopping smoking: a prospective, randomized, double-blind study comparing nortriptyline to placebo. Chest 2002; 122:403–408 [A]
1593. Covey LS, Glassman AH: A meta-analysis of double-blind placebo-controlled trials of clonidine for smoking cessation. Br J Addict 1991; 86:991–998 [E]
1594. Gourlay SG, Benowitz NL: Is clonidine an effective smoking cessation therapy? Drugs 1995; 50:197–207 [E]
1595. Cepeda-Benito A: Meta-analytical review of the efficacy of nicotine chewing gum in smoking treatment programs. J Consult Clin Psychol 1993; 61:822–830 [E]
1596. Pomerleau OF, Pomerleau CS: Neuroregulators and the reinforcement of smoking: towards a biobehavioral explanation. Neurosci Biobehav Rev 1984; 8:503–513 [F]
1597. Krishnan-Sarin S, Meandzija B, O'Malley S: Naltrexone and nicotine patch smoking cessation: a preliminary study. Nicotine Tob Res 2003; 5:851–857 [A]
1598. Sutherland G, Stapleton JA, Russell MA, Feyerabend C: Naltrexone, smoking behaviour and cigarette withdrawal. Psychopharmacology (Berl) 1995; 120:418–425 [A]
1599. Cinciripini PM, Lapitsky L, Seay S, Wallfisch A, Meyer WJ III, Van Vunakis H: A placebo-controlled evaluation of the effects of buspirone on smoking cessation: differences between high- and low-anxiety smokers. J Clin Psychopharmacol 1995; 15:182–191 [A]

1600. Schneider NG, Olmstead RE, Steinberg C, Sloan K, Daims RM, Brown HV: Efficacy of buspirone in smoking cessation: a placebo-controlled trial. Clin Pharmacol Ther 1996; 60:568–575 [A]
1601. Dwoskin LP, Crooks PA: A novel mechanism of action and potential use for lobeline as a treatment for psychostimulant abuse. Biochem Pharmacol 2002; 63:89–98 [G]
1602. Glover ED, Leischow SJ, Rennard SI, Glover PN, Daughton D, Quiring JN, Schneider FH, Mione PJ: A smoking cessation trial with lobeline sulfate: a pilot study. Am J Health Behav 1998; 22:62–74 [A]
1603. Niaura R, Spring B, Borrelli B, Hedeker D, Goldstein MG, Keuthen N, DePue J, Kristeller J, Ockene J, Prochazka A, Chiles JA, Abrams DB: Multicenter trial of fluoxetine as an adjunct to behavioral smoking cessation treatment. J Consult Clin Psychol 2002; 70:887–896 [A]
1604. Covey LS, Glassman AH, Stetner F, Rivelli S, Stage K: A randomized trial of sertraline as a cessation aid for smokers with a history of major depression. Am J Psychiatry 2002; 159:1731–1737 [A]
1605. Blondal T, Gudmundsson LJ, Tomasson K, Jonsdottir D, Hilmarsdottir H, Kristjansson F, Nilsson F, Bjornsdottir US: The effects of fluoxetine combined with nicotine inhalers in smoking cessation: a randomized trial. Addiction 1999; 94:1007–1015 [A]
1606. Killen JD, Fortmann SP, Schatzberg AF, Hayward C, Sussman L, Rothman M, Strausberg L, Varady A: Nicotine patch and paroxetine for smoking cessation. J Consult Clin Psychol 2000; 68:883–889 [A]
1607. Berlin I, Said S, Spreux-Varoquaux O, Launay JM, Olivares R, Millet V, Lecrubier Y, Puech AJ: A reversible monoamine oxidase A inhibitor (moclobemide) facilitates smoking cessation and abstinence in heavy, dependent smokers. Clin Pharmacol Ther 1995; 58:444–452 [A]
1608. George TP, Vessicchio JC, Termine A, Jatlow PI, Kosten TR, O'Malley SS: A preliminary placebo-controlled trial of selegiline hydrochloride for smoking cessation. Biol Psychiatry 2003; 53:136–143 [A]
1609. White AR, Resch KL, Ernst E: Randomized trial of acupuncture for nicotine withdrawal symptoms. Arch Intern Med 1998; 158:2251–2255 [A–]
1610. Bier ID, Wilson J, Studt P, Shakleton M: Auricular acupuncture, education, and smoking cessation: a randomized, sham-controlled trial. Am J Public Health 2002; 92:1642–1647 [A–]
1611. Rose JE, Behm FM: Inhalation of vapor from black pepper extract reduces smoking withdrawal symptoms. Drug Alcohol Depend 1994; 34:225–229 [A]
1612. Behm F, Rose JE: Reducing craving for cigarettes while decreasing smoking intake using capsaicin-enhanced low tar cigarettes. Exp Clin Psychopharmacol 1994; 2:143–153 [A]
1613. Butschky MF, Bailey D, Henningfield JE, Pickworth WB: Smoking without nicotine delivery decreases withdrawal in 12-hour abstinent smokers. Pharmacol Biochem Behav 1995; 50:91–96 [A]
1614. Westman EC, Behm FM, Rose JE: Dissociating the nicotine and airway sensory effects of smoking. Pharmacol Biochem Behav 1996; 53:309–315 [A–]
1615. Rose JE, Behm FM, Westman EC, Johnson M: Dissociating nicotine and nonnicotine components of cigarette smoking. Pharmacol Biochem Behav 2000; 67:71–81 [A–]
1616. Levin ED, Behm F, Rose JE: The use of flavor in cigarette substitutes. Drug Alcohol Depend 1990; 26:155–160 [A]
1617. Behm FM, Levin ED, Lee YK, Rose JE: Low-nicotine regenerated smoke aerosol reduces desire for cigarettes. J Subst Abuse 1990; 2:237–247 [A]
1618. Behm FM, Schur C, Levin ED, Tashkin DP, Rose JE: Clinical evaluation of a citric acid inhaler for smoking cessation. Drug Alcohol Depend 1993; 31:131–138 [A]

1619. Westman EC, Behm FM, Rose JE: Airway sensory replacement combined with nicotine replacement for smoking cessation: a randomized, placebo-controlled trial using a citric acid inhaler. Chest 1995; 107:1358–1364 [A]
1620. Glasgow RE, Lichtenstein E: Long-term effects of behavioral smoking cessation interventions. Behavior Therapy 1987; 18:297–324 [F]
1621. Glasgow RE, Klesges RC, Klesges LM, Vasey MW, Gunnarson DF: Long-term effects of a controlled smoking program: a 2 1/2 year follow-up. Behavior Therapy 1985; 16:303–307 [F]
1622. Manske S, Miller S, Moyer C, Phaneuf MR, Cameron R: Best practice in group-based smoking cessation: results of a literature review applying effectiveness, plausibility, and practicality criteria. Am J Health Promot 2004; 18:409–423 [F]
1623. Joseph AM, Rice K, An LC, Mohiuddin A, Lando H: Recent quitters' interest in recycling and harm reduction. Nicotine Tob Res 2004; 6:1075–1077 [C]
1624. Shiffman S, Dresler CM, Rohay JM: Successful treatment with a nicotine lozenge of smokers with prior failure in pharmacological therapy. Addiction 2004; 99:83–92 [A]
1625. Digiusto E, Bird KD: Matching smokers to treatment: self-control versus social support. J Consult Clin Psychol 1995; 63:290–295 [A]
1626. Zelman DC, Brandon TH, Jorenby DE, Baker TB: Measures of affect and nicotine dependence predict differential response to smoking cessation treatments. J Consult Clin Psychol 1992; 60:943–952 [A]
1627. Park EW, Schultz JK, Tudiver F, Campbell T, Becker L: Enhancing partner support to improve smoking cessation. Cochrane Database Syst Rev 2004; CD002928 [E]
1628. Lando HA, Pirie PL, Roski J, McGovern PG, Schmid LA: Promoting abstinence among relapsed chronic smokers: the effect of telephone support. Am J Public Health 1996; 86:1786–1790 [A–]
1629. Donatelle R, Hudson D, Dobie S, Goodall A, Hunsberger M, Oswald K: Incentives in smoking cessation: status of the field and implications for research and practice with pregnant smokers. Nicotine Tob Res 2004; 6(suppl 2):S163–S179 [F]
1630. Corty E, McFall RM: Response prevention in the treatment of cigarette smoking. Addict Behav 1984; 9:405–408 [A]
1631. Lowe MR, Green L, Kurtz SM, Ashenberg ZS, Fisher EB Jr: Self-initiated, cue extinction, and covert sensitization procedures in smoking cessation. J Behav Med 1980; 3:357–372 [A]
1632. Raw M, Jarvis MJ, Feyerabend C, Russell MA: Comparison of nicotine chewing-gum and psychological treatments for dependent smokers. Br Med J 1980; 281:481–482 [B]
1633. Raw M, Russell MA: Rapid smoking, cue exposure and support in the modification of smoking. Behav Res Ther 1980; 18:363–372 [A]
1634. Hajek P, Stead LF: Aversive smoking for smoking cessation. Cochrane Database Syst Rev 2000; CD000546 [E]
1635. Community intervention trial for smoking cessation (COMMIT), II: changes in adult cigarette smoking prevalence. Am J Public Health 1995; 85:193–200 [A]
1636. Marcus BH, Albrecht AE, King TK, Parisi AF, Pinto BM, Roberts M, Niaura RS, Abrams DB: The efficacy of exercise as an aid for smoking cessation in women: a randomized controlled trial. Arch Intern Med 1999; 159:1229–1234 [A–]
1637. McGovern PG, Lando HA: Reduced nicotine exposure and abstinence outcome in two nicotine fading methods. Addict Behav 1991; 16:11–20 [B]
1638. Rychtarik RG, McGillicuddy NB, Connors GJ, Whitney RB: Participant selection biases in a randomized clinical trial of alcoholism treatment settings and intensities. Alcohol Clin Exp Res 1998; 22:969–973 [A–]
1639. Annis HM: Is inpatient rehabilitation of the alcoholic cost-effective? con position, in Controversies in Alcoholism and Substance Abuse. Edited by Stimmel B. New York, Haworth Press, 1986, pp 175–190 [F]

1640. McCrady B, Longabaugh R, Fink E, Stout R, Beattie M, Ruggieri-Authelet A: Cost effectiveness of alcoholism treatment in partial hospital versus inpatient settings after brief inpatient treatment: 12-month outcomes. J Consult Clin Psychol 1986; 54:708–713 [A–]
1641. McLachlan JF, Stein RL: Evaluation of a day clinic for alcoholics. J Stud Alcohol 1982; 43:261–272 [G]
1642. Nace EP, Davis CW, Gaspari JP: Axis II comorbidity in substance abusers. Am J Psychiatry 1991; 148:118–120 [G]
1643. Bunn JY, Booth BM, Loveland Cook CA, Blow FC, Fortney JC: The relationship between mortality and intensity of inpatient alcoholism treatment. Am J Public Health 1984; 84:211–214 [C]
1644. Wiseman EJ, Henderson KL, Briggs MJ: Individualized treatment for outpatients withdrawing from alcohol. J Clin Psychiatry 1998; 59:289–293 [B]
1645. Worner TM: Propranolol versus diazepam in the management of the alcohol withdrawal syndrome: double-blind controlled trial. Am J Drug Alcohol Abuse 1994; 20:115–124 [A]
1646. Adinoff B: Double-blind study of alprazolam, diazepam, clonidine, and placebo in the alcohol withdrawal syndrome: preliminary findings. Alcohol Clin Exp Res 1994; 18:873–878 [A]
1647. Oslin DW, Berrettini W, Kranzler HR, Pettinati H, Gelernter J, Volpicelli JR, O'Brien CP: A functional polymorphism of the mu-opioid receptor gene is associated with naltrexone response in alcohol-dependent patients. Neuropsychopharmacology 2003; 28:1546–1552 [A]
1648. Pettinati HM, Volpicelli JR, Pierce JD Jr, O'Brien CP: Improving naltrexone response: an intervention for medical practitioners to enhance medication compliance in alcohol dependent patients. J Addict Dis 2000; 19:71–83 [B]
1649. Oncken C, Van Kirk J, Kranzler HR: Adverse effects of oral naltrexone: analysis of data from two clinical trials. Psychopharmacology (Berl) 2001; 154:397–402 [G]
1650. Dean RL: The preclinical development of Medisorb Naltrexone, a once a month long acting injection, for the treatment of alcohol dependence. Front Biosci 2005; 10:643–655 [G]
1651. Ciraulo DA, Barnhill J, Boxenbaum H: Pharmacokinetic interaction of disulfiram and antidepressants. Am J Psychiatry 1985; 142:1373–1374 [G]
1652. Kranzler HR, Pierucci-Lagha A, Feinn R, Hernandez-Avila C: Effects of ondansetron in early- versus late-onset alcoholics: a prospective, open-label study. Alcohol Clin Exp Res 2003; 27:1150–1155 [B]
1653. Dodes LM: Addiction and psychoanalysis. Canadian Journal of Psychoanalysis 2003; 11:123–134 [G]
1654. Emrick CD: Alcoholics Anonymous: affiliation processes and effectiveness as treatment. Alcohol Clin Exp Res 1987; 11:416–423 [G]
1655. Ito J, Donovan D: Aftercare in alcoholism treatment: a review, in Treating Addictive Behaviors: Processes of Change. Edited by Miller WR, Heather NH. New York, Plenum, 1986, pp 435–456 [F]
1656. Malison RT, Wright S, Sanacora G, Potenza M, Mechanic K, Haroon E, Carpenter L, Pelton G, Self D, Kosten T, Krystal J, Nestler EJ: Reductions in cocaine-induced craving following the selective D1 dopamine receptor agonist ABT-431 in human cocaine abusers [abstract]. Paper presented at the annual meeting of the College for Problems of Drug Dependence. Scottsdale, Az, June 1998 [B]
1657. Haney M, Collins ED, Ward AS, Foltin RW, Fischman MW: Effect of a selective dopamine D1 agonist (ABT-431) on smoked cocaine self-administration in humans. Psychopharmacology (Berl) 1999; 143:102–110 [A]

1658. Shearer J, Wodak A, Mattick RP, van Beek I, Lewis J, Hall W, Dolan K: Pilot randomized controlled study of dexamphetamine substitution for amphetamine dependence. Addiction 2001; 96:1289–1296 [A–]
1659. Shearer J, Sherman J, Wodak A, van Beek I: Substitution therapy for amphetamine users. Drug Alcohol Rev 2002; 21:179–185 [D]
1660. McCance-Katz EF, Kosten TR, Jatlow P: Disulfiram effects on acute cocaine administration. Drug Alcohol Depend 1998; 52:27–39 [A]
1661. Smelson DA, Ziedonis DM, Losonczy MF, Williams J, Kaune MA: A double-blind study comparing olanzapine to haloperidol for reducing cue-elicited craving in individuals with schizophrenia and cocaine dependence. Schizophr Res 2003; 60:303 [A]
1662. Rawson RA, Huber A, McCann M, Shoptaw S, Farabee D, Reiber C, Ling W: A comparison of contingency management and cognitive-behavioral approaches during methadone maintenance treatment for cocaine dependence. Arch Gen Psychiatry 2002; 59:817–824 [A–]
1663. Flynn PM, Craddock SG, Hubbard RL, Anderson J, Etheridge RM: Methodological overview and research design for the Drug Abuse Treatment Outcome Study (DATOS). Psychol Addict Behav 1997; 11:230–243 [G]
1664. Hartel DM, Schoenbaum EE, Selwyn PA, Kline J, Davenny K, Klein RS, Friedland GH: Heroin use during methadone maintenance treatment: the importance of methadone dose and cocaine use. Am J Public Health 1995; 85:83–88 [G]
1665. Caplehorn JR, Bell J, Kleinbaum DG, Gebski VJ: Methadone dose and heroin use during maintenance treatment. Addiction 1993; 88:119–124 [C]
1666. Newman RG, Whitehill WB: Double-blind comparison of methadone and placebo maintenance treatments of narcotic addicts in Hong Kong. Lancet 1979; 2:485–488 [A]
1667. Jaffe JH: Methadone maintenance, in Further Experience With Methadone in the Treatment of Narcotics Users. Edited by Einstein S. New York, Marcel Dekker, 1971, pp 29–43 [G]
1668. Kosten TR, Schottenfeld R, Ziedonis D, Falcioni J: Buprenorphine versus methadone maintenance for opioid dependence. J Nerv Ment Dis 1993; 181:358–364 [A]
1669. Banys P, Tusel DJ, Sees KL, Reilly PM, Delucchi KL: Low (40 mg) versus high (80 mg) dose methadone in a 180-day heroin detoxification program. J Subst Abuse Treat 1994; 11:225–232 [A]
1670. Rhoades HM, Creson D, Elk R, Schmitz J, Grabowski J: Retention, HIV risk, and illicit drug use during treatment: methadone dose and visit frequency. Am J Public Health 1998; 88:34–39 [A–]
1671. Goldstein A, Judson BA: Efficacy and side effects of three widely different methadone doses, in Proceedings of the Fifth National Conference on Methadone Treatment, March 17–19, 1973. New York, National Association for the Prevention of Addiction to Narcotics, 1973, pp 21–44 [A–]
1672. Goldstein A, Judson BA: Three critical issues in the management of methadone programs, in Addiction. Edited by Bourne PG. New York, Academic Press, 1974, pp 129–148 [G]
1673. Wieland WF, Moffett AD: Results of low dosage methadone treatment, in Proceedings of the Third National Conference on Methadone Treatment. New York, National Association for the Prevention of Addiction to Narcotics and National Institute of Mental Health, 1970, pp 48–49 [D]
1674. Sorensen JL, Hargreaves WA, Weinberg JA: Withdrawal from heroin in three or six weeks: comparison of methadyl acetate and methadone. Arch Gen Psychiatry 1982; 39:167–171 [A]

1675. Stitzer ML, Bigelow GE, Liebson IA: Comparison of three outpatient methadone detoxification procedures. NIDA Res Monogr 1982; 41:239–245 [A–]
1676. Wilson BK, Elms RR, Thomson CP: Outpatient vs hospital methadone detoxification: an experimental comparison. Int J Addict 1975; 10:13–21 [A–]
1677. Senay EC, Dorus W, Goldberg F, Thornton W: Withdrawal from methadone maintenance: rate of withdrawal and expectation. Arch Gen Psychiatry 1977; 34:361–367 [A]
1678. Sees KL, Delucchi KL, Masson C, Rosen A, Clark HW, Robillard H, Banys P, Hall SM: Methadone maintenance vs 180-day psychosocially enriched detoxification for treatment of opioid dependence: a randomized controlled trial. JAMA 2000; 283:1303–1310 [A]
1679. Strang J, Gossop M: Comparison of linear versus inverse exponential methadone reduction curves in the detoxification of opiate addicts. Addict Behav 1990; 15:541–547 [A]
1680. Green L, Gossop M: Effects of information on the opiate withdrawal syndrome. Br J Addict 1988; 83:305–309 [A]
1681. Senay EC, Dorus W, Showalter C: Methadone detoxification: self versus physician regulation. Am J Drug Alcohol Abuse 1984; 10:361–374 [A–]
1682. Robles E, Stitzer ML, Strain EC, Bigelow GE, Silverman K: Voucher-based reinforcement of opiate abstinence during methadone detoxification. Drug Alcohol Depend 2002; 65:179–189 [A–]
1683. Martin WR, Jasinski DR, Haertzen CA, Kay DC, Jones BE, Mansky PA, Carpenter RW: Methadone: a reevaluation. Arch Gen Psychiatry 1973; 28:286–295 [A/C]
1684. Kreek MJ: Medical safety and side effects of methadone in tolerant individuals. JAMA 1973; 223:665–668 [B]
1685. Kreek MJ, Dodes L, Kane S, Knobler J, Martin R: Long-term methadone maintenance therapy: effects on liver function. Ann Intern Med 1972; 77:598–602 [C]
1686. Novick DM, Richman BL, Friedman JM, Friedman JE, Fried C, Wilson JP, Townley A, Kreek MJ: The medical status of methadone maintenance patients in treatment for 11–18 years. Drug Alcohol Depend 1993; 33:235–245 [D]
1687. Krantz MJ, Lewkowiez L, Hays H, Woodroffe MA, Robertson AD, Mehler PS: Torsade de pointes associated with very-high-dose methadone. Ann Intern Med 2002; 137:501–504 [G]
1688. Gil M, Sala M, Anguera I, Chapinal O, Cervantes M, Guma JR, Segura F: QT prolongation and torsades de pointes in patients infected with human immunodeficiency virus and treated with methadone. Am J Cardiol 2003; 92:995–997 [G]
1689. Walker PW, Klein D, Kasza L: High dose methadone and ventricular arrhythmias: a report of three cases. Pain 2003; 103:321–324 [G]
1690. Kornick CA, Kilborn MJ, Santiago-Palma J, Schulman G, Thaler HT, Keefe DL, Katchman AN, Pezzullo JC, Ebert SN, Woosley RL, Payne R, Manfredi PL: QTc interval prolongation associated with intravenous methadone. Pain 2003; 105:499–506 [D]
1691. Martell BA, Arnsten JH, Ray B, Gourevitch MN: The impact of methadone induction on cardiac conduction in opiate users. Ann Intern Med 2003; 139:154–155 [C]
1692. Krantz MJ, Kutinsky IB, Robertson AD, Mehler PS: Dose-related effects of methadone on QT prolongation in a series of patients with torsade de pointes. Pharmacotherapy 2003; 23:802–805 [G]
1693. Eissenberg T, Bigelow GE, Strain EC, Walsh SL, Brooner RK, Stitzer ML, Johnson RE: Dose-related efficacy of levomethadyl acetate for treatment of opioid dependence: a randomized clinical trial. JAMA 1997; 277:1945–1951 [A]
1694. Jaffe JH, Schuster CR, Smith BB, Blachley PH: Comparison of acetylmethadol and methadone in the treatment of long-term heroin users: a pilot study. JAMA 1970; 211:1834–1836 [A]

1695. Karp-Gelernter E, Savage C, McCabe OL: Evaluation of clinic attendance schedules for LAAM and methadone: a controlled study. Int J Addict 1982; 17:805–813 [A–]
1696. Savage C, Karp EG, Curran SF, Hanlon TE, McCabe OL: Methadone/LAAM maintenance: a comparison study. Compr Psychiatry 1976; 17:415–424 [A–]
1697. Freedman RR, Czertko G: A comparison of thrice weekly LAAM and daily methadone in employed heroin addicts. Drug Alcohol Depend 1981; 8:215–222 [A–]
1698. Marcovici M, O'Brien CP, McLellan AT, Kacian J: A clinical, controlled study of L-alpha-acetylmethadol in the treatment of narcotic addiction. Am J Psychiatry 1981; 138:234–236 [A–]
1699. Resnick RB, Orlin L, Geyer G, Schuyten-Resnick E, Kestenbaum RS, Freedman AM: L-Alpha-acetylmethadol (LAAM): prognostic considerations. Am J Psychiatry 1976; 133:814–819 [B]
1700. Senay EC, Dorus W, Renault PF: Methadyl acetate and methadone: an open comparison. JAMA 1977; 237:138–142 [A–]
1701. Taintor Z, Hough G, Plumb M, Murphy BF: L-Alpha-acetylmethadol and methadone in Buffalo: safety and efficacy. Am J Drug Alcohol Abuse 1975; 2:317–330 [A–]
1702. Trueblood B, Judson BA, Goldstein A: Acceptability of methadyl acetate (LAAM) as compared with methadone in a treatment program for heroin addicts. Drug Alcohol Depend 1978; 3:125–132 [G]
1703. Wilson BK, Spannagel V, Thomson CP: The use of L-alpha-acetylmethadol in treatment of heroin addiction: an open study. Int J Addict 1976; 11:1091–1100 [B]
1704. Zaks A, Fink M, Freedman AM: Levomethadyl in maintenance treatment of opiate dependence. JAMA 1972; 220:811–813 [A–]
1705. Ling W, Klett CJ, Gillis RD: A cooperative clinical study of methadyl acetate, I: three-times-a-week regimen. Arch Gen Psychiatry 1978; 35:345–353 [A–]
1706. Judson BA, Goldstein A, Inturrisi CE: Methadyl acetate (LAAM) in the treatment of heroin addicts, II: double-blind comparison of gradual and abrupt detoxification. Arch Gen Psychiatry 1983; 40:834–840 [A]
1707. Fudala PJ, Vocci F, Montgomery A, Trachtenberg AI: Levomethadyl acetate (LAAM) for the treatment of opioid dependence: a multisite, open-label study of LAAM safety and an evaluation of the product labeling and treatment regulations. Journal of Maintenance in the Addictions 1997; 1:9–39 [B]
1708. Nath RP, Upton RA, Everhart ET, Cheung P, Shwonek P, Jones RT, Mendelson JE: Buprenorphine pharmacokinetics: relative bioavailability of sublingual tablet and liquid formulations. J Clin Pharmacol 1999; 39:619–623 [B]
1709. Schuh KJ, Johanson CE: Pharmacokinetic comparison of the buprenorphine sublingual liquid and tablet. Drug Alcohol Depend 1999; 56:55–60 [B]
1710. Strain EC, Moody DE, Stoller KB, Walsh SL, Bigelow GE: Relative bioavailability of different buprenorphine formulations under chronic dosing conditions. Drug Alcohol Depend 2004; 74:37–43 [B]
1711. Gray RF, Ferry A, Jauhar P: Emergence of buprenorphine dependence. Br J Addict 1989; 84:1373–1374 [G]
1712. O'Connor JJ, Moloney E, Travers R, Campbell A: Buprenorphine abuse among opiate addicts. Br J Addict 1988; 83:1085–1087 [G]
1713. Obadia Y, Perrin V, Feroni I, Vlahov D, Moatti JP: Injecting misuse of buprenorphine among French drug users. Addiction 2001; 96:267–272 [G]
1714. Robinson GM, Dukes PD, Robinson BJ, Cooke RR, Mahoney GN: The misuse of buprenorphine and a buprenorphine-naloxone combination in Wellington, New Zealand. Drug Alcohol Depend 1993; 33:81–86 [G]
1715. Singh RA, Mattoo SK, Malhotra A, Varma VK: Cases of buprenorphine abuse in India. Acta Psychiatr Scand 1992; 86:46–48 [G]

1716. Strang J: Abuse of buprenorphine. Lancet 1985; 2:725 [G]
1717. Thirion X, Lapierre V, Micallef J, Ronfle E, Masut A, Pradel V, Coudert C, Mabriez JC, Sanmarco JL: Buprenorphine prescription by general practitioners in a French region. Drug Alcohol Depend 2002; 65:197–204 [G]
1718. Deveaux M, Vignau J: Buprenorphine maintenance treatment in primary care: an overview of the French experience and insight into the prison setting, in Buprenorphine Therapy of Opiate Addiction. Edited by Kintz P, Marquet P. Totowa, NJ, Humana, 2002, pp 69–82 [G]
1719. Strain EC, Clark HW, Auriacombe M, Lagier G, Mallaret M, Thirion X: French experience with buprenorphine. NIDA Res Monogr 2003; 183:134–141 [G]
1720. Mendelson J, Jones RT, Fernandez I, Welm S, Melby AK, Baggott MJ: Buprenorphine and naloxone interactions in opiate-dependent volunteers. Clin Pharmacol Ther 1996; 60:105–114 [A]
1721. Mendelson J, Jones RT, Welm S, Baggott M, Fernandez I, Melby AK, Nath RP: Buprenorphine and naloxone combinations: the effects of three dose ratios in morphine-stabilized, opiate-dependent volunteers. Psychopharmacology (Berl) 1999; 141:37–46 [A]
1722. Mendelson J, Jones RT, Welm S, Brown J, Batki SL: Buprenorphine and naloxone interactions in methadone maintenance patients. Biol Psychiatry 1997; 41:1095–1101 [A]
1723. Preston KL, Bigelow GE, Liebson IA: Buprenorphine and naloxone alone and in combination in opioid-dependent humans. Psychopharmacology (Berl) 1988; 94:484–490 [A]
1724. Stoller KB, Bigelow GE, Walsh SL, Strain EC: Effects of buprenorphine/naloxone in opioid-dependent humans. Psychopharmacology (Berl) 2001; 154:230–242 [A]
1725. Ling W, Charuvastra C, Collins JF, Batki S, Brown LS Jr, Kintaudi P, Wesson DR, McNicholas L, Tusel DJ, Malkerneker U, Renner JA Jr, Santos E, Casadonte P, Fye C, Stine S, Wang RI, Segal D: Buprenorphine maintenance treatment of opiate dependence: a multicenter, randomized clinical trial. Addiction 1998; 93:475–486 [A]
1726. Johnson RE, Eissenberg T, Stitzer ML, Strain EC, Liebson IA, Bigelow GE: A placebo controlled clinical trial of buprenorphine as a treatment for opioid dependence. Drug Alcohol Depend 1995; 40:17–25 [A]
1727. Fudala PJ, Bridge TP, Herbert S, Williford WO, Chiang CN, Jones K, Collins J, Raisch D, Casadonte P, Goldsmith RJ, Ling W, Malkerneker U, McNicholas L, Renner J, Stine S, Tusel D: Office-based treatment of opiate addiction with a sublingual-tablet formulation of buprenorphine and naloxone. N Engl J Med 2003; 349:949–958 [A]
1728. Krook AL, Brors O, Dahlberg J, Grouff K, Magnus P, Roysamb E, Waal H: A placebo-controlled study of high dose buprenorphine in opiate dependents waiting for medication-assisted rehabilitation in Oslo, Norway. Addiction 2002; 97:533–542 [A]
1729. Bickel WK, Johnson RE, Stitzer ML, Bigelow GE, Liebson IA, Jasinski DR: A clinical trial of buprenorphine, I: comparison with methadone in the detoxification of heroin addicts, II: examination of its opioid blocking properties. NIDA Res Monogr 1987; 76:182–188 [A]
1730. Pani PP, Maremmani I, Pirastu R, Tagliamonte A, Gessa GL: Buprenorphine: a controlled clinical in the treatment of opioid dependence. Drug Alcohol Depend 2000; 60:39–50 [A]
1731. Uehlinger C, Deglon J, Livoti S, Petitjean S, Waldvogel D, Ladewig D: Comparison of buprenorphine and methadone in the treatment of opioid dependence: Swiss multicentre study. Eur Addict Res 1998; 4(suppl 1):13–18 [A]
1732. Mattick RP, Ali R, White JM, O'Brien S, Wolk S, Danz C: Buprenorphine versus methadone maintenance therapy: a randomized double-blind trial with 405 opioid-dependent patients. Addiction 2003; 98:441–452 [A]

1733. Fudala PJ, Jaffe JH, Dax EM, Johnson RE: Use of buprenorphine in the treatment of opioid addiction, II: physiologic and behavioral effects of daily and alternate-day administration and abrupt withdrawal. Clin Pharmacol Ther 1990; 47:525–534 [A]
1734. Johnson RE, Eissenberg T, Stitzer ML, Strain EC, Liebson IA, Bigelow GE: Buprenorphine treatment of opioid dependence: clinical trial of daily versus alternate-day dosing. Drug Alcohol Depend 1995; 40:27–35 [A]
1735. Amass L, Bickel WK, Higgins ST, Badger GJ: Alternate-day dosing during buprenorphine treatment of opioid dependence. Life Sci 1994; 54:1215–1228 [A]
1736. Gross A, Jacobs EA, Petry NM, Badger GJ, Bickel WK: Limits to buprenorphine dosing: a comparison between quintuple and sextuple the maintenance dose every 5 days. Drug Alcohol Depend 2001; 64:111–116 [A]
1737. Petry NM, Bickel WK, Badger GJ: Examining the limits of the buprenorphine interdosing interval: daily, every-third-day and every-fifth-day dosing regimens. Addiction 2001; 96:823–834 [A]
1738. Schottenfeld RS, Pakes J, O'Connor P, Chawarski M, Oliveto A, Kosten TR: Thrice-weekly versus daily buprenorphine maintenance. Biol Psychiatry 2000; 47:1072–1079 [A]
1739. Perez de los Cobos J, Martin S, Etcheberrigaray A, Trujols J, Batlle F, Tejero A, Queralto JM, Casas M: A controlled trial of daily versus thrice-weekly buprenorphine administration for the treatment of opioid dependence. Drug Alcohol Depend 2000; 59:223–233 [A]
1740. Amass L, Kamien JB, Mikulich SK: Thrice-weekly supervised dosing with the combination buprenorphine-naloxone tablet is preferred to daily supervised dosing by opioid-dependent humans. Drug Alcohol Depend 2001; 61:173–181 [B]
1741. Bickel WK, Stitzer ML, Bigelow GE, Liebson IA, Jasinski DR, Johnson RE: A clinical trial of buprenorphine: comparison with methadone in the detoxification of heroin addicts. Clin Pharmacol Ther 1988; 43:72–78 [A]
1742. Cheskin LJ, Fudala PJ, Johnson RE: A controlled comparison of buprenorphine and clonidine for acute detoxification from opioids. Drug Alcohol Depend 1994; 36:115–121 [A]
1743. Lintzeris N, Bell J, Bammer G, Jolley DJ, Rushworth L: A randomized controlled trial of buprenorphine in the management of short-term ambulatory heroin withdrawal. Addiction 2002; 97:1395–1404 [A–]
1744. Kosten TR, Kleber HD: Buprenorphine detoxification from opioid dependence: a pilot study. Life Sci 1988; 42:635–641 [B]
1745. Umbricht A, Montoya ID, Hoover DR, Demuth KL, Chiang CT, Preston KL: Naltrexone shortened opioid detoxification with buprenorphine. Drug Alcohol Depend 1999; 56:181–190 [A]
1746. Bickel WK, Amass L, Higgins ST, Badger GJ, Esch RA: Effects of adding behavioral treatment to opioid detoxification with buprenorphine. J Consult Clin Psychol 1997; 65:803–810 [A–]
1747. O'Connor PG, Carroll KM, Shi JM, Schottenfeld RS, Kosten TR, Rounsaville BJ: Three methods of opioid detoxification in a primary care setting: a randomized trial. Ann Intern Med 1997; 127:526–530 [A]
1748. Diamant K, Fischer G, Schneider C, Lenzinger E, Pezawas L, Schindler S, Eder H: Outpatient opiate detoxification treatment with buprenorphine: preliminary investigation. Eur Addict Res 1998; 4:198–202 [B]
1749. DiPaula BA, Schwartz R, Montoya ID, Barrett D, Tang C: Heroin detoxification with buprenorphine on an inpatient psychiatric unit. J Subst Abuse Treat 2002; 23:163–169 [B]

1750. Parran TV, Adelman CL, Jasinski DR: A buprenorphine stabilization and rapid-taper protocol for the detoxification of opioid-dependent patients. Am J Addict 1994; 3:306–313 [D]
1751. Resnick RB, Galanter M, Resnick E, Pycha C: Buprenorphine treatment of heroin dependence (detoxification and maintenance) in a private practice setting. J Addict Dis 2001; 20:75–83 [B]
1752. Vignau J: Preliminary assessment of a 10-day rapid detoxification programme using high dosage buprenorphine. Eur Addict Res 1998; 4(suppl 1):29–31 [B]
1753. Petry NM, Bickel WK, Piasecki D, Marsch LA, Badger GJ: Elevated liver enzyme levels in opioid-dependent patients with hepatitis treated with buprenorphine. Am J Addict 2000; 9:265–269 [B]
1754. Berson A, Fau D, Fornacciari R, Degove-Goddard P, Sutton A, Descatoire V, Haouzi D, Letteron P, Moreau A, Feldmann G, Pessayre D: Mechanisms for experimental buprenorphine hepatotoxicity: major role of mitochondrial dysfunction versus metabolic activation. J Hepatol 2001; 34:261–269 [G]
1755. Berson A, Gervais A, Cazals D, Boyer N, Durand F, Bernuau J, Marcellin P, Degott C, Valla D, Pessayre D: Hepatitis after intravenous buprenorphine misuse in heroin addicts. J Hepatol 2001; 34:346–350 [G]
1756. Lange WR, Fudala PJ, Dax EM, Johnson RE: Safety and side-effects of buprenorphine in the clinical management of heroin addiction. Drug Alcohol Depend 1990; 26:19–28 [A]
1757. Johnson RE, Cone EJ, Henningfield JE, Fudala PJ: Use of buprenorphine in the treatment of opiate addiction, I: physiologic and behavioral effects during a rapid dose induction. Clin Pharmacol Ther 1989; 46:335–343 [B]
1758. Lofwall MR, Stitzer ML, Bigelow GE, Strain EC: Comparative safety and side effect profiles of buprenorphine and methadone in the outpatient treatment of opioid dependence. Addictive Disorders and Their Treatment 2005; 4:49–64 [A]
1759. Cowan A, Lewis JW, Macfarlane IR: Agonist and antagonist properties of buprenorphine, a new antinociceptive agent. Br J Pharmacol 1977; 60:537–545 [G]
1760. Doxey JC, Everitt JE, Frank LW, MacKenzie JE: A comparison of the effects of buprenorphine and morphine on the blood gases of conscious rats. Br J Pharmacol 1982; 75(suppl):118P [G]
1761. Lizasoain I, Leza JC, Lorenzo P: Buprenorphine: bell-shaped dose-response curve for its antagonist effects. Gen Pharmacol 1991; 22:297–300 [B]
1762. Banks CD: Overdosage of buprenorphine: case report. N Z Med J 1979; 89:255–257 [G]
1763. Clark NC, Lintzeris N, Muhleisen PJ: Severe opiate withdrawal in a heroin user precipitated by a massive buprenorphine dose. Med J Aust 2002; 176:166–167 [G]
1764. Reynaud M, Petit G, Potard D, Courty P: Six deaths linked to concomitant use of buprenorphine and benzodiazepines. Addiction 1998; 93:1385–1392 [G]
1765. Tracqui A, Kintz P, Ludes B: Buprenorphine-related deaths among drug addicts in France: a report on 20 fatalities. J Anal Toxicol 1998; 22:430–434 [G]
1766. Gueye PN, Borron SW, Risede P, Monier C, Buneaux F, Debray M, Baud FJ: Buprenorphine and midazolam act in combination to depress respiration in rats. Toxicol Sci 2002; 65:107–114 [G]
1767. Kilicarslan T, Sellers EM: Lack of interaction of buprenorphine with flunitrazepam metabolism. Am J Psychiatry 2000; 157:1164–1166 [G]
1768. Navaratnam V, Jamaludin A, Raman N, Mohamed M, Mansor SM: Determination of naltrexone dosage for narcotic agonist blockade in detoxified Asian addicts. Drug Alcohol Depend 1994; 34:231–236 [A]
1769. O'Brien CP, Greenstein RA, Mintz J, Woody GE: Clinical experience with naltrexone. Am J Drug Alcohol Abuse 1975; 2:365–377 [G]

1770. Resnick RB, Volavka J, Freedman AM, Thomas M: Studies of EN-1639A (naltrexone): a new narcotic antagonist. Am J Psychiatry 1974; 131:646–650 [B]
1771. Volavka J, Resnick RB, Kestenbaum RS, Freedman AM: Short-term effects of naltrexone in 155 heroin ex-addicts. Biol Psychiatry 1976; 11:679–685 [B]
1772. Walsh SL, Sullivan JT, Preston KL, Garner JE, Bigelow GE: Effects of naltrexone on response to intravenous cocaine, hydromorphone and their combination in humans. J Pharmacol Exp Ther 1996; 279:524–538 [A–]
1773. Brahen LS, Henderson RK, Capone T, Kordal N: Naltrexone treatment in a jail work-release program. J Clin Psychiatry 1984; 45:49–52 [B]
1774. Greenstein RA, O'Brien CP, McLellan AT, Woody GE, Grabowski J, Long M, Coyle-Perkins G, Vittor A: Naltrexone: a short-term treatment for opiate dependence. Am J Drug Alcohol Abuse 1981; 8:291–300 [B]
1775. Lewis DC: The clinical usefulness of narcotic antagonists: preliminary findings on the use of naltrexone. Am J Drug Alcohol Abuse 1975; 2:403–415 [B]
1776. Resnick RB, Washton AM: Clinical outcome with naltrexone. Ann N Y Acad Sci 1978; 311:241–247 [B]
1777. Schecter A: Clinical use of naltrexone (EN 1639 A), II: experience with the first 50 patients in a New York City treatment clinic. Am J Drug Alcohol Abuse 1975; 2:433–442 [B]
1778. Taintor Z, Landsberg R, Wicks N: Experiences with naltrexone in Buffalo. Am J Drug Alcohol Abuse 1975; 2:391–401 [G]
1779. Tennant FS Jr, Rawson RA, Cohen AJ, Mann A: Clinical experience with naltrexone in suburban opioid addicts. J Clin Psychiatry 1984; 45:42–45 [B]
1780. Kahn A, Mumford JP, Rogers GA, Beckford H: Double-blind study of lofexidine and clonidine in the detoxification of opiate addicts in hospital. Drug Alcohol Depend 1997; 44:57–61 [A]
1781. Carnwath T, Hardman J: Randomised double-blind comparison of lofexidine and clonidine in the outpatient treatment of opiate withdrawal. Drug Alcohol Depend 1998; 50:251–254 [A]
1782. Lin SK, Strang J, Su LW, Tsai CJ, Hu WH: Double-blind randomised controlled trial of lofexidine versus clonidine in the treatment of heroin withdrawal. Drug Alcohol Depend 1997; 48:127–133 [A]
1783. Walsh SL, Strain EC, Bigelow GE: Evaluation of the effects of lofexidine and clonidine on naloxone-precipitated withdrawal in opioid-dependent humans. Addiction 2003; 98:427–439 [A]
1784. White R, Alcorn R, Feinmann C: Two methods of community detoxification from opiates: an open-label comparison of lofexidine and buprenorphine. Drug Alcohol Depend 2001; 65:77–83 [B]
1785. Gold MS, Redmond DE Jr, Kleber HD: Clonidine blocks acute opiate-withdrawal symptoms. Lancet 1978; 2:599–602 [B]
1786. Gold MS, Redmond DE Jr, Kleber HD: Clonidine in opiate withdrawal. Lancet 1978; 1:929–930 [A]
1787. San L, Cami J, Peri JM, Mata R, Porta M: Efficacy of clonidine, guanfacine and methadone in the rapid detoxification of heroin addicts: a controlled clinical trial. Br J Addict 1990; 85:141–147 [A]
1788. Anton RF, Hogan I, Jalali B, Riordan CE, Kleber HD: Multiple family therapy and naltrexone in the treatment of opiate dependence. Drug Alcohol Depend 1981; 8:157–168 [D]
1789. Rounsaville BJ, Glazer W, Wilber CH, Weissman MM, Kleber HD: Short-term interpersonal psychotherapy in methadone-maintained opiate addicts. Arch Gen Psychiatry 1983; 40:629–636 [A–]

PRACTICE GUIDELINE FOR THE
Treatment of Patients With Schizophrenia
Second Edition

WORK GROUP ON SCHIZOPHRENIA

Anthony F. Lehman, M.D., M.S.P.H., Chair
Jeffrey A. Lieberman, M.D., Vice-Chair
Lisa B. Dixon, M.D., M.P.H.
Thomas H. McGlashan, M.D.
Alexander L. Miller, M.D.
Diana O. Perkins, M.D., M.P.H.
Julie Kreyenbuhl, Pharm.D., Ph.D. (Consultant)

Originally published in February 2004. A guideline watch, summarizing significant developments in the scientific literature since publication of this guideline, may be available in the Psychiatric Practice section of the APA web site at www.psych.org.

CONTENTS

Guide to Using This Practice Guideline 569

Development Process 570

Part A: Treatment Recommendations for Patients With Schizophrenia 571

I. Executive Summary 571
  A. Coding System 571
  B. Formulation and Implementation of a Treatment Plan 571
  C. Establishing a Therapeutic Alliance 572
  D. Acute Phase Treatment 572
  E. Stabilization Phase 574
  F. Stable Phase 574
  G. Other Specific Treatment Issues 576
  H. Treatment Settings and Housing Options 578

II. Formulation and Implementation of a Treatment Plan 579
  A. Psychiatric Management 579
  B. Acute Phase 584
  C. Stabilization Phase 595
  D. Stable Phase 596
  E. Special Issues in Caring for Patients With Treatment-Resistant Illness 601
  F. Clinical Features Influencing the Treatment Plan 602

III. Treatment Settings and Housing Options 616
  A. Choice of Treatment Setting or Housing 616
  B. Common Treatment Settings 616

Part B: Background Information and Review of Available Evidence 623

IV. Disease Definition, Natural History and Course, and Epidemiology 623
  A. Clinical Features 623
  B. Natural History and Course 625
  C. Epidemiology 626

V. Review and Synthesis of Available Evidence 628
  A. Pharmacological Treatments 628
  B. Other Somatic Therapies 663
  C. Specific Psychosocial Interventions 666

Part C: Future Research Directions 676

Individuals and Organizations That Submitted Comments 677

References 678

GUIDE TO USING THIS PRACTICE GUIDELINE

The *Practice Guideline for the Treatment of Patients With Schizophrenia, Second Edition*, consists of three parts (Parts A, B, and C) and many sections, not all of which will be equally useful for all readers. The following guide is designed to help readers find the sections that will be most useful to them.

Part A, "Treatment Recommendations for Patients With Schizophrenia," is published as a supplement to the *American Journal of Psychiatry* and contains general and specific treatment recommendations. Section I summarizes the key recommendations of the guideline and codes each recommendation according to the degree of clinical confidence with which the recommendation is made. Section II is a guide to the formulation and implementation of a treatment plan for the individual patient. Section II.F, "Clinical Features Influencing the Treatment Plan," discusses a range of clinical considerations that could alter the general recommendations discussed in Section II. Section III describes treatment settings and housing options and provides guidance on choice of setting.

Part B, "Background Information and Review of Available Evidence," and Part C, "Future Research Directions," are not included in the *American Journal of Psychiatry* supplement but are provided with Part A in the complete guideline, which is available in print format from American Psychiatric Publishing, Inc., and online through the American Psychiatric Association (http://www.psych.org). Part B provides an overview of schizophrenia, including general information on its natural history, course, and epidemiology. It also provides a structured review and synthesis of the evidence that underlies the recommendations made in Part A. Part C draws from the previous sections and summarizes areas for which more research data are needed to guide clinical decisions.

To share feedback on this or other published APA practice guidelines, a form is available at http://www.psych.org/psych_pract/pg/reviewform.cfm.

DEVELOPMENT PROCESS

This practice guideline was developed under the auspices of the Steering Committee on Practice Guidelines. The development process is detailed in a document available from the APA Department of Quality Improvement and Psychiatric Services: the "APA Guideline Development Process." Key features of this process include the following:

- A comprehensive literature review.
- Development of evidence tables.
- Initial drafting of the guideline by a work group that included psychiatrists with clinical and research expertise in schizophrenia.
- Production of multiple revised drafts with widespread review; four organizations and 62 individuals submitted significant comments.
- Approval by the APA Assembly and Board of Trustees.
- Planned revisions at regular intervals.

Relevant literature was identified through a computerized search of PubMed for the period from 1994 to 2002. Using the keywords schizophrenia OR schizoaffective, a total of 20,009 citations were found. Limiting the search by using the ke words antipsychotic agents, antipsychotic, tranquilizing agents, aripiprazole, olanzapine, ziprasidone, quetiapine, risperidone, clozapine, glycine, beta receptor blockers, antidepressive agents, antidepressant, divalproex, valproic acid, lithium, carbamazepine, benzodiazepines, electroconvulsive therapy, community treatment, psychoeducation, family education, skills training, social support, rehabilitation, case management, community support, supported employment, sheltered workshop, family therapy, family intervention, psychosocial adjustment, cognitive behavior, cognitive training, cognitive therapy, counseling, psychotherapy, group therapy, interpersonal therapy, individual therapy, first break, first episode, new onset, early treatment, and early detection resulted in 8,609 citations. After limiting these references to clinical trials and meta-analyses published in English that included abstracts, 1,272 articles were screened by using title and abstract information. The Cochrane Database of Systematic Reviews was also searched by using the keyword schizophrenia. Additional, less formal literature searches were conducted by APA staff and individual members of the work group on schizophrenia. Sources of funding were considered when the work group reviewed the literature but are not identified in this document. When reading source articles referenced in this guideline, readers are advised to consider the sources of funding for the studies.

This document represents a synthesis of current scientific knowledge and rational clinical practice on the treatment of patients with schizophrenia. It strives to be as free as possible of bias toward any theoretical approach to treatment. In order for the reader to appreciate the evidence base behind the guideline recommendations and the weight that should be given to each recommendation, the summary of treatment recommendations is keyed according to the level of confidence with which each recommendation is made. Each rating of clinical confidence considers the strength of the available evidence and is based on the best available data. When evidence is limited, the level of confidence also incorporates clinical consensus with regard to a particular clinical decision. In the listing of cited references, each reference is followed by a letter code in brackets that indicates the nature of the supporting evidence.

PART A: TREATMENT RECOMMENDATIONS FOR PATIENTS WITH SCHIZOPHRENIA

I. EXECUTIVE SUMMARY

A. CODING SYSTEM

Each recommendation is identified as falling into one of three categories of endorsement, indicated by a bracketed Roman numeral following the statement. The three categories represent varying levels of clinical confidence regarding the recommendation:

[I] Recommended with substantial clinical confidence.
[II] Recommended with moderate clinical confidence.
[III] May be recommended on the basis of individual circumstances.

B. FORMULATION AND IMPLEMENTATION OF A TREATMENT PLAN

Because schizophrenia is a chronic illness that influences virtually all aspects of life of affected persons, treatment planning has three goals: 1) reduce or eliminate symptoms, 2) maximize quality of life and adaptive functioning, and 3) promote and maintain recovery from the debilitating effects of illness to the maximum extent possible. Accurate diagnosis has enormous implications for short- and long-term treatment planning, and it is essential to note that diagnosis is a process rather than a one-time event. As new information becomes available about the patient and his or her symptoms, the patient's diagnosis should be reevaluated, and, if necessary, the treatment plan changed.

Once a diagnosis has been established, it is critical to identify the targets of each treatment, to have outcome measures that gauge the effect of treatment, and to have realistic expectations about the degrees of improvement that constitute successful treatment [I]. Targets of treatment, and hence of assessment, may include positive and negative symptoms, depression, suicidal ideation and behaviors, substance use disorders, medical comorbidities, posttraumatic stress disorder (PTSD), and a range of potential community adjustment problems, including homelessness, social isolation, unemployment, victimization, and involvement in the criminal justice system [I].

After the initial assessment of the patient's diagnosis and clinical and psychosocial circumstances, a treatment plan must be formulated and implemented. This formulation involves the selection of the treatment modalities, the specific type(s) of treatment, and the treatment setting. Periodic reevaluation of the diagnosis and the treatment plan is essential to good clinical practice and should be iterative and evolve over the course of the patient's association with the clinician [I].

C. ESTABLISHING A THERAPEUTIC ALLIANCE

A supportive therapeutic alliance allows the psychiatrist to gain essential information about the patient and allows the patient to develop trust in the psychiatrist and a desire to cooperate with treatment. Identifying the patient's goals and aspirations and relating these to treatment outcomes fosters the therapeutic relationship as well as treatment adherence [II]. The clinician may also identify practical barriers to the patient's ability to participate in treatment, such as cognitive impairments or disorganization and inadequate social resources. Engagement of the family and other significant support persons, with the patient's permission, is recommended to further strengthen the therapeutic effort [I]. The social circumstances of the patient can have profound effects on adherence and response to treatment. Living situation, family involvement, sources and amount of income, legal status, and relationships with significant others (including children) are all areas that may be periodically explored by mental health care clinicians [II]. The psychiatrist can work with team members, the patient, and the family to ensure that such services are coordinated and that referrals for additional services are made when appropriate. The family's needs can be addressed and an alliance with family members can be facilitated by providing families with information about community resources and about patient and family organizations such as the National Alliance for the Mentally Ill (NAMI) [II].

Many patients with schizophrenia require, and should receive, a variety of treatments, often from multiple clinicians. It is therefore incumbent on clinicians to coordinate their work and prioritize their efforts. Because an accurate history of past and current treatments and responses to them is a key ingredient to treatment planning, excellent documentation is paramount [I]. Especially critical, for example, is information about prior treatment efforts and clinical response.

D. ACUTE PHASE TREATMENT

The goals of treatment during the acute phase of treatment, defined by an acute psychotic episode, are to prevent harm, control disturbed behavior, reduce the severity of psychosis and associated symptoms (e.g., agitation, aggression, negative symptoms, affective symptoms), determine and address the factors that led to the occurrence of the acute episode, effect a rapid return to the best level of functioning, develop an alliance with the patient and family, formulate short- and long-term treatment plans, and connect the patient with appropriate aftercare in the community. Efforts to engage and collaborate with family members and other natural caregivers are often successful during the crisis of an acute psychotic episode, whether it is the first episode or a relapse, and are strongly recommended [I]. Family members are often under significant stress during this time. Also, family members and other caregivers are often needed to provide support to the patient while he or she is recovering from an acute episode.

It is recommended that every patient have as thorough an initial evaluation as his or her clinical status allows, including complete psychiatric and general medical histories and physical and mental status examinations [I]. Interviews of family members or other persons knowledgeable about the patient may be conducted routinely, unless the patient refuses to grant permission, especially since many patients are unable to provide a reliable history at the first interview [I]. The most common contributors to symptom relapse are antipsychotic medication nonadherence, substance use, and stressful life events, although relapses are not uncommon as a result of the natural course of the illness despite continuing treatment. If nonadherence is suspected, it is recommended that the reasons for it be evaluated and considered in the treatment plan. General medical health as well as medical conditions that could contribute to symptom exacerbation can be evaluated by medical history, physical and neurological examination, and appropriate laboratory, electrophysiological, and radiological assessments [I]. Measurement of body weight and vital signs (heart rate, blood pressure, temperature) is also recommended [II]. Other laboratory tests to be considered to evaluate health status include a CBC; measurements of blood electrolytes, glucose, cholesterol, and triglycerides; tests of liver, renal, and thyroid function; a syphilis test; and when indicated and permissible, determination of HIV status and a test for hepatitis C [II]. Routine evaluation of substance use with a toxicology screen is also recommended as part of the medical evaluation [I]. A pregnancy test should be strongly considered for women with childbearing potential [II]. In patients for whom the clinical picture is unclear or where there are abnormal findings from a routine examination, more detailed studies (e.g., screening for heavy metal toxins, EEG, magnetic resonance imaging [MRI] scan, or computed tomography [CT] scan) may be indicated [II].

It is important to pay special attention to the presence of suicidal potential and the presence of command hallucinations and take precautions whenever there is any question about a patient's suicidal intent, since prior suicide attempts, current depressed mood, and suicidal ideation can be predictive of a subsequent suicide attempt in schizophrenia [I]. Similar evaluations are recommended in considering the likelihood of dangerous or aggressive behavior and whether the person will harm someone else or engage in other forms of violence [I].

It is recommended that pharmacological treatment be initiated promptly, provided it will not interfere with diagnostic assessment, because acute psychotic exacerbations are associated with emotional distress, disruption to the patient's life, and a substantial risk of dangerous behaviors to self, others, or property [I]. Before the patient begins treatment with antipsychotic medication, it is suggested that the treating physician, as is feasible, discuss the potential risks and benefits of the medication with the patient [I]. The selection of an antipsychotic medication is frequently guided by the patient's previous experience with antipsychotics, including the degree of symptom response, past experience of side effects, and preferred route of medication administration. In choosing among these medications, the psychiatrist may consider the patient's past responses to treatment, the medication's side effect profile (including subjective responses, such as a dysphoric response to a medication), the patient's preferences for a particular medication based on past experience, the intended route of administration, the presence of comorbid medical conditions, and potential interactions with other prescribed medications [I]. Finally, while most patients prefer oral medication, patients with recurrent relapses related to nonadherence are candidates for a long-acting injectable antipsychotic medication, as are patients who prefer this mode of administration [II].

The recommended dose is that which is both effective and not likely to cause side effects that are subjectively difficult to tolerate, since the experience of unpleasant side effects may affect long-term adherence [I]. The dose may be titrated as quickly as tolerated to the target therapeutic dose of the antipsychotic medication, and unless there is evidence that the patient is having uncomfortable side effects, monitoring of the patient's clinical status for 2–4 weeks is warranted to evaluate the patient's response to the treatment [II]. During these weeks it is often important for physicians to be patient and avoid the temptation to prematurely escalate the dose for patients who are responding slowly [I]. If the patient is not improving, it may be helpful to establish whether the lack of response can be explained by medication nonadherence, rapid medication metabolism, or poor absorption [II].

Adjunctive medications are also commonly prescribed for comorbid conditions in the acute phase. Benzodiazepines may be used to treat catatonia as well as to manage both anxiety and agitation until the antipsychotic has had time to be therapeutically effective [II]. Antidepressants can be considered for treating comorbid major depression or obsessive-compulsive disorder, although vigilance to protect against the risk of exacerbation of psychosis with some antidepressants is important [II]. Mood stabilizers and beta-blockers may be considered for reducing the severity of recurrent hostility and aggression [II]. Careful attention must be paid to potential drug-drug interactions, especially those related to metabolism by cytochrome P450 enzymes [I].

Psychosocial interventions in the acute phase are aimed at reducing overstimulating or stressful relationships, environments, or life events and at promoting relaxation or reduced arousal through simple, clear, coherent communications and expectations; a structured and predictable environment; low performance requirements; and tolerant, nondemanding, supportive relationships with the psychiatrist and other members of the treatment team. Providing information to the patient and the family on the nature and management of the illness that is appropriate to the patient's capacity to assimilate information is recommended [II]. Patients can be encouraged to collaborate with the psychiatrist in selecting and adjusting the medication and other treatments provided [II].

The acute phase is also the best time for the psychiatrist to initiate a relationship with family members, who tend to be particularly concerned about the patient's disorder, disability, and prognosis during the acute phase and during hospitalization [I]. Educational meetings, "survival workshops" that teach the family how to cope with schizophrenia, and referrals to local chapters of patient and family organizations such as NAMI may be helpful and are recommended [III]. Family members may be under considerable stress, particularly if the patient has been exhibiting dangerous or unstable behavior.

E. STABILIZATION PHASE

During the stabilization phase, the goals of treatment are to reduce stress on the patient and provide support to minimize the likelihood of relapse, enhance the patient's adaptation to life in the community, facilitate continued reduction in symptoms and consolidation of remission, and promote the process of recovery. If the patient has improved with a particular medication regimen, continuation of that regimen and monitoring are recommended for at least 6 months [I]. Premature lowering of dose or discontinuation of medication during this phase may lead to a recurrence of symptoms and possible relapse. It is also critical to assess continuing side effects that may have been present in the acute phase and to adjust pharmacotherapy accordingly to minimize adverse side effects that may otherwise lead to medication nonadherence and relapse [I].

Psychosocial interventions remain supportive but may be less structured and directive than in the acute phase [III]. Education about the course and outcome of the illness and about factors that influence the course and outcome, including treatment adherence, can begin in this phase for patients and continue for family members [II].

It is important that there be no gaps in service delivery, because patients are particularly vulnerable to relapse after an acute episode and need support in resuming their normal life and activities in the community [I]. For hospitalized patients, it is frequently beneficial to arrange an appointment with an outpatient psychiatrist and, for patients who will reside in a community residence, to arrange a visit before discharge [II]. Adjustment to life in the community for patients can be facilitated through realistic goal setting without undue pressure to perform at high levels vocationally and socially, since unduly ambitious expectations can be stressful and can increase the risk of relapse [I]. While it is critical not to place premature demands on the patient regarding engagement in community-based activities and rehabilitation services, it is equally critical to maintain a level of momentum aimed at improving community functioning in order to instill a sense of hope and progress for the patient and family [I].

F. STABLE PHASE

The goals of treatment during the stable phase are to ensure that symptom remission or control is sustained, that the patient is maintaining or improving his or her level of functioning and quality of life, that increases in symptoms or relapses are effectively treated, and that monitoring for adverse treatment effects continues. Regular monitoring for adverse effects is recommended [I]. If the patient agrees, it is helpful to maintain strong ties with persons who interact with the patient frequently and would therefore be most likely to notice any resurgence of symptoms and the occurrence of life stresses and events that may increase the risk of relapse or impede continuing functional recovery [II]. For most persons with schizophrenia in the stable phase, psychosocial interventions are recommended as a useful adjunctive treatment to pharmacological treatment and may improve outcomes [I].

Antipsychotic medications substantially reduce the risk of relapse in the stable phase of illness and are strongly recommended [I]. Deciding on the dose of an antipsychotic medication during the stable phase is complicated by the fact that there is no reliable strategy available to identify the minimum effective dose to prevent relapse. For most patients treated with first-generation antipsychotics, a dose is recommended that is around the "extrapyramidal symptom (EPS) threshold" (i.e., the dose that will induce extrapyramidal side effects with minimal rigidity detectable on physical examination), since studies indicate that higher doses are usually not more efficacious and increase the risk of subjectively intolerable side effects [II]. Lower doses of first-generation antipsychotic medications may be associated with improved adherence and better subjective state and perhaps ultimately better functioning. Second-generation antipsychotics can generally be administered at doses that are therapeutic yet well below the "EPS threshold." The advantages of decreasing antipsychotic doses to minimize side effects can be weighed against the disadvantage of a somewhat greater risk of relapse and more frequent exacerbations of schizophrenic symptoms. In general, it is more important to prevent relapse and maintain the stability of the patient [III].

The available antipsychotic medications are associated with differential risk of a variety of side effects, including neurological, metabolic, sexual, endocrine, sedative, and cardiovascular side effects. Monitoring of side effects based on the side effect profile of the prescribed antipsychotic is warranted. During the stable phase of treatment it is important to routinely monitor all patients treated with antipsychotics for extrapyramidal side effects and the development of tardive dyskinesia [I]. Because of the risk of weight gain associated with many antipsychotics, regular measurement of weight and body mass index (BMI) is recommended [I]. Routine monitoring for obesity-related health problems (e.g., high blood pressure, lipid abnormalities, and clinical symptoms of diabetes) and consideration of appropriate interventions are recommended particularly for patients with BMI in the overweight and obese ranges [II]. Clinicians may consider regular monitoring of fasting glucose or hemoglobin A1c levels to detect emerging diabetes, since patients often have multiple risk factors for diabetes, especially patients with obesity [I].

Antipsychotic treatment often results in substantial improvement or even remission of positive symptoms. However, most patients remain functionally impaired because of negative symptoms, cognitive deficits, and limited social function. It is important to evaluate whether residual negative symptoms are in fact secondary to a parkinsonian syndrome or untreated major depression, since interventions are available to address these causes of negative symptoms [II].

Most patients who develop schizophrenia and related psychotic disorders are at very high risk of relapse in the absence of antipsychotic treatment. Unfortunately, there is no reliable indicator to differentiate the minority who will not from the majority who will relapse with drug discontinuation. It is important to discuss with the patient the risks of relapse versus the long-term potential risks of maintenance treatment with the prescribed antipsychotic [I]. If a decision is made to discontinue antipsychotic medication, additional precautions to minimize the risk of a psychotic relapse are warranted. Educating the patient and family members about early signs of relapse, advising them to develop plans for action should these signs appear, and encouraging the patient to attend outpatient visits on a regular basis are warranted [I]. Indefinite maintenance antipsychotic medication is recommended for patients who have had multiple prior episodes or two episodes within 5 years [I]. In patients for whom antipsychotic medications have been prescribed, monitoring for signs and symptoms of impending or actual relapse is recommended [I].

Adjunctive medications are commonly prescribed for comorbid conditions of patients in the stable phase. Comorbid major depression and obsessive-compulsive disorder may respond to antidepressant medications [II]. Mood stabilizers may also address prominent mood lability [II]. Benzodiazepines may be helpful for managing anxiety and insomnia during the stable phase of treatment [II].

In assessing treatment resistance or partial response, it is important to carefully evaluate whether the patient has had an adequate trial of an antipsychotic medication, including whether the dose is adequate and whether the patient has been taking the medication as prescribed. An initial trial of 4–6 weeks generally is needed to determine if the patient will have any symptomatic response, and symptoms can continue to improve over 6 months or even longer periods of antipsychotic treatment [II]. Given clozapine's superior efficacy, a clozapine trial should be considered for a patient who has had no response or partial and suboptimal response to two trials of antipsychotic medication (at least one second-generation agent) or for a patient with persistent suicidal ideation or behavior that has not responded to other treatments [I].

A number of psychosocial treatments have demonstrated effectiveness during the stable phase. They include family intervention [I], supported employment [I], assertive community treatment [I], skills training [II], and cognitive behaviorally oriented psychotherapy [II]. In the same way that psychopharmacological management must be individually tailored to the needs and preferences of the patient, so too should the selection of psychosocial treatments [I]. The selection of appropriate psychosocial treatments is guided by the circumstances of the individual patient's needs and social context [II].

Interventions that educate family members about schizophrenia are needed to provide support and offer training in effective problem solving and communication, reduce symptom relapse, and contribute to improved patient functioning and family well-being [I]. The Program for Assertive Community Treatment (PACT) is a specific model of community-based care that is needed to treat patients who are at high risk for hospital readmission and who cannot be maintained by more usual community-based treatment [I]. Persons with schizophrenia who have residual psychotic symptoms while receiving adequate pharmacotherapy also may be offered cognitive behaviorally oriented psychotherapy [II].

Supported employment is an approach to improve vocational functioning among persons with various types of disabilities, including schizophrenia, and should be made available [I]. The evidence-based supported employment programs that have been found effective include the key elements of services focused on competitive employment, eligibility based on the consumer's choice, rapid job search, integration of rehabilitation and mental health care, attention to the consumer's preferences, and time-unlimited and individualized support.

Social skills training may be helpful in addressing functional impairments with social skills or activities of daily living [II]. The key elements of this intervention include behaviorally based instruction, modeling, corrective feedback, and contingent social reinforcement.

Treatment programs need to combine medications with a range of psychosocial services to reduce the need for crisis-oriented hospitalizations and emergency department visits and enable greater recovery [I].

G. OTHER SPECIFIC TREATMENT ISSUES

1. First episode

It is important to treat schizophrenia in its initial episode as soon as possible [II]. When a patient presents with a first-episode psychosis, close observation and documentation of the signs and symptoms over time are important because first episodes of psychosis can be polymorphic and evolve into a variety of specific disorders (e.g., schizophreniform disorder, bipolar disorder, schizoaffective disorder) [I]. Furthermore, in persons who meet the criteria for being prodromally symptomatic and at risk for psychosis in the near future, careful assessment and frequent monitoring are recommended until symptoms remit spontaneously, evolve into schizophrenia, or evolve into another diagnosable and treatable mental disorder [III]. The majority of first-episode patients are responsive to treatment, with more than 70% achieving remission of psychotic signs and symptoms within 3–4 months and 83% achieving stable remission at the end of 1 year. First-episode patients are generally more sensitive to the therapeutic effects and side effects of medications and often require lower doses than patients with chronic schizophrenia. Minimizing risk of relapse in a remitted patient is a high priority, given the potential clinical, social, and vocational costs of relapse [I]. Family members are especially in need of education and support at the time of the patient's first episode [I].

2. Negative symptoms

Treatment of negative symptoms begins with assessing the patient for syndromes that can cause the appearance of secondary negative symptoms [I]. The treatment of such secondary negative symptoms consists of treating their cause, e.g., antipsychotics for primary positive symptoms, antidepressants for depression, anxiolytics for anxiety disorders, or antiparkinsonian agents or antipsychotic dose reduction for extrapyramidal side effects [III]. If negative symptoms persist, they are presumed to be primary negative symptoms of the deficit state. There are no treatments with proven efficacy for primary negative symptoms.

3. Substance use disorders

Nearly one-half of patients with schizophrenia have comorbid substance use disorders, excluding nicotine abuse/dependence, which itself exceeds 50% in prevalence in this group. The goals of treatment for patients with schizophrenia who also have a substance use disorder are the same as those for treatment of patients with schizophrenia without comorbidity but with the addition of the goals for the treatment of substance use disorders, e.g., harm reduction, abstinence, relapse prevention, and rehabilitation. A comprehensive integrated treatment model is recommended in which the same clinicians or team of clinicians provide treatment for schizophrenia as well as treatment of substance use disorders [III]. This form of treatment features assertive outreach, case management, family interventions, housing, rehabilitation, and pharmacotherapy. It also includes behavioral interventions for those who are trying to attain or maintain abstinence and a stage-wise motivational approach for patients who do not recognize the need for treatment of a substance use disorder.

4. Depression

Depressive symptoms are common at all phases of schizophrenia. A careful differential diagnosis that considers the contributions of side effects of antipsychotic medications, demoralization, the negative symptoms of schizophrenia, and substance intoxication or withdrawal is recommended [I]. Depressive symptoms that occur during the acute psychotic phase usually improve as patients recover from the psychosis. There is also evidence to suggest that depressive symptoms are reduced by antipsychotic treatment, with comparison trials finding that second-generation antipsychotics may have greater efficacy for depressive symptoms than first-generation antipsychotics [II]. Antidepressants may be added as an adjunct to antipsychotics when the depressive symptoms meet the syndromal criteria for major depressive disorder or are severe, causing significant distress or interfering with function [II].

5. Suicidal and aggressive behaviors

Suicide is the leading cause of premature death among patients with schizophrenia. Some risk factors for suicide among patients with schizophrenia are the same as those for the general population: male gender, white race, single marital status, social isolation, unemployment, a family history of suicide, previous suicide attempts, substance use disorders, depression or hopelessness, and a significant recent adverse life event. Specific demographic risk factors for suicide among persons with schizophrenia are young age, high socioeconomic status background, high IQ with a high level of premorbid scholastic achievement, high aspirations and expectations, early age at onset/first hospitalization, a chronic and deteriorating course with many relapses, and greater insight into the illness.

Despite identification of these risk factors, it is not possible to predict whether an individual patient will attempt suicide or die by suicide. It is important to consider suicide risk at all stages of the illness and to perform an initial suicide risk assessment and regular evaluation of suicide risk as part of each patient's psychiatric evaluation [I]. There is evidence to suggest that both first- and second-generation antipsychotic medications may reduce the risk of suicide. However, clozapine is the most extensively studied and has been shown to reduce the rates of suicide [II] and persistent suicidal behavior [I].

During a hospitalization, use of suicide precautions and careful monitoring over time for suicidal patients are essential [I]. Upon discharge, the patient and the family members may be advised to look for warning signs and to initiate specific contingency plans if suicidal ideation recurs [I]. After a recent discharge from the hospital, a higher frequency of outpatient visits is recommended, and the number of visits may need to be increased during times of personal crisis, significant environmental changes, heightened distress, or deepening depression during the course of illness [III].

A minority of patients with schizophrenia have an increased risk for aggressive behavior. The risk for aggressive behavior increases with comorbid alcohol abuse, substance abuse, antisocial personality, or neurological impairment. Identifying risk factors for aggressive behavior and assessment of dangerousness are part of a standard psychiatric evaluation [I].

H. TREATMENT SETTINGS AND HOUSING OPTIONS

Patients with schizophrenia may receive care in a variety of settings. In general, patients should be cared for in the least restrictive setting that is likely to be safe and to allow for effective treatment [I]. Indications for hospitalization usually include the patient's being considered to pose a serious threat of harm to self or others or being unable to care for self and needing constant supervision or support [I]. Other possible indications for hospitalization include general medical or psychiatric problems that make outpatient treatment unsafe or ineffective [III] or new onset of psychosis [III]. Efforts should be made to hospitalize such patients voluntarily [I].

Treatment programs that emphasize highly structured behavioral techniques, including a token economy, point systems, and skills training that can improve patients' functioning, are recommended for patients with treatment-resistant schizophrenia who require long-term hospitalization [I].

When it is uncertain whether the patient needs to be hospitalized, alternative treatment in the community, such as day hospitalization, home care, family crisis therapy, crisis residential care, or assertive community treatment, should be considered [III]. Day hospitalization can be used as an immediate alternative to inpatient care for acutely psychotic patients or used to continue stabilization after a brief hospital stay [III].

Day treatment programs can be used to provide ongoing supportive care for marginally adjusted patients with schizophrenia in the later part of the stabilization phase and the stable phase of illness, and such programs are usually not time-limited [III]. The goals are to provide structure, support, and treatment to help prevent relapse and to maintain and gradually improve the patient's social functioning [III].

II. FORMULATION AND IMPLEMENTATION OF A TREATMENT PLAN

Because schizophrenia is a chronic illness that affects virtually all aspects of life of affected persons, treatment planning has three goals: 1) reduce or eliminate symptoms, 2) maximize quality of life and adaptive functioning, and 3) enable recovery by assisting patients in attaining personal life goals (e.g., in work, housing, and relationships). For purposes of presentation throughout this guideline, the course of treatment for persons with schizophrenia is divided into three phases: acute, stabilization, and stable. The acute phase begins with a new onset or acute exacerbation of symptoms and spans the period until these symptoms are reduced to a level considered to be the patient's expected "baseline." The stabilization period follows the acute phase and constitutes a time-limited transition to continuing treatment in the stable phase. Combined, the acute and stabilization phases generally span approximately 6 months. The stable phase represents a prolonged period of treatment and rehabilitation during which symptoms are under adequate control and the focus is on improving functioning and recovery. While these distinctions may be somewhat arbitrary, they provide a useful framework for discussion of treatment.

Many of the advances in the treatment of schizophrenia over the past two decades have come from recognition of the complexities of the manifestations and the different stages of the illness. These insights into the multiple components of psychopathology in schizophrenia and into the role of family, social, and other environmental factors in influencing both psychopathology and adaptation have resulted in development of a wide range of treatments that target specific aspects of the illness. Recognition of the different stages of the illness has led to various approaches in treatment planning, treatment selection, and drug dosing. Fragmentation of services and treatments has long been a problem in delivering comprehensive care to persons with schizophrenia. This fragmentation is determined by several factors, including the use of many different treatment settings, the necessary involvement of several professional disciplines, and the use of multiple funding streams, coupled with inadequate insurance coverage and the decline in funding for public and private mental health services, to mention just a few. It is critical, under these circumstances, that there be an overarching treatment plan that serves the short- and long-term needs of the patient and that is periodically modified as clinical circumstances change and new knowledge about treatments becomes available.

A. PSYCHIATRIC MANAGEMENT

This section is an overview of key issues in the psychiatric management of patients with schizophrenia. It highlights areas that research has shown to be important in affecting the course of illness and success of treatment. These issues arise in the management of all psychiatric illnesses. This section notes the particular ways in which they occur in the treatment of patients with schizophrenia.

1. Assessing symptoms and establishing a diagnosis

Effective and appropriate treatments are based on accurate, relevant diagnostic and clinical assessments. In the case of schizophrenia, the diagnosis has major implications for short- and long-term treatment planning. (See Part B, Section IV.A, "Clinical Features," for a description of the characteristic symptoms of schizophrenia and the DSM-IV-TR criteria for diagnosis of the illness.) It is beyond the scope of this guideline to discuss the differential diagnosis of psychotic disorders and their evaluation. However, it is important to note that diagnosis is a process rather than a one-time event. As new information becomes available about the patient and his or her symptoms, the patient's diagnosis should be reevaluated and, if necessary, the treatment plan changed.

Proper diagnosis, while essential, is insufficient to adequately guide treatment of schizophrenia. Treatments are directed at the manifestations and sequelae of schizophrenia. It is critical to identify the targets of each treatment, to have outcome measures that gauge the effect of treatment, and to have realistic expectations about the degrees of improvement that constitute successful treatment. Depression, suicide, homelessness, substance use disorders, medical comorbidities, social isolation, joblessness, criminal victimization, past sexual or physical abuse, and involvement in the criminal justice system are all far more common among persons with schizophrenia, particularly in the chronic stages of the illness, than in the general population. In addition to the core symptoms of schizophrenia, these areas need careful assessment and, as warranted, appropriate interventions.

A number of objective, quantitative rating scales to monitor clinical status in schizophrenia are available, as described in the American Psychiatric Association's (APA's) *Handbook of Psychiatric Measures* (1). They include the Structured Clinical Interview for DSM-IV (2) for establishing diagnosis, the Abnormal Involuntary Movement Scale (3) for monitoring tardive dyskinesia and other abnormal movements, and the Brief Psychiatric Rating Scale (BPRS) (4–6) and the Positive and Negative Syndrome Scale (PANSS) (7) for monitoring psychopathology. Other brief structured assessments are also available (8, 9). There are several reasons that use of rating scales is important. First, rating scales provide a record that documents the patient's response to treatment. This record is of particular value when the treatment is nonstandard (e.g., combination of antipsychotics) or expensive. Second, the ratings can be compared with the patient's, family members', and clinician's impressions of treatment effects and over time can clarify the longitudinal course of the patient's illness. This process can help temper excessive optimism when new treatments are begun and can provide useful information about the actual effects of prior treatments. Third, use of anchored scales with criteria to assess the severity and frequency of symptoms helps patients become more informed self-observers. Finally, use of the rating scales over time ensures that information about the same areas is collected at each administration and helps avoid omission of key elements of information needed to guide treatment.

2. Developing a plan of treatment

After the assessment of the patient's diagnosis and clinical and psychosocial circumstances, a treatment plan must be formulated and implemented. This process involves the selection of the treatment modalities, specific type(s) of treatment, and treatment setting. Depending on the acuity of the clinical situation and because information about the patient's history and from the clinical evaluation may only gradually become available, this process can be iterative and evolve over the course of the patient's association with the clinician. Indeed, formulation and periodic reevaluation of the treatment plan at different phases of implementation and stages of illness are essential to good clinical practice. This process is described in greater detail in the subsequent sections on the various phases of illness, treatment settings, and types of treatments.

3. Developing a therapeutic alliance and promoting treatment adherence

It is essential for the psychiatrist who is treating the patient to establish and maintain a supportive therapeutic alliance, which forms the foundation on which treatment is conducted (10). Such an alliance allows the psychiatrist to gain essential information about the patient and allows the patient to develop trust in the psychiatrist and a desire to collaborate in treatment.

To facilitate this process, continuity of care with the same psychiatrist over time is recommended, allowing the psychiatrist to learn more about the patient as a person and the individual vicissitudes of the disorder over time. However, while continuity is desirable, it does not ensure quality, and continuity of inadequate treatment can be highly problematic.

Research indicates that specific attention in the therapeutic relationship to identifying the patient's goals and aspirations and relating them to treatment outcomes increases treatment adherence (11). Moreover, evidence supports the conclusion that the most effective medication adherence strategies focus on the patient's attitudes and behaviors with respect to medication rather than taking a general psychoeducational approach (12).

Not uncommonly, patients with schizophrenia stop taking medications, miss clinic appointments, fail to report essential information to their psychiatrists, and otherwise choose to not participate in recommended treatments. To address partial or full treatment nonadherence, the clinician should first assess contributing factors. Potential factors can be broadly conceptualized under the health belief model, which assumes adherence behavior is dynamic and influenced by a patient's beliefs about need for treatment, the potential risks and benefits of treatment, barriers to treatment, and social support for adhering to treatment (13). Frequent causes of poor adherence are lack of insight (14), breakdown of the therapeutic alliance, discrimination associated with the illness, cultural beliefs, failure to understand the need to take daily medication even in the stable phase, cognitive impairment (15, 16), and experience of unpleasant medication side effects such as akathisia (17, 18). Most patients have some ambivalence about taking antipsychotic medications, all of which can be associated with unpleasant and, rarely, dangerous side effects. Even patients with good insight into their symptoms or illness may not perceive their prescribed medication as potentially or actually helpful. Patients who do experience troublesome or serious side effects may decide that these effects outweigh the benefits of medication. Finally, people important to the patient, including family and friends, may discourage the patient from taking medication or participating in other aspects of treatment.

Once the reasons for incomplete adherence are understood, clinical interventions can be implemented to address them. For example, encouraging the patient to report side effects and attempting to diminish or eliminate them can significantly improve medication adherence. Also, it is important for patients who are relatively asymptomatic in the stable phase to understand that medication may be prophylactic in preventing relapse (19, 20). If a patient stops taking medication during the stable phase, he or she may feel better, with less sedation or other side effects. As a result, the patient may come to the false conclusion that the medication is not necessary or does not have benefits. As will be described in later sections, psychotherapeutic techniques based on motivational interviewing and cognitive behavior techniques may enhance insight and treatment adherence. In situations in which patients choose not to adhere to prescribed psychosocial interventions, a careful review of the patient's perceptions of the goals of the treatment and its likelihood for success is recommended.

The clinician may also help to identify practical barriers to adherence, such as cognitive impairments or disorganization that interferes with a willing patient's regular taking of medication or participation in treatment. Use of simple aids, such as a pillbox placed in a prominent location in the home and a watch with an alarm, can enhance adherence. Family members and significant others can also be involved, for example, by helping the patient fill the pillbox and by regularly monitoring adherence. Patients without health care insurance may have difficulty affording even generic antipsychotics or basic psychosocial services. The clinician may help with access to medications by suggesting and completing the physician's sections of the application for patients' assistance programs offered by most pharmaceutical companies. Some patients may not have transportation to the pharmacy or to physician appointments and other treatment services. For patients who are parents, lack of child care may also pose a barrier to attending appointments.

For some patients, medication with a longer elimination half-life or long-acting injectable medications are options that may improve treatment adherence or minimize nonadherence. It is also important to note that the half-lives of oral antipsychotic medications vary widely. For patients who are prone to forget doses or are intermittently nonadherent to treatment, drugs with slower rates of metabolism may be used preferentially.

When a patient does not appear for appointments or is nonadherent in other ways, assertive outreach, including telephone calls and home visits, when appropriate, may be very helpful in reengaging the patient in treatment. This outreach can be carried out by the psychiatrist or other designated team member (e.g., of an assertive community treatment team), when available, in consultation with the psychiatrist. For some patients, nonadherence with care is frequent and is associated with repeated cycles of decompensation and rehospitalization. Particularly for patients who pose ongoing risks to self or others as a result of nonadherence, many states now have programs available for mandatory outpatient treatment (sometimes referred to as outpatient commitment). Although some have questioned whether mandatory outpatient treatment increases patients' reluctance to seek help voluntarily (21–23), a growing body of evidence suggests that a number of benefits may occur with mandatory outpatient treatment for appropriately selected patients when it incorporates intensive individualized outpatient services for an extended period of time. In addition to enhanced adherence, most (24–27) but not all (28) studies show mandatory outpatient treatment to be associated with benefits, including reductions in substance use and abuse, decreases in violent incidents, reductions in the likelihood of being criminally victimized, and improvements in quality of life in appropriately targeted patients. Thus, for a small subgroup of patients with repeated relapses and rehospitalizations associated with nonadherence, mandatory outpatient treatment can be a useful approach to improved adherence and enhanced outcomes (29).

4. Providing patient and family education and therapies

Working with patients to recognize early symptoms of relapse can result in preventing full-blown illness exacerbations (30). Family education about the nature of the illness and coping strategies can markedly diminish relapses and improve quality of life for patients (31). For general educational purposes, a variety of useful written materials about schizophrenia is available. The interventions that have been shown to be effective, however, involve face-to-face interactions in individual or group sessions for a total of at least 9–12 months, with the availability of crisis intervention and problem-solving tasks as a central element of the therapy.

5. Treating comorbid conditions

As already noted, a number of psychiatric, social, and other medical conditions occur far more frequently in persons with schizophrenia than in the general population. Periodic assessment of these conditions by the treatment team is important. Commonly co-occurring major depression, substance use disorders, and PTSD are usually identifiable through clinical examinations and discussions with the patient and significant others, combined with longitudinal observation of the patient's behavior patterns. Each of these conditions deserves attention and possibly treatment in its own right, with such treatment concurrent with that for schizophrenia. Substance use disorders, in particular, complicate assessment and treatment of schizophrenia, but delaying treatment of the psychotic disorder until the substance use disorder is under control is not recommended, as untreated psychosis is likely to be associated with increased substance use (32).

Section II.F.3, "Concurrent General Medical Conditions," discusses nonpsychiatric medical conditions that are commonly comorbid with schizophrenia. Certain illnesses, such as diabetes, are more common in persons with schizophrenia and have also been associated with some second-generation antipsychotic medications. Nicotine dependence is also common among persons with schizophrenia and contributes to the increased risk of physical illnesses (33, 34). It is important that patients have access to primary care clinicians who can work with the psychiatrist to diagnose and treat concurrent general medical conditions and that the psychiatrist maintain competence in screening for common medical conditions and for providing ongoing monitoring and treatment of common medical conditions in conjunction with primary care clinicians.

6. Attending to the patient's social circumstances and functioning

The social circumstances and functioning of the patient can have profound effects on adherence and response to treatment. The patient's living situation, family involvement, sources and amount of income, legal status, and relationships with significant others (including children) can both produce stress and be protective; thus, all are areas where periodic exploration by mental health care clinicians is warranted. A frequently neglected aspect of social assessment is the parenting role of patients with children (35, 36). The patient's sexuality is also often not adequately assessed, not only from the standpoint of adverse medication effects, but in terms of sexual relations and practices.

Depending on the nature of the problem in the patient's social circumstances, other mental health professionals may need to be involved in achieving its resolution. The psychiatrist can work with team members, the patient, and the family to ensure that such services are coordinated and that referrals for additional services are made when appropriate. It is important that disability income support is secured when indicated.

7. Integrating treatments from multiple clinicians

Many patients with schizophrenia require a variety of treatments, often from multiple clinicians. This requirement creates the potential for fragmentation of treatment efforts for patients who frequently have problems with planning and organizing. In many settings integration of treatments is best accomplished through designation of treatment teams, led by a psychiatrist or other skilled mental health professional, that meet periodically to review progress and goals and to identify obstacles to improvement. So-called case management, which provides the patient assistance in gaining access to community services and resources, is often useful to facilitate integration of treatments. Either several members of a team or one person can be assigned to be the case manager, ensuring that the patient receives coordinated, continuous, and comprehensive services. For example, the case manager may accompany the patient to a welfare agency, visit the patient's home if a clinical appointment is missed, or convene a meeting of workers from different agencies serving the patient to formulate an overall treatment plan in conjunction with the psychiatrist. There are a variety of educational and organizational approaches to building teams and programs that facilitate the goal of integrated treatment (37, 38).

8. Documenting treatment

Whether treated in the private or public sector, most persons with schizophrenia will have many different practitioners over the course of their illness. These transitions result from changes in treatment venues (inpatient, outpatient, assertive community treatment, etc.), program availability, insurance, the patient's locale, and clinic personnel. Because an accurate history of past and current treatments and responses to them is a key ingredient to treatment planning, excellent documentation is paramount. Especially critical, for example, is information about prior medication trials, including doses, length of time at specific doses, side effects, and clinical response. Despite the importance of an accurate history, studies of the adequacy of documentation (39) and clinical experience illustrate the extraordinary difficulty encountered in efforts to piece together a coherent story from the medical records of most patients with schizophrenia. Although actual chart documentation is the responsibility of the individual practitioner, it is typically the employing or contracting organization that is in the best position to facilitate good documentation and to effect periodic overviews of treatment. Appropriate documentation of assessment of competency, informed consent for treatment, and release of information also deserve careful attention by the clinician and the treatment organization.

Within the organization there are at least two major issues in information management. From the standpoint of information collection, the organization and its practitioners need to agree on the critical elements of information to obtain and the frequency with which they should be obtained. Recording of information may occur contemporaneously with collection or immediately thereafter. Labor-saving forms (paper or computer-based) may help in prompting data collection and easing its recording. Once information is collected, the ability to gain access to the information is essential. Thus, the organization will want to develop plans so that medical records will be available whenever and wherever the patient is seen. In addition, if the patient's care is transferred from one practitioner to another (e.g., outpatient to inpatient), necessary information will need to be transferred to the new practitioner ahead of or along with the patient. Release of a patient's information will generally require the patient's consent and should conform to applicable regulations and policies (e.g., state law, the Health Insurance Portability and Accountability Act, and *Principles of Medical Ethics: With Annotations Especially Applicable to Psychiatry* [40]).

B. ACUTE PHASE

The goals of treatment during the acute phase of a psychotic exacerbation are to prevent harm, control disturbed behavior, reduce the severity of psychosis and associated symptoms (e.g., agitation, aggression, negative symptoms, affective symptoms), determine and address the factors that led to the occurrence of the acute episode, effect a rapid return to the best level of functioning, develop an alliance with the patient and family, formulate short- and long-term treatment plans, and connect the patient with appropriate aftercare in the community. It is especially important to address the anxiety, fear, and dysphoria commonly associated with an acute episode. Efforts to engage and collaborate with family members and other natural caregivers are often successful during the crisis of an acute psychotic episode, whether it is the first episode or a relapse. Also, family members and other caregivers are often needed to provide support to the patient while he or she is recovering from an acute episode. The main therapeutic challenge for the clinician is to select and "titrate" the doses of both pharmacological and psychosocial interventions in accordance with the symptoms and sociobehavioral functioning of the patient (41). It is important to emphasize that acute-phase treatment is often but no longer necessarily associated with hospitalization. With the growth of managed care restricting the use of hospitalization and the development of alternative community-based programs, acute-phase treatment frequently occurs outside of the hospital.

1. Assessment in the acute phase

A thorough initial workup, including complete psychiatric and general medical histories and physical and mental status examinations, is recommended for all patients, as allowed by the patient's clinical status. Interviews of family members or other persons knowledgeable about the patient should be conducted routinely unless the patient refuses to grant permission, especially since many patients are unable to provide a reliable history at the first interview. In emergency circumstances, as when a patient's safety is at risk, it may be necessary and permissible to speak with others without the patient's consent.

When a patient is in an acute psychotic state, acutely agitated, or both, it may be impossible to perform an adequate evaluation at the time of the initial contact. With the patient's consent, the psychiatrist may begin treatment with an appropriate medication and perform the necessary evaluations as the patient's condition improves and permits. For acutely psychotic or agitated patients who lack the capacity or are unwilling to agree to receive medication, state regulations on involuntary treatment should be followed.

Some of the most common contributors to symptom relapse are antipsychotic medication nonadherence, substance use, and stressful life events (42–47). Medication adherence may be assessed by the patient's report, the reports of family members or other caregivers, pill counts, prescription refill counts, and, for some medications, antipsychotic blood levels. Attention needs to be given to potential drug-drug interactions that may affect blood levels and hence toxicity and adherence. Useful guides for determining potential adverse drug interactions related to the cytochrome P450 enzyme system are now available (48, 49). The reason for nonadherence should also be evaluated and considered in the treatment plan.

General medical health as well as medical conditions that could contribute to symptom exacerbation can be evaluated by medical history; physical and neurological examination; and appropriate laboratory, electrophysiological, and radiological assessments. Substance use should be routinely evaluated as part of the medical history and with a urine toxicology screen. It is important to realize that many drugs of abuse, including most designer drugs and hallucinogens, are not detected by urine toxicology screens; if use of such substances is suspected, a blood toxicology screen can detect some of them. Withdrawal from alcohol or some other substances can present as worsening psychosis, and the possibility of withdrawal should be evaluated by medical history and vital sign monitoring in all patients with acute exacerbation of symptoms. (The results of toxicology screens will usually be negative, since risk of withdrawal is often highest several days after abstinence from chronic abuse.) Body weight and vital signs (heart rate, blood pressure, temperature) should be measured. A CT or MRI scan may provide helpful information, particularly in assessing patients with a new onset of psychosis or with an atypical clinical presentation. Although imaging studies cannot establish a diagnosis of schizophrenia, specific findings from a CT or MRI scan (e.g., ventricular enlargement, diminished cortical volume) may enhance the confidence of the diagnosis and provide information that is relevant to treatment planning and prognosis. Given the subtle nature of the neuropathological findings in schizophrenia, MRI is preferred over CT.

Table 1 delineates suggested laboratory tests for evaluating health status, including studies that may be indicated when the clinical picture is unclear or when there are abnormal findings on routine examination, as well as suggested methods to monitor for side effects of treatment.

These tests may detect occult disease that is contributing to psychosis and also determine if there are comorbid medical conditions that might affect medication selection, such as impaired liver or renal function. Tests to assess other general medical needs of patients should also be considered (e.g., gynecological examination, mammogram, and rectal examination) (54). The U.S. Preventive Services Task Force has reviewed the evidence of effectiveness and developed recommendations for clinical preventive services (http://www.ahcpr.gov/clinic/uspstfix.htm).

It is also important that special precautions be taken in the presence of suicidal ideation or intent or a suicide plan, including an assessment of risk factors such as prior attempts, depressed mood, and suicidal ideation, which are the best predictors of a subsequent suicide attempt in schizophrenia (55, 56). Other predictors of suicide that also warrant close attention include the presence of command hallucinations, hopelessness, anxiety, extrapyramidal side effects, and an alcohol or other substance use disorder. Similar evaluations are necessary in considering the likelihood of dangerous or aggressive behavior and whether the person will harm someone else or engage in other forms of violence (57). The coexistence of substance use (58) significantly increases the risk of violent behavior. Because past behavior best predicts future behavior, family members and friends are often helpful in determining the risk of a patient's harming self or others and in assessing the patient's ability for self-care.

2. Psychiatric management in the acute phase

Psychosocial interventions in the acute phase are aimed at reducing overstimulating or stressful relationships, environments, or life events and at promoting relaxation or reduced arousal through simple, clear, coherent communication and expectations; a structured and predictable environment; low performance requirements; and tolerant, nondemanding, supportive relationships with the psychiatrist and other members of the treatment team.

TABLE 1. Suggested Physical and Laboratory Assessments for Patients With Schizophrenia

Assessment	Initial or Baseline	Follow-Up
Assessments to monitor physical status and detect concomitant physical conditions		
Vital signs	Pulse, blood pressure, temperature	Pulse, blood pressure, temperature, as clinically indicated, particularly as medication doses are titrated
Body weight and height	Body weight, height, and body mass index (BMI)[a]	BMI every visit for 6 months and at least quarterly thereafter[b]
Hematology	CBC	CBC, if clinically indicated, including assessment of patients treated with clozapine
Blood chemistries	Electrolytes Renal function tests (BUN/creatinine ratio) Liver function tests Thyroid function tests	Annually and as clinically indicated
Infectious diseases	Test for syphilis Tests for hepatitis C and HIV, if clinically indicated	
Pregnancy	Consider pregnancy test for women of childbearing potential	
Toxicology	Drug toxicology screen, heavy metal screen, if clinically indicated	Drug toxicology screen, if clinically indicated
Imaging/EEG	EEG, brain imaging (CT or MRI, with MRI being preferred), if clinically indicated	
Assessments related to other specific side effects of treatment[c]		
Diabetes[d]	Screening for diabetes risk factors[e]; fasting blood glucose[f]	Fasting blood glucose or hemoglobin A1c at 4 months after initiating a new treatment and annually thereafter[f]
Hyperlipidemia	Lipid panel[g]	At least every 5 years
QTc prolongation	ECG and serum potassium before treatment with thioridazine, mesoridazine, or pimozide; ECG before treatment with ziprasidone in the presence of cardiac risk factors[h]	ECG with significant change in dose of thioridazine, mesoridazine, pimozide, and, in the presence of cardiac risk factors, ziprasidone or addition of other medications that can affect QTc interval
Hyperprolactinemia	Screening for symptoms of hyperprolactinemia[i] Prolactin level, if indicated on the basis of clinical history	Screening for symptoms of hyperprolactinemia at each visit until stable, then yearly if treated with an antipsychotic known to increase prolactin[i] Prolactin level, if indicated on the basis of clinical history
Extrapyramidal side effects, including akathisia	Clinical assessment of extrapyramidal side effects	Clinical assessment of extrapyramidal side effects weekly during acute treatment until antipsychotic dose is stable for at least 2 weeks, then at each clinical visit during stable phase
Tardive dyskinesia	Clinical assessment of abnormal involuntary movements	Clinical assessment of abnormal involuntary movements every 6 months in patients taking first-generation antipsychotics and every 12 months in those taking second-generation antipsychotics In patients at increased risk, assessment should be done every 3 months and every 6 months with treatment using first- and second-generation antipsychotics, respectively[j]

TABLE 1. Suggested Physical and Laboratory Assessments for Patients With Schizophrenia *(continued)*

Assessment	Initial or Baseline	Follow-Up
Cataracts	Clinical history to assess for changes in distance vision or blurred vision; ocular examination including slit-lamp examination for patients treated with antipsychotics associated with an increased risk of cataracts	Annual clinical history to assess for visual changes; ocular examination every 2 years for patients under age 40 and every year for patients over age 40

[a]BMI may be calculated by using the formula weight in kg/(height in m)^2 or the formula 703 × weight in lb/(height in inches)^2 or by using a BMI table available from the National Institute of Diabetes and Digestive and Kidney Diseases (http://www.niddk.nih.gov/health/nutrit/pubs/statobes.htm#table). A person with a BMI >25 to 29.9 is considered overweight, and one with a BMI of 30 or higher is considered obese. As an alternative to BMI, waist size can be used as an indicator of risk (>35 inches for women and >40 inches for men).

[b]Except for patients with a BMI of <18.5, an increase in BMI of 1 BMI unit would suggest a need for intervention by monitoring weight more closely, engaging the patient in a weight management program, using an adjunctive treatment to reduce weight, or changing the antipsychotic medication.

[c]Although this practice guideline recommends that patients treated with antipsychotic medications be monitored for physical conditions and side effects on a regular basis, there are no absolute criteria for frequency of monitoring. Occurrence of conditions and side effects may be influenced by the patient's history, preexisting conditions, and use of other medications in addition to antipsychotic agents. Thus, decisions about monitoring patients for physical conditions, specific side effects, or abnormalities in laboratory test results will necessarily depend on the clinical circumstances. In general, baseline assessments related to physical conditions and specific medication-related side effects will be done at the time of initiating or changing antipsychotic medications or when adding other medications that contribute to these side effects. Information in this section of the table is adapted from the recommendations of the October 2002 Mount Sinai Conference on Health Monitoring of Patients With Schizophrenia (50).

[d]The U.S. Food and Drug Administration has requested all manufacturers of second-generation (atypical) antipsychotic medications to include a warning in their product labeling regarding hyperglycemia and diabetes mellitus. Although precise risk estimates for hyperglycemia-related adverse events are not available for each agent, epidemiological studies suggested an increased risk of treatment-emergent adverse events with second-generation antipsychotics. In some patients, this hyperglycemia was extreme and/or associated with ketoacidosis, hyperosmolar coma, or death.

[e]Factors that indicate an increased risk for undiagnosed diabetes include a BMI greater than 25, a first-degree relative with diabetes, habitual physical inactivity, being a member of a high-risk ethnic population (African American, Hispanic American, Native American, Asian American, Pacific Islander), having delivered a baby heavier than 9 lbs or having had gestational diabetes, hypertension, a high-density lipoprotein cholesterol level <35 mg/dl and/or a triglyceride level >250 mg/dl, history of abnormal findings on the glucose tolerance test or an abnormal level of fasting blood glucose, and history of vascular disease (51). Symptoms of possible diabetes include frequent urination, excessive thirst, extreme hunger, unusual weight loss, increased fatigue, irritability, and blurry vision.

[f]As an alternative to measurement of fasting blood glucose, a hemoglobin A1c level may be obtained. An abnormal value (fasting blood glucose >110 mg/dl or hemoglobin A1c >6.1%) suggests a need for medical consultation. More frequent monitoring may be indicated in the presence of weight change, symptoms of diabetes, or a random measure of blood glucose >200 mg/dl.

[g]Additional information on screening of patients for possible lipid disorders can be found in the guidelines of the National Cholesterol Education Program (52) and the U.S. Preventive Services Task Force (53).

[h]In this context, cardiac risk factors include known heart disease, a personal history of syncope, a family history of sudden death at an early age (under age 40, especially if both parents had sudden death), or prolonged QTc syndrome.

[i]Changes in libido, menstrual changes, or galactorrhea in women; changes in libido or in erectile or ejaculatory function in men.

[j]Patients at increased risk for developing abnormal involuntary movements include elderly patients and patients who experience acute dystonic reactions, other clinically significant extrapyramidal side effects, or akathisias.

The patient should be provided information on the nature and management of the illness that is appropriate to his or her ability to assimilate information. The patient should also be encouraged to collaborate with the psychiatrist in selecting and adjusting the medication and other treatments provided. Ordinarily, a hospitalized patient should be provided with some information about the disorder and the medications being used to treat it, including their benefits and side effects. As described in Section II.A.3, "Developing a Therapeutic Alliance and Promoting Treatment Adherence," the psychiatrist must realize that the degree of acceptance of medication and information about it will vary according to the patient's cognitive capacity, the extent of the patient's insight, and efforts made by the psychiatrist to engage the patient and the patient's family members in a collaborative treatment relationship.

The acute phase is also the best time for the psychiatrist to initiate a relationship with family members, who tend to be particularly concerned about the patient's disorder, disability, and prognosis during this phase and during hospitalization. Educational meetings, "survival workshops" that teach the family how to cope with schizophrenia, and referrals to the local chapter of NAMI may be helpful. The NAMI web site (http://www.nami.org) offers a wealth of useful information. Manuals, workbooks, and videotapes are also available to aid families in this process (59–64). Active efforts to involve relatives in treatment planning and implementation are often a critical component of treatment.

3. Use of antipsychotic medications in the acute phase

Treatment with antipsychotic medication is indicated for nearly all episodes of acute psychosis in patients with schizophrenia. In this guideline the term "antipsychotic" refers to several classes of medications (Table 2). These include the first-generation antipsychotic medications and the second-generation (sometimes referred to as "atypical") agents clozapine, risperidone, olanzapine, quetiapine, ziprasidone, and aripiprazole.

Pharmacological treatment should be initiated as soon as is clinically feasible, because acute psychotic exacerbations are associated with emotional distress, disruption to the patient's life, and a substantial risk of behaviors that are dangerous to self, others, or property (57, 68, 69). There are limited circumstances where it may be appropriate to delay treatment, for example, for patients who require more extensive or prolonged diagnostic evaluation, who refuse medications, or who may experience a rapid recovery because substance use or acute stress reactions are thought to be the potential cause of the symptom exacerbation.

Before treatment with antipsychotic medication is begun, baseline laboratory studies may be indicated, if they have not already been obtained as a part of the initial assessment (Table 1). In addition, the treating physician should, as is feasible, discuss the potential risks and benefits of the medication with the patient. The depth of this discussion will, of course, be determined by the patient's condition. Even with agitated patients and patients with thought disorder, however, the therapeutic alliance will be enhanced if the patient and physician can identify target symptoms (e.g., anxiety, poor sleep, and, for patients with insight, hallucinations and delusions) that are subjectively distressing and that antipsychotics can ameliorate. Acute side effects such as orthostatic hypotension, dizziness, and extrapyramidal side effects, including dystonic reactions, insomnia, or sedation, should be discussed at this stage, leaving discussion of long-term side effects to when the acute episode is resolving. Mentioning the possibility of acute side effects helps patients to identify and report their occurrence and also may help maintain a therapeutic alliance. To the extent possible, it is important to minimize acute side effects of antipsychotic medications, such as dystonia, that can significantly influence a patient's willingness to accept and continue pharmacological treatment. Patients with schizophrenia often have attentional and other cognitive impairments that may be more severe during an acute illness exacerbation, and so it is often helpful to return to the topic of identifying target symptoms and risk of acute side effects multiple times during the course of hospitalization.

TABLE 2. Commonly Used Antipsychotic Medications

Antipsychotic Medication	Recommended Dose Range (mg/day)[a]	Chlorpromazine Equivalents (mg/day)[b]	Half-Life (hours)[c]
First-generation agents			
Phenothiazines			
Chlorpromazine	300–1000	100	6
Fluphenazine	5–20	2	33
Mesoridazine	150–400	50	36
Perphenazine	16–64	10	10
Thioridazine	300–800	100	24
Trifluoperazine	15–50	5	24
Butyrophenone			
Haloperidol	5–20	2	21
Others			
Loxapine	30–100	10	4
Molindone	30–100	10	24
Thiothixene	15–50	5	34
Second-generation agents			
Aripiprazole	10–30		75
Clozapine	150–600		12
Olanzapine	10–30		33
Quetiapine	300–800		6
Risperidone	2–8		24
Ziprasidone	120–200		7

[a]Dose range recommendations are adapted from the 2003 Schizophrenia Patient Outcome Research Team recommendations (65).

[b]Chlorpromazine equivalents represent the approximate dose equivalent to 100 mg of chlorpromazine (relative potency). Chlorpromazine equivalents are not relevant to the second-generation antipsychotics; therefore, no chlorpromazine equivalents are indicated for these agents (66).

[c]The half-life of a drug is the amount of time required for the plasma drug concentration to decrease by one-half; half-life can be used to determine the appropriate dosing interval (67). The half-life of a drug does not include the half-life of its active metabolites.

Rapid initiation of emergency treatment is needed when an acutely psychotic patient is exhibiting aggressive behaviors toward self, others, or objects. When the patient is in an emergency department, inpatient unit, or other acute treatment facility, existing therapeutic protocols usually define the appropriate response. Most of these protocols recognize that the patient is usually frightened and confused and that the first intervention involves staff members talking to the patient in an attempt to calm him or her. Attempts to restrain the patient should be done only by a team trained in safe restraint procedures to minimize risk of harm to patients or staff (70). Antipsychotics and benzodiazepines are often helpful in reducing the patient's level of agitation (71). If the patient will take oral medication, rapidly dissolving forms of olanzapine and risperidone can be used for quicker effect and to reduce nonadherence. If a patient refuses oral medication, most states allow for emergency administration despite the patient's objection. Short-acting parenteral formulations of first- and second-generation antipsychotic agents (e.g., haloperidol, ziprasidone, and olanzapine), with or without a parenteral benzodiazepine (e.g., lorazepam), are available for emergency administration in acutely agitated patients (72–79). Use of rapidly dissolving oral formulations of second-generation agents (e.g., olanzapine, risperidone) or oral concentrate formulations (e.g., risperidone, haloperidol) may also be useful for

TABLE 3. Choice of Medication in the Acute Phase of Schizophrenia

	Consider Medication From			
Patient Profile	**Group 1: First-Generation Agents**	**Group 2: Risperidone, Olanzapine, Quetiapine, Ziprasidone, or Aripiprazole**	**Group 3: Clozapine**	**Group 4: Long-Acting Injectable Antipsychotic Agents**
First episode		Yes		
Persistent suicidal ideation or behavior			Yes	
Persistent hostility and aggressive behavior			Yes	
Tardive dyskinesia		Yes; all group 2 drugs may not be equal in their lower or no tardive dyskinesia liability	Yes	
History of sensitivity to extrapyramidal side effects		Yes, except higher doses of risperidone		
History of sensitivity to prolactin elevation		Yes, except risperidone		
History of sensitivity to weight gain, hyperglycemia, or hyperlipidemia		Ziprasidone or aripiprazole		
Repeated nonadherence to pharmacological treatment				Yes

acute agitation. Other medications, such as droperidol, can be used in selected clinical situations of extreme emergency or in highly agitated patients (80). However, if droperidol is used, its potential for cardiac rhythm disturbances must be considered, as indicated in its labeling by a black-box warning for QTc prolongation.

In nonemergency circumstances in which the patient is refusing medication, the physician may have limited options. When a patient refuses medication, it is often helpful to enlist family members as allies in helping the patient to accept medication. Often, patients can be helped to accept pharmacological treatment over time and with psychotherapeutic interactions that are aimed toward identifying subjectively distressing symptoms that have previously responded to treatment (12). Clinicians are encouraged to make greater use of the option of advance directives by patients in states where this option is available. Advance directives allow competent patients to state their preferences about treatment choices in the event of future decompensation and acute incapacity to make decisions. Depending on prevailing state laws, when treatment measures instituted on the basis of an advance directive fail, pharmacological treatment may be administered involuntarily even in the absence of acute dangerousness (81). In other instances, depending on state laws, a judicial hearing may need to be sought for permission to treat a patient who lacks capacity.

The process for determining pharmacological treatment in the acute phase is shown in Table 3 and Figure 1.

The selection of an antipsychotic medication is frequently guided by the patient's previous experience with antipsychotics, including the degree of symptom response, the side effect profile (including past experience of side effects such as dysphoria), and the patient's preferences for a particular medication, including the route of administration. The second-generation antipsychotics should be considered as first-line medications for patients in the acute phase of schizophrenia, mainly because of the decreased risk of extrapyramidal side effects and tardive dyskinesia (82–85), with the understanding that there continues to be debate over the relative

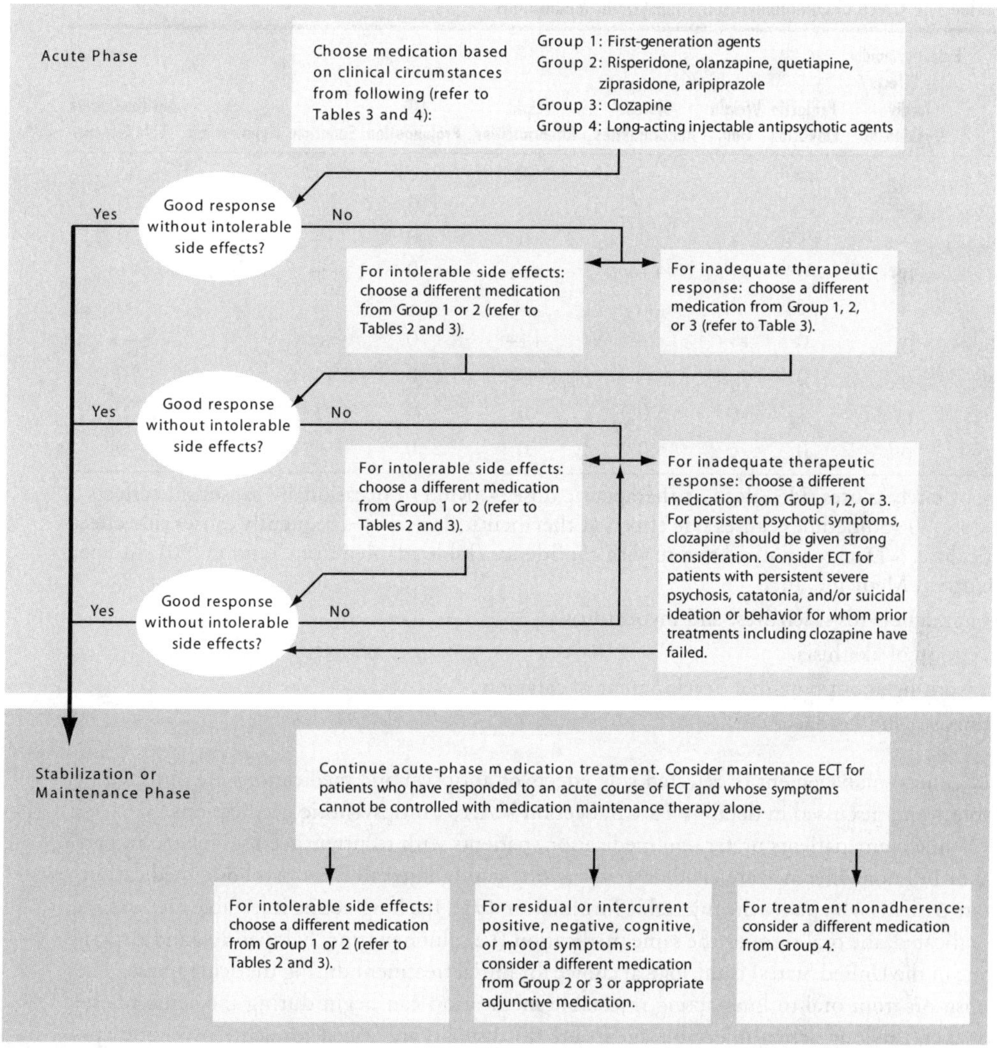

FIGURE 1. Somatic Treatment of Schizophrenia.

advantages, disadvantages, and cost-effectiveness of first- and second-generation agents (86–89). For patients who have been treated successfully in the past or who prefer first-generation agents, these medications are clinically useful and for specific patients may be the first choice. With the possible exception of clozapine for patients with treatment-resistant symptoms, antipsychotics generally have similar efficacy in treating the positive symptoms of schizophrenia, although there is emerging evidence and ongoing debate that second-generation antipsychotics may have superior efficacy in treating global psychopathology and cognitive, negative, and mood symptoms. To date, there is no definitive evidence that one second-generation antipsychotic will have superior efficacy compared with another, although in an individual patient there may be clinically meaningful differences in response (89). A patient's past history of side effects can guide antipsychotic drug selection, since there is considerable difference in side effect profiles among the available antipsychotics. Table 4 lists the relative frequency of some adverse effects associated with selected antipsychotic medications. Strategies for the monitoring

TABLE 4. Selected Side Effects of Commonly Used Antipsychotic Medications[a]

Medication	Extrapyramidal Side Effects/ Tardive Dyskinesia	Prolactin Elevation	Weight Gain	Glucose Abnormalities	Lipid Abnormalities	QTc Prolongation	Sedation	Hypotension	Anticholinergic Side Effects
Thioridazine	+	++	+	+?	+?	+++	++	++	++
Perphenazine	++	++	+	+?	+?	0	+	+	0
Haloperidol	+++	+++	+	0	0	0	++	0	0
Clozapine[b]	0[c]	0	+++	+++	+++	0	+++	+++	+++
Risperidone	+	+++	++	++	++	+	+	+	0
Olanzapine	0[c]	0	+++	+++	+++	0	+	+	++
Quetiapine[d]	0[c]	0	++	++	++	0	++	++	0
Ziprasidone	0[c]	+	0	0	0	++	0	0	0
Aripiprazole[e]	0[c]	0	0	0	0	0	+	0	0

[a]0=No risk or rarely causes side effects at therapeutic dose. +=Mild or occasionally causes side effects at therapeutic dose. ++=Sometimes causes side effects at therapeutic dose. +++=Frequently causes side effects at therapeutic dose. ?=Data too limited to rate with confidence. Table adapted from Tandon (90) with permission of Current Medicine, Inc.

[b]Also causes agranulocytosis, seizures, and myocarditis.

[c]Possible exception of akathisia.

[d]Also carries warning about potential development of cataracts.

[e]Also causes nausea and headache.

and clinical management of selected side effects of antipsychotic medications are outlined in Table 1 and discussed in detail in Part B, Section V.A.1, "Antipsychotic Medications."

While many patients prefer oral medication, patients with recurrent relapses related to partial or full nonadherence are candidates for a long-acting injectable antipsychotic medication, as are patients who prefer the injectable formulation (91). If a long-acting injectable medication is indicated, the oral form of the same medication (i.e., fluphenazine, haloperidol, and risperidone in the United States) is the logical choice for initial treatment during the acute phase. The transition from oral to long-acting injectable medication can begin during the acute phase; however, the long-acting injectable agents are not usually prescribed for acute psychotic episodes because these medications can take months to reach a stable steady state and are eliminated very slowly (92). As a result, the psychiatrist has relatively little control over the amount of medication the patient is receiving, and it is difficult to titrate the dose to control side effects and therapeutic effects. There may, however, be circumstances when it is useful to prescribe long-acting medications during acute treatment. For example, if a patient experiences an exacerbation of psychotic symptoms while receiving long-acting injectable medications, it may be useful to continue the long-acting injectable medication while temporarily supplementing it with oral medication (92).

Determining the optimal dose of antipsychotic medication in the acute phase is complicated by the fact that there is usually a delay between initiation of treatment and full therapeutic response. Patients may take between 2 and 4 weeks to show an initial response (93) and up to 6 months or longer to show full or optimal response. It is important to select a dose that is both effective and not likely to cause side effects that are subjectively difficult to tolerate, since the experience of unpleasant side effects may affect long-term adherence (see Section II.A.3, "Developing a Therapeutic Alliance and Promoting Treatment Adherence"). Some common early side effects such as sedation, postural hypotension, acute dystonia, or nausea will typically improve or resolve after the first several days or weeks of treatment, and patients can be encouraged to tolerate or temporarily manage these short-term effects. Other side effects, notably akathisia and parkinsonism, are likely to persist with long-term treatment. In general, the optimal dose (range) of medication is that which produces maximal therapeutic effects and minimal side effects. The optimal dose of first-generation antipsychotics (Table 2) is, for most patients, at the "EPS threshold," the dose that will induce extrapyramidal side effects and where a physical examination of the patient shows minimal rigidity (94). Evidence suggests that doses above this threshold increase risk of extrapyramidal and other side effects without enhancing efficacy (95–97). Second-generation antipsychotics can generally be administered at doses that are therapeutic yet well below the "EPS threshold." The target dose (Table 2) usually falls within the therapeutic dose range specified by the manufacturer and in the package labeling approved by the U.S. Food and Drug Administration (FDA). In clinical practice, however, doses of several second-generation drugs, including olanzapine, quetiapine, and ziprasidone, have extended above their recommended ranges. In determining the target dose, the psychiatrist should consider the patient's past history of response and dose needs, clinical condition, and severity of symptoms. Doses should be titrated as quickly as tolerated to the target therapeutic dose (generally sedation, orthostatic hypotension, and tachycardia are the side effects that limit the rate of increase), and unless there is evidence that the patient is having uncomfortable side effects, the patient's clinical status ideally should then be monitored for 2–4 weeks before increasing the dose or changing medications. During these weeks it is often important for the physician to be patient and avoid the temptation to prematurely escalate the dose for patients who are responding slowly. Rapid escalation can create the false impression of enhanced efficacy when time is often an important factor, and higher doses may actually be detrimental.

If the patient is not improving, consider whether the lack of response can be explained by medication nonadherence, rapid medication metabolism, or poor absorption. If the patient has been treated with one of the medications for which there are adequate data on blood level relationships with clinical response (e.g., clozapine, haloperidol), determination of the plasma concentration may be helpful. If nonadherence is a problem, behavioral tailoring (i.e., fitting taking medication into one's daily routine) (30), motivational interviewing, and other psychotherapeutic techniques may be useful in helping the patient develop an understanding of the potential benefits of medication (12, 98). In addition, surreptitious nonadherence (i.e., "cheeking") may be addressed by use of a liquid (e.g., risperidone, haloperidol), a quick-dissolving tablet (e.g., olanzapine, risperidone), or a short-acting intramuscular form (e.g., ziprasidone, haloperidol).

If the patient is adhering to treatment and has an adequate plasma concentration of medication but is not responding to the treatment, alternative treatments should be considered. If the patient is able to tolerate a higher dose of antipsychotic medication without significant side effects, raising the dose for a finite period, such as 2–4 weeks, can be tried, although the incremental efficacy of higher doses has not been well established. If dose adjustment does not result in an adequate response, a different antipsychotic medication should be considered.

4. Use of adjunctive medications in the acute phase

Other psychoactive medications are commonly added to antipsychotic medications in the acute phase to treat comorbid conditions or associated symptoms (e.g., agitation, aggression, affective symptoms), to address sleep disturbances, and to treat antipsychotic drug side effects. Therapeutic approaches to treatment resistance and residual symptoms are discussed in Section II.E, "Special Issues in Caring for Patients With Treatment-Resistant Illness."

Adjunctive medications are also commonly prescribed for residual symptoms and comorbid conditions during the acute phase. For example, benzodiazepines may be helpful in treating catatonia as well as in managing both anxiety and agitation. The most agitated patients may benefit from addition of an oral or a parenteral benzodiazepine to the antipsychotic medication. Lorazepam has the advantage of reliable absorption when it is administered either orally or parenterally (99). There is some evidence that mood stabilizers and beta-blockers may be

TABLE 5. Selected Medications for Treating Extrapyramidal Side Effects

Generic Name	Dose (mg/day)	Elimination Half-Life (hours)	Target Extrapyramidal Side Effects
Benztropine mesylate[a]	0.5–6.0	24	Akathisia, dystonia, parkinsonism
Trihexyphenidyl hydrochloride	1–15	4	Akathisia, dystonia, parkinsonism
Amantadine	100–300	10–14	Akathisia, parkinsonism
Propranolol	30–90	3–4	Akathisia
Lorazepam[a]	1–6	12	Akathisia
Diphenhydramine[a]	25–50	4–8	Akathisia, dystonia, parkinsonism

Sources. *Drug Information for the Health Care Professional* (104, p. 290) and DRUGDEX (105).
[a]Available in oral or parenteral forms.

effective in reducing the severity of recurrent hostility and aggression (100–102). Major depression and obsessive-compulsive disorder are common comorbid conditions in patients with schizophrenia and may respond to an antidepressant. However, some antidepressants (those that inhibit catecholamine reuptake) can potentially sustain or exacerbate psychotic symptoms in some patients (103). Careful attention must be paid to potential drug-drug interactions, especially those related to the cytochrome P450 enzymes (48, 49).

Sleep disturbances are common in the acute phase, and while controlled studies are lacking, there is anecdotal evidence that a sedating antidepressant (e.g., trazodone, mirtazapine) or a benzodiazepine sedative-hypnotic may be helpful.

Medications can be used to treat extrapyramidal side effects (Table 5) and other side effects of antipsychotic medications that are described in detail in Part B, Section V.A.1, "Antipsychotic Medications." Decisions to use medications to treat side effects are driven by the severity and degree of distress associated with the side effect and by consideration of other potential strategies, including lowering the dose of the antipsychotic medication or switching to a different antipsychotic medication. The following factors should be considered in decisions regarding the prophylactic use of antiparkinsonian medications in acute-phase treatment: the propensity of the antipsychotic medication to cause extrapyramidal side effects, the patient's preferences, the patient's prior history of extrapyramidal side effects, other risk factors for extrapyramidal side effects (especially dystonia), and risk factors for and potential consequences of anticholinergic side effects.

5. Use of ECT and other somatic therapies in the acute phase

ECT in combination with antipsychotic medications may be considered for patients with schizophrenia or schizoaffective disorder with severe psychotic symptoms that have not responded to treatment with antipsychotic agents. The efficacy of acute treatment with ECT in patients with schizophrenia has been described in a number of controlled trials as well as in multiple case series and uncontrolled studies (106–108). The greatest therapeutic benefits appear to occur when ECT is administered concomitantly with antipsychotic medications. The majority of studies, including several randomized studies, have shown benefit from ECT combined with first-generation antipsychotic agents (109–126). More recent findings also suggest benefit from combined treatment with ECT and second-generation antipsychotic medications (127–135). However, given the clear benefits of clozapine in patients with treatment-resistant psychotic symptoms, a trial of clozapine will generally be indicated before acute treatment with ECT.

Clinical experience, as well as evidence from case series and open prospective trials, suggests that ECT should also be considered for patients with prominent catatonic features that have not responded to an acute trial of lorazepam (136–143). For patients with schizophrenia and comorbid depression, ECT may also be beneficial if depressive symptoms are resistant to treatment or if features such as suicidal ideation and behaviors or inanition, which necessitate a rapid therapeutic response, are present.

For additional details on the assessment of patients before ECT, the informed consent process, the technical aspects of ECT administration, and the side effects associated with treatment, the reader is referred to APA's *The Practice of Electroconvulsive Therapy: Recommendations for Treatment, Training, and Privileging: A Task Force Report of the American Psychiatric Association* (107).

Although it has been suggested that repetitive transcranial magnetic stimulation (rTMS) may share beneficial features of ECT (144, 145) and several recent studies with rTMS have shown promising results in decreasing auditory hallucinations (146–148), rTMS does not have an FDA indication for the treatment of psychosis, and additional research is needed before recommending its use in clinical practice.

C. STABILIZATION PHASE

During the stabilization phase, the aims of treatment are to sustain symptom remission or control, minimize stress on the patient, provide support to minimize the likelihood of relapse, enhance the patient's adaptation to life in the community, facilitate the continued reduction in symptoms and consolidation of remission, and promote the process of recovery.

Controlled trials provide relatively little guidance for medication treatment during this phase. If the patient has achieved an adequate therapeutic response with minimal side effects or toxicity with a particular medication regimen, he or she should be monitored while taking the same medication and dose for the next 6 months. Premature lowering of dose or discontinuation of medication during this phase may lead to a relatively rapid relapse. However, it is also critical to assess continuing side effects that may have been present in the acute phase and to adjust pharmacotherapy accordingly to minimize adverse side effects that may otherwise lead to medication nonadherence and relapse. Moreover, any adjunctive medications that have been used in the acute phase should be evaluated for continuation.

Psychotherapeutic interventions remain supportive but may be less structured and directive than in the acute phase. Education about the course and outcome of the illness and about factors that influence the course and outcome, including treatment adherence, can begin in this phase for patients and continue for family members. Educational programs during this phase have been effective in teaching a wide range of patients with schizophrenia the skills of medication self-management (e.g., the benefits of maintenance antipsychotic medication, how to cope with side effects) and symptom self-management (e.g., how to identify early warning signs of relapse, develop a relapse prevention plan, and refuse illicit drugs and alcohol), as well as strategies for interacting with health care providers (149–152).

It is important that there be no gaps in service delivery, because patients are vulnerable to relapse and need support in adjusting to community life. Not uncommonly, problems in continuity of care arise when patients are discharged from hospitals to community care. It is imperative to arrange for linkage of services between hospital and community treatment before the patient is discharged from the hospital. Short lengths of hospital stay create challenges for adequately linking inpatient to outpatient care, but to the extent possible, patients should have input into selecting their postdischarge follow-up residential and treatment plans. It is frequently beneficial to arrange an appointment with an outpatient psychiatrist and, for patients who will reside in a community residence, to arrange a visit before discharge (153, 154). After discharge, patients should be helped to adjust to life in the community through realistic goal setting without undue pressure to perform at high levels vocationally and socially, since unduly ambitious expectations on the part of therapists (20), family members (155), or others, as well as an overly stimulating treatment environment (156), can be stressful to patients and can increase the risk of relapse. These principles also apply in the stable phase. Efforts should be made to actively involve family members in the treatment process. Other psychosocial treatments, discussed below in Section II.D, "Stable Phase," may be initiated during this phase depending on the patient's level of recovery and motivation. While it is critical not to place premature demands on the patient regarding engagement in community-based activities and rehabilitation services, it is equally critical to maintain a level of momentum aimed at improving community functioning in order to instill a sense of hope and progress for the patient and family. These efforts set the stage for continuing treatments during the stable phase.

D. STABLE PHASE

Treatment during the stable phase is designed to sustain symptom remission or control, minimize the risk and consequences of relapse, and optimize functioning and the process of recovery.

1. Assessment in the stable phase

Ongoing monitoring and assessment during the stable phase are necessary to determine whether the patient might benefit from alterations in the treatment program. Ongoing assessment allows patients and those who interact with them to describe any changes in symptoms or functioning and raise questions about specific symptoms and side effects.

Monitoring for adverse effects should be done regularly (Table 1). Clinicians should inquire about the course of any side effects that developed in the acute or stabilization phases (e.g., sexual side effects, sedation). Monitoring for other potential adverse effects should be guided by the particular medications chosen (see Part B, Section V.A.1, "Antipsychotic Medications").

If the patient agrees, it is helpful to maintain strong ties with persons who interact with the patient frequently and would therefore be most likely to notice any resurgence of symptoms and the occurrence of life stresses and events that may increase the risk of relapse or impede continuing functional recovery. However, the frequency of assessments by the psychiatrist or other members of the treatment team depends on the specific nature of the treatment and expected fluctuations of the illness. Frequency of contacts may range from every few weeks for patients who are doing well and are stabilized to as often as every day for those who are going through highly stressful changes in their lives.

2. Psychosocial treatments in the stable phase

For most persons with schizophrenia in the stable phase, treatment programs that combine medications with a range of psychosocial services are associated with improved outcomes. Knowledge and research regarding how best to combine treatments to optimize outcome are scarce. Nonetheless, provision of such packages of services likely reduces the need for crisis-oriented care hospitalizations and emergency department visits and enables greater recovery.

A number of psychosocial treatments have demonstrated effectiveness. These treatments include family interventions (31, 157, 158), supported employment (159–162), assertive community treatment (163–166), social skills training (167–169), and cognitive behaviorally oriented psychotherapy (158, 170). An evidence-based practices project sponsored by the Substance Abuse and Mental Health Services Administration (SAMHSA) is developing resource kits on family interventions, assertive community treatment, and supported employment (draft versions available at http://www.mentalhealthpractices.org/pdf_files/fpe_pcs.pdf; http://www.mentalhealthpractices.org/pdf_files/act_c.pdf; http://www.mentalhealthpractices.org/pdf_files/se_mhpl.pdf).

In the same way that psychopharmacological management must be individually tailored to the needs and preferences of the patient, so too should the selection of psychosocial treatments. The selection of appropriate and effective psychosocial treatments needs to be driven by the circumstances of the individual patient's needs and his or her social context. At the very least, all persons with schizophrenia should be provided with education about their illness. Beyond needing illness education, most patients will also benefit from at least some of the recommended psychosocial interventions. However, since patients' clinical and social needs will vary at different points in their illness course and since some psychosocial treatments share treatment components, it would be rare for all of these psychosocial interventions to be utilized during any one phase of illness for an individual patient.

a) Prevention of relapse and reduction of symptom severity

A major goal during the stable phase is to prevent relapse and reduce the severity of residual symptoms. Certain psychosocial interventions have demonstrated effectiveness in this regard. They include family education and support, assertive community treatment, and cognitive therapy.

Interventions that educate families about schizophrenia, provide support, and offer training in effective problem solving and communication have been subjected to numerous randomized clinical trials (171, 172). The data strongly and consistently support the value of such interventions in reducing symptom relapse, and there is some evidence that these interventions contribute to improved patient functioning and family well-being. Randomized clinical trials have reported 2-year relapse rates for patients receiving family "psychoeducation" programs in combination with medication that are 50% lower than those for patients receiving medication alone (173–180). Further, a recent study found psychoeducational programs using multiple family groups to be more effective and less expensive than individual family psychoeducational interventions for Caucasians, though not for African Americans (178). On the basis of the evidence, persons with schizophrenia and their families who have ongoing contact with each other should be offered a family intervention, the key elements of which include a duration of at least 9 months, illness education, crisis intervention, emotional support, and training in how to cope with illness symptoms and related problems.

PACT is a specific model of community-based care. Its origin is an experiment in Madison, Wisconsin, in the 1970s in which the multidisciplinary inpatient team of the state hospital was moved into the community (181, 182). The team took with it all of the functions of an inpatient team: interdisciplinary teamwork, 24-hour/7-days-per-week coverage, comprehensive treatment planning, ongoing responsibility, staff continuity, and small caseloads. PACT is designed to treat patients who are at high risk for hospital readmission and who cannot be maintained by more usual community-based treatment as well as for patients with severe psychosocial impairment who need extensive assistance to live in the community. Randomized trials comparing PACT to other community-based care have consistently shown that PACT substantially reduces utilization of inpatient services and promotes continuity of outpatient care (183, 184). Patients' satisfaction with this model is generally high, and family advocacy groups, such as NAMI in the United States, strongly support its use and dissemination.

Results are less consistent regarding the effect of PACT on other outcomes, although at least some studies have shown enhancement of clinical status, functioning, and quality of life. Cost-effectiveness studies support its value in the treatment of high-risk patients. Studies also indicate that a particular PACT program's effectiveness is related to the fidelity with which it is implemented, that is, the degree to which the program adheres to the original PACT model.

Controlled studies of cognitive behavior psychotherapy have reported benefits in reducing the severity of persistent psychotic symptoms (170). Most of the studies have been performed with individual cognitive behavior therapy of at least several months' duration; in some studies, group cognitive behavior therapy and/or therapy of a shorter duration has been used. In all of the studies clinicians who provided cognitive behavior therapy received specialized training in the approach. In addition, the key elements of this intervention include a shared understanding of the illness between the patient and therapist, identification of target symptoms, and the development of specific cognitive and behavioral strategies to cope with these symptoms. Therefore, based on the available evidence, persons with schizophrenia who have residual psychotic symptoms while receiving adequate pharmacotherapy may benefit from cognitive behaviorally oriented psychotherapy.

A variety of other approaches to counseling individual patients to help them cope better with their illness are used, although research in this area remains limited. In general, counseling that emphasizes illness education, support, and problem solving is most appropriate. A notable prototype of this approach is personal therapy, as developed by Hogarty and colleagues (185–187). Personal therapy is an individualized long-term psychosocial intervention provided to patients on a weekly to biweekly frequency within the larger framework of a treatment program that provides pharmacotherapy, family work (when a family is available), and multiple levels of support, both material and psychological. The approach is carefully tailored to the patient's phase of recovery from an acute episode and the patient's residual level of severity, disability, and vulnerability to relapse.

b) Negative symptoms

During the stable phase, negative symptoms (e.g., affective flattening, alogia, avolition) may be primary and represent a core feature of schizophrenia, or they may be secondary to psychotic symptoms, a depressive syndrome, medication side effects (e.g., dysphoria), or environmental deprivation. The effectiveness of psychosocial treatments for reducing negative symptoms is not well studied. Furthermore, most research (for both psychosocial and pharmacological treatments) does not distinguish between primary and secondary negative symptoms. Thus, the generic term "negative symptoms" is used to summarize these findings. Some studies of cognitive behavior therapy report improvements in residual negative symptoms. In a review of three studies, Rector and Beck (188) reported a large aggregated effect size favoring cognitive behavior therapy over supportive therapy for reducing negative symptoms. Also, one study of family psychoeducation reported an improvement in negative symptoms with this intervention (189).

c) Improving functional status and quality of life

A primary treatment goal during the stable phase is to enable the patient to continue the recovery process and to achieve the goals of improved functioning and quality of life. To the degree to which active positive symptoms impair functional capacity, medications that reduce positive symptoms may improve functioning. However, research indicates consistently that positive symptoms show a low correspondence with functional impairments among patients with schizophrenia (190). Rather, it is the negative symptoms and cognitive impairments that are more predictive of functional impairment (191). Because available medications have at best only modest effects on these illness dimensions, it is not surprising that there is scant evidence that medications improve functional status beyond that achieved through reduction of impairing positive symptoms. Consequently, certain psychosocial and rehabilitative interventions are essential to consider in the stable phase to enhance functional status.

Supported employment is an approach to improve vocational functioning among persons with various types of disabilities, including schizophrenia (192). The evidence-based supported employment programs that have been found effective include the key elements of individualized job development, rapid placement emphasizing competitive employment, ongoing job supports, and integration of vocational and mental health services. Randomized trials have consistently demonstrated the effectiveness of supported employment in helping persons with schizophrenia to achieve competitive employment (193, 194). Employment outcomes related to the duration of employment and to the amount of earnings also favor supported employment over traditional vocational services. Further, there is no evidence that engagement in supported employment leads to stress, increased symptoms, or other negative outcome (159). Evidence is inconsistent about the relationship between clinical and demographic variables and successful vocational performance; therefore, it is recommended that any person with schizophrenia who expresses an interest in work should be offered supported employment. Promoting job retention is a continuing challenge even for supported employment. Studies have found that persons with schizophrenia experience considerable difficulties retaining jobs achieved through supported employment (162, 194). This problem appears to be related to neurocognitive impairments (195), among other factors.

Social skills training has been found helpful in addressing functional impairments in social skills or activities of daily living. The key elements of this intervention include behaviorally based instruction, modeling, corrective feedback, and contingent social reinforcement. Clinic-based skills training should be supplemented with practice and training in the patient's day-to-day environment. The results of controlled trials indicate the benefit of skills training in improving illness knowledge, social skills, and symptom and medication management when offered with adequate pharmacotherapy (167). Evidence is strongest for the benefit of skills training in increasing the acquisition of skills assessed by situationally specific measures.

d) Patient and self-help treatment organizations

Peer support is social-emotional and sometimes instrumental support that is mutually offered or provided by persons having a mental health condition, i.e., mental health consumers, to others sharing a similar mental health condition to bring about a desired social or personal change (196). The oldest and most widely available type of peer support is self-help groups. Based largely on uncontrolled studies of self-help groups for persons with severe mental illness, Davidson et al. (197) concluded that self-help groups seem to improve symptoms and increase participants' social networks and quality of life. Additional studies of self-help groups have demonstrated other positive outcomes, including reductions in hospitalizations, improved coping, greater acceptance of the illness, improved medication adherence and illness management, improved daily functioning, lower levels of worry, and higher satisfaction with health (198–200, unpublished 1989 manuscript of M. Kennedy).

Within the realm of consumer-provided or -delivered services are consumer-run or -operated services, consumer partnership services, and consumer employees. Consumer-run or -operated services are services that are planned, operated, administered, and evaluated by consumers (201, 202). Those service programs that are not freestanding legal entities but share control of the operation of the program with nonconsumers are categorized as consumer partnerships. Consumer employees are persons who fill positions designated for consumers as well as consumers who are hired into traditional mental health positions. Reviews of peer support/consumer-provided services specifically for persons with severe mental illness have generated positive results, but the findings are somewhat tentative, given the infancy of the research area (197, 203, 204). Such services have been associated with reduced hospitalizations, reduced use of crisis services, improved social functioning, reduced substance use, and improved quality of life (205–209).

3. Use of antipsychotic medications in the stable phase

Once a patient reaches the stable or maintenance phase of treatment, it is important for the physician to develop a long-term treatment management plan that minimizes the risk of relapse, monitors for and minimizes the severity of side effects, and to the extent possible addresses residual symptoms.

Antipsychotics can reduce the risk of relapse in the stable phase of illness to less than 30% per year (210–215). Without maintenance treatment, 60%–70% of patients relapse within 1 year, and almost 90% relapse within 2 years. Strategies can be used to increase the likelihood that patients will adhere to prescribed medication regimens. Such strategies are described in Section II. A.3, "Developing a Therapeutic Alliance and Promoting Treatment Adherence."

Deciding on the dose of an antipsychotic medication during the stable phase is complicated by the fact that there is no reliable strategy available to identify the minimum effective dose to prevent relapse. Although higher doses are often more effective at reducing relapse risk than lower doses, higher doses often cause greater side effects and lessen subjective tolerability; therefore, clinicians should attempt to treat at a dose that minimizes side effects but is still in the effective range of a particular drug (refer to Table 2). For most patients treated with first-generation antipsychotics, clinicians should use a dose around the "EPS threshold" (94), since studies indicate that higher doses are usually not more efficacious and increase risk of subjectively intolerable side effects (95–97). Lower doses of first-generation antipsychotic medications may be associated with improved adherence and better subjective state and perhaps ultimately better functioning. Second-generation antipsychotics can generally be administered at doses that are therapeutic but will not induce extrapyramidal side effects. The advantages of decreasing antipsychotics to the "minimal effective dose" should be weighed against a somewhat greater risk of relapse and more frequent exacerbations of schizophrenic symptoms (216). Recent evidence suggests potentially greater efficacy in relapse prevention for the second-generation antipsychotic drugs (215, 217); however, whether this result is due to better efficacy or some other factor such as greater treatment adherence or reduced side effects is unclear.

The available antipsychotics are associated with differential risk of a variety of adverse effects, including neurological, metabolic, sexual, endocrine, sedative, and cardiovascular effects (Table 4). A suggested approach to monitoring of side effects is detailed in Table 1 and should be based on the side effect profile of the prescribed antipsychotic as detailed in Part B, Section V.A.1, "Antipsychotic Medications."

Antipsychotic treatment often results in substantial improvement or even remission of positive symptoms. However, most patients remain functionally impaired because of negative symptoms, cognitive deficits, and impaired social function. It is important to evaluate whether residual negative symptoms are in fact secondary to a parkinsonian syndrome or an untreated major depressive syndrome, since interventions are available to address these negative symptoms. There are few proven treatment options for residual positive symptoms, primary negative symptoms, cognitive deficits, or social impairments (see Section II.E, "Special Issues in Caring for Patients With Treatment-Resistant Illness").

Most patients who develop schizophrenia and related psychotic disorders (schizoaffective disorder and schizophreniform disorder) are at very high risk of relapse in the absence of antipsychotic treatment. Emerging evidence suggests this may even be true for first-episode patients; some studies (46, 218) have shown that more than 80% of such patients who do not receive antipsychotic treatment experience some recurrence of symptoms in the 5 years after remission. Unfortunately, there is no reliable indicator to differentiate the minority who will not relapse from the majority who will relapse. Antipsychotics are highly effective in the prevention of relapse in remitted first-episode patients. One-year relapse risk varies from 0% to 46% of patients who are prescribed antipsychotics (210–213). Adherence to maintenance antipsychotic medication likely has an influence on effectiveness and may contribute to varying relapse rates. The most prudent treatment options that clinicians may discuss with remitted first- or multi-episode patients include either 1) indefinite antipsychotic maintenance medication or 2) medication discontinuation (after at least 1 year of symptom remission or optimal response while taking medication) with close follow-up and with a plan to reinstitute antipsychotic treatment on symptom recurrence. However, evidence indicates that sustained treatment is associated with fewer relapses than is targeted intermittent treatment (219). In addition, intermittent treatment strategies appear to increase rather than decrease the risk of tardive dyskinesia. Clinicians should engage patients in a discussion of the long-term potential risks of maintenance treatment with the prescribed antipsychotic (see Part B, Section V.A.1, "Antipsychotic Medications") versus the risks of relapse (e.g., the effect of relapse on social and vocational functioning, the risk of dangerous behaviors with relapse, and the risk of developing chronic treatment-resistant symptoms). If a decision is made to discontinue antipsychotic medication, the discontinuation should be gradual (e.g., reducing the dose by 10% per month). Additional precautions should be taken to minimize the risk of a psychotic relapse. The physician should educate the patient and the family about early signs of relapse, advise them to develop plans for action should these signs appear, and suggest that the patient continue to be seen by a physician on a regular basis.

Indefinite maintenance antipsychotic medication is recommended for patients who have had multiple prior episodes or two episodes within 5 years. Patients taking antipsychotic medication should also be monitored for signs and symptoms of impending or actual relapse, since even in adherent patients the risk of relapse in chronic schizophrenia is about 30% per year. The treatment program should be organized to respond quickly when a patient, family member, or friend reports any symptoms that could indicate an impending or actual relapse. Early intervention using supportive therapeutic techniques and increasing medication as indicated can be very helpful in reducing the likelihood of relapse and hospitalization (220). During prodromal episodes, patients and family members should be seen more frequently for treatment, monitoring, and support, and assertive outreach, including home visits, should be used when indicated.

4. Use of adjunctive medications in the stable phase

Other psychoactive medications are commonly added to antipsychotic medications in the stable phase to treat comorbid conditions, aggression, anxiety, or other mood symptoms; to augment the antipsychotic effects of the primary drug; and to treat side effects. Other medications that may address treatment-resistant and residual psychotic symptoms are discussed in Section II.E, "Special Issues in Caring for Patients With Treatment-Resistant Illness."

Adjunctive medications are commonly prescribed for comorbid conditions. For example, major depression and obsessive-compulsive disorder are common comorbid conditions in patients with schizophrenia and may respond to antidepressant medications (221–223). However, some antidepressants (those that inhibit catecholamine reuptake) can potentially sustain or exacerbate psychotic symptoms in some patients (103). Benzodiazepines may be helpful for managing anxiety during the stable phase of treatment (224), although risk of dependence and abuse exists with chronic use of this class of medication. There is some evidence that mood stabilizers and beta-blockers (100–102) may be effective in reducing the severity of recurrent hostility and aggression. Mood stabilizers may also address prominent mood lability. As mentioned previously, attention must be given to potential drug interactions, especially related to metabolism by the cytochrome P450 enzymes (48, 49).

Patients treated with first-generation antipsychotics may require the long-term use of medications for treatment of extrapyramidal side effects (Table 5). Although the study findings are not consistent, there is some evidence that vitamin E may reduce the risk of development of tardive dyskinesia (225, 226). Given the low risk of side effects associated with vitamin E, patients may be advised to take 400–800 I.U. daily as prophylaxis.

Many other medications may be used to treat or reduce the risk of various antipsychotic side effects. These medications are discussed with each specific antipsychotic in Part B, Section V.A.1, "Antipsychotic Medications."

5. Use of ECT in the stable phase

Clinical observations (227, 228) and a single randomized clinical trial (229) suggest that maintenance ECT may be helpful for some patients who have responded to acute treatment with ECT but for whom pharmacological prophylaxis alone has been ineffective or cannot be tolerated. The frequency of treatments varies from patient to patient and depends on the degree of clinical response and side effects of treatment (107). As with acute treatment with ECT, available evidence suggests that treatment with antipsychotics should continue during the maintenance ECT course (229).

E. SPECIAL ISSUES IN CARING FOR PATIENTS WITH TREATMENT-RESISTANT ILLNESS

About 10%–30% of patients have little or no response to antipsychotic medications, and up to an additional 30% of patients have partial responses to treatment, meaning that they exhibit improvement in psychopathology but continue to have mild to severe residual hallucinations or delusions. Even if a patient's positive symptoms respond or remit with antipsychotic treatment, other residual symptoms, including negative symptoms and cognitive impairment, often persist. Treatment resistance is defined as little or no symptomatic response to multiple (at least two) antipsychotic trials of an adequate duration (at least 6 weeks) and dose (therapeutic range).

Treatment may be completely or partially unsuccessful for a variety of reasons. The patient may receive a suboptimal dose of antipsychotic, either because an inadequate dose has been prescribed or because the patient does not take some or all of the prescribed antipsychotic. The prescribed antipsychotic may be partially or fully ineffective in treating acute symptoms or in preventing relapse. Substance use may also cause or contribute to treatment resistance.

In assessing treatment resistance, clinicians should carefully evaluate whether the patient has had an adequate trial of an antipsychotic, including whether the dose is adequate and whether the patient has been taking the medication as prescribed. Strategies for improving adherence are described in Section II.A.3, "Developing a Therapeutic Alliance and Promoting Treatment Adherence."

Even when patients are taking antipsychotics, suboptimal treatment response and residual symptoms are common. There are considerable differences between patients in responsiveness to available antipsychotics. However, currently there is no reliable strategy to predict response or risk of side effects with one agent compared with another. Thus, adequate trials of multiple antipsychotics are often needed before antipsychotic treatment is optimized. Complicating the evaluation of treatment response is the fact that there is some time delay between initiation of treatment and full clinical response. An initial trial of 2–4 weeks generally is needed to determine if the patient will have any symptomatic response, and symptoms can continue to improve for up to 6 months (230, 231).

Because of clozapine's superior efficacy, a trial of clozapine should be considered for a patient with a clinically inadequate response to antipsychotic treatment or for a patient with suicidal ideation or behavior (55). Besides clozapine, there are limited options for the many patients who have severe and significant residual symptoms even after antipsychotic monotherapy has been optimized, and none have proven benefits. Various augmentation strategies that have limited or no evidence supporting their efficacy are often used. However, clinicians may consider a time-limited trial of an agent to determine if it offers any benefit to an individual patient. To avoid risking side effects and potential drug interactions, it is important that the actual efficacy of adjunctive medications is carefully evaluated and that adjunctive medications that do not produce clinical benefits are discontinued. Depending on the type of residual symptom (e.g., positive, negative, cognitive, or mood symptoms; aggressive behavior), augmentation strategies include adding another antipsychotic (232–234), anticonvulsants (102, 235–237), benzodiazepines (224), *N*-methyl-D-aspartate (NMDA) receptor allosteric agonists (e.g., D-serine [238], glycine [239–242], D-cycloserine [243–246]), and cholinergic agonists (247–249). ECT has demonstrated benefits in patients with treatment-resistant symptoms (106–108). Cognitive behavior therapy techniques may have value in improving positive symptoms with low risk of side effects (98). In addition, cognitive remediation is under investigation as a therapeutic strategy to reduce the severity of cognitive deficits (250).

F. CLINICAL FEATURES INFLUENCING THE TREATMENT PLAN

1. Psychiatric features

a) First episode

Active psychosis is dangerous to a person's safety; disrupts capacity to function, life, and reputation; and if persistent for too long can negatively affect prognosis (251). In contrast, early treatment may result in a significant reduction in morbidity and better quality of life for patients and families (252–256). Approximately 25 studies have examined this phenomenon; about two-thirds have shown a significant association between earlier treatment and better outcome on one or more measures, and none has shown a significant association between delayed treatment and better outcome on any measure (257). Despite the benefits of early treatment, there is usually a delay of 1–2 years between the onset of psychotic symptoms and the time the patient first receives adequate psychiatric treatment (252, 258–261). Thus, once psychosis is evident, it should be treated immediately.

In some persons, particularly those with a family history of schizophrenia or other factors influencing risk, prodromal symptoms may be apparent before the development of a full schizophrenia syndrome. Although empirical evidence on long-term outcome is limited, antipsychotic medication treatment may also be helpful in some persons with prodromal symptoms (262–264).

When a patient presents with a first episode of psychosis, close observation and documentation of the signs and symptoms over time are important because initial psychotic episodes can be polymorphic and evolve into a variety of specific disorders (e.g., schizophreniform disorder, bipolar disorder, schizoaffective disorder). There is controversy over whether first-episode patients should be treated as outpatients or in the hospital. Inpatient care offers both risks and protections. On the one hand, the experience of a first psychiatric hospitalization, especially in a closed setting with many chronically ill patients, can be frightening and produce its own trauma (265). On the other hand, the nature and severity of a first episode are often unknown, unpredictable, and require more than "usual" surveillance. A hospital setting also allows for careful monitoring of the psychotic symptoms as well as any side effects, including acute dystonia, akathisia, or neuroleptic malignant syndrome (266), that may arise from treatment with antipsychotic medications.

Patients with first-episode psychosis are comparatively more treatment responsive than patients with multiple episodes of psychosis but, at the same time, are quite sensitive to side effects (267–270). Up to the early 1990s, drug treatment for a first episode of psychosis was limited to first-generation antipsychotic medications that could cause severe sedation and extrapyramidal side effects. The second-generation antipsychotic medications have less propensity to cause extrapyramidal side effects, and patients are hence less likely to need concomitant anticholinergic agents (271–273).

More than 70% of first-episode patients achieve a full remission of psychotic signs and symptoms within 3–4 months, with 83% achieving stable remission at the end of 1 year (274). Studies also reveal that first-episode patients often respond to low doses of antipsychotic medications (275–279). However, predictors of poor treatment response include male gender, pre- or perinatal injury, more severe hallucinations and delusions, attentional impairments, poor premorbid function, longer duration of untreated psychosis (280), the development of extrapyramidal side effects (281), and high levels of expressed emotion in the patient's family (282–289).

Not uncommonly, symptoms of schizophrenia have their onset before adulthood, and aspects of treatment may differ in children and adolescents. For more information on treating children and adolescents, readers are referred to the American Academy of Child and Adolescent Psychiatry's *Practice Parameter for the Assessment and Treatment of Children and Adolescents With Schizophrenia* (290).

Once remission of psychotic symptoms is achieved, a high priority should be placed on minimizing risk of relapse, given its potential clinical, social, and vocational costs. In particular, recurrent episodes are associated with increasing risk of chronic residual symptoms and evidence of anatomical neuroprogression (257, 280, 291–293). Patients, their families, and treating clinicians often hope that symptom remission indicates that the disease will not become chronic, although this is true only for a minority (about 10%–20%) of patients (46, 218, 294). Thus, clinicians should candidly discuss the high risk of relapse and factors that may minimize relapse risk. Although there is very little study of factors that act to maintain recovery in remitted first-episode patients, evidence suggests that antipsychotics are highly effective in prevention of relapse. In patients for whom antipsychotics are prescribed, 1-year relapse risk varies from 0% to 46%, with relapse rates of patients who discontinue taking medication being up to five times higher than rates for those who continue treatment (46, 210–213). Since adherence to maintenance medication treatment likely influences effectiveness, it may contribute to the varying relapse rates found in these studies.

In arriving at a plan of treatment with remitted first-episode patients, clinicians should engage patients in discussion of the long-term potential risks of maintenance treatment with the prescribed antipsychotic versus risks of relapse (e.g., effect of relapse on social and vocational function, risk of dangerous behaviors with relapse, and risk of developing chronic treatment-resistant symptoms). Prudent treatment options that clinicians may discuss with remitted patients include either 1) indefinite antipsychotic maintenance medication (295) or 2) medication discontinuation with close follow-up and a plan of antipsychotic reinstitution with symptom recurrence. Medications should never be stopped abruptly, as rebound psychosis may result and may be misinterpreted as a reoccurrence. In addition to maintenance antipsychotic medication, other potential strategies to maintain recovery in remitted first-episode patients include enhancing stress management and eliminating exposure to cannabinoids and psychostimulants (296).

b) Subtypes and deficit symptoms

According to DSM-IV-TR, the classic subtypes of schizophrenia are paranoid, disorganized, catatonic, undifferentiated, and residual. There are at present no treatment strategies specific to the various subtypes, with the exception of the use of benzodiazepines for catatonia. The deficit/nondeficit categorization, or the deficit syndrome, is also important to recognize, although there are also no specific treatments (297). The negative symptoms of schizophrenia may be classified as primary or secondary. Negative symptoms may be primary and represent a core feature of schizophrenia, or they may be secondary to positive psychotic symptoms (e.g., paranoid withdrawal), medication side effects (e.g., dysphoria), depressive symptoms (e.g., anhedonia), anxiety symptoms (e.g., social phobia), demoralization, or environmental deprivation (e.g., in chronic institutionalization). Deficit schizophrenia is heavily loaded with enduring primary negative symptoms such as affective flattening, alogia, and avolition.

The prevalence of deficit states in first-episode schizophrenia has been estimated to be between 4% and 10% (298). Negative symptoms are already present in the prodromal phase (299–301), and the prevalence increases with the length of the schizophrenic illness (302–306). Male patients have been found to experience more negative symptoms than female patients (307–309). Patients with deficit schizophrenia are also found to have poorer premorbid adjustment during childhood and early adolescence. They exhibit more impairment in general cognitive abilities and have problems in sequencing of complex motor acts, which suggests frontoparietal dysfunction (310).

Treatment of negative symptoms begins with assessing the patient for factors that can cause the appearance of secondary negative symptoms (311). The treatment of such secondary negative symptoms consists of treating their cause, e.g., antipsychotics for primary positive symptoms, antidepressants for depression, anxiolytics for anxiety disorders, or antiparkinsonian agents or antipsychotic dose reduction for extrapyramidal side effects. If negative symptoms persist after such treatment, they are presumed to be primary negative symptoms of the deficit state (312).

There are no treatments with proven efficacy for primary negative symptoms. Clozapine was reported to be effective for negative symptoms in earlier short-term trials (313), but subsequent longer-term studies challenged such claims (314, 315), although clozapine treatment was associated with significant improvement in social and occupational functioning (314). The second-generation antipsychotic medications have been reported to be useful against negative symptoms (316–322), but this improvement may be accounted for by their having less propensity to cause extrapyramidal side effects (323).

c) Substance use disorders

More than one-third of patients with schizophrenia spectrum disorders also have a substance use disorder, and people with schizophrenia show six times the risk of developing a substance use disorder than do persons in the general population (324). Other research finds that between 20% and 65% of people with schizophrenia experience comorbid substance use disorders (325–328). A recent Australian study found the 6-month and lifetime prevalence of substance abuse or dependence among people with schizophrenia to be 26.8% and 59.8%, respectively (329).

Substance abuse in schizophrenia has been associated with male gender, single marital status, less education, earlier age at onset of schizophrenia and at first hospital admission, frequent and longer periods of hospitalization, more pronounced psychotic symptoms, more severe cerebral gray matter volume deficits, and negative consequences such as poor treatment adherence, depressive symptoms, suicide, violence, legal problems, incarceration, severe financial problems, family burden, housing instability, and increased risk of HIV infection (327, 330–332) and hepatitis infection, particularly hepatitis C infection (333). Substance abuse has been associated with precipitation of schizophrenia at an earlier age (334–340), and in some studies amphetamine abuse has been associated with an earlier age of onset (341). Alcohol and a variety of other substances have also been associated with symptom relapses in schizophrenia (342). Nicotine, alcohol, cannabis, and cocaine have been found to be the most commonly abused substances. Patients may also abuse prescribed medications such as benzodiazepines and antiparkinsonian agents.

The goals of treatment for patients with schizophrenia who also have a substance use disorder are the same as those for treatment of schizophrenia without comorbidity but with the addition of the goals for treatment of substance use disorders, e.g., harm reduction, abstinence, relapse prevention, and rehabilitation (343).

Evaluation of the patient with schizophrenia should always include a comprehensive inquiry into possible substance use. Self-report is often unreliable; corroborating evidence from all sources such as family members, friends, community-based case managers, and treatment personnel should be sought (330, 344). Screening instruments for substance use disorders developed for the general population, such as the Alcohol Use Disorders Identification Test (AUDIT) (345), can be used, but screening instruments specifically for patients with severe mental illnesses, such as the Dartmouth Assessment of Lifestyle Instrument (346), have been developed and may have greater sensitivity for detecting substance use disorders in people with schizophrenia. Laboratory investigations such as urine and blood toxicology for abused substances and liver function tests should be carried out. Many patients with schizophrenia do not develop the full physiological dependence syndrome associated with dependence on alcohol or other substances (330). However, even use of low levels of alcohol or other substances by patients with schizophrenia can have untoward consequences. Psychiatrists should therefore attend carefully to the presence of alcohol or other substance use and be familiar with the potential negative consequences described earlier. The rates of current substance use will likely be higher in acute settings such as the emergency department, and thus the index of suspicion and effort devoted to assessment of substance use should be especially high in such settings.

Traditionally, patients with schizophrenia and comorbid substance use disorders were treated in separate programs, either sequentially or in parallel, for the two types of disorder. Since the mid-1980s, a comprehensive integrated treatment model has been adopted to provide continuous outpatient treatment interventions and support over long periods of time (months to years), enabling patients to acquire the skills they need to manage both illnesses and to pursue functional goals. In this model, the same clinicians or teams of clinicians provide treatment both for substance use disorders and for other mental disorders. This form of treatment features assertive outreach, case management, family interventions, housing, rehabilitation, and pharmacotherapy. It also includes a stage-wise motivational approach for patients who do not recognize the need for treatment of substance use disorders and behavioral interventions for those who are trying to attain or maintain abstinence. The interventions have been associated with reduced substance use and attainment of remission (347–350).

Initially, many patients need interventions to build motivation rather than to achieve abstinence. Special efforts are made to help them recognize that their substance use is interfering with their ability to pursue personal goals and to nurture their desire to reduce and eliminate their substance use (161, 349). Such efforts represent examples of interventions during the second (persuasion) stage in a four-stage dual-diagnosis treatment model based on readiness for change; the other treatment stages are engagement, active treatment, and relapse prevention (351). Studies show that treatment programs with these characteristics can be effective in reducing substance use and in decreasing the frequency and severity of psychotic decompensations (332, 352–354). Collaboration with family members is often helpful for both the patients and the family members (64, 171, 355, 356).

In practice, treatment of substance use disorders is commonly conducted by means of a group therapy approach, usually after patients have achieved stabilization of their schizophrenic symptoms. The therapeutic approach should be an integrated one that takes into account patients' cognitive deficits and limited tolerance for stress. Generally, groups should emphasize support, psychoeducation, and skills training (344, 352, 357). The length and frequency of group sessions should be regulated according to the attention span and interactive tolerance of the patients. Therapists should be active in keeping the group structured and focused and should limit the amount of stress by avoiding the direct confrontation of patients that is common to traditional treatment programs for persons with substance use disorders. Patients should understand that they have two complex chronic disorders that together lead to a poorer prognosis than each would have separately. Patients who have not yet attained complete abstinence should be accepted into treatment, with abstinence as a treatment goal (344, 352, 358). Patients who do not view abstinence as a treatment goal may still be successfully engaged in treatment that is aimed at achieving abstinence (359). Community-based self-help and support groups such as Alcoholics Anonymous or Narcotics Anonymous can be important in the recovery of patients with substance use disorders. Such connections are, however, more effective once patients are actively pursuing abstinence (349).

Antipsychotic medications remain the mainstay of pharmacological treatment for patients with comorbid substance use disorders. They are used in the usual doses, but patients should be informed that side effects such as sedation and incoordination can be aggravated when combining antipsychotic medication with alcohol or other substances. First-generation antipsychotic medications and clozapine also have the potential to lower the seizure threshold and infrequently may precipitate seizures during alcohol or benzodiazepine withdrawal. Dysphoria associated with first-generation antipsychotic medications may precipitate or worsen the substance use (360). On the other hand, studies have demonstrated that clozapine use is associated with reductions in the use of nicotine, alcohol, cannabis, and cocaine (361–363). In some clinical trials, second-generation antipsychotics such as risperidone and olanzapine have also been shown to be effective for reducing craving in cocaine dependence (364).

There is suggestive evidence from a case series of 30 patients with schizophrenia and other severe mental illnesses and alcoholism that disulfiram in moderate doses can be used safely and is associated with clinical benefits in alcohol outcomes over 1–3 years (365). However, for patients with schizophrenia who abuse alcohol, disulfiram may pose some risk since it can precipitate psychosis at high doses (358, 366). It also has harmful physical effects when taken with alcohol, and thus it is recommended only for patients who are motivated and who have previously shown good judgment, treatment adherence, and reality testing.

d) Depressive symptoms

Depressive symptoms are common in all phases of schizophrenia (367). The proportion of patients with schizophrenia who also manifest depression ranges from 7% to 75% (368). Depression may occur in the prodromal phase (300, 301), in the first episode (369–371), during the early course (372, 373), and after remission, and it may be superimposed on the symptoms of residual schizophrenia ("postpsychotic depression") (374) or may occur in a prodrome to a psychotic relapse (375–379).

When patients with schizophrenia present with depressive features, important differential diagnostic possibilities need to be considered (368, 380). These include side effects of antipsychotic medications (including medication-induced dysphoria, akinesia, and akathisia), demoralization, and the primary negative symptoms of schizophrenia. Concurrent abuse or the sudden withdrawal of substances such as cannabis, cocaine, narcotics, alcohol, nicotine, and caffeine can also lead to depression. When the depressive symptoms are present at a syndromal level during the acute phase of the schizophrenic illness, the possibility of schizoaffective disorder should be considered.

Depressive symptoms that occur during the acute psychotic phase usually improve as the patient recovers from the psychosis. There is also evidence to suggest that depressive symptoms are reduced by antipsychotic treatment, with comparison trials finding that second-generation antipsychotics may have greater efficacy for depressive symptoms than first-generation antipsychotics (381, 382). However, there is also evidence to suggest that this apparent antidepressant effect may be related to the lower likelihood of neurological side effects with second-generation antipsychotics (222, 368, 383, 384). The approach hence is first to treat the psychosis.

If antipsychotic medication-induced dysphoria is suspected, then antipsychotic dose reduction may be effective. Alternatively, the clinician may switch the patient's medication to an antipsychotic with a lower risk of inducing extrapyramidal symptoms (Table 4). There is no evidence that medications that treat the motor symptoms of extrapyramidal side effects (e.g., benztropine, amantadine) (Table 5) are effective for the treatment of neuroleptic-induced dysphoria.

Antidepressants are added as an adjunct to antipsychotics when the depressive symptoms meet the syndromal criteria for major depressive disorder, are severe and causing significant distress (e.g., when accompanied by suicidal ideation), or are interfering with function. Tricyclic antidepressants have been extensively studied in the treatment of postpsychotic depression (103, 385). Antidepressants, including the selective serotonin reuptake inhibitors (SSRIs) and dual reuptake inhibitors, have also been found to be useful in the treatment of depression in schizophrenia (368, 384). However, very few studies have examined the effects of antidepressants in patients treated with second-generation antipsychotic medications, making it difficult to evaluate the current utility of adjunctive antidepressant agents. When prescribed, antidepressants are used in the same doses that are used for treatment of major depressive disorder. There are, however, potential pharmacokinetic interactions with certain antipsychotic medications; for example, the SSRIs (such as fluoxetine, paroxetine, and fluvoxamine) are inhibitors of cytochrome P450 enzymes and thereby increase antipsychotic plasma levels. Similarly, the blood levels of some antidepressants may be elevated by the concomitant administration of antipsychotic medications.

e) Risk of suicide

Suicide is the leading cause of premature death among persons with schizophrenia (386, 387). Compared to the general population, persons with schizophrenia are nine times more likely to die by suicide (388). Up to 30% of patients with schizophrenia attempt suicide (389), and between 4% and 10% die by suicide (390–394). The estimated rate of suicidal behavior among persons with schizophrenia is between 20% and 40% (395, 396).

Some risk factors for suicide in schizophrenia are the same as those for the general population, including being male, white, single, socially isolated, and unemployed; having a positive family history of suicide; previous suicide attempts; having a substance use disorder; being depressed or hopeless; and having a significant recent adverse life event. Specific risk factors for suicide among persons with schizophrenia are young age, high socioeconomic status background, high IQ with a high level of premorbid scholastic achievement, high aspirations and expectations, an early age at onset of illness/first hospitalization, a chronic and deteriorating course with many relapses, and greater insight into the illness (391, 397–401). A change in the environment, such as a hospital admission and discharge, may trigger suicidal behavior (402, 403). Suicide is more common within the first 6 years of the initial hospitalization and also during periods of remission after 5–10 years of illness. Other risk factors include severe depressive and psychotic symptoms, with an increase in the patient's paranoid behavior (395, 404–406). Suicidal ideation has also been shown to be predictive of suicide over the subsequent 2–4 weeks (407). As patients do not often report suicidal ideation spontaneously, clinicians are encouraged to ask patients about suicidal ideas whenever there is suggestion that they could be present (e.g., in the presence of depression or severe stress). Treatment-related factors associated with suicide include inadequate antipsychotic treatment, nonadherence to the medication regimen, and lack of response to medication (408). In several case reports, suicide has also been noted among patients with akathisia (409, 410).

Despite identification of these risk factors, it is not possible to predict whether an individual patient will attempt suicide or will die by suicide. Suicide thus must be considered at all stages of the illness, and suicide risk must be assessed initially and regularly as part of each patient's psychiatric evaluation. The patient's desire to die may be more important than the lethality of the methods used (403). Additional information may be obtained from close family members and treating therapists. Patients should be admitted to a secure inpatient unit if they are judged to be at substantial risk for suicide.

It is important to maximize the treatment of both psychosis and depression. There is suggestive evidence that both first- and second-generation antipsychotic medications may reduce the risk of suicide (411). However, clozapine is the most extensively studied and has been shown to have the greatest therapeutic effect on suicidal behavior, possibly reducing the suicide rate by as much as 75%–85% (55, 398, 399, 412). For these reasons, clozapine should be preferentially considered for patients with a history of chronic and persistent suicidal ideation or behaviors.

During the initial hospitalization, suicide precautions should be instituted, and the patient must be closely monitored to prevent escape. There should also be minimal use of ward transfers. Suicide risk should be examined carefully before a patient is granted any privileges and again before the patient is finally discharged from the hospital. The patient and the patient's family members should be advised to look for warning signs and to initiate specific contingency plans if suicidal ideation recurs. In outpatients, the frequency of visits should be higher after a recent discharge from the hospital and may need to be increased in times of personal crisis, significant environmental changes, heightened distress, or deepening depression during the course of illness.

For additional information, readers are directed to APA's *Practice Guideline for the Assessment and Treatment of Patients With Suicidal Behaviors* (56) (included in this volume).

f) Aggressive behavior

Although only a minority of patients with schizophrenia are violent, evidence does suggest that schizophrenia is associated with an increase in the risk of aggressive behavior (413–419). Sociodemographic risk factors for aggression in schizophrenia are male gender; being poor, unskilled, uneducated, or unmarried; and having a history of prior arrests or a prior history of violence (420). The risk for aggressive behavior increases with comorbid alcohol abuse, substance abuse, antisocial personality, or neurological impairment (421–427). Violent patients with schizophrenia have more positive symptoms and bizarre behaviors and may act on their delusions, especially if the delusions are distressing and the patient can find evidence to support them (428–430). Patients who experience command hallucinations to harm others are also more likely to be violent (431).

Identifying risk factors for violence and assessment of dangerousness are parts of a standard psychiatric evaluation, which should be conducted in an environment that is safe for both the patient and clinician (432). It is important to determine if use of alcohol or other substances, including use of amphetamines or other stimulants, is causing or contributing to aggressive behavior. Severe akathisia associated with prescribed medications may also cause or contribute to aggressive behavior. It is important to inquire about thoughts of violence and determine the persons to whom these thoughts are directed. Parents, for example, are frequent targets of violence when it occurs (433). When a patient is found to pose a serious threat to others (e.g., having homicidal ideation with imminent plans), the psychiatrist should consider hospitalizing the patient and must exercise his or her own best judgment, in accord with the legal requirements of the jurisdiction, to protect those people from foreseeable harm (54, 434).

If the patient is acutely aggressive, the clinician can try to calm the patient by distraction or "talking down" techniques. If restraint or seclusion is needed, it should be done with adequate numbers of well-trained professional staff (70). When sedation is indicated and the patient is unwilling to accept oral medication, intramuscular injection of a first-generation antipsychotic agent (5 mg of haloperidol) (75) or second-generation agent (e.g., ziprasidone) (76–79) can be given, with or without a concomitant dose of 1–2 mg of oral or intramuscular lorazepam (72–74). Other medications, such as 5 mg i.m. of droperidol, can be used in selected clinical situations of extreme emergency or in highly agitated patients (80, 435). However, if droperidol is used, its potential for cardiac rhythm disturbances must be considered, as indicated in its labeling by a black-box warning for QTc prolongation. After seclusion, restraint, or sedation, the mental status and vital signs of the patient should be monitored regularly. Release from seclusion or restraint can proceed in a graded fashion, as risk of harm to self or others diminishes (432).

Limit setting and behavioral approaches have been employed for the management of persistently violent patients (432, 436). Antipsychotic medications remain the mainstay of management (421, 437), with good evidence for clozapine in particular (438–440). Other agents have been used, including mood stabilizers (lithium, valproate), SSRIs (such as citalopram), benzodiazepines, and β-adrenergic blocking agents (propranolol, nadolol), but empirical evidence is lacking.

It is common for patients with schizophrenia in the community to stop taking their medications. Patients who are more likely to be violent with psychotic relapses are of particular concern and may be primary candidates for mandatory outpatient treatment programs (441) (see Section II.A.3, "Developing a Therapeutic Alliance and Promoting Treatment Adherence").

g) Psychosis-induced polydipsia

Polydipsia is compulsive water drinking, usually in excess of 3 liters per day. It can be complicated by water intoxication, i.e., severe hyponatremia (serum sodium <120 mmol/liter), which is potentially fatal, as the associated cerebral edema can result in delirium, seizures, coma, and death. About 20%–25% of chronically ill inpatients have primary polydipsia, and as many as 10% have a history of water intoxication (442–445).

The pathophysiology of the water imbalance is still unclear. It occurs most commonly in the most severely ill patients with schizophrenia and thus has been termed "psychosis-induced polydipsia." Polydipsia and water intoxication are associated with long hospitalization, high doses of antipsychotic medications, moderate doses of anticholinergic medications, and heavy smoking (442, 444). Development of hyponatremia has also been associated with use of diuretics, SSRIs and venlafaxine (446, 447), tricyclic antidepressants, and calcium antagonists (448). Polydipsia has also been known to occur prior to the introduction of antipsychotic medications (449).

The approach to psychosis-induced polydipsia is to control both the psychosis and water intake after excluding possible underlying medical causes of polydipsia, such as diabetes mellitus, diabetes insipidus, chronic renal failure, malignancy, pulmonary disease, hypocalcemia, and hypokalemia. Acute management involves water restriction and sodium replacement to prevent seizures. Clozapine appears to be effective, albeit in studies with small sample sizes

(450–452). The second-generation antipsychotics have also been examined for their role in the long-term management of the condition (453, 454). Various other medications, including demeclocycline (455, 456), naltrexone (457), enalapril (458), clonidine (458, 459), and propranolol (460), have also been used in some case studies.

2. Demographic and psychosocial variables

a) Homelessness

By current estimates, as many as 800,000 Americans are homeless on any given night; an estimated one-fourth of these people have serious mental illnesses, and more than one-half have an alcohol and/or drug problem (461). Schizophrenia is a risk factor for homelessness, as is infectious disease, alcohol and other substance use, depression, and social isolation (462, 463). Comprehensive reviews have suggested that the rate of schizophrenia in homeless persons has ranged from 2% to 45%. Methodologically superior studies have produced estimates of 4%–16%, with a weighted average prevalence of 11% (464). Factors that have been noted to contribute to the magnitude of homelessness among patients with schizophrenia include deinstitutionalization (465), limitations of public funding, problems in service integration, and lack of low-cost housing (466). Substance use disorders contribute substantially to homelessness among patients with schizophrenia. Many housing programs do not accept patients with schizophrenia who use alcohol or other substances, and treatment for substance use disorders is often lacking for these individuals (466). In addition, the illness of schizophrenia may directly predispose persons to housing difficulties through withdrawal, disorganization, and disruptive behaviors (467).

Homeless mentally ill persons are likely to have multiple impairments. Most lack basic health care, income, and any social support network. Only slightly more than one-half of the homeless persons with schizophrenia have been found to be currently receiving psychiatric treatment (464). Homeless persons with schizophrenia have been found to have elevated rates of victimization (468) and to have mortality rates that are three to four times higher than the expected rate (469). Further, a large study of mentally ill homeless veterans found that a majority of homeless veterans contacted through a national outreach program did not receive medical services within 6 months of program entry (470). Medical treatment is thus a great challenge for this population.

Given the level of need of this population, services should include provision of appropriate housing, access to medical services, treatment of substance use disorders, income support and benefits, and rehabilitation and employment assistance (466). Such services must be comprehensive, continuous, accessible, and individualized (467). A number of controlled studies have demonstrated the effectiveness of such treatment models for reducing homelessness and improving psychiatric outcomes (164, 471). The Center for Mental Health Services conducted a multisite 5-year demonstration program called Access to Community Care and Effective Services and Supports (ACCESS) to test the effect of the integration of fragmented services in treating homeless persons with serious mental illness. This study involved 18 sites in nine states from 1993 to 1998, and treatment outcomes were studied at both the system and patient levels. All project sites conducted extensive outreach efforts to engage homeless persons and provided a comprehensive range of services, including mental health treatment, medications, substance use disorder treatment or referral, job placement, housing support, social support, and primary health care. Patients served in the ACCESS program showed improved housing stability and reductions in substance use and minor criminal incidents, as well as increased use of psychiatric outpatient care, although integration of treatment did not influence these outcomes. The provision of direct community services and outreach appeared to be most important.

Clinical care of homeless mentally ill patients involves three basic stages: 1) engagement, 2) intensive care, and 3) ongoing rehabilitation (472). In introducing services into the community, psychiatrists must be prepared to work with homeless patients in nonclinical environments, including streets, shelters, subways, bus terminals, and other public spaces. In discussing outreach to homeless patients with schizophrenia, Goldfinger (467) stressed the importance of engagement. Homeless patients with schizophrenia are often fearful and distrustful of the mental health system, and they can require a combination of patience, persistence, and understanding. Depending on the needs and wants of a particular patient, the provision of food, clothing, medical attention, or simply company can be indispensable in developing a therapeutic relationship. As noted by Goldfinger (467), such provisions document one's concern, demonstrate one's reliability, and acknowledge the importance of the needs of the homeless person with schizophrenia. To engage the homeless person with schizophrenia, active outreach is usually necessary and is often performed by case managers. In particular, street outreach to homeless persons with serious mental illness is justified, as they have been found to be more severely impaired, to have more basic service needs, to be less motivated to seek treatment, and to take longer to engage than those contacted in other settings. The ACCESS program found that patients engaged from the street showed improvement on nearly all outcome measures that was equivalent to that of enrolled patients who were contacted in shelters and other service agencies (473).

Despite appropriate outreach efforts, some homeless persons with mental illness are so impaired that they remain unable to recognize their basic needs or avoid personal dangers. One program developed to address the treatment needs of this population was the Homeless Emergency Liaison Project (Project HELP), in which a mobile treatment team arranged for involuntary psychiatric emergency department evaluation of high-risk homeless patients (474). Involuntary hospitalization resulted from 93% of such evaluations, and 80% of all patients received the diagnosis of schizophrenia. At 2-year follow-up of 298 patients initially evaluated during the project, only 12% were found to be back living on the streets.

b) Cultural factors

Cultural factors are known to affect the course, diagnosis, and treatment of schizophrenia (475). There is a robust pattern of evidence that race has a substantial effect on whether persons with substantively similar symptoms receive a diagnosis of an affective disorder or a schizophrenia spectrum psychotic disorder. Compared with Caucasians, African Americans, especially men, are less likely to receive a diagnosis of a mood disorder and more likely to receive a diagnosis of schizophrenia (476–479). African Americans with schizophrenia are also less likely to receive a diagnosis of a comorbid affective or anxiety disorder (480, 481). While it is possible that such differences may reflect actual illness variation among racial/ethnic groups, there is growing evidence that cultural differences in symptom and personal presentation, help seeking, interpretation of symptoms and clinical judgments by (usually Caucasian) clinicians, and treatment referral are likely causing race-linked biases in diagnosis and therefore in treatment (e.g., see references 482–486). Additional possible causes or contributors to this pattern of disparity include low levels of cultural competence among clinicians, unbalanced research samples, inaccurate or biased pathology assessment tools, and the failure of researchers to control for socioeconomic status, education, and urbanicity (487, 488). These remarkably consistent findings suggest that clinicians should be mindful of the extent to which cultural factors influence their diagnostic approach.

c) Race

Once patients receive a diagnosis, substantial data suggest that race affects the type of pharmacological treatment they receive. For example, the Schizophrenia Patient Outcomes Research Team (PORT) (65) showed that among patients for whom psychotropic medications at doses outside the recommended range were prescribed, patients from racial/ethnic minority groups (especially African Americans) were much more likely than Caucasian patients to receive doses above recommended levels. The same patients were also more likely to receive prophylactic antiparkinsonian agents, suggesting increased rates of adverse side effects related to higher doses.

Prescription of higher doses of antipsychotic medications to African American patients has also been noted in several other reports (489–493).

However, in another PORT study, among patients with schizophrenia who were also experiencing significant depression, Caucasian patients were significantly more likely to receive adjunctive medications (494). In addition, there is growing evidence that racial/ethnic minority patients with psychotic disorders are less likely than Caucasian patients to receive second-generation antipsychotics and more likely to receive long-acting injectable agents (495–498). Other research suggests that these gaps may be decreasing over time but are still persistent and may be related to differential prescribing patterns in private versus managed health care (496, 499).

There is clearly a need for more research to describe and understand the differences in patterns of treatment by race and ethnicity. Most of the published research focuses on African Americans; the needs and treatments of other cultural groups also require attention. The observed phenomena provide little guidance about whether the care delivered is appropriate. In the meantime, the strength and consistency of these findings suggest that clinicians should consider the extent to which a patient's race and/or ethnicity are playing a role in the treatment and should ensure that care is being individualized and optimized.

To some extent, differences in drug dosing or side effect risk may be related to genetically based differences in drug metabolism. For example, the activity of the enzyme encoded by the CYP2D6 gene is very low or absent in 5%–8% of Caucasians but only 2%–5% of African Americans and Asians. Low activity of the enzyme encoded by the CYP2D6 gene may dramatically affect the metabolism of many drugs, increasing serum levels (500). There is also suggestive evidence that up to one-third of African Americans possess genetic polymorphisms of other enzymes that metabolize psychotropic agents, resulting in altered metabolism and potential for enhanced medication side effects. Ethnic factors may also confer a susceptibility to medication side effects in certain persons. For example, patients of Jewish descent have been noted to be at greater risk for clozapine-induced agranulocytosis than other patients with schizophrenia (501) and therefore may require close monitoring during clozapine treatment.

d) Gender

There are numerous gender differences in the presentation and course of schizophrenia (502–505). Men with schizophrenia have been noted to have a younger age at onset, a poorer premorbid history, more negative symptoms, a greater likelihood of having the deficit syndrome (306, 309), and a poorer overall course than women with schizophrenia (503, 506). Compared with men, women are more likely to have affective symptoms, auditory hallucinations, and persecutory delusions, but they have a better overall course and better outcomes than men, as evidenced by better social and occupational functioning, fewer hospitalizations, and less substance use and antisocial behavior (504, 505, 507). While such differences may be biologically mediated, psychosocial factors, including family and societal expectations, may also affect outcome. Haas and colleagues (507) noted that social and occupational role demands may result in unrealistic family expectations of men with schizophrenia, and this issue should be dealt with in treatment.

There are also gender differences in both response to and adverse effects of treatments for schizophrenia. Most of this research has been conducted with first-generation antipsychotic medications. Women exhibit more rapid responses to antipsychotic medications and a greater degree of improvement in both first-episode and multi-episode schizophrenia (504). It has also been observed that even after body weight is considered, women require lower antipsychotic doses (508, 509) than men, although there is suggestive evidence that postmenopausal women may require higher doses (504). Although women may show greater responsivity to antipsychotics, they also experience more neurological side effects, including acute dystonia, parkinsonism, akathisia, and tardive dyskinesia (504). Women also develop higher serum prolactin levels in response to both first-generation antipsychotics and risperidone, compared with men (504), and therefore women may be more prone to the sexual side effects of the medications. Finally, although studies of gender differences in response to psychosocial treatments are sparse, there is some evidence to suggest that social skills training may be more effective for male patients, whereas inpatient family interventions have shown greater success in families of female patients (504, 505).

e) Pregnancy

Treatment of the pregnant or lactating patient with schizophrenia must consider two issues: 1) risks of various psychotropic medications to the fetus, newborn, and breast-fed infant, and 2) adequacy of prenatal care. A general reference on medications in pregnancy and lactation is the text by Briggs et al. (510).

Controlled studies of psychotropic drug risks during pregnancy are, for obvious ethical reasons, not done. Knowledge of the risks of these agents comes from animal studies and from uncontrolled exposures in humans. Nonetheless, there is a body of information that can help guide clinicians' and patients' decision making about the use of psychotropic agents during pregnancy and lactation. Risks do vary from drug to drug and from drug class to drug class. In addition, two periods of high risk to the fetus or newborn are identifiable: teratogenic risk is highest in the first trimester, and withdrawal risk is highest at the time of birth. Only with planned pregnancies is management of first trimester psychotropic drug exposure under full control of the doctor and patient. Drug withdrawal risk at the time of parturition may be more predictable and manageable, depending on the drug(s) involved and the circumstances of delivery.

There are substantial data on fetal exposure to first-generation antipsychotic medications, with relatively little evidence of harmful effects, especially with high-potency agents (511–513). Much less information is available regarding fetal exposure to second-generation antipsychotic medications. Koren et al. (514) found that pregnant women with schizophrenia taking second-generation antipsychotic medications were frequently obese and had inadequate intake of folic acid, putting their offspring at increased risk for neural tube defects. Such an outcome would be an indirect rather than a direct effect of these medications. A limited number of reports of treatment with olanzapine during pregnancy and lactation showed that olanzapine did not appear to increase the risk of harm (515). A case report of clozapine treatment during pregnancy described development of gestational diabetes, possibly exacerbated by clozapine, but no fetal abnormalities (516). Pregnancy can be a period of decreased symptoms for women with schizophrenia, but relapses are frequent in the postpartum period (517). Thus, the clinical risks of not using antipsychotic medications may be somewhat less during pregnancy but are greater thereafter.

Compared with antipsychotic medications, mood stabilizers and benzodiazepines are much more closely associated with fetal malformations and behavioral effects (511, 513, 518). Thus, their risk/benefit ratio is different, and the need for their continuation during pregnancy and breast-feeding requires strong clinical justification.

A number of studies have shown that pregnant women with schizophrenia receive relatively poor prenatal care. These women have more obstetric complications, and their offspring are more likely to have adverse outcomes, such as low birth weight and stillbirth (519–522). There are many contributing factors to the relatively poor prenatal care and outcomes, such as low socioeconomic status, high rates of smoking and substance use disorders, and obesity. For the clinician treating a pregnant woman with schizophrenia, it is particularly important to insist on early involvement of an obstetrician who can help reduce the risks of the pregnancy and with whom risks and benefits of pharmacological treatment options can be discussed.

f) Psychosocial stressors

A variety of psychosocial stressors can precipitate the initial development or recurrence of symptoms in a vulnerable person (304, 523–526). Stressors include stressful life events (e.g., interpersonal loss, leaving home, military service), sociocultural stress (e.g., poverty, homelessness, fragmented social network), or a distressing emotional climate (e.g., hostile and critical attitudes and overprotection by others in one's living situation or high levels of expressed emotion) (282–289). While schizophrenia can emerge or worsen in the absence of environmental influences, attention to stressors frequently helps to prevent relapse and/or maximize healthy functioning. Sometimes the stress is internal, and knowledge of developmental vulnerabilities can assist in identifying and assisting with this variety of stress. Treatment strategies include preventing the development or accumulation of stressors and helping the patient develop coping strategies that keep tension levels within manageable bounds.

g) Schizophrenia in later life

With the overall increase in longevity, the number of older patients with schizophrenia is expected to increase rapidly over the next three decades (527). Among middle-aged and elderly persons with schizophrenia, approximately 80% have early-onset schizophrenia (528), with the remaining 20% including persons with late-onset schizophrenia (onset after age 40) and very-late-onset schizophrenia-like psychosis (onset after age 60) (DSM-IV, 529). The rate of aging-associated cognitive decline in older patients with schizophrenia is similar to that in age-comparable normal persons, although, as with younger patients, they have greater overall cognitive impairment (530, 531). The approach to the treatment of older persons with schizophrenia is similar to that of younger patients (532) and involves combining pharmacotherapies with psychosocial interventions.

Several age-related physiological changes may influence the approach to pharmacotherapy. These physiological changes include reduced cardiac output (and concomitant reduction in renal and hepatic blood flow, relative to younger persons), reduced glomerular filtration rate, possible reduction in hepatic metabolism, and increased fat content. These changes may alter the absorption, distribution, metabolism, and excretion of medications and may result in prolonged drug effects and greater sensitivity to medications, in terms of both therapeutic response and side effects (533). Age-related changes in receptor-site activity may further influence response to drugs in elderly patients. In general, recommended starting doses in older patients are one-quarter to one-half of the usual adult starting dose (529) (see Table 2).

The presence of concomitant medical illness or the use of multiple medications frequently complicates the treatment of older patients. In addition, age-related sensory deficits and cognitive impairment may interfere with patients' adherence to prescribed medication regimens. Elderly patients may unintentionally take incorrect doses of medications or follow erroneous dosing schedules.

Several important considerations bear on the use of antipsychotics in elderly patients. The cumulative annual incidence of tardive dyskinesia with first-generation antipsychotic medications has been found to be sixfold higher in later life than in younger adults (i.e., about 30% in later life) (534). Other side effects of particular concern in elderly patients include sedation, anticholinergic effects, and postural hypotension. Second-generation antipsychotics are generally recommended over first-generation agents because of their significantly lower risk of inducing extrapyramidal symptoms and tardive dyskinesia in older persons (534–538). However, the second-generation agents have other clinically significant and common side effects (Table 4), most notably sedation and orthostatic hypotension. Elderly patients with low cardiac output are especially vulnerable to hypotension and cardiac arrhythmia. The anticholinergic side effects of antipsychotic drugs in the presence of the age-related decrease in cholinergic function can contribute to problems such as urinary retention, confusion, and constipation or fecal impaction in the elderly patient. In some cases, elderly patients who are frail or poorly nourished may benefit from medication-induced weight gain; however, weight gain may also aggravate preexisting cardiovascular disease or osteoarthritis in this population. Elevated prolactin levels may also compromise bone-mineral density and increase osteoporosis.

Depression is not only common but also functionally disruptive in older persons with schizophrenia (539). In such instances, an antidepressant may need to be added to the treatment regimen. A wide variety of antidepressants are commonly used, although no comprehensive comparative trials in this population have been published. One small study found citalopram to be both useful and relatively safe in older patients with psychosis (540).

Psychosocial treatments are also recommended for a majority of individuals. Psychosocial evaluation may reveal a precipitating stress, such as a death in the family or a move to unfamiliar surroundings, that may explain a sudden change in the elderly person's behavior. Recent work has evaluated the benefits of integrated cognitive behavioral and social skills training (CBSST) in groups of older patients with schizophrenia (541). Results of a small randomized, controlled pilot study comparing CBSST plus pharmacotherapy to pharmacotherapy alone demonstrated the feasibility and acceptability by patients of CBSST and some improvement in psychopathology with CBSST in older patients with schizophrenia (541). Another pilot study showed the usefulness of functional adaptation skills training (542) in improving daily functioning in older patients with schizophrenia.

3. Concurrent general medical conditions

Patients with schizophrenia and related severe and persistent mental illness suffer disproportionately from a variety of comorbidities, including cardiovascular disease, respiratory disease, diabetes, infectious diseases (e.g., HIV), and substance use disorders (including nicotine, alcohol, and other substances) (543–554). A consequence of this excess comorbidity is an increased non-suicide-related mortality rate in this population (34, 388, 555). The increased frequencies of the various comorbid conditions are determined by multiple factors, including associations with schizophrenia itself (e.g., diabetes, smoking), life style (e.g., smoking, substance use, obesity, lack of exercise), environment (e.g., poverty, institutionalization), and medications (e.g., extrapyramidal syndromes, tardive dyskinesia, hyperprolactinemia, weight gain, hyperglycemia, hyperlipidemia, and cardiac arrhythmias). Thus, treatment selection and clinical management of patients with schizophrenia must consider the patient's past medical history and general medical status of the patient in determining the treatment plan. Patients should be evaluated in terms of their medical history and baseline assessments and then monitored with the relevant measures at appropriate intervals or when the patient's medical condition warrants or when a change in medication that could affect their medical condition is made, as indicated in Table 1. In the event that the patient's comorbid medical condition is affected adversely by a therapeutic agent (including an antipsychotic drug), management strategies may include helping the patient tolerate the adverse effect, treating the comorbid condition, or considering a change in the psychotropic medication to an alternative with less potential to induce side effects.

Patients with dementia and elderly patients are at very high risk of tardive dyskinesia. In addition, patients with dementia, Parkinson's disease, or other disorders associated with structural brain pathology are at increased risk of worsening of extrapyramidal side effects. Similarly, patients with psychosis and mental retardation are at increased risk for extrapyramidal side effects and tardive dyskinesia (556, 557). Thus, in these groups of patients, second-generation antipsychotics and particularly those with minimal or no risk of extrapyramidal effects (e.g., quetiapine) are recommended (558, 559). Furthermore, when such patients are treated with antipsychotic drugs, they must be monitored for side effects, and the increased risk of extrapyramidal side effects and tardive dyskinesia must be weighed against potential therapeutic benefits.

For patients with preexisting osteopenia or osteoporosis, an antipsychotic with minimal to no effects on prolactin should be prescribed. If a drug that increases prolactin is clinically indicated, then the relative safety of the antipsychotic should be discussed with the physician treating the bone demineralization. Female patients with menstrual or fertility problems should be evaluated for abnormalities in prolactin secretion, and non-prolactin-elevating medications should be considered as indicated. In addition, for women with breast cancer, antipsychotics with prolactin-elevating effects should be avoided or prescribed only after consultation with the patient's oncologist. In such instances, aripiprazole, which partially suppresses prolactin release, may be specifically indicated. However, in lactating mothers, suppression of prolactin may be detrimental, and the potential for this effect should be considered.

Obese patients and patients who have or may be at risk for diabetes and cardiovascular disease should be assessed before beginning treatment with antipsychotic drugs. Additional assessments are indicated at appropriate intervals thereafter or when warranted by a change in the patient's medical condition or medication regimen (see Table 1). Treatment selection should weigh the expected benefits of antipsychotic therapy against its potential to exacerbate or contribute to the development of specific medical conditions.

Patients with prolonged QT syndrome, bradycardia, certain electrolyte disturbances, heart failure, or recent myocardial infarction and patients who are taking drugs that prolong the QT interval should not be treated with an antipsychotic that could further prolong the QT interval or increase the risk of the arrhythmia torsades de pointes. These antipsychotics include thioridazine, droperidol, and ziprasidone. Pimozide also may prolong the QT interval.

Medications with low affinity for α-adrenergic receptors should be prescribed for patients who are vulnerable to orthostatic hypotension, including elderly patients, patients with peripheral vascular disease or compromised cardiovascular status, and other severely debilitated patients.

For patients with acute angle-closure glaucoma, severe constipation (or at risk for fecal obstruction), history of a paralytic ileus, urinary retention, prostate hypertrophy, or delirium/dementia, antipsychotics with little or no antagonism for cholinergic receptors should be prescribed.

Patients with severe dementia may be at increased risk of stroke when treated with risperidone. Clinicians treating psychosis in patients with dementia should refer to up-to-date FDA guidelines when considering the safety of risperidone in this population.

Clozapine should not be prescribed for patients with neutropenia ($<1500/mm^3$) or low white blood cell (WBC) count ($<3000/mm^3$) or a history of such sensitivities to prior medications.

III. TREATMENT SETTINGS AND HOUSING OPTIONS

A. CHOICE OF TREATMENT SETTING OR HOUSING

Patients with schizophrenia may receive care in a variety of settings. Choice of setting may be guided by a number of factors, summarized in Table 6. In general, patients should be cared for in the least restrictive setting that is likely to be safe and to allow for effective treatment.

B. COMMON TREATMENT SETTINGS

1. Hospitals

Treatment in the hospital has the advantage of providing a safe, structured, and supervised environment and reducing stress in both patients and family members. It allows the psychiatrist to closely monitor the level of the patient's symptoms, the patient's level of functioning and reactions to treatment, and side effects of treatment.

Hospitalization is usually indicated for patients who are considered to pose a serious threat of harm to themselves or others or who are so severely disorganized or under the influence of delusions or hallucinations that they are unable to care for themselves and need constant supervision or support. Other possible indications for hospitalization include general medical or psychiatric problems that make outpatient treatment unsafe or ineffective (e.g., if a patient's psychiatric status continues to deteriorate despite optimal care in the community). Patients who cannot be adequately cared for in nonhospital settings should be hospitalized voluntarily if possible. If patients decline voluntary status, they can be hospitalized involuntarily if their condition meets the criteria for involuntary admission of the local jurisdiction.

Alternative treatment settings should be considered when it is uncertain whether the patient needs to be hospitalized or when the patient does not need formal hospitalization but requires

TABLE 6. Factors Affecting Choice of Treatment Setting or Housing

Availability of the setting or housing
The patient's clinical condition
- Need for protection from harm to self or others
- Need for external structure and support
- Ability to cooperate with treatment

Patient's and family's preference
Requirements of the treatment plan
- Need for a particular treatment or a particular intensity of treatment that may be available only in certain settings
- Need for a specific treatment for a comorbid psychiatric or other general medical condition

Characteristics of the setting
- Degrees of support, structure, and restrictiveness
- Ability to protect patient from harm to self or others
- Availability of different treatment capacities, including general medical care and rehabilitation services
- Availability of psychosocial supports to facilitate the patient's receipt of treatment and to provide critical information to the psychiatrist about the patient's clinical status and response to treatments
- Capacity to care for severely agitated or psychotic patients
- Hours of operation
- Overall milieu and treatment philosophy

Patient's current environment or circumstances
- Family functioning
- Available social supports

more intensive services than can be expected in a typical outpatient setting (560). Alternative treatment settings in the community may include day or partial hospitalization, home care, family crisis therapy, crisis residential care, and assertive community treatment (see Part B, Section V.C.1.a, "Program for Assertive Community Treatment [PACT]"). A recent meta-analysis has shown that such alternatives to hospitalization for acutely ill patients can sometimes be at least as effective and sometimes more effective than hospitalization in terms of reducing loss to follow-up, reducing family burden, and increasing the patient's and family's satisfaction while being cost-neutral (561). These crisis intervention programs typically provide medication and a mobile multidisciplinary team that is available outside of traditional office hours. Other studies have demonstrated that crisis intervention can be associated with reduced symptoms, preserved role functioning, and reduced hospital readmission rates (181, 562–570).

Patients may be moved from one level of care to another on the basis of the factors summarized in Table 6, with an ongoing assessment of their readiness and ability to benefit from a different level of care. The choice of residence must be guided by the availability of housing and accompanying psychiatric support programs as well as by the patient's and family's preferences and resources.

Since a major aim of acute hospitalization is to facilitate rapid resolution of acute symptoms through the provision of a safe, nonstressful therapeutic environment, the hospital milieu should be organized to help achieve this goal. In consideration of the severe symptoms and cognitive impairment in acute schizophrenia, the hospital milieu should be highly structured; staff members should be clearly identifiable and should always wear name tags, whether they wear uniforms or street clothes; calendars and clocks should be in evidence on the ward; and ward schedules should be posted in order to provide a clear-cut external structure for the patients, who often have disorganized and impaired reality testing (571).

For acutely ill patients whose psychotic symptoms respond rapidly to antipsychotic medication, a brief hospitalization followed by day hospitalization when indicated has been shown to be as effective as or more effective than longer-term hospitalization, with no increase in rehospitalization rate and better maintenance of role functioning and less family burden at 1- and 2-year follow-up (571, 572). A number of randomized controlled studies have compared shorter and longer lengths of hospitalization. In the United States the shortest average duration of hospitalization studied was 11 days, which was compared with an average stay of 60 days for the control group (572), while in England, Hirsch et al. (573) compared outcomes for an average stay of 9 days with those for an average stay of 14 days. Other studies examined the effects of shorter and longer hospitalizations, but the general conclusion from all of the studies was that longer hospitalization conferred no additional benefit over shorter hospitalization in such areas as symptom improvement, community adjustment, and readmission rate (574–584). Brief hospitalization allows for effective treatment in the least restrictive environment but is optimal only when there is a system of community care in place and patients adhere to follow-up treatment. Thus, when there is no longer a clear-cut need for the patient to remain in the hospital and community treatment is available and accessible, the psychiatrist should consider discharging the patient from the hospital. On the other hand, if adequate community treatment and support resources are not in place, patients should not be discharged until they have achieved sufficient remission to enable them to function in the community without such supports.

2. Long-term hospitalization

Before the introduction of clozapine, 10%–20% of persons with schizophrenia remained severely psychotic with grossly impaired functioning despite optimal pharmacological and conventional care (585). The degree to which this percentage has been decreased by the availability of clozapine and other agents is unclear, but there remains a group of patients who require long-term, supervised hospitalization for their safety and protection, as well as for the protection of the family and community (586–588).

The organization of the long-stay hospital ward, the training and duties of its personnel, and the quality of care provided vary greatly and determine the therapeutic value of the hospital experience (589, 590). Studies have suggested that patients with treatment-resistant schizophrenia who require long-term hospitalization profit most from treatment programs that emphasize highly structured behavioral techniques, including a token economy, point systems, and skills training that can improve patients' functioning (591, 592). Paradoxically, despite its demonstrated efficacy, the token economy is not often used in clinical settings (593, 594). Obstacles to its implementation include resistance by staff members who hold to traditional custodial methods, increased costs (for the reinforcers backing up the tokens), lack of support from administrators, and inadequate training of clinical staff (595).

3. Crisis residential programs

The treatment of patients outside of large institutions is a fundamental objective of community psychiatry, and this objective creates the need for adequate community-based acute care as part of the comprehensive array of services needed to support persons with serious mental illness in the community. In many mental health systems, acute-care episodes involving hospitalization are the single largest cost element in the array of services needed to provide community care. Crisis residential facilities are homes in neighborhoods that are staffed and organized to accept and treat patients with serious mental illness in lieu of voluntary psychiatric admission. Crisis residential programs 1) provide short-term monitoring and crisis intervention in a residential, nonhospital setting as an alternative to inpatient care; 2) are staffed 24 hours per day/7 days per week; and 3) support patients in maintaining continuity with their outpatient caregivers and social networks during an acute-care episode. Crisis residential models have been studied as alternatives to hospitalization for patients with serious mental illness who 1) are willing to accept voluntary treatment, 2) do not require emergent medical assessment for an unstable medical condition, and 3) do not require acute substance detoxification. The findings of three randomized controlled trials indicate that crisis residential programs can deliver clinical outcomes comparable to those of hospital care at significantly less cost. In addition, crisis residential models have been successfully integrated into mental health systems in demonstration projects in a wide range of communities throughout the United States and overseas. Crisis residential models of acute care comport with community mental health practice that values the provision of needed care in the least restrictive or most integrated setting (596–600).

4. Day hospitalization or partial hospitalization

Day hospitalization can be used as an immediate alternative to inpatient care for acutely psychotic patients or to continue stabilization after a brief hospital stay. The day hospital should be staffed in a manner similar to the staffing of the day shift for an acute inpatient service, with close coordination with and involvement of family members and/or supervised residence staff. Brief overnight stays on inpatient units should be available for patients who demonstrate severe exacerbation of symptoms. As with all alternatives to inpatient care for acutely ill patients, the patient should not be considered at risk of harming self or others, should have the capacity to cooperate at least minimally in treatment, should have a significant other willing to provide care (a crisis residence can perform the same function), and should have access to appropriate community treatment resources. Treatment alternatives such as day hospitalization have the potential advantages of less disruption of the patient's life, treatment in a less restrictive and more integrated environment, and avoidance of the stigma attached to psychiatric hospitalization.

Controlled studies have shown that day hospitalization is at least as effective as acute inpatient care, and in some studies more effective, in such measures as decreasing symptoms and the rehospitalization rate and better preserving role functioning (562, 563, 573, 601–609). Meta-analyses have shown that day hospitalization has been associated with reductions in overall days of inpatient care, more rapid resolution of symptoms, and decreased overall costs with no increase in burden to family members. Social functioning did not differ across treatment settings (562, 563, 597, 598, 604, 606, 608, 610–614). The Cochrane review (609) combined data from nine studies involving acutely ill patients, the majority of whom had a diagnosis of schizophrenia. The review found that, at the most pessimistic estimate, day hospital treatment was feasible for 23% (N=2,268, 95% CI=21%–25%) of those currently admitted to inpatient care.

5. Day treatment

Generally, day treatment programs are used to provide ongoing supportive care for marginally adjusted patients with schizophrenia in the later part of the stabilization phase and the stable phase of illness. Such programs, which are usually not time limited, provide structure, support, and treatment programs to help prevent relapse and to maintain and gradually improve the patient's social functioning. Long-term day treatment attendance was thought to improve engagement (615), improve clinical outcome (615), and reduce readmission rates (616, 617). However, a Cochrane review found that there was no evidence that day care centers were better or worse than outpatient care in their effects on any clinical or social outcome variable (609). There was some evidence that day treatment might be more expensive than outpatient care (156, 618, 619).

However, the development of effective models of vocational rehabilitation and social skills training, as discussed in Part B, Sections V.C.1.c, "Supported Employment" and V.C.1.e, "Social Skills Training," respectively, renders some of the previous research on day treatment as a "setting" of care to be less relevant than research on the types of programs that should be provided to patients with schizophrenia who are in the stable phase of illness and in need of recovery-oriented services. At this point in the development of psychosocial services, the effectiveness of day programs is likely to be a function of the quality of the programming patients receive while they attend. Thus, when planning for treatment in the stable phase of illness, the clinician should carefully evaluate the available programming and help the patient implement a plan based on the patient's preferences and needs and on the availability of services that are recovery focused and consistent with evidence-based practices.

6. Housing

The advent of community-based care has produced a challenge regarding the housing of persons with severe mental illness and its connection to psychiatric care. Other than living with family, choices include hostels, group homes, therapeutic communities, and supported independent tenancies. Increasingly, people with severe mental illness are choosing to live as independently as possible in self-contained accommodations because sharing accommodation with other residents who also have mental illness can seem like living in an institution (620). Two essential paradigms have been promoted. In the transitional housing paradigm, patients live in housing that is directly connected to psychiatric treatment. The acceptance of treatment is often a contingency of using such housing. The underlying assumption is that patients "transition" through housing with decreasing levels of supervision as their mental status improves. A second paradigm is that of supported housing. In this paradigm, housing is not directly connected to treatment. Housing is typically in independent units, and mental health services are provided as needed in order to support patients in retaining their housing. Therefore, in a transitional housing model, a patient who is experiencing a relapse or worsening of symptoms would be moved to a housing setting with a higher level of supervision. In a supported housing model, such a patient would simply receive increased psychiatric services in his or her home, to facilitate housing stability.

The type of supported housing available to people with mental disorders seems to be dependent on the local availability of resources (621).

According to Budson (622), the most common types of residential facilities used currently include:

- *Transitional halfway houses.* A transitional halfway house is defined as a residential facility providing room and board and promoting socialization until suitable housing is available (623). It is used as a transitional facility between the hospital and the community for recovering patients.
- *Long-term group residences.* These facilities have on-site staff and are used for chronically functionally disabled persons. The length of stay is indefinite, in contrast to the length of stay in a halfway house, which is usually 6–8 months.
- *Cooperative apartments.* No on-site staff persons are present in cooperative apartments, but staff members make regular visits for oversight and guidance of residents.
- *Intensive-care or crisis community residences.* These facilities can be used to help prevent hospitalization or shorten the length of hospitalization. Usually, there are on-site nursing personnel and counseling staff.
- *Foster or family care.* Some patients are placed in foster or family care in private homes. There is a concern that in some situations only a custodial function may be provided (624). Close supervision of foster families is necessary to ensure that patients are living in a therapeutic environment.
- *Board-and-care homes.* These facilities are generally proprietary rooming houses. As with family care, close monitoring and supervision are necessary, since some of these facilities provide substandard environments for patients.
- *Nursing homes.* Nursing homes are suitable for some geriatric or chronically medically disabled patients, but they have been used inappropriately for other long-term patients to facilitate discharge, mainly from state hospitals. Various investigators have suggested that more developed activity programs and psychiatric supervision are needed to prevent declines in nursing home residents' social functioning and self-care.

Research on the merits of different housing programs and arrangements is inconclusive. For example, Friedrich et al. (625) examined housing preferences of persons with severe mental illness living in three types of community residences by surveying both patients and family members. Although a larger proportion of family members than patients preferred housing with more support, for both groups, current and preferred residence were consistent. For patients living independently, social isolation was perceived as a problem by patients and family members. The authors concluded that although supported housing works well for some persons, a continued need exists for an array of housing options with varying levels of structure. In contrast, a 10-site Scandinavian study (626) found that independent housing was related to a better quality of life concerning living situation and a better social network regarding availability and adequacy of emotional relations.

Dedicated programs whereby people with severe mental illness are located within one site or building with assistance from professional workers have the potential for great benefit, as they provide a safe haven for people in need of stability and support. This potential benefit, however, may be provided at the risk of increasing patients' dependence on professionals and prolonging exclusion from the community. Whether or not the benefits outweigh the risks can be only a matter of opinion in the absence of reliable evidence. Thus, there is an urgent need to investigate the effects of supported housing on people with severe mental illness within a randomized trial (627).

Newman (628) critically reviewed studies of the relationship between housing attributes and serious mental illness. Three studies found no effect of improved housing adequacy on housing satisfaction in addition to that provided by case management. Three studies found that fewer housing occupants led to better outcomes. The strongest finding from the literature on housing as a variable and as an outcome was that living in independent housing was associated with greater satisfaction with the housing and the neighborhood. However, given the methodological weaknesses of these studies, Newman pointed out the critical need for a coherent agenda built around key hypotheses and for a uniform set of measures of housing as a variable and as an outcome.

7. Correctional settings

The number of persons with schizophrenia incarcerated in prisons and jails in the United States has grown dramatically over the past two decades, paralleling the increase in incarceration among the general population (629). Generally, the rates of schizophrenia in correctional settings have been found to be significantly higher than in the general community population (630), with 1.8%–4.4% of incarcerated persons meeting the diagnostic criteria for schizophrenia (631). Consequently, screening of newly arrived detainees and inmates by correctional officers or health care staff members is important in identifying persons with schizophrenia or other psychotic disorders who will require more in-depth psychiatric assessment and treatment (632).

Since suicide is common in jails and prisons (633) and since newly incarcerated persons are at increased risk for suicide (56), screening of incarcerated persons with schizophrenia should include questions about suicidal thoughts and suicide attempts. Periodic reassessment is recommended since persons with schizophrenia may develop suicidal ideas or become more symptomatic while in a jail or prison. This worsening of symptoms can result from a number of factors, including stress related to incarceration, removal from support systems, and inadequate mental health services within the correctional setting (632).

For detainees and inmates who are identified as having schizophrenia or other serious mental illnesses, a variety of levels of mental health care may exist in the correctional system, including "outpatient" care, specialized housing, and "inpatient" care. In fact, correctional facilities are constitutionally required to provide adequate treatment to incarcerated persons with serious mental illnesses such as schizophrenia. Minimum standards for an acceptable treatment program were established in *Ruiz v. Estelle* (634) and include screening and evaluation; treatment beyond simple segregation and supervision; the use of adequate numbers of competent mental health professionals; individualized treatment; accurate, complete, and confidential medical record keeping; appropriate supervision of use of psychiatric medications; and identification, treatment, and supervision of inmates at risk for suicide. These minimum standards have been endorsed and expanded by other organizations, including APA (632).

Since jails are local facilities used for the confinement of persons awaiting trial or those convicted of minor crimes, mental health treatment of jail inmates is often limited by the short length of stay and small size of the facility. Treatment generally emphasizes prescription of psychotropic medications or crisis intervention services, which may include transfer to special housing units, special observation, and brief psychotherapy. Some longer-term psychotherapies may be available to inmates whose pretrial confinements or sentences are of a greater duration. The essential mental health services for a jail population include access to inpatient psychiatric beds; mental health care coverage that is available 7 days a week; availability of a full range of psychotropic medications that are prescribed and monitored by a psychiatrist; appropriate nursing coverage in any medical health area, including mental health; and procedures developed and monitored by psychiatrists and nurses to ensure that psychotropic medications are distributed by qualified medical personnel, whenever possible (635).

Prisons are generally under state or federal control and are used to confine persons serving longer sentences. Consequently, prison mental health systems generally provide a more comprehensive system of mental health care to persons with schizophrenia than would be available in a jail setting. In particular, the importance of a chronic care program for inmates with serious mental illness has become increasingly recognized as an essential component of prison mental health systems. These programs are often known as residential treatment units, intermediate care units, supportive living units, special needs units, psychiatric services units, or protective environments for the seriously mentally ill. Inmates appropriate for these units generally have had significant difficulty functioning in a general population environment because of symptoms related to their serious mental disorders. These units typically are designed to house 30–50 inmates per housing unit, which allows staffing to be done in a cost-effective fashion (635). A psychosocial rehabilitation approach is a frequently used treatment model. For short-term detainees and inmates, such treatments should focus on symptom management, adjustment to the correctional setting, planning for upcoming release, and reintegration into the home community. For long-term inmates, the primary foci should be symptom management, relapse prevention, and adjustment to incarceration.

If incarcerated persons with schizophrenia refuse treatment, administrative processes may permit mandated treatment to protect the safety of the person and others. For example, in all jurisdictions, emergency treatment can be instituted if psychosis results in paranoia and threats to other inmates, to staff, or to the person him- or herself. Some jurisdictions include administrative protocols for nonemergency treatment of inmates who refuse to accept medications (e.g., protocols established by *Washington v. Harper* [636]). Thus, clinicians practicing in correctional settings should become familiar with local and state law and with institutional policy on involuntary treatment.

While incarcerated, inmates with schizophrenia may show symptoms of withdrawal, disorganization, and/or disruptive behavior, which may be associated with disciplinary infractions. These infractions, in turn, may lead the inmate with schizophrenia to be placed in a locked-down setting within units that are often called "administrative segregation" or "disciplinary segregation" (637). Such units have been conceptualized as having three main characteristics: social isolation, sensory deprivation, and confinement (638). Each of these elements can vary significantly, but inmates typically spend an average of 23 hours per day in a cell, have limited human interaction and minimal or no access to programs, and are maintained in an environment that is designed to exert maximum control over the person. Inmates' responses to the segregation experience differ, and relevant scientific literature is sparse (639). Nonetheless, mental health clinicians working in such facilities frequently report that inmates without preexisting serious mental disorders develop irritability, anxiety, and other dysphoric symptoms when housed in these units for long periods of time (640). Difficulties in providing appropriate and adequate access to mental health care and treatment are especially problematic in any segregation environment and are related to logistical issues that frequently include inadequate office space and limited access to inmates because of security issues (641). In addition, because of their inherently punitive structure, such units typically provide very little support, access to relevant treatment modalities, or therapeutic milieu. Consequently, persons with schizophrenia should generally not be placed in a 23-hour/day lockdown for behaviors that directly result from the schizophrenia, because such an intervention is likely to exacerbate rather than reduce the symptoms of schizophrenia as well as increase rather than reduce disruptive behaviors (632, 642).

Before release from a correctional facility, inmates with schizophrenia should be assisted in finding a source for needed care in the community. In addition, attention should be paid to the housing and financial needs of inmates nearing release. On leaving the correctional facility, inmates should be provided with enough medication to allow them time to consult a physician and obtain a new supply.

PART B: BACKGROUND INFORMATION AND REVIEW OF AVAILABLE EVIDENCE

IV. DISEASE DEFINITION, NATURAL HISTORY AND COURSE, AND EPIDEMIOLOGY

A. CLINICAL FEATURES

Table 7 presents DSM-IV-TR diagnostic criteria for schizophrenia, which is a major psychotic disorder. Its essential features consist of characteristic signs and symptoms that have been present for a significant length of time during a 1-month period (or for a shorter time if successfully treated), with some signs of the disorder persisting for at least 6 months. No single symptom is pathognomonic of schizophrenia. Rather, the symptoms may involve multiple psychological realms, such as perception (hallucinations), ideation, reality testing (delusions), thought processes (loose associations), feeling (flatness, inappropriate affect), behavior (catatonia, disorganization), attention, concentration, motivation (avolition, impaired intention and planning), and judgment. These psychological and behavioral characteristics are associated with a variety of impairments in occupational or social functioning. Although there can be marked deterioration with impairments in multiple domains of functioning (e.g., learning, self-care, working, interpersonal relationships, and living skills), the disorder is noted for great heterogeneity across persons and variability within persons over time. It is also associated with a recurrent and progressive course (280, 643). Persons with schizophrenia also suffer disproportionately from an increased incidence of general medical illness (644) and increased mortality (34, 645–653), especially from suicide, which occurs in up to 10% of patients (643, 654–657).

TABLE 7. DSM-IV-TR Diagnostic Criteria for Schizophrenia

A. *Characteristic symptoms:* Two (or more) of the following, each present for a significant portion of time during a 1-month period (or less if successfully treated):

1. delusions
2. hallucinations
3. disorganized speech (e.g., frequent derailment or incoherence)
4. grossly disorganized or catatonic behavior
5. negative symptoms, i.e., affective flattening, alogia, or avolition

Note: Only one Criterion A symptom is required if delusions are bizarre or hallucinations consist of a voice keeping up a running commentary on the person's behavior or thoughts, or two or more voices conversing with each other.

B. *Social/occupational dysfunction:* For a significant portion of the time since the onset of the disturbance, one or more major areas of functioning, such as work, interpersonal relations, or self-care, are markedly below the level achieved prior to the onset (or when the onset is in childhood or adolescence, failure to achieve expected level of interpersonal, academic, or occupational achievement).

C. *Duration:* Continuous signs of the disturbance persist for at least 6 months. This 6-month period must include at least 1 month of symptoms (or less if successfully treated) that meet Criterion A (i.e., active-phase symptoms) and may include periods of prodromal or residual symptoms. During these prodromal or residual periods, the signs of the disturbance may be manifested by only negative symptoms or two or more symptoms listed in Criterion A present in an attenuated form (e.g., odd beliefs, unusual perceptual experiences).

D. *Schizoaffective and Mood Disorder exclusion*: Schizoaffective Disorder and Mood Disorder With Psychotic Features have been ruled out because either (1) no Major Depressive, Manic, or Mixed Episodes have occurred concurrently with the active-phase symptoms; or (2) if mood episodes have occurred during active-phase symptoms, their total duration has been brief relative to the duration of the active and residual periods.

E. *Substance/general medical condition exclusion:* The disturbance is not due to the direct physiological effects of a substance (e.g., a drug of abuse, a medication) or a general medical condition.

F. *Relationship to a Pervasive Developmental Disorder:* If there is a history of Autistic Disorder or another Pervasive Developmental Disorder, the additional diagnosis of Schizophrenia is made only if prominent delusions or hallucinations are also present for at least a month (or less if successfully treated).

Classification of longitudinal course (can be applied only after at least 1 year has elapsed since the initial onset of active-phase symptoms):

Episodic With Interepisode Residual Symptoms (episodes are defined by the reemergence of prominent psychotic symptoms); also specify if: With Prominent Negative Symptoms

Episodic With No Interepisode Residual Symptoms

Continuous (prominent psychotic symptoms are present throughout the period of observation); also specify if: With Prominent Negative Symptoms

Single Episode In Partial Remission; also specify if: With Prominent Negative Symptoms

Single Episode In Full Remission Other or Unspecified Pattern

Source. Reprinted from *Diagnostic and Statistical Manual of Mental Disorders, 4th Edition, Text Revision*. Washington, DC, American Psychiatric Association, 2000. Copyright © 2000, American Psychiatric Association.

The characteristic symptoms of schizophrenia have often been conceptualized as falling into two broad categories—positive and negative symptoms. A third category of disorganized symptoms has recently been added because statistical analyses show it to be a dimension independent of the positive symptom category, under which it was previously included. The positive symptoms include delusions and hallucinations. Disorganized symptoms include disorganized speech (658) (thought disorder), disorganized behavior, and poor attention. Negative symptoms include restricted range and intensity of emotional expression (affective flattening), reduced thought and speech productivity (alogia), anhedonia, and decreased initiation of goal-directed behavior (avolition) (659). Negative symptoms may be primary and represent a core feature of schizophrenia, or they may be secondary to psychotic symptoms, a depressive syndrome, medication side effects (e.g., dysphoria), or environmental deprivation.

According to DSM-IV-TR, subtypes of schizophrenia are defined by the predominant symptoms at the time of the most recent evaluation and therefore may change over time. These subtypes include paranoid type, in which preoccupation with delusions or auditory hallucinations is prominent; disorganized type, in which disorganized speech and behavior and flat or inappropriate affect are prominent; catatonic type, in which characteristic motor symptoms are prominent; undifferentiated type, which is a nonspecific category used when none of the other subtype features are predominant; and residual type, in which there is an absence of prominent positive symptoms but continuing evidence of disturbance (e.g., negative symptoms or positive symptoms in an attenuated form) (660). Although the prognostic and treatment implications of these subtypes vary, the disorganized type tends to be the most severe and the paranoid type to be the least severe (661).

Other mental disorders and general medical conditions may be comorbid with schizophrenia. Along with general medical conditions, the most common comorbid disorder appears to be substance use disorder. Commonly abused substances include alcohol (327); stimulants such as cocaine and amphetamines (662–664); nicotine, cannabis, phencyclidine (PCP); and LSD (665–667). Such comorbidities can worsen the illness course and complicate treatment (331, 668–670). Individuals with schizophrenia may also experience symptoms of other mental disorders, especially depression but also obsessive and compulsive symptoms, somatic concerns, dissociative symptoms, and other mood or anxiety symptoms. Whether symptoms alone are present or whether criteria for comorbid diagnoses are met, these features can significantly worsen prognosis (671) and often require specific attention and treatment planning. General medical conditions are often present, and persons with schizophrenia may be at special risk for those associated with poor self-care or institutionalization (e.g., tuberculosis, hepatitis), substance use (e.g., emphysema and other cigarette-related pathology, HIV-related disease), and antipsychotic-induced movement disorders. Some persons with schizophrenia develop psychosis-induced polydipsia, which can lead to water intoxication and hyponatremia.

B. NATURAL HISTORY AND COURSE

Schizophrenia can be viewed as a disorder that develops in phases: premorbid, prodromal, and psychotic (252, 257, 259, 260, 672). The premorbid phase encompasses a period of normative function, although the person may experience events that contribute to the development of the subsequent illness, including complications in pregnancy and delivery during the prenatal and perinatal periods and trauma and family stress during childhood and adolescence (673).

The prodromal phase involves a change from premorbid functioning and extends up to the time of the onset of frank psychotic symptoms. It may last only weeks or months, but the average length of the prodromal phase is between 2 and 5 years (252, 260, 674). During the prodromal phase the person experiences substantial functional impairment and nonspecific symptoms such as sleep disturbance, anxiety, irritability, depressed mood, poor concentration, fatigue, and behavioral deficits such as deterioration in role functioning and social withdrawal (675, 676). Positive symptoms such as perceptual abnormalities, ideas of reference, and suspiciousness develop late in the prodromal phase and herald the imminent onset of psychosis (677).

The first psychotic episode may be abrupt or insidious in its onset. In most Western countries, 1–2 years elapse on average between the onset of the first psychotic symptoms and the first adequate treatment, defined as the duration of untreated psychosis (252, 259–261, 678). This time period has been found to be significantly longer in men than in women (261).

The psychotic phase progresses through an acute phase, a recovery or stabilization phase, and a stable phase. The acute phase refers to the presence of florid psychotic features such as delusions, hallucinations, formal thought disorder, and disorganized thinking. Negative symptoms often become more severe, and patients are usually not able to care for themselves appropriately. The stabilization (recovery) phase refers to a period of 6–18 months after acute treatment. During the stable phase, negative and residual positive symptoms that may be present are relatively consistent in magnitude and usually less severe than in the acute phase. Some patients may be asymptomatic whereas others experience nonpsychotic symptoms such as tension, anxiety, depression, or insomnia.

The period after recovery from a first episode of schizophrenia and extending for up to the subsequent 5 years is known as the early course. If patients experience further deterioration in symptoms and/or function, it is most likely to occur during this time, because by 5–10 years after onset most patients experience a plateau in their level of illness and function (257, 643). This phase has also been termed "the critical period" (679) because most follow-up studies have shown that up to 80% of patients will have relapsed within this 5-year period (46). Before relapse occurs, there is usually a prodromal period in which nonpsychotic symptoms, followed by emotional disturbance and then frank psychotic symptoms develop over a period of about 4 weeks (680–682).

The long-term outcome of schizophrenia varies along a continuum between reasonable recovery and total incapacity. About 10%–15% of persons with the disorder are free of further episodes (683), but the majority display exacerbations and remissions in the context of experiencing clinical deterioration, and about 10%–15% remain chronically severely psychotic (643, 684).

Several demographic and clinical variables have value in predicting long-term outcome. For example, better outcomes are associated, on average, with female gender, family history of affective disorder, lack of family history of schizophrenia, good premorbid social and academic functioning, higher IQ, married marital status, later age of onset (685), acute onset with precipitating stress, fewer prior episodes (both number and length), a phasic pattern of episodes and remissions, advancing age, minimal comorbidity, paranoid subtype, and symptoms that are predominantly positive (delusions, hallucinations) and not disorganized (thought disorder, disorganized behavior) or negative (flat affect, alogia, avolition) (282, 303, 304, 502, 523, 660, 661, 683, 686–692). It appears that the course is influenced by cultural factors and societal complexity, with better outcomes in developing countries (689).

The excessive mortality of patients with schizophrenia has been reported to be two to four times that of the general population (34, 551, 656, 693–696). About 4%–10% of persons with schizophrenia die by suicide, and the rates are highest among males in the early course of the disorder and in industrialized countries (387, 390, 697). Severe psychotic symptoms, depression, comorbid substance use disorder, and adverse life events increase the risk of suicide in persons with schizophrenia (395, 698). Other major causes of death also include unnatural causes, such as accidents and traumatic injuries, and medical conditions, such as cardiovascular disorders and respiratory and infectious diseases (387).

C. EPIDEMIOLOGY

The lifetime morbidity risk for schizophrenia (i.e., the proportion of a population meeting the criteria for schizophrenia at any time during life provided they live through the entire age range of risk) is estimated to be 1.0% (699, 700) and appears to be the same for men and women up to age 60 years (701, 702).

The incidence of schizophrenia appears to be stable across countries and cultures and over time (701), although there is some controversy on this point, with some studies showing significant variability (703). In the World Health Organization (WHO) Determinants of Outcome Study, the median annual incidence of schizophrenia across eight participating WHO sites was 0.22 per 1,000 population (704). Earlier reports of declining incidence of schizophrenia over time have not been confirmed (699, 700, 702).

The Epidemiologic Catchment Area study in the United States reported a lifetime prevalence rate of schizophrenia of 1.5% (705). Studies of representative community samples assessed by structured diagnostic interviews in the United States yield estimates of the lifetime prevalence for schizophrenia of 0.7% (706).

Among persons age 65 years and older, the prevalence is probably 1% (528, 707, 708). There are, however, controversies about whether early-onset and late-onset schizophrenia are different or similar disorders.

About 20%–40% of patients experience their first psychotic symptoms before age 20 years (709). For men, the peak incidence of onset of schizophrenia has been determined to be between ages 15 and 25 years; for women, between ages 25 and 35 years (710). The WHO's Determinants of Outcome Study found a mean gender difference in age at onset of 3.4 years (711). Some studies (711–713), but not all (714), have demonstrated this earlier mean age of onset in men across cultures. However, this finding may not be evident in familial schizophrenia (715, 716). Women display a second peak of onset after age 40–45 years, just before menopause (674, 717–719).

Men experience more negative symptoms and women more affective symptoms (309), although acute psychotic symptoms, either in type or severity, do not differ between the two genders (508, 720). The prevalence of negative (deficit) states in first-episode schizophrenia has been estimated to be between 4% and 10% (298) and increases with the length of the schizophrenic illness (302–306, 661).

More than 80% of patients with schizophrenia have parents who do not have the disorder (721). However, the risk of having schizophrenia is greater in persons whose parents have the disorder; the lifetime risk is 13% for a child with one parent with schizophrenia and 35%–40% for a child with two affected parents (722). The risk increases with the number of affected relatives. Twin studies have found a concordance rate among monozygotic twins of about 50%, compared to 9% for dizygotic twins and siblings (721, 723).

Many studies (724–729), but not all (730–732), have reported an association between obstetric complications that involved fetal hypoxic brain damage and a subsequent increase in risk for schizophrenia. Such complications include viral infection during pregnancy (733–738); first-trimester maternal starvation (739); rhesus incompatibility (740, 741); and maternal preeclampsia (741–743), anemia (741, 743), and diabetes (743). Patients with an early onset of schizophrenia were more likely to have a history of birth complications than those with later onsets (744, 745). Persons born in the winter months are also at a higher risk (746–748).

Substance use has been associated with precipitation of symptoms of schizophrenia (334–340, 667, 749, 750). The mean age at onset of schizophrenia as well as the age at first admission was lower in patients who had a history of substance use and higher in patients without such a history (341, 751).

Recent studies examining immigration and schizophrenia have shown an increase of the disorder in second-generation African Caribbean immigrants in the United Kingdom (752–754). Other risk factors have been associated with an increased risk for schizophrenia (691, 702). They include single marital status, a lower socioeconomic class (525), being raised in an urban environment (755, 756), environmental stress (525), and advanced paternal age (757, 758).

Schizophrenia is by far the most costly mental illness (759) and has been estimated to account for 2.5% of annual health care expenditures in the United States (760). The cost of schizophrenia for American society was estimated to be $32.5 billion in 1990; by 1995, the cost was estimated to have escalated to $65 billion (761). Indirect costs to the patients, their families, other caregivers, and society must also be considered (762). In a British study, the annual indirect costs incurred through productivity loss by patients were estimated to be at least four times the direct costs (763).

V. REVIEW AND SYNTHESIS OF AVAILABLE EVIDENCE

A. PHARMACOLOGICAL TREATMENTS

This section is organized by medication. For each medication or medication class, the available data regarding efficacy are reviewed. Short-term efficacy has generally been measured by reductions in psychopathology (positive, negative, affective, and general symptoms) among treated patients during 6- to 12-week medication trials. An advantage of studies that measure psychopathological changes is that they clearly demonstrate how well a medication can achieve a reduction in the target symptoms. Less clear is how such reductions in symptoms relate to improvements in patients' functioning. Acute and long-term efficacy have also been assessed by examining effects on cognitive function as measured by neurocognitive test performance (764–766), which in turn has been related to patients' functional capacity and performance (767).

Long-term efficacy has usually been measured by reductions in either relapse or rehospitalization rates among treated patients and by levels of persisting or residual symptoms and general outcome over the course of several years. The utility of relapse rates depends on the measure that is used. Relapse rates based on symptom reemergence have varied markedly from study to study, partly because different criteria for the types and severity of symptoms have been used to define relapse. Rehospitalization rates, which may also be used to determine rates of relapse, offer the advantage of reflecting both symptoms and functioning. However, rehospitalization rates are affected by other clinical and nonclinical determinants. Thus, they tend to be more conservative estimates of relapse (occurring at a rate of 1%–10% per month after discontinuation of therapy) than are rates of reemergence of psychotic symptoms (5%–20% per month) (99). More recently, long-term efficacy has been measured in terms of quality of life, health service utilization, and social and vocational function (768–771). In addition, these measures of outcome have been used to define the level of recovery of patients.

1. Antipsychotic medications

In this guideline the term "antipsychotic" refers to multiple medications (Table 2), including the first-generation antipsychotic medications and the second-generation agents clozapine, risperidone, olanzapine, quetiapine, ziprasidone, and aripiprazole. In addition to having therapeutic effects, both first- and second-generation antipsychotic agents can cause a broad spectrum of side effects. Side effects of medications are a crucial aspect of treatment because they often determine medication choice and are a primary reason for medication discontinuation.

Side effects can complicate and undermine antipsychotic treatment in various ways. The side effects themselves may cause or worsen symptoms associated with schizophrenia, including negative, positive, and cognitive symptoms and agitation (772). In addition, these side effects may contribute to risk for other medical disorders (50, 773). Finally, these side effects often are subjectively difficult to tolerate and may affect the patient's quality of life and willingness to take the medication (17).

Most side effects of antipsychotic treatment result from actions on neurotransmitter systems and anatomic regions beyond those involved in mediating the intended therapeutic effects of the medication. Among the antipsychotic medications, differences in the risk of specific side effects are often predictable from the potencies and receptor binding profiles of the various agents. Some side effects result from receptor-mediated effects within the central nervous system (e.g., extrapyramidal side effects, hyperprolactinemia, sedation) or outside the central nervous system (e.g., constipation, hypotension), whereas other side effects are of unclear pathophysiology (e.g., weight gain, hyperglycemia). Side effects that are similar across several classes of agents, including both first- and second-generation antipsychotics, are discussed in Section V.A.1.c, "Shared Side Effects of Antipsychotic Medications." These shared side effects include neurological effects (i.e., acute and chronic extrapyramidal effects, neuroleptic malignant syndrome), sedation, cardiovascular effects (i.e., hypotension, tachycardia, and conduction abnormalities), anticholinergic and antiadrenergic effects, weight gain and glucose and lipid metabolic abnormalities, and sexual dysfunction. Side effects unique to particular agents are discussed in the respective sections concerning those agents, as are other unique implementation issues. Suggested approaches for monitoring and clinical management of the side effects of antipsychotic medications are outlined in Table 1.

a) First-generation agents

First-generation antipsychotic agents effect their therapeutic action, as well as their extrapyramidal side effects, primarily by blocking dopamine, subtype 2 (D_2), receptors in mesolimbocortical and nigrostriatal areas of the brain (774).

(1) Efficacy in the acute phase

The evidence supporting the effectiveness of first-generation antipsychotic medications in reducing psychotic symptoms in acute schizophrenia comes from studies carried out in the 1960s (775, 776) as well as numerous subsequent clinical trials (99, 777). Each of these studies compared one or more antipsychotic medications with either placebo or a sedative agent, such as phenobarbital (778), that served as a control. Nearly all of these studies found that the antipsychotic medication was superior for treating schizophrenia. These studies demonstrated the efficacy of first-generation antipsychotic medications for every subtype and subgroup of patients with schizophrenia. Moreover, in reviews of studies that compared more than one first-generation antipsychotic medication, Klein and Davis (779) and Davis et al. (777) found that, with the exception of mepazine and promazine, all of these agents were equally effective, although there were differences in dose, potency, and side effects of the different drugs.

First-generation antipsychotic medications are effective in diminishing most symptoms of schizophrenia. In a review of five large studies comparing an antipsychotic to placebo, Klein and Davis (779) found that patients who received an antipsychotic demonstrated decreases in positive symptoms, such as hallucinations, uncooperativeness, hostility, and paranoid ideation. Patients also showed improvement in thought disorder, blunted affect, withdrawal-retardation, and autistic behavior.

These findings—along with decades of clinical experience with these agents—indicate that first-generation antipsychotic treatment can reduce the positive symptoms (hallucinations, delusions, bizarre behaviors) and secondarily reduce the negative symptoms (apathy, affective blunting, alogia, avolition) associated with schizophrenic psychosis (297). In placebo-controlled comparisons (99, 776), approximately 60% of patients treated with first-generation antipsychotic medication for 6 weeks improved to the extent that they achieved complete remission or experienced only mild symptoms, compared to only 20% of patients treated with placebo. Forty percent of medication-treated patients continued to show moderate to severe psychotic symptoms, compared to 80% of placebo-treated patients. Eight percent of medication-treated patients showed no improvement or worsening, compared to nearly one-half of placebo-treated patients. A patient's prior history of a medication response is a fairly reliable predictor of how the patient will respond to a subsequent trial (780, 781).

Since the advent of second-generation antipsychotic medications, research on first-generation agents has reduced considerably. In recent years, randomized, controlled studies of the efficacy of first-generation agents for acute treatment have focused on dosing strategies and defining the most effective dose range to maximize symptom response and minimize side effects. These studies have consistently found that modest doses of first-generation agents (typically defined in haloperidol doses of less than 10 mg/day or plasma levels <18 ng/ml) are as efficacious or more efficacious than higher doses (782–784). Moderate doses of first-generation agents have been reported to improve comorbid depression (369, 785, 786), whereas higher doses are associated with greater risk of extrapyramidal side effects and dysphoria (785, 787) and may be especially problematic for patients with frontal lobe dysfunction (788).

(2) Efficacy in the stabilization and stable phases

Empirical research provides relatively little guidance for psychiatrists who are making decisions about medication and dosage during the stabilization phase. The use of first-generation antipsychotic medications during this phase is based on the clinical observation that patients relapse abruptly when medications are discontinued during this phase of treatment.

A large number of studies (789, 790) have compared relapse rates for stabilized patients who continued taking a first-generation antipsychotic medication and for those whose regimen was changed to placebo. During the first year only about 30% of those continuing to take medications relapsed, compared with about 65% of those taking placebo. Even when adherence with medication treatment was ensured by the use of long-acting injectable medications, as many as 24% of patients relapsed in a year (791). Hogarty et al. (792) found that among outpatients maintained with antipsychotic medications for 2–3 years who had been stable and judged to be at low risk of relapse, 66% relapsed in the year after medication withdrawal. Studies in which the medications of well-stabilized patients were discontinued indicate that 75% of patients relapse within 6–24 months (790). Among patients who have experienced a first episode of schizophrenia, a number of carefully designed double-blind studies indicate that 40%–60% of patients relapse if they are untreated during the year after recovery from this initial episode (211, 212, 218).

A critical issue during the stable treatment phase is adherence to the medication regimen. One strategy for improving adherence with first-generation agents is use of the long-acting injectable formulation. Studies with long-acting antipsychotics show a dose-response relationship in prophylactic efficacy, although there is a tradeoff in the relationship between dose and relapse rate on the one hand and side effects on the other (793, 794). The higher the dose used, the lower the relapse rate but the higher the rate of side effects, whereas the reverse is seen with lower doses. Although a small number of randomized trials have assessed the effectiveness of more modest doses of long-acting injectable medications than those typically used in clinical practice, evidence on this question remains inconclusive. Inderbitzen et al. (795) found no loss of clinical effectiveness when the average dose of patients already receiving long-acting injectable fluphenazine was cut gradually by 50% over a 5-month period (from an average of 23 mg every 2 weeks to 11.5 mg every 2 weeks). Similarly, Carpenter et al. (796) found a regimen of 25 mg of fluphenazine decanoate every 6 weeks to be equally effective as the same dose administered every 2 weeks. However, Schooler et al. (219) compared three medication strategies using fluphenazine decanoate: a continuous moderate dose (12.5–50 mg every 2 weeks); a continuous low dose (2.5–10 mg every 2 weeks); and targeted, early intervention (fluphenazine only when the patient was experiencing symptoms). They found that both continuous low-dose and targeted treatment increased the use of rescue medication and the rate of relapse, while only targeted treatment increased the rate of rehospitalization.

(3) *Shared side effects*

Side effects of first-generation antipsychotic medications typically vary with the potency of the agent. High-potency first-generation antipsychotics are associated with a high risk of extrapyramidal effects, a moderate risk of sedation, a low risk of orthostatic hypotension and tachycardia, and a low risk of anticholinergic and antiadrenergic effects. In contrast, low-potency first-generation antipsychotic agents are associated with a lower risk of extrapyramidal effects, a high risk of sedation, a high risk of orthostatic hypotension and tachycardia, and a high risk of anticholinergic and antiadrenergic effects. Although other side effects also vary with the specific medication, in general, the first-generation antipsychotic medications are associated with a moderate risk of weight gain, a low risk of metabolic effects, and a high risk of sexual side effects. With certain agents (thioridazine, mesoridazine, pimozide), a moderate risk of cardiac conduction abnormalities is also present. Neuroleptic malignant syndrome occurs rarely but is likely to be more often observed with first-generation agents (especially high-potency agents) than with second-generation antipsychotic medications. Details on the nature and management of each of these side effects are provided in Section V.A.1.c, "Shared Side Effects of Antipsychotic Medications."

(4) *Other side effects*

Other side effects include seizures, allergic reactions, and dermatological, hepatic, ophthalmological, and hematological effects.

Seizures

First-generation antipsychotic medications can lower the seizure threshold and result in the development of generalized tonic-clonic seizures (797). The low-potency first-generation antipsychotic medications confer the greatest risk. The frequency of seizures with low-potency antipsychotic medications is dose related, with higher doses associated with greater risk. At usual dose ranges, the seizure rates are below 1% for all first-generation antipsychotic medications, although patients with a history of an idiopathic or medication-induced seizure have a higher risk.

Allergic and dermatological effects

Cutaneous allergic reactions occur infrequently with first-generation antipsychotic medications. Medication discontinuation or administration of an antihistamine is usually effective in reversing these symptoms. Rarely, thioridazine is associated with hyperpigmentation of the skin. Photosensitivity also occurs infrequently and is most common with the low-potency phenothiazine medications; patients should be instructed to avoid excessive sunlight and use sunscreen (99).

Hepatic effects

Also occurring with this class of medications are elevation of liver enzyme levels and cholestatic jaundice. Jaundice has been noted to occur in 0.1%–0.5% of patients taking chlorpromazine (99). This side effect usually occurs within the first month after the initiation of treatment and generally requires discontinuation of treatment. However, given the relative infrequency of antipsychotic-induced jaundice, other etiologies for jaundice should be evaluated before the cause is judged to be antipsychotic medication.

Ophthalmological effects

Pigmentary retinopathies and corneal opacities can occur with chronic administration of the low-potency medications thioridazine and chlorpromazine, particularly at high doses (e.g., more than 800 mg/day of thioridazine). For this reason, patients maintained with these medications should have periodic ophthalmological examinations (approximately every 2 years for patients with a cumulative treatment of more than 10 years), and a maximum dose of 800 mg/day of thioridazine is recommended (797). With the increased use of high-potency medications in the past two decades, there has been virtually no reporting of this side effect (777).

Hematological effects

Hematological effects, including inhibition of leukopoiesis, can occur with use of first-generation antipsychotic medications. Such effects include benign leukopenia and the more serious agranulocytosis. The best data exist for chlorpromazine, with which benign leukopenia occurs in up to 10% of patients and agranulocytosis occurs in 0.32% of patients (797).

(5) Implementation

Issues in implementation of treatment with first-generation antipsychotic medications include route of administration, dosage strategy, and medication interactions.

Route of administration

First-generation antipsychotic medications can be administered in oral forms, as short-acting intramuscular preparations, or as long-acting injectable preparations. Short-acting intramuscular medications reach a peak concentration 30–60 minutes after the medication is administered, whereas oral medications reach a peak in 2–3 hours (798). As a result, the calming effect of the first-generation antipsychotic may begin more quickly when the medication is administered parenterally. However, this calming effect on agitation is different from the true antipsychotic effect of these medications, which may require several days or weeks (779). It is also worth noting that oral concentrates are typically better and more rapidly absorbed than pill preparations and often approximate intramuscular administration in their time to peak serum concentrations.

A single or twice-daily dose of an oral preparation will result in steady-state blood levels in 2–5 days (798). Long-acting injectable first-generation antipsychotic medications (fluphenazine decanoate or enanthate and haloperidol decanoate in the United States) may require up to 3–6 months to reach a steady state (92). As a result, they are seldom used alone during acute treatment, when the psychiatrist is adjusting the dose in accordance with therapeutic effects and side effects.

The advantage of long-acting injectable medications has been best demonstrated in studies such as those conducted by Johnson (799) under conditions that resemble most closely those in community clinics. In these studies, patients with histories of poor adherence were included in the study population and the amount of contact between patients and staff was limited. In the larger, more carefully controlled investigations (791, 800), patients with serious adherence problems—that is, the patients most likely to benefit from treatment with long-acting injectable medications—were commonly not included. Thus, a study by Hogarty et al. (800) showed a reduction in relapse associated with fluphenazine decanoate compared to oral fluphenazine only after 2 years of follow-up, as the effect of the drug on nonadherence and subsequent relapse took time to develop in a study population that was relatively stable and adherent at baseline.

Long-acting injectable medications are thought to be especially helpful in the stabilization and stable phases. Janicak et al. (99) examined six studies that compared the risk of psychotic relapse in patients who were randomly assigned to receive either oral or long-acting injectable medication. The longest of those studies (800) lasted 2 years and showed a relapse rate of 65% for patients taking oral medication and a rate of 40% for patients taking long-acting injectable medication. Although the remaining five studies, all of which lasted 1 year or less, had variable results, a meta-analysis of all six studies showed a significantly lower relapse rate in patients who received long-acting injectable medication ($p<0.0002$) (99).

Dosage strategy

The effective dose of a first-generation antipsychotic medication is closely related to its affinity for dopamine receptors (particularly D_2 receptors) and its tendency to cause extrapyramidal side effects (801, 802). Thus, high-potency medications have a greater affinity for dopamine receptors than do low-potency medications, and a much lower dose of high-potency medcations is required to treat psychosis. This relationship can be expressed in terms of dose equivalence (e.g., 100 mg of chlorpromazine has an antipsychotic effect that is similar to that of 2 mg of haloperidol). The dose equivalencies of commonly prescribed medications are listed in Table 2.

High-potency first-generation antipsychotic medications, such as haloperidol and fluphenazine, are more commonly prescribed than low-potency compounds (803). Although these medications have a greater tendency to cause extrapyramidal side effects than the low-potency medications, such as chlorpromazine and thioridazine, their side effects are easier to manage than the sedation and orthostatic hypotension associated with low-potency agents. High-potency medications can more safely be administered intramuscularly, since they seldom cause hypotension. In addition, because of sedation, orthostatic hypotension, and lethargy, the dose of a low-potency medication should be increased gradually, whereas an adequate dose of a high-potency medication can usually be achieved within a day or two. Finding the optimal dose of a first-generation antipsychotic is complicated by a number of factors. Patients with schizophrenia demonstrate large differences in the dose of first-generation antipsychotic they can tolerate and the dose required for an antipsychotic effect. A patient's age may influence the appropriate dose; elderly patients are more sensitive to both the therapeutic and adverse effects of first-generation antipsychotics. In addition, in studies in which dose is not fixed, it is difficult to determine dose by assessing antipsychotic effectiveness, since it may take many days at a therapeutic dose before there is an appreciable decrease in psychosis (778, 780).

A number of studies (reviewed by Davis et al. [777] and by Baldessarini et al. [95]) provide guidance about the usual doses required for acute treatment. Results of 19 controlled trials suggested that daily doses below 250 mg of chlorpromazine (or 5 mg of haloperidol or fluphenazine) are less adequate for many acutely psychotic patients than are moderate doses, between 300 and 600 mg of chlorpromazine. In the studies, response was typically measured by improvement in the score on the excitement, agitation, or psychosis subscale of the BPRS (6), and the proportions of patients responding to low doses after 1 and 2–10 days were 38% and 50%, respectively; these rates compared unfavorably with the improvement rates of 61% and 56% among patients taking moderate doses for similar periods (95). Davis et al. (777) came to similar conclusions. They found that daily doses between 540 and 940 mg of chlorpromazine were optimal. The findings of clinical trials involve groups of patients; some patients have optimal responses at doses above or below these optimal ranges. Psychiatrists have treated acutely psychotic patients with high doses of high-potency first-generation antipsychotic medications during the first days of treatment. This treatment is based on the belief that higher doses result in a more rapid improvement than that resulting from moderate doses (804). However, studies have revealed that high daily doses (more than 800 mg of chlorpromazine equivalents daily) were no more effective, or faster acting, on average than were moderate doses (500–700 mg/day) (95). After 1 day, 50% of the patients treated with high doses responded, compared to 61% of those who received moderate doses. After 2–10 days, high-dose treatment led to a slightly worse outcome: only 38% of those receiving high doses but 56% of those receiving moderate doses were improved. These studies indicate that higher doses are no more effective for acute treatment than normal doses, but higher doses are associated with a greater incidence of side effects.

Controlled trials have provided similar information regarding the effect of medication dose on outcome during the maintenance phase. In 33 randomized trials in which high doses (mean, 5200 mg/day of chlorpromazine equivalents) were compared to low doses (mean, 400 mg/day) during maintenance treatment, the lower doses were more effective in improving clinical state in more than two-thirds of the trials (95). In addition, in 95% of the studies the higher doses resulted in greater neurological side effects. Studies of doses of less than 200 mg/day of chlorpromazine equivalents tended to show that such doses were less effective than higher doses. An international consensus conference (294) made the reasonable recommendation of a reduction in first-generation antipsychotic dose of approximately 20% every 6 months until a minimal maintenance dose is reached. A minimal dose was considered to be as low as 2.5 mg of oral fluphenazine or haloperidol daily, 50 mg of haloperidol decanoate every 4 weeks, or 5 mg of fluphenazine decanoate every 2 weeks.

Concerns about the side effects of first-generation antipsychotic medications during maintenance treatment and the risk of tardive dyskinesia led to several studies that focused on methods for treating patients with the lowest effective maintenance dose. A number of investigators (19, 805–807) have studied gradual reductions in the amounts of medication given to stabilized patients until the medications are completely discontinued. Each patient was followed closely until there were signs of the beginning of a relapse. At that time, the patient's medication was reinstituted. To make this strategy work, patients and their families were trained to detect the early signs of impending psychotic breakdown. This approach used antipsychotic medications only intermittently to target symptom exacerbations and to avert anticipated exacerbations. Studies of the efficacy of this "targeted medication approach" have produced mixed results, and this approach is not recommended because of the substantial increase in the risk of relapse (19, 219, 805, 806).

Another strategy involves using much lower doses of a long-acting injectable first-generation antipsychotic than are usually prescribed. Several groups have compared low doses to moderate and high doses of fluphenazine decanoate. Initially, studies found that patients receiving very low doses (mean=2.5 mg every 2 weeks) were significantly more likely to relapse over the course of 1 year than were patients receiving standard doses (12.5–50.0 mg every 2 weeks) (56% versus 7%) (794). A subsequent study demonstrated that patients given a slightly higher dose (2.5–10.0 mg every 2 weeks) showed a nonsignificant difference in relapse after 1 year, compared with patients given standard doses (24% versus 14%) (808). Another study found no significant difference in relapse after 1 year between patients who received low doses (mean=5 mg every 2 weeks) and those who received standard doses (25–50 mg every 2 weeks) but did detect a significant difference in relapse rates after 2 years between the low-dose group and the standard-dose group (70% versus 35%) (793). Other studies, however, reported no difference in relapse rates after 2 years between patients who received low doses (mean=3.8 mg every 2 weeks) and those who received standard doses (25 mg every 2 weeks) (809). However, Schooler et al. (219) found that low-dose fluphenazine decanoate (2.5–10 mg every 2 weeks) increased the relapse rate and the use of rescue medication, compared to a continuous moderate dose (12.5–50 mg every 2 weeks). Collectively, these studies indicate that doses of fluphenazine decanoate as low as 5–10 mg every 2 weeks have been shown to be clinically effective, and some patients may respond to even lower doses, but the risk of relapse can increase significantly with these lower doses. However, consideration should be given to judicious reduction in the long-acting injectable dose over time, especially for patients with adverse side effects, in order to evaluate the optimal dose.

In considering the use of low-dose, long-acting injectable first-generation antipsychotics, the beneficial side effect profile associated with the use of lower doses should also be taken into account. Kane et al. (794) found that low-dose users had fewer early signs of tardive dyskinesia after 1 year than did standard-dose users. In a study by Marder et al. (793), lower doses were associated with significantly less discomfort (as measured with the SCL-90-R [810]), psychomotor retardation, and akathisia after 2 years. Hogarty et al. (809) reported that patients receiving minimal doses had less muscle rigidity, akathisia, and other side effects at 1 year and had greater improvements in instrumental and interpersonal role performances at 2 years.

First-generation antipsychotic medications have a very high therapeutic index for life-threatening side effects (780). Consequently, overdoses rarely are fatal unless they are complicated by preexisting medical problems or concurrent ingestion of alcohol or other medications. Symptoms of overdose are generally characterized by exaggerations of the adverse effects, with respiratory depression and hypotension presenting the greatest danger. Treatment is symptomatic and supportive and includes 1) ensuring airway patency and maintenance of respiration;

2) orally administering activated charcoal to decrease absorption and considering gastric lavage; 3) maintaining blood pressure with intravenous fluids and vasopressor agents; and 4) administering anticholinergic agents if needed to counteract extrapyramidal signs (811).

Medication interactions

A number of medication interactions can have clinically important effects for patients who are treated with antipsychotic medications (48, 49, 812). Certain heterocyclic antidepressants, most SSRIs, some beta-blockers, and cimetidine may increase antipsychotic plasma levels and increase side effects. On the other hand, barbiturates and carbamazepine decrease plasma levels through effects on cytochrome P450 enzymes.

b) Second-generation agents

The medications discussed in this section are referred to as second-generation antipsychotics primarily because the doses that are effective against the psychopathology of schizophrenia do not cause extrapyramidal side effects. Their therapeutic effects are attributed to central antagonism of both serotonin and dopamine receptors and also possibly to relatively loose binding to D_2 receptors (813–815).

Clozapine

Clozapine is a second-generation antipsychotic with antagonist activity at numerous receptors, including dopamine (D_1, D_2, D_3, D_4, D_5), serotonin (5-HT_{1A}, 5-HT_{2A}, 5-HT_{2C}), muscarinic (M_1, M_2, M_3, M_5), α_1- and α_2-adrenergic, and histamine (H_1) receptors (816–818). Clozapine is an agonist at muscarinic (M_4) receptors (819). Clozapine is also distinguished from other antipsychotic medications by its greater efficacy in treating positive symptoms in patients with treatment-resistant illness and by the absence of extrapyramidal side effects. However, it is associated with several serious and potentially fatal adverse effects, including agranulocytosis in 0.5%–1% of patients, seizures in about 2% of patients, and rare occurrences of myocarditis and cardiomyopathy.

Efficacy of clozapine

Clozapine has demonstrated superior efficacy for the treatment of general psychopathology in patients with treatment-resistant schizophrenia, compared to the first-generation antipsychotics haloperidol and chlorpromazine in six of eight published double-blind randomized trials (313, 314, 769, 820–824). A meta-analysis pooled the results of five of these studies that categorically defined subjects as "responders" based on clinically meaningful improvement in psychopathology and found that clozapine-treated patients were 2.5 times more likely to meet response criteria than those treated with a first-generation antipsychotic ($p=0.001$) (87). Clozapine also has demonstrated efficacy in reducing the frequency of suicidal ideation and suicide attempts in a randomized 2-year study of 980 patients with schizophrenia or schizoaffective disorder at high risk for suicide because of previous or current suicidal ideation or behavior (55). In this study patients were randomly assigned to receive either clozapine or olanzapine. Fewer patients who received clozapine attempted suicide (34 subjects), compared to patients who received olanzapine (55 subjects) ($p=0.03$), and a 24% reduction in risk of suicidal behaviors was found. In light of this evidence, clozapine should be preferentially considered for patients with a history of chronic and persistent suicidal ideation or behaviors. In addition, several studies suggest that clozapine may reduce the severity of hostility and aggression in patients with treatment-resistant symptoms (57, 314, 440, 821, 825–827). Open-label and double-blind studies of clozapine have produced inconsistent results with regard to effects on cognition, with some measures showing improvement and others showing no changes or even decrements in performance (828–840).

There is also preliminary evidence from open-label observational studies that clozapine may reduce risk of relapse in patients with treatment-resistant schizophrenia (841–845). Although these studies are encouraging, they are limited since some included only clozapine responders, while others did not include a comparison group. These studies are supported by the results of a large randomized open trial, in which significantly fewer hospital readmissions were observed for patients treated with clozapine, compared to those treated with usual care in a state hospital system over a 2-year period (822). The only double-blind study that measured readmission rates over a 1-year period failed to show a difference between haloperidol and clozapine for patients with treatment-resistant schizophrenia, although patients treated with clozapine stayed fewer days in the hospital (769). Taken together, the evidence is suggestive that treatment with clozapine is associated with reduced rates of relapse and rehospitalization in patients with treatment-resistant schizophrenia.

Studies of other populations, including patients with first-episode schizophrenia (846) and patients with treatment-responsive schizophrenia or schizoaffective disorder (847), demonstrate only limited or inconsistent superior efficacy for clozapine. In addition, studies comparing clozapine to other second-generation antipsychotics generally show comparable efficacy of clozapine with other second-generation antipsychotics (87, 381, 820, 848). However, since relatively low doses of clozapine were used in these studies, the results must be interpreted with caution.

In summary, a clozapine trial should be considered for patients who have shown a poor response to other antipsychotic medications. Clozapine may also be considered for patients with a history of chronic and persistent suicidal ideation or behaviors. In addition, clozapine may also be considered for patients with persistent hostility and aggression, given that superior efficacy of clozapine has been demonstrated in these patient populations.

Shared side effects of clozapine

Clozapine is associated with a very low risk of acute and chronic extrapyramidal side effects, a high risk of sedation, a high risk of orthostatic hypotension and tachycardia, a low risk of cardiac conduction abnormalities, a high risk of anticholinergic effects, a high risk of weight gain and metabolic abnormalities, and a low risk of prolactin elevation and sexual side effects. Neuroleptic malignant syndrome occurs rarely with clozapine. Details on the nature and management of each of these side effects are provided in Section V.A.1.c, "Shared Side Effects of Antipsychotic Medications."

Other side effects of clozapine

Sialorrhea and drooling occur relatively frequently and are most likely due to decreased saliva clearance related to impaired swallowing mechanisms (849), or possibly as a result of muscarinic cholinergic antagonist activity at the M_4 receptor or to α-adrenergic agonist activity (850). Interventions include use of a towel on the pillow at night to reduce discomfort. While there is little systematic information about pharmacological interventions, case reports suggest potential improvement with antimuscarinic agents and α receptor agonists (851–853). However, since clozapine also exhibits significant anticholinergic properties, use of agents with added anticholinergic effects must be approached with extreme caution to avoid potential adverse effects such as constipation or cognitive impairment.

Fever (>38°C) may occur during the first few weeks of treatment (854, 855). Generally a clozapine-associated fever is self-limiting and responds to supportive measures. However, fever is a symptom of neuroleptic malignant syndrome, agranulocytosis, and cardiomyopathy, and the presence of fever warrants evaluation for these potentially life-threatening complications of clozapine treatment.

The risk of agranulocytosis (defined as an absolute neutrophil count less than $500/mm^3$) has been estimated at 1.3% of patients per year of treatment with clozapine (99, 854, 856). The risk is highest in the first 6 months of treatment, and therefore weekly WBC and neutrophil monitoring is required. After 6 months, monitoring may occur every 2 weeks, as the risk of agranulocytosis appears to diminish considerably (an estimated rate of three cases per 1,000 patients). WBC counts must remain above $3000/mm^3$ during clozapine treatment, and absolute neutrophil counts must remain above $1500/mm^3$.

In the United States through 1989 there were 149 cases of agranulocytosis, with 48 (32%) fatalities. With the advent of systematic monitoring, fatalities have been greatly reduced (857–859). Between 1989 and 1997, among the 150,409 patients treated with clozapine who were included in the patient registry maintained by the U.S. manufacturer of the drug, 585 cases of agranulocytosis, with nine fatalities, were reported. Thus, awareness of agranulocytosis and the monitoring system have decreased the reported rate of clozapine-induced agranulocytosis to less than 0.5%.

Reports of myocarditis, with resultant cardiomyopathy and fatal heart failure, associated with clozapine use suggest a 17- to 322-fold elevation in risk in clozapine-treated patients. The absolute risk is estimated to range from 1 per 500 treated patients (860) to 1 per 10,000 treated patients (861). An immune mechanism mediated by immunoglobulin E antibodies is suspected because of reports of associated eosinophilia. Most but not all cases have occurred early in treatment, suggesting that the risk of myocarditis may be less after the first few months.

Clozapine is also associated with a dose-related risk of seizures (854). The overall seizure rate is 2.8%; with low-dose treatment (<300 mg/day) the risk is 1%, with medium doses (300–599 mg/day) the risk is 2.7%, and with high doses (>599 mg/day) the risk is 4.4%. The seizure risk for clozapine is also related to rapid increases in dose. Therefore, the rate of titration should not exceed the guidelines described in the subsequent section on implementation of treatment with clozapine.

In addition, there are case reports associating clozapine treatment with several other rare but potentially serious adverse events, including pancreatitis (862, 863), deep vein thrombosis (864, 865), pulmonary embolism, hepatitis (866, 867), and eosinophilia (863). Because of the small number of reports, the causal relationship with clozapine is unclear.

Implementation of treatment with clozapine

Before initiating treatment with clozapine, a complete blood count (CBC) with differential should be performed and the patient's general and cardiovascular health status should be evaluated. The cardiovascular side effects of clozapine should be considered in planning treatment for patients with preexisting heart disease. Treatment should be initiated at a low dose (12.5–25 mg once or twice daily) and increased gradually (by no more than 25–50 mg/day) as tolerated until a target dose is reached. Because of the risk of marked hypotension, sedation, and seizures with rapid dose escalation, dose titration should not occur more rapidly. During dose titration the patient's cardiovascular status, including orthostatic pulse, blood pressure, and subjective complaints of dizziness, should be monitored. Since the side effects of clozapine in the initial and dose-adjustment phases may be severe in some patients, admission to the hospital may be justifiable (e.g., for unstable patients who require rapid dose increases to a therapeutic level, patients with a limited social support system, or patients prone to orthostatic hypotension or seizures).

Adequate safety monitoring during treatment is important to minimize the risk of adverse events. The clozapine package label states that WBC and neutrophil counts should be evaluated before treatment is initiated, weekly during the first 6 months of treatment and at least every 2 weeks after 6 months of treatment (854). Clozapine treatment should not be initiated if the initial WBC count is <3500/mm^3, if the patient has a history of a myeloproliferative disorder, or if the patient has a history of clozapine-induced agranulocytosis or granulocytopenia.

With maintenance treatment, patients should be advised to report any sign of infection immediately (e.g., sore throat, fever, weakness, lethargy). A WBC count <2000/mm^3 or absolute neutrophil count (ANC) <1000/mm^3 indicates impending or actual agranulocytosis, and the clinician should stop clozapine treatment immediately, check WBC and differential counts daily, monitor for signs of infection, and consider bone marrow aspiration and protective isolation if granulopoiesis is deficient. A WBC count of 2000–3000/mm^3 or ANC of 1000–1500/mm^3 indicates high risk of or impending agranulocytosis, and the clinician should stop clozapine treatment immediately, check the WBC and differential counts daily, and monitor for signs of infection. Clozapine may be resumed if no infection is present, the WBC count rises to >3000, and the ANC is >1500 (resume checking WBC count twice a week until it is >3500). If the WBC count is 3000–3500/mm^3, if it falls to 3000/mm^3 over 1–3 weeks, or if immature WBC forms are present, repeat the WBC count with a differential count. If the subsequent WBC count is 3000–3500/mm^3 and the ANC is >1500/mm^3, repeat the WBC count with a differential count twice a week until the WBC count is >3500/mm^3.

Agranulocytosis is usually reversible if clozapine is discontinued immediately (868). When agranulocytosis develops, clozapine should be immediately discontinued, and patients should be given intensive treatment for the secondary complications, e.g., sepsis. Granulocyte colony stimulating factor has been used to accelerate granulopoietic function and shorten recovery time (869). Lithium has also been considered as a possible treatment for leukopenia or to prevent the development of agranulocytosis in patients who may be susceptible to this adverse effect (870, 871).

Although there have been reports of successful clozapine rechallenge after leukopenia, the risk of recurrence remains high (872). A rechallenge with clozapine should not be undertaken in patients with confirmed cases of agranulocytosis (ANC <500/mm^3), as recurrence is almost certain (872). Clinically, rechallenge should only be considered for patients whose WBC count remained greater than 2000/mm^3, whose absolute neutrophil count remained greater than 1500/mm^3, and for whom trials with multiple other antipsychotics had failed but a good clinical response to clozapine was shown.

In addition, patients should be monitored for weight gain, glucose abnormalities, and hyperlipidemias that may occur during treatment with clozapine. Table 1 outlines suggested monitoring and clinical management of such adverse effects. Patients should also be monitored for other potentially life-threatening adverse effects of clozapine, including fever and other signs of myocarditis. Patients should be advised to report any signs of myocarditis (e.g., fever, fatigue, chest pain, palpitations, tachycardia, respiratory distress, peripheral edema). Immediate clinical evaluation is warranted, and a cardiovascular evaluation is needed if these symptoms are not explained by other causes. A cardiac evaluation is thus recommended for clozapine-treated patients who experience unexplained fever, fatigue, chest pain, palpitations, tachycardia, hypotension, narrowed pulse pressure, respiratory distress, peripheral edema, ST-T wave abnormalities or arrhythmias as shown by ECG, or hypereosinophilia as shown by a CBC, especially if these symptoms are experienced during the first few months of treatment (873).

Controlled trials provide only limited guidance regarding the optimal dose of clozapine for schizophrenia. Since there have been no trials in which patients were randomly assigned to different doses of clozapine, the only available data are based on studies in which psychiatrists used what they considered the most effective dose. Fleischhacker et al. (874) reviewed 16 controlled trials from Europe and the United States. The mean dose from the European trials was 283.7 mg/day, and the U.S. mean was 444 mg/day. Plasma levels may help guide dosing, with studies suggesting that maximal clinical efficacy may be achieved when plasma levels of clozapine are between 200 and 400 ng/ml (typically associated with a dose of 300–400 mg/day) (875–878).

Although most patients whose symptoms respond to clozapine demonstrate maximal clinical improvement during the first 6–12 weeks of treatment, clinical benefits may continue to develop after 6–12 months (87, 879, 880). Twelve-week empirical trials of clozapine appear to be adequate to determine whether a patient is likely to respond to this medication (881, 882).

The elimination half-life of clozapine is approximately 12 hours, indicating that patients are likely to reach a steady-state plasma concentration after 2–3 days (883). Clozapine is metabolized primarily by the CYP1A2 enzyme. Other liver enzymes also contribute to clozapine metabolism, including CYP2C19, CYP2D6, and CYP3A4. Coadministration of drugs that inhibit cytochrome P450 enzymes (e.g., cimetidine, caffeine, erythromycin, fluvoxamine, fluoxetine, paroxetine, sertraline) may lead to a significant increase in clozapine plasma levels;

inducers of CYP1A2 (e.g., phenytoin, nicotine, rifampin) can significantly reduce clozapine levels. In particular, changes in smoking status may affect clozapine levels (500, 884). The concomitant use of medications such as carbamazepine can lower the WBC count and increase the potential danger of agranulocytosis; such medications should therefore be avoided. Some cases of respiratory or cardiac arrest have occurred among patients receiving benzodiazepines or other psychoactive medications concomitantly with clozapine. While no specific interaction between clozapine and benzodiazepines has been established, judicious use is advised when benzodiazepines or other psychotropic medications are administered with clozapine (885).

Risperidone

Risperidone is a second-generation antipsychotic with antagonist activity at dopamine (D_1, D_2, D_3, D_4), serotonin ($5\text{-}HT_{1A}$, $5\text{-}HT_{2A}$, $5\text{-}HT_{2C}$), α_1- and α_2-adrenergic, and histamine (H_1) receptors (816, 817).

Efficacy of risperidone

There are numerous published clinical trials comparing the acute efficacy of risperidone with placebo, first-generation antipsychotics (haloperidol or perphenazine), and other second-generation antipsychotics in patients with schizophrenia, schizoaffective disorder, and schizophreniform disorder. Placebo-controlled studies consistently demonstrate that for acutely relapsed patients, risperidone is efficacious in the treatment of global psychopathology and the positive symptoms of schizophrenia (886–888), as well as in increasing the likelihood of clinical response (e.g., ≥20% improvement on rating scales of global psychopathology). There is less consistent evidence that negative symptoms improve with risperidone treatment, as significant improvement compared with placebo was not found at all doses of risperidone (886, 887, 889). It is likely that the improvements in negative symptoms are due to the decreased likelihood of secondary negative symptoms (e.g., related to parkinsonism or to psychosis). Active-comparator-controlled studies demonstrate comparable or occasionally greater likelihood of clinical response and improvement of global psychopathology and positive symptoms with risperidone, compared with haloperidol (886, 887, 890–894) and perphenazine (895). Meta-analyses of these studies suggest that risperidone may have modestly better efficacy, compared with haloperidol and perphenazine, in decreasing positive symptoms (889, 896, 897) and global psychopathology and increasing the likelihood of response (82, 86, 88, 89, 889, 898–900). These studies also show less consistent evidence that negative symptoms improve with risperidone treatment, with any improvements possibly due to the decreased likelihood of secondary negative symptoms or resulting from comparison with high doses of first-generation antipsychotic agents. One study (271) found risperidone to have similar efficacy to haloperidol in the acute treatment of first-episode schizophrenia, as measured by greater response rates, improvement in global psychopathology, and improvement in positive symptoms.

Several studies have examined the efficacy of risperidone in the treatment of neurocognitive deficits of schizophrenia. Generally, these studies find that global measures of neurocognitive function improved with risperidone, although the magnitude of improvement was similar to that observed with haloperidol in two studies (901, 902). However, in one 14-week trial that included 101 patients, treatment with risperidone resulted in statistically significantly greater improvement in global neurocognition, compared with haloperidol (838). The clinical significance of this effect, however, is unclear. Thus, further investigation is required to determine the magnitude and clinical significance of risperidone effects on neurocognition.

Several studies have examined the efficacy of risperidone in patients with treatment-resistant schizophrenia. In an 8-week double-blind study, risperidone (mean dose=7.5 mg/day, N=34) and haloperidol (mean dose=19.4 mg/day, N=33) demonstrated similar efficacy in the treatment of global psychopathology (903). In a 14-week double-blind trial, treatment with risperidone (mean dose=11.6 mg/day, N=41) resulted in significant improvement in global psychopathology scores but not in positive and negative symptom subscale scores, for which the effects of risperidone were comparable to those of haloperidol (mean dose=25.7 mg/day, N=37) (820). In a 12-week double-blind study, 6 mg/day of risperidone (N=39) was superior to 20 mg/day of haloperidol (N=39) in the treatment of global psychopathology and negative symptoms (904).

Studies comparing risperidone to other second-generation antipsychotics in the treatment of acute episodes have generally found similar efficacy for treatment of psychopatholgy both in patients with treatment-responsive illness and in those with treatment-resistant illness (848, 902, 905–907).

Compared with haloperidol, risperidone has demonstrated superior efficacy in the prevention of relapse in the maintenance phase of treatment. In a study of 397 stable patients with DSM-IV schizophrenia or schizoaffective disorder, haloperidol-treated patients (mean dose= 11.7 mg/day) were 1.93 times more likely to relapse than risperidone-treated patients (mean dose=4.9 mg/day) during the 1-year follow-up period (382). In this study, the risperidone-treated patients also had significantly greater improvement in global psychopathology, compared to the haloperidol-treated patients.

Shared side effects of risperidone

Risperidone is associated with a low risk of sedation, a low to moderate risk of extrapyramidal side effects, a moderate risk of orthostatic hypotension and tachycardia, a low risk of anticholinergic effects, a moderate risk of weight gain and metabolic abnormalities, and a high risk of prolactin elevation and sexual side effects. Risperidone slightly alters cardiac conduction but not to a clinically meaningful extent. Neuroleptic malignant syndrome occurs rarely with risperidone. Details on the nature and management of each of these side effects are provided in Section V.A.1.c, "Shared Side Effects of Antipsychotic Medications."

Other side effects of risperidone

Clinical trial data suggest a small increase in the risk of stroke in patients with dementia treated with risperidone, compared with placebo-treated patients. Thus, dementia patients treated with risperidone should be carefully monitored for signs and symptoms of stroke (908). Similar increases in risk of stroke have not been reported in elderly risperidone-treated patients with schizophrenia who do not have dementia.

Implementation of treatment with risperidone

While the original efficacy studies comparing different doses of risperidone indicated optimal effectiveness at doses of around 6 mg/day, clinical investigations and subsequent studies indicate that for most adult patients optimal doses are between 2 and 6 mg/day, with a minority of patients requiring higher doses. Higher doses often lead to extrapyramidal side effects without greater effectiveness. Patients who develop parkinsonian symptoms are probably receiving too high a dose, and dose reduction is required for these patients.

During the titration and early treatment phase, risperidone-treated patients should be monitored for extrapyramidal side effects, orthostatic hypotension and reflex tachycardia, side effects associated with prolactin elevation, and sedation. In addition, patients should be monitored for weight gain, glucose abnormalities, and hyperlipidemias that may occur during treatment with risperidone. Table 1 outlines suggested strategies for monitoring and clinical management of such adverse effects. Elderly patients, particularly those with dementia, should be monitored for signs and symptoms of stroke.

Risperidone's effectiveness appears to be related to actions of both the parent compound and a major metabolite, 9-hydroxyrisperidone (909). They are therapeutically equipotent, have similar types of pharmacological activity, and, therefore, probably produce similar therapeutic effects. Although risperidone itself has an elimination half-life of only 3 hours, its metabolite has an elimination half-life of about 24 hours. As a result, most patients can be managed with a once-daily dose of risperidone. However, since risperidone can cause orthostatic hypotension, twice-daily dosing may be useful during the titration phase and for patients who may be vulnerable to orthostatic changes, such as elderly patients.

Risperidone is primarily metabolized by the hepatic CYP2D6 enzyme into the 9-hydroxyrisperidone metabolite (910). 9-Hydroxyrisperidone may also be metabolized by the CYP3A4 liver enzyme (500, 911). As a result, inducers of CYP3A4 may decrease risperidone blood levels and thus reduce therapeutic efficacy (912). In contrast, inhibitors of CYP2D6 and CYP3A4 may raise blood levels of risperidone and its active metabolite 9-hydroxyrisperidone and thus produce increased side effects, such as extrapyramidal side effects (913). In 5%–8% of Caucasians and 2%–5% of African Americans and Asians, the activity of the CYP2D6 enzyme is very low or absent. In poor metabolizers, the half-life is 17 hours for risperidone and 30 hours for 9-hydroxyrisperidone, compared to half-lives in extensive metabolizers of 3 hours for risperidone and 21 hours for 9-hydroxyrisperidone. Thus, the relative proportion of risperidone to 9-hydroxyrisperidone will be higher in patients who are slow metabolizers. In addition, drugs that inhibit the CYP2D6 enzyme (e.g., quinidine) will effectively turn extensive metabolizers into poor metabolizers. In terms of CYP liver enzymes other than CYP3A4 and CYP2D6, risperidone does not tend to produce significant inhibition or induction.

Olanzapine

Olanzapine is a second-generation antipsychotic with antagonist activity at dopamine (D_1, D_2, D_3, D_4), serotonin (5-HT_{2A}, 5-HT_{2C}), muscarinic (M_1, M_2, M_3, M_5), α_1-adrenergic, and histamine (H_1) receptors (818, 914).

Efficacy of olanzapine

There are several published clinical trials comparing the acute efficacy of olanzapine with placebo, first-generation antipsychotics (haloperidol or chlorpromazine), and other second-generation antipsychotics in patients with schizophrenia, schizoaffective disorder, and schizophreniform disorder. Placebo-controlled studies consistently demonstrate that in acutely relapsed patients olanzapine is efficacious in treating global psychopathology and the positive symptoms of schizophrenia, as well as in increasing the likelihood of clinical response (e.g., ≥20% improvement on rating scales of global psychopathology) (915–917). The evidence that negative symptoms improve with olanzapine treatment, compared with placebo, is less consistently found across doses of the drug (915–917). It is likely that any improvements in negative symptoms in these studies are due to decreased likelihood of secondary negative symptoms (e.g., related to parkinsonism or to psychosis) rather than to direct effects on primary negative symptoms (323). Active-comparator-controlled studies demonstrate similar or occasionally greater likelihood of clinical response and greater improvement of global psychopathology and positive and negative symptoms with olanzapine, compared to haloperidol (279, 319, 916–920). Meta-analyses of these studies suggest that olanzapine may have modestly better efficacy, compared with haloperidol, in the treatment of global psychopathology and positive and negative symptoms (921) and in increasing the likelihood of response (82, 86, 88). Effects on hostility are mixed, with one study (921) showing greater improvement in hostility with olanzapine than with haloperidol, and another study finding no difference in hostility response (440). In patients with a first episode of schizophrenia, one study (a subanalysis of a Lilly olanzapine database) found significantly greater improvement in global psychopathology, positive and negative symptoms, and response rate after a 6-week trial of olanzapine, compared to haloperidol (272). A second study found that a significantly larger proportion of olanzapine-treated patients, compared with haloperidol-treated patients, remained in the trial and completed the first 12 weeks of treatment (279). In addition, the study found that the olanzapine-treated patients had slight but significant improvements in global psychopathology and negative symptoms and were more likely to meet the response criteria, although this difference only approached significance ($p=0.06$).

Four studies have examined the efficacy of olanzapine in the treatment of neurocognitive deficits of schizophrenia. Two of these studies found significant improvement in neurocognition as measured by a global index in olanzapine-treated patients, compared to haloperidol-treated patients (838, 902). One 12-week analysis of treatment effects in first-episode patients found significant improvement with olanzapine, compared to haloperidol, in global neurocognition assessed with a measure derived from a principal-component analysis, but the difference only approached significance when an empirically derived a priori measure of global neurocognition was used (922). The fourth study did not find differences between haloperidol and olanzapine in effects on global neurocognition (923). Olanzapine significantly improved motor function (838, 902), verbal fluency, nonverbal fluency and construction, immediate recall (902), general executive function (838, 923), and perceptual function and attention (838). Although a relatively consistent finding is that olanzapine has beneficial effects on neurocognition in schizophrenia, findings for the specific domains affected and the clinical significance of these effects are less clear. Further study is needed to determine the magnitude and clinical significance of the effects of olanzapine on neurocognition.

Several studies have examined the efficacy of olanzapine in patients with treatment-resistant illness (i.e., patients who have shown little or no response to adequate trials of other antipsychotics). In an 8-week double-blind study, 25 mg/day of olanzapine (N=42) and 1200 mg/day of chlorpromazine (N=39) demonstrated similar efficacy in the treatment of global psychopathology (924). In a 14-week double-blind trial, treatment with a mean dose of 30.4 mg/day of olanzapine (N=39) resulted in significantly greater improvement in global psychopathology and negative symptoms, compared with a mean dose of 25.7 mg/day of haloperidol (N=37) (820). A third study that used a Lilly clinical trial database to retrospectively identify patients without response to first-generation antipsychotics found that olanzapine-treated patients, compared to haloperidol-treated patients, had significantly greater improvements in global psychopathology and positive, negative, and mood symptoms; higher response rates; and higher completion rates (925). Although higher doses of olanzapine (doses up to 60 mg/day) are being used clinically for patients with treatment-resistant illness, current evidence of improved efficacy at higher doses is inconclusive (820, 926, 927).

Studies comparing olanzapine to other second-generation antipsychotics in the treatment of acute episodes have generally found similar efficacy for treatment of psychopathology both in patients with treatment-responsive symptoms and in those with treatment-resistant symptoms (381, 820, 905, 906), with some exceptions in which olanzapine was found to be superior (820, 902).

In terms of treatment during the stabilization and stable phases, analysis of data from the double-blind extension phase of 6-week acute treatment trials suggests that olanzapine may reduce the risk of relapse, compared to haloperidol. Pooling data across three studies, the investigators found that 19.7% of olanzapine-treated patients relapsed during the 1-year follow-up period, compared to 28% of haloperidol-treated patients ($p<0.04$) (928).

Shared side effects of olanzapine

Olanzapine is associated with a low risk of extrapyramidal side effects, a low risk of sedation, a low risk of orthostatic hypotension and tachycardia, a low risk of cardiac conduction abnormalities, a moderate risk of anticholinergic effects, a high risk of weight gain and metabolic abnormalities, and a low risk of prolactin elevation and sexual side effects. Neuroleptic malignant syndrome occurs rarely with olanzapine. Details on the nature and management of each of these side effects are provided in Section V.A.1.c, "Shared Side Effects of Antipsychotic Medications."

Implementation of treatment with olanzapine

Olanzapine is an effective antipsychotic when administered in doses of 10–20 mg/day in the acute phase of schizophrenia, although higher doses, up to 60 mg/day, have been reported to be used for patients with treatment-resistant schizophrenia (820, 926, 927). With the possible exception of akathisia, parkinsonian symptoms are infrequent at any dose of olanzapine.

During the titration and early treatment phase olanzapine-treated patients should be monitored for extrapyramidal side effects, orthostatic hypotension and reflex tachycardia, and sedation. Orthostatic hypotension may be more likely if benzodiazepines are coadministered (929). Evening administration may improve tolerance of the sedation that is common early in treatment. In addition, patients should be monitored for weight gain, glucose abnormalities, and hyperlipidemias that may occur during treatment with olanzapine. Table 1 outlines suggested monitoring and clinical management of such adverse effects.

Patients are typically managed with a single daily dose of olanzapine since the elimination half-life of olanzapine is 33 hours (ranging from 21 to 54 hours) (929). Olanzapine is primarily metabolized by the hepatic CYP1A2 enzyme, with a minor metabolic pathway involving the CYP2D6 enzyme. Inducers of the CYP1A2 enzyme (such as tobacco use) may reduce olanzapine plasma levels, and so changes in smoking status may affect efficacy and side effects at a given dose (500). There is some evidence to suggest differential metabolism of olanzapine by gender, with women exhibiting higher plasma concentrations than men at equivalent doses (509).

Quetiapine

Quetiapine is a second-generation antipsychotic with antagonist activity at dopamine (D_1, D_2), serotonin ($5\text{-}HT_{1A}$, $5\text{-}HT_{2A}$, $5\text{-}HT_{2C}$), α_1-adrenergic, and histamine (H_1) receptors (818, 930).

Efficacy of quetiapine

There are several published clinical trials comparing the acute efficacy of quetiapine with that of placebo, first-generation antipsychotics (haloperidol or chlorpromazine), and other second-generation antipsychotics in patients with schizophrenia, schizoaffective disorder, and schizophreniform disorder. Placebo-controlled studies consistently demonstrate that in acutely relapsed patients quetiapine is efficacious in the treatment of global psychopathology, in improving the likelihood of clinical response (e.g., ≥20% improvement on rating scales of global psychopathology), and in improving the positive symptoms of schizophrenia (318, 931, 932). The evidence that negative symptoms improve with quetiapine treatment is less clear, as significant improvement with quetiapine, compared with placebo, is less consistently found across different doses of the drug and different studies (318, 931, 932). It is likely that the improvements in negative symptoms in these studies are due to decreased likelihood of secondary negative symptoms (e.g., related to parkinsonism or to psychosis) rather than to direct effects on primary negative symptoms. Active-comparator-controlled studies demonstrate comparable or occasionally greater improvement of global psychopathology and positive and negative symptoms, as well as an increased likelihood of clinical response with quetiapine, compared to haloperidol or chlorpromazine (933–935). Meta-analyses of these studies suggest that the efficacy of quetiapine is similar to that of first-generation antipsychotics (82, 86, 88).

In terms of relapse prevention, one 4-month randomized, open-label study compared the efficacy of quetiapine (mean dose=254 mg/day, N=553) to that of risperidone (mean dose=4.4 mg/day, N=175) (907). This study found both antipsychotics to have similar effects on global psychopathology and positive symptoms and negative symptoms, with marginally significant greater improvement in depressive symptoms in the quetiapine-treated patients. While this study lends preliminary evidence for the efficacy of quetiapine in preventing relapse, further studies using blinded methods are needed before definitive conclusions can be made.

One study compared the efficacy of 600 mg/day of quetiapine (N=143) to that of 20 mg/day of haloperidol (N=145) in patients with treatment-resistant illness and found that a significantly greater proportion of the quetiapine-treated patients met the response criteria (52%, compared to 38% of the haloperidol-treated patients) (936). However, the mean changes in global psychopathology, positive symptoms, and negative symptoms were similar for both groups.

Two studies found beneficial effects on neurocognition for quetiapine, compared to first-generation antipsychotics. In a 6-month randomized, double-blind study, significant improvement in global cognition, verbal reasoning and fluency, and immediate recall was found for subjects treated with 300–600 mg/day of quetiapine (N=13) but not for subjects treated with 10–20 mg/day of haloperidol (N=12) (937). Similarly, in a 24-week double-blind, randomized study, significantly greater improvement in global cognition, executive function, attention, and verbal memory was found for subjects treated with 600 mg/day of quetiapine, compared to subjects treated with 12 mg/day of haloperidol (938).

Shared side effects of quetiapine

Quetiapine is associated with a very low risk of extrapyramidal side effects, a high risk of sedation, a moderate risk of orthostatic hypotension and tachycardia, a low risk of cardiac conduction abnormalities, a low risk of anticholinergic effects, a moderate risk of weight gain and metabolic abnormalities, and a low risk of prolactin elevation and sexual side effects. Neuroleptic malignant syndrome occurs rarely with quetiapine. Details on the nature and management of each of these side effects are provided in Section V.A.1.c, "Shared Side Effects of Antipsychotic Medications."

Other side effects of quetiapine

Preclinical studies in beagles found associations between quetiapine and increased risk of cataracts, prompting the FDA to suggest routine screening ophthalmological examinations before and every 6 months during quetiapine treatment. This risk has not been confirmed in humans, and there is no indication from postmarketing reporting of an association between increased cataract risk and quetiapine use (939).

Implementation of treatment with quetiapine

Quetiapine is an effective antipsychotic when administered in doses of 300–800 mg/day in the acute phase of schizophrenia. Evidence suggests that the higher doses in this range (and perhaps doses greater than 800 mg/day) may be more efficacious (318). Even at doses above 800 mg/day, there are virtually no extrapyramidal side effects, with the possible exception of akathisia. During the titration and early treatment phase, quetiapine-treated patients should be monitored for orthostatic hypotension, reflex tachycardia, and sedation. Patients are typically managed with twice-daily dosing of quetiapine, since the elimination half-life is 6 hours (940). However, uneven dosing with the larger dose given at bedtime may improve tolerance of the sedation that is common early in treatment. In addition, patients should be monitored for weight gain, glucose abnormalities, and hyperlipidemias, which may occur during treatment with quetiapine. Table 1 outlines suggested strategies for the monitoring and clinical management of such adverse effects. Quetiapine is primarily metabolized by the hepatic cytochrome P450 CYP3A4 enzyme. Metabolism of the drug is minimally altered in patients with renal disease, but it may be significantly altered in patients with liver disease. Smoking does not affect the metabolism of quetiapine (500, 940). However, coadministration of phenytoin with quetiapine has been demonstrated to increase the clearance of quetiapine up to fivefold (941). Similarly potent inducers of CYP3A4 are likely to produce similar decreases in quetiapine levels, which may lead to loss of therapeutic efficacy.

Ziprasidone

Ziprasidone is a second-generation antipsychotic with antagonist activity at dopamine (D_2), serotonin (5-HT_{2A}, 5-HT_{2C}, and 5-$HT_{1B/1D}$), α_1-adrenergic, and histamine (H_1) receptors. In addition, ziprasidone has partial agonist activity at serotonin 5-HT_{1A} receptors and inhibits neuronal reuptake of serotonin and norepinephrine (942).

Efficacy of ziprasidone

There are several published clinical trials comparing the efficacy of ziprasidone with placebo and with first-generation antipsychotics in the acute treatment of patients with schizophrenia, schizoaffective disorder, and schizophreniform disorder. Placebo-controlled studies consistently demonstrate that in acutely relapsed patients ziprasidone is efficacious in the treatment of global psychopathology and the positive symptoms of schizophrenia, as well as in increasing the likelihood of clinical response (e.g., ≥20% improvement on rating scales of global psychopathology) (943, 944). The evidence that negative symptoms improve with ziprasidone treatment is less clear, as significant improvement with ziprasidone, compared with placebo, is less consistently found across doses of drug and across studies (943–945). Active-comparator-controlled studies of ziprasidone compared with haloperidol demonstrate comparable improvement in positive and negative symptoms and in global psychopathology, as well as comparable likelihood of clinical response (945, 946). It is likely that the improvements in negative symptoms in these studies are due to a decreased likelihood of secondary negative symptoms (e.g., related to parkinsonism or to psychosis) rather than to direct effects on primary negative symptoms. However, in an additional placebo-controlled study of stable, residually symptomatic patients, the time course of improvement in negative symptoms was consistent with a therapeutic effect on primary negative symptoms (947). Nonetheless, this study was conducted with environmentally deprived persons who received more attention than usual by participating in the study, which may explain (in part) the observed improvements in negative symptoms.

One 52-week study demonstrated that ziprasidone is effective in reducing risk of relapse, compared with placebo, during the maintenance phase of treatment (947). Relapse risk was 43%, 35%, and 36% for patients receiving 40 mg/day, 80 mg/day, and 160 mg/day of ziprasidone, respectively, compared to 77% for placebo-treated patients.

Several studies have demonstrated the efficacy of intramuscular administration of ziprasidone for the treatment of acute agitation in relapsed patients with schizophrenia or schizoaffective disorder (76, 948, 949).

Shared side effects of ziprasidone

Ziprasidone is associated with a low risk of extrapyramidal side effects, a low risk of sedation, a low risk of orthostatic hypotension and tachycardia, a moderate risk of cardiac conduction abnormalities, a low risk of anticholinergic effects, a low risk of weight gain and metabolic abnormalities, and a low risk of prolactin elevation and sexual side effects. Neuroleptic malignant syndrome occurs rarely with ziprasidone. Details on the nature and management of each of these side effects are provided in Section V.A.1.c, "Shared Side Effects of Antipsychotic Medications."

Other side effects of ziprasidone

While short-term clinical trials do not report insomnia as an adverse event with ziprasidone, there is some evidence from a longer-term outpatient study to suggest that stable outpatients whose medication is switched to ziprasidone may experience insomnia (945). This insomnia appears early in treatment, is typically transient, and most often responds to usual sedative-hypnotics (e.g., zolpidem, trazodone).

Implementation of treatment with ziprasidone

Ziprasidone is an effective antipsychotic when administered in doses of 80–200 mg/day in the acute phase of schizophrenia. There is emerging evidence that doses up to 320 mg/day may be safe, although there are no published data suggesting improved efficacy at high doses. Stable patients whose medication is switched to ziprasidone may report insomnia, which usually is transient and responsive to sedative-hypnotics.

Before treatment with ziprasidone is initiated in patients with preexisting cardiovascular disease and those who are at risk for electrolyte disturbances (e.g., patients taking diuretics and those with chronic diarrhea), the safety of using the medication should be evaluated. This evaluation should include laboratory assessment of electrolytes and an ECG. Preexisting prolonged QT syndrome, persistent findings of QTc interval >500 msec, history of arrhythmia, recent acute myocardial infarction, or uncompensated heart failure are contraindications to use of ziprasidone. The value of a screening ECG in apparently healthy persons to reliably detect congenital prolonged QT syndrome is not established and is of questionable utility, given the normal variability of the QT interval. During the maintenance phase of treatment, regular monitoring of electrolytes should be done for patients who are also treated with diuretics or who may be at risk for electrolyte disturbances. Patients should be monitored regularly for symptoms of possible arrhythmia, including dizziness, syncopal episodes, and palpitations. Patients with such symptoms should be referred for cardiovascular evaluation. Patients should also be warned about concomitant treatment with other drugs that also may affect the QT interval.

Patients are typically treated with twice-daily dosing of ziprasidone, since the elimination half-life is 7 hours, and steady state is reached after 1–3 days. Food increases the absorption of ziprasidone; under fasting conditions only 60% of ziprasidone will be absorbed. Two-thirds of ziprasidone is metabolized by aldehyde oxidase, and one-third by the cytochrome P450 system, primarily by the liver CYP3A4 enzyme, and to a lesser extent by CYP1A2 (950). Sex, age, smoking, and the presence of renal failure have not been found to affect the metabolism of ziprasidone, but liver disease potentially affects metabolism of the drug (951, 952). Ziprasidone has little effect on other liver enzyme systems and has not been found to affect the metabolism of other drugs.

Aripiprazole

Aripiprazole is pharmacologically distinct from other second-generation antipsychotic medications. It has partial agonist activity at dopamine (D_2) and serotonin (5-HT_{1A}) receptors and antagonist activity at dopamine (D_3), serotonin (5-HT_{2A}, 5-HT_{2C}, 5-HT_7), α_1-adrenergic, and histamine (H_1) receptors. In addition, aripiprazole inhibits neuronal reuptake of serotonin to a modest extent (953, 954).

Efficacy of aripiprazole

There are several published clinical trials comparing the acute efficacy of aripiprazole with placebo and first-generation antipsychotics in patients with schizophrenia, schizoaffective disorder, and schizophreniform disorder. Placebo-controlled studies consistently demonstrate that in acutely relapsed patients, aripiprazole is efficacious in the treatment of global psychopathology, in improving the likelihood of clinical response (e.g., ≥20% improvement on rating scales of global psychopathology), and in improving the positive symptoms of schizophrenia (955). The evidence that negative symptoms improve with aripiprazole treatment is less clear, as significant improvement with aripiprazole, compared with placebo, is less consistently found across doses of drug and studies (955). It is possible that the improvements in negative symptoms in these studies are due to decreased likelihood of secondary negative symptoms (e.g., related to parkinsonism or to psychosis) rather than to direct effects on primary negative symptoms. Active-comparator-controlled studies demonstrate comparable or occasionally greater improvement of global psychopathology and positive and negative symptoms, as well as an increased likelihood of clinical response, with aripiprazole, compared to haloperidol or chlorpromazine (955, 956).

Two studies have found aripiprazole effective in reducing risk of relapse. In a 26-week randomized, double-blind trial that included stable patients with schizophrenia or schizoaffective disorder, the time to relapse was significantly longer for patients treated with aripiprazole

(15 mg/day) than for those who received placebo, and a greater proportion of patients who received placebo (57%) than of aripiprazole-treated patients (34%) met the relapse criteria (957). In a 52-week randomized, double-blind trial that included patients with acute exacerbation of schizophrenia or schizoaffective disorder, the response rate and time to discontinuation for any reason were significantly greater for patients treated with aripiprazole (30 mg/day, N=647) than for those treated with haloperidol (10 mg/day, N=647) (unpublished 2003 manuscript of R.D. McQuade et al.). A greater proportion of aripiprazole-treated patients (43%) than of the haloperidol-treated patients (30%) completed the 52-week trial.

Shared side effects of aripiprazole

Aripiprazole is associated with a low risk of extrapyramidal side effects, a moderate risk of sedation, a low risk of orthostatic hypotension and tachycardia, a low risk of cardiac conduction abnormalities, a low risk of anticholinergic effects, a low risk of weight gain and metabolic abnormalities, and a low risk of prolactin elevation and sexual side effects. There have been no reports to date of neuroleptic malignant syndrome with aripiprazole. Details on the nature and management of each of these side effects are provided below in Section V.A.1.c, "Shared Side Effects of Antipsychotic Medications."

Other side effects of aripiprazole

Aripiprazole received FDA approval for use in the treatment of schizophrenia in late 2002, and thus experience with the drug in clinical settings and knowledge of rare side effects are limited. Insomnia was not reported as an adverse event in treatment trials involving patients with acutely exacerbated symptoms (955, 956). Trials that included stable patients found transient insomnia and acute agitation early in treatment, but these side effects typically resolved after several weeks (955, 956). While there are no systematic studies, it is reasonable to treat aripiprazole-associated insomnia with sedative-hypnotics (e.g., zolpidem, trazodone, antihistamines) and agitation with benzodiazepines.

Implementation of treatment with aripiprazole

Aripiprazole is an effective antipsychotic when administered in doses of 10–30 mg/day in the acute phase of schizophrenia. With the possible exception of akathisia, parkinsonian symptoms rarely occur within the usual dose range.

Stable patients whose medication was switched to aripiprazole may report insomnia that usually is transient and responsive to sedative-hypnotics.

Patients are typically treated with once-daily dosing of aripiprazole since the elimination half-life is 75 hours (94 hours for the active metabolite dehydro-aripiprazole), and steady state is reached after 14 days. Aripiprazole is metabolized by the cytochrome P450 system, primarily by the liver enzymes CYP2D6 and CYP3A4 (958). Sex, age, smoking, and the presence of renal or hepatic failure have not been found to significantly affect the metabolism of aripiprazole (958). Aripiprazole has little effect on other liver enzyme systems and has not been found to affect the metabolism of other drugs.

c) Shared side effects of antipsychotic medications

This section provides information on the side effects that are shared among multiple antipsychotic medications.

(1) Neurological side effects

Neurological side effects of antipsychotic medications include acute extrapyramidal side effects such as medication-induced parkinsonism, dystonia, and akathisia; chronic extrapyramidal side effects such as tardive dyskinesia and tardive dystonia; and neuroleptic malignant syndrome.

(2) Extrapyramidal side effects

Extrapyramidal side effects are especially common in patients treated with the first-generation antipsychotics and occur to varying extents with several of the second-generation agents, especially higher doses of risperidone. Of the spectrum of adverse effects of first-generation antipsychotic medications, the neurological side effects are the most common and the most troublesome (959, 960). Extrapyramidal side effects can broadly be divided into acute and chronic categories. Acute extrapyramidal side effects are signs and symptoms that occur in the first days and weeks of antipsychotic medication administration, are dose dependent, and are reversible with medication dose reduction or discontinuation. The three types of acute extrapyramidal side effects are parkinsonism, dystonia, and akathisia (961–964). Chronic extrapyramidal side effects are signs and symptoms that occur after months and years of antipsychotic medication administration, are not clearly dose dependent, and may persist after medication discontinuation. Chronic extrapyramidal side effects include tardive dyskinesia and tardive dystonia. Detailed descriptions and differential diagnoses of the extrapyramidal side effect syndromes are provided in the "Medication-Induced Movement Disorders" section of DSM-IV-TR. More than 60% of patients who receive acute treatment with first-generation antipsychotic medications develop clinically significant extrapyramidal side effects in one form or another (959, 960, 965). Some patients may develop more than one form at the same time. Second-generation drugs as a group cause fewer or no extrapyramidal side effects, relative to first-generation drugs. Studies using multiple doses of risperidone (886, 887, 890) have shown that risperidone causes a dose-related increase in extrapyramidal side effects, with risk highest in doses greater than 6 mg/day (82, 899). In any individual patient, it is likely that the maximally clinically effective dose of risperidone is lower than the dose that will cause extrapyramidal side effects. Thus, first-line intervention for extrapyramidal side effects due to risperidone should be to gradually lower the dose until symptoms resolve. The other second-generation drugs cause few or no extrapyramidal side effects, with the possible exception of akathisia. However, younger patients (children, adolescents, and young adults) may be more prone to extrapyramidal side effects from second-generation medications (unpublished 2003 manuscript of L. Sikich et al.).

Medication-induced parkinsonism is characterized by the symptoms of idiopathic Parkinson's disease (rigidity, tremor, akinesia, and bradykinesia) and is the most common form of extrapyramidal side effect caused by first-generation antipsychotics (787, 964). These symptoms arise in the first days and weeks of antipsychotic medication administration and are dose dependent. Medication-induced parkinsonism generally resolves after discontinuation of antipsychotic medication, although some cases of persisting symptoms have been reported (966, 967).

Akinesia or bradykinesia is a feature of medication-induced parkinsonism that affects both motor and cognitive function. A patient with this condition appears to be slow moving, less responsive to the environment, apathetic, emotionally constricted, and cognitively slowed. This effect has been noted alone or with other extrapyramidal side effects in almost one-half of patients treated with first-generation antipsychotics. In very severe cases, it may mimic catatonia. Akinesia is subjectively unpleasant and may be associated with poor medication adherence (968, 969). Depressive symptoms can also be present in patients with akinesia, in which case the syndrome is termed "akinetic depression" (970, 971). Symptoms of medication-induced parkinsonism, in particular the cognitive and emotional features, need to be carefully distinguished from the negative symptoms of schizophrenia. Furthermore, it is noteworthy that patients may experience these emotional and cognitive symptoms of parkinsonism in the absence of detectable motor symptoms.

The first approach to treatment of parkinsonism associated with first-generation antipsychotics should be to lower the antipsychotic dose to the EPS threshold (dose where minimal rigidity is detectable in a physical examination), since studies indicate that doses above the EPS threshold are unlikely to yield further clinical benefits (94). If dose reduction does not sufficiently improve symptoms, then a switch to a second-generation antipsychotic should be considered. Medications with anticholinergic (e.g., benztropine) or dopamine agonist (e.g., amantadine) activity often reduce the severity of parkinsonian symptoms. However, dopamine agonists carry a potential risk of exacerbating psychosis, and anticholinergic drugs can cause anticholinergic side effects. Thus, excessive doses and chronic use of these agents should be avoided or minimized (972, 973).

Acute dystonia is characterized by the spastic contraction of discrete muscle groups. Dystonic reactions occur in up to 10% of patients beginning therapy with high-potency first-generation antipsychotic agents. Although precise estimates of the incidence of dystonic reactions are not available, they appear to be less common with treatment with low-potency first-generation antipsychotic agents and relatively rare with second-generation antipsychotics. In addition to the use of high-potency medications, other risk factors for dystonic reactions include young age, male gender, high doses, and intramuscular administration. Dystonic reactions frequently arise after the first few doses of medication (90% occur within the first 3 days) (974). They can occur in various body regions but most commonly affect the muscles of the neck, larynx, eyes, and torso (963). The specific name of the reaction is derived from the specific anatomic region that is affected. Hence, the terms "torticollis," "laryngospasm," "oculogyric crisis," and "opisthotonos" are used to describe dystonic reactions in specific body regions (975). These reactions are sudden in onset, are dramatic in appearance, and can cause patients great distress. For some patients, these conditions, e.g., laryngospasm, can be dangerous and even life-threatening.

Acute dystonic reactions respond dramatically to the administration of anticholinergic or antihistaminic medication. Parenteral administration will have a more rapid onset of action than oral administration. Short-term maintenance treatment with an oral regimen of anticholinergic antiparkinsonian medication prevents the recurrence of acute dystonic reactions.

Akathisia is characterized by somatic restlessness that is manifest subjectively and objectively in up to 30% of patients treated with first-generation antipsychotics (961, 970). Although precise estimates of the incidence of akathisia are not available, it appears to be less common with low-potency first-generation antipsychotics and even more infrequent with second-generation antipsychotic agents. Patients characteristically complain of an inner sensation of restlessness and an irresistible urge to move various parts of their bodies. Objectively, this appears as increased motor activity. With mild akathisia, the patient may control body movements; in more severe forms, the patient may rock from foot to foot while standing, pace, and have difficulty sitting still. Even in mild forms in which the patient is able to control most movements, this side effect is often extremely distressing to patients, is a frequent cause of nonadherence with antipsychotic treatment, and, if allowed to persist, can produce dysphoria. Case reports suggest that akathisia may also be a possible contributor to aggressive or suicidal behavior (409). Intervention includes dose reduction or switching to a second-generation antipsychotic with less risk of akathisia. In this regard, however, it is important to note that risperidone may cause akathisia at the higher end of the dose range (887).

Effective treatments for akathisia include centrally acting beta-blockers such as a low dose of propranolol (30–90 mg/day) (972, 976). When these medications are administered, blood pressure and pulse rate should be monitored with dose changes. Benzodiazepines such as lorazepam and clonazepam are also effective in decreasing symptoms of akathisia (977). In contrast, anticholinergic antiparkinsonian medications have limited efficacy in treating akathisia (972). While there has been little systematic study, akathisia induced by risperidone or other second-generation antipsychotics is treated similarly to akathisia associated with first-generation antipsychotic treatment.

A common problem that arises in assessing patients with akathisia is distinguishing this side effect from psychomotor agitation associated with the psychosis. Mistaking akathisia for psychotic agitation and raising the dose of antipsychotic medication usually leads to a worsening of the akathisia and thus the agitation. When the etiology of agitation is unclear, the nonspecific effects of benzodiazepines on akathisia and agitation can be useful, although the dose necessary for therapeutic effects on psychotic agitation usually is higher than that required for akathisia (978).

Given the high rate of acute extrapyramidal side effects among patients receiving first-generation antipsychotic medications, and to a lesser extent risperidone, the prophylactic use of antiparkinsonian medications may be considered. The benefit of this approach has been demonstrated in several studies. For example, Hanlon et al. (979) found that only 10% of patients taking perphenazine with an antiparkinsonian medication developed an extrapyramidal side effect, in contrast to 27% of patients taking perphenazine without an antiparkinsonian medication. The risk is that some patients may be treated unnecessarily with these medications, risking anticholinergic side effects (978). However, schizophrenia is a long-term illness, and the development of a therapeutic alliance is of paramount importance. The minimization of uncomfortable, painful, and unnecessary side effects can contribute significantly to establishing such an alliance. Thus, prophylactic antiparkinsonian medication may be considered for all patients with a prior history of susceptibility to extrapyramidal side effects and for patients for whom antipsychotic agents known to induce these effects (e.g., first-generation agents, high doses of risperidone) are prescribed.

The various medications used to treat acute extrapyramidal side effects are listed in Table 5. The major differences among the anticholinergic medications are in their potencies and durations of action. Patients who are very sensitive to anticholinergic side effects (e.g., dry mouth, blurred vision, constipation) may require lower doses or less potent preparations (e.g., trihexyphenidyl, procyclidine hydrochloride). The need for anticholinergic medications should be reevaluated after the acute phase of treatment is over and whenever the dose of antipsychotic medication is changed. If the dose of antipsychotic medication is lowered, anticholinergic medication may no longer be necessary or may be given at a lower dose.

Tardive dyskinesia is a hyperkinetic abnormal involuntary movement disorder caused by sustained exposure to antipsychotic medication; tardive dyskinesia can affect neuromuscular function in any body region but is most commonly seen in the oral-facial region (980, 981). (For a description of tardive dyskinesia and its differential diagnosis, see DSM-IV-TR.) Evaluation of the risk of tardive dyskinesia is complicated by the fact that spontaneous dyskinesias are clinically indistinguishable from tardive dyskinesia and have been described in up to 20% of never-medicated patients with chronic schizophrenia, as well as in elderly patients (982, 983). Thus dyskinetic movements are part of the natural history of schizophrenia. Tardive dyskinesia occurs at a rate of approximately 4%–8% per year in adult patients treated with first-generation antipsychotics (980, 984). Various factors are associated with greater vulnerability to tardive dyskinesia, including older age, antipsychotic-induced parkinsonian symptoms, female gender combined with postmenopausal status, diagnosis of affective disorder (particularly major depressive disorder), concurrent general medical disease such as diabetes, and use of high doses of antipsychotic medications (982, 985–987). Studies comparing intermittent, targeted first-generation antipsychotic drug treatment with maintenance antipsychotic treatment have found increased risk of tardive dyskinesia with targeted treatment strategies (988).

Tardive dyskinesia has been reported after exposure to any of the available antipsychotic medications, although the risk appears to be substantially less (approximately 10-fold) with the second-generation antipsychotics, compared to first-generation antipsychotics (83, 319, 382, 989–992). One study summarizing available longitudinal clinical trial data with risperidone reports an annual risk of 0.3%, which is substantially less than the expected risk with first-generation antipsychotics of approximately 5% per year (989, 992, 993). In a 9-month study of older patients (mean age=66 years), substantially more patients treated with haloperidol (32%), compared with risperidone-treated patients (5%), developed tardive dyskinesia (535, 990). In these studies the mean dose of both antipsychotics was low, and the rates of tardive dyskinesia in the haloperidol-treated subjects were similar to those reported for older patients in other studies

(987). For olanzapine, analyses of longitudinal double-blind data from multiple studies find a 12-fold lower risk of tardive dyskinesia with olanzapine treatment, compared to haloperidol treatment (0.05% and 7.45%, respectively) (319, 992). There are few systematic data concerning quetiapine and risk of tardive dyskinesia. In a 52-week open-label study of quetiapine that included 184 patients age >65 years, there was no change in the severity of dyskinetic movements, as evaluated by rating scales (994). In addition, emerging results from studies of other second-generation antipsychotics suggest that low risk of tardive dyskinesia may be found with drugs such as quetiapine that have a low risk of extrapyramidal effects.

With clozapine, although long-term prospective incidence studies are lacking, controlled short- and long-term trials generally find that the severity of dyskinetic movements improves with clozapine treatment, compared to treatment with first-generation antipsychotics (769, 995).

Although the majority of patients who develop tardive dyskinesia have mild symptoms, a proportion (approximately 10%) develop symptoms of moderate or severe degrees. An often severe variant of tardive dyskinesia is tardive dystonia, which is characterized by spastic muscle contractions in contrast to choreoathetoid movements (996). Tardive dystonia is often associated with great distress and physical discomfort. Patients receiving antipsychotic medication treatment on a sustained basis (for more than 4 weeks) should be evaluated at a minimum of every 3 months for signs of dyskinetic movements. The occurrence of dyskinetic movements warrants a neurological evaluation (980).

Treatment options for tardive dyskinesia occurring in the context of treatment with first-generation antipsychotic agents include switching to a second-generation antipsychotic or reducing the dose of the first-generation antipsychotic. An initial increase in dyskinetic symptoms may occur after conversion to a second-generation drug or antipsychotic dose reduction (withdrawal-emergent dyskinesia). With sustained first-generation antipsychotic exposure without dose reduction after the development of tardive dyskinesia, the likelihood of reversibility diminishes but is not lost. In some patients dyskinetic movements can persist despite long periods of time without medication. Despite the fact that continued treatment with antipsychotic medication increases the chances for the persistence of tardive dyskinesia symptoms, in many patients the severity of tardive dyskinesia does not increase over time at steady, moderate doses. The documentation in the clinical record should reflect that, despite mild tardive dyskinesia, a risk-benefit analysis favored continued maintenance of antipsychotic treatment to prevent the likelihood of relapse.

A large number of agents have been evaluated as possible treatment for tardive dyskinesia with few positive results. Although not consistent, there is some evidence that vitamin E may reduce the risk of development of tardive dyskinesia (225, 226). Given the low risk of side effects associated with vitamin E, patients may be advised to take 400–800 I.U. daily as prophylaxis. Small clinical trials have investigated the potential benefits of benzodiazepines, anticholinergic agents, calcium channel blockers (997), γ-aminobutyric acid agonists (998), essential fatty acids, estrogen, and insulin, with no studies yet producing convincing data to suggest any of these agents may be effective treatments for tardive dyskinesia (225, 999–1002).

(3) Neuroleptic malignant syndrome

Neuroleptic malignant syndrome is characterized by the triad of rigidity, hyperthermia, and autonomic instability, including hypertension and tachycardia (962). In addition, neuroleptic malignant syndrome is often associated with an elevated level of serum creatine kinase. In patients treated with second-generation antipsychotic medications, this classic triad of symptoms is generally although not invariably present (1003, 1004). The prevalence of neuroleptic malignant syndrome is uncertain, but this effect probably occurs in less than 1% of patients treated with first-generation antipsychotic medications (1005–1007) and is even more rare among patients treated with second-generation antipsychotic medications (1003, 1004, 1008–1012).

Neuroleptic malignant syndrome is frequently misdiagnosed and can be fatal in 5%–20% of patients if untreated (1013). It can be sudden and unpredictable in its onset and usually occurs early in the course of treatment, often within the first week after treatment is begun or the dose is increased. Risk factors for neuroleptic malignant syndrome include acute agitation, young age, male gender, preexisting neurological disability, physical illness, dehydration, rapid escalation of antipsychotic dose, use of high-potency medications, and use of intramuscular preparations (1014, 1015). Other diagnostic considerations in patients presenting with rigidity, hyperthermia, autonomic instability, or elevated levels of serum creatine kinase include neuroleptic-induced heat stroke, lethal catatonia, serotonin syndrome (in patients also taking serotonergic drugs such as SSRIs), anticholinergic syndrome, "benign" elevations in the level of serum creatine kinase, and fever in association with clozapine treatment (855, 1015–1018).

Since neuroleptic malignant syndrome is rare, most evidence regarding treatment comes from single case reports or case series. Antipsychotic medications should always be discontinued, and supportive treatment to maintain hydration and to treat the fever and cardiovascular, renal, or other symptoms should be provided. Some case series suggest that, compared with supportive treatment alone, treatment with dopamine agonists such as bromocriptine and amantadine or with dantrolene, which directly reduces skeletal muscle rigidity, may improve the symptoms of neuroleptic malignant syndrome (1019). Based on the overlap in symptoms between catatonia and neuroleptic malignant syndrome (1020), treatment with benzodiazepines, such as lorazepam, may also be helpful (1021, 1022). In patients with severe and treatment-resistant neuroleptic malignant syndrome, ECT is reported to improve symptoms (107, 1016, 1023). After several weeks of recovery, patients may be retreated with antipsychotic medication cautiously (1024). Generally, when treatment is resumed, doses are increased gradually, and a medication other than the precipitating agent is used (usually a second-generation antipsychotic or a first-generation antipsychotic medication of lower potency).

(4) **Sedation**

Sedation is a very common side effect of first-generation antipsychotic medications, as well as several of the second-generation agents, including clozapine, risperidone, olanzapine, and quetiapine. This effect may be related to antagonist effects of those drugs on histamine, adrenergic, and dopamine receptors (777, 1025, 1026). Most patients experience some sedation, particularly with the low-potency first-generation agents such as chlorpromazine, but it occurs to some extent with virtually all antipsychotic medications. With clozapine, sedation is very common, and in many patients it may be persistent and severe. Quetiapine has a high risk of sedation that may be maximal at the low end of the dose range (e.g., maximal by 100–200 mg/day). Olanzapine has a moderate dose-related risk of sedation. Risperidone produces dose-related sedation (890); within the usual dose range (<6 mg/day) the risk of sedation is relatively low, compared to the risk with other first-generation and second-generation (e.g., olanzapine, clozapine, quetiapine) antipsychotics.

Sedation is most pronounced in the initial phases of treatment, since most patients develop some tolerance to the sedating effects with continued administration. For agitated patients, the sedating effects of these medications in the initial phase of treatment can have therapeutic benefits. However, persistent sedation, including daytime drowsiness and increased sleep time, can interfere with social, recreational, and vocational function. Lowering of the daily dose, consolidation of divided doses into one evening dose, or changing to a less sedating antipsychotic medication may be effective in reducing the severity of sedation.

There are no systematic data on specific pharmacological interventions for sedation, but caffeine is a relatively safe option (1027). Some forms of psychostimulants (e.g., modafinil) have also been used to treat daytime drowsiness (1028). However, there have been case reports of clozapine toxicity associated with modafinil and other stimulant treatments of sedation, and thus this drug combination should be carefully considered and used with caution (1029, 1030).

(5) Cardiovascular effects

Cardiovascular effects include orthostatic hypotension, tachycardia, and QTc prolongation.

Orthostatic hypotension and tachycardia

Hypotension is related to the antiadrenergic effects of antipsychotic medications. With clozapine treatment initiation and dose escalation, there is a high risk of orthostatic hypotension and compensatory tachycardia, with rare (one of 3,000 patients treated) reports of cardiovascular collapse (854). These side effects typically limit the rate of titration, and orthostatic vital signs should be regularly monitored with dose escalation. When orthostatic hypotension is severe, it can cause dizziness and syncopal episodes. Patients who experience severe postural hypotension must be cautioned against getting up quickly and without assistance. Elderly patients are particularly prone to this adverse effect, and syncopal episodes may contribute to an increased risk of falls and related hip fractures in elderly patients. Risperidone has high affinity and quetiapine has moderate affinity for α-adrenergic receptors and thus can produce orthostatic hypotension and reflex tachycardia. Clozapine has the highest affinity and greatest propensity to cause hypotension. Gradual dose titration starting with a low dose minimizes risk. Management strategies for orthostatic hypotension include decreasing or dividing doses of antipsychotic or switching to an antipsychotic without antiadrenergic effects. Supportive measures include the use of support stockings, increased dietary salt, and, as a last resort, administration of the salt/fluid-retaining corticosteroid fludrocortisone to increase intravascular volume.

Tachycardia can result from the anticholinergic effects of antipsychotic medications but may also occur as a result of postural hypotension. While healthy patients may be able to tolerate some increase in resting pulse rate, this may not be the case for patients with preexisting heart disease. Tachycardia unrelated to orthostatic blood pressure changes that result from anticholinergic effects may occur in up to 25% of patients treated with clozapine. Because of the cardiovascular side effects of clozapine, extreme care should be taken in initiating a clozapine trial in patients with heart disease. Tachycardia due to anticholinergic effects without hypotension can be managed with low doses of a peripherally acting beta-blocker (e.g., atenolol) (1031, 1032).

QTc prolongation

The length of time required for the heart ventricles to repolarize is measured by the QT interval on the electrocardiogram. The QT interval varies with heart rate; thus, a QT interval corrected for heart rate (the "QTc") is routinely used clinically. Prolongation of the QTc interval above 500 msec is associated with increased risk for a ventricular tachyarrhythmia, "torsades de pointes." Torsades de pointes is associated with syncopal episodes and may lead to life-threatening consequences (e.g., ventricular fibrillation, sudden death).

Among the first-generation antipsychotic agents, thioridazine, mesoridazine, pimozide, and high-dose intravenous haloperidol have been associated with risk of QTc prolongation (1033). Because of the clinically significant risk of torsades de pointes–type arrhythmias and the potential for related sudden death (1033), the FDA recommends that thioridazine should be used only when patients have not had a clinically acceptable response to other available antipsychotics (885). This safety warning is available online at http://www.fda.gov/medwatch/safety/2000/mellar.htm and at www.medsafe.govt.nz/Profs/PUarticles/thioridazine.htm.

Ziprasidone is associated with an average increase of 20 msec in the QTc interval; however, the clinical effects of this magnitude of QT prolongation are uncertain (1034). Unlike drugs that prolong the QTc interval to a greater extent (e.g., thioridazine) (1035), ziprasidone has not been reported to be associated with arrhythmias or sudden death (1034). Patients treated with ziprasidone should be monitored for other risk factors for torsades de pointes, including congenital prolonged QT syndrome, bradycardia, hypokalemia, hypomagnesemia, heart failure, and factors that might increase levels of a drug associated with QTc prolongation (e.g., hepatic or renal failure, overdose of ziprasidone or other drugs known to prolong the QTc interval). Concomitant treatment with other drugs known to significantly prolong the QTc interval at normal clinical doses should be avoided. A list of such drugs is available at http://www.torsades.org. Given the normal variability of the QT interval (about 100 msec), an ECG is of questionable value in screening for congenital prolonged QT syndrome or in evaluating the effects of ziprasidone on the QTc interval in individual patients. Glassman and Bigger (1036) have reviewed the literature on prolonged QTc interval, torsades de pointes, and sudden death with antipsychotic drugs, including ziprasidone.

Anticholinergic and antiadrenergic effects

The anticholinergic effects of first-generation antipsychotic medications (along with the anticholinergic effects of antiparkinsonian medications, if concurrently administered) can produce a variety of peripheral side effects, including dry mouth, blurred vision, constipation, tachycardia, urinary retention, and thermoregulatory effects. Anticholinergic side effects may occur in 10%–50% of treated patients (980, 1037). These effects are also common with the second-generation agent clozapine. Although most anticholinergic side effects are mild and tolerable, these side effects can be particularly troublesome for older patients (e.g., older men with benign prostatic hypertrophy) (1037). In rare instances, serious consequences of anticholinergic effects can occur. For example, death can result from ileus of the bowel if it is undetected. In addition, some patients can develop hyperthermia, particularly in warm weather.

Central anticholinergic effects include impaired learning and memory and slowed cognition. Symptoms of anticholinergic toxicity include confusion, delirium, somnolence, and hallucinations (1038, 1039). Such symptoms are more likely to occur with medications that have more potent anticholinergic effects (e.g., chlorpromazine, thioridazine) or from administration of anticholinergic antiparkinsonian medications and in elderly or medically debilitated patients. Clozapine is frequently associated with anticholinergic side effects, including constipation and urinary retention (1040, 1041). Rarely, these effects have been severe, resulting in fecal obstruction and paralytic ileus and enduring impairment of bladder function (1042). Because of these anticholinergic effects, patients with preexisting prostate hypertrophy require careful monitoring of urinary function, and clozapine is contraindicated in patients with narrow-angle glaucoma (1031, 1032). Olanzapine has moderate affinity for muscarinic receptors and acts as an antagonist at the M_1, M_2, M_3, and M_5 receptors; however, anticholinergic effects are infrequent. The rarity of these effects is believed to be due to a difference between the drug's in vitro binding affinities and its actions in vivo. Constipation is occasionally associated with olanzapine treatment, but generally there is a low risk of anticholinergic side effects with olanzapine. Quetiapine has moderate affinity for muscarinic receptors. Constipation and dry mouth are occasionally associated with quetiapine treatment, and elderly and medically debilitated patients may be more sensitive to its anticholinergic side effects.

Anticholinergic side effects are often dose-related and thus may improve with lowering of the dose or administration of the anticholinergic antiparkinsonian drug in divided doses. In cases of anticholinergic delirium, parenteral physostigmine (0.5–2.0 mg i.m. or i.v.) has been used to reverse the symptoms, although this treatment should be provided only under close medical monitoring.

(6) Weight gain and metabolic abnormalities

Weight gain occurs with most antipsychotic agents. Up to 40% of patients treated with first-generation agents gain weight, with the greatest risk associated with the low-potency antipsychotics (797). The most notable exception is molindone, which may not cause significant weight gain (1043). The risk of weight gain with clozapine is thought to be the highest of all antipsychotics (1043), with studies reporting that between 10% and 50% of clozapine-treated patients are obese (1044, 1045). Typically, weight gain is progressive over the first 6 months of treatment, although some patients continue to gain weight indefinitely. In a meta-analysis of available studies, the mean weight gain after 10 weeks of treatment with clozapine was estimated at 4.45 kg (1043). Weight gain also is common in patients treated with risperidone and olanzapine. With risperidone, mean weight gain is estimated at 2.1 kg over the first 10 weeks of treatment (1043) and 2.3 kg after 1 year (382). With olanzapine, mean weight gain is estimated at 4.2 kg after 10 weeks of treatment (1043), and one study observed a mean weight gain of 12.2 kg after 1 year of treatment with olanzapine (918). No appreciable weight gain was observed with ziprasidone after 10 weeks (1043) or 1 year (947). Few studies have characterized the extent of weight gain with quetiapine or aripiprazole.

While studies have not systematically examined the health consequences of antipsychotic-related weight gain, the risk of cardiovascular disease, hypertension, cancers, diabetes, osteoarthritis, and sleep apnea is likely similar to that in idiopathic obesity. The association of high cholesterol and triglycerides with weight gain further increases the risk of cardiovascular disease (1046–1052). Adolescents may be particularly vulnerable to these side effects (1053).

Prevention of weight gain should be a high priority, since weight loss is difficult for many patients. Efforts should be made to intervene proactively, since obese persons rarely lose more than 10% of body weight with weight loss regimens. When weight gain occurs, clinicians should suggest or refer patients to diet and exercise interventions (1054). If the patient has not had substantial clinical benefits of the antipsychotic medication that outweigh the health risks of weight gain, a trial of an antipsychotic with lower weight-gain liability should be considered. Few systematic studies have been done to evaluate the effectiveness of specific interventions to prevent antipsychotic-induced weight gain or to promote weight loss, although potential strategies include diet and exercise programs (1055, 1056). No pharmacological interventions have proven efficacy in treating weight gain associated with second-generation antipsychotics, although uncontrolled studies have reported possible benefit from amantadine (1057, 1058), topiramate (1059–1063), the H_2 histamine antagonist nizatidine (1064, 1065), and noradrenergic reuptake inhibitor antidepressants (1066).

Uncontrolled studies and case series suggest that clozapine and olanzapine are associated with increased risk of hyperglycemia and diabetes (1050–1052, 1067–1073). While controlled studies are lacking, one prospective study found that 30 of 82 (36%) clozapine-treated outpatients developed diabetes during the 5-year follow-up period (1050). Complicating the evaluation of antipsychotic-related risk of diabetes is that schizophrenia is associated also with increased diabetes risk (1074). In some patients obesity may contribute to diabetes risk. Other mechanisms may also be involved. For example, insulin resistance may develop early in treatment with olanzapine and contribute to abnormal regulation of glucose and subsequent diabetes (1075, 1076).

Further, some of the second-generation antipsychotic agents, olanzapine and clozapine in particular, have been associated with diabetic ketoacidosis and nonketotic hyperosmolar coma, relatively rare complications of diabetes that are extremely dangerous if untreated (1077–1081). Numerous case reports have described scenarios in which diabetic ketoacidosis appears acutely in the absence of a known diagnosis of diabetes (1082). Diabetic ketoacidosis can present with mental status changes that can be attributed to schizophrenia. The treating psychiatrist must be aware of the possibility of diabetic ketoacidosis, given its potential lethality and its often confusing presentation. The overall prevalence and mechanism of diabetic ketoacidosis associated with antipsychotics and the differential risk of specific antipsychotic agents to cause this side effect are at present unknown.

Given the rare occurrence of extreme hyperglycemia, ketoacidosis, hyperosmolar coma, or death and the suggestion from epidemiological studies of an increased risk of treatment-emergent adverse events with second-generation antipsychotics, the FDA has requested all manufacturers of second-generation antipsychotic medications to include a warning in their product labeling regarding hyperglycemia and diabetes mellitus.

There is also suggestive evidence that certain antipsychotic medications, particularly clozapine and olanzapine, may increase the risk for hyperlipidemias. Most of the evidence is derived from case reports and other uncontrolled studies (1048–1050, 1067, 1070, 1083–1087). Pharmacological treatment with lipid-lowering drugs should be considered in patients with hyperlipidemia.

Table 1 lists suggested strategies for monitoring and clinical management associated with weight gain, glucose abnormalities, and hyperlipidemias in patients with schizophrenia.

(7) **Effects on sexual function**

Disturbances in sexual function can occur with a number of antipsychotic agents, including first- and second-generation agents (1088). Several mechanisms contribute to the genesis of sexual side effects with these medications. Prolactin elevation is very common in patients treated with first-generation antipsychotics as well as risperidone (1089). Female patients appear to be more sensitive to prolactin elevation than male patients (1090). All first-generation antipsychotic medications increase prolactin secretion by blocking the inhibitory actions of dopamine on lactotrophic cells in the anterior pituitary. This prolactin elevation may be even greater with risperidone than with first-generation antipsychotics. The reason for the propensity of risperidone to elevate prolactin may be due to risperidone's relative difficulty in crossing the blood-brain barrier, with the pituitary, which is outside the blood-brain barrier, exposed to higher peripheral levels of risperidone (1091).

Effects of hyperprolactinemia may include breast tenderness, breast enlargement, and lactation. Since prolactin also regulates gonadal function, hyperprolactinemia can lead to decreased production of gonadal hormones, including estrogen and testosterone. In women decreased gonadal hormone production may disrupt or even eliminate menstrual cycles. In both men and women prolactin-related disruption of the hypothalamic-pituitary-gonadal axis can lead to decreased sexual interest and impaired sexual function (1088).

The long-term clinical consequences of chronic elevation of prolactin are poorly understood. There is some epidemiological evidence, however, that postmenopausal women may have an increased risk of breast cancer if exposed to medications that potentially elevate levels of prolactin (1092). Chronic hypogonadal states may increase risk of osteopenia and osteoporosis (1093–1097), but increased risk of these disorders has not been directly linked to antipsychotic-induced hyperprolactinemia.

If a patient is experiencing clinical symptoms of prolactin elevation, the dose of antipsychotic may be reduced or the medication regimen may be switched to an antipsychotic with less effect on prolactin (e.g., any of the second-generation antipsychotics with the exception of risperidone). When the antipsychotic must be maintained, dopamine agonists such as bromocriptine (2–10 mg/day) or amantadine may reduce prolactin levels and thus the symptoms of hyperprolactinemia (1058).

The association between the other second-generation antipsychotic medications (clozapine, olanzapine, quetiapine, ziprasidone, and aripiprazole) and sexual dysfunction is less clear. Sexual interest and function may be reduced in both men and women receiving clozapine, but generally to a lesser extent than with first-generation antipsychotics (1098, 1099). Sexual dysfunction may also occur in patients treated with olanzapine and quetiapine (1100, 1101), but there is no prospective study that might indicate whether a causal relationship exists.

Erectile dysfunction occurs in 23%–54% of men treated with first-generation medications (812). Other effects can include ejaculatory disturbances in men and loss of libido or anorgasmia in women and men. In addition, with specific antipsychotic medications, including thioridazine and risperidone, retrograde ejaculation has been reported, most likely because of antiadrenergic and antiserotonergic effects (886). Dose reduction or discontinuation usually results in improvement or elimination of symptoms. A 25–50-mg dose of imipramine at bedtime may be helpful for treating retrograde ejaculation induced by thioridazine (1102). If dose reduction or a switch to an alternative medication is not feasible, yohimbine (an α_2-antagonist) or cyproheptadine (a 5-HT_2 antagonist) can be used (797). Because retrograde ejaculation is annoying rather than dangerous, psychoeducation may also help the patient tolerate this side effect. Priapism is very rarely associated with clozapine (1103, 1104), risperidone (1104), olanzapine (1105, 1106), quetiapine (1107), and ziprasidone (1108, 1109). There have been no reports to date of priapism associated with aripiprazole.

2. Adjunctive medications

A wide variety of medications, including additional antipsychotics, have been added to antipsychotic medications, either to enhance their efficacy for the treatment of symptoms of schizophrenia or to treat other symptoms often associated with the illness. Targets of these added medications have included residual positive symptoms, negative symptoms, cognitive deficits, depression, agitation and aggression, obsessions and compulsions, and anxiety. Some medications (e.g., antidepressants) have been used for more than one symptom cluster (e.g., depression, obsessions and compulsions).

a) Anticonvulsants

A number of studies of the efficacy of carbamazepine and valproate in schizophrenia have been done. Excluding findings suggesting their use in treating patients whose illness has strong affective components, the evidence is quite convincing that neither agent, used alone, is of significant value in the long-term treatment of schizophrenia. Recent studies have tended to concentrate on use of anticonvulsants in combination with antipsychotics.

With carbamazepine, studies examining the effects of the drug in combination with first-generation antipsychotics have had negative findings (236, 1110). For valproate, on the other hand, both negative and positive results have been noted (102, 235–237, 1111). Most studies have included relatively few patients, but the study by Casey et al. (237) included 242 subjects with acutely exacerbated symptoms who were randomly assigned to receive risperidone or olanzapine, each combined with placebo or divalproex. Compared with the placebo group, the divalproex group improved significantly more rapidly over the first 2 weeks of treatment. Both groups were equally improved by the end of the study at 4 weeks. This intriguing result warrants further study and replication to establish whether divalproex augmentation shortens the time to discharge and to determine the value of longer-term divalproex augmentation.

(1) Side effects

There are generally no additional side effects from the combination of anticonvulsant and antipsychotic medications beyond those of the individual medications themselves. Carbamazepine is not recommended for use with clozapine, because of the potential of both medications to cause agranulocytosis.

(2) Implementation

For patients with schizophrenia, these medications are generally used in the same therapeutic dose ranges and blood levels that are used for the treatment of seizure disorders and bipolar disorder. Studies to determine dosing in schizophrenia have not been reported. A complicating factor is the fact that carbamazepine can decrease the blood levels of antipsychotic medications by induction of hepatic enzymes (1112–1114).

b) Antidepressants

Studies of antidepressants in schizophrenia broadly subdivide into those that have examined these agents as treatment for depression and those that have tested their efficacy for other symptoms, such as negative symptoms. These areas will be reviewed separately.

Good clinical practice dictates that clinicians be alert to the occurrence of depression in a broad spectrum of psychiatric and medical disorders and treat it when it is diagnosed. Earlier work (1115) indicated the effectiveness of a tricyclic antidepressant for symptoms of depression in schizophrenia, and 12-month follow-up showed the advantage of maintenance treatment (1116). One study found the effects of an SSRI (sertraline) to be equal to those of imipramine for treatment of postpsychotic depression (1117) and another noted positive effects of citalopram (540), but the only placebo-controlled study of an SSRI for treatment of depressed patients with schizophrenia showed a large placebo effect and no difference between groups (1118). Although the evidence is most strong for patients who meet the syndromal criteria for depression, two reviews have noted the paucity of evidence for the efficacy of antidepressants in schizophrenia (222, 1119). For clinicians, a further question, not addressed in the literature, is whether failure of an antidepressant to improve depression in a person with schizophrenia is an indication for changing antidepressants or changing antipsychotics.

A number of studies have tested the efficacy of antidepressants in treating the negative symptoms of schizophrenia. The overlap between depressive and negative symptoms has complicated study design and interpretation. In five placebo-controlled studies of SSRIs for negative symptoms, one reported a modest advantage of fluoxetine added to long-acting injectable antipsychotic medication (1120), while four found no advantage for SSRIs, compared with placebo, in patients receiving clozapine (1121) or first-generation antipsychotics (1122–1124). Several studies of adjunctive fluvoxamine have demonstrated positive results (1125–1127). An open-label study of selegiline found beneficial effects on negative symptoms (1128), but in a placebo-controlled trial both the selegiline and placebo groups improved, and there was no difference between them (1129). Overall, the evidence for efficacy of antidepressants for negative symptoms of schizophrenia is very modest. Since most of the studies have been done in combination with first-generation antipsychotics, it is possible that the findings might be different with second-generation antipsychotics, although this possibility seems unlikely.

In terms of treating other symptoms that are sometimes observed in patients with schizophrenia, two small studies found efficacy of clomipramine and fluvoxamine in treating obsessive-compulsive symptoms in schizophrenia (221, 223). In a small crossover study in which citalopram or placebo was added to first-generation antipsychotics, patients with a history of aggression had significantly fewer incidents while taking citalopram (1130).

(1) Side effects

Although the side effects of antidepressants are no different when administered to patients with schizophrenia than to patients with other disorders, combinations of antipsychotics and antidepressants have the potential for adverse, even dangerous, pharmacokinetic and pharmacodynamic interactions. In addition to prior history of response to antidepressant treatment, potential drug-drug interactions should be taken into account in selecting an antidepressant agent. Of particular concern with regard to drug toxicity are the inhibitory effects of some antidepressants on clozapine metabolism, leading to increased serum levels and risk of seizures. Fluvoxamine can cause large increases in clozapine serum levels, and the combination of the two drugs should be avoided. Some other SSRIs and nefazodone may also cause clinically significant increases in clozapine serum levels and should be used carefully in clozapine-treated patients. Clozapine serum levels should be monitored after adding one of the antidepressants discussed earlier to the medication regimen of patients treated with clozapine. Because bupropion itself is associated with a risk of seizures, a pharmacodynamic interaction with clozapine exists. Therefore, the combination of clozapine and bupropion should be avoided. There are many sources of information about drug-drug interactions. A useful, frequently updated web site maintained by D. Flockhart at Indiana University is available at http://medicine.iupui.edu/flockhart. Another useful drug interaction computer program maintained by J. Oesterheld and D. Osser is available at http://www.mhc.com/Cytochromes.

(2) Implementation

Use of antidepressants in schizophrenia generally has been studied by using the doses and titration schedules that are usually used when the agents are administered by themselves. There is no reason to think that dosing should be modified on the basis of coexisting schizophrenia. As noted earlier, however, the potential for drug-drug interactions suggests that close monitoring of side effects is warranted. Monitoring of the blood levels of the antipsychotic at baseline and after several weeks of antidepressant treatment may be helpful, particularly for clozapine, where there is evidence that high blood levels are associated with increased risk of seizures and low levels may be ineffective. The same considerations apply when an antidepressant is being discontinued.

c) Antipsychotics

Most reports on the combination of antipsychotics describe the effects of combinations with clozapine. The only randomized, controlled trial used sulpiride, a dopamine receptor antagonist similar to first-generation antipsychotics that is available in Europe but not in North America. Shiloh et al. (1131) added placebo or sulpiride, titrated up to a dose of 600 mg/day, to clozapine for 10 weeks in the treatment of 28 partially responsive patients who were taking stable doses of clozapine and who had BPRS scores >42. The sulpiride group had significantly greater decreases in BPRS (15%), Scale for the Assessment of Negative Symptoms (10%), and Scale for the Assessment of Positive Symptoms (12%) scores.

Case series show improvements in residual positive symptoms with the addition of a number of other antipsychotics to clozapine. These agents include loxapine (233), pimozide (234), and risperidone (232).

Although the quality of the evidence for augmentation of clozapine with another antipsychotic is modest, this strategy seems reasonable in treating patients whose response to clozapine is fair at best. Before taking this step, however, the clinician should be sure that the clozapine treatment has been of sufficient duration and that the patient's blood level of clozapine indicates a sufficient dose. The other alternatives—switching to monotherapy with a different antipsychotic not already tried or combining two other antipsychotics—have even less evidence to support them than does augmentation of clozapine.

Combinations of two or more antipsychotics, neither of which is clozapine, are also used frequently for treatment of schizophrenia (1132). Some of this use reflects periods of cross-titration in the transition from one antipsychotic to another, but much of it represents long-term treatment. Evidence for (or against) this practice is minimal, as there are no controlled studies in the literature. The largest case series includes six persons with inadequate responses to 20–40 mg/day of olanzapine, who had average decreases in BPRS and PANSS scores of 35% after addition of 60–600 mg/day of sulpiride for at least 10 weeks (1133). Without a control group, such results are difficult to evaluate. Moreover, sulpiride is not available in the United States, and there is no way to know if similar results might be found with other antipsychotics.

The absence of evidence for combinations of antipsychotics does not mean that there are no patients who are best treated with such a combination. However, their use should be justified by strong documentation that the patient is not equally benefited by monotherapy with either component of the combination. Practitioners should be aware of the problems inherent in combination therapies, including increased side effects and drug interactions as well as increased costs and decreased adherence (1132).

d) Benzodiazepines

Benzodiazepines have been evaluated as monotherapy for schizophrenia and as adjuncts to antipsychotic medications. Wolkowitz and Pickar (224) reviewed double-blind studies of benzodiazepines as monotherapy and found that positive effects (reductions in anxiety, agitation, global impairment, or psychotic symptoms) were reported in nine of 14 studies. Six of 10 studies that specifically examined psychotic symptoms showed greater efficacy for benzodiazepines than placebo. In a study comparing diazepam, fluphenazine, and placebo as treatments for impending psychotic relapse in patients who were taking no antipsychotic medications, the effects of diazepam and fluphenazine were equal, and both were superior to placebo (1134).

Double-blind studies evaluating benzodiazepines as adjuncts to antipsychotic medications were also reviewed by Wolkowitz and Pickar (224). Seven of 16 studies showed some positive effect on anxiety, agitation, psychosis, or global impairment; five of 13 showed efficacy in treating psychotic symptoms specifically. The reviewers concluded that benzodiazepines may improve the response to antipsychotic medications.

Some studies indicate that the effectiveness of benzodiazepines as adjuncts to antipsychotic medications is limited to the acute phase and may not be sustained. Altamura et al. (1135) found that clonazepam plus haloperidol, but not haloperidol alone or placebo, produced significant lowering of total BPRS scores after 1 week. This reduction, which was primarily due to decreases in anxiety and tension, disappeared by the end of the 4-week study. Csernansky et al. (1136) also found that when alprazolam was added to antipsychotic medication, there was a significant reduction in the BPRS withdrawal/retardation subfactor score after the first week, but this reduction disappeared by study end at week 5.

Benzodiazepines are commonly used alone or in combination with an antipsychotic for acutely agitated patients in emergency department settings. One study compared the effects of lorazepam with those of haloperidol over the first 4 hours of treatment (1137). The compounds were equal in efficacy, and the authors suggested that lorazepam may be preferable, in that delayed extrapyramidal symptoms can occur with haloperidol. Another study compared lorazepam and haloperidol alone with the combination of both over 12 hours (75). Combination treatment was modestly more effective during the first 3 hours, and there were no significant differences between groups at later times. The haloperidol alone group needed more injections and had more extrapyramidal symptoms.

Benzodiazepines are effective for treatment of acute catatonic reactions, whether associated with schizophrenia or other disorders (137, 140, 142, 1138–1141). Although most studies have used lorazepam (1–2 mg i.v. or i.m. or 2–4 mg p.o., repeated as needed over 48–72 hours), beneficial effects have also been found with clonazepam and oxazepam. One report has questioned the value of benzodiazepines in treating chronic catatonia, although patients were maintained on antipsychotic treatment during the study, and the contribution of tardive dystonia to the observed behaviors was uncertain (1142).

(1) Side effects

Benzodiazepines have some limitations in schizophrenia. Their common side effects include sedation, ataxia, cognitive impairment, and a tendency to cause behavioral disinhibition in some patients. This last side effect can be a serious problem in patients who are being treated for agitation. Reactions to withdrawal from benzodiazepines can include psychosis and seizures. In addition, patients with schizophrenia are vulnerable to both abuse of and addiction to these agents.

(2) Implementation

Evidence relating to the choice of a specific benzodiazepine is limited, since few studies have compared the effectiveness of more than one. Important considerations in selection include abuse potential and severity of withdrawal symptoms if treatment is prolonged. In general, longer-acting agents have lower abuse potential. Withdrawal of alprazolam seems more likely to be associated with seizures, compared to withdrawal of other benzodiazepines.

e) Beta-blockers

Beta-blocking agents are often used for treatment of drug-induced akathisia, discussed in Section V.A.1.c, "Shared Side Effects of Antipsychotic Medications." There are also a few controlled studies of the combination of beta-blockers with antipsychotics to treat aggression.

Pindolol in a dose of 5 mg t.i.d. reduced aggression scores significantly more than placebo in a double-blind crossover study that included 30 male patients with schizophrenia in a maximum-security facility (100). In a psychiatric intensive care setting, 80–120 mg/day of nadolol had initial beneficial effects on psychosis scores and extrapyramidal symptoms, compared with placebo (101). The difference in extrapyramidal symptoms persisted over the 3 weeks of the study. In both of these studies, most patients were taking first-generation agents. Replication of the findings with aggressive patients taking second-generation agents would be helpful. As noted earlier, clozapine is indicated as a treatment for persistently aggressive, psychotic patients.

f) Cognition enhancers

Cognitive deficits are characteristic of schizophrenia, and several studies have examined the efficacy of adding acetylcholinesterase inhibitors developed for use in dementia to treat patients with schizophrenia. One case report found substantial cognitive benefits from donepezil, compared with placebo (247), and an uncontrolled study observed positive results with donepezil on a variety of cognitive measures (249). However, a randomized, placebo-controlled trial of donepezil in 34 patients with chronic schizophrenia reported no group differences (248). As such, there is currently insufficient evidence to support the usefulness of these agents in improving cognitive performance in schizophrenia.

g) Glutamatergic agents

Because phencyclidine, which blocks ion channels associated with NMDA-type glutamate receptors, can produce a clinical state with psychotic and negative symptoms resembling schizophrenia, agents with glutamatergic properties have been tested in schizophrenia (1143). The agents that have been tested are glycine, D-cycloserine, and D-serine. Of these, only D-cycloserine is available for medicinal human use in the United States, as an antituberculosis treatment.

Five randomized, controlled trials have examined the effects of glycine in doses ranging from 0.4 to 0.8 g/kg. Most have reported beneficial effects of glycine on negative symptoms, with decreases of 15%–40% in negative symptom measures (239, 240, 242, 1144). Little effect on positive symptoms has been found in most studies. In a group of 30 patients who were taking clozapine, glycine did not produce any significant symptom changes, compared with placebo (241), confirming the result of an earlier case series report (1145). Javitt et al. (242) did, however, report robust negative symptom improvements in four patients who received clozapine plus glycine.

Results with D-cycloserine are more variable. The usual dose is 50 mg/day. Modest, but significant, decreases in negative symptoms were found by some investigators (244–246) but not others (1146, 1147). In a study of D-cycloserine added to clozapine, there was no benefit of the combination (243), which may be related to its dose-response curve.

A report by Tsai et al. (238) on adjunctive D-serine noted significant decreases in positive and negative symptoms in patients stabilized with a first-generation antipsychotic or risperidone. The same group later reported no benefit from adding D-serine to clozapine (1148).

Overall, the evidence for glutamatergic agents is encouraging, except as additions to clozapine. Most studies have used first-generation antipsychotics, risperidone, or clozapine. It remains to be seen if combinations of glutamatergic agents with other second-generation antipsychotics are helpful. Although the data seem most positive for glycine, studies directly comparing these agents are needed to determine if their effects actually differ.

h) Lithium

Lithium as a sole treatment has limited effectiveness in schizophrenia and is inferior to treatment with antipsychotic medications (1149–1152).

Earlier reports indicated that when added to antipsychotic medications, lithium augmented the antipsychotic response, in general, and improved negative symptoms specifically (1153,

1154). Other evidence indicated benefits of lithium for patients with schizophrenia with affective symptoms and for patients with schizoaffective disorder (1155–1159).

More recent literature, however, has not reported robust effects (1160). Relatively low doses of lithium over an 8-week period improved anxiety symptoms more than did placebo, but effects in other areas of psychopathology were not found (1161). Patients who had not responded to 6 months of treatment with fluphenazine decanoate showed no more improvement than the placebo group after 8 weeks of lithium augmentation at therapeutic levels (1162). There have been no reported controlled trials of lithium combined with second-generation antipsychotics. Since at least some of these agents have evidence for effects on depression, anxiety, and mood stabilization, the potential value of combining lithium with them may be limited.

(1) Side effects

The side effects of lithium include tremor, gastrointestinal distress, sedation or lethargy, impaired coordination, weight gain, cognitive problems, nephrogenic diabetes insipidus with associated polyuria and polydipsia, renal insufficiency, hair loss, benign leukocytosis, acne, and edema. These have been reviewed in detail in APA's *Practice Guideline for the Treatment of Patients With Bipolar Disorder* (1163) (included in this volume). The combination of an antipsychotic medication and lithium may increase the possibility of the development of neuroleptic malignant syndrome. However, the evidence for this association comes mainly from some debated reports of cases or series of cases, rather than from quantitative data. Most reported cases of neuroleptic malignant syndrome in patients treated with lithium plus antipsychotic medication have occurred in cases of high lithium blood levels associated with dehydration.

(2) Implementation

Generally, lithium is added to the antipsychotic medication that the patient is already receiving, after the patient has had an adequate trial of the antipsychotic medication but has reached a plateau in the level of response and has persisting residual symptoms. The dose of lithium is that required to obtain a blood level in the range of 0.8–1.2 meq/liter. Response to treatment usually appears promptly; a trial of 3–4 weeks is adequate for determining whether there is a therapeutic response, although some investigators have noted that improvements may emerge only after 12 weeks or more (1160). Patients should be monitored for adverse effects that are commonly associated with lithium (e.g., polyuria, tremor) and with its interaction with an antipsychotic medication (e.g., extrapyramidal side effects, confusion, disorientation, other signs of neuroleptic malignant syndrome) (266), particularly during the initial period of combined treatment. Given the toxicity of lithium in overdose, prescription of conservative quantities should be considered for patients at increased risk for suicidal behaviors.

i) Monoaminergic agents

Some studies have examined the efficacy of adjunctive dopaminergic and noradrenergic agents in schizophrenia. High doses of oral tyrosine added to molindone produced no clinical effects different from placebo in a crossover study of 11 patients, even though there was physiological evidence that the tyrosine had CNS effects (1164). Clonidine added to 20 mg/day of haloperidol reduced psychotic symptoms more than placebo in a small study of 12 patients (1165). The lack of an effect of clonidine on chronic polydipsia in schizophrenia has recently been reported (459).

j) Polyunsaturated fatty acids

Based on hypotheses concerning membrane stability and second messenger dysfunction in schizophrenia, several investigators have tested the efficacy of polyunsaturated fatty acids in the illness. The bulk of the evidence comes from studies of eicosapentaenoic acid (EPA). One study also examined docosahexaenoic acid and found it had no effects (1166).

In separate studies, Peet et al. (1166) found that EPA added to a stable dose of antipsychotic improved total and positive symptoms more than placebo and that EPA alone was more effective as sole treatment for unmedicated schizophrenia patients than placebo alone. By contrast, Fenton et al. (1167) found no benefit of EPA, compared with placebo, in a study of more than 80 patients. Emsley et al. (1168), in a South African cohort, noted greater decreases in PANSS and dyskinesia scores with EPA added to stable antipsychotic dose. The two phenomena were correlated; those with dyskinesia improvements were most likely to also have symptom improvements. Patients taking clozapine did not benefit from EPA treatment.

The EPA data are intriguing but far from definitive. Most data come from studies of combination therapy with first-generation antipsychotics. The compound appears to be free of side effects other than initial mild gastrointestinal upset in some patients.

B. OTHER SOMATIC THERAPIES

1. ECT

a) Efficacy

The efficacy of acute treatment with ECT in patients with schizophrenia has been described in multiple case series and uncontrolled studies as well as a number of controlled trials; detailed reviews have been provided by Fink and Sackeim (106), an APA task force (107), and Tharyan and Adams (108). Although early research used small patient samples that were not well characterized and probably included some patients with mood disorder, antipsychotic treatment alone generally produced better short-term outcomes than ECT alone. There also appeared to be no advantage to ECT, compared to sham treatment. On the other hand, combined treatment with ECT and first-generation antipsychotic medications was more effective than either treatment by itself in most (109–118) but not all (1169, 1170) studies. In patients with treatment-resistant illness, case series also suggest that ECT may augment response to first-generation antipsychotics (119–125, 229). More recent reports suggest that increased therapeutic benefit may be seen with combined use of ECT and second-generation antipsychotic medications (127–135). Thus, ECT in combination with antipsychotic medications may be considered for patients with schizophrenia or schizoaffective disorder who have severe psychotic symptoms that have not responded to treatment with antipsychotic agents.

In terms of factors that may predict a greater likelihood of response to ECT, little rigorous evidence exists. While many psychiatrists believe that mood symptoms or a diagnosis of schizoaffective disorder suggest a better response to ECT, the evidence supporting this view is inconsistent (1171–1176). However, some reports suggest that greater benefits are observed in patients with positive symptoms (1177), shorter illness and episode durations (125, 1178–1180), or fewer paranoid or schizoid premorbid personality traits (1173).

Patients with catatonic features constitute another group who have been clinically felt to derive particular benefit from treatment with ECT. Evidence in the more recent literature is limited by the inclusion of patients with mood disorder diagnoses and consists primarily of case series (139, 141, 142) and open prospective trials (136–138, 140, 143, 1141). Nonetheless, findings from these studies confirm the clinical impression that ECT is beneficial in patients with schizophrenia who have prominent catatonic features that have not responded to a trial of lorazepam.

The efficacy of ECT as a continuation/maintenance therapy has been evaluated in only one randomized, single-blind clinical trial, which assessed patients with treatment-resistant schizophrenia (229). Patients who had responded to an acute course of treatment with concomitant bilateral ECT and the first-generation antipsychotic flupenthixol (N=45) were randomly assigned to receive continuation therapy with ECT alone, flupenthixol alone, or combination treatment. Relapse rates at 6 months in those receiving combined treatment were less than half those in the other treatment groups (40% versus 93%). These findings supplement clinical observations of the benefits of maintenance ECT for some patients (227, 228) and support the use of ECT for those responding to an acute course of ECT in whom pharmacological prophylaxis alone has been ineffective or cannot be tolerated.

b) Side effects

Effects of ECT on the cardiovascular system are seen in virtually all patients but are typically benign and self-limited. With administration of the ECT stimulus, parasympathetic activation produces an initial bradycardia, and, in some instances, a brief sinus pause may be noted. The subsequent sympathetic activation that occurs with induction of a generalized seizure produces a transient rise in heart rate and blood pressure and resulting increases in cardiac workload, intracranial pressure, and blood-brain barrier permeability (107, 1181). Typically, these effects normalize spontaneously; however, when they are prolonged or occur in patients with preexisting cardiac or vascular disease, medications may be needed to minimize these physiological responses (1182, 1183). Less commonly, ECT may be associated with more serious cardiac arrhythmias, ischemia, and infarction, although the type, severity, and likelihood of cardiac complications are generally related to the type and severity of preexisting cardiac disease (1184, 1185).

Cognitive side effects may also be observed with ECT, although there is much individual variation in the extent and severity of such effects (107). In addition, the cognitive effects of ECT in persons with schizophrenia are unclear, since most studies of cognition after ECT have involved patients treated for depression. For many patients, however, the ECT treatment and its associated anesthesia are associated with a transient postictal confusional state, at times accompanied by postictal agitation (1186). Patients may also experience some difficulties with rapid forgetting of newly learned information and in recalling information, particularly for events occurring near the time of the treatment (1187–1189). This retrograde memory impairment typically resolves in a few weeks to months after cessation of treatment (1190, 1191), but, rarely, patients report more pervasive or persistent cognitive disruption that involves more distant memories (1192). On the other hand, for many patients, improvements in concentration and attention with ECT are associated with improvement rather than worsening of objective memory function (1193, 1194).

Other side effects that are commonly noted after ECT include headache, generalized muscle aches, and nausea and/or vomiting. These effects usually resolve spontaneously or with analgesic or antiemetic medications.

c) Implementation

Before initiating a course of ECT, a pre-ECT evaluation is conducted to determine the potential benefits of ECT for the patient, the potential risks of ECT based on the patient's medical and psychiatric status, and the potential modifications that could be made in medications or in the ECT or anesthetic technique to minimize those risks (107). Although there are no absolute contraindications to ECT, recent myocardial infarction, some cardiac arrhythmias, and some intracranial-space-occupying lesions may increase risk and are indications for caution and consultation. Morbidity and mortality with ECT are also increased in the presence of severe preexisting pulmonary disease and with higher levels of anesthetic risk (i.e., status 4 or 5 in the American Society of Anesthesiologists physical status classification [http://www.asahq.org/clinical/physicalstatus.htm]).

During the informed consent process, these and other potential risks of ECT will be considered along with the potential benefits of ECT and the corresponding risks and benefits of other therapeutic approaches. The informed consent process will also include a discussion of the ECT procedure, including a description of the anesthesia used for the treatment, the electrode placement being used to administer the treatment, and the likely number of ECT sessions that will be required.

In terms of electrode placement, no recent studies have assessed the effects of differing electrode placements in patients with schizophrenia or schizoaffective disorder who receive ECT. The two studies that did compare bitemporal to unilateral nondominant hemisphere electrode placements in patients with schizophrenia used a sine wave stimulus, did not measure the extent to which stimulus intensities were suprathreshold, and had high rates of patient dropout, making their findings of limited utility to present ECT practice (1195, 1196). Although findings in patients with depression suggest that unilateral (1187–1189) and perhaps bifrontal (1197, 1198) electrode placement may be associated with fewer cognitive effects and that efficacy with unilateral electrode placement may depend on the extent to which the stimulus intensity exceeds the seizure threshold, the applicability of these observations to patients with schizophrenia is uncertain. A single randomized, double-blind study assessed three different stimulus intensities in 66 patients treated with bitemporal ECT and found that rates of remission and effects on cognition were comparable (1199). However, among patients who remitted, those receiving stimulus intensities just above the seizure threshold required more treatments and had a longer time to remission than patients treated with stimulus intensities that were two to four times the seizure threshold. Thus, in making decisions about stimulus intensity and electrode placement for ECT, psychiatrists may wish to consider factors such as past responses to treatment including ECT, existing cognitive impairment, the need for a more rapid response to treatment, and medical problems or concomitant medications that may increase the seizure threshold and/or may increase the risk associated with each ECT treatment. In addition, individualization of the stimulus intensity to the patient by using either stimulus titration or a formula-based dosing strategy is advisable.

The likely number of ECT treatments required should also be reviewed with the patient. Again evidence is limited, although clinical case series primarily from the older literature suggest that achieving full clinical benefit for patients with schizophrenia may require a longer course of acute treatment than for patients with mood disorders (229, 1179, 1200). In general, ECT is given two to three times per week, although some practitioners will taper the frequency of treatments near the end of the treatment course (1201). Additional details on ECT administration can be found in the 2001 APA ECT Task Force Report (107).

2. rTMS

Repetitive transcranial magnetic stimulation (rTMS) has recently been studied as another somatic technique for ameliorating psychotic symptoms. Whereas the electrical stimulation associated with ECT produces a generalized seizure and global central nervous system excitation, rTMS permits targeted stimulation of specific brain regions that may be involved in the genesis of psychosis (144, 145). These unique features suggest that rTMS may be able to produce therapeutic effects without some of the associated side effects and the need for anesthesia with ECT. Data from one small (N=24) randomized, double-blind, sham-controlled trial (146) and two small (N=8 and N=12) randomized, double-blind, crossover trials (147, 148) suggest that improvements in auditory hallucinations occur when rTMS of the left temporal-parietal cortex is used to augment antipsychotic treatment. However, data from another small (N=25) randomized, controlled trial (1202), which stimulated the right dorsolateral prefrontal cortex, showed no such effect of rTMS on psychotic symptoms. In these studies, the effect of rTMS on more global measures of psychopathology was also variable, although no significant changes were noted in mood, anxiety, or cognition. Although these findings of potential benefits of rTMS in schizophrenia and other psychotic disorders are interesting and worthy of future research, rTMS has not been approved for use in patients with schizophrenia, and there is insufficient evidence to recommend its use in clinical practice.

C. SPECIFIC PSYCHOSOCIAL INTERVENTIONS

As part of a comprehensive treatment approach, psychosocial interventions can improve the course of schizophrenia when integrated with psychopharmacological treatments (1203, 1204). These interventions can provide additional benefits for patients in such areas as relapse prevention, improved coping skills, better social and vocational functioning, and ability to function more independently. While pharmacotherapy focuses on symptom diminution, psychosocial interventions may provide emotional support and address particular deficits associated with schizophrenia. Psychosocial treatments are interpersonal and call on various roles of the clinician: a manager to coordinate the services available within a treatment system, a teacher to provide education about the patient's disorder and how to cope with it, a friendly other to provide support and encouragement, a trained therapist to provide strategies for interpersonal enrichment, and a physician to provide biological treatments. These roles and therapeutic opportunities come in many forms and settings, e.g., individual, group, family. The choice of psychosocial approaches and particular interventions depends on the particular needs of the patient at various phases of his or her life and illness.

The goals and tasks of these treatments vary widely, depending on the individual patient, disorder, and life situation. The central components of psychosocial treatment are described in the earlier section on psychiatric management (see Section II.D.2, "Psychosocial Treatments in the Stable Phase"). The overall goals are to minimize vulnerability and stress and to maximize adaptive capacities and functioning while enhancing social supports.

The evidence supporting psychosocial treatments is quite variable and generally does not correspond well with actual patterns of practice. In order to foster a more evidence-based approach to the selection and application of psychosocial interventions, this section is organized such that the interventions with the best evidence are discussed first for emphasis, followed by discussions of treatments that may be widely used but for which scientific evidence of effectiveness is minimal or lacking.

1. Psychosocial treatments with substantial evidence bases

a) Program for Assertive Community Treatment (PACT)

PACT includes both case management and active treatment interventions by one team using a highly integrated approach. This program is designed specifically for the marginally adjusted and poorly functioning person with schizophrenia to help prevent relapse and maximize social and vocational functioning. It uses an individually tailored treatment program in the community that is based on an assessment of each person's deficits in coping skills, assets, and requirements for community living (181, 1205). Treatment takes place through teams working 24 hours a day, 7 days a week, and most treatment is delivered in patients' homes, neighborhoods, and places of work. Staff members assist patients in daily living tasks, such as clothes laundering, shopping, cooking, grooming, budgeting, and using transportation. In addition, patients are given sustained and intensive assistance in finding a job, schooling, or a sheltered workshop placement; staff members maintain their contact with the patient after these placements to resolve crises and conflicts and to help prevent relapse. Staff members also guide patients in constructive use of leisure time and in social skills.

The key elements in PACT are emphasizing the patients' strengths in adapting to community life (rather than focusing on psychopathology); providing support and consultation to patients' natural support networks (e.g., family members, employers, friends and peers, and community agencies); and providing assertive outreach to ensure that patients remain in the treatment program. Medication adherence is emphasized, as well as ready access to a psychiatrist. Persons with schizophrenia who are marginally functioning and/or poorly adherent to treatment may benefit from such a comprehensive approach. Others who are more able to function in the community and who are adherent to treatment do not need such extensive services.

Controlled studies have shown the efficacy of PACT in improving symptom severity (1206), reducing the length of hospitalizations, and improving living conditions (163–166, 181, 1207–1211). There have been replications of these results in several U.S. locales and in other countries (1212, 1213).

Although it is not clear which particular elements in the PACT program are most essential for positive outcomes, evidence is strongest for programs that closely follow the original PACT model, including maintenance of a patient-staff ratio of approximately 10:1 (1214). Other public mental health systems have attempted to apply PACT principles, but unfortunately, many do not have adequate resources to carry out such a program. Nonetheless, creative reallocation of resources within a system can strengthen PACT programs (1215, 1216). An evidence-based practices project sponsored by SAMHSA is developing a resource kit on assertive community treatment (draft version available at http://www.mentalhealthpractices.org/pdf_files/act_c.pdf).

b) Family interventions

A guiding principle is that the patient's family members should be involved and engaged in a collaborative treatment process to the greatest extent possible. Family members generally contribute to the patient's care and require education, guidance, and support, as well as training to help them optimize their caretaking role and to improve their own well-being. Clinicians must understand that families often experience considerable stress and burdens in providing such caretaking. For these purposes, "family" should be defined broadly and extend beyond blood relatives to include other patient- and self-defined caretakers.

All evidence-based approaches emphasize the value of family participation in treatment and stress the importance of working together in a collaborative endeavor. The main goal of family interventions, referred to as "psychoeducation," is to decrease the risk of the patient's relapse. More recent research has emphasized other goals, such as improving patient functioning, decreasing family burden, and improving family functioning. All effective family interventions include education about the illness and its course, training in coping and problem-solving skills within the family, improved communication, and stress reduction. These interventions use practical educative and behavioral methods to elicit family participation and collaboration in treatment planning, goal setting, and service delivery. All effective family interventions include somatic treatments, such as medication, for the patient and are intended to optimize their use.

The research variants of family psychoeducation are highly structured programs that last 9 months to 2–3 years and embed the psychiatrist's care within a multidisciplinary team approach to the patient and family. While the variations in research studies on family interventions and their control conditions make it difficult to distill the results of the more than 20 controlled studies, family programs have typically halved relapse rates (173, 174, 176, 189, 1207, 1217–1231). Meta-analyses pooling data across studies have consistently shown reductions in relapse rates (157, 158, 1232) and also reduced family burden (1233). The control treatments have included individual supportive therapy, intensive case management, and medication alone.

More recent studies have compared different family interventions. The one consistent finding is that brief interventions lasting less than 9 months have little effect and are therefore inferior to programs lasting 9 months or longer (157). In a multisite study (Treatment Strategies for Schizophrenia, sponsored by the National Institute of Mental Health) that used a less intensive, once-monthly variant of family management as a control condition for a more intensive family management approach, significant differences in relapse rates between the conditions were not found (1234). Families may be seen individually (173, 174) or in multiple-family groups (1223, 1235). McFarlane (1235) found slightly better protection against relapse from the multiple-family groups in a controlled study. However, on the whole, the critical elements of family interventions have not been precisely defined.

The acute phase or times of crisis may be the best time to engage the family in psychoeducational family meetings. When the patient is most ill, family members tend to be most motivated to reach out and make contact, ask questions, and seek information to reassure and guide them.

The practicing psychiatrist should remain flexible when considering the type of family intervention to offer, with the patient's and the family's preferences playing a large role. Structured family psychoeducation approaches may be challenging to implement at mental health agencies, and considerable organizational barriers to their implementation have been identified (1236). If a highly structured clinical program is not possible, a collaborative and supportive approach to families remains beneficial. Also helpful are referrals to family support organizations and peer-based non-clinical programs, such as the National Alliance for the Mentally Ill's widely available Family-to-Family Education Program (1237, 1238). An evidence-based practices project sponsored by SAMHSA is developing a resource kit on family interventions (draft version available at http://www.mentalhealthpractices.org/pdf_files/fpe_pcs.pdf).

c) Supported employment

Supported employment is an approach to improve vocational functioning among persons with various types of disabilities, including schizophrenia (192). A crucial influence on the conceptualization of supported employment for persons with schizophrenia and other severe mental illnesses has been the work of Becker and Drake in the development of the Individual Placement and Support (IPS) model (1239). Among the key principles defining IPS are 1) services focused on competitive employment, 2) eligibility based on the consumer's choice, 3) rapid job search, 4) integration of rehabilitation and mental health, 5) attention to consumers' preferences, and 6) time-unlimited and individualized support (1240). An evidence-based practices project sponsored by SAMHSA is developing a resource kit on supported employment (draft version available at http://www.mentalhealthpractices.org/pdf_files/se_mhpl.pdf).

Several reviewers of the supported employment literature have reached similar conclusions (193, 194, 1241, 1242). The major sources of evidence for supported employment include day treatment conversion studies and randomized, controlled studies.

Four studies have examined the effectiveness of converting day treatment services to supported employment (1243–1247). During follow-up periods ranging from 3 to 18 months, 43% of the patients in the converted supported employment sites were working competitively, compared to only 17% of the patients in the comparison sites that did not convert.

Nine randomized, controlled trials have compared supported employment to a variety of traditional vocational services for people with severe mental illnesses (160, 162, 1248–1253). These nine studies were conducted by seven independent research teams in various geographic locations, representing both urban and rural communities. The studies compared newly or relatively newly established supported employment programs to established vocational services and used a variety of measures to assess employment outcomes, including the percentage of patients who achieve competitive employment, total wages earned, and number of weeks worked. In general, most objective indicators of employment outcomes converged toward similar conclusions. The average competitive employment rate was 56% for patients in supported employment, compared to 19% for those in comparison conditions, yielding a large mean effect size of 0.85.

A continuing challenge even for supported employment is promoting job retention; studies have found that persons with schizophrenia experience considerable difficulties retaining jobs achieved through supported employment (162, 194). This problem appears to be related to neurocognitive impairments (195), among other factors.

Further, there is no evidence that engagement in supported employment leads to stress, increased symptoms, or other negative outcome (159). Evidence is inconsistent about the relationship between clinical and demographic variables and successful vocational performance; therefore, it is recommended that any person with schizophrenia who expresses an interest in work should be offered supported employment.

d) Cognitive behavior therapy

Cognitive behavior therapy was originally crafted for the treatment of depression and anxiety disorders (1254, 1255), but it has been modified for the treatment of schizophrenia in the past decade, largely by clinical investigators in the United Kingdom. The assumptions of cognitive behavior therapy are that normal psychological processes can both maintain and weaken the fixity and severity of psychotic symptoms, especially delusions and hallucinations. Cognitive behavior therapy is usually conducted in a one-to-one therapeutic relationship. Supportive elements precede and always accompany the cognitive work. An empathic and nonthreatening relationship is built during which the patient elaborates his or her experiences with schizophrenia. Specific symptoms are identified as problematic by the patient and/or therapist and become targeted for special attention in cognitive behavior therapy. The therapist does not challenge these symptoms as irrational but helps the patient through guided questions to focus on his or her own beliefs about the symptoms and the natural coping mechanisms the patient has elaborated to deal with the symptoms. Some of cognitive behavior therapy involves endorsing and strengthening natural coping mechanisms; the rest involves supportively guiding the patient to a more rational cognitive perspective about his or her symptom(s). This work may include belief modification, focusing/reattribution, and normalizing the psychotic experience, among other strategies (170).

In belief modification, evidence for a delusional belief is gently challenged in reverse order to the strength to which the delusion is held. Focusing/reattribution especially targets chronic auditory hallucinations. The therapist encourages the patient to elaborate his or her experience with the hallucination in exhaustive detail, in the process highlighting how the symptom relates to the patient's daily life and ultimately helping the patient reattribute the hallucination to an internal source. In normalizing the patient's psychotic experience, the therapist helps the patient see that his or her symptoms are embedded within the stressful vicissitudes of daily life, thus making them appear more normal and less "crazy."

Several randomized, controlled trials examining the effects of cognitive behavior therapy in schizophrenia have been conducted (356, 1256–1272). This research has been reviewed extensively (158, 168, 170, 188, 1273–1276). Overall, the data support the efficacy of cognitive behavior therapy for reducing the frequency and severity of positive symptoms and the distress associated with these symptoms. Furthermore, these gains appear to continue over time. The benefits do not appear to extend to relapse, rehospitalization, or social functioning. Further, it should be noted that treatment refusal and dropout rates are high for cognitive behavior therapy, perhaps because weekly one-to-one meetings amount to therapeutic overload for many chronic patients with high levels of negative symptoms. Persons with schizophrenia or delusional disorder who appear to benefit from cognitive behavior therapy are largely chronic outpatients with treatment-resistant (and often distressing) delusions and/or hallucinations. The intervention ranges in duration from weeks to years; usually several months are required. Cognitive behavior therapy manuals are available, but application typically requires supervised training.

e) Social skills training

Social skills training is defined by the use of behavioral techniques or learning activities that enable patients to acquire instrumental and affiliative skills in domains required to meet the interpersonal, self-care, and coping demands of community life (1277). The goal of social skills training is to remedy specific deficits in patients' role functioning. Thus, training is targeted rather than broad, and it is a highly structured approach that involves systematically teaching patients specific behaviors that are critical for success in social interactions. Social skills training can also include teaching patients how to manage antipsychotic medications, identify side effects, identify warning signs of relapse, negotiate medical and psychiatric care, express their needs to community agencies, and interview for a job. Social skills training can also be effective in increasing the use of specific social behaviors such as gaze and voice volume. Skills are taught through a combination of the therapist's modeling (demonstration); the patient's role playing, usually to try out a particular skill in a simulated interaction; positive and corrective feedback to the patient; and homework assignments, by which the patient can practice a skill outside the training session. Social skills training can be provided individually, but it is almost always conducted in small groups of six to eight patients, for cost reasons and so that patients can learn from one another. Large groups (more than 10 patients) are not advised, as patients do not have adequate opportunity to rehearse.

Clinical trials have supported the efficacy of social skills training (149, 150, 173, 542, 1217, 1277–1292). With the exception of a recent meta-analysis (168), reviews have also endorsed social skills training (167, 169, 1293, 1294).

It is evident that patients with schizophrenia can learn a wide variety of social and independent living skills. Follow-up evaluations lasting up to 1 year showed good retention of the skills that were taught earlier (149, 150, 1278, 1282). When patients attempted to document the use of skills learned in the clinic in their natural environments, the results suggested generalization, but much more research is needed (1278, 1286).

While social skills training may have a positive effect on social role functioning (1283, 1295), it is not effective for reducing symptoms or preventing relapse (169). There are several reports of controlled studies in which social skills training significantly reduced relapse rates and symptom levels (1285, 1286), but more research is needed to document the extent to which social skills training actually protects patients from relapse. In fact, a study by Hogarty et al. (173) showed a loss in prophylactic effect at 2-year follow-up.

Skills training can be implemented in individual and group settings with patients, their families, or both. Patients selected for training should have moderate to severe deficits in social functioning; better-functioning patients require other approaches. There are a number of useful tools and guides for learning how to implement social skills training, including several teaching modules with a trainer's manual, a participant's workbook, and demonstration videos (169, 1296).

f) Programs of early intervention to delay or prevent relapse

The use of early intervention with the appearance of prodromal symptoms to relapse is one part of psychiatric management that can be effective in preventing rehospitalization. Studies have shown that relapse is usually preceded by the appearance of prodromal symptoms, which may last a few days, several weeks, or longer. The prodromal phase of relapse usually consists of moderate to severe dysphoric symptoms, such as tension and nervousness, eating less, difficulty concentrating and remembering, trouble sleeping, and depression, and it may also include mild psychotic symptoms and idiosyncratic behaviors (19, 375, 377, 806, 1297–1304). Such changes preceding relapse indicate either the emergence of new symptoms or increases in symptoms that were already present at baseline. In addition to changes in symptoms, changes in observable behaviors are noted by some patients and families. Examples include social withdrawal, wearing makeup in excessive or bizarre ways, and loss of concern about one's appearance. Controlled studies have demonstrated that specific programs to educate patients and families about prodromal symptoms and early intervention when symptoms occur can be helpful in reducing relapse rates (19, 220, 682, 807, 1305–1307).

2. Psychosocial treatments with very limited evidence bases

a) Personal therapy

As developed by Hogarty and colleagues (185–187), personal therapy is an individualized long-term psychosocial intervention provided to patients with schizophrenia with a weekly to bimonthly frequency within the larger framework of a treatment program that provides pharmacotherapy, family work (when a family exists), and multiple levels of both material and psychological support. The primary objective of personal therapy is to achieve and maintain clinical stability in patients who are at risk for future relapses and functional disabilities. The approach is carefully tailored to the patient's phase of recovery from an acute episode and the patient's residual level of symptom severity, disability, and vulnerability to relapse. Personal therapy is delivered in three distinct phases that match the patient's level of clinical recovery and social/instrumental reintegration. Patients graduate to the next phase only if and when they have managed and stabilized at the prior phase. The therapy is therefore flexible, phase relevant, and sensitive to the dangers of environmental overload (including overload within the therapeutic environment). Another operational principle is that recovery requires time and disorder-appropriate treatment. As such, personal therapy is a long-term endeavor, with each phase lasting several months to 1–2 years. Although the initial results of Hogarty's seminal work on personal therapy are very promising, there have been no replications of this study.

b) Group therapies

The group therapies include a range of modalities, such as psychoeducation groups, social skills training groups, group counseling, and group psychotherapy, with some groups providing a blend of these modalities. The goals of group therapy are enhancements of problem solving, goal planning, social interactions, and medication and side effect management (1308). Kanas (1309, 1310) suggests that groups should focus on "here-and-now" issues and can be effective in increasing patients' coping skills, including the ability to cope with psychotic symptoms. In addition, group approaches may aid in teaching persons with schizophrenia interpersonal and coping skills and in providing a supportive social network for patients who tend to be socially isolated. Group meetings on a weekly basis are also a time-efficient way of monitoring patients for the onset of prodromal symptoms (19).

The evidence for the efficacy of group therapy in schizophrenia is not strong (163, 1308, 1311–1317). Most studies of outpatient and inpatient group therapy were conducted in the 1970s; there have been few recent studies. A number of well-controlled studies involving stable outpatients indicate that there is very modest evidence that group therapy can be effective in improving social adjustment (1318–1321) and coping skills (1316). For hospitalized patients in the acute phase of illness, there is no evidence for the effectiveness of insight-oriented group psychotherapy and some evidence that it may be harmful (1322). However, supportive groups may be useful in helping patients learn to cope with their symptoms, practice relating to others in a controlled environment, and develop a therapeutic alliance with the treatment team (1310, 1323, 1324).

The criteria for selection of patients for groups are derived from clinical experience; patients must have sufficient stability and enough reality testing that they can meaningfully participate (the exception may be previous group members who may benefit from group support while being stabilized after an acute episode). Exclusion criteria include constant preoccupation with hallucinations or delusions (especially paranoid), severe thought disorganization, and very poor impulse control. Higher functioning outpatients may benefit from interaction-oriented group therapy, while poorly functioning patients who may be overstimulated may benefit more from group approaches that attempt to reprogram cognitive and behavioral deficits (1325). There should be flexible use of adjunctive individual sessions, especially in times of crisis, for patients whose primary treatment mode is group therapy. It is generally recommended that a group should consist of six to eight patients (1321). A larger number of patients can be assigned to a group if some members do not attend sessions regularly (1326).

c) Programs of early detection and intervention to treat schizophrenia at or before onset

The early course of schizophrenia includes a premorbid stage, a prodromal stage, and a first-episode stage of illness. The premorbid phase refers to an asymptomatic period that may, in a minority of patients, include subtle and stable "neurodevelopmental" deficits in motor, social, and/or intellectual functioning. While deficits usually mark a vulnerability to developing psychosis, they possess little if any ability to predict later development of psychosis (unpublished 1997 manuscript by P. Jones and J. van Os).

Developmental changes usually associated with adolescence may accelerate neurobiological processes (e.g., cortical-cortical synaptic pruning) that can become expressed symptomatically as neurodegeneration leading to the prodromal phase of disorder. The first signs of disorder are usually functional, not symptomatic, and consist of deficits in social and intellectual functioning and organizational abilities. Prodromal "symptoms" ultimately emerge alongside functional decline between 1 and 24 months before onset of an initial episode of illness. Nonspecific and negative symptoms usually develop first, followed by attenuated positive symptoms. In the year before onset, especially the last 4–6 months, symptoms accelerate in number and intensity. Their characteristic schizophrenic-like phenomenology (e.g., ideas of reference, paranoid ideation, unusual or alien thoughts, unexplained sounds) becomes more apparent, and ultimately psychosis ensues (675, 676, 718, 1327–1330). Criteria that are diagnostic of a prodromal syndrome have been articulated (1331–1333). These criteria predict conversion to psychosis within a year with high frequency, e.g., between 36% and 54% of such samples (1334, 1335).

Early intervention has two aims: 1) to treat active psychotic or prodromal symptoms and 2) to prevent future deterioration and further course progression toward chronicity. Postonset, early intervention targets the duration of untreated psychosis in hopes of reducing future severity and chronicity and preventing the extensive collateral damage that results from active disorder, such as discrimination, social shunning, and poor treatment alliance and adherence (tertiary prevention). Preonset or prodromal phase intervention targets all of the previously mentioned aims plus delaying onset (secondary prevention, reducing prevalence) or preventing onset (primary prevention, reducing incidence).

Because active psychosis is sometimes lethal and often socially destructive, the rationale for treating the symptoms of psychosis as close to onset as possible is compelling (251). Evidence also suggests that existing treatments might affect the natural course of psychosis beyond controlling symptoms. Numerous studies demonstrate significant correlations of earlier intervention (medication and/or psychosocial) after onset with more rapid treatment response and better longer-term outcome (reviewed by McGlashan [254, 1336, 1337]). Not all studies find this correlation, however, and a causal relationship between postonset early intervention and better prognosis has yet to be demonstrated using controlled designs (1338, 1339).

More compelling evidence of the benefit of early intervention comes from recent studies in the prodromal phase. McGorry et al. (262) randomly assigned operationally defined, prodromally symptomatic, high-risk patients to receive one of two open-label treatments. The enriched treatment group received second-generation antipsychotics, cognitive behavior therapy emphasizing stress management, and basic support. The control group received basic support without medication. At 6 months, significantly more patients in the control group had converted to psychosis. McGlashan et al. (263) randomly assigned a similarly defined symptomatic prodromal population (1340) to receive second-generation antipsychotics or placebo in a double-blind design. The study found a significant drug effect on prodromal symptoms at 8 weeks (264) and beyond, up to 1 year (1341).

Overall, the evidence to date indicates that early intervention in psychosis has tertiary preventive benefit and suggests that it also has secondary preventive benefit. Several more studies are necessary before treatment recommendations are appropriate; however, two strategies are clear: 1) first-episode psychosis should be treated as soon as possible and 2) persons who meet the criteria for being prodromally symptomatic and at risk for psychosis in the near future should be assessed carefully and monitored frequently until their symptoms either remit spontaneously, evolve into schizophrenia, or evolve into another diagnosable and treatable mental disorder.

d) Patient education

While patient education must clearly be a part of standard medical practice and is required medicolegally as part of the informed consent process, it has not been clear just how best to provide this education and whether the provision of education actually improves patients' knowledge and changes patients' behavior (30). Over the last few years different types of patient education have been subjected to empirical study (11, 1270, 1342–1346). These so-called educational approaches employed a variety of cognitive, behavioral, and psychological strategies as well. Studies conducted to date provide modest evidence that group approaches improve social functioning (1343) and that interventions focused on medication adherence achieve their intended effect (11, 1270, 1346). However, at this point no specific educational approach can be recommended.

e) Case management

A common observation has been that patients often "fall through the cracks" between different community agencies or program elements and do not receive needed care. To remedy this situation, a case management function has been developed. Either several members of a team or one staff member can be assigned to be the case manager, ensuring that patients receive coordinated, continuous, and comprehensive services. For example, the case manager may accompany a patient to a welfare agency, visit the home if a clinical appointment is missed, or convene a meeting of workers from different agencies serving the patient to formulate an overall treatment plan in conjunction with the psychiatrist.

Results of controlled studies of the effects of case management have yielded inconsistent findings, probably because of methodological problems in design, including 1) lack of specification of the case management intervention, 2) poor characterization of the patient population, 3) inadequacy of outcome measures, 4) inadequate length of the program, and 5) lack of specification of community context (1347). A major problem that has arisen in community mental health planning is that some public programs have developed case management services without having adequate treatment resources for optimal patient care. Problems in implementation also occur when case managers function independently and are not well integrated into the treatment team.

Recent research has focused on the effectiveness of specific models of case management. One approach has been to develop "enhanced" case management programs, either by lowering the caseloads of staff members (1348–1350), emphasizing a team model (1348, 1351–1353), or augmenting the usual services of case managers with those of additional clinician experts (1354–1356). These enhancements have been found to improve outcomes in some studies.

f) Cognitive remediation and therapy

The cognitive deficits associated with schizophrenia have assumed an increasingly central role in explaining the disability associated with the disorder. Distractibility, memory problems, lack of vigilance, attentional deficits, and limitations in planning and decision making characterize these cognitive impairments. Cognitive remediation strategies have attempted to address these problems using restorative, compensatory, and environmental approaches to treatment. The restorative model emphasizes direct elimination of impairments by correction of underlying cognitive deficits. Compensatory strategies attempt to help patients "work around" their deficits, while environmental approaches manipulate the environment to decrease cognitive demands on patients (1357). An underlying premise of these cognitive approaches is that they not only will have direct benefit but will increase the ability of patients to profit from other therapeutic approaches and improve social and other aspects of functioning.

Numerous experimental trials have demonstrated that relatively brief, frequently computer-assisted training programs can improve patients' performance on neuropsychological tests (1207, 1358–1371). However, these studies, while promising, failed to demonstrate durability and generalizability, failed to control for medication use, and have involved a relatively small number of subjects overall (1207). In one study with encouraging findings, cognitive remediation was paired with work therapy and treatment was sustained over 6 months (1372). Compared with work therapy alone, cognitive remediation yielded significantly greater improvements as measured by neuropsychological tests of executive function and working memory. Working memory effects endured 6 months after the conclusion of treatment (1373). Nevertheless, cognitive remediation must still be regarded as experimental and cannot yet be recommended as part of routine practice. The few studies that focus on compensatory and environmental strategies bear similarities to psychosocial interventions that provide case management. Velligan and colleagues developed cognitive adaptation training (1374, 1375). This compensatory approach improved symptoms, motivation, and functioning, but these findings need to be replicated before such an approach can be recommended.

3. Self-help groups

Patients and their families are taking an increasingly active role in the treatment process. Their goals include increasing their influence on treatment planning and implementation, becoming less dependent on professionals, decreasing the discrimination associated with mental illness, and working to achieve adequate support for treatment and research in mental illness. Consumer organizations fall into three major categories (consumer-run or -operated services, consumer partnership services, and consumers as employees), each with its own membership, purpose, and philosophy (1376). Patients and families should be informed about the existence of these organizations.

a) Patient and self-help treatment organizations

Peer support is social, emotional, and sometimes instrumental support that is mutually offered or provided by persons having a mental health condition (e.g., consumers of mental health services) to others sharing a similar mental health condition to bring about a desired social or personal change (196). Peer support may be either financially compensated or voluntary. A consumer in this context is an individual with severe mental illness who is or was a user or recipient of mental health services and who identifies him- or herself as such (203).

The oldest and most pervasive of peer support types is self-help groups. Although there are groups that cover most mental health-related problems, the most noted ones that are relevant to schizophrenia are GROW, Recovery, Inc., Schizophrenics Anonymous, National Depressive and Manic Depressive Association groups, double-trouble groups (for those with both substance use disorders and other mental disorders), and Emotions Anonymous. Until very recently these groups were required to be face-to-face (196). However, Internet online support groups, with no face-to-face interaction, have come into existence (1377).

Based largely on uncontrolled studies of self-help groups for persons with severe mental illness, Davidson et al. (197) concluded that self-help groups seem to improve symptoms and increase participants' social networks and quality of life. Specifically, Galanter (1378) evaluated Recovery, Inc.; Kennedy evaluated GROW (unpublished 1989 manuscript of M. Kennedy); and Kurtz (1379) evaluated the National Depressive and Manic Depressive Association with regard to hospitalizations. All found reductions in hospitalizations and, in one instance, shorter hospitalization when consumers were hospitalized (unpublished 1989 manuscript of M. Kennedy). In addition, these studies, along with Raiff's (198) study of Recovery, Inc., determined that members had improved coping, greater acceptance of illness, improved medication adherence, lower levels of worry, and higher satisfaction with their health. Further, in a study by Powell et al. (200), self-help participation resulted in improved daily functioning and improved illness management. Furthermore, longer term participants have better outcomes (198, 199, and outcomes are better when participants are involved in operating the group rather than just attending the group (200).

Within the realm of consumer-provided or -delivered services are consumer-run or -operated services, consumer partnership services, and consumers as employees. Consumer-run or -operated services are services that are planned, operated, administered, and evaluated by consumers (201, 202). Examples of consumer-operated services include drop-in centers, club houses, crisis services, vocational and employment services, consumer compeer services, psychosocial educational services, and peer support programs, such as Friends Connection in Philadelphia (207), where consumers with dual diagnoses are matched with recovering consumers. Those service programs that are not freestanding legal entities but share the control of the operation of the program with nonconsumers are categorized as consumer partnerships. Consumer employees are individuals who fill positions designated for consumers as well as consumers who are hired into traditional mental health positions. When consumers are hired into existing mainstream positions, to be considered a consumer employee, the individual must fulfill the definition of a consumer, which includes publicly identifying him- or herself as a consumer. Frequently, these designated consumer positions are adjuncts to traditional mental health services, such as a case manager aid position. Examples of specially designated consumer positions are peer companion, peer advocate, consumer case manager, peer specialist, and peer counselor. The term "prosumer" has also come into use. It refers to a person who is both a consumer and a professional, such as a trained psychologist who identifies him- or herself as a consumer (1380).

Reviews of peer support/consumer-provided services specifically for persons with severe mental illness have generated positive but somewhat tentative results, given the infancy of the research area (197, 203, 204). Consumer-provided services have been found to be as effective as or more effective than services provided by nonconsumers (1381, 1382). Two studies using experimental or quasi-experimental designs found reduced use of hospitalization and/or crisis services associated with peer support (207, 208). In the study by Klein et al., recipients of the consumer-delivered services also had improved social functioning, reduced substance use, and improved quality of life. In a randomized study, consumers assigned to a condition in which a consumer assisted in postdischarge network services had fewer and shorter hospitalizations, relative to comparison subjects, and functioned in the community without utilizing mental health services (205). The addition of a peer specialist to an intensive case management team, compared to addition of a nonconsumer specialist to the team, was associated with gains in some aspects of quality of life, fewer significant life problems, and improved self-esteem and social support among consumers (1383). Other less rigorously designed studies also found fewer hospitalizations for those served by consumers (206, 209). A consumer employment program resulted in higher rates of employment, higher earnings, and a tendency toward better vocational rehabilitation outcomes for program participants, compared with consumers who did not receive peer-supported vocational services (1384). Similarly, recipients of a consumer-operated employment program obtained employment at higher rates than found in usual employment services (1385).

b) Relative organizations

Family associations have taken on very important roles in supporting research, providing education, and supporting the families of the mentally ill (1386–1388).

The myriad services provided by family associations include (but are not limited to):

- Education about mental illness—for the public, as well as for professionals who do not specialize in psychiatric disorders.
- Support for research on family services—not only by raising money directly but also by advocating for government funds (1237). The National Alliance for Research on Schizophrenia and Affective Disorders, NAMI in the United States, and other associations in Europe have helped to fund and support research projects.

- In-depth education for families. This education includes not only help lines and literature for patients and families who call with questions about medication, physicians, or community services but also information about the long-term treatment of the major psychiatric disorders. NAMI's Family-to-Family Education Program is a specific example of an organized educational program offered free to families. This program has been shown to reduce families' subjective burden of illness and improve their well-being (1238).
- Advocacy for the rights of the mentally ill by means of legal action.
- Crisis lines and web sites (1389).
- Centers where consumers can meet, find support, and share their feelings with other families without (what they perceive as) "interference" from mental health professionals. Specific support groups are available for siblings and for families of children or adolescents with schizophrenia.

Studies have suggested that helping families educate and empower themselves and helping them to become more involved in service delivery results in better outcomes for the mentally ill family members (1390, 1391).

PART C: FUTURE RESEARCH DIRECTIONS

The ultimate goal of treatment is to minimize the effects of illness and to enable patients to live full, productive, and rewarding lives. This goal remains elusive for many persons with schizophrenia. Not only do most persons not receive the full range of evidence-based treatments, but even the best treatments currently available do not enable most patients the opportunity for full and productive lives that they might have experienced without the illness. Available treatments focus primarily on the psychotic symptoms of schizophrenia and are reasonably effective at controlling these symptoms in the majority of patients. Most patients experience symptom reduction with pharmacotherapy, and relapse rates are reduced by more than half with maintenance treatment. Certain family intervention approaches further reduce relapse rates, and selected psychosocial treatments appear beneficial for occupational and social functioning. Despite efficacious treatment, most patients remain symptomatic and vulnerable to relapse. Persistent impairments are common, and long-term outcomes, while heterogeneous, still represent significant morbidity for most patients. Outcomes in other domains, especially the deficit symptoms and impaired functional status, remain unsatisfactory. This situation underscores the need for several research priorities.

Basic research is essential to provide a better understanding of the etiologies and mechanisms of these impairments and to develop treatment technologies derived from new knowledge. It is likely that the schizophrenia syndrome is heterogeneous, and hence future treatment development must be informed through a better understanding of the various components of the syndrome. In particular, attention must be directed toward understanding the deficit syndrome and neurocognitive impairments that account for many of the disabling effects of the illness. Major breakthroughs in prevention or treatment will likely depend on advances in basic knowledge about brain function.

Intervention research must be informed by advances in basic neuroscience so that new treatments more directly affect these aspects of the syndrome that remain largely resistant to current treatments. Priority must be given to pharmacological and psychosocial interventions that address functional impairments and especially to combined treatment approaches that optimize brain function as well as opportunities for patients to take advantage of improved capacity. Intervention research is needed to examine the relative efficacy of available treatments, especially options that represent substantial cost differentials. Research should continue on psychosocial interventions that show promise when added to antipsychotic medications. These interventions include family interventions, disease-specific forms of psychological treatments, skills training, cognitive therapy, supported employment, and personally tailored combinations of these modalities. Given the crucial importance of adequate housing, research is needed to examine the effectiveness of various approaches to promoting stable, high-quality housing, including the matching of patients to housing resources on the basis of clinical and social characteristics.

Research into early detection and treatment of schizophrenia is also important to determine whether applying existing pharmacological and psychosocial interventions earlier in the course of the disorder provides added efficacy or has the potential for secondary or tertiary prevention.

Clinical research should also attend to a fuller range of outcomes, beyond symptom relief, including functional status and quality of life. These outcomes represent the range of priorities by various "stakeholders": researchers, practitioners, patients, families, and payers. A more comprehensive approach to outcomes assessment will ensure that studies are viewed as relevant and informative to these various stakeholders, who function as effective advocates at various levels. Furthermore, we must ask for whom outcomes are improved. Clinical research on treatment-relevant subgroups will aid in better treatment matching and more judicious allocation of resources. Genetics research also has the potential for providing data to match patients with optimal treatments. In short, we need to know which treatments enhance which outcomes for which patients.

Clinical services research should address the translation of efficacious interventions into practice. Several questions must be addressed: To what degree are efficacious treatments used in practice? Who receives them, and what are the patient-related and provider-related determinants of these practice patterns? What is the cost-effectiveness in practice of interventions with known efficacy? What are the barriers to the adoption of efficacious treatments in practice, and how can these be overcome? What strategies for changing practices are most effective? Service systems research must tackle these questions at the system level and, in addition, address the question of which organizational and financing strategies promote services that incorporate the most effective treatments. Finally, services research needs to address the current failure of treatment systems to ensure that evidence-based treatments are properly implemented and offered to those who can benefit from them. In addition, services research needs to examine the relationships between patterns of service use and illness characteristics, especially the effect of cognitive deficits on patients' capacity to gain access to and use services. Such research should also evaluate the effects of interventions in improving patients' capacity to use services appropriately.

INDIVIDUALS AND ORGANIZATIONS THAT SUBMITTED COMMENTS

Carol L. Alter, M.D.
Allan A. Anderson, M.D.
Ross J. Baldessarini, M.D.
Karen Ballard, M.S.N., R.N.
Carl C. Bell, M.D.
Morris D. Bell, Ph.D., A.B.P.P.
Alan Bellack, Ph.D.
Gary R. Bond, Ph.D.
John J. Boronow, M.D.
Robert W. Buchanan, M.D.
Peter F. Buckley, M.D.
Michael Burke, M.D.

Robert P. Cabaj, M.D.
William T. Carpenter Jr., M.D.
Norman A. Clemens, M.D.
Carl I. Cohen, M.D.
Robert R. Conley, M.D.
Patrick W. Corrigan, Psy.D.
Francine Cournos, M.D.
John M. Davis, M.D.
Susan M. Essock, Ph.D.
Wayne Fenton, M.D.
Andrew J. Francis, M.D., Ph.D.
Alan Gelenberg, M.D.
Donald C. Goff, M.D.
Gregory E. Gray, M.D., Ph.D.
Tina Haynes, M.T.-B.C.
Elizabeth R. Hudler, M.D.
Michael Jellinek, M.D.
Dilip V. Jeste, M.D.
Nick Kanas, M.D.
John M. Kane, M.D.
Jerald Kay, M.D.
Paul Keck, M.D.
Carol Ann Kuchmak, M.D.
William B. Lawson, M.D., Ph.D.
Cheng Lee, M.D.
Sarah H. Lisanby, M.D.
Francis G. Lu, M.D.
K. Roy MacKenzie, M.D.
Harold A. Maio, M.A.
Henry Mallard, M.D.
William R. McFarlane, M.D.
Hunter L. McQuistion, M.D.
Jeffrey L. Metzner, M.D.
Henry A. Nasrallah, M.D.
Marvin Nierenberg, M.D.
Jacqueline Payne, M.S.N., R.N., N.P.-P.
Steven G. Potkin, M.D.
Michele Press, M.D.
Elliott Richelson, M.D.
Barbara Rosenfeld, M.D.
Erik Roskes, M.D.
Patricia Rowell, Ph.D., R.N., C.N.P.
Pedro Ruiz, M.D.
Neil Sandson, M.D.
S. Warren Seides, M.D.
Ann-Louise Silver, M.D.
Robert Stern, M.D., Ph.D.
Nada L. Stotland, M.D.
Marvin S. Swartz, M.D.
Martin S. Willick, M.D.
Alexander S. Young, M.D., M.S.H.S.

American Academy of Pediatrics
American Academy of Geriatric Psychiatry
American Music Therapy Association
American Nurses Association

REFERENCES

The following coding system is used to indicate the nature of the supporting evidence in the summary recommendations and references:

[A] *Double-blind, randomized clinical trial.* A study of an intervention in which subjects are prospectively followed over time; there are treatment and control groups; subjects are randomly assigned to the two groups; both the subjects and the investigators are blind to the assignments.

[A–] *Randomized clinical trial.* Same as above but not double-blind.

[B] *Clinical trial.* A prospective study in which an intervention is made and the results of that intervention are tracked longitudinally; study does not meet standards for a randomized clinical trial.

[C] *Cohort or longitudinal study.* A study in which subjects are prospectively followed over time without any specific intervention.

[D] *Case-control study.* A study in which a group of patients is identified in the present and information about them is pursued retrospectively or backward in time.

[E] *Review with secondary data analysis.* A structured analytic review of existing data, e.g., a meta-analysis or a decision analysis.

[F] *Review.* A qualitative review and discussion of previously published literature without a quantitative synthesis of the data.

[G] *Other.* Textbooks, expert opinion, case reports, and other reports not included above.

1. American Psychiatric Association: Handbook of Psychiatric Measures. Washington, DC, American Psychiatric Publishing, 2000 [G]
2. First MB, Spitzer RL, Gibbon M, Williams JBW: Structured Clinical Interview for DSM-IV Axis I Disorders (SCID), Clinician Version (User's Guide and Interview). Washington, DC, American Psychiatric Press, 1996 [G]
3. Guy W (ed): ECDEU Assessment Manual for Psychopharmacology: Publication ADM 76-338. Washington, DC, US Department of Health, Education, and Welfare, 1976 [G]
4. Ventura J, Lukoff D, Nuechterlein K: A Brief Psychiatric Rating Scale (BPRS) expanded version (4.0): scales, anchor points and administration manual. Int J Methods Psychiatr Res 1993; 3:227–243 [G]
5. Ventura J, Green MF, Shaner A, Liberman RP: Training and quality assurance in the use of the Brief Psychiatric Rating Scale: the "drift busters." Int J Methods Psychiatr Res 1993; 3:221–244 [B]
6. Overall JE, Gorham DR: The Brief Psychiatric Rating Scale. Psychol Rep 1962; 10:799–812 [G]
7. Kay SR, Fiszbein A, Opler LA: The positive and negative syndrome scale (PANSS) for schizophrenia. Schizophr Bull 1987; 13:261–276 [G]
8. Shores-Wilson K, Biggs MM, Miller AL, Carmody TJ, Chiles JA, Rush AJ, Crismon ML, Toprac MG, Witte BP, Webster JC: Itemized clinician ratings versus global ratings of symptom severity in patients with schizophrenia. Int J Methods Psychiatr Res 2002; 11:45–53 [G]
9. Miller AL, Chiles JA, Chiles JK, Crismon ML, Rush AJ, Shon SP: The Texas Medication Algorithm Project (TMAP) schizophrenia algorithms. J Clin Psychiatry 1999; 60:649–657 [G]
10. Frank AF, Gunderson JG: The role of the therapeutic alliance in the treatment of schizophrenia: relationship to course and outcome. Arch Gen Psychiatry 1990; 47:228–236 [C]
11. Kemp R, Kirov G, Everitt B, Hayward P, David A: Randomised controlled trial of compliance therapy: 18-month follow-up. Br J Psychiatry 1998; 172:413–419 [A]
12. Zygmunt A, Olfson M, Boyer CA, Mechanic D: Interventions to improve medication adherence in schizophrenia. Am J Psychiatry 2002; 159:1653–1664 [F]
13. Perkins DO: Predictors of noncompliance in patients with schizophrenia. J Clin Psychiatry 2002; 63:1121–1128 [F]
14. Weiden P, Rapkin B, Mott T, Zygmunt A, Goldman D, Horvitz-Lennon M, Frances A: Rating of medication influences (ROMI) scale in schizophrenia. Schizophr Bull 1994; 20: 297–310 [G]
15. Coldham EL, Addington J, Addington D: Medication adherence of individuals with a first episode of psychosis. Acta Psychiatr Scand 2002; 106:286–290 [G]
16. Robinson DG, Woerner MG, Alvir JM, Bilder RM, Hinrichsen GA, Lieberman JA: Predictors of medication discontinuation by patients with first-episode schizophrenia and schizoaffective disorder. Schizophr Res 2002; 57:209–219 [C]
17. Van Putten T: Why do schizophrenic patients refuse to take their drugs? Arch Gen Psychiatry 1974; 31:67–72 [G]
18. Van Putten T, May PR: Subjective response as a predictor of outcome in pharmacotherapy: the consumer has a point. Arch Gen Psychiatry 1978; 35:477–480 [B]
19. Herz MI, Glazer WM, Mostert MA, Sheard MA, Szymanski HV, Hafez H, Mirza M, Vana J: Intermittent vs maintenance medication in schizophrenia: two-year results. Arch Gen Psychiatry 1991; 48:333–339 [A]

20. Hogarty GE, Goldberg SC: Drug and sociotherapy in the aftercare of schizophrenic patients: one-year relapse rates. Arch Gen Psychiatry 1973; 28:54–64 [A]
21. Swartz MS, Swanson JW, Hannon MJ: Does fear of coercion keep people away from mental health treatment? Evidence from a survey of persons with schizophrenia and mental health professionals. Behav Sci Law 2003; 21:459–472 [G]
22. Swartz MS, Wagner HR, Swanson JW, Hiday VA, Burns BJ: The perceived coerciveness of involuntary outpatient commitment: findings from an experimental study. J Am Acad Psychiatry Law 2002; 30:207–217 [A–]
23. Hoge MA, Grottole E: The case against outpatient commitment. J Am Acad Psychiatry Law 2000; 28:165–170 [G]
24. Swanson JW, Swartz MS, Elbogen EB, Wagner HR, Burns BJ: Effects of involuntary outpatient commitment on subjective quality of life in persons with severe mental illness. Behav Sci Law 2003; 21:473–491 [A–]
25. Swartz MS, Swanson JW, Wagner HR, Burns BJ, Hiday VA: Effects of involuntary outpatient commitment and depot antipsychotics on treatment adherence in persons with severe mental illness. J Nerv Ment Dis 2001; 189:583–592 [A–]
26. Hiday VA, Swartz MS, Swanson JW, Borum R, Wagner HR: Impact of outpatient commitment on victimization of people with severe mental illness. Am J Psychiatry 2002; 159:1403–1411 [A–]
27. Swartz MS, Swanson JW, Hiday VA, Wagner HR, Burns BJ, Borum R: A randomized controlled trial of outpatient commitment in North Carolina. Psychiatr Serv 2001; 52:325–329 [A–]
28. Steadman HJ, Gounis K, Dennis D, Hopper K, Roche B, Swartz M, Robbins PC: Assessing the New York City involuntary outpatient commitment pilot program. Psychiatr Serv 2001; 52:330–336 [A–]
29. Gerbasi JB, Bonnie RJ, Binder RL: Resource document on mandatory outpatient treatment. J Am Acad Psychiatry Law 2000; 28:127–144 [G]
30. Mueser KT, Corrigan PW, Hilton DW, Tanzman B, Schaub A, Gingerich S, Essock SM, Tarrier N, Morey B, Vogel-Scibilia S, Herz MI: Illness management and recovery: a review of the research. Psychiatr Serv 2002; 53:1272–1284 [F]
31. Dixon L, McFarlane WR, Lefley H, Lucksted A, Cohen M, Falloon I, Mueser K, Miklowitz D, Solomon P, Sondheimer D: Evidence-based practices for services to families of people with psychiatric disabilities. Psychiatr Serv 2001; 52:903–910 [B/C]
32. Drake RE, Essock SM, Shaner A, Carey KB, Minkoff K, Kola L, Lynde D, Osher FC, Clark RE, Rickards L: Implementing dual diagnosis services for clients with severe mental illness. Psychiatr Serv 2001; 52:469–476 [G]
33. Daumit GL, Pratt LA, Crum RM, Powe NR, Ford DE: Characteristics of primary care visits for individuals with severe mental illness in a national sample. Gen Hosp Psychiatry 2002; 24:391–395 [G]
34. Brown S, Inskip H, Barraclough B: Causes of the excess mortality of schizophrenia. Br J Psychiatry 2000; 177:212–217 [C]
35. Benjet C, Azar ST, Kuersten-Hogan R: Evaluating the parental fitness of psychiatrically diagnosed individuals: advocating a functional-contextual analysis of parenting. J Fam Psychol 2003; 17:238–251 [G]
36. Caton CL, Cournos F, Dominguez B: Parenting and adjustment in schizophrenia. Psychiatr Serv 1999; 50:239–243 [D]
37. Corrigan PW, Giffort DW (eds): Building Teams and Programs for Effective Rehabilitation. New Dir Ment Health Serv 1998; 79:1–93 [G]
38. Corrigan PW, Steiner L, McCracken SG, Blaser B, Barr M: Strategies for disseminating evidence-based practices to staff who treat people with serious mental illness. Psychiatr Serv 2001; 52:1598–1606 [G]

39. Cradock J, Young AS, Sullivan G: The accuracy of medical record documentation in schizophrenia. J Behav Health Serv Res 2001; 28:456–465 [G]
40. American Psychiatric Association: The Principles of Medical Ethics: With Annotations Especially Applicable to Psychiatry, 12th ed. Washington, DC, American Psychiatric Publishing, 2001 [G]
41. Kopelowicz A, Liberman RP: Biobehavioral treatment and rehabilitation of schizophrenia. Harv Rev Psychiatry 1995; 3:55–64 [D]
42. Hirsch S, Bowen J, Emami J, Cramer P, Jolley A, Haw C, Dickinson M: A one year prospective study of the effect of life events and medication in the aetiology of schizophrenic relapse. Br J Psychiatry 1996; 168:49–56 [A]
43. Olfson M, Mechanic D, Boyer CA, Hansell S, Walkup J, Weiden PJ: Assessing clinical predictions of early rehospitalization in schizophrenia. J Nerv Ment Dis 1999; 187:721–729 [C]
44. Hunt GE, Bergen J, Bashir M: Medication compliance and comorbid substance abuse in schizophrenia: impact on community survival 4 years after a relapse. Schizophr Res 2002; 54:253–264 [C]
45. Ayuso-Gutierrez JL, Rio Vega JM: Factors influencing relapse in the long-term course of schizophrenia. Schizophr Res 1997; 28:199–206 [G]
46. Robinson D, Woerner MG, Alvir JM, Bilder R, Goldman R, Geisler S, Koreen A, Sheitman B, Chakos M, Mayerhoff D, Lieberman JA: Predictors of relapse following response from a first episode of schizophrenia or schizoaffective disorder. Arch Gen Psychiatry 1999; 56: 241–247 [C]
47. Gupta S, Hendricks S, Kenkel AM, Bhatia SC, Haffke EA: Relapse in schizophrenia: is there a relationship to substance abuse? Schizophr Res 1996; 20:153–156 [D]
48. Sandson NB: Drug Interactions Casebook: The Cytochrome P450 System and Beyond. Arlington, Va, American Psychiatric Publishing, 2003 [G]
49. Cozza KL, Armstrong SC, Oesterheld JO: Concise Guide to Drug Interaction Principles for Medical Practice: Cytochrome P450s, UGTs, P-Glycoproteins, 2nd Ed. Arlington, Va, American Psychiatric Publishing, 2003 [G]
50. Marder SR, Essock SM, Miller AL, Buchanan RW, Davis JM, Kane JM, Lieberman J, Schooler NR: The Mount Sinai conference on the pharmacotherapy of schizophrenia. Schizophr Bull 2002; 28:5–16 [G]
51. American Diabetes Association: Clinical Practice Recommendations 2003. Diabetes Care 2003; 26(suppl):S33–S50 [G]
52. National Cholesterol Education Program: Final Report of the National Cholesterol Education Program (NCEP) Expert Panel on Detection, Evaluation, and Treatment of High Blood Cholesterol in Adults (Adult Treatment Panel III): NIH Publication 02-5215. Bethesda, Md, National Heart, Lung, and Blood Institute, 2003. (http://www.nhlbi.nih.gov/guidelines/cholesterol/index.htm) [G]
53. Pignone MP, Phillips CJ, Atkins D, Teutsch SM, Mulrow CD, Lohr KN: Screening and treating adults for lipid disorders. Am J Prev Med 2001; 20:77–89 [G]
54. American Psychiatric Association: Practice Guideline for Psychiatric Evaluation of Adults. Am J Psychiatry 1995; 152:63–80 [F]
55. Meltzer HY, Alphs L, Green AI, Altamura AC, Anand R, Bertoldi A, Bourgeois M, Chouinard G, Islam MZ, Kane J, Krishnan R, Lindenmayer JP, Potkin S: Clozapine treatment for suicidality in schizophrenia: International Suicide Prevention Trial (InterSePT). Arch Gen Psychiatry 2003; 60:82–91 [A–]
56. American Psychiatric Association: Practice Guideline for the Assessment and Treatment of Patients with Suicidal Behaviors. Am J Psychiatry 2003; 160(Nov suppl):1–60 [G]
57. Buckley PF, Noffsinger SG, Smith DA, Hrouda DR, Knoll JL: Treatment of the psychotic patient who is violent. Psychiatr Clin North Am 2003; 26:231–272 [G]

58. Taylor PJ, Monahan J: Commentary: dangerous patients or dangerous diseases? Br Med J 1996; 312:967–969 [G]
59. Lefley HP, Johnson D: Families as Allies in the Treatment of the Mentally Ill. Washington, DC, American Psychiatric Press, 1990 [G]
60. Hatfield AB, Lefley HP: Surviving Mental Illness: Stress, Coping, and Adaptation. New York, Guilford, 1993 [G]
61. Marsh DT, Dickens R: How to Cope With Mental Illness in Your Family: A Self-Care Guide for Siblings, Offspring, and Parents. New York, Jeremy P. Tarcher/Putnam, 1998 [G]
62. Green MF: Schizophrenia Revealed. New York, WW Norton, 2001 [G]
63. Torrey EF: Surviving Schizophrenia: A Manual for Families, Consumers and Providers, 4th ed. New York, HarperTrade, 2001 [G]
64. Mueser KT, Gingerich SL: Coping With Schizophrenia: A Guide for Families. New York, Guilford, 2004 [G]
65. Lehman AF, Kreyenbuhl J, Buchanan RW, Dickerson FB, Dixon LB, Goldberg R, Green-Paden LD, Tenhula WN, Boerescu D, Tek C, Sandson N: The Schizophrenia Patient Outcomes Research Team (PORT): updated treatment recommendations 2003. Schizophr Bull (in press) [G]
66. Centorrino F, Eakin M, Bahk WM, Kelleher JP, Goren J, Salvatore P, Egli S, Baldessarini RJ: Inpatient antipsychotic drug use in 1998, 1993, and 1989. Am J Psychiatry 2002; 159: 1932–1935 [D]
67. Hardman JG, Limbird LE, Gilman AG (eds): Goodman and Gilman's The Pharmacological Basis of Therapeutics, 10th ed. New York, McGraw-Hill Professional, 2001 [G]
68. Cohen LJ, Test MA, Brown RL: Suicide and schizophrenia: data from a prospective community treatment study. Am J Psychiatry 1990; 147:602–607 [C]
69. Angermeyer MC: Schizophrenia and violence. Acta Psychiatr Scand Suppl 2000; 102:63–67 [F]
70. American Psychiatric Association, American Psychiatric Nurses Association, National Association of Psychiatric Health Systems: Learning From Each Other: Success Stories and Ideas for Reducing Restraint/Seclusion in Behavioral Health. Arlington, Va, American Psychiatric Association, 2003. (http://www.psych.org/clin_res/learningfromeachother.cfm) [G]
71. Hughes DH, Kleespies PM: Treating aggression in the psychiatric emergency service. J Clin Psychiatry 2003; 64(suppl 4):10–15 [G]
72. Salzman C, Green AI, Rodriguez-Villa F, Jaskiw GI: Benzodiazepines combined with neuroleptics for management of severe disruptive behavior. Psychosomatics 1986; 27:17–22 [B]
73. Dubin WR: Rapid tranquilization: antipsychotics or benzodiazepines? J Clin Psychiatry 1988; 49(suppl):5–12 [G]
74. Allen MH, Currier GW, Hughes DH, Reyes-Harde M, Docherty JP, Expert Consensus Panel for Behavioral Emergencies: The Expert Consensus Guideline Series: Treatment of Behavioral Emergencies. Postgrad Med 2001; 109(May special number):1–88 [G]
75. Battaglia J, Moss S, Rush J, Kang J, Mendoza R, Leedom L, Dubin W, McGlynn C, Goodman L: Haloperidol, lorazepam, or both for psychotic agitation? A multicenter, prospective, double-blind, emergency department study. Am J Emerg Med 1997; 15:335–340 [A]
76. Lesem MD, Zajecka JM, Swift RH, Reeves KR, Harrigan EP: Intramuscular ziprasidone, 2 mg versus 10 mg, in the short-term management of agitated psychotic patients. J Clin Psychiatry 2001; 62:12–18 [A]
77. Wright P, Birkett M, David SR, Meehan K, Ferchland I, Alaka KJ, Saunders JC, Krueger J, Bradley P, San L, Bernardo M, Reinstein M, Breier A: Double-blind, placebo-controlled comparison of intramuscular olanzapine and intramuscular haloperidol in the treatment of acute agitation in schizophrenia. Am J Psychiatry 2001; 158:1149–1151 [A]

78. Yildiz A, Sachs GS, Turgay A: Pharmacological management of agitation in emergency settings. Emerg Med J 2003; 20:339–346 [F]
79. Breier A, Meehan K, Birkett M, David S, Ferchland I, Sutton V, Taylor CC, Palmer R, Dossenbach M, Kiesler G, Brook S, Wright P: A double-blind, placebo-controlled dose-response comparison of intramuscular olanzapine and haloperidol in the treatment of acute agitation in schizophrenia. Arch Gen Psychiatry 2002; 59:441–448 [A]
80. Shale JH, Shale CM, Mastin WD: A review of the safety and efficacy of droperidol for the rapid sedation of severely agitated and violent patients. J Clin Psychiatry 2003; 64:500–505 [F]
81. Cournos F: Involuntary medication and the case of Joyce Brown. Hosp Community Psychiatry 1989; 40:736–740 [E]
82. Leucht S, Pitschel-Walz G, Abraham D, Kissling W: Efficacy and extrapyramidal side-effects of the new antipsychotics olanzapine, quetiapine, risperidone, and sertindole compared to conventional antipsychotics and placebo: a meta-analysis of randomized controlled trials. Schizophr Res 1999; 35:51–68 [E]
83. Correll CU, Leucht S, Kane JM: Reduced risk for tardive dyskinesia with second-generation antipsychotics: a systematic review of one-year studies. Am J Psychiatry (in press) [E]
84. Sartorius N, Fleischhacker WW, Gjerris A, Kern U, Knapp M, Leonard BE, Lieberman JA, Lopez-Ibor JJ, van Raay B, Twomey E: The Usefulness and Use of Second-Generation Antipsychotic Medications. Curr Opin Psychiatry 2002; 15(suppl 1):S1–S51 [G]
85. National Institute for Clinical Excellence: Schizophrenia: Core Interventions in the Treatment and Management of Schizophrenia in Primary and Secondary Care. London, National Institute for Clinical Excellence, 2002. (http://www.nice.org.uk) [G]
86. Geddes J, Freemantle N, Harrison P, Bebbington P: Atypical antipsychotics in the treatment of schizophrenia: systematic overview and meta-regression analysis. Br Med J 2000; 321: 1371–1376 [D]
87. Chakos M, Lieberman J, Hoffman E, Bradford D, Sheitman B: Effectiveness of second-generation antipsychotics in patients with treatment-resistant schizophrenia: a review and meta-analysis of randomized trials. Am J Psychiatry 2001; 158:518–526 [E]
88. Leucht S, Wahlbeck K, Hamann J, Kissling W: New generation antipsychotics versus low-potency conventional antipsychotics: a systematic review and meta-analysis. Lancet 2003; 361:1581–1589 [E]
89. Davis JM, Chen N, Glick ID: A meta-analysis of the efficacy of second-generation antipsychotics. Arch Gen Psychiatry 2003; 60:553–564 [E]
90. Tandon R: Antipsychotic agents, in Current Psychotherapeutic Drugs, 2nd Ed. Edited by Quitkin FM, Adams DC, Bowden CL, Heyer ES, Rifkin A, Sellers EM, Tandon R, Taylor BP. Philadelphia, Current Medicine, 1998, pp 120–154 [G]
91. Walburn J, Gray R, Gournay K, Quraishi S, David AS: Systematic review of patient and nurse attitudes to depot antipsychotic medication. Br J Psychiatry 2001; 179:300–307 [D]
92. Marder SR, Hubbard JW, Van Putten T, Midha KK: Pharmacokinetics of long-acting injectable neuroleptic drugs: clinical implications. Psychopharmacology (Berl) 1989; 98: 433–439 [E]
93. Correll CU, Malhotra AK, Kaushik S, McMeniman M, Kane JM: Early prediction of antipsychotic response in schizophrenia. Am J Psychiatry 2003; 160:2063–2065 [G]
94. McEvoy JP, Hogarty GE, Steingard S: Optimal dose of neuroleptic in acute schizophrenia: a controlled study of the neuroleptic threshold and higher haloperidol dose. Arch Gen Psychiatry 1991; 48:739–745 [A]
95. Baldessarini RJ, Cohen BM, Teicher MH: Significance of neuroleptic dose and plasma level in the pharmacological treatment of psychoses. Arch Gen Psychiatry 1988; 45:79–91 [E]
96. Van Putten T, Marder SR, Mintz J: A controlled dose comparison of haloperidol in newly admitted schizophrenic patients. Arch Gen Psychiatry 1990; 47:754–758 [A–]

97. Rifkin A, Doddi S, Karajgi B, Borenstein M, Wachspress M: Dosage of haloperidol for schizophrenia. Arch Gen Psychiatry 1991; 48:166–170 [A]
98. Cormac I, Jones C, Campbell C: Cognitive behaviour therapy for schizophrenia. Cochrane Database Syst Rev 2002; (1):CD000524 [E]
99. Janicak PG, Davis JM, Preskorn SH, Ayd FJ Jr: Principles and Practice of Psychopharmacotherapy. Baltimore, Williams & Wilkins, 1993 [G]
100. Caspi N, Modai I, Barak P, Waisbourd A, Zbarsky H, Hirschmann S, Ritsner M: Pindolol augmentation in aggressive schizophrenic patients: a double-blind crossover randomized study. Int Clin Psychopharmacol 2001; 16:111–115 [A]
101. Allan ER, Alpert M, Sison CE, Citrome L, Laury G, Berman I: Adjunctive nadolol in the treatment of acutely aggressive schizophrenic patients. J Clin Psychiatry 1996; 57:455–459 [A]
102. Afaq I, Riaz J, Sedky K, Chung DJ, Vanina Y, el Mallakh R, Lippmann S: Divalproex as a calmative adjunct for aggressive schizophrenic patients. J Ky Med Assoc 2002; 100:17–22 [B]
103. Siris S, Pollack S, Bermanzohn P, Stronger R: Adjunctive imipramine for a broader group of post-psychotic depressions in schizophrenia. Schizophr Res 2000; 44:187–192 [A]
104. United States Pharmacopeial Convention: Drug Information for the Health Care Professional, 17th ed, vol 1. Rockville, Md, United States Pharmacopeial Convention, 1997 [G]
105. Klasco RK (ed): DRUGDEX System. Greenwood Village, Col, Thomson MICROMEDEX, 2003 [G]
106. Fink M, Sackeim HA: Convulsive therapy in schizophrenia? Schizophr Bull 1996; 22:27–39 [G]
107. American Psychiatric Association: The Practice of Electroconvulsive Therapy: Recommendations for Treatment, Training, and Privileging: A Task Force Report of the American Psychiatric Association. Washington, DC, American Psychiatric Association, 2001 [G]
108. Tharyan P, Adams CE: Electroconvulsive therapy for schizophrenia. Cochrane Database Syst Rev 2002; (2):CD000076 [E]
109. Small JG, Milstein V, Klapper M, Kellams JJ, Small IF: ECT combined with neuroleptics in the treatment of schizophrenia. Psychopharmacol Bull 1982; 18:34–35 [A–]
110. Das PS, Saxena S, Mohan D, Sundaram KR: Adjunctive electroconvulsive therapy for schizophrenia. Natl Med J India 1991; 4:183–184 [G]
111. Ungvari G, Petho B: High-dose haloperidol therapy: its effectiveness and a comparison with electroconvulsive therapy. J Psychiatr Treat Eval 1982; 4:279–283 [G]
112. Ray SD: Relative efficacy of ECT and CPZ in schizophrenia. J Indian Med Assoc 1962; 38:332–333 [B]
113. Klapheke MM: Combining ECT and antipsychotic agents: benefits and risks. Convuls Ther 1993; 9:241–255 [F]
114. Childers RT Jr: Comparison of four regimens in newly admitted female schizophrenics. Am J Psychiatry 1964; 120:1010–1011 [B]
115. Smith K, Surphlis WRP, Gynther MD, Shimkunas A: ECT-chlorpromazine and chlorpromazine compared in the treatment of schizophrenia. J Nerv Ment Dis 1967; 144:284–290 [B]
116. Abraham KR, Kulhara P: The efficacy of electroconvulsive therapy in the treatment of schizophrenia: a comparative study. Br J Psychiatry 1987; 151:152–155 [A]
117. Brandon S, Cowley P, McDonald C, Neville P, Palmer R, Wellstood-Eason S: Leicester ECT trial: results in schizophrenia. Br J Psychiatry 1985; 146:177–183 [A]
118. Taylor P, Fleminger JJ: ECT for schizophrenia. Lancet 1980; 1:1380–1382 [A]
119. Rahman R: A review of treatment of 176 schizophrenic patients in the mental hospital Pabna. Br J Psychiatry 1968; 114:775–777 [G]
120. Konig P, Glatter-Gotz U: Combined electroconvulsive and neuroleptic therapy in schizophrenia refractory to neuroleptics. Schizophr Res 1990; 3:351–354 [G]
121. Milstein V, Small JG, Miller MJ, Sharpley PH, Small IF: Mechanisms of action of ECT: schizophrenia and schizoaffective disorder. Biol Psychiatry 1990; 27:1282–1292 [G]

122. Sajatovic M, Meltzer HY: The effect of short-term electroconvulsive treatment plus neuroleptics in treatment-resistant schizophrenia and schizoaffective disorder. Convuls Ther 1993; 9:167–175 [B]
123. Friedel RO: The combined use of neuroleptics and ECT in drug resistant schizophrenic patients. Psychopharmacol Bull 1986; 22:928–930 [B]
124. Gujavarty K, Greenberg LB, Fink M: Electroconvulsive therapy and neuroleptic medication in therapy-resistant positive-symptom psychosis. Convuls Ther 1987; 3:185–195 [B]
125. Chanpattana W, Chakrabhand ML: Combined ECT and neuroleptic therapy in treatment-refractory schizophrenia: prediction of outcome. Psychiatry Res 2001; 105:107–115 [B]
126. Chanpattana W, Chakrabhand ML, Kongsakon R, Techakasem P, Buppanharun W: Short-term effect of combined ECT and neuroleptic therapy in treatment-resistant schizophrenia. J ECT 1999; 15:129–139 [G]
127. Safferman AZ, Munne R: Combining clozapine with ECT. Convuls Ther 1992; 8:141–143 [G]
128. Landy DA: Combined use of clozapine and electroconvulsive therapy. Convuls Ther 1991; 7:218–221 [G]
129. Frankenburg FR, Suppes T, McLean PE: Combined clozapine and electroconvulsive therapy. Convuls Ther 1993; 9:176–180 [G]
130. Cardwell BA, Nakai B: Seizure activity in combined clozapine and ECT: a retrospective view. Convuls Ther 1995; 11:110–113 [G]
131. Benatov R, Sirota P, Megged S: Neuroleptic-resistant schizophrenia treated with clozapine and ECT. Convuls Ther 1996; 12:117–121 [G]
132. Kales HC, Dequardo JR, Tandon R: Combined electroconvulsive therapy and clozapine in treatment-resistant schizophrenia. Prog Neuropsychopharmacol Biol Psychiatry 1999; 23: 547–556 [G]
133. Kupchik M, Spivak B, Mester R, Reznik I, Gonen N, Weizman A, Kotler M: Combined electroconvulsive-clozapine therapy. Clin Neuropharmacol 2000; 23:14–16 [G]
134. James DV, Gray NS: Elective combined electroconvulsive and clozapine therapy. Int Clin Psychopharmacol 1999; 14:69–72 [G]
135. Fink M: ECT and clozapine in schizophrenia. J ECT 1998; 14:223–226 [G]
136. Abrams R, Taylor MA: Catatonia: a prospective clinical study. Arch Gen Psychiatry 1976; 33:579–581 [C]
137. Bush G, Fink M, Petrides G, Dowling F, Francis A: Catatonia, II: treatment with lorazepam and electroconvulsive therapy. Acta Psychiatr Scand 1996; 93:137–143 [B]
138. Escobar R, Rios A, Montoya ID, Lopera F, Ramos D, Carvajal C, Constain G, Gutierrez JE, Vargas S, Herrera CP: Clinical and cerebral blood flow changes in catatonic patients treated with ECT. J Psychosom Res 2000; 49:423–429 [B]
139. Pataki J, Zervas IM, Jandorf L: Catatonia in a university inpatient service (1985–1990). Convuls Ther 1992; 8:163–173 [G]
140. Petrides G, Divadeenam KM, Bush G, Francis A: Synergism of lorazepam and electroconvulsive therapy in the treatment of catatonia. Biol Psychiatry 1997; 42:375–381 [B]
141. Rohland BM, Carroll BT, Jacoby RG: ECT in the treatment of the catatonic syndrome. J Affect Disord 1993; 29:255–261 [G]
142. Rosebush PI, Hildebrand AM, Furlong BG, Mazurek MF: Catatonic syndrome in a general psychiatric inpatient population: frequency, clinical presentation, and response to lorazepam. J Clin Psychiatry 1990; 51:357–362 [B]
143. Suzuki K, Awata S, Matsuoka H: Short-term effect of ECT in middle-aged and elderly patients with intractable catatonic schizophrenia. J ECT 2003; 19:73–80 [B]
144. Hoffman RE, Cavus I: Slow transcranial magnetic stimulation, long-term depotentiation, and brain hyperexcitability disorders. Am J Psychiatry 2002; 159:1093–1102 [F]
145. Burt T, Lisanby SH, Sackeim HA: Neuropsychiatric applications of transcranial magnetic stimulation: a meta analysis. Int J Neuropsychopharmacol 2002; 5:73–103 [E]

146. Hoffman RE, Hawkins KA, Gueorguieva R, Boutros NN, Rachid F, Carroll K, Krystal JH: Transcranial magnetic stimulation of left temporoparietal cortex and medication-resistant auditory hallucinations. Arch Gen Psychiatry 2003; 60:49–56 [A]
147. Hoffman RE, Boutros NN, Hu S, Berman RM, Krystal JH, Charney DS: Transcranial magnetic stimulation and auditory hallucinations in schizophrenia. Lancet 2000; 355: 1073–1075 [B]
148. Rollnik JD, Huber TJ, Mogk H, Siggelkow S, Kropp S, Dengler R, Emrich HM, Schneider U: High frequency repetitive transcranial magnetic stimulation (rTMS) of the dorsolateral prefrontal cortex in schizophrenic patients. Neuroreport 2000; 11:4013–4015 [B]
149. Eckman TA, Wirshing WC, Marder SR, Liberman RP, Johnston-Cronk K, Zimmermann K, Mintz J: Technique for training schizophrenic patients in illness self-management: a controlled trial. Am J Psychiatry 1992; 149:1549–1555 [A]
150. Wallace CJ, Liberman RP, MacKain SJ, Blackwell G, Eckman TA: Effectiveness and replicability of modules for teaching social and instrumental skills to the severely mentally ill. Am J Psychiatry 1992; 149:654–658 [B]
151. Eckman TA, Liberman RP, Phipps CC, Blair KE: Teaching medication management skills to schizophrenic patients. J Clin Psychopharmacol 1990; 10:33–38 [G]
152. Glynn SM: Psychiatric rehabilitation in schizophrenia: advances and challenges. Clin Neuroscience Res 2003; 3:23–33 [G]
153. Olfson M, Mechanic D, Boyer CA, Hansell S: Linking inpatients with schizophrenia to outpatient care. Psychiatr Serv 1998; 49:911–917 [D]
154. Boyer CA, McAlpine DD, Pottick KJ, Olfson M: Identifying risk factors and key strategies in linkage to outpatient psychiatric care. Am J Psychiatry 2000; 157:1592–1598 [G]
155. Vaughn CE, Leff JP: Patterns of emotional response in relatives of schizophrenic patients. Schizophr Bull 1981; 7:43–44 [G]
156. Linn MW, Caffey EM Jr, Klett CJ, Hogarty GE, Lamb HR: Day treatment and psychotropic drugs in the aftercare of schizophrenic patients: a Veterans Administration cooperative study. Arch Gen Psychiatry 1979; 36:1055–1066 [B]
157. Pitschel-Walz G, Leucht S, Bauml J, Kissling W, Engel RR: The effect of family interventions on relapse and rehospitalization in schizophrenia: a meta-analysis. Schizophr Bull 2001; 27:73–92 [E]
158. Pilling S, Bebbington P, Kuipers E, Garety P, Geddes J, Orbach G, Morgan C: Psychological treatments in schizophrenia: I. meta-analysis of family intervention and cognitive behaviour therapy. Psychol Med 2002; 32:763–782 [E]
159. Lehman AF: Vocational rehabilitation in schizophrenia. Schizophr Bull 1995; 21:645–656 [G]
160. Drake RE, McHugo GJ, Becker DR, Anthony WA, Clark RE: The New Hampshire study of supported employment for people with severe mental illness. J Consult Clin Psychol 1996; 64:391–399 [A–]
161. Drake RE, Mueser KT, Clark RE, Wallach M: The course, treatment, and outcome of substance disorder in persons with severe mental illness. Am J Orthopsychiatry 1996; 66:42–51 [F]
162. Lehman AF, Goldberg R, Dixon LB, McNary S, Postrado L, Hackman A, McDonnell K: Improving employment outcomes for persons with severe mental illnesses. Arch Gen Psychiatry 2002; 59:165–172 [A]
163. Scott JE, Dixon LB: Psychological interventions for schizophrenia. Schizophr Bull 1995; 21:621–630 [G]
164. Lehman AF, Dixon LB, Kernan E, DeForge BR, Postrado LT: A randomized trial of assertive community treatment for homeless persons with severe mental illness. Arch Gen Psychiatry 1997; 54:1038–1043 [A–]
165. Salkever D, Domino ME, Burns BJ, Santos AB, Deci PA, Dias J, Wagner HR, Faldowski RA, Paolone J: Assertive community treatment for people with severe mental illness: the effect on hospital use and costs. Health Serv Res 1999; 34:577–601 [A–]

166. Rosenheck RA, Dennis D: Time-limited assertive community treatment for homeless persons with severe mental illness. Arch Gen Psychiatry 2001; 58:1073–1080 [B]
167. Heinssen RK, Liberman RP, Kopelowicz A: Psychosocial skills training for schizophrenia: lessons from the laboratory. Schizophr Bull 2000; 26:21–46 [F]
168. Pilling S, Bebbington P, Kuipers E, Garety P, Geddes J, Martindale B, Orbach G, Morgan C: Psychological treatments in schizophrenia: II. meta-analyses of randomized controlled trials of social skills training and cognitive remediation. Psychol Med 2002; 32:783–791 [E]
169. Bellack A: Social skills training, in Comprehensive Textbook of Psychiatry, 8th ed. Edited by Sadock BJ, Sadock VA. Philadelphia, Lippincott Williams & Wilkins (in press) [F]
170. Dickerson FB: Cognitive behavioral psychotherapy for schizophrenia: a review of recent empirical studies. Schizophr Res 2000; 43:71–90 [F]
171. Dixon LB, Lehman AF: Family interventions for schizophrenia. Schizophr Bull 1995; 21: 631–643 [F]
172. Dixon L, Adams C, Lucksted A: Update on family psychoeducation for schizophrenia. Schizophr Bull 2000; 26:5–20 [F]
173. Hogarty GE, Anderson CM, Reiss DJ, Kornblith SJ, Greenwald DP, Ulrich RF, Carter M, Environmental-Personal Indicators in the Course of Schizophrenia (EPICS) Research Group: Family psychoeducation, social skills training, and maintenance chemotherapy in the aftercare treatment of schizophrenia: II. two-year effects of a controlled study on relapse and adjustment. Arch Gen Psychiatry 1991; 48:340–347 [A–]
174. Falloon IR, Boyd JL, McGill CW, Williamson M, Razani J, Moss HB, Gilderman AM, Simpson GM: Family management in the prevention of morbidity of schizophrenia: clinical outcome of a two-year longitudinal study. Arch Gen Psychiatry 1985; 42:887–896 [A, B]
175. Leff J, Kuipers L, Berkowitz R, Sturgeon D: A controlled trial of social intervention in the families of schizophrenic patients: two year follow-up. Br J Psychiatry 1985; 146:594–600 [C]
176. Tarrier N, Barrowclough C, Vaughn C, Bamrah JS, Porceddu K, Watts S, Freeman H: Community management of schizophrenia: a two-year follow-up of a behavioural intervention with families. Br J Psychiatry 1989; 154:625–628 [A–]
177. Leff J, Berkowitz R, Shavit N, Strachan A, Glass I, Vaughn C: A trial of family therapy versus a relatives' group for schizophrenia: two-year follow-up. Br J Psychiatry 1990; 157: 571–577 [B]
178. McFarlane WR, Lukens E, Link B, Dushay R, Deakins SA, Newmark M, Dunne EJ, Horen B, Toran J: Multiple-family groups and psychoeducation in the treatment of schizophrenia. Arch Gen Psychiatry 1995; 52:679–687 [A–]
179. McFarlane WR, Dushay RA, Stastny P, Deakins SM, Link B: A comparison of two levels of family-aided assertive community treatment. Psychiatr Serv 1996; 47:744–750 [A–]
180. Montero I, Asencio A, Hernandez I, Masanet MJ, Lacruz M, Bellver F, Iborra M, Ruiz I: Two strategies for family intervention in schizophrenia: a randomized trial in a Mediterranean environment. Schizophr Bull 2001; 27:661–670 [A–]
181. Stein LI, Test MA: Alternative to mental hospital treatment: I. conceptual model, treatment program, and clinical evaluation. Arch Gen Psychiatry 1980; 37:392–397 [B]
182. Marx AJ, Test MA, Stein LI: Extrohospital management of severe mental illness: feasibility and effects of social functioning. Arch Gen Psychiatry 1973; 29:505–511 [B]
183. Scott JE, Dixon LB: Assertive community treatment and case management for schizophrenia. Schizophr Bull 1995; 21:657–668 [F]
184. Mueser KT, Bond GR, Drake RE, Resnick SG: Models of community care for severe mental illness: a review of research on case management. Schizophr Bull 1998; 24:37–74 [F]
185. Hogarty GE, Kornblith SJ, Greenwald D, DiBarry AL, Cooley S, Ulrich RF, Carter M, Flesher S: Three-year trials of personal therapy among schizophrenic patients living with or independent of family, I: description of study and effects on relapse rates. Am J Psychiatry 1997; 154:1504–1513 [A–]

186. Hogarty GE, Greenwald D, Ulrich RF, Kornblith SJ, DiBarry AL, Cooley S, Carter M, Flesher S: Three-year trials of personal therapy among schizophrenic patients living with or independent of family, II: effects on adjustment of patients. Am J Psychiatry 1997; 154: 1514–1524 [A–]
187. Hogarty GE: Personal Therapy for Schizophrenia and Related Disorders. New York, Guilford, 2002 [G]
188. Rector NA, Beck AT: Cognitive behavioral therapy for schizophrenia: an empirical review. J Nerv Ment Dis 2001; 189:278–287 [E]
189. Dyck DG, Short RA, Hendryx MS, Norell D, Myers M, Patterson T, McDonell MG, Voss WD, McFarlane WR: Management of negative symptoms among patients with schizophrenia attending multiple-family groups. Psychiatr Serv 2000; 51:513–519 [A–]
190. Anthony WA, Rogers ES, Cohen M, Davies RR: Relationships between psychiatric symptomatology, work skills, and future vocational performance. Psychiatr Serv 1995; 46:353–358 [C]
191. Carpenter WT Jr, Buchanan RW: Schizophrenia. N Engl J Med 1994; 330:681–690 [G]
192. Bond G, Drake RE, Becker D, Mueser K: Effectiveness of psychiatric rehabilitation approaches for employment of people with severe mental illness. J Disability Policy Studies 1999; 10:18–52 [F]
193. Bond GR, Drake RE, Mueser KT, Becker DR: An update on supported employment for people with severe mental illness. Psychiatr Serv 1997; 48:335–346 [F]
194. Bond GR, Becker DR, Drake RE, Rapp CA, Meisler N, Lehman AF, Bell MD, Blyler CR: Implementing supported employment as an evidence-based practice. Psychiatr Serv 2001; 52:313–322 [G]
195. Gold JM, Goldberg RW, McNary SW, Dixon LB, Lehman AF: Cognitive correlates of job tenure among patients with severe mental illness. Am J Psychiatry 2002; 159:1395–1402 [A–]
196. Gartner AJ, Riessman F: Self-help and mental health. Hosp Community Psychiatry 1982; 33:631–635 [G]
197. Davidson L, Chinman M, Kloos B, Weingarten R, Stayner D, Tebes J: Peer support among individuals with severe mental illness: a review of the evidence. Clinical Psychology: Science and Practice 1999; 6:165–187 [F]
198. Raiff N: Some health related outcomes of self-help participation: Recovery, Inc as a case example of a self-help organization in mental health, in The Self-Help Revolution. Edited by Gartner A, Reissman F. New York, Human Sciences Press, 1984, pp 183–193 [G]
199. Rappaport J: Narrative studies, personal stories, and identity transformation in the mutual help context. J Applied Behav Sci 1993; 29:239–256 [G]
200. Powell TJ, Yeaton W, Hill EM, Silk KR: Predictors of psychosocial outcomes for patients with mood disorders: the effects of self-help group participation. Psychiatr Rehabil J 2001; 25:3–11 [G]
201. Center for Mental Health Services: Consumer/Survivor-Operated Self-Help Programs: A Technical Report. Rockville, Md, Center for Mental Health Services, 1998 [G]
202. Stroul B: Rehabilitation in community support systems, in Psychiatric Rehabilitation in Practice. Edited by Flexer R, Solomon P. Boston, Andover Medical, 1993 [G]
203. Solomon P, Draine J: The state of knowledge of the effectiveness of consumer provided services. Psychiatr Rehabil J 2001; 25:20–27 [G]
204. Simpson EL, House AO: Involving users in the delivery and evaluation of mental health services: systematic review. Br Med J 2002; 325:1265 [F]
205. Edmunson E, Bedell J, Archer R, Gordon R: Integrating skill building and peer support in mental health treatment: the Early Intervention and Community Network Development Projects, in Community Mental Health and Behavioral Ecology. Edited by Jeger M, Slotnick R. New York, Plenum, 1982, pp 127–139 [G]
206. Nikkel RE, Smith G, Edwards D: A consumer-operated case management project. Hosp Community Psychiatry 1992; 43:577–579 [G]

207. Klein A, Cnaan RA, Whitecraft J: Significance of peer social support for dually diagnosed clients: findings from pilot study. Res Soc Work Pract 1998; 8:529–551 [G]
208. Clarke GN, Herinckx HA, Kinney RF, Paulson RI, Cutler DL, Lewis K, Oxman E: Psychiatric hospitalizations, arrests, emergency room visits, and homelessness of clients with serious and persistent mental illness: findings from a randomized trial of two ACT programs vs usual care. Ment Health Serv Res 2000; 2:155–164 [A–]
209. Chinman MJ, Weingarten R, Stayner D, Davidson L: Chronicity reconsidered: improving person-environment fit through a consumer-run service. Community Ment Health J 2001; 37:215–229 [G]
210. Rabiner CJ, Wegner JT, Kane JM: Outcome study of first-episode psychosis. I: relapse rates after 1 year. Am J Psychiatry 1986; 143:1155–1158 [C]
211. Kane JM, Rifkin A, Quitkin F, Nayak D, Ramos-Lorenzi J: Fluphenazine vs placebo in patients with remitted, acute first-episode schizophrenia. Arch Gen Psychiatry 1982; 39: 70–73 [A]
212. Crow TJ, MacMillan JF, Johnson AL, Johnstone EC: A randomised controlled trial of prophylactic neuroleptic treatment. Br J Psychiatry 1986; 148:120–127 [A–]
213. McCreadie RG, Wiles D, Grant S, Crockett GT, Mahmood Z, Livingston MG, Watt JA, Greene JG, Kershaw PW, Todd NA (Scottish Schizophrenia Research Group): The Scottish first episode schizophrenia study: VII. two-year follow-up. Acta Psychiatr Scand 1989; 80: 597–602 [C]
214. Gilbert PL, Harris MJ, McAdams LA, Jeste DV: Neuroleptic withdrawal in schizophrenic patients: a review of the literature. Arch Gen Psychiatry 1995; 52:173–188 [F]
215. Leucht S, Barnes TR, Kissling W, Engel RR, Correll C, Kane JM: Relapse prevention in schizophrenia with new-generation antipsychotics: a systematic review and exploratory meta-analysis of randomized, controlled trials. Am J Psychiatry 2003; 160:1209–1222 [A]
216. Schooler NR: Maintenance medication for schizophrenia: strategies for dose reduction. Schizophr Bull 1991; 17:311–324 [F, G]
217. Csernansky JG, Schuchart EK: Relapse and rehospitalisation rates in patients with schizophrenia: effects of second generation antipsychotics. CNS Drugs 2002; 16:473–484 [G]
218. Gitlin M, Nuechterlein K, Subotnik KL, Ventura J, Mintz J, Fogelson DL, Bartzokis G, Aravagiri M: Clinical outcome following neuroleptic discontinuation in patients with remitted recent-onset schizophrenia. Am J Psychiatry 2001; 158:1835–1842 [B]
219. Schooler NR, Keith SJ, Severe JB, Matthews SM, Bellack AS, Glick ID, Hargreaves WA, Kane JM, Ninan PT, Frances A, Jacobs M, Lieberman JA, Mance R, Simpson GM, Woerner MG: Relapse and rehospitalization during maintenance treatment of schizophrenia: the effects of dose reduction and family treatment. Arch Gen Psychiatry 1997; 54:453–463 [A]
220. Herz MI, Lamberti JS, Mintz J, Scott R, O'Dell SP, McCartan L, Nix G: A program for relapse prevention in schizophrenia: a controlled study. Arch Gen Psychiatry 2000; 57:277–283 [A–]
221. Berman I, Sapers BL, Chang HH, Losonczy MF, Schmildler J, Green AI: Treatment of obsessive-compulsive symptoms in schizophrenic patients with clomipramine. J Clin Psychopharmacol 1995; 15:206–210 [A]
222. Levinson DF, Umapathy C, Musthaq M: Treatment of schizoaffective disorder and schizophrenia with mood symptoms. Am J Psychiatry 1999; 156:1138–1148 [F]
223. Reznik I, Sirota P: An open study of fluvoxamine augmentation of neuroleptics in schizophrenia with obsessive and compulsive symptoms. Clin Neuropharmacol 2000; 23: 157–160 [C]
224. Wolkowitz OM, Pickar D: Benzodiazepines in the treatment of schizophrenia: a review and reappraisal. Am J Psychiatry 1991; 148:714–726 [B]
225. Soares KV, McGrath JJ: Vitamin E for neuroleptic-induced tardive dyskinesia. Cochrane Database Syst Rev 2001; (4):CD000209 [E]

226. Adler LA, Rotrosen J, Edson R, Lavori P, Lohr J, Hitzemann R, Raisch D, Caligiuri M, Tracy K (Veterans Affairs Cooperative Study #394 Study Group): Vitamin E treatment for tardive dyskinesia. Arch Gen Psychiatry 1999; 56:836–841 [A]
227. Swoboda E, Conca A, Konig P, Waanders R, Hansen M: Maintenance electroconvulsive therapy in affective and schizoaffective disorder. Neuropsychobiology 2001; 43:23–28 [D]
228. Stiebel VG: Maintenance electroconvulsive therapy for chronic mentally ill patients: a case series. Psychiatr Serv 1995; 46:265–268 [G]
229. Chanpattana W, Chakrabhand ML, Sackeim HA, Kitaroonchai W, Kongsakon R, Techakasem P, Buppanharun W, Tuntirungsee Y, Kirdcharoen N: Continuation ECT in treatment-resistant schizophrenia: a controlled study. J ECT 1999; 15:178–192 [A–]
230. Rosenheck R, Evans D, Herz L, Cramer J, Xu W, Thomas J, Henderson W, Charney D: How long to wait for a response to clozapine: a comparison of time course of response to clozapine and conventional antipsychotic medication in refractory schizophrenia. Schizophr Bull 1999; 25:709–719 [A]
231. Marder SR, Glynn SM, Wirshing WC, Wirshing DA, Ross D, Widmark C, Mintz J, Liberman RP, Blair KE: Maintenance treatment of schizophrenia with risperidone or haloperidol: 2-year outcomes. Am J Psychiatry 2003; 160:1405–1412 [A]
232. Henderson DC, Goff DC: Risperidone as an adjunct to clozapine therapy in chronic schizophrenics. J Clin Psychiatry 1996; 57:395–397 [C]
233. Mowerman S, Siris SG: Adjunctive loxapine in a clozapine-resistant cohort of schizophrenic patients. Ann Clin Psychiatry 1996; 8:193–197 [C]
234. Friedman J, Ault K, Powchik P: Pimozide augmentation for the treatment of schizophrenic patients who are partial responders to clozapine. Biol Psychiatry 1997; 42:522–523 [D]
235. Dose M, Hellweg R, Yassouridis A, Theison M, Emrich HM: Combined treatment of schizophrenic psychoses with haloperidol and valproate. Pharmacopsychiatry 1998; 31:122–125 [A]
236. Hesslinger B, Normann C, Langosch JM, Klose P, Berger M, Walden J: Effects of carbamazepine and valproate on haloperidol plasma levels and on psychopathologic outcome in schizophrenic patients. J Clin Psychopharmacol 1999; 19:310–315 [A]
237. Casey DE, Daniel DG, Wassef AA, Tracy KA, Wozniak P, Sommerville KW: Effect of divalproex combined with olanzapine or risperidone in patients with an acute exacerbation of schizophrenia. Neuropsychopharmacology 2003; 28:182–192 [A]
238. Tsai G, Yang P, Chung LC, Lange N, Coyle JT: d-Serine added to antipsychotics for the treatment of schizophrenia. Biol Psychiatry 1998; 44:1081–1089 [A]
239. Javitt DC, Zylberman I, Zukin SR, Heresco-Levy U, Lindenmayer JP: Amelioration of negative symptoms in schizophrenia by glycine. Am J Psychiatry 1994; 151:1234–1236 [A]
240. Heresco-Levy U, Javitt DC, Ermilov M, Mordel C, Horowitz A, Kelly D: Double-blind, placebo-controlled, crossover trial of glycine adjuvant therapy for treatment-resistant schizophrenia. Br J Psychiatry 1996; 169:610–617 [A]
241. Evins AE, Fitzgerald SM, Wine L, Rosselli R, Goff DC: Placebo-controlled trial of glycine added to clozapine in schizophrenia. Am J Psychiatry 2000; 157:826–828 [A]
242. Javitt DC, Silipo G, Cienfuegos A, Shelley AM, Bark N, Park M, Lindenmayer JP, Suckow R, Zukin SR: Adjunctive high-dose glycine in the treatment of schizophrenia. Int J Neuropsychopharmacol 2001; 4:385–391 [B]
243. Goff DC, Henderson DC, Evins AE, Amico E: A placebo-controlled crossover trial of D-cycloserine added to clozapine in patients with schizophrenia. Biol Psychiatry 1999; 45: 512–514 [A–]
244. Goff DC, Tsai G, Levitt J, Amico E, Manoach D, Schoenfeld DA, Hayden DL, McCarley R, Coyle JT: A placebo-controlled trial of D-cycloserine added to conventional neuroleptics in patients with schizophrenia. Arch Gen Psychiatry 1999; 56:21–27 [A]
245. Evins AE, Amico E, Posever TA, Toker R, Goff DC: D-Cycloserine added to risperidone in patients with primary negative symptoms of schizophrenia. Schizophr Res 2002; 56:19–23 [B]

246. Heresco-Levy U, Ermilov M, Shimoni J, Shapira B, Silipo G, Javitt DC: Placebo-controlled trial of D-cycloserine added to conventional neuroleptics, olanzapine, or risperidone in schizophrenia. Am J Psychiatry 2002; 159:480–482 [A]
247. Risch SC, McGurk S, Horner MD, Nahas Z, Owens SD, Molloy M, Gilliard C, Christie S, Markowitz JS, DeVane CL, Mintzer J, George MS: A double-blind placebo-controlled case study of the use of donepezil to improve cognition in a schizoaffective disorder patient: functional MRI correlates. Neurocase 2001; 7:105–110 [G]
248. Friedman JI, Adler DN, Howanitz E, Harvey PD, Brenner G, Temporini H, White L, Parrella M, Davis KL: A double blind placebo controlled trial of donepezil adjunctive treatment to risperidone for the cognitive impairment of schizophrenia. Biol Psychiatry 2002; 51:349–357 [A]
249. Buchanan RW, Summerfelt A, Tek C, Gold J: An open-labeled trial of adjunctive donepezil for cognitive impairments in patients with schizophrenia. Schizophr Res 2003; 59:29–33 [B]
250. Bark N, Revheim N, Huq F, Khalderov V, Ganz ZW, Medalia A: The impact of cognitive remediation on psychiatric symptoms of schizophrenia. Schizophr Res 2003; 63:229–235 [B]
251. Lieberman JA, Fenton WS: Delayed detection of psychosis: causes, consequences, and effect on public health. Am J Psychiatry 2000; 157:1727–1730 [G]
252. Loebel AD, Lieberman JA, Alvir JM, Mayerhoff DI, Geisler SH, Szymanski SR: Duration of psychosis and outcome in first-episode schizophrenia. Am J Psychiatry 1992; 149:1183–1188 [C]
253. McGlashan TH, Johannessen JO: Early detection and intervention with schizophrenia: rationale. Schizophr Bull 1996; 22:201–222 [G]
254. McGlashan TH: Duration of untreated psychosis in first-episode schizophrenia: marker or determinant of course? Biol Psychiatry 1999; 46:899–907 [G]
255. Haas GL, Garratt LS, Sweeney JA: Delay to first antipsychotic medication in schizophrenia: impact on symptomatology and clinical course of illness. J Psychiatr Res 1998; 32:151–159 [G]
256. Larsen TK, Johannessen JO, Opjordsmoen S: First-episode schizophrenia with long duration of untreated psychosis: pathways to care. Br J Psychiatry Suppl 1998; 172(33):40–45 [G]
257. Lieberman JA, Perkins D, Belger A, Chakos M, Jarskog F, Boteva K, Gilmore J: The early stages of schizophrenia: speculations on pathogenesis, pathophysiology, and therapeutic approaches. Biol Psychiatry 2001; 50:884–897 [G]
258. MacMillan JF, Crow TJ, Johnson AL, Johnstone EC: Short-term outcome in trial entrants and trial eligible patients. Br J Psychiatry 1986; 148:128–133 [G]
259. Haas GL, Sweeney JA: Premorbid and onset features of first-episode schizophrenia. Schizophr Bull 1992; 18:373–386 [G]
260. Beiser M, Erickson D, Fleming JA, Iacono WG: Establishing the onset of psychotic illness. Am J Psychiatry 1993; 150:1349–1354 [G]
261. Larsen TK, McGlashan TH, Moe LC: First-episode schizophrenia, I: early course parameters. Schizophr Bull 1996; 22:241–256 [F]
262. McGorry PD, Yung AR, Phillips LJ, Yuen HP, Francey S, Cosgrave EM, Germano D, Bravin J, McDonald T, Blair A, Adlard S, Jackson H: Randomized controlled trial of interventions designed to reduce the risk of progression to first-episode psychosis in a clinical sample with subthreshold symptoms. Arch Gen Psychiatry 2002; 59:921–928 [A–]
263. McGlashan TH, Zipursky RB, Perkins D, Addington J, Miller TJ, Woods SW, Hawkins KA, Hoffman R, Lindborg S, Tohen M, Breier A: The PRIME North America randomized double-blind clinical trial of olanzapine versus placebo in patients at risk of being prodromally symptomatic for psychosis, I: study rationale and design. Schizophr Res 2003; 61:7–18 [G]
264. Woods SW, Breier A, Zipursky RB, Perkins DO, Addington J, Miller TJ, Hawkins KA, Marquez E, Lindborg SR, Tohen M, McGlashan TH: Randomized trial of olanzapine vs placebo in the symptomatic acute treatment of the schizophrenic prodrome. Biol Psychiatry 2003; 54:453–464 [A]

265. McGorry PD, Chanen A, McCarthy E, Van Riel R, McKenzie D, Singh BS: Posttraumatic stress disorder following recent-onset psychosis: an unrecognized postpsychotic syndrome. J Nerv Ment Dis 1991; 179:253–258 [C]
266. Kaufmann CA, Wyatt RJ: Neuroleptic malignant syndrome, in Psychopharmacology: The Third Generation of Progress. Edited by Meltzer HY. New York, Raven, 1987, pp 1421–1430 [G]
267. Lieberman JA: Prediction of outcome in first-episode schizophrenia. J Clin Psychiatry 1993; 54(suppl):13–17 [C]
268. Lieberman JA, Koreen AR, Chakos M, Sheitman B, Woerner M, Alvir JM, Bilder R: Factors influencing treatment response and outcome of first-episode schizophrenia: implications for understanding the pathophysiology of schizophrenia. J Clin Psychiatry 1996; 57(suppl 9):5–9 [G]
269. Dequardo JR: Pharmacologic treatment of first-episode schizophrenia: early intervention is key to outcome. J Clin Psychiatry 1998; 59(suppl 19):9–17 [G]
270. Remington G, Kapur S, Zipursky RB: Pharmacotherapy of first-episode schizophrenia. Br J Psychiatry Suppl 1998; 172(33):66–70 [F]
271. Emsley RA, Risperidone Working Group: Risperidone in the treatment of first-episode psychotic patients: a double-blind multicenter study. Schizophr Bull 1999; 25:721–729 [A]
272. Sanger TM, Lieberman JA, Tohen M, Grundy S, Beasley C Jr, Tollefson GD: Olanzapine versus haloperidol treatment in first-episode psychosis. Am J Psychiatry 1999; 156:79–87 [A]
273. O'Toole M, Taylor T, Ohlsen RI, Jones HM, Purvis RG, Szmukler G, Pilowsky LS: Quetiapine treatment of first-episode psychosis—The Southwark First Onset Psychosis Service (FIRST)—A preliminary audit of psychotic symptoms. Schizophr Res 2002; 53(suppl 1):181–182 [B]
274. Lieberman JA, Alvir JM, Koreen A, Geisler S, Chakos M, Sheitman B, Woerner M: Psychobiologic correlates of treatment response in schizophrenia. Neuropsychopharmacology 1996; 14:13S–21S [G]
275. Zhang-Wong J, Zipursky RB, Beiser M, Bean G: Optimal haloperidol dosage in first-episode psychosis. Can J Psychiatry 1999; 44:164–167 [B]
276. Oosthuizen P, Emsley RA, Turner J, Keyter N: Determining the optimal dose of haloperidol in first-episode psychosis. J Psychopharmacol 2001; 15:251–255 [B]
277. Merlo MC, Hofer H, Gekle W, Berger G, Ventura J, Panhuber I, Latour G, Marder SR: Risperidone, 2 mg/day vs 4 mg/day, in first-episode, acutely psychotic patients: treatment efficacy and effects on fine motor functioning. J Clin Psychiatry 2002; 63:885–891 [A]
278. Kopala LC, Good KP, Honer WG: Extrapyramidal signs and clinical symptoms in first-episode schizophrenia: response to low-dose risperidone. J Clin Psychopharmacol 1997; 17:308–313 [G]
279. Lieberman JA, Tollefson G, Tohen M, Green AI, Gur RE, Kahn R, McEvoy J, Perkins D, Sharma T, Zipursky R, Wei H, Hamer RM: Comparative efficacy and safety of atypical and conventional antipsychotic drugs in first-episode psychosis: a randomized, double-blind trial of olanzapine versus haloperidol. Am J Psychiatry 2003; 160:1396–1404 [A]
280. Lieberman J, Chakos M, Wu H, Alvir J, Hoffman E, Robinson D, Bilder R: Longitudinal study of brain morphology in first episode schizophrenia. Biol Psychiatry 2001; 49:487–499 [C]
281. Robinson DG, Woerner MG, Alvir JM, Geisler S, Koreen A, Sheitman B, Chakos M, Mayerhoff D, Bilder R, Goldman R, Lieberman JA: Predictors of treatment response from a first episode of schizophrenia or schizoaffective disorder. Am J Psychiatry 1999; 156:544–549 [C]
282. McGlashan TH: The prediction of outcome in chronic schizophrenia, IV: the Chestnut Lodge follow-up study. Arch Gen Psychiatry 1986; 43:167–176 [C, D]
283. Kavanagh DJ: Recent developments in expressed emotion and schizophrenia. Br J Psychiatry 1992; 160:601–620 [F, G]

284. Mueser KT, Gingerich SL, Rosenthal CK: Familial factors in psychiatry. Curr Opin Psychiatry 1993; 6:251–257 [G]
285. Beels CC, Gutwirth L, Berkeley J, Struening E: Measurements of social support in schizophrenia. Schizophr Bull 1984; 10:399–411 [G]
286. Doane JA, West KL, Goldstein MJ, Rodnick EH, Jones JE: Parental communication deviance and affective style: predictors of subsequent schizophrenia spectrum disorders in vulnerable adolescents. Arch Gen Psychiatry 1981; 38:679–685 [E, G]
287. Leff J, Vaughn C: The role of maintenance therapy and relatives' expressed emotion in relapse of schizophrenia: a two-year follow-up. Br J Psychiatry 1981; 139:102–104 [C]
288. Vaughn CE, Snyder KS, Jones S, Freeman WB, Falloon IR: Family factors in schizophrenic relapse: replication in California of British research on expressed emotion. Arch Gen Psychiatry 1984; 41:1169–1177 [C, D]
289. Hogarty GE: Depot neuroleptics: the relevance of psychosocial factors—a United States perspective. J Clin Psychiatry 1984; 45:36–42 [F]
290. American Academy of Child and Adolescent Psychiatry: Practice Parameter for the Assessment and Treatment of Children and Adolescents With Schizophrenia. J Am Acad Child Adolesc Psychiatry 2001; 40:4S–23S [G]
291. DeLisi LE, Sakuma M, Tew W, Kushner M, Hoff AL, Grimson R: Schizophrenia as a chronic active brain process: a study of progressive brain structural change subsequent to the onset of schizophrenia. Psychiatry Res 1997; 74:129–140 [C]
292. Cahn W, Pol HE, Lems EB, van Haren NE, Schnack HG, van der Linden JA, Schothorst PF, van Engeland H, Kahn RS: Brain volume changes in first-episode schizophrenia: a 1-year follow-up study. Arch Gen Psychiatry 2002; 59:1002–1010 [C]
293. Ho BC, Andreasen NC, Nopoulos P, Arndt S, Magnotta V, Flaum M: Progressive structural brain abnormalities and their relationship to clinical outcome: a longitudinal magnetic resonance imaging study early in schizophrenia. Arch Gen Psychiatry 2003; 60:585–594 [C]
294. Kissling W: Guidelines for Neuroleptic Relapse Prevention in Schizophrenia. Berlin, Springer-Verlag, 1991 [F, G]
295. Tauscher-Wisniewski S, Zipursky RB: The role of maintenance pharmacotherapy in achieving recovery from a first episode of schizophrenia. Int Rev Psychiatry 2002; 14:284–292 [G]
296. Perkins DO, Nieri J, Kazmer J: Clinical interactions with patients and families, in Comprehensive Care of Schizophrenia: A Textbook of Clinical Management. Edited by Lieberman JA, Murray R. London, Martin Dunitz, 2001 [G]
297. Carpenter WT Jr, Heinrichs DW, Wagman AM: Deficit and nondeficit forms of schizophrenia: the concept. Am J Psychiatry 1988; 145:578–583 [G]
298. Mayerhoff DI, Loebel AD, Alvir JM, Szymanski SR, Geisler SH, Borenstein M, Lieberman JA: The deficit state in first-episode schizophrenia. Am J Psychiatry 1994; 151:1417–1422 [C]
299. McGlashan TH: The profiles of clinical deterioration in schizophrenia. J Psychiatr Res 1998; 32:133–141 [G]
300. Hafner H, Loffler W, Maurer K, Hambrecht M, an der Heiden W: Depression, negative symptoms, social stagnation and social decline in the early course of schizophrenia. Acta Psychiatr Scand 1999; 100:105–118 [C]
301. Hafner H: Onset and early course as determinants of the further course of schizophrenia. Acta Psychiatr Scand Suppl 2000; 102:44–48 [D]
302. Harris MJ, Jeste DV, Krull A, Montague J, Heaton RK: Deficit syndrome in older schizophrenic patients. Psychiatry Res 1991; 39:285–292 [D]
303. Fenton WS, McGlashan TH: Natural history of schizophrenia subtypes, II: positive and negative symptoms and long-term course. Arch Gen Psychiatry 1991; 48:978–986 [C]
304. McGlashan TH, Fenton WS: Subtype progression and pathophysiologic deterioration in early schizophrenia. Schizophr Bull 1993; 19:71–84 [C, D]

305. Hori A, Tsunashima K, Watanabe K, Takekawa Y, Ishihara I, Terada T, Uno M: Symptom classification of schizophrenia changes with the duration of illness. Acta Psychiatr Scand 1999; 99:447–452 [G]
306. Bottlender R, Jager M, Groll C, Strauss A, Moller HJ: Deficit states in schizophrenia and their association with the length of illness and gender. Eur Arch Psychiatry Clin Neurosci 2001; 251:272–278 [G]
307. Larsen TK, McGlashan TH, Johannessen JO, Vibe-Hansen L: First-episode schizophrenia, II: premorbid patterns by gender. Schizophr Bull 1996; 22:257–269 [G]
308. Schultz SK, Miller DD, Oliver SE, Arndt S, Flaum M, Andreasen NC: The life course of schizophrenia: age and symptom dimensions. Schizophr Res 1997; 23:15–23 [G]
309. Roy MA, Maziade M, Labbe A, Merette C: Male gender is associated with deficit schizophrenia: a meta-analysis. Schizophr Res 2001; 47:141–147 [E]
310. Galderisi S, Maj M, Mucci A, Cassano GB, Invernizzi G, Rossi A, Vita A, Dell'Osso L, Daneluzzo E, Pini S: Historical, psychopathological, neurological, and neuropsychological aspects of deficit schizophrenia: a multicenter study. Am J Psychiatry 2002; 159:983–990 [D]
311. Carpenter WT Jr, Heinrichs DW, Alphs LD: Treatment of negative symptoms. Schizophr Bull 1985; 11:440–452 [G]
312. Kelley ME, van Kammen DP, Allen DN: Empirical validation of primary negative symptoms: independence from effects of medication and psychosis. Am J Psychiatry 1999; 156:406–411 [G]
313. Kane J, Honigfeld G, Singer J, Meltzer H: Clozapine for the treatment-resistant schizophrenic: a double-blind comparison with chlorpromazine. Arch Gen Psychiatry 1988; 45: 789–796 [A]
314. Buchanan RW, Breier A, Kirkpatrick B, Ball P, Carpenter WT Jr: Positive and negative symptom response to clozapine in schizophrenic patients with and without the deficit syndrome. Am J Psychiatry 1998; 155:751–760 [A]
315. Rosenheck R, Dunn L, Peszke M, Cramer J, Xu W, Thomas J, Charney D (Department of Veterans Affairs Cooperative Study Group on Clozapine in Refractory Schizophrenia): Impact of clozapine on negative symptoms and on the deficit syndrome in refractory schizophrenia. Am J Psychiatry 1999; 156:88–93 [A]
316. Paillere-Martinot ML, Lecrubier Y, Martinot JL, Aubin F: Improvement of some schizophrenic deficit symptoms with low doses of amisulpride. Am J Psychiatry 1995; 152:130–134 [A]
317. Loo H, Poirier-Littre MF, Theron M, Rein W, Fleurot O: Amisulpride versus placebo in the medium-term treatment of the negative symptoms of schizophrenia. Br J Psychiatry 1997; 170:18–22 [A]
318. Small JG, Hirsch SR, Arvanitis LA, Miller BG, Link CG (Seroquel Study Group): Quetiapine in patients with schizophrenia: a high- and low-dose double-blind comparison with placebo. Arch Gen Psychiatry 1997; 54:549–557 [A]
319. Tollefson GD, Beasley CM Jr, Tran PV, Street JS, Krueger JA, Tamura RN, Graffeo KA, Thieme ME: Olanzapine versus haloperidol in the treatment of schizophrenia and schizoaffective and schizophreniform disorders: results of an international collaborative trial. Am J Psychiatry 1997; 154:457–465 [A]
320. Moller HJ: Atypical neuroleptics: a new approach in the treatment of negative symptoms. Eur Arch Psychiatry Clin Neurosci 1999; 249(suppl 4):99–107 [G]
321. Storosum JG, Elferink AJ, van Zwieten BJ, van Strik R, Hoogendijk WJ, Broekmans AW: Amisulpride: is there a treatment for negative symptoms in schizophrenia patients? Schizophr Bull 2002; 28:193–201 [E]
322. Carman J, Peuskens J, Vangeneugden A: Risperidone in the treatment of negative symptoms of schizophrenia: a meta-analysis. Int Clin Psychopharmacol 1995; 10:207–213 [E]
323. Kopelowicz A, Zarate R, Tripodis K, Gonzalez V, Mintz J: Differential efficacy of olanzapine for deficit and nondeficit negative symptoms in schizophrenia. Am J Psychiatry 2000; 157: 987–993 [B]

324. Regier DA, Farmer ME, Rae DS, Locke BZ, Keith SJ, Judd LL, Goodwin FK: Comorbidity of mental disorders with alcohol and other drug abuse: results from the Epidemiologic Catchment Area (ECA) Study. JAMA 1990; 264:2511–2518 [G]
325. Alterman AI, Erdlen DL, Laporte DJ, Erdlen FR: Effects of illicit drug use in an inpatient psychiatric population. Addict Behav 1982; 7:231–242 [D]
326. Barbee JG, Clark PD, Crapanzano MS, Heintz GC, Kehoe CE: Alcohol and substance abuse among schizophrenic patients presenting to an emergency psychiatric service. J Nerv Ment Dis 1989; 177:400–407 [G]
327. Drake RE, Osher FC, Wallach MA: Alcohol use and abuse in schizophrenia: a prospective community study. J Nerv Ment Dis 1989; 177:408–414 [C, E]
328. Mueser KT, Yarnold PR, Bellack AS: Diagnostic and demographic correlates of substance abuse in schizophrenia and major affective disorder. Acta Psychiatr Scand 1992; 85:48–55 [D]
329. Fowler IL, Carr VJ, Carter NT, Lewin TJ: Patterns of current and lifetime substance use in schizophrenia. Schizophr Bull 1998; 24:443–455 [G]
330. Drake RE, Osher FC, Noordsy DL, Hurlbut SC, Teague GB, Beaudett MS: Diagnosis of alcohol use disorders in schizophrenia. Schizophr Bull 1990; 16:57–67 [D]
331. Mathalon DH, Pfefferbaum A, Lim KO, Rosenbloom MJ, Sullivan EV: Compounded brain volume deficits in schizophrenia-alcoholism comorbidity. Arch Gen Psychiatry 2003; 60:245–252 [D]
332. Kivlahan DR, Heiman JR, Wright RC, Mundt JW, Shupe JA: Treatment cost and rehospitalization rate in schizophrenic outpatients with a history of substance abuse. Hosp Community Psychiatry 1990; 42:609–614 [D]
333. Rosenberg SD, Goodman LA, Osher FC, Swartz MS, Essock SM, Butterfield MI, Constantine NT, Wolford GL, Salyers MP: Prevalence of HIV, hepatitis B, and hepatitis C in people with severe mental illness. Am J Public Health 2001; 91:31–37 [G]
334. Addington J, Addington D: Effect of substance misuse in early psychosis. Br J Psychiatry Suppl 1998; 172:134–136 [D]
335. Alterman AI, Ayre FR, Williford WO: Diagnostic validation of conjoint schizophrenia and alcoholism. J Clin Psychiatry 1984; 45:300–303 [G]
336. Breakey WR, Goodell H, Lorenz PC, McHugh PR: Hallucinogenic drugs as precipitants of schizophrenia. Psychol Med 1974; 4:255–261 [D]
337. Erard R, Luisada PV, Peale R: The PCP psychosis: prolonged intoxication or drug-induced functional illness? J Psychedelic Drugs 1980; 12:235–251 [G]
338. Salyers MP, Mueser KT: Social functioning, psychopathology, and medication side effects in relation to substance use and abuse in schizophrenia. Schizophr Res 2001; 48:109–123 [C]
339. Tsuang MT, Simpson JC, Kronfol Z: Subtypes of drug abuse with psychosis: demographic characteristics, clinical features, and family history. Arch Gen Psychiatry 1982; 39:141–147 [D]
340. Weller MP, Ang PC, Latimer-Sayer DT, Zachary A: Drug abuse and mental illness. Lancet 1988; 1:997 [G]
341. Mueser KT, Yarnold PR, Levinson DF, Singh H, Bellack AS, Kee K, Morrison RL, Yadalam KG: Prevalence of substance abuse in schizophrenia: demographic and clinical correlates. Schizophr Bull 1990; 16:31–56 [D, F]
342. Drake RE, Brunette MF: Complications of severe mental illness related to alcohol and drug use disorders. Recent Dev Alcohol 1998; 14:285–299 [G]
343. American Psychiatric Association: Practice Guideline for the Treatment of Patients With Substance Use Disorders: Alcohol, Cocaine, Opioids. Am J Psychiatry 1995; 152(Nov suppl):1–59 [F]
344. Salloum IM, Moss HB, Daley DC: Substance abuse and schizophrenia: impediments to optimal care. Am J Drug Alcohol Abuse 1991; 17:321–336 [F]
345. Dawe S, Seinen A, Kavanagh D: An examination of the utility of the AUDIT in people with schizophrenia. J Stud Alcohol 2000; 61:744–750 [G]

346. Rosenberg SD, Drake RE, Wolford GL, Mueser KT, Oxman TE, Vidaver RM, Carrieri KL, Luckoor R: Dartmouth Assessment of Lifestyle Instrument (DALI): a substance use disorder screen for people with severe mental illness. Am J Psychiatry 1998; 155:232–238 [G]
347. Drake RE, Mercer-McFadden C, Mueser KT, McHugo GJ, Bond GR: Review of integrated mental health and substance abuse treatment for patients with dual disorders. Schizophr Bull 1998; 24:589–608 [F]
348. Drake RE, Mueser KT: Psychosocial approaches to dual diagnosis. Schizophr Bull 2000; 26:105–118 [G]
349. Drake RE, Mueser KT: Substance abuse comorbidity, in Comprehensive Care of Schizophrenia: A Textbook of Clinical Management. Edited by Lieberman JA, Murray RM. London, Martin Dunitz, 2001, pp 243–253 [G]
350. Mueser KT, Drake RE: Integrated dual disorder treatment in New Hampshire (USA), in Substance Misuse in Psychosis: Approaches to Treatment and Service Delivery. Edited by Graham HL, Copello A, Birchwood MJ, Mueser KT. West Sussex, UK, John Wiley & Sons, 2003, pp 93–106 [G]
351. Osher FC, Kofoed LL: Treatment of patients with psychiatric and psychoactive substance abuse disorders. Hosp Community Psychiatry 1989; 40:1025–1030 [G]
352. Hellerstein DJ, Meehan B: Outpatient group therapy for schizophrenic substance abusers. Am J Psychiatry 1987; 144:1337–1339 [B]
353. Drake RE, Bartels SJ, Teague GB, Noordsy DL, Clark RE: Treatment of substance abuse in severely mentally ill patients. J Nerv Ment Dis 1993; 181:606–611 [F]
354. Bennett ME, Bellack AS, Gearon JS: Treating substance abuse in schizophrenia: an initial report. J Subst Abuse Treat 2001; 20:163–175 [G]
355. Clark RE: Family support for persons with dual disorders. New Dir Ment Health Serv 1996; 70:65–78 [F]
356. Barrowclough C, Haddock G, Tarrier N, Lewis SW, Moring J, O'Brien R, Schofield N, McGovern J: Randomized controlled trial of motivational interviewing, cognitive behavior therapy, and family intervention for patients with comorbid schizophrenia and substance use disorders. Am J Psychiatry 2001; 158:1706–1713 [A–]
357. Addington J, el Guebaly N: Group treatment for substance abuse in schizophrenia. Can J Psychiatry 1998; 43:843–845 [B]
358. Kofoed L, Kania J, Walsh T, Atkinson RM: Outpatient treatment of patients with substance abuse and coexisting psychiatric disorders. Am J Psychiatry 1986; 143:867–872 [B]
359. Mueser KT, Noordsy DL, Drake RE, Fox L: Integrated Treatment for Dual Disorders: A Guide to Effective Practice. New York, Guilford, 2003 [G]
360. Voruganti LN, Heslegrave RJ, Awad AG: Neuroleptic dysphoria may be the missing link between schizophrenia and substance abuse. J Nerv Ment Dis 1997; 185:463–465 [G]
361. Green AI, Zimmet SV, Strous RD, Schildkraut JJ: Clozapine for comorbid substance use disorder and schizophrenia: do patients with schizophrenia have a reward-deficiency syndrome that can be ameliorated by clozapine? Harv Rev Psychiatry 1999; 6:287–296 [G]
362. Drake RE, Xie H, McHugo GJ, Green AI: The effects of clozapine on alcohol and drug use disorders among patients with schizophrenia. Schizophr Bull 2000; 26:441–449 [C]
363. Farren CK, Hameedi FA, Rosen MA, Woods S, Jatlow P, Kosten TR: Significant interaction between clozapine and cocaine in cocaine addicts. Drug Alcohol Depend 2000; 59:153–163 [B]
364. Smelson DA, Losonczy MF, Davis CW, Kaune M, Williams J, Ziedonis D: Risperidone decreases craving and relapses in individuals with schizophrenia and cocaine dependence. Can J Psychiatry 2002; 47:671–675 [B]
365. Mueser KT, Noordsy DL, Fox L, Wolfe R: Disulfiram treatment for alcoholism in severe mental illness. Am J Addict 2003; 12:242–252 [G]

366. Kingsbury SJ, Salzman C: Disulfiram in the treatment of alcoholic patients with schizophrenia. Hosp Community Psychiatry 1990; 41:133–134 [G]
367. Sands JR, Harrow M: Depression during the longitudinal course of schizophrenia. Schizophr Bull 1999; 25:157–171 [C]
368. Siris SG: Depression in schizophrenia: perspective in the era of "atypical" antipsychotic agents. Am J Psychiatry 2000; 157:1379–1389 [F]
369. Koreen AR, Siris SG, Chakos M, Alvir J, Mayerhoff D, Lieberman J: Depression in first-episode schizophrenia. Am J Psychiatry 1993; 150:1643–1648 [B]
370. Addington D, Addington J, Patten S: Depression in people with first-episode schizophrenia. Br J Psychiatry Suppl 1998; 172:90–92 [C]
371. Emsley RA, Oosthuizen PP, Joubert AF, Roberts MC, Stein DJ: Depressive and anxiety symptoms in patients with schizophrenia and schizophreniform disorder. J Clin Psychiatry 1999; 60:747–751 [G]
372. Bottlender R, Strauss A, Moller HJ: Prevalence and background factors of depression in first admitted schizophrenic patients. Acta Psychiatr Scand 2000; 101:153–160 [C]
373. Wassink TH, Flaum M, Nopoulos P, Andreasen NC: Prevalence of depressive symptoms early in the course of schizophrenia. Am J Psychiatry 1999; 156:315–316 [C]
374. McGlashan TH, Carpenter WT Jr: Postpsychotic depression in schizophrenia. Arch Gen Psychiatry 1976; 33:231–239 [E]
375. Herz MI, Melville C: Relapse in schizophrenia. Am J Psychiatry 1980; 137:801–805 [D]
376. Johnson DA: The significance of depression in the prediction of relapse in chronic schizophrenia. Br J Psychiatry 1988; 152:320–323 [C]
377. Subotnik KL, Nuechterlein KH: Prodromal signs and symptoms of schizophrenic relapse. J Abnorm Psychol 1988; 97:405–412 [D]
378. Green MF, Nuechterlein KH, Ventura J, Mintz J: The temporal relationship between depressive and psychotic symptoms in recent-onset schizophrenia. Am J Psychiatry 1990; 147:179–182 [C]
379. Malla AK, Norman RMG: Prodromal symptoms in schizophrenia. Br J Psychiatry 1994; 164:287–293 [C]
380. Bartels SJ, Drake RE: Depressive symptoms in schizophrenia: comprehensive differential diagnosis. Compr Psychiatry 1988; 29:467–483 [G]
381. Tollefson GD, Birkett MA, Kiesler GM, Wood AJ: Double-blind comparison of olanzapine versus clozapine in schizophrenic patients clinically eligible for treatment with clozapine. Biol Psychiatry 2001; 49:52–63 [A]
382. Csernansky JG, Mahmoud R, Brenner R: A comparison of risperidone and haloperidol for the prevention of relapse in patients with schizophrenia. N Engl J Med 2002; 346:16–22 [A]
383. Collaborative Working Group on Clinical Trial Evaluations: Atypical antipsychotics for treatment of depression in schizophrenia and affective disorders. J Clin Psychiatry 1998; 59(suppl 12):41–45 [G]
384. Shergill SS, Murray RM: Affective symptoms in schizophrenia, in Comprehensive Care of Schizophrenia: A Textbook of Clinical Management. Edited by Lieberman JA, Murray RM. London, Martin Dunitz, 2001, pp 205–218 [G]
385. Siris SG: Diagnosis of secondary depression in schizophrenia: implications for DSM-IV. Schizophr Bull 1991; 17:75–98 [F]
386. Black DW, Fisher R: Mortality in DSM-III-R schizophrenia. Schizophr Res 1992; 7:109–116 [E]
387. Simpson JC, Tsuang MT: Mortality among patients with schizophrenia. Schizophr Bull 1996; 22:485–499 [C]
388. Harris EC, Barraclough B: Excess mortality of mental disorder. Br J Psychiatry 1998; 173: 11–53 [F]

389. Radomsky ED, Haas GL, Mann JJ, Sweeney JA: Suicidal behavior in patients with schizophrenia and other psychotic disorders. Am J Psychiatry 1999; 156:1590–1595 [G]
390. Allebeck P: Schizophrenia: a life-shortening disease. Schizophr Bull 1989; 15:81–89 [F]
391. Caldwell CB, Gottesman II: Schizophrenics kill themselves too: a review of risk factors for suicide. Schizophr Bull 1990; 16:571–589 [F]
392. Harkavy-Friedman JM, Nelson EA: Assessment and intervention for the suicidal patient with schizophrenia. Psychiatr Q 1997; 68:361–375 [G]
393. Inskip HM, Harris EC, Barraclough B: Lifetime risk of suicide for affective disorder, alcoholism and schizophrenia. Br J Psychiatry 1998; 172:35–37 [E]
394. Harkavy-Friedman JM, Nelson E: Management of the suicidal patient with schizophrenia. Psychiatr Clin North Am 1997; 20:625–640 [G]
395. Fenton WS, McGlashan TH, Victor BJ, Blyler CR: Symptoms, subtype, and suicidality in patients with schizophrenia spectrum disorders. Am J Psychiatry 1997; 154:199–204 [C]
396. Drake RE, Gates C, Whitaker A, Cotton PG: Suicide among schizophrenics: a review. Compr Psychiatry 1985; 26:90–100 [F]
397. Gupta S, Black DW, Arndt S, Hubbard WC, Andreasen NC: Factors associated with suicide attempts among patients with schizophrenia. Psychiatr Serv 1998; 49:1353–1355 [D]
398. Meltzer HY: Treatment of suicidality in schizophrenia. Ann NY Acad Sci 2001; 932:44–58 [G]
399. Meltzer HY: Suicidality in schizophrenia: a review of the evidence for risk factors and treatment options. Curr Psychiatry Rep 2002; 4:279–283 [F]
400. Kim CH, Jayathilake K, Meltzer HY: Hopelessness, neurocognitive function, and insight in schizophrenia: relationship to suicidal behavior. Schizophr Res 2003; 60:71–80 [C]
401. De Hert M, McKenzie K, Peuskens J: Risk factors for suicide in young people suffering from schizophrenia: a long-term follow-up study. Schizophr Res 2001; 47:127–134 [D]
402. Heila H, Heikkinen ME, Isometsa ET, Henriksson MM, Marttunen MJ, Lonnqvist JK: Life events and completed suicide in schizophrenia: a comparison of suicide victims with and without schizophrenia. Schizophr Bull 1999; 25:519–531 [D]
403. Funahashi T, Ibuki Y, Domon Y, Nishimura T, Akehashi D, Sugiura H: A clinical study on suicide among schizophrenics. Psychiatry Clin Neurosci 2000; 54:173–179 [D]
404. Roy A: Psychiatric emergencies, in Comprehensive Textbook of Psychiatry, 6th ed. Edited by Kaplan HI, Sadock BJ. Baltimore, Williams & Wilkins, 1995, pp 1739–1752 [G]
405. Heila H, Isometsa ET, Henriksson MM, Heikkinen ME, Marttunen MJ, Lonnqvist JK: Suicide and schizophrenia: a nationwide psychological autopsy study on age- and sex-specific clinical characteristics of 92 suicide victims with schizophrenia. Am J Psychiatry 1997; 154:1235–1242 [G]
406. Saarinen PI, Lehtonen J, Lonnqvist J: Suicide risk in schizophrenia: an analysis of 17 consecutive suicides. Schizophr Bull 1999; 25:533–542 [G]
407. Young AS, Nuechterlein KH, Mintz J, Ventura J, Gitlin M, Liberman RP: Suicidal ideation and suicide attempts in recent-onset schizophrenia. Schizophr Bull 1998; 24:629–634 [C]
408. Heila H, Isometsa ET, Henriksson MM, Heikkinen ME, Marttunen MJ, Lonnqvist JK: Suicide victims with schizophrenia in different treatment phases and adequacy of antipsychotic medication. J Clin Psychiatry 1999; 60:200–208 [G]
409. Drake RE, Ehrlich J: Suicide attempts associated with akathisia. Am J Psychiatry 1985; 142: 499–501 [G]
410. Shear MK, Frances A, Weiden P: Suicide associated with akathisia and depot fluphenazine treatment. J Clin Psychopharmacol 1983; 3:235–236 [G]
411. Palmer DD, Henter ID, Wyatt RJ: Do antipsychotic medications decrease the risk of suicide in patients with schizophrenia? J Clin Psychiatry 1999; 60(suppl 2):100–103 [G]
412. Reid WH, Mason M, Hogan T: Suicide prevention effects associated with clozapine therapy in schizophrenia and schizoaffective disorder. Psychiatr Serv 1998; 49:1029–1033 [D]

413. Arseneault L, Moffitt TE, Caspi A, Taylor PJ, Silva PA: Mental disorders and violence in a total birth cohort: results from the Dunedin Study. Arch Gen Psychiatry 2000; 57:979–986 [G]
414. Bland RC, Newman SC, Thompson AH, Dyck RJ: Psychiatric disorders in the population and in prisoners. Int J Law Psychiatry 1998; 21:273–279 [D]
415. Hodgins S: Mental disorder, intellectual deficiency, and crime: evidence from a birth cohort. Arch Gen Psychiatry 1992; 49:476–483 [C]
416. Hodgins S, Cote G: Major mental disorder and antisocial personality disorder: a criminal combination. Bull Am Acad Psychiatry Law 1993; 21:155–160 [G]
417. Hodgins S, Mednick SA, Brennan PA, Schulsinger F, Engberg M: Mental disorder and crime: evidence from a Danish birth cohort. Arch Gen Psychiatry 1996; 53:489–496 [D]
418. Swanson JW, Holzer CE III, Ganju VK, Jono RT: Violence and psychiatric disorder in the community: evidence from the Epidemiologic Catchment Area surveys. Hosp Community Psychiatry 1990; 41:761–770 [G]
419. Teplin LA: The prevalence of severe mental disorder among male urban jail detainees: comparison with the Epidemiologic Catchment Area program. Am J Public Health 1990; 80:663–669 [D]
420. Glancy GD, Regehr C: The forensic psychiatric aspects of schizophrenia. Psychiatr Clin North Am 1992; 15:575–589 [G]
421. Taylor PJ: Schizophrenia and the risk of violence, in Schizophrenia. Edited by Hirsch SR, Weinberger DR. Oxford, UK, Blackwell Science, 1995, pp 163–183 [G]
422. Modestin J: Criminal and violent behavior in schizophrenic patients: an overview. Psychiatry Clin Neurosci 1998; 52:547–554 [F]
423. Rasanen P, Tiihonen J, Isohanni M, Rantakallio P, Lehtonen J, Moring J: Schizophrenia, alcohol abuse, and violent behavior: a 26-year followup study of an unselected birth cohort. Schizophr Bull 1998; 24:437–441 [C]
424. Soyka M: Substance misuse, psychiatric disorder and violent and disturbed behaviour. Br J Psychiatry 2000; 176:345–350 [F]
425. Walsh E, Buchanan A, Fahy T: Violence and schizophrenia: examining the evidence. Br J Psychiatry 2002; 180:490–495 [F]
426. Nolan KA, Volavka J, Mohr P, Czobor P: Psychopathy and violent behavior among patients with schizophrenia or schizoaffective disorder. Psychiatr Serv 1999; 50:787–792 [D]
427. Krakowski M, Czobor P, Chou JC: Course of violence in patients with schizophrenia: relationship to clinical symptoms. Schizophr Bull 1999; 25:505–517 [C]
428. Bartels SJ, Drake RE, Wallach MA, Freeman DH: Characteristic hostility in schizophrenic outpatients. Schizophr Bull 1991; 17:163–171 [C]
429. Buchanan A: The investigation of acting on delusions as a tool for risk assessment in the mentally disordered. Br J Psychiatry Suppl 1997; 170(32):12–16 [G]
430. Taylor PJ, Leese M, Williams D, Butwell M, Daly R, Larkin E: Mental disorder and violence: a special (high security) hospital study. Br J Psychiatry 1998; 172:218–226 [G]
431. McNiel DE, Eisner JP, Binder RL: The relationship between command hallucinations and violence. Psychiatr Serv 2000; 51:1288–1292 [G]
432. Tardiff K: Assessment and Management of Violent Patients, 2nd ed. Washington, DC, American Psychiatric Press, 1996 [G]
433. Estroff SE, Swanson JW, Lachicotte WS, Swartz M, Bolduc M: Risk reconsidered: targets of violence in the social networks of people with serious psychiatric disorders. Soc Psychiatry Psychiatr Epidemiol 1998; 33(suppl 1):S95–S101 [C]
434. Simon RI: Clinical Psychiatry and the Law, 2nd ed. Washington, DC, American Psychiatric Press, 1992 [G]
435. Chase PB, Biros MH: A retrospective review of the use and safety of droperidol in a large, high-risk, inner-city emergency department patient population. Acad Emerg Med 2002; 9: 1402–1410 [G]

436. Ball GG: Modifying the behavior of the violent patient. Psychiatr Q 1993; 64:359–369 [G]
437. Steinert T, Sippach T, Gebhardt RP: How common is violence in schizophrenia despite neuroleptic treatment? Pharmacopsychiatry 2000; 33:98–102 [G]
438. Hector RI: The use of clozapine in the treatment of aggressive schizophrenia. Can J Psychiatry 1998; 43:466–472 [G]
439. Volavka J: The effects of clozapine on aggression and substance abuse in schizophrenic patients. J Clin Psychiatry 1999; 60(suppl 12):43–46 [G]
440. Citrome L, Volavka J, Czobor P, Sheitman B, Lindenmayer JP, McEvoy J, Cooper TB, Chakos M, Lieberman JA: Effects of clozapine, olanzapine, risperidone, and haloperidol on hostility among patients with schizophrenia. Psychiatr Serv 2001; 52:1510–1514 [A]
441. Swanson JW, Swartz MS, Borum R, Hiday VA, Wagner HR, Burns BJ: Involuntary outpatient commitment and reduction of violent behaviour in persons with severe mental illness. Br J Psychiatry 2000; 176:324–331 [A–]
442. de Leon J, Verghese C, Tracy JI, Josiassen RC, Simpson GM: Polydipsia and water intoxication in psychiatric patients: a review of the epidemiological literature. Biol Psychiatry 1994; 35:408–419 [F]
443. de Leon J, Dadvand M, Canuso C, Odom-White A, Stanilla J, Simpson GM: Polydipsia and water intoxication in a long-term psychiatric hospital. Biol Psychiatry 1996; 40:28–34 [G]
444. de Leon J, Tracy J, McCann E, McGrory A: Polydipsia and schizophrenia in a psychiatric hospital: a replication study. Schizophr Res 2002; 57:293–301 [G]
445. de Leon J: Polydipsia: a study in a long-term psychiatric unit. Eur Arch Psychiatry Clin Neurosci 2003; 253:37–39 [C]
446. Movig KL, Leufkens HG, Lenderink AW, Egberts AC: Serotonergic antidepressants associated with an increased risk for hyponatraemia in the elderly. Eur J Clin Pharmacol 2002; 58:143–148 [D]
447. Madhusoodanan S, Bogunovic OJ, Moise D, Brenner R, Markowitz S, Sotelo J: Hyponatraemia associated with psychotropic medications: a review of the literature and spontaneous reports. Adverse Drug React Toxicol Rev 2002; 21:17–29 [F]
448. Siegler EL, Tamres D, Berlin JA, Allen-Taylor L, Strom BL: Risk factors for the development of hyponatremia in psychiatric inpatients. Arch Intern Med 1995; 155:953–957 [D]
449. Verghese C, de Leon J, Josiassen RC: Problems and progress in the diagnosis and treatment of polydipsia and hyponatremia. Schizophr Bull 1996; 22:455–464 [G]
450. Fuller MA, Jurjus G, Kwon K, Konicki PE, Jaskiw GE: Clozapine reduces water-drinking behavior in schizophrenic patients with polydipsia. J Clin Psychopharmacol 1996; 16:329–332 [G]
451. Spears NM, Leadbetter RA, Shutty MS Jr: Clozapine treatment in polydipsia and intermittent hyponatremia. J Clin Psychiatry 1996; 57:123–128 [G]
452. Canuso CM, Goldman MB: Clozapine restores water balance in schizophrenic patients with polydipsia-hyponatremia syndrome. J Neuropsychiatry Clin Neurosci 1999; 11:86–90 [B]
453. Kruse D, Pantelis C, Rudd R, Quek J, Herbert P, McKinley M: Treatment of psychogenic polydipsia: comparison of risperidone and olanzapine, and the effects of an adjunctive angiotensin-II receptor blocking drug (irbesartan). Aust NZ J Psychiatry 2001; 35:65–68 [G]
454. Kawai N, Baba A, Suzuki T: Risperidone failed to improve polydipsia-hyponatremia of the schizophrenic patients. Psychiatry Clin Neurosci 2002; 56:107–110 [G]
455. Alexander RC, Karp BI, Thompson S, Khot V, Kirch DG: A double blind, placebo-controlled trial of demeclocycline treatment of polydipsia-hyponatremia in chronically psychotic patients. Biol Psychiatry 1991; 30:417–420 [A]
456. Brookes G, Ahmed AG: Pharmacological treatments for psychosis-related polydipsia. Cochrane Database Syst Rev 2002; (3):CD003544 [E]
457. Becker JA, Goldman MB, Alam MY, Luchins DJ: Effects of naltrexone on mannerisms and water imbalance in polydipsic schizophrenics: a pilot study. Schizophr Res 1995; 17:279–282 [B]

458. Greendyke RM, Bernhardt AJ, Tasbas HE, Lewandowski KS: Polydipsia in chronic psychiatric patients: therapeutic trials of clonidine and enalapril. Neuropsychopharmacology 1998; 18:272–281 [A]
459. Delva NJ, Chang A, Hawken ER, Lawson JS, Owen JA: Effects of clonidine in schizophrenic patients with primary polydipsia: three single case studies. Prog Neuropsychopharmacol Biol Psychiatry 2002; 26:387–392 [G]
460. Kishi Y, Kurosawa H, Endo S: Is propranolol effective in primary polydipsia? Int J Psychiatry Med 1998; 28:315–325 [G]
461. National Resource Center on Homelessness and Mental Illness: Fact Sheet: Who Is Homeless? Delmar, NY, National Resource Center on Homelessness and Mental Illness, 2003. (http://www.nrchmi.samhsa.gov/facts/facts_question_2.asp) [G]
462. D'Amore J, Hung O, Chiang W, Goldfrank L: The epidemiology of the homeless population and its impact on an urban emergency department. Acad Emerg Med 2001; 8: 1051–1055 [D]
463. Martens WH: A review of physical and mental health in homeless persons. Public Health Rev 2001; 29:13–33 [F]
464. Folsom D, Jeste DV: Schizophrenia in homeless persons: a systematic review of the literature. Acta Psychiatr Scand 2002; 105:404–413 [F]
465. Bachrach LL: What we know about homelessness among mentally ill persons: an analytical review and commentary. Hosp Community Psychiatry 1992; 43:453–464 [G]
466. Schlenger WE, Kroutil LA, Roland EJ: Case management as a mechanism for linking drug abuse treatment and primary care: preliminary evidence from the ADAMHA/HRSA linkage demonstration. NIDA Res Monogr 1992; 127:316–330 [G]
467. Goldfinger SM: Homelessness and schizophrenia: a psychosocial approach, in Handbook of Schizophrenia, vol 4: Psychosocial Treatment of Schizophrenia. Edited by Herz MI, Keith SJ, Docherty JP. Amsterdam, Elsevier, 1990, pp 355–385 [G]
468. Hiday VA, Swartz MS, Swanson JW, Borum R, Wagner HR: Criminal victimization of persons with severe mental illness. Psychiatr Serv 1999; 50:62–68 [D]
469. Babidge NC, Buhrich N, Butler T: Mortality among homeless people with schizophrenia in Sydney, Australia: a 10-year follow-up. Acta Psychiatr Scand 2001; 103:105–110 [C]
470. Desai MM, Rosenheck RA, Kasprow WJ: Determinants of receipt of ambulatory medical care in a national sample of mentally ill homeless veterans. Med Care 2003; 41:275–287 [C]
471. Herman D, Opler L, Felix A, Valencia E, Wyatt RJ, Susser E: A critical time intervention with mentally ill homeless men: impact on psychiatric symptoms. J Nerv Ment Dis 2000; 188:135–140 [A–]
472. McQuistion HL, Finnerty M, Hirschowitz J, Susser ES: Challenges for psychiatry in serving homeless people with psychiatric disorders. Psychiatr Serv 2003; 54:669–676 [G]
473. Lam JA, Rosenheck R: Street outreach for homeless persons with serious mental illness: is it effective? Med Care 1999; 37:894–907 [C]
474. Cohen NL, Marcos LR: Outreach intervention models for the homeless mentally ill, in Treating the Homeless Mentally Ill: A Report of the Task Force on the Homeless Mentally Ill. Edited by Lamb RH, Bachrach LL, Kass FI. Washington, DC, American Psychiatric Association, 1992, pp 141–158 [G]
475. Karno M, Jenkins JH: Cross-cultural issues in the course and treatment of schizophrenia. Psychiatr Clin North Am 1993; 16:339–350 [G]
476. Rayburn TM, Stonecypher JF: Diagnostic differences related to age and race of involuntarily committed psychiatric patients. Psychol Rep 1996; 79:881–882 [G]
477. Kilgus MD, Pumariega AJ, Cuffe SP: Influence of race on diagnosis in adolescent psychiatric inpatients. J Am Acad Child Adolesc Psychiatry 1995; 34:67–72 [G]
478. Adebimpe VR: Race, racism, and epidemiological surveys. Hosp Community Psychiatry 1994; 45:27–31 [G]

479. Baker FM, Bell CC: Issues in the psychiatric treatment of African Americans. Psychiatr Serv 1999; 50:362–368 [G]
480. Delahanty J, Ram R, Postrado L, Balis T, Green-Paden L, Dixon L: Differences in rates of depression in schizophrenia by race. Schizophr Bull 2001; 27:29–38 [G]
481. Dixon L, Green-Paden L, Delahanty J, Lucksted A, Postrado L, Hall J: Variables associated with disparities in treatment of patients with schizophrenia and comorbid mood and anxiety disorders. Psychiatr Serv 2001; 52:1216–1222 [G]
482. Klinkenberg WD, Calsyn RJ: The moderating effects of race on return visits to the psychiatric emergency room. Psychiatr Serv 1997; 48:942–945 [G]
483. Leda C, Rosenheck R: Race in the treatment of homeless mentally ill veterans. J Nerv Ment Dis 1995; 183:529–537 [C]
484. Callan AF: Schizophrenia in Afro-Caribbean immigrants. J R Soc Med 1996; 89:253–256 [D]
485. Cole J, Pilisuk M: Differences in the provision of mental health services by race. Am J Orthopsychiatry 1976; 46:510–525 [G]
486. Cuffe SP, Waller JL, Cuccaro ML, Pumariega AJ, Garrison CZ: Race and gender differences in the treatment of psychiatric disorders in young adolescents. J Am Acad Child Adolesc Psychiatry 1995; 34:1536–1543 [G]
487. Neighbors HW, Jackson JS, Campbell L, Williams D: The influence of racial factors on psychiatric diagnosis: a review and suggestions for research. Community Ment Health J 1989; 25:301–311 [F]
488. Somervell PD, Leaf PJ, Weissman MM, Blazer DG, Bruce ML: The prevalence of major depression in black and white adults in five United States communities. Am J Epidemiol 1989; 130:725–735 [G]
489. Chung H, Mahler JC, Kakuma T: Racial differences in treatment of psychiatric inpatients. Psychiatr Serv 1995; 46:586–591 [D]
490. Glazer WM, Morgenstern H, Doucette J: Race and tardive dyskinesia among outpatients at a CMHC. Hosp Community Psychiatry 1994; 45:38–42 [G]
491. Segal SP, Bola JR, Watson MA: Race, quality of care, and antipsychotic prescribing practices in psychiatric emergency services. Psychiatr Serv 1996; 47:282–286 [G]
492. Valenstein M, Copeland L, Owen R, Blow F, Visnic S: Delays in adopting evidence-based dosages of conventional antipsychotics. Psychiatr Serv 2001; 52:1242–1244 [G]
493. Walkup JT, McAlpine DD, Olfson M, Labay LE, Boyer C, Hansell S: Patients with schizophrenia at risk for excessive antipsychotic dosing. J Clin Psychiatry 2000; 61:344–348 [G]
494. Lehman AF, Steinwachs DM: Patterns of usual care for schizophrenia: initial results from the Schizophrenia Patient Outcomes Research Team (PORT) Client Survey. Schizophr Bull 1998; 24:11–20 [G]
495. Kreyenbuhl J, Zito JM, Buchanan RW, Soeken KL, Lehman AF: Racial disparity in the pharmacological management of schizophrenia. Schizophr Bull 2003; 29:183–193 [G]
496. Copeland LA, Zeber JE, Valenstein M, Blow FC: Racial disparity in the use of atypical antipsychotic medications among veterans. Am J Psychiatry 2003; 160:1817–1822 [G]
497. Kuno E, Rothbard AB: Racial disparities in antipsychotic prescription patterns for patients with schizophrenia. Am J Psychiatry 2002; 159:567–572 [G]
498. Owen RR, Feng W, Thrush CR, Hudson TJ, Austen MA: Variations in prescribing practices for novel antipsychotic medications among Veterans Affairs hospitals. Psychiatr Serv 2001; 52:1523–1525 [G]
499. Daumit GL, Crum RM, Guallar E, Powe NR, Primm AB, Steinwachs DM, Ford DE: Outpatient prescriptions for atypical antipsychotics for African Americans, Hispanics, and whites in the United States. Arch Gen Psychiatry 2003; 60:121–128 [C]
500. Prior TI, Baker GB: Interactions between the cytochrome P450 system and the second-generation antipsychotics. J Psychiatry Neurosci 2003; 28:99–112 [G]

501. Lieberman JA, Yunis J, Egea E, Canoso RT, Kane JM, Yunis EJ: HLA-B38, DR4, DQw3 and clozapine-induced agranulocytosis in Jewish patients with schizophrenia. Arch Gen Psychiatry 1990; 47:945–948 [B]
502. Bardenstein KK, McGlashan TH: Gender differences in affective, schizoaffective, and schizophrenic disorders: a review. Schizophr Res 1990; 3:159–172 [F]
503. Goldstein JM, Tsuang MT: Gender and schizophrenia: an introduction and synthesis of findings. Schizophr Bull 1990; 16:179–344 [F]
504. Leung A, Chue P: Sex differences in schizophrenia: a review of the literature. Acta Psychiatr Scand Suppl 2000; 401:3–38 [F]
505. Tamminga CA: Gender and schizophrenia. J Clin Psychiatry 1997; 58(suppl 15):33–37 [G]
506. Castle D, Sham P, Murray R: Differences in distribution of ages of onset in males and females with schizophrenia. Schizophr Res 1998; 33:179–183 [D]
507. Haas GL, Glick ID, Clarkin JF, Spencer JH, Lewis AB: Gender and schizophrenia outcome: a clinical trial of an inpatient family intervention. Schizophr Bull 1990; 16:277–292 [B]
508. Szymanski S, Lieberman JA, Alvir JM, Mayerhoff D, Loebel A, Geisler S, Chakos M, Koreen A, Jody D, Kane J: Gender differences in onset of illness, treatment response, course, and biologic indexes in first-episode schizophrenic patients. Am J Psychiatry 1995; 152:698–703 [B]
509. Kelly DL, Conley RR, Tamminga CA: Differential olanzapine plasma concentrations by sex in a fixed-dose study. Schizophr Res 1999; 40:101–104 [G]
510. Briggs GG, Freeman RK, Yaffe SJ: Drugs in Pregnancy and Lactation: A Reference Guide to Fetal and Neonatal Risk, 6th ed. Baltimore, Williams & Wilkins, 2002 [G]
511. American Academy of Pediatrics: Use of psychoactive medication during pregnancy and possible effects on the fetus and newborn. Pediatrics 2000; 105:880–887 [G]
512. Cohen LS, Rosenbaum JF: Psychotropic drug use during pregnancy: weighing the risks. J Clin Psychiatry 1998; 59(suppl 2):18–28 [G]
513. Gold LH: Use of psychotropic medication during pregnancy: risk management guidelines. Psychiatr Ann 2000; 30:421–432 [F]
514. Koren G, Cohn T, Chitayat D, Kapur B, Remington G, Reid DM, Zipursky RB: Use of atypical antipsychotics during pregnancy and the risk of neural tube defects in infants. Am J Psychiatry 2002; 159:136–137 [D]
515. Goldstein DJ, Corbin LA, Fung MC: Olanzapine-exposed pregnancies and lactation: early experience. J Clin Psychopharmacol 2000; 20:399–403 [C]
516. Dickson RA, Hogg L: Pregnancy of a patient treated with clozapine. Psychiatr Serv 1998; 49:1081–1083 [G]
517. Grigoriadis S, Seeman MV: The role of estrogen in schizophrenia: implications for schizophrenia practice guidelines for women. Can J Psychiatry 2002; 47:437–442 [F]
518. Ernst CL, Goldberg JF: The reproductive safety profile of mood stabilizers, atypical antipsychotics, and broad-spectrum psychotropics. J Clin Psychiatry 2002; 63(suppl 4):42–55 [G]
519. Bennedsen BE: Adverse pregnancy outcome in schizophrenic women: occurrence and risk factors. Schizophr Res 1998; 33:1–26 [G]
520. Bennedsen BE, Mortensen PB, Olesen AV, Henriksen TB: Preterm birth and intra-uterine growth retardation among children of women with schizophrenia. Br J Psychiatry 1999; 175:239–245 [D]
521. Bennedsen BE, Mortensen PB, Olesen AV, Henriksen TB, Frydenberg M: Obstetric complications in women with schizophrenia. Schizophr Res 2001; 47:167–175 [D]
522. Nilsson E, Lichtenstein P, Cnattingius S, Murray RM, Hultman CM: Women with schizophrenia: pregnancy outcome and infant death among their offspring. Schizophr Res 2002; 58:221–229 [D]
523. McGlashan TH: Schizophrenia: psychosocial therapies and the role of psychosocial factors in its etiology and pathogenesis, in Psychiatry Update: The American Psychiatric Press Annual Review, vol. 5. Edited by Frances AJ, Hales RE. Washington, DC, American Psychiatric Press, 1986, pp 96–111 [F, G]

524. Spring B: Stress and schizophrenia: some definitional issues. Schizophr Bull 1981; 7:24–33 [E, G]
525. Dohrenwend BP, Egri G: Recent stressful life events and episodes of schizophrenia. Schizophr Bull 1981; 7:12–23 [C, D, E]
526. Zubin J, Spring B: Vulnerability: a new view of schizophrenia. J Abnorm Psychol 1977; 86: 103–126 [G]
527. Palmer BW, Heaton SC, Jeste DV: Older patients with schizophrenia: challenges in the coming decades. Psychiatr Serv 1999; 50:1178–1183 [F]
528. Cohen CI, Cohen GD, Blank K, Gaitz C, Katz IR, Leuchter A, Maletta G, Meyers B, Sakauye K, Shamoian C: Schizophrenia and older adults—an overview: directions for research and policy. Am J Geriatr Psychiatry 2000; 8:19–28 [F, G]
529. Howard R, Rabins PV, Seeman MV, Jeste DV (The International Late-Onset Schizophrenia Group): Late-onset schizophrenia and very-late-onset schizophrenia-like psychosis: an international consensus. Am J Psychiatry 2000; 157:172–178 [F]
530. Eyler Zorrilla LT, Heaton RK, McAdams LA, Zisook S, Harris MJ, Jeste DV: Cross-sectional study of older outpatients with schizophrenia and healthy comparison subjects: no differences in age-related cognitive decline. Am J Psychiatry 2000; 157:1324–1326 [C]
531. Heaton RK, Gladsjo JA, Palmer BW, Kuck J, Marcotte TD, Jeste DV: Stability and course of neuropsychological deficits in schizophrenia. Arch Gen Psychiatry 2001; 58:24–32 [C]
532. Sajatovic M, Madhusoodanan S, Buckley PJ: Schizophrenia in the elderly: guidelines for its recognition and treatment. CNS Drugs 2000; 13:103–115 [F]
533. Salzman C: Principles of psychopharmacology, in Verwoerdt's Clinical Geropsychiatry, 3rd ed. Edited by Bienenfeld D. Baltimore, Williams & Wilkins, 1990, pp 235–249 [G]
534. Jeste DV, Rockwell E, Harris MJ, Lohr JB, Lacro J: Conventional vs newer antipsychotics in elderly patients. Am J Geriatr Psychiatry 1999; 7:70–76 [B, F]
535. Jeste DV, Lacro JP, Bailey A, Rockwell E, Harris MJ, Caligiuri MP: Lower incidence of tardive dyskinesia with risperidone compared with haloperidol in older patients. J Am Geriatr Soc 1999; 47:716–719 [C]
536. Street JS, Clark WS, Gannon KS, Cummings JL, Bymaster FP, Tamura RN, Mitan SJ, Kadam DL, Sanger TM, Feldman PD, Tollefson GD, Breier A (The HGEU Study Group): Olanzapine treatment of psychotic and behavioral symptoms in patients with Alzheimer disease in nursing care facilities: a double-blind, randomized, placebo-controlled trial. Arch Gen Psychiatry 2000; 57:968–976 [A]
537. Dolder CR, Jeste DV: Incidence of tardive dyskinesia with typical versus atypical antipsychotics in very high risk patients. Biol Psychiatry 2003; 53:1142–1145 [B]
538. Jeste DV, Barak Y, Madhusoodanan S, Grossman F, Gharabawi G: International multisite double-blind trial of the atypical antipsychotics risperidone and olanzapine in 175 elderly patients with chronic schizophrenia. Am J Geriatr Psychiatry 2003; 11:638–647 [A]
539. Jin H, Zisook S, Palmer BW, Patterson TL, Heaton RK, Jeste DV: Association of depressive symptoms with worse functioning in schizophrenia: a study in older outpatients. J Clin Psychiatry 2001; 62:797–803 [D]
540. Kasckow JW, Mohamed S, Thallasinos A, Carroll B, Zisook S, Jeste DV: Citalopram augmentation of antipsychotic treatment in older schizophrenia patients. Int J Geriatr Psychiatry 2001; 16:1163–1167 [A]
541. Granholm E, McQuaid JR, McClure FS, Pedrelli P, Jeste DV: A randomized controlled pilot study of cognitive behavioral social skills training for older patients with schizophrenia. Schizophr Res 2002; 53:167–169 [B]
542. Patterson TL, McKibbin C, Taylor M, Goldman S, Davila-Fraga W, Bucardo J, Jeste DV: Functional adaptation skills training (FAST): a pilot psychosocial intervention study in middle-aged and older patients with chronic psychotic disorders. Am J Geriatr Psychiatry 2003; 11:17–23 [A–]

543. Green AI, Salomon MS, Brenner MJ, Rawlins K: Treatment of schizophrenia and comorbid substance use disorder. Curr Drug Target CNS Neurol Disord 2002; 1:129–139 [G]
544. Green AI, Canuso CM, Brenner MJ, Wojcik JD: Detection and management of comorbidity in patients with schizophrenia. Psychiatr Clin North Am 2003; 26:115–139 [G]
545. Folsom DP, McCahill M, Bartels SJ, Lindamer LA, Ganiats TG, Jeste DV: Medical comorbidity and receipt of medical care by older homeless people with schizophrenia or depression. Psychiatr Serv 2002; 53:1456–1460 [D]
546. Friedman JI, Harvey PD, McGurk SR, White L, Parrella M, Raykov T, Coleman T, Adler DN, Davis KL: Correlates of change in functional status of institutionalized geriatric schizophrenic patients: focus on medical comorbidity. Am J Psychiatry 2002; 159:1388–1394 [C]
547. Kilbourne AM, Justice AC, Rabeneck L, Rodriguez-Barradas M, Weissman S: General medical and psychiatric comorbidity among HIV-infected veterans in the post-HAART era. J Clin Epidemiol 2001; 54(suppl 1):S22–S28 [G]
548. Dixon L, Weiden P, Delahanty J, Goldberg R, Postrado L, Lucksted A, Lehman A: Prevalence and correlates of diabetes in national schizophrenia samples. Schizophr Bull 2000; 26:903–912 [G]
549. Goldman LS: Medical illness in patients with schizophrenia. J Clin Psychiatry 1999; 60(suppl 21):10–15 [G]
550. Dalack GW, Healy DJ, Meador-Woodruff JH: Nicotine dependence in schizophrenia: clinical phenomena and laboratory findings. Am J Psychiatry 1998; 155:1490–1501 [F]
551. Jeste DV, Gladsjo JA, Lindamer LA, Lacro JP: Medical comorbidity in schizophrenia. Schizophr Bull 1996; 22:413–430 [G]
552. Mukherjee S, Decina P, Bocola V, Saraceni F, Scapicchio PL: Diabetes mellitus in schizophrenic patients. Compr Psychiatry 1996; 37:68–73 [G]
553. de Leon J, Dadvand M, Canuso C, White AO, Stanilla JK, Simpson GM: Schizophrenia and smoking: an epidemiological survey in a state hospital. Am J Psychiatry 1995; 152:453–455 [G]
554. Vieweg V, Levenson J, Pandurangi A, Silverman J: Medical disorders in the schizophrenic patient. Int J Psychiatry Med 1995; 25:137–172 [F]
555. Newman SC, Bland RC: Mortality in a cohort of patients with schizophrenia: a record linkage study. Can J Psychiatry 1991; 36:239–245 [C]
556. Wszola BA, Newell KM, Sprague RL: Risk factors for tardive dyskinesia in a large population of youths and adults. Exp Clin Psychopharmacol 2001; 9:285–296 [D]
557. Advokat CD, Mayville EA, Matson JL: Side effect profiles of atypical antipsychotics, typical antipsychotics, or no psychotropic medications in persons with mental retardation. Res Dev Disabil 2000; 21:75–84 [G]
558. Tariot PN, Ismail MS: Use of quetiapine in elderly patients. J Clin Psychiatry 2002; 63(suppl 13):21–26 [G]
559. Friedman JH, Fernandez HH: Atypical antipsychotics in Parkinson-sensitive populations. J Geriatr Psychiatry Neurol 2002; 15:156–170 [G]
560. Warner R, Wolleson C: Alternative acute treatment settings, in Practicing Psychiatry in the Community: A Manual. Edited by Vaccaro JV, Clark GH Jr. Washington, DC, American Psychiatric Press, 1996, pp 89–115 [G]
561. Joy CB, Adams CE, Rice K: Crisis intervention for people with severe mental illnesses. Cochrane Database Syst Rev 2000; (2):CD001087 [E]
562. Wilder JF, Levin G, Zwerling I: A two-year follow-up evaluation of acute psychotic patients treated in a day hospital. Am J Psychiatry 1966; 122:1095–1101 [B]
563. Herz MI, Endicott J, Spitzer RL, Mesnikoff A: Day versus inpatient hospitalization: a controlled study. Am J Psychiatry 1971; 127:1371–1382 [B]
564. Langsley DG, Machotka P, Flomenhaft K: Avoiding mental hospital admission: a follow-up study. Am J Psychiatry 1971; 127:1391–1394 [B]

565. Pasamanick B, Scarpitti FR, Dinitz S: Schizophrenics in the Community. New York, Appleton-Century-Crofts, 1967 [B]
566. Fenton FR, Tessier L, Struening EL: A comparative trial of home and hospital psychiatric care: one-year follow-up. Arch Gen Psychiatry 1979; 36:1073–1079 [B]
567. Mosher LR, Menn A, Matthew SM: Soteria: evaluation of a home-based treatment for schizophrenia. Am J Orthopsychiatry 1975; 45:455–467 [B]
568. Ciompi L, Dauwalder HP, Maier C, Aebi E, Trutsch K, Kupper Z, Rutishauser C: The pilot project "Soteria Berne": clinical experiences and results. Br J Psychiatry Suppl 1992; 161(suppl 18):145–153 [B]
569. Sledge WH, Tebes J, Rakfeldt J: Acute respite care, in Emergency Mental Health Services in the Community. Cambridge, UK, Cambridge University Press, 1995, pp 233–258 [B]
570. Brook BD: Crisis hostel: an alternative to psychiatric hospitalization for emergency patients. Hosp Community Psychiatry 1973; 24:621–624 [B]
571. Herz MI: Short-term hospitalization and the medical model. Hosp Community Psychiatry 1979; 30:117–121 [F]
572. Herz MI, Endicott J, Spitzer RL: Brief hospitalization: a two-year follow-up. Am J Psychiatry 1977; 134:502–507 [B]
573. Hirsch SR, Platt S, Knights A, Weyman A: Shortening hospital stay for psychiatric care: effect on patients and their families. Br Med J 1979; 1:442–446 [B]
574. Johnstone P, Zolese G: Length of hospitalisation for people with severe mental illness. Cochrane Database Syst Rev 2000; (2):CD000384 [E]
575. Caffey EM Jr, Jones RD, Diamond LS, Burton E, Bowen WT: Brief hospital treatment of schizophrenia: early results of a multiple-hospital study. Hosp Community Psychiatry 1968; 19:282–287 [B]
576. Caffey EM, Galbrecht CR, Klett CJ: Brief hospitalization and aftercare in the treatment of schizophrenia. Arch Gen Psychiatry 1971; 24:81–86 [B]
577. Glick ID, Hargreaves WA, Goldfield MD: Short vs long hospitalization—a prospective controlled study, I: the preliminary results of a one-year follow-up schizophrenics. Arch Gen Psychiatry 1974; 30:363–369 [B]
578. Glick ID, Hargreaves WA, Raskin M, Kutner SJ: Short versus long hospitalization: a prospective controlled study, II: results for schizophrenic inpatients. Am J Psychiatry 1975; 132:385–390 [B]
579. Glick ID, Hargreaves WA, Drues J, Showstack JA: Short versus long hospitalization: a prospective controlled study, IV: one-year follow-up results for schizophrenic patients. Am J Psychiatry 1976; 133:509–514 [B]
580. Hargreaves WA, Glick ID, Drues J, Showstack JA, Feigenbaum E: Short vs long hospitalization: a prospective controlled study, VI: two-year follow-up results for schizophrenics. Arch Gen Psychiatry 1977; 34:305–311 [B]
581. Rosen B, Katzoff A, Carrillo C, Klein DF: Clinical effectiveness of "short" vs "long" psychiatric hospitalization, I: inpatient results. Arch Gen Psychiatry 1976; 33:1316–1322 [B]
582. Mattes JA, Rosen B, Klein DF: Comparison of the clinical effectiveness of "short" versus "long" stay psychiatric hospitalization, II: results of a 3-year posthospital follow-up. J Nerv Ment Dis 1977; 165:387–394 [B]
583. Mattes JA, Rosen B, Klein DF, Millan D: Comparison of the clinical effectiveness of "short" versus "long" stay psychiatric hospitalization, III: further results of a 3-year posthospital follow-up. J Nerv Ment Dis 1977; 165:395–402 [B]
584. Mattes JA, Klein DF, Millan D, Rosen B: Comparison of the clinical effectiveness of "short" versus "long" stay psychiatric hospitalization, IV: predictors of differential benefit. J Nerv Ment Dis 1979; 167:175–181 [B]

585. Brenner HD, Dencker SJ, Goldstein MJ, Hubbard JW, Keegan DL, Kruger G, Kulhanek F, Liberman RP, Malm U, Midha KK: Defining treatment refractoriness in schizophrenia. Schizophr Bull 1990; 16:551–561 [F]
586. Bleuler M: Schizophrenic Disorders: Long-Term Patient and Family Studies. New Haven, Conn, Yale University Press, 1978 [E]
587. Huber G, Gross G, Schuttler R, Linz M: Longitudinal studies of schizophrenic patients. Schizophr Bull 1980; 6:592–605 [C, E]
588. Ciompi L: The natural history of schizophrenia in the long term. Br J Psychiatry 1980; 136:413–420 [E]
589. Hall J, Baker R: Token economies and schizophrenia: a review, in Contemporary Issues in Schizophrenia. Edited by Kerr TA, Snaith RP. London, Gaskell, 1986, pp 410–419 [G]
590. Glynn SM: Token economy approaches for psychiatric patients: progress and pitfalls over 25 years. Behav Modif 1990; 14:383–407 [F]
591. Paul GL, Lentz RJ: Psychological Treatment of Chronic Mental Patients: Milieu Versus Social-Learning Programs. Cambridge, Mass, Harvard University Press, 1977 [B]
592. Wong SE, Flanagan SG, Kuehnel TG, Liberman RP, Hunnicut R, Adams-Badgett J: Training chronic mental patients to independently practice personal grooming skills. Hosp Community Psychiatry 1988; 39:874–879 [B]
593. Boudewyns PA, Fry TJ, Nightingale T: Token economy programs in VA medical centers: where are they today? Behav Ther 1986; 9:126–127 [E]
594. Bellack AS, Mueser KT: A comprehensive treatment program for schizophrenia and chronic mental illness. Community Ment Health J 1986; 22:175–189 [B]
595. Corrigan PW: Strategies that overcome barriers to token economies in community programs for severe mentally ill adults. Community Ment Health J 1991; 27:17–30 [G]
596. Stroul BA: Crisis Residential Services in a Community Support System. Rockville, Md, National Institute of Mental Health, 1987 [G]
597. Sledge WH, Tebes J, Rakfeldt J, Davidson L, Lyons L, Druss B: Day hospital/crisis respite care versus inpatient care, part I: clinical outcomes. Am J Psychiatry 1996; 153:1065–1073 [A–]
598. Sledge WH, Tebes J, Wolff N, Helminiak TW: Day hospital/crisis respite care versus inpatient care, part II: service utilization and costs. Am J Psychiatry 1996; 153:1074–1083 [A–]
599. Fenton WS, Mosher LR, Herrell JM, Blyler CR: Randomized trial of general hospital and residential alternative care for patients with severe and persistent mental illness. Am J Psychiatry 1998; 155:516–522 [A–]
600. Fenton WS, Hoch JS, Herrell JM, Mosher L, Dixon L: Cost and cost-effectiveness of hospital vs residential crisis care for patients who have serious mental illness. Arch Gen Psychiatry 2002; 59:357–364 [A–]
601. Herz MI, Endicott J, Gibbon M: Brief hospitalization: two-year follow-up. Arch Gen Psychiatry 1979; 36:701–705 [B]
602. Washburn S, Vannicelli M, Longabaugh R, Scheff BJ: A controlled comparison of psychiatric day treatment and inpatient hospitalization. J Consult Clin Psychol 1976; 44:665–675 [B]
603. Creed F, Black D, Anthony P: Day-hospital and community treatment for acute psychiatric illness: a critical appraisal. Br J Psychiatry 1989; 154:300–310 [F]
604. Creed F, Black D, Anthony P, Osborn M, Thomas P, Tomenson B: Randomised controlled trial of day patient versus inpatient psychiatric treatment. Br Med J 1990; 300:1033–1037 [B]
605. Creed F, Black D, Anthony P, Osborn M, Thomas P, Franks D, Polley R, Lancashire S, Saleem P, Tomenson B: Randomised controlled trial of day and in-patient psychiatric treatment, 2: comparison of two hospitals. Br J Psychiatry 1991; 158:183–189 [B]
606. Dick P, Cameron L, Cohen D, Barlow M, Ince A: Day and full time psychiatric treatment: a controlled comparison. Br J Psychiatry 1985; 147:246–249 [B]

607. Gudeman JE, Dickey B, Evans A, Shore MF: Four-year assessment of a day hospital-inn program as an alternative to inpatient hospitalization. Am J Psychiatry 1985; 142:1330–1333 [B]
608. Schene AH, van Wijngaarden B, Poelijoe NW, Gersons BP: The Utrecht comparative study on psychiatric day treatment and inpatient treatment. Acta Psychiatr Scand 1993; 87:427–436 [B]
609. Marshall M, Crowther R, Almaraz-Serrano A, Creed F, Sledge W, Kluiter H, Roberts C, Hill E, Wiersma D: Day hospital versus admission for acute psychiatric disorders. Cochrane Database Syst Rev 2003; (1):CD004026 [E]
610. Creed F, Mbaya P, Lancashire S, Tomenson B, Williams B, Holme S: Cost effectiveness of day and inpatient psychiatric treatment: results of a randomised controlled trial. Br Med J 1997; 314:1381–1385 [A–]
611. Kris EB: Day hospitals. Current Therapeutic Research 1965; 7:320–323 [G]
612. Wiersma D, Kluiter H, Nienhuis FJ, Ruphan M, Giel R: Costs and benefits of day treatment with community care for schizophrenic patients. Schizophr Bull 1991; 17:411–419 [A–]
613. Wiersma D, Kluiter H, Nienhuis FJ, Ruphan M, Giel R: Costs and benefits of hospital and day treatment with community care of affective and schizophrenic disorders. Br J Psychiatry Suppl 1995; 166(suppl 27):52–59 [A–]
614. Zwerling I, Wilder JF: An evaluation of the applicability of the day hospital in the treatment of acutely disturbed patients. Isr Ann Psychiatry Relat Discip 1964; 2:162–185 [G]
615. Lamb HR: Chronic psychiatric patients in the day hospital. Arch Gen Psychiatry 1967; 17: 615–621 [B]
616. Guidry LS, Winstead DK, Levine M, Eicke FJ: Evaluation of day treatment center effectiveness. J Clin Psychiatry 1979; 40:221–224 [G]
617. Moscowitz IS: The effectiveness of day hospital treatment: a review. J Community Psychol 1980; 8:155–164 [F]
618. Meltzoff J, Blumenthal RL: The Day Treatment Center: Principles, Application and Evaluation. Springfield, Ill, Charles C Thomas, 1966 [B]
619. Weldon E, Clarkin JE, Hennessy JJ, Frances A: Day hospital versus outpatient treatment: a controlled study. Psychiatr Q 1979; 51:144–150 [B]
620. Trainor JN, Morrell-Bellai TL, Ballantyne R, Boydell KM: Housing for people with mental illnesses: a comparison of models and an examination of the growth of alternative housing in Canada. Can J Psychiatry 1993; 38:494–501 [G]
621. McCrone P, Strathdee G: Needs not diagnosis: towards a more rational approach to community mental health resourcing in Britain. Int J Soc Psychiatry 1994; 40:79–86 [G]
622. Budson RD: Models of supportive living: community residential care, in Handbook of Schizophrenia, vol 4: Psychosocial Treatment of Schizophrenia. Edited by Herz MI, Keith SJ, Docherty JP. New York, Elsevier, 1990, pp 317–338 [F]
623. Campbell R: Psychiatric Dictionary, 7th ed. New York, Oxford University Press, 1996 [G]
624. Murphy HB, Engelsmann F, Tcheng-Laroche F: The influence of foster-home care on psychiatric patients. Arch Gen Psychiatry 1976; 33:179–183 [C]
625. Friedrich RM, Hollingsworth B, Hradek E, Friedrich HB, Culp KR: Family and client perspectives on alternative residential settings for persons with severe mental illness. Psychiatr Serv 1999; 50:509–514 [G]
626. Hansson L, Middelboe T, Sorgaard KW, Bengtsson-Tops A, Bjarnason O, Merinder L, Nilsson L, Sandlund M, Korkeila J, Vinding HR: Living situation, subjective quality of life and social network among individuals with schizophrenia living in community settings. Acta Psychiatr Scand 2002; 106:343–350 [G]
627. Chilvers R, MacDonald GM, Hayes AA: Supported housing for people with severe mental disorders. Cochrane Database Syst Rev 2002; (4):CD000453 [E]
628. Newman SJ: Housing attributes and serious mental illness: implications for research and practice. Psychiatr Serv 2001; 52:1309–1317 [F]

629. Harrison P, Karberg JC: Prison and Jail Inmates at Midyear 2002 (NCJ-198877). Washington, DC, US Department of Justice, Bureau of Justice Statistics, 2003 [G]
630. Metzner JL, Cohen F, Grossman LS, Wettstein RM: Treatment in jails and prisons, in Treatment of Offenders With Mental Disorders. Edited by Wettstein RM. New York, Guilford, 1998, pp 211–264 [G]
631. Lamb HR, Weinberger LE: Persons with severe mental illness in jails and prisons: a review. Psychiatr Serv 1998; 49:483–492 [F]
632. American Psychiatric Association: Psychiatric Services in Jails and Prisons, 2nd ed. Washington, DC, American Psychiatric Association, 2000 [G]
633. Marauschak LM: HIV in Prisons and Jails, 1999 (NCJ-187456). Washington, DC, US Department of Justice, Bureau of Justice Statistics, 2001 [G]
634. Ruiz v Estelle, 503 F Supp 1265 (SD Tex 1980) [G]
635. Metzner JL: An introduction to correctional psychiatry: Part III. J Am Acad Psychiatry Law 1998; 26:107–115 [G]
636. Washington v Harper, 494 US 210 (1990) [G]
637. Krelstein MS: The role of mental health in the inmate disciplinary process: a national survey. J Am Acad Psychiatry Law 2002; 30:488–496 [G]
638. Zubek JP, Bayer L, Shephard JM: Relative effects of prolonged social isolation and confinement: behavioral and EEG changes. J Abnorm Psychol 1969; 74:625–631 [B]
639. Zinger I, Whichmann C: The Psychological Effects of 60 Days in Administrative Segregation. Ottawa, Correctional Service of Canada, Research Branch, 1999 [G]
640. Metzner JL: Class action litigation in correctional psychiatry. J Am Acad Psychiatry Law 2002; 30:19–29 [G]
641. Metzner JL: Mental health considerations for segregated inmates, in Standards for Health Services in Prisons. Chicago, National Commission on Correctional Healthcare, 2003 [G]
642. Metzner JL: Guidelines for psychiatric services in prisons. Criminal Behav Ment Health 1993; 3:252–267 [G]
643. McGlashan TH: A selective review of recent North American long-term followup studies of schizophrenia. Schizophr Bull 1988; 14:515–542 [F, G]
644. Karasu TB, Waltzman SA, Lindenmayer JP, Buckley PJ: The medical care of patients with psychiatric illness. Hosp Community Psychiatry 1980; 31:463–472 [G]
645. Bland RC, Parker JH, Orn H: Prognosis in schizophrenia: a ten-year follow-up of first admissions. Arch Gen Psychiatry 1976; 33:949–954 [C]
646. Tsuang MT, Woolson RF: Mortality in patients with schizophrenia, mania, depression and surgical conditions: a comparison with general population mortality. Br J Psychiatry 1977; 130:162–166 [C, D, E]
647. Tsuang MT, Woolson RF: Excess mortality in schizophrenia and affective disorders: do suicides and accidental deaths solely account for this excess? Arch Gen Psychiatry 1978; 35: 1181–1185 [C]
648. Tsuang MT, Woolson RF, Fleming JA: Causes of death in schizophrenia and manic-depression. Br J Psychiatry 1980; 136:239–242 [E]
649. Tsuang MT, Woolson RF, Fleming JA: Premature deaths in schizophrenia and affective disorders: an analysis of survival curves and variables affecting the shortened survival. Arch Gen Psychiatry 1980; 37:979–983 [C, D, E]
650. Eaton WW, Day R, Kramer M: The use of epidemology for risk factor research in schizophrenia: an overview and methodologic critique, in Handbook of Schizophrenia. Edited by Tsuang MT, Simpson JC. New York, Elsevier, 1988, pp 169–204 [E, G]
651. Rasanen S, Hakko H, Viilo K, Meyer-Rochow VB, Moring J: Excess mortality among long-stay psychiatric patients in northern Finland. Soc Psychiatry Psychiatr Epidemiol 2003; 38: 297–304 [C]

652. Cohen M, Dembling B, Schorling J: The association between schizophrenia and cancer: a population-based mortality study. Schizophr Res 2002; 57:139–146 [D]
653. Hannerz H, Borga P, Borritz M: Life expectancies for individuals with psychiatric diagnoses. Public Health 2001; 115:328–337 [C]
654. Dingman CW, McGlashan TH: Discriminating characteristics of suicides: Chestnut Lodge follow-up sample including patients with affective disorder, schizophrenia and schizoaffective disorder. Acta Psychiatr Scand 1986; 74:91–97 [C, D, E]
655. Tsuang MT: Suicide in schizophrenics, manics, depressives, and surgical controls: a comparison with general population suicide mortality. Arch Gen Psychiatry 1978; 35:153–155 [C, D, E]
656. Hiroeh U, Appleby L, Mortensen PB, Dunn G: Death by homicide, suicide, and other unnatural causes in people with mental illness: a population-based study. Lancet 2001; 358: 2110–2112 [G]
657. Osby U, Correia N, Brandt L, Ekbom A, Sparen P: Mortality and causes of death in schizophrenia in Stockholm County, Sweden. Schizophr Res 2000; 45:21–28 [C]
658. Docherty NM, DeRosa M, Andreasen NC: Communication disturbances in schizophrenia and mania. Arch Gen Psychiatry 1996; 53:358–364 [E]
659. McGlashan TH, Fenton WS: The positive-negative distinction in schizophrenia: review of natural history validators. Arch Gen Psychiatry 1992; 49:63–72 [F]
660. McGlashan TH, Fenton WS: Classical subtypes for schizophrenia: literature review for DSM-IV. Schizophr Bull 1991; 17:609–632 [F]
661. Fenton WS, McGlashan TH: Natural history of schizophrenia subtypes, I: longitudinal study of paranoid, hebephrenic, and undifferentiated schizophrenia. Arch Gen Psychiatry 1991; 48:969–977 [C, D]
662. Brady K, Anton R, Ballenger JC, Lydiard RB, Adinoff B, Selander J: Cocaine abuse among schizophrenic patients. Am J Psychiatry 1990; 147:1164–1167 [E, G]
663. Janowsky DS, Davis JM: Methylphenidate, dextroamphetamine, and levamfetamine: effects on schizophrenic symptoms. Arch Gen Psychiatry 1976; 33:304–308 [G]
664. Lieberman JA, Kane JM, Alvir J: Provocative tests with psychostimulant drugs in schizophrenia. Psychopharmacology (Berl) 1987; 91:415–433 [F]
665. Dixon L, Haas G, Weiden P, Sweeney J, Frances A: Acute effects of drug abuse in schizophrenic patients: clinical observations and patients' self-reports. Schizophr Bull 1990; 16:69–79 [G]
666. McGlashan TH, Krystal JH: Schizophrenia-related disorders and dual diagnosis, in Treatments of Psychiatric Disorders. Edited by Gabbard GO. Washington, DC, American Psychiatric Press, 1995, pp 1039–1074 [F, G]
667. Linszen DH, Dingemans PM, Lenior ME: Cannabis abuse and the course of recent-onset schizophrenic disorders. Arch Gen Psychiatry 1994; 51:273–279 [C]
668. Test MA, Wallisch LS, Allness DJ, Ripp K: Substance use in young adults with schizophrenic disorders. Schizophr Bull 1989; 15:465–476 [C, D, E]
669. Zisook S, Heaton R, Moranville J, Kuck J, Jernigan T, Braff D: Past substance abuse and clinical course of schizophrenia. Am J Psychiatry 1992; 149:552–553 [C, D, E]
670. van Os J, Bak M, Hanssen M, Bijl RV, de Graaf R, Verdoux H: Cannabis use and psychosis: a longitudinal population-based study. Am J Epidemiol 2002; 156:319–327 [C]
671. Fenton WS, McGlashan TH: The prognostic significance of obsessive-compulsive symptoms in schizophrenia. Am J Psychiatry 1986; 143:437–441 [C, D]
672. Keshavan MS, Schooler NR: First-episode studies in schizophrenia: criteria and characterization. Schizophr Bull 1992; 18:491–513 [F]
673. Olin SC, Mednick SA: Risk factors of psychosis: identifying vulnerable populations premorbidly. Schizophr Bull 1996; 22:223–240 [F]

674. Hafner H, Maurer K, Loffler W, Riecher-Rossler A: The influence of age and sex on the onset and early course of schizophrenia. Br J Psychiatry 1993; 162:80–86 [G]
675. Yung AR, McGorry PD: The prodromal phase of first-episode psychosis: past and current conceptualizations. Schizophr Bull 1996; 22:353–370 [G]
676. Yung AR, McGorry PD: The initial prodrome in psychosis: descriptive and qualitative aspects. Aust N Z J Psychiatry 1996; 30:587–599 [G]
677. Woods SW, Tandy M, McGlashan TH: The "prodromal" patient: both symptomatic and at-risk. CNS Spectrum 2001; 6:223–232 [G]
678. Johnstone EC, Crow TJ, Johnson AL, MacMillan JF: The Northwick Park Study of first episodes of schizophrenia, I: presentation of the illness and problems relating to admission. Br J Psychiatry 1986; 148:115–120 [G]
679. Birchwood M, Todd P, Jackson C: Early intervention in psychosis: the critical period hypothesis. Br J Psychiatry Suppl 1998; 172:53–59 [F]
680. Birchwood M, Smith J, Macmillan F, Hogg B, Prasad R, Harvey C, Bering S: Predicting relapse in schizophrenia: the development and implementation of an early signs monitoring system using patients and families as observers, a preliminary investigation. Psychol Med 1989; 19:649–656 [G]
681. Jorgensen P: Early signs of psychotic relapse in schizophrenia. Br J Psychiatry 1998; 172: 327–330 [C]
682. Herz MI, Lamberti JS: Prodromal symptoms and relapse prevention in schizophrenia. Schizophr Bull 1995; 21:541–551 [G]
683. Fenton WS, McGlashan TH: Prognostic scale for chronic schizophrenia. Schizophr Bull 1987; 13:277–286 [C, D, E]
684. Hegarty JD, Baldessarini RJ, Tohen M, Waternaux C, Oepen G: One hundred years of schizophrenia: a meta-analysis of the outcome literature. Am J Psychiatry 1994; 151:1409–1416 [E]
685. Krausz M, Muller-Thomsen T: Schizophrenia with onset in adolescence: an 11-year followup. Schizophr Bull 1993; 19:831–841 [G]
686. McGlashan TH: Predictors of shorter-, medium-, and longer-term outcome in schizophrenia. Am J Psychiatry 1986; 143:50–55 [C, D, E]
687. McGlashan TH, Bardenstein KK: Gender differences in affective, schizoaffective, and schizophrenic disorders. Schizophr Bull 1990; 16:319–329 [C, D]
688. McGlashan TH, Williams PV: Predicting outcome in schizoaffective psychosis. J Nerv Ment Dis 1990; 178:518–520 [C, D]
689. Davidson L, McGlashan TH: The varied outcomes of schizophrenia. Can J Psychiatry 1997; 42:34–43 [F]
690. Goldstein JM: Gender differences in the course of schizophrenia. Am J Psychiatry 1988; 145:684–689 [C]
691. Bromet EJ, Fennig S: Epidemiology and natural history of schizophrenia. Biol Psychiatry 1999; 46:871–881 [C, F]
692. Craig TJ, Siegel C, Hopper K, Lin S, Sartorius N: Outcome in schizophrenia and related disorders compared between developing and developed countries: a recursive partitioning re-analysis of the WHO DOSMD data. Br J Psychiatry 1997; 170:229–233 [C]
693. Allebeck P, Wistedt B: Mortality in schizophrenia: a ten-year follow-up based on the Stockholm County inpatient register. Arch Gen Psychiatry 1986; 43:650–653 [C]
694. Morgan MG, Scully PJ, Youssef HA, Kinsella A, Owens JM, Waddington JL: Prospective analysis of premature mortality in schizophrenia in relation to health service engagement: a 7.5-year study within an epidemiologically complete, homogeneous population in rural Ireland. Psychiatry Res 2003; 117:127–135 [C]
695. Joukamaa M, Heliovaara M, Knekt P, Aromaa A, Raitasalo R, Lehtinen V: Mental disorders and cause-specific mortality. Br J Psychiatry 2001; 179:498–502 [C]

696. Druss BG, Bradford WD, Rosenheck RA, Radford MJ, Krumholz HM: Quality of medical care and excess mortality in older patients with mental disorders. Arch Gen Psychiatry 2001; 58:565–572 [C]
697. Harris EC, Barraclough B: Suicide as an outcome for mental disorders: a meta-analysis. Br J Psychiatry 1997; 170:205–228 [E]
698. Roy A: Suicide in chronic schizophrenia. Br J Psychiatry 1982; 141:171–177 [D]
699. Jablensky A: Schizophrenia: recent epidemiologic issues. Epidemiol Rev 1995; 17:10–20 [F]
700. Jablensky A: Schizophrenia: the epidemiological horizon, in Schizophrenia. Edited by Hirsch SR, Weinberger DR. Oxford, UK, Blackwell Scientific Press, 1995, pp 206–252 [G]
701. Hafner H, an der Heiden W: Epidemiology of schizophrenia. Can J Psychiatry 1997; 42: 139–151 [F]
702. Jablensky A: The 100-year epidemiology of schizophrenia. Schizophr Res 1997; 28:111–125 [F]
703. Goldner EM, Hsu L, Waraich P, Somers JM: Prevalence and incidence studies of schizophrenic disorders: a systematic review of the literature. Can J Psychiatry 2002; 47:833–843 [E]
704. Bromet EJ, Dew MA, Eaton WW: Epidemiology of psychosis with special reference to schizophrenia, in Textbook in Psychiatric Epidemiology. Edited by Tsuang M, Tohen M, Zahner G. New York, Wiley-Liss, 1995, pp 283–300 [G]
705. Eaton WW, Kessler LG: Epidemiologic Field Methods in Psychiatry: The NIMH Epidemiologic Catchment Area Program. New York, Academic Press, 1985 [G]
706. Kendler KS, Gallagher TJ, Abelson JM, Kessler RC: Lifetime prevalence, demographic risk factors, and diagnostic validity of nonaffective psychosis as assessed in a US community sample: the National Comorbidity Survey. Arch Gen Psychiatry 1996; 53:1022–1031 [G]
707. Gurland BJ, Cross PS: Epidemiology of psychopathology in old age: some implications for clinical services. Psychiatr Clin North Am 1982; 5:11–26 [F]
708. Cohen CI: Outcome of schizophrenia into later life: an overview. Gerontologist 1990; 30: 790–797 [F]
709. Loranger AW: Sex difference in age at onset of schizophrenia. Arch Gen Psychiatry 1984; 41:157–161 [D]
710. Hafner H, Maurer K, Loffler W, Fatkenheuer B, an der Heiden W, Riecher-Rossler A, Behrens S, Gattaz WF: The epidemiology of early schizophrenia: influence of age and gender on onset and early course. Br J Psychiatry Suppl 1994; 164(suppl 23):29–38 [G]
711. Hambrecht M, Maurer K, Hafner H: Gender differences in schizophrenia in three cultures: results of the WHO collaborative study on psychiatric disability. Soc Psychiatry Psychiatr Epidemiol 1992; 27:117–121 [G]
712. Lewine RR: Sex differences in schizophrenia: timing or subtypes? Psychol Bull 1981; 90: 432–434 [G]
713. Hambrecht M, Maurer K, Hafner H, Sartorius N: Transnational stability of gender differences in schizophrenia? an analysis based on the WHO study on determinants of outcome of severe mental disorders. Eur Arch Psychiatry Clin Neurosci 1992; 242:6–12 [G]
714. Jablensky A, Cole SW: Is the earlier age at onset of schizophrenia in males a confounded finding? results from a cross-cultural investigation. Br J Psychiatry 1997; 170:234–240 [G]
715. DeLisi LE, Bass N, Boccio A, Shields G, Morganti C: Age of onset in familial schizophrenia. Arch Gen Psychiatry 1994; 51:334–335 [G]
716. Albus M, Maier W: Lack of gender differences in age at onset in familial schizophrenia. Schizophr Res 1995; 18:51–57 [D]
717. Castle D, Wessely S, Der G, Murray RM: The incidence of operationally defined schizophrenia in Camberwell, 1965–84. Br J Psychiatry 1991; 159:790–794 [G]
718. Hafner H, Riecher-Rossler A, Maurer K, Fatkenheuer B, Loffler W: First onset and early symptomatology of schizophrenia: a chapter of epidemiological and neurobiological research into age and sex differences. Eur Arch Psychiatry Clin Neurosci 1992; 242:109–118 [G]

719. Lindamer LA, Lohr JB, Harris MJ, Jeste DV: Gender, estrogen, and schizophrenia. Psychopharmacol Bull 1997; 33:221–228 [G]
720. Perry W, Moore D, Braff D: Gender differences on thought disturbance measures among schizophrenic patients. Am J Psychiatry 1995; 152:1298–1301 [D]
721. Gottesman II: Schizophrenia Genesis: The Origin of Madness. New York, WH Freeman, 1991 [G]
722. Kestenbaum CJ: Children at risk for schizophrenia. Am J Psychother 1980; 34:164–177 [F]
723. Gottesman II, Shields J: Schizophrenia and Genetics: A Twin Study Vantage Point. New York, Academic Press, 1972 [G]
724. McNeil TF: Obstetric factors and perinatal injuries, in Handbook of Schizophrenia, vol 3: Nosology, Epidemiology and Genetics of Schizophrenia. Edited by Tsuang MT, Simpson JC. New York, Elsevier, 1988, pp 319–344 [G]
725. McNeil TF: Perinatal risk factors and schizophrenia: selective review and methodological concerns. Epidemiol Rev 1995; 17:107–112 [F]
726. Geddes JR, Lawrie SM: Obstetric complications and schizophrenia: a meta-analysis. Br J Psychiatry 1995; 167:786–793 [E]
727. Geddes JR, Verdoux H, Takei N, Lawrie SM, Bovet P, Eagles JM, Heun R, McCreadie RG, McNeil TF, O'Callaghan E, Stober G, Willinger U, Murray RM: Schizophrenia and complications of pregnancy and labor: an individual patient data meta-analysis. Schizophr Bull 1999; 25:413–423 [E]
728. Cannon TD: On the nature and mechanisms of obstetric influences in schizophrenia: a review and synthesis of epidemiologic studies. Int Rev Psychiatry 1997; 9:387–397 [F]
729. Cannon M, Jones PB, Murray RM: Obstetric complications and schizophrenia: historical and meta-analytic review. Am J Psychiatry 2002; 159:1080–1092 [E]
730. Byrne M, Browne R, Mulryan N, Scully A, Morris M, Kinsella A, Takei N, McNeil T, Walsh D, O'Callaghan E: Labour and delivery complications and schizophrenia: case-control study using contemporaneous labour ward records. Br J Psychiatry 2000; 176:531–536 [D]
731. Kendell RE, McInneny K, Juszczak E, Bain M: Obstetric complications and schizophrenia: two case-control studies based on structured obstetric records. Br J Psychiatry 2000; 176: 516–522 [D]
732. Westergaard T, Mortensen PB, Pedersen CB, Wohlfahrt J, Melbye M: Exposure to prenatal and childhood infections and the risk of schizophrenia: suggestions from a study of sibship characteristics and influenza prevalence. Arch Gen Psychiatry 1999; 56:993–998 [C]
733. Mednick SA, Machon RA, Huttunen MO, Bonett D: Adult schizophrenia following prenatal exposure to an influenza epidemic. Arch Gen Psychiatry 1988; 45:189–192 [D]
734. O'Callaghan E, Sham P, Takei N, Glover G, Murray RM: Schizophrenia after prenatal exposure to 1957 A2 influenza epidemic. Lancet 1991; 337:1248–1250 [D]
735. Sham PC, O'Callaghan E, Takei N, Murray GK, Hare EH, Murray RM: Schizophrenia following pre-natal exposure to influenza epidemics between 1939 and 1960. Br J Psychiatry 1992; 160:461–466 [D]
736. O'Reilly RL: Viruses and schizophrenia. Aust N Z J Psychiatry 1994; 28:222–228 [G]
737. McGrath J, Murray RM: Risk factors for schizophrenia: from conception to birth, in Schizophrenia. Edited by Hirsch SR, Weinberger DR. Oxford, UK, Blackwell Scientific Press, 1995, pp 187–205 [G]
738. Brown AS, Schaefer CA, Wyatt RJ, Goetz R, Begg MD, Gorman JM, Susser ES: Maternal exposure to respiratory infections and adult schizophrenia spectrum disorders: a prospective birth cohort study. Schizophr Bull 2000; 26:287–295 [C]
739. Susser E, Neugebauer R, Hoek HW, Brown AS, Lin S, Labovitz D, Gorman JM: Schizophrenia after prenatal famine: further evidence. Arch Gen Psychiatry 1996; 53:25–31 [G]
740. Hollister JM, Laing P, Mednick SA: Rhesus incompatibility as a risk factor for schizophrenia in male adults. Arch Gen Psychiatry 1996; 53:19–24 [C]

741. Kendell RE, Juszczak E, Cole SK: Obstetric complications and schizophrenia: a case control study based on standardised obstetric records. Br J Psychiatry 1996; 168:556–561 [D]
742. Jones PB, Rantakallio P, Hartikainen AL, Isohanni M, Sipila P: Schizophrenia as a long-term outcome of pregnancy, delivery, and perinatal complications: a 28-year follow-up of the 1966 north Finland general population birth cohort. Am J Psychiatry 1998; 155:355–364 [C]
743. Dalman C, Allebeck P, Cullberg J, Grunewald C, Koster M: Obstetric complications and the risk of schizophrenia: a longitudinal study of a national birth cohort. Arch Gen Psychiatry 1999; 56:234–240 [C]
744. Verdoux H, Geddes JR, Takei N, Lawrie SM, Bovet P, Eagles JM, Heun R, McCreadie RG, McNeil TF, O'Callaghan E, Stober G, Willinger MU, Wright P, Murray RM: Obstetric complications and age at onset in schizophrenia: an international collaborative meta-analysis of individual patient data. Am J Psychiatry 1997; 154:1220–1227 [E]
745. Cannon TD, Rosso IM, Bearden CE, Sanchez LE, Hadley T: A prospective cohort study of neurodevelopmental processes in the genesis and epigenesis of schizophrenia. Dev Psychopathol 1999; 11:467–485 [C]
746. Bradbury TN, Miller GA: Season of birth in schizophrenia: a review of evidence, methodology, and etiology. Psychol Bull 1985; 98:569–594 [F]
747. Boyd JH, Pulver AE, Stewart W: Season of birth: schizophrenia and bipolar disorder. Schizophr Bull 1986; 12:173–186 [F]
748. Hafner H, Haas S, Pfeifer-Kurda M, Eichhorn S, Michitsuji S: Abnormal seasonality of schizophrenic births: a specific finding? Eur Arch Psychiatry Neurol Sci 1987; 236:333–342 [D, F]
749. Allebeck P, Adamsson C, Engstrom A, Rydberg U: Cannabis and schizophrenia: a longitudinal study of cases treated in Stockholm County. Acta Psychiatr Scand 1993; 88:21–24 [C]
750. Zammit S, Allebeck P, Andreasson S, Lundberg I, Lewis G: Self reported cannabis use as a risk factor for schizophrenia in Swedish conscripts of 1969: historical cohort study. Br Med J 2002; 325:1199–1201 [C]
751. Hambrecht M, Hafner H: Substance abuse and the onset of schizophrenia. Biol Psychiatry 1996; 40:1155–1163 [D]
752. Harvey I, Williams M, McGuffin P, Toone BK: The functional psychoses in Afro-Caribbeans. Br J Psychiatry 1990; 157:515–522 [C]
753. Wessely S, Castle D, Der G, Murray R: Schizophrenia and Afro-Caribbeans: a case-control study. Br J Psychiatry 1991; 159:795–801 [D]
754. Bhugra D, Leff J, Mallett R, Der G, Corridan B, Rudge S: Incidence and outcome of schizophrenia in whites, African-Caribbeans and Asians in London. Psychol Med 1997; 27: 791–798 [C]
755. Lewis G, David A, Andreasson S, Allebeck P: Schizophrenia and city life. Lancet 1992; 340: 137–140 [C]
756. Freeman H: Schizophrenia and city residence. Br J Psychiatry 164(suppl 23):39–50 [F]
757. Brown AS, Schaefer CA, Wyatt RJ, Begg MD, Goetz R, Bresnahan MA, Harkavy-Friedman J, Gorman JM, Malaspina D, Susser ES: Paternal age and risk of schizophrenia in adult offspring. Am J Psychiatry 2002; 159:1528–1533 [C]
758. Malaspina D, Harlap S, Fennig S, Heiman D, Nahon D, Feldman D, Susser ES: Advancing paternal age and the risk of schizophrenia. Arch Gen Psychiatry 2001; 58:361–367 [C]
759. McGuire TG: Measuring the economic costs of schizophrenia. Schizophr Bull 1991; 17: 375–388 [F]
760. Rupp A, Keith SJ: The costs of schizophrenia: assessing the burden. Psychiatr Clin North Am 1993; 16:413–423 [G]
761. Rice DP, Miller LS: The economic burden of schizophrenia: conceptual and methodology issues and cost estimates, in Handbook of Mental Health Economics and Health Policy,

vol 1: Schizophrenia. Edited by Moscarelli M, Rupp A, Sartorius N. New York, Wiley, 1996, pp 321–334 [G]
762. Knapp MRJ, Almond S, Percudani M: Costs of schizophrenia, a review, in Schizophrenia. Edited by Maj M, Sartorius N. Chichester, UK, John Wiley & Sons, 1999, pp 407–454 [G]
763. Davies LM, Drummond MF: Economics and schizophrenia: the real cost. Br J Psychiatry 1994; 165(suppl 25):18–21 [G]
764. Harvey PD, Keefe RS: Studies of cognitive change in patients with schizophrenia following novel antipsychotic treatment. Am J Psychiatry 2001; 158:176–184 [G]
765. Meltzer HY, McGurk SR: The effects of clozapine, risperidone, and olanzapine on cognitive function in schizophrenia. Schizophr Bull 1999; 25:233–255 [F]
766. Keefe RS, Silva SG, Perkins DO, Lieberman JA: The effects of atypical antipsychotic drugs on neurocognitive impairment in schizophrenia: a review and meta-analysis. Schizophr Bull 1999; 25:201–222 [E]
767. Green MF: What are the functional consequences of neurocognitive deficits in schizophrenia? Am J Psychiatry 1996; 153:321–330 [F]
768. Rosenheck R, Cramer J, Xu W, Grabowski J, Douyon R, Thomas J, Henderson W, Charney D (Department of Veterans Affairs Cooperative Study Group on Clozapine in Refractory Schizophrenia): Multiple outcome assessment in a study of the cost-effectiveness of clozapine in the treatment of refractory schizophrenia. Health Serv Res 1998; 33:1237–1261 [A]
769. Rosenheck R, Cramer J, Xu W, Thomas J, Henderson W, Frisman L, Fye C, Charney D (Department of Veterans Affairs Cooperative Study Group on Clozapine in Refractory Schizophrenia): A comparison of clozapine and haloperidol in hospitalized patients with refractory schizophrenia. N Engl J Med 1997; 337:809–815 [A]
770. Sernyak MJ, Leslie D, Rosenheck R: Use of system-wide outcomes monitoring data to compare the effectiveness of atypical neuroleptic medications. Am J Psychiatry 2003; 160: 310–315 [C]
771. Corrigan PW, Reinke RR, Landsberger SA, Charate A, Toombs GA: The effects of atypical antipsychotic medications on psychosocial outcomes. Schizophr Res 2003; 63:97–101 [F]
772. Tandon R, Jibson MD: Extrapyramidal side effects of antipsychotic treatment: scope of problem and impact on outcome. Ann Clin Psychiatry 2002; 14:123–129 [G]
773. Nasrallah HA, Mulvihill T: Iatrogenic disorders associated with conventional vs atypical antipsychotics. Ann Clin Psychiatry 2001; 13:215–227 [G]
774. Marder SR: Antipsychotic medications, in The American Psychiatric Press Textbook of Psychopharmacology, 2nd ed. Edited by Schatzberg AF, Nemeroff CB. Washington, DC, American Psychiatric Press, 1998, pp 309–321 [G]
775. Laskey JJ, Klett CJ, Caffey EM Jr, Bennett JL, Rosenblum MP, Hollister LE: Drug treatment of schizophrenic patients: a comprehensive evaluation of chlorpromazine, chlorprothixene, fluphenazine, reserpine, thioridazine, and triflupromazine. Dis Nerv Syst 1962; 23:698–706 [A]
776. National Institutes of Health Psychopharmacology Service Center Collaborative Study Group: Phenothiazine treatment in acute schizophrenia. Arch Gen Psychiatry 1964; 10: 246–261 [A]
777. Davis JM, Barter JT, Kane JM: Antipsychotic drugs, in Comprehensive Textbook of Psychiatry, 5th ed. Edited by Kaplan HI, Sadock BJ. Baltimore, Williams & Wilkins, 1989, pp 1591–1626 [G]
778. Casey JF, Lasky JJ, Klett CJ, Hollister LE: Treatment of schizophrenic reactions with phenothiazine derivatives: a comparative study of chlorpromazine, triflupromazine, mepazine, prochlorperazine, perphenazine, and phenobarbital. Am J Psychiatry 1960; 117:97–105 [A]
779. Klein DF, Davis JM: Diagnosis and Drug Treatment of Psychiatric Disorders. Huntington, NY, Krieger, 1969 [G]

780. Baldessarini RJ: Drugs and treatment of psychiatric disorders: psychosis and anxiety, in Goodman and Gilman's The Pharmacologic Basis of Therapeutics, 9th ed. Edited by Hardman JG, Limbird LE, Molinoff PB, Ruddon RW, Gilman AG. New York, McGraw Hill, 1996, pp 447–483 [G]
781. Kolakowska T, Williams AO, Ardern M, Reveley MA, Jambor K, Gelder MG, Mandelbrote BM: Schizophrenia with good and poor outcome: I: early clinical features, response to neuroleptics and signs of organic dysfunction. Br J Psychiatry 1985; 146:229–239 [D]
782. Coryell W, Miller DD, Perry PJ: Haloperidol plasma levels and dose optimization. Am J Psychiatry 1998; 155:48–53 [A–]
783. Volavka J, Cooper TB, Czobor P, Lindenmayer JP, Citrome LL, Mohr P, Bark N: High-dose treatment with haloperidol: the effect of dose reduction. J Clin Psychopharmacol 2000; 20:252–256 [A]
784. Stone CK, Garve DL, Griffith J, Hirschowitz J, Bennett J: Further evidence of a dose-response threshold for haloperidol in psychosis. Am J Psychiatry 1995; 152:1210–1212 [A]
785. Krakowski M, Czobor P, Volavka J: Effect of neuroleptic treatment on depressive symptoms in acute schizophrenic episodes. Psychiatry Res 1997; 71:19–26 [A–]
786. Volavka J, Cooper TB, Czobor P, Meisner M: Effect of varying haloperidol plasma levels on negative symptoms in schizophrenia and schizoaffective disorder. Psychopharmacol Bull 1996; 32:75–79 [A]
787. Bollini P, Pampallona S, Orza MJ, Adams ME, Chalmers TC: Antipsychotic drugs: is more worse? a meta-analysis of the published randomized control trials. Psychol Med 1994; 24: 307–316 [G]
788. Convit A, Volavka J, Czobor P, de Asis J, Evangelista C: Effect of subtle neurological dysfunction on response to haloperidol treatment in schizophrenia. Am J Psychiatry 1994; 151:49–56 [A–]
789. Davis JM: Overview: maintenance therapy in psychiatry, I: schizophrenia. Am J Psychiatry 1975; 132:1237–1245 [E]
790. Kane JM: Treatment programme and long-term outcome in chronic schizophrenia. Acta Psychiatr Scand Suppl 1990; 358:151–157 [F]
791. Schooler NR, Levine J, Severe JB, Brauzer B, DiMascio A, Klerman GL, Tuason VB: Prevention of relapse in schizophrenia: an evaluation of fluphenazine decanoate. Arch Gen Psychiatry 1980; 37:16–24 [A–]
792. Hogarty GE, Ulrich RF, Mussare F, Aristigueta N: Drug discontinuation among long term, successfully maintained schizophrenic outpatients. Dis Nerv Syst 1976; 37:494–500 [C]
793. Marder SR, Van Putten T, Mintz J, Lebell M, McKenzie J, May PR: Low- and conventional-dose maintenance therapy with fluphenazine decanoate: two-year outcome. Arch Gen Psychiatry 1987; 44:518–521 [A]
794. Kane JM, Rifkin A, Woerner M, Reardon G, Sarantakos S, Schiebel D, Ramos-Lorenzi J: Low-dose neuroleptic treatment of outpatient schizophrenics, I: preliminary results for relapse rates. Arch Gen Psychiatry 1983; 40:893–896 [A]
795. Inderbitzin LB, Lewine RR, Scheller-Gilkey G, Swofford CD, Egan GJ, Gloersen BA, Vidan-agama BP, Waternaux C: A double-blind dose-reduction trial of fluphenazine decanoate for chronic, unstable schizophrenic patients. Am J Psychiatry 1994; 151:1753–1759 [A]
796. Carpenter WT Jr, Buchanan RW, Kirkpatrick B, Lann HD, Breier AF, Summerfelt AT: Comparative effectiveness of fluphenazine decanoate injections every 2 weeks versus every 6 weeks. Am J Psychiatry 1999; 156:412–418 [A]
797. Kane JM, Lieberman JA: Adverse Effects of Psychotropic Drugs. New York, Guilford, 1992 [G]
798. Dahl SG: Pharmacokinetics of antipsychotic drugs in man. Acta Psychiatr Scand Suppl 1990; 358:37–40 [G]
799. Johnson DA: Observations on the use of long-acting depot neuroleptic injections in the maintenance therapy of schizophrenia. J Clin Psychiatry 1984; 45:13–21 [D]

800. Hogarty GE, Schooler NR, Ulrich R, Mussare F, Ferro P, Herron E: Fluphenazine and social therapy in the aftercare of schizophrenic patients: relapse analyses of a two-year controlled study of fluphenazine decanoate and fluphenazine hydrochloride. Arch Gen Psychiatry 1979; 36:1283–1294 [A–]
801. Seeman P, Lee T, Chau-Wong M, Wong K: Antipsychotic drug doses and neuroleptic/dopamine receptors. Nature 1976; 261:717–719 [G]
802. Creese I, Burt DR, Snyder SH: Dopamine receptor binding predicts clinical and pharmacological potencies of antischizophrenic drugs. Science 1976; 192:481–483 [G]
803. Reardon GT, Rifkin A, Schwartz A, Myerson A, Siris SG: Changing patterns of neuroleptic dosage over a decade. Am J Psychiatry 1989; 146:726–729 [G]
804. Neborsky R, Janowsky D, Munson E, Depry D: Rapid treatment of acute psychotic symptoms with high- and low-dose haloperidol: behavioral considerations. Arch Gen Psychiatry 1981; 38:195–199 [E]
805. Carpenter WT Jr, Heinrichs DW, Hanlon TE: A comparative trial of pharmacologic strategies in schizophrenia. Am J Psychiatry 1987; 144:1466–1470 [A–]
806. Jolley AG, Hirsch SR, McRink A, Manchanda R: Trial of brief intermittent neuroleptic prophylaxis for selected schizophrenic outpatients: clinical outcome at one year. Br Med J 1989; 298:985–990 [A]
807. Pietzcker A, Gaebel W, Kopcke W, Linden M, Muller P, Muller-Spahn F, Schussler G, Tegeler J: A German multicentre study of the neroleptic long term therapy of schizophrenic patients: preliminary report. Pharmacopsychiatry 1986; 19:161–166 [A, B]
808. Kane JM, Woerner M, Sarantakos S: Depot neuroleptics: a comparative review of standard, intermediate, and low-dose regimens. J Clin Psychiatry 1986; 47(suppl):30–33 [F]
809. Hogarty GE, McEvoy JP, Munetz M, DiBarry AL, Bartone P, Cather R, Cooley SJ, Ulrich RF, Carter M, Madonia MJ: Dose of fluphenazine, familial expressed emotion, and outcome in schizophrenia: results of a two-year controlled study. Arch Gen Psychiatry 1988; 45:797–805 [A]
810. Derogatis LR: SCL-90-R: Administration, Scoring, and Procedures Manual, II. Towson, Md, Clinical Psychometric Research, 1983 [G]
811. Toll LL, Hurlbut KM (eds): POISINDEX® System. Greenwood Village, Col, MICROMEDEX, 2003 [G]
812. Marder SR, van Kammen DP: Dopamine receptor antagonists (typical antipsychotics), in Kaplan and Sadock's Comprehensive Textbook of Psychiatry, 7th ed. Edited by Sadock BJ, Sadock VA. Baltimore, Lippincott Williams & Wilkins, 2000 [G]
813. Kapur S, Seeman P: Antipsychotic agents differ in how fast they come off the dopamine D2 receptors: implications for atypical antipsychotic action. J Psychiatry Neurosci 2000; 25:161–166 [G]
814. Kapur S, Zipursky R, Jones C, Shammi CS, Remington G, Seeman P: A positron emission tomography study of quetiapine in schizophrenia: a preliminary finding of an antipsychotic effect with only transiently high dopamine D2 receptor occupancy. Arch Gen Psychiatry 2000; 57:553–559 [A–]
815. Kapur S, Seeman P: Does fast dissociation from the dopamine d(2) receptor explain the action of atypical antipsychotics? a new hypothesis. Am J Psychiatry 2001; 158:360–369 [G]
816. Schotte A, Janssen PF, Gommeren W, Luyten WH, Van Gompel P, Lesage AS, De Loore K, Leysen JE: Risperidone compared with new and reference antipsychotic drugs: in vitro and in vivo receptor binding. Psychopharmacology (Berl) 1996; 124:57–73 [G]
817. Richelson E, Souder T: Binding of antipsychotic drugs to human brain receptors focus on newer generation compounds. Life Sci 2000; 68:29–39 [G]
818. Kroeze WK, Hufeisen SJ, Popadak BA, Renock SM, Steinberg S, Ernsberger P, Jayathilake K, Meltzer HY, Roth BL: H1-histamine receptor affinity predicts short-term weight gain for typical and atypical antipsychotic drugs. Neuropsychopharmacology 2003; 28:519–526 [G]

819. Zeng XP, Le F, Richelson E: Muscarinic m4 receptor activation by some atypical antipsychotic drugs. Eur J Pharmacol 1997; 321:349–354 [G]
820. Volavka J, Czobor P, Sheitman B, Lindenmayer JP, Citrome L, McEvoy JP, Cooper TB, Chakos M, Lieberman JA: Clozapine, olanzapine, risperidone, and haloperidol in the treatment of patients with chronic schizophrenia and schizoaffective disorder. Am J Psychiatry 2002; 159:255–262 [A]
821. Kane JM, Marder SR, Schooler NR, Wirshing WC, Umbricht D, Baker RW, Wirshing DA, Safferman A, Ganguli R, McMeniman M, Borenstein M: Clozapine and haloperidol in moderately refractory schizophrenia: a 6-month randomized and double-blind comparison. Arch Gen Psychiatry 2001; 58:965–972 [A]
822. Essock SM, Hargreaves WA, Covell NH, Goethe J: Clozapine's effectiveness for patients in state hospitals: results from a randomized trial. Psychopharmacol Bull 1996; 32:683–697 [A–]
823. Hong CJ, Chen JY, Chiu HJ, Sim CB: A double-blind comparative study of clozapine versus chlorpromazine on Chinese patients with treatment-refractory schizophrenia. Int Clin Psychopharmacol 1997; 12:123–130 [A]
824. Kumra S, Frazier JA, Jacobsen LK, McKenna K, Gordon CT, Lenane MC, Hamburger SD, Smith AK, Albus KE, Alaghband-Rad J, Rapoport JL: Childhood-onset schizophrenia: a double-blind clozapine-haloperidol comparison. Arch Gen Psychiatry 1996; 53:1090–1097 [A–]
825. Chengappa KN, Vasile J, Levine J, Ulrich R, Baker R, Gopalani A, Schooler N: Clozapine: its impact on aggressive behavior among patients in a state psychiatric hospital. Schizophr Res 2002; 53:1–6 [D]
826. Gordon BJ, Milke DJ: Dose related response to clozapine in a state psychiatric hospital population: a naturalistic study. Psychiatr Q 1996; 67:65–74 [D]
827. Chatterjee A, Lieberman JA: Studies of biological variables in first-episode schizophrenia: a comprehensive review, in The Recognition and Management of Early Psychosis. Edited by McGorry PD, Jackson HJ. Cambridge, UK, Cambridge University Press, 1999, pp 115–152 [F]
828. Goldberg TE, Greenberg RD, Griffin SJ, Gold JM, Kleinman JE, Pickar D, Schulz SC, Weinberger DR: The effect of clozapine on cognition and psychiatric symptoms in patients with schizophrenia. Br J Psychiatry 1993; 162:43–48 [G]
829. Hagger C, Buckley P, Kenny JT, Friedman L, Ubogy D, Meltzer HY: Improvement in cognitive functions and psychiatric symptoms in treatment-refractory schizophrenic patients receiving clozapine. Biol Psychiatry 1993; 34:702–712 [B]
830. Buchanan RW, Holstein C, Breier A: The comparative efficacy and long-term effect of clozapine treatment on neuropsychological test performance. Biol Psychiatry 1994; 36: 717–725 [A]
831. Hoff AL, Faustman WO, Wieneke M, Espinoza S, Costa M, Wolkowitz O, Csernansky JG: The effects of clozapine on symptom reduction, neurocognitive function, and clinical management in treatment-refractory state hospital schizophrenic inpatients. Neuropsychopharmacology 1996; 15:361–369 [B]
832. Grace J, Bellus SB, Raulin ML, Herz MI, Priest BL, Brenner V, Donnelly K, Smith P, Gunn S: Long-term impact of clozapine and psychosocial treatment on psychiatric symptoms and cognitive functioning. Psychiatr Serv 1996; 47:41–45 [B]
833. Galletly CA, Clark CR, McFarlane AC, Weber DL: Relationships between changes in symptom ratings, neurophysiological test performance and quality of life in schizophrenic patients treated with clozapine. Psychiatry Res 1997; 72:161–166 [G]
834. Meyer-Lindenberg A, Gruppe H, Bauer U, Lis S, Krieger S, Gallhofer B: Improvement of cognitive function in schizophrenic patients receiving clozapine or zotepine: results from a double-blind study. Pharmacopsychiatry 1997; 30:35–42 [A]
835. Lindenmayer JP, Iskander A, Park M, Apergi FS, Czobor P, Smith R, Allen D: Clinical and neurocognitive effects of clozapine and risperidone in treatment-refractory schizophrenic patients: a prospective study. J Clin Psychiatry 1998; 59:521–527 [B]

836. Lee MA, Jayathilake K, Meltzer HY: A comparison of the effect of clozapine with typical neuroleptics on cognitive function in neuroleptic-responsive schizophrenia. Schizophr Res 1999; 37:1–11 [A–]
837. Manschreck TC, Redmond DA, Candela SF, Maher BA: Effects of clozapine on psychiatric symptoms, cognition, and functional outcome in schizophrenia. J Neuropsychiatry Clin Neurosci 1999; 11:481–489 [B]
838. Bilder RM, Goldman RS, Volavka J, Czobor P, Hoptman M, Sheitman B, Lindenmayer JP, Citrome L, McEvoy J, Kunz M, Chakos M, Cooper TB, Horowitz TL, Lieberman JA: Neurocognitive effects of clozapine, olanzapine, risperidone, and haloperidol in patients with chronic schizophrenia or schizoaffective disorder. Am J Psychiatry 2002; 159:1018–1028 [A]
839. Potkin SG, Fleming K, Jin Y, Gulasekaram B: Clozapine enhances neurocognition and clinical symptomatology more than standard neuroleptics. J Clin Psychopharmacol 2001; 21:479–483 [A]
840. Purdon SE, Labelle A, Boulay L: Neuropsychological change in schizophrenia after 6 weeks of clozapine. Schizophr Res 2001; 48:57–67 [G]
841. Meltzer HY, Burnett S, Bastani B, Ramirez LF: Effects of six months of clozapine treatment on the quality of life of chronic schizophrenic patients. Hosp Community Psychiatry 1990; 41:892–897 [B]
842. Miller DD, Perry PJ, Cadoret R, Andreasen NC: A two and one-half year follow-up of treatment-refractory schizophrenics treated with clozapine (abstract). Biol Psychiatry 1992; 31(March suppl):85A [E]
843. Breier A, Buchanan RW, Irish D, Carpenter WT Jr: Clozapine treatment of outpatients with schizophrenia: outcome and long-term response patterns. Hosp Community Psychiatry 1993; 44:1145–1149 [C]
844. Pollack S, Woerner MG, Howard A, Fireworker RB, Kane JM: Clozapine reduces rehospitalization among schizophrenia patients. Psychopharmacol Bull 1998; 34:89–92 [C]
845. Conley RR, Love RC, Kelly DL, Bartko JJ: Rehospitalization rates of patients recently discharged on a regimen of risperidone or clozapine. Am J Psychiatry 1999; 156:863–868 [D]
846. Lieberman JA, Phillips M, Gu H, Stroup S, Zhang P, Kong L, Ji Z, Koch G, Hamer RM: Atypical and conventional antipsychotic drugs in treatment-naive first-episode schizophrenia: a 52-week randomized trial of clozapine vs chlorpromazine. Neuropsychopharmacology 2003; 28:995–1003 [A]
847. Baldessarini RJ, Frankenburg FR: Clozapine: a novel antipsychotic agent. N Engl J Med 1991; 324:746–754 [G]
848. Klieser E, Lehmann E, Kinzler E, Wurthmann C, Heinrich K: Randomized, double-blind, controlled trial of risperidone versus clozapine in patients with chronic schizophrenia. J Clin Psychopharmacol 1995; 15:45S–51S [A]
849. Rabinowitz T, Frankenburg FR, Centorrino F, Kando J: The effect of clozapine on saliva flow rate: a pilot study. Biol Psychiatry 1996; 40:1132–1134 [D]
850. Zorn SH, Jones SB, Ward KM, Liston DR: Clozapine is a potent and selective muscarinic M4 receptor agonist. Eur J Pharmacol 1994; 269:R1–R2 [G]
851. Corrigan FM, MacDonald S, Reynolds GP: Clozapine-induced hypersalivation and the alpha 2 adrenoceptor (letter). Br J Psychiatry 1995; 167:412 [G]
852. Comley C, Galletly C, Ash D: Use of atropine eye drops for clozapine induced hypersalivation. Aust N Z J Psychiatry 2000; 34:1033–1034 [G]
853. Davydov L, Botts SR: Clozapine-induced hypersalivation. Ann Pharmacother 2000; 34:662–665 [F]
854. Novartis Pharmaceuticals Corporation: Clozaril Prescribing Information. East Hanover, NJ, Novartis Pharmaceuticals Corporation, 2003. (http://www.clozaril.com) [G]
855. Tham JC, Dickson RA: Clozapine-induced fevers and 1-year clozapine discontinuation rate. J Clin Psychiatry 2002; 63:880–884 [G]

856. Alvir JM, Lieberman JA, Safferman AZ, Schwimmer JL, Schaaf JA: Clozapine-induced agranulocytosis: incidence and risk factors in the United States. N Engl J Med 1993; 329: 162–167 [G]
857. Honigfeld G, Arellano F, Sethi J, Bianchini A, Schein J: Reducing clozapine-related morbidity and mortality: 5 years of experience with the Clozaril National Registry. J Clin Psychiatry 1998; 59(suppl 3):3–7 [G]
858. Munro J, O'Sullivan D, Andrews C, Arana A, Mortimer A, Kerwin R: Active monitoring of 12,760 clozapine recipients in the UK and Ireland: beyond pharmacovigilance. Br J Psychiatry 1999; 175:576–580 [C]
859. Lambertenghi DG: Blood dyscrasias in clozapine-treated patients in Italy. Haematologica 2000; 85:233–237 [C]
860. Killian JG, Kerr K, Lawrence C, Celermajer DS: Myocarditis and cardiomyopathy associated with clozapine. Lancet 1999; 354:1841–1845 [G]
861. Warner B, Alphs L, Schaedelin J, Koestler T: Clozapine and sudden death (letter). Lancet 2000; 355:842 [G]
862. Cerulli TR: Clozapine-associated pancreatitis. Harv Rev Psychiatry 1999; 7:61–63 [G]
863. Garlipp P, Rosenthal O, Haltenhof H, Machleidt W: The development of a clinical syndrome of asymptomatic pancreatitis and eosinophilia after treatment with clozapine in schizophrenia: implications for clinical care, recognition and management. J Psychopharmacol 2002; 16:399–400 [G]
864. Hagg S, Spigset O: Antipsychotic-induced venous thromboembolism: a review of the evidence. CNS Drugs 2002; 16:765–776 [F]
865. Kortepeter C, Chen M, Knudsen JF, Dubitsky GM, Ahmad SR, Beitz J: Clozapine and venous thromboembolism. Am J Psychiatry 2002; 159:876–877 [G]
866. Thatcher GW, Cates M, Bair B: Clozapine-induced toxic hepatitis. Am J Psychiatry 1995; 152:296–297 [G]
867. Markowitz JS, Grinberg R, Jackson C: Marked liver enzyme elevations with clozapine. J Clin Psychopharmacol 1997; 17:70–71 [G]
868. Lieberman JA, Johns CA, Kane JM, Rai K, Pisciotta AV, Saltz BL, Howard A: Clozapine-induced agranulocytosis: non-cross-reactivity with other psychotropic drugs. J Clin Psychiatry 1988; 49:271–277 [F]
869. Lamberti JS, Bellnier TJ, Schwarzkopf SB, Schneider E: Filgrastim treatment of three patients with clozapine-induced agranulocytosis. J Clin Psychiatry 1995; 56:256–259 [B]
870. Adityanjee: Modification of clozapine-induced leukopenia and neutropenia with lithium carbonate. Am J Psychiatry 1995; 152:648–649 [G]
871. Blier P, Slater S, Measham T, Koch M, Wiviott G: Lithium and clozapine-induced neutropenia/agranulocytosis. Int Clin Psychopharmacol 1998; 13:137–140 [G]
872. Safferman AZ, Lieberman JA, Alvir JM, Howard A: Rechallenge in clozapine-induced agranulocytosis. Lancet 1992; 339:1296–1297 [G]
873. Wooltorton E: Antipsychotic clozapine (Clozaril): myocarditis and cardiovascular toxicity. CMAJ 2002; 166:1185–1186 [G]
874. Fleischhacker WW, Hummer M, Kurz M, Kurzthaler I, Lieberman JA, Pollack S, Safferman AZ, Kane JM: Clozapine dose in the United States and Europe: implications for therapeutic and adverse effects. J Clin Psychiatry 1994; 55(suppl B):78–81 [E]
875. VanderZwaag C, McGee M, McEvoy JP, Freudenreich O, Wilson WH, Cooper TB: Response of patients with treatment-refractory schizophrenia to clozapine within three serum level ranges. Am J Psychiatry 1996; 153:1579–1584 [A]
876. Kronig MH, Munne RA, Szymanski S, Safferman AZ, Pollack S, Cooper T, Kane JM, Lieberman JA: Plasma clozapine levels and clinical response for treatment-refractory schizophrenic patients. Am J Psychiatry 1995; 152:179–182 [B]

877. Perry PJ: Therapeutic drug monitoring of antipsychotics. Psychopharmacol Bull 2001; 35: 19–29 [G]
878. van Kammen DP, Marder SR: Clozapine, in Comprehensive Textbook of Psychiatry, 6th ed, vol 2. Edited by Kaplan HI, Sadock BJ. Baltimore, Williams & Wilkins, 1995, pp 1979–1987 [G]
879. Meltzer HY: Treatment of the neuroleptic-nonresponsive schizophrenic patient. Schizophr Bull 1992; 18:515–542 [G]
880. Carpenter WT Jr, Conley RR, Buchanan RW, Breier A, Tamminga CA: Patient response and resource management: another view of clozapine treatment of schizophrenia. Am J Psychiatry 1995; 152:827–832 [F]
881. Lieberman JA, Safferman AZ, Pollack S, Szymanski S, Johns C, Howard A, Kronig M, Bookstein P, Kane JM: Clinical effects of clozapine in chronic schizophrenia: response to treatment and predictors of outcome. Am J Psychiatry 1994; 151:1744–1752 [F]
882. Conley RR, Carpenter WT Jr, Tamminga CA: Time to clozapine response in a standardized trial. Am J Psychiatry 1997; 154:1243–1247 [G]
883. Ackenheil M: Clozapine: pharmacokinetic investigations and biochemical effects in man. Psychopharmacology (Berl) 1989; 99(suppl):S32–S37 [B]
884. Nemeroff CB, DeVane CL, Pollock BG: Newer antidepressants and the cytochrome P450 system. Am J Psychiatry 1996; 153:311–320 [F]
885. Medical Economics Company: Physicians' Desk Reference, 57th ed. Montvale, NJ, Medical Economics Company, 2003 [G]
886. Chouinard G, Jones B, Remington G, Bloom D, Addington D, MacEwan GW, Labelle A, Beauclair L, Arnott W: A Canadian multicenter placebo-controlled study of fixed doses of risperidone and haloperidol in the treatment of chronic schizophrenic patients. J Clin Psychopharmacol 1993; 13:25–40 [A]
887. Marder SR, Meibach RC: Risperidone in the treatment of schizophrenia. Am J Psychiatry 1994; 151:825–835 [A]
888. Borison RL, Pathiraja AP, Diamond BI, Meibach RC: Risperidone: clinical safety and efficacy in schizophrenia. Psychopharmacol Bull 1992; 28:213–218 [A]
889. Marder SR, Davis JM, Chouinard G: The effects of risperidone on the five dimensions of schizophrenia derived by factor analysis: combined results of the North American trials. J Clin Psychiatry 1997; 58:538–546 [G]
890. Peuskens J, Risperidone Study Group: Risperidone in the treatment of patients with chronic schizophrenia: a multi-national, multi-centre, double-blind, parallel-group study versus haloperidol. Br J Psychiatry 1995; 166:712–726 [A]
891. Claus A, Bollen J, De Cuyper H, Eneman M, Malfroid M, Peuskens J, Heylen S: Risperidone versus haloperidol in the treatment of chronic schizophrenic inpatients: a multicentre double-blind comparative study. Acta Psychiatr Scand 1992; 85:295–305 [A]
892. Blin O, Azorin JM, Bouhours P: Antipsychotic and anxiolytic properties of risperidone, haloperidol, and methotrimeprazine in schizophrenic patients. J Clin Psychopharmacol 1996; 16:38–44 [A–]
893. Min SK, Rhee CS, Kim CE, Kang DY: Risperidone versus haloperidol in the treatment of chronic schizophrenic patients: a parallel group double-blind comparative trial. Yonsei Med J 1993; 34:179–190 [A]
894. Ceskova E, Svestka J: Double-blind comparison of risperidone and haloperidol in schizophrenic and schizoaffective psychoses. Pharmacopsychiatry 1993; 26:121–124 [A]
895. Hoyberg OJ, Fensbo C, Remvig J, Lingjaerde O, Sloth-Nielsen M, Salvesen I: Risperidone versus perphenazine in the treatment of chronic schizophrenic patients with acute exacerbations. Acta Psychiatr Scand 1993; 88:395–402 [A]
896. Czobor P, Volavka J, Meibach RC: Effect of risperidone on hostility in schizophrenia. J Clin Psychopharmacol 1995; 15:243–249 [A]

897. Aleman A, Kahn RS: Effects of the atypical antipsychotic risperidone on hostility and aggression in schizophrenia: a meta-analysis of controlled trials. Eur Neuropsychopharmacol 2001; 11:289–293 [E]
898. Glick ID, Lemmens P, Vester-Blokland E: Treatment of the symptoms of schizophrenia: a combined analysis of double-blind studies comparing risperidone with haloperidol and other antipsychotic agents. Int Clin Psychopharmacol 2001; 16:265–274 [E]
899. de Oliveira IR, Miranda-Scippa AM, de Sena EP, Pereira EL, Ribeiro MG, de Castro-e-Silva E, Bacaltchuk J: Risperidone versus haloperidol in the treatment of schizophrenia: a meta-analysis comparing their efficacy and safety. J Clin Pharm Ther 1996; 21:349–358 [E]
900. Davis JM, Janicak PG: Efficacy and safety of the new antipsychotics. Lancet 1994; 343: 476–477 [G]
901. Green MF, Marshall BD Jr, Wirshing WC, Ames D, Marder SR, McGurk S, Kern RS, Mintz J: Does risperidone improve verbal working memory in treatment-resistant schizophrenia? Am J Psychiatry 1997; 154:799–804 [A]
902. Purdon SE, Jones BD, Stip E, Labelle A, Addington D, David SR, Breier A, Tollefson GD (Canadian Collaborative Group for Research in Schizophrenia): Neuropsychological change in early phase schizophrenia during 12 months of treatment with olanzapine, risperidone, or haloperidol. Arch Gen Psychiatry 2000; 57:249–258 [A]
903. Wirshing DA, Marshall BD Jr, Green MF, Mintz J, Marder SR, Wirshing WC: Risperidone in treatment-refractory schizophrenia. Am J Psychiatry 1999; 156:1374–1379 [A]
904. Zhang XY, Zhou DF, Cao LY, Zhang PY, Wu GY, Shen YC: Risperidone versus haloperidol in the treatment of acute exacerbations of chronic inpatients with schizophrenia: a randomized double-blind study. Int Clin Psychopharmacol 2001; 16:325–330 [A]
905. Tran PV, Hamilton SH, Kuntz AJ, Potvin JH, Andersen SW, Beasley C Jr, Tollefson GD: Double-blind comparison of olanzapine versus risperidone in the treatment of schizophrenia and other psychotic disorders. J Clin Psychopharmacol 1997; 17:407–418 [A]
906. Conley RR, Mahmoud R: A randomized double-blind study of risperidone and olanzapine in the treatment of schizophrenia or schizoaffective disorder. Am J Psychiatry 2001; 158: 765–774 [A]
907. Mullen J, Jibson MD, Sweitzer D: A comparison of the relative safety, efficacy, and tolerability of quetiapine and risperidone in outpatients with schizophrenia and other psychotic disorders: the quetiapine experience with safety and tolerability (QUEST) study. Clin Ther 2001; 23:1839–1854 [A]
908. Janssen PP: Risperdal Prescribing Information. Titusville, NJ, Janssen Pharmaceutica Products, 2003. (http://www.risperdal.com) [G]
909. Borison RL, Diamond B, Pathiraja A, Meibach RC: Pharmacokinetics of risperidone in chronic schizophrenic patients. Psychopharmacol Bull 1994; 30:193–197 [D]
910. DeVane CL, Nemeroff CB: An evaluation of risperidone drug interactions. J Clin Psychopharmacol 2001; 21:408–416 [G]
911. Caccia S: New antipsychotic agents for schizophrenia: pharmacokinetics and metabolism update. Curr Opin Investig Drugs 2002; 3:1073–1080 [G]
912. de Leon J, Bork J: Risperidone and cytochrome P450 3A (letter). J Clin Psychiatry 1997; 58:450 [G]
913. Spina E, Avenoso A, Scordo MG, Ancione M, Madia A, Gatti G, Perucca E: Inhibition of risperidone metabolism by fluoxetine in patients with schizophrenia: a clinically relevant pharmacokinetic drug interaction. J Clin Psychopharmacol 2002; 22:419–423 [G]
914. Bymaster FP, Nelson DL, DeLapp NW, Falcone JF, Eckols K, Truex LL, Foreman MM, Lucaites VL, Calligaro DO: Antagonism by olanzapine of dopamine D1, serotonin 2, muscarinic, histamine H1 and alpha 1-adrenergic receptors in vitro. Schizophr Res 1999; 37:107–122 [G]

915. Beasley CM Jr, Tollefson G, Tran P, Satterlee W, Sanger T, Hamilton S: Olanzapine versus placebo and haloperidol: acute phase results of the North American double-blind olanzapine trial. Neuropsychopharmacology 1996; 14:111–123 [A]
916. Beasley CM Jr, Sanger T, Satterlee W, Tollefson G, Tran P, Hamilton S: Olanzapine versus placebo: results of a double-blind, fixed-dose olanzapine trial. Psychopharmacology (Berl) 1996; 124:159–167 [A]
917. Hamilton SH, Revicki DA, Genduso LA, Beasley CM Jr: Olanzapine versus placebo and haloperidol: quality of life and efficacy results of the North American double-blind trial. Neuropsychopharmacology 1998; 18:41–49 [A]
918. Beasley CM Jr, Hamilton SH, Crawford AM, Dellva MA, Tollefson GD, Tran PV, Blin O, Beuzen JN: Olanzapine versus haloperidol: acute phase results of the international double-blind olanzapine trial. Eur Neuropsychopharmacol 1997; 7:125–137 [A]
919. Ishigooka J, Inada T, Miura S: Olanzapine versus haloperidol in the treatment of patients with chronic schizophrenia: results of the Japan multicenter, double-blind olanzapine trial. Psychiatry Clin Neurosci 2001; 55:403–414 [A]
920. Revicki DA, Genduso LA, Hamilton SH, Ganoczy D, Beasley CM Jr: Olanzapine versus haloperidol in the treatment of schizophrenia and other psychotic disorders: quality of life and clinical outcomes of a randomized clinical trial. Qual Life Res 1999; 8:417–426 [A]
921. Tollefson GD, Sanger TM, Lu Y, Thieme ME: Depressive signs and symptoms in schizophrenia: a prospective blinded trial of olanzapine and haloperidol. Arch Gen Psychiatry 1998; 55:250–258 [A]
922. Keefe RSE, Seidman LJ, Christensen BK, Hamer RM, Sharma T, Sitskoorn MM, Lewine RRJ, Yurgelun-Todd DA, Gur RC, Tohen M, Tollefson GD, Sanger TM, Lieberman JA (HGDH Research Group): Comparative effect of atypical and conventional antipsychotic drugs on neurocognition in first-episode psychosis: a randomized double-blind trial of olanzapine versus haloperidol. Am J Psychiatry (in press) [A]
923. Smith RC, Infante M, Singh A, Khandat A: The effects of olanzapine on neurocognitive functioning in medication-refractory schizophrenia. Int J Neuropsychopharmacol 2001; 4: 239–250 [A]
924. Conley RR, Tamminga CA, Bartko JJ, Richardson C, Peszke M, Lingle J, Hegerty J, Love R, Gounaris C, Zaremba S: Olanzapine compared with chlorpromazine in treatment-resistant schizophrenia. Am J Psychiatry 1998; 155:914–920 [A]
925. Breier A, Hamilton SH: Comparative efficacy of olanzapine and haloperidol for patients with treatment-resistant schizophrenia. Biol Psychiatry 1999; 45:403–411 [G]
926. Sheitman BB, Lindgren JC, Early J, Sved M: High-dose olanzapine for treatment-refractory schizophrenia (letter). Am J Psychiatry 1997; 154:1626 [G]
927. Lerner V: High-dose olanzapine for treatment-refractory schizophrenia. Clin Neuropharmacol 2003; 26:58–61 [G]
928. Tran PV, Dellva MA, Tollefson GD, Wentley AL, Beasley CM Jr: Oral olanzapine versus oral haloperidol in the maintenance treatment of schizophrenia and related psychoses. Br J Psychiatry 1998; 172:499–505 [A]
929. Callaghan JT, Bergstrom RF, Ptak LR, Beasley CM: Olanzapine: pharmacokinetic and pharmacodynamic profile. Clin Pharmacokinet 1999; 37:177–193 [G]
930. Nemeroff CB, Kinkead B, Goldstein J: Quetiapine: preclinical studies, pharmacokinetics, drug interactions, and dosing. J Clin Psychiatry 2002; 63(suppl 13):5–11 [F]
931. Borison RL, Arvanitis LA, Miller BG (US Seroquel Study Group): ICI 204,636, an atypical antipsychotic: efficacy and safety in a multicenter, placebo-controlled trial in patients with schizophrenia. J Clin Psychopharmacol 1996; 16:158–169 [A]
932. Fabre LF Jr, Arvanitis L, Pultz J, Jones VM, Malick JB, Slotnick VB: ICI 204,636, a novel, atypical antipsychotic: early indication of safety and efficacy in patients with chronic and subchronic schizophrenia. Clin Ther 1995; 17:366–378 [A]

933. Arvanitis LA, Miller BG (The Seroquel Trial 13 Study Group): Multiple fixed doses of "Seroquel" (quetiapine) in patients with acute exacerbation of schizophrenia: a comparison with haloperidol and placebo. Biol Psychiatry 1997; 42:233–246 [A]
934. Peuskens J, Link CG: A comparison of quetiapine and chlorpromazine in the treatment of schizophrenia. Acta Psychiatr Scand 1997; 96:265–273 [A]
935. Copolov DL, Link CG, Kowalcyk B: A multicentre, double-blind, randomized comparison of quetiapine (ICI 204,636, "Seroquel") and haloperidol in schizophrenia. Psychol Med 2000; 30:95–105 [A]
936. Emsley RA, Raniwalla J, Bailey PJ, Jones AM (PRIZE Study Group): A comparison of the effects of quetiapine ("Seroquel") and haloperidol in schizophrenic patients with a history of and a demonstrated, partial response to conventional antipsychotic treatment. Int Clin Psychopharmacol 2000; 15:121–131 [A]
937. Purdon SE, Malla A, Labelle A, Lit W: Neuropsychological change in patients with schizophrenia after treatment with quetiapine or haloperidol. J Psychiatry Neurosci 2001; 26:137–149 [A]
938. Velligan DI, Newcomer J, Pultz J, Csernansky J, Hoff AL, Mahurin R, Miller AL: Does cognitive function improve with quetiapine in comparison to haloperidol? Schizophr Res 2002; 53:239–248 [A]
939. Shahzad S, Suleman MI, Shahab H, Mazour I, Kaur A, Rudzinskiy P, Lippmann S: Cataract occurrence with antipsychotic drugs. Psychosomatics 2002; 43:354–359 [G]
940. DeVane CL, Nemeroff CB: Clinical pharmacokinetics of quetiapine: an atypical antipsychotic. Clin Pharmacokinet 2001; 40:509–522 [F]
941. Wong YW, Yeh C, Thyrum PT: The effects of concomitant phenytoin administration on the steady-state pharmacokinetics of quetiapine. J Clin Psychopharmacol 2001; 21:89–93 [G]
942. Schmidt AW, Lebel LA, Howard HR Jr, Zorn SH: Ziprasidone: a novel antipsychotic agent with a unique human receptor binding profile. Eur J Pharmacol 2001; 425:197–201 [G]
943. Keck P Jr, Buffenstein A, Ferguson J, Feighner J, Jaffe W, Harrigan EP, Morrissey MR: Ziprasidone 40 and 120 mg/day in the acute exacerbation of schizophrenia and schizoaffective disorder: a 4-week placebo-controlled trial. Psychopharmacology (Berl) 1998; 140: 173–184 [A]
944. Daniel DG, Zimbroff DL, Potkin SG, Reeves KR, Harrigan EP, Lakshminarayanan M (Ziprasidone Study Group): Ziprasidone 80 mg/day and 160 mg/day in the acute exacerbation of schizophrenia and schizoaffective disorder: a 6-week placebo-controlled trial. Neuropsychopharmacology 1999; 20:491–505 [A]
945. Hirsch SR, Kissling W, Bauml J, Power A, O'Connor R: A 28-week comparison of ziprasidone and haloperidol in outpatients with stable schizophrenia. J Clin Psychiatry 2002; 63:516–523 [A]
946. Goff DC, Posever T, Herz L, Simmons J, Kletti N, Lapierre K, Wilner KD, Law CG, Ko GN: An exploratory haloperidol-controlled dose-finding study of ziprasidone in hospitalized patients with schizophrenia or schizoaffective disorder. J Clin Psychopharmacol 1998; 18:296–304 [A]
947. Arato M, O'Connor R, Meltzer HY: A 1-year, double-blind, placebo-controlled trial of ziprasidone 40, 80 and 160 mg/day in chronic schizophrenia: the Ziprasidone Extended Use in Schizophrenia (ZEUS) study. Int Clin Psychopharmacol 2002; 17:207–215 [A]
948. Brook S, Lucey JV, Gunn KP (Ziprasidone IM Study Group): Intramuscular ziprasidone compared with intramuscular haloperidol in the treatment of acute psychosis. J Clin Psychiatry 2000; 61:933–941 [A]
949. Daniel DG, Potkin SG, Reeves KR, Swift RH, Harrigan EP: Intramuscular (IM) ziprasidone 20 mg is effective in reducing acute agitation associated with psychosis: a double-blind, randomized trial. Psychopharmacology (Berl) 2001; 155:128–134 [A]

950. Prakash C, Kamel A, Cui D, Whalen RD, Miceli JJ, Tweedie D: Identification of the major human liver cytochrome P450 isoform(s) responsible for the formation of the primary metabolites of ziprasidone and prediction of possible drug interactions. Br J Clin Pharmacol 2000; 49(suppl 1):35S–42S [G]
951. Aweeka F, Jayesekara D, Horton M, Swan S, Lambrecht L, Wilner KD, Sherwood J, Anziano RJ, Smolarek TA, Turncliff RZ: The pharmacokinetics of ziprasidone in subjects with normal and impaired renal function. Br J Clin Pharmacol 2000; 49(suppl 1):27S–33S [B]
952. Everson G, Lasseter KC, Anderson KE, Bauer LA, Carithens RL Jr, Wilner KD, Johnson A, Anziano RJ, Smolarek TA, Turncliff RZ: The pharmacokinetics of ziprasidone in subjects with normal and impaired hepatic function. Br J Clin Pharmacol 2000; 49(suppl 1):21S–26S [B]
953. Burris KD, Molski TF, Xu C, Ryan E, Tottori K, Kikuchi T, Yocca FD, Molinoff PB: Aripiprazole, a novel antipsychotic, is a high-affinity partial agonist at human dopamine D2 receptors. J Pharmacol Exp Ther 2002; 302:381–389 [G]
954. Shapiro DA, Renock S, Arrington E, Chiodo LA, Liu LX, Sibley DR, Roth BL, Mailman R: Aripiprazole, a novel atypical antipsychotic drug with a unique and robust pharmacology. Neuropsychopharmacology 2003; 28:1400–1411 [G]
955. Marder SR, McQuade RD, Stock E, Kaplita S, Marcus R, Safferman AZ, Saha A, Ali M, Iwamoto T: Aripiprazole in the treatment of schizophrenia: safety and tolerability in short-term, placebo-controlled trials. Schizophr Res 2003; 61:123–136 [E]
956. Kane JM, Carson WH, Saha AR, McQuade RD, Ingenito GG, Zimbroff DL, Ali MW: Efficacy and safety of aripiprazole and haloperidol versus placebo in patients with schizophrenia and schizoaffective disorder. J Clin Psychiatry 2002; 63:763–771 [A]
957. Pigott TA, Carson WH, Saha AR, Torbeyns AF, Stock EG, Ingenito GG: Aripiprazole for the prevention of relapse in stabilized patients with chronic schizophrenia: a placebo-controlled 26-week study. J Clin Psychiatry 2003; 64:1048–1056 [A]
958. McGavin JK, Goa KL: Aripiprazole. CNS Drugs 2002; 16:779–786 [G]
959. Casey DE: Neuroleptic drug-induced extrapyramidal syndromes and tardive dyskinesia. Schizophr Res 1991; 4:109–120 [G]
960. Ayd FJ Jr: A survey of drug-induced extrapyramidal reactions. JAMA 1961; 75:1054–1060 [D]
961. Braude WM, Barnes TR, Gore SM: Clinical characteristics of akathisia: a systematic investigation of acute psychiatric inpatient admissions. Br J Psychiatry 1983; 143:139–150 [C]
962. Caroff SN: The neuroleptic malignant syndrome. J Clin Psychiatry 1980; 41:79–83 [F]
963. Rupniak NM, Jenner P, Marsden CD: Acute dystonia induced by neuroleptic drugs. Psychopharmacology (Berl) 1986; 88:403–419 [F]
964. Goetz CG, Klawans HL: Drug-induced extrapyramidal disorders: a neuropsychiatric interface. J Clin Psychopharmacol 1981; 1:297–303 [G]
965. Chakos MH, Mayerhoff DI, Loebel AD, Alvir JM, Lieberman JA: Incidence and correlates of acute extrapyramidal symptoms in first episode of schizophrenia. Psychopharmacol Bull 1992; 28:81–86 [C]
966. Melamed E, Achiron A, Shapira A, Davidovicz S: Persistent and progressive parkinsonism after discontinuation of chronic neuroleptic therapy: an additional tardive syndrome? Clin Neuropharmacol 1991; 14:273–278 [F]
967. Jeste DV, Lohr JB, Eastham JH, Rockwell E, Caligiuri MP: Adverse neurobiological effects of long-term use of neuroleptics: human and animal studies. J Psychiatr Res 1998; 32:201–214 [F]
968. Fenton WS, Blyler CR, Heinssen RK: Determinants of medication compliance in schizophrenia: empirical and clinical findings. Schizophr Bull 1997; 23:637–651 [F]
969. Weiden PJ, Miller AL: Which side effects really matter? screening for common and distressing side effects of antipsychotic medications. J Psych Pract 2001; 7:41–47 [G]

970. Van Putten T, May RP: "Akinetic depression" in schizophrenia. Arch Gen Psychiatry 1978; 35:1101–1107 [E]
971. Rifkin A, Quitkin F, Klein DF: Akinesia: a poorly recognized drug-induced extrapyramidal behavioral disorder. Arch Gen Psychiatry 1975; 32:672–674 [F]
972. Miller CH, Fleischhacker WW: Managing antipsychotic-induced acute and chronic akathisia. Drug Saf 2000; 22:73–81 [G]
973. Gelenberg AJ: Treating extrapyramidal reactions: some current issues. J Clin Psychiatry 1987; 48(suppl):24–27 [G]
974. Raja M: Managing antipsychotic-induced acute and tardive dystonia. Drug Saf 1998; 19: 57–72 [G]
975. Ayd FJJ: Early-onset neuroleptic-induced extrapyramidal reactions: a second survey, 1961–1981, in Neuroleptics: Neurochemical, Behavioral and Clinical Perspectives. Edited by Coyle JT, Enna SJ. New York, Raven Press, 1983, pp 75–92 [C]
976. Fleischhacker WW, Roth SD, Kane JM: The pharmacologic treatment of neuroleptic-induced akathisia. J Clin Psychopharmacol 1990; 10:12–21 [F]
977. Lima AR, Soares-Weiser K, Bacaltchuk J, Barnes TR: Benzodiazepines for neuroleptic-induced acute akathisia. Cochrane Database Syst Rev 2002;CD001950 [E]
978. Rifkin A, Siris S: Drug treatment of acute schizophrenia, in Psychopharmacology: The Third Generation of Progress. Edited by Meltzer HY. New York, Raven Press, 1987, pp 1095–1101 [G]
979. Hanlon TE, Schoenrich C, Freinek W, Turek I, Kurland AA: Perphenazine-benztropine mesylate treatment of newly admitted psychiatric patients. Psychopharmacologia 1966; 9: 328–339 [A]
980. Tardive Dyskinesia: A Task Force Report of the American Psychiatric Association. Washington, DC, APA, 1992 [F]
981. Tarsy D, Baldessarini RJ: Tardive dyskinesia. Annu Rev Med 1984; 35:605–623 [F]
982. Saltz BL, Woerner MG, Kane JM, Lieberman JA, Alvir JM, Bergmann KJ, Blank K, Koblenzer J, Kahaner K: Prospective study of tardive dyskinesia incidence in the elderly. JAMA 1991; 266:2402–2406 [C]
983. Fenton WS, Wyatt RJ, McGlashan TH: Risk factors for spontaneous dyskinesia in schizophrenia. Arch Gen Psychiatry 1994; 51:643–650 [C]
984. Glazer WM: Review of incidence studies of tardive dyskinesia associated with typical antipsychotics. J Clin Psychiatry 2000; 61(suppl 4):15–20 [F]
985. Ganzini L, Casey DE, Hoffman WF, Heintz RT: Tardive dyskinesia and diabetes mellitus. Psychopharmacol Bull 1992; 28:281–286 [B]
986. Woerner MG, Saltz BL, Kane JM, Lieberman JA, Alvir JM: Diabetes and development of tardive dyskinesia. Am J Psychiatry 1993; 150:966–968 [C]
987. Woerner MG, Alvir JM, Saltz BL, Lieberman JA, Kane JM: Prospective study of tardive dyskinesia in the elderly: rates and risk factors. Am J Psychiatry 1998; 155:1521–1528 [C]
988. Goldman MB, Luchins DJ: Intermittent neuroleptic therapy and tardive dyskinesia: a literature review. Hosp Community Psychiatry 1984; 35:1215–1219 [F]
989. Gutierrez-Esteinou R, Grebb JA: Risperidone: an analysis of the first three years in general use. Int Clin Psychopharmacol 1997; 12(suppl 4):S3–S10 [G]
990. Jeste DV, Okamoto A, Napolitano J, Kane JM, Martinez RA: Low incidence of persistent tardive dyskinesia in elderly patients with dementia treated with risperidone. Am J Psychiatry 2000; 157:1150–1155 [A]
991. Davidson M, Harvey PD, Vervarcke J, Gagiano CA, De Hooge JD, Bray G, Dose M, Barak Y, Haushofer M (Risperidone Working Group): A long-term, multicenter, open-label study of risperidone in elderly patients with psychosis. Int J Geriatr Psychiatry 2000; 15:506–514 [B]
992. Glazer WM: Expected incidence of tardive dyskinesia associated with atypical antipsychotics. J Clin Psychiatry 2000; 61(suppl 4):21–26 [A]

993. Glazer WM: Extrapyramidal side effects, tardive dyskinesia, and the concept of atypicality. J Clin Psychiatry 2000; 61(suppl 3):16–21 [G]
994. Tariot PN, Salzman C, Yeung PP, Pultz J, Rak IW: Long-term use of quetiapine in elderly patients with psychotic disorders. Clin Ther 2000; 22:1068–1084 [B]
995. Lieberman JA, Saltz BL, Johns CA, Pollack S, Borenstein M, Kane J: The effects of clozapine on tardive dyskinesia. Br J Psychiatry 1991; 158:503–510 [F]
996. Fernandez HH, Friedman JH: Classification and treatment of tardive syndromes. Neurolog 2003; 9:16–27 [G]
997. Soares KV, McGrath JJ: Calcium channel blockers for neuroleptic-induced tardive dyskinesia. Cochrane Database Syst Rev 2001;CD000206 [E]
998. Soares KV, McGrath JJ, Deeks JJ: Gamma-aminobutyric acid agonists for neuroleptic-induced tardive dyskinesia. Cochrane Database Syst Rev 2001;CD000203 [E]
999. McGrath JJ, Soares KV: Miscellaneous treatments for neuroleptic-induced tardive dyskinesia. Cochrane Database Syst Rev 2000;CD000208 [E]
1000. Soares KV, McGrath JJ: Diltiazem, nifedipine, nimodipine or verapamil for neuroleptic-induced tardive dyskinesia. Cochrane Database Syst Rev 2000;CD000206 [E]
1001. Alpert M, Friedhoff AJ, Marcos LR, Diamond F: Paradoxical reaction to L-dopa in schizophrenic patients. Am J Psychiatry 1978; 135:1329–1332 [E]
1002. Allen RM, Flemenbaum A: The effect of amantadine HCl on haloperidol-induced striatal dopamine neuron hypersensitivity. Biol Psychiatry 1979; 14:541–544 [A–]
1003. Caroff SN, Mann SC, Campbell EC: Atypical antipsychotics and neuroleptic malignant syndrome. Psychiatr Ann 2000; 30:314–321 [G]
1004. Farver DK: Neuroleptic malignant syndrome induced by atypical antipsychotics. Expert Opin Drug Saf 2003; 2:21–35 [F]
1005. Gelenberg AJ, Bellinghausen B, Wojcik JD, Falk WE, Sachs GS: A prospective survey of neuroleptic malignant syndrome in a short-term psychiatric hospital. Am J Psychiatry 1988; 145:517–518 [C]
1006. American Medical Association: Antipsychotic drugs, in Drug Evaluations Annual 1995. Chicago, AMA, 1995 [F]
1007. Adityanjee, Aderibigbe YA, Mathews T: Epidemiology of neuroleptic malignant syndrome. Clin Neuropharmacol 1999; 22:151–158 [F]
1008. Kontaxakis VP, Havaki-Kontaxaki BJ, Christodoulou NG, Paplos KG: Olanzapine-associated neuroleptic malignant syndrome. Prog Neuropsychopharmacol Biol Psychiatry 2002; 26:897–902 [F]
1009. Solomons K: Quetiapine and neuroleptic malignant syndrome (letter). Can J Psychiatry 2002; 47:791 [G]
1010. Sing KJ, Ramaekers GM, Van Harten PN: Neuroleptic malignant syndrome and quetiapine. Am J Psychiatry 2002; 159:149–150 [G]
1011. Bourgeois JA, Babine S, Meyerovich M, Doyle J: A case of neuroleptic malignant syndrome with quetiapine (letter). J Neuropsychiatry Clin Neurosci 2002; 14:87 [G]
1012. Murty RG, Mistry SG, Chacko RC: Neuroleptic malignant syndrome with ziprasidone. J Clin Psychopharmacol 2002; 22:624–626 [G]
1013. American Medical Association: Antipsychotic drugs, in Drug Evaluations Annual 1993. Chicago, AMA, 1993 [F]
1014. Keck PE Jr, Pope HG Jr, Cohen BM, McElroy SL, Nierenberg AA: Risk factors for neuroleptic malignant syndrome: a case-control study. Arch Gen Psychiatry 1989; 46:914–918 [D]
1015. Pelonero AL, Levenson JL, Pandurangi AK: Neuroleptic malignant syndrome: a review. Psychiatr Serv 1998; 49:1163–1172 [F]
1016. Adnet P, Lestavel P, Krivosic-Horber R: Neuroleptic malignant syndrome. Br J Anaesth 2000; 85:129–135 [F]

1017. Meltzer HY: Massive serum creatine kinase increases with atypical antipsychotic drugs: what is the mechanism and the message? Psychopharmacology (Berl) 2000; 150:349–350 [G]
1018. Jeong SH, Ahn YM, Koo YJ, Kang UG, Kim YS: The characteristics of clozapine-induced fever. Schizophr Res 2002; 56:191–193 [G]
1019. Caroff SN, Mann SC, Keck PE Jr: Specific treatment of the neuroleptic malignant syndrome. Biol Psychiatry 1998; 44:378–381 [G]
1020. Koch M, Chandragiri S, Rizvi S, Petrides G, Francis A: Catatonic signs in neuroleptic malignant syndrome. Compr Psychiatry 2000; 41:73–75 [G]
1021. Francis A, Chandragiri S, Rizvi S, Koch M, Petrides G: Is lorazepam a treatment for neuroleptic malignant syndrome? CNS Spectr 2000; 5:54–57 [G]
1022. Khalderov V: Benzodiazepines for the treatment of neuroleptic malignant syndrome. Hosp Physician Sept 2000; pp 51–55 [G]
1023. Trollor JN, Sachdev PS: Electroconvulsive treatment of neuroleptic malignant syndrome: a review and report of cases. Aust N Z J Psychiatry 1999; 33:650–659 [F]
1024. Rosebush PI, Stewart TD, Gelenberg AJ: Twenty neuroleptic rechallenges after neuroleptic malignant syndrome in 15 patients. J Clin Psychiatry 1989; 50:295–298 [B]
1025. Stahl SM: Psychopharmacology of wakefulness: pathways and neurotransmitters. J Clin Psychiatry 2002; 63:551–552 [G]
1026. Kinon BJ, Lieberman JA: Mechanisms of action of atypical antipsychotic drugs: a critical analysis. Psychopharmacology (Berl) 1996; 124:2–34 [G]
1027. Wesensten NJ, Belenky G, Kautz MA, Thorne DR, Reichardt RM, Balkin TJ: Maintaining alertness and performance during sleep deprivation: modafinil versus caffeine. Psychopharmacology (Berl) 2002; 159:238–247 [A]
1028. Makela EH, Miller K, Cutlip WD: Three case reports of modafinil use in treating sedation induced by antipsychotic medications. J Clin Psychiatry 2003; 64:485–486 [G]
1029. Narendran R, Young CM, Valenti AM, Nickolova MK, Pristach CA: Is psychosis exacerbated by modafinil? Arch Gen Psychiatry 2002; 59:292–293 [G]
1030. Dequardo JR: Modafinil-associated clozapine toxicity. Am J Psychiatry 2002; 159:1243–1244 [G]
1031. Miller DD: Review and management of clozapine side effects. J Clin Psychiatry 2000; 61(suppl 8):14–17 [F]
1032. Young CR, Bowers MB Jr, Mazure CM: Management of the adverse effects of clozapine. Schizophr Bull 1998; 24:381–390 [F]
1033. Al Khatib SM, LaPointe NM, Kramer JM, Califf RM: What clinicians should know about the QT interval. JAMA 2003; 289:2120–2127 [F]
1034. Taylor D: Ziprasidone in the management of schizophrenia: the QT interval issue in context. CNS Drugs 2003; 17:423–430 [G]
1035. Haddad PM, Anderson IM: Antipsychotic-related QTc prolongation, torsade de pointes and sudden death. Drugs 2002; 62:1649–1671 [G]
1036. Glassman AH, Bigger JT Jr: Antipsychotic drugs: prolonged QTc interval, torsade de pointes, and sudden death. Am J Psychiatry 2001; 158:1774–1782 [F]
1037. Cole JO, Davis JM: Antipsychotic drugs, in The Schizophrenic Syndrome. Edited by Bellak L, Loeb L. New York, Grune & Stratton, 1969, pp 478–568 [G]
1038. Arana GW, Santos AB: Anticholinergics and amantadine, in Comprehensive Textbook of Psychiatry, 6th ed, vol 2. Edited by Kaplan HI, Sadock BJ. Baltimore, Williams & Wilkins, 1995, pp 1919–1923 [G]
1039. Gelenberg AJ: The catatonic syndrome. Lancet 1976; 1:1339–1341 [F]
1040. Marinkovic D, Timotijevic I, Babinski T, Totic S, Paunovic VR: The side-effects of clozapine: a four year follow-up study. Prog Neuropsychopharmacol Biol Psychiatry 1994; 18:537–544 [C]

1041. Chengappa KN, Pollock BG, Parepally H, Levine J, Kirshner MA, Brar JS, Zoretich RA: Anticholinergic differences among patients receiving standard clinical doses of olanzapine or clozapine. J Clin Psychopharmacol 2000; 20:311–316 [B]
1042. Levin TT, Barrett J, Mendelowitz A: Death from clozapine-induced constipation: case report and literature review. Psychosomatics 2002; 43:71–73 [F]
1043. Allison DB, Mentore JL, Heo M, Chandler LP, Cappelleri JC, Infante MC, Weiden PJ: Antipsychotic-induced weight gain: a comprehensive research synthesis. Am J Psychiatry 1999; 156:1686–1696 [F]
1044. Umbricht DS, Pollack S, Kane JM: Clozapine and weight gain. J Clin Psychiatry 1994; 55(suppl B):157–160 [D]
1045. Frankenburg FR, Zanarini MC, Kando J, Centorrino F: Clozapine and body mass change. Biol Psychiatry 1998; 43:520–524 [B]
1046. Atmaca M, Kuloglu M, Tezcan E, Ustundag B: Serum leptin and triglyceride levels in patients on treatment with atypical antipsychotics. J Clin Psychiatry 2003; 64:598–604 [D]
1047. Atmaca M, Kuloglu M, Tezcan E, Gecici O, Ustundag B: Weight gain, serum leptin and triglyceride levels in patients with schizophrenia on antipsychotic treatment with quetiapine, olanzapine and haloperidol. Schizophr Res 2003; 60:99–100 [G]
1048. Wirshing DA, Boyd JA, Meng LR, Ballon JS, Marder SR, Wirshing WC: The effects of novel antipsychotics on glucose and lipid levels. J Clin Psychiatry 2002; 63:856–865 [D]
1049. Meyer JM: A retrospective comparison of weight, lipid, and glucose changes between risperidone- and olanzapine-treated inpatients: metabolic outcomes after 1 year. J Clin Psychiatry 2002; 63:425–433 [D]
1050. Henderson DC, Cagliero E, Gray C, Nasrallah RA, Hayden DL, Schoenfeld DA, Goff DC: Clozapine, diabetes mellitus, weight gain, and lipid abnormalities: a five-year naturalistic study. Am J Psychiatry 2000; 157:975–981 [B]
1051. Dursun SM, Szemis A, Andrews H, Reveley MA: The effects of clozapine on levels of total cholesterol and related lipids in serum of patients with schizophrenia: a prospective study. J Psychiatry Neurosci 1999; 24:453–455 [B]
1052. Spivak B, Lamschtein C, Talmon Y, Guy N, Mester R, Feinberg I, Kotler M, Weizman A: The impact of clozapine treatment on serum lipids in chronic schizophrenic patients. Clin Neuropharmacol 1999; 22:98–101 [D]
1053. Martin A, L'Ecuyer S: Triglyceride, cholesterol and weight changes among risperidone-treated youths: a retrospective study. Eur Child Adolesc Psychiatry 2002; 11:129–133 [D]
1054. Aquila R: Management of weight gain in patients with schizophrenia. J Clin Psychiatry 2002; 63(suppl 4):33–36 [G]
1055. Ball MP, Coons VB, Buchanan RW: A program for treating olanzapine-related weight gain. Psychiatr Serv 2001; 52:967–969 [B]
1056. Green AI, Patel JK, Goisman RM, Allison DB, Blackburn G: Weight gain from novel antipsychotic drugs: need for action. Gen Hosp Psychiatry 2000; 22:224–235 [G]
1057. Floris M, Lejeune J, Deberdt W: Effect of amantadine on weight gain during olanzapine treatment. Eur Neuropsychopharmacol 2001; 11:181–182 [B]
1058. Correa N, Opler LA, Kay SR, Birmaher B: Amantadine in the treatment of neuroendocrine side effects of neuroleptics. J Clin Psychopharmacol 1987; 7:91–95 [G]
1059. McElroy SL, Suppes T, Keck PE, Frye MA, Denicoff KD, Altshuler LL, Brown ES, Nolen WA, Kupka RW, Rochussen J, Leverich GS, Post RM: Open-label adjunctive topiramate in the treatment of bipolar disorders. Biol Psychiatry 2000; 47:1025–1033 [G]
1060. Levy E, Margolese HC, Chouinard G: Topiramate produced weight loss following olanzapine-induced weight gain in schizophrenia (letter). J Clin Psychiatry 2002; 63:1045 [G]
1061. Chengappa KN, Chalasani L, Brar JS, Parepally H, Houck P, Levine J: Changes in body weight and body mass index among psychiatric patients receiving lithium, valproate, or topiramate: an open-label, nonrandomized chart review. Clin Ther 2002; 24:1576–1584 [D]

1062. Lessig MC, Shapira NA, Murphy TK: Topiramate for reversing atypical antipsychotic weight gain (letter). J Am Acad Child Adolesc Psychiatry 2001; 40:1364 [G]
1063. Dursun SM, Devarajan S: Clozapine weight gain, plus topiramate weight loss (letter). Can J Psychiatry 2000; 45:198 [G]
1064. Cavazzoni P, Tanaka Y, Roychowdhury SM, Breier A, Allison DB: Nizatidine for prevention of weight gain with olanzapine: a double-blind placebo-controlled trial. Eur Neuropsychopharmacol 2003; 13:81–85 [A]
1065. Sacchetti E, Guarneri L, Bravi D: H(2) antagonist nizatidine may control olanzapine-associated weight gain in schizophrenic patients. Biol Psychiatry 2000; 48:167–168 [G]
1066. Poyurovsky M, Isaacs I, Fuchs C, Schneidman M, Faragian S, Weizman R, Weizman A: Attenuation of olanzapine-induced weight gain with reboxetine in patients with schizophrenia: a double-blind, placebo-controlled study. Am J Psychiatry 2003; 160:297–302 [A]
1067. Lindenmayer JP, Czobor P, Volavka J, Citrome L, Sheitman B, McEvoy JP, Cooper TB, Chakos M, Lieberman JA: Changes in glucose and cholesterol levels in patients with schizophrenia treated with typical or atypical antipsychotics. Am J Psychiatry 2003; 160:290–296 [A]
1068. Gianfrancesco FD, Grogg AL, Mahmoud RA, Wang RH, Nasrallah HA: Differential effects of risperidone, olanzapine, clozapine, and conventional antipsychotics on type 2 diabetes: findings from a large health plan database. J Clin Psychiatry 2002; 63:920–930 [C]
1069. Sernyak MJ, Leslie DL, Alarcon RD, Losonczy MF, Rosenheck R: Association of diabetes mellitus with use of atypical neuroleptics in the treatment of schizophrenia. Am J Psychiatry 2002; 159:561–566 [G]
1070. Lund BC, Perry PJ, Brooks JM, Arndt S: Clozapine use in patients with schizophrenia and the risk of diabetes, hyperlipidemia, and hypertension: a claims-based approach. Arch Gen Psychiatry 2001; 58:1172–1176 [D]
1071. Henderson DC: Atypical antipsychotic-induced diabetes mellitus: how strong is the evidence? CNS Drugs 2002; 16:77–89 [G]
1072. Henderson DC: Diabetes mellitus and other metabolic disturbances induced by atypical antipsychotic agents. Curr Diab Rep 2002; 2:135–140 [G]
1073. Koller EA, Doraiswamy PM: Olanzapine-associated diabetes mellitus. Pharmacotherapy 2002; 22:841–852 [G]
1074. Dynes JB: Diabetes in schizophrenia and diabetes in nonpsychotic medical patients. Dis Nerv Syst 1969; 30:341–344 [G]
1075. Newcomer JW, Haupt DW, Fucetola R, Melson AK, Schweiger JA, Cooper BP, Selke G: Abnormalities in glucose regulation during antipsychotic treatment of schizophrenia. Arch Gen Psychiatry 2002; 59:337–345 [D]
1076. Melkersson KI, Hulting AL, Brismar KE: Different influences of classical antipsychotics and clozapine on glucose-insulin homeostasis in patients with schizophrenia or related psychoses. J Clin Psychiatry 1999; 60:783–791 [G]
1077. Henderson DC: Clinical experience with insulin resistance, diabetic ketoacidosis, and type 2 diabetes mellitus in patients treated with atypical antipsychotic agents. J Clin Psychiatry 2001; 62(suppl 27):10–14 [G]
1078. Lindenmayer JP, Patel R: Olanzapine-induced ketoacidosis with diabetes mellitus (letter). Am J Psychiatry 1999; 156:1471 [G]
1079. Peterson GA, Byrd SL: Diabetic ketoacidosis from clozapine and lithium cotreatment. Am J Psychiatry 1996; 153:737–738 [G]
1080. Koval MS, Rames LJ, Christie S: Diabetic ketoacidosis associated with clozapine treatment. Am J Psychiatry 1994; 151:1520–1521 [G]
1081. Wilson DR, D'Souza L, Sarkar N, Newton M, Hammond C: New-onset diabetes and ketoacidosis with atypical antipsychotics. Schizophr Res 2003; 59:1–6 [G]

1082. Seaburg HL, McLendon BM, Doraiswamy PM: Olanzapine-associated severe hyperglycemia, ketonuria, and acidosis: case report and review of literature. Pharmacotherapy 2001; 21:1448–1454 [G]

1083. Melkersson KI, Dahl ML: Relationship between levels of insulin or triglycerides and serum concentrations of the atypical antipsychotics clozapine and olanzapine in patients on treatment with therapeutic doses. Psychopharmacology (Berl) 2003; 170:157–166 [G]

1084. Osser DN, Najarian DM, Dufresne RL: Olanzapine increases weight and serum triglyceride levels. J Clin Psychiatry 1999; 60:767–770 [B]

1085. Gaulin BD, Markowitz JS, Caley CF, Nesbitt LA, Dufresne RL: Clozapine-associated elevation in serum triglycerides. Am J Psychiatry 1999; 156:1270–1272 [D]

1086. Meyer JM: Novel antipsychotics and severe hyperlipidemia. J Clin Psychopharmacol 2001; 21:369–374 [G]

1087. Koro CE, Fedder DO, L'Italien GJ, Weiss S, Magder LS, Kreyenbuhl J, Revicki D, Buchanan RW: An assessment of the independent effects of olanzapine and risperidone exposure on the risk of hyperlipidemia in schizophrenic patients. Arch Gen Psychiatry 2002; 59:1021–1026 [D]

1088. Pollack MH, Reiter S, Hammerness P: Genitourinary and sexual adverse effects of psychotropic medication. Int J Psychiatry Med 1992; 22:305–327 [F]

1089. Perkins DO: Prolactin and endocrine related disorders, in Medical Illness in Schizophrenia. Edited by Meyer JM, Nasrallah HA. Arlington, Va, American Psychiatric Publishing, 2003, pp 215–232 [G]

1090. Kinon BJ, Gilmore JA, Liu H, Halbreich UM: Hyperprolactinemia in response to antipsychotic drugs: characterization across comparative clinical trials. Psychoneuroendocrinology 2003; 28(suppl 2):69–82 [F]

1091. Kapur S, Langlois X, Vinken P, Megens AA, De Coster R, Andrews JS: The differential effects of atypical antipsychotics on prolactin elevation are explained by their differential blood-brain disposition: a pharmacological analysis in rats. J Pharmacol Exp Ther 2002; 302:1129–1134 [G]

1092. Wang PS, Walker AM, Tsuang MT, Orav EJ, Glynn RJ, Levin R, Avorn J: Dopamine antagonists and the development of breast cancer. Arch Gen Psychiatry 2002; 59:1147–1154 [D]

1093. Sanfilippo JS: Implications of not treating hyperprolactinemia. J Reprod Med 1999; 44: 1111–1115 [G]

1094. Halbreich U, Rojansky N, Palter S, Hreshchyshyn M, Kreeger J, Bakhai Y, Rosan R: Decreased bone mineral density in medicated psychiatric patients. Psychosom Med 1995; 57:485–491 [G]

1095. Ataya K, Mercado A, Kartaginer J, Abbasi A, Moghissi KS: Bone density and reproductive hormones in patients with neuroleptic-induced hyperprolactinemia. Fertil Steril 1988; 50: 876–881 [G]

1096. Becker D, Liver O, Mester R, Rapoport M, Weizman A, Weiss M: Risperidone, but not olanzapine, decreases bone mineral density in female premenopausal schizophrenia patients. J Clin Psychiatry 2003; 64:761–766 [B]

1097. Naidoo U, Goff DC, Klibanski A: Hyperprolactinemia and bone mineral density: the potential impact of antipsychotic agents. Psychoneuroendocrinology 2003; 28(suppl 2): 97–108 [G]

1098. Hummer M, Kemmler G, Kurz M, Kurzthaler I, Oberbauer H, Fleischhacker WW: Sexual disturbances during clozapine and haloperidol treatment for schizophrenia. Am J Psychiatry 1999; 156:631–633 [C]

1099. Aizenberg D, Modai I, Landa A, Gil-Ad I, Weizman A: Comparison of sexual dysfunction in male schizophrenic patients maintained on treatment with classical antipsychotics versus clozapine. J Clin Psychiatry 2001; 62:541–544 [D]

1100. Cutler AJ: Sexual dysfunction and antipsychotic treatment. Psychoneuroendocrinology 2003; 28(suppl 1):69–82 [G]
1101. Bobes J, Garc AP, Rejas J, Hern NG, Garcia-Garcia M, Rico-Villademoros F, Porras A: Frequency of sexual dysfunction and other reproductive side-effects in patients with schizophrenia treated with risperidone, olanzapine, quetiapine, or haloperidol: the results of the EIRE study. J Sex Marital Ther 2003; 29:125–147 [D]
1102. Aizenberg D, Zemishlany Z, Dorfman-Etrog P, Weizman A: Sexual dysfunction in male schizophrenic patients. J Clin Psychiatry 1995; 56:137–141 [B, G]
1103. Compton MT, Saldivia A, Berry SA: Recurrent priapism during treatment with clozapine and olanzapine (letter). Am J Psychiatry 2000; 157:659 [G]
1104. Compton MT, Miller AH: Priapism associated with conventional and atypical antipsychotic medications: a review. J Clin Psychiatry 2001; 62:362–366 [F]
1105. Songer DA, Barclay JC: Olanzapine-induced priapism. Am J Psychiatry 2001; 158:2087–2088 [G]
1106. Kuperman JR, Asher I, Modai I: Olanzapine-associated priapism (letter). J Clin Psychopharmacol 2001; 21:247 [G]
1107. Pais VM, Ayvazian PJ: Priapism from quetiapine overdose: first report and proposal of mechanism (case report). Urology 2001; 58:462 [G]
1108. Reeves RR, Kimble R: Prolonged erections associated with ziprasidone treatment: a case report. J Clin Psychiatry 2003; 64:97–98 [G]
1109. Reeves RR, Mack JE: Priapism associated with two atypical antipsychotic agents. Pharmacotherapy 2002; 22:1070–1073 [G]
1110. Leucht S, McGrath J, White P, Kissling W: Carbamazepine augmentation for schizophrenia: how good is the evidence? J Clin Psychiatry 2002; 63:218–224 [F]
1111. Wassef AA, Dott SG, Harris A, Brown A, O'Boyle M, Meyer WJ III, Rose RM: Randomized, placebo-controlled pilot study of divalproex sodium in the treatment of acute exacerbations of chronic schizophrenia. J Clin Psychopharmacol 2000; 20:357–361 [A]
1112. Jann MW, Ereshefsky L, Saklad SR, Seidel DR, Davis CM, Burch NR, Bowden CL: Effects of carbamazepine on plasma haloperidol levels. J Clin Psychopharmacol 1985; 5:106–109 [B]
1113. Fast DK, Jones BD, Kusalic M, Erickson M: Effect of carbamazepine on neuroleptic plasma levels and efficacy. Am J Psychiatry 1986; 143:117–118 [B]
1114. Raitasuo V, Lehtovaara R, Huttunen MO: Carbamazepine and plasma levels of clozapine (letter). Am J Psychiatry 1993; 150:169 [B]
1115. Siris SG: Akinesia and postpsychotic depression: a difficult differential diagnosis. J Clin Psychiatry 1987; 48:240–243 [G]
1116. Siris SG, Bermanzohn PC, Mason SE, Shuwall MA: Maintenance imipramine therapy for secondary depression in schizophrenia: a controlled trial. Arch Gen Psychiatry 1994; 51: 109–115 [A]
1117. Kirli S, Caliskan M: A comparative study of sertraline versus imipramine in postpsychotic depressive disorder of schizophrenia. Schizophr Res 1998; 33:103–111 [A]
1118. Addington D, Addington J, Patten S, Remington G, Moamai J, Labelle A, Beauclair L: Double-blind, placebo-controlled comparison of the efficacy of sertraline as treatment for a major depressive episode in patients with remitted schizophrenia. J Clin Psychopharmacol 2002; 22:20–25 [A]
1119. Whitehead C, Moss S, Cardno A, Lewis G: Antidepressants for people with both schizophrenia and depression. Cochrane Database Syst Rev 2002;CD002305 [E]
1120. Goff DC, Midha KK, Sarid-Segal O, Hubbard JW, Amico E: A placebo-controlled trial of fluoxetine added to neuroleptic in patients with schizophrenia. Psychopharmacology (Berl) 1995; 117:417–423 [A]
1121. Buchanan RW, Kirkpatrick B, Bryant N, Ball P, Breier A: Fluoxetine augmentation of clozapine treatment in patients with schizophrenia. Am J Psychiatry 1996; 153:1625–1627 [A]

1122. Salokangas RK, Saarijarvi S, Taiminen T, Kallioniemi H, Lehto H, Niemi H, Tuominen J, Ahola V, Syvalahti E: Citalopram as an adjuvant in chronic schizophrenia: a double-blind placebo-controlled study. Acta Psychiatr Scand 1996; 94:175–180 [A]
1123. Lee MS, Kim YK, Lee SK, Suh KY: A double-blind study of adjunctive sertraline in haloperidol-stabilized patients with chronic schizophrenia. J Clin Psychopharmacol 1998; 18:399–403 [A]
1124. Arango C, Kirkpatrick B, Buchanan RW: Fluoxetine as an adjunct to conventional antipsychotic treatment of schizophrenia patients with residual symptoms. J Nerv Ment Dis 2000; 188:50–53 [A]
1125. Silver H, Shmugliakov N: Augmentation with fluvoxamine but not maprotiline improves negative symptoms in treated schizophrenia: evidence for a specific serotonergic effect from a double-blind study. J Clin Psychopharmacol 1998; 18:208–211 [A]
1126. Silver H, Barash I, Aharon N, Kaplan A, Poyurovsky M: Fluvoxamine augmentation of antipsychotics improves negative symptoms in psychotic chronic schizophrenic patients: a placebo-controlled study. Int Clin Psychopharmacol 2000; 15:257–261 [A]
1127. Silver H, Nassar A, Aharon N, Kaplan A: The onset and time course of response of negative symptoms to add-on fluvoxamine treatment. Int Clin Psychopharmacol 2003; 18:87–92 [G]
1128. Bodkin JA, Cohen BM, Salomon MS, Cannon SE, Zornberg GL, Cole JO: Treatment of negative symptoms in schizophrenia and schizoaffective disorder by selegiline augmentation of antipsychotic medication: a pilot study examining the role of dopamine. J Nerv Ment Dis 1996; 184:295–301 [C]
1129. Jungerman T, Rabinowitz D, Klein E: Deprenyl augmentation for treating negative symptoms of schizophrenia: a double-blind, controlled study. J Clin Psychopharmacol 1999; 19:522–525 [A]
1130. Vartiainen H, Tiihonen J, Putkonen A, Koponen H, Virkkunen M, Hakola P, Lehto H: Citalopram, a selective serotonin reuptake inhibitor, in the treatment of aggression in schizophrenia. Acta Psychiatr Scand 1995; 91:348–351 [A]
1131. Shiloh R, Zemishlany Z, Aizenberg D, Radwan M, Schwartz B, Dorfman-Etrog P, Modai I, Khaikin M, Weizman A: Sulpiride augmentation in people with schizophrenia partially responsive to clozapine: a double-blind, placebo-controlled study. Br J Psychiatry 1997; 171:569–573 [A]
1132. Miller AL, Craig CS: Combination antipsychotics: pros, cons, and questions. Schizophr Bull 2002; 28:105–109 [F]
1133. Raskin S, Durst R, Katz G, Zislin J: Olanzapine and sulpiride: a preliminary study of combination/augmentation in patients with treatment-resistant schizophrenia. J Clin Psychopharmacol 2000; 20:500–503 [B]
1134. Carpenter WT Jr, Buchanan RW, Kirkpatrick B, Breier AF: Diazepam treatment of early signs of exacerbation in schizophrenia. Am J Psychiatry 1999; 156:299–303 [A]
1135. Altamura AC, Mauri MC, Mantero M, Brunetti M: Clonazepam/haloperidol combination therapy in schizophrenia: a double blind study. Acta Psychiatr Scand 1987; 76:702–706 [A]
1136. Csernansky JG, Riney SJ, Lombrozo L, Overall JE, Hollister LE: Double-blind comparison of alprazolam, diazepam, and placebo for the treatment of negative schizophrenic symptoms. Arch Gen Psychiatry 1988; 45:655–659 [A]
1137. Foster S, Kessel J, Berman ME, Simpson GM: Efficacy of lorazepam and haloperidol for rapid tranquilization in a psychiatric emergency room setting. Int Clin Psychopharmacol 1997; 12:175–179 [A]
1138. Northoff G, Wenke J, Demisch L, Eckert J, Gille B, Pflug B: Catatonia: short-term response to lorazepam and dopaminergic metabolism. Psychopharmacology (Berl) 1995; 122:182–186 [B]
1139. Lee JW, Schwartz DL, Hallmayer J: Catatonia in a psychiatric intensive care facility: incidence and response to benzodiazepines. Ann Clin Psychiatry 2000; 12:89–96 [B]

1140. Schmider J, Standhart H, Deuschle M, Drancoli J, Heuser I: A double-blind comparison of lorazepam and oxazepam in psychomotor retardation and mutism. Biol Psychiatry 1999; 46:437–441 [B]
1141. Ungvari GS, Leung CM, Wong MK, Lau J: Benzodiazepines in the treatment of catatonic syndrome. Acta Psychiatr Scand 1994; 89:285–288 [B]
1142. Ungvari GS, Chiu HF, Chow LY, Lau BS, Tang WK: Lorazepam for chronic catatonia: a randomized, double-blind, placebo-controlled cross-over study. Psychopharmacology (Berl) 1999; 142:393–398 [A]
1143. Javitt DC, Zukin SR: Recent advances in the phencyclidine model of schizophrenia. Am J Psychiatry 1991; 148:1301–1308 [F]
1144. Heresco-Levy U, Javitt DC, Ermilov M, Mordel C, Silipo G, Lichtenstein M: Efficacy of high-dose glycine in the treatment of enduring negative symptoms of schizophrenia. Arch Gen Psychiatry 1999; 56:29–36 [A]
1145. Potkin SG, Jin Y, Bunney BG, Costa J, Gulasekaram B: Effect of clozapine and adjunctive high-dose glycine in treatment-resistant schizophrenia. Am J Psychiatry 1999; 156:145–147 [A]
1146. Rosse RB, Fay-McCarthy M, Kendrick K, Davis RE, Deutsch SI: d-Cycloserine adjuvant therapy to molindone in the treatment of schizophrenia. Clin Neuropharmacol 1996; 19: 444–450 [A]
1147. van Berckel BN, Evenblij CN, van Loon BJ, Maas MF, van der Geld MA, Wynne HJ, van Ree JM, Kahn RS: d-Cycloserine increases positive symptoms in chronic schizophrenic patients when administered in addition to antipsychotics: a double-blind, parallel, placebo-controlled study. Neuropsychopharmacology 1999; 21:203–210 [A]
1148. Tsai GE, Yang P, Chung LC, Tsai IC, Tsai CW, Coyle JT: d-Serine added to clozapine for the treatment of schizophrenia. Am J Psychiatry 1999; 156:1822–1825 [A]
1149. Alexander PE, van Kammen DP, Bunney WE Jr: Antipsychotic effects of lithium in schizophrenia. Am J Psychiatry 1979; 136:283–287 [B]
1150. Shopsin B, Kim SS, Gershon S: A controlled study of lithium vs. chlorpromazine in acute schizophrenics. Br J Psychiatry 1971; 119:435–440 [B]
1151. Greil W, Ludwig-Mayerhofer W, Erazo N, Engel RR, Czernik A, Giedke H, Muller-Oerlinghausen B, Osterheider M, Rudolf GA, Sauer H, Tegeler J, Wetterling T: Lithium vs carbamazepine in the maintenance treatment of schizoaffective disorder: a randomised study. Eur Arch Psychiatry Clin Neurosci 1997; 247:42–50 [A–]
1152. Schexnayder LW, Hirschowitz J, Sautter FJ, Garver DL: Predictors of response to lithium in patients with psychoses. Am J Psychiatry 1995; 152:1511–1513 [B]
1153. Growe GA, Crayton JW, Klass DB, Evans H, Strizich M: Lithium in chronic schizophrenia. Am J Psychiatry 1979; 136:454–455 [A or A–]
1154. Small JG, Kellams JJ, Milstein V, Moore J: A placebo-controlled study of lithium combined with neuroleptics in chronic schizophrenic patients. Am J Psychiatry 1975; 132:1315–1317 [B]
1155. Lerner Y, Mintzer Y, Schestatzky M: Lithium combined with haloperidol in schizophrenic patients. Br J Psychiatry 1988; 153:359–362 [A]
1156. Biederman J, Lerner Y, Belmaker RH: Combination of lithium carbonate and haloperidol in schizo-affective disorder: a controlled study. Arch Gen Psychiatry 1979; 36:327–333 [A]
1157. Johnson G: Differential response to lithium carbonate in manic depressive and schizo-affective disorders. Dis Nerv Syst 1970; 31:613–615 [B]
1158. Prien RF, Caffey EM Jr, Klett CJ: A comparison of lithium carbonate and chlorpromazine in the treatment of excited schizo-affectives: report of the Veterans Administration and National Institute of Mental Health collaborative study group. Arch Gen Psychiatry 1972; 27:182–189 [A]
1159. Carman JS, Bigelow LB, Wyatt RJ: Lithium combined with neuroleptics in chronic schizophrenic and schizoaffective patients. J Clin Psychiatry 1981; 42:124–128 [A]

1160. Hogarty GE, McEvoy JP, Ulrich RF, DiBarry AL, Bartone P, Cooley S, Hammill K, Carter M, Munetz MR, Perel J: Pharmacotherapy of impaired affect in recovering schizophrenic patients. Arch Gen Psychiatry 1995; 52:29–41 [A]
1161. Terao T, Oga T, Nozaki S, Ohta A, Ohtsubo Y, Yamamoto S, Zamami M, Okada M: Lithium addition to neuroleptic treatment in chronic schizophrenia: a randomized, double-blind, placebo-controlled, cross-over study. Acta Psychiatr Scand 1995; 92:220–224 [A]
1162. Schulz SC, Thompson PA, Jacobs M, Ninan PT, Robinson D, Weiden PJ, Yadalam K, Glick ID, Odbert CL: Lithium augmentation fails to reduce symptoms in poorly responsive schizophrenic outpatients. J Clin Psychiatry 1999; 60:366–372 [A]
1163. American Psychiatric Association: Practice Guideline for the Treatment of Patients With Bipolar Disorder (Revision). Am J Psychiatry 2002; 159(April suppl):1–50 [F]
1164. Deutsch SI, Rosse RB, Schwartz BL, Banay-Schwartz M, McCarthy MF, Johri SK: l-Tyrosine pharmacotherapy of schizophrenia: preliminary data. Clin Neuropharmacol 1994; 17:53–62 [A]
1165. Maas JW, Miller AL, Tekell JL, Funderburg L, Silva JA, True J, Velligan D, Berman N, Bowden CL: Clonidine plus haloperidol in the treatment of schizophrenia/psychosis. J Clin Psychopharmacol 1995; 15:361–364 [A]
1166. Peet M, Brind J, Ramchand CN, Shah S, Vankar GK: Two double-blind placebo-controlled pilot studies of eicosapentaenoic acid in the treatment of schizophrenia. Schizophr Res 2001; 49:243–251 [A]
1167. Fenton WS, Dickerson F, Boronow J, Hibbeln JR, Knable M: A placebo-controlled trial of omega-3 fatty acid (ethyl eicosapentaenoic acid) supplementation for residual symptoms and cognitive impairment in schizophrenia. Am J Psychiatry 2001; 158:2071–2074 [A]
1168. Emsley R, Myburgh C, Oosthuizen P, van Rensburg SJ: Randomized, placebo-controlled study of ethyl-eicosapentaenoic acid as supplemental treatment in schizophrenia. Am J Psychiatry 2002; 159:1596–1598 [A]
1169. Janakiramaiah N, Channabasavanna SM, Murthy NS: ECT/chlorpromazine combination versus chlorpromazine alone in acutely schizophrenic patients. Acta Psychiatr Scand 1982; 66:464–470 [B]
1170. Sarkar P, Andrade C, Kapur B, Das P, Sivaramakrishna Y, Harihar C, Pandey A, Anand A, Dharmendra MS: An exploratory evaluation of ECT in haloperidol-treated DSM-III-R schizophreniform disorder. Convuls Ther 1994; 10:271–278 [A]
1171. Folstein M, Folstein S, McHugh PR: Clinical predictors of improvement after electroconvulsive therapy of patients with schizophrenia, neurotic reactions, and affective disorders. Biol Psychiatry 1973; 7:147–152 [G]
1172. Wells DA: Electroconvulsive treatment for schizophrenia: a ten-year survey in a university hospital psychiatric department. Compr Psychiatry 1973; 14:291–298 [G]
1173. Dodwell D, Goldberg D: A study of factors associated with response to electroconvulsive therapy in patients with schizophrenic symptoms. Br J Psychiatry 1989; 154:635–639 [G]
1174. Black DW, Winokur G, Nasrallah A: Treatment of mania: a naturalistic study of electroconvulsive therapy versus lithium in 438 patients. J Clin Psychiatry 1987; 48:132–139 [D]
1175. Ries RK, Wilson L, Bokan JA, Chiles JA: ECT in medication resistant schizoaffective disorder. Compr Psychiatry 1981; 22:167–173 [G]
1176. Tsuang MT, Dempsey GM, Fleming JA: Can ECT prevent premature death and suicide in "schizoaffective" patients? J Affect Disord 1979; 1:167–171 [D]
1177. Landmark J, Joseph L, Merskey H: Characteristics of schizophrenic patients and the outcome of fluphenazine and of electroconvulsive treatments. Can J Psychiatry 1987; 32: 425–428 [B]
1178. Danziger L, Kendwall JA: Prediction of the immediate outcome of shock therapy in dementia praecox. Dis Nerv Syst 1946; 7:229–303 [G]

1179. Kalinowsky LB: Electric convulsive therapy, with emphasis on importance of adequate treatment. Arch Neurol Psychiatry 1943; 50:652–660 [G]
1180. Kalinowsky LB, Worthing HJ: Results with electroconvulsive therapy in 200 cases of schizophrenia. Psychiatr Q 1943; 17:144–153 [G]
1181. Dolinski SY, Zvara DA: Anesthetic considerations of cardiovascular risk during electroconvulsive therapy. Convuls Ther 1997; 13:157–164 [F]
1182. Burd J, Kettl P: Incidence of asystole in electroconvulsive therapy in elderly patients. Am J Geriatr Psychiatry 1998; 6:203–211 [D]
1183. Huuhka MJ, Seinela L, Reinikainen P, Leinonen EV: Cardiac arrhythmias induced by ECT in elderly psychiatric patients: experience with 48-hour Holter monitoring. J ECT 2003; 19:22–25 [B]
1184. Rice EH, Sombrotto LB, Markowitz JC, Leon AC: Cardiovascular morbidity in high-risk patients during ECT. Am J Psychiatry 1994; 151:1637–1641 [D]
1185. Zielinski RJ, Roose SP, Devanand DP, Woodring S, Sackeim HA: Cardiovascular complications of ECT in depressed patients with cardiac disease. Am J Psychiatry 1993; 150:904–909 [D]
1186. Devanand DP, Briscoe KM, Sackeim HA: Clinical features and predictors of postictal excitement. Convuls Ther 1989; 5:140–146 [D]
1187. Sackeim HA, Prudic J, Devanand DP, Nobler MS, Lisanby SH, Peyser S, Fitzsimons L, Moody BJ, Clark J: A prospective, randomized, double-blind comparison of bilateral and right unilateral electroconvulsive therapy at different stimulus intensities. Arch Gen Psychiatry 2000; 57:425–434 [A]
1188. McCall WV, Reboussin DM, Weiner RD, Sackeim HA: Titrated moderately suprathreshold vs fixed high-dose right unilateral electroconvulsive therapy: acute antidepressant and cognitive effects. Arch Gen Psychiatry 2000; 57:438–444 [A]
1189. Lisanby SH, Maddox JH, Prudic J, Devanand DP, Sackeim HA: The effects of electroconvulsive therapy on memory of autobiographical and public events. Arch Gen Psychiatry 2000; 57:581–590 [A]
1190. Ng C, Schweitzer I, Alexopoulos P, Celi E, Wong L, Tuckwell V, Sergejew A, Tiller J: Efficacy and cognitive effects of right unilateral electroconvulsive therapy. J ECT 2000; 16:370–379 [B]
1191. McCall WV, Dunn A, Rosenquist PB, Hughes D: Markedly suprathreshold right unilateral ECT versus minimally suprathreshold bilateral ECT: antidepressant and memory effects. J ECT 2002; 18:126–129 [A]
1192. Donahue AB: Electroconvulsive therapy and memory loss: a personal journey. J ECT 2000; 16:133–143 [G]
1193. Prudic J, Peyser S, Sackeim HA: Subjective memory complaints: a review of patient self-assessment of memory after electroconvulsive therapy. J ECT 2000; 16:121–132 [F]
1194. Brodaty H, Berle D, Hickie I, Mason C: "Side effects" of ECT are mainly depressive phenomena and are independent of age. J Affect Disord 2001; 66:237–245 [C]
1195. Bagadia VN, Abhyankar R, Pradhan PV, Shah LP: Reevaluation of ECT in schizophrenia: right temporoparietal versus bitemporal electrode placement. Convuls Ther 1988; 4:215–220 [B]
1196. Doongaji DR, Jeste DV, Saoji NJ, Kane PV, Ravindranath S: Unilateral versus bilateral ECT in schizophrenia. Br J Psychiatry 1973; 123:73–79 [A–]
1197. Bailine SH, Rifkin A, Kayne E, Selzer JA, Vital-Herne J, Blieka M, Pollack S: Comparison of bifrontal and bitemporal ECT for major depression. Am J Psychiatry 2000; 157:121–123 [B]
1198. Delva NJ, Brunet D, Hawken ER, Kesteven RM, Lawson JS, Lywood DW, Rodenburg M, Waldron JJ: Electrical dose and seizure threshold: relations to clinical outcome and cognitive effects in bifrontal, bitemporal, and right unilateral ECT. J ECT 2000; 16:361–369 [A]
1199. Chanpattana W, Chakrabhand ML, Buppanharun W, Sackeim HA: Effects of stimulus intensity on the efficacy of bilateral ECT in schizophrenia: a preliminary study. Biol Psychiatry 2000; 48:222–228 [A]

1200. Baker AA, Bird G, Lavin NI, Thorpe JG: ECT in schizophrenia. J Ment Sci 1960; 106: 1506–1511 [A–]
1201. Chanpattana W: The use of the stabilization period in ECT research in schizophrenia, I: a pilot study. J Med Assoc Thai 1999; 82:1193–1199 [G]
1202. Klein E, Kolsky Y, Puyerovsky M, Koren D, Chistyakov A, Feinsod M: Right prefrontal slow repetitive transcranial magnetic stimulation in schizophrenia: a double-blind sham-controlled pilot study. Biol Psychiatry 1999; 46:1451–1454 [A]
1203. Mojtabai R, Nicholson RA, Carpenter BN: Role of psychosocial treatments in management of schizophrenia: a meta-analytic review of controlled outcome studies. Schizophr Bull 1998; 24:569–587 [E]
1204. Marder SR: Integrating pharmacological and psychosocial treatments for schizophrenia. Acta Psychiatr Scand Suppl 2000; 102:87–90 [F]
1205. Stein LI, Diamond RJ, Factor RM: A system approach to the care of persons with schizophrenia, in Handbook of Schizophrenia, vol 4. Edited by Herz MI, Keith SJ, Docherty JP. New York, Elsevier, 1990, pp 213–246 [G]
1206. Bond GR, Drake RE, Mueser KT, Latimer E: Assertive community treatment for people with severe mental illness: critical ingredients and impact on clients. Disease Management and Health Outcomes 2001; 9:141–159 [G]
1207. Penn DL, Mueser KT: Research update on the psychosocial treatment of schizophrenia. Am J Psychiatry 1996; 153:607–617 [F, G]
1208. Group for the Advancement of Psychiatry: Implications for psychosocial interventions in patients with schizophrenia, in Beyond Symptom Suppression: Improving the Long-Term Outcomes of Schizophrenia. Report 134. Washington, DC, American Psychiatric Press, 1992, pp 59–78 [F]
1209. Burns BJ, Santos AB: Assertive community treatment: an update of randomized trials. Psychiatr Serv 1995; 46:669–675 [E]
1210. Weisbrod BA, Test MA, Stein LI: Alternative to mental hospital treatment, II: economic benefit-cost analysis. Arch Gen Psychiatry 1980; 37:400–405 [G]
1211. Wolff N, Helminiak TW, Morse GA, Calsyn RJ, Klinkenberg WD, Trusty ML: Cost-effectiveness evaluation of three approaches to case management for homeless mentally ill clients. Am J Psychiatry 1997; 154:341–348 [A–]
1212. Hoult J: Community care of the acutely mentally ill. Br J Psychiatry 1986; 149:137–144 [F]
1213. Test MA: Training in community living, in Handbook of Psychiatric Rehabilitation. Edited by Liberman RP. Boston, Allyn & Bacon, 1992, pp 153–170 [F]
1214. Taube CA, Morlock L, Burns BJ, Santos AB: New directions in research on assertive community treatment. Hosp Community Psychiatry 1990; 41:642–647 [G]
1215. Stein LI: Wisconsin's system of mental health financing. New Dir Ment Health Serv 1989; 43:29–41 [G]
1216. Stein LI: Innovating against the current. New Dir Ment Health Serv 1992; 56:5–22 [G]
1217. Hogarty GE, Anderson CM, Reiss DJ, Kornblith SJ, Greenwald DP, Javna CD, Madonia MJ: Family psychoeducation, social skills training, and maintenance chemotherapy in the aftercare treatment of schizophrenia, I: one-year effects of a controlled study on relapse and expressed emotion. Arch Gen Psychiatry 1986; 43:633–642 [B]
1218. McFarlane WR, Stastny P, Deakins S: Family-aided assertive community treatment: a comprehensive rehabilitation and intensive case management approach for persons with schizophrenic disorders. New Dir Ment Health Serv 1992; 53:43–54 [F]
1219. Tarrier N, Barrowclough C, Vaughn C, Bamrah JS, Porceddu K, Watts S, Freeman H: The community management of schizophrenia: a controlled trial of a behavioural intervention with families to reduce relapse. Br J Psychiatry 1988; 153:532–542 [A–]
1220. Leff J, Berkowitz R, Shavit N, Strachan A, Glass I, Vaughn C: A trial of family therapy v a relatives group for schizophrenia. Br J Psychiatry 1989; 154:58–66 [B]

1221. Randolph ET, Eth S, Glynn SM, Paz GG, Leong GB, Shaner AL, Strachan A, Van Vort W, Escobar JI, Liberman RP: Behavioural family management in schizophrenia: outcome of a clinic-based intervention. Br J Psychiatry 1994; 164:501–506 [B]
1222. Liberman RP, Lillie F, Falloon IR, Harpin RE, Hutchinson W, Stoute B: Social skills training with relapsing schizophrenics: an experimental analysis. Behav Modif 1984; 8:155–179 [G]
1223. Vaughn CE, Snyder KS, Freeman W, Jones S, Falloon IR, Liberman RP: Family factors in schizophrenic relapse: a replication. Schizophr Bull 1982; 8:425–426 [B]
1224. Goldstein MJ, Rodnick EH, Evans JR, May PR, Steinberg MR: Drug and family therapy in the aftercare of acute schizophrenics. Arch Gen Psychiatry 1978; 35:1169–1177 [A–]
1225. Zhang M, Yan H, Yao C, Ye J, Yu Q, Chen P, Yang J, Qu G, Zhen W, Cai J, Shen M, Hou J, Wang L, Zhang Y, Zhang B, Orley J, Gittelman M: Effectiveness of psychoeducation of relatives of schizophrenic patients: a prospective cohort study in five cities of China. Int J Ment Health 1993; 22:47–59 [C]
1226. Xiong W, Phillips MR, Hu X, Wang R, Dai Q, Kleinman J, Kleinman A: Family-based intervention for schizophrenic patients in China: a randomised controlled trial. Br J Psychiatry 1994; 165:239–247 [A–]
1227. Xiang M, Ran M, Li S: A controlled evaluation of psychoeducational family intervention in a rural Chinese community. Br J Psychiatry 1994; 165:544–548 [A–]
1228. Zhang M, Wang M, Li J, Phillips MR: Randomised-control trial of family intervention for 78 first-episode male schizophrenic patients: an 18-month study in Suzhou, Jiangsu. Br J Psychiatry Suppl 1994; 165:96–102 [A–]
1229. Dyck DG, Hendryx MS, Short RA, Voss WD, McFarlane WR: Service use among patients with schizophrenia in psychoeducational multiple-family group treatment. Psychiatr Serv 2002; 53:749–754 [A–]
1230. Tomaras V, Mavreas V, Economou M, Ioannovich E, Karydi V, Stefanis C: The effect of family intervention on chronic schizophrenics under individual psychosocial treatment: a 3-year study. Soc Psychiatry Psychiatr Epidemiol 2000; 35:487–493 [A–]
1231. Barrowclough C, Tarrier N, Lewis S, Sellwood W, Mainwaring J, Quinn J, Hamlin C: Randomised controlled effectiveness trial of a needs-based psychosocial intervention service for carers of people with schizophrenia. Br J Psychiatry 1999; 174:505–511 [A–]
1232. Mari JJ, Streiner DL: An overview of family interventions and relapse on schizophrenia: meta-analysis of research findings. Psychol Med 1994; 24:565–578 [E]
1233. Cuijpers P: The effects of family interventions on relatives' burden: a meta-analysis. J Ment Health 1999; 8:275–285 [E]
1234. Schooler NR, Keith SJ, Severe JB, Matthews SM: Maintenance treatment of schizophrenia: a review of dose reduction and family treatment strategies. Psychiatr Q 1995; 66:279–292 [F]
1235. McFarlane WR: Multiple-family groups and psychoeducation in the treatment of schizophrenia. New Dir Ment Health Serv 1994; 62:13–22 [F]
1236. Dixon L, Lyles A, Scott J, Lehman A, Postrado L, Goldman H, McGlynn E: Services to families of adults with schizophrenia: from treatment recommendations to dissemination. Psychiatr Serv 1999; 50:233–238 [G]
1237. Dixon L, Goldman H, Hirad A: State policy and funding of services to families of adults with serious and persistent mental illness. Psychiatr Serv 1999; 50:551–553 [G]
1238. Dixon L, Stewart B, Burland J, Delahanty J, Lucksted A, Hoffman M: Pilot study of the effectiveness of the family-to-family education program. Psychiatr Serv 2001; 52:965–967 [G]
1239. Becker DR, Drake RE: A Working Life for People With Severe Mental Illness. New York, Oxford University Press, 2003 [G]
1240. Bond GR: Principles of the Individual Placement and Support model: empirical support. Psychosocial Rehabilitation J 1998; 22:11–23 [G]
1241. Crowther RE, Marshall M, Bond GR, Huxley P: Helping people with severe mental illness to obtain work: systematic review. Br Med J 2001; 322:204–208 [E]

1242. Twamley EW, Jeste DV, Lehman AF: Vocational rehabilitation in schizophrenia and other psychotic disorders: a literature review and meta-analysis of randomized controlled trials. J Nerv Ment Dis 2003; 191:515–523 [E]
1243. Bailey E, Ricketts S, Becker DR, Xie H, Drake RE: Conversion of day treatment to supported employment: one-year outcomes. Psychiatr Rehabil J 1998; 22:24–29 [B]
1244. Becker DR, Bond GR, McCarthy D, Thompson D, Xie H, McHugo GJ, Drake RE: Converting day treatment centers to supported employment programs in Rhode Island. Psychiatr Serv 2001; 52:351–357 [C]
1245. Drake RE, Becker DR, Biesanz JC, Torrey WC, McHugo GJ, Wyzik PF: Rehabilitative day treatment vs supported employment, I: vocational outcomes. Community Ment Health J 1994; 30:519–532 [D]
1246. Drake RE, Becker DR, Biesanz JC, Wyzik PF, Torrey WC: Day treatment versus supported employment for persons with severe mental illness: a replication study. Psychiatr Serv 1996; 47:1125–1127 [A–]
1247. Gold M, Marrone J: Mass Bay Employent Services (a service of Bay Cove Human Services, Inc.): a story of leadership, vision, and action resulting in employment for people with mental illness, in Roses and Thorns From the Grassroots. Boston, Institute for Community Inclusion, 1998 [G]
1248. Bond GR, Dietzen LL, McGrew JH, Miller LD: Accelerating entry into supported employment for persons with severe psychiatric disabilities. Rehabil Psychol 1995; 40:91–111 [A–]
1249. Chandler D, Meisel J, Hu T, McGowen M, Madison K: A capitated model for a cross-section of severely mentally ill clients: employment outcomes. Community Ment Health J 1997; 33:501–516 [B]
1250. Drake RE, McHugo GJ, Bebout RR, Becker DR, Harris M, Bond GR, Quimby E: A randomized clinical trial of supported employment for inner-city patients with severe mental disorders. Arch Gen Psychiatry 1999; 56:627–633 [A–]
1251. Gervey R, Bedell JR: Supported employment in vocational rehabilitation, in Psychological Assessment and Treatment of Persons With Severe Mental Disorders. Edited by Bedell JR. Washington, DC, Taylor & Francis, 1994, pp 151–175 [G]
1252. McFarlane WR, Dushay RA, Deakins SM, Stastny P, Lukens EP, Toran J, Link B: Employment outcomes in family-aided assertive community treatment. Am J Orthopsychiatry 2000; 70:203–214 [A–]
1253. Mueser KT, Clark RE, Haines M, Drake RE, McHugo GJ, Bond GR, Becker DR, Essock SM, Wolfe R, Swain K: The Hartford study of supported employment for severe mental illness. J Consult Clin Psychol (in press) [A–]
1254. Ellis A: Reason and Emotion in Psychotherapy. New York, Lyle Stuart, 1962 [G]
1255. Beck AT: Cognitive Therapy and the Emotional Disorders. New York, International Universities Press, 1976 [G]
1256. Sensky T, Turkington D, Kingdon D, Scott JL, Scott J, Siddle R, O'Carroll M, Barnes TR: A randomized controlled trial of cognitive-behavioral therapy for persistent symptoms in schizophrenia resistant to medication. Arch Gen Psychiatry 2000; 57:165–172 [A–]
1257. Turkington D, Kingdon D: Cognitive-behavioural techniques for general psychiatrists in the management of patients with psychoses. Br J Psychiatry 2000; 177:101–106 [A–]
1258. Turkington D, Kingdon D, Turner T: Effectiveness of a brief cognitive-behavioural therapy intervention in the treatment of schizophrenia. Br J Psychiatry 2002; 180:523–527 [A–]
1259. Kuipers E, Garety P, Fowler D, Dunn G, Bebbington P, Freeman D, Hadley C: London-East Anglia randomised controlled trial of cognitive-behavioural therapy for psychosis, I: effects of the treatment phase. Br J Psychiatry 1997; 171:319–327 [A–]
1260. Kuipers E, Fowler D, Garety P, Chisholm D, Freeman D, Dunn G, Bebbington P, Hadley C: London-East Anglia randomised controlled trial of cognitive-behavioural therapy for

psychosis, III: follow-up and economic evaluation at 18 months. Br J Psychiatry 1998; 173: 61–68 [A–]

1261. Tarrier N, Yusupoff L, Kinney C, McCarthy E, Gledhill A, Haddock G, Morris J: Randomised controlled trial of intensive cognitive behaviour therapy for patients with chronic schizophrenia. Br Med J 1998; 317:303–307 [A–]

1262. Tarrier N, Wittkowski A, Kinney C, McCarthy E, Morris J, Humphreys L: Durability of the effects of cognitive-behavioural therapy in the treatment of chronic schizophrenia: 12-month follow-up. Br J Psychiatry 1999; 174:500–504 [A–]

1263. Tarrier N, Kinney C, McCarthy E, Humphreys L, Wittkowski A, Morris J: Two-year follow-up of cognitive-behavioral therapy and supportive counseling in the treatment of persistent symptoms in chronic schizophrenia. J Consult Clin Psychol 2000; 68:917–922 [A–]

1264. Haddock G, Tarrier N, Morrison AP, Hopkins R, Drake R, Lewis S: A pilot study evaluating the effectiveness of individual inpatient cognitive-behavioural therapy in early psychosis. Soc Psychiatry Psychiatr Epidemiol 1999; 34:254–258 [B]

1265. Drury V, Birchwood M, Cochrane R, Macmillan F: Cognitive therapy and recovery from acute psychosis: a controlled trial, I: impact on psychotic symptoms. Br J Psychiatry 1996; 169:593–601 [A–]

1266. Drury V, Birchwood M, Cochrane R, Macmillan F: Cognitive therapy and recovery from acute psychosis: a controlled trial, II: impact on recovery time. Br J Psychiatry 1996; 169: 602–607 [A–]

1267. Drury V, Birchwood M, Cochrane R: Cognitive therapy and recovery from acute psychosis: a controlled trial, 3: five-year follow-up. Br J Psychiatry 2000; 177:8–14 [A–]

1268. Bradshaw W: Integrating cognitive-behavioral psychotherapy for persons with schizophrenia into a psychiatric rehabilitation program: results of a three year trial. Community Ment Health J 2000; 36:491–500 [A–]

1269. Halperin S, Nathan P, Drummond P, Castle D: A cognitive-behavioural, group-based intervention for social anxiety in schizophrenia. Aust N Z J Psychiatry 2000; 34:809–813 [A–]

1270. Lecompte D, Pelc I: A cognitive-behavioral program to improve compliance with medication in patients with schizophrenia. Int J Ment Health 1996; 25:51–56 [B]

1271. Tarrier N, Beckett R, Harwood S, Baker A, Yusupoff L, Ugarteburu I: A trial of two cognitive-behavioural methods of treating drug-resistant residual psychotic symptoms in schizophrenic patients, I: outcome. Br J Psychiatry 1993; 162:524–532 [B]

1272. Tarrier N, Sharpe L, Beckett R, Harwood S, Baker A, Yusopoff L: A trial of two cognitive behavioural methods of treating drug-resistant residual psychotic symptoms in schizophrenic patients: II. treatment-specific changes in coping and problem-solving skills. Soc Psychiatry Psychiatr Epidemiol 1993; 28:5–10 [B]

1273. Bouchard S, Vallières A, Roy MA, Maziade M: Cognitive restructuring in the treatment of psychotic symptoms in schizophrenia: a critical analysis. Behav Ther 1996; 27:257–277 [F]

1274. Gould RA, Mueser KT, Bolton E, Mays V, Goff D: Cognitive therapy for psychosis in schizophrenia: an effect size analysis. Schizophr Res 2001; 48:335–342 [E]

1275. Norman RM, Townsend LA: Cognitive-behavioural therapy for psychosis: a status report. Can J Psychiatry 1999; 44:245–252 [F]

1276. Shergill SS, Murray RM, McGuire PK: Auditory hallucinations: a review of psychological treatments. Schizophr Res 1998; 32:137–150 [F]

1277. Liberman RP, DeRisis WJ, Mueser KT: Social Skills Training for Psychiatric Patients. Needham Heights, Mass, Allyn & Bacon, 1989 [G]

1278. Mueser KT, Wallace CJ, Liberman RP: New developments in social skills training. Behav Change 1995; 12:31–40 [G]

1279. Benton MK, Schroeder HE: Social skills training with schizophrenics: a meta-analytic evaluation. J Consult Clin Psychol 1990; 58:741–747 [E]

1280. Corrigan PW: Social skills training in adult psychiatric populations: a meta-analysis. J Behav Ther Exp Psychiatry 1991; 22:203–210 [E]
1281. Liberman RP, Vaccaro JV, Corrigan PW: Psychiatric rehabilitation, in Comphrehensive Textbook of Psychiatry, 6th ed, vol 2. Edited by Kaplan HI, Sadock BJ. Baltimore, Williams & Wilkins, 1995, pp 2696–2719 [G]
1282. Holmes MR, Hansen DJ, St Lawrence JS: Conversational skills training with aftercare patients in the community: social validation and generalization. Behav Ther 1984; 15:84–100 [B]
1283. Wallace CJ, Liberman RP: Social skills training for patients with schizophrenia: a controlled clinical trial. Psychiatry Res 1985; 15:239–247 [B]
1284. Smith TE, Hull JW, Romanelli S, Fertuck E, Weiss KA: Symptoms and neurocognition as rate limiters in skills training for psychotic patients. Am J Psychiatry 1999; 156:1817–1818 [A–]
1285. Marder SR, Wirshing WC, Mintz J, McKenzie J, Johnston K, Eckman TA, Lebell M, Zimmerman K, Liberman RP: Two-year outcome of social skills training and group psychotherapy for outpatients with schizophrenia. Am J Psychiatry 1996; 153:1585–1592 [A–]
1286. Dobson DJ, McDougall G, Busheikin J, Aldous J: Effects of social skills training and social milieu treatment on symptoms of schizophrenia. Psychiatr Serv 1995; 46:376–380 [B]
1287. Hayes RL, Halford WK, Varghese FT: Social skills training with chronic schizophrenic patients: eEffects on negative symptoms and community functioning. Behav Ther 1995; 26:433–449 [A–]
1288. Kopelowicz A, Wallace CJ, Zarate R: Teaching psychiatric inpatients to re-enter the community: a brief method of improving the continuity of care. Psychiatr Serv 1998; 49: 1313–1316 [A–]
1289. Liberman RP, Wallace CJ, Blackwell G, Kopelowicz A, Vaccaro JV, Mintz J: Skills training versus psychosocial occupational therapy for persons with persistent schizophrenia. Am J Psychiatry 1998; 155:1087–1091 [A–]
1290. Li F, Wang M: A behavioural training programme for chronic schizophrenic patients: a three-month randomised controlled trial in Beijing. Br J Psychiatry 1994; 164(suppl 24): 32–37 [A–]
1291. Roder V, Brenner HD, Muller D, Lachler M, Zorn P, Reisch T, Bosch J, Bridler R, Christen C, Jaspen E, Schmidl F, Schwemmer V: Development of specific social skills training programmes for schizophrenia patients: results of a multicentre study. Acta Psychiatr Scand 2002; 105:363–371 [B]
1292. Glynn SM, Marder SR, Liberman RP, Blair K, Wirshing WC, Wirshing DA, Ross D, Mintz J: Supplementing clinic-based skills training with manual-based community support sessions: effects on social adjustment of patients with schizophrenia. Am J Psychiatry 2002; 159: 829–837 [A–]
1293. Dilk MN, Bond GR: Meta-analytic evaluation of skills training research for individuals with severe mental illness. J Consult Clin Psychol 1996; 64:1337–1346 [E]
1294. Halford WK, Hayes RL: Psychological rehabilitation of chronic schizophrenic patients: recent findings on social skills training and family psychoeducation. Clin Psychol Rev 1991; 11:23–44 [G]
1295. Brown MA, Munford AM: Life skills training for chronic schizophrenics. J Nerv Ment Dis 1983; 171:466–470 [A–]
1296. Wallace CJ, Liberman RP: Psychiatric rehabilitation, in Treatment of Psychiatric Disorders. Edited by Gabbard GO. Washington, DC, American Psychiatric Press, 1995, pp 1019–1038 [G]
1297. Marder SR, Van Putten T, Mintz J, Lebell M, McKenzie J, Faltico G: Maintenance therapy in schizophrenia: new findings, in Drug Maintenance Strategies in Schizophrenia. Edited by Kane JM. Washington, DC, American Psychiatric Press, 1984, pp 31–49 [F]
1298. Heinrichs DW, Carpenter WT Jr: Prospective study of prodromal symptoms in schizophrenic relapse. Am J Psychiatry 1985; 142:371–373 [D]

1299. McCandless-Glimcher L, McKnight S, Hamera E, Smith BL, Peterson KA, Plumlee AA: Use of symptoms by schizophrenics to monitor and regulate their illness. Hosp Community Psychiatry 1986; 37:929–933 [C]
1300. Kumar S, Thara R, Rajkumar S: Coping with symptoms of relapse in schizophrenia. Eur Arch Psychiatry Neurol Sci 1989; 239:213–215 [D]
1301. Jolley AG, Hirsch SR, Morrison E, McRink A, Wilson L: Trial of brief intermittent neuroleptic prophylaxis for selected schizophrenic outpatients: clinical and social outcome at two years. Br Med J 1990; 301:837–842 [A]
1302. Marder SR, Mintz J, Van Putten T, Lebell M, Wirshing WC, Johnston-Cronk K: Early prediction of relapse in schizophrenia: an application of receiver operating characteristic (ROC) methods. Psychopharmacol Bull 1991; 27:79–82 [C]
1303. Tarrier N, Barrowclough C, Bamrah JS: Prodromal signs of relapse in schizophrenia. Soc Psychiatry Psychiatr Epidemiol 1991; 26:157–161 [C]
1304. Henmi Y: Prodromal symptoms of relapse in schizophrenic outpatients: retrospective and prospective study. Jpn J Psychiatry Neurol 1993; 47:753–775 [C, D]
1305. Pietzcker A, Gaebel W, Kopcke W, Linden M, Muller P, Muller-Spahn F, Tegeler J: Intermittent versus maintenance neuroleptic long-term treatment in schizophrenia: 2-year results of a German multicenter study. J Psychiatr Res 1993; 27:321–339 [B]
1306. Marder SR, Wirshing WC, Van Putten T, Mintz J, McKenzie J, Johnston-Cronk K, Lebell M, Liberman RP: Fluphenazine vs placebo supplementation for prodromal signs of relapse in schizophrenia. Arch Gen Psychiatry 1994; 51:280–287 [A]
1307. Herz MI, Lamberti JS: Prodromal symptoms and early intervention in schizophrenia. Neurol Psychiatry Brain Res 1998; 6:37–44 [A–]
1308. May PR, Simpson GM: Schizophrenia: overview of treatment methods, in Conphrehensive Textbook of Psychiatry, 3rd ed, vol 2. Edited by Kaplan HI, Freedman AM, Sadock BJ. Baltimore, Williams & Wilkins, 1980, pp 1192–1216 [F]
1309. Kanas N: Group therapy with schizophrenic patients: a short-term, homogeneous approach. Int J Group Psychother 1991; 41:33–48 [G]
1310. Kanas N: Group Therapy for Schizophrenic Patients. Washington, DC, American Psychiatric Press, 1996 [G]
1311. Luborsky L, Singer B: Comparative studies of psychotherapies: is it true that "everybody has won and all must have prizes"? in Evaluation of Psychological Therapies. Edited by Spitzer RL, Klein DF. Baltimore, John Hopkins University Press, 1976, pp 3–22 [F]
1312. Parloff MB, Dies RR: Group psychotherapy outcome research 1966–1975. Int J Group Psychother 1977; 27:281–319 [F]
1313. Mosher LR, Keith SJ: Psychosocial treatment: individual, group, family, and community support approaches. Schizophr Bull 1980; 6:10–41 [F]
1314. Keith SJ, Matthews SM: Group, family, and milieu therapies and psychosocial rehabilitation in the treatment of schizophrenic disorders, in Psychiatry 1982: The American Psychiatric Association Annual Review. Edited by Grinspoon L. Washington, DC, American Psychiatric Press, 1982, pp 166–177 [F]
1315. O'Brien CP: Group psychotherapy with schizophrenia and affective disorders, in Comphrehensive Group Psychotherapy, 2nd ed. Edited by Kaplan HI, Sadock BJ. Baltimore, Williams & Wilkins, 1983, pp 242–249 [B]
1316. Kanas N: Group therapy with schizophrenics: a review of controlled studies. Int J Group Psychother 1986; 36:339–360 [F]
1317. Schooler NR, Keith SJ: The clinical research base for the treatment of schizophrenia. Psychopharmacol Bull 1993; 29:431–446 [F]
1318. Donlon PT, Rada RT, Knight SW: A therapeutic aftercare setting for "refractory" chronic schizophrenic patients. Am J Psychiatry 1973; 130:682–684 [B]

1319. O'Brien CP, Hamm KB, Ray BA, Pierce JF, Luborsky L, Mintz J: Group vs individual psychotherapy with schizophrenics: a controlled outcome study. Arch Gen Psychiatry 1972; 27:474–478 [B]
1320. Malm U: The influence of group therapy on schizophrenia. Acta Psychiatr Scand Suppl 1982; 297:1–65 [B]
1321. Malm U: Group therapy, in Handbook of Schizophrenia, vol 4: Psychosocial Treatment of Schizophrenia. Edited by Herz MI, Keith SJ, Docherty JP. Amsterdam, Elsevier, 1990, pp 191–211 [F]
1322. Kanas N, Rogers M, Kreth E, Patterson L, Campbell R: The effectiveness of group psychotherapy during the first three weeks of hospitalization: a controlled study. J Nerv Ment Dis 1980; 168:487–492 [B]
1323. Kanas N: Group psychotherapy with schizophrenia, in Comphrehensive Group Psychotherapy, 3rd ed. Edited by Kaplan HI, Sadock BJ. Baltimore, Williams & Wilkins, 1993, pp 407–418 [G]
1324. Kibel HD: Group psychotherapy, in Less Time to Do More: Psychotherapy on the Short-Term Impatient Unit. Edited by Leibenluft E, Tasman A, Green SA. Washington, DC, American Psychiatric Press, 1993, pp 89–109 [F]
1325. Group therapy in schizophrenia, in Treatments of Psychiatric Disorders: A Task Force Report of the American Psychiatric Association, vol 2. Washington, DC, American Psychiatric Association, 1989, pp 1529–1542 [F]
1326. Stone WN: Group therapy for seriously mentally ill patients in a managed care system, in Effective Use of Group Therapy in Managed Care. Edited by MacKenzie KR. Washington, DC, American Psychiatric Press, 1995, pp 129–146 [G]
1327. Varsamis J, Adamson JD: Early schizophrenia. Can Psychiatr Assoc J 1971; 16:487–497 [C]
1328. Maurer K, Hafner H: Methodological aspects of onset assessment in schizophrenia. Schizophr Res 1995; 15:265–276 [G]
1329. Moller P, Husby R: The initial prodrome in schizophrenia: searching for naturalistic core dimensions of experience and behavior. Schizophr Bull 2000; 26:217–232 [G]
1330. Hafner H, Maurer K: The prodromal phase of psychosis, in Early Intervention in Psychotic Disorders. Edited by Miller T, Mednick SA, McGlashan TH, Libiger J, Johannessen JO. Dordrecht, Netherlands, Kluwer Academic Publishers, 2001, pp 71–100 [G]
1331. Yung AR, McGorry PD, McFarlane CA, Jackson HJ, Patton GC, Rakkar A: Monitoring and care of young people at incipient risk of psychosis. Schizophr Bull 1996; 22:283–303 [G]
1332. Miller TJ, McGlashan TH, Woods SW, Stein K, Driesen N, Corcoran CM, Hoffman R, Davidson L: Symptom assessment in schizophrenic prodromal states. Psychiatr Q 1999; 70:273–287 [G]
1333. McGlashan TH, Miller TJ, Woods SW, Hoffman RE, Davidson L: Instrument for the assessment of prodromal symptoms and states, in Early Intervention in Psychotic Disorders. Edited by Miller TJ, Mednick SA, McGlashan TH, Libiger J, Johannessen JO. Dordrecht, Netherlands, Kluwer Academic Publishers, 2001, pp 135–149 [G]
1334. Yung AR, Phillips LJ, McGorry PD, McFarlane CA, Francey S, Harrigan S, Patton GC, Jackson HJ: Prediction of psychosis: a step towards indicated prevention of schizophrenia. Br J Psychiatry Suppl 1998; 172:14–20 [C]
1335. Miller TJ, McGlashan TH, Rosen JL, Somjee L, Markovich PJ, Stein K, Woods SW: Prospective diagnosis of the initial prodrome for schizophrenia based on the Structured Interview for Prodromal Syndromes: preliminary evidence of interrater reliability and predictive validity. Am J Psychiatry 2002; 159:863–865 [G]
1336. McGlashan TH: Early detection and intervention in schizophrenia: editor's introduction. Schizophr Bull 1996; 22:197–199 [G]
1337. McGlashan TH: Treating schizophrenia earlier in life and the potential for prevention. Curr Psychiatry Rep 2000; 2:386–392 [G]

1338. McGlashan TH: Early detection and intervention in schizophrenia: research. Schizophr Bull 1996; 22:327–345 [G]
1339. Larsen TK, McGlashan TH, Johannessen JO, Friis S, Guldberg C, Haahr U, Horneland M, Melle I, Moe LC, Opjordsmoen S, Simonsen E, Vaglum P: Shortened duration of untreated first episode of psychosis: changes in patient characteristics at treatment. Am J Psychiatry 2001; 158:1917–1919 [B]
1340. Miller TJ, Zipursky RB, Perkins D, Addington J, Woods SW, Hawkins KA, Hoffman R, Preda A, Epstein I, Addington D, Lindborg S, Marquez E, Tohen M, Breier A, McGlashan TH: The PRIME North America randomized double-blind clinical trial of olanzapine versus placebo in patients at risk of being prodromally symptomatic for psychosis, II: baseline characteristics of the "prodromal" sample. Schizophr Res 2003; 61:19–30 [G]
1341. McGlashan TH, Zipursky RB, Perkins DO, Addington JM, Woods SW, Lindborg S, Breier AF: Olanzapine versus PBO for the schizophrenic prodrome: one-year results, in 2003 Annual Meeting New Research Program and Abstracts. Arlington, Va, American Psychiatric Association, 2003, number NR584 [A]
1342. Ascher-Svanum H, Whitesel J: A randomized controlled study of two styles of group patient education about schizophrenia. Psychiatr Serv 1999; 50:926–930 [A–]
1343. Atkinson JM, Coia DA, Gilmour WH, Harper JP: The impact of education groups for people with schizophrenia on social functioning and quality of life. Br J Psychiatry 1996; 168:199–204 [A–]
1344. Buchkremer G, Klingberg S, Holle R, Schulze MH, Hornung WP: Psychoeducational psychotherapy for schizophrenic patients and their key relatives or care-givers: results of a 2-year follow-up. Acta Psychiatr Scand 1997; 96:483–491 [A–]
1345. Klingberg S, Buchkremer G, Holle R, Schulze MH, Hornung WP: Differential therapy effects of psychoeducational psychotherapy for schizophrenic patients: results of a 2-year follow-up. Eur Arch Psychiatry Clin Neurosci 1999; 249:66–72 [A–]
1346. Kemp R, Hayward P, Applewhaite G, Everitt B, David A: Compliance therapy in psychotic patients: randomised controlled trial. Br Med J 1996; 312:345–349 [A–]
1347. Baker F, Intagliata J: Case management, in Handbook of Psychiatric Rehabilitation. Edited by Liberman RP. Boston, Allyn & Bacon, 1992, pp 213–243 [G]
1348. Rosenheck R, Neale M, Leaf P, Milstein R, Frisman L: Multisite experimental cost study of intensive psychiatric community care. Schizophr Bull 1995; 21:129–140 [A–]
1349. Quinlivan R, Hough R, Crowell A, Beach C, Hofstetter R, Kenworthy K: Service utilization and costs of care for severely mentally ill clients in an intensive case management program. Psychiatr Serv 1995; 46:365–371 [A–]
1350. Holloway F, Carson J: Intensive case management for the severely mentally ill: controlled trial. Br J Psychiatry 1998; 172:19–22 [A–]
1351. Sands RG, Cnaan RA: Two modes of case management: assessing their impact. Community Ment Health J 1994; 30:441–457 [D]
1352. Chandler D, Meisel J, Hu T, McGowen M, Madison K: A capitated model for a cross-section of severely mentally ill clients: hospitalization. Community Ment Health J 1998; 34:13–26 [A–]
1353. Issakidis C, Sanderson K, Teesson M, Johnston S, Buhrich N: Intensive case management in Australia: a randomized controlled trial. Acta Psychiatr Scand 1999; 99:360–367 [A–]
1354. Chan S, Mackenzie A, Jacobs P: Cost-effectiveness analysis of case management versus a routine community care organization for patients with chronic schizophrenia. Arch Psychiatr Nurs 2000; 14:98–104 [A–]
1355. Rossler W, Loffler W, Fatkenheuer B, Riecher-Rossler A: Case management for schizophrenic patients at risk for rehospitalization: a case control study. Eur Arch Psychiatry Clin Neurosci 1995; 246:29–36 [D]

1356. Tyrer P, Morgan J, Van Horn E, Jayakody M, Evans K, Brummell R, White T, Baldwin D, Harrison-Read P, Johnson T: A randomised controlled study of close monitoring of vulnerable psychiatric patients. Lancet 1995; 345:756–759 [A–]
1357. Twamley EW, Doshi RR, Nayak GV, Palmer BW, Golshan S, Heaton RK, Patterson TL, Jeste DV: Generalized cognitive impairments, ability to perform everyday tasks, and level of independence in community living situations of older patients with psychosis. Am J Psychiatry 2002; 159:2013–2020 [G]
1358. Medalia A, Revheim N, Casey M: Remediation of memory disorders in schizophrenia. Psychol Med 2000; 30:1451–1459 [G]
1359. Medalia A, Aluma M, Tryon W, Merriam AE: Effectiveness of attention training in schizophrenia. Schizophr Bull 1998; 24:147–152 [A–]
1360. Medalia A, Dorn H, Watras-Gans S: Treating problem-solving deficits on an acute care psychiatric inpatient unit. Psychiatry Res 2000; 97:79–88 [A–]
1361. van der Gaag M, Kern RS, van den Bosch RJ, Liberman RP: A controlled trial of cognitive remediation in schizophrenia. Schizophr Bull 2002; 28:167–176 [A–]
1362. Wykes T, Reeder C, Corner J, Williams C, Everitt B: The effects of neurocognitive remediation on executive processing in patients with schizophrenia. Schizophr Bull 1999; 25:291–307 [A–]
1363. Spaulding WD, Reed D, Sullivan M, Richardson C, Weiler M: Effects of cognitive treatment in psychiatric rehabilitation. Schizophr Bull 1999; 25:657–676 [A–]
1364. Hadas-Lidor N, Katz N, Tyano S, Weizman A: Effectiveness of dynamic cognitive intervention in rehabilitation of clients with schizophrenia. Clin Rehabil 2001; 15:349–359 [A–]
1365. Bellack AS, Weinhardt LS, Gold JM, Gearon JS: Generalization of training effects in schizophrenia. Schizophr Res 2001; 48:255–262 [A–]
1366. Corrigan PW, Hirschbeck JN, Wolfe M: Memory and vigilance training to improve social perception in schizophrenia. Schizophr Res 1995; 17:257–265 [A–]
1367. Kurtz MM, Moberg PJ, Mozley LH, Swanson CL, Gur RC, Gur RE: Effectiveness of an attention- and memory-training program on neuropsychological deficits in schizophrenia. Neurorehabil Neural Repair 2001; 15:75–80 [E]
1368. Vollema MG, Geurtsen GJ, van Voorst AJ: Durable improvements in Wisconsin Card Sorting Test performance in schizophrenic patients. Schizophr Res 1995; 16:209–215 [A–]
1369. Green MF: Cognitive remediation in schizophrenia: is it time yet? Am J Psychiatry 1993; 150:178–187 [F]
1370. Spaulding W, Sullivan M: From laboratory to clinic: psychological methods and principles in psychiatric rehabilitation, in Handbook of Psychiatric Rehabilitation. Edited by Liberman RP. Boston, Allyn & Bacon, 1992, pp 30–55 [G]
1371. Corrigan PW, Yudofsky SC: Cognitive Rehabilitation for Neuropsychiatric Disorders. Washington, DC, American Psychiatric Press, 1996 [B]
1372. Bell M, Bryson G, Greig T, Corcoran C, Wexler BE: Neurocognitive enhancement therapy with work therapy: effects on neuropsychological test performance. Arch Gen Psychiatry 2001; 58:763–768 [A–]
1373. Bell M, Bryson G, Wexler BE: Cognitive remediation of working memory deficits: durability of training effects in severely impaired and less severely impaired schizophrenia. Acta Psychiatr Scand 2003; 108:101–109 [A–]
1374. Velligan DI, Mahurin RK, True JE, Lefton RS, Flores CV: Preliminary evaluation of cognitive adaptation training to compensate for cognitive deficits in schizophrenia. Psychiatr Serv 1996; 47:415–417 [B]
1375. Velligan DI, Bow-Thomas CC, Huntzinger C, Ritch J, Ledbetter N, Prihoda TJ, Miller AL: Randomized controlled trial of the use of compensatory strategies to enhance adaptive functioning in outpatients with schizophrenia. Am J Psychiatry 2000; 157:1317–1323 [C/D]

1376. Vine P, Beels CC: Support and advocacy groups for the mentally ill, in Handbook of Schizophrenia, vol. 4. Edited by Herz MI, Keith SJ, Docherty JP. New York, Elsevier, 1990, pp 387–405 [G]
1377. Perron B: Online support for caregivers of people with a mental illness. Psychiatr Rehabil J 2002; 26:70–77 [G]
1378. Galanter M: Zealous self-help groups as adjuncts to psychiatric treatment: a study of Recovery, Inc. Am J Psychiatry 1988; 145:1248–1253 [G]
1379. Kurtz LF: Mutual aid for affective disorders: the Manic Depressive and Depressive Association. Am J Orthopsychiatry 1988; 58:152–155 [G]
1380. Frese F, Davis W: The consumer-survivor movement, recovery, and consumer professional. Prof Psychol Res Pr 1997; 28:243–245 [G]
1381. Solomon P, Draine J: The efficacy of a consumer case management team: 2-year outcomes of a randomized trial. J Ment Health Adm 1995; 22:135–146 [A–]
1382. Solomon P, Draine J: One year outcomes of a randomized trial of consumer case management. Eval Program Plann 1995; 18:117–127 [A–]
1383. Felton CJ, Stastny P, Shern DL, Blanch A, Donahue SA, Knight E, Brown C: Consumers as peer specialists on intensive case management teams: impact on client outcomes. Psychiatr Serv 1995; 46:1037–1044 [C]
1384. Kaufmann C: The Self Help Employment Center: some outcomes from the first year. Psychosocial Rehabilitation J 1995; 18:145–162 [A–]
1385. Miller L, Miller L: ANGELS, Inc: consumer-run supported employment agency. Psychosocial Rehabilitation J 1997; 21:160–163 [G]
1386. Hall LL, Flynn LM: In defense of families of the mentally ill. Am J Psychiatry 1996; 153: 1373–1374 [G]
1387. Burgmann FN, Panico S: Sharing the same goals. ACNP Quarterly 1996; 2:1–4 [G]
1388. Glick I, Dixon L: Patient and family support organization services should be included as part of treatment for the severely mentally ill. J Psychiatr Practice 2002; 8:1–7 [G]
1389. Ginther C: The web as resource for patient advocacy groups. Psychiatric Times, Nov 1997 [G]
1390. Lam DH: Psychosocial family intervention in schizophrenia: a review of empirical studies. Psychol Med 1991; 21:423–441 [G]
1391. Strachan A: Family intervention, in Handbook of Psychiatric Rehabilitation. Edited by Liberman RP. Boston, Allyn & Bacon, 1992, pp 183–212 [G]

GUIDELINE WATCH: PRACTICE GUIDELINE FOR THE TREATMENT OF PATIENTS WITH MAJOR DEPRESSIVE DISORDER, 2ND EDITION

Laura J. Fochtmann, M.D.
Alan J. Gelenberg, M.D.

Since the publication in 2000 of the APA's *Practice Guideline for the Treatment of Patients With Major Depressive Disorder,* 2nd Edition (1), two important safety concerns have emerged (hepatotoxicity with nefazodone and suicide risk with antidepressants), and two new antidepressants have been approved for use (escitalopram and duloxetine). This watch describes these developments as well as evidence that has accrued since 2000 in other areas related to the treatment of major depressive disorder.

ANTIDEPRESSANTS AND OTHER SOMATIC TREATMENTS

Hepatotoxicity with nefazodone

The guideline recommends the serotonin modulator nefazodone as an effective medication for the treatment of depression. However, before initiating or continuing treatment with nefazodone, consideration should be given to the recent reports of life-threatening hepatic failure in patients treated with nefazodone (2–8). These reports have led the Food and Drug Administration (FDA) to change the drug's labeling, adding a black box warning of possible liver failure leading to death and/or a need for transplant and contraindicating the drug in patients who

---

The American Psychiatric Association (APA) practice guidelines are developed by expert work groups using an explicit methodology that includes rigorous review of available evidence, broad peer review of iterative drafts, and formal approval by the APA Assembly and Board of Trustees. APA practice guidelines are intended to assist psychiatrists in clinical decision making. They are not intended to be a standard of care. The ultimate judgment regarding a particular clinical procedure or treatment plan must be made by the psychiatrist in light of the clinical data presented by the patient and the diagnostic and treatment options available. Guideline watches summarize significant developments in practice that have occurred since publication of an APA practice guideline. Watches may be authored and reviewed by experts associated with the original guideline development effort and are approved for publication by APA's Executive Committee on Practice Guidelines. Thus, watches represent the opinion of the authors and approval of the Executive Committee but not policy of the APA. This guideline watch was published in September 2005. Suggested citation: Fochtmann LJ, Gelenberg AJ: *Guideline Watch: Practice Guideline for the Treatment of Patients With Major Depressive Disorder,* 2nd Edition. Arlington, VA: American Psychiatric Association, 2005. Available online at http://www.psych.org/psych_pract/treatg/pg/prac_guide.cfm.

were withdrawn from it because of evidence of liver injury. According to the warning, the reported rate of liver failure resulting in death or transplant in the United States is about 1 case per 250,000–300,000 patient-years of nefazodone treatment. This represents a rate of about three to four times the estimated background rate of liver failure and is probably an underestimate. There are no known predictors of the development of liver toxicity and failure with nefazodone; toxicity and failure have been reported in individuals early in the course of treatment as well as in persons receiving stable dosages for many months. The FDA warns that patients with preexisting liver disease should not be treated with nefazodone and that patients should be advised to immediately report symptoms that may indicate liver dysfunction, such as jaundice, anorexia, gastrointestinal complaints, and malaise. The warning is available at http://www.fda.gov/medwatch/SAFETY/2002/serzone_deardoc.pdf.

Suicide risk and antidepressants

Because patients with major depressive disorder are at greater risk of suicide, the guideline indicates that they should be assessed for suicide risk initially and over the course of treatment. The guideline also notes that "the risk of suicide in some patients recovering from major depressive disorder increases transiently as they develop the energy and capacity to act on self-destructive plans made earlier in the course of their illness" (1). The guideline describes factors associated with an increased risk of suicide in patients with major depressive disorder but notes that "the ability to predict suicide attempts and completed suicide is poor, with both many false positives (i.e., patients who appear more likely to make attempts or complete suicide but who do not) and false negatives (i.e., patients who appear less likely to make attempts or complete suicide but who do)" (1). With respect to children and adolescents, the guideline recommends caution when basing treatment decisions on adult data. All of these general principles remain true.

Recent research has raised concern about the safety of antidepressant use for children and adolescents and has led the FDA to add additional warnings, including a black box warning, to the labeling of all antidepressant medications (9). Although the APA practice guideline focused on treatment of adults, not children and adolescents, discussion of this research is appropriate in this watch. In 23 short-term (4- to 16-week) trials involving more than 4,400 patients receiving nine antidepressant drugs (selective serotonin reuptake inhibitors [SSRIs] and others), suicidal thinking or behavior was observed in 78 individuals. The average risk of suicidal thinking or behaviors was 3.8% for participants receiving a drug compared with 2.1% for those given placebo, suggesting an approximately twofold increase in risk (10). Consequently, in the new labeling, the FDA notes that pooled analyses of placebo-controlled antidepressant trials (available at http://www.fda.gov/ohrms/dockets/ac/04/briefing/2004-4065b1.htm) have shown an increased risk of suicidal thinking or behavior in children and adolescents with major depressive disorder, obsessive-compulsive disorder, and other psychiatric disorders. However, it is important to note that no suicides occurred in any of these trials. Furthermore, according to the Centers for Disease Prevention and Control, suicidal thinking and suicide attempts are common among adolescents, occurring respectively in about 17% and 8.5% of adolescents each year. As a result of such attempts, only 0.002% of girls and 0.012% of boys ultimately die (11), highlighting the fact that suicidality (i.e., suicidal thoughts and behaviors) and suicide are not equivalent.

Although the studies reviewed by the FDA showed some variations among antidepressants, it was not clear whether the increase in suicidal thinking or behavior was specific to particular antidepressants, extended to adults, or occurred with longer-term antidepressant use (i.e., beyond several months). Thus, the FDA labeling change recommends that "all pediatric patients being treated with antidepressants for any indication should be observed closely for clinical worsening, suicidality, and unusual changes in behavior, especially during the initial few months of a course of drug therapy, or at times of dose changes, either increases or decreases" (9). To facilitate this, the FDA suggests an increased frequency of face-to-face contacts (i.e., weekly for the first 4 weeks, biweekly for the next 8 weeks), with prescriptions written for "the smallest quantity of tablets consistent with good patient management, in order to reduce the risk of overdose." The FDA also recommends that patients be screened for bipolar disorder before antidepressant therapy is initiated. Medication guides that will accompany prescriptions of antidepressant medications are intended to alert families and caregivers of pediatric and adult patients to the need to monitor patients for the emergence of agitation, irritability, hostility (aggressiveness), impulsivity, anxiety, panic attacks, insomnia, akathisia, hypomania, mania, or unusual changes in behavior so that such symptoms can be reported immediately to health care professionals.

When signs or symptoms are observed that suggest an increased suicide risk, recommendations are available for assessing and managing suicidal behaviors in children and adolescents from the American Academy of Child and Adolescent Psychiatry (12) and in adults from the APA (13).

As with all decisions about treatment for individuals with psychiatric illnesses, the choice to initiate antidepressant therapy must balance the potential risks of treatment against the potential therapeutic benefit and the risks of untreated illness (14–16). The risks of untreated depression, including suicide and other suicidal behaviors, are high and have been clearly delineated in youths and in adults (1, 12, 13, 17). In adults, the evidence for antidepressant efficacy is also clear, as reviewed in the APA guideline.

In children and adolescents, the issue has been confounded by a smaller number of clinical trials as well as by negative trials. Positive evidence includes the studies of fluoxetine that led to its receiving an FDA indication for treatment of depression in children and adolescents and the recent Treatment for Adolescents With Depression Study (TADS) sponsored by the National Institute of Mental Health. This large, yearlong community effectiveness trial (18) of youths with moderate to severe major depressive disorder found that by 12 weeks of treatment, rates of response to fluoxetine alone (60.9%) were greater than those with either placebo (35%) or cognitive behavior therapy (CBT) alone (43.2%). In combination with CBT, fluoxetine was associated with an even greater response rate (71%)—twice that seen with placebo. Furthermore, clinically significant suicidal thinking, which was observed in 29% of study subjects prior to treatment, improved in all groups.

In addition to this direct evidence of antidepressant efficacy from clinical trials, the national decreases in youth suicide and overall suicide rates, during a period when the prescribing of antidepressants has increased, might provide indirect evidence for an overall preventive effect of antidepressant treatment on suicide (14, 19, 20).

Because additional information on the issue of antidepressants and suicide risk is likely to emerge, readers are urged to seek updates on the Web sites of the FDA (http://www.fda.gov), the American Academy of Child and Adolescent Psychiatry (http://www.aacap.org), and the APA (http://www.psych.org).

Availability of new antidepressants

Two new antidepressants, escitalopram and duloxetine, have been approved by the FDA since publication of the guideline. Escitalopram, the active *S*-enantiomer of citalopram, is an SSRI antidepressant that has FDA approval for acute and maintenance treatment of major depressive disorder. Evidence from randomized, clinical trials suggests that escitalopram is superior to placebo in the short-term treatment of depression (21), with efficacy and tolerability comparable to that of other antidepressants, including venlafaxine (22, 23) and citalopram (21, 24).

Duloxetine, a dual serotonin-norepinephrine reuptake inhibitor, has also been approved for the treatment of depression. Randomized, clinical trials show duloxetine to be more efficacious than placebo (25–28) and comparable in efficacy to SSRI antidepressants (27, 28). The drug is generally well tolerated, with reported adverse effects of treatment (e.g., nausea, dry mouth, dizziness, somnolence, insomnia, constipation, and asthenia) varying across studies but typically being infrequent at total oral daily doses of 40–120 mg. In addition to ameliorating core symptoms of depression, duloxetine exhibits efficacy relative to placebo in treating painful physical symptoms (26, 28–31) and anxiety in depressed individuals (32). It also appears to ameliorate pain in the absence of depression (31), and it is FDA indicated for the management of pain associated with diabetic peripheral neuropathy.

Since publication of the guideline, the combination of fluoxetine and olanzapine has received FDA approval on the basis of a randomized, clinical trial supporting its use (33). Although the combination product (brand name Symbyax) is indicated for the treatment of episodes of bipolar depression, combined treatment with fluoxetine and olanzapine has also been found useful in treating episodes of major depression with psychotic features (34) and in treatment-resistant depression (35, 36).

Reboxetine, a selective norepinephrine reuptake inhibitor that was noted in the guideline to be possibly close to receiving approval, is not currently approved for use. Atomoxetine, another selective norepinephrine reuptake inhibitor, has recently become available but is approved for the treatment of attention deficit hyperactivity disorder. Although the possibility of using atomoxetine, either alone or in combination with an SSRI, for the treatment of depression has prompted interest among clinicians, the drug does not have an FDA indication for this use, and data on its use in the treatment of depression are limited (37–39). In addition, the FDA has just added a bolded warning to atomoxetine's labeling noting that the medication should be discontinued in patients who develop jaundice or laboratory evidence of liver injury (http://www.fda.gov/bbs/topics/ANSWERS/2004/ANS01335.html).

The evidence cited here on new medications is based on premarketing research. Clinicians are cautioned that real-world experiences after a drug is approved often bring unexpected findings, including less efficacy in some circumstances and unanticipated adverse events.

St. John's wort

Since publication of the guideline, results from additional meta-analyses and well-designed trials of St. John's wort have become available. Although some additional randomized, controlled trials have shown St. John's wort to be superior to placebo (40–42) or to comparator antidepressants (43, 44) in treating mild to moderate depression, other large trials have shown it to be no better than placebo (45–47) or comparator antidepressants in efficacy (42, 46–50). Several factors continue to confound interpretation of the literature, including trial length, adequacy of comparison treatment, and the reliability, stability, and comparability of *Hypericum* preparations. The most recent meta-analysis noted a trend for decreasing effect sizes in trials of St. John's wort over time, suggesting that it may be less effective in treating depression than previously thought (51). Although St. John's wort is generally well tolerated in clinical trials, increasing attention has been given to its tendency to compromise the effectiveness of other medications (e.g., cyclosporine, HIV protease inhibitors, oral contraceptives, digoxin, warfarin, and theophylline) by interactions mediated through cytochrome P450 enzymes (e.g., CYP3A4, CYP2C9, CYP1A2, CYP2C19) and transport protein P-glycoproteins (52–56).

Other somatic treatments

Evidence for the efficacy of electroconvulsive therapy (ECT) in treating major depressive episodes, already compelling at the time the guideline was published, has been strengthened by additional findings. Recent meta-analyses have highlighted the superior efficacy of ECT relative to sham treatment and also relative to pharmacotherapies for depression (57, 58). In depressed patients who received an acute course of ECT, data from the Consortium for Research in ECT have shown that thrice-weekly bilateral ECT is associated with rapid initial response and high rates of sustained response and remission (59). In comparison with bilateral ECT, right unilateral ECT has been associated with fewer cognitive effects (60, 61), particularly in autobiographical memory (62). However, as with bilateral ECT, cognitive effects vary with the extent to which the electrical stimulus exceeds the seizure threshold (60). In addition, the overall efficacy of unilateral ECT appears to be less than that with bilateral ECT (57). Several additional studies highlight the diminished efficacy of barely suprathreshold electrical stimulation with right unilateral electrode placement (60, 61, 63) and a corresponding need to administer right unilateral ECT at stimulus intensities that are at least six times the initial seizure threshold (64). Additional details on the clinical use of ECT in the treatment of major depression can be found in the 2001 revision of the APA's *The Practice of Electroconvulsive Therapy: Recommendations for Treatment, Training, and Privileging* (64).

Although other somatic treatments, including repetitive transcranial magnetic stimulation, magnetic seizure therapy, and vagal nerve stimulation, have also been studied over the past 5 years, evidence is not yet sufficient to recommend their use in routine clinical practice.

PSYCHOTHERAPY AND OTHER PSYCHOSOCIAL TREATMENTS

Recent studies have provided additional support for the efficacy of a number of psychosocial treatment approaches, including problem-solving treatment (65, 66), group psychoeducation (65), and the cognitive behavioral analysis system of psychotherapy (67). Additional meta-analyses have suggested that among psychotherapeutic approaches, other bona fide psychotherapies have efficacy comparable with CBT for treating depression (68, 69), although more research with CBT has been done. Given the evidence for the benefits of exercise in older depressed adults (70, 71), exercise may also be of value in other subgroups of patients with major depression.

Psychotherapy combined with pharmacotherapy

As noted in the guideline, studies examining combination treatment with psychotherapy and pharmacotherapy have shown mixed results. Although this has continued to be true in subsequently published studies (66, 67, 72, 73), a recent meta-analysis suggested that a combination of psychotherapy and pharmacotherapy is more effective than pharmacotherapy alone (74). Combination therapy may be particularly useful in improving treatment adherence (73, 74) and might be of some use in targeting particular symptoms or patient subgroups (75–77).

CONTINUATION AND MAINTENANCE TREATMENT

At the time the guideline was published, much data suggested the importance of continuation and maintenance treatment in individuals at high risk of recurrent depression, although the majority of studies on this practice examined the use of tricyclic antidepressants. Several more recent studies have confirmed the benefits of continuation and maintenance treatment with antidepressants in other classes (e.g., sertraline, venlafaxine, and mirtazapine) in decreasing the likelihood of recurrence (78–82).

Supplementing the earlier data on continuation and maintenance psychotherapy, most (83–87) but not all (88) additional studies of CBT support its use either alone or in addition to pharmacotherapy in decreasing depressive recurrence.

Inadequate response to treatment

Given the clinical importance of treatment nonresponse, it is not surprising that a number of studies and meta-analyses have examined strategies for augmenting antidepressant therapy. Although no consistently effective approach has emerged (89), pharmacotherapeutic approaches with some recent positive results include augmentation with thyroid hormone (particularly in women) (90), lithium (91, 92), buspirone (93), and lamotrigine (94). Addition of a benzodiazepine may also be helpful in some individuals after a careful weighing of potential advantages and disadvantages (95). Some studies have suggested that adjunctive treatment with omega-3 fatty acids is efficacious (96–98), although a single study using omega-3 fatty acid monotherapy showed no benefit (99). Evidence on the use of estradiol augmentation in perimenopausal or postmenopausal women is mixed (100, 101), and other potentially negative health effects of estrogen treatment are emerging. The possible adjunctive use of mifepristone in treating psychotic depression has also generated interest recently, although data are sparse (102, 103).

Modafinil has been used increasingly in depressed patients, either as an augmenting agent or to counteract symptoms of fatigue resulting from depression or sedation from other agents. Evidence for the efficacy of modafinil is limited and comes primarily from small or uncontrolled trials (104–107). A single randomized trial showed a brief period of improvement in fatigue after initiating adjunctive treatment with modafinil but no augmenting effect on depressive symptoms relative to placebo (108).

Some additional evidence suggests that response may be enhanced by increasing the dosage of antidepressant medication, although an increase in side effects may also be observed (109–111).

In terms of the choice of antidepressant medication, some studies (111–114) and meta-analyses (115–118) suggest that greater efficacy is seen with medications that act on more than one neurotransmitter system (e.g., venlafaxine and mirtazapine), although this is not invariably the case (119, 120). Despite the fact that tricyclic antidepressants are no longer typically used as first-line agents because of problems with tolerability and toxicity, they are efficacious (120–125) and may still be indicated in individuals whose illness has not responded to other treatments.

Gender may also play a role in response to and tolerability with specific antidepressants, but findings across studies are inconsistent (126–132).

As noted in the guideline, there is some evidence that addition of cognitive-behavior psychotherapy may be beneficial for patients who have had only a partial response to pharmacotherapy. However, more recent findings have been mixed, with some (87, 133) but not all (88) studies showing adjunctive psychotherapy to be beneficial. One study suggests that in women, outcomes with combined treatment may not be as good as outcomes using sequential treatment with initial interpersonal psychotherapy followed by pharmacotherapy in nonresponders (134). Although the full implications of this finding are unclear, the sequential treatment approach merits further study and may be of particular relevance to women in the childbearing years.

TREATMENT OF DEPRESSION IN OLDER ADULTS

A number of recent randomized, controlled trials have examined the treatment of depression in older adults. Comparisons of several SSRIs with the tricyclic antidepressant nortriptyline show better tolerability with SSRIs in this group of patients (135–137). Although the efficacies of nortriptyline and SSRIs generally appear to be comparable (135, 136), some data suggest that nortriptyline may be more effective in severely depressed individuals (137). An additional randomized, controlled outpatient trial showed comparable efficacy for two SSRIs, sertraline and fluoxetine, in the acute treatment of major depression (138).

Maintenance antidepressant therapy is associated with a lesser likelihood of relapse in older adults (139, 140). These data extend the findings of Reynolds et al. (141), discussed in the guideline, which showed antidepressant medication (nortriptyline) or interpersonal therapy to be effective maintenance therapy for elderly patients with recurrent major depressive disorder.

In the PROSPECT study (142), in which elderly patients were treated in primary care practices with facilitation by case managers, interventions included treatment with an antidepressant (typically citalopram) and interpersonal psychotherapy (for patients who declined antidepressant). Compared with treatment as usual, intervention was associated with more rapid and more prominent reductions in suicidal ideation and depressive symptoms, and the beneficial impact on depression extended throughout the 12-month study period. Although not all patients in the intervention group continued to receive treatment for depression throughout the study period, a greater proportion of intervention patients received ongoing treatment compared with the treatment-as-usual group, strengthening the observation that maintenance treatment is beneficial in depressed older adults.

Several studies have compared antidepressant treatment, nonpharmacological treatments, or combined treatments in older adults. Blumenthal et al. (143) found comparable rates of response in older depressed patients randomly assigned to treatment with sertraline, aerobic exercise, or combination treatment. After 10 months, greater sustained benefit was seen in the exercise-alone group, whereas response rates in the sertraline-alone and sertraline-plus-exercise groups were comparable (71). Thompson et al. (144) showed combination treatment with desipramine and CBT to be better than desipramine alone, comparable to CBT alone, and of particular benefit in elderly outpatients who were severely depressed. These findings supplement those of Reynolds et al. (141), who showed a trend for superior acute response with combined nortriptyline and interpersonal therapy. With maintenance treatment, either therapy was effective in rapid responders to treatment, but combined treatment was superior in patients who had a mixed or delayed response to initial therapy (139). In addition, combination therapy was more effective in maintaining social adjustment than either therapy alone (145).

REFERENCES

1. American Psychiatric Association: Practice guideline for the treatment of patients with major depressive disorder (revision). Am J Psychiatry 2000; 157:1–45
2. Aranda-Michel J, Koehler A, Bejarano PA, Poulos JE, Luxon BA, Khan CM, Ee LC, Balistreri WF, Weber FL Jr: Nefazodone-induced liver failure: report of three cases. Ann Intern Med 1999; 130:285–288
3. Choi S: Nefazodone (Serzone) withdrawn because of hepatotoxicity. CMAJ 2003; 169:1187
4. Conway CR, McGuire JM, Baram VY: Nefazodone-induced liver failure. J Clin Psychopharmacol 2004; 24:353–354
5. Eloubeidi MA, Gaede JT, Swaim MW: Reversible nefazodone-induced liver failure. Dig Dis Sci 2000; 45:1036–1038
6. Lucena MI, Andrade RJ, Gomez-Outes A, Rubio M, Cabello MR: Acute liver failure after treatment with nefazodone. Dig Dis Sci 1999; 44:2577–2579
7. Schirren CA, Baretton G: Nefazodone-induced acute liver failure. Am J Gastroenterol 2000; 95:1596–1597
8. Tzimas GN, Dion B, Deschenes M: Early onset, nefazodone-induced fulminant hepatic failure. Am J Gastroenterol 2003; 98:1663–1664
9. Food and Drug Administration: Labeling Change Request Letter for Antidepressant Medications. Rockville, Md, October 28, 2004. Available at: http://www.fda.gov/cder/drug/antidepressants/SSRIlabelChange.htm
10. Newman TB: A black-box warning for antidepressants in children? N Engl J Med 2004; 351:1595–1598
11. National Center for Injury Prevention and Control: Web-based Injury Statistics Query and Reporting System (WISQARS). Atlanta, Ga, Centers for Disease Control and Prevention. Available at: http://www.cdc.gov/ncipc/wisqars
12. American Academy of Child and Adolescent Psychiatry: Practice parameter for the assessment and treatment of children and adolescents with suicidal behavior. J Am Acad Child Adolesc Psychiatry 2001; 40:24S–51S
13. American Psychiatric Association: Practice guideline for the assessment and treatment of patients with suicidal behaviors. Am J Psychiatry 2003; 160(suppl 11):1–60
14. Brent DA: Antidepressants and pediatric depression: the risk of doing nothing. N Engl J Med 2004; 351:1598–1601
15. American Academy of Child and Adolescent Psychiatry: Message to Members and Supplementary Talking Points for Child and Adolescent Psychiatrists Regarding the FDA Black Box Warning on the Use of Antidepressants for Pediatric Patients Washington, DC, 2004. Available at: http://www.aacap.org/press_releases/2004/SSRIemail10_29_041.pdf

16. American Psychiatric Association: News Release: APA Statement on the FDA's Hearing on Antidepressant Use in Pediatric Patients. Arlington, Va, September 16, 2004. Available at: http://www.psych.org/news_room/press_releases/antidepressantuse09202004.pdf
17. American Academy of Child and Adolescent Psychiatry: Practice parameter for the assessment and treatment of children and adolescents with depressive disorders. J Am Acad Child Adolesc Psychiatry 1998; 37:63S–83S
18. March J, Silva S, Petrycki S, Curry J, Wells K, Fairbank J, Burns B, Domino M, McNulty S, Vitiello B, Severe J: Fluoxetine, cognitive-behavioral therapy, and their combination for adolescents with depression: Treatment for Adolescents With Depression Study (TADS) randomized controlled trial. JAMA 2004; 292:807–820
19. Grunebaum MF, Ellis SP, Li S, Oquendo MA, Mann JJ: Antidepressants and suicide risk in the United States, 1985–1999. J Clin Psychiatry 2004; 65:1456–1462
20. Olfson M, Shaffer D, Marcus SC, Greenberg T: Relationship between antidepressant medication treatment and suicide in adolescents. Arch Gen Psychiatry 2003; 60:978–982
21. Burke WJ, Gergel I, Bose A: Fixed-dose trial of the single isomer SSRI escitalopram in depressed outpatients. J Clin Psychiatry 2002; 63:331–336
22. Bielski RJ, Ventura D, Chang CC: A double-blind comparison of escitalopram and venlafaxine extended release in the treatment of major depressive disorder. J Clin Psychiatry 2004; 65:1190–1196
23. Montgomery SA, Huusom AK, Bothmer J: A randomised study comparing escitalopram with venlafaxine XR in primary care patients with major depressive disorder. Neuropsychobiology 2004; 50:57–64
24. Lepola U, Wade A, Andersen HF: Do equivalent doses of escitalopram and citalopram have similar efficacy? A pooled analysis of two positive placebo-controlled studies in major depressive disorder. Int Clin Psychopharmacol 2004; 19:149–155
25. Detke MJ, Lu Y, Goldstein DJ, McNamara RK, Demitrack MA: Duloxetine 60 mg once daily dosing versus placebo in the acute treatment of major depression. J Psychiatr Res 2002; 36:383–390
26. Detke MJ, Lu Y, Goldstein DJ, Hayes JR, Demitrack MA: Duloxetine, 60 mg once daily, for major depressive disorder: a randomized double-blind placebo-controlled trial. J Clin Psychiatry 2002; 63:308–315
27. Goldstein DJ, Mallinckrodt C, Lu Y, Demitrack MA: Duloxetine in the treatment of major depressive disorder: a double-blind clinical trial. J Clin Psychiatry 2002; 63:225–231
28. Goldstein DJ, Lu Y, Detke MJ, Wiltse C, Mallinckrodt C, Demitrack MA: Duloxetine in the treatment of depression: a double-blind placebo-controlled comparison with paroxetine. J Clin Psychopharmacol 2004; 24:389–399
29. Goldstein DJ, Lu Y, Detke MJ, Hudson J, Iyengar S, Demitrack MA: Effects of duloxetine on painful physical symptoms associated with depression. Psychosomatics 2004; 45:17–28
30. Fava M, Mallinckrodt CH, Detke MJ, Watkin JG, Wohlreich MM: The effect of duloxetine on painful physical symptoms in depressed patients: do improvements in these symptoms result in higher remission rates? J Clin Psychiatry 2004; 65:521–530
31. Arnold LM, Lu Y, Crofford LJ, Wohlreich M, Detke MJ, Iyengar S, Goldstein DJ: A double-blind, multicenter trial comparing duloxetine with placebo in the treatment of fibromyalgia patients with or without major depressive disorder. Arthritis Rheum 2004; 50:2974–2984
32. Dunner DL, Goldstein DJ, Mallinckrodt C, Lu Y, Detke MJ: Duloxetine in treatment of anxiety symptoms associated with depression. Depress Anxiety 2003; 18:53–61
33. Tohen M, Vieta E, Calabrese J, Ketter TA, Sachs G, Bowden C, Mitchell PB, Centorrino F, Risser R, Baker RW, Evans AR, Beymer K, Dube S, Tollefson GD, Breier A: Efficacy of olanzapine and olanzapine-fluoxetine combination in the treatment of bipolar I depression. Arch Gen Psychiatry 2003; 60:1079–1088

34. Rothschild AJ, Williamson DJ, Tohen MF, Schatzberg A, Andersen SW, Van Campen LE, Sanger TM, Tollefson GD: A double-blind, randomized study of olanzapine and olanzapine/fluoxetine combination for major depression with psychotic features. J Clin Psychopharmacol 2004; 24:365–373
35. Corya SA, Andersen SW, Detke HC, Kelly LS, Van Campen LE, Sanger TM, Williamson DJ, Dube S: Long-term antidepressant efficacy and safety of olanzapine/fluoxetine combination: a 76-week open-label study. J Clin Psychiatry 2003; 64:1349–1356
36. Shelton RC, Tollefson GD, Tohen M, Stahl S, Gannon KS, Jacobs TG, Buras WR, Bymaster FP, Zhang W, Spencer KA, Feldman PD, Meltzer HY: A novel augmentation strategy for treating resistant major depression. Am J Psychiatry 2001; 158:131–134
37. Berigan TR: Atomoxetine used adjunctively with selective serotonin reuptake inhibitors to treat depression. Prim Care Companion J Clin Psychiatry 2004; 6:93–94
38. Chouinard G, Annable L, Bradwejn J: An early phase II clinical trial of tomoxetine (LY139603) in the treatment of newly admitted depressed patients. Psychopharmacology (Berl) 1984; 83:126–128
39. Chouinard G, Annable L, Bradwejn J, Labonte A, Jones B, Mercier P, Belanger MC: An early phase II clinical trial with followup of tomoxetine (LY139603) in the treatment of newly admitted depressed patients. Psychopharmacol Bull 1985; 21:73–76
40. Kalb R, Trautmann-Sponsel RD, Kieser M: Efficacy and tolerability of Hypericum extract WS 5572 versus placebo in mildly to moderately depressed patients: a randomized double-blind multicenter clinical trial. Pharmacopsychiatry 2001; 34:96–103
41. Lecrubier Y, Clerc G, Didi R, Kieser M: Efficacy of St. John's wort extract WS 5570 in major depression: a double-blind, placebo-controlled trial. Am J Psychiatry 2002; 159:1361–1366
42. Philipp M, Kohnen R, Hiller KO: Hypericum extract versus imipramine or placebo in patients with moderate depression: randomised multicentre study of treatment for eight weeks. BMJ 1999; 319:1534–1538
43. Friede M, Henneicke von Zepelin HH, Freudenstein J: Differential therapy of mild to moderate depressive episodes (ICD-10 F 32.0; F 32.1) with St. John's wort. Pharmacopsychiatry 2001; 34(suppl 1):S38–S41
44. Schrader E: Equivalence of St John's wort extract (Ze 117) and fluoxetine: a randomized, controlled study in mild–moderate depression. Int Clin Psychopharmacol 2000; 15:61–68
45. Shelton RC, Keller MB, Gelenberg A, Dunner DL, Hirschfeld R, Thase ME, Russell J, Lydiard RB, Crits-Cristoph P, Gallop R, Todd L, Hellerstein D, Goodnick P, Keitner G, Stahl SM, Halbreich U: Effectiveness of St John's wort in major depression: a randomized controlled trial. JAMA 2001; 285:1978–1986
46. Hypericum Depression Trial Study Group: Effect of Hypericum perforatum (St John's wort) in major depressive disorder: a randomized controlled trial. JAMA 2002; 287:1807–1814
47. Bjerkenstedt L, Edman GV, Alken RG, Mannel M: Hypericum extract LI 160 and fluoxetine in mild to moderate depression: a randomized, placebo-controlled multi-center study in outpatients. Eur Arch Psychiatry Clin Neurosci 2004 (epub 12 Nov)
48. van Gurp G, Meterissian GB, Haiek LN, McCusker J, Bellavance F: St John's wort or sertraline? Randomized controlled trial in primary care. Can Fam Physician 2002; 48:905–912
49. Behnke K, Jensen GS, Graubaum HJ, Gruenwald J: Hypericum perforatum versus fluoxetine in the treatment of mild to moderate depression. Adv Ther 2002; 19:43–52
50. Harrer G, Schmidt U, Kuhn U, Biller A: Comparison of equivalence between the St. John's wort extract LoHyp-57 and fluoxetine. Arzneimittelforschung 1999; 49:289–296
51. Werneke U, Horn O, Taylor DM: How effective is St John's wort? The evidence revisited. J Clin Psychiatry 2004; 65:611–617
52. Henderson L, Yue QY, Bergquist C, Gerden B, Arlett P: St John's wort (Hypericum perforatum): drug interactions and clinical outcomes. Br J Clin Pharmacol 2002; 54:349–356

53. Wang LS, Zhou G, Zhu B, Wu J, Wang JG, Abd El-Aty AM, Li T, Liu J, Yang TL, Wang D, Zhong XY, Zhou HH: St John's wort induces both cytochrome P450 3A4-catalyzed sulfoxidation and 2C19-dependent hydroxylation of omeprazole. Clin Pharmacol Ther 2004; 75:191–197
54. Hennessy M, Kelleher D, Spiers JP, Barry M, Kavanagh P, Back D, Mulcahy F, Feely J: St John's wort increases expression of P-glycoprotein: implications for drug interactions. Br J Clin Pharmacol 2002; 53:75–82
55. Markowitz JS, Donovan JL, DeVane CL, Taylor RM, Ruan Y, Wang JS, Chavin KD: Effect of St John's wort on drug metabolism by induction of cytochrome P450 3A4 enzyme. JAMA 2003; 290:1500–1504
56. Obach RS: Inhibition of human cytochrome P450 enzymes by constituents of St. John's wort, an herbal preparation used in the treatment of depression. J Pharmacol Exp Ther 2000; 294:88–95
57. UK ECT Review Group: Efficacy and safety of electroconvulsive therapy in depressive disorders: a systematic review and meta-analysis. Lancet 2003; 361:799–808
58. Kho KH, van Vreeswijk MF, Simpson S, Zwinderman AH: A meta-analysis of electroconvulsive therapy efficacy in depression. J ECT 2003; 19:139–147
59. Husain MM, Rush AJ, Fink M, Knapp R, Petrides G, Rummans T, Biggs MM, O'Connor K, Rasmussen K, Litle M, Zhao W, Bernstein HJ, Smith G, Mueller M, McClintock SM, Bailine SH, Kellner CH: Speed of response and remission in major depressive disorder with acute electroconvulsive therapy (ECT): a Consortium for Research in ECT (CORE) report. J Clin Psychiatry 2004; 65:485–491
60. McCall WV, Reboussin DM, Weiner RD, Sackeim HA: Titrated moderately suprathreshold vs fixed high-dose right unilateral electroconvulsive therapy: acute antidepressant and cognitive effects. Arch Gen Psychiatry 2000; 57:438–444
61. Sackeim HA, Prudic J, Devanand DP, Nobler MS, Lisanby SH, Peyser S, Fitzsimons L, Moody BJ, Clark J: A prospective, randomized, double-blind comparison of bilateral and right unilateral electroconvulsive therapy at different stimulus intensities. Arch Gen Psychiatry 2000; 57:425–434
62. Lisanby SH, Maddox JH, Prudic J, Devanand DP, Sackeim HA: The effects of electroconvulsive therapy on memory of autobiographical and public events. Arch Gen Psychiatry 2000; 57:581–590
63. McCall WV, Dunn A, Rosenquist PB, Hughes D: Markedly suprathreshold right unilateral ECT versus minimally suprathreshold bilateral ECT: antidepressant and memory effects. J ECT 2002; 18:126–129
64. American Psychiatric Association: The Practice of Electroconvulsive Therapy: Recommendations for Treatment, Training, and Privileging. A Task Force Report of the American Psychiatric Association, 2nd Edition. Washington, DC, American Psychiatric Press, 2001
65. Dowrick C, Dunn G, Ayuso-Mateos JL, Dalgard OS, Page H, Lehtinen V, Casey P, Wilkinson C, Vazquez-Barquero JL, Wilkinson G: Problem solving treatment and group psychoeducation for depression: multicentre randomised controlled trial. Outcomes of Depression International Network (ODIN) Group. BMJ 2000; 321:1450–1454
66. Mynors-Wallis LM, Gath DH, Day A, Baker F: Randomised controlled trial of problem solving treatment, antidepressant medication, and combined treatment for major depression in primary care. BMJ 2000; 320:26–30
67. Keller MB, McCullough JP, Klein DN, Arnow B, Dunner DL, Gelenberg AJ, Markowitz JC, Nemeroff CB, Russell JM, Thase ME, Trivedi MH, Zajecka J: A comparison of nefazodone, the cognitive behavioral-analysis system of psychotherapy, and their combination for the treatment of chronic depression. N Engl J Med 2000; 342:1462–1470
68. Leichsenring F: Comparative effects of short-term psychodynamic psychotherapy and cognitive-behavioral therapy in depression: a meta-analytic approach. Clin Psychol Rev 2001; 21:401–419

69. Wampold BE, Minami T, Baskin TW, Callen TS: A meta-(re)analysis of the effects of cognitive therapy versus "other therapies" for depression. J Affect Disord 2002; 68:159–165
70. Mather AS, Rodriguez C, Guthrie MF, McHarg AM, Reid IC, McMurdo ME: Effects of exercise on depressive symptoms in older adults with poorly responsive depressive disorder: randomised controlled trial. Br J Psychiatry 2002; 180:411–415
71. Babyak M, Blumenthal JA, Herman S, Khatri P, Doraiswamy M, Moore K, Craighead WE, Baldewicz TT, Krishnan KR: Exercise treatment for major depression: maintenance of therapeutic benefit at 10 months. Psychosom Med 2000; 62:633–638
72. de Jonghe F, Hendricksen M, van Aalst G, Kool S, Peen V, Van R, van den EE, Dekker J: Psychotherapy alone and combined with pharmacotherapy in the treatment of depression. Br J Psychiatry 2004; 185:37–45
73. de Jonghe F, Kool S, van Aalst G, Dekker J, Peen J: Combining psychotherapy and antidepressants in the treatment of depression. J Affect Disord 2001; 64:217–229
74. Pampallona S, Bollini P, Tibaldi G, Kupelnick B, Munizza C: Combined pharmacotherapy and psychological treatment for depression: a systematic review. Arch Gen Psychiatry 2004; 61:714–719
75. Nemeroff CB, Heim CM, Thase ME, Klein DN, Rush AJ, Schatzberg AF, Ninan PT, McCullough JP Jr, Weiss PM, Dunner DL, Rothbaum BO, Kornstein S, Keitner G, Keller MB: Differential responses to psychotherapy versus pharmacotherapy in patients with chronic forms of major depression and childhood trauma. Proc Natl Acad Sci USA 2003; 100:14293–14296
76. Thase ME, Rush AJ, Manber R, Kornstein SG, Klein DN, Markowitz JC, Ninan PT, Friedman ES, Dunner DL, Schatzberg AF, Borian FE, Trivedi MH, Keller MB: Differential effects of nefazodone and cognitive behavioral analysis system of psychotherapy on insomnia associated with chronic forms of major depression. J Clin Psychiatry 2002; 63:493–500
77. Kool S, Dekker J, Duijsens IJ, de Jonghe F, Puite B: Efficacy of combined therapy and pharmacotherapy for depressed patients with or without personality disorders. Harv Rev Psychiatry 2003; 11:133–141
78. Kocsis JH, Schatzberg A, Rush AJ, Klein DN, Howland R, Gniwesch L, Davis SM, Harrison W: Psychosocial outcomes following long-term, double-blind treatment of chronic depression with sertraline vs placebo. Arch Gen Psychiatry 2002; 59:723–728
79. Koran LM, Gelenberg AJ, Kornstein SG, Howland RH, Friedman RA, DeBattista C, Klein D, Kocsis JH, Schatzberg AF, Thase ME, Rush AJ, Hirschfeld RM, LaVange LM, Keller MB: Sertraline versus imipramine to prevent relapse in chronic depression. J Affect Disord 2001; 65:27–36
80. Lepine JP, Caillard V, Bisserbe JC, Troy S, Hotton JM, Boyer P: A randomized, placebo-controlled trial of sertraline for prophylactic treatment of highly recurrent major depressive disorder. Am J Psychiatry 2004; 161:836–842
81. Simon JS, Aguiar LM, Kunz NR, Lei D: Extended-release venlafaxine in relapse prevention for patients with major depressive disorder. J Psychiatr Res 2004; 38:249–257
82. Thase ME, Nierenberg AA, Keller MB, Panagides J: Efficacy of mirtazapine for prevention of depressive relapse: a placebo-controlled double-blind trial of recently remitted high-risk patients. J Clin Psychiatry 2001; 62:782–788
83. Petersen T, Harley R, Papakostas GI, Montoya HD, Fava M, Alpert JE: Continuation cognitive-behavioural therapy maintains attributional style improvement in depressed patients responding acutely to fluoxetine. Psychol Med 2004; 34:555–561
84. Kocsis JH, Rush AJ, Markowitz JC, Borian FE, Dunner DL, Koran LM, Klein DN, Trivedi MH, Arnow B, Keitner G, Kornstein SG, Keller MB: Continuation treatment of chronic depression: a comparison of nefazodone, cognitive behavioral analysis system of psychotherapy, and their combination. Psychopharmacol Bull 2003; 37:73–87

85. Scott J, Palmer S, Paykel E, Teasdale J, Hayhurst H: Use of cognitive therapy for relapse prevention in chronic depression: cost-effectiveness study. Br J Psychiatry 2003; 182:221–227
86. Klein DN, Santiago NJ, Vivian D, Blalock JA, Kocsis JH, Markowitz JC, McCullough JP Jr, Rush AJ, Trivedi MH, Arnow BA, Dunner DL, Manber R, Rothbaum B, Thase ME, Keitner GI, Miller IW, Keller MB: Cognitive-behavioral analysis system of psychotherapy as a maintenance treatment for chronic depression. J Consult Clin Psychol 2004; 72:681–688
87. Paykel ES, Scott J, Teasdale JD, Johnson AL, Garland A, Moore R, Jenaway A, Cornwall PL, Hayhurst H, Abbott R, Pope M: Prevention of relapse in residual depression by cognitive therapy: a controlled trial. Arch Gen Psychiatry 1999; 56:829–835
88. Perlis RH, Nierenberg AA, Alpert JE, Pava J, Matthews JD, Buchin J, Sickinger AH, Fava M: Effects of adding cognitive therapy to fluoxetine dose increase on risk of relapse and residual depressive symptoms in continuation treatment of major depressive disorder. J Clin Psychopharmacol 2002; 22:474–480
89. Stimpson N, Agrawal N, Lewis G: Randomised controlled trials investigating pharmacological and psychological interventions for treatment-refractory depression: systematic review. Br J Psychiatry 2002; 181:284–294
90. Altshuler LL, Bauer M, Frye MA, Gitlin MJ, Mintz J, Szuba MP, Leight KL, Whybrow PC: Does thyroid supplementation accelerate tricyclic antidepressant response? A review and meta-analysis of the literature. Am J Psychiatry 2001; 158:1617–1622
91. Bauer M, Dopfmer S: Lithium augmentation in treatment-resistant depression: meta-analysis of placebo-controlled studies. J Clin Psychopharmacol 1999; 19:427–434
92. Januel D, Poirier MF, D'alche-Biree F, Dib M, Olie JP: Multicenter double-blind randomized parallel-group clinical trial of efficacy of the combination clomipramine (150 mg/day) plus lithium carbonate (750 mg/day) versus clomipramine (150 mg/day) plus placebo in the treatment of unipolar major depression. J Affect Disord 2003; 76:191–200
93. Appelberg BG, Syvalahti EK, Koskinen TE, Mehtonen OP, Muhonen TT, Naukkarinen HH: Patients with severe depression may benefit from buspirone augmentation of selective serotonin reuptake inhibitors: results from a placebo-controlled, randomized, double-blind, placebo wash-in study. J Clin Psychiatry 2001; 62:448–452
94. Normann C, Hummel B, Scharer LO, Horn M, Grunze H, Walden J: Lamotrigine as adjunct to paroxetine in acute depression: a placebo-controlled, double-blind study. J Clin Psychiatry 2002; 63:337–344
95. Furukawa TA, Streiner DL, Young LT: Is antidepressant-benzodiazepine combination therapy clinically more useful? A meta-analytic study. J Affect Disord 2001; 65:173–177
96. Nemets B, Stahl Z, Belmaker RH: Addition of omega-3 fatty acid to maintenance medication treatment for recurrent unipolar depressive disorder. Am J Psychiatry 2002; 159:477–479
97. Su KP, Huang SY, Chiu CC, Shen WW: Omega-3 fatty acids in major depressive disorder: a preliminary double-blind, placebo-controlled trial. Eur Neuropsychopharmacol 2003; 13:267–271
98. Peet M, Horrobin DF: A dose-ranging study of the effects of ethyl-eicosapentaenoate in patients with ongoing depression despite apparently adequate treatment with standard drugs. Arch Gen Psychiatry 2002; 59:913–919
99. Marangell LB, Martinez JM, Zboyan HA, Kertz B, Kim HF, Puryear LJ: A double-blind, placebo-controlled study of the omega-3 fatty acid docosahexaenoic acid in the treatment of major depression. Am J Psychiatry 2003; 160:996–998
100. Soares CN, Almeida OP, Joffe H, Cohen LS: Efficacy of estradiol for the treatment of depressive disorders in perimenopausal women: a double-blind, randomized, placebo-controlled trial. Arch Gen Psychiatry 2001; 58:529–534

101. Morrison MF, Kallan MJ, Ten Have T, Katz I, Tweedy K, Battistini M: Lack of efficacy of estradiol for depression in postmenopausal women: a randomized, controlled trial. Biol Psychiatry 2004; 55:406–412
102. Belanoff JK, Rothschild AJ, Cassidy F, DeBattista C, Baulieu EE, Schold C, Schatzberg AF: An open label trial of C-1073 (mifepristone) for psychotic major depression. Biol Psychiatry 2002; 52:386–392
103. Belanoff JK, Flores BH, Kalezhan M, Sund B, Schatzberg AF: Rapid reversal of psychotic depression using mifepristone. J Clin Psychopharmacol 2001; 21:516–521
104. Menza MA, Kaufman KR, Castellanos A: Modafinil augmentation of antidepressant treatment in depression. J Clin Psychiatry 2000; 61:378–381
105. Schwartz TL, Azhar N, Cole K, Hopkins G, Nihalani N, Simionescu M, Husain J, Jones N: An open-label study of adjunctive modafinil in patients with sedation related to serotonergic antidepressant therapy. J Clin Psychiatry 2004; 65:1223–1227
106. Ninan PT, Hassman HA, Glass SJ, McManus FC: Adjunctive modafinil at initiation of treatment with a selective serotonin reuptake inhibitor enhances the degree and onset of therapeutic effects in patients with major depressive disorder and fatigue. J Clin Psychiatry 2004; 65:414–420
107. DeBattista C, Lembke A, Solvason HB, Ghebremichael R, Poirier J: A prospective trial of modafinil as an adjunctive treatment of major depression. J Clin Psychopharmacol 2004; 24:87–90
108. DeBattista C, Doghramji K, Menza MA, Rosenthal MH, Fieve RR: Adjunct modafinil for the short-term treatment of fatigue and sleepiness in patients with major depressive disorder: a preliminary double-blind, placebo-controlled study. J Clin Psychiatry 2003; 64:1057–1064
109. Schmidt ME, Fava M, Zhang S, Gonzales J, Raute NJ, Judge R: Treatment approaches to major depressive disorder relapse, part 1: dose increase. Psychother Psychosom 2002; 71:190–194
110. Bollini P, Pampallona S, Tibaldi G, Kupelnick B, Munizza C: Effectiveness of antidepressants: meta-analysis of dose-effect relationships in randomised clinical trials. Br J Psychiatry 1999; 174:297–303
111. Mehtonen OP, Sogaard J, Roponen P, Behnke K: Randomized, double-blind comparison of venlafaxine and sertraline in outpatients with major depressive disorder. Venlafaxine 631 Study Group. J Clin Psychiatry 2000; 61:95–100
112. Rudolph RL, Feiger AD: A double-blind, randomized, placebo-controlled trial of once-daily venlafaxine extended release (XR) and fluoxetine for the treatment of depression. J Affect Disord 1999; 56:171–181
113. Schatzberg AF, Kremer C, Rodrigues HE, Murphy GM Jr: Double-blind, randomized comparison of mirtazapine and paroxetine in elderly depressed patients. Am J Geriatr Psychiatry 2002; 10:541–550
114. Tzanakaki M, Guazzelli M, Nimatoudis I, Zissis NP, Smeraldi E, Rizzo F: Increased remission rates with venlafaxine compared with fluoxetine in hospitalized patients with major depression and melancholia. Int Clin Psychopharmacol 2000; 15:29–34
115. Entsuah AR, Huang H, Thase ME: Response and remission rates in different subpopulations with major depressive disorder administered venlafaxine, selective serotonin reuptake inhibitors, or placebo. J Clin Psychiatry 2001; 62:869–877
116. Smith D, Dempster C, Glanville J, Freemantle N, Anderson I: Efficacy and tolerability of venlafaxine compared with selective serotonin reuptake inhibitors and other antidepressants: a meta-analysis. Br J Psychiatry 2002; 180:396–404
117. Stahl SM, Entsuah R, Rudolph RL: Comparative efficacy between venlafaxine and SSRIs: a pooled analysis of patients with depression. Biol Psychiatry 2002; 52:1166–1174
118. Thase ME, Entsuah AR, Rudolph RL: Remission rates during treatment with venlafaxine or selective serotonin reuptake inhibitors. Br J Psychiatry 2001; 178:234–241

119. Freemantle N, Anderson IM, Young P: Predictive value of pharmacological activity for the relative efficacy of antidepressant drugs: meta-regression analysis. Br J Psychiatry 2000; 177:292–302
120. Anderson IM: Selective serotonin reuptake inhibitors versus tricyclic antidepressants: a meta-analysis of efficacy and tolerability. J Affect Disord 2000; 58:19–36
121. Joyce PR, Mulder RT, Luty SE, McKenzie JM, Rae AM: A differential response to nortriptyline and fluoxetine in melancholic depression: the importance of age and gender. Acta Psychiatr Scand 2003; 108:20–23
122. Montgomery SA: A meta-analysis of the efficacy and tolerability of paroxetine versus tricyclic antidepressants in the treatment of major depression. Int Clin Psychopharmacol 2001; 16:169–178
123. Nelson JC, Mazure CM, Jatlow PI, Bowers MB Jr, Price LH: Combining norepinephrine and serotonin reuptake inhibition mechanisms for treatment of depression: a double-blind, randomized study. Biol Psychiatry 2004; 55:296–300
124. Robinson RG, Schultz SK, Castillo C, Kopel T, Kosier JT, Newman RM, Curdue K, Petracca G, Starkstein SE: Nortriptyline versus fluoxetine in the treatment of depression and in short-term recovery after stroke: a placebo-controlled, double-blind study. Am J Psychiatry 2000; 157:351–359
125. Guaiana G, Barbui C, Hotopf M: Amitriptyline versus other types of pharmacotherapy for depression. Cochrane Database Syst Rev 2003, CD004186
126. Baca E, Garcia-Garcia M, Porras-Chavarino A: Gender differences in treatment response to sertraline versus imipramine in patients with nonmelancholic depressive disorders. Prog Neuropsychopharmacol Biol Psychiatry 2004; 28:57–65
127. Joyce PR, Mulder RT, Luty SE, Sullivan PF, McKenzie JM, Abbott RM, Stevens IF: Patterns and predictors of remission, response, and recovery in major depression treated with fluoxetine or nortriptyline. Aust N Z J Psychiatry 2002; 36:384–391
128. Kornstein SG, Schatzberg AF, Thase ME, Yonkers KA, McCullough JP, Keitner GI, Gelenberg AJ, Davis SM, Harrison WM, Keller MB: Gender differences in treatment response to sertraline versus imipramine in chronic depression. Am J Psychiatry 2000; 157:1445–1452
129. Quitkin FM, Stewart JW, McGrath PJ, Taylor BP, Tisminetzky MS, Petkova E, Chen Y, Ma G, Klein DF: Are there differences between women's and men's antidepressant responses? Am J Psychiatry 2002; 159:1848–1854
130. Scheibe S, Preuschhof C, Cristi C, Bagby RM: Are there gender differences in major depression and its response to antidepressants? J Affect Disord 2003; 75:223–235
131. Parker G, Parker K, Austin MP, Mitchell P, Brotchie H: Gender differences in response to differing antidepressant drug classes: two negative studies. Psychol Med 2003; 33:1473–1477
132. Wohlfarth T, Storosum JG, Elferink AJ, van Zwieten BJ, Fouwels A, van den BW: Response to tricyclic antidepressants: independent of gender? Am J Psychiatry 2004; 161:370–372
133. Kennedy SH, Segal ZV, Cohen NL, Levitan RD, Gemar M, Bagby RM: Lithium carbonate versus cognitive therapy as sequential combination treatment strategies in partial responders to antidepressant medication: an exploratory trial. J Clin Psychiatry 2003; 64:439–444
134. Frank E, Grochocinski VJ, Spanier CA, Buysse DJ, Cherry CR, Houck PR, Stapf DM, Kupfer DJ: Interpersonal psychotherapy and antidepressant medication: evaluation of a sequential treatment strategy in women with recurrent major depression. J Clin Psychiatry 2000; 61:51–57
135. Mulsant BH, Pollock BG, Nebes R, Miller MD, Sweet RA, Stack J, Houck PR, Bensasi S, Mazumdar S, Reynolds CF III: A twelve-week, double-blind, randomized comparison of nortriptyline and paroxetine in older depressed inpatients and outpatients. Am J Geriatr Psychiatry 2001; 9:406–414

136. Bondareff W, Alpert M, Friedhoff AJ, Richter EM, Clary CM, Batzar E: Comparison of sertraline and nortriptyline in the treatment of major depressive disorder in late life. Am J Psychiatry 2000; 157:729–736
137. Navarro V, Gasto C, Torres X, Marcos T, Pintor L: Citalopram versus nortriptyline in late-life depression: a 12-week randomized single-blind study. Acta Psychiatr Scand 2001; 103:435–440
138. Newhouse PA, Krishnan KR, Doraiswamy PM, Richter EM, Batzar ED, Clary CM: A double-blind comparison of sertraline and fluoxetine in depressed elderly outpatients. J Clin Psychiatry 2000; 61:559–568
139. Dew MA, Reynolds CF III, Mulsant B, Frank E, Houck PR, Mazumdar S, Begley A, Kupfer DJ: Initial recovery patterns may predict which maintenance therapies for depression will keep older adults well. J Affect Disord 2001; 65:155–166
140. Klysner R, Bent-Hansen J, Hansen HL, Lunde M, Pleidrup E, Poulsen DL, Andersen M, Petersen HE: Efficacy of citalopram in the prevention of recurrent depression in elderly patients: placebo-controlled study of maintenance therapy. Br J Psychiatry 2002; 181:29–35
141. Reynolds CF III, Frank E, Perel JM, Imber SD, Cornes C, Miller MD, Mazumdar S, Houck PR, Dew MA, Stack JA, Pollock BG, Kupfer DJ: Nortriptyline and interpersonal psychotherapy as maintenance therapies for recurrent major depression: a randomized controlled trial in patients older than 59 years. JAMA 1999; 281:39–45
142. Bruce ML, Ten Have TR, Reynolds CF III, Katz II, Schulberg HC, Mulsant BH, Brown GK, McAvay GJ, Pearson JL, Alexopoulos GS: Reducing suicidal ideation and depressive symptoms in depressed older primary care patients: a randomized controlled trial. JAMA 2004; 291:1081–1091
143. Blumenthal JA, Babyak MA, Moore KA, Craighead WE, Herman S, Khatri P, Waugh R, Napolitano MA, Forman LM, Appelbaum M, Doraiswamy PM, Krishnan KR: Effects of exercise training on older patients with major depression. Arch Intern Med 1999; 159:2349–2356
144. Thompson LW, Coon DW, Gallagher-Thompson D, Sommer BR, Koin D: Comparison of desipramine and cognitive/behavioral therapy in the treatment of elderly outpatients with mild-to-moderate depression. Am J Geriatr Psychiatry 2001; 9:225–240
145. Lenze EJ, Dew MA, Mazumdar S, Begley AE, Cornes C, Miller MD, Imber SD, Frank E, Kupfer DJ, Reynolds CF III: Combined pharmacotherapy and psychotherapy as maintenance treatment for late-life depression: effects on social adjustment. Am J Psychiatry 2002; 159:466–468

PRACTICE GUIDELINE FOR THE
Treatment of Patients With Major Depressive Disorder
Second Edition

WORK GROUP ON MAJOR DEPRESSIVE DISORDER

T. Byram Karasu, M.D., Chair
Alan Gelenberg, M.D.
Arnold Merriam, M.D.
Philip Wang, M.D., Dr.P.H. (Consultant)

Originally published in April 2000. A guideline watch, summarizing significant developments in the scientific literature since publication of this guideline, may be available in the Psychiatric Practice section of the APA web site at www.psych.org.

CONTENTS

Guide to Using This Practice Guideline 767

Development Process 768

Introduction 769

Part A: Treatment Recommendations for Patients With Major Depressive Disorder 771

I. Summary of Treatment Recommendations........ 771
   A. Psychiatric Management........ 771
   B. Acute Phase 772
   C. Continuation Phase........ 777
   D. Maintenance Phase........ 777
   E. Discontinuation of Active Treatment 778

II. Formulation and Implementation of a Treatment Plan 778
   A. Psychiatric Management........ 779
   B. Acute Phase 782
   C. Continuation Phase........ 787
   D. Maintenance Phase........ 787
   E. Discontinuation of Active Treatment 788

III. Specific Clinical Features Influencing the Treatment Plan 788
   A. Psychiatric Features 788
   B. Demographic and Psychosocial Variables........ 792
   C. Treatment Implications of Concurrent General Medical Disorders 797

Part B: Background Information and Review of Available Evidence 799

IV. Disease Definition, Epidemiology, Natural History, and Course 799
   A. Specific Features of Diagnosis........ 800
   B. Epidemiology........ 800
   C. Natural History and Course........ 802

V. Review and Synthesis of Available Evidence........ 803
   A. Acute Phase Somatic Treatments........ 803
   B. Acute Phase Psychosocial Interventions 815
   C. Psychotherapy Combined With Pharmacotherapy........ 820
   D. Continuation Treatment 820
   E. Maintenance Treatment 821

Part C: Future Research Needs 822

VI. Antidepressant Medications 822

VII. Psychotherapy 823

VIII. Electroconvulsive Therapy 823

IX. Other Treatment Modalities 823

X. Individuals and Organizations That Submitted Comments 824

XI. References 824

GUIDE TO USING THIS PRACTICE GUIDELINE

This practice guideline uses available evidence to develop treatment recommendations for the care of adult patients with major depressive disorder. This guideline contains many sections, not all of which will be equally useful for all readers. The following guide is designed to help readers find the sections that will be most useful to them.

Part A contains the treatment recommendations for patients with major depressive disorder. Section I is the summary of treatment recommendations, which includes the main treatment recommendations, along with codes that indicate the degree of clinical confidence in each recommendation. Section II is a guide to the formulation and implementation of a treatment plan for the individual patient. This section includes all of the treatment recommendations. Section III, "Specific Clinical Features Influencing the Treatment Plan," discusses a range of clinical conditions that could alter the general recommendations discussed in Section II.

Part B, "Background Information and Review of Available Evidence," will be useful to understand, in detail, the evidence underlying the treatment recommendations of Part A. Section IV provides an overview of DSM-IV criteria, prevalence rates for major depressive disorder, and general information on its natural history and course. Section V is a structured review and synthesis of published literature regarding the available treatments for major depressive disorder.

Part C, "Future Research Needs," draws from the previous sections to summarize those areas in which better research data are needed to guide clinical decisions.

To share feedback on this or other published APA practice guidelines, a form is available at http://www.psych.org/psych_pract/pg/reviewform.cfm.

DEVELOPMENT PROCESS

This document is a practical guide to the management of major depressive disorder for adults over the age of 18 and represents a synthesis of current scientific knowledge and rational clinical practice. This guideline strives to be as free as possible of bias toward any theoretical posture, and it aims to represent a practical approach to treatment. Studies were identified through an extensive review of the literature by using MEDLARS for the period 1971–1999. The key words used were affective disorder, major depression, depressive disorder, seasonal affective disorder, melancholia, unipolar depression, endogenous depression, dysthymic disorder, dysthymia, postpartum depression, pseudodementia, antidepressant medications, tricyclic antidepressive agents, monoamine oxidase inhibitors, lithium, and electroconvulsive therapy and included the concepts of melancholia, neurotic depression, and major depression. In addition, the key words for the psychotherapy search were psychotherapy (not otherwise specified); behavior therapy, including aversive therapy, biofeedback (psychology), cognitive therapy, desensitization (psychologic), implosive therapy, and relaxation techniques (meditation); psychoanalytic therapy, including existentialism, free association, transactional analysis, psychotherapy (brief); and psychotherapy (group), including family therapy and marital therapy.

Major review articles and standard psychiatric texts were consulted. The Agency for Healthcare Policy Research *Evidence Report on Treatment of Depression—Newer Pharmacotherapies* (1) was reviewed in its entirety. Review articles and relevant clinical trials were reviewed in their entirety; other studies were selected for review on the basis of their relevance to the particular issues discussed in this guideline. Definitive standards are difficult to achieve, except in narrow circumstances in which multiple replicated studies and wide clinical opinion dictate certain forms of treatment. In other areas, the specific choice among two or more treatment options is left to the clinical judgment of the clinician.

The recommendations are based on the best available data and clinical consensus with regard to the particular clinical decision. The summary of treatment recommendations is keyed according to the level of confidence with which each recommendation is made. In addition, each reference is followed by a letter code in brackets that indicates the nature of the supporting evidence.

INTRODUCTION

This guideline seeks to summarize the specific forms of somatic, psychotherapeutic, psychosocial, and educational treatments that have been developed to deal with major depressive disorder. It begins at the point where the psychiatrist has diagnosed an adult patient as suffering from major depressive disorder, according to the criteria defined in DSM-IV, and has medically evaluated the patient to ascertain the presence of alcohol or substance use disorder or other somatic factors that may contribute to the disease process (e.g., hypothyroidism, pancreatic carcinoma) or complicate its treatment (e.g., cardiac disorders). The purpose of this guideline is to assist the physician faced with the task of implementing specific antidepressant treatment(s). It should be noted that many patients have coexisting conditions and their difficulties cannot be described with one DSM diagnostic category. The psychiatrist should consider, but not be limited to, the treatment guidelines for a single diagnosis. For patients found to have depressive symptoms within the context of bipolar disorder, the psychiatrist should refer to the *Practice Guideline for the Treatment of Patients With Bipolar Disorder* (2) (included in this volume).

This document concerns patients 18 years of age and older. Some comments regarding the treatment of major depressive disorders in children and adolescents can be found in Section III.B.5., along with more definitive references.

PART A:
TREATMENT RECOMMENDATIONS FOR PATIENTS WITH MAJOR DEPRESSIVE DISORDER

I. SUMMARY OF TREATMENT RECOMMENDATIONS

Each recommendation is identified as falling into one of three categories of endorsement, indicated by a bracketed Roman numeral following the statement. The three categories represent varying levels of clinical confidence regarding the recommendation:

[I] Recommended with substantial clinical confidence.
[II] Recommended with moderate clinical confidence.
[III] May be recommended on the basis of individual circumstances.

Successful treatment of patients with major depressive disorder is promoted by a thorough assessment of the patient [I]. Treatment consists of an acute phase, during which remission is induced; a continuation phase, during which remission is preserved; and a maintenance phase, during which the susceptible patient is protected against the recurrence of subsequent major depressive episodes. Psychiatrists initiating treatment for major depressive disorder have at their disposal a number of medications, a variety of psychotherapeutic approaches, electroconvulsive therapy (ECT), and other treatment modalities (e.g., light therapy) that may be used alone or in combination. The psychiatrist must determine the setting that will most likely ensure the patient's safety as well as promote improvement in the patient's condition [I].

A. PSYCHIATRIC MANAGEMENT

Psychiatric management consists of a broad array of interventions and activities that should be instituted by psychiatrists for all patients with major depressive disorder [I]. Regardless of the specific treatment modalities selected, it is important to continue providing psychiatric management through all phases of treatment. The specific components of psychiatric management that must be addressed for all patients include performing a diagnostic evaluation, evaluating safety of the patient and others, evaluating the level of functional impairments, determining a treatment setting, establishing and maintaining a therapeutic alliance, monitoring the patient's psychiatric status and safety, providing education to patients and families, enhancing treatment adherence, and working with patients to address early signs of relapse.

B. ACUTE PHASE

1. Choice of an initial treatment modality

In the acute phase, in addition to psychiatric management, the psychiatrist may choose between several initial treatment modalities, including pharmacotherapy, psychotherapy, the combination of medications plus psychotherapy, or ECT [I]. Selection of an initial treatment modality should be influenced by both clinical (e.g., severity of symptoms) and other factors (e.g., patient preference) (Figure 1).

a) Antidepressant medications

If preferred by the patient, antidepressant medications may be provided as an initial primary treatment modality for mild major depressive disorder [I]. Antidepressant medications should be provided for moderate to severe major depressive disorder unless ECT is planned [I]. A combination of antipsychotic and antidepressant medications or ECT should be used for psychotic depression [I].

b) Psychotherapy

A specific, effective psychotherapy alone as an initial treatment modality may be considered for patients with mild to moderate major depressive disorder [II]. Patient preference for psychotherapeutic approaches is an important factor that should be considered in the decision. Clinical features that may suggest the use of psychotherapeutic interventions include the presence of significant psychosocial stressors, intrapsychic conflict, interpersonal difficulties, or a comorbid axis II disorder [I].

c) Psychotherapy plus antidepressant medications

The combination of a specific effective psychotherapy and medication may be a useful initial treatment choice for patients with psychosocial issues, interpersonal problems, or a comorbid axis II disorder together with moderate to severe major depressive disorder [I]. In addition, patients who have had a history of only partial response to adequate trials of single treatment modalities may benefit from combined treatment. Poor adherence with treatments may also warrant combined treatment modalities.

d) Electroconvulsive therapy

ECT should be considered for patients with major depressive disorder with a high degree of symptom severity and functional impairment or for cases in which psychotic symptoms or catatonia are present [I]. ECT may also be the treatment modality of choice for patients in whom there is an urgent need for response, such as patients who are suicidal or refusing food and nutritionally compromised [II].

2. Choice of specific pharmacologic treatment

Antidepressant medications that have been shown to be effective are listed in Table 1 [II]. The effectiveness of antidepressant medications is generally comparable between classes and within classes of medications. Therefore, the initial selection of an antidepressant medication will largely be based on the anticipated side effects, the safety or tolerability of these side effects for individual patients, patient preference, quantity and quality of clinical trial data regarding the medication, and its cost (see Section V.A.1) [I]. On the basis of these considerations, the following medications are likely to be optimal for most patients: selective serotonin reuptake inhibitors (SSRIs), desipramine, nortriptyline, bupropion, and venlafaxine. In general, monoamine oxidase inhibitors (MAOIs) should be restricted to patients who do not respond to other treatments because of their potential for serious side effects and the necessity of dietary restrictions. Patients with major depressive disorder with atypical features are one group for whom several studies sug-

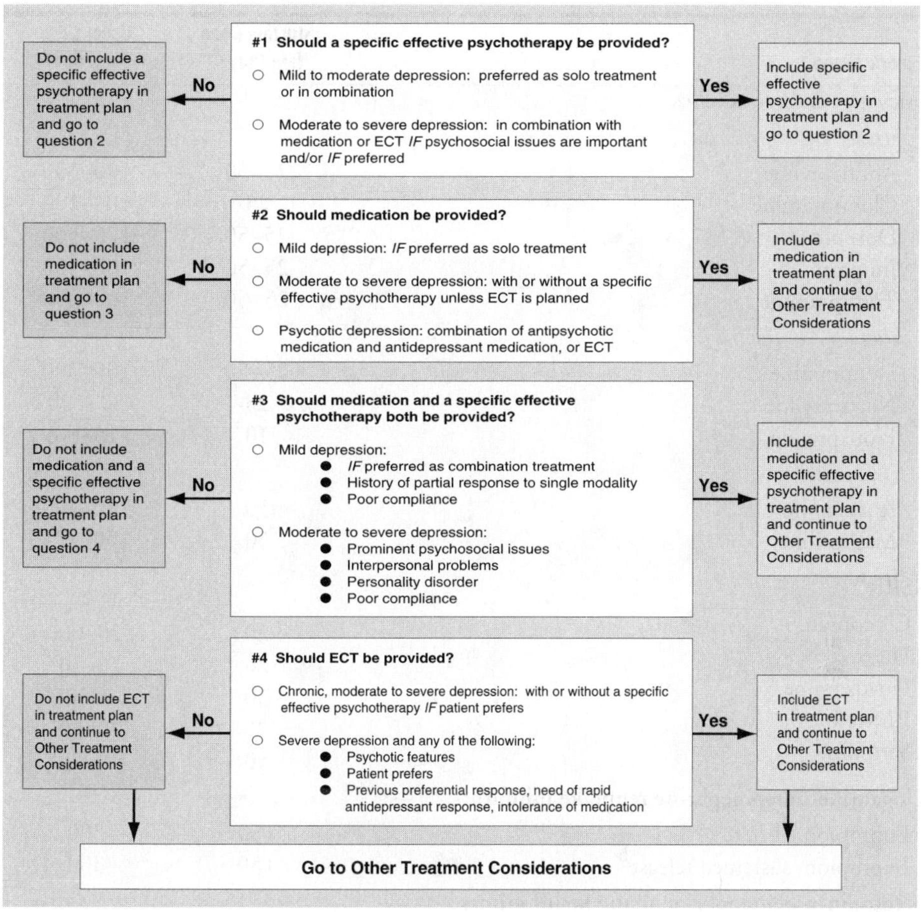

FIGURE 1. Choice of Treatment Modalities for Major Depressive Disorder.

gest MAOIs may be particularly effective; however, in clinical practice, many psychiatrists start with SSRIs in such patients because of the more favorable adverse effect profile.

a) Implementation

When pharmacotherapy is part of the treatment plan, it must be integrated with the psychiatric management and any other treatments that are being provided (e.g., psychotherapy) [I]. Once an antidepressant medication has been selected, it can be started at the dose levels suggested in Table 1 [I]. Titration to full therapeutic doses generally can be accomplished over the initial week(s) of treatment but may vary depending on the development of side effects, the patient's age, and the presence of comorbid illnesses. Patients who have started taking an antidepressant medication should be carefully monitored to assess their response to pharmacotherapy as well as the emergence of side effects, clinical condition, and safety [I] (see Figure 2). Factors to consider in determining the frequency of patient monitoring include the severity of illness, the patient's cooperation with treatment, the availability of social supports, and the presence of comorbid general medical problems. Visits should also be frequent enough to monitor and address suicidality and to promote treatment adherence. In practice, the frequency of monitoring during the acute phase of pharmacotherapy can vary from once a week in routine cases to multiple times per week in more complex cases.

TABLE 1. Commonly Used Antidepressant Medications (this list is representative, but not comprehensive)

Generic Name	Starting Dose (mg/day)[a]	Usual Dose (mg/day)
Tricyclics and tetracyclics		
Tertiary amine tricyclics		
Amitriptyline	25–50	100–300
Clomipramine	25	100–250
Doxepin	25–50	100–300
Imipramine	25–50	100–300
Trimipramine	25–50	100–300
Secondary amine tricyclics		
Desipramine[b]	25–50	100–300
Nortriptyline[b]	25	50–200
Protriptyline	10	15–60
Tetracyclics		
Amoxapine	50	100–400
Maprotiline	50	100–225
SSRIs[b]		
Citalopram	20	20–60[c]
Fluoxetine	20	20–60[c]
Fluvoxamine	50	50–300[c]
Paroxetine	20	20–60[c]
Sertraline	50	50–200[c]
Dopamine-norepinephrine reuptake inhibitors		
Bupropion[b]	150	300
Bupropion, sustained release[b]	150	300
Serotonin-norepinephrine reuptake inhibitors		
Venlafaxine[b]	37.5	75–225
Venlafaxine, extended release[b]	37.5	75–225
Serotonin modulators		
Nefazodone	50	150–300
Trazodone	50	75–300
Norepinephrine-serotonin modulator		
Mirtazapine	15	15–45
MAOIs		
Irreversible, nonselective		
Phenelzine	15	15–90
Tranylcypromine	10	30–60
Reversible MAOI-A		
Moclobemide	150	300–600
Selective noradrenaline reuptake inhibitor		
Reboxetine	—[d]	—[d]

[a]Lower starting doses are recommended for elderly patients and for patients with panic disorder, significant anxiety or hepatic disease, and general comorbidity.

[b]These medications are likely to be optimal medications in terms of the patient's acceptance of side effects, safety, and quantity and quality of clinical trial data.

[c]Dose varies with diagnosis; see text for specific guidelines.

[d]FDA approval is anticipated. When available, consult manufacturer's package insert or the Physician's Desk Reference for recommended starting and usual doses.

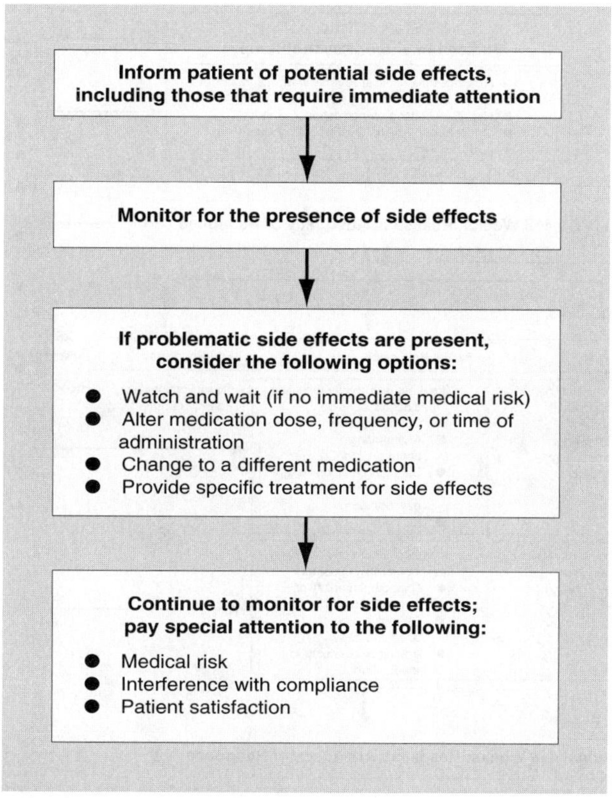

FIGURE 2. Management of Medication Side Effects.

b) Failure to respond

If at least moderate improvement is not observed following 6–8 weeks of pharmacotherapy, a reappraisal of the treatment regimen should be conducted [I]. Section II.B.2.b reviews options for adjusting the treatment regimen when necessary. Following any change in treatment, the patient should continue to be closely monitored. If there is not at least a moderate improvement in major depressive disorder symptoms after an additional 6–8 weeks of treatment, the psychiatrist should conduct another thorough review. An algorithm depicting the sequence of subsequent steps that can be taken for patients who fail to respond fully to treatment is provided in Figure 3.

3. Choice of specific psychotherapy

Cognitive behavioral therapy and interpersonal therapy are the psychotherapeutic approaches that have the best documented efficacy in the literature for the specific treatment of major depressive disorder, although rigorous studies evaluating the efficacy of psychodynamic psychotherapy have not been published [II]. When psychodynamic psychotherapy is used as a specific treatment, in addition to symptom relief, it is frequently associated with broader long-term goals. Patient preference and the availability of clinicians with appropriate training and expertise in the specific approach are also factors in the choice of a particular form of psychotherapy.

a) Implementation

When psychotherapy is part of the treatment plan, it must be integrated with the psychiatric management and any other treatments that are being provided (e.g., medication treatment) [I].

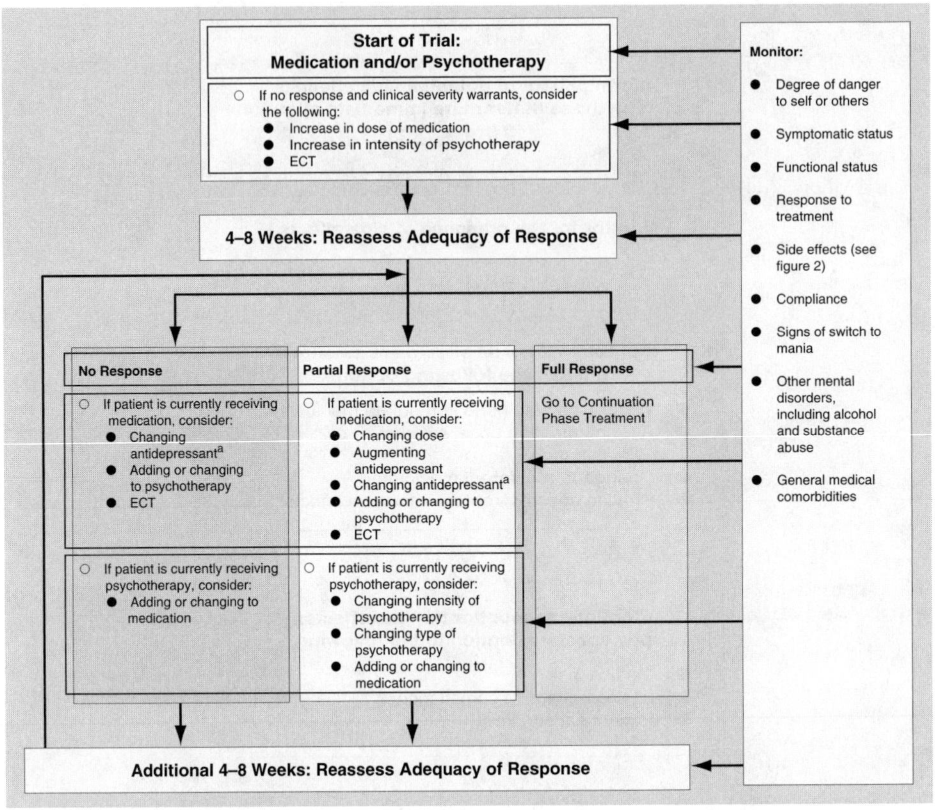

FIGURE 3. Acute Phase Treatment of Major Depressive Disorder.

[a]Choose either another antidepressant from the same class or, if two previous medication trials from the same class were ineffective, an antidepressant from a different class.

The optimal frequency of psychotherapy has not been rigorously studied in controlled trials. The psychiatrist should take into account multiple factors when determining the frequency for individual patients, including the specific type and goals of psychotherapy, the frequency necessary to create and maintain a therapeutic relationship, the frequency of visits required to ensure treatment adherence, and the frequency necessary to monitor and address suicidality. The frequency of outpatient visits during the acute phase generally varies from once a week in routine cases to as often as several times a week.

Regardless of the type of psychotherapy selected, the patient's response to treatment should be carefully monitored [I].

If more than one clinician is involved in providing the care, it is essential that all treating clinicians have sufficient ongoing contact with the patient and with each other to ensure that relevant information is available to guide treatment decisions [I].

b) Failure to respond

If after 4–8 weeks of treatment at least a moderate improvement is not observed, then a thorough review and reappraisal of the diagnosis, complicating conditions and issues, and treatment plan should be conducted [I]. Figure 3 and Section II.B.3.b review the options to consider.

TABLE 2. Considerations in the Decision to Use Maintenance Treatment

Factor	Component
Risk of recurrence	Number of prior episodes; presence of comorbid conditions; residual symptoms between episodes
Severity of episodes	Suicidality; psychotic features; severe functional impairments
Side effects experienced with continuous treatment	
Patient preferences	

4. Choice of medications plus psychotherapy

In general, the same issues that influence the specific choice of medication or psychotherapy when used alone should be considered when choosing treatments for patients receiving combined modalities [I].

5. Assessing the adequacy of response

It is not uncommon for patients to have a substantial but incomplete response in terms of symptom reduction or improvement in functioning during acute phase treatments. It is important not to conclude the acute phase of treatment for such patients, as a partial response is often associated with poor functional outcomes. When patients are found to have not fully responded to an acute phase treatment, a change in treatment should be considered as outlined in Figure 3 [II].

C. CONTINUATION PHASE

During the 16–20 weeks following remission, patients who have been treated with antidepressant medications in the acute phase should be maintained on these agents to prevent relapse [I]. In general, the dose used in the acute phase is also used in the continuation phase. Although there has been less study of the use of psychotherapy in the continuation phase to prevent relapse, there is growing evidence to support the use of a specific effective psychotherapy during the continuation phase [I]. Use of ECT in the continuation phase has received little formal study but may be useful in patients for whom medication or psychotherapy has not been effective in maintaining stability during the continuation phase [II]. The frequency of visits must be determined by the patient's clinical condition as well as the specific treatments being provided.

D. MAINTENANCE PHASE

Following the continuation phase, maintenance phase treatment should be considered for patients to prevent recurrences of major depressive disorder [I]. Factors to consider are discussed in Table 2 and in Section II.D.

In general, the treatment that was effective in the acute and continuation phases should be used in the maintenance phase [II]. In general, the same full antidepressant medication doses are employed as were used in prior phases of treatment; use of lower doses of antidepressant medication in the maintenance phase has not been well studied. For cognitive behavioral therapy and interpersonal therapy, maintenance phase treatments usually involve a decreased frequency of visits (e.g., once a month).

TABLE 3. Risk Factors for Recurrence of Major Depressive Disorder

- Prior history of multiple episodes of major depressive disorder
- Persistence of dysthymic symptoms after recovery from an episode of major depressive disorder
- Presence of an additional nonaffective psychiatric diagnosis
- Presence of a chronic general medical disorder

The frequency of visits in the maintenance phase must be determined by the patient's clinical condition as well as the specific treatments being provided. The frequency required could range from as low as once every 2–3 months for stable patients who require only psychiatric management and medication monitoring to as high as multiple times a week for those in whom psychodynamic psychotherapy is being conducted.

E. DISCONTINUATION OF ACTIVE TREATMENT

The decision to discontinue active treatment should be based on the same factors considered in the decision to initiate maintenance treatment, including the probability of recurrence, the frequency and severity of past episodes, the persistence of dysthymic symptoms after recovery, the presence of comorbid disorders, and patient preferences [I]. In addition to the factors listed in Table 2 and Table 3, patients and their psychiatrists should consider patient response, in terms of both beneficial and adverse effects, to maintenance treatments.

Specific clinical features that will influence the general treatment are discussed in Section III.

II. FORMULATION AND IMPLEMENTATION OF A TREATMENT PLAN

The following discussion regarding formulation and implementation of a treatment plan refers specifically to patients with major depressive disorder. For the treatment of patients found to have depressive symptoms within the context of bipolar disorder, readers should refer to the *Practice Guideline for the Treatment of Patients With Bipolar Disorder* (2) (included in this volume). The treatment recommendations that follow may have some relevance for patients who have depressive symptoms on the basis of other syndromes, such as dysthymia, although this cannot be fully established with the existing scientific literature.

The successful treatment of patients with major depressive disorders is promoted by an initial thorough assessment of the patient. Treatment then consists of an acute phase lasting a minimum of 6–8 weeks, during which remission is induced. Remission is defined as a return to the patient's baseline level of symptom severity and functioning and should not be confused with substantial but incomplete improvement. After achieving remission, the patient enters the continuation phase, which usually lasts 16–20 weeks, during which time the remission is preserved and relapse is prevented. Relapse is generally defined as the reemergence of significant depressive symptoms or dysfunction following a remission. Patients who successfully complete the continuation phase without relapse then enter the maintenance phase of treatment. The goal during the maintenance phase is to protect susceptible patients against recurrence of subsequent major depressive episodes; the duration of the maintenance phase will vary depending on the frequency and severity of prior major depressive episodes.

Psychiatrists initiating treatment of an episode of major depressive disorder have at their disposal a number of medications, a variety of psychotherapeutic approaches, ECT, and other treatment modalities (e.g., light therapy). These various interventions may be used alone or in combination. The psychiatrist must determine the setting that will most likely ensure the patient's safety as well as promote improvement in the patient's condition.

A. PSYCHIATRIC MANAGEMENT

Psychiatric management consists of a broad array of interventions and activities that should be instituted by psychiatrists for all patients with major depressive disorder. The specific components of psychiatric management that must be addressed for all patients are described in more detail below.

1. Perform a diagnostic evaluation

Patients with major depressive disorder symptoms should receive a thorough diagnostic evaluation both to determine whether a diagnosis of depression is warranted and to reveal the presence of other psychiatric or general medical conditions. The general principles and components of a complete psychiatric evaluation have been outlined in the American Psychiatric Association's *Practice Guideline for Psychiatric Evaluation of Adults* (3) (included in this volume). These should include a history of the present illness and current symptoms; a psychiatric history, including symptoms of mania as well as a treatment history that particularly notes current treatments and responses to previous treatments; a general medical history and history of substance use disorders; a personal history (e.g., psychological development, response to life transitions, and major life events); a social, occupational, and family history; a review of the patient's medications; a review of systems; a mental status examination; a physical examination; and diagnostic tests as indicated.

2. Evaluate the safety of patient and others

A careful assessment of the patient's risk for suicide is crucial. Some components of an evaluation for suicide risk are summarized in Table 4. An assessment of the presence of suicidal ideation is essential, including the degree to which the patient intends to act on any suicidal ideation and the extent to which the patient has made plans for or begun to prepare for suicide. The availability of means for suicide should be inquired about and a judgment made concerning the lethality of those means. Clinical factors that may increase the likelihood of a patient acting on suicidal ideation should be assessed, including the presence of psychotic symptoms, severe anxiety, panic attacks, and alcohol or substance use. Whether a patient has a history of making suicide attempts and the nature of those attempts should be evaluated. Patients should also be asked about suicide in their family history and recent exposure to suicide or suicide attempts by others. A complete assessment of suicide risk should be individualized to the particular circumstances of the patient and include an evaluation of the patient's strengths and motivation to seek help. Patients who are found to possess suicidal or homicidal ideation, intention, or plans require close monitoring. Measures such as hospitalization (involuntary when indicated) should be considered for those at significant risk. However, it should be kept in mind that the ability to predict suicide attempts and completed suicide is poor, with both many false positives (i.e., patients who appear more likely to make attempts or complete suicide but who do not) and false negatives (i.e., patients who appear less likely to make attempts or complete suicide but who do). For this reason, despite the best efforts of the psychiatrist, some patients may engage in self-harm or harm toward others.

TABLE 4. Components of an Evaluation for Suicide Risk

- Presence of suicidal or homicidal ideation, intent, or plans
- Access to means for suicide and the lethality of those means
- Presence of psychotic symptoms, command hallucinations, or severe anxiety
- Presence of alcohol or substance use
- History and seriousness of previous attempts
- Family history of or recent exposure to suicide

3. Evaluate functional impairments

Major depressive disorder is frequently associated with functional impairments, and the presence, type(s), and severity of dysfunction should be evaluated. Impairments can include deficits in interpersonal relationships, work, living conditions, and other medical or health-related needs. Identified impairments in functioning should be addressed; for example, some patients may require assistance in scheduling absences from work or other responsibilities, whereas others may require encouragement to not make any major life changes while in a major depressive disorder state. Patients should also be encouraged to set realistic, attainable goals for themselves in terms of desirable levels of functioning.

4. Determine a treatment setting

Treatment settings for patients with major depressive disorder include a continuum of possible levels of care, from involuntary hospitalizations to day programs to ambulatory settings. In general, patients should be treated in the setting that is most likely to prove safe and effective. The psychiatrist should choose an appropriate site of treatment after evaluating the patient's clinical condition, including symptom severity, comorbidity, suicidality, homicidality, level of functioning, and available support system. The determination of a treatment setting should also include consideration of patients' ability to adequately care for themselves, provide reliable feedback to the psychiatrist, and cooperate with treatment of their major depressive disorder.

Patients who exhibit suicidal or homicidal ideation, intention, or a plan require close monitoring. Hospitalization is usually indicated for patients who are considered to pose a serious threat of harm to themselves or others. If patients refuse, they can be hospitalized involuntarily if their condition meets criteria for involuntary admission of the local jurisdiction. Severely ill patients who lack adequate social support outside of a hospital setting should be considered for admission to a hospital or intensive day program. Additionally, those patients who also have complicating psychiatric or general medical conditions or who have not responded adequately to outpatient treatment may need to be hospitalized.

The optimal treatment setting and the patient's ability to benefit from a different level of care should be reevaluated on an ongoing basis throughout the course of treatment.

5. Establish and maintain a therapeutic alliance

Regardless of the treatment modalities ultimately selected for patients, it is important for the psychiatrist to establish a therapeutic alliance with the patient. Major depressive disorder is often a chronic condition that requires patients to actively participate and adhere to treatment plans for long periods. Unfortunately, features of major depressive disorder may include poor motivation, pessimism over the effectiveness of treatments, decrements in cognition such as attention or memory, decreased self-care, and possibly intentional self-harm. In addition, successful treatment may require patients to tolerate side effects. For these reasons, a strong treatment alliance between patient and psychiatrist is crucial. To establish and maintain a therapeutic alliance with patients, it is important for psychiatrists to pay attention to the concerns of patients and their families as well as their wishes for treatment. Management of the therapeutic alliance should include awareness of transference and countertransference issues, even if these are not directly addressed in treatment.

6. Monitor the patient's psychiatric status and safety

As treatment progresses, different features and symptoms of the patient's illness may emerge or subside. Monitoring the patient's status for the emergence of changes in destructive impulses toward self or others is especially crucial; additional measures such as hospitalization or more intensive treatment should be considered for patients found to be at higher risk. The psychiatrist should be vigilant to changes in the patient's psychiatric status, including major depressive disorder symptoms as well as symptoms of other potential comorbid conditions. Significant changes in a patient's psychiatric status or the emergence of new symptoms may warrant a diagnostic reevaluation of the patient.

7. Provide education to the patient and, when appropriate, to the family

Education concerning major depressive disorder and its treatments should be provided to all patients. When appropriate, education should also be provided to involved family members. Specific educational elements may be especially helpful in some circumstances; for example, emphasizing that major depressive disorder is a real illness and that effective treatments are both necessary and available may be crucial for patients who attribute their illness to a moral defect or for family members who are convinced that there is nothing wrong with the patient. Education regarding available treatment options will help patients make informed decisions, anticipate side effects, and adhere to treatments.

8. Enhance treatment adherence

The successful treatment of major depressive disorder requires close adherence to treatment plans, in some cases for long or indefinite durations. Especially while symptomatic, patients with major depressive disorder may be poorly motivated, unduly pessimistic over their chances of recovery with treatment, suffering from deficits in memory, or taking less care of themselves. In addition, the side effects or requirements of treatments may lead to nonadherence. Particularly during the maintenance phase, euthymic patients may tend to undervalue the benefits of treatment and focus on the burdens of treatment. Psychiatrists should recognize these possibilities, encourage the patient to articulate any concerns regarding adherence, and emphasize the importance of adherence for successful treatment. Specific components of a message to patients that have been shown to improve adherence include emphasizing: 1) when and how often to take the medicine; 2) the need for at least 2–4 weeks before beneficial effects may be noticed; 3) the need to take medication even after feeling better; 4) the need to consult with the doctor before discontinuing medication; and 5) what to do if problems or questions arise (4). Some patients, particularly elderly patients, have been shown to have improved adherence when both the complexity of medication regimens and the costs of treatments are minimized. Severe or persistent problems of nonadherence may represent psychological conflicts or psychopathology for which psychotherapy should be considered. When family members are involved, they can also be encouraged to play a helpful role in improving adherence.

9. Work with the patient to address early signs of relapse

Given the chronic, episodic nature of major depressive disorder, exacerbations are common. Patients, as well as their families if appropriate, should be instructed about the significant risk of relapse. They should be educated to identify early signs and symptoms of new episodes. Patients should also be instructed to seek adequate treatment as early in the course of the new episode as possible to decrease the likelihood of a full-blown exacerbation or complications.

B. ACUTE PHASE

1. Choice of initial treatment modality

In the acute phase, in addition to psychiatric management, the psychiatrist may choose between several initial treatment modalities, including pharmacotherapy, psychotherapy, the combination of medications and psychotherapy, or ECT. A discussion of the potential role of other treatments (e.g., light therapy and St. John's wort) can be found in Section V. Selection of an initial treatment modality should be influenced by both clinical (e.g., severity of symptoms) and other factors (e.g., patient preference) (Figure 1).

a) Antidepressant medications

When pharmacotherapy is part of the treatment plan, it must be integrated with the psychiatric management and any other treatments that are being provided (e.g., psychotherapy). Antidepressant medications can be used as an initial treatment modality by patients with mild, moderate, or severe major depressive disorder. Clinical features that may suggest that medications are the preferred treatment modality include history of prior positive response to antidepressant medications, severity of symptoms, significant sleep and appetite disturbances or agitation, or anticipation of the need for maintenance therapy. Other issues that may be important considerations in the decision to use antidepressant medication include patient preference or the lack of available adequate alternative treatment modalities. Patients with major depressive disorder with psychotic features require either the combined use of antidepressant and antipsychotic medications or ECT.

b) Psychotherapy

A specific, effective psychotherapy alone may be considered as an initial treatment modality for patients with mild to moderate major depressive disorder. Clinical features that may suggest the use of a specific psychotherapy include the presence of significant psychosocial stressors, intrapsychic conflict, interpersonal difficulties, or axis II comorbidity. Patient preference for psychotherapeutic approaches is an important factor that should be considered in the decision to use psychotherapy as the initial treatment modality. Pregnancy, lactation, or the wish to become pregnant may also be an indication for psychotherapy as an initial treatment.

c) Psychotherapy plus antidepressant medications

The combination of a specific effective psychotherapy and medication may be a useful initial treatment choice for patients with psychosocial issues, intrapsychic conflict, interpersonal problems, or a comorbid axis II disorder together with moderate to severe major depressive disorder. In addition, patients who have had a history of only partial response to adequate trials of single treatment modalities may benefit from combined treatment. Poor adherence with treatments may also warrant combined treatment with pharmacotherapy and psychotherapeutic approaches that focus on treatment adherence.

d) Electroconvulsive therapy

ECT should be considered for patients with major depressive disorder with a high degree of symptom severity and functional impairment as well as in cases in which psychotic symptoms or catatonia are present. ECT may also be the treatment modality of choice for patients in whom there is an urgent need for response, such as patients who are suicidal or who are refusing food and are nutritionally compromised. The presence of comorbid general medical conditions that preclude the use of antidepressant medications, a prior history of positive response to ECT, and patient preference are other important considerations that may influence the psychiatrist's decision to select ECT as a treatment modality.

TABLE 5. Factors to Consider in Choosing a First-Line Antidepressant Medication

- Anticipated side effects and their safety or tolerability
- History of prior response in patient or family member
- Patient preference
- Cost
- Quantity and quality of clinical trial data
- MAOIs: generally reserve for patients who do not respond to other treatments
- SSRIs or MAOIs: consider for patients with atypical symptoms

2. Choice of specific pharmacologic treatment

Antidepressant medications that have been shown to be effective are listed in Table 1. The effectiveness of antidepressant medications is generally comparable between classes and within classes of medications. Therefore, the initial selection of an antidepressant medication will largely be based on the anticipated side effects, the safety or tolerability of these side effects for individual patients, patient preference, quantity and quality of clinical trial data regarding the medication, and its cost (Table 5). On the basis of these considerations, the following medications are likely to be optimal agents for most patients: SSRIs, desipramine, nortriptyline, bupropion, and venlafaxine. Additional considerations that may influence the choice of antidepressant medication include a history of prior response to a medication and the presence of comorbid psychiatric or general medical conditions. For example, secondary amine tricyclic antidepressant medications may not be optimal in patients with cardiovascular conditions, cardiac conduction defects, closed-angle glaucoma, urinary retention, or significant prostatic hypertrophy. SSRIs can carry a risk of sexual side effects and may be more expensive because of the lack of currently available generic preparations. Similarly, the specific side effect profiles and higher costs should be considerations in decisions regarding use of other newer antidepressant medications. In general, MAOIs should be restricted to patients who do not respond to other treatments because of their potential for serious side effects and the necessity of dietary restrictions. Patients with major depressive disorder with atypical features are one group for whom several studies suggest MAOIs may be particularly effective; however, in clinical practice, many psychiatrists start with SSRIs in such patients because of the more favorable adverse effect profile.

a) Implementation of pharmacotherapy

Once an antidepressant medication has been selected it can be started at doses suggested in Table 1. Titration of the dose to full therapeutic doses generally can be accomplished over the initial week(s) of treatment but may vary depending on the development of side effects, the patient's age, and the presence of comorbid conditions. In elderly or medically frail patients, the starting and therapeutic doses should be reduced, generally to half of the usual adult doses.

Patients who have started taking an antidepressant medication should be carefully monitored to assess the response to pharmacotherapy as well as the emergence of side effects, clinical condition, and safety (see Figure 2). There are limited clinical trial data to guide the decision regarding the frequency of monitoring patients during pharmacotherapy. Factors to consider when determining this frequency include the severity of illness, the patient's cooperation with treatment, the availability of social supports, and the presence of comorbid general medical problems. Visits should also be frequent enough to monitor and address suicidality and to promote treatment adherence. Experienced researchers have found that patients in clinical trials appear to benefit from monitoring once a week or more to enhance adherence rates and to avoid the demoralization that may occur before the onset of beneficial effects. In clinical practice, the frequency of monitoring during the acute phase of pharmacotherapy may vary from once a week in routine cases to multiple times per week in more complex cases. The method of monitoring may vary depending upon the clinical context (e.g., face-to-face visits, telephone contact, or contact with another clinician knowledgeable about the patient and the treatment modality).

TABLE 6. Required Washout Times Between Antidepressant Trials

Antidepressant Change	Minimum Washout Period
To MAOI from drug with long-half-life metabolites (e.g., fluoxetine)	5 weeks
To MAOI from drug without long-half-life metabolites (e.g., tricyclic antidepressant, paroxetine, fluvoxamine, venlafaxine) or other MAOI	2 weeks
To non-MAOI antidepressant from MAOI	2 weeks

Improvement with pharmacotherapy can be observed after 4–8 weeks of treatment. If at least a moderate improvement is not observed in this time period, reappraisal and adjustment of the pharmacotherapy should be considered.

b) Failure to respond

If at least moderate improvement is not observed following 4–8 weeks of pharmacotherapy, a reappraisal of the treatment regimen should be conducted. An algorithm depicting the sequence of subsequent steps that can be taken and possible outcomes for patients who do not respond fully to treatment is provided in Figure 3. It is important to keep in mind when employing such algorithms that they are based largely on clinical experience and only limited clinical trial data.

First, patient adherence and pharmacokinetic/pharmacodynamic factors affecting treatment should be investigated, in some cases through determination of serum antidepressant medication levels. Following this review, the treatment plan can be revised by implementing one of several therapeutic options, including maximizing the initial medication treatment, switching to another non-MAOI antidepressant medication (Table 1 and Table 6), augmenting antidepressant medications with other agents or psychotherapy, using an MAOI, or ECT (5).

Maximizing the initial treatment regimen is perhaps the most conservative strategy. For patients who have shown a partial response, particularly those with features of personality disorders, extending the antidepressant medication trial (e.g., by 2–4 weeks) may allow some patients to respond more fully (6). Use of higher antidepressant doses may be helpful for patients who have received only modest doses or for those who for pharmacodynamic reasons have low serum drug levels despite usual doses and adherence. Patients who have had their dose increased should be monitored for an increase in the severity of side effects.

Switching to a different non-MAOI antidepressant medication is a common strategy for treatment-refractory patients, especially those who have not shown at least partial response to the initial medication regimen. Patients can be switched to a non-MAOI antidepressant medication from the same pharmacologic class (e.g., from an SSRI to another SSRI) or to one from a different pharmacologic class (e.g., from an SSRI to a tricyclic antidepressant) (see Table 1 and Table 6) (5).

Augmentation of non-MAOI antidepressant medications may be helpful, particularly for patients who have had a partial response to antidepressant monotherapy. Options include adding a second non-MAOI antidepressant medication from a different pharmacologic class, taking care to avoid drug-drug interactions, or adding another adjunctive medication such as lithium, thyroid hormone, an anticonvulsant, or psychostimulants.

Adding, changing, or increasing the intensity of psychotherapy should be considered for patients with major depressive disorder who do not respond to medication treatment. Additional strategies for patients who do not respond adequately to treatment include switching to an MAOI after allowing sufficient time between medications to avoid hazardous interactions. ECT also remains perhaps the most effective therapy for treatment-resistant patients.

Following any change in treatment, the patient should continue to be closely monitored. If there is not at least a moderate improvement in major depressive disorder symptoms after an additional 4–8 weeks of treatment, the psychiatrist should conduct another thorough review. This reappraisal should include the following: verifying the patient's diagnosis and adherence; uncovering and addressing clinical factors that may be preventing improvement, such as the presence of comorbid general medical conditions or psychiatric conditions (e.g., alcohol or substance abuse); and uncovering and addressing psychosocial issues that may be impeding recovery. If no new information is uncovered to explain the patient's lack of adequate response, other treatment options should be considered, including obtaining a consultation and possibly ECT.

3. Choice of a specific psychotherapy

Cognitive behavioral therapy and interpersonal therapy have the best-documented effectiveness in the literature for the specific treatment of major depressive disorder. When psychodynamic psychotherapy is used as a specific treatment, in addition to symptom relief, it is frequently associated with broader long-term goals. Patient preference and the availability of clinicians with appropriate training and expertise in specific psychotherapeutic approaches are also factors in the choice of a particular form of psychotherapy. Other clinical factors influencing the type of psychotherapy employed are the stage and severity of the major depressive disorder episode. For example, although some data suggest that cognitive behavioral therapy alone may be effective for patients with moderate to severe major depressive disorder, most such patients will require medication. In general, the choice among psychotherapeutic approaches is dependent on patient preference, with particular regard to whether the goals are mainly symptomatic improvement versus broader psychosocial goals.

During the initial phases of treatment for patients with moderate to severe major depressive disorder, psychiatric management will have to include support and psychoeducation for the patient and the family, permission for the patient to excuse himself or herself from duties impossible to perform, and assistance regarding the making or postponing of major personal and business decisions. Some patients at this stage may not have the emotional energy or cognitive ability required for insight-oriented psychotherapy. If indicated, this may be initiated later in the course of recovery.

a) Implementation

When psychotherapy is part of the treatment plan, it must be integrated with the psychiatric management and any other treatments that are being provided (e.g., medication treatment). The optimal frequency of psychotherapy has not been rigorously studied in controlled trials. The psychiatrist should take into account multiple factors when determining the frequency for individual patients, including the specific type and goals of the psychotherapy, the frequency necessary to create and maintain a therapeutic relationship, the frequency of visits required to ensure treatment adherence, and the frequency necessary to monitor and address suicidality. Also affecting the frequency of psychotherapy visits are the severity of illness, the patient's cooperation with treatment, the availability of social supports, cost, geographic accessibility, and presence of comorbid general medical problems. The frequency of outpatient visits during the acute phase generally varies from once a week in routine cases to as often as several times a week. Transference-focused treatments tend to require more frequent and regular visits.

Regardless of the type of psychotherapy selected, the patient's response to treatment should be carefully monitored. If after 4–8 weeks of treatment at least a moderate improvement is not observed, then a thorough review and reappraisal of the treatment plan should be conducted.

There are no definitive studies to determine when it is preferable to have the psychiatrist provide all treatments (sometimes referred to as the "integrated" model) versus when it might be preferable to have a different clinician provide the psychotherapy, with the psychiatrist providing the psychiatric management and the medication (sometimes referred to as "split" treatment). The expertise of the psychiatrist in providing the desired type of psychotherapy and the preferences of the patient are frequently factors in the decision. The integrated treatment model provides for better coordination of care. Lower costs have been used as a rationale in support of the split-treatment model. However, it is not clear that the costs of that model are actually lower than for the integrated model (7).

If the split model is used, it is essential that the psychiatrist who is providing the psychiatric management and the medication treatment meets with the patient frequently enough to monitor his or her care. It is also essential that the two (or more) treating clinicians have sufficient ongoing contact to ensure that relevant information is available to guide treatment decisions.

b) Failure to respond

The patient's condition and response to therapeutic interventions should be carefully monitored from the outset of psychotherapy. If the patient's condition fails to stabilize or is deteriorating, reassessment is indicated (8). If after 4–8 weeks of treatment at least a moderate improvement is not observed, then a thorough review and reappraisal of the diagnosis, complicating conditions and issues, and treatment plan should be conducted. In many cases, the treatment plan can be revised by the addition or substitution of pharmacotherapy (see Figure 3). Following any revision or refinement of treatment, the patient should continue to be closely monitored. If there continues to not be at least a moderate improvement in major depressive disorder symptoms after an additional 4–8 weeks of treatment, another thorough review, reappraisal, and revision of the treatment plan should be conducted.

4. Choice of medications plus psychotherapy

There are relatively few empirical data from clinical trials to help guide the selection of particular antidepressant medications and psychotherapeutic approaches for individuals who will receive the combination of both modalities. In general, the same issues that influence these decisions when choosing a monotherapy will apply, and the same doses of antidepressant medication and the same frequency and course of psychotherapy should be used for patients receiving combination modality treatments as those employed for patients receiving them as a monotherapy.

Patients receiving combined antidepressant medication and psychotherapy should also be monitored closely for treatment effect, side effects, clinical condition, and safety. If after 4–8 weeks there is not at least a moderate improvement, a thorough review should be conducted, including of the patient's adherence and pharmacokinetic/pharmacodynamic factors affecting treatment. The treatment plan can be revised by using many of the same therapeutic options described for patients who have not responded to treatment with either modality alone. Following any change in treatment, the patient should continue to be monitored, and if there is not at least a moderate improvement in major depressive disorder symptoms after an additional 4–8 weeks of treatment, another thorough review should be conducted. Other treatment options should be considered, including clinical consultation or possibly ECT.

5. Assessing the adequacy of treatment response

The goal of acute phase treatment for major depressive disorder is to return patients to their baseline levels of symptomatic and functional status. However, it is not uncommon for patients to have a substantial but incomplete response in terms of symptom reduction or improvement in functioning during acute phase treatment. It is important not to conclude the acute phase of treatment for such patients, as a partial response is often associated with poor functional outcomes.

Identifying patients who have not had a complete response to treatment and formally assessing the extent to which patients have returned to their baseline may be aided by the use of structured measures of depression symptom severity and functional status. When patients are found to have not fully responded to an acute phase treatment, a change in treatment should be considered, as outlined in Figure 3.

C. CONTINUATION PHASE

During the 16–20 weeks following remission, patients who have been treated with antidepressant medications in the acute phase should be maintained with these agents to prevent relapse. In general, the dose used in the acute phase is also used in the continuation phase. Some psychiatrists combine a decrease in the dose with careful monitoring in the continuation phase; however, there are no data to support the effectiveness of this approach. Although there has been less study of the use of psychotherapy in the continuation phase to prevent relapse, there is growing evidence to support the use of a specific effective psychotherapy during the continuation phase. Use of ECT in the continuation phase has received little formal study. The frequency of visits must be determined by the patient's clinical condition as well as the specific treatments being provided.

During the continuation phase, the frequency of visits may vary. For stable patients in whom the visits are for the purpose of providing psychiatric management, the frequency could be once every 2–3 months. For other patients, such as those in whom active psychotherapy is being conducted, the frequency required may be as high as multiple times a week. If maintenance phase treatment is not indicated for patients who remain stable following the continuation phase, patients may be considered for discontinuation of treatment. If treatment is discontinued, patients should be carefully monitored for relapse, and treatment should be promptly reinstituted if relapse occurs.

D. MAINTENANCE PHASE

On average, 50%–85% of patients with a single episode of major depressive disorder will have at least one more episode. Therefore, following the continuation phase, maintenance phase treatment should be considered for patients to prevent recurrences of major depressive episodes. Factors that should be considered when deciding whether to use maintenance treatment are summarized in Table 2.

In general, the treatment that was effective in the acute and continuation phases should be used in the maintenance phase. In general, the same full antidepressant medication doses are employed as were used in prior phases of treatment; use of lower doses of antidepressant medication in the maintenance phase has not been well studied. For cognitive behavioral therapy and interpersonal therapy, maintenance phase treatments usually involve a decrease in frequency of visits (e.g., once a month). Psychodynamic psychotherapy usually continues at the same frequency in the effort to explore the role of axis II disorders or other psychological factors in predisposing to depressive episodes.

Although the effectiveness of combinations of antidepressant medication and psychotherapy in the maintenance phase has not been well studied, such combinations may be an option for some patients. Patients who exhibit repeated episodes of moderate or severe major depressive disorder despite optimal pharmacologic treatment or patients who are medically ineligible for such treatment may be maintained with periodic ECT. There has been little formal study of other treatment modalities in the maintenance phase.

Similar to the continuation phase, the frequency of visits may vary in the maintenance phase. The frequency required could range from as low as once every several months for stable patients who require only psychiatric management and medication monitoring to as high as once or twice per week for those in whom psychodynamic psychotherapy is being conducted. Maintenance ECT is usually administered monthly; individuals for whom this is insufficient may find treatment at more frequent intervals to be beneficial. The optimal length of maintenance treatment is not known and may also vary depending on the frequency and severity of recurrences, tolerability of treatments, and patient preferences. For some patients, maintenance treatment may be required indefinitely.

E. DISCONTINUATION OF ACTIVE TREATMENT

The precise timing and method of discontinuing psychotherapy and pharmacotherapy for depression have not been systematically studied. The decision to discontinue maintenance treatment should be based on the same factors considered in the decision to initiate maintenance treatment, including the probability of recurrence, the frequency and severity of past episodes, the persistence of depressive symptoms after recovery, the presence of comorbid disorders, and patient preferences. In addition to the factors listed in Table 2 and Table 3, patients and their psychiatrists should consider patient response, in terms of both beneficial and adverse effects, to maintenance treatments.

When the decision is made to discontinue or terminate psychotherapy in the maintenance phase, the manner in which this is done should be individualized to the patient's needs and will depend on the type of psychotherapy, duration, and intensity of treatment. For example, maintenance treatment with cognitive behavioral therapy may have been of a preplanned length and not require extensive time for termination; on the other hand, a long-term psychodynamic psychotherapy may require greater time for and attention to the termination process.

When the decision is made to discontinue maintenance pharmacotherapy, it is best to taper the medication over the course of at least several weeks. Such tapering may allow for the detection of emerging symptoms or recurrences when patients are still partially treated and therefore more easily returned to full therapeutic intensity. In addition, such tapering can help minimize the risks of antidepressant medication discontinuation syndromes (9). Discontinuation syndromes are problematic because their symptoms include disturbances of mood, energy, sleep, and appetite and can be mistaken for or mask signs of relapse (10). Discontinuation syndromes have been found to be more frequent after discontinuation of medications with shorter half-lives, and patients maintained on short-acting agents should be given even longer, more gradual tapering (11).

After the discontinuation of active treatment, patients should be reminded of the potential for a depressive relapse. Early signs of major depressive disorder should be reviewed, and a plan for seeking treatment in the event of recurrence of symptoms should be established. Patients should continue to be monitored over the next several months to identify those in whom a relapse has occurred. If a patient suffers a relapse upon discontinuation of medication, treatment should be promptly reinitiated. In general, the previous treatment regimen to which the patient responded in the acute and continuation phases should be considered. Patients who relapse following discontinuation of antidepressant medication therapy should be considered to have suffered from another major depressive disorder episode and should receive another round of adequate acute phase treatment followed by continuation phase treatment and possibly maintenance phase treatment.

III. SPECIFIC CLINICAL FEATURES INFLUENCING THE TREATMENT PLAN

A. PSYCHIATRIC FEATURES

1. Suicide risk

Patients with major depressive disorder are at greater risk for suicide. Suicide risk should be assessed initially and over the course of treatment. If the patient has suicidal ideation, intention, or a plan, close surveillance is necessary. Factors to be considered in determining the nature and intensity of treatment include (but are not limited to) the nature of the doctor-patient alliance, the availability and adequacy of social supports, access to and lethality of suicide means, and past history of suicidal behavior. The risk of suicide in some patients recovering from major depressive disorder increases transiently as they develop the energy and capacity to act on self-destructive plans made earlier in the course of their illness. Clinicians must be aware of the risk of suicide throughout the course of treatment. However, the prediction of suicide attempts or suicide completion for any given patient is extremely difficult, with both many false positives (patients who appear to be at greater risk of making attempts or completing suicide but who do not) and false negatives (patients who appear to be at decreased risk but who ultimately do make attempts or complete suicide). Therefore, even with the best possible care, a small proportion of patients with major depressive disorder are likely to die by suicide.

2. Psychotic features

Major depressive disorder with psychotic features carries a higher risk of suicide than does major depressive disorder uncomplicated by psychosis (12), and it constitutes a risk factor for recurrent major depressive disorder. Major depressive disorder with psychotic features responds better to treatment with a combination of an antipsychotic medication and an antidepressant medication than to treatment with either component alone (13). Lithium augmentation is helpful in some patients who have not responded to combined antidepressant-antipsychotic medication treatment (14). ECT is highly effective in major depressive disorder with psychotic features and may be considered a first-line treatment for this disorder (15).

3. Catatonic features

Catatonic features may occur in the context of mood disorders and are characterized by at least two of the following manifestations: motoric immobility, as evidenced by catalepsy or stupor; extreme agitation; extreme negativism; peculiarities of voluntary movement, as evidenced by posturing, stereotyped movements, mannerisms, or grimacing; and echolalia or echopraxia (16). Catatonia often dominates the presentation and may be so severe as to be life-threatening, compelling the consideration of urgent biological treatment. Immediate relief may often be obtained by the intravenous administration of benzodiazepines such as lorazepam or amobarbital. For patients who show some relief, continued oral administration of lorazepam, diazepam, or amobarbital may be helpful. Concurrent antidepressant medication treatments should be considered. When relief is not immediately obtained by administering barbiturates or benzodiazepines, the urgent provision of ECT should be considered. The efficacy of ECT, usually apparent after a few treatments, is well documented; ECT may initially be administered daily. After the catatonic manifestations are relieved, treatment may be continued with antidepressant medications, lithium, antipsychotics, or a combination of these compounds, as determined by the patient's condition.

4. Atypical features

Atypical major depressive disorder features include vegetative symptoms of reversed polarity (i.e., increased rather than decreased sleep, appetite, and weight), marked mood reactivity, sensitivity to emotional rejection, phobic symptoms, and a sense of severe fatigue that creates a sensation of leaden paralysis or extreme heaviness of the arms or legs (17). Patients need not have all of these features to be diagnosed as having atypical major depressive disorder (18). There is some overlap between patients with atypical major depressive disorder and patients with anergic bipolar major depressive disorder. Although tricyclic antidepressant medications yield response rates of only 35%–50% in patients with atypical major depressive disorder, several other antidepressant classes have been found to be more effective, yielding response rates of 55%–75% (comparable to the response rate of typical forms of major depressive disorder to tricyclic therapy) (19, 20). Results of several studies suggest that SSRIs, MAOIs, and possibly bupropion may be more effective treatments for atypical major depressive disorder (21–23). The presence and severity of specific symptoms as well as safety considerations should help guide the choice of treatment for atypical major depressive disorder. For example, if a patient does not wish to, cannot, or is unlikely to adhere to the dietary and medication precautions associated with MAOI treatment, the use of an alternative antidepressant medication is indicated; on the other hand, bupropion may be anxiogenic and not preferred in cases where anxiety predominates.

5. Alcohol or substance abuse or dependence

Because of the frequent comorbidity of major depressive disorder and alcohol or other substance abuse, the psychiatrist should make every effort to obtain a detailed history of the patient's substance use. If there is suspicion that there is a problem in this area, the clinician should consider questioning a collateral for confirmation. If the patient is found to have a substance use disorder, a program to secure abstinence should be regarded as a principal priority in the treatment. A patient suffering from major depressive disorder with comorbid addiction is more likely to require hospitalization, more likely to attempt suicide, and less likely to comply with treatment than is a patient with major depressive disorder of similar severity not complicated by this factor. Some alcohol- and chemical-abusing patients reduce their consumption of these substances upon remediation of an underlying major depressive disorder, making the recognition and treatment of major depressive disorder doubly important for such individuals.

It is advisable, if other factors permit, to detoxify patients before initiating antidepressant medication therapy. Identifying the patients who should be started on a regimen of antidepressant medication therapy earlier, after initiation of abstinence, is difficult. A positive family history of major depressive disorder, a history of major depressive disorder preceding alcohol or other substance abuse, or a history of major depressive disorder during periods of sobriety raises the likelihood that the patient would benefit from antidepressant medication treatment, which may then be started earlier in treatment.

Concurrent drug abuse, especially with stimulant drugs, predisposes the patient to toxic interactions with MAOIs, although there have been few reports of such events (24). Benzodiazepines and other sedative-hypnotics carry the potential for abuse or dependence and should be used cautiously except as part of a detoxification regimen. Benzodiazepines have also been reported to contribute to major depressive disorder symptoms. Hepatic dysfunction and hepatic enzyme induction frequently complicate pharmacotherapy of patients with alcoholism and other substance abuse; these conditions may require careful monitoring of blood levels (if available), therapeutic effects, and side effects to avoid either psychotropic medication intoxication or inadequate treatment.

6. Comorbid panic or other anxiety disorder

Panic disorder complicates major depressive disorder in 15%–30% of the cases (25). Individuals with symptoms of both disorders manifest greater degrees of impairment than do patients with major depressive disorder only. In major depressive disorder with comorbid anxiety or panic disorder, both the major depressive disorder symptoms and anxiety symptoms have been shown to respond to antidepressant medication treatment (26). Although there is some evidence that MAOIs may be more effective than other classes for patients with major depressive disorder and anxiety symptoms (25), therapy should first be initiated with a non-MAOI agent because of the somewhat greater complications associated with MAOIs. Tricyclic antidepressant medications and SSRIs may initially worsen rather than alleviate anxiety and panic symptoms; these medications should therefore be introduced at a low dose and slowly increased when used to treat such patients. Bupropion has been reported as ineffective in the treatment of panic disorder (27). Alprazolam may sometimes be used with benefit in conjunction with antidepressant medications; in general, benzodiazepines should not be used as the primary pharmacologic agent for patients with major depressive disorder and anxiety symptoms, especially patients with more severe forms of major depressive disorder.

Obsessive-compulsive symptoms are also more common in patients with major depressive disorder episodes. Clomipramine and the SSRIs have demonstrated efficacy in the management of obsessive-compulsive symptoms in addition to also being effective antidepressant medications (28, 29). Such agents may be used to good effect when obsessive symptoms accompany an episode of major depressive disorder.

7. Major depressive disorder–related cognitive dysfunction (pseudodementia)

Major depressive disorder is routinely accompanied by signs and symptoms of cognitive inefficiency. Some patients have both major depressive disorder and dementia, while others have major depressive disorder that causes cognitive impairment (i.e., pseudodementia). In the latter case, the treatment of the major depressive disorder should reverse the signs and symptoms of cognitive dysfunction. Many patients complain that their thoughts are slowed and their capacity to process information is reduced; they also display diminished attention to their self-care and to their environment. Transient cognitive impairments, especially involving attention, concentration, and memory storage and retrieval, are demonstrable through neuropsychological testing (30). In extreme examples, especially in the elderly, these complaints and deficits are so prominent that patients may appear demented. Major depressive disorder–related cognitive dysfunction is a reversible condition that resolves with treatment of the underlying major depressive disorder. Several clinical features help differentiate major depressive disorder pseudodementia from true dementia. When performing cognitive tasks, pseudodemented patients generally exert relatively less effort but report more incapacity than do demented patients. The latter group, especially in more advanced stages, typically neither recognize nor complain of their cognitive failures, since insight is impaired; in comparison, pseudodemented patients characteristically complain bitterly that they cannot think or cannot remember. Major depressive disorder pseudodementia lacks the signs of cortical dysfunction (i.e., aphasia, apraxia, agnosia) encountered in degenerative dementia, such as Alzheimer's disease (31). It is vital that individuals with major depressive disorder–related cognitive disturbance not be misdiagnosed and thereby denied vigorous antidepressant medication treatment or ECT.

8. Dysthymia

Antidepressant medications have been found to be effective in the treatment of dysthymia and chronic major depressive disorder, including tricyclic antidepressants, SSRIs, other newer agents, and MAOIs; unfortunately, there is little evidence from clinical trials regarding the relative efficacies of particular agents (1, 32, 33). In general, the manner in which antidepressive agents are implemented for dysthymia is similar to that for episodes of major depressive disorder; responses to antidepressant medications by patients with dysthymia and chronic major depressive disorder have been shown to be comparable to the responses by patients with major depressive disorder episodes (34).

Psychotherapy, including interpersonal therapy, cognitive behavioral therapy, cognitive therapy, and behavior therapy, has also been shown to be effective in treating patients with dysthymia and chronic major depressive disorder, although responses have been somewhat smaller than when these modalities are used to treat patients with major depressive disorder (34, 35). Individuals with chronic major depressive disorder may also be considered for psychodynamic psychotherapy in order to examine psychological factors that may maintain the depressed disposition. The combination of psychotherapy and medication has been shown to be more effective than medication alone in patients with dysthymia (36–38).

Double depression is the term used to describe the common condition of a patient with chronic dysthymia who suffers the additional burden of a more severe and pervasive episode of major depressive disorder. Antidepressant medication treatment has been shown to reverse not only the acute major depressive disorder episode but also the underlying chronic dysthymia (39).

9. Comorbid personality disorders

People with any of a variety of personality disorders, including obsessive-compulsive, avoidant, dependent, and borderline disorders, are prone to episodes of major depressive disorder (40). Clinical experience indicates that patients with narcissistic personality disorder are also particularly vulnerable to episodes of major depressive disorder. Patients with major depressive disorder who meet criteria for borderline personality disorder frequently exhibit atypical features, including mood reactivity, and may be more likely to respond to MAOIs and SSRIs than to tricyclic antidepressants (41). Patients with virtually any form of personality disorder exhibit less satisfactory antidepressant medication treatment response, in terms of both social functioning and residual major depressive disorder symptoms, than do individuals without personality disorders (42). Psychodynamic psychotherapy, including psychoanalysis, may be beneficial in modifying the personality disorder in selected patients. Antisocial personality traits tend to interfere with treatment adherence and development of a psychotherapeutic relationship.

10. Seasonal major depressive disorder

Some individuals suffer annual episodes of major depressive disorder with onset in the fall or early winter, usually at the same time each year. Some of these patients suffer manic or hypomanic episodes as well. The major depressive disorder episodes frequently have atypical features such as hypersomnia and overeating. The entire range of treatments for major depressive disorder may also be used to treat seasonal affective disorder, either in combination with or as an alternative to light therapy. As a primary form of treatment, light therapy may be recommended as a time-limited trial (43), primarily in outpatients with clear seasonal patterns. In patients with more severe forms of seasonal major depressive disorder, its use is considered adjunctive to psychopharmacologic intervention.

B. DEMOGRAPHIC AND PSYCHOSOCIAL VARIABLES

1. Major psychosocial stressors

Major depressive disorder may follow a substantial adverse life event, especially one that involves the loss of an important human relationship or life role. Major depressive disorder episodes following life stresses are no less likely than other depressive episodes to either require or benefit from antidepressant medication treatment. Nonetheless, attention to the relationship of both prior and concurrent life events to the onset, exacerbation, or maintenance of major depressive disorder symptoms is an important aspect of the overall treatment approach. A close relationship between a life stressor and major depressive disorder suggests the potential utility of a psychotherapeutic intervention coupled, as indicated, with somatic treatment.

2. Bereavement

Bereavement is a particularly severe stressor and is commonly accompanied by the signs and symptoms of major depressive disorder. Historically, such depressive manifestations have been regarded as normative, and presentations otherwise diagnosable as major depressive disorder are therefore diagnosed in DSM-IV as uncomplicated bereavement when they begin within the first 3 months of the loss (44). Data indicate that almost one-quarter of bereaved individuals meet the criteria for major depressive disorder at 2 months and again at 7 months and that many of these people continue to do so at 13 months (45). Individuals with more prolonged major depressive disorder manifestations tend to be younger and to have a history of prior episodes of major depressive disorder. Antidepressant medications or psychotherapy should be used when the reaction to a loss is particularly prolonged and psychopathology and functional impairment persist.

3. Family distress

The recognition of a problem in the family setting is important in that such a situation constitutes an ongoing stressor that may hamper the patient's response to treatment. Ambivalent, abusive, rejecting, or highly dependent family relationships may particularly predispose an individual to major depressive disorder. Such families should be evaluated for family therapy, which may be used in conjunction with individual and pharmacologic therapies. Even for instances in which there is no apparent family dysfunction, it is important to provide the family with education about the nature of the illness and to enlist the family's support and cooperation.

4. Cultural factors

Specific cultural variables may hamper the accurate assessment of major depressive disorder symptoms. An appreciation by the therapist of cultural variables is critical in the accurate diagnosis of major depressive disorder and in the selection and conduct of psychotherapy and pharmacotherapy. There is evidence that the expression of major depressive disorder symptoms may vary among cultures, especially the tendency to manifest somatic and psychomotor symptoms (46). Ethnic groups may also differ in their pharmacotherapeutic responses to antidepressant medications (47, 48). The language barrier has also been shown to severely impede accurate psychiatric diagnosis and effective treatment (49, 50).

5. Children and adolescents

The clinical presentation of depression in children and adolescents can differ significantly from that of adults and will vary with the child's age. Younger children may exhibit behavioral problems such as social withdrawal, aggressive behavior, apathy, sleep disruption, and weight loss. Adolescents may present with somatic complaints, self-esteem problems, rebelliousness, poor performance in school, or a pattern of engaging in risky or aggressive behavior. A careful assessment of the risk of suicide is necessary and should include an evaluation of risk factors such as recent loss or termination of a relationship, especially by suicide, disciplinary action, or alcohol or other substance abuse. A variety of informants should be used in the evaluation, including parents and teachers.

While a review of medication treatment studies (1) and a number of treatment recommendations (51) for children and adolescents are available, the evidence base for guiding treatment decisions for youth with major depressive disorder is quite limited. As a result, treatment decisions are frequently based on clinical consensus and the extrapolation of data from adults. It is important to be aware, however, that the extrapolation of adult data to children and adolescents is fraught with problems. For example, medications shown to be effective in adults have not always been found to be effective in children, and medications shown to be safe in adults have raised some serious safety concerns in children.

6. Older age

Considerations that go into choosing among psychotherapy, pharmacotherapy, and ECT for the elderly are essentially the same as for younger patients (52). The elderly typically display more vegetative signs and cognitive disturbance and complain less of subjective dysphoria than do their younger counterparts; major depressive disorder may consequently be misattributed to physical illness, dementia, or the aging process itself. It is recognized, however, that major depressive disorder and general medical illness frequently coexist in this age group, and those undergoing their first major depressive disorder episode in old age should be regarded as possibly harboring an as yet undiagnosed neurological or other general medical disorder that is responsible for the major depressive disorder condition. Some medications commonly prescribed for the elderly (e.g., beta-blockers) are thought to be risk factors for the development of major depressive disorder. The clinician should carefully assess whether a given agent contributed to the major depressive disorder before prematurely altering what may be a valuable medication regimen. Major depressive disorder is a common complication of cerebral infarction, especially in the anterior left hemisphere (53).

Although elderly patients typically require a lower oral dose than younger patients to yield a particular blood level and tolerate a given blood level less well, the blood levels at which antidepressant medications are maximally effective appear to be the same as for younger patients (54). Elderly patients are particularly prone to orthostatic hypotension and cholinergic blockade; for this reason, fluoxetine, sertraline, bupropion, desipramine, and nortriptyline are frequently chosen rather than amitriptyline, imipramine, and doxepin. Weight loss may be especially problematic in the elderly. When this is the case, it might be beneficial to use an antidepressant that causes weight gain (see Table 7). Although the role of stimulants for antidepressant monotherapy is very limited, these compounds have some role in apathetic major depressive disorder in elderly patients with complicating general medical conditions. ECT should be considered for many of these patients. A recent study has shown that antidepressant medication (nortriptyline) and interpersonal therapy are effective maintenance therapies for elderly patients with recurrent major depressive disorder; a trend toward superior response was observed for combined pharmacotherapy and psychotherapy compared to pharmacotherapy alone (52).

7. Gender and pregnancy

The risks of certain adverse effects from treatments may also differ by gender. Caution is advised in the prescription of trazodone to men because of the risk of priapism. Older men are at risk for prostatic hypertrophy, making them particularly sensitive to medication effects on the bladder outlet. While both men and women may experience decreased libido or anorgasmia while taking SSRIs, men may also experience ejaculatory dysfunction. Some women who are taking birth control pills require higher doses of tricyclic antidepressant medications because of the induction of the hepatic enzymes responsible for medication metabolism.

The diagnostic assessment for women, in particular, should include a detailed inquiry regarding reproductive life history, including menstruation, menopause, birth control, and abortions. History of experiences of sexual and physical abuse, posttraumatic stress disorder, and treatment, if any, should be obtained.

Major depressive disorder occurring during pregnancy is a difficult therapeutic problem. Women of childbearing potential in psychiatric treatment should be carefully counseled as to the risks of becoming pregnant while taking psychotropic medications. Whenever possible, a pregnancy should be planned in consultation with the psychiatrist so that medication may be discontinued before conception if feasible. Antidepressant medication treatment should be considered for pregnant women who have major depressive disorder, as well as for those women who are in remission from major depressive disorder, receiving maintenance medication, and deemed to be at high risk for a recurrence if the medication is discontinued. The risks of treatment with medications must be weighed against the risks of alternative treatments, as well as the risks to the woman if the major depressive disorder is not effectively treated. These risks have recently been reviewed (55).

Specific concerns about the risks of untreated major depressive disorder in pregnancy include the possibility of low birth weight secondary to poor maternal weight gain (or frank weight loss). Suicidality, as well as the potential for long-term hospitalization, marital discord, the inability to engage in appropriate obstetrical care, and difficulty caring for other children must also be considered.

The considerations for the use of psychotherapy during pregnancy are identical to those relevant to nonpregnant patients, with the caveat that the risks of a delay in effectiveness may need to be considered in the context of the mother's safety as well as the safety of her fetus.

TABLE 7. Potential Treatments for Side Effects of Antidepressant Medications

Side Effect	Antidepressant(s) Associated With Effect	Treatment
Cardiovascular		
Orthostatic hypotension	Tricyclic antidepressants; trazodone; nefazodone; MAOIs	Lower dose; discontinue medication; fludrocortisone; add salt to diet
Reduced cardiac output	Tricyclic antidepressants	Discontinue medication
Arrhythmias	Tricyclic antidepressants	Discontinue medication
Hypertension	Venlafaxine	Lower dose; discontinue medication
Hypertensive crisis	MAOIs	Discontinue medication; intravenous phentolamine
Increase in cholesterol	Mirtazapine	Lower dose; discontinue medication
Anticholinergic		
Dry mouth	Tricyclic antidepressants; reboxetine	Pilocarpine oral rinse; gum; candy
Constipation	Tricyclic antidepressants; reboxetine	Hydration; bulk laxatives
Urinary hesitancy	Tricyclic antidepressants; reboxetine	Bethanechol
Visual changes	Tricyclic antidepressants; reboxetine	Pilocarpine eye drops
Delirium	Tricyclic antidepressants	Discontinue medication; antipsychotic medication
Sedation	Tricyclic antidepressants; trazodone; nefazodone; mirtazapine	Bedtime dosing
Weight gain	Tricyclic antidepressants; mirtazapine; MAOIs	Lower dose; change to secondary amine (if tricyclic antidepressant required); discontinue medication
Nausea, vomiting	SSRIs; bupropion, sustained release; venlafaxine, extended release	Lower dose; discontinue medication
Insomnia	SSRIs; bupropion; reboxetine	Lower dose; discontinue medication; morning dosing; trazodone at bedtime
Activation	SSRIs; venlafaxine	Lower dose; discontinue medication
Neurological		
Myoclonus	Tricyclic antidepressants; MAOIs	Lower dose; discontinue medication; clonazepam
Extrapyramidal symptoms; tardive dyskinesia	Amoxapine; SSRIs	Lower dose; discontinue medication
Seizures	Bupropion; amoxapine	Lower dose; discontinue medication; antiepileptic medication
Headaches	SSRIs; bupropion	Lower dose; discontinue medication
Sexual side effects		
Arousal, erectile dysfunction	Paroxetine; venlafaxine	Lower dose; discontinue medication; sildenafil; yohimbine; ginkgo; methylphenidate; dextroamphetamine; pemoline
	Tricyclic antidepressants; SSRIs	Lower dose; discontinue medication; sildenafil; yohimbine; ginkgo; bethanechol; neostigmine

TABLE 7. Potential Treatments for Side Effects of Antidepressant Medications *(continued)*

Side Effect	Antidepressant(s) Associated With Effect	Treatment
Sexual side effects *(continued)*		
Orgasm dysfunction	SSRIs; venlafaxine	Lower dose; discontinue medication; granisetron; amantadine; cyproheptadine; sildenafil
	MAOIs; tricyclic antidepressants	Lower dose; discontinue medication; cyproheptadine; amantadine
Priapism	Trazodone	Discontinue medication; surgical correction
Serotonin syndrome	SSRIs; MAOIs; venlafaxine	Discontinue medication
Agranulocytosis	Mirtazapine	Discontinue medication; monitor white blood cell count, granulocyte colony–stimulating factor

Wisner et al. reviewed the risks associated with the use of antidepressant medications during pregnancy (55). Potential risks that should be considered include intrauterine death, morphologic teratogenicity, growth impairment, behavioral teratogenicity, and neonatal toxicity. Wisner et al. also reviewed the limitations of the available database and the basic principles to be used in treating pregnant women with antidepressants. In particular, dose requirements change during pregnancy because of changes in volume of distribution, hepatic metabolism, protein binding, and gastrointestinal absorption. Although clinicians need to keep abreast of new data as they become available, at this time there is no evidence that tricyclic antidepressants, fluoxetine, or newer SSRIs cause either intrauterine death or major birth defects. However, in one large study (56), three or more minor physical anomalies occurred more commonly in infants exposed to fluoxetine than in a comparison group. This study also demonstrated that fetuses exposed to fluoxetine after 25 weeks' gestation had lower birth weights, which were associated with lower maternal weight gain.

The area of behavioral teratogenicity remains the major area of concern when prescribing psychoactive medications to pregnant women. Both tricyclic antidepressants and fluoxetine have been studied, and the results provide no evidence for effects on cognitive function, temperament, or general behavior. However, replication studies, as well as data regarding other newer antidepressants, are needed.

Neonatal withdrawal syndromes have been reported in babies exposed, in utero, to tricyclic antidepressants, fluoxetine, and sertraline. Given these data, it is recommended that consideration be given to using either a tricyclic antidepressant or an SSRI that has been studied in pregnant women. If a tricyclic antidepressant is to be used, nortriptyline should be particularly considered because of its relatively low anticholinergic effects, long history of use, and well-studied relationship between plasma concentration and therapeutic effect (55). When antidepressants are used, maternal weight gain should be carefully monitored, and consideration should be given to gradually tapering the medication 10–14 days before the expected date of delivery. If this is done, and the woman is considered to be at risk from her major depressive disorder, the medication can be restarted following delivery, although the dose should be readjusted to that required before pregnancy. In selected cases not responding to or unsuitable for medication, for patients with major depressive disorder with psychotic features, or for individuals electing to use this modality as a matter of preference after having weighed the relative risks and benefits, ECT may be used as an alternative treatment; the current literature supports the safety for mother and fetus, as well as the efficacy of ECT during pregnancy (57).

Several major depressive disorder conditions may follow childbirth (58). The transient 7–10-day depressive condition referred to as postpartum blues typically is too mild to meet the criteria for major depressive disorder and does not require medication. It is optimally treated by reassuring the patient of its brief nature and favorable outcome. Puerperal psychosis is a more severe disorder complicating 1–2 per 1,000 births; more than one-half of the episodes of this type meet the criteria for major depressive disorder (59), and many patients who have had episodes of this type ultimately prove to have bipolar disorder. Major depressive disorder, and especially major depressive disorder with psychotic features, can seriously interfere with the new mother's ability to provide physically and emotionally appropriate care for her baby. The woman's parenting skills for both the newborn baby and any other children in her care must be carefully assessed. Women with postpartum psychotic major depressive disorder may have homicidal impulses toward the newborn; for this reason, careful assessment of homicidal as well as suicidal ideation, intention, or plans is important. Women whose maintenance antidepressant medication treatment was discontinued during pregnancy appear to be particularly at risk for recurrence of major depressive disorder; such individuals should have their medications restored after delivery, in the absence of a contraindication.

Major depressive disorder in the postpartum period should be treated according to the same principles delineated for other types of major depressive disorder. However, when a woman decides to nurse, the potential benefits to the mother of using antidepressant medications should be balanced against the potential risks to the newborn inherent in the possibility of receiving some antidepressant in the breast milk; mothers should be counseled regarding the relative risks and benefits when making treatment decisions (60, 61).

8. Family history

The presence of a positive family history of recurrent major depressive disorder increases the chances that the patient's own illness will be recurrent and that the patient will not fully recover between episodes.

The presence in a depressed patient of a positive family history of bipolar disorder or acute psychosis probably increases the chances that the patient's own major depressive disorder is a manifestation of bipolar rather than unipolar disorder and that antidepressant medication therapy may incite a switch to mania (62). Patients with such a family history should be particularly closely questioned regarding a prior history of mania or hypomania, since lithium used alone or in conjunction with another antidepressant medication is particularly likely to exert a beneficial effect in patients with bipolar disorder who have a major depressive episode. Patients with major depressive disorder with a family history of bipolar disorder should be carefully observed for signs of a switch to mania during antidepressant medication treatment.

C. TREATMENT IMPLICATIONS OF CONCURRENT GENERAL MEDICAL DISORDERS

1. Asthma

Individuals with asthma who receive MAOIs should be cautioned regarding interactions with sympathomimetic bronchodilators, although other antiasthma agents appear to be safe. Other antidepressant medications may be used for patients with asthma without fear of interaction.

2. Cardiac disease

The presence of specific cardiac conditions complicates or contraindicates certain forms of antidepressant medication therapy, notably use of tricyclic agents; the cardiac history should therefore be carefully explored before the initiation of medication treatment. Although tricyclic antidepressants have been used effectively to treat major depressive disorder in patients with some forms of ischemic heart disease (63), psychiatrists should take particular care in using tricyclics for patients with a history of ventricular arrhythmia, subclinical sinus node dysfunction, conduction defects (including asymptomatic conduction defects), prolonged QT intervals, or a recent history of myocardial infarction (64–70). SSRIs, bupropion, and ECT appear to be safer for patients with preexisting cardiac disease, although the latter may require consultation with a specialist and treatment modification before use (63, 71–77). MAOIs do not adversely affect cardiac conduction, rhythm, or contraction but may induce orthostatic hypotension and also run the risk of interacting adversely with other medications that may be taken by such patients. There is anecdotal evidence that trazodone may induce ventricular arrhythmias, but the agent appears to be safe for the overwhelming majority of patients.

A depressed patient with a history of any cardiac problem should be monitored for the emergence of cardiac symptoms, ECG changes, or orthostatic blood pressure decrements. Consultation with the patient's cardiologist before and during antidepressant medication treatment may be advisable and is especially advisable during any treatment for a patient who has recently had a myocardial infarction.

3. Dementia

Treatment of major depressive disorder in the cognitively impaired patient requires the involvement of clinicians in the patient's pharmacotherapy, supervision, and monitoring; this involvement may entail education of home health aides, nursing home providers, and others. Individuals with dementia are particularly susceptible to the toxic effects of muscarinic blockade on memory and attention. Therefore, individuals suffering from dementia generally do best when given antidepressant medications with the lowest possible degree of anticholinergic effect, e.g., bupropion, fluoxetine, sertraline, trazodone, and, of the tricyclic agents, desipramine or nortriptyline. Alternatively, some patients do well given stimulants in small doses. ECT is also effective in major depressive disorder superimposed on dementia, and it should be used if medications are contraindicated, not tolerated, or if immediate resolution of the major depressive disorder episode is medically indicated (such as when it interferes with the patient's acceptance of food). Practitioners should be aware that a transient worsening of the patient's cognitive status may occur in such cases (72, 75, 78).

4. Epilepsy

Although many antidepressant medications lower the seizure threshold and theoretically exert a dose-dependent adverse effect on seizure control in patients with major depressive disorder with epilepsy, major depressive disorder in patients with seizure disorders can usually be safely and effectively managed according to the same principles outlined for patients without seizures. Consideration should be given to concomitant prescription of an antiepileptic (or elevating the dose of an existing antiepileptic).

5. Glaucoma

Medications with anticholinergic potency may precipitate acute narrow-angle glaucoma in susceptible individuals (i.e., those with shallow anterior chambers) (79). Patients with glaucoma receiving local miotic therapy may be treated with antidepressant medications, including those possessing anticholinergic properties, provided that their intraocular pressure is monitored during antidepressant medication treatment. Agents lacking anticholinergic activity (bupropion, sertraline, fluoxetine, and trazodone) avoid this liability.

6. Hypertension

Antihypertensive agents and tricyclic antidepressant medications may interact to either intensify or counteract the effect of the antihypertensive therapy. The action of antihypertensive agents that block alpha receptors (e.g., prazosin) may be intensified by antidepressant medications that block these same receptors, notably the tricyclic antidepressants and trazodone. Tricyclic antidepressants may antagonize the therapeutic actions of guanethidine, clonidine, or α-methyldopa. Concurrent antihypertensive treatment, especially with diuretics, increases the likelihood that tricyclic antidepressants, trazodone, or MAOIs will induce symptomatic orthostatic hypotension. Beta-blockers, especially propranolol, may be a cause of major depressive disorder in some patients; individuals who have become depressed after initiation of treatment with one of these medications should be changed to another antihypertensive regimen. Dose-dependent elevations in blood pressure with venlafaxine are usually mild, although more severe elevations have been observed (80), making this agent less preferable in patients with hypertension.

7. Obstructive uropathy

Prostatism and other forms of bladder outlet obstruction are relative contraindications to the use of antidepressant medication compounds with antimuscarinic effects. Benzodiazepines, trazodone, and MAOIs may also retard bladder emptying. The antidepressant medications with the least propensity to do this are SSRIs, bupropion, and desipramine.

8. Parkinson's disease

Amoxapine, an antidepressant medication with dopamine-receptor blocking properties, should be avoided for patients who have Parkinson's disease. Lithium may in some instances induce or exacerbate parkinsonian symptoms. Bupropion, in contrast, exerts a beneficial effect on the symptoms of Parkinson's disease in some patients but may also induce psychotic symptoms, perhaps because of its agonistic action in the dopaminergic system (81). MAOIs (other than selegiline, also known as L-deprenyl, a selective type B MAOI recommended in the treatment of Parkinson's disease) may adversely interact with L-dopa products (82). Selegiline loses its specificity for MAO-B in doses greater than 10 mg/day and may induce serotonin syndrome when given in higher doses in conjunction with serotonin-enhancing antidepressant medications. Major depressive disorder, which occurs to some degree in 40%–50% of patients with Parkinson's disease, may be related to the alterations of serotonergic and noradrenergic systems that occur in this disorder. There is no evidence favoring any particular antidepressant medication from the standpoint of therapeutic efficacy in patients with Parkinson's disease complicated by major depressive disorder. The theoretical benefits of the antimuscarinic effects of some of the tricyclic agents in the treatment of patients with major depressive disorder with Parkinson's disease are offset by the memory impairment that may result. ECT exerts a transient beneficial effect on the symptoms of idiopathic Parkinson's disease in many patients (83).

PART B: BACKGROUND INFORMATION AND REVIEW OF AVAILABLE EVIDENCE

IV. DISEASE DEFINITION, EPIDEMIOLOGY, NATURAL HISTORY, AND COURSE

DSM-IV criteria for major depressive episode and major depressive disorder are listed in Table 8.

A. SPECIFIC FEATURES OF DIAGNOSIS

1. Severity

An episode of major depressive disorder may be classified as mild, moderate, or severe. Mild episodes are characterized by little in the way of symptoms beyond the minimum required to make the diagnosis and by minor functional impairment. Moderate episodes are characterized by the presence of symptoms in excess of the bare diagnostic requirements and by greater degrees of functional impairment. Severe episodes are characterized by the presence of several symptoms in excess of the minimum requirements and by the symptoms' marked interference with social and/or occupational functioning. In the extreme, afflicted individuals may be totally unable to function socially or occupationally or even to feed or clothe themselves or to maintain minimal personal hygiene. The nature of the symptoms, such as suicidal ideation and behavior, should also be considered in assessing severity.

2. Melancholia

The melancholic subtype is a severe form of major depressive disorder with characteristic somatic symptoms, and it is believed to be particularly responsive to pharmacotherapy and ECT.

3. Psychotic features

Major depressive disorder may be accompanied by hallucinations or delusions; these may be congruent or noncongruent with the depressive mood.

4. Dysthymia

The differential diagnosis of dysthymia and major depressive disorder is particularly difficult, since the two disorders share similar symptoms and differ primarily in duration and severity. Usually major depressive disorder consists of one or more discrete major depressive episodes that can be distinguished from the person's usual functioning, whereas dysthymia is characterized by a chronic mild depressive syndrome that has been present for at least 2 years. If the initial onset of what appears to be dysthymia directly follows a major depressive episode, the appropriate diagnosis is major depressive disorder in partial remission. The diagnosis of dysthymia can be made following major depressive disorder only if there has been a full remission of the major depressive episode that has lasted at least 6 months before the development of dysthymia.

People with dysthymia frequently have a superimposed major depressive disorder, and this condition is often referred to as double major depressive disorder. Patients with double major depressive disorder are less likely to have a complete recovery than are patients with major depressive disorder without dysthymia.

B. EPIDEMIOLOGY

The Epidemiologic Catchment Area study indicates that major depressive disorder has a 1-month prevalence of 2.2% and a lifetime prevalence of 5.8% in Americans 18 years and older (84). Other studies estimate the lifetime prevalence to be as high as 26% for women and 12% for men. The illness is 1.5 to 3 times as common among those with a first-degree biological relative affected with the disorder as among the general population. Major depressive disorder is frequently accompanied by comorbid conditions. For example, in one study of patients with major depressive disorder under the care of psychiatrists in the United States, 84% had at least one comorbid condition: 61% had a co-occurring axis I condition, 30% a comorbid axis II condition, and 58% a comorbid axis III condition (85). Frequently a major depressive episode follows a psychosocial stressor, particularly death of a loved one, marital separation, or the ending of an important relationship. Childbirth sometimes precipitates a major depressive episode. Pa-

TABLE 8. DSM-IV Criteria for Major Depressive Episode and Major Depressive Disorder

Diagnosis	Criterion/Symptom Description
Major depressive episode	A. At least five of the following symptoms have been present during the same 2-week period and represent a change from previous functioning; at least one of the symptoms is either 1) depressed mood or 2) loss of interest or pleasure (do not include symptoms that are clearly due to general medical condition or mood-incongruent delusions or hallucinations) 1. Depressed mood most of the day, nearly every day, as indicated either by subjective report (e.g., feels sad or empty) or observation made by others (e.g., appears tearful) 2. Markedly diminished interest or pleasure in all, or almost all, activities most of the day, nearly every day (as indicated by either subjective account or observation made by others) 3. Significant weight loss when not dieting or weight gain (e.g., a change of more than 5% of body weight in a month), or decrease or increase in appetite nearly every day 4. Insomnia or hypersomnia nearly every day 5. Psychomotor agitation or retardation nearly every day (observable by others, not merely subjective feelings of restlessness or being slowed down) 6. Fatigue or loss of energy nearly every day 7. Feelings of worthlessness or excessive or inappropriate guilt (which may be delusional) nearly every day (not merely self-reproach or guilt about being sick) 8. Diminished ability to think or concentrate, or indecisiveness, nearly every day (either by subjective account or as observed by others) 9. Recurrent thoughts of death (not just fear of dying), recurrent suicidal ideation without a specific plan, or a suicide attempt or specific plan for committing suicide B. The symptoms do not meet criteria for a mixed episode C. The symptoms cause clinically significant distress or impairment in social, occupational, or other important areas of functioning D. The symptoms are not due to the direct physiological effects of a substance (e.g., a drug of abuse, a medication) or a general medical condition (e.g., hypothyroidism) E. The symptoms are not better accounted for by bereavement, i.e., after the loss of a loved one, the symptoms persist for longer than 2 months or are characterized by marked functional impairment, morbid preoccupation with worthlessness, suicidal ideation, psychotic symptoms, or psychomotor retardation
Major depressive disorder, single episode	A. Presence of a single major depressive episode B. The major depressive episode is not better accounted for by schizoaffective disorder and is not superimposed on schizophrenia, schizophreniform disorder, delusional disorder, or psychotic disorder not otherwise specified C. There has never been a manic episode, a mixed episode, or a hypomanic episode

TABLE 8. DSM-IV Criteria for Major Depressive Episode and Major Depressive Disorder *(continued)*

Diagnosis	Criterion/Symptom Description
Major depressive disorder, recurrent	A. Presence of two or more major depressive episodes (each separated by at least 2 months in which criteria are not met for a major depressive episode) B. The major depressive episodes are not better accounted for by schizoaffective disorder and are not superimposed on schizophrenia, schizophreniform disorder, delusional disorder, or psychotic disorder not otherwise specified C. There has never been a manic episode, a mixed episode, or a hypomanic episode

Source. Reprinted from *Diagnostic and Statistical Manual of Mental Disorders,* 4th Edition. Washington, DC, American Psychiatric Association, 1994. Copyright © 1994, American Psychiatric Association.

tients with major depressive disorder identified in psychiatric settings tend to have episodes of greater severity and to have recurrent forms of major depressive disorder and also are more likely to have other mental disorders than are subjects from the community and primary care settings.

C. NATURAL HISTORY AND COURSE

The average age at onset is the late 20s, but the disorder may begin at any age. The symptoms of major depressive disorder typically develop over days to weeks. Prodromal symptoms, including generalized anxiety, panic attacks, phobias, or depressive symptoms that do not meet the diagnostic threshold, may occur over the preceding several months. In some cases, however, a major depressive disorder may develop suddenly (e.g., when associated with severe psychosocial stress). The duration of a major depressive episode is also variable. Untreated, the episode typically lasts 6 months or longer. Some patients with major depressive disorder will eventually have a manic or hypomanic episode and will then be diagnosed as having bipolar disorder.

1. Recurrence

Although some people have only a single episode of major depressive disorder, with full return to premorbid functioning, it is estimated that from 50% to 85% of the people who have such an episode will eventually have another episode, at which time the illness will meet the criteria for recurrent major depressive disorder (86). People with major depressive disorder superimposed on dysthymia are at greater risk for having recurrent episodes of major depressive disorder than those without dysthymia.

The course of recurrent major depressive disorder is variable. Some people have episodes separated by many years of normal functioning, others have clusters of episodes, and still others have increasingly frequent episodes as they grow older.

2. Interepisode status

Functioning usually returns to the premorbid level between episodes. In 20%–35% of the cases, however, there are persistent residual symptoms and social or occupational impairment. Patients who continue to meet the criteria for a major depressive episode throughout the course of the disturbance are considered to have the chronic type, whereas those who remain symptomatic are considered to be in partial remission.

3. Seasonal pattern

A seasonal pattern of major depressive disorder is characterized by a regular temporal relationship between the onset and remission of symptoms and particular periods of the year (e.g., in the northern hemisphere, regular appearance of symptoms between the beginning of October and the end of November and regular remission from mid-February to mid-April). Patients should not receive this diagnosis if there is an obvious effect of seasonally related psychosocial stressors, e.g., seasonal unemployment.

4. Complications

The most serious complications of a major depressive episode are suicide and other violent acts. Other complications include marital, parental, social, and vocational difficulties (87). The illness, especially in its recurrent and chronic forms, may cause distress for other individuals in the patient's social network, e.g., children, spouse, and significant others. If the patient is a parent, the disorder may affect his or her ability to fulfill parental role expectations (88). Major depressive disorder episodes are associated with occupational dysfunction, including unemployment, absenteeism, and decreased work productivity (89). Major depressive disorder may also complicate recovery from other medical illnesses. Major depressive disorder has been demonstrated to be a major risk factor in the post-myocardial-infarction period.

V. REVIEW AND SYNTHESIS OF AVAILABLE EVIDENCE

Successful treatment of patients with major depressive disorder is promoted by a thorough assessment of the patient's symptoms; past general medical and psychiatric history; psychological makeup and conflicts; life stressors; family, psychosocial, and cultural environment; and preference for specific treatments or approaches.

The psychiatrist's task is both to effect and to maintain improvement. Treatment consists of an acute phase, during which remission is induced; a continuation phase, during which remission is preserved; and a maintenance phase, during which the susceptible patient is protected against the recurrence of subsequent major depressive disorder episodes. Psychiatrists initiating treatment of a major depressive disorder episode have at their disposal a number of medications, a variety of psychosocial approaches, ECT, and light therapy. These various interventions may be used alone or in combination. Furthermore, the psychiatrist must decide whether to conduct treatment on an outpatient, partial hospitalization, or inpatient basis.

A. ACUTE PHASE SOMATIC TREATMENTS

1. Antidepressant medications

a) Goals

The goal of treatment with antidepressant medications in the acute phase is the remission of major depressive disorder symptoms. For cases of first-episode major depressive disorder uncomplicated by comorbid general medical illness or by special features such as atypical, psychotic, or bipolar symptoms, many antidepressant medications are available. Systematic data from clinical trials regarding the relative efficacy of different antidepressant medications are lacking. For most patients, antidepressant medications approved by the Food and Drug Administration (FDA) are generally considered equally effective, with response rates in clinical trials ranging from 50% to 75% of patients. However, among some subgroups of patients with major depressive disorder, efficacy may differ. Antidepressant medications also differ in their potential to cause particular side effects. Antidepressant medications have been grouped as follows: 1) tricyclic antidepressant medications, which for the purposes of this review also include the tetracyclic antidepressant medication maprotiline; 2) SSRIs, which include fluoxetine, sertraline, paroxetine, fluvoxamine, and citalopram; 3) other antidepressant medications, including bupropion, nefazodone, trazodone, venlafaxine, mirtazapine, and reboxetine (for which FDA approval is anticipated); and 4) MAOIs, which include phenelzine, tranylcypromine, and isocarboxazid.

b) Efficacy

Quantitative reviews of the efficacy of antidepressant medications for major depressive disorder have been performed, including the recent *Evidence Report on Treatment of Depression—Newer Pharmacotherapies* (1). This study examined 315 trials, lasting 6 weeks or longer, of newer pharmacotherapies for patients with depressive disorders. Additional details concerning the evidence of antidepressant medication efficacy that may be beyond the scope of this guideline can be obtained from such reviews.

Interpreting data from clinical trials on the efficacy of pharmacotherapy for major depressive disorder can be complicated by several issues. First, it is important to consider whether and what type of comparison group was used (e.g., placebo or active agent). In trials of antidepressant medication treatments, high placebo response rates could explain observed treatment effects in poorly controlled trials as well as make detection of true treatment effects difficult in well-controlled trials. It is also important to consider both whether trials were blinded and whether in "blinded" trials, medication side effects could reveal the identity of active agents. Issues related to the outcomes measured in trials are important as well. A variety of different outcome measures are employed, and a report of "efficacy" could refer to symptom reduction (e.g., reduction in the frequency or severity of major depressive disorder symptoms), response (e.g., reduction in major depressive disorder symptoms below a threshold), or prevention of relapse. Data often come from short-term (6- to 12-week) efficacy trials that may not reveal whether treatments are effective over the medium and long term. Lastly, it is important to consider whether publication bias against reporting of negative studies could affect the perception of overall treatment effectiveness.

(1) Tricyclic antidepressants

Since the first trial in which a tricyclic compound (imipramine) was shown to improve major depressive disorder symptoms (90), hundreds of subsequent randomized controlled trials have demonstrated the efficacy of this class as a treatment for major depressive disorder (1). Heterocyclic antidepressant medications, including tricyclics and tetracyclics, have been found to be statistically significantly superior to placebo in approximately 75% of studies (91); several reviews suggest that approximately 50%–75% of patients with major depressive disorder treated with heterocyclic antidepressant medications respond compared to 25%–33% treated with placebo (92–95). The efficacy of individual agents and subclasses of tricyclics (e.g., secondary amines or tertiary amines) appears to be comparable.

Results of some investigations have suggested that tricyclic antidepressants may possess superior efficacy among subgroups of patients with severe major depressive disorder symptoms (91, 96–99). Some studies have also suggested that in major depressive disorder marked by melancholic features, tricyclic antidepressants may be additionally effective (100, 101) as well as superior to SSRIs (102, 103); however, not all research supports these findings (104).

(2) Selective serotonin reuptake inhibitors

SSRIs currently available include fluoxetine, sertraline, paroxetine, fluvoxamine, and citalopram. A large body of literature containing approximately 50 randomized, placebo-controlled trials supports the premise that SSRIs are superior to placebo in the treatment of major depressive disorder. In over 50 investigations the effectiveness of SSRIs has been compared to that of other antidepressant medications, mainly tricyclic antidepressants; in these trials, SSRIs have generally had comparable efficacy to antidepressant medications from other classes (1, 105, 106). In general, significant differences in efficacy between individual SSRIs have not been observed.

There is some evidence that SSRIs may be more effective than tricyclic antidepressants for subgroups of patients with atypical symptoms of major depressive disorder (e.g., mood reactivity, hypersomnia, hyperphagia, and hypersensitivity to rejections) (23). SSRIs have also been shown to be helpful for some patients who have not responded to tricyclic antidepressants (107).

(3) Other antidepressant medications

Several other antidepressant medications are available that differ structurally or in their pharmacologic action from medications in the categories just described. Trazodone is the medication from this group for which the most data on efficacy exists. In most trials, trazodone has had superior efficacy relative to placebo; however, its efficacy relative to other antidepressant medications remains controversial. Although data from some controlled trials suggest comparable efficacy to tricyclic antidepressants (108, 109), other investigations suggest trazodone may possess inferior efficacy relative to other antidepressant medications (1, 110, 111), particularly in subgroups with severe major depressive disorder symptoms or prominent psychomotor retardation (112, 113).

Nefazodone has an analogous structure to trazodone but somewhat different pharmacologic properties. In controlled trials, nefazodone has had superior efficacy to placebo; in five trials, nefazodone has been found to have comparable efficacy to tricyclic antidepressants (1, 114, 115). Some studies suggest that nefazodone may have an optimal therapeutic dose range corresponding to approximately 300–600 mg/day (115, 116).

Bupropion appears to inhibit the reuptake of both norepinephrine and dopamine, although its mechanism of action remains unclear. Trial data have shown that bupropion is superior to placebo (117) and generally comparable in efficacy to both tricyclic antidepressants (1, 118–121) and SSRIs (122).

Venlafaxine and mirtazapine appear to act through inhibition of reuptake of both norepinephrine and serotonin. Both have been demonstrated to be superior to placebo; venlafaxine and mirtazapine have each been shown in four trials to possess generally comparable efficacy to tricyclic antidepressants (1, 110, 123–128). Results from one trial suggest a positive relationship between the effective dose of venlafaxine and the severity of major depressive disorder—favorable responses were achieved with lower doses in milder major depressive disorders, whereas higher doses were more efficacious in severe major depressive disorder (129).

Reboxetine is a new selective noradrenaline reuptake inhibitor for which approval from the FDA is expected. In four trials, reboxetine has been shown to be more effective than placebo; in 6 trials against active treatment, reboxetine has been found to possess at least comparable effectiveness as tricyclic antidepressants and SSRIs (1, 130).

(4) Monoamine oxidase inhibitors

MAOIs that have been used as antidepressant medications include phenelzine, tranylcypromine, and isocarboxazid. MAOIs have also been shown in multiple trials to be effective treatments for major depressive disorder. Although some earlier comparisons employing lower doses of MAOIs found tricyclic antidepressants to be superior, MAOIs are now considered to have comparable efficacy to tricyclic antidepressants for typical cases of major depressive disorder (131–136). There are no significant differences in efficacy among the MAOIs.

Results of several investigations suggest that MAOIs may be particularly effective in treating subgroups of patients with major depressive disorder with atypical features such as reactive moods, reversed neurovegetative symptoms, and sensitivity to rejection (19, 137, 138). MAOIs have also been shown to be effective treatments for some patients who have failed other antidepressant medication trials (132, 136, 139, 140).

c) Side effects

The severity of side effects from antidepressant medications in clinical trials has been assessed both through the frequency of reported side effects and through the frequency of treatment dropout. The likelihood of different side effects varies between classes of antidepressant medications, between subclasses, and between individual agents. Prominent and clinically relevant side effects associated with particular classes, subclasses, and individual medications are reviewed in Table 7.

(1) Tricyclic antidepressants

i. Cardiovascular effects

Tricyclic antidepressants can cause a number of cardiovascular side effects through α-adrenergic blockade, including tachycardia or orthostatic hypotension. Side effects such as orthostatic hypotension may in turn lead to events such as dizziness, falls, or fractures. Secondary amines such as nortriptyline or desipramine cause less α-adrenergic blockade and may offer advantages over tertiary amines (69). Salt depletion, whether voluntary or a result of diuretic treatment, may contribute to orthostatic hypotension. If there is no medical contraindication, patients with symptomatic orthostatic hypotension should be cautioned against extreme dietary salt restriction.

Tricyclic antidepressant medications act similarly to class I antiarrhythmic agents such as quinidine, disopyramide, and procainamide by prolonging cardiac repolarization and depressing fast sodium ion channels (141). Both secondary and tertiary amines have been documented to suppress ventricular premature depolarizations (64, 67). Combinations of tricyclic antidepressants with other class I antiarrhythmic agents can exert additive toxic effects on cardiac conduction; patients with ventricular arrhythmias taking another class I antiarrhythmic agent who require tricyclic medication therapy should be under careful medical supervision. Tricyclic antidepressants may also provoke arrhythmias in patients with subclinical sinus node dysfunction; for example, in patients with tachyarrhythmias, treatment with tricyclic antidepressants may on occasion provoke bradyarrhythmias (65). Among patients with preexisting but asymptomatic conduction defects, such as interventricular conduction delay and bundle-branch block, tricyclic antidepressants may induce symptomatic conduction defects and symptomatic orthostatic hypotension (69). Individuals with prolonged QT intervals, whether preexistent or medication-induced, are predisposed to the development of ventricular tachycardia (70). It has also been reported that patients with normal pretreatment ECG results may develop atrioventricular block that reverts to normal after discontinuation of antidepressant medication treatment (69).

For most patients, tricyclic antidepressants exert no appreciable effect on ventricular ejection fraction (142); rarely (and usually in patients with marked baseline disturbances of myocardial function), tricyclic antidepressants may exert a deleterious effect on ejection fraction (66, 68).

ii. Anticholinergic side effects

All tricyclic antidepressant medications have some degree of antimuscarinic action; tertiary amine tricyclic antidepressants produce the most anticholinergic side effects, whereas the newer secondary amines, desipramine and nortriptyline, have less antimuscarinic activity. The most common undesirable consequences of muscarinic blockade are dry mouth, impaired ability to focus at close range, constipation, urinary hesitation, tachycardia, and sexual dysfunction. Although patients can develop some degree of tolerance to anticholinergic side effects, these symptoms may require treatment if they cause substantial dysfunction or interfere with adherence. Impaired visual accommodation may be counteracted through the use of pilocarpine eye drops. Urinary hesitation may be treated by prescribing bethanechol, 200 mg/day (in divided doses to avoid symptoms of cholinergic excess, principally abdominal cramps, nausea, and diarrhea). Dry mouth may be counteracted by advising the patient to use sugarless gum or candy or by prescribing an oral rinse of 1% pilocarpine used three or four times daily; oral bethanecol may also be effective. Constipation is best dealt with through adequate hydration and the use of bulk laxatives. Antidepressant medications with anticholinergic side effects should be avoided in patients with cognitive impairment, narrow-angle glaucoma, or prostatic hypertrophy. Tricyclic antidepressants may also precipitate anticholinergic delirium, particularly in patients who are elderly or medically compromised.

iii. Sedation

Tricyclic antidepressants also have affinity for histaminergic receptors and produce varying degrees of sedation. In general, tertiary amines cause greater sedation, whereas secondary amines cause less. Sedation often attenuates in the first weeks of treatment, and patients experiencing only minor difficulty from this side effect should be encouraged to allow some time to pass before changing antidepressant medications. Patients with major depressive disorder with insomnia may benefit from sedation when their medication is given as a single dose before bedtime.

iv. Weight gain

Tricyclic antidepressants have the capacity to induce weight gain, possibly through their histaminergic properties. The degree of weight gain appears to vary by agent (e.g., greater weight gain with amitriptyline and less with desipramine), be dose dependent, and be reversible with cessation of tricyclic antidepressant therapy.

v. Neurological effects

Tricyclic antidepressants can induce mild myoclonus (143). Since this may be a sign of toxicity, the clinician may wish to check the blood level (if available) to ensure that it is not excessive. If the level is nontoxic and the myoclonus is not symptomatic, the agent may be continued without a change in dose. If the myoclonus is symptomatic and the blood level is within the recommended range, the patient may be treated with clonazepam at a dose of 0.25 mg t.i.d. Alternatively, the antidepressant medication may be changed. A toxic confusional state has been identified in some patients with high blood levels of tricyclic antidepressant medications, and it responds to simply lowering the dose (144). Amoxapine, a tricyclic antidepressant with antipsychotic properties, can also cause extrapyramidal side effects and tardive dyskinesia. In overdoses, tricyclic antidepressants can precipitate seizures.

vi. Medication interactions

Medications that induce hepatic microsomal enzymes, such as carbamazepine or barbiturates, will cause a decrease in serum tricyclic antidepressant level. On the other hand, drugs such as antipsychotic medications or SSRIs can reduce the metabolism and clearance of tricyclic antidepressants and raise tricyclic antidepressant levels. Tricyclic antidepressants can also alter the pharmacokinetics or pharmacodynamics of other medications; for example, tricyclic antidepressants can cause a lowering of valproate levels and reduce the activity of clonidine. Therefore, adjustments in medication doses may be necessary when tricyclic antidepressants are administered concomitantly with other drugs for which there is an interaction. Potentially dangerous interactions, including hypertensive crises, can develop when tricyclic antidepressants are administered with MAOIs, norepinephrine, or epinephrine.

(2) Selective serotonin reuptake inhibitors

i. Gastrointestinal

SSRIs cause nausea, vomiting, and diarrhea to a greater extent than tricyclic antidepressant medications (145). These adverse events are generally dose dependent and tend to dissipate over the first few weeks of treatment.

ii. Activation/insomnia

In some patients, SSRIs may precipitate or exacerbate restlessness, agitation, and sleep disturbances. These side effects often attenuate with time. Anxiety may be minimized by introducing the agent at a low dose; insomnia may be effectively treated by the addition of trazodone, up to 100 mg at bedtime.

iii. Sexual side effects

Although loss of erectile or ejaculatory function in men and loss of libido and anorgasmia in both sexes may be complications of virtually any antidepressant medication, these side effects appear to be more common with SSRIs. The psychiatrist should ascertain whether the sexual dysfunction is a result of the antidepressant medication or the underlying major depressive disorder. If sexual dysfunction is determined to be a side effect of the antidepressant medication, a variety of strategies are available, including continuing treatment to assess whether the dysfunction will disappear with time, lowering the dose, discontinuing the antidepressant, or substituting another antidepressant such as bupropion (Table 7) (146). Specific pharmacologic treatments that can be added for arousal or erectile dysfunction include sildenafil, yohimbine, or neostigmine; specific medications that can be added for orgasm dysfunction include sildenafil, cyproheptadine, or amantadine (147).

iv. Neurological effects

SSRIs can initially exacerbate both migraine headaches and tension headaches. These effects tend to be transient and improve within the first few weeks of treatment. There is some suggestion that with continued treatment SSRIs may then actually help prevent and treat migraine headaches (148, 149). SSRIs have also been associated with extrapyramidal reactions, including akathisia, dystonia, parkinsonism, and tardive dyskinesia (150, 151). The occurrence of such extrapyramidal symptoms is generally very low but may be higher in older patients, especially those with Parkinson's disease.

v. Effects on weight

Fluoxetine has been shown to cause an initial reduction in weight but this tends to be gained back subsequently (152). The literature differs as to whether patients taking SSRIs beyond the acute phase do (153) or do not (154) experience weight gain as a medication side effect.

vi. Serotonin syndrome

SSRI use has been associated with the rare development of a syndrome due to an excess of serotonergic activity. Features of serotonin syndrome include abdominal pain, diarrhea, flushing, sweating, hyperthermia, lethargy, mental status changes, tremor and myoclonus, rhabdomyolysis, renal failure, cardiovascular shock, and possibly death (155, 156). Although serotonin syndrome can occur with the use of SSRIs alone, it is usually associated with the simultaneous use of multiple serotonergic agents such as SSRIs together with MAOIs, fenfluramine, or dexfenfluramine.

vii. Drug interactions

As previously described, there can be a potentially lethal interaction between SSRIs and MAOIs: serotonin syndrome. It has been suggested that at least five half-lives elapse between the time an SSRI is stopped and an MAOI is started; for fluoxetine discontinuation, this corresponds to waiting approximately 5 weeks before starting an MAOI, whereas for discontinuation of other SSRIs it corresponds to waiting approximately 1 week before starting an MAOI (157). A 2-week waiting period has been suggested after discontinuing an MAOI before starting an SSRI.

SSRIs can also have variable effects on hepatic microsomal enzymes and therefore cause both increases and decreases in the blood levels of other medications.

(3) Other antidepressant medications

i. Trazodone

The most common side effect with trazodone is sedation; this side effect may allow trazodone to be used to advantage in patients with initial insomnia. Trazodone can also cause cardiovascular side effects including orthostasis. Although trazodone does not prolong cardiac conduction, there have been case reports of cardiac arrhythmias developing during trazodone treatment (158, 159). Trazodone can cause sexual side effects, including erectile dysfunction in men; in rare instances, this may lead to irreversible priapism requiring surgical correction (160).

ii. Nefazodone

Side effects observed with nefazodone treatment include dry mouth, nausea, and constipation. Although nefazodone lacks anticholinergic properties, blurred vision has been noted. Nefazodone may also cause sedation and orthostasis but not as severe as that observed with trazodone. Nefazodone is known to inhibit hepatic microsomal enzymes and can raise levels of concurrently administered medications such as certain antihistamines, benzodiazepines, and digoxin.

iii. Bupropion

Neurological side effects have been observed with bupropion treatment including headaches, tremors, and seizures. Risks of seizures can be reduced by avoiding high doses (e.g., using less than 450 mg/day), using divided dosing schedules (e.g., three times a day), and avoiding bupropion use in patients with risk factors for seizures. Bupropion also possesses dopaminergic activity and has been associated with the development of psychotic symptoms, including delusions and hallucinations. For these reasons, bupropion should be used cautiously in patients with psychotic disorders. Other side effects observed with bupropion treatment include insomnia and gastrointestinal upset.

iv. Venlafaxine

The side effects of venlafaxine have been likened to those seen with SSRIs, including nausea and vomiting, sexual dysfunction, and activation; like the side effects seen with SSRIs, those with venlafaxine can attenuate with continued use. Venlafaxine can also cause an increase in blood pressure. Because this increase is dose related, venlafaxine-induced hypertension may respond to dose reduction.

v. Mirtazapine

The most common side effects from mirtazapine include sedation, dry mouth, and weight gain. These tend to occur early and may attenuate with continued treatment. Mirtazapine has also been shown to increase serum cholesterol levels in some patients (161). Although agranulocytosis has been observed to occur in patients taking mirtazapine, its occurrence has been very rare. Routine monitoring of a patient's WBC count is not needed, although checking may be advisable in patients with signs or symptoms of infection.

vi. Reboxetine

The most frequently reported side effects in trials of reboxetine have been dry mouth, constipation, increased sweating, insomnia, urinary hesitancy/retention, impotence, tachycardia, and vertigo (162). In clinical trials done to date, few serious adverse events have been reported among patients treated with reboxetine.

(4) Monoamine oxidase inhibitors

i. Hypertensive crises

A hypertensive crisis can occur when a patient taking an MAOI ingests large amounts of tyramine or other pressor amines in foods or medications. This reaction is characterized by the acute onset of severe headache, nausea, neck stiffness, palpitations, profuse perspiration, and confusion, possibly leading to stroke and death (163). Dietary restrictions include avoiding such foods as aged cheeses or meats, fermented products, yeast extracts, fava or broad beans, and overripe or spoiled foods. The list of medications that must be avoided includes all sympathomimetic and stimulant drugs as well as over-the-counter decongestants and cold remedies.

Some clinicians have recommended that patients carry nifedipine and, at the outset of a possible hypertensive crisis, take an oral dose of 10 mg before proceeding to the hospital (164); this practice has not been approved by the FDA, and further study of the safety and efficacy of this strategy is needed (165). Definitive treatment of hypertensive crises usually involves intravenous administration of phentolamine in an emergency room setting.

ii. Serotonin syndrome

This syndrome most commonly occurs when MAOIs are taken in close proximity to other serotonergic agents (166). When patients are being switched from an SSRI with a short half-life to an MAOI, a waiting period of at least 2 weeks is needed between the discontinuation of one medication and the initiation of the other. When switching from fluoxetine to an MAOI, a waiting period of at least 5 weeks is needed before the MAOI is started. The serotonin syndrome may also occur when venlafaxine is administered soon after an MAOI (167).

iii. Cardiovascular effects

Orthostatic hypotension is commonly seen during MAOI treatment. Possible treatments for this side effect include the addition of salt to increase intravascular volume or use of the steroid fludrocortisone. MAOI use can also be associated with the development of peripheral edema, which may be helped by the use of support stockings.

iv. Weight gain

Weight gain is also commonly seen in patients treated with MAOIs. The likelihood of this side effect appears to vary with the agent used, with most weight gain seen with tranylcypromine and the least with phenelzine.

v. Sexual side effects

Sexual side effects seen with MAOI therapy include anorgasmia, decreased libido, and erectile or ejaculatory dysfunction. Sexual side effects may diminish over time or with reductions in MAOI doses.

vi. Neurological effects

MAOI treatment can also be accompanied by headaches and insomnia; these side effects may diminish over time with continued use. Other neurological effects seen with MAOI use include sedation, myoclonic jerks, paresthesias, and, rarely, peripheral neuropathy.

d) Implementation

Typical starting doses and typical effective adult dose ranges that have been used in short-term efficacy trials of antidepressant medications appear in Table 1. Initial doses should be incrementally raised as tolerated until a presumably therapeutic dose is reached. For some antidepressant medications, the exact relationships between doses and major depressive disorder symptom response have not been rigorously investigated with fixed-dose studies, and minimum effective doses have not been clearly established; for other antidepressant medications, studies have failed to show dose-response relationships (168–170). Therefore, the initial doses and usual adult doses in Table 1 are intended to serve as general guidelines, and actual doses may vary from individual to individual. In general, older patients, medically frail patients, or patients with decreased ability to metabolize and clear antidepressant medications will require lower doses; in such patients, reduction of initial and therapeutic doses to 50% of usual adult doses is often recommended. Doses will also be affected by the side effect profile of medications and the patient's ability to tolerate these.

In short-term efficacy trials, all antidepressant medications appear to require 4–6 weeks to achieve their maximum therapeutic effects (171, 172) (although some patients may show partial improvement by as soon as the end of the first week [173]). Therefore, adequacy of response cannot be judged until after this period of time. Patients should be alerted to this and instructed to continue taking their antidepressant medications throughout this initial period.

For some medications, particularly the tricyclic antidepressants nortriptyline, desipramine, and imipramine, blood drug levels have been shown to correlate with both efficacy and side effects. Although in most cases monitoring of serum antidepressant medication levels is not necessary, in some circumstances this can be very useful. These circumstances can include when patients have not responded to adequate doses of an antidepressant medication given for adequate durations; when patients are particularly vulnerable to the toxic effects of a medication and require the lowest possible effective dose; when there are concerns about patient adherence; and when there is concern that drug-drug interactions are adversely affecting antidepressant medication levels.

Some antidepressant medications, especially tricyclics, can be associated with significant morbidity and potentially mortality in overdose. Ingestion of a 10-day supply of a tricyclic agent administered at a dose of 200 mg/day is often lethal. Early on in treatment, it is prudent to dispense only small quantities of such antidepressant medications and keep in mind the possibility that patients can hoard medications over time. Alternatively, in patients who are suicidal it may be preferable to employ agents that are safer in overdose such as the SSRIs, trazodone, nefazodone, bupropion, venlafaxine, or mirtazapine.

2. Failure to respond to pharmacotherapy in the acute phase

Adequate treatment with an antidepressant medication for at least 4–8 weeks is necessary before concluding that a patient is not responsive or only partially responsive to a particular medication (172). Initial treatment with antidepressant medication fails to achieve a satisfactory response in approximately 20%–30% of patients with major depressive disorder; poor treatment response has been found to be not just the result of inadequate treatment but also a consequence of inappropriate diagnoses; failure to appreciate and remedy coexisting general medical conditions, psychiatric disorders, or complicating psychosocial factors; and nonadherence (174). For these reasons a first step in the care of a patient who has not responded to medication should be a review and reappraisal of the diagnosis, adherence, and neglected contributing factors, including general medical problems, alcohol or substance abuse or dependence, other psychiatric disorders, and general psychosocial issues impeding recovery. In cases where nonadherence or complicating psychosocial stressors are prominent, the addition of psychotherapy may be effective in enhancing response (152).

For patients whose treatment failure is not readily attributable to inappropriate diagnoses, poor adherence, or complicating conditions, a variety of therapeutic options are available, including maximizing the initial treatment, switching to another non-MAOI agent, augmenting antidepressant medications with other medications or psychotherapy, using an MAOI, and ECT (5). Empirical data concerning the relative efficacies of these strategies are limited.

a) Maximizing initial treatments

There is little evidence to support extending antidepressant medication trials beyond 6 weeks in patients who have shown no response. However, for patients who have shown a partial response, particularly those with features of personality disorders and prominent psychosocial stressors, extending the antidepressant medication trial (e.g., by 2–4 weeks) may allow up to one-third of patients to respond more fully (6).

Use of higher antidepressant medication doses is another strategy to maximize an initial treatment regimen, especially for patients who have received only modest doses or those who for pharmacodynamic reasons have low serum drug levels despite adequate doses and adherence.

Unfortunately, with the exception of nortriptyline, therapeutic windows for serum drug levels of most antidepressant medications are unknown. In addition, the strategy of increasing doses is often limited by the occurrence of more frequent and severe side effects.

b) Switching to a different non-MAOI agent

With the introduction of many newer antidepressant medications, switching to a different non-MAOI antidepressant medication has been a common strategy for patients who have failed a trial of pharmacotherapy. A few trials have been conducted in which patients who failed an initial antidepressant medication were switched to a non-MAOI antidepressant medication from the same pharmacologic class (e.g., from one tricyclic antidepressant to another) or to one from a different pharmacologic class (e.g., from a tricyclic antidepressant to an SSRI). Although results from these trials have been variable, up to 50% of patients have been found to respond to a second non-MAOI antidepressant medication trial (5). Data regarding the types of treatment-refractory patients who are most likely to benefit from particular switching strategies are limited. Although their use in this context has not been extensively evaluated, mood stabilizers such as carbamazepine and valproic acid have demonstrated some benefit in the treatment of medication-resistant major depressive disorder (175, 176).

c) Augmenting antidepressant medications with other treatments

Antidepressant medication augmentation strategies often consist of the use of multiple non-MAOI antidepressant medications. An SSRI in combination with a tricyclic agent, such as desipramine, has been reported to induce a rapid antidepressant medication response (50). However, SSRIs added to a tricyclic antidepressant medication may cause an increased blood level and delayed elimination of the tricyclic medication, predisposing the patient to tricyclic medication toxicity unless the dose of the tricyclic is reduced (177).

Lithium is another medication commonly used as an adjunct; other agents in use are thyroid hormone and stimulants. Lithium is felt by many experienced clinicians to be the most effective adjunct; it is reported to be useful in up to 50% of antidepressant medication nonresponders and is usually well tolerated (178). The interval before full response to adjunctive lithium is said to be in the range of several days to 3 weeks. The blood level required in this context has not yet been determined. If effective and well tolerated, lithium should be continued for the duration of treatment of the acute episode. Lithium may also increase the antidepressant medication effectiveness of carbamazepine (179). Thyroid hormone supplementation, even in euthyroid patients, may increase the effectiveness of antidepressant medication treatment (180). The dose proposed for this purpose is 25 μg/day of triiodothyronine, increased to 50 μg/day in a week or so in the event of continued nonresponse. The duration of treatment required has not been well studied. Case reports suggest that stimulant medications may be effective adjuncts to antidepressant medication therapy (181, 182). There are no clear guidelines regarding the length of time stimulants should be coadministered.

A rarely used strategy is the combined use of a tricyclic antidepressant medication and an MAOI. This combination has been shown to be effective in alleviating some severe medication-resistant major depressive disorders; however, the risk of toxic interactions necessitates careful monitoring (183, 184). The combined use of MAOIs and other antidepressant medications has in some circumstances led to serious untoward reactions characterized by delirium, hyperthermia, hyperreflexia, myoclonus, and death; the reaction is sometimes referred to as the serotonin syndrome and is thought to be the result of overly enhanced serotonergic transmission. Use of an MAOI in combination with a tricyclic antidepressant should probably not be considered until all other strategies for treatment-refractory patients have been exhausted; psychiatrists and patients choosing to use an MAOI and a tricyclic antidepressant should be well acquainted with the potential hazards and carefully weigh the relative risks and benefits of such a strategy.

Data indicating the relative efficacies of the various adjunctive treatments are generally lacking.

d) Using a monoamine oxidase inhibitor

The role of MAOIs in major depressive disorder has largely become that of a treatment for patients who have failed other pharmacotherapies. Studies have demonstrated the effectiveness of MAOIs in patients who have failed to respond to other antidepressant medications, particularly tricyclic antidepressants (185). However, the effectiveness of MAOIs relative to other strategies for treatment-resistant patients remains unclear. Great care must be taken when switching patients from another antidepressant medication to an MAOI and from an MAOI to other antidepressant medications because of the persistence of the effects of discontinued medications and their metabolites and the potential for toxic interactions. For example, if the clinician chooses to discontinue a monoamine uptake blocking antidepressant medication and substitute an MAOI, toxic interactions can best be avoided by allowing a 1- to 2-week washout period between medication trials. The long half-life of the SSRI fluoxetine and its metabolites necessitates a 5-week washout period before the use of an MAOI.

e) Using electroconvulsive therapy

ECT has the highest rate of response of any form of antidepressant treatment and should be considered in virtually all cases of moderate or severe major depressive disorder not responsive to pharmacologic intervention. Even medication-resistant patients may show at least a 50% likelihood of a satisfactory response to ECT (186). ECT may also be the strategy of choice for patients with major depressive disorder with psychotic symptoms who have not responded to an antidepressant medication plus antipsychotic medication. ECT is generally considered to be safer than many forms of combination antidepressant medication treatment, although data to support this are lacking. There is growing use of ECT combined with antidepressant medication to potentiate response, although only a small amount of data supporting this practice presently exists (72, 187–191). The safety of combining lithium and ECT has been questioned, although there are conflicting data (72, 192–195).

3. Electroconvulsive therapy

a) Efficacy

ECT has been shown in controlled clinical trials to have efficacy that is superior to placebo, simulated ECT, and antidepressant medication therapy (196). The proportion of patients with major depressive disorder who respond to ECT is high, with 80%–90% of those treated showing improvement (197). Results of several studies indicate that ECT can be effective in over half of patients with major depressive disorder who have failed antidepressant medication therapy (198–200).

The report of the APA Task Force on Electroconvulsive Therapy identified patient populations for whom ECT may be particularly beneficial and indicated (72, 201). ECT should be considered as the treatment choice for severe major depressive disorder when it is coupled with psychotic features, catatonic stupor, severe suicidality, or food refusal leading to nutritional compromise, as well as in other situations (such as pregnancy or when a particularly rapid antidepressant response is required). ECT is also indicated as a first-line treatment for patients who have previously shown a positive response to this treatment modality or who prefer it. It should be considered for all patients with functional impairment whose illness has not responded to medication or who have a medical condition that precludes the use of an antidepressant medication.

b) Side effects

ECT is generally a very safe treatment. However, although risks of morbidity and mortality in general do not exceed those associated with anesthesia alone, some types of serious medical conditions may have an increased risk with ECT as well as with other treatment modalities (72, 202–204). The chief side effects of ECT are cognitive. Treatment is associated with a transient postictal confusional state and with a longer period of anterograde and retrograde memory interference. The anterograde memory impairment, which has been difficult to disentangle from the memory deficits accompanying major depressive disorder itself, typically resolves in a few weeks after cessation of treatment (205). Some degree of retrograde amnesia, particularly for recent memories, may continue, at least for patients receiving bilateral ECT (72, 206–209). Rarely, patients report more pervasive and persistent cognitive disruption, the basis of which is uncertain (210).

ECT may have cardiovascular side effects, mediated by changes on the autonomic nervous system. ECT can cause a transient rise in heart rate, cardiac workload, and blood pressure, which may have deleterious effects on patients with cardiovascular disease, including recent myocardial infarction, congestive heart failure, and cardiac arrhythmias (211). The presence of significant cardiovascular disease in candidates for ECT is an indication for caution and general medical or cardiology consultation.

ECT has also been associated with a transient rise in intracranial pressure and blood-brain barrier permeability (212). For these reasons, patients with evidence of increased intracranial pressure or cerebrovascular fragility are at substantially greater risk and should only receive ECT after careful general medical, neurological, or neurosurgical evaluation (72, 78).

c) Implementation

The evaluation preceding ECT should consist of a psychiatric history and examination to verify the indication for this treatment, a general medical evaluation to define risk factors (including medical history and physical examination with cognitive assessment, vital signs, and any specifically indicated laboratory tests), anesthesia evaluation addressing the nature and extent of anesthetic risk and the need for modification of medications or anesthetic technique, the obtaining of informed consent, and, finally, an evaluation that summarizes treatment indications and risks and suggests any indicated additional evaluative procedures, alterations in treatment, or modifications in ECT technique (72). In assessing cases with indications for caution (e.g., recent myocardial infarction, cardiac arrhythmias, and intracranial-space-occupying lesions), the relative risks and benefits should be carefully weighed in collaboration with an anesthesiologist and a general medical physician, cardiologist, or neurologist, as the case requires.

ECT may be administered either bilaterally or unilaterally. Compared to bilateral treatment, unilateral placement induces less cognitive interference in most patients, but in some cases it is also less effective (213). When unilateral treatment is used, stimuli that are only marginally above seizure threshold exhibit a less satisfactory antidepressant medication effect than those of higher intensity, although this effect must be balanced against the cognitive interference evoked by grossly suprathreshold stimulation. In the event that unilateral treatment is initiated and the patient does not respond satisfactorily to the initial six treatments, bilateral treatment should be considered. Stimulus parameters vary from patient to patient but should be titrated to induce an adequate generalized seizure, which is typically at least 15–25 seconds in duration (72, 214, 215).

The total course of treatment should be such that maximal remission of symptoms is achieved (i.e., the patient fully recovers or reaches a plateau); typically this involves 6 to 12 treatments and generally does not exceed 20 treatments (72, 216). ECT is typically administered every other day; less frequent administration has been associated with less cognitive impairment but also a prolonged period until onset of action (217).

Patients should be maintained on antidepressant medication therapy or lithium following acute response to ECT (218). Patients who do not respond to such maintenance medication therapies may require maintenance ECT treatment (219).

4. Light therapy

Although several trials conducted during the 1980s demonstrated that bright light therapy was more effective than a dim-light control condition, some questions have been raised concerning the adequacy of the study designs (220). However, recent trials with more adequate control conditions have also demonstrated the effectiveness of bright light therapy over nonlight control conditions (221–223). On the basis of limited trial data, bright light therapy has been suggested as a first-line treatment in subsyndromal winter "blues" and as an adjunct in chronic major depressive disorder or dysthymia with seasonal exacerbations. Patients with a history of reactivity to ambient light, hypersomnia, atypical negative symptoms, and overeating of sweet food in the afternoon have also been considered candidates for favorable response to light treatment. On the other hand, studies of the role of light therapy in premenstrual dysphoria or in older patients with nonseasonal major depressive disorder with advanced sleep phase disorder yielded equivocal results.

Side effects of light therapy include headache, eye strain, irritability, insomnia, and occasionally hypomania, which declines by decrease of exposure time and/or distance to light. Although patients with retinal diseases or ordinary photosensitivity, systemic lupus erythematosus, and history of skin cancer are vulnerable, none of these conditions is an absolute contraindication for light therapy. Each condition would require the attention and consultative supervision of the appropriate specialist if the light therapy is to be conducted.

A 10,000-lux intensity light box slanted toward the patient's face for 30 minutes/day either once or in two divided times is the preferred short-term treatment procedure. Timing may be designed to secure adherence. The late-night application is discouraged as it may cause insomnia. Duration of treatment is titrated according to the patient's reaction. Patients usually show improvement within 1 week, but at times the full response manifests over several weeks.

Patients who are responsive may be given light therapy at each episode of recurrence, presumably without any diminished efficacy. Prophylactic use of light therapy administered in the late fall and early winter is being explored. Combining light therapy with an antidepressant medication may potentiate the effectiveness of each agent. Such an approach may be useful if either or both therapies cannot be used in full therapeutic doses. The potential photosensitizing effect of antidepressant medications should be considered, and patients receiving both treatments should be advised to take appropriate precautions.

5. St. John's wort

St. John's wort is a whole plant product with antidepressant medication properties. Since it is not regulated as a drug by the FDA, preparations lack standardization regarding their contained ingredients and composition as well as potency.

A recent review of 14 short-term, double-blind (although the distinctive taste of St. John's wort extract may have caused some unblinding) trials conducted in outpatients with mild to moderate major depressive disorder symptoms demonstrated that St. John's wort had efficacy superior to placebo and generally comparable to low-dose tricyclic treatment (e.g., amitriptyline, 30–150 mg/day) (1). The proportion experiencing any side effect was lower among those taking St. John's wort than tricyclics (25% versus 40%) (1).

Although the doses of St. John's wort used in trials ranged between 300 and 1,800 mg/day, differences in extract preparations make dose comparisons and the identification of optimal doses difficult. The combined use of St. John's wort with MAOIs is contraindicated. The safety and efficacy of the combined use of St. John's wort with other antidepressant medications is not known.

B. ACUTE PHASE PSYCHOSOCIAL INTERVENTIONS

1. Goals

A range of psychosocial interventions may be useful in the acute treatment of major depressive disorder. Although various therapeutic approaches are discussed here and in the literature as distinct entities, such separate categorizations are primarily useful for heuristic or research purposes. In practice, psychiatrists use a combination or synthesis of various approaches and strategies; these in turn are determined by and individually tailored to each patient on the basis of that person's particular conditions and coping capacities. In actual application the techniques and the therapist-patient relationship are powerfully intertwined.

2. Efficacy

Evaluating the efficacy of psychotherapeutic approaches for major depressive disorder can be complicated by several problems. For some types of psychotherapeutic interventions, few or no clinical trials have been conducted. Those that have been conducted have compared psychotherapy to a variety of control conditions such as waiting lists, other forms of psychotherapy, medications, placebos, or no control group, making comparisons of the observed treatment effect sizes between trials difficult. Some trials have not examined the effects of psychotherapy exclusively among patients with major depressive disorder and may not have examined or adequately assessed, specifically, improvement in major depressive disorder as an outcome. In other trials, the nature of the psychotherapeutic intervention has involved a poor protocol or has been poorly described, thereby making generalization of the study results to psychotherapeutic approaches used in practice difficult.

a) Cognitive behavioral therapy

Cognitive behavioral therapy (also considered to include cognitive psychotherapy) maintains that irrational beliefs and distorted attitudes toward the self, the environment, and the future perpetuate depressive affects. The goal of cognitive behavioral therapy is to reduce depressive symptoms by challenging and reversing these beliefs and attitudes (224).

In the two decades since it was first evaluated as a treatment for major depressive disorder, cognitive behavioral therapy has been extensively studied in over 80 controlled trials. Based on different subsets of these trials, several meta-analytic studies have quantified the efficacy of cognitive behavioral therapy. Effect sizes for cognitive behavioral therapy compared to no treatment or minimal treatment have been fairly robust (generally near or above 1 standard deviation in the outcome measure) (53, 225–228). However, estimates from meta-analyses of the effectiveness of cognitive behavioral therapy relative to other treatments have been more inconsistent, probably because of differences in the criteria that were used to include or exclude trials (e.g., characteristics of study populations, interventions or control conditions, or outcome measures used). For example, some meta-analyses have concluded that effect sizes for cognitive behavioral therapy are larger than for pharmacotherapy (225–231), whereas others suggest they are equally effective (232). Effect sizes for cognitive behavioral therapy have generally been at least as large as, and in some cases larger than, for other forms of psychotherapy such as behavior therapy, interpersonal therapy, or brief dynamic psychotherapy (231).

There have been suggestions on the basis of individual clinical trials that the efficacy of cognitive behavioral therapy may differ on the basis of the severity of major depressive disorder. In subanalyses of the National Institute of Mental Health (NIMH) Treatment of Depression Collaborative Research Program study, cognitive behavioral therapy was observed to be less effective than imipramine plus clinical management among individuals with severe depression (defined as scores ≥20 on the Hamilton Rating Scale for Depression or ≤50 on the Global Assessment of Functioning); there was also a trend for cognitive behavioral therapy to be less effective than interpersonal therapy (233). No differences were observed between cognitive behavioral therapy, interpersonal therapy, imipramine plus clinical management, or placebo plus clinical management among less severely depressed subjects. Other trials have failed to show differential responses to treatments on the basis of initial symptom severity, possibly because of lack of statistical power (230, 234).

Several studies have used clinical trial data to identify other characteristics of patients that may be associated with differential response to cognitive behavioral therapy. Factors suggested as being associated with poor response to cognitive behavioral therapy include unemployment, male gender, comorbidity, dysfunctional attitudes, and several laboratory test values (e.g., abnormal sleep EEG results, increased hypothalamic-pituitary-adrenocortical activity, and increased T_4; 235–238). On the other hand, results from several analyses have suggested that cognitive behavioral therapy may be more effective than other treatments for depressed individuals with personality disorders (42, 239).

b) Behavior therapy

Behavior therapy of major depressive disorder is based on theoretical models drawn from behavior theory (240) and social learning theory (241). Specific behavior therapy techniques include activity scheduling (155, 242), self-control therapy (243), social skills training (244), and problem solving (245).

Although the efficacy of behavior therapy has been examined in a substantial number of trials, relatively few have employed random assignments and adequate control arms. Two meta-analyses that covered 10 of these trials have concluded that behavior therapy is superior to wait listing (observed in seven of eight trials) (92, 231). Results of individual clinical trials have suggested that behavior therapy may be superior in efficacy to brief dynamic psychotherapy (246, 247) and generally comparable in efficacy to cognitive therapy (248–251) or pharmacotherapy (252).

One post hoc examination of clinical trial data found that response to behavior therapy may be more likely in patients with less initial severity of major depressive disorder symptoms (253), whereas other studies have not (254–256). Among depressed adolescents, parental involvement has been found to predict response to behavior therapy (257).

c) Interpersonal therapy

Interpersonal therapy focuses on losses, role disputes and transitions, social isolation, deficits in social skills, and other interpersonal factors that may impact the development of depression (258). Interpersonal therapy attempts to intervene by facilitating mourning and promoting recognition of related affects, resolving role disputes and transitions, and overcoming deficits in social skills to permit the acquisition of social supports.

In one trial conducted among depressed psychiatric patients, interpersonal therapy was found to be superior to nonscheduled controls and comparable to other active treatments, including cognitive therapy or antidepressant medication (231). In the NIMH Treatment of Depression Collaborative Research Program study, interpersonal therapy was also reported to be more effective than placebo plus clinical management and comparable to cognitive behavioral therapy or imipramine plus clinical management (42). However, in subanalyses, interpersonal therapy, cognitive behavioral therapy, and imipramine plus clinical management were no different from placebo plus clinical management among those with mild depression severity (defined as scores of <20 on the Hamilton depression rating scale or >50 on the Global Assessment of Functioning); among those with more severe major depressive disorder, both interpersonal therapy and imipramine plus clinical management were more effective than either cognitive behavioral therapy or placebo plus clinical management (233, 259). A controlled trial of interpersonal therapy has also been conducted demonstrating the effectiveness of interpersonal therapy among depressed primary care patients (260). After 8 months, the proportions of patients treated with interpersonal therapy, nortriptyline, or usual care that achieved remission were 46%, 48%, and 18%, respectively.

Some recent studies have also suggested possible subgroups in whom interpersonal therapy may show differential efficacy. In one trial conducted among HIV-positive patients with major depressive disorder, significantly greater improvement was observed following interpersonal therapy than supportive therapy (261). In a subsequent study among depressed HIV-positive patients, greater improvements were observed after interpersonal therapy or interpersonal therapy plus imipramine than supportive psychotherapy or cognitive behavioral therapy (262). On the other hand, post hoc analyses of clinical trial data suggest that there may be an interaction between type of psychotherapy and dimensions of personality. Two such analyses have found that patients with major depressive disorder with personality disorders, particularly avoidant personality pathology, may be less responsive to interpersonal therapy than cognitive therapy (42, 263). Conversely, interpersonal therapy has been proposed to be more effective than cognitive therapy for patients with major depressive disorder with obsessive personality traits and for patients who are single and noncohabitating (264).

d) Psychodynamic psychotherapy

The term "psychodynamic psychotherapy" encompasses a number of psychotherapeutic interventions that may be brief or long-term in duration (265–267). These interventions share a basis in psychodynamic theories regarding the etiologic nature of psychological vulnerability, personality development, and symptom formation as shaped by developmental deficit and conflict occurring during the life cycle from earliest childhood forward (268–272). Some of these theories focus predominantly on conflicts related to guilt, shame, interpersonal relationships, the management of anxiety, and repressed or unacceptable impulses. Others are more focused on developmental psychological deficits produced by inadequacies or problems in the relationship between the child and emotional caretakers, resulting in problems of self-esteem, a sense of psychological cohesiveness, and emotional self-regulation (271, 273–277).

Psychodynamic psychotherapy is most often of longer-term duration than other psychotherapies and is usually associated with goals beyond that of immediate symptom relief. These goals are usually associated with an attempt to modify the underlying psychological conflicts and deficits that increase the patient's vulnerability to major depressive affect and the development of major depressive disorder. Psychodynamic psychotherapy is therefore much broader than most other psychotherapies, encompassing both current and past problems in interpersonal relationships, self-esteem, and developmental conflicts associated with anxiety, guilt, or shame. Time-limited, structured psychodynamic psychotherapy may focus more on understanding the psychological basis of the presenting symptoms or on a selected underlying conflict. It is often combined with psychopharmacologic intervention to reduce the major depressive disorder episode, which is consistent with the common belief that major depressive disorder is a biopsychosocial phenomenon. Sometimes a goal of psychodynamic psychotherapy, brief or extended, may be to help the patient accept or adhere to necessary pharmacotherapy (8).

Determining the efficacy of psychodynamic psychotherapy as a single modality in the treatment of major depressive disorder is complicated by two problems. First, many trials of psychodynamic psychotherapy for depression have included patients with conditions that would not meet DSM-IV criteria for major depressive disorder. Second, variations of psychodynamic psychotherapy have served in many studies as a nonspecific comparison treatment to other psychotherapeutic interventions; as a result, details of the psychodynamic psychotherapy employed have been poorly defined. Results of two meta-analyses suggest that brief psychodynamic psychotherapy for the treatment of major depressive disorder is more effective than a waiting list control condition but probably less effective than other forms of psychotherapy (92, 231). In one of these meta-analyses involving six trials (92), the proportions of patients considered to be responders to brief psychodynamic psychotherapy, cognitive therapy, interpersonal therapy, and behavioral therapy were 35%, 47%, 52%, and 55%, respectively. Research on the efficacy of combined pharmacotherapy and brief psychodynamic psychotherapy (278, 279) is also limited and inconclusive.

Although psychodynamic psychotherapy appears to be used widely in clinical practice, the efficacy of long-term psychodynamic psychotherapy in the acute phase of major depressive disorder has not been adequately studied in controlled trials.

e) Marital therapy and family therapy

Marital and family problems are common in the course of mood disorders, and comprehensive treatment often demands that these problems be assessed and addressed. Marital and family problems may be a consequence of major depressive disorder but may also increase vulnerability to major depressive disorder and in some instances retard recovery (280, 281). Techniques for using marital/family approaches for the treatment of major depressive disorder have been developed, including behavioral approaches (280), a psychoeducational approach, and a strategic marital therapy approach (9). Family therapy has also been used in the inpatient treatment of patients with major depressive disorder (282).

Studies of the efficacy of marital or family therapy, either as a primary or adjunctive treatment, have been conducted among patients with depressive symptoms and not among patients with, specifically, major depressive disorder. Based on data from 17 clinical trials of marital therapy, two reviews have concluded that it is an effective means for reducing major depressive disorder symptoms and risk of relapse (283, 284). Results from individual studies suggest that the efficacy of marital therapy and its effectiveness relative to other psychotherapies may depend on whether marital distress is present. In one study, a greater proportion of depressed subjects with marital distress responded to marital therapy than cognitive therapy (88% versus 71%); on the other hand, among depressed subjects without marital distress, a greater proportion responded to cognitive therapy than marital therapy (85% versus 55%) (285). In another study conducted among depressed subjects with marital discord, marital therapy and cognitive behavioral therapy were both equally effective and more effective than a wait list condition (286).

f) Group therapy

Specific types of psychotherapy for which there are some data to support that they may be effective in the treatment of depression when administered in a group format include cognitive behavioral therapy (287–289) and interpersonal therapy (290–291). Although there have been meta-analyses of the relative effectiveness of psychotherapeutic approaches conducted in a group format versus an individual format, these have not specifically involved studies of patients with rigorously defined major depressive disorder (292–295).

On the basis of very limited controlled studies, supportive group therapy has also been suggested to be useful in the treatment of major depressive disorder. For example, one recent study conducted among depressed outpatients found that a mutual support group and cognitive behavioral therapy in a group format were equally effective in reducing depressive symptoms among depressed outpatients (287). In another study of patients with mild to moderate major depressive disorder who were also HIV positive, treatment with structured supportive group therapy plus placebo yielded similar decreases in depressive symptoms as structured group therapy plus fluoxetine (296). Individuals experiencing bereavement or such common stressors as chronic illness may particularly benefit from the example of others who have successfully dealt with the same or similar challenges. Survivors are offered the opportunity to gain enhanced self-esteem by making themselves models for others, and they offer newer patients successful role models.

Medication maintenance support groups may also offer benefits, although data from controlled trials among patients with major depressive disorder are lacking. Such groups provide information to the patient and to family members regarding prognosis and medication issues, thereby providing a psychoeducational forum that makes a chronic mental illness understandable in the context of a medical model.

The efficacy of self-help groups led by lay members (297) in the treatment of major depressive disorder has not been well studied. However, one recent investigation of group therapies found that a higher proportion of depressed outpatients had remitted following treatment in groups led by professionals than in groups led by nonprofessionals (287). The possibility that self-help support groups comprising individuals with major depressive disorder may serve a useful role by enhancing the support network and self-esteem of participating patients and their families requires future study.

3. Side effects

In general, psychotherapeutic treatments are relatively safe and well-tolerated interventions. Psychotherapeutic approaches that may employ exposure to unpleasant situations (e.g., behavior therapy, cognitive behavioral therapy) may initially increase distress in patients. Psychotherapy that requires considerable time or patience to practice frequent exercises may be poorly tolerated.

One imperfect measure of the relative side effects and tolerability of psychotherapy can be obtained from the dropout rates in clinical trials; however, many other factors can also affect these rates (e.g., other burdens of the research trial, specific features of the clinical management provided). In the NIMH Treatment of Depression Collaborative Research Program, dropout rates during 16 weeks of treatment with interpersonal therapy, cognitive behavioral therapy, imipramine plus clinical management, or placebo plus clinical management were 23%, 32%, 33%, and 40%, respectively (259).

4. Implementation

There can be a variety of methods for conducting psychotherapeutic interventions, both between and within specific types of psychotherapy.

Clinical considerations and other patient factors should be considered in determinations of the nature and intensity of psychosocial interventions. Generally, dynamic psychotherapy is conducted in a less directive manner than behavioral psychotherapy; transference considerations and the patient's freedom to associate into unexpected material are taken into account. More behaviorally oriented psychotherapy, on the other hand, may be conducted in a more structured manner and require patients to be instructed in practice exercises and monitoring techniques.

There are little data available on optimal length of psychosocial interventions. In many trials, cognitive behavioral therapy has been delivered in approximately 12 weekly sessions and interpersonal therapy has been delivered in 16–20 weekly sessions. In a subanalysis of one clinical trial, cognitive behavioral therapy delivered in 16 weeks was more effective than cognitive behavioral therapy delivered in 8 weeks among those with severe major depressive disorder (298).

C. PSYCHOTHERAPY COMBINED WITH PHARMACOTHERAPY

Several reviews of trials of the combination of psychotherapy and pharmacotherapy for patients with mild to moderate major depressive disorder have failed to find the combination to be superior to either treatment modality alone (92, 299). On the other hand, among patients with severe or recurrent major depressive disorder, the combination of psychotherapy (including interpersonal therapy, cognitive behavioral therapy, behavior therapy, or brief dynamic therapy) and pharmacotherapy has been found to be superior to treatment with a single modality in individual studies (38, 300–304) and a meta-analysis (305).

Results from a series of recent studies provide indirect evidence that for patients who have had only a partial response to pharmacotherapy, adding a course of cognitive behavioral therapy may be an effective strategy for preventing relapse (306–309).

D. CONTINUATION TREATMENT

The continuation phase of treatment is generally considered to be the 16–20 weeks after achieving full remission. The goal of continuation treatment is to prevent relapse in the vulnerable period immediately following symptomatic recovery. Several studies have shown that if antidepressant medications are discontinued following recovery, approximately 25% of patients will relapse within 2 months (92, 310, 311). There is evidence that patients who do not completely recover during acute treatment have a significantly higher risk of relapse than those who have no residual symptoms and are especially in need of treatment in later phases (312).

Although randomized controlled trials of antidepressant medications in the continuation phase are limited, the available data indicate that patients treated for a first episode of uncomplicated major depressive disorder who exhibit a satisfactory response to an antidepressant medication should continue to receive a full therapeutic dose of that agent for at least 16–20 weeks after achieving and maintaining full remission (1, 313, 314).

There is some evidence that patients who are given cognitive behavioral therapy in the acute phase have a lower rate of relapse than those who receive and then discontinue antidepressant medications in the acute phase and an equivalent relapse rate to those who take antidepressant medication in the continuation phase (234). There have also been a few recent studies of treatment with psychotherapeutic interventions administered in the continuation phase. One study found that among patients who responded to acute treatment with cognitive therapy, those who continued this treatment over 2 years had lower relapse rates than those who did not have continuation treatment (315). Results from a series of studies (307, 309, 316) suggest that cognitive behavioral therapy may be an effective continuation treatment following antidepressant medication therapy for preventing relapse (306).

When treatments are ultimately tapered and discontinued after the continuation phase, patients should be carefully monitored during and immediately after discontinuation to ensure that remission is stable. Patients who have had multiple prior episodes of major depressive disorder should be considered for maintenance medication treatment.

E. MAINTENANCE TREATMENT

Major depressive disorder is, for many, a recurrent disorder. Among those suffering from an episode of major depressive disorder, between 50% and 85% will go on to have at least one lifetime recurrence, usually within 2 or 3 years (310). Factors that have been found to be associated with a higher risk of recurrence appear in Table 2. Factors that have been found to be associated with increased severity of subsequent episodes include a history of a prior episode complicated by serious suicide attempts, psychotic features, or severe functional impairment.

Among the therapeutic options available for maintenance treatment, antidepressant medications have received the most study. There have been over 20 trials of pharmacotherapy in the maintenance phase, and results from these have generally demonstrated the effectiveness of antidepressant medication for relapse prevention (317); these trials have mainly been of tricyclic antidepressant medications (318, 319), although six trials involved newer antidepressant medications (1). Information to assist in the full range of clinical decisions regarding medication use in the maintenance phase is more limited. Results from one study suggest that full doses are superior to lower doses in the maintenance phase, despite the fact that lower doses are less likely to produce side effects (320).

There have been fewer investigations of the effectiveness of psychotherapy in the maintenance phase. In one study, maintenance cognitive therapy delivered over 2 years was as effective as maintenance medication for recurrent major depressive disorder (228). Another report suggests that interpersonal psychotherapy during the maintenance phase may be effective in lengthening the interepisode interval in some less severely ill patients not receiving medication (318).

The combined use of psychotherapy, such as cognitive behavioral therapy, cognitive therapy, or interpersonal therapy, and pharmacotherapy in the maintenance phase has also been considered by investigators, and some results suggest that the combination of antidepressant medications plus psychotherapy may be additionally effective in preventing relapse over treatment with single modalities (307, 318, 319, 321, 322).

ECT has also been used in the maintenance phase, although evidence for its benefits comes largely from case reports (197, 219, 323, 324). The optimal frequency and duration of maintenance phase ECT treatments has not been well studied.

The timing and method of discontinuing maintenance treatment has not been systematically studied. However, the risk of cholinergic rebound observed with abrupt discontinuation of some antidepressant medications together with concerns about major depressive disorder recurrences after the discontinuation of any antidepressant medication argue in favor of gradual tapering (325).

PART C: FUTURE RESEARCH NEEDS

Notable progress has been made in our understanding of major depressive disorder and its treatment, including the introduction of a variety of therapeutic agents and treatment modalities. However, many issues remain regarding how to optimally use these treatments to achieve the best health outcomes for patients with major depressive disorder. The following are a few of the types of research questions that require future study.

VI. ANTIDEPRESSANT MEDICATIONS

In terms of the use of antidepressant medications during the acute, continuation, and maintenance phases of treatment, many important questions remain.

1. What are the specific clinical indications for the use of particular antidepressant medications?
2. What are the relative efficacies of different antidepressant medications?
3. What are the relationships between antidepressant blood levels and response?
4. What are the relative risks of toxicities (e.g., cardiotoxicity) and adverse effects for different antidepressant medications?
5. What should the duration of treatment be before a patient is considered medication-resistant, and does this duration vary among agents?
6. Does the combination of antidepressants from different pharmacologic classes (e.g., SSRIs and tricyclic antidepressants) offer greater efficacy than administration of single agents?
7. What are the comparative efficacies of different antidepressant medications in the continuation and maintenance phases?
8. What are the long-term side effects of chronic use of specific antidepressant medications?
9. What is the required duration of maintenance treatment with antidepressants?
10. What are indications for a trial of discontinuation of maintenance treatment?

VII. PSYCHOTHERAPY

Many issues concerning the use of psychotherapy in the treatment of major depressive disorder during the acute, continuation, and maintenance phases also require clarification. The disparity between the widespread use of psychodynamic psychotherapy in practice and the complete lack of rigorous studies of its efficacy must be addressed. In particular, there is a critical need to design and implement rigorous, controlled studies to evaluate the efficacy and effectiveness of psychodynamic psychotherapy for the treatment of patients with major depressive disorder.

In addition, the following are critical issues:

1. What are the relative efficacies of different psychotherapeutic approaches in the acute phase of treatment?
2. What components or aspects of specific psychotherapeutic approaches are responsible for efficacy? What common elements of all effective psychotherapeutic approaches are responsible for efficacy?
3. What are the indications (e.g., subtypes of depressive disorders) for use of various forms of psychotherapy?
4. What are the efficacies of particular psychotherapeutic approaches in the continuation and maintenance phases of treatment?
5. Is the use of multiple forms of psychotherapy, either concurrently or sequentially, effective?
6. What are the optimal frequencies of psychotherapeutic contact for the various forms of psychotherapy in the acute, continuation, and maintenance phases?

VIII. ELECTROCONVULSIVE THERAPY

Regarding ECT, additional research is needed to clarify several important issues.

1. What are indications for initial treatment with bilateral electrode placement?
2. After how many unilateral treatments without satisfactory response should a switch from unilateral to bilateral electrode placement be made?
3. Can the efficacy or tolerability of ECT be increased with adjunctive antidepressant and antipsychotic agents?
4. What are the indications and best methods for providing maintenance ECT?

IX. OTHER TREATMENT MODALITIES

In addition to research on the treatments covered above, additional rigorous investigation is needed to answer questions concerning other therapeutic modalities.

1. What are the indications, relative efficacies, and safety of specific treatments such as lithium or thyroid hormone as adjuncts to antidepressant medications for nonresponders?
2. Is light therapy effective as an adjunct in nonseasonal major depressive disorder or as a primary treatment for seasonal major depressive disorder in the maintenance phase?

X. INDIVIDUALS AND ORGANIZATIONS THAT SUBMITTED COMMENTS

David A. Adler, M.D.
Carl Bell, M.D.
Dan G. Blazer II, M.D., Ph.D.
Philip Boyce, M.D.
David S. Brody, M.D.
Robert M. Chaflin, M.D.
Margaret J. Dorfman, M.D.
Peter Ellis, Ph.D.
Aaron H. Fink, M.D.
Michael Gales, M.D.
Linda Gochfeld, M.D.
David A. Gorelick, M.D., Ph.D.
James A. Greene, M.D.
Diane Keddy, M.S., R.D.
Sidney H. Kennedy, M.D.
Donald F. Klein, M.D.
James H. Kocsis, M.D.
K. Roy Mackenzie, M.D.
John C. Markowitz, M.D.
David A. Moltz, M.D.
Vaughn I. Rickert, Psy.D.
Peter Ross
Teresa A. Rummans, M.D.
Henry L. Shapiro, M.D.
Don Smith
Michael Thase, M.D.
Richard Weiner, M.D., Ph.D.
Josef H. Weissberg, M.D.
Myrna M. Weissman, Ph.D.
Rhonda Whitson, R.R.A.
William M. Zurhellen, M.D.

American Academy of Psychoanalysis
American Association of Community Psychiatrists
American College of Emergency Physicians
American Dietetic Association
American Society of Clinical Psychopharmacology, Inc.
Black Psychiatrists of America
Royal Australian & New Zealand College of Psychiatrics
Society for Adolescent Medicine

XI. REFERENCES

The following coding system is used to indicate the nature of the supporting evidence in the references:

[A] *Randomized clinical trial.* A study of an intervention in which subjects are prospectively followed over time; there are treatment and control groups; subjects are randomly assigned to the two groups; both the subjects and the investigators are blind to the assignments.

[B] *Clinical trial.* A prospective study in which an intervention is made and the results of that intervention are tracked longitudinally; study does not meet standards for a randomized clinical trial.

[C] *Cohort or longitudinal study.* A study in which subjects are prospectively followed over time without any specific intervention.

[D] *Case-control study.* A study in which a group of patients and a group of control subjects are identified in the present and information about them is pursued retrospectively or backward in time.

[E] *Review with secondary analysis.* A structured analytic review of existing data (e.g., a meta-analysis or a decision analysis).

[F] *Review.* A qualitative review and discussion of previously published literature without a quantitative synthesis of the data.

[G] *Other.* Textbooks, expert opinion, case reports, and other reports not included above.

1. Agency for Healthcare Policy Research: Evidence Report on Treatment of Depression—Newer Pharmacotherapies. San Antonio Evidence-Based Practice Center. Washington, DC, AHCPR, Evidence-Based Practice Centers, 1999 [F]
2. American Psychiatric Association: Practice Guideline for the Treatment of Patients With Bipolar Disorder (Revised). Am J Psychiatry 2002; 159(April suppl) [G]
3. American Psychiatric Association: Practice Guideline for Psychiatric Evaluation of Adults. Am J Psychiatry 1995; 152(Nov suppl):63–80 [G]
4. Lin EHB, von Korff M, Katon W, Bush T, Simon GE, Walker E, Robinson P: The role of the primary care physician in patients' adherence to antidepressant therapy. Med Care 1995; 33:67–74 [B]
5. Thase ME, Rush AJ: Treatment-resistant depression, in Psychopharmacology: The Fourth Generation of Progress. Edited by Bloom F, Kupfer DJ. New York, Raven Press, 1995, pp 1081–1097 [F]
6. Frank E, Kupfer DJ: Axis II personality disorders and personality features in treatment-resistant and refractory depression, in Treatment Strategies for Refractory Depression. Edited by Roose SP, Glassman AH. Washington, DC, American Psychiatric Press, 1990, pp 207–221 [F]
7. Goldman W, McCulloch J, Cuffel B, Zarin DA, Suarez A, Burns BJ: Outpatient utilization patterns of integrated and split psychotherapy and pharmacotherapy for depression. Psychiatr Serv 1998; 49:477–482 [G]
8. Gray SH: Developing practice guidelines for psychoanalysis. J Psychother Pract Res 1996; 5:213–227 [F]
9. Coyne JC: Strategic therapy, in Affective Disorders and the Family: Assessment and Treatment. Edited by Clarkin JF, Haas GL, Glick JD. New York, Guilford, 1988, pp 89–113 [F]
10. Lejoyeux M, Ades J: Antidepressant discontinuation: a review of the literature. J Clin Psychiatry 1997; 58(suppl 7):11–16 [F]
11. Coupland NJ, Bell CJ, Potokar JP: Serotonin reuptake inhibitor withdrawal. J Clin Psychopharmacol 1996; 16:356–362 [D]
12. Glassman AH, Roose SP: Delusional depression. Arch Gen Psychiatry 1981; 38:424–427 [E]
13. Spiker DG, Weiss JC, Dealy RS, Griffin SJ, Hanin I, Neil JF, Perel JM, Rossi AJ, Soloff PH: The pharmacological treatment of delusional depression. Am J Psychiatry 1985; 142:430–436 [A]
14. Price LH, Conwell Y, Nelson JC: Lithium augmentation of combined neuroleptic-tricyclic treatment in delusional depression. Am J Psychiatry 1983; 140:318–322 [E]
15. Kantor SJ, Glassman AH: Delusional depression: natural history and response to treatment. Br J Psychiatry 1977; 131:351–360 [E]
16. Fink M, Taylor MA: Catatonia: a separate category for DSM-IV? Integrative Psychiatry 1991; 7:2–10 [G]
17. Liebowitz MR, Quitkin FM, Stewart JW, McGrath PJ, Harrison WM, Markowitz JS, Rabkin JG, Tricamo E, Goetz DM, Klein DF: Antidepressant specificity in atypical depression. Arch Gen Psychiatry 1988; 45:129–137 [A]
18. Davidson JR, Miller R, Turnbull CD, Sullivan JL: Atypical depression. Arch Gen Psychiatry 1982; 39:527–534 [G]

19. Quitkin FM, Harrison W, Stewart JW, McGrath PJ, Tricamo E, Ocepek-Welikson K, Rabkin JG, Wager SG, Nunes E, Klein DF: Response to phenelzine and imipramine in placebo nonresponders with atypical depression: a new application of the crossover design. Arch Gen Psychiatry 1991; 48:319–323 [A]
20. Quitkin FM, Stewart JW, McGrath PJ, Liebowitz MR, Harrison WM, Tricamo E, Klein DF, Rabkin JG, Markowitz JS, Wager SG: Phenelzine versus imipramine in the treatment of probable atypical depression: defining syndrome boundaries of selective MAOI responders. Am J Psychiatry 1988; 145:306–311 [A]
21. Goodnick PJ: Acute and long-term bupropion therapy: response and side effects. Ann Clin Psychiatry 1991; 3:311–313 [C]
22. Goodnick PJ, Extein I: Bupropion and fluoxetine in depressive subtypes. Ann Clin Psychiatry 1989; 1:119–122 [C]
23. Pande AC, Birkett M, Fechner-Bates S, Haskett RF, Greden JF: Fluoxetine versus phenelzine in atypical depression. Biol Psychiatry 1996; 40:1017–1020 [A]
24. Sands BF, Ciraulo DA: Cocaine drug-drug interactions. J Clin Psychopharmacol 1992; 12:49–55 [G]
25. Grunhaus L: Clinical and psychobiological characteristics of simultaneous panic disorder and major depression. Am J Psychiatry 1988; 145:1214–1221 [F]
26. Schatzberg AF, Ballenger JC: Decisions for the clinician in the treatment of panic disorder: when to treat, which treatment to use, and how long to treat. J Clin Psychiatry 1991; 52:26–31 [G]
27. Sheehan DV, Davidson JR, Manschreck T, Van Wyck Fleet J: Lack of efficacy of a new antidepressant (bupropion) in the treatment of panic disorder with phobias. J Clin Psychopharmacol 1983; 3:28–31 [C]
28. Clomipramine Collaborative Study Group: Clomipramine in the treatment of patients with obsessive-compulsive disorder. Arch Gen Psychiatry 1991; 48:730–738 [A]
29. Jenike MA, Buttolph L, Baer L, Ricciardi J, Holland A: Open trial of fluoxetine in obsessive-compulsive disorder. Am J Psychiatry 1989; 146:909–911 [A]
30. Stoudemire A, Hill C, Gulley LR, Morris R: Neuropsychological and biomedical assessment of depression-dementia syndromes. J Neuropsychiatry Clin Neurosci 1989; 1:347–361 [C]
31. Caine ED: Pseudodementia: current concepts and future directions. Arch Gen Psychiatry 1981; 38:1359–1364 [F]
32. Akiskal HS, Rosenthal TL, Haykal RF, Lemmi H, Rosenthal RH: Characterological depressions: clinical and sleep EEG findings separating subaffective dysthymias from character spectrum disorders. Arch Gen Psychiatry 1980; 37:777–783 [B]
33. Howland RH: Pharmacotherapy of dysthymia: a review. J Clin Psychopharmacol 1991; 11:83–92 [G]
34. Keller MD, Hanks DL, Klein DN: Summary of the DSM-IV mood disorders field trial and issue overview. Psychiatr Clin North Am 1996; 19:1–28 [F]
35. Thase ME, Reynolds CF, Frank E, Simons AD: Response to cognitive-behavioral therapy in chronic depression. J Psychotherapy Practice and Research 1994; 3:204–214 [B]
36. Conte HR, Karasu TB: A review of treatment studies of minor depression 1980–1981. Am J Psychother 1992; 46:58–74 [F]
37. Frances AJ: An introduction to dysthymia. Psychiatr Annals 1993; 23:607–608 [F]
38. Keller MD, McCullough JP, Rush AJ, Klein DF, Schatzberg AF, Gelenberg J, Thase ME: Nefazodone HCI, cognitive behavioral analysis system of psychotherapy and combination therapy for the acute treatment of chronic depression, in 1999 Annual Meeting New Research Program and Abstracts. Washington, DC, American Psychiatric Association, 1999, p 178 [A]
39. Kocsis JH, Frances AJ, Voss CB, Mann JJ, Mason BJ, Sweeney J: Imipramine treatment for chronic depression. Arch Gen Psychiatry 1988; 45:253–257 [A]
40. Shea MT, Glass DR, Pilkonis PA, Watkins J, Docherty JP: Frequency and implications of personality disorders in a sample of depressed outpatients. J Personal Disord 1987; 1:27–42 [C]

41. Parsons B, Quitkin FM, McGrath PJ, Stewart JW, Tricamo E, Ocepek-Welikson K, Harrison W, Rabkin JG, Wager SG, Nunes E: Phenelzine, imipramine, and placebo in borderline patients meeting criteria for atypical depression. Psychopharmacol Bull 1989; 25:524–534 [A]
42. Shea MT, Pilkonis PA, Beckham E, Collins JF, Elkin I, Sotsky SM, Docherty JP: Personality disorders and treatment outcome in the NIMH Treatment of Depression Collaborative Research Program. Am J Psychiatry 1990; 147:711–718 [A]
43. Rosenthal NE, Sack DA, Carpenter CJ, Parry BL, Mendelson WB, Wehr TA: Antidepressant effects of light in seasonal affective disorder. Am J Psychiatry 1985; 142:163–170 [C]
44. American Psychiatric Association: Diagnostic and Statistical Manual of Mental Disorders, 4th ed. Washington, DC, APA, 1994 [G]
45. Zisook S, Shuchter SR: Depression through the first year after the death of a spouse. Am J Psychiatry 1991; 148:1346–1352 [C]
46. Escobar JI, Gomez J, Tuason VB: Depressive phenomenology in North and South American patients. Am J Psychiatry 1983; 140:47–51 [C]
47. Escobar JI, Tuason VB: Antidepressant agents: a cross-cultural study. Psychopharmacol Bull 1980; 16:49–52 [C]
48. Marcos LR, Cancro R: Psychopharmacotherapy of Hispanic depressed patients: clinical observations. Am J Psychother 1982; 36:505–512 [F]
49. Marcos LR, Uruyo L, Kesselman M, Alpert M: The language barrier in evaluating Spanish-American patients. Arch Gen Psychiatry 1973; 29:655–659 [C]
50. Nelson JC, Mazure CM, Bowers MBJ, Jatlow PI: A preliminary, open study of the combination of fluoxetine and desipramine for rapid treatment of major depression. Arch Gen Psychiatry 1991; 48:303–307 [C]
51. American Academy of Child and Adolescent Psychiatry: Practice Parameters for the Assessment and Treatment of Children and Adolescents With Depressive Disorders. Washington, DC, AACAP, 1998 [G]
52. Reynolds CF, Frank E, Perel JM, Imber SD, Cornes C, Miller MD, Mazumdar S, Houck PR, Dew MA, Stack JA, Pollock BG, Kupfer DJ: Nortriptyline and interpersonal psychotherapy as maintenance therapies for recurrent major depression: a randomized controlled trial in patients older than 59 years. JAMA 1999; 281:39–45 [A]
53. Robinson RG, Starkstein SE: Current research in affective disorders following stroke. J Neuropsychiatry Clin Neurosci 1990; 2:1–14 [F]
54. Nelson JC, Jatlow PI, Mazure CM: Rapid desipramine dose adjustment using 24-hour levels. J Clin Psychopharmacol 1987; 7:72–77 [C]
55. Wisner KL, Gelenberg AJ, Leonard H, Zarin D, Frank E: Pharmacologic treatment of depression during pregnancy. JAMA 1999; 282:1264–1269 [F]
56. Chambers CD, Johnson KA, Dick LM, Felix RJ, Jones KL: Birth outcomes in pregnant women taking fluoxetine. N Engl J Med 1996; 335:1010–1015 [B]
57. Nurnberg HG: An overview of somatic treatment of psychosis during pregnancy and postpartum. Gen Hosp Psychiatry 1989; 11:328–338 [F]
58. Gitlin MJ, Pasnau RO: Psychiatric syndromes linked to reproductive function in women: a review of current knowledge. Am J Psychiatry 1989; 146:1413–1422 [F]
59. Brockington IF, Cernik KF, Schofield EM, Downing AR, Francis AF, Keelan C: Puerperal psychosis: phenomena and diagnosis. Arch Gen Psychiatry 1981; 38:829–833 [C]
60. Ananth J: Side effects in the neonate from psychotropic agents excreted through breast feeding. Am J Psychiatry 1978; 135:801–805 [E]
61. Altshuler LL, Cohen L, Szuba MP, Burt VK, Gitlin M, Mintz J: Pharmacologic management of psychiatric illness during pregnancy: dilemmas and guidelines. Am J Psychiatry 1996; 153: 592–606 [E]

62. Akiskal HS, Walker P, Puzantian VR, King D, Rosenthal TL, Dranon M: Bipolar outcome in the course of depressive illness: phenomenologic, familial, and pharmacologic predictors. J Affect Disord 1983; 5:115–128 [A]
63. Nelson JC, Kennedy JS, Pollock BG, Laghrissi-Thode F, Narayan M, Nobler MS, Robin DW, Gergel I, McCafferty J, Roose S: Treatment of major depression with nortriptyline and paroxetine in patients with ischemic heart disease. Am J Psychiatry 1999; 156:1024–1028 [A]
64. Bigger JT, Giardina EG, Perel JM, Kantor SJ, Glassman AH: Cardiac antiarrhythmic effect of imipramine hydrochloride. N Engl J Med 1977; 296:206–208 [G]
65. Connolly SJ, Mitchell LB, Swerdlow CD, Mason JW, Winkle RA: Clinical efficacy and electrophysiology of imipramine for ventricular tachycardia. Am J Cardiol 1984; 53:516–521 [B]
66. Dalack GW, Roose SP, Glassman AH: Tricyclics and heart failure (letter). Am J Psychiatry 1991; 148:1601 [E]
67. Giardina EG, Barnard T, Johnson L, Saroff AL, Bigger JT, Louie M: The antiarrhythmic effect of nortriptyline in cardiac patients with ventricular premature depolarizations. J Am Coll Cardiol 1986; 7:1363–1369 [E]
68. Glassman AH, Johnson LL, Giardina EG, Walsh BT, Roose SP, Cooper TB, Bigger JT: The use of imipramine in depressed patients with congestive heart failure. JAMA 1983; 250:1997–2001 [C]
69. Roose SP, Glassman AH, Giardina EG, Walsh BT, Woodring S, Bigger JT: Tricyclic antidepressants in depressed patients with cardiac conduction disease. Arch Gen Psychiatry 1987; 44:273–275 [A]
70. Schwartz P, Wolf S: QT interval prolongation as predictor of sudden death in patients with myocardial infarction. Circulation 1978; 57:1074–1077 [G]
71. Applegate RJ: Diagnosis and management of ischemic heart disease in the patient scheduled to undergo electroconvulsive therapy. Convuls Ther 1997; 13:128–144 [F]
72. The Practice of Electroconvulsive Therapy: Recommendations for Treatment, Training, and Privileging: A Task Force Report of the American Psychiatric Association. Washington, DC, APA, 1990 [G]
73. Dolinski SY, Zvara DA: Anesthetic considerations of cardiovascular risk during electroconvulsive therapy. Convuls Ther 1997; 13:157–164 [E]
74. Rayburn BK: Electroconvulsive therapy in patients with heart failure or valvular heart disease. Convuls Ther 1997; 13:145–156 [F]
75. Weiner RD, Coffey CE, Krystal AD: Electroconvulsive therapy in the medical and neurologic patient, in Psychiatric Care of the Medical Patient, 2nd ed. Edited by Stoudemire A, Fogel B, Greenberg D. New York, Oxford University Press, 1999 [F]
76. Roose SP, Dalack GW, Glassman AH, Woodring S, Walsh BT, Giardina EGV: Cardiovascular effects of bupropion in depressed patients with heart disease. Am J Psychiatry 1991; 148:512–516 [C]
77. Roose SP, Glassman AH, Giardina EG, Johnson L, Walsh BT, Bigger JT: Cardiovascular effects of imipramine and bupropion in depressed patients with congestive heart failure. J Clin Psychopharmacol 1987; 7:247–251 [A]
78. Krystal AD, Coffey CE: Neuropsychiatric considerations in the use of electroconvulsive therapy. J Neuropsychiatry Clin Neurosci 1997; 9:283–292 [F]
79. Lieberman E, Stoudemire A: Use of tricyclic antidepressants in patients with glaucoma. Psychosomatics 1987; 28:145–148 [G]
80. Thase ME: Effects of venlafaxine on blood pressure: a meta-analysis of original data on 3744 depressed patients. J Clin Psychiatry 1998; 59:502–508 [E]
81. Goetz CG, Tanner CM, Klawans HL: Bupropion in Parkinson's disease. Neurology 1984; 34:1092–1094 [C]

82. Monoamine oxidase inhibitors for depression. Med Lett Drugs Ther 1980; 22:58–60 [G]
83. Andersen K, Balldin J, Gottfries CG, Granerus AK, Modigh K, Svennerholm L, Wallin A: A double-blind evaluation of electroconvulsive therapy in Parkinson's disease with on-off phenomena. Acta Neurol Scand 1987; 76:191–199 [A]
84. Regier DA, Boyd JH, Burke JD Jr, Rae DS, Myers JK, Kramer M, Robins LN, George LK, Karno M, Locke BZ: One-month prevalence of mental disorders in the United States: based on five Epidemiologic Catchment Area sites. Arch Gen Psychiatry 1988; 45:977–986 [A]
85. Pincus HA, Zarin DZ, Tanielian TL, Johnson JL, West JC, Petit AR, Marcus SC, Kessler RC, McIntyre JS: Psychiatric patients and treatments in 1997: findings from the American Psychiatric Practice Research Network. Arch Gen Psychiatry 1999; 56:442–449 [C]
86. Mueller TI, Leon AC, Keller MB, Solomon DA, Endicott J, Coryell W, Warshaw M, Maser JD: Recurrence after recovery from major depressive disorder during 15 years of observational follow-up. Am J Psychiatry 1999; 156:1000–1006 [B]
87. Klerman GL, Weissman MM: The course, morbidity and costs of depression. Arch Gen Psychiatry 1992; 49:831–834 [G]
88. Keller MD, Beardslee WR, Dorer DJ, Lavori PW, Samuelson H, Klerman GL: Impact of severity and chronicity of parental affective illness on adaptive functioning and psychopathology in children. Arch Gen Psychiatry 1986; 43:930–937 [B]
89. Mintz J, Mintz LI, Arruda MJ, Hwang SS: Treatments of depression and the functional capacity to work. Arch Gen Psychiatry 1992; 49:761–768 [E]
90. Kuhn R: The treatment of depressive states with G22355 (imipramine hydrochloride). Am J Psychiatry 1958; 115:459–464 [B]
91. Brotman AW, Falk WE, Gelenberg AJ: Pharmacologic treatment of acute depressive subtypes, in Psychopharmacology: The Third Generation of Progress. Edited by Meltzer HY. New York, Raven Press, 1987, pp 1031–1040 [F]
92. Depression Guideline Panel: Clinical Practice Guideline Number 5: Depression in Primary Care, Treatment of Major Depression: HHS Publication 93-0551. Rockville, Md, Agency for Health Care Policy and Research, 1993 [E]
93. Klein DF, Gittelman R, Quitkin FM, Rifkin A: Diagnosis and Drug Treatment of Psychiatric Disorders: Adults and Children, 2nd ed. Baltimore, Williams & Wilkins, 1980 [G]
94. Klerman GL, Cole JO: Clinical pharmacology of imipramine and related antidepressant compounds. Int J Psychiatry 1967; 3:267–304 [F]
95. Potter WZ, Manji HK, Rudorfer MV: Tricyclics and tetracyclics, in American Psychiatric Press Textbook of Psychopharmacology, 2nd ed. Edited by Schatzberg AF, Nemeroff CB. Washington, DC, American Psychiatric Press, 1998, pp 199–218 [F]
96. Coryell W, Turner R: Outcome and desipramine therapy in subtypes of non-psychotic major depression. J Affect Disord 1985; 9:149–154 [B]
97. Fairchild CJ, Rush AJ, Vasavada N, Giles DE, Khatami M: Which depressions respond to placebo? Psychiatry Res 1986; 18:217–226 [B]
98. Joyce PR, Paykel ES: Predictors of drug response in depression. Arch Gen Psychiatry 1989; 46:89–99 [F]
99. Stewart JW, Quitkin FM, Liebowitz MR, McGrath PJ, Harrison WM, Klein DF: Efficacy of desipramine in depressed outpatients: response according to Research Diagnostic Criteria diagnoses and severity of illness. Arch Gen Psychiatry 1989; 40:220–227 [A]
100. Paykel ES: Depressive typologies and response to amitriptyline. Br J Psychiatry 1972; 120:147–156 [B]
101. Raskin A, Crook TA: The endogenous-neurotic distinction as a predictor of response to antidepressant drugs. Psychol Med 1976; 6:59–70 [G]
102. Danish University Antidepressant Group: Paroxetine: a selective serotonin reuptake inhibitor showing better tolerance but weaker antidepressant effect than clomipramine in a controlled multicenter study. J Affect Disord 1990; 18:289–299 [A]

103. Perry PJ: Pharmacotherapy for major depression with melancholic features: relative efficacy of tricyclic versus selective serotonin reuptake inhibitor antidepressants. J Affect Disord 1996; 39:1–6 [F]
104. Paykel ES: Treatment of depression: the relevance of research for clinical practice. Br J Psychiatry 1989; 155:754–763 [F]
105. Anderson IM, Tomenson BM: Treatment discontinuation with selective serotonin reuptake inhibitors compared with tricyclic antidepressants: a meta-analysis. Br Med J 1995; 310:1433–1438 [E]
106. Rickels K, Schweizer E: Clinical overview of serotonin reuptake inhibitors. J Clin Psychiatry 1990; 51:9–12 [F]
107. Delgado PL, Price LH, Charney DS, Heninger GR: Efficacy of fluvoxamine in treatment-refractory depression. J Affect Disord 1988; 15:55–60 [B]
108. Golden RN, Brown TM, Miller H, Evans DL: The new antidepressants. NC Med J 1988; 49:549–554 [F]
109. Schatzberg AF: Trazodone: a 5-year review of antidepressant efficacy. Psychopathology 1987; 20(suppl 1):48–56 [F]
110. Cunningham LA, Borison RL, Carman JS, Chouinard G, Crowder JE, Diamond BI, Fischer DE, Hearst E: A comparison of venlafaxine, trazodone, and placebo in major depression. J Clin Psychopharmacol 1994; 14:99–106 [A]
111. Weisler RH, Johnston JA, Lineberry CG, Samara B, Branconnier RJ, Billow AA: Comparison of bupropion and trazodone for the treatment of major depression. J Clin Psychopharmacol 1994; 14:170–179 [A]
112. Klein HE, Muller N: Trazodone in endogenous depressed patients: a negative report and a critical evaluation of the pertaining literature. Prog Neuropsychopharmacol Biol Psychiatry 1985; 9:173–186 [B]
113. Shopsin B, Cassano GB, Conti L: An overview of new second generation antidepressant compounds: research and treatment implications, in Antidepressants: Neurochemical, Behavioral and Clinical Perspectives. Edited by Enna SJ, Malick J, Richelson E. New York, Raven Press, 1981, pp 219–251 [F]
114. Feighner JP, Pambakian R, Fowler RC, Boyer WF, D'Amico MF: A comparison of nefazodone, imipramine, and placebo in patients with moderate to severe depression. Psychopharmacol Bull 1989; 25:219–221 [A]
115. Fontaine R, Ontiveros A, Elie R, Kensler TT, Roberts DL, Kaplita S, Ecker JA, Faludi G: A double-blind comparison of nefazodone, imipramine, and placebo in major depression. J Clin Psychiatry 1994; 55:234–241 [A]
116. Mendels J, Reimherr F, Marcus RN, Roberts DL, Francis RJ, Anton SF: A double-blind, placebo-controlled trial of two dose ranges of nefazodone in the treatment of depressed outpatients. J Clin Psychiatry 1995; 56(suppl 6):30–36 [A]
117. Pitts WM, Fann WE, Halaris AE, Dressler DM, Sajadi C, Snyder S, Ilaria RL: Bupropion in depression: a tri-center placebo-controlled study. J Clin Psychiatry 1983; 44(5, pt 2): 95–100 [A]
118. Chouinard G: Bupropion and amitriptyline in the treatment of depressed patients. J Clin Psychiatry 1983; 44:121–129 [A]
119. Davidson J, Miller R, Van Wyck Fleet J, Strickland R, Manberg P, Allen S, Parrott R: A double-blind comparison of bupropion and amitriptyline in depressed patients. J Clin Psychiatry 1983; 44:115–117 [B]
120. Feighner J, Hendrickson G, Miller L, Stern W: Double-blind comparison of doxepin vs bupropion in outpatients with major depressive disorder. J Clin Psychopharmacol 1986; 6:27–32 [A]
121. Mendels J, Amin MM, Chouinard G, Cooper AJ, Miles JE, Remick RA, Saxena B, Secunda SK, Singh AN: A comparative study of bupropion and amitriptyline in depressed outpatients. J Clin Psychiatry 1983; 44:118–120 [A]

122. Feighner JP, Gardner EA, Johnston JA, Batey SR, Khayrallah MA, Ascher JA, Lineberry CG: Double-blind comparison of bupropion and fluoxetine in depressed outpatients. J Clin Psychiatry 1991; 52:329–335 [A]
123. Claghorn JL, Lesem MD: A double-blind placebo-controlled study of Org 3770 in depressed outpatients. J Affect Disord 1995; 34:165–171 [A]
124. Guelfi JD, White C, Hackett D, Guichoux JY, Magni G: Effectiveness of venlafaxine in patients hospitalized with major depression and melancholia. J Clin Psychiatry 1995; 56:450–458 [A]
125. Holm KJ, Markham A: Mirtazapine: a review of its use in major depression. CNS Drugs 1999; 57:607–631 [F]
126. Kasper S: Clinical efficacy of mirtazapine: a review of meta-analyses of pooled data. Int Clin Psychopharmacol 1995; 10(suppl 4):25–35; correction, 1996; 11:153 [F]
127. Schweizer E, Feighner J, Mandos LA, Rickels K: Comparison of venlafaxine and imipramine in the acute treatment of major depression in outpatients. J Clin Psychiatry 1994; 55:104–108 [A]
128. Zivkov M, DeJongh G: Org 3770 versus amitriptyline: a 6-week randomized, double-blind multicentre trial in hospitalized depressed patients. Human Psychopharmacology 1995; 10:173–180 [B]
129. Kelsey JE: Dose-response relationship with venlafaxine. J Clin Psychopharmacol 1996; 16 (suppl 2):21S–28S [A]
130. Montgomery SA: Reboxetine: additional benefits to depressed patients. J Psychopharmacol 1997; 11(4 suppl):S9–S15 [F]
131. Davidson J, Raft D, Pelton S: An outpatient evaluation of phenelzine and imipramine. J Clin Psychiatry 1987; 48:143–146 [B]
132. Himmelhoch JM, Thase ME, Mallinger AG, Houck P: Tranylcypromine versus imipramine in anergic bipolar depression. Am J Psychiatry 1991; 148:910–916 [A]
133. McGrath PJ, Stewart JW, Harrison W, Wager S, Quitkin FM: Phenelzine treatment of melancholia. J Clin Psychiatry 1986; 47:420–422 [B]
134. Quitkin FM, Rifkin A, Klein DF: Monoamine oxidase inhibitors: a review of antidepressant effectiveness. Arch Gen Psychiatry 1979; 36:749–760 [F]
135. Thase ME, Trivedi MH, Rush AJ: MAOIs in the contemporary treatment of depression. Neuropsychopharmacology 1995; 12:185–219 [E]
136. White K, Razani J, Cadow B, Gelfand R, Palmer R, Simpson G, Sloane RB: Tranylcypromine vs nortriptyline vs placebo in depressed outpatients: a controlled trial. Psychopharmacology (Berl) 1984; 82:259–262 [B]
137. Quitkin FM, McGrath PJ, Stewart JW, Harrison W, Tricamo E, Wager SG, Ocepek-Welikson K, Nunes E, Rabkin JG, Klein DF: Atypical depression, panic attacks, and response to imipramine and phenelzine: a replication. Arch Gen Psychiatry 1990; 47:935–941 [A]
138. Zisook S, Braff DL, Click MA: Monoamine oxidase inhibitors in the treatment of atypical depression. J Clin Psychopharmacol 1985; 5:131–137 [A]
139. Himmelhoch JM, Fuchs CZ, Symons BJ: A double-blind study of tranylcypromine treatment of major anergic depression. J Nerv Ment Dis 1982; 170:628–634 [A]
140. Thase ME, Mallinger AG, McKnight D, Himmelhoch JM: Treatment of imipramine-resistant recurrent depression, IV: a double-blind crossover study of tranylcypromine for anergic bipolar depression. Am J Psychiatry 1992; 149:195–198 [A]
141. Stoudemire A, Atkinson P: Use of cyclic antidepressants in patients with cardiac conduction disturbance. Gen Hosp Psychiatry 1988; 10:389–397 [G]
142. Veith RC, Raskind MA, Caldwell JH, Barnes RF, Gumbrecht G, Ritchie JL: Cardiovascular effects of tricyclic antidepressants in depressed patients with chronic heart disease. N Engl J Med 1982; 306:954–959 [A]
143. Garvey MJ, Tollefson GD: Occurrence of myoclonus in patients treated with cyclic antidepressants. Arch Gen Psychiatry 1987; 44:269–272 [E]

144. Preskorn SH, Jerkovich GS: Central nervous system toxicity of tricyclic antidepressants: phenomenology, course, risk factors, and role of therapeutic drug monitoring. J Clin Psychopharmacol 1990; 10:88–95 [E]
145. Frazer A: Antidepressants. J Clin Psychiatry 1997; 58:9–25 [F]
146. Walker PW, Cole JO, Gardner EA, Hughes AR, Johnston JA, Batey SR, Lineberry CG: Improvement in fluoxetine-associated sexual dysfunction in patients switched to bupropion. J Clin Psychiatry 1993; 54:459–465 [B]
147. Pollack MH, Rosenbaum JF: Management of antidepressant-induced side effects: a practical guide for the clinician. J Clin Psychiatry 1987; 48:3–8 [G]
148. Doughty MJ, Lyle WM: Medications used to prevent migraine headaches and their potential ocular adverse effects. Optom Vis Sci 1995; 72:879–891 [F]
149. Hamilton JA, Halbreich U: Special aspects of neuropsychiatric illness in women: with a focus on depression. Annu Rev Med 1993; 44:355–364 [F]
150. Gerber PE, Lynd LD: Selective serotonin-reuptake inhibitor-induced movement disorders. Ann Pharmacother 1998; 32:692–698 [E]
151. Leo RJ: Movement disorders associated with the serotonin selective reuptake inhibitors. J Clin Psychiatry 1996; 57:449–454 [E]
152. Marcus ER, Bradley SS: Combination of psychotherapy and psychopharmacotherapy with treatment-resistant inpatients with dual diagnoses. Psychiatr Clin North Am 1990; 13:209–214 [E]
153. Bouwer CD, Harvey BH: Phasic craving for carbohydrate observed with citalopram. Int Clin Psychopharmacol 1996; 11:273–278 [B]
154. Michelson D, Amsterdam JD, Quitkin FM, Reimherr F, Rosenbaum JF, Zajecka J, Sundell KL, Kim Y, Beasley CM Jr: Changes in weight during a 1-year trial of fluoxetine. Am J Psychiatry 1999; 156:1170–1176 [A]
155. Lewinsohn PM, Antonuccio DA, Steinmetz-Breckinridge J, Teri L: The Coping With Depression Course: A Psychoeducational Intervention for Unipolar Depression. Eugene, Ore, Castalia Publishing, 1984 [G]
156. Metz A, Shader RI: Adverse interactions encountered when using trazodone to treat insomnia associated with fluoxetine. Int Clin Psychopharmacol 1990; 5:191–194 [G]
157. Beasley CM Jr, Masica DN, Heiligenstein JH, Wheadon DE, Zerbe RL: Possible monoamine oxidase inhibitor-serotonin uptake inhibitor interaction: fluoxetine clinical data and preclinical findings. J Clin Psychopharmacol 1993; 13:312–320 [F]
158. Vitullo RN, Wharton JM, Allen NB, Pritchett EL: Trazodone-related exercise-induced nonsustained ventricular tachycardia. Chest 1990; 98:247–248 [G]
159. Aronson MD, Hafez H: A case of trazodone-induced ventricular tachycardia. J Clin Psychiatry 1986; 47:388–389 [G]
160. Thompson JW Jr, Ware MR, Blashfield RK: Psychotropic medication and priapism: a comprehensive review. J Clin Psychiatry 1990; 51:430–433 [F]
161. Davis R, Wilde MI: Mirtazapine: a review of its pharmacology and therapeutic potential in the management of major depression. CNS Drugs 1996; 5:389–402 [F]
162. Mucci M: Reboxetine: a review of antidepressant tolerability. J Psychopharmacol 1997; 11(4 suppl):S33–S37 [F]
163. Gardner DM, Shulman KI, Walker SE, Tailor SAN: The making of a user friendly MAOI diet. J Clin Psychiatry 1996; 57:99–104 [F]
164. Schenk CH, Remick RA: Sublingual nifedipine in the treatment of hypertensive crisis associated with monoamine oxidase inhibitors (letter). Ann Emerg Med 1989; 18:114–115 [B]
165. Grossman E, Messerli FH, Grodzicki T, Kowey P: Should a moratorium be placed on sublingual nifedipine capsules given for hypertensive emergencies and pseudoemergencies? JAMA 1996; 276:1328–1331 [F]
166. Sternbach H: The serotonin syndrome. Am J Psychiatry 1991; 148:705–713 [F]

167. Gelenberg AJ: Serotonin syndrome update. Biological Therapies in Psychiatry Newsletter 1997; 20:33–34 [F]
168. Beasley CM Jr, Sayler ME, Cunningham GE, Weiss AM, Masica DN: Fluoxetine in tricycylic refractory major depressive disorder. J Affect Disord 1990; 20:193–200 [B]
169. Jenner PN: Paroxetine: an overview of dosage, tolerability, and safety. Int Clin Psychopharmacol 1992; 6(suppl 4):69–80 [F]
170. Montgomery SA, Pedersen V, Tanghoj P, Rasmussen C, Rioux P: The optimal dosing regimen for citalopram—a meta-analysis of nine placebo-controlled studies. Int Clin Psychopharmacol 1994; 9(suppl 1):35–40 [E]
171. Quitkin FM, Rabkin JG, Markowitz JM, Stewart JW, McGrath PJ, Harrison W: Use of pattern analysis to identify true drug response. Arch Gen Psychiatry 1987; 44:259–264 [A]
172. Quitkin FM, Rabkin JG, Ross D, McGrath PJ: Duration of antidepressant drug treatment: what is an adequate trial? Arch Gen Psychiatry 1984; 41:238–245 [G]
173. Katz MM, Koslow SH, Maas JW, Frazer A, Bowden CL, Casper R, Croughan J, Kocsis J, Redmond E Jr: The timing, specificity and clinical prediction of tricyclic drug effects in depression. Psychol Med 1987; 17:297–309 [C]
174. Guscott R, Grof P: The clinical meaning of refractory depression: a review for the clinician. Am J Psychiatry 1991; 148:695–704 [G]
175. Cullen M, Mitchell P, Brodaty H, Boyce P, Parker G, Hickie I, Wilhem K: Carbamazepine for treatment-resistant melancholia. J Clin Psychiatry 1991; 52:472–476 [C]
176. Hayes SG: Long-term use of valproate in primary psychiatric disorders. J Clin Psychiatry 1989; 50:35–39 [D]
177. Rosenstein DL, Takeshita J, Nelson JC: Fluoxetine-induced elevation and prolongation of tricyclic levels in overdose (letter). Am J Psychiatry 1991; 148:807 [E]
178. Price LH, Charney DS, Heninger GR: Variability of response to lithium augmentation in refractory depression. Am J Psychiatry 1986; 143:1387–1392 [C]
179. Kramlinger KG, Post RM: The addition of lithium to carbamazepine: antidepressant efficacy in treatment-resistant depression. Arch Gen Psychiatry 1989; 46:794–800 [C]
180. Prange AJ, Loosen PT, Wilson IC, Lipton MA: The therapeutic use of hormones of the thyroid axis in depression, in The Neurobiology of Mood Disorders. Edited by Post R, Ballenger J. Baltimore, Williams & Wilkins, 1984, pp 311–322 [G]
181. Feighner JP, Herbstein J, Damlouji N: Combined MAOI, TCA, and direct stimulant therapy of treatment-resistant depression. J Clin Psychiatry 1985; 46:206–209 [G]
182. Wharton RN, Perel JM, Dayton PG, Malitz S: A potential clinical use for methylphenidate (Ritalin) with tricyclic antidepressants. Am J Psychiatry 1971; 127:1619–1625 [E]
183. Razani J, White KL, White J, Simpson G, Sloane RB, Rebal R, Palmer R: The safety and efficacy of combined amitriptyline and tranylcypromine antidepressant treatment: a controlled trial. Arch Gen Psychiatry 1983; 40:657–661 [A]
184. Young JPR, Lader MH, Hughes WC: Controlled trial of trimipramine, monoamine oxidase inhibitors, and combined treatment in depressed outpatients. Br Med J 1979; 2:1315–1317 [A]
185. Devlin MJ, Walsh BT: Use of monoamine oxidase inhibitors in refractory depression, in American Psychiatric Press Review of Psychiatry, vol 9. Edited by Tasman A, Goldfinger SM, Kaufmann CA. Washington, DC, American Psychiatric Press, 1990, pp 74–90 [F]
186. Prudic J, Sackeim HA: Refractory depression and electroconvulsive therapy, in Treatment Strategies for Refractory Depression. Edited by Roose SP, Glassman AH. Washington, DC, American Psychiatric Press, 1990, pp 111–128 [G]
187. El-Ganzouri A, Ivankovich AD, Braverman B, McCarthy R: Monoamine oxidase inhibitors: should they be discontinued preoperatively? Anesth Analg 1985; 64:592–596 [B]
188. Klapheke MM: Combining ECT and antipsychotic agents: benefits and risks. Convuls Ther 1993; 9:241–255 [F]
189. Klapheke MM: Electroconvulsive therapy consultation: an update. Convuls Ther 1997; 13:227–241 [F]

190. Lauritzen L, Odgaard K, Clemmesen L, Lunde M, Ohrstrom J, Black C, Bech P: Relapse prevention by means of paroxetine in ECT-treated patients with major depression: a comparison with imipramine and placebo in medium-term continuation therapy. Acta Psychiatr Scand 1996; 94:241–251 [A]
191. Nelson JP, Benjamin L: Efficacy and safety of combined ECT and tricyclic antidepressant therapy in the treatment of depressed geriatric patients. Convuls Ther 1989; 5:321–329 [E]
192. Penney JF: Concurrent and close temporal administration of lithium and ECT. Convuls Ther 1990; 6:139–145 [D]
193. Hill GE, Wong KC, Hodges MR: Potentiation of succinylcholine neuromuscular blockade by lithium carbonate. Anesthesiology 1976; 44:439–442 [E]
194. Jha AK, Stein GS, Fenwick P: Negative interaction between lithium and electroconvulsive therapy—a case control study. Br J Psychiatry 1996; 168:241–243 [D]
195. Lippman SB, Tao CA: Electroconvulsive therapy and lithium: safe and effective treatment. Convuls Ther 1993; 9:54–57 [G]
196. Janicak PG, Davis JM, Gibbons RD, Ericksen S, Chang S, Gallagher P: Efficacy of ECT: a meta-analysis. Am J Psychiatry 1985; 142:297–302 [E]
197. Weiner RD: Electroconvulsive therapy, in Treatments of Psychiatric Disorders. Edited by Gabbard GO. Washington, DC, American Psychiatric Press, 1995, pp 1237–1262 [G]
198. Devanand DP, Sackeim HA, Prudic J: Electroconvulsive therapy in the treatment-resistant patient. Psychiatr Clin North Am 1991; 14:905–923 [F]
199. Avery D, Winokur G: The efficacy of electroconvulsive therapy and antidepressants in depression. Biol Psychiatry 1977; 12:507–523 [F]
200. Paul SM, Extein I, Calil HM, Potter WZ, Chodoff P, Goodwin FK: Use of ECT with treatment-resistant depressed patients at the National Institute of Mental Health. Am J Psychiatry 1981; 138:486–489 [B]
201. The Practice of Electroconvulsive Therapy: Recommendations for Treatment, Training, and Privileging: A Task Force Report of the American Psychiatric Association. Washington, DC, APA, 1990 [G]
202. Abrams R: The mortality rate with ECT. Convuls Ther 1997; 13:125–127 [G]
203. Fink M: Efficacy and safety of induced seizures (ECT) in man. Compr Psychiatry 1978; 19:1–18 [F]
204. Gomez J: Subjective side-effects of ECT. Br J Psychiatry 1975; 127:609–611 [B]
205. Stoudemire A, Hill CD, Morris R, Dalton ST: Improvement in depression-related cognitive dysfunction following ECT. J Neuropsychiatry Clin Neurosci 1995; 7:31–34 [B]
206. McElhiney MC, Moody BJ, Steif BL, Prudic J, Devanand DP, Nobler MS, Sackeim HA: Autobiographical memory and mood: effects of electroconvulsive therapy. Neuropsychology 1995; 9:501–517 [A]
207. Sobin C, Sackeim HA, Prudic J, Devanand DP, Moody BJ, McElhiney MC: Predictors of retrograde amnesia following ECT. Am J Psychiatry 1995; 152:995–1001 [A]
208. Squire LR, Slater PC, Miller PL: Retrograde amnesia and bilateral electroconvulsive therapy: long-term follow-up. Arch Gen Psychiatry 1981; 38:89–95 [C]
209. Weiner RD, Rogers HJ, Davidson JR, Squire LR: Effects of stimulus parameters on cognitive side effects. Ann NY Acad Sci 1986; 462:315–325 [B]
210. Squire LR, Slater PC: Electroconvulsive therapy and complaints of memory dysfunction: a prospective three-year follow-up study. Br J Psychiatry 1983; 142:1–8 [B]
211. Dec GW Jr, Stern TA, Welch C: The efforts of electroconvulsive therapy on serial electrocardiograms and serum cardiac enzyme values: a prospective study of depressed hospitalized inpatients. JAMA 1985; 253:2525–2529 [B]
212. Abrams R: Electroconvulsive Therapy, 3rd ed. New York, Oxford University Press, 1997 [G]
213. Sackeim HA, Prudic J, Devanand DP, Kiersky JE, Fitzsimons L, Moody BJ, McElhiney MC, Coleman EA, Settembrino JM: Effects of stimulus intensity and electrode placement

on the efficacy and cognitive effects of electroconvulsive therapy. N Engl J Med 1993; 328:839–846 [A]
214. Krystal AD, Weiner RD: ECT seizure therapeutic adequacy. Convuls Ther 1994; 10:153–164 [F]
215. Weiner RD, Coffey CE, Krystal AD: The monitoring and management of electrically induced seizures. Psychiatr Clin North Am 1991; 14:845–869 [F]
216. Hales RE, Yudofsky SC, Talbott JA (eds): The American Psychiatric Press Textbook of Psychiatry, 3rd ed. Washington, DC, American Psychiatric Press, 1999 [G]
217. Lerer B, Shapira B, Calev A, Tubi N, Drexler H, Kindler S, Lidsky D, Schwartz JE: Antidepressant and cognitive effects of twice- versus three-times-weekly ECT. Am J Psychiatry 1995; 152:564–570 [A]
218. Shapira B, Gorfine M, Lerer B: A prospective study of lithium continuation therapy in depressed patients who have responded to electroconvulsive therapy. Convuls Ther 1995; 11:80–85 [B]
219. Schwarz T, Loewenstein J, Isenberg KE: Maintenance ECT: indications and outcome. Convuls Ther 1995; 11:14–23 [B]
220. Terman M, Terman JS, Quitkin FM, McGrath PJ, Stewart JW, Rafferty B: Light therapy for seasonal affective disorder: a review of efficacy. Neuropsychopharmacology 1989; 2:1–22 [B]
221. Eastman CI, Young MA, Fogg LF, Liu L, Meaden PM: Bright light treatment of winter depression: a placebo-controlled trial. Arch Gen Psychiatry 1998; 55:883–889 [B]
222. Terman M, Terman JS, Ross DC: A controlled trial of timed bright light and negative air ionization for treatment of winter depression. Arch Gen Psychiatry 1998; 55:875–882 [B]
223. Lewy AJ, Bauer VK, Cutler NL, Sack RL, Ahmed S, Thomas KH, Blood ML, Jackson JM: Morning versus evening light treatment of patients with winter depression. Arch Gen Psychiatry 1998; 55:890–896 [B]
224. Beck AT, Rush AJ, Shaw BF, Emery G: Cognitive Therapy of Depression. New York, Guilford, 1979 [G]
225. Gloaguen V, Cottraux J, Cucherat M, Blackburn IM: A meta-analysis of the effects of cognitive therapy in depressed patients. J Affect Disord 1998; 49:59–72 [E]
226. Dobson KS: A meta-analysis of the efficacy of cognitive therapy for depression. J Consult Clin Psychol 1989; 57:414–419 [E]
227. Gaffan EA, Tsaousis I, Kemp-Wheeler SM: Researcher allegiance and meta-analysis: the case of cognitive therapy for depression. J Consult Clin Psychol 1995; 63:966–980 [E]
228. Blackburn IM, Moore RG: Controlled acute and follow-up trial of cognitive therapy and pharmacotherapy in out-patients with recurrent depression. Br J Psychiatry 1997; 171:328–334 [B]
229. DeRubeis RJ, Gelfand LA, Tang TZ, Simons AD: Medications versus cognitive behavior therapy for severely depressed outpatients: mega-analysis of four randomized comparisons. Am J Psychiatry 1999; 156:1007–1013 [E]
230. Hollon SD, DeRubeis RJ, Evans MD, Wierner MJ, Garvey MJ, Grove WM, Tuason VB: Cognitive therapy and pharmacotherapy for depression. Arch Gen Psychiatry 1992; 49:774–781 [A]
231. Jarrett RB, Rush AJ: Short-term psychotherapy of depressive disorders: current status and future directions. Psychiatry 1994; 57:115–132 [F]
232. Clark DM, Salkovskis PM, Hackmann A, Middleton H, Anastasiades P, Gelder M: A comparison of cognitive therapy, applied relaxation and imipramine in the treatment of panic disorder. Br J Psychiatry 1994; 164:759–769 [B]
233. Elkin I, Shea MT, Watkins JT, Imber SD, Sotsky SM, Collins JF, Glass DR, Pilkonis PA, Leber WR, Docherty JP: National Institute of Mental Health Treatment of Depression Collaborative Research Program: general effectiveness of treatments. Arch Gen Psychiatry 1989; 46:971–982 [F]

234. Evans MD, Hollong SD, Garvey MJ, Piasecki JM, Grove WM, Garvey MJ, Tuason VB: Differential relapse following cognitive therapy and pharmacotherapy for depression. Arch Gen Psychiatry 1992; 49:802–808 [B]
235. Joffe R, Segal Z, Singer W: Change in thyroid hormone levels following response to cognitive therapy for major depression. Am J Psychiatry 1996; 153:411–413 [B]
236. Thase ME, Dubé S, Bowler K, Howland RH, Myers JE, Friedman E, Jarrett DB: Hypothalamic-pituitary-adrenocortical activity and response to cognitive behavior therapy in unmedicated, hospitalized depressed patients. Am J Psychiatry 1996; 153:886–891 [B]
237. Thase ME, Simons AD, Reynolds CF: Abnormal electroencephalographic sleep profiles in major depression: association with response to cognitive behavior therapy. Arch Gen Psychiatry 1996; 53:99–108 [B]
238. Blatt SJ, Quinlan DM, Zuroff DC, Pilkonis PA: Interpersonal factors in brief treatment of depression: further analyses of the National Institute of Mental Health Treatment of Depression Collaborative Research Program. J Consult Clin Psychol 1996; 64:162–171 [F]
239. Patience DA, McGuire RJ, Scott AI, Freeman CP: The Edinburgh Primary Care Depression Study: personality disorders and outcome. Br J Psychiatry 1995; 167:324–330
240. Ferster CB: A functional analysis of depression. Am Psychol 1973; 10:857–870 [F]
241. Bandura A: Social Learning Theory. Englewood Cliffs, NJ, Prentice-Hall, 1977 [G]
242. Lewinsohn PM, Clarke G: Group treatment of depressed individuals: the Coping With Depression Course. Advances in Behavioral Research and Therapy 1984; 6:99–114 [F]
243. Rehm LP: Behavior Therapy for Depression. New York, Academic Press, 1979 [G]
244. Bellack AS, Hersen M: A comparison of social-skills training, pharmacotherapy and psychotherapy for depression. Behav Res Ther 1983; 21:101–107 [A]
245. Nezu AM: Efficacy of a social problem-solving therapy for unipolar depression. J Consult Clin Psychol 1986; 54:196–202 [A]
246. McLean PD, Hakstian AR: Clinical depression: comparative efficacies of outpatient treatments. J Consult Clin Psychol 1979; 47:818–836 [F]
247. Steuer JL, Mintz J, Hammen CL, Hill MA, Jarvik LF, McCarley T, Motoike P, Rosen R: Cognitive-behavioral and psychodynamic group psychotherapy in treatment of geriatric depression. J Consult Clin Psychol 1984; 52:180–189 [B]
248. Beach SR, O'Leary KD: Extramarital sex: impact on depression and commitment in couples seeking marital therapy. J Sex Marital Ther 1985; 11:99–108 [D]
249. Jacobson NS, Dobson K, Fruzetti AE, Schmaling KB, Salusky S: Marital therapy as a treatment for depression. J Consult Clin Psychol 1991; 59:547–557 [G]
250. Rabin AS, Kaslow NJ, Rehm LP: Factors influencing continuation in a behavioral therapy. Behav Res Ther 1985; 23:695–698 [C]
251. Thompson JK, Williams DE: An interpersonally based cognitive-behavioral psychotherapy. Prog Behav Modif 1987; 21:230–258 [G]
252. Miller IW, Norman WH, Keitner GI, Bishop SB: Cognitive-behavioral treatment of depressed inpatients. Behavior Therapy 1989; 20:25–47 [B]
253. Taylor S, McLean P: Outcome profiles in the treatment of unipolar depression. Behav Res Ther 1993; 31:325–330 [B]
254. McLean P, Taylor S: Severity of unipolar depression and choice of treatment. Behav Res Ther 1992; 30:443–451 [A]
255. Rohde P, Lewinsohn PM, Seeley JR: Response of depressed adolescents to cognitive-behavioral treatment: do differences in initial severity clarify the comparison of treatments? J Consult Clin Psychol 1994; 62:851–854 [B]
256. Thase ME, Simons AD, Cahalane J, McGeary J, Harden T: Severity of depression and response to cognitive behavior therapy. Am J Psychiatry 1991; 148:784–789 [B]
257. Kendall PC, Morris RJ: Child therapy: issues and recommendations. J Consult Clin Psychol 1991; 59:777–784 [F]

258. Klerman GL, Weissman MM, Rounsaville BJ, Chevron ES: Interpersonal Psychotherapy of Depression. New York, Basic Books, 1984 [G]
259. Elkin I, Shea MT, Watkins JT, Imber SD, Sotsky SM, Collins JF, Glass DR, Pilkonis PA, Leber WR, Docherty JP, Fiester SJ, Parloff MB: National Institute of Mental Health Treatment of Depression Collaborative Research Program: general effectiveness of treatments. Arch Gen Psychiatry 1989; 46:971–982 [A]
260. Schulberg HC, Block MR, Madonia MJ, Scott CP, Rodriguez E, Imber SD, Perel J, Lave J, Houck PR, Coulehan JL: Treating major depression in primary care practice: eight-month clinical outcomes. Arch Gen Psychiatry 1996; 53:913–919 [A]
261. Markowitz JC, Klerman GL, Clougherty KF, Spielman LA, Jacobsberg LB, Fishman B, Frances AJ, Kocsis JH, Perry SW III: Individual psychotherapies for depressed HIV-positive patients. Am J Psychiatry 1995; 152:1504–1509 [B]
262. Markowitz JC, Kocsis J, Fishman B, Spielman LA, Jacobsberg LB, Frances AJ, Klerman GL, Perry SW: Treatment of depressive symptoms in human immunodeficiency virus-positive patients. Arch Gen Psychiatry 1998; 55:452–457 [B]
263. Hardy GE, Barkham M, Shapiro DA, Reynolds S, Rees A, Stiles WB: Credibility and outcome of cognitive-behavioural and psychodynamic-interpersonal psychotherapy. Br J Clin Psychol 1995; 34:555–569 [F]
264. Barber JP, Muenz LR: The role of avoidance and obsessiveness in matching patients to cognitive and interpersonal psychotherapy: empirical findings from the Treatment for Depression Collaborative Research Program. J Consult Clin Psychol 1996; 64:951–958 [B]
265. Bash M: Understanding Psychotherapy: The Science Behind the Art. New York, Basic Books, 1988 [G]
266. Bibring E: Psychoanalysis and the dynamic psychotherapies. J Am Psychoanal Assoc 1954; 2:745–770 [G]
267. Gray SH: Quality assurance and utilization review of individual medical psychotherapies, in Manual of Quality Assurance Review. Edited by Mattson MR. Washington, DC, American Psychiatric Press, 1992, pp 159–166 [F]
268. Blatt SJ: Contributions of psychoanalysis to the understanding and treatment of depression. J Am Psychoanal Assoc 1998; 46:722–752 [F]
269. Brenner C: Depression, anxiety and affect theory. J Psychoanal 1974; 55:25–32 [G]
270. Freud S: Mourning and melancholia (1917 [1915]), in Complete Psychological Works, standard ed, vol 14. London, Hogarth Press, 1957, pp 243–258 [G]
271. Kohut H: Thoughts on narcissism and narcissistic rage. Psychoanal Study Child 1972; 27:360–400 [G]
272. Zetzel ER: On the incapacity to bear depression (1965), in The Capacity for Emotional Growth. New York, International Universities Press, 1970, pp 82–224 [G]
273. Loewald HW: Perspectives on memory (1972), in Papers on Psychoanalysis. New Haven, Conn, Yale University Press, 1980, pp 148–173 [G]
274. Tasman A, Kay J, Lieberman JA: Psychiatry. Philadelphia, WB Saunders, 1996 [G]
275. Brenner C: Psychoanalytic Technique and Psychic Conflict. New York, International Universities Press, 1976 [F]
276. Rado S: The problem of melancholia (1927), in Psychoanalysis of Behavior: Collected Papers. New York, Grune & Stratton, 1956 [G]
277. Karasu TB: Developmentalist metatheory of depression and psychotherapy. Am J Psychother 1992; 46:37–49 [F]
278. Covi L, Lipman RS, Derogatis LR, Smith JE III, Pattison JH: Drugs and group psychotherapy in neurotic depression. Am J Psychiatry 1974; 131:191–198 [A]
279. Daneman EA: Imipramine in office management of depressive reactions (a double-blind study). Dis Nerv Syst 1961; 22:213–217 [A]
280. Beach SRH, Sandeen EE, O'Leary KD: Depression in Marriage. New York, Guilford, 1990 [G]

281. Yager J: Mood disorders and marital and family problems, in American Psychiatric Press Review of Psychiatry, vol 11. Edited by Tasman A, Riba MB. Washington, DC, American Psychiatric Press, 1992, pp 477–493 [G]
282. Coyne JC, Kessler RC, Tal M, Turnball J, Wortman CB, Greden JF: Living with a depressed person. J Consult Clin Psychol 1987; 55:347–352 [F]
283. Hahlweg K, Markman HJ: Effectiveness of behavioral marital therapy: empirical status of behavioral techniques in preventing and alleviating marital distress. J Consult Clin Psychol 1988; 56:440–447 [F]
284. Jacobson NS, Martin B: Behavioral marriage therapy: current status. Psychol Bull 1976; 83:540–556 [F]
285. Jacobson N, Addis M: Research on couples and couple therapy: what do we know? where are we going? J Consult Clin Psychol 1993; 61:85–93 [F]
286. O'Leary KD, Beach SR: Marital therapy: a viable treatment for depression and marital discord. Am J Psychiatry 1990; 147:183–186 [A]
287. Bright JI, Baker KD, Neimeyer RA: Professional and paraprofessional group treatments for depression: a comparison of cognitive-behavioral and mutual support interventions. J Consult Clin Psychol 1999; 67:491–501 [A]
288. Neimeyer RA, Baker KD, Haykal RF, Akiskal HS: Patterns of symptomatic change in depressed patients in a private inpatient mood disorders program. Bull Menninger Clin 1995; 59:460–471 [C]
289. Neimeyer RA, Feixas G: The role of homework and skill acquisition in the outcome of group cognitive therapy for depression. Behavior Therapy 1990; 21:281–292 [B]
290. MacKenzie RR: Anti-depression interpersonal psychotherapy groups (IPT-G): preliminary effectiveness data. Society for Psychotherapy Research Conference, 1999 [B]
291. Yalom ID: The Theory and Practice of Group Psychotherapy, 4th ed. New York, Basic Books, 1995 [G]
292. Smith ML, Glass GV, Miller TI: The Benefits of Psychotherapy. Baltimore, Johns Hopkins University Press, 1980 [G]
293. Toseland RW, Siporin M: When to recommend group treatment: a review of the clinical and group literature. Int J Group Psychother 1986; 36:171–201 [F]
294. Piper WE, Joyce AS: A consideration of factors influencing utilization of time-limited short-term group therapy. Int J Group Psychother 1996; 46:311–328 [F]
295. McRoberts C, Burlingame GM, Hoag MJ: Comparative efficacy of individual and group psychotherapy: a meta-analytic perspective. Group Dynamics: Theory, Research, and Practice 1998; 2:101–117 [E]
296. Targ EF, Karasic DH, Diefenbach PN, Anderson DA, Bystritsky A, Fawzy FI: Structured group therapy and fluoxetine to treat depression in HIV-positive persons. Psychosomatics 1994; 35:132–137 [B]
297. Lieberman MA, Borman LD: Self-Help Groups for Coping With Crisis. San Francisco, Jossey-Bass, 1979 [G]
298. Shapiro DA, Barkham M, Rees A, Hardy GE, Reynolds S, Startup M: Effects of treatment duration and severity of depression on the effectiveness of cognitive-behavioral and psychodynamic-interpersonal psychotherapy. J Consult Clin Psychol 1994; 62:522–534 [B]
299. Wexler BE, Cicchetti DV: The outpatient treatment of depression: implications of outcome research for clinical practice. J Nerv Ment Dis 1992; 180:277–286 [F]
300. Beck AT, Jallon SD, Young JE: Treatment of depression with cognitive therapy and amitriptyline. Arch Gen Psychiatry 1985; 42:142–148 [D]
301. Blackburn IM, Bishop S, Glen AI, Whalley LJ, Christie JE: The efficacy of cognitive therapy in depression: a treatment trial using cognitive therapy and pharmacotherapy, each alone and in combination. Br J Psychiatry 1981; 139:181–189 [A]

302. Chaudhry HR, Najam N, Naqvi A: The value of amineptine in depressed patients treated with cognitive behavioural psychotherapy. Hum Psychopharmacol 1998; 13:419–424 [A]
303. Hersen M, Bellack AS, Himmelhoch JM, Thase ME: Effects of social skill training, amitriptyline, and psychotherapy in unipolar depressed women. Behavior Therapy 1984; 15:21–40 [B]
304. Murphy GE, Simons AD, Wetzel RD, Lustman PJ: Cognitive therapy and pharmacotherapy: singly and together in the treatment of depression. Arch Gen Psychiatry 1984; 41:33–41 [A]
305. Thase ME, Greenhouse JB, Frank E, Reynolds CF, Pilkonis PA, Hurley K, Grochocinski VJ, Kupfer DJ: Treatment of major depression with psychotherapy or psychotherapy-pharmacotherapy combinations. Arch Gen Psychiatry 1997; 54:1009–1015 [E]
306. Fava GA, Grandi S, Zielezny M, Canestrari R, Morphy MA: Cognitive behavioral treatment of residual symptoms in primary major depressive disorder. Am J Psychiatry 1994; 151:1295–1299 [B]
307. Fava M, Kaji J: Continuation and maintenance treatments of major depressive disorder. Psychiatr Annals 1994; 24:281–290 [F]
308. Fava M, Davidson KG: Definition and epidemiology of treatment-resistant depression. Psychiatr Clin North Am 1996; 19:179–200 [F]
309. Fava GA, Rafanelli C, Grandi S, Conti S, Belluardo P: Prevention of recurrent depression with cognitive behavioral therapy: preliminary findings. Arch Gen Psychiatry 1998; 55:816–820 [G]
310. Consensus Development Panel: NIMH/NIH Consensus Development Conference Statement: mood disorders: pharmacologic prevention of recurrences. Am J Psychiatry 1985; 142:469–476 [F]
311. Maj M, Veltro F, Pirozzi R, Lobrace S, Magliano L: Pattern of recurrence of illness after recovery from an episode of major depression: a prospective study. Am J Psychiatry 1992; 149:795–800 [B]
312. Thase ME, Simons AD, McGeary J, Cahalane JF, Hughes C, Harden T, Friedman E: Relapse after cognitive behavior therapy of depression: potential implications for longer courses of treatment. Am J Psychiatry 1992; 149:1046–1052 [C]
313. Keller MD, Gelenberg AJ, Hirschfeld RM, Rush AJ, Thase ME, Kocsis JH, Markowitz JC, Fawcett JA, Koran LM, Klein DN, Russell JM, Kornstein SG, McCullough JP, Davis SM, Harrison WM: The treatment of chronic depression, part 2: a double-blind, randomized trial of sertraline and imipramine. J Clin Psychiatry 1998; 59:598–607 [A]
314. Prien RF, Kupfer DJ: Continuation drug therapy for major depressive episodes: how long should it be maintained? Am J Psychiatry 1986; 143:18–23 [B]
315. Jarrett DB, Basco MR, Riser R, Ramanan J, Marwill M, Rush AJ: Is there a role for continuation phase cognitive therapy for depressed outpatients? J Consult Clin Psychol 1998; 66:1036–1040 [B]
316. Fava GA, Grandi S, Zielezny M, Rafanelli C, Canestrari R: Four-year outcome for cognitive behavioral treatment of residual symptoms in major depression. Am J Psychiatry 1996; 153:945–947 [B]
317. Solomon DA, Bauer MS: Continuation and maintenance pharmacotherapy for unipolar and bipolar mood disorders. Psychiatr Clin North Am 1993; 16:515–540 [F]
318. Frank E, Kupfer DJ, Perel JM, Cornes C, Jarrett DB, Mallinger AG, Thase ME, McEachran AB, Grochocinski VJ: Three-year outcomes for maintenance therapies in recurrent depression. Arch Gen Psychiatry 1990; 47:1093–1099 [A]
319. Kupfer DJ, Frank E, Perel JM, Cornes C, Mallinger AG, Thase ME, McEachran AB, Grochocinski VJ: Five-year outcome for maintenance therapies in recurrent depression. Arch Gen Psychiatry 1992; 49:769–773 [A]

320. Frank E, Kupfer DJ, Perel JM, Cornes C, Mallinger AG, Thase ME, McEachran AB, Grochocinski VJ: Comparison of full-dose versus half-dose pharmacotherapy in the maintenance treatment of recurrent depression. J Affect Disord 1993; 27:139–145 [A]
321. Scott J: Chronic depression: can cognitive therapy succeed when other treatments fail? Behavioural Psychotherapy 1992; 20:25–36 [B]
322. Belsher G, Costello CB: Relapse after recovery from unipolar depression: a critical review. Psychol Bull 1988; 104:84–96 [F]
323. Petrides G, Dhossche D, Fink M, Francis A: Continuation ECT: relapse prevention in affective disorders. Convuls Ther 1994; 10:189–194 [B]
324. Vanelle JM, Loo H, Galinowski A, de Carvalho W, Bourdel MC, Brochier P, Bouvet O, Brochier T, Olie JP: Maintenance ECT in intractable manic-depressive disorders. Convuls Ther 1994; 10:195–205 [C]
325. Dilsaver SC, Kronfol Z, Sackellares JC, Greden JF: Antidepressant withdrawal syndromes: evidence supporting the cholinergic overdrive hypothesis. J Clin Psychopharmacol 1983; 3:157–164 [F]

GUIDELINE WATCH: PRACTICE GUIDELINE FOR THE TREATMENT OF PATIENTS WITH BIPOLAR DISORDER, 2ND EDITION

Robert M. A. Hirschfeld, M.D.

APA's *Practice Guideline for the Treatment of Patients With Bipolar Disorder,* 2nd Edition, was published in April 2002 (1). Since that time, a number of controlled treatment studies on aspects of bipolar disorder have been completed and published or are in press, including studies of second-generation (atypical) antipsychotics as monotherapy and as adjunctive treatment (with more traditional mood stabilizers) for the acute treatment of mania, studies of antiepileptic agents for the acute treatment of mania, trials for three medications for the acute treatment of bipolar depression, four monotherapy and one combination therapy relapse prevention studies, and studies of psychosocial interventions for maintenance. The evidence from these studies supports a substantially expanded set of options for clinicians who treat patients with bipolar disorder. This guideline watch briefly reviews the most important of the studies. The majority of the studies were industry supported.

PSYCHIATRIC MANAGEMENT

Recently completed epidemiological studies have estimated the lifetime prevalence of bipolar I and II disorders in the general population to be 3.7%–3.9% (2, 3). The prevalence in samples of patients presenting with depression is much higher, ranging from 21% (4) to 26% (5) in primary care settings and from 28% (6) to 49% (7) in psychiatric clinics. Use of a screening instrument, such as the Mood Disorder Questionnaire, can substantially improve recognition of patients with bipolar disorder, particularly among depressed patients (8).

The American Psychiatric Association (APA) practice guidelines are developed by expert work groups using an explicit methodology that includes rigorous review of available evidence, broad peer review of iterative drafts, and formal approval by the APA Assembly and Board of Trustees. APA practice guidelines are intended to assist psychiatrists in clinical decision making. They are not intended to be a standard of care. The ultimate judgment regarding a particular clinical procedure or treatment plan must be made by the psychiatrist in light of the clinical data presented by the patient and the diagnostic and treatment options available. Guideline watches summarize significant developments in practice since publication of an APA practice guideline. Watches may be authored and reviewed by experts associated with the original guideline development effort and are approved for publication by APA's Executive Committee on Practice Guidelines. Thus, watches represent opinion of the authors and approval of the Executive Committee but not policy of the APA. This guideline watch was published in November 2005. Suggested citation: Hirschfeld RMA: *Guideline Watch: Practice Guideline for the Treatment of Patients With Bipolar Disorder.* Arlington, VA: American Psychiatric Association. Available online at http://www.psych.org/psych_pract/treatg/pg/prac_guide.cfm.

Acute treatment

Manic or mixed episodes

Two randomized, double-blind, controlled studies have shown olanzapine monotherapy to be significantly better than placebo for the acute treatment of patients with mania or mixed episodes, with initial dosing of either 10 mg/day or 15 mg/day (9, 10). Somnolence, dry mouth, dizziness, and weight gain occurred significantly more frequently in the olanzapine group than in the placebo group. In another randomized, double-blind study, olanzapine was equivalent to haloperidol for patients with acute mania and was superior to haloperidol for patients whose index episode did not include psychotic features (11). Olanzapine monotherapy has also been compared with divalproex monotherapy in two randomized, double-blind, controlled studies. In one there was equivalent efficacy (12), and in the other olanzapine had superior efficacy (13). However, the side-effect profile for divalproex was more benign.

Olanzapine has also been studied as an adjunctive agent to traditional mood stabilizers. In a double-blind, randomized, controlled trial, olanzapine added to divalproex or lithium was superior to divalproex or lithium alone in patients who had had an inadequate response to at least 2 weeks of lithium or valproate monotherapy (14). Side effects included somnolence, hyperkinesia, and nausea.

The efficacy of risperidone monotherapy for the acute treatment of mania has been demonstrated in three randomized, double-blind, placebo-controlled trials. Risperidone monotherapy was superior to placebo in all three studies. In the three studies patients were started on 3 mg/day of risperidone, with titration to a maximum of 6 mg/day. Onset of action in one study was seen at day 3 (15), and in another at 1 week (16). In the third study, risperidone was equivalent to haloperidol and superior to placebo (17). Side effects included somnolence, hyperkinesia, and nausea.

Two randomized, double-blind, placebo-controlled studies examined the adjunctive use of risperidone with traditional mood stabilizers (i.e., lithium or divalproex) (18, 19). In both studies the combination of risperidone with mood stabilizer outperformed mood stabilizer alone. The addition of risperidone substantially increased the prevalence of extrapyramidal symptoms.

The efficacy of ziprasidone as monotherapy in the acute treatment of patients with manic or mixed episodes was tested in two randomized, double-blind, placebo-controlled studies, with initial dosing of 40 mg twice a day (20, 21). Ziprasidone had an onset of action at day 2 in both trials and was superior to placebo at endpoint. The mean dosage in the two studies was 130 mg/day and 112 mg/day, respectively. Side effects included somnolence, dizziness, extrapyramidal syndrome, nausea, akathisia, and tremor.

Two studies of aripiprazole monotherapy in the acute treatment of mania have been published (22, 23). In a randomized, double-blind, controlled study, aripiprazole at a starting dosage of 30 mg/day was compared with placebo in patients with manic or mixed episodes (22). Aripiprazole was superior to placebo in efficacy, beginning at day 4. Side effects included nausea, dyspepsia, somnolence, vomiting, insomnia, and akathisia. A second study compared aripiprazole and haloperidol over 12 weeks (23). The drugs performed similarly regarding improvement in manic symptoms, but substantially more aripiprazole patients completed the study. Extrapyramidal symptoms were much higher for haloperidol.

The efficacy of quetiapine in patients with manic episodes has been studied in two different 12-week randomized, double-blind, placebo-controlled trials—one against lithium and the other against haloperidol (24, 25). Quetiapine was initiated at 100 mg on day 1, with an upward titration to 800 mg/day or higher. Quetiapine was equivalent in efficacy to the two active comparators, and both were superior to placebo at day 21. Side effects included dry mouth, somnolence, weight gain, and dizziness.

In another study, adjunctive quetiapine or placebo was given to acutely manic patients who were still manic after at least 7 days of treatment with lithium or divalproex. Quetiapine was initiated at 100 mg and titrated to 400 mg/day by day 4, with a target dose of 200–800 mg/day (26).

The quetiapine treatment group had a significantly higher response rate and reduction in manic symptoms. The mean last-week dosage in all patients receiving quetiapine was 504 mg/day.

There have been two recently published randomized, double-blind, placebo-controlled studies of the extended-release formulation of the anticonvulsant carbamazepine for the acute treatment of manic or mixed episodes (27, 28). In both studies, carbamazepine extended-release was initiated at 400 mg in divided doses on day 1 and increased as tolerated up to 1,600 mg/day. The mean final dosages were 756 mg/day (27) and 643 mg/day (28), respectively. An onset of action was seen at day 14 in the first trial and at day 7 in the second trial, and both trials found carbamazepine extended-release to be superior to placebo at endpoint. Side effects included dizziness, somnolence, nausea, vomiting, ataxia, blurred vision, dyspepsia, dry mouth, pruritus, and speech disorder.

The many monotherapy and adjunctive therapy studies of mania since 2002 provide a number of new options for clinicians in the acute treatment of patients with mania.

A significant clinical concern is metabolic effects associated with second-generation antipsychotics (29). Clozapine and olanzapine are associated with increased risks of developing diabetes mellitus and dyslipidemia. A recent comparative antipsychotic trial in schizophrenia suggested significantly greater weight gain for olanzapine than for the other antipsychotics studied (i.e., perphenazine, quetiapine, risperidone, and ziprasidone) (30). Clozapine and olanzapine are associated with the most weight gain, risperidone and quetiapine with moderate weight gain, and ziprasidone and aripiprazole with minimal weight change. Because of these risks, clinicians have been advised to monitor weight, waist circumference, blood pressure, glucose, and lipids at baseline and at monthly intervals in patients on these medications (31).

Depressive episodes

The impact (in terms of duration of episodes and quality of life) of depressive episodes in bipolar patients is substantially worse than the impact of manic episodes (32, 33). Unfortunately, far less research attention has been paid to the treatment of bipolar depression (34, 35). This section reviews three studies published since the 2002 publication of the second edition practice guideline.

In an 8-week placebo-controlled, double-blind study, olanzapine monotherapy and the combination of olanzapine and fluoxetine were examined in the acute treatment of bipolar I depression (36). Although both olanzapine and the combination of olanzapine and fluoxetine were superior to placebo in efficacy, the response in the combination group was much greater, and only the combination of olanzapine and fluoxetine received an indication from the Food and Drug Administration for the acute treatment of bipolar depression. The first separation from placebo occurred at week 1 and continued throughout the trial. The mean dosage in the combination group was 7.4 mg/day of olanzapine and 39.3 mg/day of fluoxetine. By the end of the study, 8 of 10 core symptoms of depression had improved relative to placebo. Side effects included somnolence, weight gain, increased appetite, dry mouth, asthenia, and diarrhea. Neither olanzapine monotherapy nor the combination of olanzapine and fluoxetine caused switching into mania or hypomania.

A large randomized, double-blind, placebo-controlled trial supported the efficacy of quetiapine monotherapy for the treatment of bipolar I or II depression (37). Quetiapine initiated at 50 mg/day and titrated to either 300 mg/day or 600 mg/day within 1 week was found to be effective compared with placebo at both doses, with no significant difference in efficacy between the two dosage groups. Onset of action occurred by 1 week and continued throughout the trial. Statistical significance was achieved at endpoint in 9 of 10 core features of depression. Side effects included dry mouth, sedation, somnolence, dizziness, and constipation and were substantially greater in the 600 mg/day group compared with the 300 mg/day group. Incidence of treatment-emergent mania did not differ from that of placebo.

A single-blind, randomized, nonplacebo-controlled comparison of venlafaxine and paroxetine was conducted with patients with bipolar disorder who were currently presenting with a major depressive episode and who were currently taking a mood stabilizer (38). Both medications yielded significant improvements in depressive symptomatology with no significant differences in safety measures. Among the patients treated with paroxetine, 3% switched to hypomania or mania, compared with 13% in the venlafaxine group.

Two small, controlled studies of the adjunctive use of the dopamine agonist pramipexole in the treatment of bipolar depression suggest efficacy (39, 40). Both studies were 6-week placebo-controlled studies of pramipexole (mean peak dosage = 1.7 mg/day) added to the therapeutic levels of traditional mood stabilizers. Results were strongly positive in both studies, with few adverse events.

In conclusion, medications having the strongest evidence for efficacy for acute treatment of depression in patients with bipolar I disorder are the olanzapine-fluoxetine combination, quetiapine, and lamotrigine. There is suggestive evidence that the adjunctive use of pramipexole may be helpful. Evidence for the efficacy of an antidepressant with adjunctive mood stabilizer is modest. Prescription of antidepressants in the absence of a mood stabilizer is not recommended for bipolar I patients.

Maintenance treatment

Since publication of the second edition practice guideline, new studies have been published on the long-term treatment of patients with bipolar disorder.

Pharmacological interventions

Two large randomized, double-blind studies examined the utility of lamotrigine in the maintenance treatment of patients with bipolar I disorder (41, 42). Both studies were placebo controlled and included lithium monotherapy as an active comparator. In one study, patients had most recently suffered a depressive episode (41) and, in the other, a manic or hypomanic episode (42). Both studies involved an open-label stabilization period of 8–16 weeks followed by an 18-month trial of lamotrigine monotherapy, lithium monotherapy, or placebo in patients who had recovered and were stable.

In the study of recently depressed patients (41), both lamotrigine (200 mg/day or 400 mg/day) and lithium (0.8–1.1 meq/liter) were superior to placebo in preventing any mood episode. Lamotrigine, but not lithium, was superior to placebo in preventing a depressive episode. Lithium, but not lamotrigine, was superior to placebo in preventing a manic, hypomanic, or mixed episode. With the exception of rash, there were no side effects of lamotrigine that exceeded placebo. There were no serious rashes. For the lithium group, the incidence of somnolence and tremor exceeded that of placebo.

In the study of recently manic or hypomanic patients (42), both lamotrigine (target dosage of 200 mg/day) and lithium (0.8–1.1 meq/liter) were superior to placebo in delaying onset of any mood episode. Lithium, but not lamotrigine, was superior to placebo in prevention of a manic episode, but neither agent was superior to placebo in preventing depressive episodes. There were no adverse events for which lamotrigine statistically exceeded placebo. Lithium exceeded placebo for diarrhea only.

When the data from both studies were pooled, lamotrigine was superior to placebo in time to intervention for any mood episode, as well as for prevention of depressive episodes and manic, hypomanic, or mixed episodes (43). Similarly, lithium was superior to placebo in time to intervention for a mood episode and for prevention of a manic, hypomanic, or mixed episode. Lithium was not superior to placebo in prevention of a depressed episode.

Given the results from these studies, both lamotrigine and lithium appear to have substantial utility in the maintenance treatment of patients with bipolar disorder. The utility of lamotrigine was somewhat greater for the prevention of depressive compared with manic episodes, and the opposite is true for lithium.

A 47-week, randomized, double-blind study of olanzapine versus divalproex for manic or mixed episodes was completed (44). The median time to remission was shorter for olanzapine than for divalproex, although the remission rates at the end of the study did not differ between agents. Adverse events for olanzapine included somnolence, dry mouth, increased appetite, weight gain, akathisia, and high alanine aminotransferase levels, while adverse events for divalproex were nausea and nervousness.

A randomized, double-blind, controlled trial compared the efficacy of olanzapine and lithium for the prevention of relapse or recurrence of a manic or mixed episode (45). In this study patients currently experiencing a manic or mixed episode were treated acutely with olanzapine and lithium for 6–12 weeks. Patients who achieved remission were randomly assigned to 52 weeks of olanzapine or lithium monotherapy. A relapse into mania or depression occurred in 30% of the olanzapine-treated patients and in 39% of the lithium-treated patients—an insignificant difference. Olanzapine was superior to lithium in rates of symptomatic recurrence of mania or mixed episodes (14% vs. 28%), but rates of depression recurrence did not differ. Treatment-emergent insomnia was higher in the lithium group than in the olanzapine group. Among the lithium group, 26% discontinued treatment because of side effects, compared with 19% of the olanzapine group.

A randomized, double-blind, controlled study examined the utility of continued combination treatment with a mood stabilizer (lithium, carbamazepine, or valproate) and a first-generation (typical) antipsychotic (perphenazine) (46). Immediately following remission from a manic episode, patients were randomly assigned to remain on the combination therapy or to receive the mood stabilizer plus placebo. Among those on continued combination therapy, there was shorter time to depressive relapse, a higher rate of discontinuation, and higher rates of dysphoria, depressive symptoms, and extrapyramidal symptoms. The study concluded that there were no short-term benefits with the continuation of the first-generation antipsychotic with a mood stabilizer; in fact, its continued use was associated with the aforementioned detrimental effects.

However, a similar study of the second-generation antipsychotic olanzapine plus mood stabilizer versus mood stabilizer plus placebo had somewhat different results (47). In this randomized, double-blind, controlled study, patients who achieved remission after 6 weeks of treatment with olanzapine plus either lithium or valproate received continued lithium or valproate plus olanzapine or plus placebo for 18 months. There were no differences in time to relapse into mania or depression between the monotherapy and combination therapy groups, but combination therapy was significantly better for prevention of symptomatic relapse. Combination therapy was associated with increased somnolence, weight gain, and tremor.

Psychosocial interventions

Knowledge of the utility of psychosocial interventions has expanded recently. Family-focused therapy is a manualized psychosocial program involving all available family members in which weekly psychoeducation, communication enhancement training, and problem-solving skills training occur adjunctively with pharmacotherapy. A 2-year randomized, controlled study of family-focused therapy plus pharmacotherapy versus a crisis management intervention and pharmacotherapy (supported by grants from the National Institute of Mental Health, the National Alliance for Research on Schizophrenia, and the MacArthur Foundation) found that postepisode symptomatic adjustment and drug adherence were enhanced with the family-focused therapy and pharmacotherapy combination compared with the other (48). Patients in the group receiving family-focused therapy had fewer relapses and longer survival intervals.

Another randomized, controlled study examined the utility of cognitive therapy in conjunction with pharmacotherapy over a 12-month period (49). Those treated with cognitive therapy and pharmacotherapy had significantly fewer bipolar episodes, days in an episode, and number of admissions.

Two controlled studies (supported by grants from the Stanley Medical Research Institute, the Instituto de Salud Carlos III, the Fundació Marató de TV3, and the Fundació María Francisca Roviralta) of a longitudinal (21-session) psychoeducational program were conducted in Spain (50, 51). In both studies psychoeducation reduced recurrences over 2 years. Psychoeducation enhanced lifestyle regularity and early syndrome detection.

A recent study (supported by grants from the National Institute of Mental Health) found that a psychosocial intervention focused on addressing interpersonal problems and regulating social rhythms during acute treatment in bipolar I patients extended the time to new episode and reduced the likelihood of recurrence (52).

CONCLUSION

Since the publication in 2002 of the *Practice Guideline for the Treatment of Patients With Bipolar Disorder,* 2nd Edition, new options for the acute treatment of manic, mixed, or depressive episodes have emerged. Knowledge of pharmacological and psychosocial interventions for maintenance has also increased.

ACKNOWLEDGMENT

The author thanks Colleen M. Sonora, M.A., for help in preparing this guideline watch.

REFERENCES

1. American Psychiatric Association: Practice guideline for the treatment of patients with bipolar disorder (revision). Am J Psychiatry 2002; 159:1–50
2. Kessler RC, Berglund P, Demler O, Jin R, Merikangas KR, Walters EE: Lifetime prevalence and age-of-onset distributions of DSM-IV disorders in the National Comorbidity Survey Replication. Arch Gen Psychiatry 2005; 62:593–602
3. Hirschfeld RM, Calabrese JR, Weissman MM, Reed M, Davies MA, Frye MA, Keck PE Jr, Lewis L, McElroy SL, McNulty JP, Wagner KD: Screening for bipolar disorder in the community. J Clin Psychiatry 2003; 64:53–59
4. Hirschfeld RM, Cass AR, Holt DC, Carlson CA: Screening for bipolar disorder in patients treated for depression in a family medicine clinic. J Am Board Fam Pract 2005; 18:233–239
5. Manning JS, Haykal RF, Connor PD, Akiskal HS: On the nature of depressive and anxious states in a family practice setting: the high prevalence of bipolar II and related disorders in a cohort followed longitudinally. Compr Psychiatry 1997; 38:102–108
6. Hantouche EG, Akiskal HS, Lancrenon S, Allilaire JF, Sechter D, Azorin JM, Bourgeois M, Fraud JP, Chatenet-Duchene L: Systematic clinical methodology for validating bipolar II disorder: data in mid-stream from a French national multi-site study (EPIDEP). J Affect Disord 1998; 50:163–173
7. Benazzi F: Prevalence of bipolar II disorder in outpatient depression: a 203-case study in private practice. J Affect Disord 1997; 43:163–166
8. Hirschfeld RM, Williams JB, Spitzer RL, Calabrese JR, Flynn L, Keck PE Jr, Lewis L, McElroy SL, Post RM, Rapport DJ, Russell JM, Sachs GS, Zajecka J: Development and validation of a screening instrument for bipolar spectrum disorder: the Mood Disorder Questionnaire. Am J Psychiatry 2000; 157:1873–1875
9. Tohen M, Sanger TM, McElroy SL, Tollefson GD, Chengappa KN, Daniel DG, Petty F, Centorrino F, Wang R, Grundy SL, Greaney MG, Jacobs TG, David SR, Toma V:

Olanzapine versus placebo in the treatment of acute mania. Olanzapine HGEH Study Group. Am J Psychiatry 1999; 156:702–709

10. Tohen M, Jacobs TG, Grundy SL, McElroy SL, Banov MC, Janicak PG, Sanger T, Risser R, Zhang F, Toma V, Francis J, Tollefson GD, Breier A : Efficacy of olanzapine in acute bipolar mania: a double-blind, placebo-controlled study. The Olanzapine HGGW Study Group. Arch Gen Psychiatry 2000; 57:841–849
11. Tohen M, Goldberg JF, Gonzalez-Pinto Arrillaga AM, Azorin JM, Vieta E, Hardy-Bayle MC, Lawson WB, Emsley RA, Zhang F, Baker RW, Risser RC, Namjoshi MA, Evans AR, Breier A: A 12-week, double-blind comparison of olanzapine vs haloperidol in the treatment of acute mania. Arch Gen Psychiatry 2003; 60:1218–1226
12. Zajecka JM, Weisler R, Sachs G, Swann AC, Wozniak P, Sommerville KW: A comparison of the efficacy, safety, and tolerability of divalproex sodium and olanzapine in the treatment of bipolar disorder. J Clin Psychiatry 2002; 63:1148–1155
13. Tohen M, Baker RW, Altshuler LL, Zarate CA, Suppes T, Ketter TA, Milton DR, Risser R, Gilmore JA, Breier A, Tollefson GA: Olanzapine versus divalproex in the treatment of acute mania. Am J Psychiatry 2002; 159:1011–1017
14. Tohen M, Chengappa KN, Suppes T, Zarate CA Jr, Calabrese JR, Bowden CL, Sachs GS, Kupfer DJ, Baker RW, Risser RC, Keeter EL, Feldman PD, Tollefson GD, Breier A: Efficacy of olanzapine in combination with valproate or lithium in the treatment of mania in patients partially nonresponsive to valproate or lithium monotherapy. Arch Gen Psychiatry 2002; 59:62–69
15. Hirschfeld RM, Keck PE Jr, Kramer M, Karcher K, Canuso C, Eerdekens M, Grossman F: Rapid antimanic effect of risperidone monotherapy: a 3-week multicenter, double-blind, placebo-controlled trial. Am J Psychiatry 2004; 161:1057–1065
16. Khanna S, Vieta E, Lyons B, Grossman F, Eerdekens M, Kramer M: Risperidone in the treatment of acute bipolar mania: double-blind, placebo-controlled study. Br J Psychiatry 2005; 187:229–234
17. Smulevich AB, Khanna S, Eerdekens M, Karcher K, Kramer M, Grossman F: Acute and continuation risperidone monotherapy in bipolar mania: a 3-week placebo-controlled trial followed by a 9-week double-blind trial of risperidone and haloperidol. Eur Neuropsychopharmacol 2005; 15:75–84
18. Sachs GS, Grossman F, Ghaemi SN, Okamoto A, Bowden CL: Combination of a mood stabilizer with risperidone or haloperidol for treatment of acute mania: a double-blind, placebo-controlled comparison of efficacy and safety. Am J Psychiatry 2002; 159:1146–1154
19. Yatham LN, Grossman F, Augustyns I, Vieta E, Ravindran A: Mood stabilisers plus risperidone or placebo in the treatment of acute mania: international, double-blind, randomised controlled trial. Br J Psychiatry 2003; 182:141–147
20. Keck PE Jr, Versiani M, Potkin S, West SA, Giller E, Ice K: Ziprasidone in the treatment of acute bipolar mania: a three-week, placebo-controlled, double-blind, randomized trial. Am J Psychiatry 2003; 160:741–748
21. Potkin SG, Keck PE Jr, Segal S, Ice K, English P: Ziprasidone in acute bipolar mania: a 21-day randomized, double-blind, placebo-controlled replication trial. J Clin Psychopharmacol 2005; 25:301–310
22. Keck PE Jr, Marcus R, Tourkodimitris S, Ali M, Liebeskind A, Saha A, Ingenito G: A placebo-controlled, double-blind study of the efficacy and safety of aripiprazole in patients with acute bipolar mania. Am J Psychiatry 2003; 160:1651–1658
23. Vieta E, Bourin M, Sanchez R, Marcus R, Stock E, McQuade R, Carson W, Abou-Gharbia N, Swanink R, Iwamoto T: Effectiveness of aripiprazole vs haloperidol in acute bipolar mania: double-blind, randomised, comparative 12-week trial. Br J Psychiatry 2005; 187:235–242

24. McIntyre RS, Brecher M, Paulsson B, Huziar K, Mullen J: Quetiapine or haloperidol as monotherapy for bipolar mania: a 12-week, double-blind, randomised, parallel-group, placebo-controlled trial. Eur Neuropsychopharmacol 2005; 15:573–585
25. Bowden CL, Grunze H, Mullen J, Brecher M, Paulsson B, Jones M, Vagero M, Svensson K: A randomized, double-blind, placebo-controlled efficacy and safety study of quetiapine or lithium as monotherapy for mania in bipolar disorder. J Clin Psychiatry 2005; 66:111–121
26. Sachs G, Chengappa KN, Suppes T, Mullen JA, Brecher M, Devine NA, Sweitzer DE: Quetiapine with lithium or divalproex for the treatment of bipolar mania: a randomized, double-blind, placebo-controlled study. Bipolar Disord 2004; 6:213–223
27. Weisler RH, Kalali AH, Ketter TA: A multicenter, randomized, double-blind, placebo-controlled trial of extended-release carbamazepine capsules as monotherapy for bipolar disorder patients with manic or mixed episodes. J Clin Psychiatry 2004; 65:478–484
28. Weisler RH, Keck PE Jr, Swann AC, Cutler AJ, Ketter TA, Kalali AH: Extended-release carbamazepine capsules as monotherapy for acute mania in bipolar disorder: a multicenter, randomized, double-blind, placebo-controlled trial. J Clin Psychiatry 2005; 66:323–330
29. Newcomer JW: Second-generation (atypical) antipsychotics and metabolic effects: a comprehensive literature review. CNS Drugs 2005; 19(suppl 1):1–93
30. Lieberman JA, Stroup TS, McEvoy JP, Swartz MS, Rosenheck RA, Perkins DO, Keefe RS, Davis SM, Davis CE, Lebowitz BD, Severe J, Hsiao JK: Effectiveness of antipsychotic drugs in patients with chronic schizophrenia. N Engl J Med 2005; 353:1209–1223
31. American Diabetes Association, American Psychiatry Association, American Association of Clinical Endocrinologists: Consensus development conference on antipsychotic drugs and obesity and diabetes. J Clin Psychiatry 2004; 65:267–272
32. Judd LL, Akiskal HS, Schettler PJ, Endicott J, Maser J, Solomon DA, Leon AC, Rice JA, Keller MB: The long-term natural history of the weekly symptomatic status of bipolar I disorder. Arch Gen Psychiatry 2002; 59:530–537
33. Calabrese JR, Hirschfeld RM, Frye MA, Reed ML: Impact of depressive symptoms compared with manic symptoms in bipolar disorder: results of a U.S. community-based sample. J Clin Psychiatry 2004; 65:1499–1504
34. Gijsman HJ, Geddes JR, Rendell JM, Nolen WA, Goodwin GM: Antidepressants for bipolar depression: a systematic review of randomized, controlled trials. Am J Psychiatry 2004; 161:1537–1547
35. Hirschfeld RM, Fochtmann LJ, McIntyre JS: Antidepressants for bipolar depression. Am J Psychiatry 2005; 162:1546–1547
36. Tohen M, Vieta E, Calabrese J, Ketter TA, Sachs G, Bowden C, Mitchell PB, Centorrino F, Risser R, Baker RW, Evans AR, Beymer K, Dube S, Tollefson GD, Breier A: Efficacy of olanzapine and olanzapine-fluoxetine combination in the treatment of bipolar I depression. Arch Gen Psychiatry 2003; 60:1079–1088
37. Calabrese JR, Keck PE Jr, Macfadden W, Minkwitz M, Ketter TA, Weisler RH, Cutler AJ, McCoy R, Wilson E, Mullen J: A randomized, double-blind, placebo-controlled trial of quetiapine in the treatment of bipolar I or II depression. Am J Psychiatry 2005; 162:1351–1360
38. Vieta E, Martinez-Aran A, Goikolea JM, Torrent C, Colom F, Benabarre A, Reinares M: A randomized trial comparing paroxetine and venlafaxine in the treatment of bipolar depressed patients taking mood stabilizers. J Clin Psychiatry 2002; 63:508–512
39. Goldberg JF, Burdick KE, Endick CJ: Preliminary randomized, double-blind, placebo-controlled trial of pramipexole added to mood stabilizers for treatment-resistant bipolar depression. Am J Psychiatry 2004; 161:564–566
40. Zarate CA Jr, Payne JL, Singh J, Quiroz JA, Luckenbaugh DA, Denicoff KD, Charney DS, Manji HK: Pramipexole for bipolar II depression: a placebo-controlled proof of concept study. Biol Psychiatry 2004; 56:54–60

41. Calabrese JR, Bowden CL, Sachs G, Yatham LN, Behnke K, Mehtonen OP, Montgomery P, Ascher J, Paska W, Earl N, DeVeaugh-Geiss J: A placebo-controlled 18-month trial of lamotrigine and lithium maintenance treatment in recently depressed patients with bipolar I disorder. J Clin Psychiatry 2003; 64:1013–1024
42. Bowden CL, Calabrese JR, Sachs G, Yatham LN, Asghar SA, Hompland M, Montgomery P, Earl N, Smoot TM, DeVeaugh-Geiss J: A placebo-controlled 18-month trial of lamotrigine and lithium maintenance treatment in recently manic or hypomanic patients with bipolar I disorder. Arch Gen Psychiatry 2003; 60:392–400
43. Goodwin GM, Bowden CL, Calabrese JR, Grunze H, Kasper S, White R, Greene P, Leadbetter R: A pooled analysis of 2 placebo-controlled 18-month trials of lamotrigine and lithium maintenance in bipolar I disorder. J Clin Psychiatry 2004; 65:432–441
44. Tohen M, Ketter TA, Zarate CA, Suppes T, Frye M, Altshuler L, Zajecka J, Schuh LM, Risser RC, Brown E, Baker RW: Olanzapine versus divalproex sodium for the treatment of acute mania and maintenance of remission: a 47-week study. Am J Psychiatry 2003; 160:1263–1271
45. Tohen M, Greil W, Calabrese JR, Sachs GS, Yatham LN, Oerlinghausen BM, Koukopoulos A, Cassano GB, Grunze H, Licht RW, Dell'Osso L, Evans AR, Risser R, Baker RW, Crane H, Dossenbach MR, Bowden CL: Olanzapine versus lithium in the maintenance treatment of bipolar disorder: a 12-month, randomized, double-blind, controlled clinical trial. Am J Psychiatry 2005; 162:1281–1290
46. Zarate CA Jr, Tohen M: Double-blind comparison of the continued use of antipsychotic treatment versus its discontinuation in remitted manic patients. Am J Psychiatry 2004; 161:169–171
47. Tohen M, Chengappa KN, Suppes T, Baker RW, Zarate CA, Bowden CL, Sachs GS, Kupfer DJ, Ghaemi SN, Feldman PD, Risser RC, Evans AR, Calabrese JR: Relapse prevention in bipolar I disorder: 18-month comparison of olanzapine plus mood stabiliser vs mood stabiliser alone. Br J Psychiatry 2004; 184:337–345
48. Miklowitz DJ, George EL, Richards JA, Simoneau TL, Suddath RL: A randomized study of family-focused psychoeducation and pharmacotherapy in the outpatient management of bipolar disorder. Arch Gen Psychiatry 2003; 60:904–912
49. Lam DH, Watkins ER, Hayward P, Bright J, Wright K, Kerr N, Parr-Davis G, Sham P: A randomized controlled study of cognitive therapy for relapse prevention for bipolar affective disorder: outcome of the first year. Arch Gen Psychiatry 2003; 60:145–152
50. Colom F, Vieta E, Reinares M, Martinez-Aran A, Torrent C, Goikolea JM, Gasto C: Psychoeducation efficacy in bipolar disorders: beyond compliance enhancement. J Clin Psychiatry 2003; 64:1101–1105
51. Colom F, Vieta E, Martinez-Aran A, Reinares M, Goikolea JM, Benabarre A, Torrent C, Comes M, Corbella B, Parramon G, Corominas J: A randomized trial on the efficacy of group psychoeducation in the prophylaxis of recurrences in bipolar patients whose disease is in remission. Arch Gen Psychiatry 2003; 60:402–407
52. Frank E, Kupfer DJ, Thase ME, Mallinger AG, Swartz HA, Fagiolini AM, Grochocinski V, Houck P, Scott J, Thompson W, Monk T: Two-year outcomes for interpersonal and social rhythm therapy in individuals with bipolar I disorder. Arch Gen Psychiatry 2005; 62:996–1004

PRACTICE GUIDELINE FOR THE
Treatment of Patients With Bipolar Disorder
Second Edition

WORK GROUP ON BIPOLAR DISORDER

Robert M.A. Hirschfeld, M.D., Chair

Charles L. Bowden, M.D.
Michael J. Gitlin, M.D.
Paul E. Keck, M.D.
Trisha Suppes, M.D., Ph.D.
Michael E. Thase, M.D.
Karen D. Wagner, M.D., Ph.D.
Roy H. Perlis, M.D. (Consultant)

Originally published in April 2002. A guideline watch, summarizing significant developments in the scientific literature since publication of this guideline, may be available in the Psychiatric Practice section of the APA web site at www.psych.org.

CONTENTS

Guide to Using This Practice Guideline 855

Introduction 856

Development Process 857

Part A: Treatment Recommendations for Patients With Bipolar Disorder 859

I. Executive Summary of Recommendations 859
   A. Psychiatric Management 859
   B. Acute Treatment 859
   C. Maintenance Treatment 861

II. Formulation and Implementation of a Treatment Plan 861
   A. Psychiatric Management 862
   B. Acute Treatment 866
   C. Maintenance Treatment 868

III. Special Clinical Features Influencing the Treatment Plan 869
   A. Psychiatric Features 869
   B. Demographic and Psychosocial Factors 871
   C. Concurrent General Medical Conditions 875

Part B: Background Information and Review of Available Evidence 876

IV. Disease Definition, Natural History and Course, and Epidemiology 876
   A. Definition of Bipolar Disorder 876
   B. Natural History and Course 877
   C. Epidemiology 880

V. Review and Synthesis of Available Evidence 881
   A. Somatic Treatments of Acute Manic and Mixed Episodes 881
   B. Somatic Treatments of Acute Depressive Episodes 892
   C. Rapid Cycling 897
   D. Maintenance Treatment 898
   E. Psychosocial Interventions 901
   F. Somatic Therapies for Children and Adolescents 905

Part C: Future Research Needs 906

VI. General Principles 907

VII. Acute Treatment 907
A. Manic and Mixed Episodes 907
B. Depressive Episodes 907
C. Rapid Cycling 907

VIII. Maintenance Treatment 908

IX. Psychosocial Interventions 908

Individuals and Organizations That Submitted Comments 909

References 909

GUIDE TO USING THIS PRACTICE GUIDELINE

This practice guideline is based on available evidence and clinical consensus and offers treatment recommendations to help psychiatrists develop plans for the care of adult patients with bipolar disorder. This guideline contains many sections, not all of which will be equally useful for all readers. The following guide is designed to help readers find the sections that will be most useful to them. Part A contains the treatment recommendations for patients with bipolar disorder. Section I is the summary of the treatment recommendations, which includes the main treatment recommendations along with codes that indicate the degree of clinical confidence in each recommendation. Section II is a guide to the formulation and implementation of a treatment plan for the individual patient. This section includes all of the treatment recommendations. Section III, "Special Clinical Features Influencing the Treatment Plan," discusses a range of clinical considerations that could alter the general recommendations discussed in Section II.

Part B, "Background Information and Review of Available Evidence," will be useful to understand, in detail, the evidence underlying the treatment recommendations of Part A. Section IV provides an overview of DSM-IV bipolar disorder criteria, features of the disorder, and general information on its natural history, course, and epidemiology. Section V is a structured review and synthesis of published literature regarding available treatments for bipolar disorder. Because of the paucity of published data on some important clinical questions, unpublished studies as well as those in press were also reviewed and included, although they were given considerably less weight than published trials.

Part C, "Future Research Needs," draws from the previous sections to summarize those areas in which better research data are needed to guide clinical decisions.

To share feedback on this or other published APA practice guidelines, a form is available at http://www.psych.org/psych_pract/pg/reviewform.cfm.

INTRODUCTION

This practice guideline summarizes data on the specific somatic and psychosocial interventions that have been studied in the treatment of bipolar disorder. It begins at the point at which a diagnostic evaluation performed by a psychiatrist has raised the concern that an adult patient may be suffering from bipolar disorder. According to the criteria defined in DSM-IV-TR (1), patients with bipolar I disorder have experienced at least one episode of mania; they may have experienced mixed, hypomanic, and depressive episodes as well. Patients with bipolar II disorder have experienced hypomanic and depressive episodes. Cyclothymic disorder may be diagnosed in those patients who have never experienced a manic, mixed, or major depressive episode but who have experienced numerous periods of depressive symptoms and numerous periods of hypomanic symptoms for at least 2 years (or 1 year for children [1]), with no symptom-free period greater than 2 months. Finally, patients with depressive symptoms and periods of mood elevation who do not meet criteria for any specific bipolar disorder may be diagnosed with bipolar disorder not otherwise specified. For patients with depressive symptoms and no history of mania or hypomania, the psychiatrist should refer to the APA *Practice Guideline for the Treatment of Patients With Major Depressive Disorder* (2; included in this volume).

In addition to looking for evidence of the existence of a mood disorder, the initial psychiatric evaluation includes an assessment for the presence of an alcohol or substance use disorder or other somatic factors that may contribute to the disease process or complicate its treatment. The evaluation also requires a judgment about the safety of the patient and those around him or her and a decision about the appropriate setting for treatment (e.g., outpatient, day program, inpatient).

The purpose of this guideline is to assist the clinician faced with the task of implementing a specific regimen for the treatment of a patient with bipolar disorder. It should be noted that many patients with bipolar disorder also suffer from comorbid psychiatric illnesses. Although this guideline provides considerations for managing comorbidity in the context of bipolar disorder, it is likely that the psychiatrist will also need to refer to treatment guidelines appropriate to other diagnoses.

This guideline concerns patients 18 years of age and older. Some comments regarding the treatment of bipolar disorder in children and adolescents can be found in sections III.B.4 and V.F as well as in more definitive references (3).

DEVELOPMENT PROCESS

This document is a practical guide to the management of patients—primarily adults 18 years of age and older—with bipolar disorder and represents a synthesis of current scientific knowledge and rational clinical practice. This guideline strives to be as free as possible of bias toward any theoretical approach to treatment.

This practice guideline was developed under the auspices of the Steering Committee on Practice Guidelines. The development process is detailed in the Appendix. Key features of this process include the following:

- A comprehensive literature review and development of evidence tables.
- Initial drafting by a work group that included psychiatrists with clinical and research expertise in bipolar disorder.
- The production of multiple drafts with widespread review; seven organizations and more than 40 individuals submitted significant comments.
- Approval by the APA Assembly and Board of Trustees.
- Planned revisions at regular intervals.

A computerized search of the relevant literature from MEDLINE and PsycINFO was conducted. Sources of funding were not considered when reviewing the literature.

The first literature search was conducted by searching MEDLINE and PsycINFO for the period from 1992 to 2000. Key words used were "bipolar disorder," "bipolar depression," "mania," "mixed states," "mixed episodes," "mixed mania," "antimanic," "hypomanic," "hypomania," "manic depression," "prophylactic," "pharmacotherapy," "mood stabilizers," "mood-stabilizing," "rapid cycling," "maintenance," "continuation," "child and adolescent," "antidepressants," "valproate," "lithium," "carbamazepine," "olanzapine," "risperidone," "gabapentin," "topiramate," "lamotrigine," "clonazepam," "divalproex," "psychotherapy," "family therapy," "psychoeducation," "course," "epidemiology," "comorbidity," "anxiety," "anxiety disorders," "attention deficit," "catatonia," "elderly," "family history," "gender," "general medical conditions," "life events," "personality disorders," "pregnancy," "psychosis," "stress," "substance-related disorders," "suicide," "homicide," and "violence." A total of 3,382 citations were found.

An additional MEDLINE search for the period from 1992 to 2001 used the key words "genetic counseling," "family functioning," "cross-cultural issues," and "pharmacokinetics." A total of 122 citations were found. A search on PubMed was also conducted through 2001 that used the search terms "electroconvulsive," "intravenous drug abuse," "treatment response," "pharmacogenetic," "attention deficit disorder," "violence," "aggression," "aggressive," "suicidal," "cognitive impairment," "sleep," "postpartum," "ethnic," "racial," "metabolism," "hyperparathyroidism," "overdose," "toxicity," "intoxication," "pregnancy," "breast-feeding," and "lactation."

Additional, less formal, literature searches were conducted by APA staff and individual members of the work group on bipolar disorder.

The recommendations are based on the best available data and clinical consensus with regard to a particular clinical decision. The summary of treatment recommendations is keyed according to the level of confidence with which each recommendation is made. In addition, each reference is followed by a letter code in brackets that indicates the nature of the supporting evidence.

PART A:
TREATMENT RECOMMENDATIONS FOR PATIENTS WITH BIPOLAR DISORDER

I. EXECUTIVE SUMMARY OF RECOMMENDATIONS

Each recommendation is identified as falling into one of three categories of endorsement, indicated by a bracketed Roman numeral following the statement. The three categories represent varying levels of clinical confidence regarding the recommendation:

[I] Recommended with substantial clinical confidence.
[II] Recommended with moderate clinical confidence.
[III] May be recommended on the basis of individual circumstances.

A. PSYCHIATRIC MANAGEMENT

At this time, there is no cure for bipolar disorder; however, treatment can decrease the associated morbidity and mortality [I]. Initially, the psychiatrist should perform a diagnostic evaluation and assess the patient's safety and level of functioning to arrive at a decision about the optimum treatment setting [I]. Subsequently, specific goals of psychiatric management include establishing and maintaining a therapeutic alliance, monitoring the patient's psychiatric status, providing education regarding bipolar disorder, enhancing treatment compliance, promoting regular patterns of activity and of sleep, anticipating stressors, identifying new episodes early, and minimizing functional impairments [I].

B. ACUTE TREATMENT

1. Manic or mixed episodes

The first-line pharmacological treatment for more severe manic or mixed episodes is the initiation of either lithium plus an antipsychotic or valproate plus an antipsychotic [I]. For less ill patients, monotherapy with lithium, valproate, or an antipsychotic such as olanzapine may be sufficient [I]. Short-term adjunctive treatment with a benzodiazepine may also be helpful [II]. For mixed episodes, valproate may be preferred over lithium [II]. Atypical antipsychotics are preferred over typical antipsychotics because of their more benign side effect profile [I], with most of the evidence supporting the use of olanzapine or risperidone [II]. Alternatives include carbamazepine or oxcarbazepine in lieu of lithium or valproate [II]. Antidepressants should be tapered and discontinued if possible [I]. If psychosocial therapy approaches are used, they should be combined with pharmacotherapy [I].

For patients who, despite receiving maintenance medication treatment, experience a manic or mixed episode (i.e., a "breakthrough" episode), the first-line intervention should be to optimize the medication dose [I]. Introduction or resumption of an antipsychotic is sometimes necessary [II]. Severely ill or agitated patients may also require short-term adjunctive treatment with a benzodiazepine [I].

When first-line medication treatment at optimal doses fails to control symptoms, recommended treatment options include addition of another first-line medication [I]. Alternative treatment options include adding carbamazepine or oxcarbazepine in lieu of an additional first-line medication [II], adding an antipsychotic if not already prescribed [I], or changing from one antipsychotic to another [III]. Clozapine may be particularly effective in the treatment of refractory illness [II]. Electroconvulsive therapy (ECT) may also be considered for patients with severe or treatment-resistant mania or if preferred by the patient in consultation with the psychiatrist [I]. In addition, ECT is a potential treatment for patients experiencing mixed episodes or for patients experiencing severe mania during pregnancy [II].

Manic or mixed episodes with psychotic features usually require treatment with an antipsychotic medication [II].

2. Depressive episodes

The first-line pharmacological treatment for bipolar depression is the initiation of either lithium [I] or lamotrigine [II]. Antidepressant monotherapy is not recommended [I]. As an alternative, especially for more severely ill patients, some clinicians will initiate simultaneous treatment with lithium and an antidepressant [III]. In patients with life-threatening inanition, suicidality, or psychosis, ECT also represents a reasonable alternative [I]. ECT is also a potential treatment for severe depression during pregnancy [II].

A large body of evidence supports the efficacy of psychotherapy in the treatment of unipolar depression [I]. In bipolar depression, interpersonal therapy and cognitive behavior therapy may be useful when added to pharmacotherapy [II]. While psychodynamic psychotherapy has not been empirically studied in patients with bipolar depression, it is widely used in addition to medication [III].

For patients who, despite receiving maintenance medication treatment, suffer a breakthrough depressive episode, the first-line intervention should be to optimize the dose of maintenance medication [II].

When an acute depressive episode of bipolar disorder does not respond to first-line medication treatment at optimal doses, next steps include adding lamotrigine [I], bupropion [II], or paroxetine [II]. Alternative next steps include adding other newer antidepressants (e.g., a selective serotonin reuptake inhibitor [SSRI] or venlafaxine) [II] or a monoamine oxidase inhibitor (MAOI) [II]. For patients with severe or treatment-resistant depression or depression with psychotic or catatonic features, ECT should be considered [I].

The likelihood of antidepressant treatment precipitating a switch into a hypomanic episode is probably lower in patients with bipolar II depression than in patients with bipolar I depression. Therefore, clinicians may elect to recommend antidepressant treatment earlier in patients with bipolar II disorder [II].

Depressive episodes with psychotic features usually require adjunctive treatment with an antipsychotic medication [I]. ECT represents a reasonable alternative [I].

3. Rapid cycling

As defined in DSM-IV-TR (1) and applied in this guideline, rapid cycling refers to the occurrence of four or more mood disturbances within a single year that meet criteria for a major depressive, mixed, manic, or hypomanic episode. These episodes are demarcated either by partial or full remission for at least 2 months or a switch to an episode of opposite polarity (e.g., from a major depressive to a manic episode). The initial intervention in patients who experience rapid cycling is to identify and treat medical conditions, such as hypothyroidism or drug or alcohol use, that may contribute to cycling [I]. Certain medications, particularly antidepressants, may also contribute to cycling and should be tapered if possible [II]. The initial treatment for patients who experience rapid cycling should include lithium or valproate [I]; an alternative treatment is lamotrigine [I]. For many patients, combinations of medications are required [II].

C. MAINTENANCE TREATMENT

Following remission of an acute episode, patients may remain at particularly high risk of relapse for a period of up to 6 months; this phase of treatment, sometimes referred to as continuation treatment, is considered in this guideline to be part of the maintenance phase. Maintenance regimens of medication are recommended following a manic episode [I]. Although few studies involving patients with bipolar II disorder have been conducted, consideration of maintenance treatment for this form of the illness is also strongly warranted [II]. The medications with the best empirical evidence to support their use in maintenance treatment include lithium [I] and valproate [I]; possible alternatives include lamotrigine [II] or carbamazepine or oxcarbazepine [II]. If one of these medications was used to achieve remission from the most recent depressive or manic episode, it generally should be continued [I]. Maintenance sessions of ECT may also be considered for patients whose acute episode responded to ECT [II].

For patients treated with an antipsychotic medication during the preceding acute episode, the need for ongoing antipsychotic treatment should be reassessed upon entering maintenance treatment [I]; antipsychotics should be discontinued unless they are required for control of persistent psychosis [I] or prophylaxis against recurrence [III]. While maintenance therapy with atypical antipsychotics may be considered [III], there is as yet no definitive evidence that their efficacy in maintenance treatment is comparable to that of agents such as lithium or valproate.

During maintenance treatment, patients with bipolar disorder are likely to benefit from a concomitant psychosocial intervention—including psychotherapy—that addresses illness management (i.e., adherence, lifestyle changes, and early detection of prodromal symptoms) and interpersonal difficulties [II].

Group psychotherapy may also help patients address such issues as adherence to a treatment plan, adaptation to a chronic illness, regulation of self-esteem, and management of marital and other psychosocial issues [II]. Support groups provide useful information about bipolar disorder and its treatment [I].

Patients who continue to experience subthreshold symptoms or breakthrough mood episodes may require the addition of another maintenance medication [II], an atypical antipsychotic [III], or an antidepressant [III]. There are currently insufficient data to support one combination over another. Maintenance sessions of ECT may also be considered for patients whose acute episode responded to ECT [II].

II. FORMULATION AND IMPLEMENTATION OF A TREATMENT PLAN

The following discussion regarding the formulation and implementation of a treatment plan refers specifically to patients with bipolar disorder. Every effort has been made to identify and highlight distinctions between bipolar I and bipolar II disorder in terms of patient response to treatment. However, with few exceptions, data from large trials have been presented in such a way that making such distinctions is difficult. For the treatment of patients with major depressive disorder, readers should refer to the APA *Practice Guideline for the Treatment of Patients With Major Depressive Disorder* (2).

Initial treatment of bipolar disorder requires a thorough assessment of the patient, with particular attention to the safety of the patient and those around him or her as well as attention to possible comorbid psychiatric or medical illnesses. In addition to the current mood state, the clinician needs to consider the longitudinal history of the patient's illness. Patients frequently seek treatment during an acute episode, which may be characterized by depression, mania, hypomania, or a mixture of depressive and manic features. Treatment is aimed at stabilization of the episode with the goal of achieving remission, defined as a complete return to baseline level of functioning and a virtual lack of symptoms. (Following remission of a depressive episode, patients may remain at particularly high risk of relapse for a period up to 6 months; this phase of treatment, sometimes referred to as continuation treatment [4], is considered in this guideline to be part of maintenance treatment.) After successfully completing the acute phase of treatment, patients enter the maintenance phase. At this point, the primary goal of treatment is to optimize protection against recurrence of depressive, mixed, manic, or hypomanic episodes. Concurrently, attention needs to be devoted to maximizing patient functioning and minimizing subthreshold symptoms and adverse effects of treatment.

Of note, in the treatment recommendations outlined in this guideline, several references are made to adding medications or offering combinations of medications. Patients with bipolar disorder often require such combinations in order to achieve adequate symptom control and prophylaxis against future episodes. However, each additional medication generally increases the side effect burden and the likelihood of drug-drug interactions or other toxicity and therefore must be assessed in terms of the risk-benefit ratio to the individual patient. This guideline has attempted to highlight medication interactions used in common clinical practice that are of particular concern (e.g., interactions between lamotrigine and valproate or between carbamazepine and oral contraceptives). In addition, for several of the medications addressed in this guideline, different preparations or forms are available (e.g., valproic acid and divalproex). Although the guideline refers to these medications in general terms, the form of medication with the best tolerability and fewest drug interactions should be preferred.

At other times in treatment, it may be necessary to discontinue a medication (e.g., because of intolerable side effects) or substitute one medication for another. It is preferable to slowly taper the medication to be discontinued rather than discontinuing it abruptly.

In this revision of the previously published *Practice Guideline for the Treatment of Patients With Bipolar Disorder* (5), the term "mood stabilizer" has been omitted. Several definitions of what constitutes a mood stabilizer have been proposed and generally include such criteria as proven efficacy for the treatment of mania or depression, absence of exacerbation of manic or mixed symptoms, or prophylactic efficacy. Because of the absence of a consensus definition, this guideline will instead generally refer to specific medications or to the phase of illness in which they may be used.

A. PSYCHIATRIC MANAGEMENT

The cross-sectional (i.e., current clinical status) and longitudinal (i.e., frequency, severity, and consequences of past episodes) context of the treatment decision should guide the psychiatrist and bipolar disorder patient in choosing from among various possible treatments and treatment settings. Such treatment decisions must be based on knowledge of the potential beneficial and adverse effects of available options along with information about patient preferences. In addition, treatment decisions should be continually reassessed as new information becomes available, the patient's clinical status changes, or both. Lack of insight or minimization is often a prominent part of bipolar disorder and may at times interfere with the patient's ability to make reasoned treatment decisions, necessitating the involvement of family members or significant others in treatment whenever possible.

At this time, there is no cure for bipolar disorder; however, treatment can significantly decrease the associated morbidity and mortality. The general goals of bipolar disorder treatment are to assess and treat acute exacerbations, prevent recurrences, improve interepisode function-

TABLE 1. Characteristics to Evaluate in an Assessment of Suicide Risk in Patients With Bipolar Disorder

Presence of suicidal or homicidal ideation, intent, or plans
Access to means for suicide and the lethality of those means
Presence of command hallucinations, other psychotic symptoms, or severe anxiety
Presence of alcohol or substance use
History and seriousness of previous attempts
Family history of or recent exposure to suicide

Source. Adapted from the APA *Practice Guideline for the Treatment of Patients With Major Depressive Disorder* (2).

ing, and provide assistance, insight, and support to the patient and family. Initially, the psychiatrist will perform a diagnostic evaluation and assess the patient's safety, level of functioning, and clinical needs in order to arrive at a decision about the optimum treatment setting. Subsequently, specific goals of psychiatric management include establishing and maintaining a therapeutic alliance, monitoring the patient's psychiatric status, providing education regarding bipolar disorder, enhancing treatment compliance, promoting regular patterns of activity and of sleep, anticipating stressors, identifying new episodes early, and minimizing functional impairments.

1. Perform a diagnostic evaluation

The evaluation for bipolar disorder requires careful and thorough attention to the clinical history. Patients with bipolar disorder most often exhibit symptoms of depression but may also exhibit substance use, impulsivity, irritability, agitation, insomnia, problems with relationships, or other concerns. Patients rarely volunteer information about manic or hypomanic episodes, so clinicians must probe about time periods with mood dysregulation, lability, or both that are accompanied by associated manic symptoms (e.g., decreased need for sleep, increased energy).

One way to improve efficiency and increase sensitivity in detecting bipolar disorder is to screen for it, particularly in patients with depression, irritability, or impulsivity. The Mood Disorder Questionnaire is a 13-item, self-report screening instrument for bipolar disorder that has been used successfully in psychiatric clinics (6) and in the general population (unpublished 2001 study of R.M.A. Hirschfeld). The general principles and components of a complete psychiatric evaluation have been outlined in the APA *Practice Guideline for Psychiatric Evaluation of Adults* (7).

2. Evaluate the safety of the patient and others and determine a treatment setting

Suicide completion rates in patients with bipolar I disorder may be as high as 10%–15% (8–13); thus, a careful assessment of the patient's risk for suicide is critical. The overwhelming majority of suicide attempts are associated with depressive episodes or depressive features during mixed episodes. The elements of an evaluation for suicide risk are summarized in Table 1. All patients should be asked about suicidal ideation, intention to act on these ideas, and extent of plans or preparation for suicide. Collateral information from family members or others is critical in assessing suicide risk. Access to means of committing suicide (e.g., medications, firearms) and the lethality of these means should also be determined. Other clinical factors that may increase the risk of a patient acting on suicidal ideation should be assessed; these may include substance abuse or other psychiatric comorbidity, such as psychosis. The nature of any prior suicide attempts, including their potential for lethality, should be considered.

The ability to predict suicide or violence risk from clinical data is somewhat limited. Consequently, patients who exhibit suicidal or violent ideas or intent require close monitoring. Whenever suicidal or violent ideas are expressed or suspected, careful documentation of the decision-making process is essential. Hospitalization is usually indicated for patients who are considered to pose a serious threat of harm to themselves or others. If patients refuse, they can be hospitalized involuntarily if their condition meets criteria of the local jurisdiction for involuntary admission. Severely ill patients who lack adequate social support outside of a hospital setting or demonstrate significantly impaired judgment should also be considered for admission to a hospital. Additionally, those patients who have psychiatric or general medical complications or who have not responded adequately to outpatient treatment may need to be hospitalized. The optimal treatment setting and the patient's ability to benefit from a different level of care should be reevaluated on an ongoing basis throughout the course of treatment.

During the manic phase of bipolar disorder, a calm and highly structured environment is optimal. Such stimuli as television, videos, music, and even animated conversations can heighten manic thought processes and activities. Patients and their families should be advised that during manic episodes, patients may engage in reckless behavior and that, at times, steps should be taken to limit access to cars, credit cards, bank accounts, and telephones or cellular phones.

3. Establish and maintain a therapeutic alliance

Bipolar disorder is a long-term illness that manifests in different ways in different patients and at different points during its course. Establishing and maintaining a supportive and therapeutic relationship is critical to the proper understanding and management of an individual patient. A crucial element of this alliance is the knowledge gained about the course of the patient's illness that allows new episodes to be identified as early as possible.

4. Monitor treatment response

The psychiatrist should remain vigilant for changes in psychiatric status. While this is true for all psychiatric disorders, it is especially important in bipolar disorder because limited insight on the part of the patient is so frequent, especially during manic episodes. In addition, small changes in mood or behavior may herald the onset of an episode, with potentially devastating consequences. Such monitoring may be enhanced by knowledge gained over time about particular characteristics of a patient's illness, including typical sequence (e.g., whether episodes of mania are usually followed by episodes of depression) and typical duration and severity of episodes.

5. Provide education to the patient and to the family

Patients with bipolar disorder benefit from education and feedback regarding their illness, prognosis, and treatment. Frequently, their ability to understand and retain this information will vary over time. Patients will also vary in their ability to accept and adapt to the idea that they have an illness that requires long-term treatment. Education should therefore be an ongoing process in which the psychiatrist gradually but persistently introduces facts about the illness. Over an extended period of time, such an approach to patient education will assist in reinforcing the patient's collaborative role in treating this persistent illness. In this capacity, the patient will know when to report subsyndromal symptoms. Printed material on cross-sectional and longitudinal aspects of bipolar illness and its treatment can be helpful, including information available on the Internet (such as that found in the Medical Library at www.medem.com). Similar educational approaches are also important for family members and significant others. They too may have difficulty accepting that the patient has an illness and may minimize the consequences of the illness and the patient's need for continuing treatment (14–17). A list of depressive and bipolar disorder resources, including associations that conduct regular educational meetings and support groups, is provided in Appendix 1.

6. Enhance treatment compliance

Bipolar disorder is a long-term illness in which adherence to carefully designed treatment plans can improve the patient's health status. However, patients with this disorder are frequently ambivalent about treatment (18). This ambivalence often takes the form of noncompliance with medication and other treatments (19, 20), which is a major cause of relapse (21, 22).

Ambivalence about treatment stems from many factors, one of which is lack of insight. Patients who do not believe that they have a serious illness are not likely to be willing to adhere to long-term treatment regimens. Patients with bipolar disorder may minimize or deny the reality of a prior episode or their own behavior and its consequences. Lack of insight may be especially pronounced during a manic episode.

Another important factor for some patients is their reluctance to give up the experience of hypomania or mania (19). The increased energy, euphoria, heightened self-esteem, and ability to focus may be very desirable and enjoyable. Patients often recall this aspect of the experience and minimize or deny entirely the subsequent devastating features of full-blown mania or the extended demoralization of a depressive episode. As a result, they are often reluctant to take medications that prevent elevations in mood.

Medication side effects, cost, and other demands of long-term treatment may be burdensome and need to be discussed realistically with the patient and family members. Many side effects can be corrected with careful attention to dosing, scheduling, and preparation. Troublesome side effects that remain must be discussed in the context of an informed assessment of the risks and benefits of the current treatment and its potential alternatives.

7. Promote awareness of stressors and regular patterns of activity and sleep

Patients and families can also benefit from an understanding of the role of psychosocial stressors and other disruptions in precipitating or exacerbating mood episodes. Psychosocial stressors are consistently found to be increased before both manic and depressive episodes (23). Although this relationship was previously thought to hold true only for the first few episodes of bipolar disorder, more recent studies have found that stressors commonly precede episodes in all phases of the illness (24). Social rhythm disruption with disrupted sleep-wake cycles may specifically trigger manic (but not depressive) episodes (25). Of course, some episodes may not be associated with any discernible life events or stressors. Clinically, the pharmacological management of manic or depressive episodes does not depend on whether stressors preceded the episode. However, patients and families should be informed about the potential consequences of sleep disruption on the course of bipolar disorder (26). To target vulnerable times and to generate coping strategies for these stressors, the unique association between specific types of life stressors and precipitating episodes for each patient should also be addressed (27). It is similarly important to recognize distress or dysfunction in the family of a patient with bipolar disorder, since such ongoing stress may exacerbate the patient's illness or interfere with treatment (14, 15, 28, 29).

Patients with bipolar disorder may benefit from regular patterns of daily activities, including sleeping, eating, physical activity, and social and emotional stimulation. The psychiatrist should help the patient determine the degree to which these factors affect mood states and develop methods to monitor and modulate daily activities. Many patients find that if they establish regular patterns of sleeping, other important aspects of life will fall into regular patterns as well.

8. Work with the patient to anticipate and address early signs of relapse

The psychiatrist should help the patient, family members, and significant others recognize early signs and symptoms of manic or depressive episodes. Such identification can help the patient enhance mastery over his or her illness and can help ensure that adequate treatment is instituted as early as possible in the course of an episode. Early markers of episode onset vary from patient to patient but are often usefully predictable across episodes for an individual patient. Many patients experience changes in sleep patterns early in the development of an episode. Other symptoms may be quite subtle and specific to the individual (e.g., participating in religious activities more or less often than usual). The identification of these early prodromal signs or symptoms is facilitated by the presence of a consistent relationship between the psychiatrist and the patient as well as a consistent relationship with the patient's family (27). The use of a graphic display or timeline of life events and mood symptoms can be very helpful in this process (30). First conceived by Kraepelin (31) and Meyer (32) and refined and advanced by Post et al. (30), a life chart provides a valuable display of illness course and episode sequence, polarity, severity, frequency, response to treatment, and relationship (if any) to environmental stressors. A graphic display of sleep patterns may be sufficient for some patients to identify early signs of episodes.

9. Evaluate and manage functional impairments

Episodes of mania or depression often leave patients with emotional, social, family, academic, occupational, and financial problems. During manic episodes, for example, patients may spend money unwisely, damage important relationships, lose jobs, or commit sexual indiscretions. Following mood episodes, they may require assistance in addressing the psychosocial consequences of their actions.

Bipolar disorder is associated with functional impairments even during periods of euthymia, and the presence, type, and severity of dysfunction should be evaluated (33–35). Impairments can include deficits in cognition, interpersonal relationships, work, living conditions, and other medical or health-related needs (36, 37). Identified impairments in functioning should be addressed. For example, some patients may require assistance in scheduling absences from work or other responsibilities, whereas others may require encouragement to avoid major life changes while in a depressive or manic state. Patients should also be encouraged to set realistic, attainable goals for themselves in terms of desirable levels of functioning. Occupational therapists may be helpful with addressing functional impairments caused by bipolar disorder.

Patients who have children may need help assessing and addressing their children's needs. In particular, children of individuals with bipolar disorder have genetic as well as psychosocial risk factors for developing a psychiatric disorder; parents may need help in obtaining a psychiatric evaluation for children who show early signs of mood instability.

B. ACUTE TREATMENT

1. Manic or mixed episodes

For patients experiencing a manic or mixed episode, the primary goal of treatment is the control of symptoms to allow a return to normal levels of psychosocial functioning. The rapid control of agitation, aggression, and impulsivity is particularly important to ensure the safety of patients and those around them.

Lithium, valproate, and antipsychotic medications have shown efficacy in the treatment of acute mania, although the time to onset of action for lithium may be somewhat slower than that for valproate or antipsychotics. The *combination* of an antipsychotic with either lithium or valproate may be more effective than any of these agents alone. Thus, the first-line pharmacological treatment for patients with severe mania is the initiation of either lithium plus an antipsychotic or valproate plus an antipsychotic. For less ill patients, monotherapy with lithium, valproate, or an antipsychotic such as olanzapine may be sufficient. Alternatives with less supporting evidence for treatment of manic and mixed states include ziprasidone or quetiapine in lieu of another antipsychotic and carbamazepine or oxcarbazepine in lieu of lithium or valproate. (Although efficacy data for oxcarbazepine remain limited, this medication may have equivalent efficacy and better tolerability than carbamazepine.) Short-term adjunctive treatment with a benzodiazepine may also be helpful. In contrast, antidepressants may precipitate or exacerbate manic or mixed episodes and generally should be tapered and discontinued if possible.

Selection of the initial treatment should be guided by clinical factors such as illness severity, by associated features (e.g., rapid cycling, psychosis), and by patient preference where possible, with particular attention to side effect profiles. A number of factors may lead the clinician to choose one particular agent over another. For example, some evidence suggests a greater efficacy of valproate compared with lithium in the treatment of mixed states. Also, severely ill and agitated patients who are unable to take medications by mouth may require antipsychotic medications that can be administered intramuscularly. Because of the more benign side effect profile of atypical antipsychotics, they are preferred over typical antipsychotics such as haloperidol and chlorpromazine. Of the atypical antipsychotics, there is presently more placebo-controlled evidence in support of olanzapine and risperidone.

If psychosocial therapies are used, they should be combined with pharmacotherapy. Perhaps the only indications for psychotherapy alone for patients experiencing acute manic or mixed episodes are when all established treatments have been refused, involuntary treatment is not appropriate, and the primary goals of therapy are focused and crisis-oriented (e.g., resolving ambivalence about taking medication).

For patients who, despite receiving the aforementioned medications, experience a manic or mixed episode (i.e., a "breakthrough" episode), the first-line intervention should be to optimize the medication dose. Optimization of dosage entails ensuring that the blood level is in the therapeutic range and in some cases achieving a higher serum level (although one still within the therapeutic range). Introduction or resumption of an antipsychotic is often necessary. Severely ill or agitated patients may require short-term adjunctive treatment with an antipsychotic agent or benzodiazepine.

With adequate dosing and serum levels, medications for the treatment of mania generally exert some appreciable clinical effect by the 10th to the 14th day of treatment. When first-line medications at optimal doses fail to control symptoms, recommended treatment options include addition of another first-line medication. Alternative treatment options include adding carbamazepine or oxcarbazepine in lieu of an additional first-line medication, adding an antipsychotic if not already prescribed, or changing from one antipsychotic to another. Of the antipsychotic agents, clozapine may be particularly effective for treatment of refractory illness. As always, caution should be exercised when combining medications, since side effects may be additive and metabolism of other agents may be affected.

ECT may also be considered for patients with severe or treatment-resistant illness or when preferred by the patient in consultation with the psychiatrist. In addition, ECT is a potential treatment for patients with mixed episodes or for severe mania experienced during pregnancy.

Patients displaying psychotic features during a manic episode usually require treatment with an antipsychotic medication. Atypical antipsychotics are favored because of their more benign side effect profile.

2. Depressive episodes

The primary goal of treatment in bipolar depression, as with nonbipolar depression, is remission of the symptoms of major depression with return to normal levels of psychosocial functioning. An additional focus of treatment is to avoid precipitation of a manic or hypomanic episode.

The first-line pharmacological treatment for bipolar depression is the initiation of either lithium or lamotrigine. The better supported of these is lithium. While standard antidepressants such as SSRIs have shown good efficacy in the treatment of unipolar depression, for bipolar disorder they generally have been studied as add-ons to medications such as lithium or valproate; antidepressant monotherapy is not recommended, given the risk of precipitating a switch into mania. For severely ill patients, some clinicians will initiate treatment with lithium and an antidepressant simultaneously, although there are limited data to support this approach. In patients with life-threatening inanition, suicidality, or psychosis, ECT also represents a reasonable alternative. In addition, ECT is a potential treatment for severe depression during pregnancy. Selection of the initial treatment should be guided by clinical factors such as illness severity, by associated features (e.g., rapid cycling, psychosis), and by patient preference, with particular attention to side effect profiles.

Small studies have suggested that interpersonal therapy and cognitive behavior therapy may also be useful when added to pharmacotherapy during depressive episodes in patients with bipolar disorder. There have been no definitive studies to date of psychotherapy in lieu of antidepressant treatment for bipolar depression. However, a larger body of evidence supports the efficacy of psychotherapy in the treatment of unipolar depression (2).

For patients who, despite receiving maintenance medication treatment, suffer a breakthrough depressive episode, the first-line intervention should be to optimize the dose of the maintenance medication. Optimization of dosage entails ensuring that the serum drug level is in the therapeutic range and in some cases achieving a higher serum level (although one still within the therapeutic range).

For patients who do not respond to optimal maintenance treatment, next steps include adding lamotrigine, bupropion, or paroxetine. Alternative next steps include adding other newer antidepressants (e.g., another SSRI or venlafaxine) or an MAOI. Although there are few empirical data that directly compare risk of switch or efficacy among antidepressants in the treatment of bipolar disorder, tricyclic antidepressants may carry a greater risk of precipitating a switch into hypomania or mania. Also, while MAOIs have generally demonstrated good efficacy, their side effect profile may make other agents preferable as initial interventions (2). ECT should be considered for patients with severe or treatment-resistant depressive episodes or for those episodes with catatonic features.

Patients with psychotic features during a depressive episode usually require adjunctive treatment with an antipsychotic medication. ECT represents a reasonable alternative.

Studies of bipolar depression rarely separate results for patients with bipolar I disorder from those of patients with bipolar II disorder. It is not known whether specific pharmacotherapy regimens differ in efficacy for treatment of bipolar I versus bipolar II depression. However, existing data suggest that for patients with bipolar II disorder, antidepressant treatment—either alone or in combination with a maintenance medication—is less likely to result in a switch into a hypomanic episode relative to those with bipolar I disorder (38).

3. Rapid cycling

The initial intervention for patients who experience rapid-cycling episodes of illness is to identify and treat medical conditions that may contribute to cycling, such as hypothyroidism or drug or alcohol use. Since antidepressants may also contribute to cycling, the need for continued antidepressant treatment should be reassessed; antidepressants should be tapered if possible. The initial treatment for patients who experience rapid-cycling episodes of illness should include lithium or valproate; an alternative treatment is lamotrigine. In many instances, combinations of medications are required (39, 40); possibilities include combining two of these agents or combining one of them with an antipsychotic. Because of their more benign side effect profile, atypical antipsychotics are preferred over typical antipsychotics.

C. MAINTENANCE TREATMENT

Maintenance medication treatment is generally recommended following a single manic episode. Although few studies have been conducted involving patients with bipolar II disorder, consideration of maintenance treatment for this form of the illness is also warranted. Primary goals of treatment include relapse prevention, reduction of subthreshold symptoms, and reduction of suicide risk. Goals also need to include reduction of cycling frequency and mood instability as well as improvement in overall functioning. Pharmacotherapy must be employed in ways that yield good tolerability and do not predispose the patient to nonadherence.

Options with the best empirical evidence to support their use as maintenance treatments include lithium or valproate; possible alternatives include lamotrigine, carbamazepine, or oxcarbazepine. Despite limited data, oxcarbazepine is included—as it was for acute treatment of mania—because its efficacy may be similar to that of carbamazepine but with better tolerability. In general, if one of these medications was used to achieve remission from the most recent depressive or manic episode, it should be continued. Maintenance ECT may also be considered for patients whose acute episode responded to ECT. Selection of the initial treatment should be guided by clinical factors such as illness severity, by associated features (e.g., rapid cycling, psychosis), and by patient preference, with particular attention to side effect profiles.

For patients treated with an antipsychotic medication during the preceding acute episode, the need for ongoing antipsychotic treatment should be reassessed upon entering the maintenance phase. Since antipsychotic agents, particularly typical antipsychotics, may cause tardive dyskinesia with long-term use, antipsychotics should be slowly tapered and discontinued unless they are required to control persistent psychosis or provide prophylaxis against recurrence. While maintenance therapy with atypical antipsychotics may be considered, there is as yet no definitive evidence that their efficacy in maintenance is comparable to that of agents such as lithium or valproate.

Patients with bipolar disorder are likely to gain some additional benefit during the maintenance phase from a concomitant psychosocial intervention that addresses illness management (i.e., adherence, lifestyle changes, and early detection of prodromal symptoms) and interpersonal difficulties. Although not adequately studied to provide evidence-based documentation, supportive and psychodynamic psychotherapy are widely used in addition to medication.

Group psychotherapy, in conjunction with appropriate medication, may also help patients address such issues as adherence to a treatment plan, adaptation to a chronic illness, regulation of self-esteem, and management of marital as well as other psychosocial issues.

Support groups provide useful information about bipolar disorder and its treatment. Patients in these groups often benefit from hearing the experiences of others who are struggling with such issues as denial versus acceptance of the need for medication, problems with side effects, and how to shoulder other burdens associated with the illness and its treatment. Advocacy groups such as the National Depressive and Manic-Depressive Association and the National Alliance for the Mentally Ill (Appendix 1) have many local chapters that provide both support and educational material to patients and their families.

Although maintenance medication combinations are often associated with increases in side effects, use of such regimens should be considered for patients who have not responded adequately to simpler regimens. The addition of another maintenance medication, an atypical antipsychotic, or an antidepressant may be necessary for patients who experience either continuing high levels of subthreshold symptoms or a breakthrough episode of illness. There are currently insufficient data to support one combination over another. Maintenance ECT may also be considered for patients whose acute episode responded to ECT.

III. SPECIAL CLINICAL FEATURES INFLUENCING THE TREATMENT PLAN

A. PSYCHIATRIC FEATURES

1. Psychosis

Psychotic symptoms (e.g., delusions, hallucinations) are commonly seen during episodes of either mania or depression but are more common in the former, appearing in over one-half of manic episodes (41). Mood-congruent features during a manic episode probably are not predictive of a poorer outcome, although early onset (before age 21) of psychotic mania may predict a more severe disorder (42). Mood-incongruent features have been identified in some (43) but not all (44) studies to be a predictor of a shorter time in remission. The presence of psychotic features during a manic episode may not require an antipsychotic medication, although most clinicians prescribe them in addition to a maintenance agent (45).

2. Catatonia

Catatonic features may develop in up to one-third of patients during a manic episode (46). The most commonly observed symptoms of catatonia in mania are motor excitement, mutism, and stereotypic movements. Because catatonic symptoms are seen in other psychiatric and neurological disorders, a careful assessment is indicated for an accurate diagnosis. In addition, patients who exhibit catatonic stupor may go on to show more typical signs and symptoms of mania during the same episode of illness (47). The presence of catatonic features during the course of a manic episode is associated with greater episode severity, mixed states, and somewhat poorer short-term outcomes (46). In treating catatonia, neuroleptics have generally exhibited poor efficacy (48). In contrast, prospective studies have demonstrated the efficacy of lorazepam in the treatment of catatonic syndromes, including those associated with mania (49–52). Since ECT is probably the most effective treatment for catatonic syndromes regardless of etiology, ECT should be considered if benzodiazepines do not result in symptom resolution (48).

3. Risk of suicide, homicide, and violence

Like those suffering from major depression, patients with bipolar disorder are at high risk for suicide (53, 54). The frequency of suicide attempts appears similar for the bipolar I and bipolar II subtypes (55, 56). Individuals with bipolar disorder repeatedly have been shown to have greater overall mortality than the general population (41). Although much of this risk reflects the higher rate of suicide, cardiovascular and pulmonary mortality among patients with untreated bipolar disorder is also high (41, 57).

Known general risk factors for suicide also apply to patients with bipolar disorder. These include a history of suicide attempts, suicidal ideation, comorbid substance abuse, comorbid personality disorders (58), agitation, pervasive insomnia, impulsiveness (59), and family history of suicide. Among the phases of bipolar disorder, depression is associated with the highest suicide risk, followed by mixed states and presence of psychotic symptoms, with episodes of mania being least associated with suicide (8, 56). Suicidal ideation during mixed states has been correlated with the severity of depressive symptoms (10). In general, a detailed evaluation of the individual patient is necessary to assess suicide risk (Table 1). Judgment of suicide risk is inherently imperfect; therefore, risks and benefits of intervention should be carefully weighed and documented.

Long-term treatment with lithium has been associated with reduction of suicide risk (56, 60). Whether this reflects an anti-impulsivity factor beyond lithium's mood-stabilizing effect is not yet clear. Lithium may also diminish the greater mortality risk observed among bipolar disorder patients from causes other than suicide (61). It is unknown whether prolonged survival is also seen with the anticonvulsant maintenance agents.

Clinical experience attests to the presence of violent behavior in some patients with bipolar disorder, and violence may be an indication for hospitalization (41). Comorbid substance abuse and psychosis may contribute to the threat of criminal violence or aggression (62–64).

4. Substance use disorders

Bipolar disorder with a comorbid substance use disorder is a very common presentation, with bipolar disorder patients of both sexes showing much higher rates of substance use than the general population (65). For example, the Epidemiologic Catchment Area study found rates of alcohol abuse or dependence in 46% of patients with bipolar disorder compared with 13% for the general population. Comparable drug abuse and dependence figures are 41% and 6%, respectively (66, 67). Substance abuse may obscure or exacerbate endogenous mood swings. Conversely, comorbid substance use disorder may be overlooked in patients with bipolar disorder (68, 69). Substance abuse may also precipitate mood episodes or be used by patients to ameliorate the symptoms of such episodes. Comorbid substance use is typically associated with fewer and slower remissions, greater rates of suicide and suicide attempts, and poorer outcome (70–73).

Treatment for substance abuse and bipolar disorder should proceed concurrently when possible. It is also helpful to obtain consultation from an addiction expert, such as an addiction psychiatrist, or to arrange for concomitant treatment of the bipolar disorder and the substance use disorder in a dual-diagnosis program.

Alcohol abuse and its effects may affect bipolar disorder pharmacotherapy. For instance, alcohol-related dehydration may raise lithium levels to toxicity. Hepatic dysfunction from chronic alcohol abuse or from hepatitis associated with intravenous substance use may alter plasma levels of valproate and carbamazepine (74). If the hepatic dysfunction is severe, the use of these hepatically metabolized medications may be problematic. In these cases, coordination with the patient's primary care physician or gastroenterologist is recommended (75).

5. Comorbid psychiatric conditions

Patients with comorbid personality disorders pose complicated diagnostic pictures. They are clearly at greater risk for experiencing intrapsychic and psychosocial stress that can precipitate or exacerbate mood episodes. Patients with comorbid personality disorders generally have greater symptom burden, lower recovery rates from episodes, and greater functional impairment (76). In addition, these patients may have particular difficulty adhering to long-term treatment regimens (77).

Relative to the general population, individuals with bipolar disorder are at greater risk for comorbid anxiety disorders, especially panic disorder and obsessive-compulsive disorder. Comorbid anxiety disorders may predict a longer time to recovery of mood episodes (78). Treatment for the bipolar disorder and the comorbid anxiety disorder should proceed concurrently.

The presence of comorbid attention-deficit/hyperactivity disorder (ADHD) in adults and children with bipolar disorder may make it difficult to monitor changes in mood states. Of note, adults with bipolar disorder and comorbid ADHD are likely to have experienced a much earlier age at onset of their mood disorder relative to those without comorbid ADHD (79).

B. DEMOGRAPHIC AND PSYCHOSOCIAL FACTORS

1. Gender

A number of issues related to gender must be considered when treating patients with bipolar disorder. Hypothyroidism is more common in women, and women may be more susceptible to the antithyroid effects of lithium (80). Additionally, rapid cycling is more common in women (81, 82). Treatment with antipsychotics and, to a lesser extent, SSRIs may elevate serum levels of prolactin and result in galactorrhea, sexual dysfunction, menstrual disorders, and impaired fertility (83, 84).

2. Pregnancy

Because many medications used to treat bipolar disorder are associated with a higher risk of birth defects, the psychiatrist should encourage effective contraceptive practices for all female patients of childbearing age who are receiving pharmacological treatment (85, 86). Since carbamazepine, oxcarbazepine, and topiramate increase the metabolism of oral contraceptives, women taking these medications should not rely on oral contraceptives for birth control (87–89). This effect does not occur with other medications used to treat bipolar disorder.

Multiple clinical issues arise in relationship to pregnancy in bipolar disorder patients. In order to permit discussion of the risks and benefits of therapeutic options, a pregnancy should be planned in consultation with the psychiatrist whenever possible. Because of the higher genetic risk for bipolar disorder (90–92), patients with bipolar disorder who are considering having children may also benefit from genetic counseling (22).

a) Continuing/discontinuing medications

Around the time of pregnancy, the risks and benefits of continuing versus discontinuing treatment require the most thoughtful judgment and discussion among the patient, the psychiatrist, the obstetrician, and the father. Specific options include continuing medication throughout pregnancy, discontinuing medications at the beginning of pregnancy or before conception, and discontinuing the medication only for the first trimester.

In clinical decision making, the potential teratogenic risks of psychotropic medications must be balanced against the risk of no prophylactic treatment, with the attendant risks of illness (93). Although the course of bipolar disorder during pregnancy is still unclear, some evidence suggests that pregnancy does not alter the rate of mood episodes compared with other times (94). However, in patients who have been stable on a regimen of lithium, the rate of recurrent mood episodes is clearly increased by lithium discontinuation, particularly when discontinuation is abrupt (94). Should the decision be made to discontinue medication, the woman should be advised about the potentially greater risk of mood episode recurrence with rapid discontinuation of lithium (and possibly other maintenance agents) compared with a slower taper over many weeks (95).

Although direct evidence of a negative effect of untreated psychiatric disorders on fetal development is lacking, antenatal stress, depression, and anxiety are linked with a variety of abnormalities in newborns (96–101). Additionally, during a manic episode, women are at risk of increasing their consumption of alcohol and other drugs, thus conferring additional dangers to the fetus.

b) Prenatal exposure to medications

First-trimester exposure to lithium, valproate, or carbamazepine is associated with a greater risk of birth defects. With lithium exposure the absolute risk for Ebstein's anomaly, a cardiovascular defect, is 1–2 per 1,000. This is approximately 10–20 times greater than the risk in the general population (102). Exposure to carbamazepine and valproate during the first trimester is associated with neural tube defects at rates of up to 1% and 3%–5%, respectively (85). Both carbamazepine and valproate exposure have also been associated with craniofacial abnormalities (103, 104). Other congenital defects that have been observed with valproate include limb malformations and cardiac defects (104). Little is known about the potential teratogenicity of lamotrigine, gabapentin, or other newer anticonvulsants.

No teratogenic effects have been demonstrated with tricyclic antidepressants. Near term, however, their use has been associated with side effects in the neonate (105). The SSRIs seem to be relatively benign in their risks to exposed fetuses (106), with safety data being strongest for fluoxetine and citalopram. Although data with bupropion, mirtazapine, nefazodone, trazodone, and venlafaxine are limited (105), none of the newer antidepressants has been shown to be teratogenic (106, 107). Nonetheless, caution must be exercised if they are prescribed to treat bipolar depression in pregnant women (93).

Antipsychotic agents may be needed to treat psychotic features of bipolar disorder during pregnancy, but they may also represent an alternative to lithium for treating symptoms of mania (105). High-potency antipsychotic medications are preferred during pregnancy, since they are less likely to have associated anticholinergic, antihistaminergic, or hypotensive effects. In addition, there is no evidence of teratogenicity with exposure to haloperidol, perphenazine, thiothixene, or trifluoperazine (105). When high-potency antipsychotic medications are used near term, neonates may show extrapyramidal side effects, but these are generally short-lived

(108). To limit the duration of such effects, however, long-acting depot preparations of antipsychotic medications are not recommended during pregnancy (105). For newer antipsychotic agents such as risperidone, olanzapine, clozapine, quetiapine, and ziprasidone, little is known about the potential risks of teratogenicity or the potential effects in the neonate.

The risk of teratogenicity with benzodiazepines is not clear (108). Early studies, primarily with diazepam and chlordiazepoxide, suggested that first-trimester exposure may have led to malformations, including facial clefts, in some infants. Later studies showed no significant increases in specific defects or in the overall incidence of malformations (108). A recent meta-analysis of the risk of oral cleft or major malformations showed no association with fetal exposure to benzodiazepines in pooled data from cohort studies, but a greater risk was reported on the basis of pooled data from case-control studies (109). In general, however, teratogenic risks are thought likely to be small with benzodiazepines (105). Near term, use of benzodiazepines may be associated with sedation in the neonate. Withdrawal symptoms resulting from dependence may also be seen in the neonate (108). As a result, if benzodiazepines are used during pregnancy, lorazepam is generally preferred (105).

ECT is also a potential treatment for severe mania or depression during pregnancy (110). In terms of teratogenicity, the short-term administration of anesthetic agents with ECT may present less risk to the fetus than pharmacological treatment options (111). The APA Task Force Report on ECT contains additional details on the use of ECT during pregnancy (110).

c) Prenatal monitoring

Women who choose to remain on regimens of lithium, valproate, or carbamazepine during pregnancy should have maternal serum α-fetoprotein screening for neural tube defects before the 20th week of gestation, with amniocentesis as well as targeted sonography performed for any elevated α-fetoprotein values (105). Women should also be encouraged to undergo high-resolution ultrasound examination at 16–18 weeks gestation to detect cardiac abnormalities in the fetus. Since hepatic metabolism, renal excretion, and fluid volume are altered during pregnancy and the perinatal period, serum levels of medications should be monitored and doses adjusted if indicated. At delivery, the rapid fluid shifts in the mother will markedly increase lithium levels unless care is taken to either lower the lithium dose, ensure hydration, or both (112). Discontinuing lithium on the day of delivery is probably not necessary and may be unwise given the high risk for postpartum mood episodes and the greater risk of recurrence if lithium is discontinued in women with bipolar disorder (94, 112).

d) Postpartum issues

The postpartum period is consistently associated with a markedly greater risk for relapse into mania, depression, or psychosis. For women with bipolar disorder, the rate of postpartum relapse is as high as 50% (86, 94). Women who have had severe postpartum affective episodes in the past are at highest risk to have another episode of illness after subsequent pregnancies. Despite a paucity of studies, it is generally considered that prophylactic medications such as lithium or valproate may prevent postpartum mood episodes in women with bipolar disorder (113). Also, since changes in sleep are common in the postpartum period, women should be educated about the need to maintain normal sleep patterns to avoid precipitating episodes of mania.

e) Infant medication exposure through breast-feeding

All medications used in the treatment of bipolar disorder are secreted in breast milk in varying degrees, thereby exposing the neonate to maternally ingested medication (114). However, as with the risks of medications during pregnancy, risks of breast-feeding with psychotropic medications must be weighed against the benefits of breast-feeding (115, 116). Because lithium is secreted in breast milk at 40% of maternal serum concentration, most experts have recommended against its use in mothers who choose to breast-feed (105). Fewer data on breast-feeding are available for carbamazepine and valproate. Although it is generally considered safe, potential risks should always be considered. Little is known about lamotrigine exposure in breast-fed neonates; however, levels in the infant may reach 25% of maternal serum levels (117). Consequently, the potential for pharmacological effects, including a risk for life-threatening rash, should be taken into consideration (118). With other psychotropic medications (including antipsychotics, antidepressants, and benzodiazepines), there are few reports of specific adverse effects in breast-feeding infants. Nonetheless, these drugs are found in measurable quantities in breast milk and could conceivably affect central nervous system functioning in the infant (118).

3. Cross-cultural issues

Culture can influence the experience and communication of symptoms of depression and mania. Underdiagnosis or misdiagnosis, as well as delayed detection of early signs of recurrence, can be reduced by being alert to specific ethnic and cultural differences in reporting complaints of a major mood episode. Specifically, minority patients (particularly African and Hispanic Americans) with bipolar disorder are at greater risk for being misdiagnosed with schizophrenia (119, 120). This greater risk appears to result from clinicians failing to elicit affective symptoms in minority patients with affective psychoses (121).

Ethnicity and race must also be taken into consideration when prescribing medications, since ethnic and racial groups may differ in their metabolism of some medications (122, 123). For example, relative to Caucasian patients, Chinese patients have a lower average activity of the cytochrome P-450 isoenzyme 2D6 (123). As a result, they typically require lower doses of antidepressants and antipsychotics that are metabolized by this enzyme (122). Similar deficits in average activity of the cytochrome P-450 isoenzyme 2C19 have been found in Chinese, Japanese, and Korean patients compared with Caucasians (123).

4. Children and adolescents

The prevalence of bipolar disorder in a community sample of children and adolescents was 1%; an additional 5.7% had mood symptoms that met criteria for bipolar disorder not otherwise specified (124). Although DSM-IV-TR criteria are used to diagnose bipolar disorder in childhood and adolescence, the clinical features of childhood bipolar disorder differ from bipolar disorder in adults. Children with bipolar disorder often have mixed mania, rapid cycling, and psychosis (125). Child and adolescent bipolar disorder is often comorbid with attention deficit and conduct disorders (126–128). For children and adolescents in a current manic episode, 1-year recovery rates of 37.1% and relapse rates of 38.3% have been reported (1, 129). In a 5-year prospective follow-up of adolescents experiencing bipolar disorder, relapse rates of 44% were found (130). Despite the severity and chronicity of this disorder in children and adolescents and its devastating impact on social, emotional, and academic development, treatment research has lagged far behind that of adult bipolar disorder.

Although there is more information available about the use of lithium and divalproex in children and adolescents with bipolar disorder, other medication treatment options include atypical antipsychotics, carbamazepine, and combinations of these medications.

Treatment with a maintenance agent should continue for a minimum of 18 months after stabilization of a manic episode. There is evidence that ultimate stabilization takes a number of years (131). In addition, lithium discontinuation has been shown to increase relapse rates in adolescents with bipolar disorder: relapse occurred within 18 months in 92% of those who discontinued lithium versus 37% of those who continued lithium (132). Consequently, medication discontinuation should be done gradually at a time when there are no major anticipated stressors.

Psychiatric comorbidity may complicate the diagnosis and treatment of bipolar disorder in children and adolescents. The presence of ADHD, especially in children and adolescents, confounds the assessment of mood changes in patients with bipolar disorder. Early manifestations of mania and hypomania can be particularly difficult to distinguish from the ongoing symptoms of ADHD. Careful tracking of symptoms and behaviors is helpful. In addition, the presence of ADHD is associated with higher rates of learning disabilities, which should be addressed in treatment planning.

Youths with bipolar disorder are at greater risk for substance use disorders (133, 134). Comorbid substance use has been shown to complicate the course of bipolar disorder and its treatment (135). Short-term treatment with lithium (136) and divalproex (137) may be useful in these conditions. However, in a 2-year follow-up of hospitalized manic adolescents, the bipolar disorder patients who continued to abuse substances had more manic episodes and poorer functioning than early-onset bipolar disorder patients who did not exhibit comorbid substance abuse. In contrast, cessation of substance use was associated with fewer episodes and greater functional improvement at the 4-year follow-up point (135).

5. Geriatric patients

In patients over 65 years of age, prevalence rates of bipolar disorder range from 0.1% to 0.4% (138). In addition, 5%–12% of geriatric psychiatry admissions are for bipolar disorder (138). Relative to patients with onset of mania at a younger age, those with onset at an older age tend to have less of a family history of bipolar disorder. They may also have longer episode durations or more frequent episodes of illness (139). Of individuals with onset of mania at older ages, one-half have had previous depressive episodes, often with a long latency period before the first manic episode (140).

Manic syndromes in geriatric patients may also be associated with general medical conditions, medications used to treat those conditions, or substance use (138–140). The new onset of mania in later life is particularly associated with high rates of medical and neurological diseases (139–141). Right hemispheric cortical or subcortical lesions are especially common. Relative to elderly patients with multiple episodes of mania, geriatric patients with a first episode of mania have a higher risk of mortality (141). Therefore, any patient with a late onset of manic symptoms should be evaluated carefully for general medical and neurological causes (138–140).

General principles for treating geriatric mania are similar to those for younger adults. Older patients will usually require lower doses of medications, since aging is associated with reductions in renal clearance and volume of distribution (142). Concomitant medications and medical conditions may also alter the metabolism or excretion of psychotropic medications (139). Older patients may also be more sensitive to side effects because of greater end-organ sensitivity. Many elderly patients tolerate only low serum levels of lithium (e.g., 0.4–0.6 meq/liter) (138) and can respond to these levels. Those who tolerate low serum lithium levels but who are not showing benefit should have slow dose increases to yield serum levels in the usual therapeutic range.

Older patients may be more likely to develop cognitive impairment with medications such as lithium or benzodiazepines (138). They may also have difficulty tolerating antipsychotic medications and are more likely to develop extrapyramidal side effects and tardive dyskinesia than younger individuals (143). With some antipsychotics and antidepressants, orthostatic hypotension may be particularly problematic and increases the risk of falls. Use of benzodiazepines and of neuroleptics also has been associated with greater risks of falls and hip fractures in geriatric patients (144).

C. CONCURRENT GENERAL MEDICAL CONDITIONS

In the presence of a severe medical disorder, the disorder itself or the medications used to treat it should always be considered as possible causes of a manic episode. Neurological conditions commonly associated with secondary mania are multiple sclerosis, lesions involving right-side subcortical structures, and lesions of cortical areas with close links to the limbic system (145). L-Dopa and corticosteroids are the most common medications associated with secondary mania (146).

The presence of a general medical condition may also exacerbate the course or severity of bipolar disorder or complicate its treatment (147). For example, the course of bipolar disorder may be exacerbated by any condition that requires intermittent or regular use of steroids (e.g., asthma, inflammatory bowel disease) or that leads to abnormal thyroid functioning. In addition, treatment of patients with bipolar disorder may be complicated by conditions requiring the use of diuretics, angiotensin-converting enzyme inhibitors, nonsteroidal anti-inflammatory drugs, cyclooxygenase-2 inhibitors, or salt-restricted diets, all of which affect lithium excretion. Conditions or their treatments that are associated with abnormal cardiac conduction or rhythm or that affect renal or hepatic function may further restrict the choice or dosage of medications. In HIV-infected patients, lower doses of medications are often indicated because of patients' greater sensitivity to side effects and because of the potential for drug-drug interactions. Special considerations in the treatment of HIV-infected patients are presented in the APA *Practice Guideline for the Treatment of Patients With HIV/AIDS* (148).

Whenever patients are taking more than one medication, the possibility of adverse drug-drug interactions should always be considered. Patients should be educated about the importance of informing their psychiatrist and other physicians about their current medications whenever new medications are prescribed. Clinicians should also inquire about patient use of herbal preparations and over-the-counter medications.

PART B: BACKGROUND INFORMATION AND REVIEW OF AVAILABLE EVIDENCE

IV. DISEASE DEFINITION, NATURAL HISTORY AND COURSE, AND EPIDEMIOLOGY

A. DEFINITION OF BIPOLAR DISORDER

According to DSM-IV-TR (1), patients with bipolar I disorder have had at least one episode of mania (criteria for a manic episode are presented in Table 2). Some patients have had previous depressive episodes (Table 3), and most patients will have subsequent episodes that can be either manic or depressive. Hypomanic and mixed episodes (Table 4 and Table 5, respectively) can occur, as well as significant subthreshold mood lability between episodes. Patients meeting criteria for bipolar II disorder have a history of major depressive episodes and hypomanic episodes only. Patients may also exhibit significant evidence of mood lability, hypomania, and depressive symptoms but fail to meet duration criteria for bipolar II disorder, thereby leading to a diagnosis of bipolar disorder not otherwise specified. Finally, cyclothymic disorder may be diagnosed in those patients who have never experienced a manic, mixed, or major depressive episode but who experience numerous periods of depressive symptoms and numerous periods of hypomanic symptoms for at least 2 years (1 year in children), with no symptom-free period greater than 2 months. The subtypes of bipolar disorder, as well as selected other affective illnesses, are summarized and compared in Table 6.

TABLE 2. Diagnostic Criteria for a Manic Episode

A. A distinct period of abnormally and persistently elevated, expansive, or irritable mood, lasting at least 1 week (or any duration if hospitalization is necessary).

B. During the period of mood disturbance, three (or more) of the following symptoms have persisted (four if the mood is only irritable) and have been present to a significant degree:

1) Inflated self-esteem or grandiosity
2) Decreased need for sleep (e.g., feels rested after only 3 hours of sleep)
3) More talkative than usual or pressure to keep talking
4) Flight of ideas or subjective experience that thoughts are racing
5) Distractibility (i.e., attention too easily drawn to unimportant or irrelevant external stimuli)
6) Increase in goal-directed activity (either socially, at work or school, or sexually) or psychomotor agitation
7) Excessive involvement in pleasurable activities that have a high potential for painful consequences (e.g., engaging in unrestrained buying sprees, sexual indiscretions, or foolish business investments)

C. The symptoms do not meet criteria for a mixed episode.

D. The mood disturbance 1) is sufficiently severe to cause marked impairment in occupational functioning, usual social activities, or relationships with others, 2) necessitates hospitalization to prevent harm to self or others, or 3) has psychotic features.

E. The symptoms are not due to the direct physiological effects of a substance (e.g., a drug of abuse, a medication, or other treatment) or a general medical condition (e.g., hyperthyroidism).

Source. Adapted from DSM-IV-TR; manic-like episodes that are clearly caused by somatic antidepressant treatment (e.g., medication, ECT, light therapy) should not count toward a diagnosis of bipolar I disorder.

In addition to providing definitions of bipolar disorder, DSM-IV-TR also includes specifiers describing the course of recurrent episodes, such as seasonal pattern, longitudinal course (with or without full interepisode recovery), and rapid cycling.

Some investigators have advocated moving from a categorical to a more dimensional perspective in characterizing bipolar disorder. In particular, this perspective includes the concept of a bipolar spectrum that would encompass a range of presentations not currently considered bipolar (149). For example, a patient with antidepressant-induced hypomanic symptoms would be considered to have a form of bipolar disorder under the spectrum conceptualization.

B. NATURAL HISTORY AND COURSE

Bipolar disorder is generally an episodic, lifelong illness with a variable course. The first episode of bipolar disorder may be manic, hypomanic, mixed, or depressive. Men are more likely than women to be initially manic, but both are more likely to have a first episode of depression. Patients with untreated bipolar disorder may have more than 10 total episodes of mania and depression during their lifetime, with the duration of episodes and interepisode periods stabilizing after the fourth or fifth episode (150). Often, 4 years or more may elapse between the first and second episodes, but the intervals between subsequent episodes usually narrow. However, it must be emphasized that variability is the hallmark of this illness. Thus, when taking a history, a number of longitudinal issues must be considered, including the number of prior episodes, the average length and severity of episodes, average interepisode duration, and the interval since the last episode of mania or depression.

TABLE 3. Diagnostic Criteria for a Major Depressive Episode

A. Five (or more) of the following symptoms have been present nearly every day during the same 2-week period and represent a change from previous functioning; at least one of the symptoms is either depressed mood or loss of interest or pleasure:

1) Depressed mood[a] most of the day as indicated by either subjective report (e.g., feels sad or empty) or observation made by others (e.g., appears tearful)
2) Markedly diminished interest or pleasure in all, or almost all, activities most of the day (as indicated by either subjective account or observation made by others)
3) Significant weight loss when not dieting,[b] weight gain (e.g., a change of more than 5% of body weight in a month), or a decrease or increase in appetite
4) Insomnia or hypersomnia
5) Psychomotor agitation or retardation (observable by others, not merely subjective feelings of restlessness or being slowed down)
6) Fatigue or loss of energy
7) Feelings of worthlessness or excessive or inappropriate guilt (which may be delusional)[c]
8) Diminished ability to think or concentrate or indecisiveness (either by subjective account or as observed by others)
9) Recurrent thoughts of death (not just fear of dying), recurrent suicidal ideation without a specific plan, or previous suicide attempt or a specific plan for committing suicide

B. The symptoms do not meet criteria for a mixed episode.

C. The symptoms cause clinically significant distress or impairment in social, occupational, or other important areas of functioning.

D. The symptoms are not due to the direct physiological effects of a substance (e.g., a drug of abuse, a medication) or a general medical condition (e.g., hypothyroidism).

E. The symptoms are not better accounted for by bereavement (i.e., after the loss of a loved one) and have persisted for longer than 2 months or are characterized by marked functional impairment, morbid preoccupation with worthlessness, suicidal ideation, psychotic symptoms, or psychomotor retardation.

Source. Adapted from DSM-IV-TR; mood-incongruent delusions, hallucinations, and symptoms that are clearly due to a general medical condition should not count toward a diagnosis of major depressive disorder.

[a]In children and adolescents, mood can also be irritable.

[b]In children, can also include failure to make expected weight gains.

[c]Symptoms extend beyond mere self-reproach or guilt about being sick.

Frequently, a patient will experience several episodes of depression before a manic episode occurs (34, 151). Consequently, bipolar disorder should always be considered in the differential diagnosis of depression. Patients very often do not report prior episodes of mania and hypomania and instead seek treatment for complaints of depression, delaying correct diagnosis (5, 152–157). For a patient who is not educated about bipolar disorder, symptoms of dysphoric hypomania may not be recognized or reported. Therefore, the psychiatrist needs to ask explicitly about prior manic or hypomanic episodes, since knowledge of their presence can influence treatment decisions. The psychiatrist should also ask about a family history of mood disorders, including mania and hypomania. Consultation with family members and significant others may be extremely useful in establishing family history and identifying prior affective episodes.

In addition to substance abuse and risk-taking behavior, other cross-sectional features that can have an impact on diagnosis and treatment planning include the presence of psychotic symptoms or cognitive impairment and the risk of suicide or violence to persons or property (41).

TABLE 4. Diagnostic Criteria for a Hypomanic Episode

A. A distinct period of persistently elevated, expansive, or irritable mood, lasting at least 4 days, that is clearly different from the usual nondepressed mood.

B. During the period of mood disturbance, three (or more) of the following symptoms have persisted (four if the mood is only irritable) and have been present to a significant degree:

1) Inflated self-esteem or grandiosity
2) Decreased need for sleep (e.g., feels rested after only 3 hours of sleep)
3) More talkative than usual or pressure to keep talking
4) Flight of ideas or subjective experience that thoughts are racing
5) Distractibility (i.e., attention too easily drawn to unimportant or irrelevant external stimuli)
6) Increase in goal-directed activity (either socially, at work or school, or sexually) or psychomotor agitation
7) Excessive involvement in pleasurable activities that have a high potential for painful consequences (e.g., engaging in unrestrained buying sprees, sexual indiscretions, or foolish business investments)

C. The episode is associated with an unequivocal change in functioning that is uncharacteristic of the person when not symptomatic.

D. The disturbance in mood and the change in functioning are observable by others.

E. The episode 1) is not severe enough to cause marked impairment in social or occupational functioning, 2) does not necessitate hospitalization, and 3) does not have psychotic features.

F. The symptoms are not due to the direct physiological effects of a substance (e.g., a drug of abuse, a medication, or other treatment) or a general medical condition (e.g., hyperthyroidism).

Source. Adapted from DSM-IV-TR; hypomanic-like episodes that are clearly caused by somatic antidepressant treatment (e.g., medication, ECT, light therapy) should not count toward a diagnosis of bipolar II disorder.

Suicide rates are high among bipolar disorder patients. Completed suicide occurs in an estimated 10%–15% of individuals with bipolar I disorder. Suicide is more likely to occur during a depressive or a mixed episode (8–13). Pharmacotherapy may substantially reduce the risk of suicide (56, 60, 153). For example, in an 11-year follow-up study of 103 patients with bipolar disorder who were receiving lithium, death rates were well below those expected for this group on the basis of age and sex (154).

Bipolar disorder causes substantial psychosocial morbidity, frequently affecting patients' relationships with spouses or partners, children, and other family members as well as their occupation and other aspects of their lives. Even during periods of euthymia, patients may experience impairments in psychosocial functioning or residual symptoms of depression or mania/hypomania. It is estimated that as many as 60% of people diagnosed with bipolar I disorder experience chronic interpersonal or occupational difficulties and subclinical symptoms between acute episodes (13, 33, 34, 158–164). Divorce rates are substantially higher in patients with bipolar disorder, approaching two to three times the rate of comparison subjects (152). The occupational status of patients with bipolar disorder is twice as likely to deteriorate as that of comparison subjects (152). Patients' ability to care for themselves, degree of disability or distress, childbearing status or plans, availability of supports such as family or friends, and resources such as housing and finances also bear on treatment plans.

TABLE 5. Diagnostic Criteria for a Mixed Episode

A. The criteria are met both for a manic episode and for a major depressive episode (except for duration) nearly every day during at least a 1-week period.

B. The mood disturbance 1) is sufficiently severe to cause marked impairment in occupational functioning, usual social activities, or relationships with others, 2) necessitates hospitalization to prevent harm to self or others, or 3) has psychotic features.

C. The symptoms are not due to the direct physiological effects of a substance (e.g., a drug of abuse, a medication, or other treatment) or a general medical condition (e.g., hyperthyroidism).

Source. Adapted from DSM-IV-TR; mixed-like episodes that are clearly caused by somatic antidepressant treatment (e.g., medication, ECT, light therapy) should not count toward a diagnosis of bipolar I disorder.

C. EPIDEMIOLOGY

Bipolar I disorder affects approximately 0.8% of the adult population, with estimates from community samples ranging between 0.4% and 1.6%. These rates are consistent across diverse cultures and ethnic groups (165). Bipolar II disorder affects approximately 0.5% of the population (156). While bipolar II disorder is apparently more common in women (81), bipolar I disorder affects men and women fairly equally. These estimates of prevalence are considered conservative. Reasons for this underestimate may include differences in diagnostic definitions and inclusion of persons who fall within the bipolar spectrum but who do not meet DSM-IV-TR criteria for bipolar I or bipolar II disorder (166).

The Epidemiologic Catchment Area study reported a mean age at onset of 21 years for bipolar disorder (6). When studies examining age at onset are stratified into 5-year intervals, the peak age at onset of first symptoms falls between ages 15 and 19, followed closely by ages 20–24. There is often a 5- to 10-year interval, however, between age at onset of illness and age at first treatment or first hospitalization (34, 151). Onset of mania before age 15 has been less well studied (167). Bipolar disorder may be difficult to diagnose in this age group because of its atypical presentation with ADHD (13, 157–163). Thus, the true age at onset of bipolar disorder is still unclear and may be younger than reported for the full syndrome, since there is uncertainty about the symptom presentation in children. Research that follows cohorts of offspring of patients with bipolar disorder may help to clarify early signs in children.

Onset of mania after age 60 is less likely to be associated with a family history of bipolar disorder and is more likely to be associated with identifiable general medical factors, including stroke or other central nervous system lesion (34, 155, 168).

Evidence from epidemiological and twin studies strongly suggests that bipolar disorder is a heritable illness (164, 169). First-degree relatives of patients with bipolar disorder have significantly higher rates of mood disorder than do relatives of nonpsychiatrically ill comparison groups. However, the mode of inheritance remains unknown. In clinical practice, a family history of mood disorder, especially of bipolar disorder, provides strong corroborative evidence of the potential for a primary mood disorder in a patient with otherwise predominantly psychotic features.

Likewise, the magnitude of the role played by environmental stressors, particularly early in the course of the illness, remains uncertain. However, there is growing evidence that environmental and lifestyle features can have an impact on severity and course of illness (170–172). Stressful life events, changes in sleep-wake schedule, and current alcohol or substance abuse may affect the course of illness and lengthen the time to recovery (26, 71, 73, 173–175).

TABLE 6. Summary of Manic and Depressive Symptom Criteria in DSM-IV-TR Mood Disorders

Disorder	Manic Symptom Criteria	Depressive Symptom Criteria
Major depressive disorder	No history of mania or hypomania	History of major depressive episodes (single or recurrent)
Dysthymic disorder	No history of mania or hypomania	Depressed mood, more days than not, for at least 2 years (but not meeting criteria for a major depressive episode)
Bipolar I disorder	History of manic or mixed episodes	Major depressive episodes typical but not required for diagnosis
Bipolar II disorder	One or more episodes of hypomania; no manic or mixed episodes	History of major depressive episodes
Cyclothymic disorder	For at least 2 years, the presence of numerous periods with hypomanic symptoms	Numerous periods with depressive symptoms that do not meet criteria for a major depressive episode
Bipolar disorder not otherwise specified	Manic symptoms present, but criteria not met for bipolar I, bipolar II, or cyclothymic disorder	Not required for diagnosis

V. REVIEW AND SYNTHESIS OF AVAILABLE EVIDENCE

A. SOMATIC TREATMENTS OF ACUTE MANIC AND MIXED EPISODES

In general, the primary goal of treatment for patients experiencing a manic or mixed episode is symptom control to allow a return to normal levels of psychosocial functioning. The rapid control of symptoms such as agitation and aggression may be particularly important for the safety of the patient and others.

1. Lithium

Lithium has been used for the treatment of acute bipolar mania for over 50 years. Five studies have demonstrated that lithium is superior to placebo (176–180). Pooled data from these studies reveal that 87 (70%) of 124 patients displayed at least partial reduction of mania with lithium. However, the use of a crossover design in four of these trials (176–179), nonrandom assignment in two studies (177, 178), and variations in diagnostic criteria and trial duration limit interpretation of the results of all but one trial (180). Nevertheless, in the only placebo-controlled, parallel-design trial in which lithium served as an active comparator to divalproex, lithium and divalproex exerted comparable efficacy (180). In active comparator trials, lithium displayed efficacy comparable to that of carbamazepine (181, 182), risperidone (183), olanzapine (184), and chlorpromazine and other typical antipsychotics (185–190). Among active comparator trials, however, only three (185, 186, 189) were likely to be of sufficient size to detect possible differences in efficacy between treatments. Open studies (191–194) and randomized, active comparator-controlled studies (195–197) indicate that lithium is likely to be effective for treatment of pure or elated mania but is less often effective in the treatment of mixed states.

a) Side effects

Up to 75% of patients treated with lithium experience some side effects (41, 198). These side effects vary in clinical significance; most are either minor or can be reduced or eliminated by lowering the lithium dose or changing the dosage schedule. For example, Schou (199) reported a 30% reduction in side effects among patients treated with an average lithium level of 0.68 meq/liter compared with those treated with an average level of 0.85 meq/liter. Side effects that appear to be related to peak serum levels (e.g., tremor that peaks within 1 to 2 hours of a dose) may be reduced or eliminated by using a slow-release preparation or changing to a single bedtime dose.

Dose-related side effects of lithium include polyuria, polydipsia, weight gain, cognitive problems (e.g., dulling, impaired memory, poor concentration, confusion, mental slowness), tremor, sedation or lethargy, impaired coordination, gastrointestinal distress (e.g., nausea, vomiting, dyspepsia, diarrhea), hair loss, benign leukocytosis, acne, and edema (200). Side effects that persist despite dosage adjustment may be managed with other medications (e.g., beta-blockers for tremor; diuretics for polyuria, polydipsia, or edema; topical antibiotics or retinoic acid for acne). Gastrointestinal disturbances can be managed by administering lithium with meals or changing lithium preparations (especially to lithium citrate).

Lithium may cause benign ECG changes associated with repolarization. Less commonly, cardiac conduction abnormalities have been associated with lithium treatment. Anecdotal reports have linked lithium with other ECG changes, including the exacerbation of existing arrhythmias and, less commonly, the development of new arrhythmias (201).

The most common renal effect of lithium is impaired concentrating capacity caused by reduced renal response to ADH, manifested as polyuria, polydipsia, or both (202, 203). Although the polyuria associated with early lithium treatment may resolve, persistent polyuria (ranging from mild and well tolerated to severe nephrogenic diabetes insipidus) may occur. Polyuria can frequently be managed by changing to a once-daily bedtime dose. If the polyuria persists, management includes ensuring that fluid intake is adequate and that the lithium dose is as low as possible. If these measures do not ameliorate the problem, then concurrent administration of a thiazide diuretic (e.g., hydrochlorothiazide at a dose of 50 mg/day) may be helpful. The lithium dose will usually need to be decreased (typically by 50%) to account for the increased reabsorption induced by thiazides (198). In addition, potassium levels will need to be monitored, and potassium replacement may be necessary. Amiloride, a potassium-sparing diuretic, is reported to be effective in treating lithium-induced polyuria and polydipsia (203). Its advantages are that it does not alter lithium levels and does not cause potassium depletion. Amiloride may be started at 5 mg b.i.d. and may be increased to 10 mg b.i.d. as needed (204).

Hypothyroidism occurs in 5%–35% of patients treated with lithium. It occurs more frequently in women, tends to appear after 6–18 months of lithium treatment, and may be associated with rapid cycling (41, 80, 198, 205). Lithium-induced hypothyroidism is not a contraindication to continuing lithium and is easily treated by the administration of levothyroxine (198, 205). In addition to the other signs and symptoms of hypothyroidism, patients with bipolar disorder are at risk of developing depression or rapid cycling. If these symptoms occur in the presence of laboratory evidence of suboptimal thyroid functioning, then thyroid supplementation, discontinuation of lithium, or both should be considered (206–208). Hyperparathyroidism has also been noted with lithium treatment (209–211).

A small number of case reports have described exacerbation or first occurrences of psoriasis associated with lithium treatment (212). Some of these patients improved with appropriate dermatologic treatment or when the lithium dose was lowered. In some cases, however, lithium seemed to block the effects of dermatologic treatment, with psoriasis clearing only after lithium was discontinued. In addition, patients occasionally experience severe pustular acne that does not respond well to standard dermatologic treatments and only resolves once the lithium treatment is discontinued (212). This is in contrast to the more common mild to moderate acne that can occur with lithium treatment, which is usually responsive to standard treatments (198).

Approximately 10%–20% of patients receiving long-term lithium treatment (i.e., for more than 10 years) display morphological kidney changes—usually interstitial fibrosis, tubular atrophy, and sometimes glomerular sclerosis. These changes may be associated with impairment of water reabsorption but not with reduction in glomerular filtration rate or development of renal insufficiency (41, 198, 213–216). Although irreversible renal failure caused by lithium has not been unequivocally established, there are a number of case reports of probable lithium-induced renal insufficiency (215, 217, 218). Additionally, several studies have shown that a small percentage of patients treated with lithium may develop rising serum creatinine concentrations after 10 years or more of treatment (215, 218).

b) Toxicity/overdose

Toxic effects of lithium become more likely as the serum level rises (219). Most patients will experience some toxic effects with levels above 1.5 meq/liter; levels above 2.0 meq/liter are commonly associated with life-threatening side effects. For many patients, the therapeutic range within which beneficial effects outweigh toxic effects is quite narrow, so that small changes in serum level may lead to clinically significant alterations in the beneficial and harmful effects of lithium. Elderly patients may experience toxic effects at lower levels and have a correspondingly narrower therapeutic window (138).

Signs and symptoms of early intoxication (with levels above 1.5 meq/liter) include marked tremor, nausea and diarrhea, blurred vision, vertigo, confusion, and increased deep tendon reflexes. With levels above 2.5 meq/liter, patients may experience more severe neurological complications and eventually experience seizures, coma, cardiac dysrhythmia, and permanent neurological impairment. The magnitude of the serum level and the duration of exposure to a high level of lithium are both correlated with risk of adverse effects (219). Therefore, rapid steps to reduce the serum level are essential. In addition, during treatment for severe intoxication, patients may experience "secondary peaks" during which the serum level rises after a period of relative decline; the clinician must therefore continue to monitor serum levels during treatment for severe intoxication. The patient with lithium intoxication should be treated with supportive care (e.g., maintenance of fluid and electrolyte balance), and steps should be taken to prevent further absorption of the medication (e.g., gastric lavage or, in the alert patient, induction of emesis).

Hemodialysis is the only reliable method of rapidly removing excess lithium from the body and is more effective than peritoneal dialysis for this purpose (220). Criteria for the use of hemodialysis in lithium intoxication are not firmly established, and the decision to dialyze must take into account both the patient's clinical status and the serum lithium level (219, 221). When serum lithium levels are below 2.5 meq/liter, hemodialysis usually is unnecessary. The need for hemodialysis differs in patients who have developed toxicity after an acute overdose compared with those who have developed gradual toxicity or have an acute overdose superimposed on long-term lithium treatment. In acute poisoning, hemodialysis is generally required with serum lithium levels over 6–8 meq/liter, whereas hemodialysis may be needed with serum levels over 4 meq/liter in those who have been on long-term regimens of lithium treatment. Hemodialysis may also be necessary at lower serum levels in patients who are more susceptible to complications because of underlying illnesses (e.g., cardiac disease, renal impairment). Regardless of serum lithium level, hemodialysis is generally indicated in patients with progressive clinical deterioration or severe clinical signs of intoxication such as coma, convulsions, cardiovascular symptoms, or respiratory failure (219, 221). Because serum levels of lithium may rebound after initial hemodialysis, repeat dialysis may be needed (219, 222).

In cases of overdose with sustained-release preparations of lithium, development of toxicity is likely to be delayed, and the duration of toxicity is likely to be prolonged (223, 224). This should be taken into consideration in decisions about the need for initial or repeat hemodialysis (219).

c) Implementation and dosing

Before beginning lithium treatment, the patient's general medical history should be reviewed, with special reference to those systems that might affect or be affected by lithium therapy (e.g., renal, thyroid, and cardiac functioning). In addition, pregnancy or the presence of a dermatologic disorder must be ascertained. Patient education should address potential side effects of lithium treatment as well as the need to avoid salt-restricted diets or concomitant medications that could elevate serum lithium levels (e.g., diuretics, angiotensin-converting enzyme inhibitors, nonsteroidal anti-inflammatory drugs, cyclooxygenase-2 inhibitors). Patients should be cautioned, particularly if nephrogenic diabetes insipidus is present, that lithium toxicity might occur with dehydration from environmental heat, gastrointestinal disturbance, or inadequate fluid intake.

Laboratory measures and other diagnostic tests are generally recommended on the basis of pathophysiological knowledge and anticipated clinical decisions rather than on empirical evidence of their clinical utility. The decision to recommend a test is based on the probability of detecting a finding that would alter treatment as well as the expected benefit of such alterations in treatment. Recommended tests fall into three categories: 1) baseline measures to facilitate subsequent interpretation of laboratory tests (e.g., ECG, CBC); 2) tests to determine conditions requiring different or additional treatments (e.g., pregnancy, thyroid-stimulating hormone level); and 3) tests to determine conditions requiring alteration of the standard dosage regimen of lithium (e.g., creatinine level).

On the basis of these considerations, the following procedures are generally recommended before beginning lithium therapy: a general medical history, a physical examination, BUN and creatinine level measurement, a pregnancy test, thyroid function evaluation, and, for patients over age 40, ECG monitoring with rhythm strip. Some authorities also suggest a CBC.

Lithium is usually started in low, divided doses to minimize side effects (e.g., 300 mg t.i.d. or less, depending on the patient's weight and age), with the dose titrated upward (generally to serum concentrations of 0.5–1.2 meq/liter) according to response and side effects (225). Lithium levels should be checked after each dose increase and before the next. Steady-state levels are likely to be reached approximately 5 days after dose adjustment, but levels may need to be checked sooner if a rapid increase is necessary (e.g., in the treatment of acute mania) or if toxicity is suspected. As levels approach the upper limits of the therapeutic range (i.e., ≥1.0 meq/liter), they should be checked at shorter intervals after each dose increase to minimize the risk of toxicity.

Serum concentrations required for prophylaxis may be, in some cases, as high as those required for treatment of the acute episode. A controlled study by Gelenberg et al. (225) found that patients randomly assigned to a "low" lithium level (0.4–0.6 meq/liter) had fewer side effects but more illness episodes than patients in the "standard" lithium group (0.8–1.0 meq/liter). However, the lithium levels of some of the patients in the low-lithium group decreased relatively rapidly from their previous treatment levels, a decrease that could have increased their risk of relapse. Although the prophylactic efficacy of lithium levels between 0.6 and 0.8 meq/liter has not been formally studied, this range is commonly chosen by patients and their psychiatrists (226). Despite the lack of formal study, it is likely that for many patients, increases in maintenance lithium levels will result in a trade-off between greater protection from illness episodes at the cost of an increase in side effects. The "optimal" maintenance level may therefore vary somewhat from patient to patient. Some patients find that a single, daily dose facilitates treatment compliance and reduces or does not change side effects.

The clinical status of patients receiving lithium needs to be monitored especially closely. The frequency of monitoring depends on the individual patient's clinical situation but generally should be no less than every 6 months for stable patients. The optimal frequency of serum level monitoring in an individual patient depends on the stability of lithium levels over time for that patient and the degree to which the patient can be relied upon to notice and report symptoms.

In general, renal function should be tested every 2–3 months during the first 6 months of treatment, and thyroid function should be evaluated once or twice during the first 6 months of lithium treatment. Subsequently, renal and thyroid function may be checked every 6 months to 1 year in stable patients or whenever clinically indicated (e.g., in the presence of breakthrough affective symptoms, changes in side effects, or new medical or psychiatric signs or symptoms) (198, 214).

2. Divalproex/valproate/valproic acid

Divalproex and its sodium valproate and valproic acid formulations have been studied in four randomized, placebo-controlled trials: two small crossover trials (227, 228) and two parallel-group trials (180, 229). All four studies found significantly greater efficacy for valproate compared with placebo, with response rates ranging from 48% to 53%. Secondary analyses (150, 197) of data from the largest parallel-group trial (180) suggested that patients with prominent depressive symptoms during mania and with multiple prior mood episodes were more likely to respond to acute treatment with divalproex than with lithium. An additional randomized comparison also reported valproate to be more efficacious than lithium among manic patients with mixed symptoms (195). In patients with acute mania, divalproex was comparable in efficacy to haloperidol in an open trial (230) and to olanzapine in a randomized, controlled trial (231) in the reduction of symptoms of mania and psychosis. In contrast, in a second head-to-head comparison trial (232), olanzapine was superior to divalproex in the mean reduction of manic symptoms and in the proportion of patients in remission at the end of the study.

a) Side effects

Minor side effects of valproate, such as sedation or gastrointestinal distress, are common initially and typically resolve with continued treatment or dose adjustment. In addition, valproate has a wide therapeutic window. Inadvertent overdose is uncommon, and purposeful overdose is less likely to be lethal than it is with lithium. However, in rare instances, valproate can cause life-threatening side effects, and patients must be relied upon to report the often subtle symptoms of these reactions promptly.

Common dose-related side effects of valproate include gastrointestinal distress (e.g., anorexia, nausea, dyspepsia, vomiting, diarrhea), benign hepatic transaminase elevations, osteoporosis (233, 234), tremor, and sedation. Patients with past or current hepatic disease may be at greater risk for hepatotoxicity (235). Mild, asymptomatic leukopenia and thrombocytopenia occur less frequently and are reversible upon drug discontinuation. Other side effects that are often bothersome to the patient include hair loss (236, 237), increased appetite, and weight gain. Persistent gastrointestinal distress associated with valproate can be alleviated by dose reduction, change of preparation (use of the divalproex sodium formulation rather than valproic acid), or by administration of a histamine-2 antagonist (e.g., famotidine or cimetidine) (238–242). Tremor can be managed with dose reduction or coadministration of beta-blockers. Cases of mild, asymptomatic leukopenia (total WBC count $>3000/mm^3$ and polymorphonuclear leukocyte count $>1500/mm^3$) are usually reversible upon dose reduction or discontinuation. Similarly, if mild, asymptomatic thrombocytopenia occurs, a decrease in valproate dose will usually restore the platelet count to normal. However, more severe cases of thrombocytopenia have been reported (243).

The relationship between polycystic ovarian syndrome and valproate treatment is unclear (244–246). One uncontrolled report indicated that 80% of women receiving long-term valproate treatment for epilepsy before the age of 20 had polycystic ovaries or hyperandrogenism (247). Other cross-sectional studies have demonstrated higher rates of polycystic ovaries and polycystic ovarian syndrome in women with epilepsy (244–246). However, none of the studies examined whether the polycystic ovarian syndrome began before or after the development of epilepsy or the initiation of valproate therapy (246). Furthermore, women with bipolar disorder may differ from women with epilepsy in their rates of polycystic ovarian syndrome independent of treatment. An accurate assessment of risk will require a longitudinal study of women with bipolar disorder before and after initiation of valproate treatment (246). Consequently, although the risks are unclear, psychiatrists should be aware that polycystic ovarian syndrome may be possible with valproate treatment, and thus patients should be monitored accordingly (244).

Rare, idiosyncratic, but potentially fatal adverse events with valproate include irreversible hepatic failure, hemorrhagic pancreatitis, and agranulocytosis. Thus, patients taking valproate need to be instructed to contact their psychiatrist or primary care physician immediately if they develop symptoms of these conditions.

b) Toxicity/overdose

Valproate has a wide therapeutic window, so unintentional overdose is uncommon (248). Signs of overdose include somnolence, heart block, and eventually coma. Deaths have been reported. Overdose can be treated with hemodialysis (249, 250).

c) Implementation and dosing

Before initiating valproate treatment, a general medical history should be taken, with special attention to hepatic, hematologic, and bleeding abnormalities. Results of liver function tests and hematologic measures should be obtained at baseline to evaluate general medical health.

Data from a number of open trials (230, 251–253) and one randomized controlled trial (254) indicate that divalproex can be administered at a therapeutic initial starting dose of 20–30 mg/kg per day in inpatients. This strategy appears to be well tolerated and may be more rapidly efficacious than more gradual titration from a lower starting dose (254). After a serum valproate level is obtained, the dose is then adjusted downward to achieve a target level between 50 and 125 mcg/ml.

Among outpatients, elderly patients, or patients who are hypomanic or euthymic, valproate may be initiated in low, divided doses to minimize gastrointestinal and neurological toxicity. Valproate should generally be started at 250 mg t.i.d., with the dose increased every few days as side effects allow (204). Depending upon clinical response and side effects, the dose is then titrated upward by 250–500 mg/day every few days, generally to a serum concentration of 50–125 mcg/ml, with a maximum adult daily dose of 60 mg/kg per day (250). Once the patient is stable, valproate regimens can be simplified to enhance convenience and compliance, since many patients do well with once- or twice-a-day dosing.

Extended-release divalproex, a new formulation that allows for once-a-day dosing, has become available. Bioavailability is approximately 15% lower than the immediate-release formulation (hence usually requiring slightly higher doses), and side effect profiles appear to be better than that of the immediate-release formulation (255). Demonstration of efficacy in patients with bipolar disorder is limited to open studies (255–257).

Asymptomatic hepatic enzyme elevations, leukopenia, and thrombocytopenia do not reliably predict life-threatening hepatic or bone marrow failure. In conjunction with careful monitoring of clinical status, educating patients about the signs and symptoms of hepatic and hematologic dysfunction and instructing them to report these symptoms if they occur are essential. Some investigators believe that in otherwise healthy patients with epilepsy receiving long-term valproate treatment, routine monitoring of hematologic and hepatic function is not necessary (258). Nevertheless, most psychiatrists perform clinical assessments, including tests of hematologic and hepatic function, at a minimum of every 6 months for stable patients who are taking valproate (252, 259, 260). Patients who cannot reliably report signs or symptoms of toxicity need to be monitored more frequently.

Psychiatrists should be alert to the potential for interactions between valproate and other medications (261). For example, valproate displaces highly protein-bound drugs from their protein binding sites. In addition, valproate inhibits lamotrigine metabolism and more than doubles its elimination half-life by competing for glucuronidation enzyme sites in the liver (262, 263). Consequently, in patients treated with valproate, lamotrigine must be initiated at a dose that is less than half that used in patients who are not receiving concomitant valproate.

3. Carbamazepine

Many controlled trials of carbamazepine have been conducted in the treatment of acute bipolar mania, but interpretation of the results of a number of these studies is difficult because of the confounding effects of other medications administered as part of study protocols (264). Carbamazepine was superior to placebo in one randomized, crossover trial (265). Carbamazepine was less effective and associated with more need for adjunctive "rescue medication" than valproate in a randomized, blind, parallel-group trial of 30 hospitalized manic patients (266). Carbamazepine was comparable to lithium in two randomized comparison trials (181, 182) and comparable to chlorpromazine in two other randomized trials (267, 268).

a) Side effects

Up to 50% of patients receiving carbamazepine experience side effects, and the drug is associated with potentially serious adverse reactions (258, 269, 270).

The most common dose-related side effects of carbamazepine include neurological symptoms, such as diplopia, blurred vision, fatigue, nausea, and ataxia. These effects are usually transient and often reversible with dose reduction. Elderly patients, however, may be more sensitive to side effects. Less frequent side effects include skin rashes (271), mild leukopenia, mild thrombocytopenia, hyponatremia, and (less commonly) hypo-osmolality. Mild liver enzyme elevations occur in 5%–15% of patients. Mild asymptomatic leukopenia is not related to serious idiopathic blood dyscrasias and usually resolves spontaneously with continuation of carbamazepine treatment or with dose reduction. In the event of asymptomatic leukopenia, thrombocytopenia, or elevated liver enzymes, the carbamazepine dose can be reduced or, in the case of severe changes, discontinued. Hyponatremia may be related to water retention caused by carbamazepine's antidiuretic effect (272). Hyponatremia occurs in 6%–31% of patients, is rare in children but probably more common in the elderly, occasionally develops many months after the initiation of carbamazepine treatment, and sometimes necessitates carbamazepine discontinuation. In addition, carbamazepine may decrease total and free thyroxine levels and increase free cortisol levels, but these effects are rarely clinically significant. Weight gain is also a common side effect of carbamazepine.

Rare, idiosyncratic, but serious and potentially fatal side effects of carbamazepine include agranulocytosis, aplastic anemia, thrombocytopenia, hepatic failure, exfoliative dermatitis (e.g., Stevens-Johnson syndrome), and pancreatitis (243, 258, 273–275). Although these side effects usually occur within 3–6 months of carbamazepine initiation, they have also occurred after more extended periods of treatment. Routine blood monitoring does not reliably predict blood dyscrasias, hepatic failure, or exfoliative dermatitis. Thus, in addition to careful monitoring of clinical status, it is essential to educate patients about the signs and symptoms of hepatic, hematologic, or dermatologic reactions and instruct them to report symptoms if they occur. Other rare side effects include systemic hypersensitivity reactions, cardiac conduction disturbances, psychiatric symptoms (including sporadic cases of psychosis), and, very rarely, renal effects (including renal failure, oliguria, hematuria, and proteinuria).

b) Toxicity/overdose

Carbamazepine may be fatal in overdose; deaths have been reported with ingestions of more than 6 g. Signs of impending carbamazepine toxicity include dizziness, ataxia, sedation, and diplopia. Acute intoxication can result in hyperirritability, stupor, or coma. The most common symptoms of carbamazepine overdose are nystagmus, ophthalmoplegia, cerebellar and extrapyramidal signs, impaired consciousness, convulsions, and respiratory dysfunction. Cardiac symptoms may include tachycardia, arrhythmia, conduction disturbances, and hypotension. Gastrointestinal and anticholinergic symptoms may also occur. Management of carbamazepine intoxication includes symptomatic treatment, gastric lavage, and hemoperfusion.

c) Implementation and dosing

A pretreatment evaluation for carbamazepine should include a general medical history and physical examination, with special emphasis on prior history of blood dyscrasias or liver disease. Most authorities recommend that the minimum baseline evaluation include a CBC with differential and platelet count, a liver profile (evaluation of LDH, SGOT, SGPT, bilirubin, and alkaline phosphatase), and renal function tests (204). Serum electrolyte levels may also be obtained, especially in the elderly, who may be at higher risk for hyponatremia.

Although doses can range from 200 to 1800 mg/day, the relationships among dose, serum concentration, response, and side effects are variable. Therefore, the dose should be titrated upward according to response and side effects. In patients over the age of 12, carbamazepine is usually begun at a total daily dose of 200–600 mg, given in three to four divided doses. In hospitalized patients with acute mania, the dose may be increased in increments of 200 mg/day up to 800–1000 mg/day (unless side effects develop), with slower increases thereafter as indicated. In less acutely ill outpatients, dose adjustments should be slower, since rapid increases may cause patients to develop nausea and vomiting or mild neurological symptoms such as drowsiness, dizziness, ataxia, clumsiness, or diplopia. Should such side effects occur, the dose can be decreased temporarily and then increased again more slowly once these side effects have passed.

While therapeutic serum levels of carbamazepine have not been established for patients with bipolar disorder, serum concentrations established for treatment of seizure disorders (4–12 mcg/ml) are generally applied. Trough levels are most meaningful for establishing an effective level for a given patient and are conveniently drawn before the first morning dose. Serum levels should be determined 5 days after a dose change or sooner if toxicity or noncompliance is suspected. Maintenance doses average about 1000 mg/day but may range from 200–1600 mg/day in routine clinical practice (204). Doses higher than 1600 mg/day are not recommended.

CBCs, platelet measurements, and liver function tests should be performed every 2 weeks during the first 2 months of carbamazepine treatment. Thereafter, if results of laboratory tests remain normal and no symptoms of bone marrow suppression or hepatitis appear, blood counts and liver function tests should be performed at least every 3 months (204). More frequent monitoring is necessary in patients with laboratory findings, signs, or symptoms consistent with hematologic or hepatic abnormalities. Life-threatening reactions, however, are not always detected by routine monitoring. The psychiatrist should educate patients about signs and symptoms of hepatic, hematologic, or dermatologic reactions and instruct patients to report these symptoms if they occur. More frequent clinical and laboratory assessments are needed for those patients who cannot reliably report symptoms.

Psychiatrists should be aware that carbamazepine is able to induce drug metabolism, including its own, through cytochrome P-450 oxidation and conjugation (261, 263, 276). This enzymatic induction may decrease levels of concomitantly administered medications such as valproate, lamotrigine, oral contraceptives, protease inhibitors, benzodiazepines, and many antipsychotic and antidepressant medications. In addition, carbamazepine has an active epoxide metabolite and is metabolized primarily through a single enzyme, cytochrome P-450 isoenzyme 3A3/4, making drug-drug interactions even more likely. Consequently, carbamazepine levels may be increased by medications that inhibit the cytochrome P-450 isoenzyme 3A3/4, such as fluoxetine, fluvoxamine, cimetidine, and some antibiotics and calcium channel blockers. Thus, in patients treated with carbamazepine, more frequent clinical and laboratory assessments may be needed with addition or dose adjustments of other medications.

4. Other anticonvulsants

Oxcarbazepine, the 10-keto analog of carbamazepine, was comparable in efficacy to lithium and haloperidol in two small trials (277, 278). However, these studies lacked sufficient power to detect possible drug-drug differences. While direct comparisons with carbamazepine in studies of bipolar disorder are lacking, studies of epilepsy suggest that oxcarbazepine may have a lower rate of severe side effects (279) and be well tolerated overall (280), although it has been associated with clinically significant hyponatremia (281). Moreover, unlike carbamazepine, oxcarbazepine does not induce its own metabolism (282). However, it may still decrease plasma concentrations of oral contraceptives and dihydropyridine calcium channel blockers, requiring medication change or dose adjustment. (For a more complete review, see the bipolar disorder treatment algorithm of the Texas Medication Algorithm Project [283].)

Three controlled studies, all with methodological limitations, have evaluated lamotrigine in the treatment of bipolar mania. In the first trial, 28 patients with bipolar I or bipolar II disorder were assessed in a double-blind, randomized, crossover series of three 6-week monotherapy trials of lamotrigine, gabapentin, or placebo (284). The response rate for manic symptom improvement, as measured by the Clinical Global Impression Scale for Bipolar Illness, did not differ significantly among the three treatment groups. However, the low mean Young Mania Rating Scale scores at baseline, the crossover design, and the small number of subjects may have limited the findings. In the second study, 16 outpatients with mania, hypomania, or mixed episodes who were inadequately responsive to or unable to tolerate lithium were randomly assigned to lamotrigine or placebo as mono- or adjunctive therapy (285). There were no significant differences between lamotrigine and placebo groups on changes in Young Mania Rating Scale scores or response rates. Limitations of this study included the small study group size and high (50%) placebo response rate. In the third study, 30 inpatients were randomly assigned to lamotrigine or lithium for 4 weeks (286). Both treatment groups displayed significant and comparable reductions in manic symptoms from baseline to endpoint. Limitations of this study included lack of a placebo group, small patient group size, and use of relatively low lithium levels (mean plasma concentration of 0.7 meq/liter at study endpoint). Adverse events and implementation and dosing issues associated with lamotrigine treatment are described in detail in Section V.B.2.c.

Two controlled studies have evaluated the efficacy of gabapentin in the treatment of bipolar manic symptoms. In the first study (284), there were no significant differences in efficacy between gabapentin monotherapy and placebo in improvement in manic symptoms. The second controlled trial (287) compared gabapentin with placebo added to lithium, valproate, or both in 114 outpatients with manic, hypomanic, or mixed symptoms. Both treatment groups displayed a decrease in Young Mania Rating Scale scores from baseline to endpoint, but this decrease was significantly greater in the placebo group.

Finally, one small placebo-controlled trial also suggested efficacy for the anticonvulsant phenytoin in the treatment of mania when added to haloperidol treatment (288).

5. Olanzapine

Olanzapine was superior to placebo in the treatment of acute bipolar mania in two large, multicenter randomized controlled trials. In the first trial (289), olanzapine versus placebo differences did not reach statistical significance until the third week of treatment. In the second study (290), significant reductions in manic symptoms were apparent in olanzapine-treated patients compared with those receiving placebo at the first assessment point (after 1 week). These differences were probably due to differences in initial starting dose, since the initial olanzapine dose was 10 mg/day in the first study and 15 mg/day in the second trial. In a secondary analysis of data from the second trial, in which sufficient proportions of patients with mixed episodes or rapid cycling were included for comparison, olanzapine response was comparable in patients with or without these features (291). In other randomized, controlled trials, olanzapine exerted comparable efficacy to lithium (184), divalproex (231), and haloperidol (292) in the reduction of manic symptoms. Olanzapine was superior to divalproex in a randomized comparison trial (232). Last, olanzapine was superior to placebo as adjunctive therapy to lithium or divalproex in a randomized, controlled acute treatment trial (292).

a) Side effects

In short-term, placebo-controlled clinical trials, somnolence was the most common side effect associated with olanzapine. Other common side effects included constipation, dry mouth, increased appetite, and weight gain (291). Especially during initial dose titration, olanzapine may induce orthostatic hypotension associated with dizziness, tachycardia, and, in some patients, syncope. Syncope was reported in 0.6% of olanzapine-treated patients in phase II and III trials.

In clinical trials, seizures occurred in 0.9% of olanzapine-treated patients. Although confounding factors may have contributed to seizures in many instances, olanzapine should be used cautiously in patients with a history of seizure disorder or in clinical conditions associated with lowered seizure threshold. Transient elevations in plasma prolactin concentrations were also observed in short-term trials (293). These elevations typically remained within the normal physiological range and decreased with continued treatment. Clinically significant hepatic transaminase elevations (≥3 times the upper limit of the normal range) were observed in 2% of olanzapine-treated patients.

In long-term studies, 56% of olanzapine-treated patients gained >7% of their baseline weight. In retrospective analyses of patients followed for a median of 2.54 years, the mean and median weight gains were 6.26 kg and 5.9 kg, respectively (294). Weight gain did not appear to be dose related, occurred most rapidly within the first 39 weeks of treatment, was greatest in patients with the lowest baseline body mass index, and was not correlated with increases in serum glucose. Increases in serum glucose in olanzapine-treated patients did not differ significantly from those in patients treated with haloperidol (294). Weight gain and hyperglycemia in patients treated with atypical antipsychotics have been reviewed in detail elsewhere (295, 296).

In short-term trials, there were no significant differences in the incidence of dystonic reactions, parkinsonism, akathisia, or dyskinetic events among patients receiving placebo or olanzapine (291). Also, extrapyramidal side effects with olanzapine were substantially less than those seen with conventional antipsychotic medications such as haloperidol (297). In a 1-year haloperidol-controlled trial, the incidence of dyskinetic movements among olanzapine-treated patients with schizophrenia was 0.6% compared with 7.5% in patients receiving haloperidol (298). This incidence rate is confounded by prior treatment with typical antipsychotics and the rate of spontaneous dyskinesia in patients with schizophrenia. In 98 patients with bipolar disorder who received olanzapine for 1 year, some in combination with lithium or fluoxetine, no patients developed dyskinetic movements (291).

b) Implementation and dosing

In the two placebo-controlled studies of olanzapine in patients with bipolar mania, the mean final dose was approximately 15 mg/day. In the first study in which olanzapine was initiated at 10 mg/day and then titrated according to response and side effects, olanzapine did not differentiate from placebo until the third week of the trial (289). The second trial used a starting dose of 15 mg/day and found a significant difference in efficacy in favor of olanzapine at 1 week (the time of the first rating) (290). Taken together, the results of these trials suggest that for inpatients with acute mania, a starting dose of 15 mg/day may be more rapidly efficacious. For outpatients, lower starting doses of 5–10 mg/day may be indicated (299).

6. Other antipsychotics

Only one randomized, placebo-controlled study of typical antipsychotic medications has been reported in the treatment of acute bipolar mania (300). In this study, chlorpromazine was superior to placebo in global improvement of manic symptoms. Typical antipsychotics were comparable to lithium in reducing manic and psychotic symptoms in acute treatment comparison trials (185–190).

Among the atypical antipsychotic agents, risperidone and ziprasidone have also been studied in the treatment of acute bipolar mania with randomized, placebo-controlled trials. As an adjunct to treatment with lithium or divalproex, risperidone was comparable to haloperidol and superior to placebo (301). Ziprasidone was also superior to placebo in a large, multicenter monotherapy trial, with significant differences in favor of ziprasidone apparent at the time of the first rating, day 2 of treatment (302). While no placebo-controlled trials exist for the use of clozapine in the treatment of bipolar disorder, one randomized 1-year trial in patients with refractory bipolar or schizoaffective disorder showed greater clinical improvement with the addition of clozapine than with treatment as usual (303). An open trial of clozapine in the treatment of refractory mania was also associated with improvement in manic symptoms (304, 305). In general, these trials have used dose ranges similar to those used in schizophrenia trials, with similar rates of adverse events.

7. Combination therapy

Controlled trials of lithium plus an antipsychotic and of valproate plus an antipsychotic suggest greater efficacy or more rapid onset of action with these combinations than with any of these agents alone. All of these studies involved patients who were currently being treated but who experienced breakthrough episodes of mania or incomplete response to monotherapy. The studies compared combination therapies: an antipsychotic combined with either valproate or placebo (306); lithium or valproate combined with either olanzapine or placebo (290); lithium or valproate combined with either risperidone or placebo (301); or lithium, valproate, or carbamazepine combined with either risperidone or placebo (307). This last trial supported combination therapy only when the carbamazepine-treated group was excluded.

8. ECT

Three prospective studies have assessed clinical outcomes of treatment of acute mania with ECT. In a prospective, randomized controlled trial (308), patients who received ECT followed by lithium maintenance treatment exhibited greater improvement after 8 weeks than did patients who received lithium as both acute and maintenance treatment. Clinical outcomes with ECT were also found to be superior to outcomes with a combination of lithium and haloperidol (309). In a third study (310), 30 manic patients were all treated with chlorpromazine but were randomly assigned to receive a course of either six ECT sessions or six sham ECT sessions. Patients treated with sham ECT did significantly worse than those treated with real ECT. Although all of these studies had small study group sizes, the results were consistent with other earlier retrospective comparisons of outcome in mania (311, 312) and with earlier naturalistic case series (see Mukherjee et al. [309] and the APA Task Force Report on ECT [110] for reviews).

Although there are no prospective, randomized controlled studies of the use of ECT in the treatment of mixed states, in the aforementioned trial of ECT for treatment of mania (308), the strongest predictor of clinical response was the baseline rating of depressive symptoms. Case reports also suggest that ECT may be efficacious in treatment of mixed states (313–315).

Information on side effects and implementation of ECT can be found in the APA Task Force Report on ECT (110).

9. Novel treatments

A number of new agents are under active investigation as potential treatments for patients with acute bipolar mania, but data regarding their efficacy from randomized controlled trials are not yet available. These agents include the atypical antipsychotics quetiapine and aripiprazole; the antiepileptics zonisamide, acamprosate, and levetiracetam; and omega-3 fatty acids (316).

Two other medication classes, benzodiazepines and calcium channel blockers, have been studied in randomized controlled trials for treatment of acute bipolar mania. Among the benzodiazepines, clonazepam and lorazepam have been studied alone and in combination with lithium (317–322). Interpretation of many of these studies is confounded by small study group sizes, short treatment durations, concomitant antipsychotic use, and difficulties in distinguishing putative antimanic effects from nonspecific sedative effects. Taken together, however, these studies suggest that the sedative effects of benzodiazepines may make them effective treatment adjuncts while awaiting the effects of a primary antimanic agent to become evident. The fact that lorazepam, unlike other benzodiazepines, is well absorbed after intramuscular injection has made it particularly useful for the management of agitation. However, intramuscular olanzapine was superior to intramuscular lorazepam in ameliorating agitation in patients with bipolar mania (322).

Two randomized, controlled trials found little support for the efficacy of the calcium channel antagonist verapamil in the treatment of acute mania. In the first study, verapamil was compared with lithium in 40 patients hospitalized for an acute manic episode (323). The mean reduction in manic symptoms was significantly greater in the group of patients receiving lithium compared with the verapamil-treated group. The second trial, a 3-week double-blind study involving 32 patients with acute mania (324), showed no significant differences in efficacy between verapamil and placebo. These studies indicate that lithium was superior to verapamil and that verapamil, in turn, was not superior to placebo as an antimanic agent. In contrast, in a crossover trial involving 12 patients with refractory ultrarapid-cycling bipolar disorder (325), the calcium channel antagonist nimodipine was superior to placebo in ameliorating mood cycling.

B. SOMATIC TREATMENTS OF ACUTE DEPRESSIVE EPISODES

Somatic treatments that have been studied in bipolar depression include lithium, anticonvulsants, antidepressants, and ECT. Open studies and case reports comprise most of the literature on the treatment of bipolar depression, with the best-controlled data relating to treatment with lithium, lamotrigine, and paroxetine.

In general, the goals for treatment of acute depression in a patient with bipolar disorder are identical to those for patients with nonbipolar depression. The primary goal is remission of the symptoms of major depression and a return to normal levels of psychosocial functioning. Concerns about precipitation of a manic or hypomanic episode introduce management issues in the treatment of bipolar depression that do not exist for unipolar depression. This section will present efficacy data on lithium, anticonvulsants, antidepressants, ECT, and novel treatments. Information on side effects and implementation and dosing issues for lithium and the anticonvulsants are presented in this guideline in their respective sections under "Somatic Treatments of Acute Manic and Mixed Episodes" (Section V.A). Information on side effects and implementation and dosing issues for the antidepressants is provided in the APA *Practice Guideline for the Treatment of Patients With Major Depressive Disorder* (2).

1. Lithium

There have been eight placebo-controlled studies of lithium in the treatment of bipolar depression that had five or more subjects. All of these studies employed crossover designs, and all were completed before 1980 (for a review, see Zornberg and Pope [326]). Among a total of 160 patients, the overall rate of response to lithium, regardless of the degree of improvement or relapse with placebo, was 79%. However, the "unequivocal" lithium response rate, defined as a good or moderate response to lithium with a subsequent relapse when given placebo, was much lower (36%). An additional consideration in the use of lithium as an antidepressant is its time to onset (6–8 weeks), which is later than its antimanic effect (326).

2. Anticonvulsants

a) Divalproex and sodium valproate

There have been no published controlled studies of valproate in the treatment of bipolar depression. In an unpublished study, 43 subjects with bipolar I or bipolar II depression were entered into an 8-week, double-blind, placebo-controlled trial of divalproex. Forty-three percent of divalproex-treated patients and 27% of placebo-treated patients achieved recovery, defined as an improvement of ≥50% in score on the 16-item Hamilton Depression Rating Scale in the absence of hypomania (Young Mania Rating Scale score <10). This difference was not statistically significant (Gary Sachs and Michelle Collins, personal communication). While these results suggest that divalproex may be useful in the treatment of bipolar depression, a more definitive study is needed.

b) Carbamazepine

In a double-blind, placebo-controlled crossover study (327), four of nine patients with bipolar depression showed significant improvement from baseline in depressive symptoms with carbamazepine treatment.

In an open study of carbamazepine (328), there were significant reductions from baseline in 17-item Hamilton depression scale scores among 27 patients with bipolar depression and nine patients with mixed episodes. Patients with mixed episodes were significantly less likely to have a remission than those with bipolar depression.

c) Lamotrigine

Lamotrigine at doses of 50 mg/day and 200 mg/day was compared with placebo in a 7-week double-blind trial in 195 patients with bipolar I disorder with major depression (329). Both lamotrigine groups reported significantly better response rates on the Montgomery-Åsberg Depression Rating Scale but not on the Hamilton depression scale. The first significant lamotrigine versus placebo difference in Hamilton depression scale scores occurred at week 5 in the patients receiving 200 mg/day, whereas it occurred at week 7 in those given 50 mg/day. Switches into manic or hypomanic episodes occurred at equivalent rates (3%–8%) among the three groups.

In a flexible-dose, placebo-controlled study of lamotrigine in 206 patients with bipolar I or bipolar II major depression (330), both treatment groups improved significantly (response rate to lamotrigine was 50%, response rate to placebo was 49%), but lamotrigine did not distinguish itself from placebo. Lamotrigine was started at 25 mg/day and titrated over 5–6 weeks to the target dose of 400 mg/day. In a subgroup analysis, the patients with bipolar I disorder given lamotrigine did respond significantly better than those given placebo in terms of Montgomery-Åsberg Depression Rating Scale score (mean change of 13.5 versus 10.1, respectively).

In a double-blind, crossover study of patients with refractory, rapid-cycling bipolar I or bipolar II disorder who were treated with lamotrigine, gabapentin, or placebo, 45% of the depressed patients responded to lamotrigine, compared with response rates of 26% for gabapentin and 19% for placebo (284).

Finally, in an open study of patients with refractory bipolar disorder, 48% of 40 depressed patients treated with lamotrigine showed a marked response, and 20% showed a moderate response (331).

The most common side effects of lamotrigine in the treatment of depression are headache, nausea, infection, and xerostomia (39, 329). However, none of these occurred at significantly higher percentage than with placebo (332).

The risk of serious rash, including Stevens-Johnson syndrome and toxic epidermal necrolysis, was found to be higher in patients treated for epilepsy in the first year after the introduction of lamotrigine in Europe (333). In clinical trials for epilepsy, the incidence of serious rash was approximately 0.3% in adults and approximately 1% in children (334, 335). However, with a slow titration schedule, the risk of serious rash was reduced to 0.01% in adults (329), which is comparable to that of other anticonvulsant medications. Rash can occur at any time during treatment but is more likely to occur early in treatment. It may also be more likely if lamotrigine and valproate are administered concomitantly (334, 335). Whenever lamotrigine is prescribed, patients should be apprised of the risk of rash and urged to contact the psychiatrist or primary care physician immediately if a rash occurs. At rash onset, it is difficult to distinguish between a serious and a more benign rash. Particularly worrisome are rashes accompanied by fever or sore throat, those that are diffuse and widespread, and those with prominent facial or mucosal involvement. In such circumstances lamotrigine (and concurrent valproate) should be discontinued.

Lamotrigine should be administered at 25 mg/day for the first 2 weeks, then 50 mg/day for weeks 3 and 4. After that, 50 mg can be added per week as clinically indicated. With concurrent valproate treatment, pharmacokinetic interactions lead to lamotrigine levels that are approximately twice normal. To minimize the risk of potentially serious rash in patients who are receiving valproate, the dose schedule should be cut in half (i.e., 12.5 mg/day or 25 mg every other day for 2 weeks, then 25 mg/day for weeks 3 and 4). Similarly, concurrent carbamazepine treatment leads to an increase in lamotrigine metabolism and requires dosing to be doubled. Further details of lamotrigine dosing and adverse effects can be found in several reviews (262, 334–337).

d) Topiramate

There are no placebo-controlled trials of topiramate in the treatment of bipolar depression, but several trials have suggested its efficacy as an add-on therapy. McIntyre et al. (338) conducted a single-blind, add-on study of topiramate and sustained-release bupropion in depressed patients with bipolar I or bipolar II disorder. Both groups had significant baseline-to-endpoint reduction in 17-item Hamilton depression scale and Clinical Global Impression (CGI) improvement scores, with no difference between the two groups. Thirty-three percent of patients receiving cotreatment with topiramate discontinued treatment because of adverse events compared with 22% of the patients receiving bupropion alone. The most common adverse events were sweating, blurred vision, difficulty sleeping, tremors, and paresthesia.

Hussain (339) conducted an open-label, add-on, 6-month study with topiramate in depressed patients with bipolar I or bipolar II disorder. Of 45 patients, 19 fully responded (Hamilton depression scale score=3–7), and 12 partially responded (Hamilton depression scale score=8–12). Five patients discontinued treatment because of lack of efficacy, and nine discontinued because of adverse events.

Conversely, in an open study of patients with bipolar I or bipolar II disorder, the 11 patients who were initially depressed and received add-on topiramate treatment had no significant improvements in either CGI or Inventory of Depressive Symptomatology scores (316).

3. MAOI antidepressants

a) Tranylcypromine

The efficacy of tranylcypromine was compared with that of imipramine in 56 outpatients with bipolar I or bipolar II depression (340). Compared with imipramine (at doses of at least 150 mg/day), tranylcypromine (at doses of at least 30 mg/day) produced significantly superior outcomes in terms of lower attrition, greater symptomatic improvement, and higher global response without a greater risk of treatment-emergent hypomania or mania.

In a second study (341), tranylcypromine was compared with imipramine in a double-blind crossover fashion for the 16 nonresponsive patients with bipolar I or bipolar II disorder from the previous trial. Tranylcypromine had comparatively better results, including lower attrition, greater symptomatic improvement, higher global response, and no greater risk of precipitating a switch into hypomania or mania.

b) Moclobemide

Moclobemide was compared to imipramine in a 4-week, multicenter, randomized study of 381 patients (342). No significant differences in efficacy were observed between the groups (both had response rates of 58%). The number of patients with adverse events and the total number of adverse events were greater in the imipramine group.

4. SSRIs and other newer antidepressant agents

a) Fluoxetine

Fluoxetine was compared with imipramine and placebo in 89 patients with bipolar depression. Twenty-two of the 89 patients were also taking lithium during the study. Eighty-six percent of the patients receiving fluoxetine over 6 weeks improved compared with 57% receiving imipramine and 38% given placebo. The response rate with fluoxetine was significantly better than that of both imipramine ($p<0.05$) and placebo ($p=0.005$). There were significantly fewer fluoxetine patients who discontinued treatment because of adverse events (343).

b) Paroxetine

Paroxetine was studied as an add-on treatment in three double-blind studies of patients with bipolar depression. In one study (344), depressed patients with bipolar I or bipolar II disorder maintained on regimens of lithium or divalproex were randomly assigned either to addition of paroxetine or a combination of lithium and divalproex in a 6-week outpatient trial. In terms of improvement from baseline in 17-item Hamilton depression scale scores, both treatments were equally effective at week 6: the mean scores of 6 and 9 in the subjects given lithium plus divalproex and those treated with adjunctive paroxetine, respectively, represented a decrease of 50%–70% ($p<0.001$). There were more dropouts among those treated with the combination of lithium and divalproex.

In a placebo-controlled multicenter trial of paroxetine and imipramine in the treatment of patients with bipolar I depression maintained on a regimen of lithium (345), imipramine and paroxetine were found to be superior to placebo in patients whose serum lithium level was ≤0.8 meq/liter. In those patients with serum lithium levels >0.8 meq/liter, there were no differences among the groups. Of the patients receiving imipramine, treatment-induced switches into manic or hypomanic episodes occurred in 6% of those with lithium levels >0.8 meq/liter and 11% of those with lithium levels ≤0.8 meq/liter. Switches occurred in none of the paroxetine-treated patients and in 2% of the placebo group (all of whom had lithium levels ≤0.8 meq/liter).

Paroxetine and venlafaxine were studied in the treatment of patients with bipolar depression on a maintenance medication regimen (346). Forty-three percent of the paroxetine group and 48% of the venlafaxine group were rated as having responded (difference not significant). Whereas switches to episodes of mania or hypomania occurred in 3% of those treated with paroxetine, the rate of switching in the venlafaxine group was 13%.

c) Citalopram

In a 24-week, open-label trial, the use of citalopram as an add-on treatment was studied in 45 patients with bipolar depression (30 [67%] with bipolar I disorder) who were receiving lithium, valproate, or carbamazepine (347). Of the 33 patients who completed the 8-week acute phase, 64% responded, and most of these patients continued to improve through the 16-week continuation phase.

d) Bupropion

There have been two controlled studies of bupropion in the treatment of bipolar depression. In a double-blind, 8-week study (348), patients who had been maintained on regimens of lithium, valproate, or carbamazepine were randomly assigned to bupropion or desipramine treatment. The response rate was 55% for bupropion and 50% for desipramine, a nonsignificant difference. In the first 8 weeks, 30% of the patients receiving desipramine switched into a manic episode, whereas 11% of those receiving bupropion did. Over the entire study, with follow-up to 1 year, the observed rate of switching into manic or hypomanic episodes in patients receiving desipramine was 50%, whereas the rate was 11% with bupropion.

In a 6-week, double-blind study of bupropion versus idazoxan (a selective α_2 antagonist) in 16 patients with bipolar I disorder—some of whom were also on a maintenance regimen of lithium—no significant differences were seen between the groups (349).

e) Venlafaxine

In addition to the aforementioned double-blind study that compared venlafaxine with paroxetine (346), another study reported on 15 depressed women with bipolar II disorder who were treated with venlafaxine (350). Sixty-three percent of the patients experienced a ≥50% reduction from baseline in scores on the 21-item Hamilton depression scale. Two patients (13%) discontinued treatment because of adverse events.

5. Tricyclic antidepressants

Imipramine and desipramine have been used as active control treatments in studies of tranylcypromine, fluoxetine, paroxetine, and bupropion. In general, the tricyclic antidepressants had response rates that were equivalent to or poorer than that of the active comparator (yet superior to placebo). In addition, treatment with tricyclic antidepressants was associated with higher rates of switching into manic or hypomanic episodes.

6. Antipsychotics

In an 8-week, double-blind study of olanzapine monotherapy, olanzapine and fluoxetine combination therapy, and placebo in the treatment of 833 patients with acute bipolar I depression, olanzapine monotherapy and combination therapy were both significantly better than placebo at endpoint (M. Tohen, personal communication, 2001). Furthermore, both of these treatment regimens showed significant separation from placebo at week 1.

7. ECT

Several controlled studies of ECT in patients with bipolar depression were conducted several decades ago (326). All found ECT to be as or more effective than MAOIs, tricyclic antidepressants, or placebo. ECT is a viable option for patients with severe bipolar depression, especially if psychotic features are present (110). For information on side effects and implementation of ECT, see the APA Task Force Report on ECT (110).

8. Novel treatments

Several studies have suggested that sleep deprivation has an antidepressant effect in patients with bipolar depression, although its effect is usually short-lived (351). It has been studied in conjunction with pindolol in a placebo-controlled protocol (352). Forty patients with bipolar depression were randomly assigned to receive either pindolol or placebo in combination with total sleep deprivation. Fourteen of 20 patients who underwent total sleep deprivation while receiving pindolol were rated as having responded (Hamilton depression scale score <8), whereas only one patient receiving placebo and pindolol responded. No switches into manic episodes were observed. Another study examined the value of phototherapy or lithium in conjunction with total sleep deprivation among 115 patients with bipolar depression (353). The authors reported that each adjunctive treatment improved total sleep-deprivation response rates, but the combination of all three added nothing.

Thyroid hormones, particularly thyroxine (T_4), have been reported to be useful in the treatment of bipolar disorder, particularly rapid cycling (205). In patients with nonbipolar depression, triiodothyronine (T_3) augmentation is associated with an antidepressant effect. The use of thyroid hormones in patients with bipolar depression remains to be studied.

The use of other agents, such as risperidone, olanzapine, ziprasidone, omega-3 fatty acids (354), pramipexole (355), or interventions such as phototherapy (353), vagus nerve stimulation (356), or repetitive transcranial magnetic stimulation (357) requires further study.

C. RAPID CYCLING

Rapid cycling is generally difficult to treat (358, 359). An important first step is to assess for and treat medical conditions that may contribute to cycling, such as hypothyroidism or drug or alcohol use. Medications, particularly antidepressants, may also contribute to cycling. Such medications should be discontinued if possible. Increases in cycling frequency or precipitation of hypomanic or manic episodes have been reported in association with essentially all currently approved antidepressants (340, 343, 360). Use of some form of mood chart can aid in identifying a link between a medication and cycling frequency.

Rapid cycling is relatively unresponsive to lithium or carbamazepine (358, 361–363). Among 41 lithium-treated patients with rapid-cycling bipolar disorder followed for 5 years, all patients experienced at least one recurrence. Twenty-six percent derived limited or no prophylactic benefit (364). The limited benefit of lithium in rapid cycling may be a function of its lack of efficacy for depressive symptoms, despite its efficacy for manic symptoms (365, 366). In the open-stabilization phase of a study of lithium and divalproex in patients with rapid-cycling bipolar disorder, those who failed to meet criteria for random assignment were more likely to have refractory depression (76%) than manic or mixed states (24%) (40). These results suggest that 1) the major benefit of treatment with lithium or lithium combined with divalproex is on the manic aspects of rapid-cycling bipolar disorder and 2) rapid cycling is principally characterized by recurrent depression.

In a randomized, blind, placebo-controlled study of 182 patients with rapid-cycling bipolar I or bipolar II disorder who were receiving maintenance treatment (39), lamotrigine was superior to placebo on overall study survival ($p<0.04$) but not on the primary measure, which was the time elapsed until the onset of a mood episode that required additional pharmacotherapy. The lamotrigine over placebo advantage was greatest ($p=0.01$) among the 52 patients with bipolar II disorder: the median time to discontinuation for any reason among patients with bipolar II disorder was 17 weeks for the patients receiving lamotrigine and 7 weeks for those given placebo (the discontinuation times among the entire group were 18 weeks and 12 weeks for the lamotrigine-treated and placebo-treated patients, respectively). Similarly, the rate of study completion without relapse in patients receiving medication monotherapy was significantly greater among the lamotrigine-treated than among the placebo-treated patients with bipolar II disorder (46% versus 18%, $p=0.04$); this difference was not seen among those with bipolar I disorder (39). An open study comparing response to lamotrigine in patients with rapid-cycling versus non-rapid-cycling bipolar disorder also indicated efficacy, with some evidence that rapid-cycling patients with more severe manic symptoms at the start of treatment respond less well (367).

Divalproex was effective as monotherapy or as an add-on therapy in an open study of 107 rapid-cycling patients followed for a mean of 17 months. Marked benefit occurred among 77% of the patients who entered the study when manic or hypomanic. However, only 38% of those who entered the study depressed reached the maintenance stage (368, 369).

These limited data provide support for the use of lamotrigine in rapid-cycling bipolar disorder—especially for depressive features, which appear to dominate the bipolar II form of rapid cycling—and suggest that combination drug therapy is often superior to use of a single drug.

D. MAINTENANCE TREATMENT

Maintenance treatment of patients with bipolar disorder has multiple goals. In addition to relapse prevention, reduction of subthreshold symptoms, and reduction of suicide risk, aims need to include reduction of cycling frequency and mood instability as well as improvement of functioning. Maintenance medication is generally recommended following a manic episode (370, 371). Although few studies involving patients with bipolar II disorder have been conducted in this area, consideration of maintenance treatment for this form of the illness is also strongly warranted.

Maintenance studies pose two difficulties not central to acute episode studies. The multiple treatment goals make it impractical to select a single goal as an adequate index of efficacy. Also, because of risks associated with full relapse and of suicidal behavior, few placebo-controlled studies have been conducted, and many of those have enrolled somewhat less severely ill patients than seen in the spectrum of clinical practice with bipolar disorder (372).

This section will present efficacy data on lithium, anticonvulsants, antipsychotics, and ECT as maintenance treatment agents. Information on side effects and implementation and dosing issues for lithium and the anticonvulsants are presented in this guideline in their respective sections under "Somatic Treatments of Acute Manic and Mixed Episodes" (Section V.A), with the exception of lamotrigine, the data for which are presented under "Somatic Treatment of Acute Depressive Episodes" (Section V.B.2.c).

1. Lithium

Studies conducted over 25 years ago consistently reported lithium to be more effective than placebo with regard to the proportion of patients who did not relapse (373–377). Most of these studies used discontinuation study designs, in which patients taking stable doses of lithium were abruptly discontinued from lithium if randomly assigned to placebo. It has subsequently become clear that such discontinuation of lithium increases early relapse into mania or depression (378). These studies had additional design limitations, including enrollment of both unipolar and bipolar depressed patients, lack of specification of diagnostic criteria, reporting of results only for patients who completed the study, and failure to report reasons for premature discontinuation. These studies raised expectations for lithium therapy unrealistically.

In large, open, naturalistic studies on the effectiveness of lithium as a maintenance treatment agent in patients with bipolar disorder, good outcomes (e.g., no relapse and only mild symptoms) were seen in approximately one-third of the subjects (226, 364, 379–382). At a 2-year follow-up evaluation, Markar and Mander (379) reported no difference in the rate of hospital readmissions between patients who received lithium and those who did not. Harrow et al. (380) reported equivalent 1-year outcomes for patients receiving lithium and those not taking medication, with 40% of patients taking lithium for the year developing manic episodes. Coryell et al. (381) reported a lower risk of relapse during the first 32 weeks of treatment for patients taking lithium than for those receiving no prophylactic medication, but no difference in relapse risk was seen for weeks 33–96. Other large, open studies that have employed varying methods have reported similar results (226, 364, 383, 384). In general, these studies have also reported high dropout rates.

However, two recent randomized, double-blind, parallel-group studies have indicated evidence of efficacy for lithium compared with placebo in extending time until a new manic episode (385, 386). Each study enrolled patients who were currently experiencing or recently had experienced a manic episode. Symptoms were initially controlled through open treatment with medications (including those to which the subjects would be randomly assigned). Subjects were then randomly assigned either to treatment with lithium, placebo, or divalproex (385) or treatment with lithium, placebo, or lamotrigine (386). The first study measured the time until 25% of subjects undergoing 1 year of maintenance lithium treatment suffered recurrent mania. In this study, lithium extended the time until recurrence by 55% compared with placebo (385).

In the second study, an 18-month trial that enrolled patients during or shortly after a manic episode, lithium significantly extended time until intervention for a recurrent manic episode relative to placebo (p=0.006). The relapse rate into mania was 17% for lithium-treated patients, compared with 41% for placebo-treated patients (386). However, lithium did not significantly extend time until a new depressive episode in either study and tended to worsen subthreshold depressive symptoms in the first study (385). These two studies were the first maintenance studies to use modern methods, enroll patients during an index manic episode, and taper lithium taken during the open phase for those patients entering the randomized, placebo-controlled maintenance phase. Earlier randomized, placebo-controlled studies and a crossover study also have reported efficacy for lithium with regard to manic, but not depressive, symptoms (362, 365, 366).

A randomized, open 2.5-year study compared lithium maintenance treatment with that of carbamazepine (387). The primary efficacy measure, time until hospitalization, did not indicate a significant difference between the treatments. However, broader secondary analyses, such as time until relapse or need for concomitant medication, favored lithium (44% versus 67%, p=0.04). Rapid cycling is associated with relatively poor response to lithium (358); however, in a small prospective study, both rapid-cycling and non-rapid-cycling patients had fewer manic episodes with lithium therapy than did those receiving placebo (365). In addition, one small study has suggested that combining lithium and carbamazepine improves the proportion of response among rapid-cycling patients to a rate equivalent to that of non-rapid-cycling patients (362).

Serum-level guidelines are not well established for maintenance treatment with lithium. In clinical settings, doses and serum levels somewhat lower than those employed for treatment of acute mania are generally used (316). One randomized study of high- and low-dose lithium ranges indicated better efficacy for lithium at 0.8–1.0 meq/liter than at 0.4–0.6 meq/liter in the prevention of manic, but not depressed, episodes (225). However, tolerability was much worse at the higher range. An open study similarly reported rates of rehospitalization lower than those before treatment for the subset of patients whose serum levels were consistently above 0.5 meq/liter (364).

2. Divalproex or valproate

Valproate has been studied in one placebo-controlled, double-blind, randomized trial (385) and two randomized comparisons with lithium (254, 388). In the placebo-controlled study, there was no significant difference in the primary efficacy measure (time until development of any mood episode) among patients treated with divalproex, lithium, and placebo, although there was a nonsignificant difference favoring divalproex over lithium (p=0.06). Divalproex was superior to placebo on rate of early termination for any mood episode (24% versus 38%, respectively; p<0.02), early termination for depression (6% versus 16%; p<0.02), and termination due to failure to adhere to protocol, intercurrent illness, or administrative reasons (16% versus 25%; p<0.02). Early termination for intolerance or noncompliance favored divalproex over lithium (22% versus 35%, respectively; p<0.03). The divalproex advantage over placebo was greater in the subset of 149 patients who had received divalproex treatment for their manic episode during the open period, with rates of early termination for any mood episode of 29% and 50%, respectively (p<0.04). One randomized, 18-month open study of valproate (formulated as valpromide) versus lithium reported a 20% lower rate of new episodes among valpromide-treated patients than among lithium-treated patients (388). Relative to patients given lithium, a lower proportion of patients given valpromide had their treatment discontinued because of intolerance or lack of efficacy. Divalproex and lithium were comparably effective in a 1-year, open, naturalistic, longitudinal study that allowed addition of any needed medication (254). Finally, divalproex was effective both as monotherapy and when added to lithium therapy in a large, open maintenance trial of patients with rapid-cycling presentations (368). These findings indicate efficacy and generally good tolerability of divalproex in maintenance treatment, with effectiveness at least comparable to lithium.

As with lithium, dosing guidelines for maintenance treatment are less evidence-based than for acute treatment of mania, and lower levels are sometimes used for maintenance treatment. A 1-year study of divalproex found an association between higher serum levels and increased appetite, reduced platelet counts, and reduced WBC counts (371).

3. Lamotrigine

Lamotrigine has been studied in one large, 18-month, randomized, double-blind, placebo-controlled study of patients who had experienced a manic or hypomanic episode within 60 days of entry into an open treatment phase (386). Patients who improved during the open treatment phase were randomly assigned to maintenance treatment with lamotrigine, lithium, or placebo. For the primary outcome measure (time until additional pharmacotherapy required for treatment of a mood episode), both lamotrigine and lithium were superior to placebo ($p<0.02$ and $p=0.003$, respectively). The median time until one-quarter of the patients in each treatment group developed a mood episode was 72 weeks for those given lamotrigine, 58 weeks for those receiving lithium, and 35 weeks for those given placebo. On a secondary outcome measure (time until discontinuation for any reason), lamotrigine was superior to placebo, but lithium was not ($p=0.03$ and $p=0.07$, respectively). Lamotrigine did not significantly prolong the time until a manic episode but was superior to placebo in prolonging the time until a depressive episode ($p<0.02$), whereas lithium was not ($p<0.17$). Lamotrigine was also superior to placebo in a 26-week study of rapid-cycling patients with bipolar I or bipolar II disorder (39). The primary efficacy measure, time until additional medication required for treatment of a mood episode, did not differ significantly ($p=0.07$). However, among patients with bipolar II disorder, the median time until additional pharmacotherapy was required was significantly greater for those receiving lamotrigine than for those given placebo (17 weeks versus 7 weeks, $p=0.01$). Time until additional pharmacotherapy was required did not differ significantly among patients with bipolar I disorder. Also, the proportion of patients who completed the study without requiring additional medication was greater among those treated with lamotrigine than for those given placebo (41% versus 26%, $p=0.03$). Among patients requiring additional pharmacotherapy, 80% required medication for depressive symptoms; 20% required medication for manic, hypomanic, or mixed symptoms (39). These results are consistent with those of an open study of patients with bipolar disorder treated with lamotrigine for up to 48 weeks either as monotherapy or as part of combination therapy (329).

4. Carbamazepine

The effectiveness of carbamazepine for maintenance treatment of bipolar disorder is unclear (362). Carbamazepine was inferior to lithium on most outcome measures in one randomized, open, 2.5-year study (387). Carbamazepine was nonsignificantly better than lithium among patients with mood-incongruent illnesses, comorbidity, mixed states, and bipolar II disorder (389). Crossover studies have reported carbamazepine somewhat less effective than lithium in maintenance treatment of bipolar disorder (362, 390). The proportion of time spent in a manic episode dropped from 25% before treatment to 19% in patients treated with carbamazepine and 9% in patients treated with lithium ($p<0.01$). The proportion of time spent in a depressive episode did not change after initiation of either drug (before treatment: 32%, in patients treated with carbamazepine: 26%, in patients treated with lithium: 31%) (362).

5. Antipsychotic medications

The one placebo-controlled study of prophylactic treatment with an antipsychotic drug did not show an advantage of flupentixol plus lithium compared with lithium alone (391). Open case reports and one randomized, open study of clozapine plus usual care compared with usual care alone have indicated benefits of maintenance clozapine treatment over 1 year (303).

6. ECT

The use of ECT on a maintenance basis to prevent mood episodes in patients with bipolar disorder was initially described over 50 years ago (392, 393). While efficacy of maintenance ECT for bipolar disorder patients has never been assessed in a randomized, controlled trial, multiple case reports and case series have suggested its utility (51, 356, 394–403). A more extensive naturalistic review (404) identified 56 patients, including nine with bipolar disorder, who received maintenance ECT following successful index treatment. Of the patients with bipolar disorder, 78% showed at least some improvement, and 33% were much improved.

Vanelle et al. (405) prospectively followed 22 medication-resistant or medication-intolerant patients for more than 18 months of maintenance ECT treatment. Seven of these individuals were diagnosed with bipolar disorder, and four had shown a rapid-cycling course. When the study period was compared with the 1-year period before ECT initiation, the maintenance ECT group as a whole showed a significant decrease in time spent in the hospital and in the number of episodes of illness that necessitated hospitalization. For the patients with bipolar disorder, as well as in those with major depressive disorder, the mean number of mood episodes significantly decreased during the maintenance ECT course. None of the bipolar disorder patients failed to show a response to maintenance ECT.

Schwarz et al. (406), using a case-control approach, compared depressed patients who responded to an acute course of ECT and then received maintenance ECT to patients who responded to acute ECT but received no maintenance ECT. A third comparison group received only pharmacotherapy. In each group, four of the 21 patients had a diagnosis of bipolar disorder. Although this number was too small to permit subgroup analysis, the rate of rehospitalization decreased by 67% for the study patients as a whole with implementation of maintenance ECT. In depressed patients who had responded to an acute course of ECT, Gagné et al. (407) also used a case-control approach to compare patients who received maintenance pharmacotherapy alone with those who received maintenance ECT in combination with maintenance pharmacotherapy. The two groups differed only in the number of "adequate" pharmacotherapy trials before ECT, with patients receiving maintenance ECT showing greater resistance to pharmacotherapy. Of the 58 depressed patients in the study, 12 had a diagnosis of bipolar disorder. For the group as a whole, patients receiving maintenance ECT had a greater cumulative probability of surviving without relapse or recurrence at 2 years than patients receiving only pharmacotherapy after the index ECT course (93% versus 52%, respectively). At 5 years, the difference in survival between the two groups was even more striking (73% versus 18%, respectively). Proportional hazards regression did not demonstrate statistically significant rate differences between patients with bipolar disorder and those with major depressive disorder.

Thus, in studies of maintenance ECT, study group sizes have been small, and patients with bipolar disorder have made up a small proportion of those groups, making subgroup analyses impossible. Nonetheless, the findings suggest that maintenance ECT may be helpful for individual patients with severe bipolar illness who are unable to tolerate or do not respond to maintenance pharmacotherapy.

E. PSYCHOSOCIAL INTERVENTIONS

Although psychiatric management and pharmacotherapy are essential components of bipolar disorder treatment, specific forms of psychotherapy also are critical components of the treatment plan for many patients. Patients with bipolar disorder suffer from the psychosocial consequences of past episodes, the ongoing vulnerability to future episodes, and the burdens of adhering to a long-term treatment plan that may involve unpleasant side effects. In addition, many patients have clinically significant residual symptoms or mood instability between major episodes. The primary goals of psychotherapeutic treatments are to reduce distress and improve the patient's functioning between episodes as well as decrease the likelihood and severity of future episodes (408).

Most patients with bipolar disorder struggle with some of the following issues: 1) emotional consequences of episodes of mania and depression; 2) coming to terms with having a potentially chronic mental illness; 3) problems associated with stigmatization; 4) delays or major deviations in development; 5) fears of recurrence and consequent inhibition of more autonomous functioning; 6) interpersonal difficulties, including issues pertaining to marriage, family, childbearing, and parenting; 7) academic and occupational problems; and 8) other legal, social, and emotional problems that arise from reckless, inappropriate, withdrawn, or violent behavior that may occur during episodes. Although a specific psychotherapeutic approach (in addition to psychiatric management) may be needed to address these issues, the form, intensity, and focus of psychotherapy will vary over time for each patient.

There are now a range of specific psychotherapeutic interventions that have been shown to be helpful when used in combination with pharmacotherapy and psychiatric management for treatment of bipolar disorder. The best-studied treatment approaches have been developed around psychoeducational, interpersonal, family, and cognitive behavior therapies. Formal studies have been conducted for these treatments, and additional investigations are underway. Further, psychodynamic and other forms of therapy may be indicated for some patients. The available psychotherapeutic treatments are discussed as separate entities, even though psychiatrists commonly use a combination or synthesis of different approaches depending on both training and the patient's needs and preferences.

1. Efficacy

Evidence concerning the utility of specific psychosocial interventions for patients with bipolar disorder is slowly building. The research summarized here involves the specific forms of psychotherapy that have been studied in randomized, controlled clinical trials.

Perry et al. (27) evaluated a relatively brief (average: seven sessions) individual psychoeducational intervention that focused on illness management, recognition of risk factors, and prevention of relapses. When compared with a group randomly assigned to a treatment-as-usual condition, patients receiving psychoeducation (in addition to pharmacotherapy) experienced a significant reduction in risk of manic relapses as well as improved social and vocational functioning.

A brief (approximately six sessions) inpatient family intervention (409) has been developed for patients with schizophrenia or bipolar disorder. Goals include accepting the reality of the illness, identifying precipitating stressors and likely future stressors inside and outside the family, elucidating family interactions that produce stress on the patient, planning strategies for managing or minimizing future stressors, and bringing about the patient's family's acceptance of the need for continued treatment after hospital discharge. In the initial study (410), the family intervention resulted in improved outcomes for female patients with affective disorders but not for male patients. In a subsequent study by this group (410), ongoing couples therapy (extending for up to 11 months after hospitalization) was found to significantly enhance treatment adherence and improve global functioning. Unfortunately, this study was too small (intent-to-treat N=42) to reliably detect more modest effects, such as a reduction of relapse risk.

When the functional impairments of bipolar disorder are severe and persistent, other services may be necessary, such as case management, assertive community treatment, psychosocial rehabilitation, and supported employment. These approaches, which have traditionally been studied in patients with schizophrenia, also show effectiveness for certain individuals with bipolar disorder.

Family-focused treatment was developed for patients who have recently had an episode of mania or depression (411). Family-focused therapy is behaviorally based and includes psychoeducation, communication skills training, and problem-solving skills training. One adequately sized trial of behavioral family treatment has been completed; the investigators found that behavioral family management (in concert with adequate pharmacotherapy) resulted in a substantial decrease in depressive relapse rates when compared with a treatment-as-usual control condition (412).

A cognitive behavior therapy program for patients with bipolar disorder has been developed by Basco and Rush (413). The goals of the program are to educate the patient regarding bipolar disorder and its treatment, teach cognitive behavior skills for coping with psychosocial stressors and attendant problems, facilitate compliance with treatment, and monitor the occurrence and severity of symptoms. A large study of the impact of cognitive behavior therapy for prophylaxis against bipolar recurrences is underway. Preliminary studies suggest that this approach may help reduce depressive symptoms (414), improve longer-term outcomes (415), and improve treatment adherence (416).

The observation that many patients with bipolar disorder experience less mood lability when they maintain a regular pattern of daily activities (including sleeping, eating, physical activity, and emotional stimulation) has led to the development of a formalized psychotherapy called interpersonal and social rhythm therapy (417). This form of psychotherapy builds upon the traditional focus of interpersonal psychotherapy by incorporating a behavioral self-monitoring program intended to help patients with bipolar disorder initiate and maintain a lifestyle characterized by more regular sleep-wake cycles, meal times, and other so-called social zeitgebers. The ultimate goal is to help regulate circadian disturbances that may provoke or exaggerate episodes of mood disorder.

Frank and colleagues have reported several findings from their ongoing study of interpersonal and social rhythm therapy. First, interpersonal and social rhythm therapy (in combination with pharmacotherapy) was associated with significant increases in targeted lifestyle regularities when compared with a clinical management plus pharmacotherapy control group (418). However, interpersonal and social rhythm therapy was not associated with a faster time to recovery from manic (419) or depressive (420) episodes. The withdrawal of interpersonal and social rhythm therapy after stabilization was associated with a significant increase in relapse rates (421). Across 2 years of maintenance treatment, interpersonal and social rhythm therapy led to a reduction of both depressive symptoms and manic/hypomanic symptoms and an increase in days of euthymia when compared with treatment as usual (unpublished 2001 study by E. Frank and D.J. Kupfer).

Finally, preliminary results of a trial comparing group psychoeducation to standard medical care alone among a group of patients with bipolar disorder suggest that patients receiving psychoeducation had significantly fewer manic episodes, depressive episodes, and hospitalizations (422).

2. Psychotherapeutic treatment of mania

Psychosocial therapies alone are generally not useful treatments for acute mania. Perhaps the only indications for psychotherapy alone are when all established treatments have been refused, involuntary treatment is not appropriate, and the primary focus of therapy is focused and crisis-oriented (e.g., resolving ambivalence about taking medication). In one study of bipolar I disorder patients with acute mania or hypomania, treatment with the combination of interpersonal and social rhythm therapy and pharmacotherapy did not produce an additive effect on manic symptoms or reduce time to remission when compared with an intensive clinical paradigm plus medication (419). Moreover, patients withdrawn from this psychotherapy after completion of acute treatment had a poorer prognosis when compared with those who either received monthly maintenance psychotherapy sessions or recovered with intensive clinical management and pharmacotherapy (421).

3. Psychotherapeutic treatment of depression

Several psychotherapeutic approaches, including cognitive behavior therapy (423) and interpersonal therapy (424–426), have demonstrated efficacy in patients with unipolar depression, either in lieu of or in addition to pharmacotherapy. Efficacy data are discussed in the APA *Practice Guideline for the Treatment of Patients With Major Depressive Disorder* (2).

For unipolar depression, the application of a specific, effective psychotherapy in lieu of pharmacotherapy may be considered for patients with mild to moderate symptoms. For bipolar depression, the use of focused psychotherapy instead of antidepressant pharmacotherapy has potential appeal, particularly with respect to avoiding antidepressant side effects and minimizing the risk of treatment-emergent mania or induction of rapid cycling. However, only a handful of reports have described such an approach, and there have been no definitive studies to date.

Cole et al. (420) evaluated the impact of a modified form of interpersonal psychotherapy as part of a larger study relating thyroid function to clinical course in 65 patients with bipolar I depression. Patients were randomly assigned to receive weekly interpersonal and social rhythm therapy sessions or treatment as usual. All patients received pharmacotherapy (principally lithium salts); about two-thirds of the patients also received antidepressants. Cole et al. found that the addition of weekly psychotherapy did not enhance depressive symptom reduction or accelerate time to remission in comparison with treatment as usual across up to 6 months of treatment.

Zaretsky et al. (414) treated 11 patients with bipolar depression with individual cognitive behavior therapy (20 weekly sessions) in addition to ongoing pharmacotherapy. They compared their patients' outcomes to a contemporaneous group of age and sex-matched patients with unipolar depression. Among the eight completers in the bipolar depression group (seven with bipolar I disorder, one with bipolar II disorder), improvements were comparable to those in the unipolar depression group. Further, no depressed patient receiving cognitive behavior therapy developed treatment-emergent mania or hypomania.

4. Maintenance treatment

Since the 1994 publication of the first APA practice guideline for bipolar disorder (5), a number of reports on the value of concomitant psychosocial treatment during the maintenance phase of treatment for bipolar disorder have been published. All studies used "add-on" designs, with patients continuing pharmacotherapies such as lithium and divalproex. Many of these reports described preliminary or pilot studies; nevertheless, results of three larger, more definitive studies have been published for psychoeducation (27), interpersonal and social rhythm therapy (427), and family-focused (412) interventions.

Overall, these studies demonstrated that the addition of a time-limited individual psychosocial intervention appropriately modified for bipolar disorder is likely to improve outcomes across 1–2 years of follow-up. When feasible, group psychoeducational interventions also appear useful (428), which may improve the cost efficiency of treatment. Despite these promising results, however, improvements have not been consistently documented across studies on the full range of syndromal, functional, adherence, and interpersonal domains. On the basis of a methodological review of the more numerous studies of unipolar depression (429), such inconsistencies in findings are more likely to be attributable to differences in patient populations and statistical power than true therapeutic specificity.

Nevertheless, the weight of the evidence suggests that patients with bipolar disorder are likely to gain some additional benefit during the maintenance phase from a concomitant psychosocial intervention, including psychotherapy, that addresses illness management (i.e., adherence, lifestyle changes, and early detection of prodromal symptoms) and interpersonal difficulties. The more commonly practiced supportive and dynamic-eclectic therapies have not been studied in randomized, controlled trials as maintenance treatments for patients with bipolar disorder.

5. Addressing comorbid disorders and psychosocial consequences

Patients in remission from bipolar disorder suffer from the psychosocial consequences of past episodes and ongoing vulnerability to future episodes. In addition, patients with this disorder remain vulnerable to other psychiatric disorders, including, most commonly, substance use disorders (66) and personality disorders (430, 431). Each of these comorbid disorders has particular consequences and increases the overall psychosocial vulnerability of the patient with bipolar disorder. Psychosocial treatments, including psychotherapy, should address issues of comorbidity and complications that are present.

F. SOMATIC THERAPIES FOR CHILDREN AND ADOLESCENTS

To date, there has been only one double-blind, placebo-controlled, randomized study of pharmacotherapy in the treatment of adolescents with bipolar disorder (432). The majority of information available about pharmacological treatments for bipolar disorder in youth relies upon open studies, case series, and case reports.

1. Lithium

There are more data available for lithium than for any other medication in the treatment of bipolar disorder in children and adolescents. Geller et al. (432) conducted the only double-blind, placebo-controlled, parallel-group study of lithium treatment in 25 adolescent outpatients with comorbid bipolar disorder and substance dependence. Subjects were randomly assigned to lithium or placebo for a 6-week trial. There was significantly greater improvement in global functioning with lithium treatment than with placebo. Significantly more patients in the lithium-treatment group experienced thirst, polyuria, nausea, vomiting, and dizziness.

In four double-blind, placebo-controlled, crossover studies of children with bipolar disorder, significant improvement in mood lability, explosive outbursts, aggressive behavior, and psychosis was found with lithium compared with placebo (433–436). However, small study group sizes, diagnostic issues, and short treatment durations limit the interpretation of these findings. There have also been open studies, case series, and case reports with clinical responses ranging from 50% to 100% (437–455).

2. Valproate/divalproex

There have been no placebo-controlled studies of divalproex in the treatment of bipolar disorder in children and adolescents, but divalproex response rates in four open studies ranged from 60% to 83% (127, 456–458).

In the only multisite open study of divalproex treatment for children and adolescents with bipolar disorder (458), 40 subjects ages 7–17 years received divalproex for 2–8 weeks. Sixty-one percent of the subjects showed a ≥50% improvement from baseline scores on the Young Mania Rating Scale. Twenty-three patients (58%) discontinued the study, of whom 16 had a comorbid psychiatric diagnosis such as ADHD, conduct disorder, or oppositional defiant disorder. The most commonly occurring side effects (>10% incidence) were headache, nausea, vomiting, diarrhea, and somnolence. No significant laboratory abnormalities were noted.

There have also been four case reports or series of divalproex sodium treatment of bipolar disorder in youth. Response rates have ranged from 66% to 100% in these reports (459–462).

Divalproex also showed efficacy in an active-comparator study in which 42 children and adolescents (ages 8–18 years) with bipolar disorder were randomly assigned to 6 weeks of open treatment with lithium, divalproex, or carbamazepine (463). No significant differences in response rates (>50% change from baseline to last Young Mania Rating Scale score) were found among the patients receiving divalproex (53%), lithium (38%), or carbamazepine (38%). There were no serious adverse events reported with any of these medications.

In the continuation phase of this study, 35 patients received open treatment for an additional 16–18 weeks (463). Response during the continuation phase was defined as a score of 1 or 2 on the Bipolar Clinical Global Improvement Scale. Thirty patients (85%) were classified as having responded at the end of the continuation phase. Only 13 patients (37%) were receiving a single study drug (lithium, divalproex, or carbamazepine) and no other psychotropic medication at the end of the continuation phase. For the 22 patients who required additional psychotropic medication, 11 received a second study drug (lithium, divalproex, or carbamazepine), and 11 received a stimulant.

3. Carbamazepine

Information about the use of carbamazepine in the treatment of adolescent bipolar disorder is limited to case reports. Woolston (464) described three cases of carbamazepine monotherapy for adolescents with bipolar disorder in whom clinical improvement of manic symptoms was demonstrated. A positive response was reported with the combination of carbamazepine and lithium in seven adolescents with bipolar disorder (192, 449).

4. Atypical antipsychotics

There are two case series and one open trial of olanzapine as primary or adjunctive treatment for children and adolescents with bipolar disorder. In an open study, 23 children ages 5–14 years with bipolar disorder received olanzapine 2.5–20 mg/day for 8 weeks (465). Response was defined as ≥30% improvement in score on the Young Mania Rating Scale, and the response rate was 61%. There were no significant side effects reported except weight gain (mean=5 kg). In case reports of three youths (ages 9–19 years) with bipolar disorder, olanzapine was used as an adjunctive treatment in addition to existing medication regimens (466). Within a week, CGI scores were rated markedly improved. Sedation and weight gain were the common side effects. Finally, in a report of seven cases of adolescents with bipolar disorder (467), olanzapine was used as adjunctive treatment to existing psychotropic medication regimens. Seventy-one percent of adolescents showed marked to moderate response on CGI scores with adjunctive olanzapine treatment.

A retrospective chart review of 28 outpatient children and adolescents ages 4–17 years with bipolar disorder assessed adjunctive risperidone treatment (468). These subjects received risperidone over an average of 6 months. Improvement (CGI score ≤2) in manic and aggressive symptoms was seen in 82% of the patients, and 69% exhibited improvement in psychotic symptoms. No serious adverse effects were reported, although common side effects were weight gain and sedation.

5. Newer antiepileptics

There are few reports of the use of the newer antiepileptic agents in the treatment of children and adolescents with bipolar disorder. In a retrospective study of 18 adolescents for whom prior medication trials had failed (469), subjects with bipolar disorder not otherwise specified (N= 15), bipolar II disorder (N=1), or schizoaffective disorder (N=2) received gabapentin at doses between 900 and 2400 mg/day. Sixteen of the adolescents who continued gabapentin treatment had cessation of cycling. Of these patients, six reported improved mood. Gabapentin was also reported to be effective in the treatment of an adolescent patient with mania (470).

6. ECT

ECT has been used to treat refractory mania in two prepubertal children (471). A review of literature on ECT use in young people (472) reported its efficacy for mania in adolescents.

PART C:
FUTURE RESEARCH NEEDS

While a number of large, double-blind, controlled trials in bipolar disorder have been conducted since the publication of the first guideline on the treatment of bipolar disorder in 1994 (5), many significant questions remain regarding optimal use of the available treatments. The introduction of new pharmacotherapies, including newer anticonvulsants and atypical antipsychotics, has also led to a need to directly compare traditional and newer interventions. Moreover, fundamental questions remain to be addressed about the nature of bipolar disorder itself.

VI. GENERAL PRINCIPLES

1. Is there a more clinically and scientifically useful definition of a "mood stabilizer"? Do newer agents (e.g., atypical antipsychotics and anticonvulsants) have true "mood-stabilizing" properties?
2. What is the relationship of bipolar I disorder, bipolar II disorder, and possible "bipolar spectrum" illnesses?
3. To what extent do patients with bipolar I or bipolar II disorder respond differentially to treatment?

VII. ACUTE TREATMENT

A. MANIC AND MIXED EPISODES

1. What medication dosage and treatment duration can be considered an adequate trial?
2. In what circumstances is combination therapy favored over monotherapy?
3. Do different atypical antipsychotics exert different antimanic effects? Which combinations are most efficacious?
4. Can true antimanic properties of medications be distinguished from sedative properties of medications?

B. DEPRESSIVE EPISODES

1. How effective are newer antidepressants, such as SSRIs, in treating bipolar depression? How and when can they best be combined with other pharmacotherapies, such as lithium and valproate?
2. Do the different antidepressants have different relative efficacies?
3. What medication dosage and treatment duration can be considered an adequate trial?
4. In treating an episode of bipolar depression, at what point in time is the addition of an antidepressant appropriate?

C. RAPID CYCLING

1. Which pharmacotherapy regimens are most effective in the treatment of rapid cycling?
2. Do newer antidepressants or other medications truly differ in their propensity to induce rapid cycling or switches into hypomanic episodes?

VIII. MAINTENANCE TREATMENT

1. What is the efficacy of newer agents in maintenance pharmacotherapy?
2. What are the predictors of response or nonresponse to maintenance pharmacotherapy?
3. What is the optimum treatment of residual or subthreshold symptoms?
4. How can the side effects seen with all maintenance pharmacotherapies be minimized?
5. To what extent do interventions in bipolar disorder improve functional status rather than symptoms?

IX. PSYCHOSOCIAL INTERVENTIONS

1. What are the relative efficacies of (and indications for) different psychotherapeutic approaches in the acute and maintenance phases of treatment?
2. What are the elements of psychotherapy that are critical to its efficacy?

APPENDIX 1. Educational Sources for Depression and Bipolar Disorder

Internet Mental Health
www.mentalhealth.org

National Alliance for the Mentally Ill
Colonial Place Three, 2107 Wilson Blvd.
Suite 300
Arlington, VA 22201
(703) 524-7600
NAMI HelpLine: (800) 950-NAMI [6264]
www.nami.org

National Depressive and Manic-Depressive Association
730 N. Franklin St., Suite 501
Chicago, IL 60610-7204
(312) 642-0049
(800) 826-3632
www.ndmda.org

National Foundation for Depressive Illness, Inc.
P.O. Box 2257
New York, NY 10116
(800) 239-1265
www.depression.org

NIMH Public Inquiries
Depression Information Program
6001 Executive Blvd., Rm. 8184
MSC 9663
Bethesda, MD 20892-9663
(301) 443-4513
TTY Line: (301) 443-8431
www.nimh.nih.gov

National Mental Health Association
1021 Prince St.
Alexandria, VA 22314-2971
(703) 684-7722
TTY Line: (800) 433-5959
www.nmha.org

INDIVIDUALS AND ORGANIZATIONS THAT SUBMITTED COMMENTS

Martin Alda, M.D.
Michael H. Allen, M.D.
Jay D. Amsterdam, M.D.
Ross Baldessarini, M.D.
Joseph Biederman, M.D.
Jack Bonner, M.D.
M.L. Bourgeois, M.D.
Joseph Calabrese, M.D.
James E. Campbell, M.D.
Gabrielle A. Carlson, M.D.
Norman A. Clemens, M.D.
Greg Crosby, M.A., L.C.P., C.G.P.
Dave M. Davis, M.D.
Diana L. Dell, M.D.
Himasiri De Silva, M.D.
David L. Dunner, M.D.
Anita S. Everett, M.D.
Ellen Frank, Ph.D.
Valentim Gentil, M.D., Ph.D.
S. Nasir Ghaemi, M.D.
William M. Greenberg, M.D.
Joseph F. Hagan, M.D.
William Hankin, M.D.
Kay Redfield Jamison, M.D.
David Janowsky, M.D.
Gordon Johnson, M.D.
Tadafumi Kato, M.D.
Matcheri S. Keshavan, M.D.
Edward Kim, M.D.
David J. Kupfer, M.D.
Mario Maj, M.D.
John C. Markowitz, M.D.
Theresa Miskimen, M.D.
Rodrigo A. Muñoz, M.D.
Jim Nininger, M.D.
Willem Nolen, M.D.
Herb Peyne, M.D.
June Powell, M.D.
Lawrence H. Price, M.D.
Marian Scheinholtz, M.S., O.T.R.L.
Robert Stern, M.D., Ph.D.
Nada Stotland, M.D., M.P.H.
Stephen M. Strakowski, M.D.
Mauricio F. Tohen, M.D., Ph.D.
Eduard Vieta, M.D., Ph.D.
Myrna Weissman, Ph.D.
Barbara Yarn, M.D.

American Academy of Family Physicians
American Academy of Pediatrics
American College of Obstetricians and Gynecologists
American Group Psychotherapy Association
American Occupational Therapy Association
Brain Science Institute
New Jersey Psychiatric Association

REFERENCES

The following coding system is used to indicate the nature of the supporting evidence in the references:

[A] *Randomized clinical trial.* A study of an intervention in which subjects are prospectively followed over time; there are treatment and control groups; subjects are randomly assigned to the two groups; both the subjects and the investigators are blind to the assignments.

[B] *Clinical trial.* A prospective study in which an intervention is made and the results of that intervention are tracked longitudinally; study does not meet standards for a randomized clinical trial.
[C] *Cohort or longitudinal study.* A study in which subjects are prospectively followed over time without any specific intervention.
[D] *Control study.* A study in which a group of patients and a group of control subjects are identified in the present and information about them is pursued retrospectively or backward in time.
[E] *Review with secondary data analysis.* A structured analytic review of existing data, e.g., a meta-analysis or a decision analysis.
[F] *Review.* A qualitative review and discussion of previously published literature without a quantitative synthesis of the data.
[G] *Other.* Textbooks, expert opinion, case reports, and other reports not included above.

1. American Psychiatric Association: Diagnostic and Statistical Manual of Mental Disorders, Fourth Edition (text revision). Washington, DC, APA, 2000 [G]
2. American Psychiatric Association: Practice Guideline for the Treatment of Patients With Major Depressive Disorder (Revision). Am J Psychiatry 2000; 157(April suppl) [G]
3. American Academy of Child and Adolescent Psychiatry: AACAP official action: practice parameters for the assessment and treatment of children and adolescents with bipolar disorder. J Am Acad Child Adolesc Psychiatry 1997; 36:138–157 [G]
4. Frank E, Prien RF, Jarrett RB, Keller MB, Kupfer DJ, Lavori PW, Rush AJ, Weissman MM: Conceptualization and rationale for consensus definitions of terms in major depressive disorder: remission, recovery, relapse, and recurrence. Arch Gen Psychiatry 1991; 48:851–855 [F]
5. American Psychiatric Association: Practice Guideline for the Treatment of Patients With Bipolar Disorder. Am J Psychiatry 1994; 151(Dec suppl) [G]
6. Hirschfeld RMA, Williams JBW, Spitzer RL, Calabrese JR, Flynn L, Keck PE Jr, Lewis L, McElroy SL, Post RM, Rapport DJ, Russell JM, Sachs GS, Zajecka J: Development and validation of a screening instrument for bipolar spectrum disorder: the Mood Disorder Questionnaire. Am J Psychiatry 2000; 157:1873–1875 [G]
7. American Psychiatric Association: Practice Guideline for Psychiatric Evaluation of Adults. Am J Psychiatry 1995; 152(Nov suppl) [G]
8. Isometsa ET, Henriksson MM, Aro HM, Lonnqvist JK: Suicide in bipolar disorder in Finland. Am J Psychiatry 1994; 151:1020–1024 [D]
9. Dilsaver SC, Chen YW, Swann AC, Shoaib AM, Krajewski KJ: Suicidality in patients with pure and depressive mania. Am J Psychiatry 1994; 151:1312–1315 [D]
10. Strakowski SM, McElroy SL, Keck PE Jr, West SA: Suicidality among patients with mixed and manic bipolar disorder. Am J Psychiatry 1996; 153:674–676 [C]
11. Muller-Oerlinghausen B, Wolf T, Ahrens B, Glaenz T, Schou M, Grof E, Grof P, Lenz G, Simhandl C, Thau K, Vestergaard P, Wolf R: Mortality of patients who dropped out from regular lithium prophylaxis: a collaborative study by the International Group for the Study of Lithium-Treated Patients (IGSLI). Acta Psychiatr Scand 1996; 94:344–347 [C]
12. Baldessarini RJ, Tondo L, Hennen J: Effects of lithium treatment and its discontinuation on suicidal behavior in bipolar manic-depressive disorders. J Clin Psychiatry 1999; 60(suppl 2):77–84 [E]
13. Angst J, Preisig M: Outcome of a clinical cohort of unipolar, bipolar and schizoaffective patients: results of a prospective study from 1959 to 1985. Schweiz Arch Neurol Psychiatr 1995; 146:17–23 [C]
14. Rosenfarb IS, Miklowitz DJ, Goldstein MJ, Harmon L, Nuechterlein KH, Rea MM: Family transactions and relapse in bipolar disorder. Fam Process 2001; 40:5–14 [C]

15. Mino Y, Shimodera S, Inoue S, Fujita H, Tanaka S, Kanazawa S: Expressed emotion of families and the course of mood disorders: a cohort study in Japan. J Affect Disord 2001; 63:43–49 [C]
16. Tompson MC, Rea MM, Goldstein MJ, Miklowitz DJ, Weisman AG: Difficulty in implementing a family intervention for bipolar disorder: the predictive role of patient and family attributes. Fam Process 2000; 39:105–120 [G]
17. Simoneau TL, Miklowitz DJ, Saleem R: Expressed emotion and interactional patterns in the families of bipolar patients. J Abnorm Psychol 1998; 107:497–507 [G]
18. Jamison KR, Gerner RH, Goodwin FK: Patient and physician attitudes toward lithium: relationship to compliance. Arch Gen Psychiatry 1979; 36:866–869 [G]
19. Gutheil TG: The psychology of psychopharmacology. Bull Menninger Clin 1982; 46:321–330 [G]
20. Jamison KR: Manic-depressive illness: the overlooked need for psychotherapy, in Integrating Pharmacotherapy and Psychotherapy. Washington, DC, American Psychiatric Press, 1991 [F]
21. Jamison KR, Akiskal HS: Medication compliance in patients with bipolar disorder. Psychiatr Clin North Am 1983; 6:175–192 [F]
22. Pardes H, Kaufmann CA, Pincus HA, West A: Genetics and psychiatry: past discoveries, current dilemmas, and future directions. Am J Psychiatry 1989; 146:435–443 [G]
23. Johnson SL, Roberts JE: Life events and bipolar disorder: implications from biological theories. Psychol Bull 1995; 117:434–449 [F]
24. Hammen C, Gitlin M: Stress reactivity in bipolar patients and its relation to prior history of disorder. Am J Psychiatry 1997; 154:856–857 [D]
25. Malkoff-Schwartz S, Frank E, Anderson B, Sherrill JT, Siegel L, Patterson D, Kupfer DJ: Stressful life events and social rhythm disruption in the onset of manic and depressive bipolar episodes: a preliminary investigation. Arch Gen Psychiatry 1998; 55:702–707 [D]
26. Leibenluft E, Suppes T: Treating bipolar illness: focus on treatment algorithms and management of the sleep-wake cycle (case conf). Am J Psychiatry 1999; 156:1976–1986 [G]
27. Perry A, Tarrier N, Morriss R, McCarthy E, Limb K: Randomised controlled trial of efficacy of teaching patients with bipolar disorder to identify early symptoms of relapse and obtain treatment. Br Med J 1999; 318:149–153 [A]
28. Butzlaff RL, Hooley JM: Expressed emotion and psychiatric relapse: a meta-analysis. Arch Gen Psychiatry 1998; 55:547–552 [E]
29. Miklowitz DJ, Goldstein MJ, Nuechterlein KH, Snyder KS, Mintz J: Family factors and the course of bipolar affective disorder. Arch Gen Psychiatry 1988; 45:225–231 [C]
30. Post RM, Roy-Byrne PP, Uhde TW: Graphic representation of the life course of illness in patients with affective disorder. Am J Psychiatry 1988; 145:844–848 [G]
31. Kraepelin E: Manic-Depressive Insanity and Paranoia (1921). Translated by Barclay RM. Salem, NH, Ayer, 1976 [G]
32. Meyer A: The Collected Papers of Adolph Meyer. Baltimore, Johns Hopkins University Press, 1950 [G]
33. Tohen M, Hennen J, Zarate CM Jr, Baldessarini RJ, Strakowski SM, Stoll AL, Faedda GL, Suppes T, Gebre-Medhin P, Cohen BM: Two-year syndromal and functional recovery in 219 cases of first-episode major affective disorder with psychotic features. Am J Psychiatry 2000; 157:220–228 [D]
34. Suppes T, Leverich GS, Keck PE Jr: The Stanley Foundation Bipolar Network: demographics and illness characteristics of the first 261 patients with bipolar disorder. J Affect Disord (in press) [C]
35. Keck PE Jr, McElroy SL, Strakowski SM, West SA, Sax KW, Hawkins JM, Bourne ML, Haggard P: 12-month outcome of patients with bipolar disorder following hospitalization for a manic or mixed episode. Am J Psychiatry 1998; 155:646–652 [C]

36. Rossi A, Arduini L, Daneluzzo E, Bustini M, Prosperini P, Stratta P: Cognitive function in euthymic bipolar patients, stabilized schizophrenic patients, and healthy controls. J Psychiatr Res 2000; 34:333–339 [G]
37. Bearden CE, Hoffman KM, Cannon TD: The neuropsychology and neuroanatomy of bipolar affective disorder: a critical review. Bipolar Disord 2001; 3:106–150 [F]
38. Howland RH: Induction of mania with serotonin reuptake inhibitors. J Clin Psychopharmacol 1996; 16:425–427 [B]
39. Calabrese JR, Suppes T, Bowden CL, Sachs GS, Swann AC, McElroy SL, Kusumakar V, Ascher JA, Earl NL, Greene PL, Monaghan ET (Lamictal 614 Study Group): A double-blind, placebo-controlled, prophylaxis study of lamotrigine in rapid-cycling bipolar disorder. J Clin Psychiatry 2000; 61:841–850 [A]
40. Calabrese JR, Shelton MD, Bowden CL, Rapport DJ, Suppes T, Shirley ER, Kimmel SE, Caban SJ: Bipolar rapid cycling: focus on depression as its hallmark. J Clin Psychiatry 2001; 62(suppl 14):34–41 [F]
41. Goodwin FK, Jamison KR: Manic-Depressive Illness. New York, Oxford University Press, 1990 [G]
42. Carlson GA, Bromet EJ, Sievers S: Phenomenology and outcome of subjects with early- and adult-onset psychotic mania. Am J Psychiatry 2000; 157:213–219 [C]
43. Tohen M, Tsuang MT, Goodwin DC: Prediction of outcome in mania by mood-congruent or mood-incongruent psychotic features. Am J Psychiatry 1992; 149:1580–1584 [C]
44. Fennig S, Bromet EJ, Karant MT, Ram R, Jandorf L: Mood-congruent versus mood-incongruent psychotic symptoms in first-admission patients with affective disorder. J Affect Disord 1996; 37:23–29 [D]
45. McElroy SL, Keck PE Jr, Strakowski SM: Mania, psychosis, and antipsychotics. J Clin Psychiatry 1996; 57(suppl 3):14–26 [F]
46. Braunig P, Kruger S, Shugar G: Prevalence and clinical significance of catatonic symptoms in mania. Compr Psychiatry 1998; 39:35–46 [D]
47. Taylor MA, Abrams R: Catatonia: prevalence and importance in the manic phase of manic-depressive illness. Arch Gen Psychiatry 1977; 34:1223–1225 [C]
48. Hawkins JM, Archer KJ, Strakowski SM, Keck PE: Somatic treatment of catatonia. Int J Psychiatry Med 1995; 25:345–369 [F]
49. Rosebush PI, Hildebrand AM, Furlong BG, Mazurek MF: Catatonic syndrome in a general psychiatric inpatient population: frequency, clinical presentation, and response to lorazepam. J Clin Psychiatry 1990; 51:357–362 [B]
50. Northoff G, Wenke J, Demisch L, Eckert J, Gille B, Pflug B: Catatonia: short-term response to lorazepam and dopaminergic metabolism. Psychopharmacology (Berl) 1995; 122:182–186 [B]
51. Bush G, Fink M, Petrides G, Dowling F, Francis A: Catatonia, II: treatment with lorazepam and electroconvulsive therapy. Acta Psychiatr Scand 1996; 93:137–143 [B]
52. Lee JW: Serum iron in catatonia and neuroleptic malignant syndrome. Biol Psychiatry 1998; 44:499–507 [B]
53. Cooper TB, Bergner PE, Simpson GM: The 24-hour serum lithium level as a prognosticator of dosage requirements. Am J Psychiatry 1973; 130:601–603 [C]
54. Simpson SG, Jamison KR: The risk of suicide in patients with bipolar disorders. J Clin Psychiatry 1999; 60(suppl 2):53–56 [F]
55. Lester D: Suicidal behavior in bipolar and unipolar affective disorders: a meta-analysis. J Affect Disord 1993; 27:117–121 [E]
56. Tondo L, Baldessarini RJ: Reduced suicide risk during lithium maintenance treatment. J Clin Psychiatry 2000; 61(suppl 9):97–104 [F]
57. Norton B, Whalley LJ: Mortality of a lithium-treated population. Br J Psychiatry 1984; 145: 277–282 [F]

58. Vieta E, Colom F, Martinez-Aran A, Benabarre A, Gasto C: Personality disorders in bipolar II patients. J Nerv Ment Dis 1999; 187:245–248 [G]
59. Fawcett J: Treating impulsivity and anxiety in the suicidal patient. Ann NY Acad Sci 2001; 932:94–102 [F]
60. Tondo L, Jamison KR, Baldessarini RJ: Effect of lithium maintenance on suicidal behavior in major mood disorders. Ann NY Acad Sci 1997; 836:339–351 [E]
61. Ahrens B, Muller-Oerlinghausen B, Schou M, Wolf T, Alda M, Grof E, Grof P, Lenz G, Simhandl C, Thau K: Excess cardiovascular and suicide mortality of affective disorders may be reduced by lithium prophylaxis. J Affect Disord 1995; 33:67–75 [D]
62. Brennan PA, Mednick SA, Hodgins S: Major mental disorders and criminal violence in a Danish birth cohort. Arch Gen Psychiatry 2000; 57:494–500 [D]
63. Barlow K, Grenyer B, Ilkiw-Lavalle O: Prevalence and precipitants of aggression in psychiatric inpatient units. Aust NZ J Psychiatry 2000; 34:967–974 [C]
64. Asnis GM, Kaplan ML, Hundorfean G, Saeed W: Violence and homicidal behaviors in psychiatric disorders. Psychiatr Clin North Am 1997; 20:405–425 [F]
65. Hendrick V, Altshuler LL, Gitlin MJ, Delrahim S, Hammen C: Gender and bipolar illness. J Clin Psychiatry 2000; 61:393–396 [D]
66. Regier DA, Farmer ME, Rae DS, Locke BZ, Keith SJ, Judd LL, Goodwin FK: Comorbidity of mental disorders with alcohol and other drug abuse: results from the Epidemiologic Catchment Area (ECA) study. JAMA 1990; 264:2511–2518 [D]
67. Regier DA, Boyd JH, Burke JD Jr, Rae DS, Myers JK, Kramer M, Robins LN, George LK, Karno M, Locke BZ: One-month prevalence of mental disorders in the United States: based on five Epidemiologic Catchment Area sites. Arch Gen Psychiatry 1988; 45:977–986 [D]
68. Tohen M, Waternaux CM, Tsuang MT, Hunt AT: Four-year follow-up of twenty-four first-episode manic patients. J Affect Disord 1990; 19:79–86 [C]
69. Tohen M, Waternaux CM, Tsuang MT: Outcome in mania: a 4-year prospective follow-up of 75 patients utilizing survival analysis. Arch Gen Psychiatry 1990; 47:1106–1111 [C]
70. Potash JB, Kane HS, Chiu Y-F, Simpson SG, MacKinnon DF, McInnis MG, McMahon FJ, DePaulo JR Jr: Attempted suicide and alcoholism in bipolar disorder: clinical and familial relationships. Am J Psychiatry 2000; 157:2048–2050 [D]
71. Goldberg JF, Garno JL, Leon AC, Kocsis JH, Portera L: A history of substance abuse complicates remission from acute mania in bipolar disorder. J Clin Psychiatry 1999; 60:733–740 [D]
72. Sonne SC, Brady KT: Substance abuse and bipolar comorbidity. Psychiatr Clin North Am 1999; 22:609–627 [F]
73. Tondo L, Baldessarini RJ, Hennen J, Minnai GP, Salis P, Scamonatti L, Masia M, Ghiani C, Mannu P: Suicide attempts in major affective disorder patients with comorbid substance use disorders. J Clin Psychiatry 1999; 60(suppl 2):63–69 [C]
74. Hagan H, Des J: HIV and HCV infection among injecting drug users. Mt Sinai J Med 2000; 67:423–428 [F]
75. American Psychiatric Association: Practice Guideline for the Treatment of Patients With Substance Use Disorders: Alcohol, Cocaine, Opioids. Am J Psychiatry 1995; 152(Nov suppl) [G]
76. Dunayevich E, Sax KW, Keck PE Jr, McElroy SL, Sorter MT, McConville BJ, Strakowski SM: Twelve-month outcome in bipolar patients with and without personality disorders. J Clin Psychiatry 2000; 61:134–139 [C]
77. Colom F, Vieta E, Martinez-Aran A, Reinares M, Benabarre A, Gasto C: Clinical factors associated with treatment noncompliance in euthymic bipolar patients. J Clin Psychiatry 2000; 61:549–555 [D]
78. Feske U, Frank E, Mallinger AG, Houck PR, Fagiolini A, Shear MK, Grochocinski VJ, Kupfer DJ: Anxiety as a correlate of response to the acute treatment of bipolar I disorder. Am J Psychiatry 2000; 157:956–962 [D]

79. Sachs GS, Baldassano CF, Truman CJ, Guille C: Comorbidity of attention deficit hyperactivity disorder with early- and late-onset bipolar disorder. Am J Psychiatry 2000; 157:466–468 [G]
80. Johnston AM, Eagles JM: Lithium-associated clinical hypothyroidism: prevalence and risk factors. Br J Psychiatry 1999; 175:336–339 [C]
81. Leibenluft E: Women with bipolar illness: clinical and research issues. Am J Psychiatry 1996; 153:163–173 [F]
82. Tondo L, Baldessarini RJ, Hennen J, Floris G, Silvetti F, Tohen M: Lithium treatment and risk of suicidal behavior in bipolar disorder patients. J Clin Psychiatry 1998; 59:405–414 [B]
83. Dickson RA, Seeman MV, Corenblum B: Hormonal side effects in women: typical versus atypical antipsychotic treatment. J Clin Psychiatry 2000; 61(suppl 3):10–15 [F]
84. Goodnick PJ, Chaudry T, Artadi J, Arcey S: Women's issues in mood disorders. Expert Opin Pharmacother 2000; 1:903–916 [F]
85. Viguera AC, Cohen LS: The course and management of bipolar disorder during pregnancy. Psychopharmacol Bull 1998; 34:339–346 [F]
86. Altshuler LL, Hendrick V, Cohen LS: Course of mood and anxiety disorders during pregnancy and the postpartum period. J Clin Psychiatry 1998; 59(suppl 2):29–33 [F]
87. Rosenfeld WE, Doose DR, Walker SA, Nayak RK: Effect of topiramate on the pharmacokinetics of an oral contraceptive containing norethindrone and ethinyl estradiol in patients with epilepsy. Epilepsia 1997; 38:317–323 [B]
88. Wilbur K, Ensom MH: Pharmacokinetic drug interactions between oral contraceptives and second-generation anticonvulsants. Clin Pharmacokinet 2000; 38:355–365 [F]
89. Spina E, Pisani F, Perucca E: Clinically significant pharmacokinetic drug interactions with carbamazepine: an update. Clin Pharmacokinet 1996; 31:198–214 [F]
90. Potash JB, DePaulo JR Jr: Searching high and low: a review of the genetics of bipolar disorder. Bipolar Disord 2000; 2:8–26 [F]
91. Berrettini WH: Genetics of psychiatric disease. Annu Rev Med 2000; 51:465–479 [F]
92. Duffy A, Grof P, Robertson C, Alda M: The implications of genetics studies of major mood disorders for clinical practice. J Clin Psychiatry 2000; 61:630–637 [F]
93. Wisner KL, Zarin D, Holmboe E, Appelbaum P, Gelenberg AJ, Leonard HL, Frank E: Risk-benefit decision making for treatment of depression during pregnancy. Am J Psychiatry 2000; 157:1933–1940 [F]
94. Viguera AC, Nonacs R, Cohen LS, Tondo L, Murray A, Baldessarini RJ: Risk of recurrence of bipolar disorder in pregnant and nonpregnant women after discontinuing lithium maintenance. Am J Psychiatry 2000; 157:179–184 [D]
95. Viguera AC, Tondo L, Baldessarini RJ: Sex differences in response to lithium treatment. Am J Psychiatry 2000; 157:1509–1511 [D]
96. Hoffman S, Hatch MC: Depressive symptomatology during pregnancy: evidence for an association with decreased fetal growth in pregnancies of lower social class women. Health Psychol 2000; 19:535–543 [C]
97. Paarlberg KM, Vingerhoets AJ, Passchier J, Dekker GA, Heinen AG, van Geijn HP: Psychosocial predictors of low birthweight: a prospective study. Br J Obstet Gynaecol 1999; 106:834–841 [C]
98. Spielvogel A, Wile J: Treatment and outcomes of psychotic patients during pregnancy and childbirth. Birth 1992; 19:131–137 [D]
99. Coverdale JH, Chervenak FA, McCullough LB, Bayer T: Ethically justified clinically comprehensive guidelines for the management of the depressed pregnant patient. Am J Obstet Gynecol 1996; 174:169–173 [F]
100. Stocky A, Lynch J: Acute psychiatric disturbance in pregnancy and the puerperium. Baillieres Best Pract Res Clin Obstet Gynaecol 2000; 14:73–87 [F]
101. Cohen LS, Rosenbaum JF: Psychotropic drug use during pregnancy: weighing the risks. J Clin Psychiatry 1998; 59(suppl 2):18–28 [F]

102. Cohen LS, Friedman JM, Jefferson JW, Johnson EM, Weiner ML: A reevaluation of risk of in utero exposure to lithium. JAMA 1994; 271:146–150 [F]
103. Holmes LB, Harvey EA, Coull BA, Huntington KB, Khoshbin S, Hayes AM, Ryan LM: The teratogenicity of anticonvulsant drugs. N Engl J Med 2001; 344:1132–1138 [C]
104. Arpino C, Brescianini S, Robert E, Castilla EE, Cocchi G, Cornel MC, de Vigan C, Lancaster PA, Merlob P, Sumiyoshi Y, Zampino G, Renzi C, Rosano A, Mastroiacovo P: Teratogenic effects of antiepileptic drugs: use of an International Database on Malformations and Drug Exposure (MADRE). Epilepsia 2000; 41:1436–1443 [C]
105. American Academy of Pediatrics Committee on Drugs: Use of psychoactive medication during pregnancy and possible effects on the fetus and newborn. Pediatrics 2000; 105:880–887 [F]
106. Wisner KL, Gelenberg AJ, Leonard H, Zarin D, Frank E: Pharmacologic treatment of depression during pregnancy. JAMA 1999; 282:1264–1269 [F]
107. Ericson A, Kallen B, Wiholm B: Delivery outcome after the use of antidepressants in early pregnancy. Eur J Clin Pharmacol 1999; 55:503–508 [C]
108. McElhatton PR: The effects of benzodiazepine use during pregnancy and lactation. Reprod Toxicol 1994; 8:461–475 [F]
109. Dolovich LR, Addis A, Vaillancourt JM, Power JD, Koren G, Einarson TR: Benzodiazepine use in pregnancy and major malformations or oral cleft: meta-analysis of cohort and case-control studies. Br Med J 1998; 317:839–843 [E]
110. American Psychiatric Association: The Practice of Electroconvulsive Therapy: Recommendations for Treatment, Training, and Privileging: A Task Force Report of the American Psychiatric Association, 2nd ed. Washington, DC, American Psychiatric Press, 2001 [G]
111. Shnider SM, Levinson G: Anesthesia for Obstetrics, 3rd ed. Baltimore, Williams & Wilkins, 1993 [G]
112. Llewellyn A, Stowe ZN, Strader JR Jr: The use of lithium and management of women with bipolar disorder during pregnancy and lactation. J Clin Psychiatry 1998; 59(suppl 6):57–64 [F]
113. Cohen LS, Sichel DA, Robertson LM, Heckscher E, Rosenbaum JF: Postpartum prophylaxis for women with bipolar disorder. Am J Psychiatry 1995; 152:1641–1645 [D]
114. Yoshida K, Smith B, Kumar R: Psychotropic drugs in mothers' milk: a comprehensive review of assay methods, pharmacokinetics and of safety of breast-feeding. J Psychopharmacol 1999; 13:64–80 [F]
115. Chaudron LH, Jefferson JW: Mood stabilizers during breastfeeding: a review. J Clin Psychiatry 2000; 61:79–90 [F]
116. Burt VK, Suri R, Altshuler L, Stowe Z, Hendrick VC, Muntean E: The use of psychotropic medications during breast-feeding. Am J Psychiatry 2001; 158:1001–1009 [F]
117. Tomson T, Ohman I, Vitols S: Lamotrigine in pregnancy and lactation: a case report. Epilepsia 1997; 38:1039–1041 [G]
118. American Academy of Pediatrics Committee on Drugs: Transfer of drugs and other chemicals into human milk. Pediatrics 2001; 108:776–789 [F]
119. Strakowski SM, McElroy SL, Keck PE Jr, West SA: Racial influence on diagnosis in psychotic mania. J Affect Disord 1996; 39:157–162 [D]
120. Strakowski SM, Flaum M, Amador X, Bracha HS, Pandurangi AK, Robinson D, Tohen M: Racial differences in the diagnosis of psychosis. Schizophr Res 1996; 21:117–124 [D]
121. Strakowski SM, Hawkins JM, Keck PE Jr, McElroy SL, West SA, Bourne ML, Sax KW, Tugrul KC: The effects of race and information variance on disagreement between psychiatric emergency service and research diagnoses in first-episode psychosis. J Clin Psychiatry 1997; 58:457–463 [D]
122. Lin KM, Anderson D, Poland RE: Ethnicity and psychopharmacology: bridging the gap. Psychiatr Clin North Am 1995; 18:635–647 [F]

123. Bertilsson L: Geographical/interracial differences in polymorphic drug oxidation: current state of knowledge of cytochromes P450 (CYP) 2D6 and 2C19. Clin Pharmacokinet 1995; 29:192–209 [F]
124. Lewinsohn PM, Klein DN, Seeley JR: Bipolar disorders in a community sample of older adolescents: prevalence, phenomenology, comorbidity, and course. J Am Acad Child Adolesc Psychiatry 1995; 34:454–463 [C]
125. Geller B, Zimerman B, Williams M, Bolhofner K, Craney JL, DelBello MP, Soutullo CA: Diagnostic characteristics of 93 cases of a prepubertal and early adolescent bipolar disorder phenotype by gender, puberty and comorbid attention deficit hyperactivity disorder. J Child Adolesc Psychopharmacol 2000; 10:157–164 [C]
126. Kovacs M, Pollock M: Bipolar disorder and comorbid conduct disorder in childhood and adolescence. J Am Acad Child Adolesc Psychiatry 1995; 34:715–723 [C]
127. West SA, McElroy SL, Strakowski SM, Keck PE Jr, McConville BJ: Attention deficit hyperactivity disorder in adolescent mania. Am J Psychiatry 1995; 152:271–273 [D]
128. Faraone SV, Biederman J, Wozniak J, Mundy E, Mennin D, O'Donnell D: Is comorbidity with ADHD a marker for juvenile-onset mania? J Am Acad Child Adolesc Psychiatry 1997; 36:1046–1055 [D]
129. Altshuler LL, Cohen LS, Moline ML, Kahn DA, Carpenter D, Docherty JP: The Expert Consensus Guideline Series: Treatment of Depression in Women. New York, McGraw-Hill Companies, 2001 [F]
130. Strober M, Schmidt-Lackner S, Freeman R, Bower S, Lampert C, DeAntonio M: Recovery and relapse in adolescents with bipolar affective illness: a five-year naturalistic, prospective follow-up. J Am Acad Child Adolesc Psychiatry 1995; 34:724–731 [C]
131. Biederman J, Mick E, Bostic JQ, Prince J, Daly J, Wilens TE, Spencer T, Garcia-Jetton J, Russell R, Wozniak J, Faraone SV: The naturalistic course of pharmacologic treatment of children with maniclike symptoms: a systematic chart review. J Clin Psychiatry 1998; 59: 628–637 [B]
132. Strober M, Morrell W, Lampert C, Burroughs J: Relapse following discontinuation of lithium maintenance therapy in adolescents with bipolar I illness: a naturalistic study. Am J Psychiatry 1990; 147:457–461 [C]
133. Biederman J, Faraone SV, Wozniak J, Monuteaux MC: Parsing the association between bipolar, conduct, and substance use disorders: a familial risk analysis. Biol Psychiatry 2000; 48:1037–1044 [C]
134. Wilens TE, Biederman J, Millstein RB, Wozniak J, Hahesy AL, Spencer TJ: Risk for substance use disorders in youths with child- and adolescent-onset bipolar disorder. J Am Acad Child Adolesc Psychiatry 1999; 38:680–685 [C]
135. Carlson GA, Lavelle J, Bromet EJ: Medication treatment in adolescents vs adults with psychotic mania. J Child Adolesc Psychopharmacol 1999; 9:221–231 [C]
136. Geller B, Luby J: Child and adolescent bipolar disorder: a review of the past 10 years. J Am Acad Child Adolesc Psychiatry 1997; 36:1168–1176; correction, 36:1642 [F]
137. Donovan SJ, Nunes EV: Treatment of comorbid affective and substance use disorders: therapeutic potential of anticonvulsants. Am J Addict 1998; 7:210–220 [F]
138. Van Gerpen MW, Johnson JE, Winstead DK: Mania in the geriatric patient population: a review of the literature. Am J Geriatr Psychiatry 1999; 7:188–202 [F]
139. Young RC, Klerman GL: Mania in late life: focus on age at onset. Am J Psychiatry 1992; 149:867–876 [F]
140. Shulman KI, Herrmann N: The nature and management of mania in old age. Psychiatr Clin North Am 1999; 22:649–665 [F]
141. Tohen M, Shulman KI, Satlin A: First-episode mania in late life. Am J Psychiatry 1994; 151: 130–132 [C]

142. Sproule BA, Hardy BG, Shulman KI: Differential pharmacokinetics of lithium in elderly patients. Drugs Aging 2000; 16:165–177 [F]
143. Caligiuri MR, Jeste DV, Lacro JP: Antipsychotic-induced movement disorders in the elderly: epidemiology and treatment recommendations. Drugs Aging 2000; 17:363–384 [F]
144. Leipzig RM, Cumming RG, Tinetti ME: Drugs and falls in older people: a systematic review and meta-analysis, I: psychotropic drugs. J Am Geriatr Soc 1999; 47:30–39 [E]
145. Strakowski SM, McElroy SL, Keck PW Jr, West SA: The co-occurrence of mania with medical and other psychiatric disorders. Int J Psychiatry Med 1994; 24:305–328 [F]
146. Peet M, Peters S: Drug-induced mania. Drug Saf 1995; 12:146–153 [F]
147. Cozza KL, Armstrong SC (eds): Concise Guide to the Cytochrome P450 System: Drug Interaction Principles for Medical Practice. Washington, DC, American Psychiatric Press, 2001, pp 103–200 [G]
148. American Psychiatric Association: Practice Guideline for the Treatment of Patients With HIV/AIDS. Am J Psychiatry 2000; 157(Nov suppl) [G]
149. Akiskal HS, Pinto O: The evolving bipolar spectrum: prototypes I, II, III, and IV. Psychiatr Clin North Am 1999; 22:517–534 [F]
150. Swann AC, Bowden CL, Calabrese JR, Dilsaver SC, Morris DD: Differential effect of number of previous episodes of affective disorder on response to lithium or divalproex in acute mania. Am J Psychiatry 1999; 156:1264–1266 [E]
151. Lish JD, Dime-Meenan S, Whybrow PC, Price RA, Hirschfeld RM: The National Depressive and Manic-Depressive Association (DMDA) survey of bipolar members. J Affect Disord 1994; 31:281–294 [G]
152. Manning JS, Haykal RF, Connor PD, Akiskal HS: On the nature of depressive and anxious states in a family practice setting: the high prevalence of bipolar II and related disorders in a cohort followed longitudinally. Compr Psychiatry 1997; 38:102–108 [D]
153. Perugi G, Akiskal HS, Lattanzi L, Cecconi D, Mastrocinque C, Patronelli A, Vignoli S, Bemi E: The high prevalence of "soft" bipolar (II) features in atypical depression. Compr Psychiatry 1998; 39:63–71 [G]
154. Benazzi F: Prevalence of bipolar II disorder in outpatient depression: a 203-case study in private practice. J Affect Disord 1997; 43:163–166 [G]
155. Akiskal HS, Maser JD, Zeller PJ, Endicott J, Coryell W, Keller M, Warshaw M, Clayton P, Goodwin F: Switching from "unipolar" to bipolar II: an 11-year prospective study of clinical and temperamental predictors in 559 patients. Arch Gen Psychiatry 1995; 52:114–123 [C]
156. Mitchell PB, Wilhelm K, Parker G, Austin MP, Rutgers P, Malhi GS: The clinical features of bipolar depression: a comparison with matched major depressive disorder patients. J Clin Psychiatry 2001; 62:212–216 [D]
157. Ghaemi SN, Sachs GS, Chiou AM, Pandurangi AK, Goodwin K: Is bipolar disorder still underdiagnosed? are antidepressants overutilized? J Affect Disord 1999; 52:135–144 [G]
158. Fogarty F, Russell JM, Newman SC, Bland RC: Epidemiology of psychiatric disorders in Edmonton: mania. Acta Psychiatr Scand Suppl 1994; 376:16–23 [G]
159. Faedda GL, Baldessarini RJ, Suppes T, Tondo L, Becker I, Lipschitz DS: Pediatric-onset bipolar disorder: a neglected clinical and public health problem. Harv Rev Psychiatry 1995; 3:171–195 [F]
160. Winokur G, Coryell W, Akiskal HS, Endicott J, Keller M, Mueller T: Manic-depressive (bipolar) disorder: the course in light of a prospective ten-year follow-up of 131 patients. Acta Psychiatr Scand 1994; 89:102–110 [C]
161. Dion GL, Tohen M, Anthony WA, Waternaux CS: Symptoms and functioning of patients with bipolar disorder six months after hospitalization. Hosp Community Psychiatry 1988; 39:652–657 [C]
162. Goodnick PJ, Fieve RR, Schlegel A, Baxter N: Predictors of interepisode symptoms and relapse in affective disorder patients treated with lithium carbonate. Am J Psychiatry 1987; 144:367–369 [B]

163. Goldberg JF, Harrow M, Grossman LS: Course and outcome in bipolar affective disorder: a longitudinal follow-up study. Am J Psychiatry 1995; 152:379–384 [C]
164. Coryell W, Scheftner W, Keller M, Endicott J, Maser J, Klerman GL: The enduring psychosocial consequences of mania and depression. Am J Psychiatry 1993; 150:720–727 [C]
165. Weissman MM, Bland RC, Canino GJ, Faravelli C, Greenwald S, Hwu HG, Joyce PR, Karam EG, Lee CK, Lellouch J, Lepine JP, Newman SC, Rubio-Stipec M, Wells JE, Wickramaratne PJ, Wittchen H, Yeh EK: Cross-national epidemiology of major depression and bipolar disorder. JAMA 1996; 276:293–299 [E]
166. Angst J: The emerging epidemiology of hypomania and bipolar II disorder. J Affect Disord 1998; 50:143–151 [C]
167. Geller B, Craney JL, Bolhofner K, DelBello MP, Williams M, Zimerman B: One-year recovery and relapse rates of children with a prepubertal and early adolescent bipolar disorder phenotype. Am J Psychiatry 2001; 158:303–305 [C]
168. McDonald WM, Nemeroff CB: The diagnosis and treatment of mania in the elderly. Bull Menninger Clin 1996; 60:174–196 [F]
169. Tohen M, Bromet E, Murphy JM, Tsuang MT: Psychiatric epidemiology. Harvard Rev Psychiatry 2000; 8:111–125 [G]
170. Leverich GS, McElroy SL, Suppes T: Early physical or sexual abuse and the course of bipolar illness. Biological Psychiatry (in press) [G]
171. Johnson SL, Miller I: Negative life events and time to recovery from episodes of bipolar disorder. J Abnorm Psychol 1997; 106:449–457 [C]
172. Frank E, Thase ME: Natural history and preventative treatment of recurrent mood disorders. Annu Rev Med 1999; 50:453–468 [F]
173. Colombo C, Benedetti F, Barbini B, Campori E, Smeraldi E: Rate of switch from depression into mania after therapeutic sleep deprivation in bipolar depression. Psychiatry Res 1999; 86:267–270 [B]
174. Ashman SB, Monk TH, Kupfer DJ, Clark CH, Myers FS, Frank E, Leibenluft E: Relationship between social rhythms and mood in patients with rapid cycling bipolar disorder. Psychiatry Res 1999; 86:1–8 [C]
175. Strakowski SM, DelBello MP: The co-occurrence of bipolar and substance use disorders. Clin Psychol Rev 2000; 20:191–206 [F]
176. Schou M, Juel-Nielson, Stroomgren E, Voldby H: The treatment of manic psychoses by administration of lithium salts. J Neurol Neurosurg Psychiatry 1954; 17:250–260 [B]
177. Goodwin FK, Murphy DL, Bunney WE Jr: Lithium-carbonate treatment in depression and mania: a longitudinal double-blind study. Arch Gen Psychiatry 1969; 21:486–496 [B]
178. Stokes PE, Shamoian CA, Stoll PM, Patton MJ: Efficacy of lithium as acute treatment of manic-depressive illness. Lancet 1971; 1:1319–1325 [B]
179. Maggs R: Treatment of manic illness with lithium carbonate. Br J Psychiatry 1963; 109: 56–65 [B]
180. Bowden CL, Brugger AM, Swann AC, Calabrese JR, Janicak PG, Petty F, Dilsaver SC, Davis JM, Rush AJ, Small JG (Depakote Mania Study Group): Efficacy of divalproex vs lithium and placebo in the treatment of mania. JAMA 1994; 271:918–924 [A]
181. Lerer B, Moore N, Meyendorff E, Cho SR, Gershon S: Carbamazepine versus lithium in mania: a double-blind study. J Clin Psychiatry 1987; 48:89–93 [A]
182. Small JG, Klapper MH, Milstein V, Kellams JJ, Miller MJ, Marhenke JD, Small IF: Carbamazepine compared with lithium in the treatment of mania. Arch Gen Psychiatry 1991; 48:915–921 [A]
183. Segal J, Berk M, Brook S: Risperidone compared with both lithium and haloperidol in mania: a double-blind randomized controlled trial. Clin Neuropharmacol 1998; 21:176–180 [A]
184. Berk M, Ichim L, Brook S: Olanzapine compared to lithium in mania: a double-blind randomized controlled trial. Int Clin Psychopharmacol 1999; 14:339–343 [A]

185. Takahashi R, Sakuma A, Itoh K, Itoh H, Kurihara M: Comparison of efficacy of lithium carbonate and chlorpromazine in mania: report of collaborative study group on treatment of mania in Japan. Arch Gen Psychiatry 1975; 32:1310–1318 [A]
186. Platman SR: A comparison of lithium carbonate and chlorpromazine in mania. Am J Psychiatry 1970; 127:351–353 [A]
187. Spring G, Schweid D, Gray C, Steinberg J, Horwitz M: A double-blind comparison of lithium and chlorpromazine in the treatment of manic states. Am J Psychiatry 1970; 126: 1306–1310 [A]
188. Johnson G, Gershon S, Burdock EI, Floyd A, Hekimian L: Comparative effects of lithium and chlorpromazine in the treatment of acute manic states. Br J Psychiatry 1971; 119:267–276 [A]
189. Prien RF, Caffey EM Jr, Klett CJ: Comparison of lithium carbonate and chlorpromazine in the treatment of mania: report of the Veterans Administration and National Institute of Mental Health Collaborative Study Group. Arch Gen Psychiatry 1972; 26:146–153 [A]
190. Shopsin B, Gershon S, Thompson H, Collins P: Psychoactive drugs in mania: a controlled comparison of lithium carbonate, chlorpromazine, and haloperidol. Arch Gen Psychiatry 1975; 32:34–42 [A]
191. Secunda SK, Katz MM, Swann A, Koslow SH, Maas JW, Chuang S, Croughan J: Mania: diagnosis, state measurement and prediction of treatment response. J Affect Disord 1985; 8:113–121 [E]
192. Himmelhoch JM, Garfinkel ME: Sources of lithium resistance in mixed mania. Psychopharmacol Bull 1986; 22:613–620 [C]
193. Prien RF, Himmelhoch JM, Kupfer DJ: Treatment of mixed mania. J Affect Disord 1988; 15:9–15 [B]
194. Kramlinger KG, Post RM: Adding lithium carbonate to carbamazepine: antimanic efficacy in treatment-resistant mania. Acta Psychiatr Scand 1989; 79:378–385 [B]
195. Freeman TW, Clothier JL, Pazzaglia P, Lesem MD, Swann AC: A double-blind comparison of valproate and lithium in the treatment of acute mania. Am J Psychiatry 1992; 149:108–111 [A]
196. Bowden CL: Predictors of response to divalproex and lithium. J Clin Psychiatry 1995; 56(suppl 3):25–30 [E]
197. Swann AC, Bowden CL, Morris D, Calabrese JR, Petty F, Small J, Dilsaver SC, Davis JM: Depression during mania: treatment response to lithium or divalproex. Arch Gen Psychiatry 1997; 54:37–42 [E]
198. Jefferson JW, Greist JH, Acherman DL, Carroll JA: Lithium Encyclopedia for Clinical Practice, 2nd ed. Washington, DC, American Psychiatric Press, 1987 [F]
199. Schou M: Lithium prophylaxis: myths and realities. Am J Psychiatry 1989; 146:573–576 [F]
200. Peet M, Pratt JP: Lithium: current status in psychiatric disorders. Drugs 1993; 46:7–17 [F]
201. Burggraf GW: Are psychotropic drugs at therapeutic levels a concern for cardiologists? Can J Cardiol 1997; 13:75–80 [F]
202. Gitlin M: Lithium and the kidney: an updated review. Drug Saf 1999; 20:231–243 [F]
203. Bendz H, Aurell M: Drug-induced diabetes insipidus: incidence, prevention and management. Drug Saf 1999; 21:449–456 [F]
204. Arana GW, Hyman SE: Handbook of Psychiatric Drug Therapy, 2nd ed. Boston, Little, Brown, 1991 [F]
205. Bauer MS, Whybrow PC: Rapid cycling bipolar affective disorder, II: treatment of refractory rapid cycling with high-dose levothyroxine: a preliminary study. Arch Gen Psychiatry 1990; 47:435–440 [A]
206. Kleiner J, Altshuler L, Hendrick V, Hershman JM: Lithium-induced subclinical hypothyroidism: review of the literature and guidelines for treatment. J Clin Psychiatry 1999; 60: 249–255 [F]
207. Smigan L, Wahlin A, Jacobsson L, von Knorring L: Lithium therapy and thyroid function tests: a prospective study. Neuropsychobiology 1984; 11:39–43 [B]

208. Bocchetta A, Bernardi F, Burrai C, Pedditzi M, Loviselli A, Velluzzi F, Martino E, Del Zompo M: The course of thyroid abnormalities during lithium treatment: a two-year follow-up study. Acta Psychiatr Scand 1992; 86:38–41 [C]
209. Haden ST, Stoll AL, McCormick S, Scott J, Fuleihan GE-H: Alterations in parathyroid dynamics in lithium-treated subjects. J Clin Endocrinol Metab 1997; 82:2844–2848 [B]
210. Kallner G, Petterson U: Renal, thyroid and parathyroid function during lithium treatment: laboratory tests in 207 people treated for 1–30 years. Acta Psychiatr Scand 1995; 91:48–51 [C]
211. Mak TW, Shek CC, Chow CC, Wing YK, Lee S: Effects of lithium therapy on bone mineral metabolism: a two-year prospective longitudinal study. J Clin Endocrinol Metab 1998; 83: 3857–3859 [B]
212. Chan HH, Wing Y, Su R, Van Krevel C, Lee S: A control study of the cutaneous side effects of chronic lithium therapy. J Affect Disord 2000; 57:107–113 [D]
213. Vestergaard P, Schou M, Thomsen K: Monitoring of patients in prophylactic lithium treatment: an assessment based on recent kidney studies. Br J Psychiatry 1982; 140:185–187 [C]
214. Schou M: Effects of long-term lithium treatment on kidney function: an overview. J Psychiatr Res 1988; 22:287–296 [F]
215. Gitlin MJ: Lithium-induced renal insufficiency. J Clin Psychopharmacol 1993; 13:276–279 [C]
216. Bendz H, Sjodin I, Aurell M: Renal function on and off lithium in patients treated with lithium for 15 years or more: a controlled, prospective lithium-withdrawal study. Nephrol Dial Transplant 1996; 11:457–460 [B]
217. von Knorring L, Walton SA, Okuma T, Bohman SO: Uraemia induced by long-term lithium treatment. Lithium 1990; 1:251–253 [G]
218. Markowitz GS, Radhakrishnan J, Kambham N, Valeri AM, Hines WH, D'Agati VD: Lithium nephrotoxicity: a progressive combined glomerular and tubulointerstitial nephropathy. J Am Soc Nephrol 2000; 11:1439–1448 [G]
219. Ellenhorn MJ: Lithium, in Ellenhorn's Medical Toxicology: Diagnosis and Treatment of Human Poisoning. Baltimore, Williams & Wilkins, 1997, pp 1579–1585 [G]
220. Scharman EJ: Methods used to decrease lithium absorption or enhance elimination. J Toxicol Clin Toxicol 1997; 35:601–608 [F]
221. Jaeger A, Sauder P, Kopferschmitt J, Tritsch L, Flesch F: When should dialysis be performed in lithium poisoning? a kinetic study in 14 cases of lithium poisoning. J Toxicol Clin Toxicol 1993; 31:429–447 [B]
222. van Bommel EF, Kalmeijer MD, Ponssen HH: Treatment of life-threatening lithium toxicity with high-volume continuous venovenous hemofiltration. Am J Nephrol 2000; 20: 408–411 [G]
223. Friedberg RC, Spyker DA, Herold DA: Massive overdoses with sustained-release lithium carbonate preparations: pharmacokinetic model based on two case studies. Clin Chem 1991; 37:1205–1209 [G]
224. Bosse GM, Arnold TC: Overdose with sustained-release lithium preparations. J Emerg Med 1992; 10:719–721 [G]
225. Gelenberg AJ, Kane JM, Keller MB, Lavori P, Rosenbaum JF, Cole K, Lavelle J: Comparison of standard and low serum levels of lithium for maintenance treatment of bipolar disorder. N Engl J Med 1989; 321:1489–1493 [A]
226. Vestergaard P, Licht RW, Brodersen A, Rasmussen NA, Christensen H, Arngrim T, Gronvall B, Kristensen E, Poulstrup I, Wentzer LR: Outcome of lithium prophylaxis: a prospective follow-up of affective disorder patients assigned to high and low serum lithium levels. Acta Psychiatr Scand 1998; 98:310–315 [B]
227. Emrich HM, von Zerssen D, Kissling W: On a possible role of GABA in mania: therapeutic efficacy of sodium valproate, in GABA and Benzodiazepine Receptors. Edited by Costa E, Dicharia G, Gessa GL. New York, Raven Press, 1981, pp 287–296 [B]

228. Brennan MJW, Sandyk R, Borsook D: Use of sodium valproate in the management of affective disorders: basic and clinical aspects, in Anticonvulsants in Affective Disorders. Edited by Emrich HM, Okuma T, Muller AA. Amsterdam, Excerpta Medica, 1984, pp 56–65 [A]
229. Pope HG Jr, McElroy SL, Keck PE Jr, Hudson JI: Valproate in the treatment of acute mania: a placebo-controlled study. Arch Gen Psychiatry 1991; 48:62–68 [A]
230. McElroy SL, Keck PE, Stanton SP, Tugrul KC, Bennett JA, Strakowski SM: A randomized comparison of divalproex oral loading versus haloperidol in the initial treatment of acute psychotic mania. J Clin Psychiatry 1996; 57:142–146 [B]
231. Zajecka JM, Weisler R, Swann AC: Divalproex sodium versus olanzapine for the treatment of mania in bipolar disorder, in American College of Neuropsychopharmacology Annual Meeting Poster Abstracts. Nashville, Tenn, ACNP, 2000 [A]
232. Tohen MF, Milton DR, Davis AR: Olanzapine versus divalproex for the treatment of acute mania, in Congress Poster Abstracts. Munich, European College of Neuropsychopharmacology, 2000 [A]
233. Sheth RD, Wesolowski CA, Jacob JC, Penney S, Hobbs GR, Riggs JE, Bodensteiner JB: Effect of carbamazepine and valproate on bone mineral density. J Pediatr 1995; 127:256–262 [D]
234. Tannirandorn P, Epstein S: Drug-induced bone loss. Osteoporos Int 2000; 11:637–659 [F]
235. Davis R, Peters DH, McTavish D: Valproic acid: a reappraisal of its pharmacological properties and clinical efficacy in epilepsy. Drugs 1994; 47:332–372 [F]
236. Mercke Y, Sheng H, Khan T, Lippmann S: Hair loss in psychopharmacology. Ann Clin Psychiatry 2000; 12:35–42 [F]
237. Gautam M: Alopecia due to psychotropic medications. Ann Pharmacother 1999; 33:631–637 [F]
238. Stoll AL, Walton SA, McElroy SL: Histamine-2-receptor antagonists for the treatment of valproate-induced gastrointestinal distress. Ann Clin Psychiatry 1991; 3:301–304 [G]
239. Spiller HA, Krenzelok EP, Klein-Schwartz W, Winter ML, Weber JA, Sollee DR, Bangh SA: Multicenter case series of valproic acid ingestion: serum concentrations and toxicity. J Toxicol Clin Toxicol 2000; 38:755–760 [G]
240. Loscher W: Valproate: a reappraisal of its pharmacodynamic properties and mechanisms of action. Prog Neurobiol 1999; 58:31–59 [F]
241. Bryant AE III, Dreifuss FE: Valproic acid hepatic fatalities, III: US experience since 1986. Neurology 1996; 46:465–469 [B]
242. Gidal B, Spencer N, Maly M, Pitterle M, Williams E, Collins M, Jones J: Valproate-mediated disturbances of hemostasis: relationship to dose and plasma concentration. Neurology 1994; 44:1418–1422 [C]
243. Finsterer J, Pelzl G, Hess B: Severe, isolated thrombocytopenia under polytherapy with carbamazepine and valproate. Psychiatry Clin Neurosci 2001; 55:423–426 [G]
244. Chappell KA, Markowitz JS, Jackson CW: Is valproate pharmacotherapy associated with polycystic ovaries? Ann Pharmacother 1999; 33:1211–1216 [F]
245. Genton P, Bauer J, Duncan S, Taylor AE, Balen AH, Eberle A, Pedersen B, Salas-Puig X, Sauer MV: On the association between valproate and polycystic ovary syndrome. Epilepsia 2001; 42:295–304 [F]
246. Joffe H, Taylor AE, Hall JE: Polycystic ovarian syndrome—relationship to epilepsy and antiepileptic drug therapy. J Clin Endocrinol Metab 2001; 86:2946–2949 [F]
247. Isojarvi JI, Laatikainen TJ, Pakarinen AJ, Juntunen KT, Myllyla VV: Polycystic ovaries and hyperandrogenism in women taking valproate for epilepsy. N Engl J Med 1993; 329:1383–1388 [G]
248. Ellenhorn MJ: Valproate, in Ellenhorn's Medical Toxicology: Diagnosis and Treatment of Human Poisoning. Baltimore, Williams & Wilkins, 1997, pp 610–612 [G]
249. Janicak P, Davis JM, Preskorn SH, Ayd FJ: Principles and Practice of Psychopharmacotherapy. Baltimore, Williams & Wilkins, 1993 [F]

250. Gilman AG, Rall TW, Nies AS, Taylor P (eds): Goodman and Gilman's The Pharmacological Basis of Therapeutics, 8th ed. New York, Pergamon Press, 1990 [G]
251. Keck PE Jr, McElroy SL, Tugrul KC, Bennett JA: Valproate oral loading in the treatment of acute mania. J Clin Psychiatry 1993; 54:305–308 [B]
252. McElroy SL, Keck PE Jr, Tugrul KC, Bennett JA: Valproate as a loading treatment in acute mania. Neuropsychobiology 1993; 27:146–149 [G]
253. Martinez JM, Russell JM, Hirschfeld RM: Tolerability of oral loading of divalproex sodium in the treatment of acute mania. Depress Anxiety 1998; 7:83–86 [D]
254. Hirschfeld RM, Allen MH, McEvoy JP, Keck PE Jr, Russell JM: Safety and tolerability of oral loading divalproex sodium in acutely manic bipolar patients. J Clin Psychiatry 1999; 60:815–818 [A]
255. Longo LP: Divalproex sodium for alcohol withdrawal and relapse prevention: a case report. J Clin Psychiatry 2000; 61:947–948 [G]
256. Horne M, Lindley SE: Divalproex sodium in the treatment of aggressive behavior and dysphoria in patients with organic brain syndromes (letter). J Clin Psychiatry 1995; 56: 430–431 [G]
257. Miller PR: Clozapine therapy for a patient with a history of Hodgkin's disease (letter). Psychiatr Serv 2001; 52:110–111 [G]
258. Pellock JM, Willmore LJ: A rational guide to routine blood monitoring in patients receiving antiepileptic drugs. Neurology 1991; 41:961–964 [G]
259. McElroy SL, Keck PE Jr, Pope HG Jr, Hudson JI: Valproate in the treatment of bipolar disorder: literature review and clinical guidelines. J Clin Psychopharmacol 1992; 12:42S–52S [F]
260. McElroy SL, Keck PE Jr, Pope HG Jr, Hudson JI, Faedda GL, Swann AC: Clinical and research implications of the diagnosis of dysphoric or mixed mania or hypomania. Am J Psychiatry 1992; 149:1633–1644 [F]
261. Riva R, Albani F, Contin M, Baruzzi A: Pharmacokinetic interactions between antiepileptic drugs: clinical considerations. Clin Pharmacokinet 1996; 31:470–493 [F]
262. Matsuo F: Lamotrigine. Epilepsia 1999; 40(suppl 5):S30–S36 [F]
263. Tanaka E: Clinically significant pharmacokinetic drug interactions between antiepileptic drugs. J Clin Pharmacol Ther 1999; 24:87–92 [F]
264. Keck PE Jr, McElroy SL, Nemeroff CB: Anticonvulsants in the treatment of bipolar disorder. J Neuropsychiatry Clin Neurosci 1992; 4:395–405 [F]
265. Ballenger JC, Post RM: Therapeutic effects of carbamazepine in affective illness: a preliminary report. Commun Psychopharmacol 1978; 2:159–175 [A]
266. Vasudev K, Goswami U, Kohli K: Carbamazepine and valproate monotherapy: feasibility, relative safety and efficacy, and therapeutic drug monitoring in manic disorder. Psychopharmacology (Berl) 2000; 150:15–23 [A]
267. Grossi E, Sacchetti E, Vita A: Anticonvulsants in affective disorders, in Carbamazepine Versus Chlorpromazine in Mania: A Double-Blind Trial. Edited by Emirch HM, Okuma T, Muller AA. Amsterdam, Excerpta Medica, 1984, pp 177–187 [B]
268. Okuma T, Inanaga K, Otsuki S, Sarai K, Takahashi R, Hazama H, Mori A, Watanabe M: Comparison of the antimanic efficacy of carbamazepine and chlorpromazine: a double-blind controlled study. Psychopharmacology (Berl) 1979; 66:211–217 [A]
269. Rimmer EM, Richens A: An update on sodium valproate. Pharmacotherapy 1985; 5:171–184 [F]
270. Smith MC, Bleck TP: Convulsive disorders: toxicity of anticonvulsants. Clin Neuropharmacol 1991; 14:97–115 [F]
271. Kramlinger KG, Phillips KA, Post RM: Rash complicating carbamazepine treatment. J Clin Psychopharmacol 1994; 14:408–413 [C]
272. Van Amelsvoort T, Bakshi R, Devaux CB, Schwabe S: Hyponatremia associated with carbamazepine and oxcarbazepine therapy: a review. Epilepsia 1994; 35:181–188 [F]

273. Seetharam MN, Pellock JM: Risk-benefit assessment of carbamazepine in children. Drug Saf 1991; 6:148–158 [F]
274. Knowles SR, Shapiro LE, Shear NH: Anticonvulsant hypersensitivity syndrome: incidence, prevention and management. Drug Saf 1999; 21:489–501 [F]
275. Schweiger FJ, Kelton JG, Messner H, Klein M, Berger S, McIlroy WJ, Falk J, Keating A: Anticonvulsant-induced marrow suppression and immune thrombocytopenia. Acta Haematol 1988; 80:54–58 [G]
276. Ketter TA, Frye MA, Cora-Locatelli G, Kimbrell TA, Post RM: Metabolism and excretion of mood stabilizers and new anticonvulsants. Cell Mol Neurobiol 1999; 19:511–532 [F]
277. Muller AA, Stoll KD: Anticonvulsants in affective disorders, in Carbamazepine and Oxcarbazepine in the Treatment of Manic Syndromes: Studies in Germany. Edited by Emrich HM, Okuma T, Muller AA. Amsterdam, Exerpta Medica, 1984, pp 134–147 [B]
278. Emrich HM, Zihl J, Raptis C, Wendl A: Reduced dark-adaptation: an indication of lithium's neuronal action in humans. Am J Psychiatry 1990; 147:629–631 [G]
279. Dam M, Ekberg R, Loyning Y, Waltimo O, Jakobsen K: A double-blind study comparing oxcarbazepine and carbamazepine in patients with newly diagnosed, previously untreated epilepsy. Epilepsy Res 1989; 3:70–76 [A]
280. Glauser TA, Nigro M, Sachdeo R, Pasteris LA, Weinstein S, Abou-Khalil B, Frank LM, Grinspan A, Guarino T, Bettis D, Kerrigan J, Geoffroy G, Mandelbaum D, Jacobs T, Mesenbrink P, Kramer L, D'Souza J (Oxcarbazepine Pediatric Study Group): Adjunctive therapy with oxcarbazepine in children with partial seizures. Neurology 2000; 54:2237–2244 [A]
281. Smith PE: Clinical recommendations for oxcarbazepine. Seizure 2001; 10:87–91 [F]
282. Wellington K, Goa KL: Oxcarbazepine: an update of its efficacy in the management of epilepsy. CNS Drugs 2001; 15:137–163 [F]
283. Suppes T, Swann AC, Dennehy EB, Habermacher ED, Mason M, Crismon ML, Toprac MG, Rush AJ, Shon SP, Altshuler KZ: Texas Medication Algorithm Project: development and feasibility testing of a treatment algorithm for patients with bipolar disorder. J Clin Psychiatry 2001; 62:439–447 [B]
284. Frye MA, Ketter TA, Kimbrell TA, Dunn RT, Speer AM, Osuch EA, Luckenbaugh DA, Cora-Locatelli G, Leverich GS, Post RM: A placebo-controlled study of lamotrigine and gabapentin monotherapy in refractory mood disorders. J Clin Psychopharmacol 2000; 20: 607–614 [A]
285. Anand A, Oren DA, Berman RM: Lamotrigine treatment of lithium failure in outpatient mania: a double-blind, placebo-controlled trial, in Abstract Book, Third International Bipolar Conference. Edited by Soares JC, Gershon S. Pittsburgh, Munksgaard, 1999, p 23 [A]
286. Ichim L, Berk M, Brook S: Lamotrigine compared with lithium in mania: a double-blind randomized controlled trial. Ann Clin Psychiatry 2000; 12:5–10 [A]
287. Pande AC, Crockatt JG, Janney CA, Werth JL, Tsaroucha G (Gabapentin Bipolar Disorder Study Group): Gabapentin in bipolar disorder: a placebo-controlled trial of adjunctive therapy. Bipolar Disord 2000; 2:249–255 [A]
288. Mishory A, Yaroslavsky Y, Bersudsky Y, Belmaker RH: Phenytoin as an antimanic anticonvulsant: a controlled study. Am J Psychiatry 2000; 157:463–465 [B]
289. Tohen M, Sanger TM, McElroy SL, Tollefson GD, Chengappa KNR, Daniel DG, Petty F, Centorrino F, Wang R, Grundy SL, Greaney MG, Jacobs TG, David SR, Toma V (Olanzapine HGEH Study Group): Olanzapine versus placebo in the treatment of acute mania. Am J Psychiatry 1999; 156:702–709 [A]
290. Tohen M, Jacobs TG, Grundy SL, McElroy SL, Banov MC, Janicak PG, Sanger T, Risser R, Zhang F, Toma V, Francis J, Tollefson GD, Breier A (Olanzapine HGGW Study Group): Efficacy of olanzapine in acute bipolar mania: a double-blind, placebo-controlled study. Arch Gen Psychiatry 2000; 57:841–849 [A]

291. Sanger TM, Grundy SL, Gibson PJ, Namjoshi MA, Greaney MG, Tohen MF: Long-term olanzapine therapy in the treatment of bipolar I disorder: an open-label continuation phase study. J Clin Psychiatry 2001; 62:273–281 [E]
292. Tohen M, Zhang F, Feldman PD, Evans AR, Brier A: Olanzapine versus haloperidol in the treatment of acute mania, in 1998 Annual Meeting Syllabus and Proceedings Summary. Washington, DC, American Psychiatric Association, 1998 [A]
293. Crawford AM, Beasley CM Jr, Tollefson GD: The acute and long-term effect of olanzapine compared with placebo and haloperidol on serum prolactin concentrations. Schizophr Res 1997; 26:41–54 [A]
294. Kinon BJ, Basson BR, Gilmore JA, Tollefson GD: Long-term olanzapine treatment: weight change and weight-related health factors in schizophrenia. J Clin Psychiatry 2001; 62:92–100 [A]
295. Allison DB, Casey DE: Antipsychotic-induced weight gain: a review of the literature. J Clin Psychiatry 2001; 62(suppl 7):22–31 [F]
296. Lindenmayer JP, Nathan AM, Smith RC: Hyperglycemia associated with the use of atypical antipsychotics. J Clin Psychiatry 2001; 62(suppl 23):30–38 [F]
297. Leucht S, Pitschel-Walz G, Abraham D, Kissling W: Efficacy and extrapyramidal side-effects of the new antipsychotics olanzapine, quetiapine, risperidone, and sertindole compared to conventional antipsychotics and placebo: a meta-analysis of randomized controlled trials. Schizophr Res 1999; 35:51–68 [E]
298. Beasley CM, Dellva MA, Tamura RN, Morgenstern H, Glazer WM, Ferguson K, Tollefson GD: Randomised double-blind comparison of the incidence of tardive dyskinesia in patients with schizophrenia during long-term treatment with olanzapine or haloperidol. Br J Psychiatry 1999; 174:23–30 [A]
299. Chou JC, Czobor P, Charles O, Tuma I, Winsberg B, Allen MH, Trujillo M, Volavka J: Acute mania: haloperidol dose and augmentation with lithium or lorazepam. J Clin Psychopharmacol 1999; 19:500–505 [A]
300. Klein DF: Importance of psychiatric diagnosis in prediction of clinical drug effects. Arch Gen Psychiatry 1967; 16:118–126 [A]
301. Sachs GS: Emerging data: atypical antipsychotics in bipolar disorder, in Program and Abstracts of the 52nd Institute on Psychiatric Services. Washington, DC, American Psychiatric Association, 2001 [A]
302. Keck PE Jr: Atypical antipsychotics in the treatment of aggressive behaviors, in 2001 Annual Meeting Syllabus and Proceedings Summary. Washington, DC, American Psychiatric Association, 2001 [A]
303. Suppes T, Webb A, Paul B, Carmody T, Kraemer H, Rush AJ: Clinical outcome in a randomized 1-year trial of clozapine versus treatment as usual for patients with treatment-resistant illness and a history of mania. Am J Psychiatry 1999; 156:1164–1169 [B]
304. Calabrese JR, Kimmel SE, Woyshville MJ, Rapport DJ, Faust CJ, Thompson PA, Meltzer HY: Clozapine for treatment-refractory mania. Am J Psychiatry 1996; 153:759–764 [B]
305. Green AI, Tohen M, Patel JK, Banov M, DuRand C, Berman I, Chang H, Zarate C Jr, Posener J, Lee H, Dawson R, Richards C, Cole JO, Schatzberg AF: Clozapine in the treatment of refractory psychotic mania. Am J Psychiatry 2000; 157:982–986 [B]
306. Muller-Oerlinghausen B, Retzow A, Henn FA, Giedke H, Walden J (European Valproate Mania Study Group): Valproate as an adjunct to neuroleptic medication for the treatment of acute episodes of mania: a prospective, randomized, double-blind, placebo-controlled, multicenter study. J Clin Psychopharmacol 2000; 20:195–203 [A]
307. Yatham LN: Safety and efficacy of risperidone as combination therapy for the manic phase of bipolar disorder: preliminary findings of a randomized double blind study (RIS-INT-46). Int J Neuropsychopharmacol 2000; 3(suppl 1):S142 [A]
308. Small JG, Klapper MH, Kellams JJ, Miller MJ, Milstein V, Sharpley PH, Small IF: Electroconvulsive treatment compared with lithium in the management of manic states. Arch Gen Psychiatry 1988; 45:727–732 [A]

309. Mukherjee S, Sackeim HA, Schnur DB: Electroconvulsive therapy of acute manic episodes: a review of 50 years' experience. Am J Psychiatry 1994; 151:169–176 [F]
310. Sikdar S, Kulhara P, Avasthi A, Singh H: Combined chlorpromazine and electroconvulsive therapy in mania. Br J Psychiatry 1994; 164:806–810 [A]
311. Black DW, Winokur G, Nasrallah A: Treatment of mania: a naturalistic study of electroconvulsive therapy versus lithium in 438 patients. J Clin Psychiatry 1987; 48:132–139 [C]
312. Thomas J, Reddy B: The treatment of mania: a retrospective evaluation of the effects of ECT, chlorpromazine, and lithium. J Affect Disord 1982; 4:85–92 [D]
313. Ciapparelli A, Dell'Osso L, Tundo A, Pini S, Chiavacci MC, Di Sacco I, Cassano GB: Electroconvulsive therapy in medication-nonresponsive patients with mixed mania and bipolar depression. J Clin Psychiatry 2001; 62:552–555 [B]
314. Devanand DP, Polanco P, Cruz R, Shah S, Paykina N, Singh K, Majors L: The efficacy of ECT in mixed affective states. J ECT 2000; 16:32–37 [B]
315. Gruber NP, Dilsaver SC, Shoaib AM, Swann AC: ECT in mixed affective states: a case series. J ECT 2000; 16:183–188 [G]
316. McElroy SL, Keck PE Jr: Pharmacologic agents for the treatment of acute bipolar mania. Biol Psychiatry 2000; 48:539–557 [F]
317. Lenox RH, Newhouse PA, Creelman WL, Whitaker TM: Adjunctive treatment of manic agitation with lorazepam versus haloperidol: a double-blind study. J Clin Psychiatry 1992; 53:47–52 [A]
318. Edwards R, Stephenson U, Flewett T: Clonazepam in acute mania: a double blind trial. Aust NZ J Psychiatry 1991; 25:238–242 [A]
319. Chouinard G, Young SN, Annable L: Antimanic effect of clonazepam. Biol Psychiatry 1983; 18:451–466 [B]
320. Chouinard G: Clonazepam in acute and maintenance treatment of bipolar affective disorder. J Clin Psychiatry 1987; 48(Oct suppl):29–37 [B]
321. Chouinard G, Annable L, Turnier L, Holobow N, Szkrumelak N: A double-blind randomized clinical trial of rapid tranquilization with IM clonazepam and IM haloperidol in agitated psychotic patients with manic symptoms. Can J Psychiatry 1993; 38(suppl 4):S114–S121 [A]
322. Meehan K, Zhang F, David S, Tohen M, Janicak P, Small J, Koch M, Rizk R, Walker D, Tran P, Breier A: A double-blind, randomized comparison of the efficacy and safety of intramuscular injections of olanzapine, lorazepam, or placebo in treating acutely agitated patients diagnosed with bipolar mania. J Clin Psychopharmacol 2001; 21:389–397 [A]
323. Walton SA, Berk M, Brook S: Superiority of lithium over verapamil in mania: a randomized, controlled, single-blind trial. J Clin Psychiatry 1996; 57:543–546 [A]
324. Janicak PG, Sharma RP, Pandey G, Davis JM: Verapamil for the treatment of acute mania: a double-blind, placebo-controlled trial. Am J Psychiatry 1998; 155:972–973 [A]
325. Pazzaglia PJ, Post RM, Ketter TA, George MS, Marangell LB: Preliminary controlled trial of nimodipine in ultra-rapid cycling affective dysregulation. Psychiatry Res 1993; 49:257–272 [A]
326. Zornberg GL, Pope HG Jr: Treatment of depression in bipolar disorder: new directions for research. J Clin Psychopharmacol 1993; 13:397–408 [F]
327. Ballenger JC, Post RM: Carbamazepine in manic-depressive illness: a new treatment. Am J Psychiatry 1980; 137:782–790 [B]
328. Dilsaver SC, Swann SC, Chen YW, Shoaib A, Joe B, Krajewski KJ, Gruber N, Tsai Y: Treatment of bipolar depression with carbamazepine: results of an open study. Biol Psychiatry 1996; 40:935–937 [G]
329. Calabrese JR, Bowden CL, Sachs GS, Ascher JA, Monaghan E, Rudd GD (Lamictal 602 Study Group): A double-blind placebo-controlled study of lamotrigine monotherapy in outpatients with bipolar I depression. J Clin Psychiatry 1999; 60: 79–88 [A]
330. Bowden CL: Novel treatments for bipolar disorder. Expert Opin Investig Drugs 2001; 10: 661–671 [F]

331. Calabrese JR, Bowden CL, McElroy SL, Cookson J, Andersen J, Keck PE Jr, Rhodes L, Bolden-Watson C, Zhou J, Ascher JA: Spectrum of activity of lamotrigine in treatment-refractory bipolar disorder. Am J Psychiatry 1999; 156:1019–1023 [B]
332. Deveaugh-Geiss J, Ascher J, Brrok S, Cedrone J, Earl N, Emsley R, Frangou S, Huffman R: Safety and tolerability of lamotrigine in controlled monotherapy, in American College of Neuropsychopharmacology Annual Meeting Poster Abstracts. Nashville, Tenn, ACNP, 2000 [G]
333. Sullivan JR, Shear NH: The drug hypersensitivity syndrome: what is the pathogenesis? Arch Dermatol 2001; 137:357–364 [G]
334. Guberman AH, Besag FM, Brodie MJ, Dooley JM, Duchowny MS, Pellock JM, Richens A, Stern RS, Trevathan E: Lamotrigine-associated rash: risk/benefit considerations in adults and children. Epilepsia 1999; 40:985–991 [G]
335. Messenheimer J, Mullens EL, Giorgi L, Young F: Safety review of adult clinical trial experience with lamotrigine. Drug Saf 1998; 18:281–296 [F]
336. Fitton A, Goa KL: Lamotrigine: an update of its pharmacology and therapeutic use in epilepsy. Drugs 1995; 50:691–713 [F]
337. Rambeck B, Wolf P: Lamotrigine clinical pharmacokinetics. Clin Pharmacokinet 1993; 25: 433–443 [F]
338. McIntyre RS, Mancini D, McCann JM: Randomized, single-blind comparison of topiramate and bupropion SR as add-on therapy in bipolar depression (abstract). Acta Neuropsychiatrica 2000; 12:163 [B]
339. Hussein MZ: Treatment of bipolar depression with topiramate (abstract). Eur Neuropsychopharmacol 1999; 9(suppl 5):S222 [B]
340. Himmelhoch JM, Thase ME, Mallinger AG, Houck P: Tranylcypromine versus imipramine in anergic bipolar depression. Am J Psychiatry 1991; 148:910–916 [A]
341. Thase ME, Mallinger AG, McKnight D, Himmelhoch JM: Treatment of imipramine-resistant recurrent depression, IV: a double-blind crossover study of tranylcypromine for anergic bipolar depression. Am J Psychiatry 1992; 149:195–198 [A]
342. Baumhackl U, Biziere K, Fischbach R, Geretsegger C, Hebenstreit G, Radmayr E, Stabl M: Efficacy and tolerability of moclobemide compared with imipramine in depressive disorder (DSM-III): an Austrian double-blind, multicentre study. Br J Psychiatry Suppl 1989; 6:78–83 [A]
343. Cohn JB, Collins G, Ashbrook E, Wernicke JF: A comparison of fluoxetine, imipramine, and placebo in patients with bipolar depressive disorder. Int Clin Psychopharmacol 1989; 4:313–322 [A]
344. Young LT, Joffe RT, Robb JC, MacQueen GM, Marriott M, Patelis-Siotis I: Double-blind comparison of addition of a second mood stabilizer versus an antidepressant to an initial mood stabilizer for treatment of patients with bipolar depression. Am J Psychiatry 2000; 157:124–126 [A]
345. Nemeroff CB, Evans DL, Gyulai L, Sachs GS, Bowden CL, Gergel IP, Oakes R, Pitts CD: Double-blind, placebo-controlled comparison of imipramine and paroxetine in the treatment of bipolar depression. Am J Psychiatry 2001; 158:906–912 [A]
346. Vieta E: Martinez-Arán A, Goikolea JM: A randomized trial comparing paroxetine and venlafaxine in the treatment of bipolar depressed patients taking mood stabilizers. J Clin Psychiatry (in press) [A]
347. Kupfer DJ, Chengappa KN, Gelenberg AJ, Hirschfeld RM, Goldberg JF, Sachs GS, Grochochinski VJ, Houck PR, Kolar KB: Citalopram as adjunctive therapy in bipolar depression. J Clin Psychiatry 2001; 62:985–990 [B]
348. Sachs GS, Lafer B, Stoll AL, Banov M, Thibault AB, Tohen M, Rosenbaum JF: A double-blind trial of bupropion versus desipramine for bipolar depression. J Clin Psychiatry 1994; 55:391–393 [A]

349. Grossman F, Potter WZ, Brown EA, Maislin G: A double-blind study comparing idazoxan and bupropion in bipolar depressed patients. J Affect Disord 1999; 56:237–243 [A]
350. Amsterdam JD, Garcia-Espana F: Venlafaxine monotherapy in women with bipolar II and unipolar major depression. J Affect Disord 2000; 59:225–229 [A]
351. Wehr TA, Sack DA, Rosenthal NE: Sleep reduction as a final common pathway in the genesis of mania. Am J Psychiatry 1987; 144:201–204; correction, 144:542 [F]
352. Smeraldi E, Benedetti F, Barbini B, Campori E, Colombo C: Sustained antidepressant effect of sleep deprivation combined with pindolol in bipolar depression: a placebo-controlled trial. Neuropsychopharmacology 1999; 20:380–385 [A]
353. Colombo C, Lucca A, Benedetti F, Barbini B, Campori E, Smeraldi E: Total sleep deprivation combined with lithium and light therapy in the treatment of bipolar depression: replication of main effects and interaction. Psychiatry Res 2000; 95:43–53 [A]
354. Stoll AL, Severus WE, Freeman MP, Rueter S, Zboyan HA, Diamond E, Cress KK, Marangell LB: Omega 3 fatty acids in bipolar disorder: a preliminary double-blind, placebo-controlled trial. Arch Gen Psychiatry 1999; 56:407–412 [A]
355. Sporn J, Ghaemi SN, Sambur MR, Rankin MA, Recht J, Sachs GS, Rosenbaum JF, Fava M: Pramipexole augmentation in the treatment of unipolar and bipolar depression: a retrospective chart review. Ann Clin Psychiatry 2000; 12:137–140 [D]
356. George MS, Sackeim HA, Rush AJ, Marangell LB, Nahas Z, Husain MM, Lisanby S, Burt T, Goldman J, Ballenger JC: Vagus nerve stimulation: a new tool for brain research and therapy. Biol Psychiatry 2000; 47:287–295 [F]
357. Nahas Z, Molloy MA, Hughes PL, Oliver NC, Arana GW, Risch SC, George MS: Repetitive transcranial magnetic stimulation: perspectives for application in the treatment of bipolar and unipolar disorders. Bipolar Disord 1999; 1:73–80 [F]
358. Cole AJ, Scott J, Ferrier IN, Eccleston D: Patterns of treatment resistance in bipolar affective disorder. Acta Psychiatr Scand 1993; 88:121–123 [C]
359. Dunner DL, Fieve RR: Clinical factors in lithium carbonate prophylaxis failure. Arch Gen Psychiatry 1974; 30:229–233 [F]
360. Peet M: Induction of mania with selective serotonin re-uptake inhibitors and tricyclic antidepressants. Br J Psychiatry 1994; 164:549–550 [E]
361. Okuma T, Inanaga K, Otsuki S, Sarai K, Takahashi R, Hazama H, Mori A, Watanabe S: A preliminary double-blind study on the efficacy of carbamazepine in prophylaxis of manic-depressive illness. Psychopharmacology (Berl) 1981; 73:95–96 [A]
362. Denicoff KD, Smith-Jackson EE, Disney ER, Ali SO, Leverich GS, Post RM: Comparative prophylactic efficacy of lithium, carbamazepine, and the combination in bipolar disorder. J Clin Psychiatry 1997; 58:470–478 [B]
363. Bauer MS, Whybrow PC, Gyulai L, Gonnel J, Yeh HS: Testing definitions of dysphoric mania and hypomania: prevalence, clinical characteristics and inter-episode stability. J Affect Disord 1994; 32:201–211 [C]
364. Maj M, Pirozzi R, Magliano L, Bartoli L: Long-term outcome of lithium prophylaxis in bipolar disorder: a 5-year prospective study of 402 patients at a lithium clinic. Am J Psychiatry 1998; 155:30–35 [C]
365. Dunner DL, Stallone F, Fieve RR: Lithium carbonate and affective disorders, V: a double-blind study of prophylaxis of depression in bipolar illness. Arch Gen Psychiatry 1976; 33: 117–120 [A]
366. Shapiro DR, Quitkin FM, Fleiss JL: Response to maintenance therapy in bipolar illness: effect of index episode. Arch Gen Psychiatry 1989; 46:401–405 [E]
367. Bowden CL, Calabrese JR, McElroy SL, Rhodes LJ, Keck PE Jr, Cookson J, Anderson J, Bolden-Watson C, Ascher J, Monaghan E, Zhou J: The efficacy of lamotrigine in rapid cycling and non-rapid cycling patients with bipolar disorder. Biol Psychiatry 1999; 45:953–958 [G]

368. Calabrese JR, Delucchi GA: Spectrum of efficacy of valproate in 55 patients with rapid-cycling bipolar disorder. Am J Psychiatry 1990; 147:431–434 [G]
369. Calabrese JR, Woyshville MJ, Kimmel SE, Rapport DJ: Predictors of valproate response in bipolar rapid cycling. J Clin Psychopharmacol 1993; 13:280–283 [E]
370. Sachs GS, Printz DJ, Kahn DA, Carpenter D, Docherty JP: The Expert Consensus Guideline Series: Medication Treatment of Bipolar Disorder. Postgrad Med Special Issue 2000; 1:1–104 [G]
371. Bowden CL, Lecrubier Y, Bauer M, Goodwin G, Greil W, Sachs G, von Knorring L: Maintenance therapies for classic and other forms of bipolar disorder. J Affect Disord 2000; 59(suppl 1):S57–S67 [F]
372. Baldessarini RJ, Tohen M, Tondo L: Maintenance treatment in bipolar disorder. Arch Gen Psychiatry 2000; 57:490–492 [G]
373. Baastrup PC, Poulsen JC, Schou M, Thomsen K, Amdisen A: Prophylactic lithium: double blind discontinuation in manic-depressive and recurrent-depressive disorders. Lancet 1970; 2:326–330 [A]
374. Melia PI: Prophylactic lithium: a double-blind trial in recurrent affective disorders. Br J Psychiatry 1970; 116:621–624 [A]
375. Coppen A, Peet M, Bailey J, Noguera R, Burns BH, Swani MS, Maggs R, Gardner R: Double-blind and open prospective studies on lithium prophylaxis in affective disorders. Psychiatr Neurol Neurochir 1973; 76:501–510 [F]
376. Cundall RL, Brooks PW, Murray LG: A controlled evaluation of lithium prophylaxis in affective disorders. Psychol Med 1972; 2:308–311 [B]
377. Prien RF, Caffey EM Jr, Klett CJ: Prophylactic efficacy of lithium carbonate in manic-depressive illness: report of the Veterans Administration and National Institute of Mental Health collaborative study group. Arch Gen Psychiatry 1973; 28:337–341 [A]
378. Suppes T, Baldessarini RJ, Faedda GL, Tohen M: Risk of recurrence following discontinuation of lithium treatment in bipolar disorder. Arch Gen Psychiatry 1991; 48:1082–1088 [E]
379. Markar HR, Mander AJ: Efficacy of lithium prophylaxis in clinical practice. Br J Psychiatry 1989; 155:496–500 [F]
380. Harrow M, Goldberg JF, Grossman LS, Meltzer HY: Outcome in manic disorders: a naturalistic follow-up study. Arch Gen Psychiatry 1990; 47:665–671 [C]
381. Coryell W, Winokur G, Solomon D, Shea T, Leon A, Keller M: Lithium and recurrence in a long-term follow-up of bipolar affective disorder. Psychol Med 1997; 27:281–289 [C]
382. Gitlin MJ, Swendsen J, Heller TL, Hammen C: Relapse and impairment in bipolar disorder. Am J Psychiatry 1995; 152:1635–1640 [C]
383. Licht RW, Vestergaard P, Rasmussen NA, Jepsen K, Brodersen A, Hansen PE: A lithium clinic for bipolar patients: 2-year outcome of the first 148 patients. Acta Psychiatr Scand 2001; 104:387–390 [B]
384. Peselow ED, Fieve RR, Difiglia C, Sanfilipo MP: Lithium prophylaxis of bipolar illness: the value of combination treatment. Br J Psychiatry 1994; 164:208–214 [D]
385. Bowden CL, Calabrese JR, McElroy SL, Gyulai L, Wassef A, Petty F, Pope HG Jr, Chou JC, Keck PE Jr, Rhodes LJ, Swann AC, Hirschfeld RM, Wozniak PJ (Divalproex Maintenance Study Group): A randomized, placebo-controlled 12-month trial of divalproex and lithium in treatment of outpatients with bipolar I disorder. Arch Gen Psychiatry 2000; 57:481–489 [A]
386. Calabrese JR, Bowden CL, DeVeaugh-Geiss J, Earl NL, Gyulai L, Sachs GS, Montgomery P: Lamotrigine demonstrates long-term mood stabilization in manic patients, in 2001 Annual Meeting New Research Program and Abstracts. Washington, DC, American Psychiatric Association, 2001, p 110 [A]
387. Greil W, Ludwig-Mayerhofer W, Erazo N, Schochlin C, Schmidt S, Engel RR, Czernik A, Giedke H, Muller-Oerlinghausen B, Osterheider M, Rudolf GA, Sauer H, Tegeler J, Wetterling T: Lithium versus carbamazepine in the maintenance treatment of bipolar disorders—a randomised study. J Affect Disord 1997; 43:151–161 [B]

388. Lambert PA, Venaud G: [Comparative study of valpromide versus lithium as prophylactic treatment in affective disorders.] Nervure 1992; 5:57–65 (French) [B]
389. Greil W, Kleindienst N, Erazo N, Muller-Oerlinghausen B: Differential response to lithium and carbamazepine in the prophylaxis of bipolar disorder. J Clin Psychopharmacol 1998; 18:455–460 [E]
390. Stromgren LS: The combination of lithium and carbamazepine in treatment and prevention of manic-depressive disorder: a review and a case report. Compr Psychiatry 1990; 31:261–265 [E]
391. Esparon J, Kolloori J, Naylor GJ, McHarg AM, Smith AH, Hopwood SE: Comparison of the prophylactic action of flupenthixol with placebo in lithium treated manic-depressive patients. Br J Psychiatry 1986; 148:723–725 [A]
392. Stevenson GH, Geoghegan JJ: Prophylactic electroshock; a five-year study. Am J Psychiatry 1951; 107:743–748 [B]
393. Geoghegan JJ, Stevenson GH: Prophylactic electroshock. Am J Psychiatry 1949; 105:494–496 [B]
394. Godemann F, Hellweg R: [20 years unsuccessful prevention of bipolar affective psychosis recurrence.] Nervenarzt 1997; 68:582–585 (German) [F]
395. Chanpattana W: Combined ECT and clozapine in treatment-resistant mania. J ECT 2000; 16:204–207 [G]
396. Decina P, Schlegel AM, Fieve RR: Lithium poisoning. NY State J Med 1987; 87:230–231 [G]
397. Kramer BA: A naturalistic review of maintenance ECT at a university setting. J ECT 1999; 15:262–269 [G]
398. Rhodes LJ: Maintenance ECT replaced with lamotrigine (letter). Am J Psychiatry 2000; 157:2058 [G]
399. Gupta S, Austin R, Devanand DP: Lithium and maintenance electroconvulsive therapy. J ECT 1998; 14:241–244 [G]
400. Barnes RC, Hussein A, Anderson DN, Powell D: Maintenance electroconvulsive therapy and cognitive function. Br J Psychiatry 1997; 170:285–287 [G]
401. Jaffe R, Dubin WR: Oral versus intravenous caffeine augmentation of ECT (letter). Am J Psychiatry 1992; 149:1610 [G]
402. Karliner W: Accidental convulsion induced by atropine. Am J Psychiatry 1965; 122:578–579 [G]
403. Clarke L: Psychiatric nursing and electroconvulsive therapy. Nurs Ethics 1995; 2:321–331 [F]
404. Kramer BA: A seasonal schedule for maintenance ECT. J ECT 1999; 15:226–231 [G]
405. Vanelle JM, Loo H, Galinowski A, de Carvalho W, Bourdel MC, Brochier P, Bouvet O, Brochier T, Olie JP: Maintenance ECT in intractable manic-depressive disorders. Convuls Ther 1994; 10:195–205 [B]
406. Schwarz T, Loewenstein J, Isenberg KE: Maintenance ECT: indications and outcome. Convuls Ther 1995; 11:14–23 [B]
407. Gagné GG Jr, Furman MJ, Carpenter LL, Price LH: Efficacy of continuation ECT and antidepressant drugs compared to long-term antidepressants alone in depressed patients. Am J Psychiatry 2000; 157:1960–1965 [B]
408. Kahn DA: The use of psychodynamic psychotherapy in manic-depressive illness. J Am Acad Psychoanal 1993; 21:441–455 [A]
409. Haas GL, Glick ID, Clarkin JF, Spencer JH, Lewis AB, Peyser J, DeMane N, Good-Ellis M, Harris E, Lestelle V: Inpatient family intervention: a randomized clinical trial, II: results at hospital discharge. Arch Gen Psychiatry 1988; 45:217–224 [A]
410. Clarkin JF, Carpenter D, Hull J, Wilner P, Glick I: Effects of psychoeducational intervention for married patients with bipolar disorder and their spouses. Psychiatr Serv 1998; 49:531–533 [A]

411. Miklowitz DJ, Goldstein MJ: Bipolar Disorder: A Family-Focused Treatment Approach. New York, Guilford Press, 1997 [G]
412. Miklowitz DJ, Simoneau TL, George EL, Richards JA, Kalbag A, Sachs-Ericsson N, Suddath R: Family-focused treatment of bipolar disorder: 1-year effects of a psychoeducational program in conjunction with pharmacotherapy. Biol Psychiatry 2000; 48:582–592 [A]
413. Basco MR, Rush AJ: Cognitive-Behavioral Therapy for Bipolar Disorder. New York, Guilford Press, 1996 [G]
414. Zaretsky AE, Segal ZV, Gemar M: Cognitive therapy for bipolar depression: a pilot study. Can J Psychiatry 1999; 44:491–494 [B]
415. Fava GA, Bartolucci G, Rafanelli C, Mangelli L: Cognitive-behavioral management of patients with bipolar disorder who relapsed while on lithium prophylaxis. J Clin Psychiatry 2001; 62:556–559 [B]
416. Cochran SD: Preventing medical noncompliance in the outpatient treatment of bipolar affective disorders. J Consult Clin Psychol 1984; 52:873–878 [A]
417. Ehlers CL, Frank E, Kupfer DJ: Social zeitgebers and biological rhythms: a unified approach to understanding the etiology of depression. Arch Gen Psychiatry 1988; 45:948–952 [F]
418. Frank E, Hlastala S, Ritenour A, Houck P, Tu XM, Monk TH, Mallinger AG, Kupfer DJ: Inducing lifestyle regularity in recovering bipolar disorder patients: results from the maintenance therapies in bipolar disorder protocol. Biol Psychiatry 1997; 41:1165–1173 [A]
419. Frank E, Swartz HA, Kupfer DJ: Interpersonal and social rhythm therapy: managing the chaos of bipolar disorder. Biol Psychiatry 2000; 48:593–604 [F]
420. Cole DP, Thase ME, Mallinger AG, Soares JC, Luther JF, Kupfer DJ, Frank E: Slower treatment response in bipolar depression predicted by lower pretreatment thyroid function. Am J Psychiatry 2002; 159:116–121 [A]
421. Frank E, Swartz HA, Mallinger AG, Thase ME, Weaver EV, Kupfer DJ: Adjunctive psychotherapy for bipolar disorder: effects of changing treatment modality. J Abnorm Psychol 1999; 108:579–587 [A]
422. Colom F, Vieta E, Benabarre A, Martinez-Aran A, Reinares M, Corbella B, Gasto C: Topiramate abuse in a bipolar patient with an eating disorder. J Clin Psychiatry 2001; 62: 475–476 [G]
423. Beck AT, Rush AJ, Shaw BF, Emery G: Cognitive Therapy of Depression. New York, Guilford, 1979 [G]
424. Klerman GL, Weissman MM, Rounsaville BJ, Chevron ES: Interpersonal Psychotherapy of Depression. New York, Basic Books, 1984 [G]
425. Frank E, Kupfer DJ, Perel JM, Cornes C, Jarrett DB, Mallinger AG, Thase ME, McEachran AB, Grochocinski VJ: Three-year outcomes for maintenance therapies in recurrent depression. Arch Gen Psychiatry 1990; 47:1093–1099 [A]
426. Weissman MM, Markowitz JC, Klerman GL: Comprehensive Guide to Interpersonal Psychotherapy. New York, Basic Books, 2000 [G]
427. Frank E, Kupfer DJ, Gibbons R, Houck P, Kostelnik B, Mallinger AG, Swartz HA, Thase ME: Interpersonal and social rhythm therapy prevents depressive symptomatology in patients with bipolar I disorder. Arch Gen Psychiatry (in press) [A]
428. Bauer MS, McBride L, Chase C, Sachs G, Shea N: Manual-based group psychotherapy for bipolar disorder: a feasibility study. J Clin Psychiatry 1998; 59:449–455 [B]
429. Rush AJ, Thase ME: Psychotherapies for depressive disorders: a review, in Evidence and Experience in Psychiatry, vol 1: Depressive Disorders. Edited by Maj M, Sartorious N. Chichester, UK, John Wiley & Sons, 1999, pp 161–206 [G]
430. Blacker D, Tsuang MT: Contested boundaries of bipolar disorder and the limits of categorical diagnosis in psychiatry. Am J Psychiatry 1992; 149:1473–1483 [F]
431. Akiskal HS, Hirschfeld RM, Yerevanian BI: The relationship of personality to affective disorders. Arch Gen Psychiatry 1983; 40:801–810 [F]

432. Geller B, Cooper TB, Sun K, Zimerman B, Frazier J, Williams M, Heath J: Double-blind and placebo-controlled study of lithium for adolescent bipolar disorders with secondary substance dependency. J Am Acad Child Adolesc Psychiatry 1998; 37:171–178 [A]
433. Gram LF, Rafaelsen OJ: Lithium treatment of psychotic children and adolescents: a controlled clinical trial. Acta Psychiatr Scand 1972; 48:253–260 [A]
434. Lena B: Lithium in child and adolescent psychiatry. Arch Gen Psychiatry 1979; 36:854–855 [A]
435. McKnew DH, Cytryn L, Buchsbaum MS, Hamovit J, Lamour M, Rapoport JL, Gershon ES: Lithium in children of lithium-responding parents. Psychiatry Res 1981; 4:171–180 [A]
436. DeLong GR, Nieman GW: Lithium-induced behavior changes in children with symptoms suggesting manic-depressive illness. Psychopharmacol Bull 1983; 19:258–265 [A]
437. Annell AL: Manic-depressive illness in children and effect of treatment with lithium carbonate. Acta Paedopsychiatr 1969; 36:292–301 [G]
438. Dyson WL, Barcai A: Treatment of children of lithium-responding parents. Curr Ther Res Clin Exp 1970; 12:286–290 [G]
439. Dugas M, Gueriot C, Frohwirth C: [Has lithium a value in child psychiatry]. Rev Neuropsychiatr Infant 1975; 23:365–372 (French) [B]
440. Watanabe S, Ishino H, Otsuki S: Double-blind comparison of lithium carbonate and imipramine in treatment of depression. Arch Gen Psychiatry 1975; 32:659–668 [A]
441. Brumback RA, Weinberg WA: Mania in childhood, II: therapeutic trial of lithium carbonate and further description of manic-depressive illness in children. Am J Dis Child 1977; 131: 1122–1126 [B]
442. Horowitz HA: Lithium and the treatment of adolescent manic depressive illness. Dis Nerv Syst 1977; 38:480–483 [G]
443. Carlson GA, Strober M: Manic-depressive illness in early adolescence: a study of clinical and diagnostic characteristics in six cases. J Am Acad Child Psychiatry 1978; 17:138–153 [C]
444. Davis RE: Manic-depressive variant syndrome of childhood: a preliminary report. Am J Psychiatry 1979; 136:702–706 [G]
445. Hassanyeh F, Davison K: Bipolar affective psychosis with onset before age 16 years: report of 10 cases. Br J Psychiatry 1980; 137:530–539 [G]
446. Rogeness GA, Riester AE, Wicoff JS: Unusual presentation of manic depressive disorder in adolescence. J Clin Psychiatry 1982; 43:37–39 [G]
447. Sylvester CE, Burke PM, McCauley EA, Clark CJ: Manic psychosis in childhood: report of two cases. J Nerv Ment Dis 1984; 172:12–15 [G]
448. DeLong GR, Aldershof AL: Long-term experience with lithium treatment in childhood: correlation with clinical diagnosis. J Am Acad Child Adolesc Psychiatry 1987; 26:389–394 [B]
449. Hsu LK, Starzynski JM: Mania in adolescence. J Clin Psychiatry 1986; 47:596–599 [C]
450. Hsu LK: Lithium-resistant adolescent mania. J Am Acad Child Psychiatry 1986; 25:280–283 [G]
451. Varanka TM, Weller RA, Weller EB, Fristad MA: Lithium treatment of manic episodes with psychotic features in prepubertal children. Am J Psychiatry 1988; 145:1557–1559 [B]
452. Tomasson K, Kuperman S: Bipolar disorder in a prepubescent child. J Am Acad Child Adolesc Psychiatry 1990; 29:308–310 [F]
453. Carlson GA, Rapport MD, Pataki CS, Kelly KL: Lithium in hospitalized children at 4 and 8 weeks: mood, behavior and cognitive effects. J Child Psychol Psychiatry 1992; 33:411–425 [A]
454. Kafantaris V, Coletti DJ, Dicker R, Padula G, Pollack S: Are childhood psychiatric histories of bipolar adolescents associated with family history, psychosis, and response to lithium treatment? J Affect Disord 1998; 51:153–164 [A]
455. Strober M, DeAntonio M, Schmidt-Lackner S, Freeman R, Lampert C, Diamond J: Early childhood attention deficit hyperactivity disorder predicts poorer response to acute lithium therapy in adolescent mania. J Affect Disord 1998; 51:145–151 [B]

456. Papatheodorou G, Kutcher SP: Divalproex sodium treatment in late adolescent and young adult acute mania. Psychopharmacol Bull 1993; 29:213–219 [B]
457. Papatheodorou G, Kutcher SP, Katic M, Szalai JP: The efficacy and safety of divalproex sodium in the treatment of acute mania in adolescents and young adults: an open clinical trial. J Clin Psychopharmacol 1995; 15:110–116 [B]
458. Wagner KD: Safety and efficacy of divalproex in childhood bipolar disorder, in Abstracts of Posters Presented at the 2000 Annual Meeting of the American Academy of Child and Adolescent Psychiatry. Washington, DC, AACAP, 2000 [G]
459. Kastner T, Friedman DL: Verapamil and valproic acid treatment of prolonged mania. J Am Acad Child Adolesc Psychiatry 1992; 31:271–275 [D]
460. Kastner T, Friedman DL, Plummer AT, Ruiz MQ, Henning D: Valproic acid for the treatment of children with mental retardation and mood symptomatology. Pediatrics 1990; 86:467–472 [G]
461. Whittier MC, West SA, Galli VB, Raute NJ: Valproic acid for dysphoric mania in a mentally retarded adolescent. J Clin Psychiatry 1995; 56:590–591 [G]
462. Deltito JA, Levitan J, Damore J, Hajal F, Zambenedetti M: Naturalistic experience with the use of divalproex sodium on an in-patient unit for adolescent psychiatric patients. Acta Psychiatr Scand 1998; 97:236–240 [E]
463. Kowatch RA, Suppes T, Carmody TJ, Bucci JP, Hume JH, Kromelis M, Emslie GJ, Weinberg WA, Rush AJ: Effect size of lithium, divalproex sodium, and carbamazepine in children and adolescents with bipolar disorder. J Am Acad Child Adolesc Psychiatry 2000; 39:713–720 [A]
464. Woolston JL: Case study: carbamazepine treatment of juvenile-onset bipolar disorder. J Am Acad Child Adolesc Psychiatry 1999; 38:335–338 [G]
465. Frazier JA, Biederman J, Jacobs TG, Tohen MF, Toma V, Feldman PD, Rater MA, Tarazi RA, Kim GA, Garfield SB, Gonzalez-Heydrich J, Nowlin ZM: Olanzapine in the treatment of bipolar disorder in juveniles, in New Clinical Drug Evaluation Unit 2000 Program Abstracts. Washington, DC, NCDEU, 2000, poster 46 [G]
466. Chang KD, Ketter TA: Mood stabilizer augmentation with olanzapine in acutely manic children. J Child Adolesc Psychopharmacol 2000; 10:45–49 [G]
467. Soutullo CA, Sorter MT, Foster KD, McElroy SL, Keck PE: Olanzapine in the treatment of adolescent acute mania: a report of seven cases. J Affect Disord 1999; 53:279–283 [E]
468. Frazier JA, Meyer MC, Biederman J, Wozniak J, Wilens TE, Spencer TJ, Kim GS, Shapiro S: Risperidone treatment for juvenile bipolar disorder: a retrospective chart review. J Am Acad Child Adolesc Psychiatry 1999; 38:960–965 [F]
469. Ryback RS, Brodsky L, Munasifi F: Gabapentin in bipolar disorder (letter). J Neuropsychiatry Clin Neurosci 1997; 9:301 [G]
470. Soutullo CA, Casuto LS, Keck PE Jr: Gabapentin in the treatment of adolescent mania: a case report. J Child Adolesc Psychopharmacol 1998; 8:81–85 [G]
471. Hill MA, Courvoisie H, Dawkins K, Nofal P, Thomas B: ECT for the treatment of intractable mania in two prepubertal male children. Convuls Ther 1997; 13:74–82 [G]
472. Rey JM, Walter G: Half a century of ECT use in young people. Am J Psychiatry 1997; 154: 595–602 [F]

GUIDELINE WATCH: PRACTICE GUIDELINE FOR THE TREATMENT OF PATIENTS WITH PANIC DISORDER

Laura Campbell-Sills, Ph.D.
Murray B. Stein, M.D., M.P.H.

This guideline watch summarizes evidence that has accrued since publication in 1998 of APA's *Practice Guideline for the Treatment of Patients With Panic Disorder* (1). The major topics covered are safety issues, U.S. Food and Drug Administration (FDA) approvals, availability of new medications (including generics), efficacy of pharmacological and psychosocial treatments, efficacy of combined treatments, predictors of treatment response, and treatment of panic disorder in primary care settings.

SAFETY ISSUES

Liver failure associated with nefazodone treatment

The practice guideline cited one open-label trial that used the serotonin modulator nefazodone in the treatment of panic disorder. Nefazodone significantly reduced symptoms of panic disorder in this study (2). Since publication of the guideline, cases of liver failure associated with nefazodone administration have been reported (3–9). The FDA now requires that nefazodone carry a black box warning stating that cases of life-threatening liver failure have occurred in patients treated with the drug. According to the warning, the reported rate of liver failure resulting in death or transplant is approximately 1 case per 250,000–300,000 patient-years of nefazodone treatment. This represents a rate of three to four times the estimated background rate and is likely an underestimate due to incomplete reporting.

The American Psychiatric Association (APA) practice guidelines are developed by expert work groups using an explicit methodology that includes rigorous review of available evidence, broad peer review of iterative drafts, and formal approval by the APA Assembly and Board of Trustees. APA practice guidelines are intended to assist psychiatrists in clinical decision making. They are not intended to be a standard of care. The ultimate judgment regarding a particular clinical procedure or treatment plan must be made by the psychiatrist in light of the clinical data presented by the patient and the diagnostic and treatment options available. Guideline watches summarize significant developments in practice since publication of an APA practice guideline. Watches may be authored and reviewed by experts associated with the original guideline development effort and are approved for publication by APA's Executive Committee on Practice Guidelines. Thus, watches represent opinion of the authors and approval of the Executive Committee but not policy of the APA. This guideline watch was published in April 2006. Suggested citation: Campbell-Sills L, Stein MB: *Guideline Watch: Practice Guideline for the Treatment of Patients With Panic Disorder.* Arlington, VA: American Psychiatric Association, 2006. Available online at http://www.psych.org/psych_pract/treatg/pg/prac_guide.cfm.

The FDA warning (available at http://www.fda.gov/medwatch/SAFETY/2002/serzone_deardoc.pdf) includes the following recommendations:

1. Although there is at present no way to predict who might develop liver failure, nefazodone should not be initiated in patients with acute liver disease or elevated baseline levels of serum transaminases.
2. Patients taking nefazodone should be informed of the risk, signs, and symptoms of liver dysfunction and told to contact their doctors immediately if any signs or symptoms occur (e.g., jaundice, anorexia, gastrointestinal complaints, malaise).
3. Clinicians may consider the value of liver function testing in patients taking nefazodone.
4. Nefazodone should be discontinued if liver toxicity is suspected.
5. Nefazodone is contraindicated in cases in which the drug was previously discontinued because of evidence of liver injury.

Although the practice guideline does not recommend nefazodone as a first-line treatment for panic disorder, there may be instances in which it is considered as a treatment for panic disorder or a co-occurring psychiatric condition in patients without a history of liver disease. In these cases, the increased risk of liver toxicity must be weighed against the possible benefit of pharmacotherapy. Other medications with fewer risks and more efficacy data supporting their use in panic disorder should be considered as alternatives to nefazodone.

Suicidality and antidepressant use in children and adolescents

The practice guideline reports that selective serotonin reuptake inhibitors (SSRIs), tricyclic antidepressants (TCAs), and monoamine oxidase inhibitors (MAOIs) are effective for treating panic disorder in adults. Controlled studies of pharmacological treatment of pediatric patients with panic disorder were not available when the 1998 guideline was developed; however, the guideline notes that anecdotal reports and case series suggest that antidepressants are useful in treating pediatric panic disorder (1). In 2004 the FDA issued a warning that "antidepressants increased the risk of suicidal thinking and behavior (suicidality) in short-term studies of children and adolescents with major depressive disorder (MDD) and other psychiatric disorders" (http://www.fda.gov/cder/drug/antidepressants/PI_template.pdf). It is unknown whether a risk of suicidality extends to longer-term use of antidepressants in children and adolescents.

The FDA warning is based on pooled analyses of 24 placebo-controlled trials of nine antidepressants in pediatric patients with a variety of psychiatric disorders (10). These analyses showed that patients receiving antidepressants displayed a risk of suicidal thinking and behavior that was approximately twice that of patients receiving placebo during the first few months of treatment (4% in the active treatment groups vs. 2% in the placebo groups). It is important to note that no completed suicides occurred in any of the clinical trials.

With respect to suicidality and panic disorder, APA's practice guideline reports that individuals with panic disorder demonstrate a higher than average rate of suicidal ideation and suicide attempts (although this is less clear for individuals with uncomplicated panic disorder without agoraphobia) and that the presence of co-occurring conditions such as major depression, substance use disorders, and personality disorders increases the risk of suicide attempts (1). The guideline states that clinicians should assess all patients with panic disorder for suicidal ideation and risk, regardless of age or treatment regimen. The FDA warning, which advises increased monitoring for suicidal ideation and behavior in pediatric patients treated with antidepressants, further supports this recommendation.

The FDA black box warning applies to all antidepressants and indicates that the risk of increased suicidal thinking and behavior in pediatric patients must be balanced with the clinical need for pharmacotherapy. It further states that pediatric patients taking antidepressants should be observed closely for clinical worsening, suicidality, or unusual changes in behavior—

particularly in the initial few months of treatment and at times of dose changes. The black box warning advises that caregivers should observe the patient closely and communicate any concerns to the prescribing clinician. Medication guides that describe signs of clinical worsening and suicidality are available for families (http://www.fda.gov/cder/drug/antidepressants/ MG_template.pdf). Finally, the warning clarifies for which pediatric conditions the antidepressant has received approval (if any).

No antidepressant currently has FDA approval for treatment of pediatric panic disorder. However, these medications are used often enough in clinical practice that it is appropriate to review the following FDA recommendations for psychiatric management of children and adolescents taking antidepressants.

The FDA recommends a specific schedule of face-to-face clinical contacts for the first 12 weeks of treatment for all pediatric patients taking antidepressants. The schedule involves weekly contacts for the initial 4 weeks, biweekly contacts for the next 4 weeks, and a contact at 12 weeks. The warning indicates that prescriptions are to be written for "the smallest quantity of tablets consistent with good patient management, in order to reduce the risk of overdose" (http://www.fda.gov/cder/drug/antidepressants/PI_template.pdf). A similar approach is recommended for adult patients with MDD who are starting antidepressants; therefore, these guidelines are also relevant for adult patients with co-occurring panic disorder and depression.

In addition to monitoring patients for signs of general clinical worsening and suicidality, the FDA recommends that patients be assessed for risk of bipolar disorder; this assessment should include inquiring about family history of mood disorders and suicide. According to the FDA, patients at higher risk for bipolar disorder who are prescribed antidepressants should be monitored for signs of transition to hypomanic, manic, or mixed mood states. The FDA further advises that clinicians be alert for signs of increased anxiety or panic, agitation, insomnia, irritability, hostility, aggressiveness, impulsivity, mania, hypomania, akathisia, and other unusual changes in behavior. Although these signs and symptoms are not conclusively linked to suicidal thoughts and behavior, there is concern that they might be precursors to emerging suicidality. Particular concern would be warranted if these symptoms were abrupt in onset, severe, or not previously part of the patient's presenting complaint. In the event that any of these potential signs of deterioration occur, the FDA recommends that the clinician consider changing the treatment regimen and possibly discontinuing the antidepressant.

It is important to balance the FDA warnings regarding antidepressant use in children against the potential therapeutic benefit of these drugs and the risks of untreated psychiatric illness. Some concern exists that the FDA warnings will deter clinicians from prescribing in cases in which the risk-benefit ratio strongly favors antidepressant treatment. The American Psychiatric Association (http://www.psych.org/news_room/press_releases/04-55apaonfdablack boxwarning.pdf; http://www.psych.org/news_room/press_releases/05-53APAonPsychNews Analysis%20_3_.pdf) and American Academy of Child and Adolescent Psychiatry (http://www.aacap.org/press_releases/2004/1101.htm) have commented on this issue.

It is not known whether adults taking antidepressants are at increased risk of suicidality. In adults, published meta-analyses of data from short-term clinical trials have not demonstrated differences in rates of suicide or attempted suicide between individuals treated with antidepressants and those receiving placebo (11, 12). Recent research using population-based computerized health plan records also showed no significant increase in the risk of a serious suicide attempt for patients treated with antidepressants (13). For individuals treated with older antidepressants (e.g., TCAs, trazodone), the risk in the month prior to treatment was comparable to that in the first month of treatment and then declined. For individuals treated with newer antidepressants, the risk was greatest in the month prior to treatment, dropped in the first month of treatment, and continued to decline thereafter. Although numbers of deaths by suicide were small, this risk remained stable over the 6-month period after antidepressant treatment was begun.

The FDA is currently investigating the relationship between suicidality and antidepressant use in adult patients with psychiatric disorders. A public health advisory was released in June 2005 indicating that adults being treated with antidepressant medications, particularly those being treated for depression, should be monitored closely for clinical worsening and suicidality. Monitoring early in treatment and at times of dose changes is emphasized. If clinical worsening or increased suicidality occurs in conjunction with antidepressant treatment, the FDA advises that adult patients be promptly evaluated by the prescribing clinician.

The FDA continues to update its recommendations regarding antidepressants, and their Web site provides several documents that may be of interest to clinicians, including the required warnings for antidepressants (http://www.fda.gov/cder/drug/antidepressants/PI_template.pdf), the public health advisory regarding antidepressant use in children and adolescents (http://www.fda.gov/cder/drug/antidepressants/SSRIPHA200410.htm), and the public health advisory regarding antidepressant use in adults (http://www.fda.gov/cder/drug/advisory/SSRI200507.htm). Additional information may be found at the Web sites of the APA (http://www.psych.org) and the American Academy of Child and Adolescent Psychiatry (http://www.aacap.org).

FDA APPROVALS AND AVAILABILITY OF GENERICS

At the time of the practice guideline's publication, paroxetine and alprazolam had obtained FDA approval for treatment of panic disorder. The following medications have obtained approval for treatment of panic disorder since that time: alprazolam XR (extended release), clonazepam, fluoxetine, paroxetine CR (controlled release), sertraline, and venlafaxine ER (extended release). More information about the efficacy of these medications is included in the next section.

The 1998 guideline indicated that use of SSRIs to manage panic disorder might be more expensive than use of other efficacious medications because of the lack of generic preparations. This potential disadvantage of SSRI treatment no longer applies, as generic preparations of citalopram, fluoxetine, fluvoxamine, and paroxetine are now available.

ADDITIONAL RESEARCH ON DRUG EFFICACY

Specific medication classes

SSRIs

Clinical trials have continued to support the efficacy and tolerability of SSRIs in the treatment of panic disorder. At the time of the guideline's publication, four SSRIs were available in the United States: fluoxetine, paroxetine, sertraline, and fluvoxamine. Two more SSRIs (citalopram and escitalopram) and a controlled-release preparation of paroxetine are now available.

Since 1998, several additional large-scale randomized, controlled trials (RCTs) have shown fluoxetine (14–16); paroxetine (17, 18), including its controlled-release preparation (19); and sertraline (20–22) to be safe and effective for the treatment of panic disorder. Dose-response investigations suggest that therapeutic dosages are generally about 20 mg/day for fluoxetine (14, 16), 40 mg/day for paroxetine (17), and 50 mg/day for sertraline (20, 21, 23), although it is important to note that some patients may respond to lower doses and others may require significantly higher doses. Since the guideline's publication, fluvoxamine has been the least studied of the older SSRIs; however, its efficacy was supported in one RCT (24) and partially supported in a second, smaller RCT (25), in which it was superior to placebo on several outcome variables but not frequency of full panic attacks.

Citalopram and its *S*-enantiomer, escitalopram, have been approved for treatment of depression since the publication of the practice guideline. Although several RCTs have been conducted to evaluate the efficacy of these medications for panic disorder, neither has been approved for this indication in the United States. Available studies suggest that both citalopram and escitalopram are effective, well tolerated, and safe in the treatment of panic disorder (26–28). Dosages of 20–30 mg/day appear to be most effective for citalopram (26–28), whereas 10 mg/day appears to be an effective dosage for escitalopram (29).

Other antidepressants

TCAs and MAOIs are also effective medications for treatment of panic disorder (1). Because these are older agents, little evidence has accrued since 1998 that would alter or add to the recommendations provided in the practice guideline. Of the "dual" (serotonin and norepinephrine) reuptake inhibitors, venlafaxine ER at dosages of 75–225 mg/day was found to be effective in treating panic disorder (30), and this medication recently obtained FDA approval for this indication. Duloxetine is new to the market, and its efficacy for panic disorder has not been tested.

Benzodiazepines

Benzodiazepines are effective for treatment of panic disorder (1), and the guideline noted that alprazolam had the best evidence base for its antipanic efficacy. Since the guideline's publication, an extended-release preparation of alprazolam (alprazolam XR) became available and received FDA approval for treatment of panic disorder. The extended-release preparation requires less frequent dosing and may reduce the likelihood of "breakthrough anxiety" that can occur with missed doses of short-acting benzodiazepines (31). Additional studies have shown clonazepam to be a safe and effective treatment for panic disorder (32, 33). Daily dosages of clonazepam in the range of 1–2 mg are effective while minimizing side effects such as somnolence and ataxia (33), and discontinuation of clonazepam is well tolerated if accomplished with a slow taper schedule (32).

Relative efficacy and tolerability of medications

The literature that has accumulated over the past 8 years generally suggests that the large number of SSRIs, TCAs, and benzodiazepines used to treat panic disorder are equivalent in their efficacy (34–38). Early studies of SSRIs with small samples may have overestimated their efficacy in treating panic disorder; the majority of recent research suggests that SSRIs are effective but not superior in efficacy to older antidepressants in treating panic disorder. Two meta-analyses that compared SSRIs with other antidepressants showed that all classes of medications had similar effects on panic, agoraphobia, depression, and general anxiety (34, 37).

Although one meta-analysis found no difference in dropout rates for SSRIs and other antidepressants (37), the majority of studies suggest that SSRIs are better tolerated than TCAs (34, 37, 39–41). Many patients taking TCAs endure side effects such as increased heart rate, dry mouth, constipation, sweating, and weight gain, even with long-term use (42, 43).

Maintenance treatment

A common theme emerging from the last decade of research is the importance of maintenance pharmacotherapy. Studies of fluoxetine (15), paroxetine (44, 45), sertraline (46), imipramine (47), and clomipramine (48) all have demonstrated a benefit of continuing medication 6–12 months after acute treatment. Maintenance pharmacotherapy should be considered for most patients as a means of preventing recurrence of panic disorder symptoms and promoting continued symptom relief and better functioning.

Psychosocial treatment

Cognitive behavior therapy (CBT) has continued to demonstrate short- and long-term efficacy in clinical trials (49–54) and meta-analyses (55). The effects of CBT have been shown to be at least as robust as those of first-line pharmacotherapies (49, 50, 52, 56), and patients receiving CBT may have less risk for relapse following treatment withdrawal (49). The efficacy of CBT has been established in both individual and group modalities (56), and across clinical research (49), community mental health (57), and primary care settings (52, 53, 58).

CBT is a relatively underutilized treatment given its substantial evidence base for treatment of panic disorder (59). A considerable amount of recent research on CBT has focused on enhancing the efficiency and accessibility of this intervention. For example, one RCT showed that a five-session CBT protocol was comparable in efficacy to a standard-length protocol (51). Studies also have been conducted that evaluate the impact of self-administered CBT treatments for panic disorder. One RCT failed to find differences between fully self-administered CBT-oriented bibliotherapy, self-monitoring, and wait-list control groups on measures of panic disorder severity (60). Moreover, many patients dropped out of the study, suggesting that they had difficulty completing a course of CBT without any support of a professional. Results are more encouraging when self-directed CBT is combined with minimal therapist contact (61). Minimal therapist contact typically includes brief phone calls, meetings, or email to provide encouragement, clarify treatment concepts, and troubleshoot problems. Several clinical trials have shown that CBT-oriented bibliotherapy plus minimal therapist contact (61) and Internet-delivered CBT plus minimal therapist contact (62) are superior to control approaches. In some cases, primarily self-administered versions of CBT even may produce results that approximate those of therapist-administered CBT (63–65). More research is needed to determine for which patients primarily self-administered treatment is sufficient.

Other psychotherapies either have not been tested in a controlled manner or have failed to demonstrate efficacy comparable to that of CBT and pharmacotherapy. An RCT of eye movement desensitization and reprocessing (EMDR) found that EMDR was comparable to an attention-placebo control condition in reducing symptoms of panic disorder (66). In addition, an emotion-focused psychotherapy that featured exploration, empathic listening, and supportive strategies was inferior to CBT and imipramine and comparable to placebo in its effects on panic disorder (67). Psychodynamic psychotherapy remains a widely used treatment for panic disorder (59), although more research is needed to determine its utility in controlled trials. Panic-focused psychodynamic psychotherapy has been described (68) and tested in one pilot uncontrolled trial (69), with 16 of 21 patients achieving criteria for remission.

Combination treatments

Prescribing a combination of a benzodiazepine and an antidepressant is a common acute treatment of panic disorder. Recent studies suggest that administering a benzodiazepine in conjunction with an antidepressant confers a short-term benefit of quicker stabilization of panic disorder symptoms. This has been demonstrated with a clonazepam/sertraline combination (70) and a clonazepam/paroxetine combination (18). It appears that benzodiazepines facilitate early improvement of panic disorder symptoms; however, the advantage of the combination wears off quickly (i.e., individuals receiving SSRIs alone "catch up" to those receiving the benzodiazepine/SSRI combination after the first few weeks of treatment). The benefit of quicker stabilization of panic disorder symptoms should be weighed against the possibility of an increased side-effect burden when benzodiazepines are added to antidepressant therapy.

Studies that have combined medication and psychosocial treatment have failed to show a clear and lasting advantage for the combination treatment (49, 50). One small study found some benefit of combining an SSRI with very brief CBT for panic (71). The interactions between medication and CBT are complex, as demonstrated by a large RCT that compared acute and maintenance treatment using CBT, imipramine, CBT plus imipramine, CBT plus placebo, and placebo alone (49). All active treatment groups in this study were superior to pill placebo, and there were no significant differences between CBT alone and imipramine alone in the acute or maintenance phase of the study. CBT plus imipramine was equivalent to CBT plus placebo at posttreatment and superior to CBT plus placebo at 6-month follow-up. However, CBT plus imipramine also was associated with the highest rate of relapse after treatment withdrawal. The researchers concluded that addition of CBT did not help reduce relapse following imipramine discontinuation, and addition of imipramine actually appeared to reduce the durability of CBT's effects. At best, combination treatment produced a superior response in the 6 months of maintenance treatment, but this was at the expense of greater relapse following withdrawal of CBT. It is important to note that these results are specific to the CBT/imipramine combination, and more investigation of combining alternative medications and psychosocial treatments for panic disorder is needed.

Predictors of treatment response

Factors that affect response to pharmacological and psychosocial treatments for panic disorder remain poorly understood. Virtually all investigations of characteristics that contribute to treatment response have been undertaken post hoc and with relatively small samples. Some studies suggest that comorbidity affects response to standard treatments. Presence of co-occurring social phobia in patients with panic disorder has been associated with decreased response to paroxetine treatment and a paroxetine/CBT combination (72). In addition, fears of social catastrophes that could result from panic attacks predicted poorer response to both imipramine and CBT (73). Studies examining the impact of co-occurring axis II diagnoses on treatment response have shown mixed results; most (72, 74) but not all (75) suggest that co-occurring personality disorders are associated with poorer response to treatment.

The issue of treating individuals who fail to respond to their first prescribed medication or psychosocial treatment also has been left largely unexplored. One small study showed that adding paroxetine to CBT in patients who failed a trial of CBT led to significant improvements in anxiety and agoraphobic behavior (76). However, considerably more research is needed to address the issue of treatment-resistant panic disorder and the role of sequenced treatments.

Treatment of panic disorder in primary care

One advance in clinical research over the last decade has been the focus on "effectiveness" research that is conducted in real-world clinical settings as opposed to clinical research centers. Studies in primary care settings have shown that collaborative care improves outcomes for patients with panic disorder. One study demonstrated that a collaborative care intervention that included enhanced patient education, two visits with a psychiatrist, and telephone follow-ups improved outcomes for patients with panic disorder (77). Relative to treatment as usual, individuals receiving collaborative care were more likely to receive adequate medication treatment, adhere to medication recommendations, and improve significantly on measures of anxiety, depression, and disability. The collaborative care intervention also was associated with significantly more anxiety-free days and good cost-effectiveness (78).

Use of CBT in primary care settings also improves outcomes for patients with panic disorder (58). Patients who were randomly assigned to an intervention that provided up to six sessions of CBT and algorithm-based pharmacotherapy achieved higher rates of remission, response, and functioning compared with patients who received treatment as usual. These advantages were observed through the final assessment point in the study, which was 12 months postbaseline. The superior outcome of the intervention group was attributed to CBT, since most patients in the treatment-as-usual group received medication consistent with the study algorithm.

CONCLUSION

The clinical research that has been conducted since publication of the APA's *Practice Guideline for the Treatment of Patients With Panic Disorder* (1) does not contradict any of the guideline's basic recommendations. Clinicians treating patients with panic disorder should be aware of the safety issues associated with antidepressants, the availability of a broader range of new efficacious medications, and the likely benefit of maintenance pharmacotherapy. Cognitive behavior therapy remains the psychosocial treatment with the largest research base and most demonstrated efficacy for treatment of panic disorder. A clear benefit of adding medication to CBT has yet to be established, and there is a paucity of data examining the addition of CBT to medication. Other psychotherapies either have proved inferior to medication and CBT or have not been evaluated in controlled trials. Finally, more research is needed on assessing the long-term impact of medications and psychosocial treatments, combining medication and psychosocial treatments, identifying factors that predict treatment response, and ameliorating treatment-resistant panic disorder.

REFERENCES

1. American Psychiatric Association: Practice guideline for the treatment of patients with panic disorder. Am J Psychiatry 1998; 155(5 suppl):1–34
2. DeMartinis NA, Schweizer E, Rickels K: An open-label trial of nefazodone in high comorbidity panic disorder. J Clin Psychiatry 1996; 57:245–248
3. Aranda-Michel J, Koehler A, Bejarano PA, Poulos JE, Luxon BA, Khan CM, Ee LC, Balistreri WF, Weber FL Jr: Nefazodone-induced liver failure: report of three cases. Ann Intern Med 1999; 130:285–288
4. Choi S: Nefazodone (Serzone) withdrawn because of hepatotoxicity. CMAJ 2003; 169: 1187
5. Conway CR, McGuire JM, Baram VY: Nefazodone-induced liver failure. J Clin Psychopharmacol 2004; 24:353–354
6. Eloubeidi MA, Gaede JT, Swaim MW: Reversible nefazodone-induced liver failure. Dig Dis Sci 2000; 45:1036–1038
7. Lucena MI, Andrade RJ, Gomez-Outes A, Rubio M, Cabello MR: Acute liver failure after treatment with nefazodone. Dig Dis Sci 1999; 44:2577–2579
8. Schirren CA, Baretton G: Nefazodone-induced acute liver failure. Am J Gastroenterol 2000; 95:1596–1597
9. Tzimas GN, Dion B, Deschenes M: Early onset, nefazodone-induced fulminant hepatic failure. Am J Gastroenterol 2003; 98:1663–1664
10. Leslie LK, Newman TB, Chesney PJ, Perrin JM: The Food and Drug Administration's deliberations on antidepressant use in pediatric patients. Pediatrics 2005; 116:195–204
11. Khan A, Khan S, Kolts R, Brown WA: Suicide rates in clinical trials of SSRIs, other antidepressants, and placebo: analysis of FDA reports. Am J Psychiatry 2003; 160:790–792
12. Storosum JG, van Zwieten BJ, van den Brink W, Gersons BPR, Broekmans AW: Suicide risk in placebo-controlled studies of major depression. Am J Psychiatry 2001; 158:1271–1275
13. Simon GE, Savarino J, Operskalski B, Wang PS: Suicide risk during antidepressant treatment. Am J Psychiatry 2006; 163(1):41–47
14. Michelson D, Lydiard RB, Pollack MH, Tamura RN, Hoog SL, Tepner R, Demitrack MA, Tollefson GD: Outcome assessment and clinical improvement in panic disorder: evidence from a randomized controlled trial of fluoxetine and placebo. The Fluoxetine Panic Disorder Study Group. Am J Psychiatry 1998; 155:1570–1577

15. Michelson D, Pollack M, Lydiard RB, Tamura RN, Tepner R, Tollefson G: Continuing treatment of panic disorder after acute response: randomised, placebo-controlled trial with fluoxetine. Br J Psychiatry 1999; 174:213–218
16. Michelson D, Allgulander C, Dantendorfer K, Knezevic A, Maierhofer D, Micev V, Paunovic VR, Timotijevic I, Sarkar N, Skoglund L, Pemberton SC: Efficacy of usual antidepressant dosing regimens of fluoxetine in panic disorder: randomised, placebo-controlled trial. Br J Psychiatry 2001; 179:514–518
17. Ballenger JC, Wheadon DE, Steiner M, Bushnell W, Gergel IP: Double-blind, fixed-dose, placebo-controlled study of paroxetine in the treatment of panic disorder. Am J Psychiatry 1998; 155:36–42
18. Pollack MH, Simon NM, Worthington JJ, Doyle AL, Peters P, Toshkov F, Otto MW: Combined paroxetine and clonazepam treatment strategies compared to paroxetine monotherapy for panic disorder. J Psychopharmacol 2003; 17:276–282
19. Sheehan DV, Burnham DB, Iyengar MK, Perera P: Efficacy and tolerability of controlled-release paroxetine in the treatment of panic disorder. J Clin Psychiatry 2005; 66:34–40
20. Londborg PD, Wolkow R, Smith WT, DuBoff E, Englang D, Ferguson J, Rosenthal M, Weise C: Sertraline in the treatment of panic disorder: a multi-site, double-blind, placebo-controlled, fixed-dose investigation. Br J Psychiatry 1998; 173:54–60
21. Pohl RB, Wolkow RM, Clary CM: Sertraline in the treatment of panic disorder: a double-blind multicenter trial. Am J Psychiatry 1998; 155:1189–1195
22. Pollack MH, Otto MW, Worthington JJ, Manfro GG, Wolkow R: Sertraline in the treatment of panic disorder: a flexible-dose multicenter trial. Arch Gen Psychiatry 1998; 55:1010–1016
23. Sheikh JI, Londborg P, Clary CM, Fayyad R: The efficacy of sertraline in panic disorder: combined results from two fixed-dose studies. Int Clin Psychopharmacol 2000; 15:335–342
24. Asnis GM, Hameedi FA, Goddard AW, Potkin SG, Black D, Jameel M, Desagani K, Woods SW: Fluvoxamine in the treatment of panic disorder: a multi-center, double-blind, placebo-controlled study in outpatients. Psychiatry Res 2001; 103:1–14
25. Sandmann J, Lorch B, Bandelow B, Hartter S, Winter P, Hiemke C, Benkert O: Fluvoxamine or placebo in the treatment of panic disorder and relationship to blood concentrations of fluvoxamine. Pharmacopsychiatry 1998; 31:117–121
26. Leinonen E, Lepola U, Koponen H, Turtonen J, Wade A, Lehto H: Citalopram controls phobic symptoms in patients with panic disorder: randomized controlled trial. J Psychiatry Neurosci 2000; 25:25–32
27. Lepola UM, Wade AG, Leinonen EV, Koponen HJ, Frazer J, Sjodin I, Penttinen JT, Pedersen T, Lehto HJ: A controlled, prospective, 1-year trial of citalopram in the treatment of panic disorder. J Clin Psychiatry 1998; 59:528–534
28. Wade AG, Lepola U, Koponen HJ, Pedersen V, Pedersen T: The effect of citalopram in panic disorder. Br J Psychiatry 1997; 170:549–553
29. Stahl SM, Gergel I, Li D: Escitalopram in the treatment of panic disorder: a randomized, double-blind, placebo-controlled trial. J Clin Psychiatry 2003; 64:1322–1327
30. Bradwejn J, Ahokas A, Stein DJ, Salinas E, Emilien G, Whitaker T: Venlafaxine extended-release capsules in panic disorder: flexible-dose, double-blind, placebo-controlled study. Br J Psychiatry 2005; 187:352–359
31. Rickels K: Alprazolam extended-release in panic disorder. Expert Opin Pharmacother 2004; 5:1599–1611
32. Moroz G, Rosenbaum JF: Efficacy, safety, and gradual discontinuation of clonazepam in panic disorder: a placebo-controlled, multicenter study using optimized dosages. J Clin Psychiatry 1999; 60:604–612

33. Rosenbaum JF, Moroz G, Bowden CL: Clonazepam in the treatment of panic disorder with or without agoraphobia: a dose-response study of efficacy, safety, and discontinuance. Clonazepam Panic Disorder Dose-Response Study Group. J Clin Psychopharmacol 1997; 17:390–400
34. Bakker A, Van Balkom AJ, Spinhoven P: SSRIs vs TCAs in the treatment of panic disorder: a meta-analysis. Acta Psychiatr Scand 2002; 106:163–167
35. Bakker A, Van Balkom AJ, Spinhoven P, Blaauw BM, van Dyck R: Follow-up on the treatment of panic disorder with or without agoraphobia: a quantitative review. J Nerv Ment Dis 1998; 186:414–419
36. Lepola U, Arato M, Zhu Y, Austin C: Sertraline versus imipramine treatment of comorbid panic disorder and major depressive disorder. J Clin Psychiatry 2003; 64:654–662
37. Otto MW, Tuby KS, Gould RA, McLean RY, Pollack MH: An effect-size analysis of the relative efficacy and tolerability of serotonin selective reuptake inhibitors for panic disorder. Am J Psychiatry 2001; 158:1989–1992
38. Perna G, Bertani A, Caldirola D, Smeraldi E, Bellodi L: A comparison of citalopram and paroxetine in the treatment of panic disorder: a randomized, single-blind study. Pharmacopsychiatry 2001; 34:85–90
39. Lecrubier Y, Bakker A, Dunbar G, Judge R: A comparison of paroxetine, clomipramine and placebo in the treatment of panic disorder. Collaborative Paroxetine Panic Study Investigators. Acta Psychiatr Scand 1997; 95:145–152
40. Mavissakalian MR: Imipramine vs sertraline in panic disorder: 24-week treatment completers. Ann Clin Psychiatry 2003; 15:171–180
41. Toni C, Perugi G, Frare F, Mata B, Vitale B, Mengali F, Recchia M, Serra G, Akiskal HS: A prospective naturalistic study of 326 panic-agoraphobic patients treated with antidepressants. Pharmacopsychiatry 2000; 33:121–131
42. Mavissakalian MR, Perel JM: The side effects burden of extended imipramine treatment of panic disorder. J Clin Psychopharmacol 2000; 20:547–555
43. Mavissakalian M, Perel J, Guo S: Specific side effects of long-term imipramine management of panic disorder. J Clin Psychopharmacol 2002; 22:155–161
44. Ballenger JC: Remission rates in patients with anxiety disorders treated with paroxetine. J Clin Psychiatry 2004; 65:1696–1707
45. Lecrubier Y, Judge R: Long-term evaluation of paroxetine, clomipramine and placebo in panic disorder. Collaborative Paroxetine Panic Study Investigators. Acta Psychiatr Scand 1997; 95:153–160
46. Rapaport MH, Wolkow R, Rubin A, Hackett E, Pollack M, Ota KY: Sertraline treatment of panic disorder: results of a long-term study. Acta Psychiatr Scand 2001; 104:289–298
47. Mavissakalian MR, Perel JM: Long-term maintenance and discontinuation of imipramine therapy in panic disorder with agoraphobia. Arch Gen Psychiatry 1999; 56:821–827
48. Lotufo-Neto F, Bernik M, Ramos RT, Andrade L, Gorenstein C, Cordas T, Melo M, Gentil V: A dose-finding and discontinuation study of clomipramine in panic disorder. J Psychopharmacol 2001; 15:13–17
49. Barlow DH, Gorman JM, Shear MK, Woods SW: Cognitive-behavioral therapy, imipramine, or their combination for panic disorder: a randomized controlled trial. JAMA 2000; 283:2529–2536
50. Loerch B, Graf-Morgenstern M, Hautzinger M, Schlegel S, Hain C, Sandmann J,Benkert O: Randomised placebo-controlled trial of moclobemide, cognitive-behavioural therapy and their combination in panic disorder with agoraphobia. Br J Psychiatry 1999; 174:205–212
51. Clark DM, Salkovskis PM, Hackmann A, Wells A, Ludgate J, Gelder M: Brief cognitive therapy for panic disorder: a randomized controlled trial. J Consult Clin Psychol 1999; 67:583–589

52. Sharp DM, Power KG, Simpson RJ, Swanson V, Anstee JA: Global measures of outcome in a controlled comparison of pharmacological and psychological treatment of panic disorder and agoraphobia. Br J Gen Pract 1997; 47:150–155
53. Addis ME, Hatgis C, Krasnow AD, Jacob K, Bourne L, Mansfield A: Effectiveness of cognitive-behavioral treatment for panic disorder versus treatment as usual in a managed care setting. J Consult Clin Psychol 2004; 72:625–635
54. Ost LG, Thulin U, Ramnero J: Cognitive behavior therapy vs exposure in vivo in the treatment of panic disorder with agoraphobia. Behav Res Ther 2004; 42:1105–1127
55. Westen D, Morrison K: A multidimensional meta-analysis of treatments for depression, panic disorder, and generalized anxiety disorder: an empirical examination of the status of empirically supported therapies. J Consult Clin Psychol 2001; 69:875–899
56. Dannon PN, Gon-Usishkin M, Gelbert A, Lowengrub K, Grunhaus L: Cognitive behavioral group therapy in panic disorder patients: the efficacy of CGBT versus drug treatment. Ann Clin Psychiatry 2004; 16:41–46
57. Wade WA, Treat TA, Stuart GL: Transporting an empirically supported treatment for panic disorder to a service clinic setting: a benchmarking strategy. J Consult Clin Psychol 1998; 66:231–239
58. Roy-Byrne PP, Craske MG, Stein MB, Sullivan G, Bystritsky A, Katon W, Golinelli D, Sherbourne CD: A randomized effectiveness trial of cognitive-behavioral therapy and medication for primary care panic disorder. Arch Gen Psychiatry 2005; 62:290–298
59. Goisman RM, Warshaw MG, Keller MB: Psychosocial treatment prescriptions for generalized anxiety disorder, panic disorder, and social phobia, 1991–1996. Am J Psychiatry 1999; 156:1819–1821
60. Febbraro GAR, Clum GA, Roodman AA, Wright JH: The limits of bibliotherapy: a study of differential effectiveness of self-administered interventions in individuals with panic attacks. Behav Ther 1999; 30:209–222
61. Newman MG, Erikson T, Przeworski A, Dzus E: Self-help and minimal-contact therapies for anxiety disorders: is human contact necessary for therapeutic efficacy? J Clin Psychol 2003; 59:251–274
62. Carlbring P, Westling BE, Ljungstrand P, Ekselius L, Anderson G: Treatment of panic disorder via the Internet: a randomized trial of a self-help program. Behav Ther 2001; 32:751–764
63. Newman MG, Kenardy J, Herman S, Taylor CB: Comparison of palmtop-computer-assisted brief cognitive-behavioral treatment to cognitive-behavioral treatment for panic disorder. J Consult Clin Psychol 1997; 65:178–183
64. Marks IM, Kenwright M, McDonough M, Whittaker M, Mataix-Cols D: Saving clinician's time by delegating routine aspects of therapy to a computer: a randomized controlled trial in phobia/panic disorder. Psychol Med 2004; 34:9–17
65. Kenardy JA, Dow MG, Johnston DW, Newman MG, Thomson A, Taylor CB: A comparison of delivery methods of cognitive-behavioral therapy for panic-disorder: an international multicenter trial. J Consult Clin Psychol 2003; 71:1068–1075
66. Goldstein AJ, de Beurs E, Chambless DL, Wilson KA: EMDR for panic disorder with agoraphobia: comparison with waiting list and credible attention-placebo control conditions. J Consult Clin Psychol 2000; 68:947–956
67. Shear MK, Houck P, Greeno C, Masters S: Emotion-focused psychotherapy for patients with panic disorder. Am J Psychiatry 2001; 158:1993–1998
68. Busch FN, Milrod BL, Singer MB: Theory and technique in psychodynamic treatment of panic disorder. J Psychother Pract Res 1999; 8:234–242
69. Milrod BL, Busch FN, Leon AC, Aronson A, Roiphe J, Rudden M, Singer M, Shapiro T, Goldman H, Richter D, Shear MK: A pilot open trial of brief psychodynamic psychotherapy for panic disorder. J Psychother Pract Res 2001; 10:239–245

70. Goddard AW, Brouette T, Almai A, Jetty P, Woods SW, Charney DS: Early coadministration of clonazepam with sertraline for panic disorder. Arch Gen Psychiatry 2001; 58:681–686
71. Stein MB, Norton GR, Walker JR, Chartier MJ, Graham R: Do selective serotonin reuptake inhibitors enhance the efficacy of very brief cognitive behavioral therapy for panic disorder? A pilot study. Psychiatry Res 2000; 94:191–200
72. Berger P, Sachs G, Amering M, Holzinger A, Bankier B, Katschnig H: Personality disorder and social anxiety predict delayed response in drug and behavioral treatment of panic disorder. J Affect Disord 2004; 80:75–78
73. Hicks TV, Leitenberg H, Barlow DH, Gorman JM, Shear MK, Woods SW: Physical, mental, and social catastrophic cognitions as prognostic factors in cognitive-behavioral and pharmacological treatments for panic disorder. J Consult Clin Psychol 2005; 73:506–514
74. Seivewright H, Tyrer P, Johnson T: Prediction of outcome in neurotic disorder: a 5-year prospective study. Psychol Med 1998; 28:1149–1157
75. Hofmann SG, Shear MK, Barlow DH, Gorman JM, Hershberger D, Patterson M, Woods SW: Effects of panic disorder treatments on personality disorder characteristics. Depress Anxiety 1998; 8:14–20
76. Kampman M, Keijsers GP, Hoogduin CA, Hendriks GJ: A randomized, double-blind, placebo-controlled study of the effects of adjunctive paroxetine in panic disorder patients unsuccessfully treated with cognitive-behavioral therapy alone. J Clin Psychiatry 2002; 63: 772–777
77. Roy-Byrne PP, Katon W, Cowley DS, Russo J: A randomized effectiveness trial of collaborative care for patients with panic disorder in primary care. Arch Gen Psychiatry 2001; 58: 869–876
78. Katon W, Roy-Byrne PP, Russo J, Cowley D: Cost-effectiveness and cost of a collaborative care intervention for primary care patients with panic disorder. Arch Gen Psychiatry 2002; 59:1098–1104

PRACTICE GUIDELINE FOR THE Treatment of Patients With Panic Disorder

WORK GROUP ON PANIC DISORDER

Jack Gorman, M.D., Co-Chair

Katherine Shear, M.D., Co-Chair

Deborah Cowley, M.D.
C. Deborah Cross, M.D.
John March, M.D.
Walton Roth, M.D.
Michael Shehi, M.D.
Philip S. Wang, M.D., Dr.P.H. (Consultant)

Originally published in May 1998. A guideline watch, summarizing significant developments in the scientific literature since publication of this guideline, may be available in the Psychiatric Practice section of the APA web site at www.psych.org.

CONTENTS

Introduction 949

Development Process 950

I. Summary of Recommendations 951
- A. Coding System 951
- B. General Considerations 951

II. Disease Definition, Natural History, and Epidemiology 954
- A. Diagnosis of Panic Disorder 954
- B. Specific Features of Panic Disorder 954
- C. Natural History and Course 954
- D. Epidemiology and Associated Features 955

III. Treatment Principles and Alternatives 955
- A. Psychiatric Management 955
- B. Interpreting Results From Studies of Treatments for Panic Disorder 959
- C. Specific Psychosocial Interventions 959
- D. Pharmacologic Interventions 965

IV. Development of a Treatment Plan for the Individual Patient 976
- A. Choosing a Site of Treatment 976
- B. Formulation of a Treatment Plan 977

V. Clinical Features Influencing Treatment 981
- A. Psychiatric Factors 981
- B. Concurrent General Medical Conditions 983
- C. Demographic Variables 984

VI. Research Directions 986

VII. Individuals and Organizations That Submitted Comments 987

VIII. References 989

INTRODUCTION

This guideline summarizes data to inform the psychiatrist of the care of patients with panic disorder. It begins at the point where the psychiatrist has diagnosed an adult patient as suffering from this disorder according to the criteria in DSM-IV (1) and has evaluated the patient for the existence of coexisting mental disorders. It also assumes that the psychiatrist or other physician has evaluated the patient for general medical conditions or other factors that may be causing or exacerbating the panic or that may affect its treatment. The guideline also briefly addresses issues specific to the treatment of panic disorder in children and adolescents.

The purpose of this guideline is to assist the psychiatrist in caring for a patient with panic disorder. It should be noted that many patients have conditions that cannot be completely described by the DSM-IV diagnostic category. The psychiatrist caring for a patient with panic disorder should consider, but not be limited to, the treatments recommended in this practice guideline. Psychiatrists care for patients with panic disorders in many different settings and serve a variety of functions; the recommendations in this guideline are primarily intended for psychiatrists who provide, or coordinate, the overall care of the patient with panic disorder.

To share feedback on this or other published APA practice guidelines, a form is available at http://www.psych.org/psych_pract/pg/reviewform.cfm.

DEVELOPMENT PROCESS

This practice guideline was developed under the auspices of the Steering Committee on Practice Guidelines. The process is detailed in the Appendix to this volume. Key features of the process include the following:

- a comprehensive literature review (description follows) and development of evidence tables
- initial drafting by a work group that included psychiatrists with clinical and research expertise in panic disorder
- the production of multiple drafts with widespread review, in which 20 organizations and over 100 individuals submitted comments (see section VII)
- approval by the APA Assembly and Board of Trustees
- planned revisions at 3- to 5-year intervals

The following computerized searches of relevant literature were conducted.

The first literature search was conducted by using MEDLINE and Psychological Abstracts, for the period of 1980–1994. The keywords for the search were "panic disorder," "agoraphobia," "drug treatment," "non-drug treatment," and "combined modality treatment." A total of 825 citations were found.

A second search was conducted in MEDLINE for the period of 1980–1994 and used the keywords "panic disorder" and "tricyclics," "MAO inhibitors," "benzodiazepines," "SSRIs and anticonvulsants," "behavioral and/or cognitive," "all other psychotherapy/psychoanalysis," and "children without adults and combined child and adult." In Psychological Abstracts the key words "panic disorder" and "psychosocial treatment" were used.

A third search was completed in MEDLINE for the period 1992–1996 and used the following keywords: "panic disorder," "agoraphobia," "antidepressive agents," "tricyclic," "MAO inhibitors," "benzodiazepine," "anti-anxiety agents," "anticonvulsants," "behavior therapy," "psychotherapy/psychoanalysis," "children," and "psychosocial treatment."

I. SUMMARY OF RECOMMENDATIONS

A. CODING SYSTEM

Each recommendation is identified as falling into one of three categories of endorsement, indicated by a bracketed Roman numeral following the statement. The three categories represent varying levels of clinical confidence regarding the recommendation:

[I] Recommended with substantial clinical confidence.
[II] Recommended with moderate clinical confidence.
[III] May be recommended on the basis of individual circumstances.

B. GENERAL CONSIDERATIONS

Panic disorder, with or without agoraphobia, is a common psychiatric illness that can have a chronic course and be associated with significant morbidity. The care of patients with panic disorder involves a comprehensive array of approaches that are designed to reduce the frequency and severity of panic episodes, reduce morbidity, and improve patient functioning [I]. Modalities for which there is considerable evidence of efficacy in the treatment of panic disorder include psychotherapy, specifically cognitive behavioral therapies, and pharmacotherapy [I]. Other psychotherapies, including psychodynamic, are widely employed in conjunction with medication and/or elements of cognitive behavioral therapies on the basis of a clinical consensus that they are effective for some patients [II]. Considerations for choosing specific treatments among the various options are presented.

1. Choice of treatment setting

For most patients with panic disorder, treatment can be conducted on an outpatient basis and rarely requires hospitalization [I]. Examples of patients who may require inpatient treatment include individuals with comorbid depression who are at risk of suicide attempts or patients with comorbid substance use disorders who require detoxification.

Sometimes the first contact between patient and psychiatrist occurs in the emergency room or hospital to which a patient has been admitted for an acute panic episode. The psychiatrist may be able to make the diagnosis of panic disorder and initiate treatment in this setting after general medical conditions have been ruled out.

2. Formulation of a treatment plan

A comprehensive general medical and psychiatric evaluation should precede treatment to determine whether potential general medical and substance-induced conditions may be causing the panic symptoms, complicate treatment, or require specific interventions, especially with a patient who has a new onset of symptoms [I]. In addition, the assessment of developmental factors, psychosocial stressors and conflicts, social supports, and general living situation will aid the treatment [I]. The psychiatrist's evaluation of the patient's condition and the intended treatment should guide the choice of laboratory and diagnostic studies [I].

3. Psychiatric management

Psychiatric management forms the foundation of psychiatric treatment for patients with panic disorder and should be instituted for all patients in combination with specific treatments, such as medications and psychotherapy. The following are important components of psychiatric management for patients with panic disorder [I]: establishing and maintaining a therapeutic alliance; educating and reassuring the patient concerning panic disorder; evaluating particular symptoms and monitoring them over time; evaluating types and severity of functional impairment; identifying and addressing comorbid conditions; working with other health professionals; educating family members and enlisting their help when appropriate; enhancing treatment compliance; and working with the patient to address early signs of relapse. Many patients with panic disorder require a reliable treatment relationship because they relapse or have partial responses and benefit from extended periods of treatment, or because they intensely fear abandonment. For these reasons, it is helpful to be able to assure the patient of the continued availability of his or her psychiatrist.

4. Choice of treatment modalities to be used in conjunction with psychiatric management

Psychotherapy, specifically panic-focused cognitive behavioral therapy (CBT), and medications have both been shown to be effective treatments for panic disorder [I]. There is no convincing evidence that one modality is superior for all patients or for particular subpopulations of patients. The choice between psychotherapy and pharmacotherapy depends on an individualized assessment of the efficacy, benefits, and risks of each modality and the patient's personal preferences (including costs) [I]. In every case, the patient should be fully informed by the psychiatrist about the availability and relative advantages and disadvantages of CBT, antipanic medications, and other forms of treatment.

a) Cognitive behavioral therapy and other psychotherapies

CBT encompasses a range of treatments, each consisting of several elements, including psychoeducation, continuous panic monitoring, development of anxiety management skills, cognitive restructuring, and in vivo exposure. In practice, the types of therapy encompassed by CBT are often quite diverse. It is unknown whether certain elements are more effective for all patients or for specific patients. The efficacy of CBT for the treatment of panic disorder is supported by extensive and high-quality data. Other psychotherapies may be considered in conjunction with psychiatric management [III], but supplementation with (or replacement by) either CBT or an antipanic medication should be strongly considered if there is no significant improvement within 6–8 weeks.

b) Pharmacotherapy

There are four classes of medications that have been shown to be effective: selective serotonin reuptake inhibitors (SSRIs), tricyclic antidepressants (TCAs), benzodiazepines, and monoamine oxidase inhibitors (MAOIs) [I]. Medications from all four classes have been found to have roughly comparable efficacy [II]. Choosing a medication from among these classes is generally guided by considerations of adverse effects and the physician's understanding of the patient's personal preferences (including costs) and other aspects of the clinical situation [I]. For many patients, SSRIs are likely to have the most favorable balance of efficacy and adverse effects. Although SSRIs carry a risk of sexual side effects, they lack the cardiovascular side effects, anticholinergic side effects, and toxicity associated with overdose that occur with TCAs and MAOIs. SSRIs also lack the potential for physiologic dependency associated with benzodiazepines. TCAs can be tolerated by most patients, although generally not as well as SSRIs. The risks of cardiovascular and anticholinergic side effects of TCAs should be considered, especially for the elderly or patients with general medical problems. Benzodiazepines may be used preferentially in situations in which very rapid control of symptoms is critical (e.g., the patient is about to quit school, lose a job, or require hospitalization). However, the risks of long-term benzodiazepine use, including physiologic dependence, should also be considered. Benzodiazepine use is generally contraindicated for patients with a history of substance use disorder. Although MAOIs are effective, they are generally reserved for patients who do not respond to other treatments because of the risk of hypertensive crises and necessary dietary restrictions. SSRIs are likely to be more expensive than TCAs or benzodiazepines because of the lack of generic preparations.

5. Other treatment considerations

a) Combined medication and psychotherapy

Studies comparing the efficacy of combined antipanic medication and CBT with the efficacy of either modality alone have produced conflicting results. Currently, it is not possible to identify which patients might benefit more from combination therapy. Combined antipanic medication and CBT may be especially useful for patients with severe agoraphobia and those who show an incomplete response [III].

b) Determining the length of treatment

With either CBT or antipanic medication, the acute phase of treatment lasts approximately 12 weeks [II]. After this time, many clinicians reduce the frequency of CBT and then gradually discontinue treatment when the patient is judged to be stable. It is not known whether a second round of CBT is effective for patients who relapse or whether "booster" CBT sessions may prevent relapse.

If a medication has been used, a trial of discontinuation may be attempted after 12–18 months of maintenance therapy if the patient has experienced significant or full improvement [III]. Many patients will partially or fully relapse when medication is discontinued and may benefit from prolonged periods of treatment [III]. Although data on the percentage of patients that remain well after medication discontinuation have been widely divergent, evidence suggests that it is between 30% and 45% (2). Patients who relapse are generally given medication again and/or offered CBT. Patients who remain panic free should be encouraged to contact their psychiatrists in the future at the first sign of the reemergence of panic attacks.

Patients who show no improvement within 6–8 weeks with a particular treatment should be reevaluated with regard to diagnosis, the need for a different treatment, or the need for a combined treatment approach [III]. Patients who do not respond as expected to medication or CBT or who have repeated relapses should be evaluated for possible addition of a psychodynamic or other psychotherapeutic intervention.

c) Use of benzodiazepines for early symptom control, in combination with another treatment modality

It may take several weeks of treatment before patients begin to experience noticeable benefits from either CBT or pharmacotherapy. For some patients with severe panic attacks or high levels of anticipatory anxiety, concomitant benzodiazepine use may be helpful [III]. It may be appropriate to minimize the dose and duration when benzodiazepines are used in this manner, because of potential risks (e.g., physiologic dependence).

d) Comorbidities and other clinical features influencing treatment

Comorbid psychiatric illness, concurrent general medical illnesses, and certain demographic or psychosocial features of patients with panic disorder may have important influences on treatment. Prevalent comorbid psychiatric factors that should be considered include suicidality, substance use, mood disorders, other anxiety disorders, personality disorders, and significant dysfunction in personal, social, or vocational areas. Specific psychosocial therapies (including psychodynamic psychotherapy) may be useful to address comorbid disorders or environmental or psychosocial stressors in patients with panic disorder and are frequently used in conjunction with CBT and/or antipanic medications. Important general medical conditions that may be seen with, or confused with, panic disorder include an array of cardiovascular, pulmonary, neurologic, endocrinologic, and gastrointestinal conditions. Special treatment considerations are necessary for pediatric and geriatric patients with panic disorder. Details concerning the influence of these factors on the treatment of patients with panic disorder are found in Section V.

II. DISEASE DEFINITION, NATURAL HISTORY, AND EPIDEMIOLOGY

A. DIAGNOSIS OF PANIC DISORDER

The essential features of panic disorder consist of a mixture of characteristic signs and symptoms that persist for at least 1 month. The symptoms include recurrent panic attacks and persistent concern about having another attack or worry about the implications and consequences of the attacks. Panic attacks are discrete periods of intense fear or discomfort, accompanied by at least 4 of the 13 somatic or cognitive symptoms defined by DSM-IV. An attack has an abrupt onset and reaches a peak usually within 10 minutes. It is often accompanied by a sense of imminent danger and an urge to escape.

Panic disorder must be distinguished from other conditions that can have panic symptoms as an associated feature. These conditions include other mental disorders (e.g., specific phobias, posttraumatic stress disorder, or separation anxiety disorder), the direct effects of substances, including over-the-counter medications (e.g., caffeine or stimulants), withdrawal from a substance (e.g., withdrawal from sedative-hypnotics), or certain general medical conditions (e.g., hyperthyroidism). For further discussion of these issues, see DSM-IV.

B. SPECIFIC FEATURES OF PANIC DISORDER

1. Cross-sectional issues

There are a number of important clinical and psychosocial features to consider in a cross-sectional evaluation. First, because there is such variance in the types and duration of attacks that may occur with panic disorder, the psychiatrist should consider other possible diagnoses. The psychiatrist should assess the patient for the presence of life-threatening behaviors, the degree to which the panic disorder interferes with the patient's ability to conduct his or her daily routine or to care for self and others, and the presence of a substance use disorder or a depressive disorder.

2. Longitudinal issues

Because of the variable nature of panic disorder, it is necessary to consider a number of longitudinal issues when evaluating the patient. These include the fluctuations in this chronic condition, the development of complications, and the response to prior treatments.

C. NATURAL HISTORY AND COURSE

Several types of panic attacks may occur. The most common is the unexpected attack, defined as one not associated with a known situational trigger. Individuals may also experience situationally predisposed panic attacks (which are more likely to occur in certain situations but do not necessarily occur there) or situationally bound attacks (which occur almost immediately on exposure to a situational trigger). Other types of panic attacks include those that occur in particular emotional contexts, those involving limited symptoms, and nocturnal attacks.

Patients with panic disorder may also have agoraphobia, in which case they experience anxiety and avoidance of places or situations where escape or help may be unavailable if they have panic symptoms. Typical situations eliciting agoraphobia include traveling on buses, subways, or other public transportation and being on bridges, in tunnels, or far from home. Many patients who develop agoraphobia find that situational attacks become more common than unexpected attacks.

Panic attacks vary in their frequency and intensity. It is not uncommon for an individual to experience numerous moderate attacks for months at a time or to experience frequent attacks daily for a short period (e.g., a week), with months separating subsequent periods of attack.

Individuals with panic disorder commonly have anxiety about the recurrence of panic attacks or symptoms or about the implications or consequences. Panic disorder, especially with agoraphobia, may lead to the loss or disruption of interpersonal relationships, especially as individuals struggle with the impairment or loss of social role functioning and the issue of responsibility for symptoms.

Examples of the disrupting nature of panic disorder include the fear that an attack is the indicator of a life-threatening illness despite medical evaluation indicating otherwise or the fear that an attack is a sign of emotional weakness. Some individuals experience the attacks as so severe that they take such actions as quitting a job to avoid a possible attack. Others may become so anxious that they eventually avoid most activities outside their homes. Evidence from one naturalistic follow-up study of patients in a tertiary-care setting suggests that at 4–6 years posttreatment about 30% of individuals are well, 40%–50% are improved but symptomatic, and the remaining 20%–30% have symptoms that are the same or slightly worse (3, 4).

D. EPIDEMIOLOGY AND ASSOCIATED FEATURES

Epidemiologic data collected from a variety of countries have documented similarities in lifetime prevalence (1.6%–2.2%), age at first onset (20s), higher risk in females (about twofold), and symptom patterns of panic disorder (5). While the full-blown syndrome is usually not present until early adulthood, limited symptoms often occur much earlier. Several investigators have documented cases of panic disorder prepubertally (6).

One-third to one-half of individuals diagnosed with panic disorder in community samples also have agoraphobia, although a much higher rate of agoraphobia is encountered in clinical samples (5). Among individuals with panic disorder, the lifetime prevalence of major depression is 50%–60% (7). For individuals with both panic disorder and depression, the onset of depression precedes the onset of panic disorder in one-third of this population, while the onset of depression coincides with or follows the onset of panic disorder in the remaining two-thirds. Approximately one-third of patients with panic disorder are depressed when they present for treatment (7).

Epidemiologic studies have clearly documented the morbidity associated with panic disorder. In the Epidemiologic Catchment Area study, subjects with panic symptoms or disorders, as compared to other disorders, were the most frequent users of emergency medical services and were more likely to be hospitalized for physical problems (8). Patients with panic disorder, especially with comorbid depression, were at higher risk for suicide attempts (9), impaired social and marital functioning, use of psychoactive medication, and substance abuse (10).

Family studies using direct interviews of relatives and family history studies have shown that panic disorder is highly familial. Results from studies conducted in different countries (United States, Belgium, Germany, Australia) have shown that the median risk of panic disorder is eight times as high in the first-degree relatives of probands with panic disorder as in the relatives of control subjects (11). A recent family data analysis showed that forms with early onsets (at age 20 or before) were the most familial, carrying a more than 17 times greater risk (12). Results from twin studies have suggested a genetic contribution to the disorder (13, 14).

III. TREATMENT PRINCIPLES AND ALTERNATIVES

A. PSYCHIATRIC MANAGEMENT

Psychiatric management consists of a comprehensive array of activities and interventions that should be instituted by psychiatrists for all patients with panic disorder, in combination with specific treatment modalities. Patients with panic disorder frequently fear that panic attacks represent catastrophic medical events. In addition, they may live in a nearly constant state of apprehension and may be severely limited by phobic avoidance. For such reasons, reassurance, education, and support are important components of psychiatric management, along with accurate diagnosis that takes into account all the elements of a patient's individual symptom pattern. The psychiatrist should help the patient cope with the effects that panic disorder sometimes has on family members and with the possibility that the disorder may be chronic, requiring long-term treatment.

The specific components of psychiatric management include performing a diagnostic evaluation; evaluating the particular symptoms; evaluating types and severity of functional impairment of the individual patient; establishing and maintaining a therapeutic alliance; monitoring the patient's psychiatric status; providing education to the patient and, when appropriate, to the family about panic disorder; working with nonpsychiatric physicians the patient consults; enhancing treatment compliance; and working with the patient to address early signs of relapse.

1. Performing a diagnostic evaluation

Patients with panic symptoms should receive a thorough diagnostic evaluation both to determine whether a diagnosis of panic disorder is warranted and to reveal the presence of other psychiatric or general medical conditions. Evaluation of a patient with panic disorder frequently involves a number of physicians. The psychiatrist with responsibility for the care of the patient should oversee the evaluation. The general principles and components of a complete psychiatric evaluation have been outlined in the American Psychiatric Association's *Practice Guideline for Psychiatric Evaluation of Adults* (15; included in this volume). This should include a history of the present illness and current symptoms; past psychiatric history; general medical history and history of substance use disorders; personal history (e.g., psychological development, response to life transitions and major life events); social, occupational, and family history; review of the patient's medications; review of systems; mental status examination; physical examination; and diagnostic tests as indicated.

2. Evaluating particular symptoms

Although patients with panic disorder share common features of the illness, there are important interindividual differences. The frequency of panic attacks varies widely among patients, and the constellation of symptoms for each attack also differs. Some patients complain, for example, of attacks that primarily involve cardiovascular symptoms, such as palpitations, chest pain, and paresthesia, while others are more overwhelmed by cognitive symptoms, such as depersonalization and the fear of "losing one's mind." The amount of anticipatory anxiety and the degree of phobic avoidance also vary from patient to patient. Many patients with panic disorder are not highly avoidant; at the opposite extreme are patients who will not leave the house without a trusted companion. It is critical to be sensitive to these individual differences in the elements of panic disorder among patients for two reasons. First, it is important for the patient to feel that the psychiatrist understands accurately the patient's individual experience of panic. Second, treatment may be influenced by the particular constellation of symptoms and other problems of a given patient.

Therefore, it is important to carefully assess the frequency and nature of a patient's panic attacks. It is helpful for patients to monitor their panic attacks, using techniques such as keeping a daily diary, in order to gather data regarding the relationship of panic symptoms to internal stimuli (e.g., emotions) and external stimuli (e.g., substances, particular situations or settings). Such monitoring can be therapeutic.

3. Evaluating types and severity of functional impairment

The degree of functional impairment varies considerably among patients with panic disorder. It is increasingly recognized that resolution of panic attacks, even though they are the core symptom of panic disorder, may be insufficient to warrant the term "clinical remission." As already mentioned, some patients have such high levels of anticipatory anxiety that even when the panic attacks are gone they continue to live restricted lives because of fear. Varying levels of phobic avoidance also determine the degree of impairment experienced by patients with panic disorder. The avoidance of common situations and places, such as driving, restaurants, shopping malls, and elevators, is a cardinal symptom of panic disorder and obviously leads to considerable inability to function in both social and work roles. Sometimes a patient is more focused on the attacks themselves and relegates phobic avoidance to secondary importance. There are situations in which phobic avoidance becomes such a routine part of the patient's life that both the patient and the family are actually reluctant to see it remit. A patient who is homebound because of panic disorder, for example, may have assumed all of the household chores for the family for years. Remission of this kind of phobic avoidance leads to the desire to engage in activities outside of the home, thus leaving a gap. Without recognizing this, family members can tacitly undermine a potentially successful treatment to avoid disrupting their ingrained patterns. In dealing with phobic avoidance and the range of functional impairment seen in patients with panic disorder, it is critical to determine exactly what the patient defines as a satisfactory outcome. The patient should be encouraged to define a desirable level of functioning for himself or herself. Treatment of panic disorder should include substantial effort to alleviate or minimize phobic avoidance. Even after the panic attacks have subsided, the patient may continue to have significant limitations in activities that need to be addressed in treatment.

4. Establishing and maintaining a therapeutic alliance

By the very nature of the illness, many patients with panic disorder are extremely anxious about all treatment interventions. Panic disorder is usually a chronic, long-term condition for which adherence to a treatment plan is important. Hence, a strong treatment alliance is crucial. It is often the case that the treatment of panic disorder involves asking the patient to do things that may be frightening and uncomfortable, such as confronting phobic situations. Here again, a strong treatment alliance is necessary to support the patient in doing these things. Patients with panic disorder are generally very sensitive to separations and need to know that the psychiatrist will be available to answer questions in case of emergencies. Careful attention to the patient's fears and wishes with regard to his or her treatment is essential in establishing and maintaining the therapeutic alliance. Management of the therapeutic alliance should include an awareness of transference and countertransference phenomena and requires sensitive management by the psychiatrist, even if not directly addressed.

5. Monitoring the patient's psychiatric status

As treatment progresses, the different elements of panic disorder often resolve at different points. Usually, panic attacks are controlled first, but subthreshold panic attacks may linger and require further treatment. The fear that attacks may occur in the future often continues even after the attacks themselves appear to have ceased. The psychiatrist should continue to monitor the status of all of the symptoms with which the patient originally presented and should monitor the success of the treatment plan on an ongoing basis.

Finally, many illnesses, including depression and substance use disorders, co-occur with panic disorder at higher rates than are seen in the general population. Depression can develop even during successful treatment of panic disorder. Failure to recognize an emergent depression can seriously compromise therapeutic outcome.

6. Providing education to the patient and, when appropriate, to the family

Many patients with panic disorder believe they are suffering from a disorder of an organ system other than the central nervous system. They may fervently believe they have heart or lung disease. On the other hand, the significant others of patients with panic disorder frequently insist that absolutely nothing is wrong with the patient, using as evidence the fact that extensive medical testing has yielded unremarkable results (16). Under these circumstances, the patient becomes demoralized and isolated while the family can become angry or rejecting. Educating both the family and the patient and emphasizing that panic disorder is a real illness requiring support and treatment can be critical in some situations. Regardless of the method of treatment selected, successful therapies of panic disorder usually begin by explaining to the patient that the attacks themselves are not life threatening; the family may be helped to understand that panic attacks are terrifying to the patient and that the disorder, unless treated, is debilitating.

7. Working with other physicians

Patients with panic disorder often have long-standing relationships with other physicians. Because the patient is often convinced that the panic attacks represent serious abnormalities of other organ systems, a variety of general medical physicians may be involved. Psychiatric management usually requires two approaches in such cases. First, the psychiatrist may be called on to educate nonpsychiatric physicians about the ability of panic attacks to masquerade as many other general medical conditions. Although a general medical evaluation is necessary to rule out important treatable general medical conditions, there is usually little to be gained from extensive medical testing. Attempting to diagnose and treat a variety of nonspecific medical complaints sometimes only delays initiation of treatment of the panic disorder itself. Second, nonpsychiatric physicians can become frustrated with patients with panic disorder. The psychiatrist may need to intervene to ensure that the patient with panic disorder continues to receive an appropriate level of medical care from the primary care physician and medical specialists.

8. Enhancing treatment compliance

The treatment of panic disorder involves confronting many things that the patient fears. Patients are often afraid of medically adverse events; hence, they fear taking medication and are very sensitive to all somatic sensations induced by them. Some psychotherapies require the patient to confront phobic situations and often to keep careful records of anxious thoughts. These can also cause an initial increase in anxiety for the patient. The anxiety produced by treatment may lead to noncompliance. Patients stop taking medication abruptly or fail to complete required assignments during behavioral therapy. Recognition of this possibility guides the physician to design an approach to treatment that encourages the patient to articulate his or her fears. The treatment must be conducted in a completely supportive environment so that missed sessions and lapses in taking medication or carrying out behavioral and cognitive tasks are understood as part of the illness or as manifestations of issues in the therapist-patient relationship.

Family members may play a helpful role in improving treatment compliance. If compliance is not improved with discussion of fears, reassurance, nonpunitive acceptance, educational measures, and similar measures, it may be an indication of more complex resistance that is out of the patient's awareness and may be an indication for a psychodynamic treatment approach.

9. Working with the patient to address early signs of relapse

Studies have shown that panic disorder can be a chronic illness. Sometimes, an exacerbation of symptoms can occur even while the patient is undergoing treatment. This can be disconcerting and needs to be dealt with in two ways: by reassuring the patient that fluctuations in symptom levels can occur during treatment before an acceptable level of remission is reached and by evaluating whether changes in the treatment plan are warranted. Although treatment works for most patients to reduce the burden of panic disorder, patients may continue to have lingering symptoms, including occasional panic attacks of minor severity and residual avoidance. Depression can occur at any time. Relapse following treatment cessation is also always possible. Patients need to be instructed that panic disorder sometimes recurs and that if it does it is important to initiate treatment quickly to avoid the onset of complications such as phobic avoidance (17). The patient should know that he or she is welcome to contact the psychiatrist and that rapid reinitiation of treatment almost always results in improvement.

B. INTERPRETING RESULTS FROM STUDIES OF TREATMENTS FOR PANIC DISORDER

1. Measurement of outcomes

In the following sections the available data on the efficacy of treatments for panic disorder are reviewed. Short-term efficacy has usually been evaluated in 6–12-week clinical trials by observing the change in symptom ratings over the course of treatment. These outcome measures all assess a variety of panic and phobia symptoms, generally derived from the DSM-IV definition of panic attacks. Both the patient and the clinician can be asked to rate the presence and severity of a patient's symptoms. Patients have been designated as "panic free" if they do not have a sufficient number of panic symptoms to meet the DSM-IV criteria for panic disorder. However, patients labeled as "panic free" may not necessarily be free of all panic symptoms (i.e., symptom free). Another outcome measure that has been employed to assess short-term treatment response is the proportion of patients achieving remission (usually defined as the absence of panic attacks within a specified period of time).

The long-term efficacy of treatments has been measured in terms of relapse rates among panic-free or symptom-free patients receiving treatment over the course of several years. A variety of definitions of relapse have been used, based on the emergence of a certain number of symptoms or based on the percentage of change in scores on symptom rating scales. In some studies, requests for or use of additional treatment have been considered indicative of relapse; while such outcome measures may reflect an intervention's effect on patient functioning, as well as symptoms, they may also be affected by other clinical and nonclinical factors.

2. Issues in study design and interpretation

When evaluating clinical trials of medications for panic disorder, it is important to take into consideration whether a placebo group was used, the type of placebo, and the response rate in the placebo group. Response rates as high as 75% have been observed among patients receiving placebo in clinical trials of patients with panic disorder (18). High placebo response rates could explain much of the observed treatment effect in uncontrolled trials or make significant treatment effects more difficult to detect in controlled trials. It is also important to consider the dose of medication(s) employed in pharmacologic trials.

When evaluating studies of psychosocial treatments, such as CBT, which consist of multiple elements, it may be difficult to know which elements are responsible for producing beneficial outcomes. It is also important to consider the nature of the elements that were used. For example, although the types of CBT used in recent trials have been rigorously defined and have been similar, they have not been identical (19–21).

Another factor to consider is the use of medications that are not prescribed as part of the treatment protocol. For example, patients in studies of CBT may be using prescription medications that are not controlled for. In addition, patients in medication studies may be taking additional doses of the tested medications or other antipanic medications (either explicitly, as doses taken as needed, or surreptitiously). Studies that monitor such occurrences have shown rates as high as 33% (22).

C. SPECIFIC PSYCHOSOCIAL INTERVENTIONS

Psychosocial interventions, such as psychotherapy, have traditionally been the predominant psychiatric treatment for patients with panic disorder. However, unlike medication therapies, it has been more difficult to clearly define aspects of psychosocial therapies, such as the elements they consist of and the "doses." Only recently have some psychosocial treatments been more formally operationalized and evaluated.

At the present time, cognitive behavioral treatments for panic disorder have been the most well studied. Other forms of psychotherapy are widely used for patients with panic disorder but have undergone less empirical testing. These treatments may be very different from cognitive behavioral interventions. One important difference is that many forms of psychotherapy focus broadly on the patient's current life and history, rather than more narrowly on panic-related symptoms.

1. Cognitive behavioral therapy

a) Goals

CBT is a symptom-oriented approach to the treatment of panic disorder. The treatments employed in recent clinical trials contain the following key components:

- psychoeducation
- continuous panic monitoring
- breathing retraining
- cognitive restructuring focused on correction of catastrophic misinterpretation of bodily sensations
- exposure to fear cues

The types of therapy encompassed by CBT are likely to be more diverse, and such diverse approaches have not been studied.

(1) Psychoeducation

CBT always begins with one or more sessions for the purpose of psychoeducation. The aims of such sessions are to identify and name the patient's symptoms, provide a direct explanation of the basis for the symptoms, and outline a plan for the treatment. The initial education for patients is generally imparted in a didactic fashion. Exercises that actually evoke panic symptoms, such as hyperventilation, may be useful for illustrating the role of interoceptive (i.e., internal) cues in panic disorder.

(2) Continuous panic monitoring

Patients are also instructed to continuously monitor their panic attacks and record their anxious cognitions, using techniques such as keeping a daily diary. Patients are informed that this will help in the assessment of the frequency and nature of their panic attacks and provide data regarding the relationship of panic symptoms to internal stimuli (e.g., emotions) and external stimuli (e.g., substances).

(3) Breathing retraining

Next, the therapist introduces an anxiety management technique, such as abdominal breathing, to control the physiologic reactivity. The patient is asked to practice this technique daily.

(4) Cognitive restructuring

These techniques are used to identify and counter fear of bodily sensations. Most commonly, such thinking involves overestimation of the probability of a negative consequence and catastrophic thinking about the meaning of such sensations. Patients are encouraged to consider the evidence and to think of alternative possible outcomes following the experience of the bodily cue. Part of this process involves identifying the likely origin of the feared sensations and/or any misinformation about the meaning of the sensations. The cognitive restructuring component of CBT is usually conducted by using a Socratic teaching method.

(5) Exposure to fear cues

The final and central component of the treatment involves actual exposure to fear cues. In order to conduct such exposure, the therapist frequently works with the patient to identify a hi-

TABLE 1. Results of 12 Randomized Controlled Studies of Cognitive Behavioral Therapy for Patients With Panic Disorder

Treatment	Response Rate (%)
Cognitive behavioral therapy (12–15 weeks)	
Intent to treat	66
Completers	78
Control treatments	
Wait list	26
Relaxation only	
Intent to treat	45
Completers	56
Placebo	
Intent to treat	34
Completers	33
Supportive psychotherapy completers	
16 weeks	78
8 weeks	25
4 weeks	8

erarchy of fear-evoking situations. The degree of anxiety elicited in each of these situations is graded on a 0–10 scale, and several situations that evoke anxiety at each level are documented. The patient is then asked to enter situations, usually at the low end of the hierarchy, on a regular (usually daily) basis until the fear has attenuated. The situation that arouses the next level of anxiety is then targeted. Employing more intense initial exposures and not proceeding in a graduated manner, referred to as "flooding," has also been used (23). Examples of exposures to panic cues are having patients run in place, spin in a desk chair, and breathe through a straw. The cues for panic attacks are generally interoceptive, while those for agoraphobia may be either interoceptive or environmental (24). Interoceptive exposures are usually conducted in the therapist's office and at home in naturalistic situations. Agoraphobic exposure is best carried out in the actual situation(s).

b) Efficacy

CBT efficacy studies have generally involved either cognitive behavioral treatment (as just described) or cognitive therapy. Studies of agoraphobia use behavioral exposure treatment (25, 26). A recent presentation of data from 26 subjects supports the efficacy of combining these approaches (27).

Twelve randomized controlled trials of CBT for panic disorder were identified and reviewed (19–21, 28–36). The length of treatment varied from 4 weeks to 16 weeks, and the number of subjects per cell varied from 9 to 34. The degree of agoraphobia was none to mild in most of the studies. The control treatment was a wait list in five of these, a relaxation component alone in five, supportive psychotherapy in three, and a placebo medication in two. The results are shown in Table 1. The results in the control conditions suggest that length of treatment and perhaps the specific interventions used may be important in determining efficacy. However, more data are necessary before firm conclusions can be drawn. Also of note, 38% of the patients in the eight studies for which medication data were given were taking some medications that were not specifically part of the study protocols (range, 0%–70%).

Several studies have examined the use of one component of CBT, behavioral exposure, for specifically agoraphobia symptoms in patients with panic disorder (35, 37–41). These studies support the efficacy of behavioral treatment in reducing phobic symptoms for patients who are able and willing to complete a treatment program of a few months. Patients who were virtually homebound were included in some of these studies, indicating that there is no need to reserve this treatment for milder or less chronic cases.

Long-term follow-ups of panic disorder range from 6 months to 8 years (20, 29, 33, 36–38, 42, 43). The three studies that included at least 1 year of follow-up showed promising results, with an average of 88% of subjects remaining panic free. However, a closer look at the results in one study indicates that the percentage of patients who remained panic free throughout the 24-month period was only about 50%, and only 21% were panic free and had achieved "high end-state functioning" consistently throughout the follow-up period (43). "High end-state functioning" refers to a low severity of overall panic disorder symptoms, including anticipatory anxiety, limited-symptom episodes, and phobic symptoms in addition to panic attacks. These follow-up results are comparable to those found in medication treatment follow-up studies. One review of a series of studies also indicated that the improvement in agoraphobia and in disability after exposure therapy persists for 4 to 8 years (44).

c) Adverse effects

Cognitive behavioral exposure is a relatively benign type of intervention. However, exposure to feared situations does initially increase anxiety, and this could be considered an adverse effect. Sometimes the patient develops dependence on the therapist, which may need to be addressed. Another limitation of CBT is that it may not address other psychological problems that patients with panic disorder may have. While these problems may be less prominent than the panic disorder symptoms for many patients, some patients present with serious current and/or ongoing environmental stresses and/or other comorbid psychiatric disorders. For these patients, panic symptom relief may be less helpful, or even relatively unimportant, as a focus of treatment.

d) Implementation issues

(1) Patient acceptance

CBT requires considerable time and discipline on the part of the patient. Exercises must be practiced daily, and monitoring must be done continuously. In addition, patients must be willing to confront feared situations. Approximately 10%–30% of patients are unable or unwilling to complete these requirements (19, 29, 30, 33). The treatment is far less effective for these patients. Despite these limitations, however, data from several studies (39, 45, 46) indicate that more patients with panic disorder who seek treatment are willing to accept a nonmedication approach than medication.

(2) Group treatment

CBT for panic disorder is usually provided individually, in approximately 12 sessions, but there is evidence that group treatments may be equally effective (33, 47–51). Exposure treatments for patients with agoraphobia are often conducted in groups, and this approach has been used in many studies documenting efficacy. In addition, the inclusion of the spouse or significant other in agoraphobic treatment has been studied and found to enhance treatment efficacy (52). In this couples approach, the support person is included in psychoeducation sessions and is given a role as an assistant in exposure exercises.

(3) Withdrawal of anxiolytics

The discontinuation of benzodiazepines, such as alprazolam or clonazepam, for patients with panic disorder is often accompanied by withdrawal symptoms and relapse into panic disorder. Several studies have shown that using adjunctive CBT in this clinical situation results in successful discontinuation of the benzodiazepine for significantly more patients (53–55).

2. Psychodynamic psychotherapy

a) Goals

Psychodynamic psychotherapy is based on the concept that symptoms result from mental processes that may be outside of the patient's conscious awareness and that elucidating these processes can lead to remission of symptoms (56, 57). Moreover, in order to lessen vulnerability to panic, the psychodynamic therapist considers it necessary to identify and alter core conflicts (56). The goals of psychodynamic psychotherapy range considerably and may be more ambitious and require more time to achieve than those of a more symptom-focused treatment approach. There are some case reports of brief dynamic psychotherapies that took no longer than CBT to achieve reasonable treatment goals for patients with panic disorder (58–61). One recent study compared CBT to an emotion-focused brief psychotherapy and showed them to be equivalent (62). When combined with short-term symptomatic treatment, this approach may produce optimal long-term outcome for some patients.

b) Efficacy

There are no published reports of randomized controlled trials evaluating the efficacy of this approach for panic disorder. Studies documenting a role for both recent and early life events in the development of panic disorder, as well as a number of studies showing that patients with panic disorder remember the behavior and attitudes of their parents as more overprotective and less caring than do control subjects, provide indirect support for some aspects of the theory. One study documented the usefulness of psychodynamic psychotherapy as an adjunct to medication for outpatients with and without agoraphobia (63). In a second study (35), the control treatment of reflective listening produced results equivalent to those for CBT. In addition, a number of anecdotal case reports of successful psychodynamic treatment appear in the literature. Most of these are reports of isolated cases rather than systematic consecutive case series, and reliable, validated outcome measures were not used. Milrod et al. (56) have published a treatment manual for panic-focused psychodynamic psychotherapy, and a pilot test of outcome and of the ability of trained psychoanalysts to follow this manual is currently under way. An ongoing randomized controlled trial uses a manualized psychodynamically informed approach called “emotion-focused treatment.” However, this treatment also contains cognitive, behavioral, and experiential components and differs substantially from the treatment described by Milrod et al.

c) Adverse effects

In general, psychodynamic psychotherapy has relatively few side effects. As with any psychotherapy, psychological dependency must be skillfully managed so as to facilitate treatment rather than prolong it unduly.

d) Implementation issues

In psychodynamic psychotherapy, the successful emotional and cognitive understanding of the various elements of psychic conflict (impulses, conscience and internal standards that are often excessively harsh, psychological defensive patterns, and realistic concerns) and reintegration of these elements in a more realistic and adaptive way may result in symptom resolution and fewer relapses. To achieve this insight and acceptance, the therapist places the symptoms in the context of the patient’s life history and current realities and extensively uses the therapeutic relationship to focus on unconscious symptom determinants.

There are a variety of methods for conducting dynamic psychotherapy (64). Generally, the clinical approach of dynamic psychiatrists is less directive than that of behavioral therapists or psychopharmacologists. In psychodynamic psychotherapy, it is important to consider the risks and benefits of substituting the therapist’s executive functions for those of the patient. Transference considerations and the patient’s freedom to associate into unexpected material must be taken into account. Some CBT techniques can be combined with psychodynamic techniques (56, 65). Clinically, as with other treatment approaches, patient factors are important determinants of the length and intensity of appropriate treatment and of specific interventions the psychiatrist may employ.

3. Combined treatments

Investigators have examined use of the combination of medication and CBT for patients with panic disorder and agoraphobia. Several short-term treatment studies have shown that the combination of the TCA imipramine with one component of CBT, behavioral exposure, may be superior to either treatment alone (66–72). Another study showed that the SSRI paroxetine plus cognitive therapy worked significantly better for patients with panic disorder than cognitive therapy plus placebo (73).

There has been one study of the combination of psychodynamic psychotherapy with medication (63). This study suggested that psychodynamic psychotherapy may improve the long-term outcome of medication-treated patients.

4. Group therapy

Reports in the literature of group therapy in the treatment of panic disorder have consisted primarily of cognitive behavioral approaches. Telch et al. (33) found a greater proportion of panic-free subjects among those who had been given group CBT than among delayed-treatment control subjects (85% versus 30%); the authors concluded that the improvements with group CBT were comparable to those in studies of individually administered CBT and pharmacologic treatment. Fifteen patients who had incomplete responses to pharmacotherapy were treated by Pollack et al. (74) with 12 weeks of group CBT and had subsequent improvements in the number of panic attacks and in scores on the Clinical Global Impression. CBT was also used concurrently with medication in a group setting for acute treatment of panic disorder (75).

Mindfulness meditation is an additional treatment proposed for panic disorder (76). This treatment is administered in a group format and includes an attention-focusing component and relaxation strategies. In one study, an 8-week trial of mindfulness meditation resulted in significant reductions in ratings of anxiety symptoms and panic attacks (77). However, it has not been compared to other, proven treatments. A 3-year follow-up showed continued beneficial effects. Other types of groups, such as medication support groups and consumer-run self-help groups, can also provide useful adjunctive experiences for patients with panic disorder.

5. Marital and family therapy

Some of the earliest theories of agoraphobia postulated an interpersonal basis for the symptoms, and some researchers have investigated the possibility that the results of behavioral treatment of agoraphobia can be enhanced by treatment of the couple or family system. While the issue has not been studied directly, patients with panic disorder without agoraphobia have symptoms that can disrupt day-to-day patterns of relationships and may place a family member in a caretaker or rescuer role. Increased dependency needs of patients with panic disorder may lead to frustration in family members, and relationships may be jeopardized. Empirical studies of the quality of marital relationships have provided mixed results; some investigators have reported that patients with agoraphobia and their spouses are not different from happily married couples (78, 79), while others show problems (80). Several studies have documented increased marital distress in some patients following successful treatment for agoraphobia (81, 82), although in general these investigators found treatment to improve marital satisfaction. In summary, there seems to be a subgroup of these patients who experience marital and/or other family distress and may benefit from a family intervention (83).

There is no published research on the use of marital or family therapy alone or with medication for the treatment of panic or agoraphobia, so no conclusions can be drawn about the potential efficacy of such an approach. Education of family members about the nature of the illness and inclusion of the spouse in the treatment may be helpful. There is a small literature exploring the benefits of including the spouse in treatment. Overall, it is clear that such a strategy is not detrimental, and results are mixed as to whether it helps. Two studies by the same research group (84, 85) show the superiority of treatment that includes the spouse as co-therapist over treatment without spouse involvement. One study (86) documented further improvement by addition of communication skills training.

6. Patient support groups

Patient support groups are very helpful for some patients suffering from panic disorder. Patients have the opportunity to learn that they are not unique in experiencing panic attacks and to share ways of coping with the illness. Support groups may also have a positive effect in encouraging patients to confront phobic situations. Finally, family members of patients with panic disorder may benefit from the educational aspects of patient support groups. In deciding to refer a patient to a support group, however, it is imperative that the psychiatrist obtain information about the nature of the group and the credentials of its leader(s). Support groups are not a substitute for effective treatment; rather, they are complementary.

D. PHARMACOLOGIC INTERVENTIONS

Medications have been known to be useful in the treatment of panic disorder for over 30 years. Most studies have focused on their ability to stop or reduce the frequency of panic attacks, but many have also addressed the effect of medication on anticipatory anxiety, phobic avoidance, associated depression, and global function. Medications from several classes have been shown to be effective. As discussed in Section III.B, when interpreting results from trials of pharmacologic interventions, it is important to consider whether a placebo group was used and the response rate in the placebo group.

1. Selective serotonin reuptake inhibitors

a) Goals

The primary goals of SSRI therapy of panic disorder are to reduce the intensity and frequency of panic attacks, to reduce anticipatory anxiety, and to treat associated depression. Often, successful therapy with SSRIs also leads to a reduction in phobic avoidance.

b) Efficacy

Four SSRIs are now available in the United States: fluoxetine, sertraline, paroxetine, and fluvoxamine. Clinical trials indicating that each of them is effective for panic disorder have now been completed.

Results of one multicenter double-blind, randomized trial that compared two doses of fluoxetine (10 mg/day and 20 mg/day) with placebo have been presented (87). Reductions in panic symptoms, measured by using several instruments, were significantly greater for patients treated with 20 mg/day of fluoxetine than those given placebo. Fluoxetine at 10 mg/day showed superiority over placebo for only a few assessments of panic symptoms. Two open studies of fluoxetine treatment for panic disorder have been published. Gorman et al. (88) found that of 16 patients whose fluoxetine dose began at 10 mg/day and was raised in 10-mg/day increments each week, only 44% eventually responded to fluoxetine (mean dose among responders was 27.1 mg/day); however, 90% of the nonresponders had been unable to tolerate the side effects. Schneier et al. (89), initiating fluoxetine treatment at 5 mg/day and using a more conservative titration schedule with 25 patients, found that 76% had moderate to marked improvements (median dose among responders was 20 mg/day).

Results from two multicenter randomized, double-blind, placebo-controlled trials of sertraline have been presented at recent public meetings but had not been published by 1996. Wolkow et al. (90) reported that patients treated with sertraline had a significantly greater reduction in panic attack frequency than those given placebo (79% versus 59% reduction). Similarly, Baumel et al. (91) found a significantly greater reduction in panic attack frequency for patients given sertraline than for those given placebo (77% versus 51% reduction).

Paroxetine, which has received approval from the U.S. Food and Drug Administration (FDA) for treatment of panic disorder, has been studied in several placebo-controlled trials. One double-blind trial compared paroxetine plus cognitive therapy to placebo plus cognitive therapy; significantly more patients in the paroxetine group (82% versus 50%) achieved a 50% reduction in panic attack frequency (73). Ballenger et al. (92) compared placebo to three doses of paroxetine; the percentages of patients given paroxetine at daily doses of 40 mg, 20 mg, and 10 mg and patients given placebo who were subsequently panic free were 86%, 65%, 67%, and 50%, respectively (only the difference between 40-mg paroxetine and placebo was statistically significant). In another double-blind trial (93), 367 patients were randomly assigned to paroxetine, clomipramine, or placebo. Paroxetine (at a mean final dose of 39 mg/day) was found to be superior to placebo and comparable to clomipramine (mean final dose of 92 mg/day).

Several controlled trials of fluvoxamine for panic disorder have also been published. In one (94), more patients who had been given fluvoxamine than placebo were panic free (61% versus 36%). Black et al. (32) compared fluvoxamine to a modified form of cognitive therapy and to placebo; there were more panic-free patients in the fluvoxamine group (81%) than in either the cognitive therapy (50%) or placebo (39%) group (only the difference between fluvoxamine and placebo was significant). In other studies fluvoxamine has proved to be better than maprotiline and an experimental serotonin-blocking medication, ritanserin (95, 96). Citalopram, an SSRI available in Europe, was studied in one double-blind trial in which 475 patients were randomly assigned to citalopram (10–15 mg/day, 20–30 mg/day, or 40–60 mg/day), clomipramine (60–90 mg/day), or placebo (97). Citalopram at 20–30 or 40–60 mg/day was significantly superior to placebo; citalopram at 20–30 mg/day was more effective than 40–60 mg/day and comparable to clomipramine.

Although the database for SSRI therapy of panic disorder is not yet as extensive as that for either imipramine or alprazolam, there are sufficient controlled trials available to state that these medications have demonstrated short-term efficacy in treating panic attacks. A meta-analysis (98) of 27 studies involving 2,348 patients in randomized, prospective, double-blind, placebo-controlled trials suggested that the effect size for improvement with SSRIs in panic disorder is significantly greater than for alprazolam or imipramine.

c) Side effects

SSRIs are safer than TCAs. They are not lethal in overdose and have few serious effects on cardiovascular function. Because they lack clinically significant anticholinergic effects, they can be prescribed to patients with prostatic hypertrophy or narrow-angle glaucoma. Because elimination of SSRIs involves hepatic metabolism, doses need to be adjusted for patients with liver disease and dysfunction.

The main side effects of SSRIs are headaches, irritability, nausea and other gastrointestinal complaints, insomnia, sexual dysfunctions, increased anxiety, drowsiness, and tremor. There are scattered reports in the literature of extrapyramidal side effects, but these have not been observed in large multicenter trials and may be idiosyncratic. There is no evidence that SSRIs increase suicidal or violent behavior.

There are a number of published case reports of a withdrawal syndrome caused by the abrupt discontinuation of SSRIs (99). Black et al. (32) abruptly withdrew fluvoxamine from patients with panic disorder after 8 months of treatment. A withdrawal syndrome characterized by dizziness, incoordination, headache, irritability, and nausea began within 24 hours, peaked at day 5 after withdrawal, and was generally resolved by day 14.

d) Implementation issues

(1) Dose

As is the case with tricyclics, some patients with panic disorder experience an initial feeling of increased anxiety, jitteriness, shakiness, and agitation when beginning treatment with an SSRI. For that reason, the initial dose should be lower than that usually prescribed to patients with depression. Louie et al. (100), for example, found that patients with both panic disorder and major depression were less tolerant of higher doses of fluoxetine than patients with major depression alone. The recommended starting doses for SSRIs are as follows: fluoxetine, 10 mg/day or less; sertraline, 25 mg/day; paroxetine, 10 mg/day; and fluvoxamine, 50 mg/day. In the few published studies, fluoxetine has been found to be effective at doses ranging between 5 and 80 mg/day. Recent case reports suggest that for some patients fluoxetine taken in doses as low as 1–2 mg/day may be effective (101). For paroxetine, in a clinical trial the lowest dose that was significantly superior to placebo was 40 mg/day, although some patients did respond to lower doses (92). For sertraline, a fixed-dose study suggests that doses of 50, 100, and 200 mg/day are equally effective for panic disorder (102). Fluvoxamine has been found effective in doses up to 300 mg/day. It is recommended that the initial low dose of the SSRI be maintained for several days and then increased to a more standard daily dose (e.g., 20 mg of fluoxetine or paroxetine, 50 mg of sertraline, 150 mg of fluvoxamine). Patients who fail to respond after several weeks may then do better with a further dose increase.

(2) Length of treatment

Studies of SSRI therapy for panic disorder have been conducted over 6–12 weeks and even longer periods. It is generally accepted that response does not occur for at least 4 weeks, and some patients will not realize full response for 8–12 weeks.

There are few data on the optimum length of treatment following response. Gergel et al. (103) selected patients who had responded to paroxetine in an acute-phase trial and randomly assigned them to placebo or 10, 20, or 40 mg/day of paroxetine for a 12-week maintenance period. After the maintenance phase, there was a significantly higher rate of relapse among the responders who had crossed over to placebo than those whose paroxetine treatment had been maintained (30% versus 5%).

LeCrubier et al. (93) evaluated the efficacy of paroxetine, clomipramine, and placebo for patients who completed a 12-week double-blind trial and then chose to continue receiving the randomly assigned treatment for an additional 36 weeks. Compared with the placebo-treated patients, the paroxetine patients experienced significantly greater reductions in panic symptoms, and a larger proportion remained free of panic attacks throughout the long-term study. There were no significant differences in efficacy between paroxetine and clomipramine.

If the medications are to be discontinued after prolonged use, it is recommended that the SSRI dose be tapered over several weeks. It is not clear whether this is necessary for fluoxetine, which has the longest half-life of any medication in the class.

2. Tricyclic antidepressants

a) Goals

The primary goals of TCA therapy of panic disorder are to reduce the intensity and frequency of panic attacks, to reduce anticipatory anxiety, and to treat associated depression. Successful tricyclic therapy also leads to a reduction in phobic avoidance.

b) Efficacy

The first controlled study documenting the efficacy of the tricyclic imipramine in blocking panic attacks was conducted by Klein and published in 1964 (104). In this study, imipramine was superior to placebo for antipanic effect and for change in the Clinical Global Impression (CGI). Since then, 15 controlled trials (16, 66, 105–117) have shown that imipramine is effective in reducing panic. After treatment with imipramine, 45%–70% of the patients were found to be panic free, compared to 15%–50% of those receiving placebo. In addition, patients with panic disorder who were treated with imipramine had less phobic avoidance and anticipatory anxiety than those receiving placebo. Typically, patients treated with imipramine realize a substantial reduction in panic after a minimum of 4 weeks of treatment; antipanic effect may not be fully experienced until 8–12 weeks of therapy. Anticipatory anxiety usually responds after the panic attacks have been reduced, and phobic avoidance is the last to be affected.

Given the equivalency of tricyclic agents in treating depression, there is little reason to expect tricyclics other than imipramine to work less well for panic disorder. However, very few controlled studies have evaluated other tricyclics for panic disorder. Lydiard et al. (18) found desipramine to be superior to placebo for a global measure of phobic avoidance and score on the Hamilton Rating Scale for Anxiety, but there was only a trend toward superiority ($p<0.09$) on the CGI. Although 85% of the desipramine-treated patients had reductions in panic attacks, this was not significantly different from the 76% for the placebo-treated patients. One double-blind comparative study showed the tricyclic maprotiline to be less effective than the SSRI fluvoxamine (118).

Two studies have shown that clomipramine is at least as effective as imipramine. There are anecdotal reports that clomipramine is actually somewhat more effective than imipramine; however, the evidence from the few studies that have directly compared the two is equivocal. In one double-blind, placebo-controlled study (106), clomipramine (mean dose, 109 mg/day) was superior to both imipramine (mean dose, 124 mg/day) and placebo in panic reduction and decrease in score on the Hamilton anxiety scale. In a nonblind, uncontrolled trial, Cassano et al. (119) did not find significant differences between clomipramine (mean dose, 128 mg/day) and imipramine (mean dose, 144 mg/day).

c) Side effects

The major adverse side effects common to all tricyclic medications and reported in studies of panic disorder treatment are 1) anticholinergic: dry mouth, constipation, difficulty urinating, increased heart rate, and blurry vision; 2) increased sweating; 3) sleep disturbance; 4) orthostatic hypotension and dizziness; 5) fatigue and weakness; 6) cognitive disturbance; 7) weight gain, especially for long-term users; and 8) sexual dysfunction (120). Higher doses are associated with a higher dropout rate in research studies. For example, Mavissakalian and Perel (110) reported that among subjects treated with an average of 35, 99, and 200 mg/day of imipramine, the dropout rates due to drug side effects were 6%, 15%, and 36%, respectively. TCAs should not be prescribed for patients with panic disorder who also have acute narrow-angle glaucoma or clinically significant prostatic hypertrophy. Patients with cardiac conduction abnormalities may experience a severe or fatal arrhythmia with tricyclics. Overdoses with TCAs can lead to significant cardiac toxicity and fatality; for this reason, TCAs may be suboptimal for suicidal patients. Elderly patients may be at increased risk of falls because of orthostatic hypotension caused by tricyclics.

d) Implementation issues

(1) Dose

Clinicians have often noticed, and research studies have occasionally shown, that some patients with panic disorder are exquisitely sensitive to both the beneficial and adverse effects of tricyclics. Zitrin et al. (66) found that 20% of the patients in their study could not tolerate doses higher than 10 mg/day but still experienced panic blockade. Lydiard et al. (18) also reported an initial supersensitivity in some patients with panic disorder. Patients sometimes experience a stimulant-like response, including anxiety, agitation, or insomnia, when treatment with antidepressant medication of any class is initiated. For this reason, it is recommended that tricyclics be started for patients with panic disorder at doses substantially lower than those for patients with depression or other psychiatric conditions. One common strategy is to begin with only 10 mg/day of imipramine and gradually titrate the dose upward over the ensuing weeks.

Few studies have rigorously addressed the optimum dose of tricyclic medication for panic disorder. In most research studies, the mean final dose is approximately 150 mg/day and the maximum final dose is up to 300 mg/day. Mavissakalian and Perel (110) randomly assigned patients with panic disorder to low-dose (mean, 35 mg/day), medium-dose (mean, 99 mg/day), and high-dose (mean, 200 mg/day) imipramine. They found that both the medium and high doses were superior to placebo in reducing panic and not significantly different from each other; the low dose was no more effective than placebo. Given these findings, it is reasonable to titrate the imipramine dose of patients with panic disorder to approximately 100 mg/day and wait for at least 4 weeks to see whether there is a response. If tolerated, the dose can then be increased to as high as 300 mg/day if initial response is either absent or inadequate.

There is a suggestion in the literature that clomipramine may be effective in somewhat lower doses than imipramine. Clomipramine can generally be used effectively with doses less than 150 mg/day. Given the results of the studies by Modigh et al. (106) and Cassano et al. (119), it may be reasonable to administer clomipramine in a dose range of 25–150 mg/day.

(2) Length of treatment

Most controlled trials of tricyclics for the treatment of panic disorder were for a minimum of 8 weeks, and exactly when the patients began to respond has not always been reported. There is general clinical agreement that, similar to the situation with treatment of depression, it may take at least 4 weeks of tricyclic treatment for onset of antipanic effects; patients may not respond until 6 or even 8 weeks, and some additional response has been seen through 12 or more weeks. It is reasonable to wait for at least 6 weeks from initiation of tricyclic treatment, with at least 2 of those weeks at full dose, before deciding whether a tricyclic is effective for a patient with panic disorder. If there is some response at this point, the clinician and patient may wait longer to see how full the response will be by 8–12 weeks.

There are few long-term studies of tricyclic treatment for panic disorder in the literature. Cassano et al. (112) continued to treat patients with imipramine or placebo for 6 months after an acute phase 8-week study and found that imipramine was still superior to placebo for panic reduction. Curtis et al. (113) also maintained patients on a regimen of placebo or imipramine for up to 8 months after acute 8-week treatment and found that the placebo-treated patients had more panic attacks and phobic avoidance and were more likely to drop out of treatment during the maintenance phase. In two small studies, Mavissakalian and Perel (121, 122) assessed the relapse rates of patients nonrandomly assigned to either a) discontinuation of imipramine following 6 months of full-dose imipramine plus 1 year of half-dose imipramine maintenance treatment or b) discontinuation following 6 months of acute imipramine treatment alone. They found significantly less relapse among the patients who had been in treatment for 18 months than among those who had been treated for 6 months. These studies suggest that maintenance treatment is beneficial for at least a year after a patient has achieved a response to a tricyclic. The exact relapse rate following discontinuation of imipramine or other tricyclic therapy is also not known (123, 124).

3. Benzodiazepines

a) Goals

The primary goals of benzodiazepine therapy of panic disorder are to reduce the intensity and frequency of panic attacks and to reduce anticipatory anxiety. Often, successful benzodiazepine therapy also leads to a reduction in phobic avoidance.

b) Efficacy

Alprazolam has been studied more extensively than any other benzodiazepine for the treatment of panic disorder and is approved by the FDA for the treatment of panic disorder. Eleven trials of alprazolam treatment of panic disorder were reviewed, including the Cross-National Collaborative Panic Study, which involved more than 1,000 patients randomly assigned to imipramine, alprazolam, or placebo (125). Nine of the trials were double blind, and seven were placebo controlled. Two meta-analyses of studies on alprazolam treatment for panic disorder were also reviewed.

In six of the seven double-blind, placebo-controlled trials, alprazolam was found to be superior to placebo in the treatment of panic attacks (113, 126–130), while the other one did not assess panic attacks as an outcome measure (131). The percentages of patients who were panic free (generally assessed over a 1-week period) at end point were 55%–75% for alprazolam (at doses of 5–6 mg/day) and 15%–50% for placebo. These percentages represent the "intention to treat" proportions (i.e., the panic-free proportion of the patients who were originally assigned to receive active treatment or placebo at the start of the trial); the differences between the completers were less striking or nonsignificant because of higher dropout rates for the nonresponders in the placebo groups. Alprazolam was superior to placebo in reducing phobic avoidance in five of the six studies in which it was assessed, disability in five of five studies, anticipatory anxiety in three of three studies, and Hamilton anxiety scale scores in six of seven studies. In most of the studies, patients with primary current major depression were excluded and the level of phobic avoidance was moderate.

Four of the 11 trials compared alprazolam to imipramine. Three of these were double blind. Alprazolam and imipramine were comparable in efficacy for panic attacks, phobias, Hamilton anxiety scores, disability, and CGI ratings. There were more dropouts in the imipramine group in three of the four studies.

These data support the efficacy of alprazolam (especially in the 5–6 mg/day range) in treating multiple dimensions of illness in patients with panic disorder who do not have primary current major depression.

Twelve studies regarding other benzodiazepines were also reviewed (126, 128, 132–141), and they support the short-term efficacy of other benzodiazepines for panic disorder. The agents studied include clonazepam (effective in the one double-blind, placebo-controlled trial), diazepam (effective in two of two trials, both double blind and one placebo controlled), and lorazepam (equivalent to alprazolam in three of three double-blind trials). One study showed superiority of imipramine over chlordiazepoxide.

These studies suggest that other benzodiazepines (at least diazepam, clonazepam, and lorazepam), when given in equivalent doses, may be as effective as alprazolam in the treatment of panic disorder.

There was one controlled trial of alprazolam as an adjunct to imipramine for the first 4–6 weeks of treatment (115). The subjects taking alprazolam showed a more rapid therapeutic response, but this was not associated with a lower percentage of treatment dropout. In addition, 10 of 17 patients taking alprazolam were unable to taper from 1.5 mg/day to discontinuation in 2 weeks after 4–6 weeks of treatment.

c) Side effects

The adverse effects of benzodiazepines in patients with panic disorder appear similar to those reported when benzodiazepines are used for other indications and include primarily sedation, fatigue, ataxia, slurred speech, memory impairment, and weakness. Some sedation or drowsiness occurred in 38%–75% of alprazolam-treated subjects and 11%–21% of those taking placebo. Memory problems were reported by up to 15% of patients taking alprazolam and 8.5% of patients taking placebo in the Cross-National Collaborative Panic Study. However, patients may not recognize their own cognitive impairment. It is prudent to be cautious about prescribing benzodiazepines to elderly patients or those with pretreatment cognitive impairment. The risk of falls for the elderly and the increased risk of motor vehicle accidents related to benzodiazepine use should also be considered. Among patients with histories of substance abuse or dependence, benzodiazepine use may aggravate symptoms and should be avoided. In general, however, benzodiazepines seem to be well tolerated in patients with panic disorder with very few serious side effects.

Major concerns about benzodiazepine tolerance and withdrawal have been raised. According to the report of the APA Task Force on Benzodiazepine Dependence, Toxicity, and Abuse, "There are no data to suggest that long-term therapeutic use of benzodiazepines by patients commonly leads to dose escalation or to recreational abuse" (142). However, benzodiazepines may still be underused because of an inappropriate fear of addiction. The studies of long-term alprazolam treatment for panic disorder show that the doses patients use at 32 weeks of treatment are similar to those used at 8 weeks, indicating that, as a group, patients with panic disorder do not escalate alprazolam doses or display tolerance to alprazolam's therapeutic effects, at least in the first 8 months of treatment. However, studies of dose escalation following longer periods of benzodiazepine use are generally lacking.

Six studies regarding discontinuation of alprazolam for patients with panic disorder were reviewed. These studies demonstrated that significant numbers of these patients (ranging from 33% to 100%) are unable to complete a taper of the medication after 6 weeks to 22 months of treatment. One study (143) showed that alprazolam causes significantly more withdrawal symptoms, recurrent panic attacks, and failure to complete the taper than imipramine, and another (144) suggested that patients with panic disorder have more difficulty during tapering of alprazolam than do those with generalized anxiety disorder, even when the patients in both groups are treated with similar doses. Difficulties during taper seem most severe during the last half of the taper period and the first week after the taper is completed. In many instances, it is difficult to determine the extent to which symptoms are due to withdrawal, rebound, or relapse.

The one study comparing diazepam to alprazolam for panic disorder indicated that both are no different from placebo during gradual tapering of the first half of the dose (145). With abrupt discontinuation of the remaining dose, however, alprazolam caused significantly more anxiety, relapse, and rebound. In general, apart from this one study, the issue of discontinuation of benzodiazepines with short versus long half-lives or high versus low potency has not been adequately addressed in relation to panic disorder. The APA task force report on benzodiazepines (142) suggests that there are more difficulties with short-half-life, high-potency compounds. However, studies by Schweizer, Rickels, Weiss, and Zavodnick (129, 143) of benzodiazepine-treated patients showed no significant effect of half-life on the results of a gradual taper but greater withdrawal severity after abrupt discontinuation with compounds having shorter half-lives and with higher daily doses. These studies, although not involving patients with panic disorder specifically, suggest that half-life is less of a factor, or in fact may not be important, given a gradual taper schedule.

Thus, there is no evidence for significant dose escalation in patients with panic disorder (75). However, withdrawal symptoms and symptomatic rebound are commonly seen with discontinuation of alprazolam after as little as 6–8 weeks of treatment. These discontinuation effects appear more severe than those following taper of imipramine and may be more severe in patients with panic disorder than in those with generalized anxiety disorder. This would argue for tapering benzodiazepines very slowly for patients with panic disorder, probably over 2–4 months and at rates no higher than 10% of the dose per week (2, 146). Withdrawal symptoms can occur throughout the taper and may be especially severe toward the end of the taper. The decision of when to attempt a benzodiazepine taper may be influenced by factors such as the presence of psychosocial stressors or supports, the stability of comorbid conditions, and the availability of alternative treatment options.

d) Implementation issues

(1) Dose

The manufacturer's recommendation for alprazolam treatment of panic disorder notes that doses above 4 mg/day are usually necessary and that doses up to 10 mg/day are sometimes required. However, very few studies have empirically evaluated dose requirements. Two studies (22, 105) compared alprazolam doses of 6 mg/day and 2 mg/day. The study by Uhlenhuth et al. (105) showed a significant advantage for the higher dose in producing a panic-free state. The study by Lydiard et al. (22) showed very little difference between the higher and lower doses (absence of panic attacks at study end in 65% of patients taking higher dose, 50% taking lower dose, but only 15% taking placebo). However, the rates of surreptitious benzodiazepine use for the lower-dose (23%) and placebo (35%) patients were considerably greater than the rate for the patients taking the higher alprazolam dose (4%), perhaps suggesting that the patients did not find the lower dose or placebo clinically effective. Lydiard and colleagues found that adverse side effects were more pronounced at the higher dose than at the lower dose of alprazolam. Given these findings, it is necessary to be flexible in choosing the alprazolam dose for an individual patient. Most patients require three to four doses per day to avoid breakthrough or rebound symptoms, although some may achieve symptom control with two doses of alprazolam per day. The dose should be titrated up to 2–3 mg/day at first, but an increase to 5–6 mg/day will be necessary for some patients.

In one multicenter dose-ranging trial (147), patients with panic disorder were randomly assigned to placebo or one of five fixed doses (0.5, 1.0, 2.0, 3.0, or 4.0 mg/day) of clonazepam. During 6 weeks of treatment, the minimum effective dose was 1.0 mg/day, and daily doses of 1.0 mg/day and higher were equally effective in reducing the number of panic attacks. The investigators concluded that daily doses of 1.0–2.0 mg of clonazepam offered the best balance of therapeutic benefits and side effects. Because of its relatively long half-life, clonazepam can usually be administered once or twice a day.

The dosing of other benzodiazepines in the treatment of panic disorder is less well established. In controlled studies, lorazepam has been given at doses of about 7 mg/day, usually two or three times daily. Diazepam doses ranged from 5 to 40 mg/day in two published trials.

Results of several studies suggest a relationship between alprazolam blood levels and treatment response (148, 149). Monitoring blood levels of alprazolam may be useful for dose adjustment, although this is not routinely done.

(2) Length of treatment

Alprazolam had an earlier onset of action than imipramine in three controlled trials. Clinicians and patients often note some reduction in panic within the first week of treatment, although full blockade of panic attacks can take several weeks.

As with TCA treatment of panic disorder, there are very few data indicating the optimum length of maintenance therapy for responders to benzodiazepines. Two published trials have compared maintenance imipramine, alprazolam, and placebo treatment, and both suggest that imipramine may be superior. In the study by Cassano et al. (112), imipramine and alprazolam patients fared equally well in terms of panic reduction during a 6-month maintenance phase, but the imipramine-treated patients had less phobic avoidance. There were more alprazolam dropouts during the maintenance phase than during the 8-week acute treatment phase, while the number of imipramine dropouts did not differ between the two phases. Curtis et al. (113) found that from month 4 through the end of an 8-month maintenance phase patients taking imipramine had virtually no panic attacks, while alprazolam-treated patients continued to experience infrequent panic attacks. On all other measures, however, the two medications performed equally well. In a third investigation, by Lepola et al. (150), patients who had been treated with alprazolam (N=27) and imipramine (N=28) in a 9-week trial were then followed for 3 years in a naturalistic study. Significantly more alprazolam users than imipramine users were found to be still using their original medication after 3 years (74% versus 32%). The authors pointed out that it is difficult to know whether this difference is attributable to a better long-term response among the imipramine users than among the alprazolam users, a greater degree of intolerable side effects for the imipramine users, or greater difficulty in discontinuing treatment among the alprazolam users due to physiologic dependence.

4. Monoamine oxidase inhibitors

a) Goals

The primary goals of MAOI therapy of panic disorder are to reduce the intensity and frequency of panic attacks, to reduce anticipatory anxiety, and to treat associated depression. Often, successful therapy with MAOIs also leads to a reduction in phobic avoidance.

b) Efficacy

There have been virtually no studies involving the use of MAOIs since the introduction of the panic disorder diagnosis in DSM-III in 1980. It is therefore nearly impossible to cite controlled trials in which MAOIs that are approved for use in the United States and currently manufactured (i.e., phenelzine and tranylcypromine) have been used for the specific treatment of panic disorder with or without agoraphobia. Even the most modern and rigorous study (151) involved the use of phenelzine for the treatment of "phobic neurosis" (152). The commonly held belief that MAOIs are actually more potent antipanic agents than tricyclics has never been convincingly proven in the scientific literature and is only supported by clinical anecdote.

Two studies have looked at the effectiveness of a reversible inhibitor of monoamine oxidase A (RIMA) for panic disorder. No medication in the RIMA class is currently approved for use in the United States, but at least one, moclobemide, is widely used in Europe and Canada. These medications do not generally require adherence to the tyramine-free diet that is mandatory for patients treated with phenelzine or tranylcypromine. Both studies, one a double-blind comparison of brofaromine to clomipramine (153) and the other an open study of brofaromine (154), showed antipanic and antiphobic efficacy.

c) Side effects

Adverse side effects are clearly a major concern with MAOI therapy. The complexity of these medications suggests that they should be prescribed by physicians with experience in monitoring MAOI treatment.

The main risk of taking an MAOI is hypertensive crisis secondary to ingestion of tyramine. Hence, patients taking phenelzine or tranylcypromine must adhere to the special low-tyramine diet. Certain medications, including but not limited to sympathomimetic amines, decongestants, the over-the-counter medication dextromethorphan, and meperidine, must not be used with MAOIs. Another serious drug-drug interaction to be avoided is the "serotonergic syndrome" that can occur from the use of MAOIs with SSRIs (155). Even when the risk of hypertensive crisis is obviated by strict adherence to dietary and medication restrictions, MAOIs have substantial adverse effects. These include hypotension (sometimes leading to syncope), weight gain, hypomania, sexual dysfunction, paresthesia, sleep disturbance, myoclonic jerks, dry mouth, and edema.

d) Implementation issues

(1) Dose

Doses of phenelzine in controlled trials for panic-disorder-like illnesses have tended to be low, often no higher than 45 mg/day. Some authors have commented that higher doses may be more effective. Doses of phenelzine up to 90 mg/day and of tranylcypromine up to 70 mg/day are said by experienced clinicians to be necessary for some patients with panic disorder.

(2) Length of treatment

The onset of the antipanic effect of MAOIs generally follows the same time course as that for tricyclics. Patients rarely get significant benefit before several weeks have elapsed, and periods up to 12 weeks may be necessary before the full effectiveness of the medication can be judged.

No maintenance studies of MAOIs for panic disorder have been published. Hence, the optimal length of treatment, to provide the least chance of relapse, is not established.

5. Other antidepressants

a) Venlafaxine

One small controlled trial at a single site, drawn from a larger multicenter trial, showed that venlafaxine (mean dose, 150 mg/day) was effective for treating panic disorder (156). A published series of four cases of patients with panic disorder indicated that venlafaxine at relatively low doses (50–75 mg/day) may be effective and well tolerated (157).

b) Trazodone

One double-blind study (158) in which 74 patients with panic disorder were assigned to trazodone, imipramine, or alprazolam showed trazodone to be less effective than either imipramine or alprazolam. However, in a single-blind study (159) in which 11 patients with panic disorder were treated with trazodone, panic symptoms improved significantly from a baseline period of placebo treatment.

c) Bupropion

Bupropion has been found to be effective in the treatment of depression. Proposed mechanisms of action include dopaminergic and noradrenergic agonist effects. Although there have been several small clinical trials using bupropion for patients with panic disorder, there is general consensus that it is not effective in alleviating either the somatic or psychological symptoms of panic attacks. It may have a role as an adjunctive treatment for patients with panic disorder who suffer sexual dysfunction as a side effect of other antidepressant medications, but it nevertheless may be potentially "overenergizing" for this specific patient group (160).

d) Nefazodone

One retrospective analysis of a randomized, placebo-controlled trial evaluated the effectiveness of nefazodone and imipramine among patients with comorbid panic disorder and major depression (161). Patients treated with nefazodone experienced significantly greater reductions in panic symptoms than placebo-treated patients; imipramine treatment was not found to be significantly better than placebo. An open-label trial examined nefazodone treatment among patients with panic disorder and concurrent depression or depressive symptoms (162). Panic symptoms were judged to be much or very much improved in 71% of the patients treated with nefazodone.

6. Anticonvulsants

There are limited data concerning the use of anticonvulsant medication in the treatment of panic disorder. In case reports, carbamazepine has been reported to improve panic attacks in patients with EEG abnormalities (163). However, the only controlled trial of carbamazepine suggested that it is not superior to placebo in reducing panic attack frequency (164). One crossover study showed significantly greater improvement in panic symptoms during periods of treatment with valproate than during treatment with placebo (165). A few reports, mostly findings from small numbers of subjects in uncontrolled studies or anecdotal reports on a few subjects, also suggest that valproate is an effective treatment for panic disorder (166). In these studies, valproate was well tolerated, but the adverse side effects included gastrointestinal dysfunction, weight gain, dizziness, nausea, sedation, and alopecia. A single case report indicated that gabapentin was effective for a patient with panic disorder.

7. Other agents

a) Conventional antipsychotic medications

Conventional antipsychotic medications are rarely appropriate in the treatment of uncomplicated panic disorder. There is no evidence that they are effective, and the risk of neurological side effects outweighs any potential benefit. There is interest in, but no evidence of, the possibility that clozapine may be useful for extremely refractory cases of panic disorder. At present, however, this cannot be recommended.

b) Beta-blockers

The limited number of controlled trials that have been conducted with β-adrenergic blocking agents in panic disorder have provided mixed results. Noyes et al. (133) compared the efficacy of diazepam and propranolol for 21 patients with panic disorder in a double-blind crossover study. Findings revealed that 18 of the 21 patients responded "moderately" to diazepam but only 7 of the 21 responded to propranolol. As the sole agent, the beta-blocker did not appear to be effective in alleviating phobic symptoms or panic attacks, despite adequate peripheral blockade. Munjack et al. (167) compared the effectiveness of alprazolam, propranolol, and placebo for 55 patients with panic disorder and agoraphobia. This study also showed superiority of alprazolam over propranolol: 75% of the alprazolam patients met the criterion of zero panic attacks after 5 weeks, compared with 37% of the propranolol group and 43% of the placebo patients. Ravaris et al. (168) also compared propranolol with alprazolam, but the results demonstrated that alprazolam and propranolol provided similar effects in suppressing panic attacks and reducing avoidance behaviors; the only difference in this study was the more rapid onset of action of alprazolam. One open-label, case report study (169) indicated a possible additive effect of the combination of propranolol and alprazolam. No subsequent clinical trials have addressed the issue of combination therapy with these agents.

c) Calcium channel blockers

The cardiovascular symptoms associated with panic attacks include palpitations, facial flushing, light-headedness, paresthesia, presyncopal disturbances, and tachycardia, which have been attributed to autonomic instability. Calcium channel blockers have been used increasingly to offset these physical manifestations in anxious patients. Successful results have been achieved with regard to complaints of palpitations and hyperventilation. Calcium channel blockers have particular potential for patients with mitral valve prolapse, especially when echocardiographic data are correlated with physical manifestations of autonomic hyperactivity. Data from controlled clinical studies that delineate a specific efficacy of calcium channel blockers in panic disorder or other anxiety disorders are very limited. Klein and Uhde (170) conducted one double-blind crossover study of verapamil involving 11 patients with panic disorder. When treated with verapamil, the patients had statistically significant, although clinically modest, reductions in the number of panic attacks and severity of anxiety symptoms. Use of these agents as anxiety treatments is mostly based on empirical assumptions related to cardiovascular effects or on case study reports. More investigation is needed to determine their role in panic amelioration, whether as a first-line treatment or as an adjunctive modality.

d) Inositol

Benjamin et al. (171) reported efficacy for inositol in a small, placebo-controlled trial involving 21 patients. The dose was 12 g/day, and the side effects were reported as minimal.

e) Clonidine

Few clinical trials with clonidine for the treatment of panic disorder and other anxiety disorders have been conducted. The controlled trials that have been done were limited to relatively small groups, and the results were equivocal with regard to efficacy. Uhde et al. (172) evaluated clonidine for patients with panic disorder and noted that it was more effective than placebo in reducing anxiety as measured by the Spielberger State-Trait Anxiety Inventory (173), Zung Anxiety Scale (174), and patient reports of frequency of anxiety symptoms. Hoehn-Saric et al. (175) studied the effect of clonidine on 23 patients with generalized anxiety disorder and panic disorder. They observed that clonidine was superior to placebo in relieving psychic and somatic symptoms, but of the 14 patients with panic disorder, 3 worsened with this agent. Hoehn-Saric et al. also noted that clonidine was not "as good as classical anxiety agents." There was a high frequency of side effects; 95% of the patients reported undesirable effects by week 12. Results from another study indicate that if there are therapeutic effects of clonidine for patients with panic disorder, they may be transient. Uhde et al. (172) gave intravenous clonidine or placebo to patients with panic disorder and healthy control subjects. After 1 hour, they found that clonidine was significantly more effective at reducing anxiety symptoms than placebo and that patients with panic disorder had a significantly greater reduction in anxiety symptoms than the control subjects. However, among 18 patients with panic disorder given oral clonidine for an average of 10 weeks, there was no difference in anxiety symptom scores assessed before and at the end of treatment.

f) Buspirone

Buspirone has been demonstrated to be effective in the long-term treatment of psychic and somatic symptoms of generalized anxiety disorder. Thus far, however, very limited information is available regarding the efficacy of buspirone for panic disorder. Sheehan et al. (176) reported that buspirone was not superior to placebo on any outcome measure in patients with panic disorder. This study was similar in outcome to a previous study (177), which also showed that buspirone did not seem to affect the symptoms of panic disorder.

IV. DEVELOPMENT OF A TREATMENT PLAN FOR THE INDIVIDUAL PATIENT

A. CHOOSING A SITE OF TREATMENT

The treatment of panic disorder is generally conducted entirely on an outpatient basis, and the condition by itself rarely warrants hospitalization. Occasionally, the first contact between patient and psychiatrist occurs in the emergency room or the hospital when the patient has been admitted in the midst of an acute panic episode. The patient may even be admitted by emergency room staff to rule out myocardial infarction or other serious general medical events. In such cases, the psychiatrist may be able to make the diagnosis of panic disorder and initiate treatment once other general medical conditions have been ruled out. Because panic disorder is frequently comorbid with depression and appears to elevate the risk of suicide attempts by depressed patients, it may also be necessary to hospitalize the depressed patient with panic disorder when suicidal ideation is of clinical concern. The treatment of panic disorder along with the treatment of depression is then initiated on an inpatient basis. Similarly, patients with panic disorder frequently have comorbid substance use disorders, which can occasionally require inpatient detoxification. Once again, the treatment of panic can be initiated in the hospital before discharge to outpatient care. Rarely, hospitalization is required in very severe cases of panic disorder with agoraphobia when administration of outpatient treatment has been ineffective or is impractical. For example, a housebound patient may require more intensive and closely supervised CBT in the initial phase of therapy than that provided by outpatient care (178, 179).

B. FORMULATION OF A TREATMENT PLAN

Before treatment for panic disorder is initiated, a general medical and psychiatric evaluation should be conducted (15). Psychiatrists should consider potential general medical and substance-induced causes of panic symptoms, especially when caring for patients who have a new onset of symptoms. Diagnostic studies and laboratory tests should be guided by the psychiatrist's evaluation of the patient's condition and by the choice of treatment. Attention should be given to the patient's psychosocial stressors, social supports, and general living situation.

1. Psychiatric management

Once the diagnosis of panic disorder is made, the patient is informed of the diagnosis and educated about panic disorder, its clinical course, and its complications. Regardless of the ultimate treatment modality selected, it is important to reassure the patient that panic attacks reflect real physiologic events (e.g., the heart rate does increase, blood pressure usually goes up, and other physical changes occur) but that these changes are not dangerous acutely. To evaluate the frequency and nature of a patient's panic attacks, patients may be encouraged to monitor their symptoms by using techniques such as keeping a daily diary.

It is also extremely important when formulating the treatment plan to address the presence of any of the many conditions that are frequently comorbid with panic disorder. Continuing medical evaluation and management are a crucial part of the treatment plan. In some cases, treatment of these comorbid conditions may even take precedence over treatment of the panic attacks. For example, patients with serious substance abuse may need detoxification and substance abuse treatment before it is possible to institute treatment for panic disorder.

Regardless of the treatment modality, it is often helpful to involve family members and significant others when appropriate and possible. In many cases, panic disorder is not well understood by family members, who may accuse the patient of overreacting or even of malingering. In other cases, supportive and understanding family members may wish to participate in treatment by, for example, helping with exposure exercises. Educating family members and enlisting their help and support can be very helpful.

Family and supportive therapy may also be employed along with other psychosocial and pharmacologic treatments for panic disorder. This provides the necessary environment for improvement and helps resolve interpersonal issues that may have arisen as a direct result of panic attacks and avoidance behaviors.

Because patients with panic disorder often fear separations and being alone, many experience great comfort from having easy access to the treating psychiatrist. It is often important for a psychiatrist who treats patients with panic disorder to be very available to patients in the early phase of treatment, before the panic resolves. In general, these patients are very reassured by knowing their physicians are available. If the patient becomes overly dependent on the psychiatrist, the dependency should be addressed directly and nonjudgmentally in the treatment, rather than through physician unavailability. The psychiatrist should attend to the treatment of personality disorders in patients with panic disorder. Sometimes the symptoms of comorbid personality disorders are so prominent that they interfere with symptom-based treatment of panic disorder. In this case, psychodynamic psychotherapy may be indicated.

2. Choice of specific treatment modalities

As noted earlier, there are two methods that have been extensively studied and proven to be effective treatments for panic disorder: CBT and antipanic medication. Considerations that may help guide the choice between CBT and medication as the treatment modality include their comparable efficacies, differences in risks and benefits, differences in costs, the availability of clinicians trained in CBT, and patient preferences. The psychiatrist should remember that the best-studied treatments for panic disorder target specific symptoms, whereas the physician must treat the patient. This means that in some cases, less well studied psychosocial treatment (e.g., psychodynamic psychotherapy, family therapy) may be the treatment of choice, for example, when symptoms of a personality disorder or extensive psychological conflicts are prominent in the clinical picture.

a) Considerations in choice of modality

(1) Efficacy

Direct comparisons of the efficacy of CBT and antipanic medications have been conducted, and some CBT researchers have found CBT to be superior (30, 39), while some pharmacotherapy studies have shown medication to be superior (32). Results from a large four-site study documented that the two treatments perform equally well (180). This is in line with the conclusions of the NIMH consensus development panel in 1991 that either of these treatments could be considered standard and that there was not sufficient evidence that either was superior to the other (181).

(2) Risks and benefits

The specific advantages and risks associated with CBT and pharmacotherapy may help guide the choice of which treatment to initiate. CBT lacks the adverse side effects of medications and the danger of developing physiologic dependency on certain drugs. However, CBT requires patients to perform "homework" or confront feared situations, which approximately 10%–30% of patients have been found to be unwilling or unable to complete (19, 29, 30, 33). In addition, CBT may not be readily available to patients in some areas.

The advantages of pharmacotherapies include their ready availability, the need for less effort by the patient, and their more rapid onset (especially for benzodiazepines). Medications may be associated with a lower likelihood of psychological dependence on the therapist. Each class of antipanic medications (TCAs, MAOIs, SSRIs, and benzodiazepines) is associated with specific side effects, which must be considered (see discussion of choosing among the medication classes in Section IV.B.2.b.2).

(3) Costs

Several factors influence the costs of treatment. In the case of CBT, these factors include the duration and frequency of treatment, the ability to maintain treatment gains, and any requirements for additional psychosocial or pharmacologic treatment. For antipanic medications, factors affecting cost include the choice and dose of antipanic agent, the availability of generic preparations, duration of treatment, the probability of relapse following discontinuation, requirements for additional pharmacotherapy or psychosocial treatment, and costs of treating medication-related side effects.

(4) Patient preferences

In most cases, the decision to use medication, CBT, another form of psychotherapy, or a combination of treatments is highly individualized. Informed patients may consider the evidence for a treatment's efficacy, particular advantages, risks and side effects, or costs.

b) Types of modalities

(1) CBT and other psychotherapies

Specific elements of CBT are reviewed in Section III.C.1.a. Panic-focused CBT is generally administered in weekly sessions for approximately 12 weeks. The patient must be willing to fulfill "homework" assignments that include breathing exercises, recording anxious cognitions, and confronting phobic situations.

Clinicians have often reported that sessions with significant others help to relieve stress on families caused by panic attacks and phobias in the patient and thereby promote a supportive environment for the patient, which may facilitate compliance with CBT and other treatments. Cognitive behavioral approaches have been conducted in group formats with results similar to those for individual treatment.

There is evidence that many patients with panic disorder have complicating comorbid axis I and/or axis II conditions. Psychodynamic psychotherapy may be useful in reducing symptoms or maladaptive behaviors in these associated conditions. Such a treatment may also be a helpful adjunct for patients with panic disorder treated with medication who continue to experience difficulty with psychosocial stressors.

Using other psychosocial treatments in conjunction with psychiatric management may be helpful in addressing certain comorbid disorders or environmental or psychosocial stressors. However, there have been no controlled studies to support the efficacy of psychosocial treatments other than CBT, when used alone, for the treatment of panic disorder. Therefore, supplementation with or replacement by either CBT or antipanic medications should be strongly considered if no significant improvement in the panic symptoms occurs within 6–8 weeks.

(2) Medications

When pharmacotherapy has been selected, the choice of which class of medication to use may be informed by consideration of the relative efficacies of the various medication classes, differences in risks and benefits, differences in costs, and patient preferences, including the wish to conceive a child or continue with a pregnancy or nursing experience.

Because medications from all four classes—SSRIs, TCAs, benzodiazepines, and MAOIs—are roughly comparable in efficacy, the decision about which medication to choose for panic disorder mainly involves considerations of adverse side effects and cost. SSRIs are likely to be the best choice of pharmacotherapy for many patients with panic disorder because they lack significant cardiovascular and anticholinergic side effects and have no liability for physical dependency and subsequent withdrawal reactions.

The SSRIs carry a risk of sexual side effects and are also more expensive than tricyclics and benzodiazepines because generic preparations are not yet available. If cost is a consideration, it is important to note that tricyclics (particularly imipramine and clomipramine, for which most research has been conducted) and high-potency benzodiazepines (including alprazolam and clonazepam) are effective for panic disorder and that most patients can tolerate them. With tricyclics, consideration must be given to the possibility of cardiovascular and anticholinergic side effects. These are particularly troublesome for older patients and for patients with other medical problems. With benzodiazepines, consideration must be given to the fact that all of them will produce physical dependency in most patients. This may make it difficult for the patient to discontinue treatment. Also, benzodiazepines are generally contraindicated for patients with current or past substance use disorders.

Because many patients with panic disorder are hypersensitive to antidepressant medications at treatment initiation, it is recommended that doses approximately half of those given to depressed patients at the beginning of treatment be used for patients with panic disorder initially. The dose is then increased to a full therapeutic dose over subsequent days and as tolerated by the patient. TCAs, SSRIs, and MAOIs generally take 4–6 weeks to become effective for panic disorder. For this reason, high-potency benzodiazepines may be useful in situations where very rapid control of symptoms is critical. Because of their side effects and the need for dietary restrictions, MAOIs are generally reserved for patients who do not respond to other treatments.

(3) Combined medication and psychosocial treatment

The data regarding the efficacy of the combination of medications and CBT versus that of either modality alone are conflicting (66). Currently, it is not possible to identify which patients will benefit more from such combination therapy. Combining medication and CBT can be especially useful for patients with severe agoraphobia and for those who show an incomplete response to either treatment alone. In one study, combining psychodynamic psychotherapy with medication improved the long-term outcome of medication-treated patients (63). Psychodynamic psychotherapy is commonly used in conjunction with medication on the basis of a clinical consensus that it is effective for some patients.

3. Determining length of treatment

The acute phase of treatment with either CBT or medication generally lasts about 12 weeks. At the end of a successful acute phase, the patient should have markedly fewer and less intense panic attacks than before treatment. Ideally, panic attacks should be eliminated entirely. In addition, the patient should worry less about panic attacks and should experience minimal or no phobic avoidance. This is roughly the time required to realize the full benefit of either treatment.

After the acute phase of treatment with CBT, the frequency of visits is generally decreased, and they are eventually discontinued within several months. Some, but not all, studies indicate that long-term remission is possible, lasting several years after the completion of successful CBT. The efficacy of a second round of CBT for patients who relapse or "booster" CBT sessions for preventing relapse has not been studied.

There are very few systematic studies that indicate the optimal length of antipanic medication therapy. There is evidence that response to antipanic medication continues while the patient continues to take medication. Studies vary in the rate of relapse following medication discontinuation, but most show that relapse is common. It is generally believed, although not yet documented with research findings, that reinstitution of medication aborts relapse. The general recommendation has been to maintain medication treatment for at least 1 year after response and then to attempt discontinuation, with close follow-up of the patient from this point. Relapsing patients should then begin taking medication again. There is preliminary evidence that longer periods of initial treatment with medication may decrease the risk of relapse when the medication is stopped. It is not known whether continuing treatment with medication indefinitely for patients who relapse after discontinuation is beneficial.

Patients are likely to show some improvement with either medication or CBT within 6–8 weeks (although full response may take longer). Patients who show no improvement within 6–8 weeks with a particular treatment should be reevaluated with regard to diagnosis, the need for a different treatment, or the need for combined treatment. Patients who do not respond as expected to medication or CBT, or who have repeated relapses, should be evaluated for possible addition of a psychodynamic or other psychosocial intervention.

4. Use of benzodiazepines for early symptom control, in combination with a different treatment modality

Nonbenzodiazepine antipanic medication and CBT often take weeks before beneficial effects are realized, and some patients express an urgent need for a diminution of high levels of anticipatory anxiety and for some reduction in the severity of panic attacks. This can usually be accomplished by administering a benzodiazepine.

However, the potential benefits of benzodiazepines during the initial stages of treatment with another modality should be balanced against the potential risks. First, the patient may attribute all of the response he or she obtains in the course of treatment for panic disorder to the initial administration of the benzodiazepine. Even when antipanic medication or CBT has probably started to work, the patient may still believe that the benzodiazepine is the effective agent. The patient may then have difficulty discontinuing the benzodiazepine. Second, cognitive behavioral therapists and other clinicians are concerned that benzodiazepines may relieve anxiety to such an extent that the patient loses motivation to follow all of the steps of CBT.

Finally, even after relatively brief periods of benzodiazepine treatment—often only a few weeks—some patients experience withdrawal reactions upon discontinuation. Such patients may believe that they are experiencing a relapse into panic disorder and have great difficulty stopping use of the benzodiazepine.

For these reasons, when benzodiazepines are used during the initial stages of treatment with another modality, patients should be reassured that more definitive treatment will be likely to work in a few weeks. Avoiding unnecessarily high doses of benzodiazepines and asking the patient to take these medications only when needed may help avoid the development of steady-state benzodiazepine levels and the risk of dependency.

V. CLINICAL FEATURES INFLUENCING TREATMENT

The following sections review data pertinent to the treatment of individuals with panic disorder who have specific clinical features that may alter the general treatment considerations that are discussed in Section IV. These sections are necessarily brief and are not intended to stand alone as a set of treatment recommendations. The recommendations reviewed in Section IV, including the use of psychiatric management, generally apply unless otherwise indicated.

A. PSYCHIATRIC FACTORS

1. Suicidality

Both older follow-up studies of anxiety disorders and more recent investigations of panic disorder have demonstrated a higher than average rate of suicide attempts in patients with a lifetime history of these disorders (9, 182, 183). In a large epidemiological study of over 18,000 adults, Weissman et al. (9) found that 20% of individuals with a history of panic disorder and 12% of those with a history of panic attacks had attempted suicide. A high risk of suicidal ideation and attempts in patients with panic disorder has been confirmed in several studies (184–186) but not in others examining uncomplicated panic disorder or controlling for comorbid conditions (187, 188). In addition, Fawcett et al. (189), in a study of 954 patients with major depression, found that the presence of comorbid panic attacks was one determinant of suicide in the first year of follow-up.

It remains unclear whether uncomplicated panic disorder, especially panic without agoraphobia, is associated with a high risk of suicide attempts (186–188, 190) and whether suicide attempts by individuals with panic disorder are actually related to or caused by panic symptoms, as opposed to being a result of comorbid conditions. Comorbid psychiatric disorders clearly increase the risk of suicide in patients with panic disorder. In particular, comorbid lifetime major depression, alcohol or substance abuse or dependence, personality disorders, and brief depressive symptoms increase the risk of suicide attempts, as do younger age, earlier onset of illness, greater severity of illness, and a past history of suicide attempts or psychiatric hospitalization (9, 183–185, 191, 192).

The high rate of suicide attempts by patients with panic disorder is of considerable clinical significance, even if most or all of the increased risk is attributable to lifetime comorbidity. The vast majority of patients with panic disorder have current or past comorbid axis I or axis II disorders. Thus, uncomplicated panic disorder is relatively uncommon. Furthermore, comorbid conditions may go undetected in busy clinical settings. Thus, it is important to be aware that patients presenting with panic disorder are at high risk for lifetime suicidal ideation and attempts. All patients presenting with panic attacks should be asked about suicidal ideation and past suicide attempts and about conditions likely to increase risk and to require specific treatment, such as depression and substance abuse. When significant depression and/or suicidal ideation exist, appropriate antidepressant therapy should be initiated and a decision made about whether the patient can be safely treated as an outpatient. When substance abuse is present, this must become a primary focus of clinical attention, and every effort to treat the substance abuse must be made.

2. Comorbid substance use disorder

In clinical and epidemiological studies, patients with panic disorder with or without agoraphobia have higher than average rates of cocaine, alcohol, and sedative abuse and dependence (193–196). Cocaine, other stimulants, and marijuana have been reported to precipitate panic attacks in adolescents and adults (197–199). Some individuals may self-medicate panic and anxiety symptoms by using alcohol and sedatives. However, heavy alcohol use, acute alcohol withdrawal, and more prolonged subacute withdrawal may cause or exacerbate panic (193, 200). Individuals who are ataxic and tremulous may not venture out because of their embarrassment, insecurity, or disability. These actions may mimic panic disorder or agoraphobia. Patients with both panic disorder and substance abuse or dependence have a poorer prognosis than those with either disorder alone (193, 200).

Since a significant proportion of patients presenting with panic attacks or agoraphobia have a history of substance abuse or dependence, which may cause or aggravate their symptoms, clinicians should be careful to screen for substance use disorders in this population. Flashbacks induced by current or past use of inhalants or hallucinogens can cause panic-disorder-type symptoms. Treatment of the substance use disorder is essential. It is unclear whether specific antipanic treatment is necessary for patients with primary substance abuse. Several panic attacks during the early weeks of abstinence, decreasing in frequency, often warrant no treatment other than support and reassurance until the attacks abate (201, 202). However, if the panic attacks continue and increase over several weeks, the diagnosis of panic disorder is warranted. If a patient is not relieved of ongoing panic attacks, it is likely that he or she will resume substance abuse (203–207). In treating panic symptoms in dually diagnosed patients, benzodiazepines should be avoided whenever possible, in favor of psychotherapy and/or antidepressants. A history of abuse of other substances, both licit and illicit, is associated with a higher prevalence of benzodiazepine abuse, a greater euphoric response to benzodiazepines, and a higher rate of unauthorized use of alprazolam during treatment for panic disorder (208, 209). The potential benefits of other medications for panic should be weighed against possible interactions with alcohol and other medications, resulting in, for instance, lowering of the seizure threshold (for tricyclics) or hyper- or hypotensive reactions (for MAOIs).

The use of a number of legal substances, such as nicotine, caffeine, and sympathomimetics (e.g., nasal decongestants), may also worsen panic attacks and interfere with treatment response (210–212).

3. Comorbid mood disorder

Panic disorder often coexists with bipolar disorder or unipolar depression. Bowen et al. (213) reported that of 108 patients with panic disorder, 11% had comorbid unipolar depression and 23% had comorbid bipolar disorder. Savino et al. (214) found that of 140 patients with panic, 23% had comorbid unipolar depression and 11% had comorbid bipolar disorder.

Many studies indicate that patients with panic disorder and comorbid mood disorders exhibit greater impairment, more hospitalizations, a higher rate of suicide attempts, and generally more psychopathology than patients with pure panic disorder (213). In addition, patients with panic disorder and comorbid affective disorders generally respond less well to traditional treatments for panic disorder.

A significant proportion of patients with panic disorder complain of overstimulation when treated with antidepressants (both tricyclics and SSRIs), and the attrition rate due to side effects or nonresponse is high. Such medications, therefore, are most efficaciously introduced at low doses and slowly increased. If both panic disorder and depression are present, it is important that a patient's treatment regimen include specific antipanic treatments.

4. Other anxiety disorders

Panic attacks are part of the hallmark cluster of symptoms in panic disorder, but they do occur in other illnesses. Patients with posttraumatic stress disorder (PTSD), obsessive-compulsive disorder (OCD), generalized anxiety disorder, and specific and social phobias also sometimes report occasional panic attacks. Identification of triggers for panic attacks is important, since a patient can be misdiagnosed with panic disorder and considered treatment resistant if this is not done.

Other comorbid anxiety disorders complicate the picture as well. PTSD, as just mentioned, may present with a series of panic attacks (215, 216), and PTSD patients may meet specific criteria for panic disorder concomitantly. In addition, patients with PTSD often present with PTSD, panic disorder, and a third or fourth disorder (217–223). More specific treatments may be required to offset other profound symptoms in PTSD. OCD is yet another anxiety disorder that may present concomitantly with panic disorder (224) and is frequently a diagnostic oversight, in part because of the reticence of patients to talk about their experiences. Because phobias and avoidant behavior are common in panic disorder, phobic disorders and panic disorder also frequently occur as comorbid conditions. They have similar responses to MAOIs, SSRIs, and perhaps other antidepressants. Specific phobias are more responsive to specific cognitive behavioral treatments than is the phobic avoidance associated with panic disorder. In summary, panic attacks may be experienced in several anxiety disorders, either as a response to specific triggers or as part of a complicated pattern of comorbid conditions that would require very specific, tailored multimodal therapy for optimal recovery. Although the pharmacotherapeutic considerations may be similar in these conditions, specificity of treatment may make the difference between full response, partial response, and perceived refractoriness.

5. Comorbid personality disorders

About 40%–50% of patients with the diagnosis of panic disorder additionally meet the criteria for one or more axis II disorders (225–227).

The personality disorders most frequently observed in panic disorder patients are three from the anxious cluster: avoidant, obsessive-compulsive, and dependent (228–230). In addition, patients with panic disorder often show traits from other personality disorders, such as affective instability (from borderline personality disorder) and hypersensitivity to people (from paranoid personality disorder) (225).

Some studies suggest that patients with panic disorder and comorbid personality disorders may improve less or be subject to greater relapse following medication treatment (225, 228–231) or exposure therapy (42, 232–234). However, in one study (235), patients with panic disorder and comorbid personality disorders benefited as much from CBT as did patients with panic disorder without comorbid personality disorders, and in another study (236), there were no differences in treatment effect between patients with and without comorbid personality disorders after statistical adjustment for agoraphobic avoidance and frequency of panic attacks.

The therapist may need to spend more time with patients who have personality disorders in order to strengthen the therapeutic relationship and to develop a hierarchy of specific treatment goals. Psychodynamically informed management and/or formal psychodynamic treatment may be helpful for patients with panic disorder and personality disorders who have not responded to panic-focused treatments alone.

B. CONCURRENT GENERAL MEDICAL CONDITIONS

Panic attacks are associated with prominent physical symptoms and may be misinterpreted as general medical conditions by patients and/or physicians. Some general medical conditions (and/or effects of medications prescribed to treat them) may manifest themselves as panic symptoms, and general medical illness may be associated with comorbid panic disorder. A complete assessment for patients with panic disorder includes a general medical evaluation as delineated in the *Practice Guideline for Psychiatric Evaluation of Adults* (15; included in this volume). Such careful assessment, when results are negative, is reassuring for patients who fear serious physical illness. In the case of a patient who is diagnosed with a general medical condition, a decision must be made regarding the relationship between that condition and the panic disorder. If the medical condition or treatment is considered to be involved in the etiology of the panic symptoms, the treatment of panic disorder should be delayed until the general medical condition is treated and/or the medication discontinued. However, there may be a general medical condition that is not directly causing the panic disorder. Studies show that panic and other anxiety disorders are more prevalent in medically ill patients than in the population at large. Conditions that have been specifically associated with panic disorder, but not etiologically, include irritable bowel syndrome, migraine, and pulmonary disease (237–239). Acute onset of a wide range of medical conditions may also be associated with the development of an anxiety disorder. When a coexisting general medical condition is present, it is important to treat the panic disorder, since panic symptoms may exacerbate the associated general medical condition. Data from some studies suggest that panic disorder and phobic anxiety may increase the risk of mortality in patients with cardiovascular disease (182, 240). In general, treatment of panic disorder in patients with irritable bowel syndrome, pulmonary disease, or migraine is not different from treatment of uncomplicated panic disorder. In fact, studies have documented improvement in respiratory symptoms and amelioration of irritable bowel symptoms upon treatment with SSRIs, even when full-blown panic disorder is not present. If renal or liver damage is present or if there is general debilitation from general medical illness, the medication dose should be adjusted appropriately.

C. DEMOGRAPHIC VARIABLES

1. Child and adolescent population

The following section contains a brief overview of the available data regarding the treatment of children and adolescents with panic disorder. Unless stated otherwise, the general considerations discussed in Section IV of this guideline apply to children; this is especially true of the importance of psychiatric management. Information and recommendations regarding the etiology, diagnosis, and assessment of panic disorder are beyond the scope of this section. The reader is referred to the American Academy of Child and Adolescent Psychiatry's *Practice Parameters for the Assessment and Treatment of Children and Adolescents With Anxiety Disorders* (241) for a more detailed discussion. Finally, the treatments reviewed are those for which the results of formal clinical trials have been published. Given the paucity of such data in the child and adolescent literature, many treatment plans will necessarily include components that are not well studied. For example, child and adolescent psychiatrists frequently find that a treatment plan requires attention to developmental issues (from psychological and physiologic perspectives) and the involvement of multiple systems (e.g., schools, family, and community).

Panic disorder occurs in children and, more commonly, adolescents; panic disorder often is preceded by or co-occurs with separation anxiety disorder. This section reviews the literature on the treatment of pediatric panic disorder.

The literature on panic disorder in youth is considerably less robust than that for adults (242), and much controversy attends the relationship between separation anxiety disorder and panic disorder (243–245). Experts generally agree that treatment of panic disorder in children is similar to treatment of panic disorder in adults: cognitive behavioral psychotherapy and, where necessary, pharmacotherapy. Because family involvement in symptoms is common, family-based treatment strategies are often necessary. The literature regarding the psychodynamic treatment of children and adolescents tends to be focused on broader categories of anxiety disorders.

In one study of adolescents (246), panic disorder was reported to have a prevalence of 0.6% (girls, 0.7%; boys, 0.4%). Fewer than half of the young persons with panic disorder in this study had received treatment for panic disorder symptoms. The incidence of so-called limited-symptom panic attacks in young adolescents is somewhat greater and shows a steep increase with the onset of puberty (247). Panic disorder also occurs before puberty, although the true prevalence is unknown. Whether prepubertal or postpubertal, the presentation of panic disorder in young persons appears to be quite similar to that in adults, with the caveat that younger children show more separation anxiety symptoms (6).

Panic disorder is commonly accompanied by a variety of specific phobias, including fear of the dark, monsters, kidnappers, bugs, small animals, heights, and open or closed-in spaces. Nighttime fears, resistance to going to bed, difficulty falling asleep alone or sleeping through the night alone, and nightmares involving separation themes are not uncommon. These specific phobic symptoms may be common triggers for panic or separation anxiety and therefore are responsible for many of the avoidance and ritualized anxiety-reducing behaviors seen in patients with both separation anxiety disorder and panic disorder (242). Children with panic disorder also show high rates of comorbidity with other anxiety disorders and with depression (248). In younger children, separation anxiety disorder precedes depression in approximately two-thirds of the cases and may form the nidus for recurrent affective illness and panic disorder if left untreated (249).

The terms "school phobia" and "school refusal" are sometimes treated as reflecting panic disorder, even though not all children with school refusal show panic disorder and not all children with panic disorder manifest school refusal (250, 251). Moreover, while many school-refusing children do show significant separation anxiety, others are "phobic" school refusers, i.e., they are phobic of something within the school context and not fearful of leaving home or family (252, 253). Children also may refuse to go to school because of depressive disorders, conduct disorder, family problems, learning disabilities, or unrecognized mild retardation.

There is limited empirical research supporting the efficacy of any type of treatment of panic disorder in the pediatric population (242). Unfortunately, the pediatric literature primarily comprises uncontrolled studies, which are reviewed here.

Only a few published studies have addressed the treatment of panic disorder in children with cognitive behavioral techniques, and of these, there are no studies of contrasting groups. Only one study used a single-case design. Ollendick (254) applied standard treatments for panic disorder in adults (36, 255) to four adolescents with DSM-III-R panic disorder using a multiple-baseline-across-subjects design. In all cases, the panic attacks were eliminated, agoraphobia was reduced, and the ability to handle future "panicogenic" situations was enhanced.

Medication management strategies that are effective for adults with panic disorder have received anecdotal support for use with children and adolescents, but no treatment has shown conclusive support. Scattered case reports (256, 257) and case series (258, 259) suggest that standard TCAs, SSRIs, and the high-potency benzodiazepines alprazolam and clonazepam may be useful in treating pediatric panic disorder.

2. Geriatric population

Although anxiety symptoms and disorders are among the most common psychiatric ailments experienced by older adults, epidemiologic studies suggest that the prevalence of panic disorder in later life may be lower than that for midlife (260). A vigorous search for alternative and comorbid diagnoses, especially general medical conditions and effects of general medical pharmacologic agents, should be undertaken for elderly patients presenting with new panic symptoms. There have been few prospective clinical trials of anxiety disorder treatments for the elderly to document systematically the efficacy of standard medications and/or psychosocial treatments for this age group. If medication is used, the required dose may be lower than that for younger patients. The medication dose should be very low to begin, and medication increases should be slower and more limited than with younger adults. (Additional information will be provided in the forthcoming practice guideline on geriatric psychiatry.)

3. Gender

Panic disorder is more common in women for reasons that are not yet fully understood. In the Epidemiologic Catchment Area study, the lifetime prevalence of panic disorder was twice as high in women as in men (261). The treatment of pregnant and nursing women raises certain specific concerns regarding the use of antipanic medications. A careful evaluation of the risks associated with frequently used medications has recently been reviewed by Altshuler et al. (262).

4. Cultural issues

Relatively little research has been done on anxiety disorders in African Americans. The National Institute of Mental Health Epidemiologic Catchment Area study (263) and the National Comorbidity Survey (264) provide somewhat conflicting data on the prevalence of anxiety disorders. The Epidemiologic Catchment Area study indicated that African Americans have a higher lifetime prevalence of agoraphobia but not panic disorder, while the National Comorbidity Survey found no racial differences in the prevalence of any anxiety disorder (264–266). Although the prevalences may be similar, racial differences in help seeking and symptom presentation may result in underrecognition and misdiagnosis. In one study (267), researchers identified panic disorder in 25% of a group of minority psychiatric outpatients of whom none had received this diagnosis from their clinicians. There is some evidence of a different clinical presentation of panic disorder in African Americans; specifically, there are associations with isolated sleep paralysis (268) and hypertension (269, 270). Studies show that African American patients in primary care report more severe somatic symptoms and have a higher prevalence of panic disorder than whites (271) and that African Americans are more likely to seek help in medical than in mental health facilities (272, 273).

VI. RESEARCH DIRECTIONS

A substantial amount of research has been devoted to the description of the phenomenology and treatment of panic disorder in recent years. Because of this, treatment of panic disorder is generally quite successful. These guidelines reveal, however, a number of areas in which further research would be most desirable.

Although the diagnosis of panic disorder is fairly straightforward, it is increasingly clear that a large proportion of patients with panic disorder also suffer from other anxiety disorders, depression, substance use disorders, and personality disorders. We have relatively little information on the optimal ways of treating these combinations of conditions or the extent to which comorbidity affects prognosis and whether the observed high rates of comorbidity are due to chance or fundamental overlaps in psychopathology. Hence, a thorough understanding of the relationship between panic disorder and other psychiatric disorders is needed.

In addition, while the start of a successful treatment for a patient with panic disorder may include reassurance that panic attacks are not medically catastrophic events, there are emerging data indicating that patients with phobic anxiety may have higher long-term rates of cardiovascular morbidity and mortality. It is not yet clear whether this association applies to individuals with a true diagnosis of panic disorder and, if it does, whether treatment diminishes the risk. Clearly, research about the long-term health risks that may be associated with panic disorder is needed.

We have very little scientifically accumulated information about panic disorder in childhood. It has been argued that separation anxiety in childhood is a precursor for panic disorder, but this has not been systematically substantiated. The epidemiology of panic disorder in childhood has not been well studied, nor has the optimal therapeutic approach been established.

These guidelines review a number of effective interventions for panic disorder, including pharmacotherapy and psychotherapy. Treatments are highly successful when measured in terms of the rate of panic attack blockade. On the other hand, studies continue to show that blocking panic attacks is only part of the solution to panic disorder and that many patients continue to suffer from associated features of the illness, including anticipatory anxiety and phobic avoidance. Very few long-term studies have been conducted to inform clinicians about how long treatment should last before there can be a reasonable certainty that response can be sustained. It is not known, for example, whether there is a length of medication exposure after which the patient with panic disorder will have a low chance for relapse. Similarly, it is not clear whether "booster" sessions of CBT are useful.

Even in selecting the first treatment for a new patient with panic disorder, there is uncertainty. Rigorous studies have shown that both medications and CBT are better than control treatments for panic disorder and approximately equal to each other. We do not yet know whether some individuals respond better to either CBT or medications and, if so, how to identify them. Further, it is not yet known whether combinations of medication and CBT are more effective than either treatment alone. Within the pharmacotherapy options, many medications have been shown to be effective, but few studies have elucidated whether there are advantages of one class over another, how benzodiazepines should properly be used if combined with antidepressants, or the best options for patients with refractory cases. CBT generally involves a "package" of several techniques, but it is not certain whether all of them are necessary or even beneficial.

Psychodynamic therapies and psychoanalysis are widely used for patients with panic disorder. Research is clearly needed to document the rates of response of patients with panic disorder to psychodynamically based treatments. This kind of research is clearly possible and deserves attention. Furthermore, whether psychodynamic treatments combined with medication or CBT offer any advantage over any of these treatments alone needs to be explored.

Finally, the treatment of any medical illness has a greater likelihood of success if it addresses fundamental pathological processes. Preclinical science is rapidly providing important insights into the biology of fear, and these findings must be translated into the clinical arena. This promises to open the way to highly specific antipanic therapies that will be improvements even over the very successful treatments we already have.

VII. INDIVIDUALS AND ORGANIZATIONS THAT SUBMITTED COMMENTS

David A. Adler, M.D.
Dick Baldwin, M.D.
James Ballenger, M.D.
Richard Balon, M.D.
Patricia L. Baltazar, Ph.D.
David H. Barlow, M.D., Ph.D.
Monica A. Basco, Ph.D.
William Bebchuk, M.D.
J. Gayle Beck, Ph.D.
Bernard D. Beitman, M.D.
Carl C. Bell, M.D.
Dinesh Bhugra, M.D.
Charles H. Blackinton, M.D.
Jack Blaine, M.D.
Barton J. Blinder, M.D., Ph.D.
David Brook, M.D.
Oliver G. Cameron, M.D., Ph.D.
Carlyle Chan, M.D.
Norman A. Clemens, M.D.
Christopher C. Colenda, M.D., M.P.H.
Michelle G. Craske, Ph.D.
Dorynne Czechowicz, M.D.
Jonathan Davidson, M.D.
Dave M. Davis, M.D.

Ted Dinan, M.D., Ph.D.
Kim A. Eagle, M.D.
James M. Ellison, M.D., M.P.H.
Frederick Engstrom, M.D.
Ann Maxwell Eward, Ph.D.
Harvey H. Falit, M.D.
Edward D. Frohlich, M.D.
Glen Gabbard, M.D.
David T. George, M.D.
William Goldman, M.D.
Sheila Hafter Gray, M.D.
Michael K. Greenberg, M.D.
William M. Greenberg, M.D.
George T. Grossberg, M.D.
Daniel W. Hicks, M.D.
Mac Horton, M.D.
Richard Justman, M.D.
Nalani V. Juthani, M.D.
Gary Kaplan, M.D.
Robert A. Kimmich, M.D.
Donald F. Klein, M.D.
Lawrence Kline, M.D.
Ronald R. Koegler, M.D.
Barry J. Landau, M.D.
Susan Lazar, M.D.
Henrietta Leonard, M.D.
Robert Liberman, M.D.
Francis G. Lu, M.D.
Henry Mallard, M.D.
Barton J. Mann, M.D.
V. Manohar, M.D.
John C. Markowitz, M.D.
Isaac Marks, M.D.
Ronald L. Martin, M.D.
Matis Mavissakalian, M.D.
Joseph Mawhinney, M.D.
Michael Mayo-Smith, M.D.
Christopher J. McLaughlin, M.D.
Barbara Milrod, M.D.
Jerome Motto, M.D.
Marvin Nierenberg, M.D.
Philip T. Ninan, M.D.
Russell Noyes, M.D.
David Osser, M.D.
Mark H. Pollack, M.D.
C. Alec Pollard, Ph.D.
Charles W. Portney, M.D.
Elizabeth Rahdert, Ph.D.
Penny Randall, M.D.
Michelle Riba, M.D.
Vaughn Rickert, Psy.D.
Barbara Rosenfeld, M.D.
Peter Roy-Byrne, M.D.
Pedro Ruiz, M.D.
Carlotta Schuster, M.D.
John J. Schwab, M.D.
Warren Seides, M.D.
Susan Simmons-Alling, M.S., R.N., C.S.
William Sledge, M.D.
Herbert Smokler, M.D.
David Spiegel, M.D.
Roger F. Suchyta, M.D.
Eva Szigethy, M.D., Ph.D.
Gerald Tarlow, Ph.D.
William R. Tatomer, M.D.
David M. Tobolowsky, M.D.
Mauricio Tohen, M.D., Dr.P.H.
Samuel M. Turner, Ph.D.
Robert M. Ward, M.D.
Naimah Weinberg, M.D.
Myrna Weissman, Ph.D.
Joseph Westermeyer, M.D., M.P.H., Ph.D.
R. Reid Wilson, Ph.D.
Thomas Wise, M.D.
Earl Witenberg, M.D.
Sherwyn Woods, M.D., Ph.D.
Jesse H. Wright, M.D.
Roberto Zarate, M.D.
Howard Zonana, M.D.

American Academy of Addiction Psychiatry
American Academy of Child and Adolescent Psychiatry
American Academy of Neurology
American Academy of Pediatrics
American Association of Suicidology
American College of Cardiology
American Geriatric Society
American Nurses Association
American Psychoanalytic Association
American Psychosomatic Society

American Society of Addiction Medicine
American Society of Clinical Pathologists
Association for Academic Psychiatry
Association for the Advancement of Behavior Therapy
Association of Gay and Lesbian Psychiatrists
Baltimore/Washington Society for Psychoanalysis
Group for the Advancement of Psychiatry
National Institute on Drug Abuse
Royal College of Psychiatrists
Society for Adolescent Medicine

VIII. REFERENCES

The following coding system is used to indicate the nature of the supporting evidence in the summary recommendations and references:

[A] *Randomized clinical trial.* A study of an intervention in which subjects are prospectively followed over time; there are treatment and control groups; subjects are randomly assigned to the two groups; both the subjects and the investigators are blind to the assignments.
[B] *Clinical trial.* A prospective study in which an intervention is made and the results of that intervention are tracked longitudinally; study does not meet standards for a randomized clinical trial.
[C] *Cohort or longitudinal study.* A study in which subjects are prospectively followed over time without any specific intervention.
[D] *Case-control study.* A study in which a group of patients is identified in the present and information about them is pursued retrospectively or backward in time.
[E] *Review with secondary data analysis.* A structured analytic review of existing data, e.g., a meta-analysis or a decision analysis.
[F] *Review.* A qualitative review and discussion of previously published literature without a quantitative synthesis of the data.
[G] *Other.* Textbooks, expert opinion, case reports, and other reports not included above.

1. American Psychiatric Association: Diagnostic and Statistical Manual of Mental Disorders, 4th ed (DSM-IV). Washington, DC, APA, 1994 [G]
2. Ballenger JC, Pecknold J, Rickels K, Sellers EM: Medication discontinuation in panic disorders. J Clin Psychiatry 1993; 54(Oct suppl):15–21, discussion 22–24 [F]
3. Katschnig H, Amering M, Stolk JM, Ballenger JC: Predictors of quality of life in a long-term follow-up study of panic disorder patients after a clinical drug trial. Psychopharmacol Bull 1996; 32:149–155 [C]
4. Roy-Byrne PP, Cowley DS: Course and outcome in panic disorder: a review of recent follow-up studies. Anxiety 1995; 1:150–160 [F]
5. Weissman MM, Bland RC, Canino GJ, Faravelli C, Greenwald S, Hwu HG, Joyce PR, Karam EG, Lee CK, Lellouch J, Lepine JP, Newman SC, Oakley-Browne MA, Rubio-Stipec M, Wells JE, Wickramaratne PJ, Wittchen HA, Yeh EK: The cross-national epidemiology of panic disorder. Arch Gen Psychiatry 1997; 54:305–309 [E]
6. Moreau D, Weissman MM: Panic disorder in children and adolescents: a review. Am J Psychiatry 1992; 149:1306–1314 [F]

7. Lesser IM, Rubin RT, Rifkin RP, Swinson RP, Ballenger JC, Burrows GD, DuPont RL, Noyes R, Pecknold JC: Secondary depression in panic disorder and agoraphobia, II: dimensions of depression symptomatology and their response to treatment. J Affect Disord 1989; 16:49–58 [B]
8. Klerman G, Weissman MM, Ouellette R, Johnson J, Greenwald S: Panic attacks in the community: social morbidity and health care utilization. JAMA 1991; 265:742–746 [E]
9. Weissman MM, Klerman GL, Markowitz JS, Ouellette R: Suicidal ideation and attempts in panic disorder and attacks. N Engl J Med 1989; 321:1209–1214 [C]
10. Markowitz JS, Weissman MM, Ouellette R, Lish JD, Klerman GL: Quality of life in panic disorder. Arch Gen Psychiatry 1989; 46:984–992 [B]
11. Knowles JA, Weissman MM: Panic disorder and agoraphobia, in American Psychiatric Press Review of Psychiatry, vol 14. Edited by Oldham JM, Riba MB. Washington, DC, American Psychiatric Press, 1995, pp 383–404 [G]
12. Goldstein RB, Wickramarante PJ, Horwath E, Weissman MM: Familial aggregation and phenomenology of "early"-onset (at or before age 20 years) panic disorder. Arch Gen Psychiatry 1997; 54:271–278 [C]
13. Kendler KS, Neale MC, Kessler RC, Heath AC, Eaves LJ: A test of the equal-environment assumption in twin studies of psychiatric illness. Behav Genet 1993; 23:21–27 [D]
14. Kendler KS, Neale MC, Kessler RC, Heath AC, Eaves LJ: Panic disorder in women: a population-based twin study. Psychol Med 1993; 23:387–406 [D]
15. American Psychiatric Association: Practice Guideline for Psychiatric Evaluation of Adults. Am J Psychiatry 1995; 152(Nov suppl):63–80 [G]
16. Cross-National Collaborative Panic Study SPI: Drug treatment of panic disorder: comparative efficacy of alprazolam, imipramine, and placebo. Br J Psychiatry 1992; 160:191–202, discussion 202–205; correction 1993; 161:724 [A]
17. Barlow DH, Craske MG: Mastery of Your Anxiety and Panic II. Albany, NY, Graywind Publications, 1994 [G]
18. Lydiard RB, Morton WA, Emmanuel NP, Zealberg JJ, Laraia MT, Stuart GW, O'Neil PM, Ballenger JC: Preliminary report: placebo-controlled, double-blind study of the clinical and metabolic effects of desipramine in panic disorder. Psychopharmacol Bull 1993; 29:183–188 [A]
19. Barlow DH, Craske MG, Cerney JA, Klosko JS: Behavioral treatment of panic disorder. Behavior Therapy 1989; 20:261–282 [A]
20. Clark DM, Salkovskis PM, Hackmann A, Middleton H, Anastasiades P, Gelder M: A comparison of cognitive therapy, applied relaxation and imipramine in the treatment of panic disorder. Br J Psychiatry 1994; 164:759–769 [A]
21. Beck AT, Sokol L, Clark DA, Berchick R, Wright F: A crossover study of focused cognitive therapy for panic disorder. Am J Psychiatry 1992; 149:778–783 [A]
22. Lydiard RB, Lesser IM, Ballenger JC, Rubin RT, Laraia M, DuPont R: A fixed-dose study of alprazolam 2 mg, alprazolam 6 mg, and placebo in panic disorder. J Clin Psychopharmacol 1992; 12:96–103 [A]
23. Fiegenbaum W: Long-term efficacy of ungraded versus graded massed exposure in agoraphobics, in Panic and Phobias 2: Treatments and Variables Affecting Course and Outcome. Edited by Hand I, Wittchen H-U. Berlin, Springer-Verlag, 1988, pp 83–88 [G]
24. Barlow DH: Anxiety and Its Disorders: The Nature and Treatment of Anxiety and Panic. New York, Guilford, 1988 [G]
25. Chambless DL, Gillis MM: Cognitive therapy of anxiety disorders. J Consult Clin Psychol 1993; 61:248–260 [E]
26. Clum GA, Suris R: A meta-analysis of treatments for panic disorder. J Consult Clin Psychol 1993; 61:317–326 [E]

27. Hofmann SG, Lehman CL, Barlow DH: How specific are specific phobias? J Behav Ther Exp Psychiatry 1997; 28:233–240 [C]
28. Margraf J, Gobel M, Schneider S: Cognitive-Behavioral Treatments for Panic Disorder, vol 5. Amsterdam, Swets and Zeitlinger, 1990 [G]
29. Craske MG, Brown TA, Barlow DH: Behavioral treatment of panic disorder: a two-year follow-up. Behavior Therapy 1991; 22:289–304 [D]
30. Klosko JS, Barlow DH, Tassinari R, Cerny JA: A comparison of alprazolam and behavior therapy in treatment of panic disorder. J Consult Clin Psychol 1990; 58:77–84 [A]
31. Clark DB, Agras WS: The assessment and treatment of performance anxiety in musicians. Am J Psychiatry 1991; 148:598–605 [A]
32. Black DW, Wesner R, Bowers W, Gabel J: A comparison of fluvoxamine, cognitive therapy and placebo in the treatment of panic disorder. Arch Gen Psychiatry 1993; 50:44–50 [A]
33. Telch MJ, Lucas JA, Schmidt NB, Hanna HH, Jaimez LT, Lucas RA: Group cognitive-behavioral treatment of panic disorder. Behav Res Ther 1993; 31:279–287 [A]
34. Craske MG, Rodriguez BI: Behavioral treatment of panic disorders and agoraphobia. Prog Behav Modif 1994; 29:1–26 [A]
35. Shear MK, Pilkonis PA, Cloitre M, Leon AC: Cognitive behavioral treatment compared with nonprescriptive treatment of panic disorder. Arch Gen Psychiatry 1994; 51:395–401 [A]
36. Ost LG, Westling BE: Applied relaxation vs cognitive behavior therapy in the treatment of panic disorder. Behav Res Ther 1995; 33:145–158 [A]
37. Ost LG, Westling BE, Hellstrom K: Applied relaxation exposure in vivo and cognitive methods in the treatment of panic disorder with agoraphobia. Behav Res Ther 1993; 31:383–394 [A]
38. van den Hout M, Arntz A, Hoekstra R: Exposure reduced agoraphobia but not panic and cognitive therapy reduced pain but not agoraphobia. Behav Res Ther 1994; 32:447–451 [A]
39. Marks IM, Swinson RP, Basoglu M: Alprazolam and exposure alone and combined in panic disorder with agoraphobia. Br J Psychiatry 1993; 162:776–787 [B]
40. Swinson RP, Soulios C, Cox BJ, Kuch K: Brief treatment of emergency room patients with panic attacks. Am J Psychiatry 1992; 149:944–946 [A]
41. Swinson RP, Fergus KD, Cox BJ, Wickwire K: Efficacy of telephone-administered behavioral therapy for panic disorder. Behav Res Ther 1995; 33:465–469 [B]
42. Fava GA, Zielezny M, Savron G, Grandi S: Long-term effects of behavioural treatment for panic disorder with agoraphobia. Br J Psychiatry 1995; 166:87–92 [B]
43. Brown TA, Barlow DH: Long term outcome of cognitive behavioral treatment of panic disorder. J Consult Clin Psychol 1995; 63:754–765 [B]
44. O'Sullivan G, Marks IM: Long-term outcome of phobic and obsessive compulsive disorders after exposure: a review chapter, in The Treatment of Anxiety: Handbook of Anxiety, vol 4. Edited by Noyes R, Roth M, Burrows G. Amsterdam, Elsevier, 1990, pp 82–108 [G]
45. Barlow DH: Cognitive-behavioral therapy for panic disorder: current status. J Clin Psychiatry 1997; 58(suppl 2):32–36 [F]
46. Shear MK, Barlow D, Gorman J, Woods S: Multicenter treatment study of panic disorder. Presented at the 36th annual meeting of the American College of Neuropsychopharmacology, Kamuela, Hawaii, Dec 8–12, 1997 [A]
47. Neron S, Lacroix D, Chaput Y: Group vs individual cognitive behaviour therapy in panic disorder: an open clinical trial with a six month follow-up. Can J Behavioral Sci 1995; 27:379–392 [C]
48. Cerny JA, Barlow DH, Craske MG, Himadi WG: Couples treatment of agoraphobia: a two-year follow-up. Behavior Therapy 1987; 18:401–415 [C]
49. Craske MG, Rowe M, Lewin M, Noriega-Dimitri R: Interoceptive exposure versus breathing retraining within cognitive-behavioural therapy for panic disorder with agoraphobia. Br J Clin Psychol 1997; 36(part 1):85–99 [A]

50. Hoffart A, Thornes K, Hedley LM: DSM-III-R axis I and II disorders in agoraphobic inpatients before and after psychosocial treatment. Psychiatry Res 1995; 56:1–9 [C]
51. Lidren D, Watkins P, Gould R, Clum G, Asterino M, Tulloch H: A comparison of bibliotherapy and group therapy in the treatment of panic disorder. J Consult Clin Psychol 1994; 62:865–869 [B]
52. Carter MM, Turovsky J, Barlow DH: Interpersonal relationships in panic disorder with agoraphobia: a review of empirical evidence. Clin Psychol: Science and Practice 1994; 1:25–34 [F]
53. Spiegel DA, Bruce TJ, Gregg SF, Nuzzarello A: Does cognitive behavior therapy assist slow-taper alprazolam discontinuation in panic disorder? Am J Psychiatry 1994; 151: 876–881 [A]
54. Otto MW, Pollack MH, Sachs GS, Reiter SR, Meltzer-Brody S, Rosenbaum JF: Discontinuation of benzodiazepine treatment: efficacy of cognitive-behavioral therapy for patients with panic disorder. Am J Psychiatry 1993; 150:1485–1490 [A]
55. Spiegel DA, Bruce TJ: Benzodiazepines and exposure-based cognitive behavior therapies for panic disorder: conclusion from combined treatment trials. Am J Psychiatry 1997; 154:773–781 [F]
56. Milrod B, Busch F, Cooper A, Shapiro T: Manual of Panic-Focused Psychodynamic Psychotherapy. Washington, DC, American Psychiatric Press, 1997 [G]
57. Kohut H: Thoughts on narcissism and narcissistic rage. Psychoanal Study Child 1972; 27:360–400 [G]
58. Bash M: Doing Brief Psychotherapy. New York, Basic Books, 1995 [G]
59. Gray JA: The neuropsychiatry of anxiety. Br J Psychol 1978; 69:417–434 [G]
60. Sifneos PE: The current status of individual short-term dynamic psychotherapy and its future: an overview. Am J Psychother 1984; 38:472–483 [G]
61. Sifneos PE: Short-term dynamic psychotherapy for patients with physical symptomatology. Psychother Psychosom 1984; 42:48–51 [F]
62. Shear MK: Psychotherapeutic issues in long-term treatment of anxiety disorder patients. Psychiatr Clin North Am 1995; 18:885–894 [F]
63. Wiborg IM, Dahl AA: Does brief dynamic psychotherapy reduce the relapse rate of panic disorder? Arch Gen Psychiatry 1996; 53:689–694 [A]
64. Beitman BD, Goldfried MR, Norcross JC: The movement toward integrating the psychotherapies: an overview. Am J Psychiatry 1989; 146:138–147 [G]
65. Shear MK, Weiner K: Psychotherapy for panic disorder. J Clin Psychiatry 1997; 58(suppl 2):38–43 [G]
66. Zitrin CM, Klein DF, Woerner MG: Treatment of agoraphobia with group exposure in vivo and imipramine. Arch Gen Psychiatry 1980; 37:63–72 [A]
67. Zitrin CM, Klein DF, Woerner MG, Ross DC: Treatment of phobias, I: comparison of imipramine hydrochloride and placebo. Arch Gen Psychiatry 1983; 40:125–138 [A]
68. Marks IM, Gray S, Cohen D, Hill R, Mawson D, Ramm E, Stern RS: Imipramine and brief therapist-aided exposure in agoraphobics having self-exposure homework. Arch Gen Psychiatry 1983; 40:153–162 [A]
69. Mavissakalian M, Michelson L, Dealy RS: Pharmacological treatment of agoraphobia: imipramine vs imipramine with programmed practice. Br J Psychiatry 1983; 143:348–355 [A]
70. Telch MJ, Agras WS, Taylor CB, Roth WT, Gallen CC: Combined pharmacological and behavioral treatment for agoraphobia. Behav Res Ther 1985; 23:325–335 [A]
71. Mavissakalian M, Michelson L: Relative and combined effectiveness of therapist-assisted in vivo exposure and imipramine. J Clin Psychiatry 1986; 47:117–122 [B]
72. Mavissakalian M, Michelson L: Two-year follow-up of exposure and imipramine treatment of agoraphobia. Am J Psychiatry 1986; 143:1106–1112 [B]
73. Oehrberg S, Christiansen PE, Behnke K: Paroxetine in the treatment of panic disorder: a randomized double-blind placebo-controlled study. Br J Psychiatry 1995; 167:374–379 [A]

74. Pollack MH, Otto MW, Kaspi SP, Hammerness PG, Rosenbaum JF: Cognitive behavior therapy for treatment-refractory panic disorder. J Clin Psychiatry 1994; 55:200–205 [B]
75. Nagy LM, Krystal JH, Woods SW: Clinical and medication outcome after short-term alprazolam and behavioral group treatment of panic disorder: 2.5 year naturalistic follow-up. Arch Gen Psychiatry 1989; 46:993–999 [B, C]
76. Kabat-Zinn J, Massion AO, Kristeller J, Peterson LG, Fletcher KE, Pbert L, Lenderking WR, Santorelli SF: Effectiveness of a meditation-based stress reduction program in the treatment of anxiety disorders. Am J Psychiatry 1992; 149:936–943 [B]
77. Miller JJ, Fletcher K, Kabat-Zinn J: Three-year follow-up and clinical implications of a mindfulness meditation-based stress reduction intervention in the treatment of anxiety disorders. Gen Hosp Psychiatry 1995; 17:192–200 [D]
78. Buglass D, Clarke J, Henderson AS, Kreitman N: A study of agoraphobic housewives. Psychol Med 1977; 7:73–86 [D]
79. Arrindell WA, Emmelkamp PM: Marital adjustment, intimacy and needs in female agoraphobics and their partners: a controlled study. Br J Psychiatry 1986; 149:592–602; correction 1987; 150:273 [D]
80. Lange A, van Dyck R: The function of agoraphobia in the marital relationship. Acta Psychiatr Scand 1992; 85:89–93 [E]
81. Hafner RJ: Predicting the effects on husbands of behaviour therapy for wives' agoraphobia. Behav Res Ther 1984; 22: 217–226 [C]
82. Milton F, Hafner J: The outcome of behavior therapy for agoraphobia in relation to marital adjustment. Arch Gen Psychiatry 1979; 36:807–811 [B]
83. Jacobson NS, Holtzworth-Monroe A, Schmaling KB: Marital therapy and spouse involvement in the treatment of depression, agoraphobia, and alcoholism. J Consult Clin Psychol 1989; 57:5–10 [F]
84. Himadi WG, Cerny JA, Barlow DH, Cohen S, O'Brien GT: The relationship of marital adjustment to agoraphobia treatment outcome. Behav Res Ther 1986; 24:107–115 [C]
85. Barlow DH, O'Brien GT, Last CG: Couples treatment of agoraphobia. Behavior Therapy 1984; 15:41–58 [C]
86. Arnow BA, Taylor CB, Agras WS: Enhancing agoraphobia treatment outcome by changing couple communication patterns. Behavior Therapy 1985; 16:452–467 [C]
87. Lydiard RB, Pollack MH, Judge R, Michelson D, Tamura R: Fluoxetine in panic disorder: a placebo-controlled study. Presented at the 10th Congress of the European College of Neuropsychopharmacology, Vienna, Sept 13–17, 1997 [A]
88. Gorman JM, Liebowitz MR, Fyer AJ, Goetz D, Campeas RB, Fyer MR, Davies SO, Klein DF: An open trial of fluoxetine in the treatment of panic disorder. J Clin Psychopharmacol 1987; 7:319–332 [B]
89. Schneier FR, Liebowitz MR, Davies SO, Fairbanks J, Hollander E, Campeas R, Klein DF: Fluoxetine in panic disorder. J Clin Psychopharmacol 1990; 10:119–121 [B]
90. Wolkow R, Apter J, Clayton A, Coryell W, Cunningham L, McEntee W, O'Hair D, Pollack M, Rausch J, Stewart R, Weisler R: Double-blind flexible dose study of sertraline and placebo in patients with panic disorder. Presented at the XX Congress of the Collegium Internationale Neuro-Psychopharmacologicum, Melbourne, Australia, June 23–27, 1996 [A]
91. Baumel B, Bielski R, Carman J, Hegel M, Houck C, Linden R, Nakra B, Ota K, Pohl R, Wolkow R: Double-blind comparison of sertraline and placebo in patients with panic disorder. Ibid [A]
92. Ballenger JC, Wheadon DE, Steiner M, Bushnell W, Gergel IP: Double-blind, fixed-dose, placebo-controlled study of paroxetine in the treatment of panic disorder. Am J Psychiatry 1998; 155:36–42 [A]
93. LeCrubier Y, Bakker A, Dunbar G, Judge R: A comparison of paroxetine, clomipramine and placebo in the treatment of panic disorder. Acta Psychiatr Scand 1997; 95:145–152 [A]

94. Hoehn-Saric R, McLeod DR, Hipsley PA: Effect of fluvoxamine on panic disorder. J Clin Psychopharmacol 1993; 13:321–326 [B]
95. de Beurs E, van Balkom AJ, Lange A, Koele P, van Dyck R: Treatment of panic disorder with agoraphobia: comparison of fluvoxamine, placebo, and psychological panic management combined with exposure and of exposure in vivo alone. Am J Psychiatry 1995; 152:683–691 [B]
96. Westenberg HG, den Boer JA: Selective monoamine uptake inhibitors and a serotonin antagonist in the treatment of panic disorder. Psychopharmacol Bull 1989; 25:119–123 [B]
97. Wade AG, Lepola U, Koponen HJ, Pedersen V, Pedersen T: The effect of citalopram in panic disorder. Br J Psychiatry 1997; 170:549–553 [A]
98. Boyer W: Serotonin uptake inhibitors are superior to imipramine and alprazolam in alleviating panic attacks: a meta-analysis. Int Clin Psychopharmacol 1995; 10:45–49 [E]
99. Lejoyeux M, Ades J: Antidepressant discontinuation: a review of the literature. J Clin Psychiatry 1997; 58(July suppl):11–16 [G]
100. Louie AK, Lewis TB, Lannon RA: Use of low-dose fluoxetine in major depression and panic disorder. J Clin Psychiatry 1993; 54:435–438 [C]
101. Emmanuel NP, Crosby C, Ware MR, Lydiard RB: The efficacy of once-a-week fluoxetine dosing in the treatment of panic disorder, in 1996 Annual Meeting New Research Program and Abstracts. Washington, DC, American Psychiatric Association, 1996, p 252 [G]
102. DuBoff E, England D, Ferguson JM, Londborg PD, Rosenthal MH, Smith W, Weise C, Wolkow RM: Sertraline in the treatment of panic disorder. Presented at the 8th Congress of the European College of Neuropsychopharmacology, Venice, Sept 30 to Oct 4, 1995 [A]
103. Gergel I, Burnham D, Kumar R: Treatment of panic disorder with paroxetine. Presented at the 6th World Congress of Biological Psychiatry, Nice, France, June 22–27, 1997 [A]
104. Klein D: Delineation of two drug-responses for anxiety syndromes. Psychopharmacologia 1964; 5:397–408 [A]
105. Uhlenhuth EH, Matuzas W, Glass RM, Easton C: Response of panic disorder to fixed doses of alprazolam or imipramine. J Affect Disord 1989; 17:261–270 [A]
106. Modigh K, Westberg P, Eriksson E: Superiority of clomipramine over imipramine in the treatment of panic disorder: a placebo-controlled trial. J Clin Psychopharmacol 1992; 12:251–261 [A]
107. Andersch S, Rosenberg NK, Kullingsjo H, Ottoson JQ, Hanson L, Lorentzen K, Mellergard M, Rasmussen S, Rosenberg R: Efficacy and safety of alprazolam, imipramine, and placebo in treating panic disorder: a Scandinavian multicenter study. Acta Psychiatr Scand Suppl 1991; 365:18–27 [A]
108. Mavissakalian M, Perel J: Imipramine in the treatment of agoraphobia: dose-response relationships. Am J Psychiatry 1985; 142:1032–1036 [A]
109. Mavissakalian MR, Perel JM: Imipramine dose-response relationship in panic disorder with agoraphobia. Arch Gen Psychiatry 1989; 46:127–131 [A]
110. Mavissakalian MR, Perel JM: Imipramine treatment of panic disorder with agoraphobia: dose ranging and plasma level-response relationships. Am J Psychiatry 1995; 152:673–682 [A]
111. Maier W, Roth SM, Argyle N, Buller R, Lavori P, Brandon S, Benkert O: Avoidance behaviour: a predictor of the efficacy of pharmacotherapy in panic disorder? Eur Arch Psychiatry Clin Neurosci 1991; 241:151–158 [A]
112. Cassano GB, Toni C, Musetti L: Treatment of panic disorder, in Synaptic Transmission. Edited by Biggio G, Concas A, Costa E. New York, Raven Press, 1992, pp 449–461 [A]
113. Curtis GC, Massana J, Udina C, Ayuso JL, Cassano GB, Perugi G: Maintenance drug therapy of panic disorder. J Psychiatr Res 1993; 27(suppl 1):127–142 [A]
114. Keller MB, Lavori PW, Goldenberg IM, Baker LA, Pollack MH, Sachs GS, Rosenbaum JF, Deltito JA, Leon A, Shear K, Klerman GL: Influence of depression on the treatment of panic disorder with imipramine, alprazolam, imipramine. J Affect Disord 1993; 28:27–38 [A]

115. Woods S, Nagy LM, Koleszar AS, Krystal JH, Heninger GR, Charney DS: Controlled trial of alprazolam supplementation during imipramine treatment of panic disorder. J Clin Psychopharmacol 1991; 12:32–38 [A]
116. Mellergard M, Lorentzen K, Bech P, Ottoson JQ, Rosenberg R: A trend analysis of changes during treatment of panic disorder with alprazolam and imipramine. Acta Psychiatr Scand Suppl 1991; 365:28–32 [A]
117. Pollack MH, Otto MW, Sachs GS, Leon A, Shear MK, Deltito JA, Keller MB, Rosenbaum JF: Anxiety psychopathology predictive of outcome in patients with panic disorder and depression treated with imipramine, alprazolam, and placebo. J Affect Disord 1994; 30:273–281 [A]
118. Den Boer JA, Westenberg HG: Effect of a serotonin and noradrenaline uptake inhibitor in panic disorder: a double-blind comparative study with fluvoxamine and maprotiline. Int Clin Psychopharmacol 1988; 3:59–74 [B]
119. Cassano GB, Petracca A, Perugi G, Nisita C, Musetti L, Mengali F, McNair DM: Clomipramine for panic disorder, I: the first 10 weeks of a long-term comparison with imipramine. J Affect Disord 1988; 14:123–127 [B]
120. Monteiro WO, Noshirvani HF, Marks IM: Anorgasmia from clomipramine in obsessive-compulsive disorder: a controlled trial. Br J Psychiatry 1987; 151:107–112 [B]
121. Mavissakalian M, Perel JM: Clinical experiments in maintenance and discontinuation of imipramine therapy in panic disorder with agoraphobia. Arch Gen Psychiatry 1992; 49:318–323 [B]
122. Mavissakalian M, Perel JM: Protective effects of imipramine maintenance treatment in panic disorder with agoraphobia. Am J Psychiatry 1992; 149:1053–1057 [B]
123. Sheehan DV: Tricyclic antidepressants in the treatment of panic and anxiety disorders. Psychosomatics 1986; 27:10–16 [F]
124. Fyer AJ, Liebowitz MR, Gorman JM, Campeas R, Levin A, Davies SO, Goetz D, Klein DF: Discontinuation of alprazolam treatment in panic patients. Am J Psychiatry 1987; 144:303–308 [B]
125. Klerman GL: Overview of the Cross-National Collaborative Panic Study. Arch Gen Psychiatry 1988; 45:407–412 [F]
126. Dunner DL, Ishiki D, Avery DH, Wilson LG, Hyde TS: Effect of alprazolam and diazepam in anxiety and panic attacks in panic disorder: a controlled study. J Clin Psychiatry 1986; 47:458–460 [B]
127. Ballenger JC, Burrows GD, DuPont RL Jr, Lesser IM, Noyes R Jr, Pecknold JC, Rifkin A, Swinson RP: Alprazolam in panic disorder and agoraphobia: results from a multicenter trial, I: efficacy in short-term treatment. Arch Gen Psychiatry 1988; 45:413–422 [A]
128. Tesar GE, Rosenbaum JF, Pollack MH, Otto MW, Sachs GS, Herman JB, Cohen LS, Spier SA: Double-blind, placebo-controlled comparison of clonazepam and alprazolam for panic disorder. J Clin Psychiatry 1991; 52:69–76 [A]
129. Schweizer E, Rickels K, Weiss S, Zavodnick S: Maintenance drug treatment of panic disorder, I: results of a prospective, placebo-controlled comparison of alprazolam and imipramine. Arch Gen Psychiatry 1993; 50:51–60 [A]
130. Dager SR, Roy-Byrne P, Hendrickson H, Cowley DS, Avery DH, Hall KC, Dunner DL: Long-term outcome of panic states during double-blind treatment and after withdrawal of alprazolam and placebo. Ann Clin Psychiatry 1992; 4:251–258 [A]
131. Chouinard G, Annable L, Fontaine R, Solyom L: Alprazolam in the treatment of generalized anxiety and panic disorders: a double-blind placebo-controlled study. Psychopharmacology (Berl) 1982; 77:229–233 [B]
132. McNair DM, Kahn RJ: Imipramine compared with a benzodiazepine for agoraphobia, in Anxiety: New Research and Changing Concepts. Edited by Klein DF, Rabkin J. New York, Raven Press, 1981, pp 69–80 [B]

133. Noyes RJ, Anderson DJ, Clancy J, Crowe RR, Slymen DJ, Ghoneim MM, Hinrichs JV: Diazepam and propranolol in panic disorder and agoraphobia. Arch Gen Psychiatry 1984; 41:287–292 [A]
134. Schweizer E, Rickels K: Failure of buspirone to manage benzodiazepine withdrawal. Am J Psychiatry 1986; 143:1590–1592 [B]
135. Schweizer E, Case WG, Rickels K: Benzodiazepine dependence and withdrawal in elderly patients. Am J Psychiatry 1989; 146:529–531 [B]
136. Schweizer E, Clary C, Dever AI, Mandos LA: The use of low-dose intranasal midazolam to treat panic disorder: a pilot study. J Clin Psychiatry 1992; 53:19–22 [B]
137. Charney DS, Woods SW: Benzodiazepine treatment of panic disorder: a comparison of alprazolam and lorazepam. J Clin Psychiatry 1989; 50:418–423 [B]
138. Pyke RE, Greenberg HS: Double-blind comparison of alprazolam and adinazolam for panic and phobia disorders. J Clin Psychopharmacol 1989; 9:15–21 [B]
139. Savoldi F, Somenzini G, Ecari U: Etizolam versus placebo in the treatment of panic disorder with agoraphobia: a double-blind study. Curr Med Res Opin 1990; 12:185–190 [A]
140. Beaudry P, Fontaine R, Chouinard G: Bromazepam, another high-potency benzodiazepine for panic attacks (letter). Am J Psychiatry 1984; 141:464–465 [G]
141. Noyes R, Borrows GD, Reich JH, Judd FK, Garvey M, Morman TR, Cook BL, Marriot P: Diazepam versus alprazolam for the treatment of panic disorder. J Clin Psychiatry 1996; 57:349–355 [A]
142. Benzodiazepine Dependence, Toxicity, and Abuse: A Task Force Report of the American Psychiatric Association. Washington, DC, APA, 1990 [G]
143. Rickels K, Schweizer E, Weiss S, Zavodnick S: Maintenance drug treatment for panic disorder, II: short- and long-term outcome after drug taper. Arch Gen Psychiatry 1993; 50:61–68 [B]
144. Klein E, Colin V, Stolk J, Lenox RH: Alprazolam withdrawal in patients with panic disorder and generalized anxiety disorder: vulnerability and effect of carbamazapine. Am J Psychiatry 1994; 151:1760–1766 [A]
145. Noyes R Jr, Garvey MJ, Cook B, Suelzer M: Controlled discontinuation of benzodiazepine treatment for patients with panic disorder. Am J Psychiatry 1991; 148:517–523 [B]
146. Pecknold JC, Swinson RP: Taper withdrawal studies with alprazolam inpatients with panic disorder and agoraphobia. Psychopharmacol Bull 1986; 22:173–176 [A]
147. Rosenbaum JF, Moroz G, Bowden CL: Clonazepam in the treatment of panic disorder with or without agoraphobia: a dose-response study of efficacy, safety, and discontinuance. J Clin Psychopharmacol 1997; 17:390–400 [A]
148. Lesser IM, Lydiard RB, Antal E, Rubin RT, Ballenger JC, DuPont R: Alprazolam plasma concentrations and treatment response in panic disorder and agoraphobia. Am J Psychiatry 1992; 149:1556–1562 [A]
149. Greenblatt DJ, Harmatiz JS, Shader RI: Plasma alprazolam concentrations: relation to efficacy and side effects in the treatment of panic disorder. Arch Gen Psychiatry 1993; 50: 715–722 [B]
150. Lepola UM, Rimon RH, Riekkinen PJ: Three-year follow-up of patients with panic disorder after short-term treatment with alprazolam and imipramine. Int Clin Psychopharmacol 1993; 8:115–118 [B]
151. Sheehan DV, Claycomb JB, Kouretas N: Monoamine oxidase inhibitors: prescription and patient management. Int J Psychiatry Med 1980–1981; 10:99–121 [G]
152. American Psychiatric Association: Diagnostic and Statistical Manual of Mental Disorders, 2nd ed (DSM-II). Washington, DC, APA, 1968 [G]
153. Bakish D, Saxena BM, Bowen R, D'Souza J: Reversible monoamine oxidase-A inhibitors in panic disorder. Clin Neuropsychopharmacol 1993; 16(suppl 2):S77–S82 [A]

154. Garcia-Borreguero D, Lauer CJ, Ozdaglar A, Wiedemann K, Holsboer F, Krieg JC: Brofaromine in panic disorder: a pilot study with a new reversible inhibitor of monoamine oxidase-A. Pharmacopsychiatry 1992; 25:261–264 [B]
155. van Harten J: Clinical pharmacokinetics of selective serotonin reuptake inhibitors. Clin Pharmacokinet 1993; 24:203–220 [F]
156. Pollack MH, Worthington JJ, Otto MW, Maki KM, Smoller JW, Manfro GG, Rudolph R, Rosenbaum JF: Venlafaxine for panic disorder: results from a double-blind, placebo-controlled study. Psychopharmacol Bull 1996; 32:667–670 [A]
157. Geracioti JD: Venlafaxine treatment of panic disorder: a case series. J Clin Psychiatry 1995; 56:408–410 [G]
158. Charney DS, Woods SW, Goodman WK, Rifkin B, Kinch M, Aiken B, Quadrino LM, Heninger GR: Drug treatment of panic disorder: the comparative efficacy of imipramine, alprazolam, and trazodone. J Clin Psychiatry 1986; 47:580–586 [B]
159. Mavissakalian M, Perel J, Bowler K, Dealy R: Trazodone in the treatment of panic disorder and agoraphobia with panic attacks. Am J Psychiatry 1987; 144:785–787 [B]
160. Sheehan DV, Davidson J, Manschreck T, Van Wyck Fleet J: Lack of efficacy of a new antidepressant (bupropion) in the treatment of panic disorder with phobias. J Clin Psychopharmacol 1983; 3:28–31 [G]
161. Zajecka JM: The effect of nefazodone on comorbid anxiety symptoms associated with depression: experience in family practice and psychiatric outpatient settings. J Clin Psychiatry 1996; 57(2 suppl):10–14 [A]
162. DeMartinis NA, Schweizer E, Rickels K: An open-label trial of nefazodone in high comorbidity panic disorder. J Clin Psychiatry 1996; 57:245–248 [B]
163. Keck PE Jr, McElroy SL, Friedman LM: Valproate and carbamazepine in the treatment of panic and posttraumatic stress disorders, withdrawal states, and behavioral dyscontrol syndromes. J Clin Psychopharmacol 1992; 12(1 suppl):36S–41S [F]
164. Uhde TW, Stein MB, Post RM: Lack of efficacy of carbamazepine in the treatment of panic disorder. Am J Psychiatry 1988; 145:1104–1109 [B]
165. Lum M, Fontaine R, Elie R, Ontiveros A: Divalproex sodium's antipanic effect in panic disorder: a placebo-controlled study. Biol Psychiatry 1990; 27(9A):164A [A, B]
166. Woodman CL, Noyes R: Panic disorder: treatment with valproate. J Clin Psychiatry 1994; 55:134–136 [B]
167. Munjack DJ, Crocker B, Cabe D, Brown R, Usigli R, Zulueta A, McManus M, McDowell D, Palmer R, Leonard M: Alprazolam, propranolol, and placebo in the treatment of panic disorder and agoraphobia with panic attacks. J Clin Psychopharmacol 1989; 9:22–27 [A]
168. Ravaris CL, Friedman MJ, Hauri PJ, McHugo GJ: A controlled study of alprazolam and propranolol in panic-disordered and agoraphobic outpatients. J Clin Psychopharmacol 1991; 11:344–350 [A]
169. Shehi M, Patterson WM: Treatment of panic attacks with alprazolam and propranolol. Am J Psychiatry 1984; 141:900–901 [B]
170. Klein E, Uhde TW: Controlled study of verapamil for treatment of panic disorder. Am J Psychiatry 1988; 145:431–434 [A]
171. Benjamin J, Levine J, Fux M, Aviv A, Levy D, Belmaker RH: Double-blind, placebo-controlled, crossover trial of inositol treatment for panic disorder. Am J Psychiatry 1995; 152:1084–1086 [A]
172. Uhde TW, Stein MB, Vittone BJ, Siever LJ, Boulenger JP, Klein E, Mellman TA: Behavioral and physiologic effects of short-term and long-term administration of clonidine in panic disorder. Arch Gen Psychiatry 1989; 46:170–177 [A, B]
173. Spielberger CD: State-Trait Anxiety Inventory. Palo Alto, Calif, Consulting Psychologists Press, 1985 [G]
174. Zung WWK: A rating instrument for anxiety disorders. Psychosomatics 1971; 12:371–379 [G]

175. Hoehn-Saric R, Merchant AF, Keyser ML, Smith VK: Effects of clonidine on anxiety disorders. Arch Gen Psychiatry 1981; 38:1278–1282 [B]
176. Sheehan DV, Raj AB, Harnett-Sheehan K, Soto S, Knapp E: The relative efficacy of high-dose buspirone and alprazolam in the treatment of panic disorder: a double-blind placebo-controlled study. Acta Psychiatr Scand 1993; 88:1–11 [A]
177. Sheehan DV, Raj A, Sheehan KH, Soto S: Is buspirone effective for panic disorder? J Clin Psychopharmacol 1990; 10:3–11 [A]
178. Pollard CA: Inpatient treatment of complicated agoraphobia and panic disorder. Hosp Community Psychiatry 1987; 38:951–958 [B]
179. Pollard HJ, Pollard CA: Follow-up study of an inpatient program for complicated agoraphobia and panic disorder. Anxiety Disorders Practice J 1993; 1:37–40 [C]
180. Cottraux J, Note ID, Cungi C, Legeron P, Heim F, Chneiweiss L, Bernard G, Bouvard M: A controlled study of cognitive behaviour therapy with buspirone or placebo in panic disorder with agoraphobia. Br J Psychiatry 1995; 167:635–641 [A]
181. Wolfe BE, Maser JD (eds): Treatment of Panic Disorder: A Consensus Development Conference. Washington, DC, American Psychiatric Press, 1994 [G]
182. Coryell W, Noyes R, Clancy J: Excess mortality in panic disorder. Arch Gen Psychiatry 1982; 39:701–703 [D]
183. Noyes R: Suicide and panic disorder: a review. J Affect Disord 1991; 22:1–11 [F]
184. Warshaw MG, Massion AO, Peterson LG, Pratt LA, Keller MB: Suicidal behavior in inpatients with panic disorder: retrospective and prospective data. J Affect Disord 1995; 34:235–247 [C, D]
185. Lepine JP, Chignon M, Teherani M: Suicide attempts in patients with panic disorder. Arch Gen Psychiatry 1993; 50:144–149 [D]
186. Johnson J, Weissman MM, Klerman GL: Panic disorder comorbidity and suicide attempts. Arch Gen Psychiatry 1990; 47:805–808 [D]
187. Beck AT, Steer RA, Snaderson WC, Skeie TM: Panic disorder and suicidal ideation and behavior: discrepant findings in psychiatric outpatients. Am J Psychiatry 1991; 148:1195–1199 [D]
188. Hornig CD, McNally RJ: Panic disorder and suicide attempt: a reanalysis of data from the Epidemiologic Catchment Area study. Br J Psychiatry 1995; 167:76–79 [D]
189. Fawcett J, Scheftner WA, Fogg L, Clark DC, Young MA, Hedeker D, Gibbons R: Time-related predictors of suicide in major affective disorder. Am J Psychiatry 1990; 147:1189–1194 [C]
190. Mannuzza S: Panic disorder and suicide attempts. J Anxiety Disord 1992; 6:261–274 [D]
191. Cox BJ, Direnfeld DM, Swinson RP, Norton GR: Suicidal ideation and suicide attempts in panic disorder and social phobia. Am J Psychiatry 1994; 151:882–887 [D]
192. Friedman S, Jones JC, Chernen L, Barlow DH: Suicidal ideation and suicide attempts among patients with panic disorder: a survey of two outpatient clinics. Am J Psychiatry 1992; 149:680–685 [D]
193. Kushner MG, Sher KJ, Beitman BD: The relation between alcohol problems and the anxiety disorders. Am J Psychiatry 1990; 147:685–695 [F]
194. Anthony JC, Tien AY, Petronis KR: Epidemiological evidence on cocaine use and panic attacks. Am J Epidemiol 1989; 129:543–549 [C]
195. Mirin SM, Weiss RD, Griffin ML, Michael JL: Psychopathology in drug users and their families. Compr Psychiatry 1991; 32:36–51 [E]
196. Nunes E, Quitkin B, Berman C: Panic disorder and depression in female alcoholics. J Clin Psychiatry 1988; 49:441–443 [F]
197. Aronson TA, Craig TJ: Cocaine precipitation of panic disorder. Am J Psychiatry 1986; 143:643–645 [D]

198. Pallanti S, Mazzi D: MDMA (Ecstasy) precipitation of panic disorder. Biol Psychiatry 1992; 32:91–95 [G]
199. Moran C: Depersonalization and agoraphobia associated with marijuana use. Br J Med Psychol 1986; 59:187–196 [B]
200. Cowley DS: Alcohol abuse, substance abuse, and panic disorder. Am J Med 1992; 92(suppl 1A):41S–48S [F]
201. Brown SA, Irwin M, Schuckit MA: Changes in anxiety among abstinent male alcoholics. J Stud Alcohol 1991; 52:55–61 [B]
202. Thevos AK, Johnston AL, Latham PK, Randall CL, Adinoff B, Malcolm R: Symptoms of anxiety in inpatient alcoholics with and without DSM-III-R anxiety diagnoses. Alcohol Clin Exp Res 1991; 15:102–105 [B]
203. George DT, Nutt DJ, Dwyer BA, Linnoila M: Alcoholism and panic disorder: is the comorbidity more than coincidence? Acta Psychiatr Scand 1990; 81:97–107 [F]
204. Cox BJ, Norton GR, Swinson RP, Endler NS: Substance abuse and panic-related anxiety: a critical review. Behav Res Ther 1990; 28:385–393 [E]
205. Anthenelli RM, Schuckit MA: Affective and anxiety disorders and alcohol and drug dependence: diagnosis and treatment. J Addict Dis 1993; 12:73–87 [F]
206. Tucker P, Westermeyer J: Substance abuse in patients with comorbid anxiety disorder. Am J Addictions 1995; 4:226–233 [C]
207. Westermeyer J, Tucker P: Comorbid anxiety disorder and substance disorder. Am J Addictions 1995; 4:97–106 [C]
208. Ciraulo DA, Sands BF, Shader RI: Critical review of liability for benzodiazepine abuse among alcoholics. Am J Psychiatry 1988; 145:1501–1506 [F]
209. Shelton RC, Harvey DS, Stewart PM, Loosen PT: Alprazolam in panic disorder: a retrospective analysis. Prog Neuropsychopharmacol Biol Psychiatry 1993; 17:423–434 [E]
210. Lucas PB, Pickar D, Kelsoe J, Rapaport M, Pato C, Hommer D: Effects of the acute administration of caffeine in patients with schizophrenia. Biol Psychiatry 1990; 28:35–40 [B]
211. Leibenluft E, Fiero PL, Bartko JJ, Moul DE, Rosenthal NE: Depressive symptoms and the self-reported use of alcohol, caffeine, and carbohydrates in normal volunteers and four groups of psychiatric outpatients. Am J Psychiatry 1993; 150:294–301 [E]
212. Boulenger J-P, Uhde TW, Wolff EA, Post RM: Increased sensitivity to caffeine in patients with panic disorder. Arch Gen Psychiatry 1984; 41:1067–1071 [D]
213. Bowen R, South M, Hawkes J: Mood swings in patients with panic disorder. Can J Psychiatry 1994; 39:91–94 [G]
214. Savino M, Perugi G, Simonini E, Soriani A, Cassano GB, Akiskal HS: Affective comorbidity in panic disorder: is there a bipolar connection? J Affect Disord 1993; 28:155–163 [D, G]
215. Marks IM: Fears, Phobias, and Rituals. New York, Oxford University Press, 1987 [G]
216. Marks IM: Agoraphobia, panic disorder and related conditions in the DSM-IIIR and ICD-10. J Psychopharmacol 1987; 1:6–12 [G]
217. Herve C, Gaillard M, Roujas F, Huguenard P: Alcoholism in polytrauma. J Trauma 1986; 26:1123–1126 [E]
218. Boudewyns PA, Woods MG, Hyer L, Albrecht JW: Chronic combat-related PTSD and concurrent substance abuse: implications for treatment of this frequent "dual diagnosis." J Trauma Stress 1991; 4:549–560 [D]
219. Davidson J, Kudler H, Smith R: Treatment of posttraumatic stress disorder with amitriptyline and placebo. Arch Gen Psychiatry 1990; 47:259–266 [A]
220. Davidson JR, Kudler HS, Saunders WB, Smith RD: Symptom and comorbidity patterns in World War II and Vietnam veterans with posttraumatic stress disorder. Compr Psychiatry 1990; 31:162–170 [D]
221. Pitman RK, Altman B, Greenwald E: Psychiatric complications during flooding therapy for posttraumatic stress disorder. J Clin Psychiatry 1991; 52:17–20 [G]

222. Dansky BS, Roitzsch JC, Brady KT, Saladin ME: Posttraumatic stress disorder and substance abuse: use of research in a clinical setting. J Trauma Stress 1997; 10:141–148 [C]
223. Cottler LB, Compton WM III, Mager D, Spitznagel EL, Janca A: Posttraumatic stress disorder among substance users from the general population. Am J Psychiatry 1992; 149:664–670 [E]
224. Greist JH, Jefferson JW: Panic Disorder and Agoraphobia: A Guide, 2nd revised ed. Middleton, Wis, Dean Foundation for Health, Research, and Education, 1993 [G]
225. Mavissakalian M: The relationship between panic disorder/agoraphobia and personality disorders. Psychiatr Clin North Am 1990; 13:661–684 [F]
226. Brooks RB, Baltazar PL, McDowell DE, Munjack DJ, Bruns JR: Personality disorders co-occurring with panic disorder with agoraphobia. J Personality Disorders 1991; 5:328–336 [D]
227. Pollack MH, Otto MW, Rosenbaum JF, Sachs GS: Personality disorders in patients with panic disorder: association with childhood anxiety disorders, early trauma, comorbidity, and chronicity. Compr Psychiatry 1992; 33:78–83 [C]
228. Reich JH: DSM-III personality disorders and the outcome of treated panic disorder. Am J Psychiatry 1988; 145:1149–1152 [B]
229. Reich J, Troughton E: Frequency of DSM-III personality disorders in patients with panic disorder: comparison with psychiatric and normal control subjects. Psychiatry Res 1988; 26:89–100 [A]
230. Reich JH, Vasile RG: Effect of personality disorders on the treatment outcome of axis I conditions: an update. J Nerv Ment Dis 1993; 181:475–484 [F]
231. Green M, Curtis GC: Personality disorders and panic patients: response to termination of antipanic medication. J Personal Disord 1988; 2:303–314 [B]
232. Chambless DL, Renneberg B, Goldstein A, Gracely EJ: MCMI-diagnosed personality disorders among agoraphobic outpatients: prevalence and relationship of severity and treatment outcome. J Anxiety Disord 1992; 6:195–211 [D]
233. Marchand A, Goyer LR, Mainguy N: L'impact de la presence de troubles de la personnalité, sur la réponse au traitement behavioral-cognitif du trouble panique avec agoraphobie. Science et Comportement 1992; 22:149–161 [B]
234. Black DW, Wesner RB, Gabel J, Bowers W, Monahan P: Predictors of short-term treatment response in 66 patients with panic disorder. J Affect Disord 1994; 30:233–241 [A]
235. Dreessen L, Arntz A, Luttels C, Sallaerts S: Personality disorders do not influence the results of cognitive behavioral therapies for anxiety disorders. Compr Psychiatry 1994; 35:265–274 [B]
236. Keijsers GPJ, Hoogduin CAL, Schapp CPDR: Prognostic factors in the behavioral treatment of panic disorder with and without agoraphobia. Behavior Therapy 1994; 25:689–708 [B]
237. Karajgi B, Rifkin A, Doddi S, Kolli R: The prevalence of anxiety disorders in patients with chronic obstructive pulmonary disease. Am J Psychiatry 1990; 147:200–201 [D]
238. Kaplan DS, Masand PS, Gupta S: The relationship of irritable bowel syndrome (IBS) and panic disorder. Ann Clin Psychiatry 1996; 8:81–88 [D]
239. Lydiard RB, Greenwald S, Weissman MM, Johnson J, Drossman DA, Ballenger JC: Panic disorder and gastrointestinal symptoms: findings from the NIMH Epidemiologic Catchment Area project. Am J Psychiatry 1994; 151:64–70 [E]
240. Kawachi I, Colditz GA, Ascherio A, Rimm E, Giovannucci E, Stampfer MJ, Willett WC: Prospective study of phobic anxiety and risk of coronary heart disease in men. Circulation 1994; 89:1992–1997 [C]
241. American Academy of Child and Adolescent Psychiatry: Practice Parameters for the Assessment and Treatment of Children and Adolescents With Anxiety Disorders. J Am Acad Child Adolesc Psychiatry 1997; 36(10 suppl):69S–84S [G]
242. Black B: Separation anxiety disorder and panic disorder, in Anxiety Disorders in Children and Adolescents. Edited by March J. New York, Guilford, 1995, pp 212–234 [G]

243. Black B, Robbins D: Panic disorder in children and adolescents. J Am Acad Child Adolesc Psychiatry 1990; 29:36–44 [F]
244. Kearney CA, Silverman WK: The panic disorder controversy continues. J Am Acad Child Adolesc Psychiatry 1991; 30:852–853 [G]
245. Kearney CA, Silverman WK: Let's not push the "panic" button: a critical analysis of panic and panic disorder in adolescents. Clin Psychol Rev 1992; 12:293–305 [E]
246. Whitaker A, Johnson J, Shaffer D, Rapoport JL, Kalikow K, Walsh BT, Davies M, Braiman S, Dolinsky A: Uncommon troubles in young people: prevalence estimates of selected psychiatric disorders in a nonreferred adolescent population. Arch Gen Psychiatry 1990; 47:487–496 [D]
247. Hayward C, Killen JD, Hammer LD, Lift IF, Wilson DM, Simmonds B, Taylor CB: Pubertal stage and panic attack history in sixth- and seventh-grade girls. Am J Psychiatry 1992; 149:1239–1243 [D]
248. Curry J, Murphy L: Comorbidity of anxiety disorders, in Anxiety Disorders in Children and Adolescents. Edited by March J. New York, Guilford, 1995, pp 301–317 [G]
249. Kovacs M, Feinberg TL, Crouse-Novak MA, Paulauskas SL, Finkelstein R: Depressive disorders in childhood, I: a longitudinal prospective study of characteristics and recovery. Arch Gen Psychiatry 1984; 41:229–237 [B]
250. Bernstein GA: Comorbidity and severity of anxiety and depressive disorders in a clinic sample. J Am Acad Child Adolesc Psychiatry 1991; 30:43–50 [C]
251. Last CG, Francis G, Hersen M, Kazdin AE, Strauss CC: Separation anxiety and school phobia: a comparison using DSM-III criteria. Am J Psychiatry 1987; 144:653–657 [D]
252. Last CG, Strauss CC: School refusal in anxiety-disordered children and adolescents. J Am Acad Child Adolesc Psychiatry 1990; 29:31–35 [D]
253. Gittelman-Klein R, Klein DF: School phobia: diagnostic considerations in the light of imipramine effects. J Nerv Ment Dis 1973; 156:199–215 [B]
254. Ollendick TH: Cognitive behavioral treatment of panic disorder and agoraphobia in adolescents: a multiple baseline design analysis. Behavior Therapy 1995; 26:517–531 [E]
255. Barlow DH: Effectiveness of behavior treatment for panic disorder with and without agoraphobia, in Treatment of Panic Disorder: A Consensus Development Conference. Edited by Wolfe BE, Maser JD. Washington, DC, American Psychiatric Press, 1994, pp 105–120 [G]
256. Ballenger JC, Carek DJ, Steele JJ, Cornish-McTighe D: Three cases of panic disorder with agoraphobia in children. Am J Psychiatry 1989; 146:922–924 [G]
257. Biederman J: Clonazepam in the treatment of prepubertal children with panic-like symptoms. J Clin Psychiatry 1987; 48(Oct suppl):38–42 [B]
258. Birmaher B, Waterman GS, Ryan N, Cully M: Fluoxetine for childhood anxiety disorders. J Am Acad Child Adolesc Psychiatry 1994; 33:993–999 [B]
259. Kutcher SP, MacKenzie S: Successful clonazepam treatment of adolescents with panic disorder. J Clin Psychopharmacol 1988; 8:299–301 [G]
260. Blazer D, George LK, Hughes D: The epidemiology of anxiety disorders: an age comparison, in Anxiety and the Elderly: Treatment and Research. Edited by Salzman C, Lebowitz BD. New York, Springer, 1991, pp 17–30 [G]
261. Eaton WW, Dryman A, Weissman MM: Panic and phobia, in Psychiatric Disorders in America. Edited by Robins LN, Regier DA. New York, Free Press, 1991, pp 155–179 [G]
262. Altshuler LL, Cohen L, Szuba MP, Burt VK, Gitlin M, Mintz J: Pharmacologic management of psychiatric illness during pregnancy: dilemmas and guidelines. Am J Psychiatry 1996; 153:592–606 [F]
263. Regier DA, Myers JK, Kramer M, Robins LN, Blazer DG, Hough RL, Eaton WW, Locke BZ: The NIMH Epidemiologic Catchment Area program: historical context, major objectives, and study population characteristics. Arch Gen Psychiatry 1984; 41:934–941 [G]

264. Kessler RC, McGonagle KA, Zhao S, Nelson CB, Hughes M, Eshleman S, Wittchen HU, Kendler KS: Lifetime and 12 month prevalence of DSM-III-R psychiatric disorders in the United States: results from the National Comorbidity Survey. Arch Gen Psychiatry 1994; 51:8–19 [C]
265. Blazer D, George LK, Landerman R, Pennybacker M, Melville ML, Woodbury M, Manton KG, Jordan K, Locke B: Psychiatric disorders: a rural/urban comparison. Arch Gen Psychiatry 1985; 42:651–656; correction 1986; 43:1142 [G]
266. Horwath E, Johnson J, Hornig CD: Epidemiology of panic disorder in African-Americans. Am J Psychiatry 1993; 150:465–469 [D]
267. Paradis CM, Friedman S, Lazar RM, Grubea J, Kesselman M: Use of a structured interview to diagnose anxiety disorders in a minority population. Hosp Community Psychiatry 1992; 43:61–64 [G]
268. Bell CC, Shakoor B, Thompson B, Dew D, Hughley E, Mays R, Shorter-Gooden K: Prevalence of isolated sleep paralysis in black subjects. J Natl Med Assoc 1984; 76:501–508 [D]
269. Neal AM, Smucker WD: The presence of panic disorder among African American hypertensives: a pilot study. J Black Psychol 1994; 20:29–35 [D]
270. Bell CC, Hildreth CJ, Jenkins EJ, Carter C: The relationship of isolated sleep paralysis and panic disorder to hypertension. J Natl Med Assoc 1988; 80:289–294 [D]
271. Brown C, Schulberg HC, Madonia MJ: Clinical presentations of major depression by African Americans and whites in primary medical care practice. J Affect Disord 1996; 41:181–191 [A]
272. Neighbors HW: Seeking help for personal problems: black Americans' use of health and mental health services. Community Ment Health J 1985; 21:156–166 [D]
273. Cooper-Patrick L, Crum RM, Ford DE: Characteristics of patients with major depression who received care in general medical and specialty mental health settings. Med Care 1994; 32:15–24 [E]

PRACTICE GUIDELINE FOR THE
Treatment of Patients With Acute Stress Disorder and Posttraumatic Stress Disorder

WORK GROUP ON ASD AND PTSD

Robert J. Ursano, M.D., Chair
Carl Bell, M.D.
Spencer Eth, M.D.
Matthew Friedman, M.D., Ph.D.
Ann Norwood, M.D.
Betty Pfefferbaum, M.D., J.D.
Robert S. Pynoos, M.D.
Douglas F. Zatzick, M.D.
David M. Benedek, M.D., Consultant

Originally published in November 2004. A guideline watch, summarizing significant developments in the scientific literature since publication of this guideline, may be available in the Psychiatric Practice section of the APA web site at www.psych.org.

This guideline is dedicated to Rebecca M. Thaler Schwebel (1972–2004), Senior Project Manager at APA when this guideline was initiated. Becca's humor, generous spirit, and optimism will be missed.

CONTENTS

Guide to Using This Practice Guideline 1007

Development Process 1008

Introduction 1010

Part A: Treatment Recommendations 1011

I. Executive Summary 1011
  A. Coding System 1011
  B. Summary of Recommendations 1011

II. Formulation and Implementation of a Treatment Plan 1014
  A. Initial Assessment 1014
  B. Principles of Psychiatric Management 1021
  C. Principles of Treatment Selection 1026
  D. Specific Treatment Strategies 1029

III. Specific Clinical Features Influencing the Treatment Plan 1034
  A. Age 1034
  B. Gender 1034
  C. Ethnic and Cross-Cultural Factors 1034
  D. Medical and Other Psychiatric Comorbidity 1036
  E. History of Previous Traumas 1037
  F. Aggressive Behavior 1038
  G. Self-Injurious and Suicidal Behaviors 1038

Part B: Background Information and Review of Available Evidence 1039

IV. Disease Definition, Epidemiology, and Natural History 1039
  A. Core Clinical Features 1039
  B. Associated Features 1043
  C. Differential Diagnosis 1043
  D. Epidemiology 1045
  E. Natural History and Course 1051

V. Review and Synthesis of Available Evidence 1051
  A. Issues in Interpreting the Literature 1051
  B. Psychosocial Interventions 1052
  C. Pharmacotherapies 1063

Part C: Future Research Needs 1067

Individuals and Organizations That Submitted Comments 1070

References 1071

GUIDE TO USING THIS PRACTICE GUIDELINE

The *Practice Guideline for the Treatment of Patients With Acute Stress Disorder and Posttraumatic Stress Disorder* consists of three parts (Parts A, B, and C) and many sections, not all of which will be equally useful for all readers. The following guide is designed to help readers find the sections that will be most useful to them.

Part A, "Treatment Recommendations," is published as a supplement to *The American Journal of Psychiatry* and contains general and specific treatment recommendations. Section I summarizes the key recommendations of the guideline and codes each recommendation according to the degree of clinical confidence with which the recommendation is made. Section II provides further discussion of the formulation and implementation of a treatment plan as it applies to the individual patient. Section III, "Specific Clinical Features Influencing the Treatment Plan," discusses a range of clinical considerations that could alter the general recommendations discussed in Section I.

Part B, "Background Information and Review of Available Evidence," and Part C, "Future Research Needs," are not included in *The American Journal of Psychiatry* supplement but are provided with Part A in the complete guideline, which is available in print format, in guideline compendiums, from American Psychiatric Publishing, Inc. (http://www.appi.org), and online through the American Psychiatric Association (http://www.psych.org). Part B provides an overview of ASD and PTSD, including general information on natural history, course, and epidemiology. It also provides a structured review and synthesis of the evidence that underlies the recommendations made in Part A. Part C draws from the previous sections and summarizes areas for which more research data are needed to guide clinical decisions.

To share feedback on this or other published APA practice guidelines, a form is available at http://www.psych.org/psych_pract/pg/reviewform.cfm.

DEVELOPMENT PROCESS

This practice guideline was developed under the auspices of the Steering Committee on Practice Guidelines. The development process is detailed in a document available from the APA Department of Quality Improvement and Psychiatric Services: the "APA Guideline Development Process." Key features of this process include the following:

- A comprehensive literature review to identify all relevant randomized clinical trials as well as less rigorously designed clinical trials and case series when evidence from randomized trials was unavailable.
- Development of evidence tables that reviewed the key features of each identified study, including funding source, study design, sample sizes, subject characteristics, treatment characteristics, and treatment outcomes.
- Initial drafting of the guideline by a work group that included psychiatrists with clinical and research expertise in ASD and PTSD.
- Production of multiple revised drafts with widespread review; 11 organizations and 55 individuals submitted significant comments.
- Approval by the APA Assembly and Board of Trustees.
- Planned revisions at regular intervals.

Relevant literature was identified through a computerized search of MEDLINE and the Published International Literature on Traumatic Stress (PILOTS) database, produced by the National Center for Post-Traumatic Stress Disorder and available online (http://www.ncptsd.org//publications/pilots/index.html). An initial search of PubMed was conducted for the period from 1966 to 2002. Key words used were posttraumatic stress, stress disorder, acute stress disorder, posttraumatic stress disorder, and PTSD. Additional citations were identified by using key words emotional trauma, psychic trauma, posttraumatic, disaster, terrorism, rape, assault, physical abuse, sexual abuse, childhood abuse, combat, traumatic event, and traumatic incident and then limited to citations that included the key words stress, psychological sequelae, anxiety, and dissociation. In determining which of the identified citations related to treatment, key words used were treatment, management, therapy, psychotherapy, antidepressive agents, tranquilizing agents, anticonvulsants, debriefing, critical incident, eye movement desensitization, and EMDR. Citations were further limited to clinical trials or meta-analyses published in the English language and accompanied by abstracts. A total of 316 citations were found. When applied to the PILOTS database, this search strategy yielded a total of 587 citations, many of which were duplicates of those obtained in the PubMed search. Additional, less formal literature searches were conducted by APA staff and individual work group members. Other published guidelines for the treatment of ASD and PTSD were also reviewed (1, 2).

This guideline presents recommendations for the evaluation and treatment of adult patients with ASD or PTSD. The *Practice Parameters for the Assessment and Treatment of Children and Adolescents With Posttraumatic Stress Disorder* of the American Academy of Child and Adolescent Psychiatry (3) may be consulted for guidelines relating to the evaluation and treatment of children and adolescents.

This document represents a synthesis of current scientific knowledge and rational clinical practice. It strives to be as free as possible of bias toward any theoretical approach to treatment. Articles identified in the initial literature search were prioritized for review according to methodological strength. Highest priority was given to randomized, placebo-controlled trials of psychotherapeutic and psychopharmacological interventions for individuals with a diagnosis of ASD or PTSD. The work group review process identified further citations that included randomized and open trials, literature reviews, meta-analyses, and other studies that were incorporated into evidence tables in an iterative manner. In interpreting the conclusions of these studies, consideration was given to factors that could limit the generalizability of the findings, including differences between individuals enrolled in well-controlled efficacy trials and individuals seen in clinical practice. Consequently, the recommendations for any particular clinical decision are based on the best available data and clinical consensus. The summary of treatment recommendations is keyed according to the level of confidence with which each recommendation is made. In addition, each reference is followed by a letter code in brackets that indicates the nature of the supporting evidence.

INTRODUCTION

It has long been recognized that stressful life events may cause emotional and behavioral effects. In addition, the clinical phenomenon of PTSD has been known by various names, studied, and treated for centuries. In 1980, DSM-III delineated distinct criteria for the diagnosis of PTSD. The diagnosis of ASD was added to DSM-IV in 1995 to distinguish individuals with PTSD-like symptoms that lasted less than 1 month from persons who experienced milder or more transient difficulties following a stressor. The DSM-IV-TR diagnostic criteria for both disorders can be found in Section II.A.2.

Although 50% to 90% of the population may be exposed to traumatic events during their lifetimes (4, 5), most exposed individuals do not develop ASD or PTSD. ASD was introduced into DSM in an effort to prospectively characterize the subpopulation of traumatically exposed persons with early symptoms and identify those at risk for the development of PTSD. Research and clinical experience show that those with high levels of symptoms early on, including those with ASD, are at risk of subsequent PTSD; however, some patients with ASD do not develop PTSD, and a proportion of patients develop PTSD without first having met the criteria for ASD (6–8). Although research shows that individuals who are most highly exposed to a traumatic event are at greatest risk, there is still uncertainty about the patient- or trauma-specific factors that will predict the development of ASD (9) and about interventions that will mitigate against the evolution of ASD into PTSD.

The lifetime prevalence of ASD is unclear, but in the National Comorbidity Survey the estimated lifetime prevalence of PTSD was 7.8% (4). The prevalence of both disorders is considerably higher among patients who seek general medical care (10) and among persons exposed to sexual assault (4, 5) or mass casualties such as those occurring in wars or natural disasters (11–13). The lifetime prevalence of PTSD is also higher in women than in men and is higher in the presence of underlying vulnerabilities such as adverse childhood experiences or comorbid diagnoses (11, 12, 14, 15). Given the prevalence of ASD and PTSD and their associated distress and disability, psychiatrists must be prepared to recognize and treat these disorders.

PART A
TREATMENT RECOMMENDATIONS

I. EXECUTIVE SUMMARY

A. CODING SYSTEM

Each recommendation is identified as falling into one of three categories of endorsement, indicated by a bracketed Roman numeral following the statement. The three categories represent varying levels of clinical confidence regarding the recommendation:

[I] Recommended with substantial clinical confidence.
[II] Recommended with moderate clinical confidence.
[III] May be recommended on the basis of individual circumstances.

B. SUMMARY OF RECOMMENDATIONS

1. Initial assessment

The initial step in identifying individuals with ASD or PTSD involves screening for recent or remote trauma exposure, although the clinical approach may vary depending on the recency of the traumatic event [I]. If eliciting vivid and detailed recollections of the traumatic event immediately after exposure enhances the patient's distress, the interview may be limited to gathering information that is essential to provide needed medical care [I]. The first interventions in the aftermath of an acute trauma consist of stabilizing and supportive medical care and supportive psychiatric care and assessment [I]. After large-scale catastrophes, initial psychiatric assessment includes differential diagnosis of physical and psychological effects of the traumatic event (e.g., anxiety resulting from hemodynamic compromise, hyperventilation, somatic expressions of psychological distress, fatigue) and identification of persons or groups who are at greatest risk for subsequent psychiatric disorders, including ASD or PTSD [I]. This identification may be accomplished through individual evaluation, group interviews, consultation, and use of surveillance instruments [I].

Diagnostic evaluation may be continued after the initial period has passed and a physically and psychologically safe environment has been established, the individual's medical condition has been stabilized, psychological reassurance has been provided, and, in disaster settings, necessary triage has been accomplished. It is important for this diagnostic assessment to include a complete psychiatric evaluation that specifically assesses for the symptoms of ASD and PTSD, including dissociative, reexperiencing, avoidance/numbing, and hyperarousal symptom clusters and their temporal sequence relative to the trauma (i.e., before versus after 1 month from the traumatic event) [I]. Other important components of the assessment process include functional assessment, determining the availability of basic care resources (e.g., safe housing, social support network, companion care, food, clothing), and identifying previous traumatic experiences and comorbid physical or psychiatric disorders, including depression and substance use disorders [I].

2. Psychiatric management

Psychiatric management for all patients with ASD or PTSD includes instituting interventions and activities to ensure physical and psychological safety, required medical care, and availability of needed resources for self-care and recovery [I]. The patient's level of functioning and safety, including his or her risk for suicide and potential to harm others, are always important to evaluate during initial assessment and may determine the treatment setting [I]. The goals of psychiatric management for patients with ASD and PTSD also include establishing a therapeutic alliance with the patient; providing ongoing assessment of safety and psychiatric status, including possible comorbid disorders and response to treatment; and increasing the patient's understanding of and active adaptive coping with psychosocial effects of exposure to the traumatic event, such as injury, job loss, or loss of loved ones [I]. Additional goals of psychiatric management include providing education regarding ASD and PTSD, enhancing treatment adherence, evaluating and managing physical health and functional impairments, and coordinating care to include collaborating with other clinicians [I].

3. General principles of treatment selection

The goals of treatment for individuals with a diagnosis of ASD or PTSD include reducing the severity of ASD or PTSD symptoms, preventing or treating trauma-related comorbid conditions that may be present or emerge, improving adaptive functioning and restoring a psychological sense of safety and trust, limiting the generalization of the danger experienced as a result of the traumatic situation(s), and protecting against relapse [I].

Patients assessed within hours or days after an acute trauma may present with overwhelming physiological and emotional symptoms (e.g., insomnia, agitation, emotional pain, dissociation). Limited clinical trial evidence is available in this area, as randomized designs are difficult to implement; however, clinical experience suggests that these acutely traumatized individuals may benefit from supportive psychotherapeutic and psychoeducational interventions [II]. Pharmacotherapy may be the first-line intervention for acutely traumatized patients whose degree of distress precludes new verbal learning or nonpharmacological treatment strategies [II]. Research has not consistently identified patient- or trauma-specific factors that predict the development of ASD or interventions that will alter the evolution of ASD into PTSD. However, early after a trauma, once the patient's safety and medical stabilization have been addressed, supportive psychotherapy, psychoeducation, and assistance in obtaining resources such as food and shelter and locating family and friends are useful [II].

Effective treatments for the symptoms of ASD or PTSD encompass psychopharmacology, psychotherapy, and psychoeducation and other supportive measures [I]. Although studies using a combination of these approaches for ASD and PTSD are not presently available, combination treatment is widely used and may offer advantages for some patients [II]. The psychotropic medications used in clinical practice and research for the treatment of ASD and PTSD were not specifically developed for these disorders but have been used in doses similar to those recommended or approved for other psychiatric illnesses.

For patients with ASD or PTSD, choice of treatment includes consideration of age and gender, presence of comorbid medical and psychiatric illnesses, and propensity for aggression or self-injurious behavior [I]. Other factors that may influence treatment choice include the recency of the precipitating traumatic event; the severity and pattern of symptoms; the presence of particularly distressing target symptoms or symptom clusters; the development of interpersonal or family issues or occupational or work-related problems; preexisting developmental or psychological vulnerabilities, including prior trauma exposure; and the patient's preferences [I].

When the patient's symptoms do not respond to a plan of treatment, selection of subsequent interventions will depend on clinical judgment, as there are limited data to guide the clinician. It is important to systematically review factors that may contribute to treatment nonresponse, including the specifics of the initial treatment plan and its goals and rationale, the patient's perceptions of the effects of treatment, the patient's understanding of and adherence to the treatment plan, and the patient's reasons for nonadherence if nonadherence is a factor [I]. Other factors that may need to be addressed in patients who are not responding to treatment include problems in the therapeutic alliance; the presence of psychosocial or environmental difficulties; the effect of earlier life experiences such as childhood abuse or previous trauma exposures; and comorbid psychiatric disorders, including substance-related disorders and personality disorders [I].

4. Specific treatment strategies

(a) Psychopharmacology

Although it has been hypothesized that pharmacological treatment soon after trauma exposure may prevent the development of ASD and PTSD, existing evidence is limited and preliminary. Thus, no specific pharmacological interventions can be recommended as efficacious in preventing the development of ASD or PTSD in at-risk individuals.

For patients with ASD, there are few studies of pharmacological interventions. However, selective serotonin reuptake inhibitors (SSRIs) [II] and other antidepressants [III] represent reasonable clinical interventions that are supported by limited findings in ASD as well as by findings of therapeutic benefits in patients with PTSD.

SSRIs are recommended as first-line medication treatment for PTSD [I]. In both male and female patients, treatment with SSRIs has been associated with relief of core PTSD symptoms in all three symptom clusters (reexperiencing, avoidance/numbing, hyperarousal). Other antidepressants, including tricyclic antidepressants and monoamine oxidase inhibitors (MAOIs), may also be beneficial in the treatment of PTSD [II].

Benzodiazepines may be useful in reducing anxiety and improving sleep [III]. Although their efficacy in treating the core symptoms of PTSD has not been established, benzodiazepines are often used in trauma-exposed individuals and patients with PTSD. However, clinical observations include the possibility of dependence, increased incidence of PTSD after early treatment with these medications, or worsening of PTSD symptoms after withdrawal of these medications. Thus, benzodiazepines cannot be recommended as monotherapy in PTSD.

In addition to being indicated in patients with comorbid psychotic disorders, second-generation antipsychotic medications (e.g., olanzapine, quetiapine, risperidone) may be helpful in individual patients with PTSD [III]. Anticonvulsant medications (e.g., divalproex, carbamazepine, topiramate, lamotrigine), α_2-adrenergic agonists, and β-adrenergic blockers may also be helpful in treating specific symptom clusters in individual patients [III].

(b) Psychotherapeutic interventions

Some evidence is available about the effectiveness of psychotherapeutic intervention immediately after trauma in preventing development of ASD or PTSD. Studies of cognitive behavior therapy in motor vehicle and industrial accident survivors as well as in victims of rape and interpersonal violence suggest that cognitive behavior therapies may speed recovery and prevent PTSD when therapy is given over a few sessions beginning 2–3 weeks after trauma exposure [II].

Early supportive interventions, psychoeducation, and case management appear to be helpful in acutely traumatized individuals, because these approaches promote engagement in ongoing care and may facilitate entry into evidence-based psychotherapeutic and psychopharmacological treatments [II]. Encouraging acutely traumatized persons to first rely on their inherent strengths, their existing support networks, and their own judgment may also reduce the need for further intervention [II]. In populations of patients who have experienced multiple recurrent traumas, there is little evidence to suggest that early supportive care delivered as a stand-alone treatment will result in lasting reductions in PTSD symptoms. However, no evidence suggests that early supportive care is harmful. In contrast, psychological debriefings or single-session techniques are not recommended, as they may increase symptoms in some settings and appear to be ineffective in treating individuals with ASD and in preventing PTSD.

No controlled studies of psychodynamic psychotherapy, eye movement desensitization and reprocessing (EMDR), or hypnosis have been conducted that would establish data-based evidence of their efficacy as an early or preventive intervention for ASD or PTSD.

For patients with a diagnosis of ASD or PTSD, available evidence and clinical experience suggest that a number of psychotherapeutic interventions may be useful. Patients with ASD may be helped by cognitive behavior therapy and other exposure-based therapies [II]. In addition, cognitive behavior therapy is an effective treatment for core symptoms of acute and chronic PTSD [I]. EMDR is also effective [II]. Stress inoculation, imagery rehearsal, and prolonged exposure techniques may also be indicated for treatment of PTSD and PTSD-associated symptoms such as anxiety and avoidance [II]. The shared element of controlled exposure of some kind may be the critical intervention.

Psychodynamic psychotherapy may be useful in addressing developmental, interpersonal, or intrapersonal issues that relate to the nature, severity, symptoms, or treatment of ASD and PTSD and that may be of particular importance to social, occupational, and interpersonal functioning [II].

Case management, psychoeducation, and other supportive interventions may be useful in facilitating entry into ongoing treatment, appear not to exacerbate PTSD symptoms, and in some pilot investigations have been associated with PTSD symptom reduction [II]. Present-centered and trauma-focused group therapies may also reduce PTSD symptom severity [III].

II. FORMULATION AND IMPLEMENTATION OF A TREATMENT PLAN

A. INITIAL ASSESSMENT

1. Initial clinical approach to the patient

The timing and nature of initial assessments will be influenced by the type of the traumatic event (e.g., sexual assault versus natural disaster) and the scope of any destruction caused by the event. In large-scale catastrophes, the initial assessment may be the triage of individuals based on the presence of physical injury or psychological effects of the traumatic event, followed by the identification of individuals at greatest risk for psychiatric sequelae, including ASD or PTSD. Group interviews, consultation, or the administration of surveillance instruments may be part of this process. If local resources are overwhelmed by the catastrophe, psychiatric assessment will need to be prioritized so that the most severely affected individuals are seen first. Several self-rated and observer-based rating scales have been developed and validated to facilitate screening for possible PTSD; however, study of these scales in community-wide disasters with highly diverse populations has been limited. Such rating scales are most likely to be helpful after the acute event, when physical and cognitive functioning allow for a more complex assessment (16–18).

With individual traumas, the timing and nature of the first mental health contact may also vary. For individuals who have been sexually assaulted, for example, supportive psychological interventions may be initiated even before formal psychiatric assessment (e.g., use of educational materials on what to expect in the rape examination). In evaluations that occur shortly after exposure to the traumatic event, particularly in emergency settings, the initial clinical response consists of stabilizing and supportive medical care as well as supportive psychiatric care and assessment, including assessment of potential dangerousness to self or others. Addressing the individual's requirements for medical care, rest, nutrition, and control of injury-related pain is important for assuring the patient's physical health, enhancing the patient's experience of safety, and initiating the therapeutic relationship. Such interactions with trauma-exposed individuals will always entail sensitivity to the patient's wishes and to the changing symptoms, fears, and interpersonal needs that unfold after trauma exposure.

Whenever possible, care should be given within a safe environment. This may not be feasible after large-scale traumatic events in which there may be additional or ongoing exposures (e.g., earthquakes, war zones, ongoing gang warfare). With other types of traumatic events, further assurances of safety may be possible and necessary. For example, with traumatic events such as domestic violence, specific efforts or engagement of law enforcement or social service agencies may be needed to address the patient's safety and reduce the likelihood of repeat traumatization.

During the first 48–72 hours after a traumatic event, some individuals may be very aroused, anxious, or angry, whereas others may appear minimally affected or "numb" as a result of injury, pain, or dissociative phenomena (19). In triage or emergency department settings, an in-depth exploration of the traumatic event and the patient's experiences may increase distress but may be required for medical or safety reasons. For example, after physical or sexual assault, recounting events in response to the evaluator's questions or the mere gender of the evaluator may have a distressing effect in some individuals. Similarly, after an event involving death or injury to a family member, a clinician may need to obtain or disclose upsetting information, while gauging the patient's response as part of the evaluation. Insensitive or premature exploration of recent life-threatening events or losses can be counterproductive, leading the patient to avoid medical care, whereas other individuals may find in-depth exploration of recent events helpful. Therefore, evaluators must respond to the patient's needs and capabilities. After mass disasters, triage assessments in a group setting may be used effectively to identify those in need of intervention. However, discussion of distressing memories and events in heterogeneously exposed groups may adversely affect those with little or no exposure when they hear of the frightening and terrifying experiences of others.

2. Assessing exposure to a traumatic event and establishing a diagnosis of ASD or PTSD

By definition, ASD and PTSD are psychiatric disorders consisting of physiological and psychological responses resulting from exposure to an event or events involving death, serious injury, or a threat to physical integrity. Events such as natural disasters, explosions, physical or sexual assaults, motor vehicle accidents, or involvement with naturally occurring or terrorist-related disease epidemics are examples of events that may elicit the physiological and psychological response required by the diagnostic criteria of ASD and PTSD. Thus, screening for acute or remote event exposure is a necessary first step in identifying persons with either ASD or PTSD.

Table 1 and Table 2 provide the full criteria for the diagnosis of ASD and PTSD, respectively. For both disorders, DSM-IV-TR defines criterion A as exposure to a traumatic event in which both of the following conditions are present:

1. The person experienced, witnessed, or was confronted with an event or events that involved actual or threatened death or serious injury, or a threat to the physical integrity of self or others.
2. The person's response involved intense fear, helplessness, or horror.

Thus, for both ASD and PTSD, establishing a diagnosis requires consideration of the individual's response to the event as well as the nature of the event itself. It is important to note that for some individuals, initial assessment may occur in a triage setting immediately after the trauma and before all symptoms related to the trauma exposure are manifest. In addition, the presence of dissociative symptoms may prevent patients from recalling feelings of fear, helplessness, or horror and may require that clinical judgment be used in determining whether criterion A for diagnosis has been satisfied (20–22).

Clinical evaluation for ASD or PTSD requires assessment of symptoms within each of three symptom clusters: reexperiencing, avoidance/numbing, and hyperarousal. In addition, to meet the diagnostic criteria for ASD, a patient must exhibit dissociative symptoms either during or

TABLE 1. DSM-IV-TR Diagnostic Criteria for Acute Stress Disorder (DSM-IV-TR code 308.3)

A. The person has been exposed to a traumatic event in which both of the following were present:
   1. the person experienced, witnessed, or was confronted with an event or events that involved actual or threatened death or serious injury, or a threat to the physical integrity of self or others
   2. the person's response involved intense fear, helplessness, or horror

B. Either while experiencing or after experiencing the distressing event, the individual has three (or more) of the following dissociative symptoms:
   1. a subjective sense of numbing, detachment, or absence of emotional responsiveness
   2. a reduction in awareness of his or her surroundings (e.g., "being in a daze")
   3. derealization
   4. depersonalization
   5. dissociative amnesia (i.e., inability to recall an important aspect of the trauma)

C. The traumatic event is persistently reexperienced in at least one of the following ways: recurrent images, thoughts, dreams, illusions, flashback episodes, or a sense of reliving the experience; or distress on exposure to reminders of the traumatic event.

D. Marked avoidance of stimuli that arouse recollections of the trauma (e.g., thoughts, feelings, conversations, activities, places, people).

E. Marked symptoms of anxiety or increased arousal (e.g., difficulty sleeping, irritability, poor concentration, hypervigilance, exaggerated startle response, motor restlessness).

F. The disturbance causes clinically significant distress or impairment in social, occupational, or other important areas of functioning or impairs the individual's ability to pursue some necessary task, such as obtaining necessary assistance or mobilizing personal resources by telling family members about the traumatic experience.

G. The disturbance lasts for a minimum of 2 days and a maximum of 4 weeks and occurs within 4 weeks of the traumatic event.

H. The disturbance is not due to the direct physiological effects of a substance (e.g., a drug of abuse, a medication) or a general medical condition, is not better accounted for by Brief Psychotic Disorder, and is not merely an exacerbation of a preexisting Axis I or Axis II disorder.

Source. Reprinted from *Diagnostic and Statistical Manual of Mental Disorders,* 4th Edition, Text Revision. Washington, DC, American Psychiatric Association, 2000. Copyright 2000, American Psychiatric Association. Used with permission.

immediately after the traumatic event. In PTSD, dissociative symptoms (e.g., inability to recall important aspects of the trauma) are not necessary to the diagnosis but are often observed.

By definition, ASD occurs within 4 weeks of the trauma and lasts for a minimum of 2 days. Consequently, it can be diagnosed within 2 days after the trauma exposure continuing to 4 weeks after the traumatic event. If symptoms are present 1 month after the trauma exposure, PTSD is diagnosed. Since diagnostic assessment may occur at any time following a traumatic event, the clinician must bear these essential distinctions in mind when evaluating the trauma-exposed individual.

3. Additional features of the initial assessment

After it has been determined that the traumatically exposed individual is able to tolerate more extensive evaluation, it is important to obtain a detailed history of the exposure and the pa-

TABLE 2. DSM-IV-TR Diagnostic Criteria for Posttraumatic Stress Disorder (DSM-IV-TR code 309.81)

A. The person has been exposed to a traumatic event in which both of the following were present:
   1. the person experienced, witnessed, or was confronted with an event or events that involved actual or threatened death or serious injury, or a threat to the physical integrity of self or others
   2. the person's response involved intense fear, helplessness, or horror. Note: In children, this may be expressed instead by disorganized or agitated behavior

B. The traumatic event is persistently reexperienced in one (or more) of the following ways:
   1. recurrent and intrusive distressing recollections of the event, including images, thoughts, or perceptions. Note: In young children, repetitive play may occur in which themes or aspects of the trauma are expressed.
   2. recurrent distressing dreams of the event. Note: In children, there may be frightening dreams without recognizable content.
   3. acting or feeling as if the traumatic event were recurring (includes a sense of reliving the experience, illusions, hallucinations, and dissociative flashback episodes, including those that occur on awakening or when intoxicated). Note: In young children, trauma-specific reenactment may occur.
   4. intense psychological distress at exposure to internal or external cues that symbolize or resemble an aspect of the traumatic event
   5. physiological reactivity on exposure to internal or external cues that symbolize or resemble an aspect of the traumatic event

C. Persistent avoidance of stimuli associated with the trauma and numbing of general responsiveness (not present before the trauma), as indicated by three (or more) of the following:
   1. efforts to avoid thoughts, feelings, or conversations associated with the trauma
   2. efforts to avoid activities, places, or people that arouse recollections of the trauma
   3. inability to recall an important aspect of the trauma
   4. markedly diminished interest or participation in significant activities
   5. feeling of detachment or estrangement from others
   6. restricted range of affect (e.g., unable to have loving feelings)
   7. sense of a foreshortened future (e.g., does not expect to have a career, marriage, children, or a normal life span)

D. Persistent symptoms of increased arousal (not present before the trauma), as indicated by two (or more) of the following:
   1. difficulty falling or staying asleep
   2. irritability or outbursts of anger
   3. difficulty concentrating
   4. hypervigilance
   5. exaggerated startle response

E. Duration of the disturbance (symptoms in Criteria B, C, and D) is more than 1 month.

TABLE 2. DSM-IV-TR Diagnostic Criteria for Posttraumatic Stress Disorder (DSM-IV-TR code 309.81) *(continued)*

F. The disturbance causes clinically significant distress or impairment in social, occupational, or other important areas of functioning.

Specify if:

Acute: if duration of symptoms is less than 3 months

Chronic: if duration of symptoms is 3 months or more

Specify if:

With Delayed Onset: if onset of symptoms is at least 6 months after the stressor.

Source. Reprinted from *Diagnostic and Statistical Manual of Mental Disorders,* 4th Edition, Text Revision. Washington, DC, American Psychiatric Association, 2000. Copyright 2000, American Psychiatric Association. Used with permission.

tient's early responses to the trauma as well as the responses of significant others. This history can provide important information for treatment and prognosis. Often, individuals provide negative responses to all-inclusive questions (e.g., "Have you ever been abused?"), and responses may also be affected by the timing and context of questioning. Consequently, it is helpful to ask more specific questions (e.g., "Have you ever been hit, beaten, or choked?") and attempt to elicit a history of trauma exposure at various points during the evaluation.

During the evaluation, the clinician obtains a longitudinal history of all traumatic experiences, including age at the time of exposure, duration of exposure (e.g., single episode, recurrent, or ongoing), type of trauma (e.g., motor vehicle accident, natural disaster, physical or sexual assault), relationship between the patient and the perpetrator (in cases of interpersonal violence), and the patient's perception of the effect of these experiences (on self and significant others). Other factors or interventions that may have intensified or mitigated the traumatic response should also be identified.

Clinical interviews may be combined with a variety of validated self-rated measures, including the PTSD Checklist (23), the Impact of Event Scale (24, 25) (available online at www.mardihorowitz.com), and the Davidson Trauma Scale (26), to assess the full range, frequency, and severity of posttraumatic symptoms and the related distress and impairment. Structured diagnostic interviews such as the Clinician-Administered PTSD Scale (27) and the Structured Interview for PTSD (28) have been used extensively in clinical research and are well-validated instruments for the diagnosis of PTSD.

In addition, a complete psychiatric evaluation should be conducted in accordance with the general principles and components outlined in APA's *Practice Guideline for the Psychiatric Evaluation of Adults* (29). These components include a history of the present illness and current symptoms; a psychiatric history, including a substance use history; medical history; review of systems and a review of prescribed and over-the-counter medications (including herbal products and supplements); personal history (e.g., psychological development, response to life transitions and major life events); social, occupational, and family history; history of prior treatments or interventions and their degree of success; mental status examination; physical examination; and diagnostic tests as indicated. Developmental and preexisting psychodynamic issues may make the patient especially vulnerable or reactive to a traumatic event. Old and dormant concerns may resurface and complicate or otherwise intensify the emotional response to a new trauma. Past exposure to traumatic events as well as previous patient and support network responses may affect the evaluation process and choice of and response to treatment. In the context of this complete psychiatric evaluation, certain areas of inquiry should receive additional attention and are described below. Table 3 summarizes the clinical domains relevant to the comprehensive assessment of ASD and PTSD.

a) Military and war-related traumatic event history

Evaluation of exposure to traumatic events during military service or in war-torn areas is an important and often difficult part of clinical assessment. Past exposure to war environments increases the probability of exposure to traumatic events. In addition, past exposures to traumatic events or past PTSD may increase the likelihood of current PTSD from a new exposure (31–34). Persons who come from nations with past or ongoing histories of war and war atrocities may have substantial exposure to traumatic events. Military support troops in rear areas as well as combat troops are vulnerable to attacks and other life-threatening experiences. Those serving in the military or involved in humanitarian assistance may have been massively exposed to death and the dead and can have high rates of ASD and PTSD. Military service members may also be involved in or witness training accidents, including motor vehicle accidents or aircraft crashes.

For those with military service, it is often helpful to begin the evaluation by exploring why the patient joined the military and what he or she hoped to do. Specific data to be gathered that can assist in the evaluation of traumatic event exposures include the length of service (and whether this length of time was broken or unbroken), the presence or absence of any disciplinary charges, and military awards received. The patient should also be asked if he or she was ever referred for alcohol or other substance use counseling, family violence counseling, or a psychiatric evaluation. If the patient had a family while in the service, it is important to explore the frequency and effects of family separation on the service member, the spouse, and the children. With service members or veterans who report having been in combat, a description of the location and the events should be obtained. It is often helpful to obtain copies of service records to verify combat exposures.

Witnessing atrocities, seeing the death of children, seeing friends killed and wounded, and feeling responsible for the death of a friend are especially disturbing elements of some combat and war environments for both military and civilian persons. As in all traumas, the recovery environment (that is, whether family, friends, and the nation are welcoming or ashamed) plays a large role in how the experience is recalled and managed. Some immigrants have previously lived in war zones or have served as members of military, paramilitary, or insurgent units before immigration. Some may also have been victims of torture, maltreatment, or rape as part of a war environment. Immigrants who may have served for regimes that espoused strong anti-American politics may fear repercussions from an unsympathetic country. These contextual issues require clear and supportive discussion in the evaluation and assessment in order to obtain necessary clinical information.

b) Victims of crime and effects of legal system involvement

Individuals with ASD or PTSD may be involved in legal actions either because they are involved in a civil case (e.g., motor vehicle accident) related to their psychiatric condition or because they were a victim of a crime. Some individuals may express distress through a variety of symptoms that may abate after the conclusion of legal proceedings or payment of damages. This pattern may represent the effects of retraumatization resulting from exposure to a perpetrator or recollection of traumatic events during depositions, trial preparation, or testimony, followed by the (at times, only transient) sense of "closure" that these proceedings provide. If the perpetrator is incarcerated as a result of legal proceedings, symptoms may reoccur when the victim learns of the perpetrator's parole or release. Some persons may demonstrate waxing and waning symptoms regardless of the status of legal proceedings. Individuals may also fabricate or embellish symptoms. By raising the possibility that secondary gain, symptom exaggeration, or malingering may be part of the clinical picture, these factors can complicate assessment and treatment planning, as well as research (35). Confidentiality can also be compromised if the treating psychiatrist is in a dual role and is also required to communicate with members of the legal system. Some of the complexity of these cases can be managed by having the treatment and forensic evaluations performed by different psychiatrists, if possible (36, 37). As noted in DSM-IV-TR, the psychiatric assessment should address the possibility of malingering in situ-

TABLE 3. Clinical Domains of Assessment for Acute Stress Disorder (ASD) and Posttraumatic Stress Disorder (PTSD)

Clinical Domain	Component
Trauma history	Type, age, and duration
Safety	Threat of harm from others and dangerousness to self or others
Dissociative symptoms	Necessary for diagnosis of ASD: numbing, detachment, derealization/depersonalization, dissociative amnesia in acute response to trauma
ASD/PTSD symptoms	Reexperiencing, avoidance and numbing, hyperarousal as a consequence of trauma (PTSD is diagnosed if symptom onset is >30 days after the traumatic event; if <30 days and if dissociative symptoms are present, ASD is diagnosed)
Military history	Prior exposure(s), training and preparedness for exposure
Behavioral and health risks	Substance use/abuse, sexually transmitted diseases, preexisting mental illness, nonadherence to treatment, impulsivity, and potential for further exposure to violence
Personal characteristics	Coping skills, resilience, interpersonal relatedness/attachment, history of developmental trauma or psychodynamic conflict(s), motivation for treatment
Psychosocial situation	Home environment, social support, employment status, ongoing violence (e.g., interpersonal, disaster/war), parenting/caregiver skills or burdens
Stressors	Acute and/or chronic trauma, poverty, loss, bereavement
Legal system involvement	Meaning of symptoms, compensation based on disability determination or degree of distress

Source. Adapted with permission from "Posttraumatic Stress Disorder," by Kathryn M. Connor and Marian I. Butterfield. *Focus* 2003; 1:247–262 (30). Copyright © 2003. American Psychiatric Association.

ations in which financial remuneration or benefit eligibility is at issue or when forensic determinations play a role in establishing the diagnosis of PTSD. Determining the temporal course of symptoms relative to the timing of legal initiatives is helpful in this process (38).

c) Identification of ASD and PTSD in the presence of common comorbid conditions

In patients who present for evaluation after a traumatic event, exacerbations or relapse of preexisting comorbid disorders may occur and require evaluation and treatment (see Section III.D, "Medical and Other Psychiatric Comorbidity") (39, 40). Exacerbations or relapse of preexisting PTSD may also occur with subsequent traumas or reminders of trauma.

For many individuals who have experienced a traumatic event but are presenting with other clinical needs, the diagnosis of ASD or PTSD may be missed entirely without a detailed evaluation. For example, individuals hospitalized on medical or surgical services after motor vehicle accidents, severe burns, or other major physical trauma have high rates of symptomatic distress, including ASD or PTSD, that often go unrecognized (34, 41–44). Patients with serious mental illness are exposed to high rates of physical assault and sexual abuse as well as other traumas (45–49). Mental health clinicians may fail to obtain this information unless they specifically inquire (50). Seriously mentally ill persons also have higher rates of PTSD (47–49, 51), compared to the general population (5). Individuals with psychotic disorders (48) and with borderline personality disorder (50, 52–54) are particularly likely to have experienced victimization in childhood and in adulthood. The associated PTSD often goes unrecognized. Histories of victimization and PTSD are also common among individuals with substance-related disorders (55–58) and eating disorders (59–61). In addition, family members—particularly spouses—who present with symptoms of bereavement after the traumatic loss of a family member should be assessed for PTSD (62).

High rates of comorbid psychiatric and other medical diagnoses are observed in those with ASD and PTSD. For a number of reasons, the medical and neurological effects of traumatic events may not be immediately apparent. Acute psychological responses to trauma such as dissociation may also diminish the initial experience of physical pain. In the presence of overwhelming anxiety and distress, individuals may not be able to describe their mental and physical state to medical professionals in an articulate fashion. Individuals exposed to traumatic events, particularly events that include interpersonal assault and violence, can find the motives of well-intentioned evaluators suspect. Without the establishment of trust, patients may be unwilling or unable to provide a complete medical or psychiatric history.

Patients with PTSD often have comorbid major depressive disorders, anxiety disorders, and substance use disorders (use of alcohol, tobacco, and other substances). Physical complaints, which may result from injury, may also represent comorbid somatization disorder or other somatoform disorders (12, 63). Similarly, patients with preexisting personality disorders or maladaptive character traits, as well as those with unresolved psychodynamic developmental concerns or histories of childhood traumatic events, may be at higher risk for an accentuated response to further traumatic events. In the presence of prominent depressive symptoms, social withdrawal and avoidance may be increased, and suicide risk may be heightened. Thus, identification and treatment of comorbid psychiatric and other medical illnesses are important to an integrated treatment plan that addresses all of the patient's needs and contributes to recovery from PTSD.

B. PRINCIPLES OF PSYCHIATRIC MANAGEMENT

Psychiatric management consists of a broad array of interventions and activities that may be instituted by psychiatrists for patients who have been exposed to extreme trauma. The specific components of psychiatric management that appear to mitigate the sequelae of trauma exposure and that are important to the treatment of patients with ASD or PTSD are described in more detail below.

1. Evaluating the safety of the patient and others

As with all psychiatric patients, for patients exposed to trauma it is crucial to assess the risk for suicide and nonlethal self-injurious behavior as well as the risk for harm to others. Details of suicide assessment and estimation of suicide risk are described in APA's *Practice Guideline for the Assessment and Treatment of Patients With Suicidal Behaviors* (64). Although many factors have been associated with an increased risk of suicide attempts and suicide in groups of individuals, it is not possible to predict suicide in a given individual at a given point in time. Nonetheless, a number of factors should be taken into consideration in evaluating and estimating the patient's potential for self-injury or suicide.

In assessing suicide risk, it is essential to determine whether the patient has had thoughts of death, self-harm, or suicide and the degree to which the patient intends to act on any suicidal ideation, the extent of planning or preparation for suicide, and the relative lethality of any suicide methods that the patient has considered. The availability of the means for suicide, including firearms, should also be explored, and a judgment should be made concerning the lethality of those means.

Risk for suicide and for suicide attempts is also increased by the presence of previous suicide attempts, including aborted attempts. Thus, if a patient has a history of previous suicide attempts, the nature of those attempts should be determined. Individuals who experienced childhood abuse and who may have PTSD as a result of that experience sometimes exhibit self-harming behavior that is often repetitive but occurs in the absence of suicidal intent (65, 66).

Such behavior may progress to more serious forms of nonlethal self-harm but also confers an increased risk of suicidal behaviors. Patients should also be asked about suicide in their family and recent exposure to suicide or suicide attempts by others.

Depression, substance use, panic attacks, and severe anxiety are commonly present in individuals with ASD or PTSD and are associated with increased risk for suicide and suicidal behaviors. Other factors that deserve specific attention in individuals with ASD or PTSD include the presence of dissociative symptoms; high levels of shame or stigma (e.g., after rape); loss of family, friends, or employment as a result of the traumatic event; specific neurovegetative symptoms, including insomnia or weight/appetite loss; social withdrawal; social or cultural isolation with relocation or immigration; and preexisting psychological issues, personality traits, or patterns of coping that may indicate a heightened response to a specific trauma. Individuals who feel trapped within an inescapable and abusive relationship (e.g., situations involving domestic violence, marital rape, or child abuse) or who anticipate continued, imminent exposure to traumatic experiences or stimuli may be more likely to act on suicidal ideas. An association has also been observed between the number of previous traumatic events and the likelihood that an individual will attempt suicide (67, 68). Thus, a complete assessment of suicide risk should be individualized to the particular circumstances of the patient and should also include an evaluation of the patient's strengths, social support, and motivation to seek help (69–71).

Less is known about the risk factors for harm to others in the context of PTSD. Nonetheless, it is important to assess thoughts, plans, or intentions of harming others as part of the psychiatric evaluation. As with assessment of suicide risk, it is important to determine whether firearms or other lethal weapons are available that could be used for harming others. The presence of hallucinations, persecutory delusions about a particular individual or group, or the feeling of being trapped in a dangerous, abusive, and inescapable situation may augment risk of dangerousness to others.

2. Determining a treatment setting

Treatment settings for patients with ASD or PTSD include the full continuum of levels of care. Treatment should be delivered in the setting that is least restrictive, yet most likely to prove safe and effective. In determining the appropriate treatment setting, multiple patient-specific factors are considered: symptom severity, comorbidity, suicidal ideation or behavior, homicidal ideation or behavior, level of functioning, and available support system. The determination of a treatment setting should also include consideration of the patient's personal safety, ability to adequately care for him- or herself, ability to provide reliable feedback to the psychiatrist, and willingness to participate in treatment. Here also, an important consideration is the patient's ability to trust clinicians and the treatment process; this ability may be limited as a consequence of traumatic events themselves, cultural barriers, or other factors. The choice of treatment setting and the patient's ability to benefit from a different level of care should be reevaluated on an ongoing basis throughout the course of treatment, as efficacy does not necessarily increase with increasing duration of treatment in a specific setting or level of care (72).

For the majority of individuals with ASD or PTSD, treatment on an outpatient basis is the most appropriate treatment setting. However, some patients, particularly those with comorbid psychiatric and other medical diagnoses, may require treatment on an inpatient basis. Patients who exhibit suicidal or homicidal ideation, plans, or intent require close assessment and monitoring. Hospitalization is generally indicated for patients who are considered to pose a serious threat of harm to themselves or others. If such patients refuse admission, they may be hospitalized involuntarily when their condition meets local jurisdictional criteria for emergency detention or involuntary hospitalization. Severely ill patients who lack adequate social support outside a hospital setting should also be considered for hospital admission, residential treatment, or participation in an intensive outpatient or day treatment program. For severely ill patients with repeated hospitalizations related to nonadherence, assertive community treatment may also be considered.

3. Establishing and maintaining a therapeutic alliance

The therapeutic alliance is important and at times challenging to establish with patients who have experienced traumatic events.

Attention to the physician-patient interaction is important, even in settings such as emergency departments where the clinician may have only a single contact with the patient. Although more than 80% of victims of recent sexual or physical assault surveyed in an emergency department setting indicated interest in further mental health treatment (73), other studies have indicated that those with PTSD underuse or avoid mental health services (74). A positive experience may also make the patient more receptive to future evaluation or follow-up.

Evaluation and treatment should always be conducted with sensitivity and in a safe environment that facilitates the development of trust. The presence of ASD or PTSD may challenge the clinician's ability to ensure that the patient feels safe in the therapeutic relationship. Clinicians must acknowledge the patient's worst fears about reexposure to intolerable traumatic memories and recognize that treatment itself may be perceived as threatening or overly intrusive. The patient is often relieved when the therapist indicates that talking about traumatic life events can be distressing and that the patient will decide how deeply to explore the difficult events and feelings. This suggestion of flexibility helps the patient to maintain or restore a sense of control, which is often lost after exposure to traumatic events. In chronic PTSD, avoidant/numbing behaviors may have been present for many years or decades. Therefore, clinicians must be patient and ensure that therapy proceeds at a tolerable pace.

Many other components of the treatment of ASD and PTSD also require trust in the doctor-patient relationship as well as particular attention to the therapeutic alliance. Effective treatment of both of these disorders requires that patients understand educational or treatment plans and return for follow-up assessment and treatment. In addition, successful treatment may require patients to tolerate intense affect and/or disruptive or unpleasant medication side effects. To establish and maintain a therapeutic alliance, it is important for the psychiatrist to address the patient's concerns as well as treatment preferences. Developing a therapeutic alliance with a patient who has experienced significant traumatic events—particularly in childhood—may require considerable psychotherapeutic effort and require lengthening of treatment. Cultural factors may also impose barriers to developing a therapeutic relationship, since many non-Western cultures do not value traditional Western psychiatric interventions. Management of the therapeutic alliance also includes awareness of transference and countertransference issues, even if these issues are not directly addressed in treatment (75).

4. Coordinating the treatment effort

Providing optimal treatment for patients with ASD and PTSD may require a team approach involving the coordinated effort of several clinicians. Patients may have a wide variety of comorbid psychiatric and/or physical disorders that need to be addressed. Family intervention or coordination of support services is often needed. One team member must assume the primary overall responsibility for the patient's treatment. This individual serves as the coordinator of the treatment plan, advocates for the appropriate level of care, oversees the family involvement, makes decisions regarding which potential treatment modalities are useful and which should be discontinued, helps assess the effects of medications, and monitors the patient's safety. Because of the diversity and depth of medical knowledge and expertise required for this oversight function, a psychiatrist may be optimal for this role, although this staffing pattern may not be possible in some health care settings. Ongoing coordination of the overall treatment plan is enhanced by clear role definitions, plans for the management of crises, and regular communication among the clinicians who are involved in the treatment. If team members work collaboratively with each other, with the patient, and with the patient's family and other social supports, the treatment has a better chance of helping the patient distinguish safe from dangerous and potentially retraumatizing situations, develop self-monitoring skills and coping strategies for anxiety states related to reminders of his or her trauma, avoid abusive relationships, minimize alcohol and other drug misuse, and control impulsive, aggressive, or self-destructive behaviors.

Those who have experienced an acute traumatic injury or assault often require ongoing medical attention. Collaborating with physicians who are providing additional medical treatment to the patient is an important part of psychiatric treatment. Individuals with PTSD also often have high rates of somatic and somatoform (i.e., medically unexplained) symptoms that are not directly related to the traumatic event but that prompt visits to primary care physicians (76–79). In such settings, collaboration between the psychiatrist and the primary caregiver may facilitate appropriate medical assessment and management.

5. Monitoring treatment response

During treatment, different features and symptoms of the patient's illness may emerge or subside. Monitoring the patient's status for the emergence of changes in destructive impulses toward self or others is especially crucial. For patients whose risk of such behaviors is found to be increased, additional measures such as hospitalization or more intensive treatment should be considered. Emergence of new symptoms, significant deterioration in functional status, or significant periods without response to treatment may suggest a need for diagnostic reevaluation. The psychiatrist should be particularly vigilant for comorbid medical conditions or substance-related disorders, for the emergence of symptoms such as interpersonal withdrawal or avoidance, and for the development or progression of symptoms of other disorders, including anxiety disorders or major depression.

6. Providing education

For persons who seek care after traumatic events, it is helpful to provide education concerning the natural course of and interventions for ASD and PTSD as well as for the broad range of normal stress-related reactions. The APA Disaster Psychiatry web site (http://www.psych.org/disasterpsych/) provides educational materials and links to other online resources. Education should also be given to involved family members or significant members of the patient's support network. It is important to help patients understand that their symptoms may be exacerbated by reexposure to traumatic stimuli, perceiving themselves to be in unsafe situations, or remaining in abusive relationships and that they can learn methods for better managing their feelings when they are reminded of the traumatic event. Emphasizing that ASD and PTSD are conditions for which effective treatments are available may be crucial in educating patients who attribute their illness to a moral defect or in educating family members who are convinced that nothing is wrong with the patient. Education regarding available treatment options can also help patients (and family members) make informed decisions, anticipate side effects, and adhere to treatment regimens.

For individuals or groups whose occupation entails likely exposure to traumatic events (e.g., military personnel, police, firefighters, emergency medical personnel, journalists), ongoing educational efforts may decrease exposure to trauma (by reducing risk behaviors) or improve the likelihood that an individual in need will seek care. Awareness of the predictable initial psychological and physiological responses to traumatic events may also be reassuring when these responses occur and may vitiate new fears or expectations of disability. Such education can also aid in the accurate identification and support of colleagues who develop symptoms of ASD or PTSD (80, 81).

7. Enhancing adherence to treatment

For patients who develop chronic PTSD, a long or indefinite duration of treatment may be needed. During acute exacerbations, patients with chronic PTSD may be easily discouraged and unduly pessimistic about their chances of recovery. In addition, the side effects or requirements of treatments may lead to nonadherence. Patients with PTSD who appear to have achieved a stable and positive clinical response and those who appear to have recovered from ASD may exhibit sudden relapse when new events reactivate traumatic concerns and fears about the safety of their families or themselves. For patients involved in ongoing litigation related to the traumatic event and subsequent impairment, legal proceedings may similarly reactivate concerns or emotions surrounding the event and its aftermath. The patient's motivation for participating in PTSD treatment may also be altered by ongoing legal actions. Psychiatrists should recognize these possibilities, address them in therapy, and encourage the patient to discuss any concerns regarding adherence, personal safety, or reexposure to traumatic reminders.

Medication adherence may be improved by emphasizing to the patient 1) when and how often to take the medicine, 2) the expected time interval before beneficial effects of treatment may be noticed, 3) the necessity to take medication even after feeling better, 4) the need to consult with the physician before discontinuing medication, and 5) steps to take if problems or questions arise (82). Some patients, particularly those who are elderly, have achieved improved adherence when both the complexity of the medication regimen and the cost of treatments are minimized. Severe or persistent problems of nonadherence may represent psychological concerns, psychopathology, or disruptions in the doctor-patient relationship, for which additional psychotherapy should be considered. Family members who are supportive of medication and/or other treatment can also play an important role in improving adherence. Although models of care such as assertive community treatment have not been specifically studied in individuals with PTSD, they have demonstrated efficacy in decreasing symptom severity, reducing length of hospitalization, and improving living conditions in individuals with serious and persistent mental illness (83–86). Consequently, such approaches may be useful in improving adherence in individuals with PTSD who have repeated hospitalizations related to nonadherence, particularly in the presence of significant psychiatric comorbidity.

8. Increasing understanding of and adaptation to the psychosocial effects of the disorder

While trauma itself often results in detrimental social, familial, academic, occupational, and financial phenomena, further effects may also stem from the symptoms of ASD or PTSD and may perpetuate these illnesses. For example, if one loses employment as a result of a disaster or because of missed work secondary to symptoms of ASD, the additional stressor of unemployment may increase the risk of developing PTSD (87). Consequently, the psychiatrist should assist the patient in addressing issues that may arise in various life domains, including family and social relationships, living conditions, general health, and academic and occupational performance, and help the patient to consider options that may be available to address such problems (e.g., consideration of alternative school or work schedules, other vocational options, financial or social supports). Working in collaboration with patients to set realistic and achievable short- and long-term goals can be useful. Patients can increase their sense of self-worth through achieving these goals, thereby reducing the demoralization that exacerbates or perpetuates illness. It may also be important to help the patient with ASD or PTSD obtain clinical assistance for family problems or for family members who may themselves require clinical intervention. Patients who have children may need help in assessing and meeting their children's needs, both during and in the wake of acute episodes.

Resilience has been alternately defined (by various researchers) as an individual trait or quality, an outcome, or a process. The concept of resilience may also encompass the ability to negotiate psychosocial and emotional changes after trauma exposure and in this way increase recovery possibilities. However, studies to date have identified no universal resilience factor or outcome (88, 89). Barnes and Bell (90) suggested that factors involved in resilience include 1) biological factors (intellectual and physical ability, toughness), 2) psychological factors (adaptive mechanisms such as ego resilience, motivation, humor, hardiness, and perceptions of self; emotional attributes such as emotional well-being, hope, life satisfaction, optimism, happiness, and trust; cognitive attributes such as cognitive styles, causal attribution such as an internal locus of control and blame, world view or philosophy of life, and wisdom), 3) spiritual attributes, 4) atributes of posttraumatic growth, 5) social attributes (interpersonal skills, interpersonal relationships, connectedness, and social support), and 6) environmental factors such as positive life events and socioeconomic status. Some studies show that optimism can buffer the effects of life stress (91–97) and enable some individuals to mobilize protective factors such as adaptive coping skills, increased self-efficacy, ways of reinterpreting adverse experiences in a positive manner, and strategies for seeking social support (98–101). Although no published studies have assessed the effect of optimism training on the development or outcome of ASD or PTSD, a school-based community-wide screening followed by psychosocial intervention was able to effectively identify and reduce disaster-related trauma symptoms and facilitate psychological recovery in children (102). Thus, efforts to improve psychosocial functioning and resilience may help to minimize symptoms and enhance recovery and remission.

9. Evaluating and managing physical health and functional impairments

Because ASD and PTSD are often the result of physically traumatic events, they are frequently associated with physical health problems and with functional impairments. Other mechanisms (e.g., hyperarousal, hypothalamic-pituitary-adrenal [HPA] axis dysregulation, poor self-care) may contribute to this association (103). In those who have experienced a trauma, medical problems may affect many aspects of health. Consequently, the presence, type(s), and severity of medical symptoms should be monitored continuously. Medical symptoms, symptoms of ASD or PTSD, and psychosocial or interpersonal relationship problems are each associated with impairments in a patient's ability to function. For such impairments to be addressed, level of functioning should also be assessed on an ongoing basis. For example, some patients may require assistance in scheduling absences from work or other responsibilities, whereas others may require encouragement to avoid major life changes during intensification of symptoms.

C. PRINCIPLES OF TREATMENT SELECTION

1. Goals of treatment

The goals of treatment for individuals who have experienced a traumatic event and have received a diagnosis of ASD or PTSD include the following.

a) Reduce the severity of ASD or PTSD symptoms

Treatment aims include reducing the patient's overall level of emotional distress as well as reducing specific target symptoms that may impair social or occupational function. In general, the clinician attempts to assist the patient to better tolerate and manage the immediate distress of the memories of the traumatic experience(s) and to decrease distress over time. In addition, the clinician works to enhance the patient's ability to discriminate trauma cues and reminders from the original traumatic experience(s) by promoting adaptive coping with reexperiencing states and instilling the belief that the current response to triggers results from recall of a past danger that is no longer present. Thus, the aim of treatment is to prevent, ameliorate, and promote recovery from the presumed neurobiological alterations associated with ASD and PTSD. Symptom-specific goals include helping the patient reduce intrusive reexperiencing, psychological and physiological reactivity to reminders, trauma-related avoidant behaviors, nightmares and sleep disturbance, and anxieties related to fears of recurrence. Other targeted goals include reducing behaviors that unduly restrict daily life, impair functioning, interfere with decision making, and contribute to engagement in high-risk behavior.

b) Prevent or reduce trauma-related comorbid conditions

Little is known about the effects of comorbid disorders on the course of ASD. Depression, substance abuse, and other conditions can impede recovery in PTSD and carry additional risks for psychiatric morbidity and functional impairment (4, 104). Medical disorders and somatic complaints are also common in war veterans (79, 105, 106) and persons with a history of sexual abuse (107–114). Thus, a major goal of treatment is to prevent secondary disorders and to appropriately diagnose and treat other concurrent conditions when present.

c) Improve adaptive functioning and restore or promote normal developmental progression

ASD and particularly PTSD are associated with a range of functional impairments in various areas of daily life (10, 12, 115–122). In addition to interventions that may be needed to address such impairments, related goals are to foster resilience and assist patients in adaptively coping with trauma-related stresses and adversities.

Traumatic experiences at any stage in the life cycle may impede the normal developmental progression. Posttraumatic stress symptoms can curtail current developmental achievements (for example, in dating, friendship, marriage, parenthood, educational achievement, occupational advancement, and retirement). Fears of event or symptom recurrence, avoidant behaviors, and restrictions on interpersonal life can also lead to lost developmental opportunities. As patients recover from PTSD, a therapeutic goal is to help identify and develop strategies to restore and promote normal developmental progression.

d) Protect against relapse

The course of acute and posttraumatic stress reactions can vary with symptomatic exacerbation relating to reminders of trauma or loss, additional life stresses or adversities, subsequent encounters with situations of danger or trauma, or discontinuation of psychotropic medication (123). Relapse prevention assists patients in anticipating such situations and in developing skills such as problem solving, emotional regulation, and the appropriate use of interpersonal support and professional help.

e) Integrate the danger experienced as a result of the traumatic situation(s) into a constructive schema of risk, safety, prevention, and protection

The danger or consequences associated with the original traumatic experience can skew personal beliefs, expectations, and constructs about the future, the risks of life, and safety. In addition, patients often search for the meaning of their life experience. The treatment of PTSD may include strategies to assist patients to constructively address these issues. As PTSD often evolves into a chronic illness, the meaning of the precipitating trauma in terms of its connections to past experience and its effects on subsequent perceptions of self-worth and interpersonal relationships may need to be addressed. Psychodynamic approaches and other psychotherapies may facilitate this integration (124–127).

2. Choice of initial treatment modality

Patients assessed within hours or days after an acute trauma may present with overwhelming posttraumatic physiological and emotional symptoms that would appear to prevent or severely limit psychotherapeutic interchanges. Such presentations do not necessarily indicate impending development of ASD or PTSD. However, pharmacological intervention to relieve overwhelming physical or psychological pain, impairing insomnia, or extremes of agitation, rage, or dissociation may restore baseline function or may be a useful temporizing measure as the clinician monitors for the development of additional symptoms and considers additional psychotherapeutic intervention and/or medication treatment.

Treatment of ASD or PTSD symptoms includes three broad categories of intervention: pharmacological treatment, psychotherapeutic intervention, and education and supportive measures. While cognitive and behavior therapies and pharmacological intervention (particularly with SSRIs) have reasonable clinical evidence to support their efficacy in treating the core symptoms of PTSD (see Section II.D, "Specific Treatment Strategies"), few direct comparisons of specific interventions or studies of combinations of support/education, pharmacological intervention, and psychotherapies are available. Nonetheless, consensus suggests that several factors, including the presence of specific target symptoms and individual patient characteristics, may guide decisions regarding initial treatment; these factors are reviewed in Section II.D, "Specific Treatment Strategies."

For patients with ASD as well as for those without overt symptoms, single-session individual debriefing does not prevent PTSD and may impede recovery (128, 129). In ASD, early after a trauma, once the patient's safety and medical stabilization have been addressed, supportive psychotherapy, case management, and assistance in obtaining resources such as food or shelter are useful (130, 131). Furthermore, in contrast to the findings for debriefing, there is no evidence to suggest that early supportive care is harmful (131–134). Preliminary evidence also suggests that ASD patients may be helped by cognitive behavior psychotherapy that incorporates exposure (135–137). Although there are few studies of pharmacological interventions in patients with ASD, treatment with SSRIs and possibly other antidepressants may represent reasonable initial clinical interventions.

In individuals with PTSD, evidence from randomized, controlled trials supports both psychotherapeutic and medication-based approaches to initial treatment. SSRIs are recommended as first-line medication treatment for PTSD, and other antidepressants may also be beneficial. In terms of psychotherapies, cognitive behavior therapy is an effective treatment for core symptoms of acute and chronic PTSD. EMDR is also effective. Stress inoculation, imagery rehearsal, and prolonged exposure techniques may also be employed in treating PTSD as well as associated symptoms such as anxiety and avoidance. The use of psychodynamic psychotherapy in treating PTSD is supported by a considerable number of descriptive studies and process-to-outcome analyses as well as substantial clinical experience. It may be useful in addressing developmental, interpersonal, or intrapersonal issues that may be of particular importance to social, occupational, and interpersonal functioning. It also appears to be useful in addressing the patient's changes in beliefs, world expectations, generalization of threat experiences to other life events, and attempts to find meaning in her or his experience. Interpersonal issues that develop as a result of ASD or PTSD, including changes in interpersonal relationships, fears, avoidance, loss of trust, anger and aggression, and increasing generalization of fears and threat, should also be addressed psychotherapeutically.

The presence of a comorbid psychiatric disorder may also guide initial intervention. For example, substance misuse is a common concomitant of ASD or PTSD and signals a need for specific treatment for substance use disorder. In addition, individuals who are depressed may be at greater risk for further exposures to trauma. For example, when domestic partner violence is ongoing, low self-esteem or decreased energy accompanying depression may produce increased violence in the abusive partner or inadequate self-protective efforts in the patient. Thus, direct and vigorous treatment of underlying depression with psychotherapy and/or specific antidepressant pharmacotherapy may minimize the risk for additional trauma and development or prolongation of PTSD.

3. Approaches for patients who do not respond to initial treatment

Because of the paucity of high-quality evidence-based studies of interventions for patients with treatment-resistant PTSD, treatment nonresponse cannot be addressed algorithmically. However, a systematic review of the factors that may be contributing to treatment nonresponse is possible. Since the initial treatment plan will have detailed each selected treatment, the rationale for its use, and the goals for treatment outcome, a review of this initial plan of care should help determine the extent to which therapeutic goals have been met. If interventions have been introduced sequentially, it will be easier to discern their individual effects. In reviewing the original plan, the clinician should explore with the patient which (if any) symptoms have improved, worsened, or remained the same. It is also important to determine whether the patient understands the plan and is adhering to it and, if nonadherence is present, the reasons for nonadherence. For example, has the patient failed to do homework assignments or discontinued medications or skipped doses because of side effects or financial difficulties? The potential of other psychological disorders or underlying personality traits to interfere with the treatment should be reconsidered and addressed as needed. The therapist should inquire about any new psychosocial or other environmental factors that may be hindering therapy, such as a conflict at work or with family members.

If it appears that the therapist-patient relationship is not at issue and that the patient is adhering to the treatment, the therapist should explore other options. One strategy for nonresponse is to augment the initial treatment with another—for example, adding pharmacotherapy to psychotherapy, psychotherapy to a pharmacological intervention, or couples therapy to an individual psychotherapy. Generally, the therapist should first exhaust the treatments for which there is the best evidence of efficacy before trying more novel treatments. In some cases, the original treatment may need to be discontinued and a different modality selected, as in the case of a patient who is too overwhelmed by anxiety to tolerate exposure therapy. Because most therapies used for the treatment of PTSD or ASD are also indicated for other psychiatric conditions, a review of the literature on strategies for improving response in those situations may also be helpful. However, there are limited data to guide the clinician in the treatment of patients with treatment-resistant PTSD and ASD, and, at present, clinical judgment must prompt the selection of one path rather than another.

D. SPECIFIC TREATMENT STRATEGIES

Since patients with a diagnosis of ASD or PTSD experience a broad and complex range of symptoms, caring for patients with these disorders involves an array of approaches and should include consideration of the biopsychosocial diversity of the patient's clinical presentation. When choosing a specific strategy to treat ASD or PTSD, it is important to consider the weight of scientific evidence supporting each treatment option as well as the limitations of the current evidence base. There have been relatively few double-blind, randomized, controlled trials of treatments for patients with PTSD and even fewer such trials for patients with ASD. Many promising results still require replication, and some interventions that are commonly used, based on extensive clinical experience and consensus, have yet to be examined in more methodologically rigorous studies. In the studies that are available, treatment and follow-up durations are typically short, sample sizes are frequently small, and the possibility of a placebo response is often inadequately addressed (138). Furthermore, measured outcomes have often concentrated on more readily quantifiable changes in specific symptoms rather than focusing on the diagnosis of ASD and PTSD per se or on important short- and long-term outcomes such as social, occupational, and interpersonal functioning.

It is also likely that responses to specific treatments may differ depending on the type of trauma experienced (e.g., acute versus ongoing or cumulative, natural disaster versus interpersonal violence, community-wide versus individual traumatic event, presence versus absence of simultaneous physical injury) and the timing of treatment relative to the occurrence of the traumatic event. Since ASD, by definition, occurs in the 4 weeks immediately after a traumatic event, studies of treatment interventions during this period should be considered as treatment of ASD and potentially as preventive strategies for PTSD. Treatment strategies for symptoms occurring between 1 and 3 months after trauma exposure (acute PTSD) may be different than those for symptoms occurring (or reoccurring) more than 3 months after the traumatic event(s) (chronic PTSD), although the differential efficacies of specific strategies for treating acute versus chronic PTSD have not been well studied. Throughout the first 3 months after a traumatic event, recovery is the general rule (139), and this natural recovery period may extend up to 6 months (34, 140). Here, the clinician is guided by the expectation of recovery, the relief of suffering, and the use of interventions to speed recovery and to prevent additional exposure to the traumatic event, chronicity of symptoms, and relapse.

In choosing a specific treatment strategy, consideration should also be given to the patient's age, gender, and previous history (e.g., developmental history, past traumatic experiences, substance use disorders, other psychiatric diagnoses), current comorbid medical and psychiatric illnesses, propensity for aggression or self-injurious behavior (see Section III, "Specific Clinical Features Influencing the Treatment Plan"), or other factors that may vary widely across individuals. Although systematic study of these factors is rare, clinical experience suggests that these factors may also necessitate modification of the individual treatment plan. Specific treatment strategies should be selected to target the symptoms or symptom clusters (i.e., reexperiencing, avoidance/numbing, or hyperarousal) that are most disruptive for the patient and to take into account the time interval between trauma exposure and symptom development. Personality style and family interactions may affect symptom expression, persistence, or exacerbation.

Treatment for the symptoms of ASD or PTSD involves three approaches either alone or in combination: psychopharmacology, psychotherapy, and education and supportive measures. To date, no psychotropic medications have been developed specifically for use in ASD or PTSD. Therefore, in clinical practice and in pharmacotherapy research, medications have been used in doses similar to those recommended or approved for other psychiatric illnesses. While the clinical evidence to date for each of these interventions is limited, the efficacy of combinations of education/support, psychotherapy, and psychopharmacology has been even less well characterized. Clinical practice and consensus support combinations of these approaches based on several factors, such as specifically identified target symptoms, psychiatric and other medical comorbidity, and the patient's preferences. Medication therapy may also be initiated to address symptoms (e.g., physical pain, agitation, severe insomnia, or psychosis) that might otherwise limit the efficacy of psychotherapy. The sections that follow summarize specific psychopharmacological, psychotherapeutic, and educational and supportive approaches to the treatment of ASD and PTSD. Where efficacy has been established to a greater degree with regard to particular symptoms or clinical features or at particular time intervals after the trauma exposure, these findings are highlighted.

1. Psychopharmacology

a) SSRIs

Evidence from several large randomized, double-blind controlled trials suggests that SSRIs are first-line medication treatment for both men and women with PTSD (123, 141–147). There are four reasons that SSRIs are the current medications of choice for PTSD: 1) they ameliorate all three PTSD symptom clusters (i.e., reexperiencing, avoidance/numbing, and hyperarousal), 2) they are effective treatments for psychiatric disorders that are frequently comorbid with PTSD (e.g., depression, panic disorder, social phobia, and obsessive-compulsive disorder), 3) they may reduce clinical symptoms (such as suicidal, impulsive, and aggressive behaviors) that often complicate management of PTSD, and 4) they have relatively few side effects.

Reductions in the severity of core PTSD symptoms have been shown with fluoxetine, sertraline, and paroxetine in studies that were of relatively short duration (8–12 weeks) and included predominantly women with chronic PTSD resulting from rape or assault (123, 141–146, 148). While symptom reduction was generally observed within 2–4 weeks of treatment, symptoms of anger and irritability were reduced within the first week (149). In studies of fluoxetine, improvement in arousal, numbing, and avoidance (but not reexperiencing) and overall response were greater in women than in men. Other studies have demonstrated efficacy for these agents in intrusive, avoidance/numbing, and arousal symptoms. Smaller open-label studies of fluvoxamine have shown efficacy in sleep-related symptoms (including nightmares) in combat veterans (147, 150). Head-to-head comparisons between any of the SSRIs for ASD or PTSD symptoms have not been published; however, clinical consensus holds that these agents differ primarily in their pharmacokinetics, metabolic effects on other medications, and side effects rather than in their efficacy in treating ASD or PTSD.

b) Tricyclic antidepressants and MAOIs

Studies of tricyclic antidepressants demonstrated efficacy for amitriptyline and imipramine (151, 152) but not desipramine (153). With the MAOIs, limited data suggest the efficacy of phenelzine and brofaromine (an MAOI available in Europe) (154, 155). In all of the trials, subjects were primarily male combat veterans, which limits the generalizability of findings. There do not appear to be studies of the effects of either MAOIs or tricyclic antidepressants specifically in women with PTSD or ASD.

c) Benzodiazepines

While benzodiazepines can reduce anxiety and improve sleep, their efficacy in preventing PTSD or treating the core symptoms of PTSD has been neither established nor adequately evaluated (156, 157). Concerns about addictive potential in individuals with comorbid substance use disorders may prompt additional caution regarding the use of benzodiazepines. Worsening of symptoms with benzodiazepine discontinuation has also been reported (158). However, in a naturalistic study of more than 300 veterans with PTSD and comorbid substance abuse, treatment with benzodiazepines was not associated with adverse effects on outcome (159).

d) Anticonvulsants

Open-label studies of divalproex, carbamazepine, and topiramate have demonstrated mixed or limited efficacy with regard to specific symptom clusters of PTSD (160–162), but these studies, as well as a single controlled trial of lamotrigine (163), have indicated benefit with regard to the reexperiencing symptoms.

e) Antipsychotics

Psychotic symptoms are not included in the diagnostic criteria for either ASD or PTSD. Nonetheless, patients with these illnesses may also experience psychotic symptoms as part of a comorbid disorder. Before initiating antipsychotic treatment, careful diagnostic evaluation is required to appropriately address the potential contributions of delirium, dementia, primary thought disorders, brief psychotic reactions, delusional disorder, substance abuse, closed head injury, or other comorbid general medical conditions. Preliminary studies of the second-generation antipsychotic agents olanzapine (164–166), quetiapine (167), and risperidone (168) in patients with PTSD suggest a potential role for these medications in pharmacological treatment, particularly when concomitant psychotic symptoms are present or when first-line approaches have been ineffective in controlling symptoms.

f) Adrenergic inhibitors

Agents acting on adrenergic receptors have also been proposed for the treatment of PTSD. Preliminary evidence has shown possible benefits with the α_1 antagonist prazosin (169) and with the α_2 agonist clonidine in combination with imipramine (170). However, there have been no large controlled studies of these agents to date.

While β-adrenergic blockers are at times prescribed for PTSD (171) and have been used in the treatment of performance anxiety, there have been no controlled studies of these agents for PTSD. Preliminary results suggest that acute administration of propranolol after trauma may reduce some later symptoms of PTSD (137, 172). Further controlled studies are necessary to evaluate this practice before it can be considered a part of the therapeutic armamentarium.

2. Psychotherapeutic interventions

a) Cognitive and behavior therapies

Cognitive behavior therapy in ASD or PTSD targets the distorted threat appraisal process (in some instances through repeated exposure and in others through techniques focusing on information processing without repeated exposure) in an effort to desensitize the patient to trauma-related triggers. Distinctions may be drawn between psychotherapies that focus principally on aspects of cognitive processing and those that emphasize behavioral techniques. However, aspects of both are frequently combined, and studies that identify the effective components of these therapies or that distinguish one from another are not available. A course of cognitive behavior therapy generally begins with education about the symptoms of the disorder, as well as a rationale for asking the patient to recall painful experiences and relaxation training. After the therapist assesses the patient's ability to tolerate within-session anxiety and temporary exacerbations of symptoms, the patient is led through a series of sessions in which the traumatic event and its aftermath are imagined and described, and the patient is asked to focus on the negative affect and arousal until they subside. Reassurance and relaxation exercises aid the patient in progressing through these sessions, and homework assignments allow the patient to practice outside the sessions or while confronting triggers of anxiety (specific places or activities) in vivo (125, 173, 174). A limited number of well-designed studies demonstrate some success not only in speeding recovery but also in preventing PTSD when cognitive behavior therapy is given over a few sessions beginning 2–3 weeks after trauma exposure (135, 173, 175–178). Both stress inoculation and prolonged exposure techniques have demonstrated efficacy in women with PTSD resulting from assault or rape (179–181). Prolonged exposure (through imaginal and in vivo exposure to avoided situations associated with previous trauma) has been shown to be effective, particularly in the PTSD-associated symptoms of anxiety and avoidance (179, 182). However, several studies have noted that exposure may increase rather than decrease symptoms in some individuals (178, 183). Stress inoculation training involving breathing exercises, relaxation training, thought stopping, role playing, and cognitive restructuring has also proven effective alone and in combination with prolonged exposure in reducing PTSD symptoms (179). Survivors of rape, crime victims, and combat veterans have demonstrated improvement in overall PTSD symptoms and nightmares in response to imagery rehearsal (i.e., imaginal prolonged exposure) (184, 185). Clinical improvement (but not recovery) was also demonstrated in a group of PTSD patients with diverse trauma exposures who received either imaginal exposure or cognitive behavior therapy (186, 187). In group settings, cognitive processing therapy designed to correct distortions related to threat appraisal and safety through a facilitated study of the patient's written narrative of his or her traumatic experience has shown promise (188). Most of these trials have been short-term, and the extent to which improvement is maintained over time has not been assessed through follow-up study.

b) Eye movement desensitization and reprocessing (EMDR)

EMDR is a form of psychotherapy that includes an exposure-based therapy (with multiple brief, interrupted exposures to traumatic material), eye movement, and recall and verbalization of traumatic memories of an event or events. It therefore combines multiple theoretical perspectives and techniques, including cognitive behavior therapy. Some point to the use of directed eye movements as a feature markedly distinguishing this form of therapy from other cognitive behavior approaches. Others point to the fact that traumatic material need not be verbalized; instead, patients are directed to think about their traumatic experiences without having to discuss them. Like many of the studies of other cognitive behavior and exposure therapies, most of the well-designed EMDR studies have been small, but several meta-analyses have demonstrated efficacy similar to that of other forms of cognitive and behavior therapy (189–192). Studies also suggest that the eye movements are neither necessary nor sufficient to the outcome (193–195), but these findings remain controversial (196, 197). Although it appears that efficacy may be related to the components of the technique common to other exposure-based cognitive therapies, as in the previously described cognitive behavior therapies, further study is necessary to clearly identify the effective subcomponents of combined techniques. Follow-up studies are also needed to determine whether observed improvements are maintained over time.

c) Psychodynamic psychotherapy

Psychodynamic therapy has, from its beginnings, been concerned with responses to traumatic events (198–200). There is an extensive body of research that includes descriptive designs, process-to-outcome correlational studies, and case studies. However, randomized, controlled research on psychodynamic psychotherapy in patients with ASD or PTSD is extremely limited. One controlled trial of psychodynamic therapy versus hypnotherapy or desensitization versus no therapy showed all interventions were superior to the control condition (no treatment) in decreasing avoidance and intrusive symptoms (201). Other controlled trials of hypnotherapy for ASD or PTSD have not been published, but descriptive studies and clinical consensus support its use—by appropriately trained individuals—in reducing symptoms of anxiety associated with acute distress and traumatic event cues and as a nonpharmacological adjunctive approach to anxiety reduction (202). A meta-analysis of controlled psychotherapy trials (including the study by Brom et al. [201]) also suggested the efficacy of hypnosis—particularly at the end of therapy (203).

The clinical research and narrative-based literatures on psychodynamic psychotherapy outline two major approaches to the treatment of traumatic stress disorders. The first views an individual's defenses and coping skills as a product of his or her biopsychosocial development and focuses on the meaning of the trauma for the individual in terms of prior psychological conflicts and developmental experience and relationships, as well as the particular developmental time of the traumatic occurrence(s). This approach examines the person's overall capacity to cope with memories of traumatic event(s) and their triggers and the coping style he or she uses to manage these memories (204, 205). The second approach focuses on the effect of traumatic experience on the individual's prior self-object experiences, overwhelmed self-esteem, altered experience of safety, and loss of self-cohesiveness and self-observing functions and helps the person identify and maintain a functional sense of self in the face of trauma (206, 207). Both approaches appear to be useful in addressing the subjective and interpersonal sustaining factors of the illness (e.g., shattered assumptions about attachments, issues of trust), as well as the changes in beliefs and world view and the widely altered threat perceptions often seen in chronic PTSD (21, 208, 209). Psychodynamic psychotherapists employ a mixture of supportive and insight-oriented interventions based on an assessment of the individual patient's symptoms, developmental history, personality, and available social supports as well as an ongoing assessment of the patient's ability to tolerate exploration of the trauma (210, 211). In chronic PTSD, issues of transference are often explored to help the patient understand conscious and unconscious concerns surrounding the meaning of recent and more remote traumatic events in his or her life as they appear in the treatment (212). Awareness of countertransference is a central component of treatment of traumatic experience in psychodynamic psychotherapy and in other therapies. The therapist's emotional response on hearing the patient describe the traumatic events can either facilitate or disrupt the therapeutic alliance, making ongoing attention to countertransference of particular importance in treating patients with ASD and PTSD.

d) Psychological debriefing

Psychological debriefing was developed as an intervention aimed at preventing the development of the negative emotional sequelae of traumatic events, including ASD and PTSD. This staged, semistructured group (or, as often administered, individual) interview and educational process includes education about trauma experiences in general and about the chronological facts of the recently experienced traumatic event and exploration of the emotions associated with the event. Since debriefing has received considerable publicity, it may be expected (or specifically requested) by leaders or managers when a group confronts disaster. In the military, for example, group debriefings have been used as a means for describing normative responses to trauma exposures and educating individuals about pursuing further assistance if symptoms persist or cause significant dysfunction or distress. However, well-controlled studies of debriefing that have used single-session, individual, and group debriefing have not demonstrated efficacy

(128, 129, 213–216). Although some trauma survivors have reported that they experienced such debriefings as helpful, there is no evidence at present that establishes psychological debriefing as effective in preventing PTSD or improving social and occupational functioning. In some settings, it has been shown to increase symptoms (217–219). Its use may be most problematic with groups of unknown individuals who have widely varying trauma exposures or when it is administered early after trauma exposure, before safety and decreased arousal are established. Immediately after exposure, persons may not be able to listen attentively, absorb new information, or appreciate the nuances of the demands ahead in a manner that promotes recovery (220, 221). Also, in heterogeneous groups, some individuals will be increasing their exposure through group participation and obtain no added support after the group session, thereby potentially increasing their likelihood of later distress (19).

3. Psychoeducation and support

Supportive interventions are often used as the control intervention in studies of more specific treatments. However, clinical experience indicates that both support and psychoeducation appear to be helpful as early interventions to reduce the psychological sequelae of exposure to mass violence or disaster. When access to expert care is limited by environmental conditions or reduced availability of medical resources, rapid dissemination of educational materials may help many persons to deal effectively with subsyndromal manifestations of trauma exposure. Such educational materials often focus on 1) the expected physiological and emotional response to traumatic events, 2) strategies for decreasing secondary or continuous exposure to the traumatic event, 3) stress-reduction techniques such as breathing exercises and physical exercise, 4) the importance of remaining mentally active, 5) the need to concentrate on self-care tasks in the aftermath of trauma, and 6) recommendations for early referral if symptoms persist. Encouraging persons who are acutely traumatized to first rely on their inherent strengths, their existing support networks, and their own judgment may reduce the need for further intervention. Although the efficacy of these measures alone in prevention of ASD or PTSD is unproven, emphasis on self-reliance and self-care should augment other strategies when and if they become necessary.

III. SPECIFIC CLINICAL FEATURES INFLUENCING THE TREATMENT PLAN

A. AGE

Trauma exposure, and therefore ASD and PTSD, occurs in individuals of all ages, including infants. For all types of trauma, exposure varies with age (5), peaking in late adolescence. Although findings on the relationship between age and risk for developing PTSD are inconsistent (4, 33, 222), age and developmental stage may be important considerations in treatment. The meaning of the exposure to a traumatic event will differ depending on the developmental stage as well as the extent of any preexisting emotional problems or age-specific concerns of the patient. For example, an injury that causes a loss of a limb in early adulthood can raise issues of how to establish long-term intimate relations with a disability, while a similar injury late in life may raise fears of dependency, loss of mobility, and needs for care that may not be available in the family. Confrontation with the threat of the loss of one's life will also raise different concerns depending on the time of life. Since these meanings affect the patient in life planning, they should be addressed in psychotherapy or supportive treatment. Advancing age increases the probability of comorbid medical disorders (e.g., hypertension, renal failure, heart disease) and concomitant medication use that will influence psychopharmacological decisions.

B. GENDER

Although overall exposure to trauma may be somewhat greater in men than in women (4, 5, 223), men and women differ in the types of traumatic events to which they are most likely to be exposed (4, 5, 223–226). That men are more likely to be exposed to combat and physical violence, whereas women are more likely to be exposed to rape and sexual assault, only partly accounts for the significantly higher lifetime prevalence rates of PTSD among women in the general population (4, 5, 222, 223, 226) as well as the longer duration of PTSD among women (5, 226). Differences in trauma exposures between men and women may also affect treatment considerations.

Initial assessment after sexual assault or rape requires a willingness to listen to the patient with an open mind to obtain necessary medical and investigative information and establish trust. Early attention to the therapeutic alliance may enhance the degree to which support and psychotherapy may be helpful in addressing later difficulties such as sexually transmitted diseases, pregnancy, difficult contraceptive choices, and feelings of loss of self-esteem, anger, rage, or guilt. Research neither supports nor refutes the prevalent notion that a treating clinician who is experienced as "different" from the perpetrator will more rapidly be accepted early on after the traumatic event. However, the gender of the treating clinician may be an issue for a specific patient under specific circumstances; therefore, the potential influence of the clinician's gender on treatment response should be considered.

C. ETHNIC AND CROSS-CULTURAL FACTORS

The likelihood of being exposed to traumatic events, as well as the likelihood of receiving a lifetime diagnosis of PTSD, differs by ethnic group. In general, clinicians who understand the importance of social and cultural dynamics will be sensitive to the need to treat patients with ASD and PTSD in such a manner as to not alienate them from their families and communities. Treatment must be knowledgeable and respectful of the culture, the cultural meaning of symptoms or illness, and cultural values of the patient and the patient's family. Treatment must also recognize that the "cultural context" in which treatment occurs may affect the development of symptoms. That Central American refugees are viewed as immigrants rather than persons escaping combat and that Vietnam veterans were viewed with disdain rather than welcomed as heroes may help explain different aspects of these traumatized populations or their response to treatment, compared to others entering the United States in the aftermath of war. Clinicians must be sensitive to the idea that such societal views may also shape treatment response. An individual's culture may be protective and contain a supportive system of values, roles, lifestyles, and knowledge that may buffer some of the effects of traumatic events (227). Protective influences of culture and social systems occur in part through provision of an acceptable context in which social support can be experienced and the traumatic event interpreted. The social and cultural context has the potential to provide a positive evaluation of the self, as well as to provide social support, both of which buffer the negative effects of stressful events (228). In other situations, cultural norms may contribute to the perception of an experience as traumatic (e.g., a rape victim may be shunned by family members for having "shamed" them). In addition, a disruption of social and cultural foundations can result in drastic changes in people's expectations and views of the meaning of life, thus making individuals potentially more vulnerable to traumatic events. Consequently, therapy must be conducted in a manner that does not estrange the individual from his or her family and community (229). Thus, while psychosocial treatments that attempt to identify and process traumatic experiences may be effective for individuals from Western cultures, they may be contraindicated for some Southeast Asian populations and persons from other non-Western cultures (229).

No controlled studies have explored the extent to which specific religious groups or subgroups within the United States may be more or less likely to seek care for psychiatric symptoms related to trauma exposure. However, African American veterans may be less likely than European American veterans to use psychosocial care outside Department of Veterans Affairs (VA) clinical programs, even though both ethnic groups appear to respond similarly to treatment for PTSD (230).

Ethnicity is also relevant to the pharmacological treatment of patients with ASD or PTSD. Cultural values may affect a patient's decision to take medication or a patient's adherence to medication regimens. Moreover, genetic polymorphisms in hepatic cytochrome P450 (CYP) enzymes occur at varying frequencies across ethnic groups (231–234). Since most psychotropic medications are metabolized through the CYP system, polymorphisms will affect the likelihood that an individual patient will experience therapeutic benefits or adverse effects at a given dose of medication. For example, about 7% of Caucasians are poor metabolizers of CYP 2D6 substrates, and 3%–6% are poor metabolizers of CYP 2C19 substrates (233, 234). These patients would be expected to have disproportionately high blood levels of medications that are metabolized through these routes. In contrast, ultrarapid metabolism by means of CYP 2D6 enzymes is observed in 1%–3% of Middle Europeans but up to 29% of Ethiopians (232). Finally, because ethnic groups also differ in genetic polymorphisms affecting sites of psychotropic action (e.g., serotonin transporters), a drug's pharmacodynamic properties may also vary with ethnicity (235, 236). These findings emphasize the need to take ethnic and cultural factors into consideration in developing a plan of therapy with the patient.

D. MEDICAL AND OTHER PSYCHIATRIC COMORBIDITY

Individuals with ASD or PTSD present with a complex array of symptoms and comorbid conditions. Physical injury is common as a result of the exposure to traumatic events. Patients with PTSD may present with medical or somatic concerns. Indeed, a history of childhood physical and/or sexual abuse has been associated with a greater number of hospital admissions and surgical procedures, somatization, and hypochondriasis in adulthood (237). Victimization, particularly exposure to chronic trauma, has also been associated with chronic gastrointestinal symptoms (111, 114, 238–242), chronic pain syndromes (107–114), and fibromyalgia (243, 244). Thus, gender differences in the rates of childhood physical and/or sexual victimization may contribute to gender differences in associated medical comorbidity. In addition, physical disorders such as cardiac or neurological illnesses may mimic symptoms of traumatic stress (229), resulting in underdiagnosis of either ASD or PTSD. This confusion may result in inadequate treatment of posttraumatic anxiety disorders but may also result in inappropriate provision of medical or surgical care, including unnecessary prescribing of potentially addictive substances. Thus, in treating individuals with ASD or PTSD, coordination of care with other physicians is important in developing an appropriate plan of diagnostic assessment and therapy for concomitant somatic symptoms and medical disorders.

In intensive care and rehabilitation settings, ASD and later PTSD may be part of the complex medical picture of patients recovering from injuries ranging from burns and amputations to traumatic brain injury. Consideration of the patient's physical function, concurrent medications, and need for medical intervention is required for appropriate pharmacological management and psychotherapy. In the emergency department, life-sustaining measures as well as hydration, sleep, and nutrition must take precedence over psychosocial treatments. However, the longer the stay in the hospital, the more likely that ASD or PTSD symptoms will become a focus for treatment, as sleep disturbances, anxiety, depression, or fears of planning for the future become evident. Family members may also have substantial reactions to the traumatic events their loved ones have experienced. Family members should be afforded opportunities to discuss their concerns in an environment that fosters trust. They should receive available information about the condition or prognosis of loved ones, including discussion of the range of behavioral and emotional responses that may arise in the injured person(s) and in other family members. Often, indirectly affected family members will request advice about how to discuss or whether to discuss certain topics with the patient (e.g., death of a husband or wife in the same motor vehicle collision). These issues may further complicate the evaluation and management of traumatized patients and must be taken into consideration when developing a treatment plan. Complicated evaluations may, by necessity, be initiated in an inpatient (intensive care or rehabilitative) setting but continue into outpatient care.

Patients who develop ASD or PTSD are also more likely to have other comorbid psychiatric disorders, including mood, dissociative, anxiety, substance-related, and personality disorders (171, 242, 245–254). Somatization disorder may also co-occur with ASD or PTSD, and in some individuals posttraumatic symptoms may represent somatization disorder psychopathology rather than ASD or PTSD (12). Thus, integrated treatment of ASD or PTSD and other psychiatric disorders is often required.

Among individuals with ASD or PTSD, depression and suicidal ideation or behavior require particular attention both pharmacologically and psychotherapeutically. Associated symptoms of depression, such as interpersonal withdrawal, survivor guilt, or shame, may be more amenable to psychosocial interventions than psychopharmacological interventions. Suicide risk may increase as the individual adjusts to physical losses or experiences guilt, shame, anger, or grief related to the loss of loved ones who may have been injured or may have died in the same traumatic event. While treatment targeted to specific symptoms of ASD or PTSD may also address these associated depressive features, such treatment may need to be continued beyond the time frame necessary to address ASD or PTSD alone.

Substance use may have a complex relation to ASD or PTSD after trauma. At times, substance use may contribute to the traumatic event itself (e.g., industrial or motor vehicle accident). Substance use may also be part of a preexisting substance use disorder or may reflect the patient's attempt to treat posttraumatic symptoms (e.g., sleep disturbance or anxiety). In fact, a period of increased substance (alcohol, tobacco, or drug of abuse) use often occurs early in ASD or PTSD, even when no substance use disorder existed before the trauma. In studies of large populations that have been exposed to trauma, higher rates of alcohol and tobacco use are observed after the event (255). Other studies of traumatized adults have reported high rates of alcohol and substance use (247, 250, 256, 257). Although increased usage does not equate to the presence of a substance use disorder, it remains a potential health concern and risk factor for other medical comorbidity. Substance misuse may also complicate psychiatric treatment of ASD or PTSD by producing symptoms that decrease the patient's ability to make use of psychotherapeutic treatments. Substance use also complicates pharmacological management and increases the risk of inadvertent patient overdose, somnolence, and behavioral problems. Thus, after a traumatic event, increased use of substances should be addressed as part of the treatment of ASD or PTSD, regardless of whether the criteria for a substance use disorder are met.

Patients with a large number of comorbid psychiatric and medical disorders are likely to have a greater severity of symptoms and a higher likelihood of developing a chronic course. It is prudent to realize that such individuals will often require long periods of treatment related to comorbid conditions and situational crises generated from these other illnesses. In addition, as a result of debilitation from both physical and mental conditions, these patients may require high levels of management and support to accomplish activities of daily living. They may be fragile, and some treatment interventions may prove either too exhausting or more disabling. Consequently, patients with chronic PTSD accompanied by comorbid medical and other psychiatric disorders need a graduated plan of treatment that begins with a primarily supportive approach and evolves into treatment that is more directed at restoring previous function. Very fragile patients may need hospitalization if they become dangerous to themselves or others or if they become so affectively labile that they experience significant functional impairment (229).

E. HISTORY OF PREVIOUS TRAUMAS

Exposure to previous trauma may modify vulnerability to subsequent trauma (32, 33), influence the development of PTSD (32, 33, 223), and complicate treatment and recovery. Recent loss—particularly if sudden or unexpected—is also associated with an increased prevalence of PTSD and may also complicate treatment (62). Although immediate illness may be precipitated by a recent trauma, symptoms of ASD or PTSD (sleep disturbance, irritability, hyperarousal) may in fact be directly related to the more remote traumatic experience(s), including childhood sexual abuse. Psychotherapeutic interventions aimed at integrating traumatic experience and diminishing the effect of intrusive recollections must therefore target not only the precipitating trauma but the remote trauma as well.

F. AGGRESSIVE BEHAVIOR

More than a half-century ago, Kardiner (198) noted that some patients with PTSD had problems with aggressive behavior that was frequently impulsive and episodic. More recent studies have documented increases in domestic violence, child abuse, and delinquency after disasters (15, 258–260). It has been postulated that with the development of PTSD, an increased expectation of danger and potential trauma occurs and results in an "anticipatory bias" (261) or an increased readiness for "flight, fight, or freeze." This increased readiness for aggression, as well as decreased sleep associated with PTSD, may produce a reduced ability to tolerate mild or moderate slights, resulting in acts of aggression that are disproportionate to the level of provocation (262).

Little evidence addresses the treatment of heightened aggressiveness in individuals with PTSD. Based on the use of SSRI antidepressants in treating PTSD, there is reason to suggest use of these medications in patients with aggression in the context of PTSD. Observation for symptomatic exacerbations is warranted in the early phases of treatment, before the therapeutic benefits of pharmacotherapy are manifest. Anticonvulsants are sometimes suggested for management of irritability and aggression, but evidence for their efficacy is similarly sparse, with only a single small-scale open-label trial that found a modest effect of carbamazepine on irritability/aggression (160).

To the extent that aggressive behavior occurs in the context of reexperiencing symptoms (e.g., flashbacks), treatment approaches targeting this symptom cluster may also reduce aggression. Since aggressive behaviors are associated with states of both intoxication and withdrawal, concurrent treatment of comorbid substance use disorders may also reduce the likelihood of aggressive behavior.

G. SELF-INJURIOUS AND SUICIDAL BEHAVIORS

Both acute and chronic response to trauma exposure may include self-harming behaviors that range from self-mutilation to disordered eating behaviors to abuse of alcohol and other substances (256, 257, 263–270). This response may occur particularly when the trauma induces stigma, shame, or guilt. Children and adults who have been traumatized are likely to redirect onto themselves the feelings of aggression they have toward others (267, 271, 272). Furthermore, studies consistently show a significant relationship between childhood sexual abuse and various forms of self-injury later in life, particularly self-starving, cutting, and suicide attempts (267). In fact, PTSD has demonstrated the strongest association with suicidal behaviors of any of the anxiety disorders (273, 274). Specifically, PTSD is associated with a sixfold increase in the likelihood of an initial suicide attempt, an odds ratio that is double that for other anxiety disorders and about half that for mood disorders (275). In addition, individuals with PTSD appear to have an equal or greater odds ratio for making a suicide plan and for making impulsive suicide attempts, compared to those with mood disorders or other anxiety disorders (275). Anxiety disorders including PTSD are also associated with an increased risk for suicide per se (276, 277). Thus, it is apparent that patients with PTSD are at increased risk for developing self-harming and suicidal behaviors (269).

The possible utility of SSRI antidepressants in treating self-harming or suicidal behaviors in individuals with PTSD is suggested by the utility of SSRIs in treating PTSD in general (123, 141, 144–146, 148, 150, 278–280). Observation for symptomatic exacerbations is warranted in the early phases of treatment, before the therapeutic benefits of pharmacotherapy are manifest. Other pharmacotherapies may also be useful, although evidence for their efficacy is sparse. For example, one study showed carbamazepine to be effective for treatment of self-destructive behaviors (281), and a single, relatively small study suggested that lithium carbonate may also be helpful (282). Finally, although opiate receptor blockers have not been studied specifically in patients with ASD or PTSD, limited evidence suggests that such agents may decrease self-destructive behaviors in other populations (283).

Regarding psychological treatments for suicidal behavior in patients with PTSD, few studies are available. In addition, most studies of PTSD specifically exclude acutely suicidal patients; therefore, clinical judgment must augment the research to date. Thus, although many studies show that cognitive behavior therapy is effective in treating psychiatric disorders such as depression and PTSD, which can increase the risk for suicide, few studies have shown cognitive behavior therapy to be effective for reducing actual suicidal behavior and intent (284). As in other mental disorders associated with suicidal behavior, involving the patient's family members and other sources of support in the treatment plan may increase awareness of and vigilance for indications of the potential for deliberate self-harm or suicide.

PART B
BACKGROUND INFORMATION AND REVIEW OF AVAILABLE EVIDENCE

IV. DISEASE DEFINITION, EPIDEMIOLOGY, AND NATURAL HISTORY

A. CORE CLINICAL FEATURES

The DSM-IV-TR criteria for ASD and PTSD are shown in Table 1 and Table 2, respectively. Table 4 compares the specific criteria used in making these diagnoses. For both ASD and PTSD, essential features are exposure to a traumatic event that need not be outside the normal range of human experience but that arouses "intense fear, helplessness, or horror" (DSM-IV-TR, p. 463), followed by development of characteristic symptoms. Exposure can occur through direct experience or through witnessing or learning about a traumatic event that caused "actual or threatened death," "serious injury," or "threat to the physical integrity" of oneself or others (DSM-IV-TR, p. 463). Both natural and human-made traumatic events have the potential to evoke these symptoms. Naturally occurring stressors include, for example, tornadoes, earthquakes, and medical illnesses. Human-made events include accidents, domestic and community violence, rape, assault, terrorism, and war. Some of these are singular events; others involve chronic or repeated exposure. In general, human-made events have been believed to cause more frequent and more persistent psychiatric symptoms and distress.

TABLE 4. Comparison of DSM-IV-TR Diagnostic Criteria for Acute Stress Disorder (ASD) and Posttraumatic Stress Disorder (PTSD)

Description of Criterion	ASD Criterion	PTSD Criterion
Characteristics of traumatic exposure	Criterion A	Criterion A
Exposure to a traumatic event in which both of the following conditions were present:		
1. the person experienced, witnessed, or was confronted with an event or events that involved actual or threatened death or serious injury, or a threat to the physical integrity of self or others		
2. the person's response involved intense fear, helplessness, or horror		
Dissociative symptom cluster	Criterion B	—[a]
Either while experiencing or after experiencing the distressing event, the individual has three (or more) of the following symptoms:		
1. a subjective sense of numbing, detachment, or absence of emotional responsiveness		
2. a reduction in awareness of his or her surroundings (e.g., "being in a daze")		
3. derealization		
4. depersonalization		
5. dissociative amnesia (i.e., inability to recall an important aspect of the trauma)		
Reexperiencing cluster	Criterion C (except item 5)	Criterion B
The traumatic event is persistently reexperienced in one (or more) of the following ways:		
1. recurrent and intrusive distressing recollections of the event, including images, thoughts, or perceptions		
2. recurrent distressing dreams of the event		
3. acting or feeling as if the traumatic event were recurring (includes a sense of reliving the experience, illusions, hallucinations, and dissociative flashback episodes, including those that occur on awakening or when intoxicated)		
4. intense psychological distress at exposure to internal or external cues that symbolize or resemble an aspect of the traumatic event		
5. physiological reactivity on exposure to internal or external cues that symbolize or resemble an aspect of the traumatic event		

TABLE 4. Comparison of DSM-IV-TR Diagnostic Criteria for Acute Stress Disorder (ASD) and Posttraumatic Stress Disorder (PTSD) *(continued)*

Description of Criterion	ASD Criterion	PTSD Criterion
Avoidance/numbing of response cluster	Criterion D (requires only marked avoidance of stimuli that arouse recollections of the trauma)	Criterion C
Persistent avoidance of stimuli associated with the trauma and numbing of general responsiveness (not present before the trauma), as indicated by three (or more) of the following characteristics:		
1. efforts to avoid thoughts, feelings, or conversations associated with the trauma		
2. efforts to avoid activities, places, or people that arouse recollections of the trauma		
3. inability to recall an important aspect of the trauma		
4. markedly diminished interest or participation in significant activities		
5. feeling of detachment or estrangement from others		
6. restricted range of affect (e.g., unable to have loving feelings)		
7. sense of a foreshortened future (e.g., does not expect to have a career, marriage, children, or a normal life span)		
Arousal cluster	Criterion E (requires only marked symptoms of anxiety or increased arousal)	Criterion D
Persistent symptoms of increased arousal (not present before the trauma), as indicated by two (or more) of the following symptoms:		
1. difficulty falling or staying asleep		
2. irritability or outbursts of anger		
3. difficulty concentrating		
4. hypervigilance		
5. exaggerated startle response		

TABLE 4. Comparison of DSM-IV-TR Diagnostic Criteria for Acute Stress Disorder (ASD) and Posttraumatic Stress Disorder (PTSD) *(continued)*

Description of Criterion	ASD Criterion	PTSD Criterion
Duration of disturbance	Minimum of 2 days, maximum of 4 weeks	Greater than 1 month (acute PTSD is diagnosed if duration is less than 3 months; chronic PTSD if duration is 3 months or greater)
Temporal relationship to traumatic event	Occurs within 4 weeks	Usually occurs within 3 months (if onset occurs more than 6 months after stressor, delayed onset is specified)
Distress or impairment in functioning: The disturbance causes clinically significant distress or impairment in social, occupational, or other important areas of functioning (or inability to pursue some necessary task in ASD)	Criterion F	Criterion F
Exclusion of other conditions	Criterion H	—[a]
Not due to the direct physiological effects of a substance (e.g., a drug of abuse, a medication) or a general medical condition		
Not better accounted for by brief psychotic disorder		
Not an exacerbation of a preexisting axis I or axis II disorder		

[a]Not included in PTSD criteria.

The criteria for ASD overlap substantially with but are not identical to those for PTSD (Table 4). Although core symptoms fall into characteristic symptom clusters for both diagnoses, ASD and PTSD differ in the numbers of symptoms from each cluster that are required to establish a diagnosis. For example, in addition to three or more dissociative symptoms and "marked avoidance of stimuli that arouse recollections of the trauma," the diagnosis of ASD requires at least one reexperiencing symptom as well as "marked" anxiety or increased arousal. On the other hand, for a diagnosis of PTSD to be made, DSM-IV-TR stipulates that there be at least one reexperiencing symptom, two arousal symptoms, and three avoidance/numbing symptoms and that these symptoms be temporally related to the stressor. Symptoms in the reexperiencing cluster include "recurrent and intrusive recollections" of the event, recurrent distressing trauma-related dreams, acting or feeling as if the event were reoccurring, "intense psychological distress" with exposure to trauma cues, and physiological reactivity to traumatic cues (DSM-IV-TR, p. 464). Within the avoidance/numbing cluster, purposeful actions as well as unconscious mechanisms may be present and may include efforts to avoid trauma-related thoughts, feelings, or conversations; efforts to avoid activities, places, or people reminiscent of the trauma; inability to recall important aspects of the trauma; greatly decreased "interest or participation in previously enjoyed activities"; feeling detached or estranged; restricted range of affect; and a "sense of a foreshortened future" (DSM-IV-TR, p. 464). Increased arousal includes sleep disturbance, "irritability or outbursts of anger," difficulty concentrating, hypervigilance, and exaggerated startle response (DSM-IV-TR, p. 464), all of which are generalized arousal responses and are not precipitated by reminders of the stressor.

The two disorders also differ in the duration of the disturbance and its temporal relationship to the traumatic stressor. For ASD, the disturbance occurs within 4 weeks of the traumatic event and is from 2 days to 4 weeks in duration. To qualify for a diagnosis of PTSD, symptoms must be present for more than 1 month. If symptom duration is less than 3 months, acute PTSD is diagnosed, whereas chronic PTSD is diagnosed when symptoms persist for 3 months or longer. Although symptoms of PTSD usually begin within 3 months of exposure, DSM-IV-TR also allows for delayed onset with symptoms that appear months or even years after the event. Finally, for both ASD and PTSD, the severity of symptoms must be sufficient to cause "clinically significant distress" or impaired functioning (DSM-IV-TR, pp. 468, 472).

B. ASSOCIATED FEATURES

A number of additional features may be associated with PTSD. According to DSM-IV-TR, these features include somatic complaints, shame, despair, hopelessness, impaired affect modulation, social withdrawal, survivor guilt, anger, impulsive and self-destructive behavior, difficulties in interpersonal relationships, changed beliefs, and changed personality. Difficulty seeking and sustaining medical care has also been observed (285). Symptoms such as inappropriate guilt, shame, or hopelessness may be indicative of comorbid depression that requires separate intervention, and other symptoms, such as somatic complaints, may represent common phenomena that are associated with anxiety disorders but are not necessary for the diagnosis of either ASD or PTSD. Finally, symptoms of trauma-related dissociation are essential to the diagnosis of ASD but are not necessary for the diagnosis of PTSD. Nonetheless, a previous history of peritraumatic dissociation (and ASD) may be of clinical significance in patients with PTSD, as studies have demonstrated that such a history predicts greater severity and chronicity of PTSD (7, 286, 287).

C. DIFFERENTIAL DIAGNOSIS

The differential diagnosis of ASD and PTSD includes a broad range of psychiatric and physical diagnoses as well as normative responses to traumatic events. Individuals who are exposed to events that fulfill criterion A for ASD or PTSD often experience some transient symptoms that differ from those of ASD or PTSD only in their duration or in the associated level of dysfunction or distress. In some professions (e.g., military, firefighters, police, emergency medical personnel), exposure to criterion A events is inevitable. If symptoms do not meet the criteria for ASD or PTSD but are persistent or associated with dysfunction or distress, a V code diagnosis (e.g., V62.2, occupational problem) may be appropriate.

Establishing a differential diagnosis also requires that ASD be differentiated from PTSD. For a single discrete traumatic event, ASD and PTSD can be readily distinguished from one another based on the time that has passed since the trauma. However, for less discrete or reoccurring traumas such as repetitive domestic violence, the distinctions between ASD and PTSD may be less clear. Although no convention or consensus exists regarding the classification of recurrent symptoms (for more than 1 month) during the course of repetitive episodic trauma, it may be best to conceptualize this symptom presentation as PTSD rather than as recurrent episodes of ASD. Clearly, eliminating the source or threat of continued violence and injury is critical to ultimate resolution of posttraumatic symptoms, regardless of diagnostic classification. As noted earlier, beyond duration of symptoms, the major distinguishing feature between ASD and PTSD is the emphasis in the former on dissociative symptoms. Although persons with ASD often develop PTSD, this is not invariably true. PTSD may also occur in persons who manifest few or even no symptoms of ASD in the period immediately after trauma (6, 7, 9). In patients with subthreshold or full symptoms of PTSD for less than 1 month who do not experience dissociative symptoms sufficient to meet the DSM-IV-TR criteria for ASD, the illness would be best characterized as an adjustment disorder in DSM terms. Such patients would also meet the diagnostic criteria for acute stress reaction, as defined by ICD-10. The differential diagnosis also includes medical disorders as well as a number of other psychiatric disorders (Table 5).

The fact that many of these disorders occur comorbidly with ASD or PTSD further complicates diagnosis. For example, a substantial proportion of trauma-exposed veterans (20, 247), refugees (292), and civilians (12, 293) develop symptoms consistent with major depressive disorder. Mood disorders are also an established risk factor for the development of PTSD in newly exposed individuals (12, 14, 34). Symptoms such as insomnia, poor concentration, and diminished interest in activities may be present with ASD and PTSD as well as with major depression. In addition, the restricted affective range that may accompany the numbing of responses with PTSD may resemble the restricted affect seen in depressed patients. It is important to note that if the DSM-IV-TR criteria are met, a major depressive episode can be diagnosed in conjunction with ASD or PTSD.

Trauma-exposed populations and patients with PTSD frequently experience comorbid substance-related disorders (256, 257, 294–299). Patients with PTSD also manifest increased physical complaints (76–79, 300, 301) and comorbid medical conditions (302). Although DSM-IV excluded complicated or prolonged grief as an axis I diagnosis (because of a lack of empirical evidence regarding symptoms), some investigators have proposed criteria for a diagnosis of complicated grief disorder based on patterns of prolonged bereavement characterized by persistence, intensity, intrusive recollections or images of the death, preoccupation with the loss, and avoidance of reminders (303). Furthermore, there is evidence that these symptoms may be more distressing after an unnatural or violent death. Such symptoms overlap with both major depressive disorder and PTSD, but persons may acknowledge these symptoms without meeting the criteria for either diagnosis. Here, preoccupation with the suddenness, violence, or catastrophic aspects of traumatic loss may be independent from and may interfere with the normal bereavement process (304). Consensus criteria for "traumatic grief" have been developed; these criteria overlap with those of complicated grief but incorporate additional symptoms of distress related to cognitive reenactment of the death, terror, and avoidance of reminders (289). Once again, studies that address treatment for these phenomena distinct from treatment for PTSD or depression are presently lacking. Nonetheless, complicated or traumatic grief as well as bereavement must be considered in the differential diagnosis for persons who have experienced a traumatic loss.

Finally, since childhood trauma may be a common antecedent to the development of personality (particularly cluster B) disorders in adulthood, and associated features of personality disorders and PTSD overlap (e.g., difficulty with affect modulation, impulsivity, irritability, comorbid substance abuse), PTSD symptoms may be "masked" by an underlying personality disorder. Numerous reports describe childhood trauma in adults with borderline personality disorder, and other reports describe childhood trauma as a root cause of adult PTSD. However, the extent to which symptoms may be misattributed to either PTSD or a personality disorder has not been well studied. Therefore, personality disorders must be considered in the differential diagnosis either as the primary etiology for symptoms or as comorbid illnesses.

D. EPIDEMIOLOGY

Exposure to a traumatic event, the essential element for development of ASD or PSTD, is a relatively common experience, although the specific rates of such experiences within a population sample will vary with the criteria used to define a potential trauma as well as with the sample characteristics and the interviewing method (e.g., telephone survey versus face-to-face interview, clinician versus lay interviewer, structured versus unstructured interview), as reviewed by Brewin and colleagues (222). For example, using DSM-III-R criteria, which required that the event be outside the range of normal human experience, researchers in the National Comorbidity Survey (4) assessed 5,877 individuals ages 15–54 years with the Diagnostic Interview Schedule (DIS) and the Composite International Diagnostic Interview, administered by experienced nonclinician interviewers. They found that more than one-half of the subjects had experienced a traumatic event during their lifetime, with most people having experienced more than one. Giaconia and colleagues (305) also used the DSM-III-R version of the DIS and found that by age 18 years, more than two-fifths of youths in a community sample had been exposed to an event that was severe enough to qualify for a diagnosis of PTSD. Using structured telephone interviews in a national sample of 4,008 adult women, Resnick and colleagues (306) found a lifetime rate of exposure to any type of traumatic event of 69%. Using the DSM-IV version of the DIS, Breslau and colleagues (5) examined trauma exposure and the diagnosis of PTSD in a telephoned community sample of 2,181 individuals in the Detroit area and found that the lifetime prevalence of trauma exposure was 89.6%. The most prevalent types of events were the sudden unexpected death of a close relative or friend (60.0%) or learning of trauma to a close relative or friend (62.4%).

Overall exposure to traumatic events may be somewhat greater in men than in women (4, 5), although the gender difference in the lifetime prevalence of such exposure is relatively small (60.7% for men versus 51.2% for women in the study of Kessler and colleagues [4], and 92.2% for men versus 87.1% for women in the study of Breslau and colleagues [5]). In addition, men and women differ in the types of events to which they are exposed. For example, in the National Comorbidity Survey, 0.7% of men versus 9.2% of women had a lifetime experience of being raped, whereas 19.0% of men but only 6.8% of women had been threatened with a weapon and 6.6% of men but no women had experienced combat (4). In the Detroit Area Survey of Trauma (5), a similar pattern was noted, with women being more likely than men to report rape (9.4% versus 1.1%) or other sexual assault (9.4% versus 2.8%) and men being more likely than women to report other types of assaultive violence, including being mugged or threatened with a weapon (34.0% versus 16.4%) and being shot or stabbed (8.2% versus 1.8%).

Exposure to traumatic events also varies with age, showing consistent declines with age across multiple studies. For example, Norris (307) found a strong trend for decreases in both past-year and lifetime exposure with increasing age in a nonrandom sample of 1,000 individuals from four cities in southeastern states. Bromet and colleagues (14) analyzed data from the National Comorbidity Survey and found that the risk of experiencing a traumatic event was greatest in the 15- to 24-year-old cohort and decreased in subsequent age cohorts. Similarly, Breslau and colleagues (5)

TABLE 5. Psychiatric Diagnoses Often Applicable to Injured Trauma Survivors Treated in the Acute Care Medical Setting

	Diagnostic Considerations			
Diagnosis[a]	**Symptomatic Criteria**	**Functional Criteria**	**Time Course**	**Acute Care Considerations**
Acute stress disorder (ASD)	A. Exposure to a traumatic event in which the person experienced or witnessed a life-threatening event that was associated with intense emotions (e.g., physical injury) B. Either while experiencing the event or after, the person experiences three or more dissociative symptoms. C. The event is reexperienced. D. Avoidance of reminders of the event E. Symptoms of arousal	Symptoms are associated with clinically significant impairments in social, occupational, or physical function.	Diagnosis can be made between 2 and 30 days after the event.	Not all injured patients with immediate distress will experience three dissociative symptoms.
Posttraumatic stress disorder (PTSD)	A. Exposure to a traumatic event in which the person experienced or witnessed a life-threatening event that was associated with intense emotions (e.g., physical injury) B. The event is persistently reexperienced C. Persistent avoidance of reminders of the event D. Persistent arousal symptoms	Symptoms are associated with clinically significant impairments in social, occupational, or physical function.	Diagnosis must be made at least 1 month after the event.	Patient's symptoms frequently appear before the 1-month point.
Major depressive episode	Five or more of the following symptoms: depressed mood,[b] diminished interest in pleasurable activities,[b] weight loss or gain, insomnia or hypersomnia, agitation or retardation, fatigue or energy loss, feelings of worthlessness, poor concentration, and suicidal ideation	Symptoms are associated with clinically significant impairment in social, occupational, or physical function.	Symptoms must be present for 2 weeks.	Major depressive episode can be diagnosed in conjunction with ASD or PTSD. Injured trauma survivors frequently present with multiple symptoms of a depressive episode early on (i.e., before 2 weeks after the traumatic injury).

TABLE 5. Psychiatric Diagnoses Often Applicable to Injured Trauma Survivors Treated in the Acute Care Medical Setting *(continued)*

	Diagnostic Considerations			
Diagnosis[a]	**Symptomatic Criteria**	**Functional Criteria**	**Time Course**	**Acute Care Considerations**
Traumatic grief	This evolving diagnostic category can be used when the events that lead to a patient's or relative's visit to the acute care setting involve sudden unanticipated loss. The symptoms of traumatic grief involve distressing thoughts and experiences related to reunion, longing, and searching for the deceased loved one (289–291).	The disturbance causes clinically significant impairment in social, occupational, or other important areas of functioning.	Duration of disturbance is at least 2 months.	Traumatic grief is applicable to patients who have experienced the death of a significant other.
Adjustment disorder	A. Development of emotional or behavioral symptoms in response to an identifiable stressor. Symptoms can include depression, anxiety, conduct disturbance, or other emotional disturbance. B. The symptoms or behaviors are clinically significant, as evidenced by marked distress.	Emotional or behavioral symptoms are associated with marked impairment in social, role, or physical function.	Onset occurs within 3 months after the traumatic injury.	DSM-IV-TR suggests that the adjustment disorder diagnosis be used for patients who develop a symptom pattern that is not entirely consistent with the criteria for ASD/PTSD. Nonspecific symptomatic requirements make adjustment disorder a useful diagnosis for the many patients who experience posttraumatic behavioral and emotional disturbances that include symptoms that do not fit into other diagnostic rubrics (e.g., patients who present with marked somatic symptom amplification).

Source. Adapted with permission from *Diagnostic and Statistical Manual of Mental Disorders,* 4th Edition, Text Revision. Washington, DC, American Psychiatric Association, 2000. Copyright 2000. American Psychiatric Association; and from *Seminars in Clinical Neuropsychiatry*, vol. 8, Zatzick D., "Posttraumatic stress, functional impairment, and service utilization after injury: a public health approach," pp. 149–157, Copyright 2003, with permission from Elsevier.

[a]Often, posttraumatic symptoms may be present that are insufficient to meet criteria for the diagnoses listed in this table. In such cases, V code diagnoses would be indicated, as would supportive therapy, psychoeducation, and continued monitoring for the development of further psychiatric disorder(s). [b]At least one of the five symptoms must be either depressed mood or diminished interest in pleasurable activities and shall not be due to a general medical condition or mood-incongruent delusions or hallucinations.

found that in all classes of traumas studied, peak exposures to traumatic events occurred in persons ages 16–20 years, with subsequent declines in exposure rates with age.

The lifetime prevalence of ASD is unclear, but a number of community-based studies have examined the prevalence of PTSD. Here, too, the reported rates vary with the specific diagnostic criteria employed, the interviewing method, and the sample characteristics. For example, in a study of the data for 2,985 participants from a central North Carolina community who were assessed as part of the Epidemiologic Catchment Area (ECA) survey, Davidson and colleagues (242) found a lifetime prevalence for DSM-III PTSD of 1.3%. Helzer and colleagues (308) found a lifetime PTSD prevalence of 1% in the St. Louis ECA sample. Using DSM-III-R criteria, Kessler and colleagues (4) found an estimated lifetime prevalence of PTSD of 7.8% in the National Comorbidity Survey, whereas Giaconia and colleagues (305) found that more than 6% of youths in a community sample met the criteria for a lifetime diagnosis of PTSD.

The likelihood of developing PTSD after having been exposed to a traumatic event (i.e., the conditional risk of PTSD) varies widely with the specific experience. Overall in the Detroit Area Survey of Trauma, for example, 9.2% of trauma-exposed persons developed PTSD, but PTSD developed in about half of those who were raped or held captive, tortured, or kidnapped, compared to only 2.2% of those who learned of the rape, attack, or injury of a close relative (5). In the women studied by Resnick and colleagues (306), rates of PTSD were significantly greater in crime victims that in noncrime victims (25.8% versus 9.4%).

General population studies typically find a significantly higher lifetime prevalence of PTSD in women, with rates that are consistently about twice those seen in men (4, 5, 222, 242, 308). The absolute rates for a lifetime diagnosis of PTSD again vary with the definition and severity of the traumatic stressor. Using the DSM-III criteria as part of the ECA survey, Helzer and colleagues (308) found that 1.3% of women and 0.5% of men met the criteria for a lifetime diagnosis of PTSD, and Davidson and colleagues (242) found lifetime rates of PTSD of 1.8% in women and 0.9% in men. In contrast, using the DSM-III-R criteria in the National Comorbidity Survey, Kessler and colleagues (4) found a lifetime prevalence for PTSD of 10.4% in women and 5.0% in men, and Breslau and colleagues (5, 223), using the DSM-IV criteria, found the lifetime prevalence of PTSD to be 13.0% in women, compared to 6.2% in men. In terms of the relative likelihood of developing PTSD after having experienced a traumatic event, Kessler and colleagues (4) found more than a twofold increase in the conditional risk of PTSD in women, compared with men (20.4% versus 8.1%). These gender differences in rates of PTSD do not necessarily imply that women are more likely to develop PTSD, per se; the differences may be explained by other factors that increase risk for women (15), such as the greater likelihood of women's experiencing rape and other sexual assaults, which carry a high conditional risk of developing PTSD. In addition, since a history of mood disorder increases the subsequent risk of developing PTSD in response to a stressor (14), the greater prevalence of such disorders among women may influence their likelihood of developing PTSD. Furthermore, specific aspects of the traumatic event, such as fear, threat, surprise, and meaning, may influence the victim's response (309).

The literature provides inconsistent information on the relationship between age and the risk of developing PTSD. Breslau and colleagues (33), in a representative community sample in southeast Michigan, found no relationship between age and risk of PTSD. In the National Comorbidity Survey, Kessler and colleagues (4) found some variations in the lifetime prevalence of PTSD by birth cohort, but men had the highest rates in the 45- to 54-year-old cohort, whereas women had the highest rates in the 25- to 34-year-old cohort. In terms of the conditional risk of developing PTSD after adjustment for the type of trauma exposure, a subsequent analysis of the National Comorbidity Survey data also showed variations in risk with age among men but a greater risk for PTSD among women in younger age cohorts (14). Brewin and colleagues (222) found weak effects of age in a meta-analysis of risk factors for PTSD but suggested that the differences may reflect confounding factors.

The prevalence of exposure to traumatic events as well as the development of PTSD also varies across racial and ethnic groups, with high rates of exposure to violence among African Americans, American Indians, and Alaska Natives, compared to members of more economically advantaged groups (310, 311). For example, in one study, 82% of American Indians and Alaska Natives had been exposed to one traumatic event, and the prevalence of PTSD was 22% (4). American Indians have a rate of violent victimization that is more than twice the national average (312), whereas rates of PTSD among American Indians and Alaska Natives are about threefold higher than in the general population. An investigation of Northern Plains Indian youths in grades 8 through 11 found that 61% had been exposed to some kind of traumatic event (313). These adolescents were reported to have more trauma-related symptoms but not substantially higher rates of diagnosable PTSD (3%), compared to the general population (313). A study of a Southwestern American Indian community found even higher rates of experience of one or more traumatic events but also noted a higher prevalence of lifetime PTSD in this community, compared with the general U.S. population (314).

Because members of some racial and ethnic groups are more likely to have lower socioeconomic status, live in an inner-city area, or be U.S. combat veterans (315), and because such status is associated with an increased likelihood of experiencing undesirable life events (316), some racial and ethnic groups are more likely to experience ASD and PTSD (4, 314). Among veterans, an increased likelihood of traumatic early experiences (310–312, 317) may contribute to the increased rates of PTSD seen in African Americans, Hispanics, and American Indian/Alaska Natives after combat-related trauma (247, 310).

Differences in the rates of previous exposure to traumas may account, in part, for differences observed in rates of PTSD among U.S. veterans of differing ethnic and racial backgrounds. However, greater war zone exposure to traumatic experiences among African Americans (315) and American Indians (318, 319) is likely to play a large role as well. In terms of racial differences in rates of PTSD among U.S. veterans, the National Vietnam Veterans Readjustment Study found that although 10% of U.S. soldiers in Vietnam were black and 85% were white, more African American (21%) than European American (14%) veterans experienced PTSD (247). In the American Indian Vietnam Veterans Project (319), evaluation of random samples of Vietnam combat veterans from three Northwestern Plains reservations and one Southwest reservation between 1992 and 1995 showed that approximately one-third of the Northern Plains (31%) and Southwestern (27%) American Indian participants had PTSD at the time of the study. Approximately one-half had experienced the disorder in their lifetime (57% and 45%, respectively). This rate was far in excess of rates of current PTSD observed in the European American or African American veterans (247).

Hispanics also have been found to be at higher risk for war-related PTSD than their European American counterparts (247). Because the risk for Hispanics was higher than that for black veterans, minority status must not be the only risk factor (320). Of the Hispanic subgroups, Puerto Rican veterans have been found to have a higher probability of experiencing PTSD than others with similar levels of war zone stressor exposure (321). Because these differences in prevalence were not explained by exposure to stressors or acculturation and were not accompanied by significant reductions in levels of functioning, it has been proposed that differences in symptom reporting may reflect features of expressive style rather than different levels of illness (320).

National variations in rates of PTSD development have been reported across populations exposed to traumatic events. For instance, less than 5% of hospitalized European survivors of unintentional injuries (e.g., motor vehicle crashes, job-related injuries) appear to develop PTSD (322, 323). However, between 10% and 40% of survivors of both intentional (e.g., injuries associated with human malice, such as physical assaults) and unintentional injuries treated within acute care settings in the United States, England, and Australia appear to develop symptoms consistent with the disorder (34, 117, 293, 324–328). The explanations for these different rates include methodological differences, cultural differences, and diagnostic accuracy (329).

The prevalence of PTSD in countries where war and disease are endemic is substantially higher and has been reported to range between 9.4% and 37.0% of the population. For example, Bleich and colleagues (330), in a telephone survey of a representative sample of 512 Israeli adults, found that after 19 months of ongoing terrorist attacks, 16.4% had been directly exposed to a terrorist attack, 37.3% had an exposed family member or friend, and 9.4% of the sample met the symptom criteria for PTSD. Sabin and colleagues (331) found similar rates in a cross-sectional survey of Mayan refugees living in Mexico, of whom 11.8% met the symptom criteria for PTSD, as measured by the Harvard Trauma Questionnaire and Hopkins Symptom Checklist-25, 20 years after fleeing the civil conflict in Guatemala. De Jong et al. (332) used the Composite International Diagnostic Interview to assess for PTSD in community populations of four postconflict low-income countries and found a prevalence rate of PTSD of 37.4% in Algeria, 28.4% in Cambodia, 15.8% in Ethiopia, and 17.8% in Gaza.

Treatment-seeking refugees may have even higher rates of PTSD, ranging from 55% to 90% (333). Studies have revealed alarming rates of PTSD in immigrant communities with a high degree of preimmigration exposure to potentially traumatic experiences (e.g., Asian Americans and Hispanic Americans). For example, in some samples, up to 70% of refugees from Vietnam, Cambodia, and Laos met the diagnostic criteria for PTSD, in contrast to prevalence rates of about 4% for the U.S. population as a whole (334).

Studies of Southeast Asian refugees receiving mental health care have uniformly found high rates of PTSD. One study found that 70% of the subjects met the diagnostic criteria for PTSD, with Mien from the highlands of Laos and Cambodians having the highest rates (333). Another mental health study of Southeast Asian refugees (Hmong, Laotian, Cambodian, and Vietnamese) in Minnesota found that 73% had major depression, 14% had PTSD, and 6% had anxiety or somatoform disorders (335). A random community sample of Cambodian adults revealed that 45% had PTSD, and 81% experienced five or more symptoms of PTSD (336). Similarly, 43% of parents recruited from a community of resettled Cambodian refugees in Massachusetts reported the death of between one and six of their children (337). Child loss was associated with an increased likelihood of health-related concerns, a variety of somatic symptoms, and culture-bound conditions of emotional distress such as deep worrying and sadness not visible to others (337). Finally, Kinzie et al. (338) found that nearly one-half of a sample of Cambodian adolescents who survived Pol Pot's concentration camps as children had PTSD approximately 10 years after this traumatic period. Thus, many Southeast Asian refugees are at risk for PTSD associated with the events they experienced before they immigrated to the United States (311). A large community sample of Southeast Asian refugees in the United States found that preimmigration and refugee camp experiences were significant predictors of psychological distress even 5 or more years after migration (339). In this study, significant subgroup differences were found: Cambodians reported the highest levels of distress, Laotians were next, then Vietnamese. While trauma treatments may be effective for persons from Western cultures, in some Southeast Asian populations, it may be contraindicated to attempt to identify and process traumatic experiences (229).

Central American immigrants to the United States may be at risk for PTSD as a result of their preimmigration exposure to war-related trauma (340), even though they are not recognized as political refugees (311). For example, a study of Los Angeles adults who were examined for symptoms of PTSD and depression found that one-half of the Central American participants reported symptoms that were consistent with a diagnosis of PTSD (341). In comparison with recent Mexican immigrants, a greater proportion of Central American refugees reported symptoms of PTSD (50% versus 25%) (341). In another study, 60% of adult Central American refugee patients received a diagnosis of PTSD (342). Central American immigrant children seeking care at refugee service centers also had high rates of PTSD (33%) (343). In a more recent study of a systematic sample of 638 adult Latino primary care patients living in Los Angeles, Eisenman and colleagues (344) found that 54% of the sample had experienced political violence before migration, and of these, 18% had symptoms of PTSD. Those who had experienced political violence had a 3.4-fold greater risk of meeting the criteria for a PTSD diagnosis, compared to those who had not experienced political violence.

E. NATURAL HISTORY AND COURSE

Prospective studies suggest that symptomatic distress peaks in the days and weeks after a trauma and then gradually declines over the course of the year after injury (139). In the National Comorbidity Survey, symptoms also decreased most rapidly in the first 12 months after trauma exposure (4). However, approximately one-third of persons who developed PTSD had chronic symptoms that did not remit. Although this issue is not settled (309), rates of recovery from PTSD may vary by gender. Although gender differences in the duration of PTSD are in part explained by gender differences in the type of trauma experienced, Breslau and colleagues (5, 226) found a median time to remission of symptoms of 12 months in men and 48 months in women. However, studies of motor vehicle accident victims have shown initial rates of approximately 35%, decreasing nearly 50% by 12 months postaccident (34, 345).

The responses of traumatized patients fall on a continuum, and the natural course of ASD and PTSD may vary with personality and other individual characteristics. Some individuals are relatively resistant to developing posttraumatic symptoms or report interpersonal growth experiences as a result of their traumatic exposure (229, 346). For other individuals with PTSD, however, long-lasting personality change may occur (252, 347–349). Problems of impaired affect modulation; self-destructive and impulsive behavior; dissociative symptoms; somatic complaints; feelings of ineffectiveness, shame, and despair or hopelessness; feelings of being permanently damaged; a loss of previously supportive beliefs; hostility; social withdrawal; feeling constantly threatened and being in an alert status; and impaired relationships with others all portend personality change from the individual's previous characteristics.

Investigations have also shown symptoms of PTSD to be associated with functional impairment and diminished quality of life (115, 117, 122, 293, 327, 350–353). Across veteran (122), refugee (292), and injured civilian (117, 293, 327) populations, PTSD makes an independent contribution to diminished functioning and quality of life above and beyond the effects of comorbid medical conditions and injury severity. Posttraumatic stress is also coupled with a spectrum of physical health problems and medical disorders (103, 354, 355). These considerations make the treatment of PTSD important not just from the standpoint of individual suffering but also from the perspective of the potential societal costs associated with the disorder (273, 356).

Individuals who have been exposed to trauma may also be vulnerable to subsequent traumas and have an increased likelihood of developing PTSD with repeated traumatic experiences (32, 33, 223). In individuals with a first hospitalization for psychosis, a similar pattern was observed, with exposure to multiple traumatic events being associated with greater rates of PTSD than exposure to a single trauma (48). These findings suggest that in trauma-exposed individuals, interventions should include efforts to decrease the risk for subsequent exposures to traumatic events.

V. REVIEW AND SYNTHESIS OF AVAILABLE EVIDENCE

A. ISSUES IN INTERPRETING THE LITERATURE

The empirical research on the efficacy of treatments for ASD and PTSD is not as extensive at present as that for other disorders such as major depressive disorder, schizophrenia, or bipolar disorder. Most of the randomized clinical trials of ASD and PTSD treatments have a relatively small number of subjects, and their inclusion in the study is often determined by their having experienced one type of index trauma. In addition, exact replications of methods are the exception rather than the rule. Further study is needed to better establish the generalizability of findings across populations and various traumatic event exposures. For example, many studies are limited to combat veterans with chronic PTSD or to rape victims. Treatment for ASD has only just begun to be examined. Effectiveness studies of ASD and PTSD treatments are also limited.

The rapid recovery rate of patients with ASD and acute PTSD means that outcomes studies need to examine closely the timing of treatment administration and the rates of recovery as well as remission and relapse. Treatment studies that specifically examine critical symptoms (such as sleep disturbance or withdrawal or arousal) are also needed. Gender differences in the rates of PTSD suggest that close attention should be paid to gender differences in treatment outcomes. The widespread nature of traumatic exposures in some subpopulations, including persons living in urban environments in major cities, also means that PTSD may have gone undetected but may have existed long before the index disorder is diagnosed.

The high comorbidity of PTSD with major depression and substance abuse also complicates the interpretation of efficacy studies.

With psychosocial interventions, measuring the efficacy of one treatment may be confounded by the effects of other simultaneous treatments.

B. PSYCHOSOCIAL INTERVENTIONS

1. Individual psychotherapies

In general, psychotherapy, examined across all types of interventions and for different types of victims, is an effective intervention for PTSD. Sherman (203) conducted a meta-analysis of 17 controlled clinical trials of psychotherapy for PTSD that included behavioral, cognitive, and psychodynamic individual and group therapy with veterans, female assault victims, and victims of other traumatic events. Psychotherapy was found to have a significant beneficial effect on PTSD.

Prediction of success in psychotherapy of PTSD, however, is in its infancy. For instance, beliefs about mistrust, helplessness, meaninglessness, and unjustness of the world predict baseline PTSD symptom severity but not treatment outcome (357). Little is known about the relationship of the type of traumatic event to the type or duration of psychotherapy likely to be effective.

a) Psychodynamic psychotherapy

Psychodynamic psychotherapy for either ASD or PTSD has not been well studied by means of randomized, controlled trials. Given the fact that ASD, by definition, is an illness of relatively brief duration, long-term therapy would seem unnecessary. However, ASD may be associated with or may aggravate preexisting psychological problems, and a remote history of repeated trauma (including childhood abuse) predicts the development of PTSD. In the face of an acute trauma, dormant issues may at times become more apparent or more amenable to treatment. Considerable clinical literature and case studies comment on this phenomenon, but the extent to which such intervention might prevent the development of PTSD remains untested. For PTSD, one controlled trial by Brom et al. (201) compared psychodynamic therapy to trauma desensitization, hypnotherapy, and a control condition. All three treatments were significantly effective in reducing intrusive and avoidance symptoms. A meta-analysis of psychotherapies—including psychodynamic psychotherapy—also supports this mode of treatment (203). Other less rigorous studies and reviews also suggest the efficacy of psychodynamic therapy in PTSD (21, 208, 358). Again, despite a lack of randomized, controlled trials, clinical consensus reflects the idea that a psychodynamic approach is useful in helping the patient integrate past traumatic experience(s) into a more adaptive or constructive schema of risk, safety, prevention, and protection (359, 360), thereby reducing core symptoms of PTSD.

b) Cognitive and behavior therapies

The cognitive and behavior therapies are applied in the individual, family, or group treatment forms. Although particular behavior therapies have been used as stand-alone treatment, it is more common for behavior therapy to be used in conjunction with other forms of therapy, such as cognitive approaches (e.g., cognitive behavior therapy). These complex treatments may have more than one efficacious component, and in many studies it is somewhat difficult to "dismantle" the specific contributions of the various elements of such combined treatments. Cognitive approaches to the treatment of ASD or PTSD target the distorted threat appraisal process in an effort to desensitize the patient to trauma-related triggers. These approaches often include a component of repeated exposure, either in talking about the trauma or in processing the traumatic experience.

Behavior therapy is derived from psychological models of learning that emphasize the role of environmental cues and consequences in patterning behavior. A behavioral assessment of the PTSD patient would focus on the traumatic event, the reexperiencing symptoms, the maladaptive avoidance and numbing strategies, and the pathological arousal responses that drive the disorder.

Systematic desensitization has been used to reduce anxiety associated with the traumatic stressor. The essential ingredient of systematic desensitization is the gradual and progressive exposure of the patient to feared stimuli while steps are taken to reduce elicited anxiety by displacing it with a sense of relaxation (reciprocal inhibition of the fear response). Improvements in active coping and reductions in traumatic anxiety can occur both inside and outside the sessions through the learning of relaxation techniques such as progressive muscle relaxation, diaphragmatic or meditative breathing, and guided imagery. Progressive muscle relaxation involves alternating the tensing and releasing of muscle groups throughout the body, sometimes proceeding in a head-to-toe direction. Breathing exercises concentrate on exhaling in order to generalize a calming effect, while guided imagery promotes relaxation though visualizing enjoyable places or activities. Biofeedback may be used to augment relaxation by providing the patient with instantaneous feedback on physiological variables, such as blood flow and muscle contraction. These phenomena are not normally sensed, but their continuous presentation permits the patient to exert some degree of voluntary control over variables related to tension and anxiety.

Therapeutic use of prolonged and repeated exposure to traumatic cues, either in a gradual fashion or intensively through flooding or implosion, is based on the principle that traumatic anxiety will decrease in the absence of real danger. Direct therapeutic exposure can be accomplished in vivo (directly) or in imagination. Typically, a course of exposure-based treatment begins with relaxation training and education about the symptoms of PTSD and about the rationale for having participants reexpose themselves to painful experiences. The therapist assesses the patient's ability to tolerate within-session emotion and temporary exacerbations of symptoms before implementing further treatment. If these experiences are acceptable, the patient is then led through a series of sessions in which the traumatic event and its aftermath are imagined and described and patients are asked to focus on the intense negative affects and arousal that are elicited, until they subside. Relaxation exercises and reassurance permit the patient to continue without feeling overwhelmed and abandoning the therapy. Homework assignments allow the patient to practice outside the session. In addition, the treatment may be enhanced if the patient is encouraged to confront specific places or activities in vivo. Success can be measured as complete or partial extinction of PTSD symptoms (173, 174).

Early exposure research was frequently conducted with Vietnam veterans with chronic, combat-related PTSD. Peniston's 1986 randomized, controlled study of biofeedback-assisted systematic desensitization (361) provided preliminary evidence for the potential effectiveness of high-frequency exposure therapy. In one of the early studies, which used flooding, Keane et al. (362) randomly assigned 24 combat veterans with PTSD to 14–16 sessions of flooding (N=11) or to a waiting list (N=13). Assessments at pretreatment, posttreatment, and 6-month follow-up showed improvement in reexperiencing symptoms, startle response, and memory/concentration. No improvement was seen in numbing or social avoidance. Cooper and Clum (363) studied imaginal flooding as a supplementary treatment to standard VA care. All 26 subjects completed the study, which showed that exposure increased the effectiveness of the usual treatment. Boudewyns et al. (364, 365) compared 58 Vietnam veteran inpatients with severe PTSD randomly assigned to either direct therapeutic exposure (flooding) or standard therapy. At 3-month follow-up, significantly more successes than failures were in the exposure group. In a review of the limited clinical literature on flooding, implosion, and direct therapeutic exposure for PTSD in Vietnam combat veterans, Foy et al. (183) noted the significant reductions in symptoms of intrusion and arousal but did register concern regarding reports of decompensation, distress, depletion of emotional reserves, and symptom exacerbation in some patients.

Richards et al. (366) tested four weekly sessions of imaginal exposure followed by four weekly sessions of real-life exposure (or vice versa) in 14 civilian patients with PTSD. Both groups showed a 65%–80% reduction in symptoms, with only a few differences noted, suggesting the salience of imaginal and in vivo forms of exposure. Rothbaum and Hodges (367) published a single case study of the use of a virtual reality mode of exposure for PTSD in a Vietnam veteran. The patient showed a 34% reduction in clinician-rated PTSD symptoms, which was maintained at 6-month follow-up. An open clinical trial also showed promise (368). Thus, imaginal, virtual, and in vivo exposures may each represent useful methods of delivering exposure therapy to PTSD patients.

Imagery rehearsal is another behavior therapy designed to ameliorate traumatic nightmares by having the patient recall the distressing content of recurring nightmares and repetitively envision (rehearse) a different outcome. Krakow et al. (184, 369) published two reports of a controlled study of imagery rehearsal for chronic nightmares in 168 sexual assault survivors with moderate to severe PTSD. The subjects were randomly assigned to an imagery rehearsal treatment group or to a waiting-list control group. A total of 114 subjects completed follow-up at 3 and/or 6 months. The treatment groups experienced significant reductions in the number of nightmares per week and significant improvement in sleep, relative to the control group. These improvements were noted at the 3-month follow-up and were sustained without further intervention or contact between 3 and 6 months. Furthermore, PTSD symptoms decreased in a majority of treated subjects but remained the same or worsened in a majority of control subjects. Forbes et al. (185) employed the same intervention for combat-related nightmares in 12 Vietnam veterans with PTSD and found significant reductions in targeted nightmares and improvements in PTSD symptoms. These changes persisted at 12-month follow-up (370). Similar success in female rape victims with chronic PTSD was reported in a study comparing cognitive processing therapy (another non-exposure-based cognitive therapy) to prolonged exposure and a waiting-list condition (181).

Group exposure therapy has also been found to be more effective than minimal attention groups. Falsetti et al. (371) reported on the results of a pilot study of a manualized treatment that included multiple cognitive and behavioral strategies, which they called multiple channel exposure therapy (M-CET), for patients with PTSD and comorbid panic disorder. They compared M-CET with a minimal attention group. Subjects recruited from an outpatient department and a local rape crisis center were randomly assigned to either 12 weeks of once-weekly M-CET group therapy or to a minimal attention group that received bimonthly supportive telephone counseling. Women in the control condition were offered free treatment after completing their participation in that condition. Posttreatment, only 8.3% of the subjects in the M-CET condition met the Clinician-Administered PTSD Scale diagnostic criteria for PTSD, compared with 66.7% of the control subjects. Ninety-three percent of the control group reported at least one panic attack in the past month, compared with only 50% of the treatment group. Glynn et al. (372) examined a behavioral family therapy for 42 Vietnam veterans with combat-related PTSD and a family member for each veteran (typically the veteran's wife). Three conditions were used: a course of twice-weekly direct exposure therapy, the same course of exposure followed by 16 sessions of behavioral family therapy, or a waiting-list condition.

Participation in exposure therapy was associated with a decrease in positive (e.g., intrusive and hyperarousal) symptoms of PTSD but not negative (e.g., avoidance/numbing) symptoms. There were no additional therapeutic gains from the family sessions.

Cognitive behavior therapy has often been combined with exposure therapy and shown to be effective. In a randomized, controlled study by Fecteau and Nicki (373) of cognitive behavior therapy (N=10) versus a waiting-list condition (N=10), adults (14 women) with PTSD were treated approximately 18 months after motor vehicle accidents with physical injury. The treatment consisted of four weekly 2-hour sessions of cognitive behavior therapy, including education, relaxation training, imaginal exposure, self-directed in vivo practice, and cognitive restructuring. Five of the 10 cognitive behavior therapy subjects no longer had diagnosable PTSD after treatment, while all 10 of the waiting-list group continued to meet the criteria for PTSD. PTSD symptoms improved significantly, with the Clinician-Administered PTSD Scale (CAPS-2) score decreasing from an average of 70.9 (high/PTSD present) to 37.5 (moderate). In contrast, the subjects' Beck Depression Inventory scores did not show significant improvement, suggesting a specific effect on PTSD rather than merely a nonspecific improvement in comorbid depression. The weak response in depression measures may also have been related to chronic pain and disability status. Follow-up at 3 and 6 months showed persistent improvements in PTSD symptoms.

Cognitive therapy techniques have not always been combined with exposure techniques, allowing for some comparison of these techniques. Foa et al. (374) randomly assigned 55 female rape victims with PTSD to one of four conditions: 17 were assigned to stress inoculation training, 14 to prolonged exposure, 14 to supportive counseling (to control for nonspecific therapy effects), and 10 to a waiting-list control group. PTSD diagnoses were made by an outside clinician who used DSM-III-R criteria. The range of time since the assault varied from 3 months to 12 years, with a mean of 6.2 years (SD=6.7). Treatment consisted of nine biweekly 90-minute individual sessions conducted by a female therapist. PTSD symptoms, rape-related distress, general anxiety, and depression were measured pretreatment, posttreatment, and at follow-up (mean=3.5 months posttreatment). Of the 55 patients who started the study, 10 dropped out, with no significant differences in dropout rates across the three treatment groups. However, the 10 noncompleters differed from the completers on three variables: a greater percentage of the noncompleters earned an annual income of less than $10,000, a greater percentage were blue-collar workers, and they scored higher on the Rape Aftermath Symptom Test. Immediately after treatment, stress inoculation therapy was the most effective treatment in reducing PTSD symptoms, and prolonged exposure was also an effective treatment. The supportive counseling and waiting-list conditions improved arousal symptoms of PTSD but not the intrusion and avoidance symptoms. Three and one-half months after treatment, however, prolonged exposure appeared to be the superior treatment. Thus, although stress inoculation therapy appeared to be the most effective treatment in the short term, prolonged exposure appeared to be the most effective treatment in the long term. Furthermore, the superiority of stress inoculation therapy and prolonged exposure over supportive counseling and waiting-list placement was found only for PTSD symptoms.

Marks et al. (177) showed that cognitive therapy, exposure therapy, and exposure plus cognitive therapy were better than relaxation treatment in 87 subjects randomly assigned to ten 90-minute sessions of the four treatment groups. It is important to note that all three cognitive behavior therapy approaches were markedly better than relaxation at 1, 3, and 6 months but no better than each other in decreasing PTSD symptoms or symptom severity, producing remission of PTSD, or improving functioning at the end of the study. Similarly, Echeburua et al. (375) tested progressive relaxation training versus cognitive restructuring and self-exposure in 20 victims of sexual aggression. Most treated patients improved, but the cognitive restructuring and exposure treatment was more successful on all measures than relaxation alone. In contrast, Silver et al. (376) treated inpatient Vietnam veterans with additional EMDR, biofeedback, or relaxation training and found no statistically significant differences between cognitive restructuring and exposure treatment.

Given the similarities between cognitive behavior therapy and exposure therapy, it is not surprising that comparisons of these two modalities have shown similar treatment outcomes. In a randomized, double-blind trial of cognitive behavior therapy versus exposure therapy for chronic PTSD, Tarrier et al. (178) found that the two treatments were equally effective in reducing symptoms in a diverse group of 72 trauma patients but that neither therapy produced complete symptom remission. It is important to note that nine patients in the exposure condition versus three patients in the cognitive behavior therapy condition showed worsening symptoms. Subsequent studies showed that improvements were maintained at 6 months (186) and 12 months (187), again with no significant differences between therapies.

Similarly, in a small, randomized study of 16 refugee outpatients with PTSD, both cognitive behavior therapy and exposure therapy resulted in large improvement on all measures, and this improvement was maintained at follow-up (377). The two treatments did not differ on any measure, but cognitive behavior therapy required relatively more and longer sessions to obtain significant results.

Studies of cognitive behavior therapy for PTSD have also examined outcomes for factors other than PTSD symptoms, such as anger. In a randomized trial, Chemtob et al. (378) assigned 15 Vietnam combat veterans with PTSD to routine VA care or to routine VA care plus 12 sessions of cognitive behavior therapy focused on anger. The 1-hour individual cognitive behavior therapy sessions involved self-monitoring of anger, devising an anger hierarchy, relaxation, cognitive restructuring skills training, and skills practice (role playing in anger-provoking situations). The anger therapy subjects had increased capacity to control anger at completion and 18-month follow-up, although there were no differences between groups on measures of psychophysiological reactions to anger provocation at treatment end. This study showed the specific clinical utility of a cognitive behavior treatment for anger as an adjunct to routine care, although no information was given on PTSD symptoms.

A few studies have indicated that a brief cognitive behavior therapy intervention in the acute posttraumatic phase can prevent PTSD while simultaneously treating ASD. Although these studies are few and included only a small number of subjects, the measured outcome of prevention of PTSD makes them very important, and their findings should be replicated. Bryant et al. (135) examined 45 civilian trauma survivors with ASD treated with five sessions of either prolonged exposure, prolonged exposure plus anxiety management, or supportive counseling begun within 2 weeks of the traumatic event. After treatment, the criteria for PTSD were met by significantly fewer of the patients who received prolonged exposure (14%) and prolonged exposure plus anxiety management (20%) than of those who received supportive counseling (56%). The effect of the two active treatments was maintained at 6-month follow-up after the traumatic event. In contrast to previous reports that 80% of patients who initially meet the criteria for ASD will have chronic PTSD 6 months after the trauma, this study found that patients who received supportive counseling had a rate of PTSD of 67%, indicating that supportive counseling may be somewhat helpful in ameliorating symptoms of PTSD. However, substantially fewer individuals met the criteria for PTSD after either prolonged exposure plus anxiety management (23%) or prolonged exposure (15%), suggesting even greater efficacy of these treatments. There were no differences in outcome between the prolonged exposure and prolonged exposure plus anxiety management interventions, indicating that anxiety management did not contribute to treatment efficacy.

Similarly, Foa et al. (379) treated female victims of recent rape or aggravated assault with a brief prevention program consisting of four 2-hour sessions of cognitive behavior therapy and education, compared with a matched assessment control group. Two months after the assault, only 10% of the brief prevention group met the PTSD criteria, in contrast to 70% of the control group. The brief prevention group did significantly better on measures of depression and reexperiencing symptoms than did the control group members, with an effect size for brief prevention of 1.22.

Gillespie et al. (380) found a similar effect size in a case series treated with cognitive therapy. In this study, a consecutive series of 91 patients were treated within 2 weeks after exposure to a car bomb in Omagh, Northern Ireland, with cognitive therapy along the lines advocated by Ehlers and Clark (381). Neither comorbidity nor the presence or absence of a supportive relationship predicted treatment response. Those who were physically injured improved less significantly than witnesses or those who were not injured. Witnesses and emergency personnel did not differ in their degree of improvement. It is interesting to note that there was a nonsignificant trend for patients who were treated later to improve more than those who were treated earlier, which highlights a need to better understand the timing of treatment interventions. Generalization from these findings is limited by the fact that patients received varying numbers of sessions, there was no control group, and the therapy was not manualized.

c) Eye movement desensitization and reprocessing (EMDR)

EMDR is generally seen as a combination of elements of cognitive behavior therapy, exposure therapy (albeit brief and interrupted exposures), and a unique attention to eye movements. Since cognitive behavior therapy and exposure therapy have been shown to have efficacy in treatment of PTSD, a major question about EMDR has been whether the eye movements contribute to therapy outcome. A number of factors have contributed to the difficulty in establishing whether EMDR effects are distinct from those of cognitive behavior therapy and exposure therapy. Studies of EMDR have included a range of trauma types, weighted toward persons with combat exposure but also including adults with histories of childhood sexual abuse, adults with adult sexual assault, adults after a major hurricane, and (for a few studies) adults with mixed civilian traumas. There is great variation in the protocols, from one 90-minute session to 8–10 sessions. The number of subjects in the studies has also varied widely. Several studies compared EMDR to waiting-list, supportive counseling, or active listening control groups. Others compared EMDR to different forms of prolonged exposure, while several employed dismantling designs that compared EMDR with or without eye movement or finger tapping procedures. Outcome variables primarily included self-report PTSD scales (often, the Impact of Event Scale), with a few using more general symptom checklists or depression inventories. No study has included structured or systematic functional outcome measures. Thus, because of the substantial variability in study design and other methodological shortcomings, it is difficult to draw firm conclusions about the independent effective elements of EMDR.

EMDR appears to be effective in ameliorating symptoms of both acute and chronic PTSD. For example, Marcus (382) compared EMDR to standard care for 67 demographically diverse patients at a health maintenance organization who had developed PTSD after assault, rape, incest, accidents, or witnessing of a trauma. Subjects were randomly assigned to a treatment condition, but evaluations were not conducted in a fully blinded fashion, and standard care differed from therapist to therapist. Treatment sessions continued until PTSD symptoms had remitted or until the end of the study, at which point 75% of the EMDR-treated subjects and 50% of subjects who received standard care no longer met the criteria for PTSD. Significant improvements, which were more rapid in the EMDR-treated group, were also noted in PTSD symptoms as measured by the Mississippi PTSD Rating Scale and the Impact of Event Scale as well as in depressive symptoms as measured by the Beck Depression Inventory.

Rothbaum (383) randomly assigned 20 female rape victims either to three weekly 90-minute sessions of EMDR or to a waiting-list control group. The subjects all met the DSM-III-R criteria for PTSD, and most had had symptoms for years. At 4 weeks after the completion of treatment, 90% of the EMDR-treated subjects no longer met the criteria for PTSD. Unblinded symptom ratings for PTSD and depression showed significant improvements, although the duration of these benefits was unclear, since the waiting-list subjects were subsequently treated.

Scheck et al. (384) randomly assigned women (ages 16–25 years) with a self-reported traumatic memory to either EMDR or active listening, which was delivered in two 90-minute sessions

1 week apart. Although immediately after the intervention both groups showed improvements on measures of depression and anxiety, including symptoms of PTSD, greater effect sizes were noted for the EMDR group. However, the study was limited by the fact that only one-half of those eligible to participate enrolled in the study, and of those who enrolled, only 70% completed the study. In addition, only 77% of subjects met the criteria for a diagnosis of PTSD at study entry.

Wilson et al. (385) randomly assigned 80 subjects to receive either EMDR or delayed treatment with EMDR. Subjects included equal numbers of men and women who had experienced a variety of traumas that occurred from 3 months to 54 years before treatment. Only one-half of the subjects met the DSM-IV criteria for PTSD, and only one-third of the sample had not received previous therapy for their symptoms. EMDR treatment consisted of three 90-minute sessions, and follow-up assessments were conducted. The subjects who received delayed treatment showed no change in symptoms in the 30 days before EMDR was begun, whereas the subjects who received EMDR showed significant improvements on measures of PTSD symptoms, somatization, interpersonal sensitivity, depression, and anxiety. Similar improvements were seen in the delayed-treatment EMDR group after treatment initiation, with improvements in both groups maintained at 90-day follow-up and again at 15-month follow-up (386).

Ironson et al. (387) compared the efficacy of EMDR and prolonged exposure in 22 civilian patients. Both approaches produced a significant reduction in PTSD and depression symptoms that was maintained at a 3-month follow-up. Successful treatment was faster, better tolerated, and more complete in the EMDR group (387). EMDR also resulted in reduced anxiety on process measures that was disproportionate to overall symptom improvement on outcome measures, with some evidence for sustainable symptom improvement for up to 3 months.

One study with a more extended follow-up period found that treatment gains were lost by 6 months (388). In this EMDR dismantling study, 51 Australian male combat veterans with PTSD were assigned to one of three conditions. Subjects were assigned to groups that received two sessions of EMDR, two sessions of reactive eye dilation desensitization and reprocessing (REDDR), or no intervention. REDDR was the same method as EMDR, except "eye movement" was replaced by "eye dilation," and a black box with a flashing light (opticator) was substituted for the eye movement stimuli. All subjects continued to receive standard care. No statistically significant changes were found from pre- to posttreatment on any of the outcome measures for the three conditions. At 3 months, all three treatment groups had improved somewhat, but there was no statistically significant difference among them. By 6 months, changes from pretreatment were no longer statistically significant for trait anxiety, depression, or PTSD (effect sizes at 6-month follow-up for EMDR plus standard care versus REDDR plus standard care=0.25). However, these findings must be interpreted in light of the brevity of both the EMDR and REDDR conditions. In a 5-year follow-up that compared 13 Vietnam combat veterans who received EMDR to a demographically matched control group of 14 combat veterans with PTSD who did not receive EMDR, both groups showed an overall worsening of PTSD symptoms over the 5-year period and loss of the modest to moderate early benefit of EMDR (389).

In another study, Devilly and Spence (35) compared nine sessions of a cognitive behavior therapy variant with up to eight sessions of EMDR in a total of 23 subjects with mixed trauma histories. The trauma treatment protocol (TTP) used prolonged exposure, in-depth cognitive therapy, and a variant of Foa's stress inoculation training. Compared to EMDR, TTP was more effective from pre- to posttreatment and had a reasonable effect size and high power. TTP's superiority became more pronounced at 3-month follow-up, at which time 83% of the TTP patients no longer met the PTSD criteria, compared to 36% of the EMDR subjects. However, in interpreting these data, it should be noted that the study was not randomized in a conventional manner, as most of the non-EMDR subjects were grouped in an initial block and EMDR was administered in a second block.

Cusack and Spates (390) randomly assigned 38 subjects to three 90-minute sessions of either standard EMDR or eye movement desensitization, which included all components of EMDR except the cognitive reprocessing elements. Of the 27 individuals (23 women and four men) who completed the study, two-thirds had met the criteria for a DSM-IV diagnosis of PTSD at study entry and half had experienced either a physical or sexual assault. At posttreatment, both groups showed statistically significant decreases in symptoms as measured by the revised SCL-90, the Impact of Event Scale, the Structured Interview for PTSD, a behavioral assessment of speech anxiety, and a subjective unit-of-discomfort scale. However, both treatment groups showed comparable levels of improvement, suggesting that the imaginal exposure component of EMDR and not the cognitive reprocessing element is important to clinical efficacy.

Meta-analyses of the various controlled trials have generally concluded that EMDR represents an effective treatment. A 1997 review by Foa and Meadows (190) included studies of persons exposed to highly stressful events as well as those who met the criteria for PTSD. Many of the reviewed studies indicated no difference between EMDR and no-treatment or waiting-list control conditions, but one study indicated superiority of EMDR. The authors noted that because of methodological problems, further research to determine effectiveness was needed. Davidson and Parker (194) compared EMDR with no treatment, cognitive behavior therapy, exposure approaches (not involving in vivo exposure), variants of EMDR (e.g., dismantling studies), and "nonspecific" treatments. EMDR was more effective than no treatment and comparable to other active treatments. In this analysis, the dismantling studies appeared to provide comparable effectiveness across variant EMDR protocols. Maxfield and Hyer's meta-analysis (193) compared EMDR to waiting-list conditions, cognitive behavior therapy, and other treatments. EMDR was superior to the waiting-list conditions and either comparable or superior to other treatments (with considerable variability across studies). Although the meta-analysis by Shepherd et al. (191) included traumatized patients who did not all meet the DSM-IV or DSM-III-R criteria for PTSD, the researchers found that EMDR was comparable to a variety of psychotherapies and antidepressant therapy.

In summary, EMDR belongs within a continuum of exposure-related and cognitive behavior treatments. EMDR employs techniques that may give the patient more control over the exposure experience (since EMDR is less reliant on a verbal account) and provides techniques to regulate anxiety in the apprehensive circumstance of exposure treatment. Consequently, it may prove advantageous for patients who cannot tolerate prolonged exposure as well as for patients who have difficulty verbalizing their traumatic experiences. Comparisons of EMDR with other treatments in larger samples are needed to clarify such differences. The dismantling studies, in general, show no incremental effect from the use of eye movement or other proxies during the treatment sessions. Despite the demonstrable efficacy of EMDR, these studies call into question EMDR's theoretical rationale. It would therefore appear that it is the common sharing of trauma exposure techniques and emotional reprocessing that is principally responsible for treatment gains. Thus, EMDR is better than no treatment or supportive counseling and may be as effective as cognitive behavior therapy and other exposure-based techniques. As with the other therapies, the extent to which gains are maintained over the long term requires further evaluation.

2. Group psychotherapy for PTSD

There is a paucity of randomized, controlled treatment outcome studies for group treatment approaches among adults. The studies that have been done have not included groups that receive control or comparison treatments. Drawing conclusions across studies is difficult, since group protocols vary widely and include supportive therapy, psychoeducation, psychodynamic therapy, and various types of cognitive behavior therapy, including anxiety management, stress inoculation, assertiveness training, prolonged exposure, and cognitive restructuring. The patients treated in group psychotherapy studies have predominately been combat veterans and women with histories of childhood sexual abuse. Length of treatment has varied from 10 to 24 sessions that extend over 3 to 6 months. Some treatments have included booster sessions that extend over a year. Most studies have lacked sufficiently structured protocols, specific PTSD diagnostic assessments, and functional outcome measures.

Of five randomized, controlled trials, one showed modest improvement (combining trauma-focused and present-focused group data) in 64 women who received supportive-expressive group therapy, compared to 61 women in a waiting-list condition, decades after the trauma occurred (391). In another randomized, controlled trial of individuals who experienced childhood trauma and abuse, group therapy as an adjunct to individual therapy produced a decrease in PTSD symptoms (392). Schnurr et al. (393), in a well-designed multisite study of combat veterans with chronic PTSD, used methods that blended efficacy and effectiveness designs and found modest effects of both trauma-focused and present-focused group therapy but no difference between the two treatments (although the dropout rate for the trauma-focused therapy was about twice that for the present-centered treatment). The higher dropout rate highlights a concern that exposure-based therapies—whether group or individual—may prove intolerable for some patients (394, 395). A randomized study of a two-stage group therapy for incarcerated women showed reductions in PTSD, mood, and interpersonal symptoms in subjects who received dialectical behavior therapy skills training and writing assignments, although participants were not all identified as having PTSD before study entry (396). The only randomized, controlled trial that involved more recent trauma investigated group treatment among Serbian concentration camp survivors within 3 months of release from the camps (397). At study entry, 44% of the 120 men in the study met the DSM-III-R criteria for PTSD and were randomly assigned to receive group therapy, group therapy plus medication (anxiolytics and tricyclic antidepressants, but no SSRIs), or medication alone over a 6-month treatment course. The study also followed subjects who refused treatment. Although there were significant differences between treated and untreated groups at 6 months (with a much greater percentage of resolution of PTSD among the treated subjects), a 3-year follow-up among randomly selected subjects revealed the paradoxical finding that the untreated group was improved, relative to the treatment groups, in scores on the Watson Questionnaire for PTSD.

Of the six nonrandomized studies, four related to treatment of women with histories of childhood sexual abuse (180, 398–400), one was a structured inpatient group treatment of Gulf War veterans (401), and one targeted adults after the traumatic loss of an adolescent or young adult child (402). In three of the four group interventions for individuals who had experienced childhood sexual abuse, no measurements of PTSD were used. Group interventions were associated with improvement in various global symptom measures, including measures of self-concept and social adjustment. The one study that examined effects of a psychoeducation group for multiply traumatized women reported mixed and conflicting outcome findings regarding PTSD. Thus, these studies do not provide sufficient strength, in methods or outcomes, to adequately judge the usefulness of group interventions with adults who have been sexually abused in childhood.

The British Gulf War veteran group study, which examined a treatment format that was markedly different from other group interventions, provided an intensive 12-day structured inpatient group therapy, with day-group follow-up sessions for 1 year (401). The intervention included some form of ongoing psychological debriefing. There was a robust decrease in the percentage of patients who met the criteria for PTSD (from 100% to 14.7%) 1 year posttreatment. It is noteworthy that there was no reported use of drugs of abuse or increased alcohol use during the follow-up period. These findings suggest that an intensive, structured 2-week group intervention with extended booster follow-up sessions may provide a useful modality for treatment of combat-related PTSD.

The only group intervention study for traumatic bereavement in adults combined problem solving and emotional support over 12 weeks and found that mothers improved somewhat in PTSD-related reactions, while fathers worsened (402). Those with lower levels of initial PTSD symptoms worsened, while there was mild improvement among those with higher levels of initial PTSD symptoms. This study strongly points to the need for caution in selecting group membership, even among spouses, where there may be varying degrees of exposure and pretreatment levels of PTSD symptoms.

An additional nonrandomized comparison study compared two cognitive behavior approaches—stress inoculation and assertiveness training—to supportive group therapy in a group of 24 rape victims (180). Relative to 13 subjects in a waiting-list control group, all three treatments, each of which included six 2-hour sessions, did equally well in producing moderate improvements in PTSD, depression, anxiety, and self-esteem. In addition, in the active treatment groups, therapeutic benefits were maintained at 3- and 6-month follow-up.

As discussed by Foy et al. (403), the supportive groups tend to place primary emphasis on addressing current life issues, while psychodynamic or cognitive behavior-oriented groups are primarily "trauma-focused," with major work directed at specific traumatic experiences and memories. In group psychotherapy, there is the advantage of being able to provide services to large numbers of individuals in response to a shared traumatic experience or because of shared PTSD symptoms. In regard to trauma-focused group psychotherapy, most of the evidence for efficacy and effectiveness is in the treatment of children and adolescents (304, 404–407). In a study of adults, Schnurr et al. (393) randomly assigned 360 combat veterans into groups of six and compared trauma-focused group therapy in 30 weekly sessions followed by five monthly boosters to a present-centered comparison treatment. Relative to baseline, significant improvements were noted on posttreatment measures of PTSD severity in both groups, but intent-to-treat analysis showed no differences between therapy groups on any outcome measure. These studies together provide evidence that group sessions in conjunction with assigned homework can achieve sufficient prolonged trauma-focused exposure to be a bona fide treatment approach.

The trauma-focused group psychotherapies just described typically share certain principles. The first sessions provide general psychoeducation regarding PTSD, coping skills for trauma reminders and posttraumatic stress reactions, and either anxiety-regulating or emotion-regulating techniques. They also provide group process exercises to improve group cohesion, openness, and tolerance. The trauma exposure sessions utilize different versions of prolonged narrative or imaginal exposure, moving from more general accounts to the most intense traumatic moments. They rely on group members' assisting each other in this difficult task. These sessions are generally followed by problem-solving sessions that address avoidant and aggressive behavior, secondary or current adversities, and developmental hindrances. Group studies would suggest that the group format is especially effective in addressing this latter group of functional impairments.

There are as yet no clear guidelines regarding the contribution of group process to group psychotherapy outcomes in PTSD. Davies et al. (408) provided general guidelines that will need to be specifically adapted for this work. In a study that has important implications for group process, Cloitre and Koenen (398) examined the effects of interpersonal therapy groups for women who had experienced childhood sexual abuse. In mixed groups that included at least one individual with a diagnosis of borderline personality disorder, the group therapy process was no different from a waiting-list control group in symptom diminution but did induce a significant increase in posttreatment anger. In contrast, in groups that did not contain patients with borderline personality disorder, there were significant reductions in anger, depression, and symptoms of PTSD. Thus, the study results raise caution about the diagnostic composition of interpersonal therapy groups.

3. Other early psychosocial intervention strategies

There is substantial evidence that single-session, individual psychological debriefing in the immediate aftermath of a broad range of traumatic exposures (e.g., motor vehicle crashes, combat, physical assaults, burn injury) does not reduce psychological distress or prevent the onset of chronic PTSD (128–130). A series of randomized, controlled trials have assessed the efficacy of debriefing across trauma-exposed populations (213, 217–219, 409). Bisson et al. (217) randomly assigned 43 hospitalized burn survivors to 30–120 minutes of single-session debriefing versus control conditions 2–19 days after traumatic injury. Sixteen percent of the debriefed group versus 9% of the intervention group had PTSD at 13-month follow-up, a difference that was statistically significant. It is noteworthy that the subjects who were randomly assigned to debriefing had significantly greater injury severity and had more frequent involvement of others in the injury event. Carlier et al. (410) debriefed police officers within 24 hours after exposure to a variety of traumas and found no symptomatic improvement in debriefed subjects, compared with control subjects. Conlon et al. (213) performed a 30-minute debriefing with motor vehicle crash victims and found no PTSD symptom improvement in the intervention group, compared with control subjects who received an advice leaflet and follow-up telephone contact number. Hobbs et al. (218) performed a 1-hour critical incident stress debriefing in randomly selected, symptomatic subjects 24–48 hours after motor vehicle crashes. Patients who received the debriefing demonstrated either similar or worsened symptomatic outcomes, compared to control subjects at 4 months (218) and 36 months (219) posttrauma. Rose et al. (409) delivered a 1-hour critical incident stress debriefing to victims of violent crime within 1 month after the trauma and found no significant differences in PTSD symptoms in intervention patients, relative to control subjects, at the 11-month follow-up assessment.

A handful of randomized and open trials of debriefing suggest limited benefit of group debriefing. In an open trial, Shalev et al. (20) performed group debriefings (emphasizing clarification of individuals' roles, time sequences, and facts surrounding the traumatic event, without exploring emotions) with soldiers 48–72 hours after exposure to combat and found reductions in anxiety, improvement in self-efficacy, and increased homogeneity of the group immediately after the debriefing. Deahl et al. (411) randomly assigned soldiers to a postdeployment debriefing/predeployment stress prevention intervention or to predeployment stress intervention alone. Although PTSD symptoms across the two groups showed no significant differences at 6- and 12-month follow-up, there was evidence of significantly reduced alcohol use in soldiers who received the debriefing. Campfield and Hills (412) randomly assigned robbery victims to immediate (<10 hour) versus delayed (>48 hour) critical incident stress debriefing group conditions. Victims in the immediate debriefing condition demonstrated improved symptom outcomes 2 weeks after the debriefing.

Although the debriefing models that have been investigated generally do not appear to be efficacious, there is only preliminary evidence that other psychosocial interventions with established efficacy for the treatment of PTSD can be effectively delivered as early interventions in complex real-world settings such as postdisaster environments and acute care medical settings. One study suggests that cognitive behavior interventions can be effectively delivered after mass attack, although the number of treatment sessions may need to be extended and high-risk groups of trauma survivors such as the physically injured may be less responsive (380). Preliminary evidence suggests that early psychosocial intervention strategies such as in-person/telephone case management may be effective in both engaging trauma survivors in treatment and reducing acute distress (131–134). Gidron et al. (133) randomly assigned 17 patients who had had motor vehicle crash injuries and elevated heart rates during acute care to receive a telephone-based memory restructuring intervention or a supportive listening control intervention within several days of the accident. Patients who received the active telephone-based intervention demonstrated significantly decreased PTSD symptoms. Zatzick et al. (134) delivered a collaborative care intervention that included posttraumatic concern elicitation and support to 34 randomly selected survivors of intentional and unintentional injuries. At 1-month postinjury, the patients receiving the intervention had significantly diminished PTSD and depressive symptoms, compared with control patients, yet treatment gains were not maintained at the 4-month assessment. In a follow-up randomized effectiveness trial with 120 injured trauma survivors, Zatzick et al. (131) extended the stepped care procedure to include case management and evidence-based cognitive behavior therapy and medication treatment targeting PTSD. Compared with control subjects who received usual care, patients who received the combined intervention demonstrated modest and statistically significant prevention of PTSD, which coincided with the initiation of the evidence-based treatments. In a nonrandomized design, Bordow and Porritt (132) delivered a case management intervention to 70 male motor vehicle crash survivors. Intervention patients demonstrated less symptomatic distress than control groups of patients who received no intervention, immediate intervention, or delayed contact 3 months after the injury. More research is needed to determine if these initial engagement interventions will require augmentation with other proven psychotherapeutic and psychopharmacological interventions to prevent development of chronic PTSD.

4. Other psychotherapies

New psychotherapeutic approaches continue to be developed and applied to the treatment of trauma survivors with PTSD. As with previously developed interventions, it is essential that initial small-scale trials be followed by larger-scale randomized, controlled trials to establish efficacy. Recent small-scale trials of Internet-based therapies (413, 414) and Outward Bound group recreational therapies (415, 416) suggest potential beneficial effects on symptoms and functional outcomes.

In a pilot study, Gidron et al. (417) assessed the effects of written emotional disclosure on mental and physical health in Israeli patients with PTSD. One to 3 years after their trauma, subjects were randomly assigned either to the disclosure condition or to a casual writing control condition. Disclosure condition patients were asked to write for 20 minutes for 3 consecutive days about their most traumatic experiences and then, in a brief structured format, to talk about the most severe events about which they had written. Control subjects wrote about their daily agenda without affective content and then discussed one daily activity. The investigators found that a brief return to traumatic narrative may be counterproductive. Disclosure patients reported higher levels of negative affect immediately after writing than did the control patients and also reported larger increases in avoidance symptoms. The proportion of emotional words in the trauma narratives was associated with intrusive and avoidance symptoms of PTSD. The proportion of words on physical health predicted a greater number of health care visits at follow-up.

Monitoring of intrusions has also been suggested as a treatment intervention (418) and was studied in six individuals, all with PTSD. The subjects were given instructions to monitor intrusions—e.g., "try to not think of it," "think your way through," "cope with it"—over a 2-month period; then they were followed up immediately thereafter and again 3 months afterward. Of the six individuals treated with this approach, only one still met the criteria for PTSD at the end of the study, whereas four recovered. Although the small sample size limited the authors' ability to evaluate differences statistically, this innovative treatment of specific symptoms highlights future directions for possible public health interventions that may limit the need for specialty care.

With regard to novel techniques, a key question is whether they contain active components of efficacy-proven PTSD interventions. For instance, a review of case studies of Native American healing rituals that have been applied to the treatment of trauma survivors, such as sweat lodge and shamanic healing ceremonies, suggests that these interventions may contain an imaginal exposure component (419, 420). These "culturally sensitive" interventions may therefore combine "active" PTSD intervention components with socially accepted service delivery modalities that enhance adherence and reduce dropout.

C. PHARMACOTHERAPIES

1. Antidepressants

a) SSRIs

SSRIs are the most extensively studied medications in PTSD treatment research. Eight randomized, controlled trials have investigated SSRIs. These trials were often large, industry-sponsored clinical studies with hundreds of subjects. The general finding is that SSRIs are significantly more effective than placebo. In a 12-week randomized, controlled trial of sertraline, Davidson et al. (421) randomly assigned 208 civilian men and women to receive either medication or placebo. Subjects treated with the SSRI were more likely to show a significant clinical response consisting of at least a 30% reduction in PTSD symptoms and were also more likely to experience a global improvement in symptoms (improvement was found in 60% of sertraline-treated subjects, compared to 38% of the placebo group subjects). In a similarly designed study, in which a separate sample of 187 civilian subjects were randomly assigned to receive sertraline or placebo, responder rates were 55% in the SSRI group, in contrast to 35% for the placebo subjects (144). Two randomized clinical trials with the SSRI paroxetine have also had favorable results. In one, 551 civilian men and women were randomly assigned to receive 20 mg/day of paroxetine (N=183), 40 mg/day of paroxetine (N=182), or placebo (N=186). Subjects in the two medication groups did not differ from one another but demonstrated significant improvement on all three PTSD symptom clusters, global improvement, and improvement in social and occupational functioning (141). In the second large paroxetine study, 307 civilian subjects were randomly assigned to receive medication or placebo with similar positive results; the medication group showed significantly greater improvement with regard to all three clusters of PTSD symptoms, global improvement, and improvement of functional capacity (e.g., in work, social interactions, and family life) (145). Unlike the sertraline results, which were positive for women but not for men (possibly because so few men participated in these trials), paroxetine was equally effective for men and women. As a result of these large-scale multisite randomized, clinical trials, SSRIs are currently considered first-line pharmacotherapeutic treatment for PTSD, and both sertraline and paroxetine have received the approval of the U.S. Food and Drug Administration as indicated treatments for PTSD. A randomized clinical trial with fluoxetine has also had favorable results. In this study, in which 301 mostly white, male non-American veterans of United Nations peacekeeping deployments were randomly assigned to receive medication or placebo, the SSRI subjects exhibited significantly greater improvement in PTSD symptom severity and global functioning than did the placebo group (146). Open-label trials with two other SSRIs—citalopram (278) and fluvoxamine (150)—were also promising.

A few long-term continuation and discontinuation studies with sertraline are also noteworthy. Fifty-five percent of patients who failed to respond positively to sertraline after 12 weeks of treatment did exhibit a favorable response when treatment was extended for an additional 24 weeks (279). Discontinuation of sertraline treatment in patients who had previously responded favorably was six times more likely to lead to clinical relapse than was continuation of sertraline treatment (123).

In addition to finding reduction of PTSD symptoms, studies with sertraline and fluoxetine have suggested that SSRI treatment also promotes improvement in functional status and quality of life and that discontinuation of medication is associated with decreased quality of life and functional measures in addition to symptom relapse (148, 280).

To summarize, in short- and intermediate-term trials, SSRIs have proven efficacy for PTSD symptoms and related functional problems. Patients who respond favorably will generally need to continue taking medication in order to maintain clinical gains.

b) Other second-generation antidepressants

Despite high utilization of second-generation antidepressants to treat depression and other anxiety disorders, no randomized, controlled trials of these medications have been carried out in patients with PTSD. The most extensively tested medication, nefazodone, might be expected to have a favorable effect on PTSD symptoms since, like the SSRIs, it promotes serotonergic activity. Indeed, several open-label trials with nefazodone suggest that this medication may have efficacy for treatment of all three PTSD symptom clusters, especially for patients with treatment-resistant symptoms (422–426). Nefazodone is also an attractive possibility because it is often better tolerated than SSRIs, although caution must be taken given its association with irreversible and life-threatening hepatic failure.

Positive reports from small open-label trials with trazodone (427), bupropion (428), venlafaxine (429), and mirtazapine (430) do not provide sufficient evidence to justify endorsing any of these medications for PTSD patients at this time; one double-blind, placebo-controlled pilot study with mirtazapine also suggests efficacy (431). Trazodone may have a unique niche in treatment because its serotonergic action is synergistic with SSRIs while its sedative properties are often an effective antidote to SSRI-induced insomnia, and sleep disturbance is often central to the clinical picture in ASD and PTSD. Efficacy of such agents in ASD or in acutely traumatized individuals who do not meet the full diagnostic criteria for PTSD warrants further investigation.

c) Tricyclic antidepressants

In three randomized, controlled trials conducted with tricyclic antidepressants, all subjects were Vietnam veterans seeking PTSD treatment in VA hospital settings. In a study in which 60 veterans in a VA setting were randomly assigned to receive the tricyclic antidepressant imipramine (N=23, mean dose=225 mg/day), the MAOI phenelzine (N=19, mean dose=68 mg/day), or placebo (N=18), imipramine produced significantly more improvement than placebo but not as much as phenelzine (151) (see further details in the next section, Section V.C.1.d, "MAOIs"). In an 8-week trial in which 40 veterans in a VA setting were randomly assigned to receive either the tricyclic antidepressant amitriptyline (N=22, mean dose=169 mg/day) or placebo (N=18), the response rate was 47% for the patients who received amitriptyline, compared to 19% for placebo subjects; this difference was statistically significant (152). Taken together, both studies indicated that tricyclic antidepressant treatment produced global improvement and reduction of reexperiencing symptoms. It should be noted, however, that in the third published randomized, controlled trial, which included only 18 veterans randomly assigned to receive the tricyclic antidepressant desipramine (mean dose=165 mg/day) or placebo for 4 weeks, no response by either group was found (153). A quantitative analysis of all trials (randomized, controlled trials and open-label trials) with these medications indicated that tricyclic antidepressants in general produce global improvement and reductions in reexperiencing symptoms (432). Thus, although clinical management with tricyclic antidepressants may be more complicated than that with newer agents, the tricyclic antidepressants are effective medications that still have a potential role in PTSD treatment.

Robert et al. (433) compared imipramine with chloral hydrate as treatment in a randomized clinical trial. Twenty-five children, ages 2–19 years, with symptoms of ASD and hospitalized on a burn unit for severe injury (with a mean total burn surface area of 45%), received either imipramine (1 mg/kg, with a maximum dose of 100 mg/day) or chloral hydrate (25 mg/kg, with a maximum dose of 500 mg/day). After 7 days of treatment, ASD symptoms remitted in 83% of the patients treated with imipramine, compared with 38% of those treated with chloral hydrate. Stated differently, 10 of the 12 children who received imipramine were considered to have a positive treatment response. Unfortunately, there was no long-term follow-up, so it is unclear whether this early tricyclic antidepressant treatment prevented later development of PTSD. This study stands as the best demonstration that acute pharmacotherapy can be an effective treatment for acutely traumatized subjects.

d) MAOIs

Two randomized, controlled trials have been carried out with the MAOI phenelzine. In the 8-week study with American Vietnam veterans in a VA setting mentioned in the previous section, 60 subjects were randomly assigned to receive the MAOI phenelzine (N=19), the tricyclic antidepressant imipramine (N=23), or placebo (N=18) (151). In assessments with the Impact of Event Scale, both medication groups did significantly better than the placebo group, with 44% improvement among the phenelzine subjects, compared with 25% improvement among the imipramine subjects. The difference between the MAOI and tricyclic antidepressant groups was statistically significant (151). A single report of a successful open trial of the reversible monoamine oxidase type A inhibitor moclobemide (434) also supported the use of MAOIs as a class in treatment of PTSD. Moclobemide, which is not presently available in the United States, was tested in a 12-week open trial with 20 subjects and yielded promising results (434). At the end of the trial, 11 subjects no longer met the PTSD diagnostic criteria, and there was a significant reduction in PTSD symptom severity and significant improvement in global function. In addition to studies with phenelzine, two randomized, controlled trials that used brofaromine, a unique MAOI/SSRI medication that is not available commercially, showed some improvement in PTSD symptoms (155, 435). Finally, there are two reports of meta-analyses that synthesized results from a number of published reports (432, 436). Although there have been some negative reports, MAOIs have generally been shown to produce global clinical improvement and reductions in PTSD symptom severity, with specific effectiveness for reexperiencing symptoms. In the only head-to-head comparison of an MAOI (phenelzine) and a tricyclic antidepressant (imipramine), as noted earlier, the MAOI was more effective, although the tricyclic antidepressant was still more effective than placebo (151). Clinicians' reluctance to prescribe MAOIs generally relates to concerns about the capacity of patients to adhere to tyramine-free diets or to abstain from alcohol, certain drugs of abuse, and contraindicated prescription medications (e.g., SSRIs, CNS stimulants, decongestants, and meperidine). However, it must be emphasized that MAOIs are clinically effective and that many patients can adhere to such constraints. Finally, reversible monoamine oxidase type A inhibitors are much easier to manage clinically because patients need not observe such dietary or pharmacological restrictions.

2. Benzodiazepines

Benzodiazepines cannot be recommended as monotherapy for PTSD patients, despite their proven efficacy in generalized anxiety disorder. Despite widespread use in treatment of PTSD, their utility in PTSD has not been adequately evaluated. In the only pertinent randomized, controlled trial, alprazolam was tested with 10 civilians and veterans who received treatment for 5 weeks (437). The benzodiazepine was ineffective against PTSD reexperiencing and avoidant/numbing symptoms, although it did improve sleep and general anxiety. Rebound anxiety related to alprazolam treatment was also observed during this trial. In addition, a postdiscontinuation benzodiazepine withdrawal syndrome has been described that was characterized by a profound exacerbation of PTSD symptoms (158). Although a limited open-label case series also suggested improvement in insomnia and core PTSD symptoms in acutely traumatized individuals (438), positive long-term outcome data have not been reported, and a controlled study did not show advantage over placebo (156). Indeed, early administration of benzodiazepines was associated with a higher incidence of PTSD at 1- and 6-month follow-up in one study (157).

3. Miscellaneous medications

A variety of classes of psychopharmacological agents have been tested for the treatment of PTSD. Initial open and randomized trials of carbamazepine (160), valproic acid (161, 162), and lamotrigine (163) suggested that these agents may be efficacious in targeting discrete PTSD symptom clusters. Two small open-label trials showed promising results with the serotonergic anxiolytic buspirone (439, 440), but the data are insufficient to recommend it for use at this time. Two studies (169, 441) suggested that prazosin may be effective in treating nightmares and other PTSD symptoms in male combat veterans.

Olanzapine, a second-generation antipsychotic agent, when prescribed to augment ongoing sertraline treatment, was shown to produce improvement in PTSD, depressive, and sleep-related symptoms in Vietnam veterans (166). Open-label studies of adjunctive olanzapine and quetiapine have demonstrated symptom reduction in veterans with PTSD (165, 167). However, olanzapine alone did not show an effect in a small randomized, double-blind, placebo-controlled trial in female veterans (164). A small controlled study of risperidone in chronic combat-related PTSD was similarly disappointing for core PTSD symptoms, although reexperiencing and global psychotic symptoms were reduced (168).

Early case reports suggested that cyproheptadine, a serotonin antagonist, might ameliorate PTSD flashbacks and traumatic nightmares, but a randomized, controlled trial by Jacobs-Rebhun et al. (442) and a large open-label trial by Clark et al. (443) disconfirmed these findings. In the randomized trial by Jacobs-Rebhun et al., 69 veteran subjects in a VA setting were randomly assigned to receive either cyproheptadine or placebo. After 2 weeks of treatment, the cyproheptadine subjects exhibited a (nonsignificant) worsening of PTSD symptom severity, sleep quality, and traumatic nightmare severity (442). The large open-label trial of cyproheptadine by Clark et al. (443) also failed to produce positive results. Therefore, cyproheptadine cannot be recommended for PTSD treatment.

Inositol is a second messenger with limited evidence supporting efficacy in treating depression and panic disorder. However, in a small randomized, crossover study, with 13 subjects randomly assigned to receive medication or placebo for a 4-week trial, inositol was ineffective in alleviating PTSD symptom severity (444).

A number of agents have been pilot tested in the secondary prevention of PTSD. There is preliminary evidence from two studies that steroid administration during inpatient medical/surgical hospitalization may diminish PTSD symptom development in patients with critical medical illness (445, 446). One observational study among youths hospitalized after burn injury suggested that patients who received the highest doses of opiate analgesics exhibited the lowest PTSD symptom severity after discharge from the hospital (447). As mentioned previously, another randomized investigation on a pediatric burn unit suggested that imipramine is efficacious in ameliorating ASD (433). A single investigation pilot tested the use of propranolol among injured patients seen in an emergency department after a motor vehicle accident and had interesting findings; although no significant improvement in PTSD was detected and high dropout rates were observed in the intervention group, subjects who received propranolol had a significant reduction in physiological reactivity that persisted for 3 months after acute treatment (137). In addition, a recent controlled but nonblind, nonrandomized study reported that acute administration of propranolol posttrauma reduced subsequent PTSD symptoms (172). These findings will also be important to pursue further in larger randomized trials.

PART C
FUTURE RESEARCH NEEDS

Research over the past decade has led to considerable advances in our understanding of the epidemiology of the acute and long-term neurobiological and psychological changes that occur after highly stressful experiences. Research has also identified a variety of treatment approaches for pathological responses to traumatic events, including ASD and PTSD. Although much has been accomplished, future study is required to expand current understanding and inform future assessment, prevention, and treatment strategies. The following future research needs are not presented in any effort to prioritize, nor are they intended to be exhaustive. They serve to illustrate the fact that our understanding of the range of human response to traumatic stress is in its infancy and only beginning to evolve.

- **Early interventions/posttrauma treatment.** In early intervention (in the hours or days after a traumatic event), the aim is to reduce immediate distress, but ideally it might also be to prevent the development of ASD or PTSD. However, relatively little is known about prevention. Small, controlled studies of psychotherapy suggest efficacy (135, 136, 448), as do the studies of early case management interventions (131–134). In addition, a few small controlled studies suggest that early pharmacological interventions may reduce development of posttraumatic symptoms (137, 172, 433). However, larger controlled trials and long-term follow-up studies are needed to fully address the efficacy and effectiveness of psychotherapeutic, psychopharmacological, psychoeducational, and supportive interventions in reducing initial distress and later development of ASD or PTSD, as well as in improving social and occupational functioning.

- **Identification of risk factors for development of ASD or PTSD.** Given the wide variability of human response to traumatic events, future intervention strategies would be aided by a greater understanding of the extent to which ASD or other diagnoses or factors are associated with subsequent development of PTSD. Elucidation of markers or risk factors (e.g., biological or genetic markers, psychological traits, other life experiences, or ethnocultural variables) that specifically relate to the development or severity of ASD or PTSD after initial or subsequent exposures to potentially traumatic events would be valuable (179, 449, 450). Neurobiological markers are being identified, for example, that are associated with reduced susceptibility to developing disorders after exposure (or exposures) to potentially traumatic events (451). Further study of markers for both vulnerability and resilience may help explain variability in the development of ASD or PTSD within populations exposed to similar traumatic events and may contribute to a better understanding of the natural history of these conditions. Better identification of at-risk populations within groups similarly exposed may also guide future preventive and acute intervention strategies. In addition to the independent effects of specific markers or risk factors, interactions among identified biological, psychological, and social factors may further alter the likelihood of developing ASD or PTSD and also merit additional study.
- **Subthreshold and complex PTSD.** Persons may develop significant symptoms in one or more of the three ASD or PTSD symptom clusters but not meet the full diagnostic criteria for ASD or PTSD (452–454). These individuals may be significantly impaired (452, 455), raising questions about the appropriateness of current threshold criteria for PTSD. Similar questions may be raised about the current DSM-IV-TR criterion that to be considered traumatic, a person's response to an event must include "intense fear, helplessness, or horror," since this criterion excludes many persons who report feeling numb or who demonstrate dissociative responses (19). Further study is needed to determine whether such individuals, who might otherwise qualify for these diagnoses, would benefit from treatment.

Randomized, controlled trials of therapy and medications have focused on reducing readily identifiable core symptoms that are outlined in the current diagnostic criteria for PTSD; these symptoms lend themselves to quantification with available severity scales. Clinicians recognize that PTSD and ASD are associated with changes in belief systems, view of self, and ability to trust others, as well as related changes in social, occupational, and interpersonal functioning that may affect patients' lives to a far greater extent than more readily quantifiable core clinical features. The extent to which these issues rather than the more easily recognized or reliably reported reexperiencing phenomena or hyperarousal represent the more disabling aspects of the illnesses also bears further investigation. Another question for further study is whether these often-observed changes represent symptoms that should be included in refined diagnostic criteria for PTSD or should signify a separate diagnostic entity (e.g., occurring perhaps as a consequence of earlier or repeated exposure to trauma). More difficult to assess is the extent to which deterioration in spheres of functioning is mitigated by currently available treatments and which approaches may be most effective for addressing the illnesses' effects on functioning.

Whether or not traumatic grief and complicated bereavement should be recognized as separate diagnostic entities, response to loss is often a focus for persons seeking treatment (303, 456). Since traumatic loss is common, further study of potential treatments for prolonged or disabling grief is warranted.

- **Medication treatments and psychotherapies.** For the most part, studies of psychotherapy and medication treatment for ASD and PTSD have been small and of relatively brief duration. While larger, well-controlled studies of SSRIs have been conducted, similar studies are lacking and are needed for virtually all other available medication treatments. Newer medications such as tiagabine (457) have been pilot tested but will also require larger-scale controlled studies to establish efficacy.

  Benzodiazepines are a widely used and effective treatment for other psychiatric disorders, including anxiety disorders. Although they may improve sleep in ASD or PTSD, some evidence suggests that benzodiazepines also may increase the likelihood of developing PTSD (157, 438). Given the widespread use and prescription of these medications in emergency settings, well-controlled studies are needed in patients with ASD and PTSD.

  Studies of pharmacological treatments are also needed to provide evidence on stepwise or algorithmic approaches to treatment choice and to define the role of adjunctive medications in patients with partial responses to first-line agents. Pharmacokinetic or pharmacodynamic properties of medications within subclasses have yet to be studied with regard to their effect on efficacy in treatment of PTSD, nor have the effects of ethnic or cultural considerations on treatment response been clearly delineated.

  At the neurobiological level, the mechanisms by which specific medications alter putative disease processes remain unclear. Studies of the neurobiological effects of specific interventions may provide clues to the pathophysiology of these disorders and suggest other avenues of treatment.

  Cognitive and behavioral therapies—particularly as early interventions—have demonstrated efficacy largely in victims of sexual assault, interpersonal violence, and industrial or vehicular accidents. Replication of these studies in combat veterans or other victims of mass violence is also important. Preliminary findings with innovative psychotherapies (368, 413, 415–417) require further study in larger controlled trials. Manualizing both emerging and traditional psychotherapies is one approach that may promote more rigorous study. Given the widespread use of psychodynamic psychotherapy, it is particularly important to encourage controlled studies to examine the techniques used and their efficacy.

  In the clinical setting, psychotherapeutic approaches are most often used in combination with one another. Regardless of theoretical orientation, clinicians use elements of psychodynamic therapy, supportive therapy, cognitive behavior therapy, or other approaches incorporating various degrees of imaginal or in vivo exposure. Identification of the effective subcomponents of various cognitive and behavior therapies and EMDR in the research setting has not been accomplished, and even less is known about effective subcomponents of these therapies in typical clinical populations. Investigations of combinations of various psychotherapies are few (177, 397, 458). Effectiveness trials that assess whether efficacious psychotherapeutic and psychopharmacological interventions can be adapted beneficially to typical clinical settings are similarly necessary (25).
- **Treatment of specific symptoms or clinical concerns.** Given mixed results with benzodiazepines and the prominence of sleep disturbance in traumatized individuals (459–461), it is critical to identify medications or therapies that can target nightmares and insomnia without increasing the patient's likelihood of developing other symptoms (426, 462). Further study may also help to identify particular interventions that reduce other specific symptoms in patients with ASD or PTSD, such as self-injurious, deliberately self-harmful, or suicidal behaviors (277). The role of active involvement of family members and community supports in enhancing adherence—as has been applied to other severe mental disorders—requires further exploration (84). There are few studies of the potential of family or couples therapy for reducing symptoms or dysfunction in PTSD (372). The effect of other treatments on reducing functional impairment is another broad area that requires further investigation.

- **Generalization of research trials to clinical populations.** As for most disorders, the generalizability of medication trials and therapy studies for the treatment of ASD and PTSD is frequently limited by high levels of subject exclusion because of comorbidity, high subject dropout rates, and relatively short durations of follow-up periods (277). Consequently, the robust treatment responses observed in research settings may not always be seen in typical patients treated in clinical practice. Longer-term follow-up studies must also be conducted to determine whether initial gains made in therapy or with medication are long-lasting and whether maintenance treatment is necessary. More studies are needed to clarify potential adverse effects of treatment and patient factors that reduce adherence to specific regimens (463). Effectiveness trials are also necessary to assess whether efficacious therapeutic and/or psychopharmacological interventions for ASD or PTSD can produce meaningful and lasting changes in patients who typically present in community settings. The importance of PTSD as a comorbid disorder in serious and persistent mental disorders such as schizophrenia or bipolar disorder highlights a particular need for study of PTSD treatment in these patient groups.

The fact that stressful life events may cause emotional and behavioral effects has long been recognized. Psychiatrists concerned themselves with the consequences of traumatic experience decades before the diagnoses of ASD and PTSD were specifically identified. Clinical experience, descriptive literature, and case study guided treatment of persons suffering from the effects of traumatic exposure long before randomized, controlled trials were conceptualized or became a standard for evaluating new evidence. Disregarding clinical experience accumulated before these advances in research design would be as imprudent as believing that research conducted under current standards has adequately demonstrated the full range of effective treatment. Standards for gathering and evaluating new evidence are evolving and should inform the development of future guidelines for assessing and treating mental disorders that arise in the aftermath of exposure to traumatic events.

INDIVIDUALS AND ORGANIZATIONS THAT SUBMITTED COMMENTS

Jon G. Allen, Ph.D.
William Arroyo, M.D.
J. Wesson Ashford, M.D., Ph.D.
Donald Banzhaf, M.D.
Romano Biancoli, Ph.D.
Evelyn Bromet, Ph.D.
David W. Brook, M.D.
Bonnie J. Buchele, Ph.D.
Fredric Busch, M.D.
Peter Roy Byrne, M.D.
Judy Cohen, M.D.
Mary Ann Cohen, M.D.
Mirean Coleman, M.S.W., L.I.C.S.W., C.T.
Joan Cook, M.D.
Jonathan Davidson, M.D.
Cleto DiGiovanni, Jr., M.D.
Lois T. Flaherty, M.D.
Jane Meschan Foy, M.D.
Terry Fullerton, Ph.D.
Leslie Hartley Gise, M.D.
Robert M. Goisman, M.D.
Michael Good, M.D.
Tina Haynes, M.T.-B.C.
Al Herzog, M.D.
Mardi Horowitz, M.D.
Craig L. Katz, M.D.
Harold Kudler, M.D.
Barry Landau, M.D.
Melvin Lansky, M.D.
Dori Laub, M.D.

Fred M. Levin, M.D., S.C.
Brett Litz, Ph.D.
John Markowitz, M.D.
Julia Matthews, Ph.D., M.D.
Miles McFall, Ph.D.
Thomas A. Mellman, M.D.
Thomas Neylan, M.D.
Carol S. North, M.D.
Andrei Novac, M.D.
John D. O'Brien, M.D.
Herbert S. Peyser, M.D.
Roger Pitman, M.D.
Charles W. Portney, M.D.
Murray Raskind, M.D.
Barbara R. Rosenfeld, M.D.
Barbara O. Rothbaum, M.D.
Patricia Rowell, R.N., Ph.D., C.N.P.
Diane H. Schetky, M.D.
David Servan-Schreiber, M.D., Ph.D.
Jonathan Shay, M.D., Ph.D.
Bradley D. Stein, M.D., Ph.D.
Robert Stern, M.D., Ph.D.
Nicholas E. Stratas, M.D.
Elisa G. Triffleman, M.D.
Bessel A. van der Kolk, M.D.
Sidney Zisook, M.D.

American Academy of Child and Adolescent Psychiatry
American Academy of Clinical Psychiatrists
American Academy of Pediatrics
American Academy of Psychoanalysis and Dynamic Psychiatry
American Association of Community Psychiatrists
American Group Psychotherapy Association
American Music Therapy Association
American Nurses Association
International Federation of Psychoanalytic Societies
National Association of Social Workers
National Center for Post-Traumatic Stress Disorder

REFERENCES

The following coding system is used to indicate the nature of the supporting evidence in the references:

[A] *Randomized double-blind clinical trial.* A study of an intervention in which subjects are prospectively followed over time; there are treatment and control groups; subjects are randomly assigned to the two groups; both the subjects and the investigators are blind to the assignments.

[A–] *Randomized clinical trial.* Same as above but not double-blind.

[B] *Clinical trial.* A prospective study in which an intervention is made and the results of that intervention are tracked longitudinally; study does not meet standards for a randomized clinical trial.

[C] *Cohort or longitudinal study.* A study in which subjects are prospectively followed over time without any specific intervention.

[D] *Control study.* A study in which a group of patients and a group of control subjects are identified in the present and information about them is pursued retrospectively or backward in time.

[E] *Review with secondary data analysis.* A structured analytic review of existing data, e.g., a meta-analysis or a decision analysis.

[F] *Review.* A qualitative review and discussion of previously published literature without a quantitative synthesis of the data.

[G] *Other.* Textbooks, expert opinion, case reports, and other reports not included above.

1. Veterans Health Administration: Management of Post-Traumatic Stress. Office of Quality and Performance publication 10Q-CPG/PTSD-04. Washington, DC, VA/DoD Clinical Practice Guideline Working Group, Veterans Health Administration, Department of Veterans Affairs and Health Affairs, Department of Defense, 2003. http://www.oqp.med.va.gov/cpg/PTSD/PTSD_Base.htm [G]
2. Foa EB, Keane TM, Friedman MJ (eds): Effective Treatments for PTSD: Practice Guidelines From the International Society for Traumatic Stress Studies. New York, Guilford, 2000 [G]
3. American Academy of Child and Adolescent Psychiatry: Summary of the Practice Parameters for the Assessment and Treatment of Children and Adolescents With Posttraumatic Stress Disorder. J Am Acad Child Adolesc Psychiatry 1998; 37:997–1001 [G]
4. Kessler RC, Sonnega A, Bromet E, Hughes M, Nelson CB: Posttraumatic stress disorder in the National Comorbidity Survey. Arch Gen Psychiatry 1995; 52:1048–1060 [G]
5. Breslau N, Kessler RC, Chilcoat HD, Schultz LR, Davis GC, Andreski P: Trauma and posttraumatic stress disorder in the community: the 1996 Detroit Area Survey of Trauma. Arch Gen Psychiatry 1998; 55:626–632 [G]
6. Harvey AG, Bryant RA: The relationship between acute stress disorder and posttraumatic stress disorder: a 2-year prospective evaluation. J Consult Clin Psychol 1999; 67:985–988 [C]
7. Marshall RD, Spitzer R, Liebowitz MR: Review and critique of the new DSM-IV diagnosis of acute stress disorder. Am J Psychiatry 1999; 156:1677–1685 [F]
8. Staab JP, Grieger TA, Fullerton CS, Ursano RJ: Acute stress disorder, subsequent posttraumatic stress disorder and depression after a series of typhoons. Anxiety 1996; 2:219–225 [G]
9. Bryant RA, Harvey AG, Guthrie RM, Moulds ML: A prospective study of psychophysiological arousal, acute stress disorder, and posttraumatic stress disorder. J Abnorm Psychol 2000; 109:341–344 [C]
10. Stein MB, McQuaid JR, Pedrelli P, Lenox R, McCahill ME: Posttraumatic stress disorder in the primary care medical setting. Gen Hosp Psychiatry 2000; 22:261–269 [G]
11. Silver RC, Holman EA, McIntosh DN, Poulin M, Gil-Rivas V: Nationwide longitudinal study of psychological responses to September 11. JAMA 2002; 288:1235–1244 [G]
12. North CS, Nixon SJ, Shariat S, Mallonee S, McMillen JC, Spitznagel EL, Smith EM: Psychiatric disorders among survivors of the Oklahoma City bombing. JAMA 1999; 282:755–762 [G]
13. Weine SM, Becker DF, McGlashan TH, Laub D, Lazrove S, Vojvoda D, Hyman L: Psychiatric consequences of "ethnic cleansing": clinical assessments and trauma testimonies of newly resettled Bosnian refugees. Am J Psychiatry 1995; 152:536–542 [G]
14. Bromet E, Sonnega A, Kessler RC: Risk factors for DSM-III-R posttraumatic stress disorder: findings from the National Comorbidity Survey. Am J Epidemiol 1998; 147:353–361 [G]
15. Breslau N, Davis GC, Andreski P, Peterson EL, Schultz LR: Sex differences in posttraumatic stress disorder. Arch Gen Psychiatry 1997; 54:1044–1048 [G]
16. Meltzer-Brody S, Churchill E, Davidson JR: Derivation of the SPAN, a brief diagnostic screening test for post-traumatic stress disorder. Psychiatry Res 1999; 88:63–70 [G]
17. Breslau N, Peterson EL, Kessler RC, Schultz LR: Short screening scale for DSM-IV posttraumatic stress disorder. Am J Psychiatry 1999; 156:908–911 [G]
18. Brewin CR, Rose S, Andrews B, Green J, Tata P, McEvedy C, Turner S, Foa EB: Brief screening instrument for post-traumatic stress disorder. Br J Psychiatry 2002; 181:158–162 [G]
19. Shalev AY: Acute stress reactions in adults. Biol Psychiatry 2002; 51:532–543 [F]
20. Shalev AY, Peri T, Rogel-Fuchs Y, Ursano RJ, Marlowe D: Historical group debriefing after combat exposure. Mil Med 1998; 163:494–498 [B]
21. Marmar CR, Weiss DS, Pynoos RS: Dynamic psychotherapy of post-traumatic stress disorder, in Neurobiological and Clinical Consequences of Stress: From Normal Adaptation to Post-Traumatic Stress Disorder. Edited by Friedman MJ, Charney DS, Deutch AY. Philadelphia, Lippincott-Raven, 1995, pp 495–506 [F]

22. Marmar CR, Weiss DS, Schlenger WE, Fairbank JA, Jordan BK, Kulka RA, Hough RL: Peritraumatic dissociation and posttraumatic stress in male Vietnam theater veterans. Am J Psychiatry 1994; 151:902–907 [G]
23. Weathers FW, Litz BT, Huska J, Keane TM: PTSD Checklist (PCL) for DSM-IV. Boston, National Center for PTSD, Behavioral Science Division, 1994 [G]
24. Horowitz M, Wilner N, Alvarez W: Impact of Event Scale: a measure of subjective stress. Psychosom Med 1979; 41:209–218 [G]
25. Horowitz MJ: Treatment of Stress Response Syndromes. Arlington, VA, American Psychiatric Publishing, 2003 [G]
26. Davidson JR, Book SW, Colket JT, Tupler LA, Roth S, David D, Hertzberg M, Mellman T, Beckham JC, Smith RD, Davison RM, Katz R, Feldman ME: Assessment of a new self-rating scale for post-traumatic stress disorder. Psychol Med 1997; 27:153–160 [G]
27. Weathers FW, Keane TM, Davidson JR: Clinician-Administered PTSD Scale: a review of the first ten years of research. Depress Anxiety 2001; 13:132–156 [E]
28. Davidson JR, Malik MA, Travers J: Structured Interview for PTSD (SIP): psychometric validation for DSM-IV criteria. Depress Anxiety 1997; 5:127–129 [G]
29. American Psychiatric Association: Practice Guideline for Psychiatric Evaluation of Adults, 2nd ed. Am J Psychiatry (in press) [G]
30. Connor KM, Butterfield MI: Posttraumatic stress disorder. Focus 2003; 1:247–262 [F]
31. Scurfield RM, Blank AS: A guide to obtaining a military history from Viet Nam veterans, in The Trauma of War: Stress and Recovery in Viet Nam Veterans. Edited by Sonnenberg SM, Blank AS Jr, Talbott JA. Washington, DC, American Psychiatric Press, 1985, pp 263–291 [G]
32. Ballenger JC, Davidson JR, Lecrubier Y, Nutt DJ, Foa EB, Kessler RC, McFarlane AC, Shalev AY: Consensus statement on posttraumatic stress disorder from the International Consensus Group on Depression and Anxiety. J Clin Psychiatry 2000; 61(suppl 5):60–66 [G]
33. Breslau N, Chilcoat HD, Kessler RC, Davis GC: Previous exposure to trauma and PTSD effects of subsequent trauma: results from the Detroit Area Survey of Trauma. Am J Psychiatry 1999; 156:902–907 [G]
34. Ursano RJ, Fullerton CS, Epstein RS, Crowley B, Kao TC, Vance K, Craig KJ, Dougall AL, Baum A: Acute and chronic posttraumatic stress disorder in motor vehicle accident victims. Am J Psychiatry 1999; 156:589–595 [C]
35. Devilly GJ, Spence SH: The relative efficacy and treatment distress of EMDR and a cognitive-behavior trauma treatment protocol in the amelioration of posttraumatic stress disorder. J Anxiety Disord 1999; 13:131–157 [A–]
36. Strasburger LH, Gutheil TG, Brodsky A: On wearing two hats: role conflict in serving as both psychotherapist and expert witness. Am J Psychiatry 1997; 154:448–456 [G]
37. Gutheil TG, Hilliard JT: The treating psychiatrist thrust into the role of expert witness. Psychiatr Serv 2001; 52:1526–1527 [G]
38. Vallabhajosula B, van Gorp WG: Post-Daubert admissibility of scientific evidence on malingering of cognitive deficits. J Am Acad Psychiatry Law 2001; 29:207–215 [F]
39. Beckham JC, Lytle BL, Vrana SR, Hertzberg MA, Feldman ME, Shipley RH: Smoking withdrawal symptoms in response to a trauma-related stressor among Vietnam combat veterans with posttraumatic stress disorder. Addict Behav 1996; 21:93–101 [B]
40. Beckham JC: Smoking and anxiety in combat veterans with chronic posttraumatic stress disorder: a review. J Psychoactive Drugs 1999; 31:103–110 [F]
41. Silverman JJ, Peed SF, Goldberg S, Hamer RM, Stockman SJ: Surgical staff recognition of psychopathology in trauma patients. J Trauma 1985; 25:544–546 [C]
42. Whetsell LA, Patterson CM, Young DH, Schiller WR: Preinjury psychopathology in trauma patients. J Trauma 1989; 29:1158–1161 [C]
43. Cerda G, Zatzick D, Wise M, Greenhalgh D: Computerized registry recording of psychiatric disorders of pediatric patients with burns. J Burn Care Rehabil 2000; 21:368–370 [C]

44. Zatzick DF, Kang SM, Kim SY, Leigh P, Kravitz R, Drake C, Sue S, Wisner D: Patients with recognized psychiatric disorders in trauma surgery: incidence, inpatient length of stay, and cost. J Trauma 2000; 49:487–495 [C]
45. Coverdale JH, Turbott SH: Sexual and physical abuse of chronically ill psychiatric outpatients compared with a matched sample of medical outpatients. J Nerv Ment Dis 2000; 188:440–445 [D]
46. Goodman LA, Rosenberg SD, Mueser KT, Drake RE: Physical and sexual assault history in women with serious mental illness: prevalence, correlates, treatment, and future research directions. Schizophr Bull 1997; 23:685–696 [F]
47. Mueser KT, Goodman LB, Trumbetta SL, Rosenberg SD, Osher C, Vidaver R, Auciello P, Foy DW: Trauma and posttraumatic stress disorder in severe mental illness. J Consult Clin Psychol 1998; 66:493–499 [G]
48. Neria Y, Bromet EJ, Sievers S, Lavelle J, Fochtmann LJ: Trauma exposure and posttraumatic stress disorder in psychosis: findings from a first-admission cohort. J Consult Clin Psychol 2002; 70:246–251 [G]
49. Switzer GE, Dew MA, Thompson K, Goycoolea JM, Derricott T, Mullins SD: Posttraumatic stress disorder and service utilization among urban mental health center clients. J Trauma Stress 1999; 12:25–39 [G]
50. Rose SM, Peabody CG, Stratigeas B: Undetected abuse among intensive case management clients. Hosp Community Psychiatry 1991; 42:499–503 [D]
51. Mueser KT, Salyers MP, Rosenberg SD, Goodman LA, Essock SM, Osher FC, Swartz MS, Butterfield MI, 5 Site Health and Risk Study Research Committee: Interpersonal trauma and posttraumatic stress disorder in patients with severe mental illness: demographic, clinical, and health correlates. Schizophr Bull 2004; 30:45–57 [D]
52. Famularo R, Kinscherff R, Fenton T: Posttraumatic stress disorder among children clinically diagnosed as borderline personality disorder. J Nerv Ment Dis 1991; 179:428–431 [G]
53. Goldman SJ, D'Angelo EJ, DeMaso DR, Mezzacappa E: Physical and sexual abuse histories among children with borderline personality disorder. Am J Psychiatry 1992; 149:1723–1726 [D]
54. Yen S, Shea MT, Battle CL, Johnson DM, Zlotnick C, Dolan-Sewell R, Skodol AE, Grilo CM, Gunderson JG, Sanislow CA, Zanarini MC, Bender DS, Rettew JB, McGlashan TH: Traumatic exposure and posttraumatic stress disorder in borderline, schizotypal, avoidant, and obsessive-compulsive personality disorders: findings from the collaborative longitudinal personality disorders study. J Nerv Ment Dis 2002; 190:510–518 [G]
55. Bonin MF, Norton GR, Asmundson GJ, Dicurzio S, Pidlubney S: Drinking away the hurt: the nature and prevalence of PTSD in substance abuse patients attending a community-based treatment program. J Behav Ther Exp Psychiatry 2000; 31:55–66 [G]
56. Epstein JN, Saunders BE, Kilpatrick DG, Resnick HS: PTSD as a mediator between childhood rape and alcohol use in adult women. Child Abuse Negl 1998; 22:223–234 [G]
57. Duncan RD, Saunders BE, Kilpatrick DG, Hanson RF, Resnick HS: Childhood physical assault as a risk factor for PTSD, depression, and substance abuse: findings from a national survey. Am J Orthopsychiatry 1996; 66:437–448 [D]
58. Brady KT, Wohlreich M: Victimization, PTSD, and substance abuse. Women's Psychiatric Health 1994; 3:12–14 [D]
59. deGroot JM, Kennedy S, Rodin G, McVey G: Correlates of sexual abuse in women with anorexia nervosa and bulimia nervosa. Can J Psychiatry 1992; 37:516–518 [G]
60. McFarlane AC, McFarlane CM, Gilchrist PN: Posttraumatic bulimia and anorexia nervosa. Int J Eat Disord 1988; 7:705–708 [G]
61. Herzog DB, Staley JE, Carmody S, Robbins WM, van der Kolk BA: Childhood sexual abuse in anorexia nervosa and bulimia nervosa: a pilot study. J Am Acad Child Adolesc Psychiatry 1993; 32:962–966 [G]

62. Zisook S, Chentsova-Dutton Y, Shuchter SR: PTSD following bereavement. Ann Clin Psychiatry 1998; 10:157–163 [B]
63. Dobie DJ, Kivlahan DR, Maynard C, Bush KR, Davis TM, Bradley KA: Posttraumatic stress disorder in female veterans: association with self-reported health problems and functional impairment. Arch Intern Med 2004; 164:394–400 [G]
64. American Psychiatric Association: Practice Guideline for the Assessment and Treatment of Patients With Suicidal Behaviors. Am J Psychiatry 2003; 160(Nov suppl) [G]
65. Morgan HG, Burns-Cox CJ, Pocock H, Pottle S: Deliberate self-harm: clinical and socio-economic characteristics of 368 patients. Br J Psychiatry 1975; 127:564–574 [G]
66. Pattison EM, Kahan J: The deliberate self-harm syndrome. Am J Psychiatry 1983; 140:867–872 [G]
67. Anderson PL, Tiro JA, Price AW, Bender MA, Kaslow NJ: Additive impact of childhood emotional, physical, and sexual abuse on suicide attempts among low-income African American women. Suicide Life Threat Behav 2002; 32:131–138 [G]
68. Windle M, Windle RC, Scheidt DM, Miller GB: Physical and sexual abuse and associated mental disorders among alcoholic inpatients. Am J Psychiatry 1995; 152:1322–1328 [D]
69. Friedman MJ: Post Traumatic Stress Disorder: The Latest Assessment and Treatment Strategies. Kansas City, Mo, Compact Clinicals, 2000 [G]
70. Wilson JP, Friedman MJ, Lindy JD (eds): Treating Psychological Trauma and PTSD. New York, Guilford, 2001 [G]
71. Williams MB, Sommer JF Jr: Handbook of Post-Traumatic Therapy. Westport, Conn, Greenwood Press, 1994 [G]
72. Rosenheck R, Fontana A: Impact of efforts to reduce inpatient costs on clinical effectiveness: treatment of posttraumatic stress disorder in the Department of Veterans Affairs. Med Care 2001; 39:168–180 [D]
73. Roy-Byrne P, Berliner L, Russo J, Zatzick D, Pitman RK: Treatment preferences and determinants in victims of sexual and physical assault. J Nerv Ment Dis 2003; 191:161–165 [G]
74. Weisaeth L: The stressors and the post-traumatic stress syndrome after an industrial disaster. Acta Psychiatr Scand Suppl 1989; 355:25–37 [D]
75. Wilson JP, Lindy JD (eds): Countertransference in the Treatment of PTSD. New York, Guilford, 1994 [G]
76. Kimerling R, Calhoun KS: Somatic symptoms, social support, and treatment seeking among sexual assault victims. J Consult Clin Psychol 1994; 62:333–340 [C]
77. McFarlane AC, Atchison M, Rafalowicz E, Papay P: Physical symptoms in post-traumatic stress disorder. J Psychosom Res 1994; 38:715–726 [C]
78. Andreski P, Chilcoat H, Breslau N: Post-traumatic stress disorder and somatization symptoms: a prospective study. Psychiatry Res 1998; 79:131–138 [C]
79. Engel CC Jr, Liu X, McCarthy BD, Miller RF, Ursano R: Relationship of physical symptoms to posttraumatic stress disorder among veterans seeking care for Gulf War-related health concerns. Psychosom Med 2000; 62:739–745 [D]
80. Ghahramanlou M, Boradbeck C: Predictors of secondary trauma in sexual assault counselors. Int J Emerg Ment Health 2000; 4:229–240 [D]
81. Figley C (ed): Compassion Fatigue: Coping With Secondary Traumatic Stress Disorders in Those Who Treat the Traumatized. New York, Brunner-Routledge, 1995 [G]
82. Lin EH, Von Korff M, Katon W, Bush T, Simon GE, Walker E, Robinson P: The role of the primary care physician in patients' adherence to antidepressant therapy. Med Care 1995; 33:67–74 [B]
83. Zygmunt A, Olfson M, Boyer CA, Mechanic D: Interventions to improve medication adherence in schizophrenia. Am J Psychiatry 2002; 159:1653–1664 [E]

84. Phillips SD, Burns BJ, Edgar ER, Mueser KT, Linkins KW, Rosenheck RA, Drake RE, McDonel Herr EC: Moving assertive community treatment into standard practice. Psychiatr Serv 2001; 52:771–779 [F]
85. Marshall M, Lockwood A: Assertive community treatment for people with severe mental disorders. Cochrane Database Syst Rev 2000; (2):CD001089 [E]
86. American Psychiatric Association: Practice Guideline for the Treatment of Patients With Schizophrenia, Second Edition. Am J Psychiatry 2004; 161(Feb suppl) [G]
87. Galea S, Resnick H, Ahern J, Gold J, Bucuvalas M, Kilpatrick D, Stuber J, Vlahov D: Posttraumatic stress disorder in Manhattan, New York City, after the September 11th terrorist attacks. J Urban Health 2002; 79:340–353 [D]
88. Glantz MD, Sloboda Z: Analysis and reconceptualization of resilience, in Resilience and Development: Positive Life Adaptations. Edited by Glantz MD, Johnson JL. New York, Kluwer Academic/Plenum, 1999, pp 109–126 [G]
89. Kaplan HB: Toward an understanding of resilience: a critical review of definitions and models, in Resilience and Development: Positive Life Adaptations. Edited by Glantz MD, Johnson JL. New York, Kluwer Academic/Plenum, 1999, pp 17–84 [F]
90. Barnes DH, Bell CC: Paradoxes of black suicide. Preventing Suicide: The National Journal 2003; 2:2–4 [F]
91. Beck AT, Weissman A, Kovacs M: Alcoholism, hopelessness and suicidal behavior. J Stud Alcohol 1976; 37:66–77 [D]
92. Linehan MM, Goodstein JL, Nielsen SL, Chiles JA: Reasons for staying alive when you are thinking of killing yourself: the reasons for living inventory. J Consult Clin Psychol 1983; 51:276–286 [F]
93. Range LM, Penton SR: Hope, hopelessness, and suicidality in college students. Psychol Rep 1994; 75:456–458 [G]
94. Scheier M, Carver C: Effects of optimism on psychological and physical well-being: theoretical overview and empirical update. Cognitive Therapy and Research 1992; 16:201–228 [F]
95. Taylor SE, Kemeny ME, Reed GM, Bower JE, Gruenewald TL: Psychological resources, positive illusions, and health. Am Psychol 2000; 55:99–109 [G]
96. Werner EE: Vulnerable but invincible: high risk children from birth to adulthood. Eur Child Adolesc Psychiatry 1996; 5(suppl 1):47–51 [G]
97. Wyman PA, Cowen EL, Work WC, Kerley JH: The role of children's future expectations in self-esteem functioning and adjustment to life stress: a prospective study of urban at-risk children. Dev Psychopathol 1993; 5:649–661 [C]
98. Antoni MH, Lehman JM, Kilbourn KM, Boyers AE, Culver JL, Alferi SM, Yount SE, McGregor BA, Arena PL, Harris SD, Price AA, Carver CS: Cognitive-behavioral stress management intervention decreases the prevalence of depression and enhances benefit finding among women under treatment for early-stage breast cancer. Health Psychol 2001; 20:20–32 [D]
99. Brissette I, Scheier MF, Carver CS: The role of optimism in social network development, coping, and psychological adjustment during a life transition. J Pers Soc Psychol 2002; 82:102–111 [C]
100. Jaycox LH, Reivich KJ, Gillham J, Seligman ME: Prevention of depressive symptoms in school children. Behav Res Ther 1994; 32:801–816 [B]
101. Gillham JE, Reivich KJ, Jaycox LH, Seligman MEP: Prevention of depressive symptoms in school children: two-year follow-up. Psychol Sci 1995; 6:343–351 [A–]
102. Chemtob CM, Nakashima JP, Hamada RS: Psychosocial intervention for postdisaster trauma symptoms in elementary school children: a controlled community field study. Arch Pediatr Adolesc Med 2002; 156:211–216 [A]

103. Friedman M, Schnurr PP: The relationship between trauma, post-traumatic stress disorder and physical health, in Neurobiological and Clinical Consequences of Stress: From Normal Adaptation to Post-Traumatic Stress Disorder. Edited by Friedman M, Charney DS, Deutch AY. Philadelphia, Lippincott-Raven, 1995, pp 507–524 [G]
104. Breslau N, Davis GC, Peterson EL, Schultz L: Psychiatric sequelae of posttraumatic stress disorder in women. Arch Gen Psychiatry 1997; 54:81–87 [D]
105. McCarroll JE, Ursano RJ, Fullerton CS, Liu X, Lundy A: Somatic symptoms in Gulf War mortuary workers. Psychosom Med 2002; 64:29–33 [G]
106. Schnurr PP, Friedman MJ, Sengupta A, Jankowski MK, Holmes T: PTSD and utilization of medical treatment services among male Vietnam veterans. J Nerv Ment Dis 2000; 188:496–504 [D]
107. Benedikt RA, Kolb LC: Preliminary findings on chronic pain and posttraumatic stress disorder. Am J Psychiatry 1986; 143:908–910 [G]
108. Geisser ME, Roth RS, Bachman JE, Eckert TA: The relationship between symptoms of post-traumatic stress disorder and pain, affective disturbance and disability among patients with accident and non-accident related pain. Pain 1996; 66:207–214 [D]
109. Pecukonis EV: Childhood sex abuse in women with chronic intractable back pain. Soc Work Health Care 1996; 23:1–16 [C]
110. Badura AS, Reiter RC, Altmaier EM, Rhomberg A, Elas D: Dissociation, somatization, substance abuse, and coping in women with chronic pelvic pain. Obstet Gynecol 1997; 90:405–410 [G]
111. Drossman DA: Sexual and physical abuse and gastrointestinal illness. Scand J Gastroenterol Suppl 1995; 208:90–96 [G]
112. Plichta SB, Abraham C: Violence and gynecologic health in women <50 years old. Am J Obstet Gynecol 1996; 174:903–907 [G]
113. Walling MK, O'Hara MW, Reiter RC, Milburn AK, Lilly G, Vincent SD: Abuse history and chronic pain in women, II: a multivariate analysis of abuse and psychological morbidity. Obstet Gynecol 1994; 84:200–206 [D]
114. Walker EA, Gelfand AN, Gelfand MD, Green C, Katon WJ: Chronic pelvic pain and gynecological symptoms in women with irritable bowel syndrome. J Psychosom Obstet Gynaecol 1996; 17:39–46 [G]
115. Amaya-Jackson L, Davidson JR, Hughes DC, Swartz M, Reynolds V, George LK, Blazer DG: Functional impairment and utilization of services associated with posttraumatic stress in the community. J Trauma Stress 1999; 12:709–724 [C]
116. Booth BM, Blow FC, Cook CA: Functional impairment and co-occurring psychiatric disorders in medically hospitalized men. Arch Intern Med 1998; 158:1551–1559 [D]
117. Holbrook TL, Anderson JP, Sieber WJ, Browner D, Hoyt DB: Outcome after major trauma: 12-month and 18-month follow-up results from the Trauma Recovery Project. J Trauma 1999; 46:765–771 [C]
118. Holbrook TL, Hoyt DB, Stein MB, Sieber WJ: Perceived threat to life predicts posttraumatic stress disorder after major trauma: risk factors and functional outcome. J Trauma 2001; 51:287–292 [G]
119. Mollica RF, Donelan K, Tor S, Lavelle J, Elias C, Frankel M, Blendon RJ: The effect of trauma and confinement on functional health and mental health status of Cambodians living in Thailand-Cambodia border camps. JAMA 1993; 270:581–586 [G]
120. Momartin S, Silove D, Manicavasagar V, Steel Z: Dimensions of trauma associated with posttraumatic stress disorder (PTSD) caseness, severity and functional impairment: a study of Bosnian refugees resettled in Australia. Soc Sci Med 2003; 57:775–781 [G]
121. Schnurr PP, Ford JD, Friedman MJ, Green BL, Dain BJ, Sengupta A: Predictors and outcomes of posttraumatic stress disorder in World War II veterans exposed to mustard gas. J Consult Clin Psychol 2000; 68:258–268 [G]

122. Zatzick DF, Marmar CR, Weiss DS, Browner WS, Metzler TJ, Golding JM, Stewart A, Schlenger WE, Wells KB: Posttraumatic stress disorder and functioning and quality of life outcomes in a nationally representative sample of male Vietnam veterans. Am J Psychiatry 1997; 154:1690–1695 [C]
123. Davidson J, Pearlstein T, Londborg P, Brady KT, Rothbaum B, Bell J, Maddock R, Hegel MT, Farfel G: Efficacy of sertraline in preventing relapse of posttraumatic stress disorder: results of a 28-week double-blind, placebo-controlled study. Am J Psychiatry 2001; 158:1974–1981 [A]
124. Kudler HS, Blank AS, Krupnick JL: The psychodynamic treatment of PTSD, in Effective Treatments for PTSD: Practice Guidelines From the International Society for Traumatic Stress Studies. Edited by Foa EB, Keane TM, Friedman MJ. New York, Guilford, 2000, pp 176–198 [F]
125. Harvey AG, Bryant RA, Tarrier N: Cognitive behaviour therapy for posttraumatic stress disorder. Clin Psychol Rev 2003; 23:501–522 [F]
126. Plichta S: Violence and abuse, in Women's Health: The Commonwealth Fund Survey. Edited by Falik M, Collins KS. Baltimore, Johns Hopkins University Press, 1996, pp 237–270 [D]
127. Holloway HC, Ursano RJ: The Vietnam veteran: memory, social context, and metaphor. Psychiatry 1984; 47:103–108 [G]
128. Wessely S, Bisson J, Rose S: A systematic review of brief psychological interventions ("debriefing") for the treatment of immediate trauma related symptoms and the prevention of posttraumatic stress disorder, in The Cochrane Library 1998, issue 3. Oxford, UK, Update Software (http://www.update-software.com/cochrane) [E]
129. van Emmerik AA, Kamphuis JH, Hulsbosch AM, Emmelkamp PM: Single session debriefing after psychological trauma: a meta-analysis. Lancet 2002; 360:766–771 [E]
130. Litz BT, Gray M: Early intervention for trauma in adults, in Early Intervention for Trauma and Traumatic Loss. Edited by Litz BT. New York, Guilford, 2004, pp 87–111 [G]
131. Zatzick D, Roy-Byrne P, Russo J, Rivara F, Droesh R, Wagner A, Dunn C, Jurkovich G, Uehara E, Katon W: A randomized effectiveness trial of stepped collaborative care for acutely injured trauma survivors. Arch Gen Psychiatry 2004; 61:498–506 [A–]
132. Bordow S, Porritt D: An experimental evaluation of crisis intervention. Soc Sci Med 1979; 13A:251–256 [B]
133. Gidron Y, Gal R, Freedman S, Twiser I, Lauden A, Snir Y, Benjamin J: Translating research findings to PTSD prevention: results of a randomized-controlled pilot study. J Trauma Stress 2001; 14:773–780 [A–]
134. Zatzick DF, Roy-Byrne P, Russo JE, Rivara FP, Koike A, Jurkovich GJ, Katon W: Collaborative interventions for physically injured trauma survivors: a pilot randomized effectiveness trial. Gen Hosp Psychiatry 2001; 23:114–123 [A–]
135. Bryant RA, Sackville T, Dang ST, Moulds M, Guthrie R: Treating acute stress disorder: an evaluation of cognitive behavior therapy and supportive counseling techniques. Am J Psychiatry 1999; 156:1780–1786 [A]
136. Bryant RA, Harvey AG, Dang ST, Sackville T, Basten C: Treatment of acute stress disorder: a comparison of cognitive-behavioral therapy and supportive counseling. J Consult Clin Psychol 1998; 66:862–866 [B]
137. Pitman RK, Sanders KM, Zusman RM, Healy AR, Cheema F, Lasko NB, Cahill L, Orr SP: Pilot study of secondary prevention of posttraumatic stress disorder with propranolol. Biol Psychiatry 2002; 51:189–192 [A]
138. Rehm LP: How can we better disentangle placebo and drug effects? Commentary on The emperor's new drugs: an analysis of antidepressant medication data submitted to the US Food and Drug Administration. Prevention & Treatment 2002, volume 5. Washington, DC, American Psychological Association (http://journals.apa.org/prevention/volume5/pre0050031c.html) [G]

139. Rothbaum B, Foa E: Subtypes of posttraumatic stress disorder and duration of symptoms, in Posttraumatic Stress Disorder: DSM-IV and Beyond. Edited by Davidson J, Foa E. Washington, DC, American Psychiatric Press, 1994, pp 23–35 [F]
140. Blanchard EB, Hickling EJ: Acute stress disorder among MVA survivors, in After the Crash: Assessment and Treatment of Motor Vehicle Accident Survivors. Washington, DC, American Psychological Association, 1997, pp 187–196 [G]
141. Marshall RD, Beebe KL, Oldham M, Zaninelli R: Efficacy and safety of paroxetine treatment for chronic PTSD: a fixed-dose, placebo-controlled study. Am J Psychiatry 2001; 158:1982–1988 [A]
142. Connor KM, Sutherland SM, Tupler LA, Malik ML, Davidson JR: Fluoxetine in posttraumatic stress disorder: randomised, double-blind study. Br J Psychiatry 1999; 175:17–22 [A]
143. van der Kolk BA, Dreyfuss D, Michaels M, Shera D, Berkowitz R, Fisler R, Saxe G: Fluoxetine in posttraumatic stress disorder. J Clin Psychiatry 1994; 55:517–522 [A]
144. Brady K, Pearlstein T, Asnis GM, Baker D, Rothbaum B, Sikes CR, Farfel GM: Efficacy and safety of sertraline treatment of posttraumatic stress disorder: a randomized controlled trial. JAMA 2000; 283:1837–1844 [A]
145. Tucker P, Zaninelli R, Yehuda R, Ruggiero L, Dillingham K, Pitts CD: Paroxetine in the treatment of chronic posttraumatic stress disorder: results of a placebo-controlled, flexible-dosage trial. J Clin Psychiatry 2001; 62:860–868 [A]
146. Martenyi F, Brown EB, Zhang H, Prakash A, Koke SC: Fluoxetine versus placebo in posttraumatic stress disorder. J Clin Psychiatry 2002; 63:199–206 [A]
147. Neylan TC, Metzler TJ, Schoenfeld FB, Weiss DS, Lenoci M, Best SR, Lipsey TL, Marmar CR: Fluvoxamine and sleep disturbances in posttraumatic stress disorder. J Trauma Stress 2001; 14:461–467 [B]
148. Rapaport MH, Endicott J, Clary CM: Posttraumatic stress disorder and quality of life: results across 64 weeks of sertraline treatment. J Clin Psychiatry 2002; 63:59–65 [A]
149. Davidson JR, Landerman LR, Farfel GM, Clary CM: Characterizing the effects of sertraline in post-traumatic stress disorder. Psychol Med 2002; 32:661–670 [A]
150. Marmar CR, Schoenfeld F, Weiss DS, Metzler T, Zatzick D, Wu R, Smiga S, Tecott L, Neylan T: Open trial of fluvoxamine treatment for combat-related posttraumatic stress disorder. J Clin Psychiatry 1996; 57(suppl 8):66–70 [B]
151. Kosten TR, Frank JB, Dan E, McDougle CJ, Giller EL Jr: Pharmacotherapy for posttraumatic stress disorder using phenelzine or imipramine. J Nerv Ment Dis 1991; 179:366–370 [G]
152. Davidson J, Kudler H, Smith R, Mahorney SL, Lipper S, Hammett E, Saunders WB, Cavenar JO Jr: Treatment of posttraumatic stress disorder with amitriptyline and placebo. Arch Gen Psychiatry 1990; 47:259–266 [A]
153. Reist C, Kauffmann CD, Haier RJ, Sangdahl C, DeMet EM, Chicz-DeMet A, Nelson JN: A controlled trial of desipramine in 18 men with posttraumatic stress disorder. Am J Psychiatry 1989; 146:513–516 [A]
154. Katz RJ, Lott MH, Arbus P, Crocq L, Herlobsen P, Lingjaerde O, Lopez G, Loughrey GC, MacFarlane DJ, McIvor R, Mehlum L, Nugent D, Turner SW, Waisaeth L, Yule W: Pharmacotherapy of post-traumatic stress disorder with a novel psychotropic. Anxiety 1994–1995; 1:169–174 [G]
155. Baker DG, Diamond BI, Gillette GM, Hamner MB, Katzelnick D, Keller TW, Mellman TA, Pontius EB, Rosenthal M, Tucker P, van der Kolk BA, Katz RJ: A double-blind, randomized, placebo-controlled, multi-center study of brofaromine in the treatment of post-traumatic stress disorder. Psychopharmacology (Berl) 1995; 122:386–389 [A]
156. Mellman TA, Bustamante V, David D, Fins AI: Hypnotic medication in the aftermath of trauma. J Clin Psychiatry 2002; 63:1183–1184 [G]
157. Gelpin E, Bonne O, Peri T, Brandes D, Shalev AY: Treatment of recent trauma survivors with benzodiazepines: a prospective study. J Clin Psychiatry 1996; 57:390–394 [B]

158. Risse SC, Whitters A, Burke J, Chen S, Scurfield RM, Raskind MA: Severe withdrawal symptoms after discontinuation of alprazolam in eight patients with combat-induced posttraumatic stress disorder. J Clin Psychiatry 1990; 51:206–209 [B]
159. Kosten TR, Fontana A, Sernyak MJ, Rosenheck R: Benzodiazepine use in posttraumatic stress disorder among veterans with substance abuse. J Nerv Ment Dis 2000; 188:454–459 [C]
160. Lipper S, Davidson JR, Grady TA, Edinger JD, Hammett EB, Mahorney SL, Cavenar JO Jr: Preliminary study of carbamazepine in post-traumatic stress disorder. Psychosomatics 1986; 27:849–854 [B]
161. Clark RD, Canive JM, Calais LA, Qualls CR, Tuason VB: Divalproex in posttraumatic stress disorder: an open-label clinical trial. J Trauma Stress 1999; 12:395–401 [B]
162. Fesler FA: Valproate in combat-related posttraumatic stress disorder. J Clin Psychiatry 1991; 52:361–364 [B]
163. Hertzberg MA, Butterfield MI, Feldman ME, Beckham JC, Sutherland SM, Connor KM, Davidson JR: A preliminary study of lamotrigine for the treatment of posttraumatic stress disorder. Biol Psychiatry 1999; 45:1226–1229 [A]
164. Butterfield MI, Becker ME, Connor KM, Sutherland S, Churchill LE, Davidson JR: Olanzapine in the treatment of post-traumatic stress disorder: a pilot study. Int Clin Psychopharmacol 2001; 16:197–203 [A]
165. Petty F, Brannan S, Casada J, Davis LL, Gajewski V, Kramer GL, Stone RC, Teten AL, Worchel J, Young KA: Olanzapine treatment for post-traumatic stress disorder: an open-label study. Int Clin Psychopharmacol 2001; 16:331–337 [B]
166. Stein MB, Kline NA, Matloff JL: Adjunctive olanzapine for SSRI-resistant combat-related PTSD: a double-blind, placebo-controlled study. Am J Psychiatry 2002; 159:1777–1779 [A]
167. Hamner MB, Deitsch SE, Brodrick PS, Ulmer HG, Lorberbaum JP: Quetiapine treatment in patients with posttraumatic stress disorder: an open trial of adjunctive therapy. J Clin Psychopharmacol 2003; 23:15–20 [B]
168. Hamner MB, Faldowski RA, Ulmer HG, Frueh BC, Huber MG, Arana GW: Adjunctive risperidone treatment in post-traumatic stress disorder: a preliminary controlled trial of effects on comorbid psychotic symptoms. Int Clin Psychopharmacol 2003; 18:1–8 [A]
169. Raskind MA, Peskind ER, Kanter ED, Petrie EC, Radant A, Thompson CE, Dobie DJ, Hoff D, Rein RJ, Straits-Troster K, Thomas RG, McFall MM: Reduction of nightmares and other PTSD symptoms in combat veterans by prazosin: a placebo-controlled study. Am J Psychiatry 2003; 160:371–373 [A]
170. Kinzie JD, Leung P: Clonidine in Cambodian patients with posttraumatic stress disorder. J Nerv Ment Dis 1989; 177:546–550 [B]
171. Faustman WO, White PA: Diagnostic and psychopharmacological treatment characteristics of 536 inpatients with posttraumatic stress disorder. J Nerv Ment Dis 1989; 177:154–159 [D]
172. Vaiva G, Ducrocq F, Jezequel K, Averland B, Lestavel P, Brunet A, Marmar CR: Immediate treatment with propranolol decreases posttraumatic stress disorder two months after trauma. Biol Psychiatry 2003; 54:947–949 [B]
173. Foa EB, Rothbaum BO: Treating the Trauma of Rape: Cognitive-Behavioral Therapy for PTSD. New York, Guilford, 1997 [G]
174. Keane TM, Gerarali RJ, Quinn SJ, Litz BT: Behavioral treatment of posttraumatic stress disorder, in Handbook of Clinical Behavior Therapy, 2nd ed. Edited by Turner SM, Calhoun KS, Adams HE. New York, Wiley, 1992, pp 87–97 [G]
175. Bryant RA, Moulds ML, Nixon RV: Cognitive behaviour therapy of acute stress disorder: a four-year follow-up. Behav Res Ther 2003; 41:489–494 [A]
176. Solomon SD, Johnson DM: Psychosocial treatment of posttraumatic stress disorder: a practice-friendly review of outcome research. J Clin Psychol 2002; 58:947–959 [F]

177. Marks I, Lovell K, Noshirvani H, Livanou M, Thrasher S: Treatment of posttraumatic stress disorder by exposure and/or cognitive restructuring: a controlled study. Arch Gen Psychiatry 1998; 55:317–325 [A]
178. Tarrier N, Pilgrim H, Sommerfield C, Faragher B, Reynolds M, Graham E, Barrowclough C: A randomized trial of cognitive therapy and imaginal exposure in the treatment of chronic posttraumatic stress disorder. J Consult Clin Psychol 1999; 67:13–18 [A]
179. Hembree EA, Foa EB: Posttraumatic stress disorder: psychological factors and psychosocial interventions. J Clin Psychiatry 2000; 61(suppl 7):33–39 [F]
180. Resick PA, Jordan CG, Girelli SA, Hutter CK, Marhoefer-Dvorak S: A comparative victim study of behavioral group therapy for sexual assault victims. Behav Ther 1988; 19:385–401 [B]
181. Resick PA, Nishith P, Weaver TL, Astin MC, Feuer CA: A comparison of cognitive-processing therapy with prolonged exposure and a waiting condition for the treatment of chronic posttraumatic stress disorder in female rape victims. J Consult Clin Psychol 2002; 70:867–879 [A–]
182. Foa EB: Trauma and women: course, predictors, and treatment. J Clin Psychiatry 1997; 58(suppl 9):25–28 [E]
183. Foy DW, Ruzek JI, Glynn SM, Riney SA, Gusman FD: Trauma focus group therapy for combat-related PTSD. Psychotherapy in Practice 1996; 3(4):59–73 [G]
184. Krakow B, Hollifield M, Johnston L, Koss M, Schrader R, Warner TD, Tandberg D, Lauriello J, McBride L, Cutchen L, Cheng D, Emmons S, Germain A, Melendrez D, Sandoval D, Prince H: Imagery rehearsal therapy for chronic nightmares in sexual assault survivors with posttraumatic stress disorder: a randomized controlled trial. JAMA 2001; 286:537–545 [A–]
185. Forbes D, Phelps A, McHugh T: Treatment of combat-related nightmares using imagery rehearsal: a pilot study. J Trauma Stress 2001; 14:433–442 [B]
186. Tarrier N, Sommerfield C, Pilgrim H, Faragher B: Factors associated with outcome of cognitive-behavioural treatment of chronic post-traumatic stress disorder. Behav Res Ther 2000; 38:191–202 [A]
187. Tarrier N, Sommerfield C, Pilgrim H, Humphreys L: Cognitive therapy or imaginal exposure in the treatment of post-traumatic stress disorder: twelve-month follow-up. Br J Psychiatry 1999; 175:571–575 [A]
188. Resick PA, Schnicke MK: Cognitive processing therapy for sexual assault victims. J Consult Clin Psychol 1992; 60:748–756 [A–]
189. PTSD Treatment Guidelines Task Force: Guidelines for treatment of PTSD: eye movement desensitization and reprocessing. J Trauma Stress 2000; 13:539–588 [E]
190. Foa EB, Meadows EA: Psychosocial treatments for posttraumatic stress disorder: a critical review. Annu Rev Psychol 1997; 48:449–480 [F]
191. Shepherd J, Stein K, Milne R: Eye movement desensitization and reprocessing in the treatment of post-traumatic stress disorder: a review of an emerging therapy. Psychol Med 2000; 30:863–871 [F]
192. Van Etten M, Taylor S: Comparative efficacy of treatments for post-traumatic stress disorder: a meta-analysis. Clinical Psychology and Psychotherapy 1998; 5:126–144 [E]
193. Maxfield L, Hyer L: The relationship between efficacy and methodology in studies investigating EMDR treatment of PTSD. J Clin Psychol 2002; 58:23–41 [E]
194. Davidson PR, Parker KC: Eye movement desensitization and reprocessing (EMDR): a meta-analysis. J Consult Clin Psychol 2001; 69:305–316 [E]
195. Hembree EA, Foa EB, Dorfan NM, Street GP, Kowalski J, Tu X: Do patients drop out prematurely from exposure therapy for PTSD? J Trauma Stress 2003; 16:555–562 [F]
196. Herbert JD, Lilienfeld SO, Lohr JM, Montgomery RW, O'Donohue WT, Rosen GM, Tolin DF: Science and pseudoscience in the development of eye movement desensitization and reprocessing: implications for clinical psychology. Clin Psychol Rev 2000; 20:945–971 [F]

197. Lipke H: Comment on Hembree and Foa (2003) and EMDR. J Trauma Stress 2003; 16:573–574 [G]
198. Kardiner A: The Traumatic Neurosis of War. New York, Hoeber, 1941 [G]
199. Grinker RR Sr, Spiegel JP: Men Under Stress. Philadelphia, Blakiston, 1945 [G]
200. Grinker RR Sr, Spiegel JP: A psychodynamic view of character pathology in Vietnam combat veterans. Bull Menninger Clin 1983; 47:472–474 [G]
201. Brom D, Kleber RJ, Defares PB: Brief psychotherapy for posttraumatic stress disorders. J Consult Clin Psychol 1989; 57:607–612 [B]
202. Regarding Hypnosis: Position Statement [APA Document Reference No. 610001]. Washington, DC, American Psychiatric Association, Feb 1961. http://www.psych.org/edu/other_res/lib_archives/archives/610001.pdf [G]
203. Sherman JJ: Effects of psychotherapeutic treatments for PTSD: a meta-analysis of controlled clinical trials. J Trauma Stress 1998; 11:413–435 [E]
204. Freud A: Comments on trauma, in Psychic Trauma. Edited by Furst SS. New York, Basic Books, 1967, pp 235–245 [G]
205. Weiss J, Sampson H, Mount Zion Psychotherapy Research Group: The Psychoanalytic Process: Theory, Clinical Observations, and Empirical Research. New York, Guilford, 1986 [E]
206. Modlin HC: The trauma in "traumatic neurosis." Bull Menninger Clin 1960; 24:49–56 [F]
207. Shaw JA: Unmasking the illusion of safety: psychic trauma in war. Bull Menninger Clin 1987; 51:49–63 [F]
208. Lindy JD, Green BL, Grace M, Titchener J: Psychotherapy with survivors of the Beverly Hills Supper Club fire. Am J Psychother 1983; 37:593–610 [D]
209. Marmar CR: Brief dynamic psychotherapy of post-traumatic stress disorder. Psychiatr Ann 1991; 21:405–414 [F]
210. Gabbard GO: Psychodynamic Psychiatry in Clinical Practice, 3rd ed. Washington, DC, American Psychiatric Press, 2000 [G]
211. Ursano RJ, Silberman EK: Psychoanalysis, psychoanalytic psychotherapy, and supportive psychotherapy, in The American Psychiatric Publishing Textbook of Clinical Psychiatry, 4th ed. Edited by Hales RE, Yudofsky SC. Arlington, VA, American Psychiatric Publishing, 2003, pp 1177–1203 [F]
212. Chertoff J: Psychodynamic assessment and treatment of traumatized patients. J Psychother Pract Res 1997; 7:35–46 [F]
213. Conlon L, Fahy TJ, Conroy R: PTSD in ambulant RTA victims: a randomized controlled trial of debriefing. J Psychosom Res 1999; 46:37–44 [A]
214. Lee C, Slade P, Lygo V: The influence of psychological debriefing on emotional adaptation in women following early miscarriage: a preliminary study. Br J Med Psychol 1996; 69(pt 1): 47–58 [B]
215. Rose S, Brewin CR, Andrews B, Kirk M: A randomized controlled trial of individual psychological debriefing for victims of violent crime. Psychol Med 1999; 29:793–799 [A–]
216. Raphael B: Early interventions and the debriefing debate, in Terrorism and Disaster: Individual and Community Mental Health Interventions. Edited by Ursano RJ, Fullerton CS, Norwood AE. Cambridge, UK, Cambridge University Press, 2003, pp 146–161 [F]
217. Bisson JI, Jenkins PL, Alexander J, Bannister C: Randomised controlled trial of psychological debriefing for victims of acute burn trauma. Br J Psychiatry 1997; 171:78–81 [A–]
218. Hobbs M, Mayou R, Harrison B, Worlock P: A randomised controlled trial of psychological debriefing for victims of road traffic accidents. BMJ 1996; 313:1438–1439 [A–]
219. Mayou RA, Ehlers A, Hobbs M: Psychological debriefing for road traffic accident victims: three-year follow-up of a randomised controlled trial. Br J Psychiatry 2000; 176:589–593 [C]
220. Litz BT, Gray MJ, Bryant R, Adler AB: Early intervention for trauma: current status and future directions. Clinical Psychology: Science and Practice 2002; 9:112–134 [F]

221. Suzanna R, Jonathan B, Simon W: Psychological debriefing for preventing post traumatic stress disorder (PTSD). Cochrane Database Syst Rev 2001; (3):CD000560 [E]
222. Brewin CR, Andrews B, Valentine JD: Meta-analysis of risk factors for posttraumatic stress disorder in trauma-exposed adults. J Consult Clin Psychol 2000; 68:748–766 [E]
223. Breslau N: The epidemiology of posttraumatic stress disorder: what is the extent of the problem? J Clin Psychiatry 2001; 62(suppl 17):16–22 [F]
224. Russell DE: The incidence and prevalence of intrafamilial and extrafamilial sexual abuse of female children. Child Abuse Negl 1983; 7:133–146 [G]
225. Finkelhor D, Hotaling G, Lewis IA, Smith C: Sexual abuse in a national survey of adult men and women: prevalence, characteristics, and risk factors. Child Abuse Negl 1990; 14:19–28 [D]
226. Breslau N: Gender differences in trauma and posttraumatic stress disorder. J Gend Specif Med 2002; 5:34–40 [G]
227. de Vries MW: Trauma in cultural perspective, in Traumatic Stress: The Effects of Overwhelming Experience on Mind, Body, and Society. Edited by van der Kolk BA, McFarlane AC, Weisaeth L. New York, Guilford, 1996, pp 398–413 [F]
228. Lazarus RS, Folkman S: Stress, Appraisal, and Coping. New York, Springer, 1984 [G]
229. Kluft RP, Bloom SL, Kinzie JD: Treating traumatized patients and victims of violence. New Dir Ment Health Serv 2000; 86:79–102 [F]
230. Rosenheck R, Fontana A: Utilization of mental health services by minority veterans of the Vietnam era. J Nerv Ment Dis 1994; 182:685–691 [E]
231. Lin KM, Smith MW, Ortiz V: Culture and psychopharmacology. Psychiatr Clin North Am 2001; 24:523–538 [F]
232. Cascorbi I: Pharmacogenetics of cytochrome p4502D6: genetic background and clinical implication. Eur J Clin Invest 2003; 33(suppl 2):17–22 [G]
233. Poolsup N, Li Wan Po A, Knight TL: Pharmacogenetics and psychopharmacotherapy. J Clin Pharm Ther 2000; 25:197–220 [F]
234. Bertilsson L, Dahl ML, Tybring G: Pharmacogenetics of antidepressants: clinical aspects. Acta Psychiatr Scand Suppl 1997; 391:14–21 [F]
235. Gelernter J, Kranzler H, Cubells JF: Serotonin transporter protein (SLC6A4) allele and haplotype frequencies and linkage disequilibria in African- and European-American and Japanese populations and in alcohol-dependent subjects. Hum Genet 1997; 101:243–246 [G]
236. Williams RB, Marchuk DA, Gadde KM, Barefoot JC, Grichnik K, Helms MJ, Kuhn CM, Lewis JG, Schanberg SM, Stafford-Smith M, Suarez EC, Clary GL, Svenson IK, Siegler IC: Serotonin-related gene polymorphisms and central nervous system serotonin function. Neuropsychopharmacology 2003; 28:533–541 [G]
237. Salmon P, Calderbank S: The relationship of childhood physical and sexual abuse to adult illness behavior. J Psychosom Res 1996; 40:329–336 [G]
238. Fukudo S, Nomura T, Muranaka M, Taguchi F: Brain-gut response to stress and cholinergic stimulation in irritable bowel syndrome: a preliminary study. J Clin Gastroenterol 1993; 17:133–141 [A–]
239. Irwin C, Falsetti SA, Lydiard RB, Ballenger JC, Brock CD, Brener W: Comorbidity of posttraumatic stress disorder and irritable bowel syndrome. J Clin Psychiatry 1996; 57:576–578 [G]
240. Leserman J, Drossman DA, Li Z, Toomey TC, Nachman G, Glogau L: Sexual and physical abuse history in gastroenterology practice: how types of abuse impact health status. Psychosom Med 1996; 58:4–15 [F]
241. Walker EA, Katon WJ, Hansom J, Harrop-Griffiths J, Holm L, Jones ML, Hickok L, Jemelka RP: Medical and psychiatric symptoms in women with childhood sexual abuse. Psychosom Med 1992; 54:658–664 [E]

242. Davidson JR, Hughes D, Blazer DG, George LK: Post-traumatic stress disorder in the community: an epidemiological study. Psychol Med 1991; 21:713–721 [G]
243. Amir M, Kaplan Z, Neumann L, Sharabani R, Shani N, Buskila D: Posttraumatic stress disorder, tenderness and fibromyalgia. J Psychosom Res 1997; 42:607–613 [D]
244. Walker EA, Gelfand A, Katon WJ, Koss MP, Von Korff M, Bernstein D, Russo J: Adult health status of women with histories of childhood abuse and neglect. Am J Med 1999; 107:332–339 [D]
245. Fierman EJ, Hunt MF, Pratt LA, Warshaw MG, Yonkers KA, Peterson LG, Epstein-Kaye TM, Norton HS: Trauma and posttraumatic stress disorder in subjects with anxiety disorders. Am J Psychiatry 1993; 150:1872–1874 [D]
246. Green BL, Lindy JD, Grace MC, Leonard AC: Chronic posttraumatic stress disorder and diagnostic comorbidity in a disaster sample. J Nerv Ment Dis 1992; 180:760–766 [C]
247. Kulka RA, Schlenger WE, Fairbank JA, Hough RL, Jordan BK, Marmar CR, Weiss DS: Trauma and the Vietnam War Generation: Report of Findings From the National Vietnam Veterans Readjustment Study. New York, Brunner/Mazel, 1990 [G]
248. Boudewyns PA, Albrecht JW, Talbert FS, Hyer LA: Comorbidity and treatment outcome of inpatients with chronic combat-related PTSD. Hosp Community Psychiatry 1991; 42:847–849 [C]
249. Davidson JET, Fairbank JA: The epidemiology of posttraumatic stress disorder, in Posttraumatic Stress Disorder: DSM-IV and Beyond. Edited by Davidson JET, Foa EB. Washington, DC, American Psychiatric Press, 1993, pp 147–169 [F]
250. Keane TM, Wolfe J: Comorbidity in post-traumatic stress disorder: an analysis of community and clinical studies. J Appl Soc Psychol 1990; 20:1776–1788 [F]
251. Jordan BK, Schlenger WE, Hough R, Kulka RA, Weiss D, Fairbank JA, Marmar CR: Lifetime and current prevalence of specific psychiatric disorders among Vietnam veterans and controls. Arch Gen Psychiatry 1991; 48:207–215 [D]
252. Southwick SM, Yehuda R, Giller EL Jr: Personality disorders in treatment-seeking combat veterans with posttraumatic stress disorder. Am J Psychiatry 1993; 150:1020–1023 [G]
253. Solomon SD, Davidson JR: Trauma: prevalence, impairment, service use, and cost. J Clin Psychiatry 1997; 58(suppl 9):5–11 [F]
254. Breslau N, Davis GC, Andreski P, Peterson E: Traumatic events and posttraumatic stress disorder in an urban population of young adults. Arch Gen Psychiatry 1991; 48:216–222 [G]
255. Smith DW, Christiansen EH, Vincent R, Hann NE: Population effects of the bombing of Oklahoma City. J Okla State Med Assoc 1999; 92:193–198 [G]
256. Vlahov D, Galea S, Resnick H, Ahern J, Boscarino JA, Bucuvalas M, Gold J, Kilpatrick D: Increased use of cigarettes, alcohol, and marijuana among Manhattan, New York, residents after the September 11th terrorist attacks. Am J Epidemiol 2002; 155:988–996 [C]
257. Galea S, Ahern J, Resnick H, Kilpatrick D, Bucuvalas M, Gold J, Vlahov D: Psychological sequelae of the September 11 terrorist attacks in New York City. N Engl J Med 2002; 346:982–987 [C]
258. Goenjian A: A mental health relief programme in Armenia after the 1988 earthquake: implementation and clinical observations. Br J Psychiatry 1993; 163:230–239 [C]
259. Curtis T, Miller BC, Berry EH: Changes in reports and incidence of child abuse following natural disasters. Child Abuse Negl 2000; 24:1151–1162 [C]
260. Reijneveld SA, Crone MR, Verhulst FC, Verloove-Vanhorick SP: The effect of a severe disaster on the mental health of adolescents: a controlled study. Lancet 2003; 362:691–696 [D]
261. Kagan J: A conceptual analysis of the affects. J Am Psychoanal Assoc 1991; 39(suppl):109–130 [G]
262. Ornitz EM, Pynoos RS: Startle modulation in children with posttraumatic stress disorder. Am J Psychiatry 1989; 146:866–870 [C]

263. van der Kolk BA, Fisler RE: Childhood abuse and neglect and loss of self-regulation. Bull Menninger Clin 1994; 58:145–168 [G]
264. Briere J, Runtz M: Symptomatology associated with childhood sexual victimization in a nonclinical adult sample. Child Abuse Negl 1988; 12:51–59 [G]
265. Hall RC, Tice L, Beresford TP, Wooley B, Hall AK: Sexual abuse in patients with anorexia nervosa and bulimia. Psychosomatics 1989; 30:73–79 [D]
266. Palmer RL, Oppenheimer R, Dignon A, Chaloner DA, Howells K: Childhood sexual experiences with adults reported by women with eating disorders: an extended series. Br J Psychiatry 1990; 156:699–703 [G]
267. van der Kolk BA, Perry JC, Herman JL: Childhood origins of self-destructive behavior. Am J Psychiatry 1991; 148:1665–1671 [C]
268. Browne A, Finkelhor D: Impact of child sexual abuse: a review of the research. Psychol Bull 1986; 99:66–77 [F]
269. Amir M, Kaplan Z, Efroni R, Kotler M: Suicide risk and coping styles in posttraumatic stress disorder patients. Psychother Psychosom 1999; 68:76–81 [B]
270. Grieger TA, Fullerton CS, Ursano RJ: Posttraumatic stress disorder, alcohol use, and perceived safety after the terrorist attack on the Pentagon. Psychiatr Serv 2003; 54:1380–1382 [G]
271. Lewis DO: Neuropsychiatric and experiential correlates of violent juvenile delinquency. Neuropsychol Rev 1990; 1:125–136 [F]
272. Lewis DO: From abuse to violence: psychophysiological consequences of maltreatment. J Am Acad Child Adolesc Psychiatry 1992; 31:383–391 [F]
273. Kessler RC: Posttraumatic stress disorder: the burden to the individual and to society. J Clin Psychiatry 2000; 61(suppl 5):4–12 [E]
274. Molnar BE, Berkman LF, Buka SL: Psychopathology, childhood sexual abuse and other childhood adversities: relative links to subsequent suicidal behaviour in the US. Psychol Med 2001; 31:965–977 [F]
275. Kessler RC, Borges G, Walters EE: Prevalence of and risk factors for lifetime suicide attempts in the National Comorbidity Survey. Arch Gen Psychiatry 1999; 56:617–626 [C]
276. Allgulander C: Psychiatric aspects of suicidal behavior: anxiety disorders, in The International Handbook of Suicide and Attempted Suicide. Edited by Hawton K, van Herringen K. Chichester, UK, John Wiley & Sons, 2000, pp 179–192 [F]
277. Institute of Medicine: Reducing Suicide: A National Imperative. Washington, DC, National Academies Press, 2002 [E]
278. Seedat S, Lockhat R, Kaminer D, Zungu-Dirwayi N, Stein DJ: An open trial of citalopram in adolescents with post-traumatic stress disorder. Int Clin Psychopharmacol 2001; 16:21–25 [B]
279. Londborg PD, Hegel MT, Goldstein S, Goldstein D, Himmelhoch JM, Maddock R, Patterson WM, Rausch J, Farfel GM: Sertraline treatment of posttraumatic stress disorder: results of 24 weeks of open-label continuation treatment. J Clin Psychiatry 2001; 62:325–331 [B]
280. Malik ML, Connor KM, Sutherland SM, Smith RD, Davison RM, Davidson JR: Quality of life and posttraumatic stress disorder: a pilot study assessing changes in SF-36 scores before and after treatment in a placebo-controlled trial of fluoxetine. J Trauma Stress 1999; 12:387–393 [A]
281. Cowdry RW, Gardner DL: Pharmacotherapy of borderline personality disorder: alprazolam, carbamazepine, trifluoperazine, and tranylcypromine. Arch Gen Psychiatry 1988; 45:111–119 [A]
282. Wickham EA, Reed JV: Lithium for the control of aggressive and self-mutilating behavior. Int Clin Psychopharmacol 1987; 2:181–190 [F]
283. Herman BH, Hammock MK, Arthur-Smith A, Egan J, Chatoor I, Werner A, Zelnik N: Naltrexone decreases self-injurious behavior. Ann Neurol 1987; 22:550–552 [B]

284. Linehan MM: Behavioral treatments of suicidal behaviors: definitional obfuscation and treatment outcomes. Ann N Y Acad Sci 1997; 836:302–328 [G]
285. Mellman L: Consequences of violence against women, in Women's Health: A Lifelong Guide. New York, Scientific American Digital, 1998 [G]
286. Ursano RJ, Fullerton CS, Epstein RS, Crowley B, Vance K, Kao TC, Baum A: Peritraumatic dissociation and posttraumatic stress disorder following motor vehicle accidents. Am J Psychiatry 1999; 156:1808–1810 [C]
287. Epstein RS, Fullerton CS, Ursano RJ: Posttraumatic stress disorder following an air disaster: a prospective study. Am J Psychiatry 1998; 155:934–938 [C]
288. Zatzick D: Posttraumatic stress, functional impairment, and service utilization after injury: a public health approach. Semin Clin Neuropsychiatry 2003; 8:149–157 [F]
289. Rynearson EK, Favell J: Manual for Criminal Death Support Groups. Seattle, Virginia Mason Medical Center, 2000 [F]
290. Prigerson HG, Shear MK, Jacobs SC, Reynolds CF 3rd, Maciejewski PK, Davidson JR, Rosenheck R, Pilkonis PA, Wortman CB, Williams JB, Widiger TA, Frank E, Kupfer DJ, Zisook S: Consensus criteria for traumatic grief: a preliminary empirical test. Br J Psychiatry 1999; 174:67–73 [G]
291. Shear MK, Smith-Caroff K: Traumatic loss and the syndrome of complicated grief. PTSD Research Quarterly 2002; 13:1–8 [G]
292. Mollica RF, Sarajlic N, Chernoff M, Lavelle J, Vukovic IS, Massagli MP: Longitudinal study of psychiatric symptoms, disability, mortality, and emigration among Bosnian refugees. JAMA 2001; 286:546–554 [C]
293. Zatzick DF, Jurkovich GJ, Gentilello L, Wisner D, Rivara FP: Posttraumatic stress, problem drinking, and functional outcomes after injury. Arch Surg 2002; 137:200–205 [C]
294. Soderstrom CA, Smith GS, Dischinger PC, McDuff DR, Hebel JR, Gorelick DA, Kerns TJ, Ho SM, Read KM: Psychoactive substance use disorders among seriously injured trauma center patients. JAMA 1997; 277:1769–1774 [F]
295. Dunn C, Zatzick D, Russo J, Rivara F, Roy-Byrne P, Ries R, Wisner D, Gentilello L: Hazardous drinking by trauma patients during the year after injury. J Trauma 2003; 54:707–712 [C]
296. Rivara FP, Jurkovich GJ, Gurney JG, Seguin D, Fligner CL, Ries R, Raisys VA, Copass M: The magnitude of acute and chronic alcohol abuse in trauma patients. Arch Surg 1993; 128:907–912 [C]
297. Brown PJ, Wolfe J: Substance abuse and post-traumatic stress disorder comorbidity. Drug Alcohol Depend 1994; 35:51–59 [F]
298. McFarlane AC: Epidemiological evidence about the relationship between PTSD and alcohol abuse: the nature of the association. Addict Behav 1998; 23:813–825 [E]
299. Jacobsen LK, Southwick SM, Kosten TR: Substance use disorders in patients with posttraumatic stress disorder: a review of the literature. Am J Psychiatry 2001; 158:1184–1190 [F]
300. Engel CC Jr, Ursano R, Magruder C, Tartaglione R, Jing Z, Labbate LA, Debakey S: Psychological conditions diagnosed among veterans seeking Department of Defense care for Gulf War-related health concerns. J Occup Environ Med 1999; 41:384–392 [G]
301. Zatzick DF, Russo JE, Katon W: Somatic, posttraumatic stress, and depressive symptoms among injured patients treated in trauma surgery. Psychosomatics 2003; 44:479–484 [C]
302. Schnurr PP, Green BL: Trauma and Health: Physical Health Consequences of Exposure to Extreme Stress. Washington, DC, American Psychological Association, 2004 [G]
303. Horowitz MJ, Siegel B, Holen A, Bonanno GA, Milbrath C, Stinson CH: Diagnostic criteria for complicated grief disorder. Am J Psychiatry 1997; 154:904–910 [C]
304. Layne CM, Pynoos RS, Saltzman WR, Arslanagic B, Black M, Savjak N, Popovic T, Durakovic E, Music M, Campara N, Djapo N, Houston R: Trauma/grief-focused group

psychotherapy: school-based postwar intervention with traumatized Bosnian adolescents. Group Dynamics 2001; 5:277–290 [B]
305. Giaconia RM, Reinherz HZ, Silverman AB, Pakiz B, Frost AK, Cohen E: Traumas and posttraumatic stress disorder in a community population of older adolescents. J Am Acad Child Adolesc Psychiatry 1995; 34:1369–1380 [G]
306. Resnick HS, Kilpatrick DG, Dansky BS, Saunders BE, Best CL: Prevalence of civilian trauma and posttraumatic stress disorder in a representative national sample of women. J Consult Clin Psychol 1993; 61:984–991 [G]
307. Norris FH: Epidemiology of trauma: frequency and impact of different potentially traumatic events on different demographic groups. J Consult Clin Psychol 1992; 60:409–418 [G]
308. Helzer JE, Robins LN, McEvoy L: Post-traumatic stress disorder in the general population: findings of the Epidemiologic Catchment Area survey. N Engl J Med 1987; 317:1630–1634 [G]
309. Freedman SA, Gluck N, Tuval-Mashiach R, Brandes D, Peri T, Shalev AY: Gender differences in responses to traumatic events: a prospective study. J Trauma Stress 2002; 15:407–413 [C]
310. Jenkins EJ, Bell CC: Exposure and response to community violence among children and adolescents, in Children in a Violent Society. Edited by Osofsky J. New York, Guilford, 1997, pp 9–31 [G]
311. US Department of Health and Human Services: Mental Health: Culture, Race, Ethnicity—A Supplement to Mental Health: Report of the Surgeon General. Rockville, Md, US Department of Health and Human Services, Substance Abuse and Mental Health Services Administration, Center for Mental Health Services, 2001 [G]
312. Greenfeld LA, Smith SK: American Indians and Crime. Washington, DC, US Department of Justice, Office of Justice Programs, Bureau of Justice Statistics, 1999 [G]
313. Jones MC, Dauphinais P, Sack WH, Somervell PD: Trauma-related symptomatology among American Indian adolescents. J Trauma Stress 1997; 10:163–173 [G]
314. Robin RW, Chester B, Rasmussen JK, Jaranson JM, Goldman D: Prevalence and characteristics of trauma and posttraumatic stress disorder in a southwestern American Indian community. Am J Psychiatry 1997; 154:1582–1588 [G]
315. Fairbank JA, Friedman MJ, Southwick SM: Veterans of armed conflicts, in The Mental Health Consequences of Torture. Edited by Gerrity ET, Keane TM, Tuma F. New York, Kluwer Academic/Plenum, 2001, pp 121–131 [G]
316. McLeod JD, Kessler RC: Socioeconomic status differences in vulnerability to undesirable life events. J Health Soc Behav 1990; 31:162–172 [C]
317. Bremner JD, Southwick SM, Johnson DR, Yehuda R, Charney DS: Childhood physical abuse and combat-related posttraumatic stress disorder in Vietnam veterans. Am J Psychiatry 1993; 150:235–239 [D]
318. Matsunaga Vietnam Veterans Project. White River Junction, Vt, National Center for Post-Traumatic Stress Disorder and the National Center for American Indian and Alaska Native Mental Health Research, 1996 [C]
319. Beals J, Manson SM, Shore JH, Friedman M, Ashcraft M, Fairbank JA, Schlenger WE: The prevalence of posttraumatic stress disorder among American Indian Vietnam veterans: disparities and context. J Trauma Stress 2002; 15:89–97 [F]
320. Ruef AM, Litz BT, Schlenger WE: Hispanic ethnicity and risk for combat-related posttraumatic stress disorder. Cultur Divers Ethnic Minor Psychol 2000; 6:235–251 [F]
321. Ortega AN, Rosenheck R: Posttraumatic stress disorder among Hispanic Vietnam veterans. Am J Psychiatry 2000; 157:615–619 [E]
322. Schnyder U, Moergeli H, Klaghofer R, Buddeberg C: Incidence and prediction of posttraumatic stress disorder symptoms in severely injured accident victims. Am J Psychiatry 2001; 158:594–599 [C]

323. Malt U: The long-term psychiatric consequences of accidental injury: a longitudinal study of 107 adults. Br J Psychiatry 1988; 153:810–818 [C]
324. Harvey AG, Bryant RA: The relationship between acute stress disorder and posttraumatic stress disorder: a prospective evaluation of motor vehicle accident survivors. J Consult Clin Psychol 1998; 66:507–512 [C]
325. Shalev AY, Peri T, Canetti L, Schreiber S: Predictors of PTSD in injured trauma survivors: a prospective study. Am J Psychiatry 1996; 153:219–225 [C]
326. Mayou R, Bryant B, Duthie R: Psychiatric consequences of road traffic accidents. BMJ 1993; 307:647–651 [C]
327. Michaels AJ, Michaels CE, Moon CH, Smith JS, Zimmerman MA, Taheri PA, Peterson C: Posttraumatic stress disorder after injury: impact on general health outcome and early risk assessment. J Trauma 1999; 47:460–466 [C]
328. Mellman TA, David D, Bustamante V, Fins AI, Esposito K: Predictors of post-traumatic stress disorder following severe injury. Depress Anxiety 2001; 14:226–231 [C]
329. O'Donnell ML, Creamer M, Bryant RA, Schnyder U, Shalev A: Posttraumatic disorders following injury: empirical and methodological review. Clin Psychol Rev 2003; 23:587–603 [E]
330. Bleich A, Gelkopf M, Solomon Z: Exposure to terrorism, stress-related mental health symptoms, and coping behaviors among a nationally representative sample in Israel. JAMA 2003; 290:612–620 [G]
331. Sabin M, Lopes Cardozo B, Nackerud L, Kaiser R, Varese L: Factors associated with poor mental health among Guatemalan refugees living in Mexico 20 years after civil conflict. JAMA 2003; 290:635–642 [G]
332. de Jong JT, Komproe IH, Van Ommeren M, El Masri M, Araya M, Khaled N, van De Put W, Somasundaram D: Lifetime events and posttraumatic stress disorder in 4 postconflict settings. JAMA 2001; 286:555–562 [C]
333. Kinzie JD, Boehnlein JK, Leung PK, Moore LJ, Riley C, Smith D: The prevalence of posttraumatic stress disorder and its clinical significance among Southeast Asian refugees. Am J Psychiatry 1990; 147:913–917 [G]
334. US Department of Health and Human Services: Mental Health: A Report of the Surgeon General. Rockville, Md, US Department of Health and Human Services, 1999 [C]
335. Kroll J, Habenicht M, Mackenzie T, Yang M, Chan S, Vang T, Nguyen T, Ly M, Phommasouvanh B, Nguyen H, Vang Y, Souvannasoth L, Cabugao R: Depression and posttraumatic stress disorder in Southeast Asian refugees. Am J Psychiatry 1989; 146:1592–1597 [C]
336. Blair RG: Risk factors associated with PTSD and major depression among Cambodian refugees in Utah. Health Soc Work 2000; 25:23–30 [C]
337. Caspi Y, Poole C, Mollica RF, Frankel M: Relationship of child loss to psychiatric and functional impairment in resettled Cambodian refugees. J Nerv Ment Dis 1998; 186:484–491 [G]
338. Kinzie JD, Sack W, Angell R, Clarke G, Ben R: A three-year follow-up of Cambodian young people traumatized as children. J Am Acad Child Adolesc Psychiatry 1989; 28:501–504 [C]
339. Chung RC, Kagawa-Singer M: Predictors of psychological distress among Southeast Asian refugees. Soc Sci Med 1993; 36:631–639 [G]
340. Farias P: Central and South American refugees: some mental health challenges, in Amidst Peril and Pain: The Mental Health and Well Being of the World's Refugees. Edited by Marsella AJ, Bornemann T, Ekblad S, Orley J. Washington, DC, American Psychological Association, 1994, pp 101–113 [G]
341. Cervantes RC, Salgado de Snyder VN, Padilla AM: Posttraumatic stress in immigrants from Central America and Mexico. Hosp Community Psychiatry 1989; 40:615–619 [D]
342. Michultka D, Blanchard EB, Kalous T: Responses to civilian war experiences: predictors of psychological functioning and coping. J Trauma Stress 1998; 11:571–577 [G]

343. Arroyo W, Eth S: Children traumatized by Central American warfare, in Posttraumatic Stress Disorder in Children. Edited by Eth S, Pynoos RS. Washington, DC, American Psychiatric Press, 1984, pp 103–117 [G]
344. Eisenman DP, Gelberg L, Liu H, Shapiro MF: Mental health and health-related quality of life among adult Latino primary care patients living in the United States with previous exposure to political violence. JAMA 2003; 290:627–634 [G]
345. Blanchard EB, Hickling EJ, Barton KA, Taylor AE, Loos WR, Jones-Alexander J: One-year prospective follow-up of motor vehicle accident victims. Behav Res Ther 1996; 34:775–786 [C]
346. Tedeschi RG, Calhoun LG: The Posttraumatic Growth Inventory: measuring the positive legacy of trauma. J Trauma Stress 1996; 9:455–471 [G]
347. Herman JL, Perry JC, van der Kolk BA: Childhood trauma in borderline personality disorder. Am J Psychiatry 1989; 146:490–495 [D]
348. Perry JC, Herman HL, van der Kolk BA, Holk LA: Psychotherapy and psychological trauma in borderline personality disorder. Psychiatr Ann 1990; 20:33–43 [G]
349. Pollack MH, Otto MW, Rosenbaum JF, Sachs GS: Personality disorders in patients with panic disorder: association with childhood anxiety disorders, early trauma, comorbidity, and chronicity. Compr Psychiatry 1992; 33:78–83 [C]
350. Zatzick DF, Weiss DS, Marmar CR, Metzler TJ, Wells K, Golding JM, Stewart A, Schlenger WE, Browner WS: Post-traumatic stress disorder and functioning and quality of life outcomes in female Vietnam veterans. Mil Med 1997; 162:661–665 [C]
351. Mendlowicz MV, Stein MB: Quality of life in individuals with anxiety disorders. Am J Psychiatry 2000; 157:669–682 [F]
352. Bryant RA, Marosszeky JE, Crooks J, Baguley IJ, Gurka JA: Posttraumatic stress disorder and psychosocial functioning after severe traumatic brain injury. J Nerv Ment Dis 2001; 189:109–113 [C]
353. Zayfert C, Dums AR, Ferguson RJ, Hegel MT: Health functioning impairments associated with posttraumatic stress disorder, anxiety disorders, and depression. J Nerv Ment Dis 2002; 190:233–240 [C]
354. Beckham JC, Moore SD, Feldman ME, Hertzberg MA, Kirby AC, Fairbank JA: Health status, somatization, and severity of posttraumatic stress disorder in Vietnam combat veterans with posttraumatic stress disorder. Am J Psychiatry 1998; 155:1565–1569 [C]
355. Boscarino JA: Diseases among men 20 years after exposure to severe stress: implications for clinical research and medical care. Psychosom Med 1997; 59:605–614 [C]
356. Greenberg PE, Sisitsky T, Kessler RC, Finkelstein SN, Berndt ER, Davidson JR, Ballenger JC, Fyer AJ: The economic burden of anxiety disorders in the 1990s. J Clin Psychiatry 1999; 60:427–435 [E]
357. Livanou M, Basoglu M, Marks IM, De SP, Noshirvani H, Lovell K, Thrasher S: Beliefs, sense of control and treatment outcome in post-traumatic stress disorder. Psychol Med 2002; 32:157–165 [A]
358. Krupnick JL: Brief psychodynamic treatment of PTSD. J Clin Psychol 2002; 58:919–932 [G]
359. Plakun EM, Shapiro ER: Psychodynamic psychotherapy for PTSD. J Clin Psychiatry 2000; 61:787–788 [F]
360. Lansky MR: The transformation of affect in posttraumatic nightmares. Bull Menninger Clin 1991; 55:470–490 [G]
361. Peniston EG: EMG biofeedback-assisted desensitization treatment for Vietnam combat veterans' post-traumatic stress disorder. Clinical Biofeedback and Health 1986; 9:35–41 [A–]
362. Keane TM, Fairbank JA, Caddell JM, Zimering RT: Implosive (flooding) therapy reduces symptoms of PTSD in Vietnam combat veterans. Behav Ther 1989; 20:245–260 [A–]
363. Cooper NA, Clum GA: Imaginal flooding as a supplementary treatment for PTSD in combat veterans: a controlled study. Behav Ther 1989; 20:381–391 [B]

364. Boudewyns PA, Hyer L: Physiological response to combat memories and preliminary treatment outcome in Vietnam veteran PTSD patients treated with direct therapeutic exposure. Behav Ther 1990; 21:63–87 [A–]
365. Boudewyns PA, Hyer L, Woods MG, Harrison WR, McCranie E: PTSD among Vietnam veterans: an early look at treatment outcome using direct therapeutic exposure. J Trauma Stress 1990; 3:359–368 [B]
366. Richards DA, Lovell K, Marks IM: Post-traumatic stress disorder: evaluation of a behavioral treatment program. J Trauma Stress 1994; 7:669–680 [A–]
367. Rothbaum BO, Hodges LF: The use of virtual reality exposure in the treatment of anxiety disorders. Behav Modif 1999; 23:507–525 [G]
368. Rothbaum BO, Hodges LF, Ready D, Graap K, Alarcon RD: Virtual reality exposure therapy for Vietnam veterans with posttraumatic stress disorder. J Clin Psychiatry 2001; 62:617–622 [B]
369. Krakow B, Hollifield M, Schrader R, Koss M, Tandberg D, Lauriello J, McBride L, Warner TD, Cheng D, Edmond T, Kellner R: A controlled study of imagery rehearsal for chronic nightmares in sexual assault survivors with PTSD: a preliminary report. J Trauma Stress 2000; 13:589–609 [A–]
370. Forbes D, Phelps AJ, McHugh AF, Debenham P, Hopwood M, Creamer M: Imagery rehearsal in the treatment of posttraumatic nightmares in Australian veterans with chronic combat-related PTSD: 12-month follow-up data. J Trauma Stress 2003; 16:509–513 [B]
371. Falsetti SA, Resnick HS, Davis HJ, Gallagher NG: Treatment of posttraumatic stress disorder with comorbid panic attacks: combining cognitive processing therapy with panic control treatment techniques. Group Dynamics 2001; 5:252–260 [A]
372. Glynn SM, Eth S, Randolph ET, Foy DW, Urbaitis M, Boxer L, Paz GG, Leong GB, Firman G, Salk JD, Katzman JW, Crothers J: A test of behavioral family therapy to augment exposure for combat-related posttraumatic stress disorder. J Consult Clin Psychol 1999; 67:243–251 [A–]
373. Fecteau G, Nicki R: Cognitive behavioural treatment of posttraumatic stress disorder after motor vehicle accident. Behavioural and Cognitive Psychotherapy 1999; 27:201–214 [E]
374. Foa EB, Rothbaum BO, Riggs DS, Murdock TB: Treatment of posttraumatic stress disorder in rape victims: a comparison between cognitive-behavioral procedures and counseling. J Consult Clin Psychol 1991; 59:715–723 [A]
375. Echeburua E, de Corral P, Zubizarreta I, Sarasua B: Psychological treatment of chronic posttraumatic stress disorder in victims of sexual aggression. Behav Modif 1997; 21:433–456 [A–]
376. Silver SM, Brooks A, Obenchain J: Treatment of Vietnam War veterans with PTSD: a comparison of eye movement desensitization and reprocessing, biofeedback, and relaxation training. J Trauma Stress 1995; 8:337–342 [B]
377. Paunovic N, Ost LG: Cognitive-behavior therapy vs exposure therapy in the treatment of PTSD in refugees. Behav Res Ther 2001; 39:1183–1197 [A–]
378. Chemtob CM, Novaco RW, Hamada RS, Gross DM: Cognitive-behavioral treatment for severe anger in posttraumatic stress disorder. J Consult Clin Psychol 1997; 65:184–189 [A–]
379. Foa EB, Hearst-Ikeda D, Perry KJ: Evaluation of a brief cognitive-behavioral program for the prevention of chronic PTSD in recent assault victims. J Consult Clin Psychol 1995; 63:948–955 [B]
380. Gillespie K, Duffy M, Hackmann A, Clark DM: Community based cognitive therapy in the treatment of posttraumatic stress disorder following the Omagh bomb. Behav Res Ther 2002; 40:345–357 [B]
381. Ehlers A, Clark D: Early psychological interventions for adult survivors of trauma: a review. Biol Psychiatry 2003; 53:817–826 [F]

382. Marcus SV: Controlled study of treatment of PTSD using EMDR in an HMO setting. Psychotherapy 1997; 34:307–315 [A–]
383. Rothbaum BO: A controlled study of eye movement desensitization and reprocessing in the treatment of posttraumatic stress disordered sexual assault victims. Bull Menninger Clin 1997; 61:317–334 [A–]
384. Scheck MM, Schaeffer JA, Gillette C: Brief psychological intervention with traumatized young women: the efficacy of eye movement desensitization and reprocessing. J Trauma Stress 1998; 11:25–44 [A–]
385. Wilson SA, Becker LA, Tinker RH: Eye movement desensitization and reprocessing (EMDR) treatment for psychologically traumatized individuals. J Consult Clin Psychol 1995; 63:928–937 [A–]
386. Wilson SA, Becker LA, Tinker RH: Fifteen-month follow-up of eye movement desensitization and reprocessing (EMDR) treatment for posttraumatic stress disorder and psychological trauma. J Consult Clin Psychol 1997; 65:1047–1056 [C]
387. Ironson G, Freund B, Strauss JL, Williams J: Comparison of two treatments for traumatic stress: a community-based study of EMDR and prolonged exposure. J Clin Psychol 2002; 58:113–128 [A–]
388. Devilly GJ, Spence SH, Rapee RM: Statistical and reliable change with eye movement desensitization and reprocessing: treating trauma within a veteran population. Behav Ther 1998; 29:435–455 [A]
389. Macklin ML, Metzger LJ, Lasko NB, Berry NJ, Orr SP, Pitman RK: Five-year follow-up study of eye movement desensitization and reprocessing therapy for combat-related posttraumatic stress disorder. Compr Psychiatry 2000; 41:24–27 [B]
390. Cusack K, Spates CR: The cognitive dismantling of eye movement desensitization and reprocessing (EMDR) treatment of posttraumatic stress disorder (PTSD). J Anxiety Disord 1999; 13:87–99 [A–]
391. Classen C, Butler LD, Koopman C, Miller E, DiMiceli S, Giese-Davis J, Fobair P, Carlson RW, Kraemer HC, Spiegel D: Supportive-expressive group therapy and distress in patients with metastatic breast cancer: a randomized clinical intervention trial. Arch Gen Psychiatry 2001; 58:494–501 [F]
392. Zlotnick C, Shea TM, Rosen K, Simpson E, Mulrenin K, Begin A, Pearlstein T: An affect-management group for women with posttraumatic stress disorder and histories of childhood sexual abuse. J Trauma Stress 1997; 10:425–436 [A]
393. Schnurr PP, Friedman MJ, Foy DW, Shea MT, Hsieh FY, Lavori PW, Glynn SM, Wattenberg M, Bernardy NC: Randomized trial of trauma-focused group therapy for posttraumatic stress disorder: results from a Department of Veterans Affairs cooperative study. Arch Gen Psychiatry 2003; 60:481–489 [A–]
394. Zoellner LA, Feeny NC, Cochran B, Pruitt L: Treatment choice for PTSD. Behav Res Ther 2003; 41:879–886 [C]
395. Foa EB, Zoellner LA, Feeny NC, Hembree EA, Alvarez-Conrad J: Does imaginal exposure exacerbate PTSD symptoms? J Consult Clin Psychol 2002; 70:1022–1028 [D]
396. Bradley RG, Follingstad DR: Group therapy for incarcerated women who experienced interpersonal violence: a pilot study. J Trauma Stress 2003; 16:337–340 [A–]
397. Drozdek B: Follow-up study of concentration camp survivors from Bosnia-Herzegovina: three years later. J Nerv Ment Dis 1997; 185:690–694 [G]
398. Cloitre M, Koenen KC: The impact of borderline personality disorder on process group outcome among women with posttraumatic stress disorder related to childhood abuse. Int J Group Psychother 2001; 51:379–398 [A–]
399. Vaa G, Egner R, Sexton H: Sexually abused women after multimodal group therapy: a long-term follow-up study. Nord J Psychiatry 2002; 56:215–221 [B]

400. Vandeusen KM, Carr JL: Recovery from sexual assault: an innovative two-stage group therapy model. Int J Group Psychother 2003; 53:201–223 [G]
401. Busuttil W, Turnbull GJ, Neal LA, Rollins J, West AG, Blanch N, Herepath R: Incorporating psychological debriefing techniques within a brief group psychotherapy programme for the treatment of post-traumatic stress disorder. Br J Psychiatry 1995; 167:495–502 [B]
402. Murphy SA: A bereavement intervention for parents following the sudden, violent deaths of their 12–28-year-old children: description and applications to clinical practice. Can J Nurs Res 1997; 29:51–72 [B]
403. Foy DW, Glynn SM, Schnurr PP, Jankowski MK, Wattenberg MS, Weiss DS, Marmar CR, Gusman GD: Group psychotherapy, in Effective Treatments for PTSD: Practical Guidelines From the International Society for Traumatic Stress Studies. Edited by Foa EB, Keane TM, Friedman MJ. New York, Guilford, 2000, pp 155–175 [F]
404. Cohen JA, Mannarino AP: A treatment outcome study for sexually abused preschool children: initial findings. J Am Acad Child Adolesc Psychiatry 1996; 35:42–50 [A]
405. Cohen JA, Mannarino AP: Factors that mediate treatment outcome of sexually abused preschool children: six- and 12-month follow-up. J Am Acad Child Adolesc Psychiatry 1998; 37:44–51 [B]
406. March JS, Amaya-Jackson L, Murray MC, Schulte A: Cognitive-behavioral psychotherapy for children and adolescents with posttraumatic stress disorder after a single-incident stressor. J Am Acad Child Adolesc Psychiatry 1998; 37:585–593 [B]
407. Saltzman WR, Pynoos RS, Layne CM, Steinberg A, Aisenberg E: School-based trauma/grief group psychotherapy program for youth exposed to community violence. Group Dynamics 2001; 5:291–303 [B]
408. Davies DR, Burlingame GM, Layne CM: Integrating small group process principles into trauma-focused group psychotherapy: what should a group trauma therapist know? in Group Approaches for Psychological Effects of Terrorist Disasters. Edited by Schein LA, Burlingame GM, Spitz HI, Muskin PR. New York, Haworth (in press) [G]
409. Rose S, Brewin CR, Andrews B, Kirk M: A randomized controlled trial of individual psychological debriefing for victims of violent crime. Psychol Med 1999; 29:793–799 [A–]
410. Carlier IV, Voerman AE, Gersons BP: The influence of occupational debriefing on posttraumatic stress symptomatology in traumatized police officers. Br J Med Psychol 2000; 73(pt 1):87–98 [A]
411. Deahl M, Srinivasan M, Jones N, Thomas J, Neblett C, Jolly A: Preventing psychological trauma in soldiers: the role of operational stress training and psychological debriefing. Br J Med Psychol 2000; 73(pt 1):77–85 [A]
412. Campfield KM, Hills AM: Effect of timing of critical incident stress debriefing (CISD) on posttraumatic symptoms. J Trauma Stress 2001; 14:327–340 [B]
413. Lange A, van de Ven JP, Schrieken B, Emmelkamp PM: Interapy, treatment of posttraumatic stress through the Internet: a controlled trial. J Behav Ther Exp Psychiatry 2001; 32:73–90 [A]
414. Lange A, Rietdijk D, Hudcovicova M, van de Ven JP, Schrieken B, Emmelkamp PM: Interapy: a controlled randomized trial of the standardized treatment of posttraumatic stress through the Internet. J Consult Clin Psychol 2003; 71:901–909 [A]
415. Ragsdale KG, Cox RD, Finn P, Eisler RM: Effectiveness of short-term specialized inpatient treatment for war-related posttraumatic stress disorder: a role for adventure-based counseling and psychodrama. J Trauma Stress 1996; 9:269–283 [B]
416. Hyer L, Boyd S, Scurfield R, Smith D, Burke J: Effects of Outward Bound experience as an adjunct to inpatient PTSD treatment of war veterans. J Clin Psychol 1996; 52:263–278 [B]
417. Gidron Y, Peri T, Connolly JF, Shalev AY: Written disclosure in posttraumatic stress disorder: is it beneficial for the patient? J Nerv Ment Dis 1996; 184:505–507 [A]
418. Reynolds M, Tarrier N: Monitoring of intrusions in post-traumatic stress order: a report of single case studies. Br J Med Psychol 1996; 69(pt 4):371–379 [G]

419. Silver SM, Wilson JP: Native American healing and purification rituals for war stress, in Human Adaptation to Extreme Stress: From the Holocaust to Vietnam. Edited by Wilson JP, Kahana B. New York, Plenum, 1989, pp 337–355 [G]
420. Zatzick DF, Johnson FA: Alternative psychotherapeutic practice among middle class Americans, I: case studies and follow-up. Cult Med Psychiatry 1997; 21:53–88 [G]
421. Davidson JR, Rothbaum BO, van der Kolk BA, Sikes CR, Farfel GM: Multicenter, double-blind comparison of sertraline and placebo in the treatment of posttraumatic stress disorder. Arch Gen Psychiatry 2001; 58:485–492 [A]
422. Davis LL, Nugent AL, Murray J, Kramer GL, Petty F: Nefazodone treatment for chronic posttraumatic stress disorder: an open trial. J Clin Psychopharmacol 2000; 20:159–164 [B]
423. Hidalgo R, Hertzberg MA, Mellman T, Petty F, Tucker P, Weisler R, Zisook S, Chen S, Churchill E, Davidson J: Nefazodone in post-traumatic stress disorder: results from six open-label trials. Int Clin Psychopharmacol 1999; 14:61–68 [E]
424. Zisook S, Chentsova-Dutton YE, Smith-Vaniz A, Kline NA, Ellenor GL, Kodsi AB, Gillin JC: Nefazodone in patients with treatment-refractory posttraumatic stress disorder. J Clin Psychiatry 2000; 61:203–208 [B]
425. Neylan TC, Lenoci M, Maglione ML, Rosenlicht NZ, Leykin Y, Metzler TJ, Schoenfeld FB, Marmar CR: The effect of nefazodone on subjective and objective sleep quality in posttraumatic stress disorder. J Clin Psychiatry 2003; 64:445–450 [B]
426. Mellman TA, David D, Barza L: Nefazodone treatment and dream reports in chronic PTSD. Depress Anxiety 1999; 9:146–148 [B]
427. Hertzberg MA, Feldman ME, Beckham JC, Davidson JR: Trial of trazodone for posttraumatic stress disorder using a multiple baseline group design. J Clin Psychopharmacol 1996; 16:294–298 [B]
428. Canive JM, Clark RD, Calais LA, Qualls C, Tuason VB: Bupropion treatment in veterans with posttraumatic stress disorder: an open study. J Clin Psychopharmacol 1998; 18:379–383 [B]
429. Smajkic A, Weine S, Djuric-Bijedic Z, Boskailo E, Lewis J, Pavkovic I: Sertraline, paroxetine, and venlafaxine in refugee posttraumatic stress disorder with depression symptoms. J Trauma Stress 2001; 14:445–452 [B]
430. Connor KM, Davidson JR, Weisler RH, Ahearn E: A pilot study of mirtazapine in post-traumatic stress disorder. Int Clin Psychopharmacol 1999; 14:29–31 [B]
431. Davidson JR, Weisler RH, Butterfield MI, Casat CD, Connor KM, Barnett S, van Meter S: Mirtazapine vs placebo in posttraumatic stress disorder: a pilot trial. Biol Psychiatry 2003; 53:188–191 [A]
432. Southwick SM, Yehuda R, Giller EL Jr, Charney DS: Use of tricyclics and monoamine oxidase inhibitors in the treatment of PTSD: a quantitative review, in Catecholamine Function in Post-Traumatic Stress Disorder: Emerging Concepts. Edited by Murburg MM. Washington, DC, American Psychiatric Press, 1994, pp 293–305 [E]
433. Robert R, Blakeney PE, Villarreal C, Rosenberg L, Meyer WJ 3rd: Imipramine treatment in pediatric burn patients with symptoms of acute stress disorder: a pilot study. J Am Acad Child Adolesc Psychiatry 1999; 38:873–882 [A]
434. Neal LA, Shapland W, Fox C: An open trial of moclobemide in the treatment of post-traumatic stress disorder. Int Clin Psychopharmacol 1997; 12:231–237 [B]
435. Katz RJ, Lott MH, Arbus P, Crocq L, Herlobsen P, Lingjaerde O, Lopez G, Loughrey GC, MacFarlane DJ, McIvor R, Mehlum L, Nugent D, Turner SW, Weisaeth L, Yule W: Pharmacotherapy of post-traumatic stress disorder with a novel psychotropic. Anxiety 1994–1995; 1:169–174 [A]
436. Connor KM, Hidalgo RB, Crockett B, Malik M, Katz RJ, Davidson JR: Predictors of treatment response in patients with posttraumatic stress disorder. Prog Neuropsychopharmacol Biol Psychiatry 2001; 25:337–345 [E]

437. Braun P, Greenberg D, Dasberg H, Lerer B: Core symptoms of posttraumatic stress disorder unimproved by alprazolam treatment. J Clin Psychiatry 1990; 51:236–238 [A]
438. Mellman TA, Byers PM, Augenstein JS: Pilot evaluation of hypnotic medication during acute traumatic stress response. J Trauma Stress 1998; 11:563–569 [B]
439. Duffy JD, Malloy PF: Efficacy of buspirone in the treatment of posttraumatic stress disorder: an open trial. Ann Clin Psychiatry 1994; 6:33–37 [B]
440. Wells BG, Chu CC, Johnson R, Nasdahl C, Ayubi MA, Sewell E, Statham P: Buspirone in the treatment of posttraumatic stress disorder. Pharmacotherapy 1991; 11:340–343 [B]
441. Raskind MA, Thompson C, Petrie EC, Dobie DJ, Rein RJ, Hoff DJ, McFall ME, Peskind ER: Prazosin reduces nightmares in combat veterans with posttraumatic stress disorder. J Clin Psychiatry 2002; 63:565–568 [B]
442. Jacobs-Rebhun S, Schnurr PP, Friedman MJ, Peck R, Brophy M, Fuller D: Posttraumatic stress disorder and sleep difficulty. Am J Psychiatry 2000; 157:1525–1526 [A]
443. Clark RD, Canive JM, Calais LA, Qualls C, Brugger RD, Vosburgh TB: Cyproheptadine treatment of nightmares associated with posttraumatic stress disorder. J Clin Psychopharmacol 1999; 19:486–487 [B]
444. Kaplan Z, Amir M, Swartz M, Levine J: Inositol treatment of post-traumatic stress disorder. Anxiety 1996; 2:51–52 [A]
445. Schelling G: Effects of stress hormones on traumatic memory formation and the development of posttraumatic stress disorder in critically ill patients. Neurobiol Learn Mem 2002; 78:596–609 [E]
446. Schelling G, Briegel J, Roozendaal B, Stoll C, Rothenhausler HB, Kapfhammer HP: The effect of stress doses of hydrocortisone during septic shock on posttraumatic stress disorder in survivors. Biol Psychiatry 2001; 50:978–985 [B]
447. Saxe G, Stoddard F, Courtney D, Cunningham K, Chawla N, Sheridan R, King D, King L: Relationship between acute morphine and the course of PTSD in children with burns. J Am Acad Child Adolesc Psychiatry 2001; 40:915–921 [D]
448. Ehlers A, Clark DM, Hackmann A, McManus F, Fennell M, Herbert C, Mayou R: A randomized controlled trial of cognitive therapy, a self-help booklet, and repeated assessments as early interventions for posttraumatic stress disorder. Arch Gen Psychiatry 2003; 60:1024–1032 [A–]
449. Heim C, Newport DJ, Heit S, Graham YP, Wilcox M, Bonsall R, Miller AH, Nemeroff CB: Pituitary-adrenal and autonomic responses to stress in women after sexual and physical abuse in childhood. JAMA 2000; 284:592–597 [G]
450. Heim C, Nemeroff CB: The role of childhood trauma in the neurobiology of mood and anxiety disorders: preclinical and clinical studies. Biol Psychiatry 2001; 49:1023–1039 [F]
451. Charney DS: Psychobiological mechanisms of resilience and vulnerability: implications for successful adaptation to extreme stress. Am J Psychiatry 2004; 161:195–216 [G]
452. Zlotnick C, Franklin CL, Zimmerman M: Does "subthreshold" posttraumatic stress disorder have any clinical relevance? Compr Psychiatry 2002; 43:413–419 [D]
453. Weiss DS, Marmar CR, Schlenger WE, Fairbank JA, Jordan BK, Hough RL, Kulka RA: The prevalence of lifetime and partial post-traumatic stress disorder in Vietnam theater veterans. J Trauma Stress 1992; 5:365–376 [D]
454. Schutzwohl M, Maercker A: Effects of varying diagnostic criteria for posttraumatic stress disorder are endorsing the concept of partial PTSD. J Trauma Stress 1999; 12:155–165 [G]
455. Stein MB, Walker JR, Hazen AL, Forde DR: Full and partial posttraumatic stress disorder: findings from a community survey. Am J Psychiatry 1997; 154:1114–1119 [G]
456. Shear MK, Zuckoff A, Frank E: The syndrome of traumatic grief. CNS Spectrums 2001; 6:339–346 [G]
457. Taylor FB: Tiagabine for posttraumatic stress disorder: a case series of 7 women. J Clin Psychiatry 2003; 64:1421–1425 [G]

458. Foa EB, Rothbaum BO, Furr JM: Augmenting exposure therapy with other CBT procedures. Psychiatr Ann 2003; 33:47–53 [F]
459. Ross RJ, Ball WA, Dinges DF, Kribbs NB, Morrison AR, Silver SM, Mulvaney FD: Rapid eye movement sleep disturbance in posttraumatic stress disorder. Biol Psychiatry 1994; 35:195–202 [D]
460. Ross RJ, Ball WA, Sullivan KA, Caroff SN: Sleep disturbance as the hallmark of posttraumatic stress disorder. Am J Psychiatry 1989; 146:697–707 [G]
461. Pitman RK, Orr SP, Shalev AY, Metzger LJ, Mellman TA: Psychophysiological alterations in post-traumatic stress disorder. Semin Clin Neuropsychiatry 1999; 4:234–241 [G]
462. Rothbaum BO, Mellman TA: Dreams and exposure therapy in PTSD. J Trauma Stress 2001; 14:481–490 [F]
463. Foa EB, Riggs DS, Massie ED, Yarczower M: The impact of fear activation and anger on the efficacy of exposure treatment for posttraumatic stress disorder. Behav Ther 1995; 26:487–499 [C]

PRACTICE GUIDELINE FOR THE
Treatment of Patients With Eating Disorders
Third Edition

WORK GROUP ON EATING DISORDERS

Joel Yager, M.D., Chair
Michael J. Devlin, M.D.
Katherine A. Halmi, M.D.
David B. Herzog, M.D.
James E. Mitchell III, M.D.
Pauline Powers, M.D.
Kathryn J. Zerbe, M.D.

This practice guideline was approved in December 2005 and published in June 2006. A guideline watch, summarizing significant developments in the scientific literature since publication of this guideline, may be available in the Psychiatric Practice section of the APA web site at www.psych.org.

CONTENTS

Guide to Using This Practice Guideline 1101

Development Process 1102

Introduction 1103

Part A: Treatment Recommendations for Patients With Eating Disorders 1105

I. Executive Summary 1105
  A. Coding System 1105
  B. Executive Summary 1105

II. Formulation and Implementation of a Treatment Plan 1116
  A. Psychiatric Management 1116
  B. Developing a Treatment Plan for the Individual Patient 1129

III. Clinical Features Influencing the Treatment Plan 1151
  A. Chronicity of Eating Disorders 1151
  B. Other Psychiatric Factors 1152
  C. Concurrent General Medical Conditions 1154
  D. Demographic Variables 1155

Part B: Background Information and Review of Available Evidence 1160

IV. Disease Definition, Epidemiology, and Natural History 1160
  A. Disease Definition 1160
  B. Epidemiology 1163
  C. Natural History and Course 1164
  D. Genetic Factors 1167

V. Review and Synthesis of Available Evidence 1168
  A. Treatment of Anorexia Nervosa 1169
  B. Treatment of Bulimia Nervosa 1175
  C. Treatment of Binge Eating Disorder 1179

Part C: Future Research Needs 1181

Individuals and Organizations That Submitted Comments 1184

References 1185

GUIDE TO USING THIS PRACTICE GUIDELINE

The *Practice Guideline for the Treatment of Patients With Eating Disorders,* Third Edition, consists of three parts (A, B, and C) and many sections, not all of which will be equally useful for all readers. The following guide is designed to help readers find the sections that will be most useful to them.

Part A, "Treatment Recommendations," is published as a supplement to the *American Journal of Psychiatry* and contains general and specific treatment recommendations. Section I summarizes the key recommendations of the guideline and codes each recommendation according to the degree of clinical confidence with which the recommendation is made. Section II provides further discussion of the formulation and implementation of a treatment plan as it applies to the individual patient. Section III, "Clinical Features Influencing the Treatment Plan," discusses a range of clinical considerations that could alter the general recommendations discussed in Section I.

Part B, "Background Information and Review of Available Evidence," and Part C, "Future Research Needs," are not included in the *American Journal of Psychiatry* supplement but are provided with Part A in the complete guideline, which is available in print format from American Psychiatric Publishing, Inc. (http://www.appi.org), and online through the American Psychiatric Association (http://www.psych. org). Part B provides an overview of eating disorders, including general information on their natural history, course, and epidemiology. It also provides a structured review and synthesis of the evidence that underlies the recommendations made in Part A. Part C draws from the previous sections and summarizes areas for which more research data are needed to guide clinical decisions.

To share feedback on this or other published APA practice guidelines, a form is available at http:// www.psych.org/psych_pract/pg/reviewform.cfm.

DEVELOPMENT PROCESS

This practice guideline was developed under the auspices of the Steering Committee on Practice Guidelines. The development process is detailed in "APA Guideline Development Process," which is available from the APA Department of Quality Improvement and Psychiatric Services. The key features of this process include the following:

- A comprehensive literature review to identify all relevant randomized clinical trials as well as less rigorously designed clinical trials and case series when evidence from randomized trials was unavailable
- Development of evidence tables that summarized the key features of each identified study, including funding source, study design, sample sizes, subject characteristics, treatment characteristics, and treatment outcomes
- Initial drafting of the guideline by a work group that included psychiatrists with clinical and research expertise in eating disorders
- Production of multiple revised drafts with widespread review (10 organizations and 58 individuals submitted significant comments)
- Approval by the APA Assembly and Board of Trustees
- Planned revisions at regular intervals

A MEDLINE search, using PubMed, of "anorexia nervosa OR bulimia OR binge eating disorder OR binge eating disorders OR eating disorder OR eating disorders" yielded 15,561 citations, of which 3,596 were published between 1998 and 2004, were written in English, and contained abstracts. Of these, 334 were reports of clinical trials (including randomized controlled trials) or meta-analyses. Abstracts for these articles as well as abstracts for an additional 634 review articles were screened individually for their relevance to the guideline. The Cochrane Library was also searched for relevant abstracts. Additional, less formal literature searches were conducted by APA staff and individual members of the Work Group on Eating Disorders.

The recommendations contained in this practice guideline are based on the best available data and clinical consensus. The summary of treatment recommendations is keyed according to the level of confidence with which each recommendation is made (indicated by bracketed Roman numeral). In addition, each reference is followed by a bracketed letter that indicates the nature of the supporting evidence.

INTRODUCTION

As this practice guideline was developed and then reviewed by psychiatrists, researchers, and other clinicians throughout North America and Europe, a number of important general themes emerged. So that readers may better appreciate the recommendations of this guideline, the following points merit emphasis:

- **A diagnosis is presumed before the recommendations of this practice guideline apply.** Considerations for performing a detailed differential diagnosis are not included in this guideline. Special attention, however, is given to the treatment of eating disorders and common co-occurring conditions and clinical features (Section III).
- **The evidence base (including data and clinical experience) for the treatment of children and adolescents differs from that for adults.** APA practice guidelines are intended for the care of adults. However, because anorexia nervosa and bulimia nervosa often begin during adolescence and because clinicians commonly treat all ages spanning from childhood to adulthood, this guideline includes recommendations that apply to both age groups and notes if any recommendation applies exclusively to a certain age group.
- **There is a growing evidence base for the treatment of eating disorders; at the same time, there are many situations that arise in clinical care for which recommendations must be based on expert opinion and experience in the absence of data from randomized controlled trials or other systematic research studies.** This perspective is also recognized in guidelines for eating disorders available from other groups, notably the National Institute for Clinical Excellence (NICE) in England (1), the Royal Australian and New Zealand College of Psychiatrists (2), and the Society for Adolescent Medicine (3).
- **Well-conducted, small-scale studies that demonstrate the feasibility and effectiveness of a particular intervention cannot define community standards until clinicians trained in the application of that intervention are generally available.** For example, some innovative, university-based programs have demonstrated that specialized interventions can avert or reduce the length of inpatient stays for some patients with anorexia nervosa. However, the availability of such programs is limited, and it is unclear if results of small-scale studies of these interventions are generalizable to other settings and patient groups. The recommendations of this practice guideline are made with the recognition that it is inappropriate to refuse patients and families access to a more intensive treatment simply because a less intensive treatment has been demonstrated to be effective in a few small-scale studies.
- **Medical testing should be limited to that required for making clinical decisions for the individual patient.** Clinicians differ in their test-ordering patterns for various reasons. In general, this practice guideline recommends the performance of only those laboratory tests and procedures most likely needed for clinical decision making. In patients with eating disorders, many clinical parameters are likely to be abnormal; however, they typically normalize without specific attention as the patient's clinical condition improves. This guideline does not suggest ordering tests for all parameters.
- **Good clinical decisions regarding anorexia nervosa should not rely primarily on simplistic, artificial categories based on body weight percentages.** In making a diagnosis of anorexia nervosa, body weight is one of the factors that is taken into consideration. Various diagnostic criteria have suggested specific weight values that can be used as estimated thresholds for diagnosis. For example, DSM-IV-TR offers a weight of "less than 85% of that expected," whereas ICD-10 specifies weight "15% below that expected for health." Despite their

potential utility in defining reliable and valid diagnostic categories, such criteria are not strict or absolute, nor are they designed for use as thresholds in clinical care. This practice guideline concurs with the NICE guideline that states, "In anorexia nervosa, although weight and BMI are important indicators they should not be considered the sole indicators of physical risk (as they are unreliable in adults and especially in children)" (1, p. 10).

PART A

TREATMENT RECOMMENDATIONS FOR PATIENTS WITH EATING DISORDERS

I. EXECUTIVE SUMMARY

A. CODING SYSTEM

Each recommendation is identified as meriting one of three categories of endorsement, based on the level of clinical confidence regarding the recommendation, as indicated by a bracketed Roman numeral after the statement. The three categories are as follows:

[I] Recommended with substantial clinical confidence
[II] Recommended with moderate clinical confidence
[III] May be recommended on the basis of individual circumstances

B. EXECUTIVE SUMMARY

1. Psychiatric management

Psychiatric management begins with the establishment of a therapeutic alliance, which is enhanced by empathic comments and behaviors, positive regard, reassurance, and support [I]. Basic psychiatric management includes support through the provision of educational materials, including self-help workbooks; information on community-based and Internet resources; and direct advice to patients and their families (if they are involved) [I]. A team approach is the recommended model of care [I].

a) Coordinating care and collaborating with other clinicians

In treating adults with eating disorders, the psychiatrist may assume the leadership role within a program or team that includes other physicians, psychologists, registered dietitians, and social workers or may work collaboratively on a team led by others. For the management of acute and ongoing medical and dental complications, it is important that psychiatrists consult other physician specialists and dentists [I].

When a patient is managed by an interdisciplinary team in an outpatient setting, communication among the professionals is essential to monitoring the patient's progress, making necessary adjustments to the treatment plan, and delineating the specific roles and tasks of each team member [I].

b) Assessing and monitoring eating disorder symptoms and behaviors

A careful assessment of the patient's history, symptoms, behaviors, and mental status is the first step in making a diagnosis of an eating disorder [I]. The complete assessment usually requires at least several hours and includes a thorough review of the patient's height and weight history; restrictive and binge eating and exercise patterns and their changes; purging and other compensatory behaviors; core attitudes regarding weight, shape, and eating; and associated psychiatric conditions [I]. A family history of eating disorders or other psychiatric disorders, including alcohol and other substance use disorders; a family history of obesity; family interactions in relation to the patient's disorder; and family attitudes toward eating, exercise, and appearance are all relevant to the assessment [I]. A clinician's articulation of theories that imply blame or permit family members to blame one another or themselves can alienate family members from involvement in the treatment and therefore be detrimental to the patient's care and recovery [I]. It is important to identify family stressors whose amelioration may facilitate recovery [I]. In the assessment of children and adolescents, it is essential to involve parents and, whenever appropriate, school personnel and health professionals who routinely work with the patient [I].

c) Assessing and monitoring the patient's general medical condition

A full physical examination of the patient is strongly recommended and may be performed by a physician familiar with common findings in patients with eating disorders. The examination should give particular attention to vital signs, physical status (including height and weight), cardiovascular and peripheral vascular function, dermatological manifestations, and evidence of self-injurious behaviors [I]. Calculation of the patient's body mass index (BMI) is also useful (see http://www.cdc.gov/nccdphp/dnpa/bmi/00binaries/bmi-tables.pdf [for ages 2–20] and http://www.cdc.gov/nccdphp/dnpa/bmi/00binaries/bmi-adults.pdf [for adults]) [I]. Early recognition of eating disorder symptoms and early intervention may prevent an eating disorder from becoming chronic [I]. During treatment, it is important to monitor the patient for shifts in weight, blood pressure, pulse, other cardiovascular parameters, and behaviors likely to provoke physiological decline and collapse [I]. Patients with a history of purging behaviors should also be referred for a dental examination [I]. Bone density examinations should be obtained for patients who have been amenorrheic for 6 months or more [I].

In younger patients, examination should include growth pattern, sexual development (including sexual maturity rating), and general physical development [I]. The need for laboratory analyses should be determined on an individual basis depending on the patient's condition or the laboratory tests' relevance to making treatment decisions [I].

d) Assessing and monitoring the patient's safety and psychiatric status

The patient's safety will be enhanced when particular attention is given to suicidal ideation, plans, intentions, and attempts as well as to impulsive and compulsive self-harm behaviors [I]. Other aspects of the patient's psychiatric status that greatly influence clinical course and outcome and that are important to assess include mood, anxiety, and substance use disorders, as well as motivational status, personality traits, and personality disorders [I]. Assessment for suicidality is of particular importance in patients with co-occurring alcohol and other substance use disorders [I].

e) Providing family assessment and treatment

For children and adolescents with anorexia nervosa, family involvement and treatment are essential [I]. For older patients, family assessment and involvement may be useful and should be considered on a case-by-case basis [II]. Involving spouses and partners in treatment may be highly desirable [II].

2. Choosing a treatment site

Services available for treating eating disorders can range from intensive inpatient programs (in which general medical care is readily available) to residential and partial hospitalization programs to varying levels of outpatient care (in which the patient receives general medical treatment, nutritional counseling, and/or individual, group, and family psychotherapy). Because specialized programs are not available in all geographic areas and their financial requirements are often significant, access to these programs may be limited; petition, explanation, and follow-up by the psychiatrist on behalf of patients and families may help procure access to these programs. Pretreatment evaluation of the patient is essential in choosing the appropriate treatment setting [I].

In determining a patient's initial level of care or whether a change to a different level of care is appropriate, it is important to consider the patient's overall physical condition, psychology, behaviors, and social circumstances rather than simply rely on one or more physical parameters, such as weight [I]. Weight in relation to estimated individually healthy weight, the rate of weight loss, cardiac function, and metabolic status are the most important physical parameters to be considered when choosing a treatment setting; other psychosocial parameters are also important [I]. Healthy weight estimates for a given individual must be determined by that person's physicians [I]. Such estimates may be based on historical considerations (often including that person's growth charts) and, for women, the weight at which healthy menstruation and ovulation resume, which may be higher than the weight at which menstruation and ovulation became impaired. Admission to or continuation of an intensive level of care (e.g., hospitalization) may be necessary when access to a less intensive level of care (e.g., partial hospitalization) is absent because of geography or a lack of resources [I].

Generally, adult patients who weigh less than approximately 85% of their individually estimated healthy weights have considerable difficulty gaining weight outside of a highly structured program [II]. Such programs, including inpatient care, may be medically and psychiatrically necessary even for some patients who are above 85% of their individually estimated healthy weight [I]. Factors suggesting that hospitalization may be appropriate include rapid or persistent decline in oral intake, a decline in weight despite maximally intensive outpatient or partial hospitalization interventions, the presence of additional stressors that may interfere with the patient's ability to eat, knowledge of the weight at which instability previously occurred in the patient, co-occurring psychiatric problems that merit hospitalization, and the degree of the patient's denial and resistance to participate in his or her own care in less intensively supervised settings [I].

Hospitalization should occur before the onset of medical instability as manifested by abnormalities in vital signs (e.g., marked orthostatic hypotension with an increase in pulse of 20 bpm or a drop in standing blood pressure of 20 mmHg, bradycardia <40 bpm, tachycardia >110 bpm, or an inability to sustain core body temperature), physical findings, or laboratory tests [I]. To avert potentially irreversible effects on physical growth and development, many children and adolescents require inpatient medical treatment, even when weight loss, although rapid, has not been as severe as that suggesting a need for hospitalization in adult patients [I].

Patients who are physiologically stabilized on acute medical units will still require specific inpatient treatment for eating disorders if they do not meet biopsychosocial criteria for less intensive levels of care and/or if no suitable less intensive levels of care are accessible because of geographic or other reasons [I]. Weight level per se should never be used as the sole criterion for discharge from inpatient care [I]. Assisting patients in determining and practicing appropriate food intake at a healthy body weight is likely to decrease the chances of their relapsing after discharge [I].

In shifting between levels of care, it is important to establish continuity of care [II]. If the patient is going from one treatment setting or locale to another, transition planning requires that the care team in the new setting or locale be identified and that specific patient appointments be made [I]. It is preferable that a specific clinician on the team be designated as the primary coordinator of care to ensure continuity and attention to important aspects of treatment [II].

Most patients with uncomplicated bulimia nervosa do not require hospitalization; indications for the hospitalization of such patients include severe disabling symptoms that have not responded to adequate trials of outpatient treatment, serious concurrent general medical problems (e.g., metabolic abnormalities, hematemesis, vital sign changes, uncontrolled vomiting), suicidality, psychiatric disturbances that would warrant the patient's hospitalization independent of the eating disorder diagnosis, or severe concurrent alcohol or drug dependence or abuse [I].

Legal interventions, including involuntary hospitalization and legal guardianship, may be necessary to address the safety of treatment-reluctant patients whose general medical conditions are life threatening [I].

The decision about whether a patient should be hospitalized on a psychiatric versus a general medical or adolescent/pediatric unit should be made based on the patient's general medical and psychiatric status, the skills and abilities of local psychiatric and general medical staff, and the availability of suitable programs to care for the patient's general medical and psychiatric problems [I]. There is evidence to suggest that patients with eating disorders have better outcomes when treated on inpatient units specializing in the treatment of these disorders than when treated in general inpatient settings where staff lack expertise and experience in treating eating disorders [II].

Outcomes from partial hospitalization programs that specialize in eating disorders are highly correlated with treatment intensity. The more successful programs involve patients in treatment at least 5 days/week for 8 hours/day; thus, it is recommended that partial hospitalization programs be structured to provide at least this level of care [I].

Patients who are considerably below their healthy body weight and are highly motivated to adhere to treatment, have cooperative families, and have a brief symptom duration may benefit from treatment in outpatient settings, but only if they are carefully monitored and if they and their families understand that a more restrictive setting may be necessary if persistent progress is not evident in a few weeks [II]. Careful monitoring includes at least weekly (and often two to three times a week) weight determinations done directly after the patient voids and while the patient is wearing the same class of garment (e.g., hospital gown, standard exercise clothing) [I]. In patients who purge, it is important to routinely monitor serum electrolytes [I]. Urine specific gravity, orthostatic vital signs, and oral temperatures may need to be measured on a regular basis [II].

In an outpatient setting, patients can remain with their families and continue to attend school or work. Inpatient care may interfere with family, school, and work obligations; however, it is important to give priority to the safe and adequate treatment of a rapidly progressing or otherwise unresponsive disorder for which hospital care might be necessary [I].

3. Choice of specific treatments for anorexia nervosa

The aims of treating anorexia nervosa are to 1) restore patients to a healthy weight (associated with the return of menses and normal ovulation in female patients, normal sexual drive and hormone levels in male patients, and normal physical and sexual growth and development in children and adolescents); 2) treat physical complications; 3) enhance patients' motivation to cooperate in the restoration of healthy eating patterns and participate in treatment; 4) provide education regarding healthy nutrition and eating patterns; 5) help patients reassess and change core dysfunctional cognitions, attitudes, motives, conflicts, and feelings related to the eating disorder; 6) treat associated psychiatric conditions, including deficits in mood and impulse regulation and self-esteem and behavioral problems; 7) enlist family support and provide family counseling and therapy where appropriate; and 8) prevent relapse.

a) Nutritional rehabilitation

The goals of nutritional rehabilitation for seriously underweight patients are to restore weight, normalize eating patterns, achieve normal perceptions of hunger and satiety, and correct biological and psychological sequelae of malnutrition [I]. For patients age 20 years and younger, an individually appropriate range for expected weight and goals for weight and height may be determined by considering measurements and clinical factors, including current weight, bone age estimated from wrist X-rays and nomograms, menstrual history (in adolescents with secondary amenorrhea), mid-parental heights, assessments of skeletal frame, and benchmarks from Centers for Disease Control and Prevention (CDC) growth charts (available at http://www.cdc.gov/growthcharts/) [I].

For individuals who are markedly underweight and for children and adolescents whose weight has deviated below their growth curves, hospital-based programs for nutritional rehabilitation should be considered [I]. For patients in inpatient or residential settings, the discrepancy between healthy target weight and weight at discharge may vary depending on patients' ability to feed themselves, their motivation and ability to participate in aftercare programs, and the adequacy of aftercare, including partial hospitalization [I]. It is important to implement refeeding programs in nurturing emotional contexts [I]. For example, it is useful for staff to convey to patients their intention to take care of them and not let them die even when the illness prevents the patients from taking care of themselves [II]. It is also useful for staff to communicate clearly that they are not seeking to engage in control battles and have no punitive intentions when using interventions that the patient may experience as aversive [I].

In working to achieve target weights, the treatment plan should also establish expected rates of controlled weight gain. Clinical consensus suggests that realistic targets are 2–3 lb/week for hospitalized patients and 0.5–1 lb/week for individuals in outpatient programs [II]. Registered dietitians can help patients choose their own meals and can provide a structured meal plan that ensures nutritional adequacy and that none of the major food groups are avoided [I]. Formula feeding may have to be added to the patient's diet to achieve large caloric intake [II]. It is important to encourage patients with anorexia nervosa to expand their food choices to minimize the severely restricted range of foods initially acceptable to them [II]. Caloric intake levels should usually start at 30–40 kcal/kg per day (approximately 1,000–1,600 kcal/day). During the weight gain phase, intake may have to be advanced progressively to as high as 70–100 kcal/kg per day for some patients; many male patients require a very large number of calories to gain weight [II].

Patients who require much lower caloric intakes or are suspected of artificially increasing their weight by fluid loading should be weighed in the morning after they have voided and are wearing only a gown; their fluid intake should also be carefully monitored [I]. Urine specimens obtained at the time of a patient's weigh-in may need to be assessed for specific gravity to help ascertain the extent to which the measured weight reflects excessive water intake [I]. Regular monitoring of serum potassium levels is recommended in patients who are persistent vomiters [I]. Hypokalemia should be treated with oral or intravenous potassium supplementation and rehydration [I].

Physical activity should be adapted to the food intake and energy expenditure of the patient, taking into account the patient's bone mineral density and cardiac function [I]. Once a safe weight is achieved, the focus of an exercise program should be on the patient's gaining physical fitness as opposed to expending calories [I].

Weight gain results in improvements in most of the physiological and psychological complications of semistarvation [I]. It is important to warn patients about the following aspects of early recovery [I]: As they start to recover and feel their bodies getting larger, especially as they approach frightening, magical numbers on the scale that represent phobic weights, they may experience a resurgence of anxious and depressive symptoms, irritability, and sometimes suicidal thoughts. These mood symptoms, non-food-related obsessional thoughts, and compulsive behaviors, although often not eradicated, usually decrease with sustained weight gain and weight maintenance. Initial refeeding may be associated with mild transient fluid retention, but patients who abruptly stop taking laxatives or diuretics may experience marked rebound fluid retention for several weeks. As weight gain progresses, many patients also develop acne and breast tenderness and become unhappy and demoralized about resulting changes in body shape. Patients may experience abdominal pain and bloating with meals from the delayed gastric emptying that accompanies malnutrition. These symptoms may respond to pro-motility agents [III]. Constipation may be ameliorated with stool softeners; if unaddressed, it can progress to obstipation and, rarely, to acute bowel obstruction.

When life-preserving nutrition must be provided to a patient who refuses to eat, nasogastric feeding is preferable to intravenous feeding [I]. When nasogastric feeding is necessary, continuous feeding (i.e., over 24 hours) may be better tolerated by patients and less likely to result in metabolic abnormalities than three to four bolus feedings a day [II]. In very difficult situations, where patients physically resist and constantly remove their nasogastric tubes, feeding through surgically placed gastrostomy or jejunostomy tubes may be an alternative to nasogastric feeding [II]. In determining whether to begin involuntary forced feeding, the clinician should carefully think through the clinical circumstances, family opinion, and relevant legal and ethical dimensions of the patient's treatment [I]. The general principles to be followed in making the decision are those directing good, humane care; respecting the wishes of competent patients; and intervening respectfully with patients whose judgment is severely impaired by their psychiatric disorders when such interventions are likely to have beneficial results [I]. For cooperative patients, supplemental overnight pediatric nasogastric tube feeding has been used in some programs to facilitate weight gain [III].

With severely malnourished patients (particularly those whose weight is <70% of their healthy body weight) who undergo aggressive oral, nasogastric, or parenteral refeeding, a serious refeeding syndrome can occur. Initial assessments should include vital signs and food and fluid intake and output, if indicated, as well as monitoring for edema, rapid weight gain (associated primarily with fluid overload), congestive heart failure, and gastrointestinal symptoms [I]. Patients' serum levels of phosphorus, magnesium, potassium, and calcium should be determined daily for the first 5 days of refeeding and every other day for several weeks thereafter, and electrocardiograms should be performed as indicated [II]. For children and adolescents who are severely malnourished (weight <70% of healthy body weight), cardiac monitoring, especially at night, may be desirable [II]. Phosphorus, magnesium, and/or potassium supplementation should be given when indicated [I].

b) Psychosocial interventions

The goals of psychosocial interventions are to help patients with anorexia nervosa 1) understand and cooperate with their nutritional and physical rehabilitation, 2) understand and change the behaviors and dysfunctional attitudes related to their eating disorder, 3) improve their interpersonal and social functioning, and 4) address comorbid psychopathology and psychological conflicts that reinforce or maintain eating disorder behaviors.

(i) Acute anorexia nervosa

During acute refeeding and while weight gain is occurring, it is beneficial to provide anorexia nervosa patients with individual psychotherapeutic management that is psychodynamically informed and provides empathic understanding, explanations, praise for positive efforts, coaching, support, encouragement, and other positive behavioral reinforcement [I]. Attempts to conduct formal psychotherapy with starving patients who are often negativistic, obsessional, or mildly cognitively impaired may be ineffective [II].

For children and adolescents, the evidence indicates that family treatment is the most effective intervention [I]. In methods modeled after the Maudsley approach, families become actively involved, in a blame-free atmosphere, in helping patients eat more and resist compulsive exercising and purging. For some outpatients, a short-term course of family therapy using these methods may be as effective as a long-term course; however, a shorter course of therapy may not be adequate for patients with severe obsessive-compulsive features or nonintact families [II].

Most inpatient-based nutritional rehabilitation programs create a milieu that incorporates emotional nurturance and a combination of reinforcers that link exercise, bed rest, and privileges to target weights, desired behaviors, feedback concerning changes in weight, and other observable parameters [II]. For adolescents treated in inpatient settings, participation in family group psychoeducation may be helpful to their efforts to regain weight and may be equally as effective as more intensive forms of family therapy [III].

(ii) Anorexia nervosa after weight restoration

Once malnutrition has been corrected and weight gain has begun, psychotherapy can help patients with anorexia nervosa understand 1) their experience of their illness; 2) cognitive distortions and how these have led to their symptomatic behavior; 3) developmental, familial, and cultural antecedents of their illness; 4) how their illness may have been a maladaptive attempt to regulate their emotions and cope; 5) how to avoid or minimize the risk of relapse; and 6) how to better cope with salient developmental and other important life issues in the future. Clinical experience shows that patients may often display improved mood, enhanced cognitive functioning, and clearer thought processes after there is significant improvement in nutritional intake, even before there is substantial weight gain [II].

To help prevent patients from relapsing, emerging data support the use of cognitive-behavioral psychotherapy for adults [II]. Many clinicians also use interpersonal and/or psychodynamically oriented individual or group psychotherapy for adults after their weight has been restored [II]. For adolescents who have been ill <3 years, after weight has been restored, family therapy is a necessary component of treatment [I]. Although studies of different psychotherapies focus on these interventions as distinctly separate treatments, in practice there is frequent overlap of interventions [II].

It is important for clinicians to pay attention to cultural attitudes, patient issues involving the gender of the therapist, and specific concerns about possible abuse, neglect, or other developmental traumas [II]. Clinicians need to attend to their countertransference reactions to patients with a chronic eating disorder, which often include beleaguerment, demoralization, and excessive need to change the patient [I]. At the same time, when treating patients with chronic illnesses, clinicians need to understand the longitudinal course of the disorder and that patients can recover even after many years of illness [I]. Because of anorexia nervosa's enduring nature, psychotherapeutic treatment is frequently required for at least 1 year and may take many years [I].

Anorexics and Bulimics Anonymous and Overeaters Anonymous are not substitutes for professional treatment [I]. Programs that focus exclusively on abstaining from binge eating, purging, restrictive eating, or excessive exercising (e.g., 12-step programs) without attending to nutritional considerations or cognitive and behavioral deficits have not been studied and therefore cannot be recommended as the sole treatment for anorexia nervosa [I]. It is important for programs using 12-step models to be equipped to care for patients with the substantial psychiatric and general medical problems often associated with eating disorders [I].

Although families and patients are increasingly accessing worthwhile, helpful information through online web sites, newsgroups, and chat rooms, the lack of professional supervision within these resources may sometimes lead to users' receiving misinformation or create unhealthy dynamics among users. It is recommended that clinicians inquire about a patient's or family's use of Internet-based support and other alternative and complementary approaches and be prepared to openly and sympathetically discuss the information and ideas gathered from these sources [I].

(iii) Chronic anorexia nervosa

Patients with chronic anorexia nervosa generally show a lack of substantial clinical response to formal psychotherapy. Nevertheless, many clinicians report seeing patients with chronic anorexia nervosa who, after many years of struggling with their disorder, experience substantial remission, so clinicians are justified in maintaining and extending some degree of hope to patients and families [II]. More extensive psychotherapeutic measures may be undertaken to engage and help motivate patients whose illness is resistant to treatment [II] or, failing that, as compassionate care [I]. For patients who have difficulty talking about their problems, clinicians have reported that a variety of nonverbal therapeutic methods, such as the creative arts, movement therapy programs, and occupational therapy, can be useful [III]. Psychosocial programs designed for patients with chronic eating disorders are being implemented at several treatment sites and may prove useful [II].

c) Medications and other somatic treatments

(i) Weight restoration

The decision about whether to use psychotropic medications and, if so, which medications to choose will be based on the patient's clinical presentation [I]. The limited empirical data on malnourished patients indicate that selective serotonin reuptake inhibitors (SSRIs) do not appear to confer advantage regarding weight gain in patients who are concurrently receiving inpatient treatment in an organized eating disorder program [I]. However, SSRIs in combination with psychotherapy are widely used in treating patients with anorexia nervosa. For example, these medications may be considered for those with persistent depressive, anxiety, or obsessive-compulsive symptoms and for bulimic symptoms in weight-restored patients [II]. A U.S. Food and Drug Administration (FDA) black box warning concerning the use of bupropion in patients with eating disorders has been issued because of the increased seizure risk in these patients. Adverse reactions to tricyclic antidepressants and monoamine oxidase inhibitors (MAOIs) are more pronounced in malnourished individuals, and these medications should generally be avoided in this patient population [I]. Second-generation antipsychotics, particularly olanzapine, risperidone, and quetiapine, have been used in small series and individual cases for patients, but controlled studies of these medications are lacking. Clinical impressions suggest that they may be useful in patients with severe, unremitting resistance to gaining weight; severe obsessional thinking; and denial that assumes delusional proportions [III]. Small doses of older antipsychotics such as chlorpromazine may be helpful prior to meals in very disturbed patients [III]. Although the risks of extrapyramidal side effects are less with second-generation antipsychotics than with first-generation antipsychotics, debilitated anorexia nervosa patients may be at a higher risk for these than expected. Therefore, if these medications are used, it is recommended that patients be carefully monitored for extrapyramidal symptoms and akathisia [I]. It is also important to routinely monitor patients for potential side effects of these medications, which can result in insulin resistance, abnormal lipid metabolism, and prolongation of the QTc interval [I]. Because ziprasidone has not been studied in individuals with anorexia nervosa and can prolong QTc intervals, careful monitoring of serial electrocardiograms and serum potassium measurements is needed if anorexic patients are treated with ziprasidone [I]. Antianxiety agents used selectively before meals may be useful to reduce patients' anticipatory anxiety before eating [III], but because eating disorder patients may have a high propensity to become dependent on benzodiazepines, these medications should be used routinely only with considerable caution [I]. Pro-motility agents such as metoclopramide may be useful for bloating and abdominal pains that occur during refeeding in some patients [II]. Electroconvulsive therapy (ECT) has generally not been useful except in treating severe co-occurring disorders for which ECT is otherwise indicated [I].

Although no specific hormone treatments or vitamin supplements have been shown to be helpful [I], supplemental calcium and vitamin D are often recommended [III]. Zinc supplements have been reported to foster weight gain in some patients, and patients may benefit from daily zinc-containing multivitamin tablets [II].

(ii) Relapse prevention

Some data suggest that fluoxetine in dosages of up to 60 mg/day may help prevent relapse [II]. For patients receiving cognitive-behavioral therapy (CBT) after weight restoration, adding fluoxetine does not appear to confer additional benefits with respect to preventing relapse [II]. Antidepressants and other psychiatric medications may be used to treat specific, ongoing psychiatric symptoms of depressive, anxiety, obsessive-compulsive, and other comorbid disorders [I]. Clinicians should attend to the black box warnings in the package inserts relating to antidepressants and discuss the potential benefits and risks of antidepressant treatment with patients and families if such medications are to be prescribed [I].

(iii) Chronic anorexia nervosa

Although hormone replacement therapy (HRT) is frequently prescribed to improve bone mineral density in female patients, no good supporting evidence exists either in adults or in adolescents to demonstrate its efficacy [II]. Hormone therapy usually induces monthly menstrual bleeding, which may contribute to the patient's denial of the need to gain further weight [II]. Before estrogen is offered, it is recommended that efforts be made to increase weight and achieve resumption of normal menses [I]. There is no indication for the use of bisphosphonates such as alendronate in patients with anorexia nervosa [II]. Although there is no evidence that calcium or vitamin D supplementation reverses decreased bone mineral density, when calcium dietary intake is inadequate for growth and maintenance, calcium supplementation should be considered [I], and when the individual is not exposed to daily sunlight, vitamin D supplementation may be used [I]. However, large supplemental doses of vitamin D may be hazardous [I].

4. Choice of specific treatments for bulimia nervosa

The aims of treatment for patients with bulimia nervosa are to 1) reduce and, where possible, eliminate binge eating and purging; 2) treat physical complications of bulimia nervosa; 3) enhance patients' motivation to cooperate in the restoration of healthy eating patterns and participate in treatment; 4) provide education regarding healthy nutrition and eating patterns; 5) help patients reassess and change core dysfunctional thoughts, attitudes, motives, conflicts, and feelings related to the eating disorder; 6) treat associated psychiatric conditions, including deficits in mood and impulse regulation, self-esteem, and behavior; 7) enlist family support and provide family counseling and therapy where appropriate; and 8) prevent relapse.

a) Nutritional rehabilitation counseling

A primary focus for nutritional rehabilitation is to help the patient develop a structured meal plan as a means of reducing the episodes of dietary restriction and the urges to binge and purge [I]. Adequate nutritional intake can prevent craving and promote satiety [I]. It is important to assess nutritional intake for all patients, even those with a normal body weight (or normal BMI), as normal weight does not ensure appropriate nutritional intake or normal body composition [I]. Among patients of normal weight, nutritional counseling is a useful part of treatment and helps reduce food restriction, increase the variety of foods eaten, and promote healthy but not compulsive exercise patterns [I].

b) Psychosocial interventions

It is recommended that psychosocial interventions be chosen on the basis of a comprehensive evaluation of the individual patient that takes into consideration the patient's cognitive and psychological development, psychodynamic issues, cognitive style, comorbid psychopathology, and preferences as well as patient age and family situation [I]. For treating acute episodes of bulimia nervosa in adults, the evidence strongly supports the value of CBT as the most effective single intervention [I]. Some patients who do not respond initially to CBT may respond when switched to either interpersonal therapy (IPT) or fluoxetine [II] or other modes of treatment such as family and group psychotherapies [III]. Controlled trials have also shown the utility of IPT in some cases [II].

In clinical practice, many practitioners combine elements of CBT, IPT, and other psychotherapeutic techniques. Compared with psychodynamic or interpersonal therapy, CBT is associated with more rapid remission of eating symptoms [I], but using psychodynamic interventions in conjunction with CBT and other psychotherapies may yield better global outcomes [II]. Some patients, particularly those with concurrent personality pathology or other co-occurring disorders, require lengthy treatment [II]. Clinical reports suggest that psychodynamic and psychoanalytic approaches in individual or group format are useful once bingeing and purging improve [III].

Family therapy should be considered whenever possible, especially for adolescent patients still living with their parents [II] or older patients with ongoing conflicted interactions with parents [III]. Patients with marital discord may benefit from couples therapy [II].

A variety of self-help and professionally guided self-help programs have been effective for some patients with bulimia nervosa [I]. Several innovative online programs are currently under investigation and may be recommended in the absence of alternative treatments [III]. Support groups and 12-step programs such as Overeaters Anonymous may be helpful as adjuncts in the initial treatment of bulimia nervosa and for subsequent relapse prevention, but they are not recommended as the sole initial treatment approach for bulimia nervosa [I].

Issues of countertransference, discussed above with respect to the treatment of patients with anorexia nervosa, also apply to the treatment of patients with bulimia nervosa [I].

c) Medications

(i) Initial treatment

Antidepressants are effective as one component of an initial treatment program for most bulimia nervosa patients [I], with SSRI treatment having the most evidence for efficacy and the fewest difficulties with adverse effects [I]. To date, fluoxetine is the best studied of these and is the only FDA-approved medication for bulimia nervosa. Sertraline is the only other SSRI that has been shown to be effective, as demonstrated in a small, randomized controlled trial. In the absence of therapists qualified to treat bulimia nervosa with CBT, fluoxetine is recommended as an initial treatment [I]. Dosages of SSRIs higher than those used for depression (e.g., fluoxetine 60 mg/day) are more effective in treating bulimic symptoms [I]. Evidence from a small open trial suggests fluoxetine may be useful for adolescents with bulimia [II].

Antidepressants may be helpful for patients with substantial concurrent symptoms of depression, anxiety, obsessions, or certain impulse disorder symptoms or for patients who have not benefited from or had only a suboptimal response to appropriate psychosocial therapy [I]. Tricyclic antidepressants and MAOIs have been rarely used with bulimic patients and are not recommended as initial treatments [I]. Several different antidepressants may have to be tried sequentially to identify the specific medication with the optimum effect [I].

Clinicians should attend to the black box warnings relating to antidepressants and discuss the potential benefits and risks of antidepressant treatment with patients and families if such medications are to be prescribed [I].

Small controlled trials have demonstrated the efficacy of the anticonvulsant medication topiramate, but because adverse reactions to this medication are common, it should be used only when other medications have proven ineffective [III]. Also, because patients tend to lose weight on topiramate, its use is problematic for normal or underweight individuals [III].

Two drugs that are used for mood stabilization, lithium and valproic acid, are both prone to induce weight gain in patients [I] and may be less acceptable to patients who are weight preoccupied. However, lithium is not recommended for patients with bulimia nervosa because it is ineffective [I]. In patients with co-occurring bulimia nervosa and bipolar disorder, treatment with lithium is more likely to be associated with toxicity [I].

(ii) Maintenance phase

Limited evidence supports the use of fluoxetine for relapse prevention [II], but substantial rates of relapse occur even with treatment. In the absence of adequate data, most clinicians recommend continuing antidepressant therapy for a minimum of 9 months and probably for a year in most patients with bulimia nervosa [II]. Case reports indicate that methylphenidate may be helpful for bulimia nervosa patients with concurrent attention-deficit/hyperactivity disorder (ADHD) [III], but it should be used only for patients who have a very clear diagnosis of ADHD [I].

(iii) Combining psychosocial interventions and medications
In some research, the combination of antidepressant therapy and CBT results in the highest remission rates; therefore, this combination is recommended initially when qualified CBT therapists are available [II]. In addition, when CBT alone does not result in a substantial reduction in symptoms after 10 sessions, it is recommended that fluoxetine be added [II].

(iv) Other treatments
Bright light therapy has been shown to reduce binge frequency in several controlled trials and may be used as an adjunct when CBT and antidepressant therapy have not been effective in reducing bingeing symptoms [III].

5. Eating disorder not otherwise specified

Patients with subsyndromal anorexia nervosa or bulimia nervosa who meet most but not all of the DSM-IV-TR criteria (e.g., weight >85% of expected weight, binge and purge frequency less than twice per week) merit treatment similar to that of patients who fulfill all criteria for these diagnoses [II].

a) Binge eating disorder

(i) Nutritional rehabilitation and counseling
Behavioral weight control programs incorporating low- or very-low-calorie diets may help with weight loss and usually with reduction of symptoms of binge eating [I]. It is important to advise patients that weight loss is often not maintained and that binge eating may recur when weight is gained [I]. It is also important to advise them that weight gain after weight loss may be accompanied by a return of binge eating patterns [I]. Various combinations of diets, behavior therapies, interpersonal therapies, psychodynamic psychotherapies, non-weight-directed psychosocial treatments, and even some "nondiet/health at every size" psychotherapy approaches may be of benefit for binge eating and weight loss or stabilization [III]. Patients with a history of repeated weight loss followed by weight gain ("yo-yo" dieting) or patients with an early onset of binge eating may benefit from following programs that focus on decreasing binge eating rather than on weight loss [II].

There is little empirical evidence to suggest that obese binge eaters who are primarily seeking weight loss should receive different treatment than obese individuals who do not binge eat [I].

(ii) Other psychosocial treatments
Substantial evidence supports the efficacy of individual or group CBT for the behavioral and psychological symptoms of binge eating disorder [I]. IPT and dialectical behavior therapy have also been shown to be effective for behavioral and psychological symptoms and can be considered as alternatives [II]. Patients may be advised that some studies suggest that most patients continue to show behavioral and psychological improvement at their 1-year follow-up [II]. Substantial evidence supports the efficacy of self-help and guided self-help CBT programs and their use as an initial step in a sequenced treatment program [I]. Other therapies that use a "nondiet" approach and focus on self-acceptance, improved body image, better nutrition and health, and increased physical movement have been tried, as have addiction-based 12-step approaches, self-help organizations, and treatment programs based on the Alcoholics Anonymous model, but no systematic outcome studies of these programs are available [III].

(iii) Medications
Substantial evidence suggests that treatment with antidepressant medications, particularly SSRI antidepressants, is associated with at least a short-term reduction in binge eating behavior but, in most cases, not with substantial weight loss [I]. The medication dosage is typically at the high end of the recommended range [I]. The appetite-suppressant medication sibutramine is effective for binge suppression, at least in the short term, and is also associated with significant weight loss [II].

The anticonvulsant medication topiramate is effective for binge reduction and weight loss, although adverse effects may limit its clinical utility for some individuals [II]. Zonisamide may produce similar effects regarding weight loss and can also cause side effects [III].

(iv) Combining psychosocial and medication treatments

For most eating disorder patients, adding antidepressant medication to their behavioral weight control and/or CBT regimen does not have a significant effect on binge suppression when compared with medication alone. However, medications may induce additional weight reduction and have associated psychological benefits [II]. Adding the weight loss medication orlistat to a guided self-help CBT program may yield additional weight reduction [II]. Fluoxetine in conjunction with group behavioral treatment may not aid in binge cessation or weight loss but may reduce depressive symptoms [II].

b) Night eating syndrome

Progressive muscle relaxation has been shown to reduce symptoms associated with night eating syndrome [III]. Sertraline has also been shown to reduce these symptoms [II].

II. FORMULATION AND IMPLEMENTATION OF A TREATMENT PLAN

A. PSYCHIATRIC MANAGEMENT

Psychiatric management includes a broad range of therapeutic actions that are performed by the psychiatrist or that the psychiatrist ensures are provided to all patients with eating disorders in combination with other specific treatment modalities. Psychiatric management begins with the establishment of a therapeutic alliance, which is then enhanced by empathic comments and behaviors, positive regard, reassurance, and support. Basic psychiatric management includes support through the provision of educational materials, including self-help workbooks (4), information on community and Internet resources (5, 6), and direct advice to patients and their families (when they are involved) (7). It is important to caution patients and families about Internet sites that encourage eating disorder lifestyles ("pro-ana" sites). Although many service providers have made attempts to police and encourage elimination of these sites, they still continue to appear, to the concern of families and professionals (8, 9). In some settings, judicious use of e-mail contact with patients has been increasingly used (5, 10). Some resources for patients and families are presented in Table 1.

1. Establish and maintain a therapeutic alliance

At the very outset and through ongoing interactions with the patient, it is important for clinicians to attempt to build trust, establish mutual respect, and develop a therapeutic relationship that will serve as the basis for ongoing exploration and treatment of the problems associated with the eating disorder. Eating disorders are frequently long-term illnesses that can manifest themselves in different ways at different points during their course; treating them often requires the psychiatrist to adapt and modify therapeutic strategies. Many patients with anorexia nervosa are initially reluctant to enter treatment and may feel invested in their symptoms. Many are secretive and may withhold information about their behavior because of shame. During the course of treatment, they may resist looking beyond immediate symptoms to possible coexisting psychiatric disorders, comorbid psychopathology, and underlying psychodynamic issues. Conversely, some patients may resist discussing eating disorder symptoms and want to focus on only "core

TABLE 1. Self-Help Books and Internet Resources on Eating Disorders

CBT-oriented workbooks	Agras WS, Apple RF: *Overcoming Eating Disorders: A Cognitive-Behavioral Treatment for Bulimia Nervosa and Binge-Eating Disorder.* New York, Oxford University Press, 1997 (client workbook) Agras WS, Apple RF: *Overcoming Eating Disorders: A Cognitive-Behavioral Treatment for Bulimia Nervosa and Binge-Eating Disorder.* New York, Oxford University Press, 1997 (therapist workbook) Cash TF: *The Body Image Workbook: An 8-Step Program for Learning to Like Your Looks.* Oakland, CA, New Harbinger, 1997 Fairburn C: *Overcoming Binge Eating.* New York, Guilford, 1995 Goodman LJ, Villapiano M: *Eating Disorders: The Journey to Recovery Workbook.* New York, Brunner-Routledge, 2001 (client workbook) Goodman LJ, Villapiano M: *Eating Disorders: Time for Change. Plans, Strategies, and Worksheets.* New York, Brunner-Routledge, 2001 (therapist workbook) Schmidt U, Treasure J: *Getting Better Bit(e) by Bit(e): A Survival Kit for Sufferers of Bulimia Nervosa and Binge Eating Disorder.* East Sussex, UK, Psychology Press, 1993
Other books reported to be helpful by patients/families	Bulik CM, Taylor N: *Runaway Eating: The 8-Point Plan to Conquer Adult Food and Weight Obsessions.* New York, Rodale Books, 2005 Ellis A, Abrams M, Dengelegi L: *The Art and Science of Rational Eating.* Fort Lee, NJ, Barricade Books, 1992 Goodman LJ, Villapiano M: *Eating Disorders: The Journey to Recovery Workbook.* New York, Brunner-Routledge, 2001 (client workbook) Hall L: *Full Lives: Women Who Have Freed Themselves From Food and Weight Obsessions.* Carlsbad, CA, Gürze Books, 1993 Lock J, le Grange D: *Help Your Teenager Beat an Eating Disorder.* New York, Guilford, 2005 Michel DM, Willard SG: *When Dieting Becomes Dangerous.* New Haven, CT, Yale University Press, 2003 Walsh BT, Cameron VL: *If Your Child Has an Eating Disorder: An Essential Resource for Parents.* New York, Guilford, 2005 Zerbe K: *The Body Betrayed: A Deeper Understanding of Women, Eating Disorders, and Treatment.* Carlsbad, CA, Gürze Books, 1995
Books reported to be helpful for male patients	Andersen AE, Cohn L, Holbrook T: *Making Weight: Men's Conflicts With Food, Weight, Shape and Appearance.* Carlsbad, CA, Gürze Books, 2000
Internet resources for health care professionals	Academy for Eating Disorders (http://www.aedweb.org)
Internet resources for patients, families, and professionals	National Eating Disorders Association (http://www.nationaleatingdisorders.org) National Association of Anorexia Nervosa and Associated Disorders (http://www.anad.org/site/anadweb/) Eating Disorder Referral and Information Center (http://www.edreferral.com) Something Fishy (http://www.something-fishy.org; a well-monitored advocacy site)

issues," apparently to avoid relinquishing their symptoms. Psychiatrists should be mindful of the fact that the recommended interventions create extreme anxieties for individuals with anorexia nervosa. Encouraging patients to gain weight asks them to do the very thing of which they are most frightened. Patients may believe that the psychiatrist just wants to make them fat and does not understand or empathize with their underlying emotions. Consequently, by recognizing and acknowledging an awareness of patient anxieties, psychiatrists can assist in building the therapeutic alliance. The clinician may foster rapport by letting patients know that eating disorder symptoms often serve a number of important functions, such as providing a sense of accomplishment or a way to feel looked after or protected (11, 12). Addressing patients' resistance to treatment and enhancing their motivation for change may be important in allowing therapy to proceed through impasses as well as helping to ameliorate factors that serve to aggravate and maintain eating disorders (13–18). Finally, letting patients know that full recovery from anorexia nervosa takes time (19) may help build rapport, as the patient senses that the clinician is not expecting a magical, rapid turnaround, which the patient may sense is unrealistic.

2. Coordinate care and collaborate with other clinicians

Professionals from several disciplines may collaborate in the patient's care. The specific role of each professional may vary with the organizational structure of the eating disorders program and the professional qualifications of those working within the program. The psychiatrist may assume the leadership role in the patient's treatment program or the patient's treatment team or work collaboratively on a team led by other health professionals, including other physicians or psychologists. Registered dietitians with specialized training in eating disorders often provide nutritional counseling. Therapists from a variety of professional fields may provide family, individual, or group psychotherapy, including CBT. Other physician specialists and dentists may be consulted for management of acute and ongoing medical and dental complications. Often in the treatment of children and adolescents, school coaches, teachers, and school counselors may be asked to collaborate in a patient's treatment. In treatment settings where staff do not have the training or experience to deal with patients with eating disorders, the provision of education, supervision, and leadership by a qualified psychiatrist can be crucial to the success of treatment.

Although a variety of management models are used for adult patients with eating disorders, no data exist on their comparative efficacies. Psychiatrists who choose to manage both general medical and psychiatric issues should have appropriate medical backup to treat the medical complications associated with eating disorders. Some programs routinely arrange for interdisciplinary teams to manage treatment (sometimes called *split management*). In this model, the psychiatrist handles administrative and general medical requirements, prescribes medications when clinically necessary and appropriate, and recommends interventions aimed at normalizing disturbed cognitions and eating and weight-reducing behaviors. Other clinicians then provide individual and/or group psychotherapeutic interventions (e.g., CBT, psychodynamic psychotherapy, family therapy). For this management model to be effective and to avoid reinforcing some patients' tendencies to play staff off each other (i.e., split the staff), all personnel must work closely together and maintain open communication and mutual respect.

For children and adolescents, the recommended treatment model is the team approach (3). In this interdisciplinary management approach, general medical care clinicians (e.g., specialists in internal medicine, pediatrics, adolescent medicine, or nutrition) manage general medical issues, such as nutrition, weight gain, exercise, and eating patterns, whereas the psychiatrist addresses the psychiatric issues (3, 20, 21). The biopsychosocial nature of anorexia nervosa and bulimia nervosa dictates the need for interdisciplinary treatment, and each aspect of care must be developmentally tailored to the treatment of adolescents (22). In unusual circumstances, psychiatrists may be qualified to act as the primary provider of comprehensive medical care.

TABLE 2. DSM-IV-TR Diagnostic Criteria for Anorexia Nervosa

Criterion	Description
A	Refusal to maintain body weight at or above a minimally normal weight for age and height (e.g., weight loss leading to maintenance of body weight less than 85% of that expected; or failure to make expected weight gain during period of growth, leading to body weight less than 85% of that expected).
B	Intense fear of gaining weight or becoming fat, even though underweight.
C	Disturbance in the way in which one's body weight or shape is experienced, undue influence of body weight or shape on self-evaluation, or denial of the seriousness of the current low body weight.
D	In postmenarcheal females, amenorrhea, i.e., the absence of at least three consecutive menstrual cycles. (A woman is considered to have amenorrhea if her periods occur only following hormone, e.g., estrogen, administration.)
Specify type:	
Restricting type: During the current episode of anorexia nervosa, the person has not regularly engaged in binge-eating or purging behavior (i.e., self-induced vomiting or the misuse of laxatives, diuretics, or enemas).	
Binge-eating/purging type: During the current episode of anorexia nervosa, the person has regularly engaged in binge-eating or purging behavior (i.e., self-induced vomiting or the misuse of laxatives, diuretics, or enemas).	

Source. Reprinted from American Psychiatric Association: *Diagnostic and Statistical Manual of Mental Disorders,* 4th Edition, Text Revision. Washington, DC, American Psychiatric Association, 2000. Copyright 2000, American Psychiatric Association. Used with permission.

When a patient is managed by an interdisciplinary team in an outpatient setting, communication among the professionals is essential so that all team members have a clear understanding of each other's responsibilities and approaches. For example, in team management of outpatients with anorexia nervosa, one professional must be designated to consistently monitor weights so that this essential function is not inadvertently omitted from care.

3. Assess and monitor eating disorder symptoms and behaviors

It is important for the psychiatrist to carefully assess the patient's eating disorder symptoms and behaviors (23). Such an assessment will assist the clinician in identifying target symptoms and behaviors that will be addressed in the treatment plan as well as determining whether a DSM-IV-TR diagnosis of anorexia nervosa or bulimia nervosa is present (Tables 2 and 3).

It is important to note that a significant number of patients are relegated to the heterogeneous diagnostic group referred to as eating disorders not otherwise specified because they have not been amenorrheic for 3 months and consequently do not meet current criteria for anorexia nervosa. In terms of their clinical course, treatment response, or level of impairment, such patients do not differ from those who fulfill the DSM-IV-TR criteria for anorexia nervosa (24, 25). These observations have important implications with respect to making clinical treatment decisions. They also imply that patients with continued menses who fulfill other criteria for anorexia nervosa should be eligible for the same levels of care as patients with anorexia nervosa.

Obtaining a detailed report of food intake during a single day in the patient's life or using a calendar as a prompt may help elicit specific information about a patient's eating behaviors, particularly regarding perceived intake. A clinician may also obtain useful information by sharing a meal with the patient or observing the patient eating a meal; in this way, the clinician can observe any difficulties the patient may have in eating particular foods, anxieties that erupt in the course of a meal, and rituals concerning food (such as cutting, separating, or mashing) that the patient feels compelled to perform.

TABLE 3. DSM-IV-TR Diagnostic Criteria for Bulimia Nervosa

Criterion	Description
A	Recurrent episodes of binge eating. An episode of binge eating is characterized by both of the following: (1) Eating, in a discrete period of time (e.g., within any 2-hour period), an amount of food that is definitely larger than most people would eat during a similar period of time and under similar circumstances. (2) A sense of lack of control over eating during the episode (e.g., a feeling that one cannot stop eating or control what or how much one is eating).
B	Recurrent inappropriate compensatory behavior in order to prevent weight gain, such as self-induced vomiting; misuse of laxatives, diuretics, enemas, or other medications; fasting; or excessive exercise.
C	The binge eating and inappropriate compensatory behaviors both occur, on average, at least twice a week for 3 months.
D	Self-evaluation is unduly influenced by body shape and weight.
E	The disturbance does not occur exclusively during episodes of anorexia nervosa.
Specify type:	
Purging type: During the current episode of bulimia nervosa, the person has regularly engaged in self-induced vomiting or the misuse of laxatives, diuretics, or enemas.	
Nonpurging type: During the current episode of bulimia nervosa, the person has used other inappropriate compensatory behaviors, such as fasting or excessive exercise, but has not regularly engaged in self-induced vomiting or the misuse of laxatives, diuretics, or enemas.	

Source. Reprinted from American Psychiatric Association: *Diagnostic and Statistical Manual of Mental Disorders,* 4th Edition, Text Revision. Washington, DC, American Psychiatric Association, 2000. Copyright 2000, American Psychiatric Association. Used with permission.

It is important to explore the patient's understanding of how the illness developed and the effects of any interpersonal problems at the onset of the eating disorder. A family history should be obtained regarding eating disorders and other psychiatric disorders, alcohol and other substance use disorders, obesity, family interactions in relation to the patient's disorder, and family attitudes toward eating, exercise, and appearance. It is essential that the clinician avoid articulating theories that imply blame or permit family members to blame one another or themselves for the patient's disorder. No evidence exists to prove that families cause eating disorders. Furthermore, blaming family members harms their psychological well-being and often impairs their desire, willingness, and capacity to be helpful to patients and to participate actively and constructively in treatment and recovery. Rather, the point is to identify family stressors whose amelioration may facilitate recovery.

In the assessment of young patients, it is always helpful to involve parents and, whenever appropriate, school and health professionals who routinely work with children. The complete assessment usually requires several hours. Even when directly questioned, patients and their families may not initially reveal pertinent information about sensitive issues; important information may be uncovered only after a trusting relationship has been established and the patient is better able to accurately identify inner emotional states.

Formal measures are available for the assessment of eating disorders, including self-report questionnaires and semistructured interviews. Examples are listed in Table 4. Clinical decisions about a diagnosis cannot be made on the basis of self-report screening instruments. Patients who are identified on initial screening as likely to have an eating disorder must be followed up in a second-stage determination by trained clinical interviewers. The instruments shown in Table 4, used by clinicians to interview patients in a structured format, are generally taken as "gold standards" to determine clinical diagnoses.

TABLE 4. Representative Instruments for the Assessment of Eating Disorders

Instrument	Completion Time (min)	Comments
Clinician-administered measures		
Eating Disorder Examination (EDE) (26)	30–60	Measures the presence and severity of eating disorder features and provides operational DSM-IV diagnoses
Yale-Brown-Cornell Eating Disorder Scale (YBC-EDS) (27, 28)	10–15	Includes a 65-item symptom checklist plus 19 questions, covering 18 general categories of rituals and preoccupations; requires a trained administrator
Self-report measures		
Diagnostic Survey for Eating Disorders (DSED) (29)	30–40	Has 12 sections covering demographics, weight history and body image, dieting, binge eating, purging, exercise, related behaviors, sexual functioning, menstruation, medical and psychiatric history, life adjustment, and family history
Bulimia Test—Revised (BULIT-R) (30)		Brief (36-item) measure designed to assess eating behaviors and attitudes related to bulimia
Eating Attitudes Test (EAT) (31, 32)	5–10	Brief (26-item), standardized self-report screening test of symptoms and concerns characteristic of eating disorders
Eating Disorder Examination—Questionnaire (EDE-Q) (33)	8–10	Self-report version of the EDE, designed for situations in which an interview cannot be used; validated against the EDE
Eating Disorders Inventory–2 (EDI-2) (34–36)	15–20	Standardized measure of psychological traits and symptom clusters presumed to have relevance to understanding and treating eating disorders; 11 subscales presented in 6-point, forced-choice format; three scales assess attitudes and behaviors concerning eating, weight, and shape; eight assess more general psychological traits
Eating Disorders Questionnaire (EDQ) (37)	45–60	Addresses eating disorder and associated symptoms, time course, and treatment
Questionnaire on Eating and Weight Patterns (QEWP) (38, 39)	5–15	Measures the nature and quantity of binge eating episodes to assess binge eating disorder

4. Assess and monitor the patient's general medical condition

A full physical examination should be performed by a physician familiar with common findings in patients with eating disorders, with particular attention to vital signs; physical status (including height and weight); heart rate and rhythm; jugular venous pressure; heart sounds (especially midsystolic clicks or murmurs from mitral valve prolapse); acrocyanosis; delayed capillary refill; lanugo; salivary gland enlargement; scarring on the dorsum of the hands (Russell's sign); evidence of self-injurious behaviors, such as ecchymoses, linear scars, and cigarette burns; muscular weakness; indications of muscular irritability due to hypocalcemia, such as in Chvostek's and Trousseau's signs; and gait and eye abnormalities (40–43). The patient should also be referred for a dental examination if necessary or indicated by the patient's history (44). In younger patients, examination should include growth pattern and sexual development, including sexual maturity rating, as well as general physical development. The use of a growth chart of standardized values for pediatric populations may allow the clinician to identify patients who have failed to gain weight and have growth retardation (3, 45); such charts are available on the web site of the CDC (http://www.cdc.gov/growthcharts/).

BMI, in conjunction with weight and height, has gained increasing attention in research and clinical settings as a tool for assessing eating disorder patients. BMI is calculated as weight (in kilograms) divided by height (in meters squared) and is particularly useful for comparing groups according to index percentiles that take into account height, sex, and age (46). It is important to remember that BMI is a calculation based only on height and weight and does not provide any further measure of body composition. Except in individuals who are extremely under- or overweight, it is often not useful in estimating nutritional status. Furthermore, considerable debate in the scientific community exists about appropriate BMI ranges for various ethnic groups. Among Caucasian women, for example, the range of a healthy BMI may be higher than for some groups of Asian women (47). Adults with a BMI <18.5 kg/m^2 are considered to be underweight. In addition, abnormal muscularity, body frame size, fluid status, marked constipation, and fluid loading can decrease the validity of BMI as an indicator of the patient's nutritional status (48–52). In children and adolescents, an age-adjusted BMI is used (see http://www.cdc.gov/nccdphp/dnpa/bmi/00binaries/bmi-tables.pdf). Children with a BMI <5th percentile for age are considered to be underweight.

Commonly found signs, symptoms, and associated laboratory abnormalities for anorexia nervosa and bulimia nervosa are shown in Table 5 and Table 6, respectively. Although patients treated in outpatient practice may report few symptoms and show few obvious physical signs or abnormal laboratory test results, significant occult abnormalities may be present (e.g., in bone, heart, and brain).

The need for laboratory analyses should be determined on an individual basis depending on the patient's condition or when necessary for making treatment decisions (43). Some of the laboratory assessments that may be indicated for patients with eating disorders appear in Table 7.

5. Assess and monitor the patient's psychiatric status and safety

In addition to assessing patients' physiological and nutritional status as well as their behaviors, cognitions, and emotions associated with eating and exercise, it is essential that clinicians attend to the overall psychiatric status and safety of patients. Associated psychiatric issues that bear close monitoring include historical evidence, signs, and symptoms related to psychiatric conditions that are often comorbid with eating disorders (e.g., mood, anxiety, and substance use disorders) as well as personality traits and personality disorders that greatly influence patients' clinical course and outcome (78–82). Patients' motivational status also bears monitoring, as it is likely to determine their capacity to engage in treatment (15). Safety issues for patients with eating disorders include both physiological and psychiatric parameters. Many of the physiological safety parameters are described in Section II.B.1, "Choosing a Treatment Site." Clinicians must be vigilant regarding shifts in patients' weight, blood pressure, pulse, other cardiovascular parameters, and behaviors that are likely to provoke physiological decline and collapse. General psychiatric safety issues that bear constant attention include suicidal ideation and suicide attempts as well as impulsive and compulsive self-harm behaviors (83, 84).

6. Provide family assessment and treatment

The available evidence affirms the importance of family involvement and treatment in the management of children and adolescents with anorexia nervosa (85–87). In addition, clinical consensus supports the value of family assessment and involvement in the treatment of both younger and older patients with other eating disorders (88, 89). Since eating is a quintessential family activity, the opportunity to observe patterns of family interaction around the eating and particularly

TABLE 5. Physical Complications of Anorexia Nervosa

Organ System	Symptoms	Signs	Laboratory Test Results
Whole body	Increased symptoms with degree of malnutrition; include weakness and lassitude	Low body weight, dehydration, hypothermia, cachexia	*Weight:* Low weight and BMI *Anthropometrics:* Low body fat percentage by anthropometrics or underwater weighing[a]
Cardiovascular and peripheral vascular	Palpitations, faintness, weakness, dizziness, shortness of breath, chest pain, cold extremities	Most common: bradycardia, orthostatic hypotension, weak irregular pulse, acrocyanosis	*ECG:* Bradycardia or arrhythmias, QTc prolongation,[b] QT dispersion correlated with weight loss, increased PR interval, first-degree heart block, ST-T wave abnormalities *Echocardiogram:* Mitral valve prolapse,[c] pericardial effusion[d] *Chest X-ray:* Small heart
Central nervous system	Apathy, poor concentration	Cognitive impairment; anxious, depressed, irritable mood; in severe cases, seizures, peripheral neuropathy	*CT scan:* Enlarged ventricles *MRI:* Decreased gray and white matter *EEG:* Nonspecific changes, seizures (rare)[e]
Endocrine, metabolic	Fatigue, cold intolerance, diuresis	Low body temperature (hypothermia)	*Complete metabolic panel:* Electrolyte abnormalities, including hypokalemia, hypomagnesemia, hypophosphatemia (especially on refeeding), hypoglycemia (rare), hypercholesterolemia *Thyroid testing:* Decreased T_3; increase in reverse T_3 *Serum cortisol:* Increased serum cortisol *Vitamin assays:* In severe cases, folate, B_{12}, niacin, and thiamine deficiencies
Gastrointestinal	Vomiting, abdominal pain, bloating, obstipation, constipation	Abdominal distension with meals; abnormal bowel sounds; acute gastric distension (rare); in purging patients, benign parotid hyperplasia, caries, or gingivitis; in patients with vitamin deficiencies, angular stomatitis, glossitis, diarrhea	*Liver function and associated tests:* Occasionally abnormal liver function test results, increased serum amylase in purging patients; abnormal results rarely due to pancreatitis *Gastric motility testing:* Delayed gastric emptying, increased whole bowel and colonic transit time, anorectal dysfunction *Endoscopy:* Occasional inflammation or Barrett's esophagus *Radiography:* Rarely, superior mesenteric artery syndrome, pancreatitis *Stool for guaiac:* Occasionally positive because of purging or laxative abuse[f]

TABLE 5. Physical Complications of Anorexia Nervosa *(continued)*

Organ System	Symptoms	Signs	Laboratory Test Results
Genitourinary	Decreased or increased urinary volume[g]		*Renal function tests:* Increased blood urea nitrogen, decreased glomerular filtration rate, decreased serum creatinine because of low lean body mass (normal creatinine may indicate azotemia), renal failure (rare) *Other renal findings:* Greater formation of renal calculi, hypovolemic nephropathy, hypokalemic nephropathy
Hematologic	Fatigue, cold intolerance	Bruising/clotting abnormalities (rare)	*Complete blood count:* Anemia (may be normocytic, microcytic, or macrocytic); leukopenia with relative lymphocytosis; low erythrocyte sedimentation rate; thrombocytopenia; clotting factor abnormalities (rare) *Other hematologic abnormalities:* Decreased serum ferritin, B_{12}, folate
Immune system	Fewer than expected viral infections	None (during weight restoration may develop viral infections), reduced febrile response to bacterial infection	Multiple unexplained immune system abnormalities; abnormalities in tumor necrosis factor–α and interleukin subtypes[h]
Integument	Change in hair, including hair loss and dry and brittle hair; yellowing of skin	Lanugo, self-injury marks, numerous integumentary abnormalities, including xerosis, carotenoderma, and acne[i]	*Vitamin assays:* Increased serum carotene; in severe cases, vitamin deficiencies (e.g., niacin)[j]
Muscular	Symptoms are unusual; with severe malnutrition or ipecac-associated myopathy, muscle weakness, muscle aches, cramps	In severe cases, muscle wasting	*Enzyme tests:* With severe malnutrition, creatine kinase and other muscle enzyme abnormalities; creatine kinase isoenzymes for skeletal vs. cardiac source
Pulmonary	With severe malnutrition, reduced aerobic capacity	In severe states, wasting of respiratory muscles	*Pulmonary function tests:* Decreased pulmonary capacity[k]

TABLE 5. Physical Complications of Anorexia Nervosa *(continued)*

Organ System	Symptoms	Signs	Laboratory Test Results
Reproductive	Arrested development of secondary sex characteristics and psychosexual maturation or interest, loss of libido	Loss of menses or primary amenorrhea, arrested sexual development or regression of secondary sex characteristics, fertility problems, higher rates of pregnancy complications and neonatal complications; deficiencies in the mother can result in deficiencies in the fetus	*Serum gonadotropins:* Decreased serum estrogen in female patients; decreased serum testosterone in male patients; prepubertal patterns of luteinizing hormone, follicle-stimulating hormone secretion *Pelvic ultrasound:* Lack of follicular development and/or lack of dominant follicle
Skeletal	Bone pain with exercise	Point tenderness; in severe cases, short stature and arrested skeletal growth	*Radiography and bone scans:* Increased rate of pathological stress fractures; delayed bone age in some cases *DEXA:* Osteopenia or osteoporosis, especially in hip and lumbar spine

Note. More information on the physical complications of anorexia nervosa is available in Birmingham CL, Beumont PJV: *Medical Management of Eating Disorders.* Cambridge, Cambridge University Press, 2004. CT = computed tomography; DEXA = dual-energy X-ray absorptiometry; ECG = electrocardiogram; EEG = electroencephalogram; MRI = magnetic resonance imaging.

[a]Anthropometrics estimate only peripheral fat. Underwater weighing assesses total body fat.

[b]QTc prolongation in patients with anorexia nervosa has been associated with sudden death (53, 54), but QTc intervals typically normalize with refeeding (54, 55). If QTc prolongation is present, other medications known to prolong QTc intervals should generally be avoided and any electrolyte abnormalities (e.g., hypokalemia) and hypomagnesemia should be corrected (56).

[c]Powers et al. (57). [d]Frolich et al. (58). [e]Prousky (59); Winston et al. (60). [f]Waldholtz (61).

[g]Some chronically ill patients have renal abnormalities associated with decreased urinary volume. Some drink excessive amounts of fluids to assuage hunger, producing increased urinary volume.

[h]Brown et al. (62).

[i]Birmingham and Beumont (40); Strumia (63); Glorio et al. (64).

[j]Prousky (59).

[k]Birmingham and Tan (65).

TABLE 6. Physical Complications of Bulimia Nervosa

Organ System	Symptoms	Signs	Laboratory Test Results
Cardiovascular	Weakness, palpitations	Arrhythmias	*ECG:* Hypokalemia-associated depressed ST segment, QT prolongation.[a] In severe cases, hypokalemia-widened QRS complex, increased P-wave amplitude, increased PR interval, increased supraventricular and ventricular ectopic rhythms; torsade de pointes correlated with hypokalemia; autonomic dysfunction on spectral analysis *Cardiac function testing:* Cardiomyopathy in ipecac abusers
Central nervous system	Apathy, poor concentration	In severe cases, cognitive impairment; anxious, depressed, irritable mood; seizures; peripheral neuropathy	*CT scan:* Cortical atrophy, ventricular enlargement *PET, fMRI:* Abnormal cerebral blood flow and metabolism *MRI:* Decreased gray and white matter *EEG:* Nonspecific abnormalities[b]
Gastrointestinal	Heartburn, reflux, occasional blood streaking in vomitus, abdominal pain and discomfort in vomiters; occasional involuntary vomiting, obstipation, constipation, bowel irregularities; bloating in laxative abusers; acute gastric or esophageal rupture, perforation, necrosis (rare)	Enlarged salivary glands, occasional blood-streaked vomitus; in vomiters, possibly gastritis, esophagitis, gastroesophageal erosions, esophageal dysmotility patterns (including gastroesophageal reflux and, rarely, Mallory-Weiss [esophageal] or gastric tears), increased rates of pancreatitis; in chronic laxative abusers, possibly colonic dysmotility or melanosis coli	*Serum amylase:* Increased serum amylase (if fractionation is available, usually salivary gland isoenzymes); increased pancreatic amylase (rare), possibly indicating laxative abuse or other causes for pancreatic inflammation or pancreatitis
Integument		Scarring on dorsum of hand (Russell's sign), petechia, conjunctival hemorrhages shortly after vomiting	
Metabolic	Weight fluctuation; rarely, proximal weakness, irritability, muscle cramping	Poor skin turgor; pitting edema; Chvostek's and Trousseau's signs (rare)	*Urinalysis:* Dehydration (increased urine specific gravity, osmolality) *Serum electrolyte abnormalities:* Hypokalemic, hypochloremic alkalosis in vomiters; hypomagnesemia and hypophosphatemia in vomiters and laxative abusers

TABLE 6. Physical Complications of Bulimia Nervosa *(continued)*

Organ System	Symptoms	Signs	Laboratory Test Results
Muscular	In ipecac abusers, weakness, palpitations	Muscle weakness, peripheral myopathy	*EMG:* Nonspecific abnormalities
Oropharyngeal	Dental decay, pain in pharynx, swollen cheeks and neck (usually painless)	Dental caries with erosion of dental enamel, particularly the lingular surface of incisors; erythema of pharynx; palatal scratches; enlarged salivary glands	*Radiography:* Erosion of dental enamel *Serum amylase:* Increased serum amylase associated with benign parotid hyperplasia
Reproductive	Fertility problems	Spotty/scanty menstrual periods, oligomenorrhea or amenorrhea	*Serum gonadotropins:* May be hypoestrogenemic
Skeletal[c]	Bone pain with exercise	Point tenderness, short stature, arrested skeletal growth	*Radiography and bone scans:* Possible pathological stress fractures; delayed bone age in some cases *DEXA:* Possible osteopenia or osteoporosis,[c] especially in hip and lumbar spine

Note. CT = computed tomography; DEXA = dual-energy X-ray absorptiometry; ECG = electrocardiogram; EEG = electroencephalogram; EMG = electromyogram; fMRI = functional magnetic resonance imaging; MRI = magnetic resonance imaging; PET = positron emission tomography.

[a]Because QTc prolongation may be associated with sudden death, other medications known to prolong QTc intervals should generally be avoided, and any electrolyte abnormalities (e.g., hypokalemia) and hypomagnesemia should be corrected if QTc prolongation is present.

[b]Frank et al. (66); Doraiswamy et al. (67); Hoffman et al. (68, 69).

[c]Although patients with bulimia nervosa who are of normal weight may not need extensive evaluation for osteopenia or osteoporosis, those who have had previous episodes of anorexia nervosa may be at higher risk for these abnormalities (70) and require a similar assessment to that recommended for patients with anorexia nervosa.

TABLE 7. Laboratory Assessments for Patients With Eating Disorders

Assessment	Patient Indication
Basic analyses	All patients with eating disorders
Blood chemistry studies	
Serum electrolytes	
Blood urea nitrogen	
Serum creatinine (interpretations must incorporate assessments of weight)	
Thyroid-stimulating hormone test; if indicated, free T_4, T_3	
Complete blood count including differential	
Erythrocyte sedimentation rate	
Aspartate aminotransferase, alanine aminotransferase, alkaline phosphatase	
Urinalysis	
Additional analyses	Malnourished and severely symptomatic patients (serum magnesium should be obtained prior to administering certain medications if QTc is prolonged)[b]
Complement component 3[a]	
Blood chemistry studies	
Serum calcium	
Serum magnesium	
Serum phosphorus	
Serum ferritin	
Electrocardiogram	
24-hour urine for creatinine clearance[c]	
Osteopenia and osteoporosis assessments	Patients amenorrheic for >6 months
Dual-energy X-ray absorptiometry	
Serum estradiol in female patients	
Serum testosterone in male patients	
Nonroutine assessments	
Toxicology screen	Patients with suspected substance use, particularly those with anorexia nervosa, binge/purge subtype, or patients with bulimia nervosa
Serum amylase (fractionated for salivary gland isoenzyme if available to rule out pancreatic involvement)	Patients with suspected surreptitious vomiting
Serum luteinizing hormone, follicle-stimulating hormone, β-human chorionic gonadotropin, prolactin	Patients with persistent amenorrhea but who are normal weight
Brain magnetic resonance imaging, computed tomography	Patients with significant cognitive deficits, other neurological soft signs, unremitting course, or other atypical features
Stool for guaiac	Patients with suspected GI bleeding
Stool or urine for bisacodyl, emodin, aloe-emodin, rhein	Patients with suspected laxative abuse[d]

[a]Some experts recommend the routine use of complement component 3 as a sensitive marker that may indicate nutritional deficiencies even when other laboratory test results are apparently in the normal range (71, 72).

[b]During hospital refeeding, it is recommended that serum potassium, magnesium, and phosphorus levels be determined daily for 5 days and thereafter at least three times/week for 3 weeks (73, 74).

[c]Boag et al. (75). Creatinine clearance should be calculated using equations that involve body surface using assessments of height and weight. [d]Duncan and Phillips (76); Turner et al. (77).

around the eating problems can be useful in assessment (89a). Family members can provide useful perspectives on factors contributing to the onset of the disorders and issues that may aid or hamper efforts at recovery. Family members are often distressed by difficulties in understanding and interacting with the patient. Clinicians need to empathically listen to family members, advise them on their interactions with the patient, and, when indicated, involve them in conjoint or individual treatment so that the patient and family all stand the best chance of achieving a good outcome (90). Patients with anorexia nervosa who are in a relationship may present with a higher motivation to change (91), and the involvement of spouses and partners in treatment may be highly desirable. Families of adolescents with anorexia nervosa may be directed to the Maudsley approach, which focuses on the family as a resource for recovery and puts parents in charge of refeeding their affected child (87, 92, 93). Although this approach is promising, additional data are required to determine if it is the best approach for adolescents with anorexia nervosa.

B. DEVELOPING A TREATMENT PLAN FOR THE INDIVIDUAL PATIENT

1. Choice of a treatment site

Services available for the treatment of eating disorders can range from intensive inpatient settings (in which subspecialty general medical consultation is readily available) to residential and partial hospitalization programs to varying levels of outpatient care (in which the patient can receive general medical treatment, nutritional counseling, and/or individual, group, and family psychotherapy). Because specialized programs are not available in all geographic areas and financial considerations are often significant, access to these programs may be difficult. The resources listed in Table 1 may provide guidance to patients and families for accessing suitable programs.

Pretreatment evaluation of the patient is essential for determining the appropriate treatment setting. Patient weight, rate of weight loss, cardiac function, and metabolic status are the most important physical parameters for making this choice. Eating disorders should be recognized and early treatment implemented as soon as possible after the onset of symptoms. This is especially true in children, adolescents, and young adults, to avoid the disorder becoming chronic.

As a general rule, patients who weigh less than approximately 85% of their individually estimated healthy weights have considerable difficulty gaining weight outside of a highly structured program that includes inpatient care; such a program may be medically and psychiatrically necessary even for patients above that weight level. It is important to underscore that these are individually estimated healthy weights, not weights simply listed in a standard insurance table. Healthy weight estimates for a given individual must be determined by that person's physicians on the basis of historical data (e.g., growth charts) (3) and, for women, the weight at which healthy menstruation and ovulation resume, which may be higher than the weight at which menstruation and ovulation became impaired (94–96).

It is equally important that the decision to hospitalize a patient be based on psychiatric and behavioral factors, including a rapid or persistent decline in oral intake; a decline in weight despite maximally intensive outpatient or partial hospitalization intervention; the presence of additional stressors, such as dental procedures, that may interfere with the patient's ability to eat; the weight at which the patient was medically unstable in the past; and co-occurring psychiatric problems that merit hospitalization. The degree of a patient's denial and resistance to participate in his or her own care in less supervised settings is critical in deciding whether to hospitalize the patient. Once weight loss is severe enough to indicate the need for immediate hospitalization, treatment may be less effective, refeeding may entail greater risks, and prognosis may be more problematic than if intervention had been provided earlier. Because cortical gray matter deficits result from malnutrition and persist after refeeding (97–99), earlier (rather than later) interventions may be important to minimize the persistent effects of these physiological impairments. Therefore, hospitalization should occur before the onset of medical instability as manifested by vital signs, physical findings, or laboratory test results outside of the normal range.

Vital sign changes that indicate a need for immediate medical hospitalization include marked orthostatic hypotension, with an increase in pulse of 20 bpm or a drop in blood pressure of 20 mmHg standing; bradycardia, with a heart rate <40 bpm; tachycardia, with a heart rate >110 bpm; or the patient's inability to sustain his or her body core temperature (e.g., body temperatures <97.0°F) (3). Most severely underweight patients, particularly those with physiological instability, require inpatient medical management and comprehensive treatment to support their weight-gaining efforts. To avert potentially irreversible effects on physical growth and development, many children and adolescents require inpatient medical treatment, even when weight loss, although rapid, has not been as severe as that suggesting a need for hospitalization in adult patients (3). If children refuse fluids or food out of concern about gaining weight, they may become dehydrated quickly. Also, a child's small size may mean that relatively smaller reductions in weight will result in greater physiological danger.

In determining a patient's initial level of care or suitability for change to a different level of care, expert consensus indicates that it is important to consider a patient's overall clinical and social picture rather than simply rely on weight criteria. Furthermore, weight level per se should never be used as the sole criterion for discharge from inpatient care. Patients need to both gain healthy body weight and learn to maintain that weight prior to discharge; patients who reach a healthy body weight but are discharged before this learning occurs are likely to immediately decrease their caloric intake to excessively low levels that are often insufficient to sustain their healthy body weight. Assisting patients in determining and practicing appropriate food intake at a healthy body weight is likely to decrease the chances of their relapsing. Patients who are medically stabilized on acute medical units will still require inpatient treatment for eating disorders if they do not meet biopsychosocial criteria for partial hospitalization programs or if no suitable partial hospitalization program for eating disorders treatment is accessible because of geographic or other reasons. Patients with inadequate motivation or support who are discharged from inpatient to partial hospitalization programs before they are clinically ready often have high rates of early relapse, greater struggles with recovery, and slower rates of progress, necessitating longer future inpatient stays.

In shifting between levels of care, it is important to establish continuity of care. Stepping down from one level of care to a less intensive level may be destabilizing for a patient and can be even more so when this involves a change in physician, therapist, or treatment team. At times, patients may erroneously conclude that moving to a less restrictive treatment setting means that they are suddenly fully improved. The patient's ability to continue treatment with familiar and trusted staff in a partial hospitalization or outpatient setting may contribute to the success of aftercare planning. Consequently, if the patient is moving from one treatment setting or locale to another, transition planning requires that the care team in the new setting or locale be identified and that specific patient appointments be made. It is preferable that a specific clinician on the team be designated as the primary coordinator of care to ensure continuity and attention to important aspects of treatment. Guidelines for treatment settings are provided in Table 8.

Although most patients with uncomplicated bulimia nervosa do not require hospitalization, indications for hospitalization can include severe disabling symptoms that have not responded to adequate trials of outpatient treatment, serious concurrent general medical problems (e.g., metabolic abnormalities, hematemesis, vital sign changes, uncontrolled vomiting), suicidality, psychiatric disturbances that would warrant patients' hospitalization independent of the eating disorder diagnosis, or severe concurrent substance use.

Legal interventions, including involuntary hospitalization and legal guardianship, may be necessary to address the safety of patients who are reluctant to receive treatment but whose general medical conditions are life threatening (102). On a short-term basis at least, outcomes for

TABLE 8. Level of Care Guidelines for Patients With Eating Disorders

	Level 1: Outpatient	Level 2: Intensive Outpatient	Level 3: Partial Hospitalization (Full-Day Outpatient Care)[a]	Level 4: Residential Treatment Center	Level 5: Inpatient Hospitalization
Medical status	Medically stable to the extent that more extensive medical monitoring, as defined in levels 4 and 5, is not required			Medically stable to the extent that intravenous fluids, nasogastric tube feedings, or multiple daily laboratory tests are not needed	*For adults:* Heart rate <40 bpm; blood pressure <90/60 mmHg; glucose <60 mg/dl; potassium <3 mEq/L; electrolyte imbalance; temperature <97.0°F; dehydration; hepatic, renal, or cardiovascular organ compromise requiring acute treatment; poorly controlled diabetes *For children and adolescents:* Heart rate near 40 bpm, orthostatic blood pressure changes (>20 bpm increase in heart rate or >10 mmHg to 20 mmHg drop), blood pressure <80/50 mmHg, hypokalemia,[b] hypophosphatemia, or hypomagnesemia
Suicidality[c]	If suicidality is present, inpatient monitoring and treatment may be needed depending on the estimated level of risk				Specific plan with high lethality or intent; admission may also be indicated in patient with suicidal ideas or after a suicide attempt or aborted attempt, depending on the presence or absence of other factors modulating suicide risk
Weight as percentage of healthy body weight[d]	Generally >85%	Generally >80%	Generally >80%	Generally <85%	Generally <85%; acute weight decline with food refusal even if not <85% of healthy body weight

TABLE 8. Level of Care Guidelines for Patients With Eating Disorders *(continued)*

	Level 1: Outpatient	Level 2: Intensive Outpatient	Level 3: Partial Hospitalization (Full-Day Outpatient Care)[a]	Level 4: Residential Treatment Center	Level 5: Inpatient Hospitalization
Motivation to recover, including cooperativeness, insight, and ability to control obsessive thoughts	Fair-to-good motivation	Fair motivation	Partial motivation; cooperative; patient preoccupied with intrusive, repetitive thoughts[e] >3 hours/day	Poor-to-fair motivation; patient preoccupied with intrusive repetitive thoughts[e] 4–6 hours a day; patient cooperative with highly structured treatment	Very poor to poor motivation; patient preoccupied with intrusive repetitive thoughts[e]; patient uncooperative with treatment or cooperative only in highly structured environment
Co-occurring disorders (substance use, depression, anxiety)	Presence of comorbid condition may influence choice of level of care				Any existing psychiatric disorder that would require hospitalization
Structure needed for eating/gaining weight	Self-sufficient	Self-sufficient	Needs some structure to gain weight	Needs supervision at all meals or will restrict eating	Needs supervision during and after all meals or nasogastric/special feeding modality
Ability to control compulsive exercising	Can manage compulsive exercising through self-control	Some degree of external structure beyond self-control required to prevent patient from compulsive exercising; rarely a sole indication for increasing the level of care			
Purging behavior (laxatives and diuretics)	Can greatly reduce incidents of purging in an unstructured setting; no significant medical complications, such as electrocardiographic or other abnormalities, suggesting the need for hospitalization			Can ask for and use support from others or use cognitive and behavioral skills to inhibit purging	Needs supervision during and after all meals and in bathrooms; unable to control multiple daily episodes of purging that are severe, persistent, and disabling, despite appropriate trials of outpatient care, even if routine laboratory test results reveal no obvious metabolic abnormalities

TABLE 8. Level of Care Guidelines for Patients With Eating Disorders *(continued)*

	Level 1: Outpatient	Level 2: Intensive Outpatient	Level 3: Partial Hospitalization (Full-Day Outpatient Care)[a]	Level 4: Residential Treatment Center	Level 5: Inpatient Hospitalization
Environmental stress	Others able to provide adequate emotional and practical support and structure		Others able to provide at least limited support and structure	Severe family conflict or problems or absence of family so patient is unable to receive structured treatment in home; patient lives alone without adequate support system	
Geographic availability of treatment program	Patient lives near treatment setting			Treatment program is too distant for patient to participate from home	

Source. Adapted and modified from La Via et al. (100).

Note. In general, a given level of care should be considered for patients who meet one or more criteria under a particular level. These guidelines are not absolutes, however, and their application requires physician judgment.

[a]This level of care is most effective if administered for at least 8 hours/day, 5 days/week; less intensive care is demonstrably less effective (101).

[b]If the patient is dehydrated, whole-body potassium values may be low even if the serum potassium value is in the normal range; determine concurrent urine specific gravity to assess for dehydration.

[c]Determining suicide risk is a complex clinical judgment, as is determining the most appropriate treatment setting for patients at risk for suicide. Relevant factors to consider are the patient's concurrent medical conditions, psychosis, substance use, other psychiatric symptoms or syndromes, psychosocial supports, past suicidal behaviors, and treatment adherence and the quality of existing physician-patient relationships. These factors are described in greater detail in the APA's *Practice Guideline for the Assessment and Treatment of Patients With Suicidal Behaviors* (84).

[d]Although this table lists percentages of expected healthy body weight in relation to suggested levels of care, these are only approximations and do not correspond to percentages based on standardized values for the population as a whole. For any given individual, differences in body build, body composition, and other physiological variables may result in considerable differences as to what constitutes a healthy body weight in relation to "norms." For example, for some patients, a healthy body weight may be 110% of the standardized value for the population, whereas for other individuals it may be 98%. Each individual's physiological differences must be assessed and appreciated. For children, also consider the rate of weight loss. Finally, weight level per se should never be used as the sole criterion for discharge from inpatient care. Many patients require inpatient admission at higher weights and should not be automatically discharged just because they have achieved a certain weight level unless all other factors are appropriately considered. See text for further discussion regarding weight.

[e]Individuals may experience these thoughts as consistent with their own deeply held beliefs (in which case they seem to be ego-syntonic and "overvalued") or as unwanted and ego-alien repetitive thoughts, consistent with classic obsessive-compulsive disorder phenomenology.

those patients who are hospitalized involuntarily are comparable with outcomes of those hospitalized voluntarily with respect to rates of weight restoration (103). The decision to hospitalize on a psychiatric versus a general medical or adolescent/pediatric unit depends on the patient's general medical status, the skills and abilities of local psychiatric and general medical staff, and the availability of suitable programs to care for the patient's general medical and psychiatric problems (104). There is evidence to suggest that patients treated in specialized inpatient eating disorder units have better outcomes than patients treated in general inpatient settings where staff lack expertise and experience in treating patients with eating disorders (105).

Partial hospitalization and day hospital programs are being increasingly used in attempts to decrease the length of inpatient stays or even in lieu of hospitalization for individuals with milder symptoms. However, such programs may not be appropriate for patients with lower initial weights. The failure of outpatient treatment is one of the most frequent indications for the more intensive treatment provided in a day, partial hospitalization, or inpatient program. In deciding whether a patient requires a partial hospitalization program, the patient's motivation to participate in treatment and ability to work in a group setting should be considered (106, 107). A growing body of evidence suggests that partial hospitalization outcomes are highly correlated with treatment intensity and that more successful programs involve patients at least 5 days/week for 8 hours/day (101).

Patients who are considerably below their healthy body weight but who are highly motivated to adhere to treatment, have cooperative families, and have brief symptom duration may benefit from treatment in outpatient settings, but only if they are carefully monitored and if they and their families understand that a more restrictive setting may be necessary if persistent progress is not evident within a few weeks (108, 109). Careful monitoring includes at least weekly (and often twice or thrice weekly) weight determinations done immediately after the patient voids and while the patient is wearing the same class of garment (e.g., hospital gown, standard exercise clothing). Measurement of urine specific gravity, orthostatic vital signs, oral body temperature, and, in purging patients, electrolytes may also need to be monitored on a regular basis. Although child and adolescent patients treated in the outpatient setting can remain with their families and continue to attend school or work, these advantages must be balanced against the risks of failure to progress in recovery.

2. Choice of specific treatments for anorexia nervosa

Anorexia nervosa is a complex, serious, and often chronic condition that may require a variety of treatment modalities at different stages of illness and recovery. Specific treatments include nutritional rehabilitation, psychosocial interventions, and medications. The aims of treatment are to 1) restore the patient to a healthy weight (associated with the return of menses and normal ovulation in female patients, normal sexual drive and hormone levels in male patients, and normal physical and sexual development in children and adolescents); 2) treat the patient's physical complications; 3) enhance the patient's motivation to cooperate in the restoration of healthy eating patterns and participate in treatment; 4) educate the patient regarding healthy nutrition and eating patterns; 5) help the patient reassess and change core dysfunctional cognitions, attitudes, motives, conflicts, and feelings related to the eating disorder; 6) treat the patient's associated psychiatric conditions, including deficits in mood and impulse regulation, self-esteem, and behavior; 7) enlist family support and provide family counseling and therapy where appropriate; and 8) prevent the patient from relapsing.

a) Nutritional rehabilitation

The goals of nutritional rehabilitation for seriously underweight patients are to restore weight, normalize eating patterns, achieve normal perceptions of hunger and satiety, and correct biological and psychological sequelae of malnutrition (110, 111).

Healthy target weights should be established as part of the initial treatment plan and discussed explicitly with the patient, but with considerable sensitivity to how generally fearful patients are of gaining weight. On occasion it may be judicious to delay this discussion until the patient is less likely to be terrified of his or her ultimate weight goal. In general, a healthy goal weight for female patients is the weight at which normal menstruation and ovulation are restored and, for male patients, the weight at which normal testicular function is resumed. For female patients who previously had a healthy menses and ovulation, the clinician can estimate their healthy weight as approximately the same weight at which full physical and psychological vigor were present. In one study of 100 adolescent patients with anorexia nervosa (94), the resumption of menses occurred at a weight approximately 4.5 pounds greater than the weight at which menses was lost; at 90% of healthy weight, 86% of patients resumed menses. In children and adolescents, growth curves should be followed and are most useful when longitudinal data are available, given that extrapolations from cross-sectional data at one point in time can be misleading. Therefore, for most clinical work, it is reasonable to simply weigh patients and gauge how far they are from their individually estimated healthy body weight (112). Bone age may be accurately estimated from wrist X-rays and nomograms. In conjunction with bone measurements, menstrual history in adolescents with secondary amenorrhea, mid-parental heights, and assessments of skeletal frame, CDC growth charts (available at http://www.cdc.gov/growthcharts/) may be used to accurately estimate individually appropriate ranges for "expected" weights for current age and to set individually realistic expectations and goals for weight and height for patients up to age 20 years.

For individuals who are markedly underweight and for children and adolescents whose growth is substantially less than that predicted by growth curves, hospital-based programs for nutritional rehabilitation should be considered. For those in inpatient or residential settings, the weight at which it is appropriate to discharge a patient may vary in relation to the patient's healthy target weight and will depend on the patient's ability to feed him- or herself, the patient's motivation and ability to participate in aftercare programs, and the adequacy of aftercare, including partial hospitalization. In general, the closer a patient is to his or her healthy body weight before discharge, the less the risk he or she has of relapsing and being readmitted. Having patients maintain their weight for a period of time before they are discharged from inpatient treatment probably decreases the risk of their relapsing as well.

Refeeding programs should be implemented in nurturing emotional contexts. Staff should convey to patients their intention to take care of them and not let them die even when the illness prevents the patients from taking care of themselves. Staff should clearly communicate that they are not seeking to engage in control battles and have no punitive intentions when using interventions that the patient may experience as aversive. Some positive reinforcements (e.g., privileges) and negative reinforcements (e.g., required bed rest, exercise restrictions, restrictions of off-unit privileges) should be built into the program; negative reinforcements can then be reduced or terminated and positive reinforcements accelerated as target weights and other goals are achieved.

As patients work to achieve their target weights, their treatment plan should also establish expected rates of controlled weight gain. Clinical consensus suggests that realistic targets are 2–3 lb/week for hospitalized patients and 0.5–1 lb/week for individuals in outpatient programs, although an intensive partial hospitalization, stepped-down program has reported gains of up to 2 lb/week (113). Occasionally some patients may gain as much as 4–5 lb/week, but these individuals must be carefully monitored for refeeding syndrome and fluid retention. Dietitians can help patients choose their own meals and provide a structured meal plan that ensures nutritional adequacy and inclusion of all the major food groups. Formula feeding may have to be added to achieve large caloric intake. Some authorities advocate that the amount of solid food eaten should not exceed the amount that patients would ordinarily be eating at their target weight. Expanding cuisine options is important to avoid the severely restricted food choices frequently seen in eating disorder patients. Legitimate food allergies and patients' religious and cultural practices must be considered and discussed to limit patient rationalizations for restricted eating. Intake levels should usually start at 30–40 kcal/kg per day (approximately 1,000–1,600 kcal/day). During the weight gain phase, intake may have to be advanced progressively to as high as 70–100 kcal/kg per day for some patients; many male patients require a very large number of calories to gain weight. Patients who require significantly higher caloric intakes may be discarding food, vomiting, or exercising frequently or they may engage in more nonexercise motor activity such as fidgeting; others may have a truly elevated metabolic rate. Patients requiring much lower caloric intakes or those suspected of artificially increasing their weight by fluid loading should be weighed in the morning after voiding while they are wearing only a gown; their fluid intake also should be carefully monitored. Assessing urine specimens obtained at the time of weigh-in for specific gravity may help ascertain the extent to which the measured weight reflects excessive water intake.

Particularly in residential or hospital treatment programs, it may initially be difficult to obtain the cooperation of patients who do not wish to be there. In addition, many patients have delayed gastric emptying that initially impairs their ability to tolerate 1,000 calories/day. Under such circumstances, it is often more effective to begin with 200–300 calories above the patient's usual caloric intake (e.g., a patient consuming 400 calories/day may need to start at 600–700 calories/day). During hospitalization, giving patients a liquid feeding formula in the early stages of weight gain and then gradually exposing them to food and slowly increasing their activity level can be a very effective strategy for inducing weight gain (114). As patients are able and as their cooperation improves, a 2–3 lb/week gain in residential or hospital programs can be expected without compromising the patients' safety.

In addition to an increased caloric intake, patients also benefit from vitamin and mineral supplements. Serum potassium levels should be regularly monitored in patients who are persistent vomiters. Hypokalemia should be treated with oral or intravenous potassium supplementation and rehydration.

Physical activity should be adapted to the food intake and energy expenditure of the patient, taking into account bone mineral density and cardiac function. For the severely underweight patient, exercise should be restricted and always carefully supervised and monitored. Once a safe weight is achieved, the focus of an exercise program should be on physical fitness as opposed to expending calories. The focus on fitness should be balanced with restoring patients' positive relationship with their bodies—helping them to take back control and get pleasure from physical activities rather than being compulsively enslaved to them. An exercise program should involve exercises that are not solitary, are enjoyable, and have endpoints that are not determined by time spent expending calories or changing weight and shape. Sports such as soccer, basketball, volleyball, or tennis are examples (115).

Staff should help patients deal with their concerns about weight gain and body image changes, given that these are particularly difficult adjustments for patients to make. In fact, there is general agreement among clinicians that distorted attitudes about weight and shape are the least likely to change and that excessive and compulsive exercise may be one of the last of the behaviors associated with an eating disorder to abate. Although it is by no means certain that patients' abnormal eating habits will improve simply as a function of weight gain (116), there is considerable evidence to suggest that other eating disorder symptoms diminish as weight is restored with nutritional rehabilitation. For example, clinical experience indicates that with weight restoration, food choices increase, food hoarding decreases, and obsessions about food decrease in frequency and intensity, although they do not necessarily disappear.

Providing anorexia nervosa patients who have associated binge eating and purging behaviors with regular structured meal plans may also enable them to improve. For some patients, however, giving up severe dietary restrictions and restraints appears to increase binge-eating behavior, which is often accompanied by compensatory purging.

As weight is regained, changes in associated mood and anxiety symptoms as well as in physical status can be expected (117). Clinicians should advise patients of what changes they can anticipate as they start to regain weight. In the initial stages, the apathy and lethargy associated with malnourishment may abate. However, as patients start to recover and feel their bodies becoming larger, and especially as they approach frightening magical numbers on the scale that represent phobic weights, they may experience a resurgence of anxious and depressive symptoms, irritability, and sometimes suicidal thoughts. These mood symptoms, non-food-related obsessional thoughts, and compulsive behaviors, although often not eradicated, usually decrease with sustained weight gain.

Weight gains result in improvement in most of the physiological complications of semistarvation, including improvement in electrolyte levels, heart and kidney function, and attention and concentration. Initial refeeding may be associated with mild transient fluid retention, and patients who abruptly stop taking laxatives or diuretics may experience marked rebound fluid retention for several weeks, presumably from salt and water retention caused by elevated aldosterone levels associated with chronic dehydration. Refeeding edema and bloating occur frequently.

Patients may experience abdominal pain and bloating with meals from the delayed gastric emptying that accompanies malnutrition. Constipation, which may be ameliorated with stool softeners, can progress to obstipation and, rarely, acute bowel obstruction. As weight gain progresses, many patients also develop acne and breast tenderness. Many patients become unhappy and demoralized about resulting changes in body shape. Management strategies for dealing with these milder adverse effects include careful refeeding, frequent physical examinations, and forewarnings to patients about mild refeeding edema.

A severe refeeding syndrome may occur when severely malnourished patients (generally those weighing <70% of their healthy body weight) are re-fed too rapidly, particularly in the context of enteral or parenteral feedings but also with vigorous oral refeeding regimens. This syndrome consists of hypophosphatemia, hypomagnesemia, hypocalcemia, and fluid retention. Thiamine deficiency may also be seen as a feature of this syndrome. In some case series, the refeeding syndrome has been reported to occur in roughly 6% of hospitalized adolescents (118). Excessively rapid refeeding and nasogastric or parenteral feeding may be particularly dangerous because of their potential for inducing severe fluid retention, cardiac arrhythmias, cardiac failure, respiratory insufficiency, delirium, seizures, rhabdomyolysis, red cell dysfunction, and even sudden death, especially in the lowest-weight patients (118, 119). In such cases, phosphorus, magnesium, and/or potassium supplementation will be necessary (118, 120). In one series of hospitalized adolescents, moderate hypophosphatemia occurred in 5.8% and mild hypophosphatemia in 21.7% of patients, requiring some degree of phosphorus replacement in 27.5% of these patients (120).

Besides monitoring of mineral and electrolyte levels, general medical monitoring during refeeding should include assessment of vital signs, monitoring of food and fluid intake and output (if indicated), and observation for edema, rapid weight gain (associated primarily with fluid overload), congestive heart failure, and gastrointestinal symptoms. For children and adolescents who are severely malnourished (weigh <70% of their standard body weight), cardiac monitoring, especially at night, may be advisable (120).

Some patients are completely unable to recognize their illness, accept the need for treatment, or tolerate the guilt that would accompany eating, even when performed to sustain their lives. On the rare occasions when staff have to take over the responsibilities for providing life-preserving care, nasogastric feedings are preferable to intravenous feedings. In some programs, supplemental overnight pediatric nasogastric tube feedings have been used to facilitate weight gain in cooperative patients. This practice is not routinely recommended at present, although it appears to be well tolerated, may slightly decrease hospital stays in children, and may be experienced positively by some patients, particularly younger patients, who may feel relieved to know that they are being cared for and who, while they cannot bring themselves to eat, are willing to allow physicians to feed them (121). If used, such interventions should never supplant expectations that the patient will resume normal eating patterns on his or her own. Total parenteral feeding is required only rarely and for brief periods in life-threatening situations.

Forced nasogastric or parenteral feeding can each be accompanied by substantial dangers. When nasogastric feeding is necessary, clinical experience suggests that continuous feeding (i.e., over 24 hours) may be less likely than three to four bolus feedings a day to result in metabolic abnormalities or patient discomfort and may be better tolerated by patients. As an alternative to nasogastric feedings, in very difficult situations where patients physically resist and constantly remove their nasogastric tubes, gastrostomy or jejunostomy tubes may be surgically inserted. As described above, rapid refeeding can be associated with the severe refeeding syndrome, and infection is always a risk with parenteral feedings in emaciated and potentially immunocompromised patients with anorexia nervosa. Consequently, these interventions should not be used routinely but should be considered only when patients are unwilling or unable to cooperate with oral feedings or when the patients' health, physical safety, and recovery are being threatened. In situations where involuntary forced feeding is considered, careful thought should be given to clinical circumstances, family opinion, and relevant legal and ethical dimensions of the patient's treatment.

If using interventions that patients with anorexia nervosa may experience as coercive, the clinician should consider the potential impact on the therapeutic relationship, especially since maintaining a sense of control is often a key dynamic in these patients. The setting of limits is developmentally appropriate in the management of children and adolescents and may help shape the patient's behavior in a healthy direction. It is essential for caregivers to be clear about their own intentions and empathic capacities regarding the patient's impression of being coerced. Caregivers should not be seen as using techniques intended to be coercive. Rather, caregivers' interventions should always be clearly seen as components of a general medical treatment required for the patient's health and survival.

During the last few years, there has been considerable debate about the ethics of involuntarily feeding patients with anorexia nervosa (122, 123). There is general agreement that children and adolescents who are severely malnourished and in grave medical danger should be refed, involuntarily if necessary, but that every effort should be made to gain their cooperation as cognitive function improves.

Ethical as well as clinical dilemmas often confront clinicians dealing with adult patients with chronic anorexia nervosa and their families. The general principles to be followed are those directing good, humane care; respecting the wishes of competent patients; and intervening respectfully with patients whose judgment is severely impaired by their psychiatric disorders when such interventions are likely to have beneficial results (124, 125).

b) Psychosocial interventions

The goals of psychosocial interventions in patients with anorexia nervosa are to help them 1) understand and cooperate with their nutritional and physical rehabilitation, 2) understand and change the behaviors and dysfunctional attitudes related to their eating disorder, 3) improve their interpersonal and social functioning, and 4) address comorbid psychopathology and psychological conflicts that reinforce or cause them to maintain eating disorder behaviors. Efforts to achieve these goals often benefit from an initial enhancement of a patient's motivation to change along with ongoing efforts to sustain this motivation.

(i) Acute anorexia nervosa

Few controlled studies offer guidance for the psychosocial treatment of anorexia nervosa. Clinical consensus suggests that during the acute refeeding and weight gain stages, it is beneficial to provide patients with individual psychotherapeutic management that is psychodynamically informed and that provides empathic understanding, explanations, praise for positive efforts, coaching, support, encouragement, and other positive behavioral reinforcement. During all phases of treatment, seeing patients' families is also helpful, particularly for children and adolescents, for whom controlled trials suggest that family treatment is the most effective intervention (86, 126). For patients who initially lack motivation, their awareness and desire for recovery may be increased by psychotherapeutic techniques based on motivational enhancement, although solid evidence for this contention is lacking.

At the same time, clinical consensus suggests that psychotherapy alone is generally not sufficient to treat severely malnourished patients with anorexia nervosa. Although the value of establishing and maintaining a psychotherapeutically informed relationship is clearly beneficial and psychotherapeutic sessions to enhance patient motivation and further patient weight gain are likely to be helpful, the value of formal psychotherapy during the acute refeeding stage is uncertain (127). Attempts to conduct formal psychotherapy may be ineffective with starving patients, who are often negativistic, obsessional, or mildly cognitively impaired, presumably in relation to the known cortical atrophy seen in nutritionally compromised patients. One study documented the difficulty researchers have had in initiating and sustaining cognitive-behavioral therapies for patients with anorexia nervosa (128).

Most nutritional rehabilitation programs incorporate emotional nurturance and one of a variety of behavioral interventions that link exercise, bed rest, and privileges with target weights, desired behaviors, and informational feedback. Several studies of individual therapy have shown modest success, sometimes in only a small percentage of patients (7, 85). In one controlled trial, nonspecific supportive clinical management appeared to be at least as effective as CBT or IPT in some patients. However, 70% of patients either did not complete or made only small gains from the active psychotherapies they received (7). In this study, clinical management included education, care, support, and the fostering of a therapeutic relationship designed to promote adherence to treatment through the use of praise, reassurance, and advice.

The accumulated evidence strongly supports the value of family therapy for the acute treatment of children and adolescents in outpatient settings. Studies show that whether patients and parents are seen together or are treated separately in ongoing treatment, the results are better than when families are not involved at all (86, 126). This approach begins with the therapist's attempting to unite the parents in developing a consistent approach to refeeding, sympathizing with their plight, and explicitly disclaiming the notion that the parents have caused the eating problem. When families are involved in treatment, sibling subsystems can be engaged to support the affected sibling. Parents can determine for themselves how best to refeed their child with anorexia nervosa with the therapist's ongoing support and consultation. For some outpatients, a short-term course of family therapy may be as effective as a long-term course; however, a shorter course of therapy may not be adequate for patients with severe obsessive-compulsive features or nonintact families (129). In these studies (129), inpatient care was used briefly for medical stabilization. For adolescents treated in inpatient settings, participation in family group psychoeducation may help promote weight gain and may be as effective as more intensive forms of family therapy (130).

(ii) Anorexia nervosa after weight restoration

Clinical consensus suggests that psychotherapy can be helpful for patients with anorexia nervosa once their malnutrition has been corrected and they have begun gaining weight (131). Because of the enduring nature of many of the psychopathological features of anorexia nervosa and the patient's need for support during recovery, ongoing individual psychotherapeutic treatment is frequently required for at least 1 year and may take many years (132, 133).

Although there have been few formal studies of its effectiveness (134, 135), psychotherapy is generally thought to help patients understand 1) what they have been through; 2) developmental, familial, and cultural antecedents of their illness; 3) how their illness may have been a maladaptive attempt to cope and emotionally self-regulate; 4) how to avoid or minimize the risk of relapse; and 5) how to better deal with salient developmental and other important life issues in the future. At present there is no absolute weight or percentage of body fat that indicates when a patient is actually ready to begin formal psychotherapy. In addition, patients often display improved mood, enhanced cognitive functioning, and clearer thought processes once their nutritional status has significantly improved and even before they make substantial weight gains.

Little evidence from controlled studies exists to guide clinicians in the use of specific therapies for adults with anorexia nervosa. Nonetheless, some data are emerging in support of individual CBT (136–138) for helping patients maintain healthy eating behaviors and CBT or IPT for inducing cognitive restructuring and promoting more effective coping (139, 140). After a patient has begun to gain weight, CBT may be helpful in reducing the risk of relapse and improving outcome, as demonstrated in a small randomized controlled trial (136). In that study, patients who received CBT were more likely to remain in treatment (78%) and have a good outcome after a year (44%) than those assigned to nutritional counseling (7%).

Many clinicians also use psychodynamically oriented individual or group psychotherapy to address underlying personality disorders that may hamper treatment and help sustain the illness and to foster psychological insight and maturation in patients who have made strides toward weight restoration (141–148). Clinical consensus suggests that psychosocial interventions should incorporate an understanding of the patient's developmental traumas, cognitive development, psychodynamic conflict and defense styles, disorders of self-esteem, self-regulation, and "sense of self," as well as other psychological deficits, the presence of other psychiatric disorders, and the complexity of family relationships (149–152). Although studies of psychotherapies focus on different interventions as distinctly separate treatments, in practice there is frequent overlap among treatments. Indeed, most experienced clinicians report using interventions that cross theoretical boundaries when treating patients with eating disorders (153).

In adolescents, controlled studies have shown that for patients who are younger than age 19 years, have been ill for 3 years or less, and have restored their weight, family therapy is more beneficial than individual therapy, whereas individual therapy is more beneficial for patients with later-onset disorders (154). At 5-year follow-up of patients who received these therapies, much of the improvement could be attributed to the natural outcome of the illness, but it was still possible to detect long-term benefits of the psychological therapies (155).

Regardless of the clinical or theoretical approach used in treatment, some patients with eating disorders challenge clinicians' understanding and in some instances provoke countertransference reactions, particularly in response to patients' communications of aggression and defiance (140, 147, 156–162). Clinical consensus suggests that eating disorders are often difficult to ameliorate with short-term interventions, at least in older adolescents and adults; for this reason, clinicians often feel they have not done enough to change the patient's plight. Countertransference feelings often include beleaguerment, demoralization, and excessive need to change patients with a chronic eating disorder. At the same time, when treating patients with chronic illnesses, clinicians need to understand the longitudinal course of the disorder and that patients can recover even after many years of symptoms. Such awareness may help clinicians maintain a degree of therapeutic optimism and deal with the feelings of pessimistic demoralization that may arise (13, 163).

Some observations suggest that the gender of the clinician may play a role in the particular kind of countertransference reactions that come into play (156, 157). A patient's concerns about the gender of a clinician may be tied to concerns about potential boundary violations and should be attended to when selecting clinicians, including psychiatrists (164, 165). In addition, cultural differences between patients and clinicians or patients and other aspects of the care system may also influence the course and conduct of treatment and require attention. Ongoing processing of one's countertransference reactions, sometimes with the help of a supervisor or consultant, can be useful in helping the clinician persevere and reconcile intense, troublesome countertransference reactions.

When a patient with an eating disorder has been sexually abused or has felt helpless in other situations of boundary violations, this may stir up needs in the clinician to rescue the patient, which can occasionally result in a loosening of the therapeutic structure, the loss of therapeutic boundary keeping, and a sexualized countertransference reaction. In some cases, these countertransference responses have led to overt sexual acting out and unethical treatment on the part of the clinician that have not only compromised treatment but also severely harmed the patient (166). The maintenance of clear boundaries is critical in treating all patients with eating disorders, not only those who have been sexually abused but also those who may have experienced other types of boundary intrusions regarding their bodies, eating behaviors, and other aspects of the self by family members or others. Regular meetings with other team members and/or formal supervision can also help clinicians avoid boundary violations with eating disorder patients. Particularly with some adolescents, a clinician's obvious warmth and direct educational approach may facilitate initiating and sustaining the patient's trust. However, the license to be informal may create a climate in which a clinician is at a greater risk to violate therapeutic boundaries; such an occurrence must be consistently and carefully prevented. At the same time, according to some clinicians, a clinician's excessively rigid, cold manner and formal distancing behaviors (e.g., avoiding even benign pats on the shoulder that a patient might seek for reassurance) may be disconcerting to some patients and inhibit them from fully engaging in treatment.

Some clinicians use group psychotherapy as an adjunctive treatment for anorexia nervosa; in such cases, however, caution must be taken that patients do not compete to be the thinnest or sickest patient in the group or become excessively demoralized by observing the ongoing struggles of other patients in the group. For that reason, clinicians sometimes prefer heterogeneous groups that combine patients with bulimia nervosa and those with anorexia nervosa. Although there has been little formal study of group psychotherapy in the treatment of anorexia nervosa, one naturalistic study suggests that CBT may have promise (137).

Some clinicians consider that eating disorders may be usefully treated through addiction models, but no data from short- or long-term outcome studies using these methods have been reported. Literature from Anorexics and Bulimics Anonymous and Overeaters Anonymous emphasizes that these programs are not substitutes for professional treatment. These organizations specifically recommend that members seek appropriate medical and nutritional guidance. Nevertheless, there are concerns about zealous and narrow application of the 12-step philosophy in addiction-oriented programs for eating disorders. Programs that focus exclusively on abstaining from binge eating, purging, restrictive eating, and exercise (e.g., 12-step programs) without attending to nutritional considerations or cognitive and behavioral deficits have not been studied and therefore cannot be recommended as the sole treatment for anorexia nervosa. Clinicians frequently report encountering patients who, while attempting to resolve anorexia nervosa by means of a 12-step program alone, might have been greatly helped by concurrent conventional treatment approaches such as nutritional counseling and rehabilitation, medications, and psychodynamic or cognitive-behavioral approaches. By limiting their attempts to recover to their participation in a 12-step program alone, patients not only deprive themselves of the potential benefits of conventional treatments but also may expose themselves to misinformation about nutrition and eating disorders offered by well-intended nonprofessionals participating in and sometimes running these groups. Attempts have been made to integrate traditional and 12-step approaches into treatment; such approaches can offer a strong sense of community, but the effectiveness and potential adverse effects of these combined interventions have not been systematically studied (167). It is important for programs using a 12-step model to be equipped to care for patients with the substantial psychiatric and general medical problems often associated with eating disorders.

Selective support groups led by professionals and advocacy organizations may be beneficial as adjuncts to other psychosocial treatment modalities. However, clinicians should remain cognizant of the idiosyncratic recommendations made in some self-help groups. Sometimes, participants or leaders will eschew clinician-recommended treatments such as psychotropic medication or insist that a participant follow a particular kind of meal structure. These recommendations may conflict with other treatment recommendations and potentially increase the patient's resistance to treatment.

Patients and their families are increasingly using online web sites, news groups, and chat rooms as resources. Although substantial amounts of worthwhile information and support are available in this fashion, the lack of professional supervision of these sources may sometimes lead to misinformation and unhealthy dynamics among users. Clinicians should ask patients about their use of electronic support and other alternative and complementary approaches and be prepared to openly and sympathetically discuss the information and ideas they and their families have gathered from these sources.

As with any form of intervention, various psychosocial interventions may generate adverse effects; however, these have not been systematically studied with regard to treating anorexia nervosa. Some that have been observed by clinicians, patients, and families include 1) fostering negative attitudes in patients and/or families toward health care professionals without adequate discussion and reflection, thereby increasing the risk that patients will drop out of treatment and become less willing to seek or engage in professional treatment; 2) delaying referral to more appropriate interventions; and 3) generating burdensome costs without reasonable or expected benefits (13, 168).

Patients often have difficulty with certain elements of psychotherapy. For example, among patients receiving CBT, some are quite resistant to self-monitoring, whereas others have difficulty mastering cognitive restructuring. Most patients are initially resistant to changing their eating behaviors, particularly when it comes to increasing their caloric intake or reducing exercise. However, the complete lack of acceptance of a psychotherapeutic approach appears to be rare, although this has not been systematically studied.

Management strategies to deal with potential negative effects of psychotherapeutic interventions include 1) conducting a careful pretreatment evaluation, during which the therapist must assess and enhance the patient's level of motivation for change and determine the most appropriate therapeutic approach and format (e.g., individual versus group); 2) being alert to a patient's reactions to and attitudes about the proposed treatment and listening to and discussing the patient's concerns in a supportive fashion; 3) ongoing monitoring of the quality of the therapeutic relationship; and 4) identifying patients for whom another treatment should be co-administered or given before psychotherapy begins (e.g., substance use disorder treatment for those actively abusing alcohol or other drugs, antidepressant treatment for patients whose depression makes them unable to become actively involved, more intensive psychotherapy for those with severe personality disorders, group therapy for those not previously participating). Alternative strategies may be necessary to facilitate the therapeutic process and prevent the abrupt termination of therapy (13). As with all therapeutic interventions, it is essential that the therapist be alert to potential countertransference phenomena toward these often difficult-to-treat patients. If unresolved, these reactions have a high potential for disrupting or hastening the termination of treatment.

(iii) Chronic anorexia nervosa

Available studies of patients with chronic anorexia nervosa typically show a lack of substantial clinical response to psychotherapy. For example, in the study of Dare et al. (85), 84 patients, ill for an average of 6.3 years and with an initial average BMI of 15.4 kg/m^2, were assigned to one of three individual psychotherapies or a control group. The results after 1 year of psychotherapy were modest in all groups, although the psychoanalytic psychotherapy and family therapy groups fared better than those in the low-contact, routine-care control group. Nevertheless, many clinicians report seeing patients with chronic anorexia nervosa who, after many years of struggling with their disorder, experience substantial remission; thus clinicians are justified in maintaining and extending some degree of hope to patients and families.

For patients whose anorexia nervosa continues to be resistant to treatment despite substantial trials of nutritional rehabilitation, medications, and hospitalizations, more extensive psychotherapeutic measures may be undertaken in a further effort to engage and help motivate them or, failing that, as compassionate care. This difficult-to-treat subgroup may represent an as-yet poorly understood group of patients with malignant, chronic anorexia nervosa. Efforts to understand the unique plight of such patients may sometimes lead to engagement in the therapeutic alliance, thereby allowing the nutritional protocol to be initiated (125, 141, 142, 169, 170). With patients who have difficulty talking about their problems, clinicians have reported a variety of nonverbal therapeutic methods, such as creative arts and movement therapy programs, to be useful (171), but these methods have not been formally studied. At various stages of recovery, occupational therapy programs may also enhance self-concept and self-efficacy (172, 173), but again these programs have not been formally studied.

c) Medications

Although psychotropic medications should not be used as the sole or primary treatment for anorexia nervosa, they have been used as an adjunct treatment when nutritional rehabilitation programs alone are ineffective in restoring patients' normal weight or when patients demonstrate significant comorbid psychopathology such as disabling obsessive-compulsive, depressive, or anxiety symptoms. However, because anorexia nervosa symptoms and associated features such as depression may remit with weight gain, decisions concerning the use of medications should be deferred if possible until patients' weight has been restored. The decisions about whether to use psychotropic medications and which medications to choose will be determined by the remaining symptom picture (e.g., antidepressants are usually considered for those with persistent depression, anxiety, or obsessive-compulsive symptoms and for bulimic symptoms in weight-restored patients; second-generation antipsychotics are usually considered for those with severe, unremitting resistance to gaining weight, severe obsessional thinking, and denial that assumes delusional proportions). Many patients with anorexia nervosa are extremely reluctant to take medications and often refuse those that they know to specifically affect weight. These issues must be discussed sympathetically and comprehensively with patients and, for children and adolescents, with their families.

(i) Antidepressants

The efficacy of SSRI antidepressants for anorexia nervosa appears to vary with the phase of treatment. On the basis of several studies, fluoxetine does not appear to confer significant benefits during weight restoration (174, 175), nor did citalopram increase the rate of weight gain in a small study (176). In contrast, in weight-restored patients, fluoxetine in dosages of up to 60 mg/day may decrease relapse episodes and has been associated with better maintenance of weight and fewer symptoms of depression (177). However, for weight-restored patients with anorexia nervosa who are receiving CBT to help prevent relapse, adding fluoxetine to their treatment does not further decrease the risk of relapse (138).

Although higher dosages of fluoxetine have been found to impair appetite and cause weight loss in normal-weight and obese patients, this effect has not been reported in anorexia nervosa patients treated with lower dosages. Many clinicians report that malnourished depressed patients are less responsive to the beneficial effects of tricyclics, SSRIs, and other antidepressant medications than normal-weight depressed patients. These findings are consistent with those showing that SSRIs are not as effective for depression, when patients without an eating disorder undergo dietary restrictions (178, 179).

Malnourished patients are also much more prone to the side effects of medications. For example, the use of tricyclic antidepressants may be associated with greater risk of hypotension, increased cardiac conduction times, and arrhythmia, particularly in purging patients whose hydration may be inadequate and whose cardiac status may be nutritionally compromised. Given the availability of other antidepressant treatments, tricyclic antidepressants should be avoided, particularly in underweight patients and in patients who are at risk for suicide. In patients for whom there is a concern regarding potential cardiovascular effects of medication, medical specialty consultation can help evaluate the patient's status and advise on the use of medication. With all antidepressants, strategies to manage side effects include limiting the use of medications to patients with persistent depression, anxiety, or obsessive-compulsive symptoms; using low initial doses in underweight patients; and remaining vigilant about early manifestations of side effects.

Several other antidepressants have also been associated with significant side effects that are of relevance to the treatment of anorexia nervosa patients. Bupropion has been associated with an increased likelihood of seizures in patients with bulimia nervosa (180, 181); although the reason for this is unknown, it is suspected that patients with anorexia nervosa, binge-purge type, may also be at increased risk for seizures. Thus, this medication is not recommended for patients with anorexia nervosa, particularly those who purge. Mirtazapine, an antidepressant associated with weight gain, has also been associated with neutropenia. In addition, the only published case report of using mirtazapine to treat anorexia nervosa described a patient also taking fluvoxamine who developed the serotonin syndrome (182). Thus, mirtazapine may not be suitable for use in underweight anorexia nervosa patients.

Clinicians must attend to the black box warnings concerning antidepressants and conduct appropriate informed consent with patients and families if antidepressants are to be prescribed (183–189).

(ii) Antipsychotics

It has been suggested that antipsychotic medications, particularly second-generation antipsychotics, can be potentially useful during the weight-restoration phase or in treatment of other associated symptoms of anorexia nervosa, such as marked obsessionality, anxiety, limited insight, and psychotic-like thinking. Although no controlled studies have been reported in patients with anorexia nervosa, controlled trials of olanzapine and risperidone are under way. Evidence from case reports, case series, and open-label uncontrolled trials suggests that the second-generation antipsychotic olanzapine may promote weight gain in adults and in adolescent patients (190–193) and that olanzapine (190–194) and quetiapine may improve other associated symptoms (195–197). A small open-label study of low-dose haloperidol also showed improved insight and weight gain in severely ill patients (198). The quality of the available evidence on using antipsychotic medications is also limited by the fact that studies rarely include male patients and have included only small numbers of adolescents; in addition, only case reports are available regarding prepubertal children. If antipsychotic medications are used, the possibility of extrapyramidal symptoms, especially in debilitated patients, should be considered and routinely assessed. Also, appropriate attention must be given to the potential adverse impact of these medications on insulin sensitivity, lipid metabolism, and length of QTc interval.

(iii) Other medications and somatic treatments

Other somatic treatments, ranging from vitamin and hormone treatments to ECT, have been tried in uncontrolled studies. None has been shown to have specific value in the treatment of anorexia nervosa symptoms (199).

Other medications have been used to address associated features of anorexia nervosa. For example, antianxiety agents have been used selectively before meals to reduce anticipatory anxiety concerning eating (200, 201), and pro-motility agents, such as metoclopramide, are commonly offered for the bloating and abdominal pains that result from gastroparesis and that contribute to the premature satiety seen in some patients. However, before prescribing metoclopramide, clinicians should consider the fact that extrapyramidal symptoms are more likely to be seen in underweight anorexia nervosa patients.

In anorexia nervosa patients with prolonged amenorrhea, hormone replacement therapy (HRT) is frequently prescribed to improve patients' bone mineral density. However, no good supporting evidence exists to demonstrate the efficacy of this treatment (202, 203). In women with anorexia nervosa, the evidence supporting the use of HRT is marginal at best. HRT has not been demonstrated to increase bone mineral density over and above standard treatment in adults (204) or in adolescents (203). Only in a subset of very-low-weight women (<70% average body weight) did it prevent further bone loss (204). Estrogen can cause the fusion of the epiphyses and should not be administered to girls before their growth is completed (3). HRT usually induces monthly menstrual bleeding, obscuring the major sign that indicates weight normalization in women. This, in turn, may cause the patient to misunderstand that her body is functioning normally and therefore contribute to denial of the need to gain more weight. Clinicians stress that efforts should be made to allow patients to increase their weight and achieve resumption of normal menses before they are offered estrogen (205). There is no indication for the use of biphosphonates such as alendronate in patients with anorexia nervosa. In fact, long-term use of alendronate may oversuppress bone turnover (206). Thus, the recommended treatment for low bone mineral density includes weight gain and calcium with vitamin D supplementation (207).

3. Choice of specific treatments for bulimia nervosa

The aims of treatment for patients with bulimia nervosa are to 1) reduce and, where possible, eliminate binge eating and purging; 2) treat physical complications of bulimia nervosa; 3) enhance the patient's motivation to cooperate in the restoration of healthy eating patterns and participate in treatment; 4) provide education regarding healthy nutrition and eating patterns; 5) help the patient reassess and change core dysfunctional thoughts, attitudes, motives, conflicts, and feelings related to the eating disorder; 6) treat associated psychiatric conditions, including deficits in mood and impulse regulation, self-esteem, and behavior; 7) enlist family support and provide family counseling and therapy where appropriate; and 8) prevent relapse.

a) Nutritional rehabilitation and counseling

Bulimia nervosa is associated with nutritional chaos characterized by alternating cycles of dietary restriction, bingeing, and purging. A primary focus for nutritional rehabilitation is to help patients develop a structured meal plan that will allow them to reduce the episodes of dietary restriction and the urge to binge and purge. Nutritional intake should be sufficient to promote satiety. Because most bulimia nervosa patients who have been studied are of normal weight, nutritional restoration will not be a central focus of treatment. However, normal body weight (or normal BMI) does not ensure normal body composition, nor does it ensure that nutritional intake is appropriate. In addition, even if their weight is within statistically normal ranges, many patients with bulimia nervosa weigh less than their appropriate biologically determined set points (or ranges) and may have to gain some weight to achieve physiological and emotional stability. Although many patients with bulimia nervosa report irregular menses, improvement in menstrual function has not been systematically assessed in the available outcome studies. Thus, even among patients of normal weight, nutritional counseling may be a useful adjunct to other treatment modalities in reducing behaviors related to the eating disorder, minimizing food restrictions, increasing the variety of foods eaten, and encouraging healthy but not compulsive exercise patterns (208). Those patients for whom some weight gain is indicated similarly require the establishment of a pattern of regular, non-binge meals, with attention on increasing their caloric intake and expanding macronutrient selection. Patients with bulimia nervosa who are overweight or obese have not been well studied.

b) Psychosocial interventions

The goals of psychosocial interventions for patients with bulimia nervosa vary and can include the following: reducing or eliminating binge eating and purging behaviors; improving attitudes related to the eating disorder; minimizing food restriction; increasing the variety of foods eaten; encouraging healthy but not compulsive exercise patterns; treating co-occurring conditions and clinical features associated with eating disorders; and addressing themes that may underlie eating disorder behaviors such as developmental issues, identity formation, body image concerns, self-esteem in areas outside of those related to weight and shape, sexual and aggressive difficulties, affect regulation, sex role expectations, family dysfunction, coping styles, and problem solving. Consequently, psychosocial interventions should be chosen on the basis of a comprehensive evaluation of the individual patient and take into consideration the patient's cognitive and psychological development, psychodynamic issues, cognitive style, comorbid psychopathology, and preferences as well as age and family situation.

With respect to short-term interventions for treating acute episodes of bulimia nervosa in adults, the available evidence indicates that CBT is the most efficacious. CBT may effect improvements in psychological functioning of bulimia nervosa patients as well as ameliorate binge eating and purging symptoms. For example, studies have shown that bulimia nervosa patients who improved with CBT also showed improvements in self-directedness and harm avoidance (209, 210). Among patients who do not initially respond to CBT, a small number do respond to IPT or fluoxetine (211) or other modes of treatment such as family and group psychotherapies. Some controlled trials (212) have also shown the effectiveness of IPT as an initial therapy. Behavioral techniques, such as planned meals and self-monitoring, may also be helpful for managing initial symptoms and interrupting binge-purge behaviors (213, 214). It should be pointed out that these study results may not be generalizable to typical clinical situations. For example, to maximize the "clean" experimental nature of some of the CBT/IPT controlled studies mentioned above, the CBT intentionally avoided dealing with interpersonal issues and the IPT intentionally avoided talking about eating issues, which is quite different than how these therapies are conducted in clinical practice (215). It is also possible that the narrow inclusion criteria of some studies limit the generalizability of the study results (216).

Some clinical reports indicate that psychodynamic and psychoanalytic approaches in individual or group format are useful once bingeing and purging symptoms improve (217–219). These approaches address developmental issues; identity formation; body image concerns; self-esteem; conflicts surrounding sexuality, anger, or aggression; affect regulation; gender role expectations; interpersonal conflicts; family dysfunction; coping styles; and problem solving. In a recent naturalistic study of treatment as practiced by experienced clinicians in the community, both CBT and psychodynamic psychotherapy led to decreased rates of bingeing and purging similar to those seen in controlled trials (roughly 50%). However, although CBT has been reported to be associated with a more rapid remission of eating symptoms, some therapists note that more integrative treatments that include psychodynamic approaches are useful in targeting both eating symptoms and broader personality, comorbidity, and quality-of-life issues (153).

Some bulimia nervosa patients, particularly those with concurrent personality pathology or other co-occurring disorders, may require substantially longer treatment. In one study, the clinicians reported that their average CBT treatment for bulimia nervosa lasted 69 sessions (81). However, just how closely these clinicians adhered to formal CBT methods is unknown. Also unknown is how the length and characteristics of the treatments varied according to other clinical dimensions of these patients. Exactly what is required over the long run to best help patients resolve lingering preoccupations with body image and the more subtle but impairing psychological dimensions that may be associated with eating disorders requires additional study. These concerns are often approached in practice through a variety of longer-term psychotherapies.

Family therapy should be considered whenever possible, especially for adolescents still living with parents or for older patients with ongoing conflicted interactions with parents. Patients with marital discord may benefit from couples therapy.

A variety of self-help and professionally guided self-help programs have been effective for a small number of patients with bulimia nervosa (220–222) and have been piloted in some stepped-care approaches. Several innovative online programs are currently being studied (5). Support groups and 12-step programs such as Overeaters Anonymous may be helpful as adjuncts to initial treatment of bulimia nervosa and for subsequent relapse prevention but are not recommended as the sole initial treatment approach for bulimia nervosa (168, 223). As noted above, these support organizations emphasize in their literature that their programs are not substitutes for professional treatment and specifically recommend that members seek appropriate medical and nutritional guidance. However, clinicians should remain cognizant of the idiosyncratic recommendations made in some self-help groups.

Patients with bulimia nervosa occasionally have difficulties with certain elements of psychotherapy similar to what was discussed above for patients with anorexia nervosa. Possible adverse effects of psychotherapeutic and psychosocial interventions, steps that clinicians might take to minimize negative therapeutic reactions, and issues concerning countertransference (as discussed in Section II.B.2.b) apply to the treatment of patients with bulimia nervosa.

c) Medications

Antidepressants are effective as one component of an initial treatment program for most bulimia nervosa patients. Although various classes of antidepressant medications can reduce symptoms of binge eating and purging, SSRIs have the most evidence for efficacy and the fewest difficulties with adverse effects (224–226). To date, the only medication approved by the FDA for the treatment of bulimia nervosa is fluoxetine. The only other SSRI shown to be effective is sertraline, which was studied in a small randomized controlled trial (227). Available studies also suggest that antidepressants may be helpful for patients with substantial symptoms of depression or anxiety, obsessions, or certain impulse disorder symptoms or for patients who have not responded or had a suboptimal response to previous attempts at appropriate psychosocial therapy (228, 229). Dosages of SSRIs that are higher than those used for depression (e.g., fluoxetine 60 mg/day) are more effective in treating bulimic symptoms (224, 226, 230), but high dropout rates may also be seen in patients using these drugs (226). A small open trial demonstrated the safety and effectiveness of 60 mg/day of fluoxetine for treating bulimia nervosa in adolescents (225). Thus, many clinicians initiate fluoxetine treatment for bulimia nervosa at the higher dosage, titrating downward if necessary to manage side effects. Tricyclic and MAOI antidepressants are rarely used to treat bulimia nervosa, but if they are used, the dosages are similar to those used to treat depression (231).

Often, several different antidepressants may have to be tried sequentially to identify the specific medication with the optimum effect in a particular patient. In the bulimia nervosa patient whose symptoms do not respond to medication, it is important to assess whether the patient has taken the medication shortly before vomiting. Correlations between serum levels and response have not been identified; however, if serum levels of the medication are available, they may help determine whether presumably effective levels of the drug have actually been achieved. Treatment adherence will also enhance the patient's response to treatment, and subtle interpersonal and psychodynamic factors in the physician-patient relationship may contribute to treatment resistance if left unaddressed (232).

As in most clinical situations, careful education of the patient regarding possible side effects of medications and their symptomatic management (e.g., stool softeners for constipation) is important. Side effects vary widely across studies depending on the type of antidepressant medication used. In the multicenter fluoxetine trials (224, 230), sexual side effects were common, and at the dosage of 60 mg/day, insomnia, nausea, and asthenia were seen in 25%–33% of patients. For the tricyclic antidepressants, common side effects include sedation, constipation, dry mouth, and, with amitriptyline, weight gain (233–238).

The toxicity and potential lethality of tricyclic antidepressant overdosage also dictate caution in prescribing this class of drug for patients who are at risk for suicide. Practitioners should also avoid prescribing MAOIs to patients with chaotic binge eating and purging behaviors. The risk of spontaneous hypertensive crises in patients with bulimia nervosa taking MAOIs is not insignificant (239). This risk and the importance of eating a tyramine-free diet while taking MAOIs should be discussed with patients for whom this type of medication is contemplated.

There are few reports on the use of antidepressant medications in the maintenance phase of treating bulimia nervosa patients. Although there are data indicating that fluoxetine can be effective in preventing relapse in these patients (226), other data suggest that high rates of relapse occur while antidepressants are being taken and possibly higher rates are seen when the medication is withdrawn (240). In the absence of more systematic data, most clinicians recommend continuing antidepressant therapy for a minimum of 9 months and probably for 1 year in most patients with bulimia nervosa.

Clinicians must attend to the black box warnings concerning antidepressants and conduct appropriate informed consent with patients and families if these medications are to be prescribed (183–189).

For patients with bulimia nervosa who require mood stabilizers, the use of lithium carbonate is problematic, because lithium levels may shift markedly with rapid volume changes. Lithium is not effective in the treatment of bulimia nervosa (241). Both lithium carbonate and valproic acid frequently lead to undesirable weight gains that may limit their acceptability to bulimia nervosa patients. Selecting a mood stabilizer that avoids these problems may result in better patient adherence and medication effectiveness. Topiramate is not an effective mood stabilizer but may be potentially useful for bulimia nervosa and binge eating disorder (242, 243). However, in contrast to the low rates of adverse effects observed in clinical trials with topiramate, practitioners have reported several patients experiencing adverse effects with the drug, such as word-finding difficulties and paresthesias in a sizable minority of patients, although these may have been related to excessively rapid rates of dosage increases (242, 243). Also of note, patients receiving topiramate for bulimia nervosa lost an average of 1.8 kilograms, so this medication may be problematic for normal- to lower-weight individuals (243). No data are available regarding the use of these medications for treating bulimia nervosa or binge eating in children or adolescents, but safety and tolerability data have been reported for children and adolescents with other disorders for which lithium (244), valproic acid (245), and topiramate (246) have been prescribed.

Several case reports indicate that methylphenidate may be helpful for bulimia nervosa patients with concurrent ADHD (247–249). In these situations, particular attention should be given to a range of potential adverse effects, including abuse.

d) Combinations of psychosocial interventions and medications

Although not all psychotherapies have been well studied, there is general consensus among clinicians regarding the efficacy of a combined psychotherapeutic/medication approach; such an approach is worth considering when initiating treatment. In some research, the combination of antidepressant therapy and CBT has resulted in the highest remission rates of bulimia nervosa (250–252). Other studies suggest that target symptoms such as binge eating and purging and attitudes related to the eating disorder generally respond better to CBT than to pharmacotherapy (253–255), with at least two studies (251, 254) showing that the combination of CBT and medication is superior to either alone. Two of the studies suggested a greater improvement in mood and anxiety variables when antidepressant therapy is added to CBT (251, 253, 256). Of note, some experienced clinicians do not find rigidly defined and doctrinally practiced CBT to be as useful as methods that integrate CBT with other psychotherapeutic techniques. This may be due to several factors, including clinician inexperience or discomfort with the methods of CBT or differences among patients seen in the community and those who have participated as research subjects in these studies (81, 153).

e) Other treatments

Bright light therapy has been shown to reduce binge frequency in several controlled trials (257–259). Case reports suggest that repeated transcranial magnetic stimulation may be effective in treating patients with major depression and bulimia nervosa (260, 261). One controlled trial (719) showed odansetron, a peripheral 5-hydroxytryptamine type-3 (5-HT_3) receptor antagonist that reduces vagus nerve activity, to be effective in decreasing symptoms of bulimia nervosa, and its use may be considered in unusual circumstances.

4. Eating disorder not otherwise specified

The eating disorder not otherwise specified (EDNOS) category is a conceptually problematic one and comprises a clinically heterogeneous group of diagnoses (262, 263). This "everything else" category currently consists largely of individuals with subsyndromal anorexia nervosa or bulimia nervosa who do not meet DSM-IV-TR criteria of being 15% below expected weight or who binge and purge slightly less than twice per week. Such individuals merit treatment similar to that of full-syndrome patients. In addition, the EDNOS category lumps together normal-weight patients who purge, individuals who chew and spit out their food without swallowing it to prevent weight gain, and patients with binge eating disorder. Also perhaps suitable for this "other" category are individuals who experience psychiatric impairment related to the abuse of diet pills and diuretics (264), individuals who are obsessively preoccupied with liposuction (265) to deal with issues of shape and weight, and certain new-onset postgastrectomy eating disorder patients (266). The EDNOS diagnosis covers a wide spectrum, so no easily generalizable comments can be made for the entire group regarding course or prognosis (267). In addition, over time, considerable movement occurs from one eating disorder diagnostic category to another, including EDNOS (263).

Binge eating disorder is the most discrete and well-studied EDNOS subgroup. Although binge eating disorder is currently not an approved DSM-IV-TR diagnosis, research criteria listed in DSM-IV-TR consist of disturbances in one or more of the following spheres: behavioral (e.g., binge eating), somatic (obesity is common, although not required), and psychological (e.g., body image dissatisfaction, low self-esteem, depression). Empirically supported strategies for the treatment of binge eating disorder include nutritional counseling and dietary management; individual or group behavioral, cognitive behavioral, dialectical behavioral, psychodynamic, or interpersonal psychotherapy; and medications. In reviewing the available information on treating binge eating disorder, it is important to consider the focus of treatment. Most programs using nutritional rehabilitation and counseling focus on weight loss as the primary outcome, whereas studies of psychotherapy and medication generally consider reduction of binge eating as the primary outcome measure, with weight loss as a secondary outcome. Clinical consensus suggests that psychodynamic psychotherapy may also be helpful to reduce binge eating in some patients.

a) Nutritional rehabilitation and counseling: effect of diet programs on weight and binge eating symptoms

The literature on treating binge eating disorder suggests that 1) behavioral weight control programs incorporating low- or very-low-calorie diets may help patients lose weight and usually reduce symptoms of binge eating; 2) at least some degree of weight gain often follows weight loss; 3) weight gain after weight loss may be accompanied by a return of binge eating patterns; and 4) various combinations of diets, behavior therapies, non-weight-directed psychosocial treatments, and even some "nondiet/health at every size" psychotherapy approaches may be of benefit in reducing binge eating and promoting weight loss or stabilization in various circumstances (268).

Some believe that patients with a history of repeated weight loss followed by weight gain ("yo-yo" dieting) or patients with an early onset of binge eating might benefit from following programs that focus on decreasing binge eating rather than losing weight (269, 270). However, at this point, there is little empirical evidence to suggest that obese binge eaters who are primarily seeking weight loss should receive different treatment than obese individuals who do not binge eat.

b) Other psychosocial treatments: effects on binge eating disorder

CBT is the most widely studied treatment for binge eating disorder, and there is substantial evidence supporting its efficacy for behavioral and psychological symptoms, whether it is delivered in the individual or group format. IPT and dialectical behavior therapy have also been shown to be effective for behavioral and psychological symptoms and can be considered as alternative therapies. There is less consensus regarding the long-term effects of treatment; however, some studies suggest that most patients continue to show behavioral and psychological improvement at 1-year follow-up (271, 272). There is a substantial body of evidence supporting the efficacy of self-help and guided self-help CBT treatment programs (273–277) and their use as an initial low-burden step in a sequenced treatment program.

Because severe dieting may disinhibit eating and lead to compensatory overeating and binge eating (278), and because chronic calorie restriction can also increase symptoms of depression, anxiety, and irritability (279), alternative therapies have been developed that use a "nondiet" approach and focus on self-acceptance, improved body image, better nutrition and health, and increased physical movement (280–282). Addiction-based 12-step approaches, self-help organizations, and treatment programs based on the Alcoholics Anonymous model have been tried, but no systematic outcome studies of these programs are available.

In sum, there appear to be several good psychotherapeutic options for treating binge eating disorder when a reduction in binge eating is the primary goal. Weight loss, particularly in the long term, is a much more elusive goal, not only for obese patients with binge eating disorder but for obese patients in general. However, several studies suggest that at least for some patients at certain stages of recovery, behavioral weight control may be a useful treatment component. Also, because studies have found that binge eating may begin before obesity or dieting (283), specific approaches are needed for nonobese patients struggling with binge eating symptoms. The optimal sequencing of treatments—that is, whether the treatment of binge eating should precede or occur concurrently with weight control treatment—has yet to be definitively determined.

c) Medications

There is substantial evidence to suggest that treatment with antidepressant medications, particularly SSRI antidepressants, is associated with at least a short-term reduction in binge eating, in most cases without substantial weight loss. The dosage of medication is typically at the high end of the recommended range. The appetite-suppressant medication sibutramine also appears to be effective in suppressing binge eating, at least in the short term, and is additionally associated with significant weight loss (284). Heart rate and blood pressure need to be monitored closely in patients taking sibutramine, and the medication should be discontinued if there are significant elevations in these parameters, although these side effects seem to be uncommon (285). Finally, the anticonvulsant medication topiramate appears to be effective in reducing binge eating and promoting weight loss in the short (286) and long (287) term, although side effects such as cognitive problems, paresthesias, and somnolence may limit its clinical utility for some individuals. The anticonvulsant zonisamide may produce similar effects (288). Dexfenfluramine, although effective for reducing binge eating (289), has been removed from the market because of increased risk of primary pulmonary hypertension and heart valve abnormalities. Patients who report having used fenfluramine and phentermine in the past should be screened for potential cardiac and pulmonary complications.

It is important to note that in several studies, the placebo response rate has been reported to be quite high. The clinical implications of this finding are that controlled studies are extremely important, as a positive response in an open study may be nonspecific, and short-term beneficial responses to treatment should be viewed cautiously, given that a transient "honeymoon" effect of initiating treatment is common.

d) Combined psychosocial and medication treatment strategies

There have been few studies of combined treatment for binge eating disorder, so the clinical recommendations are preliminary. Overall, it appears that for most patients, the addition of antidepressant medication to behavioral weight control and/or CBT does not significantly augment binge suppression but may confer additional benefits in weight reduction (290–294). One study reported that the addition of the weight-loss medication orlistat to a guided self-help CBT program yielded additional weight loss (295). Another study found that fluoxetine in the setting of group behavioral treatment did not augment binge cessation or weight loss but did reduce depressive symptoms (294). Thus, the addition of medication to psychotherapy for binge eating disorder is not, in most cases, associated with additional benefit on the core symptom of binge eating, perhaps because psychosocial treatments are quite effective for this symptom. However, medication augmentation may have additional benefits.

e) Treatment strategies for night eating syndrome

The phenomenon of wakeful nighttime eating, variously characterized as night eating syndrome, nocturnal eating/drinking syndrome, or nocturnal sleep-related eating disorders, is currently an area of active research (296). Although formal agreed-upon definitions for these syndromes do not yet exist, the construct of night eating syndrome, first described by Stunkard et al. (297), generally includes morning anorexia, evening hyperphagia, and insomnia. In contrast, the construct of nocturnal eating/drinking syndrome emphasizes a sleep disorder with recurrent awakenings often accompanied by eating or drinking, and the construct of nocturnal sleep-related eating disorders adds to this a reduced level of awareness or recall of nocturnal eating episodes. Sleep-related eating disorders, including somnambulism, have reportedly been induced by risperidone, olanzapine, and bupropion, among other medications (298–300). The literature does not, at this point, support the recommendation of particular treatments for these disorders. However, there is preliminary evidence supporting the utility of progressive muscle relaxation (301) and sertraline (302, 303). Further studies of the phenomenology and treatment of these disorders are needed.

III. CLINICAL FEATURES INFLUENCING THE TREATMENT PLAN

A. CHRONICITY OF EATING DISORDERS

In some patients with eating disorders, the illness course becomes chronic, lasting for a decade or more. The care of chronically ill patients is challenging, and modifications in treatment goals may be needed for these patients to benefit. For example, the goals of psychological interventions may be to make small, progressive gains and achieve fewer relapses. Throughout the outpatient care of such patients, communication among professionals is especially important. In addition, more frequent outpatient contact and other supports may sometimes help prevent hospitalizations.

Among patients with a chronic course of anorexia nervosa, many are unable to maintain a healthy weight and experience chronic depression, obsessionality, and social withdrawal. Treatment may require consultation with other specialists; repeated hospitalizations, partial hospitalizations, or residential care; individual or group therapy; other social therapies; trials of various medications; and, occasionally, ECT for patients with severe or treatment-resistant depression. During hospitalizations, expectations for weight gain may be more modest; achieving a safe weight compatible with the patient's life rather than a healthy weight may be all that is possible. The focus of treatment may be on addressing quality-of-life issues (rather than on weight changes or more normal eating habits) and providing compassionate care, with the recognition that patients can realistically achieve only limited goals (125, 304, 305).

Even for patients who have been ill for 20–30 years, there is some evidence that significant benefits can still be derived from treatment. Here too the clinician's approach may need to be modified by relying more on the emotional resources of the patient and much less on the resources of the family. Therapy may need to focus on patients' recognition that their eating disorder has cost them decades of their lives; their therapists may then help them use their energy to improve the remainder of their lives. Some older patients maintain accurate images of their body and recognize that they are too thin but still need significant help with actually gaining the needed weight or relinquishing a strongly established habit of binge eating or purging. The family work often revolves around helping the family adjust to the positive changes that occur with symptom and behavioral changes in the patient (306).

B. OTHER PSYCHIATRIC FACTORS

1. Substance use disorders

Substance use disorders are common among both women and men with eating disorders (106, 307, 308). Among individuals with bulimia nervosa, 22.9% meet criteria for alcohol abuse (309). Alcohol and other substance use disorders appear to be less common among patients with the restricting type of anorexia nervosa than among those with the binge eating/purging type (310, 311). Binge eating disorder is also associated with high rates of lifetime co-occurring substance abuse, which is more prevalent in male (57%) than in female (28%) patients (313). Patients with co-occurring substance abuse and anorexia or bulimia nervosa appear to have more severe problems with impulsivity in general, including greater risk of shoplifting, suicidal behaviors, self-injurious behaviors, and laxative abuse (83, 314–316). The relation between bulimia nervosa and alcohol abuse/dependence may be indirect and may be influenced by associations with major depression and posttraumatic stress disorder (PTSD) (317).

Available data indicate that patients with eating disorders who have a history of prior but currently inactive substance use disorder respond to standard therapies in the same manner as those without such a history (318–320) and do not appear to experience exacerbation of their substance use after their eating disorder is successfully treated (319). Furthermore, co-occurring alcohol abuse increases the risk of mortality in anorexia nervosa (321). The presence of an active substance use disorder does have implications for the treatment of eating disorders. Patients with co-occurring eating and substance use disorders require longer inpatient stays and are less adherent with treatment after hospitalization than those with substance use disorders alone (322). In everyday clinical practice, substance use shows a strong association with length of treatment required for remission (81). A study of 70 patients with co-occurring eating disorders and substance abuse found that the associated axis III medical disorders reflected complications of both eating and substance use disorders. Where treatment staff are skilled in treating both disorders, concurrent treatment should be attempted.

2. Mood and anxiety disorders

A high percentage of treatment-seeking patients with eating disorders report a lifetime history of major depression (313, 323–327). Nutritional insufficiency and weight loss often predispose these patients to symptoms of depression (279). Depressed individuals with an eating disorder experience higher levels of anxiety, guilt, and obsessionality but lower levels of social withdrawal and lack of interest than depressed individuals without eating disorders (328). The presence of co-occurring depression at initial presentation has minimal or no predictive value for treatment outcome (329). Although antidepressant medications may be relatively ineffective in treating depressive symptoms before a patient has gained weight (174) and are typically not helpful in weight restoration (see Section II.B.2.c.1.), their use has sometimes been associated with reduced symptoms of depression and anxiety during the weight restoration phase (176). In addition, the experience of many clinicians suggests that severe depression can impair a patient's ability to become meaningfully involved in psychotherapy and may dictate the need for medication treatment for the mood symptoms from the beginning of treatment.

Lifetime prevalence rates for anxiety disorders also appear to be higher for patients with anorexia or bulimia nervosa. In a controlled study with a large sample, 71% of women with anorexia or bulimia nervosa had at least one anxiety disorder, a rate significantly higher than that found in the control group (330), although rates for specific anxiety disorders varied (331). Social phobia and obsessive-compulsive disorder (OCD) are the anxiety disorders most commonly described in patients with anorexia nervosa. For those with bulimia nervosa, co-occurring presentations of social phobia, OCD, PTSD, or simple phobia are most often described (332, 333). Patients with binge eating disorder also have high rates of lifetime anxiety disorders (29%), with simple phobia and panic disorder being the most commonly described (334–340). Overanxious disorders of childhood are also common in conjunction with anorexia and bulimia nervosa, and anxiety disorders often precede the onset of these eating disorders (82, 341). Youngsters with anorexia nervosa may have co-occurring OCD more frequently than adults with anorexia nervosa (342). Although there is no clear evidence that co-occurring anxiety disorders significantly affect eating disorder treatment outcome, such comorbid problems should be addressed in treatment planning.

Available data on the extent of PTSD among patients with eating disorders suggest an association between childhood trauma and bulimia nervosa (333, 343–346). Although specific causal links have not been demonstrated and the mechanisms of association and potential transmission remain unclear, it is thought that early trauma may sensitize some individuals to later traumatic experiences and an array of impulsive behaviors, including eating disorder symptoms. The lifetime rate of PTSD among women with bulimia nervosa reported in studies has varied between 6% and 45% (330, 332, 346, 347). Clinical consensus suggests that the extent of trauma history and the possible presence of PTSD should be taken into consideration in treatment planning.

3. Personality disorders

Temperament, genetics, family pathologies, and other dimensions of personality appear to be involved in the occurrence and manifestations of eating disorders (348–350). In all cases, personality types and the extent of personality pathology have implications for treatment (79, 351, 352). As with mood and anxiety disorders, the presence of comorbid personality pathology (whether or not it is severe enough to meet DSM criteria for a personality disorder) is the norm rather than the exception (353). Patients with eating disorders should routinely be assessed for concurrent personality disorders. The reported prevalence of personality disorders has varied widely across eating disorders and studies. Individuals with anorexia nervosa tend to have higher rates of Cluster C personality disorders, particularly obsessive-compulsive, perfectionistic, and avoidant and histrionic traits, whereas normal-weight patients with bulimia nervosa are more likely to display features of Cluster B disorders, particularly impulsive, affective, and narcissistic traits (354–361). The presence of borderline personality disorder seems to be associated with a greater disturbance in eating attitudes, a history of more frequent hospitalizations, and the presence of other problems such as suicidal behaviors and self-injurious behaviors (356, 360). The presence of borderline personality disorder is also associated with poorer treatment outcome and higher levels of psychopathology at follow-up (362, 363). The improvement of axis I eating disorder symptoms may produce concurrent improvement in traits associated with these personality disturbances (364). Although this approach has not yet been systematically studied, clinical consensus strongly suggests that the presence of a co-occurring personality disorder, particularly borderline personality disorder, dictates the need for longer-term therapy that focuses on the underlying personality structure, coping strategies, and interpersonal relationships in addition to the symptoms of the eating disorder. Recent naturalistic research documents the generally poorer outcome and longer treatment required for bulimia nervosa patients with borderline, avoidant, or more broadly emotionally dysregulated personality pathology, although many such patients do improve substantially with longer-term treatment (365).

C. CONCURRENT GENERAL MEDICAL CONDITIONS

1. Type 1 diabetes

Eating disorders may be more common among patients with type 1 or type 2 diabetes than among nondiabetic patients (366, 367), but this contention is not strongly supported by research (368). It has been suggested that type 1 diabetic patients are more likely to have anorexia nervosa or bulimia nervosa (368a) and type 2 diabetic patients are more likely to have binge eating disorder (367). Although patients with both an eating disorder and diabetes are more likely to be female, males with both disorders are also commonly found, particularly among type 2 diabetic patients. The presentation of eating disorders in the context of diabetes may be substantially more complex than that seen with an eating disorder alone. In addition, these concurrent diagnoses may present as numerous general medical crises before the presence of the eating disorder is diagnosed and treated, particularly among patients with type 1 diabetes. Evidence suggests that rates of diabetic complications are higher when insulin-dependent diabetes mellitus co-occurs with bulimia nervosa or EDNOS (369). Mortality rates are much higher with combined anorexia nervosa and type 1 diabetes than with either condition alone (370). Patients with uncontrolled diabetes who also have bulimia nervosa may require a period of inpatient treatment for stabilization of both illnesses (371, 372). Treatment of these concurrent disorders may also require more interaction with general medical specialists. Lengthy inpatient treatment for adult diabetic patients with eating disorders (primarily bulimia nervosa) is promising but has been studied in only a few patients (373).

Diabetic patients with eating disorders often underdose their insulin to lose weight. Throughout the studies undertaken to date, insulin omission has been found to be common (374). It has been suggested that insulin omission be considered a specific type of purging behavior in the next DSM revision.

2. Pregnancy

Eating disorders may begin de novo during pregnancy, but many patients become pregnant even while they are actively symptomatic with an eating disorder. Behaviors associated with eating disorders, including inadequate nutritional intake, binge eating, purging by various means, and the use or misuse of some teratogenic medications (e.g., lithium, benzodiazepines, divalproex, diet pills), can all result in fetal or maternal complications (375). The care of a pregnant patient with an eating disorder is difficult and usually requires the collaboration of a psychiatrist and an obstetrician who specializes in high-risk pregnancies (376–379).

In a recent study of 49 nulliparous women previously diagnosed with an eating disorder (24 with anorexia nervosa, 20 with bulimia nervosa, 5 with EDNOS), 22% had a verified relapse of eating disorder during pregnancy. Compared with a control group, women with past or current eating disorders were at increased risk of hyperemesis, infants with significantly lower birth weight, smaller head circumference (including microcephaly), and small-for-gestational-age infants (380). Women with active symptoms of anorexia or bulimia nervosa are at higher risk for Cesarean section and postpartum depression (381). Yet another study linked the presence of an eating disorder before pregnancy or an eating disorder (or dieting or fasting) during the first trimester with an increased risk to the infant, including a greater risk of low birth weight, preterm delivery, a small-for-gestational-age size, and neural tube defects (382).

Data on the impact of pregnancy on eating disorder symptoms are conflicting. One study has shown that among treated bulimia nervosa patients, childbirth is not associated with increased symptoms (383). Another study found that anorexia and bulimia nervosa patients had a decreased severity of eating disorder symptoms during pregnancy and that patients with bulimia nervosa, but not patients with anorexia nervosa, maintained this improvement through 9 months postpartum (384).

Prepregnancy counseling of eating disorder patients and their families should be detailed and cautionary. Although some patients may be able to eat normally and decrease binge eating and purging during their pregnancy, it is best for the eating disorder to be treated before the pregnancy if possible. Although women with a lifetime history of anorexia nervosa may not have reduced fertility, they do appear to be at risk for a greater number of birth complications than comparison subjects and of giving birth to babies of lower birth weight, whether or not the anorexia nervosa is active at the time of pregnancy (312). Mothers with eating disorders may have more difficulties than others in feeding their babies and young children than mothers without eating disorders and may need additional guidance, assistance, and monitoring of their mothering (385–388). In one study, primiparous mothers with an episode of eating disorder during the first postpartum year often expressed negative emotions toward their infants during meals, the infants' emotional tone was more negative, and the infants' mealtimes were more conflictual than those of control infants (388).

Active bulimia nervosa may be associated with polycystic ovaries or other follicular abnormalities. In a study of eight women with bulimia nervosa, six of the seven women with active bulimic symptoms showed polycystic ovaries; at follow-up, the five who continued to have bulimic symptoms all had polycystic ovaries, whereas normal ovaries were seen in the three whose bulimia nervosa had remitted (389).

Some patients with an eating disorder may present to fertility clinics and request medications to facilitate conception. Although little is known about the consequences of fertility drugs in patients with anorexia nervosa, the simultaneous multiple pregnancies that often occur with these drugs may be even more difficult for patients with an eating disorder to contend with than for women without an eating disorder.

D. DEMOGRAPHIC VARIABLES

1. Male gender

Although eating disorders are more prevalent in women, males with eating disorders are not rare, and case series often report on hundreds of male patients (390, 391). The stereotype that eating disorders are female illnesses may limit a full understanding of the scope and nature of problems faced by male patients with eating disorders.

There continues to be a paucity of information regarding males with eating disorders (392). However, more males may be seeking treatment (393). The most common form of eating disorders among males may be EDNOS (394).

In community samples, males with eating disorders have more psychiatric comorbidity and psychosocial morbidity than females with eating disorders (395). Studies of national samples of girls and boys exposed to physical and sexual abuse have shown that although binge and purge behaviors were nearly twice as prevalent among girls (13%) as boys (7%), boys who had experienced both physical and sexual abuse were nearly twice as likely as girls to report these behaviors (odds ratios 8.25 and 4.28, respectively) (396). Especially in the bulimia nervosa and binge eating disorder subgroups, males with eating disorders who present to tertiary care centers may have greater rates of co-occurring substance use disorders and more frequently have a history of having premorbid obesity or being overweight (397). As in women, there is a higher risk of osteoporosis in men with eating disorders (398, 399).

Although many similarities exist between males and females with different types of eating disorders, notable differences have been reported. Females with anorexia or bulimia nervosa score higher on the Drive for Thinness subscale than do males, and this appears to be a real difference; females also score higher on the body dissatisfaction subscale than do males, but this may result from a failure of these scales to address the specific ways in which males are dissatisfied with their bodies (e.g., males seem to be more concerned with upper torso and muscular development than are females). Studies of binge eating disorder patients demonstrate that women have greater body image dissatisfaction and are more likely to cope with negative affect by binge eating, whereas men have higher rates of drug and alcohol use disorder histories (400).

Body dysmorphic disorder (BDD), a severe form of body image disturbance seemingly related to OCD, is common among patients with anorexia nervosa (401) and appears to be increasing in prevalence. Although BDD is nearly as common in men as in women, the focus of body preoccupations may differ by gender (402, 403). Muscle dysmorphia, a distressing or impairing preoccupation with the idea that one's body is not sufficiently lean and muscular, is a form of BDD that occurs primarily in men, often involves abnormal eating behavior, and appears to overlap in other ways with eating disorders. The relation of BDD to eating disorders other than anorexia nervosa is poorly understood (404). In one small inpatient study, anorexia nervosa patients with BDD were found to have significantly poorer functioning, more episodes of psychiatric hospitalization, and three times the rate of lifetime suicide attempts compared with anorexia nervosa patients without BDD (401).

Although a patient's gender per se does not appear to influence the outcome of treatment, some aspects of treatment may need to be modified on the basis of gender. For example, with regard to personality traits, males with eating disorders have somewhat less perfectionism, harm avoidance and reward dependence behaviors, and cooperativeness than females (405). Open-blind studies suggest that bringing testosterone levels to within normal ranges in males during nutritional rehabilitation for anorexia nervosa may be helpful in increasing lean muscle mass, but definitive studies on this have not been completed.

Although studies in clinical samples have suggested that a higher prevalence of homosexuality may exist among males with eating disorders (390), this finding has not yet been confirmed epidemiologically. Nevertheless, because issues concerning sexual orientation are not uncommon among males with eating disorders seen in clinical settings, these issues should be considered in treatment (390).

Where possible, therapy groups restricted to male patients may address some of these patients' specific needs and help them deal with potential stigmatization of male patients by female patients in treatment. Male patients with anorexia nervosa may require higher energy intakes (up to 4,000–4,500 kcal/day) during nutritional rehabilitation because they normally have higher lean body mass and lower fat mass compared with female patients. Further, because they are generally taller and larger framed to begin with, males with anorexia nervosa often require much larger weight gains to return to a healthy weight (391, 399).

2. Age

Although most eating disorders start while patients are in their teens and 20s, earlier and later onsets have been observed as well. Among the youngest patients with early onset (i.e., ages 7–12 years), obsessional behavior and depression are common (406). Children often present with physical symptoms such as having nausea, experiencing abdominal pain, feeling full, or being unable to swallow (all conditions requiring evaluation to investigate a variety of potential etiologies) (407). Their weight loss can be rapid and dramatic. Similarly, their lack of expected weight gain is problematic. Food avoidance for primarily psychological reasons that results in weight loss (food avoidance emotional disorder [FAED]) has been delineated and differentiated from anorexia nervosa in young children. These young patients know that they are underweight, would like to be heavier, may not know why this goal is hard to achieve, and usually show more generalized anxiety unrelated to food. A small number of FAED patients go on to develop eating disorders, but direct continuity between the two types of disorders has not been demonstrated (408). Other syndromes to be considered are selective eating disorder, functional dysphasia, and pervasive refusal syndrome (407).

Children with early-onset anorexia nervosa may have delayed growth (3, 97, 98, 409–412) and be especially prone to osteopenia and osteoporosis (413, 414). In a few cases, exacerbations of anorexia nervosa and OCD-like symptoms have been associated with pediatric infection-triggered autoimmune neuropsychiatric disorders (415), but further research is needed to determine the nature of this association (416). Bulimia nervosa is rarely seen in children under age 12 years (417–420).

With respect to middle-aged patients, case reports and clinical consensus now suggest that as the baby boomer generation grows older, body image concerns and eating disorders are becoming more prevalent. One case report from an established residential program noted a shift in the age of its patients and reported treating more middle-aged women than a decade ago (417–420).

At the other end of the age spectrum, incidence rates for anorexia nervosa among women over age 50 years are low, accounting for <1% of patients with newly diagnosed anorexia nervosa (421). Anorexia nervosa has been reported in elderly patients in their 70s and 80s; these are generally women in whom the illness has been present for 40 or 50 years. In many cases, the illness started after age 25 (so-called anorexia tardive). In some case reports, adverse life events such as deaths, a marital crisis, or a divorce have been found to trigger these older-onset syndromes. The fear of aging has also been described as a major precipitating factor in some patients (142, 422). Rates of co-occurring depression have been reported to be higher among these patients in some studies but not in others (423). Regardless of the age at onset, concerns about comorbid medical conditions, especially osteopenia and osteoporosis, take on greater significance with older patients.

3. Cultural factors

Specific pressures and values concerning weight and shape vary among different cultures. The quest for beauty and acceptance in accordance with the stereotypes women perceive in contemporary media is leading increasing numbers of women around the world to develop attitudes and eating behaviors associated with eating disorders. Despite initially higher prevalence rates of this phenomenon in Western and postindustrial societies, disordered eating behaviors now appear to be globally distributed (424–427).

Popkin and Gordon-Larsen (428) have described a phenomenon called the "nutritional transition" in economically emerging countries. In some Asian and Middle Eastern countries, the decrease in activity levels and increase in access to high-fat, high-calorie foods have occurred much more rapidly than in the United States; likewise, this trend has led to a faster rate of increase in the number of individuals becoming overweight or obese than that seen in the United States. Consequently, the pressure to lose weight or remain slender may ultimately affect an even wider group of people more quickly in these regions than it has in the United States. Emerging population data suggest that transnational migration and modernization may increase the risk of disordered eating and body dissatisfaction across diverse ethnic and social contexts (427, 429–432).

Clinicians should engage female patients from non-Western cultures in informed and sensitive discussions regarding their struggles, experiences, and personal perceptions about what it means to be attractive and satisfied with their bodies (433). Clinicians should be sensitive to and inquire about how weight and shape concerns are experienced by patients, especially those who are from minority populations or non-Western or other cultural backgrounds or are transitioning and assimilating into Western societies. Transcultural differences in the meanings of terms and concepts are considerable (434). It is not uncommon to find Asian patients with atypical behaviors, such as denying a fear of weight gain, appraising their bodies as malnourished, denying distorted perceptions of their bodies, and specifically denying a drive for thinness (435). (Atypical patients who specifically deny a drive for thinness are also seen among North American and European populations [436].)

Although little information exists on cross-cultural differences among males with regard to eating disorders, male patients with anorexia nervosa, bulimia nervosa, and binge eating disorder have been described in non-Western populations. Some population differences across cultures among males have been found with regard to attitudes about eating, body shape, and weight (437, 438).

4. Eating disorders in athletes

The risk for eating disorders is greater among competitive athletes than in the general age-matched population (439–441). Female athletes in competitive sports that emphasize a thin body or appearance, such as gymnastics, figure skating, and distance running, are especially at risk, as are female ballet dancers. Male athletes in sports such as bodybuilding and wrestling are also at greater risk. Certain antecedent factors such as cultural preoccupation with thinness, performance anxiety, and athlete self-appraisal may predispose a female athlete to body dissatisfaction, which may mediate the development of eating disorder symptoms (442). Parents and coaches of young athletes may support distorted shape and eating attitudes in the service of guiding the athlete to be more competitive. Although competitive college athletes appear to be at greater risk for eating disorders than nonathlete peers, this has not been demonstrated among high school athletes (443). Girls as young as age 5 years who participate in aesthetic sports, such as ballet or figure skating, have exhibited greater weight concerns than girls who participate in nonaesthetic sports or who do not participate in sports (444). Participation in sports may protect some young athletes from developing eating disorders if, for example, they approach their sports in a sensible way and derive appropriate pride and self-esteem from their achievements (443, 445).

Physicians working with adolescent and young adult athletes, particularly competitive athletes participating in the at-risk sports mentioned above, must be alert to early symptoms of eating disorders. Simple screening questions about weight, possible dissatisfaction with appearance, amenorrhea, and nutritional intake on the day before a physical evaluation may help identify an athlete who is developing an eating disorder. Early general medical and psychiatric intervention is key to prompt recovery from the disorder.

Extreme exercise appears to be a risk factor for developing anorexia nervosa, especially when combined with dieting (446–448). A "female athlete triad" has been identified, consisting of disordered eating (including the full spectrum of eating-related problems from simple dieting to clinical eating disorders), amenorrhea, and osteoporosis (449). The exact relation between the triad and clinical eating disorders is not fully understood, but athletes with the triad would meet diagnostic criteria for EDNOS. The prevalence of the triad among collegiate athletes has been studied; menstrual irregularity has been found in nearly one-third of female athletes not using oral contraceptives, and athletes participating in aesthetic sports (e.g., gymnastics) have higher scores on the 26-item Eating Attitudes Test (31, 32) than athletes in endurance or team sports (450). Similarly, an "overtraining syndrome," described as a state of exhaustion, depression, and irritability in which athletes continue to train but their performance diminishes, has been observed (451, 452). Both the female athlete triad and the overtraining syndrome parallel the "activity anorexia" syndrome that has been observed in animal models (453, 454).

5. Eating disorders in high school and college students

Eating disorders are common among female high school and college students. From a primary prevention perspective, health professionals may be called on to provide information and education about eating disorders in classrooms, athletic programs, and other extracurricular venues. However, the efficacy of such educational programs in reducing eating disorders is still uncertain (455, 456). Health professionals who serve as trainers, coordinators, and professional supports for peer counseling efforts conducted at school, in dormitories, and through other campus institutions may help in early intervention. Through student health and psychological services, health professionals may serve as initial screeners and diagnosticians and help manage the treatment of students with eating disorders of varying levels of severity (457).

Psychiatrists may be occasionally called on as clinicians and agents of the school administration to offer guidance in the management of impaired students with serious eating disorders. In such situations, the suggested guidelines for levels of care described in Table 8 should be followed. According to the guidelines, students must be treatable as outpatients to stay in school. It is advisable that students be required to take a leave of absence if they are severely ill (457, 458). Students should be directed to inpatient hospital care if their weight is considerably below an expected healthy weight and they meet the other indications for hospitalization listed in Table 8.

For students with serious eating disorders who remain in school, it is useful for the psychiatrist and other health care professionals to work with the school's administration toward developing policies and programs that make student attendance contingent on participation in a suitable treatment program. When the psychiatrist and other health care professionals serve as "dual agents" for the school and whenever information must be shared among health care professionals, appropriate consents must be obtained and the requirements of the Health Insurance Portability and Accountability Act followed. For severely ill students, the clinical team must include a general medical clinician who can gauge patients' physical safety and monitor their weight, vital signs, and laboratory indicators. For the student to be permitted to continue in school, these clinicians may require a minimum weight and other physical, behavioral, or laboratory target measures to ensure basic medical safety. An explicit policy should be developed specifying that clinicians have the final say regarding the student's participation in physically demanding activities (e.g., organized athletics). Restrictions must be based on actual medical concerns. Procedures should be in compliance with the school's policies regarding management of students with psychiatric disabilities and the Americans With Disabilities Act (458).

6. Identification of risk and protective factors

Many efforts have been made to understand how eating disorders develop. Overall, our understanding of risk and vulnerability still outweighs our knowledge of protective factors and resilience. Temperamental factors, eating dysregulation, attachment issues, deficient self-regulation, childhood abuse in the case of bulimia nervosa, and sociocultural ideals of health and beauty may all contribute to risk and pathogenesis (367, 459, 460). High rates of childhood anxiety disorders precede eating disorders, especially overanxious disorder and OCD for anorexia nervosa and overanxious disorder and social phobia for bulimia nervosa; this could be of potential clinical relevance, especially when treating children and adolescents (341). A history of childhood obsessive-compulsive traits—notably perfectionism, rigidity, and rule-bound behavior—may also be associated with an increased risk for the development of an eating disorder (461). Richly documented clinical histories of patients with anorexia nervosa followed over 30 years from infancy to early midlife suggest several potential risk factors related to early perceived body image distortions, body regulatory problems, and academic and interpersonal problems (146).

Because it is well known that the risk of eating disorders is transmitted in families, it is important to offer particular help to patients with eating disorders who are themselves mothers. Attention should be paid to their mothering skills and attachment styles and to their offspring to minimize the risk of eating disorders being transmitted (386–388, 462, 463).

In some patients, increasingly compulsive exercise may precipitate anorexia and bulimia nervosa (447, 464). Female athletes in certain physical activities such as ballet and gymnastics are especially vulnerable (465). Unlike habitual runners, ballet dancers exhibit eating pathology similar to that of individuals with eating disorders (466). Male bodybuilders are also at risk, although the symptom picture often differs because bodybuilders may emphasize a wish to "get bigger" and may also abuse anabolic steroids to reach their goal (467, 468). This has been called the "Adonis complex" (469, 470).

Programs have been designed to influence these risk factors and thus prevent eating disorders. A recent meta-analysis (471) of prevention programs suggests that programs vary significantly in their impact, ranging from an absence of any effect to a reduction in current and future eating pathology. Some effects persist as long as 2 years and are superior to minimal-intervention control conditions. Larger effects occur for selected (versus universal), interactive (versus didactic), and multisession (versus single-session) programs; programs offered solely to female patients and to participants over age 15 years; programs without psychoeducational content; and trials that use validated measures. Several of these programs have resulted in enhanced knowledge about eating disorders and healthy eating. A few have resulted in improved attitudes toward size, shape, eating, and weight, and some have addressed self-esteem and "weightism" and stressed normal/healthy attitudes and behaviors. Other approaches have resulted in modest changes in eating- and weight-related behaviors (472–474), but these changes are not always sustained (455, 456, 475). Because some studies even suggest that certain preventive efforts actually increase the likelihood that maladaptive eating behaviors would be attempted, particularly among adolescents (455), caution is recommended in selecting target populations for such intervention and proper follow-up is necessary.

PART B

BACKGROUND INFORMATION AND REVIEW OF AVAILABLE EVIDENCE

IV. DISEASE DEFINITION, EPIDEMIOLOGY, AND NATURAL HISTORY

A. DISEASE DEFINITION

The DSM-IV-TR criteria for establishing the diagnosis of anorexia or bulimia nervosa appear in Tables 2 and 3, respectively.

Although DSM-IV-TR criteria allow clinicians to diagnose patients with a specific eating disorder, eating disorder symptoms frequently occur along a continuum between those of anorexia nervosa and those of bulimia nervosa. Weight preoccupation and excessive self-evaluation of weight and shape are primary symptoms in both disorders, and many patients demonstrate a mixture of both anorexic and bulimic behaviors. For example, 50%–64% of patients with anorexia nervosa develop bulimic symptoms, and some patients who are initially bulimic develop anorexic symptoms (476, 477). Patients with atypical features who deny a fear of weight gain, accurately appraise their bodies as malnourished, and deny distorted perceptions of their body constituted about 20% of the patients admitted to a specialty eating disorder program (478). Denial of a fear of weight gain was found in 28% of anorexia nervosa patients assessed via a structured interview (479).

Anorexia nervosa appears in two subtypes: restricting and binge eating/purging; this classification into subtypes is based on the presence or absence of binge eating or purging symptoms. Patients with anorexia nervosa can alternate between the bulimic and restricting subtypes at different periods of their illness (480–483). Among patients with the binge eating/purging subtype of anorexia nervosa, further distinctions can be made between those who both binge and purge and those who purge but do not objectively binge. Patients with bulimia nervosa can be subclassified into the purging or nonpurging subtype. Patients with the nonpurging subtype use inappropriate methods to compensate for binge eating, including fasting and excessive exercising, as opposed to patients with binge eating disorder, who do not use inappropriate compensatory strategies. Many patients, particularly younger patients, have combinations of eating disorder symptoms that cannot be strictly categorized as anorexia or bulimia nervosa and are technically diagnosed as EDNOS (484). The value of requiring persistent amenorrhea as a criterion for diagnosing anorexia nervosa has been questioned (24).

Patients with anorexia and bulimia nervosa often experience associated psychiatric symptoms and behaviors. Social isolation is common in patients with anorexia nervosa. Depressive, anxious, and obsessional symptoms; perfectionistic traits; rigid cognitive styles; and a lack of interest in sex are often present among patients with the restricting type of anorexia nervosa (363). Early in the course of their illness, patients with anorexia nervosa often have limited recognition of their disorder and experience their symptoms as intrusive repetitive thoughts; sometimes there is a corresponding limited recognition of the disorder by patients' families. Depressive, anxious, and impulsive symptoms, as well as sexual conflicts and disturbances with intimacy, are often associated with bulimia nervosa. Although patients with bulimia nervosa are likely to recognize their disorder, shame or guilt frequently prevents them from seeking treatment for it at an early stage (485). In one subgroup of patients with bulimia nervosa (the "multi-impulsive" bulimic patients), significant degrees of impulsivity have been observed and are manifested as stealing, self-harm behaviors, suicidality, substance use, and sexual promiscuity (486, 487). Patients with anorexia nervosa of the binge eating/purging subtype may also be suicidal and engage in self-harming behaviors.

In the psychodynamic literature, patients with anorexia nervosa have been described as having difficulties with separation and autonomy (often manifested as enmeshed relationships with parents), affect regulation (including the direct expression of anger and aggression), and negotiation of psychosexual development. These deficits may make women who are predisposed to anorexia nervosa more vulnerable to cultural pressures for achieving a stereotypic body image (142, 169, 488, 489).

Psychodynamic issues in bulimic patients have been understood in a number of ways, ranging from viewing bulimic symptoms as manifestations of impulsivity or problems with emotion regulation and dissociative states to viewing them along a spectrum of self-harming behaviors commonly seen in patients with borderline personality organization (363, 490–492).

Some of the clinical features associated with eating disorders may result from malnutrition or semistarvation (493, 494). Studies of volunteers who have submitted to semistarvation experiments and semistarved prisoners of war report the development of food preoccupation, food hoarding, abnormal taste preferences, binge eating, and other disturbances of appetite regulation as well as symptoms of depression, obsessionality, apathy and irritability, and other personality changes (279). In patients with anorexia nervosa, some of these starvation-related phenomena, such as abnormal taste preference, may completely reverse with refeeding, although it may take considerable time after weight restoration for them to abate completely. However, some of these symptoms may reflect both preexisting and enduring traits, such as obsessive-compulsiveness, which are then further exacerbated by semistarvation. Such symptoms, therefore, may be only partially reversed with nutritional rehabilitation (82, 495). Complete psychological assessments may not be possible until some degree of weight restoration is achieved. Although patients with bulimia nervosa may appear to be physically within the standards of healthy weight, they may also show psychological and biological correlates of semistarvation, such as depression, irritability, and obsessionality, and may be below their personally optimum weight range, even at a weight considered to be "normal" according to population norms (496, 497). Furthermore, even at normal weight, body composition may be abnormal.

Common physical complications of anorexia nervosa are listed in Table 5. Amenorrhea of even a few months may be associated with osteopenia, which may progress to potentially irreversible osteoporosis and a correspondingly higher rate of pathological fractures (498, 499). If fracture risk is substantial, patients should be cautioned to avoid high-impact exercises. Pain in the extremities may signal stress fractures that may not be evident on X-rays but may be detected in abnormal bone scan results. Patients with anorexia nervosa who develop hypoestrogenemic amenorrhea in their teenage years that persists into young adulthood are at greatest risk for osteoporosis because they not only lose bone mass but also fail to form bone at a critical development phase (207). Osteopenia may be present in women who have been recovered from anorexia nervosa for up to 21 years (500). In addition, prepubertal and early pubertal patients are also at risk for permanent growth stunting (501, 502).

Acute complications of anorexia nervosa include dehydration, electrolyte disturbances (with purging), cardiac compromise with various arrhythmias (including conduction defects and ventricular arrhythmias), gastrointestinal motility disturbances, renal problems, infertility, premature births, other perinatal complications, hypothermia, and other evidence of hypometabolism (43). Death from anorexia nervosa is often proximally due to cardiac arrest secondary to arrhythmias (503).

Common physical complications of bulimia nervosa are listed in Table 6. The most serious physical complications occur in patients with chronic, severe patterns of binge eating and purging and are of most concern in very-low-weight patients (504).

Laboratory abnormalities in anorexia nervosa may include leukopenia with relative lymphocytosis, abnormal liver function, hypoglycemia, hypercortisolemia, hypercholesterolemia, hypercarotenemia (the latter two findings attributed to reduced catabolism), low serum zinc levels, electrolyte disturbances, and widespread disturbances in endocrine function. Low potassium levels may result from purging by any of several methods and can lead to potentially fatal cardiac arrhythmias. Sometimes abnormalities in serum chloride or bicarbonate levels precede low potassium levels. Electrolyte abnormalities can occur quickly and require ongoing monitoring in patients with extensive vomiting or laxative and/or diuretic abuse alone or in combination with low weight. In such patients, electrolyte levels should be repeated periodically to assess for abnormalities. Thyroid abnormalities may include low T_4 levels, even though thyroid-stimulating hormone levels are in the normal range; the low T_4 levels reverse with weight restoration and generally should not be treated with hormone replacement therapy (200, 505–507). Normal serum phosphorus values may be misleading because they do not reflect total body phosphorus depletion (which is usually reflected in serum phosphorus only after refeeding has begun). In early malnutrition, when many other laboratory measures may still be within normal limits, serum complement component 3 and 4 and serum transferrin may be abnormally low and serve as indicators of nutritional status (71).

Abnormal findings on magnetic resonance images reflect changes in the brain (508). White matter and cerebrospinal fluid volumes appear to return to the normal range after weight restoration. However, gray matter volume deficits, which correlate with the patient's lowest recorded BMI, may persist even after weight restoration (99, 509, 510). Some patients show persistent deficits in their neuropsychological testing results that have been shown to be associated with poorer outcomes (511).

It is important to consider that laboratory findings in anorexia nervosa may be normal in spite of a patient's profound malnutrition. For example, patients may have low total body potassium levels even when serum electrolytes are normal and thus may be prone to unpredictable cardiac arrhythmias (512).

Laboratory abnormalities in bulimia nervosa may include electrolyte imbalances such as hypokalemia, hypochloremic alkalosis, mild elevations of serum amylase (most often salivary in origin), and hypomagnesemia and hypophosphatemia, especially in patients who abuse laxatives (513–515).

B. EPIDEMIOLOGY

Estimates of the incidence or prevalence of eating disorders vary depending on the sampling and assessment methods, and many gaps exist in our current knowledge base. The reported lifetime prevalence of anorexia nervosa among women has ranged from 0.3% for narrowly defined to 3.7% for more broadly defined anorexia nervosa (25, 516, 517). With regard to bulimia nervosa, estimates of the lifetime prevalence among women have ranged from 1% to 4.2% (516, 518, 519). Some studies suggest that the prevalence of bulimia nervosa in the United States may have decreased slightly in recent years (520), whereas the prevalence of anorexia nervosa may have increased slightly (421, 521). Eating disorders are more commonly seen among girls and women, with estimates of the male-female prevalence ratio ranging from 1:6 to 1:10 (516). The prevalence of anorexia nervosa and bulimia nervosa in American children and younger adolescents is not well documented.

In the United States, eating disorders appear to be about as common in young Hispanic and Native American women as in Caucasian women and less common among African American and Asian women (522–524). Although studies have shown that preadolescent African American girls report a higher drive for thinness than Caucasian girls (525, 526), the drive for thinness increases significantly in Caucasian girls during puberty and remains unchanged in African American girls (527). Disordered eating is prevalent in many other countries. In a Scandinavian study of girls and boys ages 14–15 years, 0.7% of the girls and 0.2% of the boys reported a lifetime prevalence of anorexia nervosa, and 1.2% of the girls and 0.4% of the boys reported a lifetime prevalence of bulimia nervosa (528). Studies in Japan suggest that the prevalence of eating disorders is on the rise there. Recent data indicate that >50% of female college students report a history of significant and persistent dieting, 40% use diet pills or drinks to lose weight, and 18% report a BMI <18.5 kg/m^2 (529). However, the latter finding requires cautious interpretation, because appropriate BMI ranges might vary by ethnic grouping; for example, the normal range of BMI might actually be lower in Asian populations than in North American and European populations (530). Eating disorder concerns and symptoms do appear to be increasing among Chinese women exposed to Western culture and modernization in cities such as Hong Kong (531–533). The prevalence of disturbed eating disorders attitudes, as assessed by surveys, also appears to be high in other non-Western countries such as Iran, nonwhite South Africa, and Fiji (429, 534, 535).

First-degree female relatives of patients with anorexia and bulimia nervosa have higher rates of eating disorders compared with relatives of control subjects (536–539). In addition, relatives of individuals with anorexia and bulimia nervosa have increased rates of eating disorders that do not meet full diagnostic criteria compared with relatives of control subjects (538, 539). Identical twin siblings of patients with anorexia or bulimia nervosa also have higher rates of these disorders, with monozygotic twins having higher concordance than dizygotic twins. Families of patients with bulimia nervosa have been found to have higher rates of substance abuse (particularly alcohol use disorders), affective disorders, and certain personality traits, including elevated levels of perfectionism and an increased sense of ineffectiveness (540, 541). In Fiji, the prevalence of binge eating disorder is comparable to that in the United States (542).

High rates of co-occurring psychiatric illness are found in patients seeking treatment at tertiary-level psychiatric treatment centers. Lifetime co-occurring major depression or dysthymia has been reported in 50%–75% of patients with anorexia (323, 324) and bulimia (324, 331) nervosa. Estimates of the prevalence of bipolar disorder among patients with anorexia or bulimia nervosa are usually around 4%–6% but have been reported to be as high as 13% (325).

The lifetime prevalence of OCD among anorexia nervosa patients has been as high as 25% (82, 323, 543), with OCD frequently predating the onset of anorexia nervosa (341, 461). Obsessive-compulsive symptomatology has been found in a large majority of weight-restored patients with anorexia nervosa treated in tertiary-level care centers (544). OCD is also common among patients with bulimia nervosa (82, 331, 543). Co-occurring anxiety disorders, particularly social phobias, are common among patients with anorexia and bulimia nervosa (82, 310, 323, 331, 543). Substance abuse has been found in as many as 23%–40% of patients with bulimia nervosa. Among patients with anorexia nervosa, estimates of those with substance abuse have ranged from 12% to 18%, with this problem occurring primarily among those with the binge eating/purging subtype (308, 310, 323, 545).

Co-occurring personality disorders are frequently found among patients with eating disorders, with estimates ranging from 42% to 75%. The associations between bulimia nervosa and Cluster B and C disorders (particularly borderline personality disorder and avoidant personality disorder) and between anorexia nervosa and Cluster C disorders (particularly avoidant personality disorder and obsessive-compulsive personality disorder) have been reported (546, 547). Eating disorder patients with personality disorders are more likely than those without personality disorders to also have concurrent mood or substance use disorders (308, 331). Co-occurring personality disorders are significantly more common among patients with the binge eating/purging subtype of anorexia nervosa than among patients with the restricting subtype or in normal-weight patients with bulimia nervosa (349).

Sexual abuse has been reported in 20%–50% of patients with bulimia (346) and anorexia (221, 548) nervosa, although sexual abuse may be more common in patients with bulimia nervosa than in those with the restricting subtype of anorexia nervosa (346, 549). Childhood sexual abuse histories are reported more often in women with all psychiatric disorders, including eating disorders, than in women from the general population (549). Women who have eating disorders in the context of sexual abuse appear to have higher rates of comorbid psychiatric conditions than other women with eating disorders (314, 346). Furthermore, individuals with bulimia nervosa are reported to have experienced higher rates of other types of trauma besides childhood sexual abuse, including adult rape and molestation, aggravated assault, and physical neglect (332, 550, 551).

C. NATURAL HISTORY AND COURSE

1. Anorexia nervosa

Although the overall percentage of individuals who fully recover from anorexia nervosa is modest, it is well established that younger patients who receive prompt and appropriate intervention have a much better full recovery rate. For example, in the study by Strober et al. (19), >70% of adolescents had a full and lasting recovery 5 years after the onset of comprehensive treatment. Although some patients improve symptomatically over time, a substantial proportion continue to have body image disturbances, disordered eating, and other psychiatric difficulties (163, 324, 552). In one 10-year follow-up study, a relapse rate of 42% was seen during the first posthospitalization year for patients with anorexia nervosa (553). A review of a large number of studies of patients who were hospitalized or who received tertiary-level care and were followed up at least 4 years after the onset of illness indicates that "good" outcomes occurred in 44% of the patients (i.e., weight restored to within 15% of recommended weight for height and regular menstruation established), although these criteria are clearly insufficient to consider a patient as recovered or even as having restored weight to an adequate level. Poor outcomes occurred in about 24% (weight never reached within 15% of recommended weight for height; menstruation absent or at best sporadic), and intermediate outcomes occurred in about 28% (163). Approximately 5% of the patients died. Overall, about two-thirds of anorexia nervosa patients continue to have enduring morbid food and weight preoccupation, and up to 40%

have bulimic symptoms. Even among those who have good outcomes as defined by restoration of weight and menses, many have other persistent psychiatric symptoms, including dysthymia, social phobia, obsessive-compulsive symptoms, and substance abuse (323, 554).

Among adolescents with anorexia nervosa, approximately 50%–70% recover, 20% are improved but continue to have residual symptoms, and 10%–20% develop chronic anorexia nervosa (163). In a 10- to 15-year follow-up study of adolescent patients hospitalized for anorexia nervosa—76% of whom met criteria for full recovery—time to recovery was quite protracted, ranging from 57 to 79 months depending on the definition of recovery (19, 478). Anorexia nervosa patients with atypical features, such as denying a fear of gaining weight or denying distorted perceptions of their bodies, had a somewhat better course (478). Although good outcomes were observed in only 35% of 80 patients in Eisler et al.'s 5-year follow-up study (155), outcomes were good in 62% of the 21 patients who had been ill for <3 years and whose illness began before age 19.

Diagnostic migration occurs in patients with anorexia nervosa, reflecting the development of binge eating and/or purging behavior. The most frequent change among diagnostic categories is from anorexia nervosa, restricting type, to anorexia nervosa, binge eating/purging type; most changes occur by the fifth year after the onset of illness (477, 553). In one study, >50% of patients with anorexia nervosa, restricting type (both adolescents and adults) developed bulimic symptomatology over the course of follow-up, and only a small fraction of patients with anorexia nervosa, restricting type remained in that diagnostic subtype (555). Factors leading to the development of bulimic symptoms among patients with anorexia nervosa, restricting type are not well understood, nor is the precise time course of this development.

Mortality rates in eating disorders, specifically anorexia nervosa, are among the highest in the mental disorders. The prognosis of anorexia nervosa does not appear to have improved during the 20th century (163, 556, 557). Harris and Barraclough (558) calculated the standardized mortality ratios (SMRs) for all causes of death in 152 English language reports from a MEDLINE search on the mortality of mental disorder. The highest risk of premature death from natural and unnatural causes was related to eating disorders and substance abuse. Another study analyzing 10 large samples of individuals with eating disorders found strong evidence for an elevated SMR in eight of these samples, with a definitely elevated SMR for anorexia nervosa and no conclusion for bulimia nervosa. Lower weight at presentation was associated with a higher SMR. Mortality also varied with age at presentation, with an SMR of 3.6 for those presenting under age 20 years; 9.9, for ages 20–29 years; and 5.7, for age 30 years or older. Among female patients, the risk of death was 0.59% per year (559).

Deaths among male patients from anorexia nervosa have also been studied. In a recent report, two national registers, the National Patient Register (NPR) and the Causes of Death Register (CODR), were examined in Norway for deaths related to anorexia nervosa that occurred during a 9-year period (1992–2000). The medical record or death certificate listed anorexia nervosa as a diagnosis or cause of death for 66 individuals. Rates of death related to anorexia nervosa were 6.46 and 9.93 per 100,000 deaths for the NPR and the CODR, respectively. A substantial percentage of deaths (43.9%) in both registers occurred at or above age 65 years. For the NPR, the mean age at the time of death was 61 years, and 31% of deaths occurred among men. For the CODR, the mean age at the time of death was 49 years, and 18% of deaths occurred among men (560).

In other analyses, approximately 5.6% of patients diagnosed with anorexia nervosa die per decade of illness (561), and female anorexia nervosa patients are reportedly 12 times more likely to die than women of a similar age in the general population (321). The most common causes of death are suicide and starvation-related effects. The suicide rate among women with anorexia nervosa is up to 57 times higher than that for women of a similar age in the general population (321). Lower weight at presentation, longer duration of illness, and severe alcohol use appear to be associated with higher risk of mortality (321, 562).

Nielsen (563) conducted a literature review of mortality studies in eating disorders and concluded that methodological problems created biases to the eating disorder mortality data. The major problems with these studies were small sample sizes and loss of patients to follow-up.

Mortality and morbidity for anorexia nervosa, bulimia nervosa, and related disorders are likely to be underreported because they go unrecognized by clinicians. Patients' denial of illness may result in their avoidance of treatment at an early phase and the later development of multiple chronic physical problems, with associated morbidity and mortality (321, 563).

A shorter duration of illness and younger age at onset have been associated with a better outcome; lower initial minimum weights, vomiting, binge eating, purgative abuse, chronicity of illness, and obsessive-compulsive personality symptoms are reported to be unfavorable prognostic features (163). However, many of these prognostic indicators have not been consistently replicated and may be more reliable predictors of short-term but not long-term outcomes. In general, adolescents have better outcomes than adults and younger adolescents have better outcomes than older adolescents.

2. Bulimia nervosa

Although the literature on the long-term course and prognosis of bulimia nervosa remains limited, studies over the last decade have begun to clarify these issues. First, studies have shown that in untreated community samples, there are modest degrees of spontaneous improvement over a 1- to 2-year period, with roughly a 25%–30% reduction in binge eating, purging, and laxative abuse (564, 565). The overall short-term success rate for patients receiving psychosocial treatment or medication has been reported to be 50%–70% (324). Relapse rates of 30%–85% have been reported for successfully treated patients at 6 months to 6 years of follow-up (329, 566).

In a 5-year period, most individuals with bulimia nervosa in the community continue to have some form of an eating disorder of clinical severity, with about 33% remitting each year and another 33% relapsing to full diagnostic criteria, which suggests a relatively poor prognosis for this untreated group (567). In a naturalistic longitudinal study of 110 treatment-seeking women with bulimia nervosa, 73% achieved full recovery (no bingeing or purging for at least 8 consecutive weeks) at some point during a median of 7 years of follow-up, and 36% of those relapsed (568). A 6-year follow-up of patients treated for bulimia nervosa found that 60% of the patients were rated as having a good outcome, 29% as having an intermediate outcome, and 10% as having a poor outcome; 1% were reported as having died (569). A review of the treatment literature by this same group (570) found that, over time, social adjustment tended to normalize in some patients but that a fairly large group experienced chronic symptomatology and impairment; there was little crossover to anorexia nervosa or binge eating disorder. The longest follow-up study to date (562), with a mean follow-up of 11.5 years, found that the number of women who continued to meet full diagnostic criteria for bulimia nervosa declined over time. At long-term follow-up, 30% continued to engage in recurrent binge eating and purging behaviors. Subsequent analysis of this data set concluded that although menstrual irregularities were common at follow-up, the baseline presence of illness appeared to have little impact on these patients' later ability to achieve pregnancy (571). The results of this follow-up were interpreted to indicate that treatments with demonstrated efficacy for short-term outcome appeared to improve psychosocial functioning at long-term outcome among women with bulimia nervosa (572). A review of other literature in this area concluded that no consistent evidence exists to support the idea that early intervention implies a better long-term outcome (573).

A variety of factors have been examined as possible predictors of outcome. The available literature suggests that outcomes for patients with illness onset in adolescence are better than for those with later onsets (556). Although the data are highly variable, evidence suggests that comorbidity with OCD may be associated with a longer duration of illness (574) and that comorbidity with personality disorders may alter the natural course of illness (575). Overevaluation of shape and weight and a history of childhood obesity may be negative predictor factors (576), whereas a history of substance use disorders at intake or misuse of laxatives during the follow-up period may predict suicide attempts (577). The overall conclusion is that considerable variability occurs in the natural course of this illness, with persistence of symptoms at long-term follow-up in a significant subgroup of patients.

3. Eating disorders not otherwise specified

EDNOS is a commonly used diagnosis, being given to >50% of patients with eating disorders who present to outpatient treatment settings (263). EDNOS variants consisting of mixtures of anorexia and bulimia nervosa symptoms appear to be particularly common among adolescents. This heterogeneous group of patients consists largely of subsyndromal cases of anorexia or bulimia nervosa (e.g., those who fail to meet one criterion, such as not having 3 months of amenorrhea or having fewer binge eating episodes per week than required for a strictly defined diagnosis) as well as the substantial group of patients with binge eating disorder.

Because the diagnosis of EDNOS includes individuals with diverse eating disorder presentations, it is predictable that the course of EDNOS will be highly variable. Indeed, an early study of an unselected EDNOS population found a varied course of illness and low rate of recovery over 30 months (267). In addition, in patients with a variety of eating disorders who were followed over time, it appears that considerable movement occurred from one eating disorder diagnostic category to another, including EDNOS (263).

Binge eating disorder occurs in about 2% of community cohorts and is common among patients seeking treatment for obesity at hospital-affiliated weight programs (1.3%–30.1% prevalence), with studies using more rigorous interview-based measures typically reporting lower rates (578, 579). About 33% of these patients are male. Binge eating disorder typically begins in adolescence (at least by retrospective recall) or early adulthood and occurs more frequently in adults than in adolescents, but patients generally do not present for treatment until adulthood. (580). A well-established concomitant feature of binge eating disorder is that obese individuals who binge eat are more likely than those who do not binge eat to display comorbid axis I psychopathology, particularly major depressive disorder, with lifetime rates of 46%–58% (313, 334, 335, 337, 581).

Important observations have been made regarding the course of binge eating disorder. A 5-year community study of young women with binge eating disorder reported that a majority of the women had recovered spontaneously by 5-year follow-up. However, the age of participants in this study was considerably younger than that of most patients presenting for binge eating disorder treatment, making the generalizability of these findings uncertain (567). Another community study that followed patients over a 6-month period reported that about half of patients remaining in the study continued to meet binge eating disorder criteria, whereas symptoms of the other half partially remitted (567, 582). A 6-year study (583) that followed intensively treated binge eating disorder patients found that approximately 57% had a good outcome, 35% an intermediate outcome, and 6% a poor outcome; 1% of the patients had died. Although shorter-term remission is not necessarily maintained on a longer-term basis, clinical samples and shorter-term studies of binge eating disorder treatment have often reported high rates of response to minimal interventions (e.g., placebo) (584). Taken together, these lines of evidence suggest that the course of binge eating disorder is rather unstable over time. Treatment appears to be associated with a fairly positive long-term response, but it is difficult to know how many patients might have recovered without specific treatment.

The presence of binge eating may be predictive of weight gain over time. The aforementioned study of Fairburn et al. (567) reported that the prevalence of obesity in that group of patients had nearly doubled by the end of the follow-up period. Follow-up data from several treatment studies (271, 272, 585, 586) suggest that the persistence of binge eating may be associated with weight gain over time.

D. GENETIC FACTORS

Family and twin studies suggest a strong genetic component in the development of anorexia and bulimia nervosa (587–589), but the specifics of exactly what vulnerabilities are transferred and the mechanisms whereby they contribute to the pathogenesis of eating disorders need to be identified. The evidence also suggests that anorexia and bulimia nervosa may share genetic transmission with anxiety disorders and major depression (590, 591).

Further investigation of genetic contributions to vulnerability for eating disorders has occurred with two types of analyses: linkage studies and association studies for polymorphisms of specific genes. Evidence from a large international, multisite study suggests the presence of an anorexia nervosa susceptibility locus on chromosome 1p (592) and a susceptibility locus for bulimia nervosa on chromosome 10p (593). In affected sibling pairs who ranked high for "drive for thinness" and "obsessionality" traits, suggestive linkages were found on chromosomes 1, 2, and 13 (594). Association studies for polymorphisms of specific genes with specific behavioral covariates have produced many contradictory findings. For example, four studies were positive for a polymorphism of −1438 G/A in the promoter *5HT2A* gene, and three studies were negative for this polymorphism (reviewed by Hinney et al. [595]). A meta-analysis of all the association studies of the *5HT2A* gene in anorexia nervosa showed a persistent significant effect of the −1438 allele (596).

Preliminary evidence suggests that the norepinephrine transporter gene (*NET*) and monoamine oxidase A gene (*MAOA*) contribute to the increased risk for anorexia nervosa, restricting type. A serotonin transporter gene (*SERT*), known to be associated with anxiety, is preferentially transmitted to children with anorexia nervosa when the more active *MAOA* variant is also transmitted (597). The findings regarding these three genes (*MAOA*, *SERT*, and *NET*) in relation to susceptibility to anorexia nervosa require replication. Other studies suggest significant associations between anorexia nervosa and the serotonin gene *HTR1D* and the opioid gene *OPRD1* (598).

V. REVIEW AND SYNTHESIS OF AVAILABLE EVIDENCE

In the following sections, the available data on the efficacy of treatments for eating disorders are reviewed. For several reasons, interpreting the meanings and significance of these studies for patients seen in clinical practice is often difficult. Most studies have consisted of 6- to 12-week trials designed to evaluate the short-term efficacy of treatments. Unfortunately, few data exist on the long-term efficacy of treatment for patients with eating disorders, who often have a chronic course and variable long-term prognosis. Many studies also inadequately characterize the phase of illness when patients were first treated (e.g., early or late), which may have an impact on outcomes. Particularly for studies of psychosocial therapies that may consist of multiple elements, the precise interventional elements responsible for treatment effects may be difficult to identify. Furthermore, in comparing the effects of psychosocial treatments among studies, important variations may exist in the nature of the treatments delivered to patients. In addition, most studies have examined the efficacy of treatments only on eating disorder symptoms, with few reporting the efficacy on associated features and comorbid conditions such as the persistent mood, anxiety, and personality disorders that are common in "real world" populations.

A variety of outcome measures are used in trials for patients with eating disorders. Outcome measures used in studies of patients with anorexia nervosa often include the amount of weight gained within specified time intervals or the proportion of patients achieving a specified percentage of expected body weight, as well as whether those with secondary amenorrhea experience a return of menses. Measures of the severity or frequency of eating disorder behaviors have also been reported. In studies of bulimia nervosa, outcome measures include reductions in the frequency or severity of eating disorder behaviors such as binge eating, vomiting, and laxative use and the proportion of patients achieving remission from or a specific reduction in eating disorder behaviors.

A. TREATMENT OF ANOREXIA NERVOSA

1. Nutritional rehabilitation

With regard to approaches to promoting weight gain, the evidence does not show that giving a patient a warming treatment or growth hormone injections significantly increases weight gain or decreases the length of hospitalization. In a randomized controlled trial by Birmingham et al. (599), 10 female patients with anorexia nervosa received a warming therapy, consisting of a heating vest set at medium heat for 3 hours/day for 21 days, and a control group of 11 patients received the vest when it was not turned on. Among the 18 patients who completed the study, there was no difference in change in BMI; the study authors concluded that warming did not increase the rate of weight gain. In a double-blind study by Hill et al. (600), 15 inpatients with anorexia nervosa, ages 12–18 years, were randomly assigned to receive recombinant human growth hormone (0.05 mg/kg, s.c.) or an equivalent volume of placebo daily for 28 days. At the end of the study, the growth hormone and placebo groups did not differ significantly in admission weight, BMI, or daily caloric intake.

For weight maintenance, Kaye et al. (601) found that weight-restored patients with anorexia nervosa often require 200–400 calories more than sex-, age-, weight-, and height-matched control subjects to maintain weight. The energy wasting of malnourished anorexia nervosa patients results in higher than normal resting energy expenditure (REE; measured in kilocalories per kilogram per day) (602), resulting in resistance to weight gain. In malnourished anorexia nervosa patients, a high REE has been independently linked to anxiety level; abdominal pain and vomiting; physical activity, including exercise, fidgeting, and other non-exercise-related energy expenditure; and cigarette smoking (603, 604). Of note, REE measured as kilocalories per day is lower in patients with anorexia nervosa and returns to normal with refeeding (604). These different measurement and reporting techniques may be the source of some confusion among study results, and reports concerning REE must be read carefully to fully understand exactly what is being measured (602).

Research that addresses the optimal length of hospitalization or the optimal setting for weight restoration is sparse. There is no available evidence to show that brief stays for anorexia nervosa are associated with good long-term outcomes. Several studies have reported that hospitalized patients who are discharged at a weight lower than their target weight subsequently relapse and are rehospitalized at higher rates than those who achieve their target weight before discharge (605). Baran et al. (606) assessed weight, height, eating disorder symptoms, and severity of depressive and anxiety symptoms in 22 women with anorexia nervosa at hospital admission and at follow-up occurring a mean of 29 months after patient discharge. The patients who were discharged while severely underweight reported significantly higher rates of rehospitalization and endorsed more symptoms than those who had achieved normal weight before discharge. Commerford et al. (607) had similar observations in their 5-year follow-up study (by telephone interview) of 31 patients with anorexia nervosa and bulimia nervosa who met specific criteria for discharge. That group reported that patients being discharged while at a low weight was associated with brief lengths of stay and that the closer patients were to a healthy weight at the time of discharge from the hospital, the lower their risk of relapse.

In a study by Watson et al. (103) of 397 patients admitted to an inpatient service over a 7-year period, patients who were admitted involuntarily showed the same short-term rates of weight gain as those who were admitted voluntarily. Moreover, most of those who were involuntarily treated later affirmed the need for and exhibited a better attitude toward the treatment process.

In ambulatory settings, most programs find weight gain goals of 0.5–1 lb/week to be realistic, although gains of up to 2 lb/week have been reported in a partial hospitalization step-down program in which patients previously treated as inpatients are treated 12 hours/day, 7 days/week (113). The opinion of the clinicians running this program is that it would not be as effective for never-hospitalized patients.

2. Psychosocial treatments

Although psychosocial interventions, including psychoeducation, individual therapy, family therapy, and (in some settings) group therapy, are considered to be the mainstay of effective treatment for anorexia nervosa, supporting evidence is sparse. Instead, this perspective is derived primarily from considerable clinical experience (608) and patient reports. In a review of 23 studies reporting surveys of people who have had an eating disorder to determine which treatments patients find helpful, support, understanding, and empathic relationships were rated as critically important, psychological approaches were rated as the most helpful, and medical interventions focused exclusively on weight were viewed as not helpful (609).

The concept of "readiness for change," which is widely used in the treatment of substance use disorders (610), has garnered increasing interest and use with patients with anorexia nervosa to improve their motivation for treatment and potentially improve treatment efficacy. The Anorexia Nervosa Stages of Change Questionnaire, developed with a population of patients age 14 years and older, has been designed to be specific for anorexia nervosa. It is reliable and valid (611, 612) but has not yet been used to study treatment effectiveness at various stages. The Readiness and Motivation Interview, which was developed as an assessment tool for adult patients (613), has been shown to predict clinical outcomes, such as the decision to enroll in treatment, dropping out from intensive residential treatment, posttreatment symptom change, and relapse (613–615); however, it has not yet been evaluated to determine its effectiveness in helping patients move from precontemplation stages to higher stages of readiness for treatment. After a quantitative and qualitative analysis of results from a survey of 278 patients with anorexia nervosa, Jordan et al. (616) attempted to develop a staging measure associated with recovery from anorexia nervosa; they concluded that the most meaningful measure was one that measured progress in readiness to stop restricting, bingeing, and purging behaviors. The development and use of validated tools that assess readiness are important because clinicians have been shown to be poor at estimating patients' readiness for change (617) and consequently are ill-equipped to make treatment recommendations tailored to patients' readiness status.

a) Structured inpatient and partial hospitalization programs

Most inpatient programs use one of many behaviorally formulated interventions, individual and family psychotherapy, empathic nursing approaches, nutritional counseling, and several group therapies designed to improve the patient's knowledge about and attitude toward eating, exercise, and body image (618, 619). These behavioral programs implement a variety of strategies derived from social learning theory that include reinforcement and contingency management (e.g., empathic praise, exercise-related limits and rewards, bed rest, privileges linked to achieving weight goals and desired behaviors). Behavioral programs have been shown to produce good short-term therapeutic effects (620). One review comparing behavioral psychotherapy programs with medication treatment alone found that behavior therapy resulted in more consistent weight gain among patients with anorexia nervosa as well as shorter hospital stays (620). Studies of consecutively admitted inpatients with anorexia nervosa (621, 622) found that "lenient" behavioral programs that use initial bed rest and the warning of returning the patient to bed if weight gain does not continue are as effective as, and in some situations possibly more effective than, "strict" programs in which meal-by-meal caloric intake or daily weight is tied precisely to a schedule of privileges (e.g., time out of bed, time off the unit, permission to exercise or receive visitors). Some evidence suggests that the use of a supervised graded exercise program, such as nonaerobic yoga, may be of benefit in the inpatient treatment of anorexia nervosa (623–625).

Although there is debate about the value of supplemental feedings and formula feedings during the early weight-gain phase in anorexia nervosa, emerging evidence suggests that this strategy may sometimes be helpful. In a short-term study of 100 adolescent Caucasian female patients, one center reported that over a comparable period of time, patients voluntarily treated during hospitalization with supplemental nocturnal nasogastric refeeding had greater and more rapid weight gain than patients treated with traditional oral refeeding alone (121). Other centers have reported similar experiences (626). High-calorie supplements have also been shown to lead to more rapid weight gain (627). However, further study is needed to assess the short- and long-term effectiveness of this approach (121, 628).

Adolescents with anorexia nervosa may have the best outcomes after structured inpatient or partial hospitalization treatment. For example, one study in Norway (629) found that among 55 patients who had received systematic (usually inpatient) treatment based on close cooperation among parents and the pediatric and child and adolescent psychiatry departments, outcome after 3–14 years was good. No patient had died and 82% of the patients had no eating disorder; however, 41% had other axis I diagnoses (most commonly depression or anxiety disorders).

Among adults with anorexia nervosa who receive inpatient treatment, outcome is not usually as favorable. For example, in another report from Norway of 24 adult patients, 42% of patients had improved by the 1-year follow-up, whereas the outcome was poor in 58% (630).

Attempts have been made to determine factors that predict relapse after hospitalization, but identifying such features with certainty has proved challenging. Strober et al. (19) were unable to clearly identify factors associated with posthospitalization relapse among adolescents. One study (631) found that a young age (<15 years), markedly abnormal eating attitudes at admission, and a low rate of weight gain during hospitalization predicted readmission.

b) Individual psychotherapy

During the acute phase of treatment, the efficacy of specific psychotherapeutic interventions for facilitating weight gain remains uncertain. A randomized controlled trial by McIntosh et al. (7) of 56 acutely ill adult women with anorexia nervosa treated as outpatients showed that 20 weekly sessions of nonspecific clinical management (a manual-based therapy delivered by individuals knowledgeable about the treatment of eating disorders and consisting of advice, support, and education) were as effective as or more effective than 20 weekly sessions of CBT or IPT. Of the 56 women, 70% either did not complete treatment or made small or no gains; only about 10% had a very good outcome and 20% improved considerably by the end of these treatments.

With regard to psychotherapy after weight gain, in the first clear demonstration of the efficacy of CBT, 33 adult patients with anorexia nervosa were randomly assigned after weight gain to 1 year of outpatient CBT or nutritional counseling (136). The group receiving nutritional counseling relapsed significantly earlier and at a higher rate than the group receiving CBT, and modified Morgan Russell criteria for "good outcome" were met by significantly more of the patients receiving CBT (44%) than those receiving nutritional counseling (7%).

In another study of outpatient treatment by Dare et al. (85), 84 adult outpatients with anorexia nervosa were randomized to one of four treatments: 1 year of focal psychoanalytic psychotherapy, 7 months of cognitive-analytic therapy, 1 year of family therapy, or low-contact, routine treatment as usual. At 1-year follow-up, only modest symptomatic improvement was seen in the whole group of patients, and several patients remained significantly undernourished. Although improvements were quite modest for all groups, psychoanalytic psychotherapy and family therapy were superior to the control treatment; cognitive-analytic therapy (which was shorter in duration) tended to show benefits over the control treatment as well.

In practice, individual psychotherapies, family therapies, nutritional counseling, and group therapies are often combined during hospital treatment and in comprehensive follow-up care. As of yet, no systematic data have been published regarding outcomes of using these combined approaches, which experienced clinicians often view as superior to a single-therapy approach.

c) Family psychotherapy

Evidence suggests that family therapy is frequently useful for reducing symptoms and dealing with family relational problems that may contribute to an eating disorder's persistence, particularly in adolescents. Russell et al. (154) demonstrated family therapy to be superior to individual therapy in adolescents with anorexia nervosa for <3 years. Follow-up studies showed that this superiority was maintained 5 years later (155). In an outpatient study by Eisler et al. (86), 40 adolescent patients were randomly assigned to conjoint family therapy or separated family therapy. Both therapies were found to be equally effective on global measures of outcome, but symptomatic change was more marked in the separated family group, but only if the parents were highly critical of the patient, whereas psychological change was more prominent in those receiving conjoint family therapy.

In a randomized inpatient trial, Geist et al. (130) compared the effects of two family-oriented treatments, family therapy and family group psychoeducation, on 25 girls with newly diagnosed anorexia, restrictive type. At 4 months, significant improvement in weight was noted in both groups compared with baseline—77.7% versus 89.1% for family therapy and 77.2% versus 90.4% for family group psychoeducation—with no significant difference between the two groups. In all patients, no significant changes were noted on any self-report measures of specific or nonspecific eating disorder psychopathology. This study was uncontrolled, so it is also difficult to determine the specific results of the treatments in the context of other treatments received by the patients. However, the study results suggest that family therapy and family psychoeducation may be equally helpful with respect to weight gain in the course of IPT in patients with anorexia nervosa.

In a randomized study of 37 adolescents with anorexia nervosa by Robin et al. (126), behavioral family systems therapy (BFST), in which eating and distorted beliefs are targeted during family therapy, was compared with ego-oriented individual therapy (EOIT). At the end of treatment and at 1-year follow-up, groups receiving either treatment had significant weight gain, resumed menstruation, and showed improvements in eating attitudes, depression, and eating-related family conflict. BFST produced a quicker response initially, but by 1-year follow-up, the outcome in the two groups was similar. This study was uncontrolled, and the loss of participants at follow-up could have biased the results. However, the study suggests that both BFST and EOIT may be helpful.

Systematic studies of the Maudsley model of family therapy that are currently under way are receiving considerable interest (87). In these interventions, families are "put in charge" of their children's eating. Lock et al. (87, 129) found that short-term family therapy was as helpful as longer-term family therapy and that, overall, adolescents with anorexia nervosa did well. The results suggested that those who had high levels of OCD symptoms or a nonintact family tended to need longer courses of more intense therapy. A multisite study of this approach is currently being conducted.

For adults, family therapy is less promising. Russell et al. (154) found that individual therapy tended to be superior to family therapy by the end of active treatment but that this difference disappeared at follow-up. Dare et al. (85) observed that specific treatments, including family therapy, were superior to generic treatments and treatments rendered by inexperienced clinicians. Family therapy was no less effective than the other types of therapy, but, as mentioned above, in this study results were modest for all active treatments.

d) Psychosocial interventions based on addiction models

Some programs attempt to blend features of addiction models, such as the 12 steps, with medical model programs that use cognitive-behavioral approaches (632). However, no systematic data exist regarding the effectiveness of these approaches for patients with anorexia nervosa.

e) Support groups

Expert opinion suggests that benefits are likely to accrue from support groups; however, at present no data are available that systematically assess the contribution of support groups led by professionals or advocacy organizations that provide patients and their families with mutual support, advice, and education about eating disorders.

3. Medications

a) Antidepressants

Studies of the effectiveness of antidepressants on weight restoration are limited. In two studies (174, 175), the addition of fluoxetine to the nutritional and psychosocial treatment of hospitalized, malnourished patients with anorexia nervosa did not appear to provide any advantage with respect to either the amount or the speed of weight recovery. Attia et al. (174) conducted a randomized, placebo-controlled, double-blind study of fluoxetine at a target daily dose of 60 mg in 31 women with anorexia nervosa receiving treatment for their eating disorder on a clinical research unit. At 7 weeks, there were no significant differences in body weight or measures of eating behavior or psychological state between patients receiving fluoxetine and those receiving placebo. Similar results were reported in a 6-week open-label trial by Strober et al. (175), in which the response to fluoxetine in adolescents hospitalized for the treatment of anorexia nervosa was investigated. Patients were drawn from consecutive admissions to a specialty treatment service and received fluoxetine as an add-on to their multidisciplinary treatment regimen at 3 weeks to 1 month after intake. Analyses of global clinical severity ratings of eating behaviors and weight phobia failed to show any beneficial or detrimental effect of fluoxetine in the patients when compared with matched historical case-control subjects. An uncontrolled trial by Gwirtsman et al. (633) of six patients with chronic, refractory anorexia nervosa treated with fluoxetine reported positive results, including weight restoration. Overall, however, the little evidence that is available does not support the use of antidepressant medications for weight restoration in severely malnourished patients with anorexia nervosa who are being treated in well-structured hospital-based eating disorder programs.

After patients have gained weight and when the psychological effects of malnutrition are resolving, preliminary evidence suggests that SSRI antidepressants may be helpful with weight maintenance. In a double-blind, placebo-controlled trial by Kaye et al. (177), 35 patients with restricting-type anorexia nervosa were randomly assigned to receive fluoxetine (n = 16; average 40 mg/day) or placebo (n = 19) after they had gained weight in an inpatient hospital program and were discharged; they were then observed as outpatients for 1 year. The dropout rate from the trial was much higher in the placebo (84%) than in the fluoxetine (37%) group. Patients continuing to take fluoxetine for 1 year had a reduced rate of relapse, as determined by a significant increase in weight and a reduction in symptoms. They also showed a reduction in depression, anxiety, and obsessions and compulsions. However, these study results are problematic because some patients' weight had not been restored when the study started and the study design was complex, with many exceptions and multiple raters. In contrast, preliminary analysis of data from a 5-year two-site study funded by the National Institute of Mental Health on relapse prevention for anorexia nervosa involving 93 patients ages 16 years and older did not favor fluoxetine when CBT was administered (138). After weight restoration to at least 90% of ideal body weight, all patients received CBT and were also randomized to either fluoxetine 60 mg/day or placebo. The survival analysis showed no difference between those receiving CBT plus medication and those receiving CBT alone with respect to time to relapse (138).

In an open outpatient study by Bergh et al. (634), underweight adolescent patients with anorexia nervosa treated with psychotherapy plus citalopram did worse (losing several kilograms) than did patients treated with psychotherapy alone (losing about 0.2 kg during the period of observation). Another study by Fassino et al. (176) compared 52 adult female patients with anorexia nervosa, restricting type, who received citalopram (n = 26) or were assigned to a waiting-list control group (n = 26). The randomization method in this study was not clearly defined. After 13 patients dropped out, 19 and 20 patients remained in the citalopram and control groups, respectively. Although no differences were found in weight gain between the groups, after 3 months of treatment, those receiving citalopram showed modest advantages regarding symptoms of depression, obsessive-compulsive symptoms, impulsiveness, and trait anger, as assessed by rating scales.

Data on the efficacy of tricyclic antidepressants are even more limited. In a study by Halmi et al. (635), 72 patients with anorexia nervosa were randomly assigned to receive cyproheptadine hydrochloride, a weight-inducing drug; amitriptyline hydrochloride, a tricyclic antidepressant; or placebo, using a double-blind method. Lower-weight patients with the restricting subtype of anorexia who were receiving intensive inpatient treatment seemed to benefit more, albeit to a modest degree, from either amitriptyline or cyproheptadine, compared with patients who were receiving placebo. In another double-blind, controlled study by Lacey and Crisp (636) of 16 patients with anorexia nervosa, no significant beneficial effect was observed from adding clomipramine to the usual treatment (although dosages of only 50 mg/day were used).

b) Antipsychotics

Small open-label studies in adults suggest that low doses of second-generation antipsychotic medications such as olanzapine may improve weight gain and psychological indicators, but controlled studies are needed to confirm this. Barbarich et al. (190) reported that 17 hospitalized patients with anorexia nervosa given open-label treatment with olanzapine for up to 6 weeks had a significant reduction in depression, anxiety, and core eating disorder symptoms and a significant increase in weight. Malina et al. (191) retrospectively questioned 18 patients with anorexia nervosa about their response to open treatment with olanzapine; the patients reported a significant reduction in anxiety, difficulty eating, and core eating disorder symptoms after taking olanzapine. Powers et al. (192) reported that of 14 patients with anorexia nervosa who completed a 10-week open-label study of olanzapine at 10 mg/day in an outpatient setting, 10 gained an average of 8.75 pounds, with 3 of those attaining their healthy body weight, and 4 lost a mean of 2.25 pounds. The patients also received weekly drug monitoring sessions and weekly group medication adherence sessions in which psychoeducation was provided.

The second-generation antipsychotic quetiapine, examined in an open-label study, had only a small benefit in terms of weight gain but some benefit in eating disorders–related preoccupation and depression (195, 196, 637).

In an open trial, 13 severely ill outpatients with anorexia nervosa, restricting type received low-dose (1–2 mg) haloperidol in addition to standard treatment and were reported to benefit (significant weight gain and improved insight) (198). Another study suggested no significant benefit for pimozide (638).

Although these pilot studies of antipsychotic medications are promising and suggest that these medications may be useful during the weight restoration phase, no controlled studies have been reported. In addition, few of the available studies have included male patients, only limited numbers of adolescents have been studied, and only case reports are available regarding prepubertal children. Again, controlled studies are needed.

c) Other medications and somatic treatments

Few controlled studies have been published on the use of other psychotropic medications for the treatment of anorexia nervosa. In one study (639), the use of lithium carbonate resulted in no substantial benefit. Uncontrolled studies of other somatic treatments, including vitamins, hormone treatments, and ECT, have also demonstrated no specific benefit (199).

In addressing associated features of anorexia nervosa, other medications have been used with apparent benefit, although evidence for their effect is limited. For example, antianxiety agents have been used selectively before meals to reduce anticipatory anxiety concerning eating (200, 201).

Although supplemental estrogen-progestins, calcium, and vitamin D are often prescribed in routine practice in an effort to minimize or ameliorate osteopenia or osteoporosis (203), they have not been shown to meaningfully prevent or reverse skeletal deterioration. Rather, nutritional rehabilitation during the period of bone growth is the only practical intervention shown to potentially reverse bone loss (413, 502, 640). The only controlled trial to date that has examined the effects of estrogen administration on adult women with anorexia nervosa (n=44) showed that estrogen-treated patients had no significant change in bone mass density compared with control patients (204). However, the six estrogen-treated patients whose initial body weight was <70% of their healthy weight had a 4.0% increase in mean bone density, whereas the 10 subjects of comparable body weight not treated with estrogen had a further 20.1% decrease in bone density. This finding suggests that hormone replacement therapy may help a subset of low-weight women with anorexia nervosa. At the same time, artificially inducing menses carries the risk of supporting or reinforcing a patient's denial that she does not need to gain weight.

Experimental approaches to bone revitalization using recombinant human insulin-like growth factor, bone growth factors (641), and biphosphonates (642) have also been attempted, but these approaches cannot be recommended for routine practice. Studies concerning these agents and other investigative treatments are now under way.

B. TREATMENT OF BULIMIA NERVOSA

1. Psychosocial treatments

a) Individual psychotherapy

CBT specifically directed at the eating disorder symptoms and underlying cognitions in patients with bulimia nervosa is the psychosocial intervention that has been most intensively studied in adults and for which there is the most evidence of efficacy (209, 212, 643–654). Although there has been considerable variation in the way in which CBT has been implemented, several controlled trials used short-term, time-limited interventions, such as 20 individual psychotherapy sessions over 16 weeks, with two scheduled visits per week for the first 4 weeks (212, 643, 644, 653, 655–662). Significant decrements in binge eating, vomiting, and laxative abuse have been documented among some patients receiving CBT; however, the percentage of patients who achieve full abstinence from bingeing/purging behavior is variable and often includes only a small number of patients (212, 643, 646, 648–655, 663–668). Among studies with control arms, CBT has been shown to be superior to waiting list (663–665, 667), minimal intervention (668), nutritional counseling alone (652), or nondirective control (666) conditions. In most of the published CBT trials, significant improvements in either self-reported (665, 669) or clinician-rated (670) mood have been reported. To date, there are no published treatment trials of adolescents with bulimia nervosa, although two studies are nearing completion (unpublished study of U. Schmidt et al. in London and unpublished study of D. le Grange et al. in the United States). Case series concerning CBT treatment for adolescents with bulimia nervosa are now available or in press (671, 672).

In practice, many other types of individual psychotherapy are used in the treatment of bulimia nervosa, such as interpersonal, psychodynamically oriented, or psychoanalytic approaches. Clinical experience and naturalistic survey research suggest that these approaches can help in the treatment of the co-occurring mood, anxiety, personality, interpersonal, and trauma- or abuse-related disorders that frequently accompany bulimia nervosa (153, 673). Evidence for the efficacy of these treatments for bulimia nervosa comes mainly from case reports and case series. Some modes of therapy, including the interpersonal and psychodynamic approaches, have been studied in randomized trials as comparison treatments for CBT or in separate trials (212, 643, 645, 674). In general, these and other studies have shown IPT to be helpful as an acute treatment. However, one trial examined the efficacy of IPT in patients who did not respond to CBT and found a low response rate coupled with a high dropout rate (211).

Although the specific forms of focused psychodynamic psychotherapy that have been studied in direct comparison with CBT have generally not been as effective as CBT in short-term trials (656, 657), it must be understood that in these studies the therapists were proscribed from undertaking any discussion of the patients' symptoms in the 20 sessions of psychodynamic treatment they provided.

The behavioral technique of exposure (e.g., to bingeing foods) plus response prevention (e.g., inhibiting vomiting after eating) has also been considered as treatment for bulimia nervosa. However, data on the efficacy of this approach are conflicting, as studies have reported enhanced (675), not significantly altered (676), and reduced (655) responses to CBT when this type of behavioral therapy was used as an adjunct. On the basis of results from a large clinical trial, and given the trial's logistical complexity, exposure treatment does not appear to have additive benefits over a solid core of CBT (648, 649), a finding supported by a recent authoritative meta-analysis (651).

Few studies have directly compared the effectiveness of various types of individual psychotherapy in the treatment of bulimia nervosa. One study by Fairburn et al. (643) that compared CBT, IPT, and behavior therapy showed that all three treatments were effective in reducing binge eating symptoms by the end of treatment but that CBT was most effective in improving disturbed attitudes toward shape and weight and restrictive dieting . However, at long-term follow-up (mean of 5.8 years), the study found equal efficacy for IPT and CBT on eating variables, attitudes about shape and weight, and restrictive dieting (659), which suggests that the IPT patients had "caught up" in terms of benefits over time. A second multicenter study that compared CBT with IPT suggested that CBT worked more rapidly (653) and showed greater efficacy than IPT at the end of 20 weeks of treatment (212). However, at 1-year follow-up, no significant difference was noted between the two treatment groups (212).

Another trial reported the efficacy of dialectical behavior therapy (677), and an ongoing multicenter study (678) has reported similar findings. In a 6-week controlled study involving 50 patients assigned to guided affective imagery therapy or a control group, those receiving the active treatment showed substantially more improvement in binge eating and purging behaviors and eating disorder–related attitudes (679).

b) Group psychotherapy

Group psychotherapy approaches have also been used to treat bulimia nervosa. Many clinicians favor a combination of individual and group psychotherapy. Psychodynamic and cognitive-behavioral approaches may also be combined. Group therapy may help patients to more effectively deal with the shame surrounding their disease as well as provide additional peer-based feedback and support. A meta-analysis of 40 group treatment studies suggested moderate efficacy for group therapy, with those studies that provided 1-year follow-up data reporting that improvement was typically maintained (680). There is some evidence that group treatment programs that include dietary counseling and management as part of the program are more effective than those that do not (208) and that more frequent visits (e.g., sessions several times a week) throughout treatment (646) or early in treatment (644, 646) result in improved outcome.

A direct comparison of group and individual CBT failed to find evidence of substantially different outcomes, with patients in both treatments doing equally well at follow-up (681). However, in a meta-analysis, the data showed clear advantages of delivering CBT in an individual versus a group format (216).

c) Family and marital therapy

Family therapy has been reported to be helpful in the treatment of bulimia nervosa in a large case series of adults (682), but more systematic studies are not available. A systematic study of family therapy for adolescents with bulimia nervosa is currently under way (89), but no results have been reported yet.

Family therapy should be considered whenever possible, especially for adolescents who still live with their parents, older patients with ongoing conflicted interactions with parents, or patients with marital discord. For women with eating disorders who are mothers, parenting help and interventions aimed at assessing and, if necessary, aiding their children should be included (386–388).

d) Support groups/12-step programs

Some patients have found Overeaters Anonymous and similar groups to be helpful as adjuncts to initial treatments or for prevention of subsequent relapses (223, 683), but no data from short- or long-term outcome studies of these programs have been reported.

e) Self-help approaches

A growing body of literature has suggested that CBT can be administered successfully through self-help or guided self-help manuals, at times in association with pharmacotherapy (220, 222, 651, 684–689). A review of self-help treatments with or without guidance by a professional has recently been published (690). Although such techniques are not yet sufficiently developed to recommend their acceptance as a primary treatment strategy, developments in this area may prove of great importance in providing treatment to patients who otherwise might not have access to adequate care. Clinicians unfamiliar with the CBT approach may benefit from acquainting themselves with these CBT treatment manuals and obtaining specialized training in CBT to further help their bulimia nervosa patients (656, 691–696).

2. Medications

a) Antidepressants

Early observations that individuals with bulimia nervosa exhibit an elevated lifetime prevalence of mood disorders, together with an elevated prevalence of mood disorders in their first-degree relatives, prompted initial trials of antidepressants for the acute treatment of bulimia nervosa (233). In these trials, antidepressants appeared to be effective for bulimia nervosa regardless of whether or not the patient was clinically depressed. Subsequent randomized trials confirmed that nondepressed patients responded to these medications and that the baseline presence of depression was not a predictor of medication response (234, 235, 697, 698). Although wide variability exists across studies, reductions in binge eating and vomiting rates in the range of 50%–75% have been achieved with active medication (181, 224, 230, 241, 699–714).

Specific antidepressant agents that have demonstrated efficacy among patients with bulimia nervosa in double-blind, placebo-controlled studies include trazodone (708); tricyclic compounds such as imipramine (233, 236), desipramine (234, 237, 238, 240), and amitriptyline (for mood but not eating variables) (235); the SSRIs fluoxetine (224, 230, 698, 703) and sertraline (227) but not fluvoxamine (715); and several MAOIs, including phenelzine (697) and isocarboxazid (716) but not moclobemide (717). Treatment with bupropion was also efficacious (181), but its use is not recommended because of the association between bupropion treatment and seizures in purging bulimic patients. The results of one study (709) suggest that patients with atypical depression and bulimia nervosa may preferentially respond to phenelzine in comparison with imipramine. However, because MAOIs are potentially dangerous in patients with chaotic eating and purging habits, they should be used cautiously in bulimia nervosa patients.

Dosages of tricyclic and MAOI antidepressants for treating patients with bulimia nervosa parallel those used to treat patients with depression, although fluoxetine at dosages higher than those used for depression may be more effective for bulimic symptoms (e.g., 60–80 mg/day). The first multicenter fluoxetine study (230) demonstrated that 60 mg/day was clearly superior to 20 mg/day on most variables, and in a second study (224) all subjects receiving active medication started with 60 mg/day. A third trial used 60 mg/day as a maintenance therapy, but the dropout rate from the study was very high (226). The medication was surprisingly well tolerated at this dosage, and many clinicians initiate treatment for bulimia nervosa with fluoxetine at a higher dosage, titrating downward if necessary to manage side effects.

Three trials have examined the effectiveness of antidepressant maintenance therapy. One trial with fluvoxamine (701) demonstrated an attenuated relapse rate versus placebo in patients with bulimia nervosa who were on a maintenance regimen of the medication after leaving an inpatient treatment program. However, in the continuation arm of a clinical trial with desipramine (240), 29% of the patients entering that phase experienced a relapse within 4 months. A 1-year maintenance trial using fluoxetine or placebo found evidence for a lower relapse rate on active drug, but the dropout rate was quite high in both treatment arms (226). An open-label trial found evidence that fluoxetine could be effective in adolescents (225).

Two studies have examined the efficacy of medication in patients who did not respond to IPT and/or CBT (211, 250). The results were somewhat inconsistent in that one study found medication to be quite useful, whereas the other found low rates of response and high dropout rates.

b) Other medications

A number of other medications have been used experimentally for bulimia nervosa without evidence of efficacy, including fenfluramine (700) and lithium carbonate (241). Fenfluramine has now been taken off the market because of links between its use (mainly in combination with phentermine) and cardiac valvular abnormalities. Lithium may occasionally be used concurrently for the treatment of co-occurring conditions. The opiate antagonist naltrexone has been studied in three randomized trials at dosages used for treating narcotic addiction and preventing relapse among alcohol-dependent patients (50–120 mg/day). The results consistently show that the medication is not superior to placebo in reducing bulimic symptoms (699, 704, 707). In a small double-blind, crossover study involving higher dosages (e.g., 200–300 mg/day), naltrexone did appear to have some efficacy. Further studies using these dosage ranges are needed. However, there have been mixed reports concerning the risk of hepatotoxicity with the use of high dosages of naltrexone (705, 706, 718).

Other agents that have been shown to be efficacious in treating bulimia nervosa symptoms in randomized trials are topiramate, an anti-epileptic agent (242, 243), and ondansetron, an antinausea drug that decreases afferent vagal neurotransmission through its action as a 5-HT_3 antagonist (719); however, odansetron requires multiple daily administrations and is quite expensive. In a randomized controlled trial, carbamazepine showed efficacy in only one patient, and that patient had a history of bipolar disorder (720).

3. Combinations of psychosocial and medication treatments

The relative efficacy of psychotherapy, medication, or both in the treatment of bulimia nervosa has been examined in six studies. In the first study (253), intensive group cognitive psychotherapy (45 hours of therapy over 10 weeks) was superior to imipramine alone in reducing binge eating/purging and depressive symptoms. Imipramine plus intensive group CBT did not improve the outcome on eating variables but did improve depression and anxiety variables. In the second study (254), patients in group CBT improved more than those receiving desipramine alone. Some advantage was also seen for combination therapy on some variables, such as dietary restraint. The results of the third study (255), which compared fluoxetine treatment, CBT, and combination therapy, favored CBT alone and suggested little benefit for combination therapy. These results, however, are difficult to interpret because of the high attrition rate (50% by the 1-month follow-up). In the fourth study (251), CBT was superior to supportive psychotherapy, and active medication (consisting of desipramine followed by fluoxetine if abstinence from binge eating and purging was not achieved) was superior to placebo in reducing eating disorder behaviors. The combination of CBT and active medication resulted in the highest abstinence rates. The use of sequential medication in this study addressed a limitation of earlier studies in that when one antidepressant fails, a clinician typically tries other agents that often result in better antidepressant efficacy than the first medication alone. In the fifth study (702), no advantage was found for the use of fluoxetine over placebo in an inpatient setting, although both groups improved significantly. In the sixth study (721), combination treatment with desipramine and CBT was terminated prematurely because of a high dropout rate. A recent review concluded that the combination treatment was superior on some variables (711).

In general, studies show the importance of achieving abstinence from binge eating and vomiting regardless of the interventions used in the treatment of bulimia nervosa, and they confirm that longer-term outcome is better when abstinence is achieved after short-term interventions (722).

C. TREATMENT OF BINGE EATING DISORDER

1. Nutritional rehabilitation and counseling: effect of diet programs on weight and binge eating symptoms

Some studies of treatments for binge eating disorder have prioritized weight loss as the primary goal, whereas others have prioritized cessation of binge eating. Both types of studies will be addressed below.

a) Weight loss

In patients with binge eating disorder, very-low-calorie diets alone have been associated with substantial initial weight losses, with >33% of these patients maintaining their weight loss 1 year after treatment (723–726). In some studies using low-calorie diets, either significant weight loss did not occur (727) or weight was partially regained during the first year (290, 728). The pattern of weight regain after initial weight loss is common in all general medical and psychological treatments for obesity and not only for obesity associated with binge eating disorder. In one study, the presence of subthreshold or full syndrome binge eating disorder at baseline did not appear to adversely affect weight loss in programs using behavioral weight control, a low-calorie diet, and aerobic and strength training (729). Likewise, in a study using telephone- and mail-based behavioral weight control for obesity, binge eating status at baseline was not associated with outcome (730). Treatments with psychotherapies that do not specifically address weight control, such as CBT, IPT, and dialectical behavior therapy, ordinarily do not yield significant weight reduction (see below), but adding exercise and 6-month biweekly maintenance to CBT may improve weight loss in patients with binge eating disorder (731).

b) Binge eating symptoms

Binge eating is substantially reduced in programs using very-low-calorie diets, but a small number of individuals may experience a reemergence of binge eating when regular meals are reintroduced (585, 723, 724, 726). Among individuals who do not manifest binge eating prior to treatment, behavioral weight control with a low-calorie diet does not appear to promote the emergence of binge eating (732). There is as yet little evidence regarding patient characteristics (e.g., age at onset of binge eating, magnitude and frequency of weight fluctuation) that predict differential response to programs that prioritize weight versus those that prioritize binge cessation.

2. Other psychosocial treatments: effects on binge eating disorder

CBT, behavior therapy, dialectical behavior therapy, and IPT have all been associated with binge frequency reduction rates of 67% or more and significant abstinence rates during active treatment (272, 276, 733–739). Deterioration during the follow-up period has been observed with all three forms of psychotherapy; however, in some cases, maintenance of change at 1-year follow-up has been substantial (271, 272, 731). Several studies have examined various treatments intended to augment standard CBT. The addition of exercise appears to augment both binge and weight reduction (731), whereas spouse involvement in treatment does not significantly improve outcome (88). One group reported promising effects on binge eating with a novel virtual reality modification of standard treatment (739, 740).

Nondiet approaches that focus on self-acceptance and healthy lifestyle rather than weight loss per se may reduce binge eating, depression, anxiety, bulimia, the drive for thinness, body dissatisfaction, total and LDL cholesterol, and systolic blood pressure while increasing moderate physical activity levels (741, 742). One study failed to find a difference between dieting and nondieting approaches in reducing binge eating and weight. In an expected observation, however, even the dieting treatment did not yield significant weight loss in this study, calling into question the integrity of the treatments (742, 743).

Self-help programs using self-guided, professionally designed manuals have been effective in reducing the symptoms of binge eating disorder in the short run for some patients and may have long-term benefit (273–277). One recent study found that guided self-help CBT was superior to guided self-help behavioral weight loss treatment for binge remission (46% vs. 18%, respectively), although neither treatment produced significant weight loss (277).

3. Medications

A variety of SSRIs (citalopram, fluoxetine, fluvoxamine, and sertraline) (744–747) and tricyclic antidepressants (desipramine and imipramine) (699, 748) have been found to be associated with significantly greater decreases in binge frequency than placebo. Fluvoxamine was not superior to placebo in a controlled study, in part due to a high placebo response (749). A retrospective chart review study of the serotonin-norepinephrine reuptake inhibitor venlafaxine in obese patients with binge eating disorder reported beneficial effects on eating, weight, and mood (750). As is the case for bulimia nervosa, in most studies using SSRIs for binge eating disorder, the dosages used have been at or near the high end of the recommended dosage range. Where follow-up data were reported, it appears that patients tend to relapse after medication is discontinued (289, 748); however, most medication studies to date do not report follow-up data. For the most part, treatment with antidepressants has not been demonstrated to yield clinically significant weight loss in this population, although one study reported an estimated weight loss of 5.6 kg with sertraline treatment compared with 2.4 kg in the placebo group (747). It should be noted that the treatment of other psychiatric disorders (e.g., depression) with SSRIs has at times been associated with weight gain, particularly in the long term (751).

The appetite-suppressant medication sibutramine has also shown promise in the treatment of binge eating disorder. In a randomized controlled trial (284), sibutramine was shown to have significant beneficial effects on binge eating and weight loss, with remission rates of 40% and 27% in the sibutramine and placebo groups, respectively, and a weight decrease of 7.4 kg versus a weight increase of 1.4 kg in these groups, respectively. A laboratory feeding study reported that subjects with binge eating disorder treated with sibutramine versus placebo for 4 weeks in a crossover design consumed less in a laboratory binge meal and lost more weight (3.2 vs. 0.5 kg) after sibutramine than after placebo treatment (752). Although the appetite-suppressant medications fenfluramine and dexfenfluramine have also been found to significantly reduce binge frequency (289), their use has been associated with serious adverse events, including a 23-fold increase in the risk of developing primary pulmonary hypertension when used for >3 months (753). Studies have suggested that patients taking the combination of fenfluramine and phentermine may be at greater risk of heart valve deformation and pulmonary hypertension; as a result, fenfluramine has been withdrawn from the market (753–756).

Most recently, the anticonvulsants topiramate and zonisamide have been studied in patients with binge eating disorder. Two open studies, one a retrospective review of patients with affective disorders and co-occurring binge eating disorder (757) and the other an open-label prospective study (758), as well as one randomized, double-blind, placebo-controlled study (286), found topiramate to be effective for both binge suppression and weight loss. The latter study reported remission in 64% of the topiramate group versus 30% of the placebo group, with weight loss of 5.9 and 1.2 kg in the topiramate and placebo groups, respectively. A 1-year open-label extension of this study (287) found that these effects were largely maintained over the study period; however, only a small number of the patients (10 of 61) remained in the study for the full year, and adverse effects, including paresthesias, dry mouth, cognitive problems, headache, dizziness, somnolence, fatigue, and dyspepsia, led to discontinuation in about 33%

of patients. An open-label study of the anticonvulsant zonisamide (288) suggests that it may have similar effects, both in clinical response and in adverse events.

Finally, naltrexone has been associated with a decrease in binge frequency similar to that reported with antidepressant medications, although the response rate did not differ from that of placebo (699). This observation underscores the fact that high placebo response rates are found in many studies of binge eating disorder, so caution is required in evaluating the claims of effective treatments, particularly those using a waiting-list control condition (289, 699, 749).

4. Combined psychosocial and medication treatment strategies

In some studies, coadministration of medication with psychotherapy or dietary counseling has been found to be associated with significantly more weight loss than has psychotherapy or dietary counseling alone (290–292). A recent study found that in patients receiving guided self-help CBT for binge eating disorder, the addition of orlistat yielded significantly higher rates of binge remission after active treatment but not at 3-month follow-up and significantly greater weight loss both after treatment and at 3-month follow-up compared with placebo (295). However, other studies suggest that concomitant administration of SSRI antidepressants adds little benefit in binge reduction or weight loss for patients treated with CBT for binge eating disorder (293, 294, 759). One recent study in which subjects with binge eating disorder received individual CBT plus fluoxetine, individual CBT plus placebo, fluoxetine, or placebo found that individual CBT but not fluoxetine demonstrated efficacy for reducing binge eating but not weight (293). A similar study, in which subjects with binge eating disorder were randomized to receive the same four treatments as adjuncts to group behavioral treatment, found that adjunctive individual CBT, but not fluoxetine, resulted in significant additional binge reduction, whereas fluoxetine appeared to augment the reduction in depressive symptoms. Although neither adjunctive treatment contributed significantly to weight loss, the 54 subjects who achieved binge remission lost an average of 6.2 kg, whereas the 62 subjects who did not achieve remission gained 0.7 kg (294).

5. Treatment strategies for night eating syndrome

There are few available studies of treatments for night eating syndrome. One open-label study of sertraline at dosages of up to 200 mg/day for night eating syndrome found improvements in both the number of awakenings and the nocturnal ingestions, with full remission in 29% of subjects (302). A subsequent double-blind study of sertraline for night eating syndrome reported that in a group of 24 patients, 75% of those treated with sertraline versus 25% of those who received placebo were considered to have responded to the treatment. Response was sustained during the 6-month open-label follow-up period (760). A small case series of four patients, two with night eating syndrome and two with the related condition of nocturnal sleep-related eating disorder, reported that topiramate treatment was helpful (761). Abbreviated progressive muscle relaxation training may be useful in treating night eating syndrome (301). Finally, other treatments reported to be helpful in sleep-related eating disorder are carbidopa/L-dopa, bromocriptine, codeine, and clonazepam (762, 763).

PART C
FUTURE RESEARCH NEEDS

Future research needs for eating disorders have been described by various authors (6, 764, 765). With respect to interventions, studies are needed on the following:

1. Primary prevention programs are needed in schools and through the media. Studies are required to clarify the benefits versus potential risks of such programs.
2. Targeted prevention through screenings and risk-factor early intervention programs could be beneficial. Studies are needed to better delineate the value of working with children and adolescents regarded to be at greatest risk for developing eating disorders.
3. Improved evidence is needed regarding the choice of treatment setting, selection of specific treatments, and likely length and intensity of treatments to achieve optimal outcomes (immediate and long-term follow-up) based on clearly defined clinical indicators and a more precise delineation of the stages of these disorders.
4. Newer medications affecting hunger, satiety, and energy expenditure as well as commonly associated psychiatric symptoms and conditions need to be developed and tested.
5. Adequate methods for treating osteopenia, osteoporosis, and other long-term medical sequelae of anorexia nervosa are needed.
6. The development and testing of various individually administered and "bundled" individual and group psychotherapies, including CBT, IPT, psychodynamic therapy, psychoanalytic therapy, and family therapy, as well as nutritional therapies and other psychosocial therapies (creative arts, 12-step models, professional- or layperson-led support groups, and self-help groups for patients and families), would be helpful. For anorexia nervosa, specific treatments for younger patients, who are likely to be more treatment responsive, may differ from those for older, more chronically ill patients, given that other illness characteristics and treatment responses are likely to vary between these groups. Furthermore, given the difficulties of recruiting and retaining patients with anorexia nervosa into controlled treatment studies and high dropout rates, large multisite, adequately powered studies are required.
7. For bulimia nervosa, the field requires well-conducted studies that examine "transtheoretical" and other treatment approaches, particularly those involving psychodynamically informed therapies, and studies of longer-term results of psychotherapies. Better studies are needed for psychotherapeutically treating the clinically complex patients with multiple comorbid conditions often seen in practice.
8. For binge eating disorder found in combination with obesity, studies are needed of the optimal sequencing of treatments (i.e., whether the treatment of binge eating should precede or occur concurrently with weight control treatment) and the long-term benefits of treatment with respect to both the eating disorder and weight-related symptoms. Studies are also needed comparing traditional behavioral weight loss with nondiet approaches in obese patients with and without binge eating disorder and examining both behavioral and weight-related outcomes.
9. Development and testing of better treatments are required for night eating and nocturnal eating syndromes.
10. Further development and testing of professionally designed self-administered treatments by manuals and computer-based treatment programs would be useful.
11. Further development and testing of Web-, telephone-, and other distance-based therapies for eating disorders are needed.
12. Research into the modifications of treatment required by the presence of various co-occurring conditions would be beneficial.
13. The impact of commonly used "alternative" and "complementary" therapies on the course of illness should be investigated.
14. More data are needed from treatment outcome studies related to various systems or settings of care, including fee-for-service, HMO, and other managed care payment models; limitations of hospital or other intensive treatment resources due to managed care and other resource constraints; treatment in eating disorder specialty units versus general psychiatry treatment units; and impact of staff composition, professional background of

clinicians, system or setting characteristics, and roles of primary care versus mental health professionals in treating eating disorders.

15. Further delineation of proper education and training required for psychiatrists and other health care professionals to better treat patients with eating disorders and the development of specialized institution-based and distance-based training programs to disseminate training for the necessary clinical competencies are required.

In studying treatment outcomes and developing new approaches to treatment, it is important to have a clear understanding of the underlying causes and the factors that influence the course of eating disorders. Also, greater knowledge of eating disorder diagnoses and the epidemiology of these disorders will help in identifying subgroups of patients who may be more likely to respond to particular treatments. Areas of specific concern include the following:

1. **Diagnostic studies:** Further delineating and defining diagnostic categories for eating disorders, based on advances in pathophysiological classification, developmental sciences, personality disorders and relational (interpersonal) disorders, and cultural issues, all areas of focus for DSM-V. In this regard, many of the issues mentioned below are highly relevant.
2. **Risk factors:**
   a. Genetic and other biological risk factors that contribute to the risk for and nature of eating disorders. Careful and appropriate phenotyping is required for the genetic analysis of eating disorders. Specific behavioral features that may indicate a particular phenotype and that merit attention include perfectionism, obsessive symptoms associated with symmetry, and compulsions associated with ordering and hoarding, among others.
   b. Further clarification of risk factors, morbidity, course, and prognosis for the range of eating disorders, including anorexia nervosa, bulimia nervosa, binge eating disorder, night eating and nocturnal eating syndromes, and other syndromes now encompassed under EDNOS
   c. Gender-related, developmental, psychological, familial, social, and cultural risk factors that contribute to the appearance and course of specific eating disorders
3. **Biological correlates:**
   a. More neuroimaging studies to better delineate structure-function relations associated with predisposing vulnerabilities, nutritional changes associated with eating disorders, and changes resulting from specific treatments and in recovery
   b. Animal and human studies of regulatory mechanisms governing food ingestion versus energy expenditure
   c. Linkages between physiological and psychological processes of puberty and the onset of typical eating disorders
   d. Effects of exercise, including the role of extreme exercise, and food restriction in precipitating and maintaining eating disorders; conversely, the possible protective effect of contemporary women's athletics on girls' eating and weight attitudes
4. **Clinical studies:** The impact of various comorbid conditions (including mood, anxiety, substance use, obsessive-compulsive, and personality disorders; cognitive impairments; and other commonly encountered concurrent disorders) on course and treatment response
5. **Family studies:** Includes factors associated with the onset and maintenance of eating disorders and the impact of eating disorders on other family members

INDIVIDUALS AND ORGANIZATIONS THAT SUBMITTED COMMENTS

W. Stewart Agras, M.D.
Arnold E. Andersen, M.D.
Rena L. Appel, M.D.
Evelyn Attia, M.D.
Anne E. Becker, M.D., Ph.D., Sc.M.
Laird Birmingham, M.D., M.H.Sc., F.R.C.P.
Barton Blinder, M.D.
Francesca Brambilla, M.D.
Timothy D. Brewerton, M.D., D.F.A.P.A., F.A.E.D.
Cynthia M. Bulik, Ph.D.
Robert Cabaj, M.D.
Joshua W. Calhoun, M.D.
Regina C. Casper, M.D.
Scott Crow, M.D.
Elke D. Eckert, M.D.
Judith Feldman, M.D.
Fernando Fernandez-Aranda, Ph.D., F.A.E.D.
Aaron H. Fink, M.D.
Stanley E. Fischman, M.D.
Josie Geller, Ph.D.
Neville H. Golden, M.D.
Richard Gordon, Ph.D.
Richard K. Harding, M.D.
James I. Hudson, M.D., Sc.D.
David Jimerson, M.D.
Allan S. Kaplan, M.D., M.Sc., F.R.C.P.C.
Debra K. Katzman, M.D., F.R.C.P.C.
Diane Keddy, M.S., R.D., F.A.E.D.
Urszula Kelley, M.D.
Nathan E. Lavid, M.D.
Daniel le Grange, Ph.D.
James Lock, M.D., Ph.D.
Henry C. Mallard, M.D.
Marsha D. Marcus, Ph.D.
Beth Hartman McGilley, Ph.D., F.A.E.D.
Diane Mickley, M.D., F.A.C.P., F.A.E.D.
Charles A. Murkofsky, M.D.
Marvin A. Nierenberg, M.D.
Marion P. Olmsted, Ph.D., C.Psych.
Shirley B. Papilsky, M.D.
Katharine A. Phillips, M.D.
Amir Qaseem, M.D., Ph.D., M.H.A.
Randy A. Sansone, M.D.
Patricia Santucci, M.D.
Deborah C. Schwartz, M.D., F.R.C.P.C., C.G.P.
S. Warren Seides, M.D.
Mae S. Sokol, M.D.
Hans Steiner, M.D.
Robert Stern, M.D., Ph.D.
Erin Stucky, M.D.
Mary Tantillo, Ph.D., R.N., C.S.
B. Timothy Walsh, M.D.
Drew Westen, Ph.D.
Denise E. Wilfley, Ph.D., F.A.E.D.
Susan Willard, M.S.W., L.C.S.W.
Barbara E. Wolfe, Ph.D., A.P.R.N., F.A.A.N.
Stephen Wonderlich, Ph.D.
Blake Woodside, M.D.

Academy for Eating Disorders
American College of Physicians
American Group Psychotherapy Association
American Psychiatric Nurses Association
Association for Academic Psychiatry
Eating Disorders Research Society
National Association of Anorexia Nervosa and Associated Disorders
National Eating Disorders Association
National Institute of Mental Health
The Society for Adolescent Medicine

REFERENCES

The following coding system is used to indicate the nature of the supporting evidence in the summary recommendations and references:

[A] *Double-blind, randomized clinical trial.* A study of an intervention in which subjects are prospectively followed over time; there are treatment and control groups; subjects are randomly assigned to the two groups; both the subjects and the investigators are blind to the assignments.

[A–] *Randomized clinical trial.* Same as above but not double-blind.

[B] *Clinical trial.* A prospective study in which an intervention is made and the results of that intervention are tracked longitudinally; study does not meet standards for a randomized clinical trial.

[C] *Cohort or longitudinal study.* A study in which subjects are prospectively followed over time without any specific intervention.

[D] *Control study.* A study in which a group of patients and a group of control subjects are identified in the present and information about them is pursued retrospectively or backward in time.

[E] *Review with secondary data analysis.* A structured analytic review of existing data, e.g., a meta-analysis or a decision analysis.

[F] *Review.* A qualitative review and discussion of previously published literature without a quantitative synthesis of the data.

[G] *Other.* Textbooks, expert opinion, case reports, and other reports not included above.

1. National Institute for Clinical Excellence: Eating Disorders: Core Interventions in the Treatment and Management of Anorexia Nervosa, Bulimia Nervosa and Related Eating Disorders: Clinical Guideline 9. London, National Institute for Clinical Excellence, 2004. http://www.nice.org.uk/pdf/ cg009niceguidance.pdf [G]
2. Beumont P, Hay P, Beumont D, Birmingham L, Derham H, Jordan A, Kohn M, McDermott B, Marks P, Mitchell J, Paxton S, Surgenor L, Thornton C, Wakefield A, Weigall S: Australian and New Zealand clinical practice guidelines for the treatment of anorexia nervosa. Aust N Z J Psychiatry 2004; 38:659–670 [G]
3. Golden NH, Katzman DK, Kreipe RE, Stevens SL, Sawyer SM, Rees J, Nicholls D, Rome ES: Eating disorders in adolescents: position paper of the Society for Adolescent Medicine. J Adolesc Health 2003; 33:496–503 [G]
4. Pritchard BJ, Bergin JL, Wade TD: A case series evaluation of guided self-help for bulimia nervosa using a cognitive manual. Int J Eat Disord 2004; 36:144–156 [B]
5. Myers TC, Swan-Kremeier L, Wonderlich S, Lancaster K, Mitchell JE: The use of alternative delivery systems and new technologies in the treatment of patients with eating disorders. Int J Eat Disord 2004; 36:123–143 [F]
6. Yager J: Future directions in the management of eating disorders, in Clinical Handbook of Eating Disorders: An Integrated Approach. Edited by Brewerton TD. New York, Marcel Dekker, 2004, pp 547–568 [G]
7. McIntosh VV, Jordan J, Carter FA, Luty SE, McKenzie JM, Bulik CM, Framptom CMA, Joyce PR: Three psychotherapies for anorexia nervosa: a randomized controlled trial. Am J Psychiatry 2005; 162:741–747 [A–]
8. Song S: Starvation on the Web. Time, Jul 18, 2005, p 57 [G]
9. Wilson JL, Peebles R: Hardy KK, Mulvihill LC, Kretzschmar AY, Litt I: Pro-eating disorder website usage and health outcomes in an eating disordered population. Poster presented at the annual meeting of the Pediatric Academic Societies, Washington, DC, May 14–17, 2005 [G]

10. Yager J: Clinical computing: monitoring patients with eating disorders by using e-mail as an adjunct to clinical activities. Psychiatr Serv 2003; 54:1586–1588 [G]
11. Serpell L, Treasure J, Teasdale J, Sullivan V: Anorexia nervosa: friend or foe? Int J Eat Disord 1999; 25:177–186 [G]
12. Serpell L, Treasure J: Bulimia nervosa: friend or foe? the pros and cons of bulimia nervosa. Int J Eat Disord 2002; 32:164–170 [G]
13. Kaplan AS, Garfinkel PE: Difficulties in treating patients with eating disorders: a review of patient and clinician variables. Can J Psychiatry 1999; 44:665–670 [G]
14. Feld R, Woodside DB, Kaplan AS, Olmsted MP, Carter JC: Pretreatment motivational enhancement therapy for eating disorders: a pilot study. Int J Eat Disord 2001; 29:393–400 [B]
15. Treasure J, Bauer B: Assessment and motivation, in Handbook of Eating Disorders. Edited by Treasure J, Schmidt U, van Furth E. West Sussex, UK, Wiley, 2003, pp 219–232 [G]
16. Geller J, Williams K, Srikameswaran S: Clinician stance in the treatment of chronic eating disorders. Eur Eating Disorders Rev 2001; 9:1–9 [G]
17. Vitousek K, Watson S, Wilson GT: Enhancing motivation for change in treatment-resistant eating disorders. Clin Psychol Rev 1998; 18:391–420 [G]
18. Vitousek K, Gray J: Eating disorders, in Oxford Textbook of Psychotherapy. Edited by Gabbard GO, Beck UJS, Holmes J. Oxford, UK, Oxford University Press, 2005, pp 177–202 [G]
19. Strober M, Freeman R, Morrell W: The long-term course of severe anorexia nervosa in adolescents: survival analysis of recovery, relapse, and outcome predictors over 10–15 years in a prospective study. Int J Eat Disord 1997; 22:339–360 [C]
20. Rome ES: Eating disorders. Obstet Gynecol Clin North Am 2003; 30:353–377, vii [G]
21. Kreipe RE, Yussman SM: The role of the primary care practitioner in the treatment of eating disorders. Adolesc Med 2003; 14:133–147 [G]
22. Fisher M, Golden NH, Katzman DK, Kreipe RE, Rees J, Schebendach J, Sigman G, Ammerman S, Hoberman HM: Eating disorders in adolescents: a background paper. J Adolesc Health 1995; 16:420–437 [F]
23. Kaplan AS: Medical and nutritional assessment, in Medical Issues and the Eating Disorders: The Interface. Edited by Kaplan AS, Garfinkel PE. New York, Brunner/Mazel, 1993, pp 1–16 [G]
24. Watson TL, Andersen AE: A critical examination of the amenorrhea and weight criteria for diagnosing anorexia nervosa. Acta Psychiatr Scand 2003; 108:175–182 [D]
25. Garfinkel PE, Lin E, Goering P, Spegg C, Goldbloom D, Kennedy S, Kaplan AS, Woodside DB: Should amenorrhoea be necessary for the diagnosis of anorexia nervosa? evidence from a Canadian community sample. Br J Psychiatry 1996; 168:500–506 [G]
26. Fairburn CG, Cooper Z: The Eating Disorder Examination (12th Edition), in Binge Eating: Nature, Assessment and Treatment. Edited by Fairburn CG, Wilson GT. New York, Guilford, 1993, pp 317–360 [G]
27. Mazure CM, Halmi KA, Sunday SR, Romano SJ, Einhorn AM: The Yale-Brown-Cornell Eating Disorder Scale: development, use, reliability and validity. J Psychiatr Res 1994; 28:425–445 [G]
28. Sunday SR, Halmi KA, Einhorn A: The Yale-Brown-Cornell Eating Disorder Scale: a new scale to assess eating disorder symptomatology. Int J Eat Disord 1995; 18:237–245 [G]
29. Johnson C: Diagnostic Survey for Eating Disorders (DSED), in The Etiology and Treatment of Bulimia Nervosa: A Biopsychosocial Perspective. Edited by Johnson C, Connors M. New York, Basic Books, 1987, pp 174–194 [G]
30. Thelen MH, Mintz LB, Vander Wal JS: The Bulimia Test, Revised: validation with DSM-IV criteria for bulimia nervosa. Psychol Assess 1996; 8:219–221 [G]
31. Garner DM, Olmsted MP, Bohr Y, Garfinkel PE: The Eating Attitudes Test: psychometric features and clinical correlates. Psychol Med 1982; 12:871–878 [G]

32. Garner DM: Psychoeducational principles in treatment, in Handbook of Treatment for Eating Disorders, 2nd ed. Edited by Garner DM, Garfinkel PE. New York, Guilford, 1997, pp 145–177 [G]
33. Fairburn CG, Beglin SJ: Assessment of eating disorders: interview or self-report questionnaire? Int J Eat Disord 1994; 16:363–370 [G]
34. Garner DM, Olmstead MJ, Polivy J: Development and validation of a multidimensional eating disorder inventory for anorexia nervosa and bulimia. Int J Eat Disord 1983; 2:15–34 [G]
35. Garner DM: The Eating Disorders Inventory–2: Professional Manual. Odessa, FL, Psychological Assessment Resources, 1991 [G]
36. Garner DM: The Eating Disorders Inventory–2 (EDI-2), in Outcomes Assessments in Clinical Practice. Edited by Sederer LI, Dicky B. Baltimore, Williams & Wilkins, 1996, pp 92–96 [G]
37. Mitchell JE, Hatsukami D, Eckert E, Pyle RL: The Eating Disorders Questionnaire. Psychopharmacol Bull 1985; 21:1025–1043 [G]
38. Yanovski SZ: Binge eating disorder: current knowledge and future directions. Obes Res 1993; 1:306–320 [F]
39. Nangle DW, Johnson WG, Carr-Nangle RE, Engler LB: Binge eating disorder and the proposed DSM-IV criteria: psychometric analysis of the Questionnaire on Eating and Weight Patterns. Int J Eat Disord 1994; 16:147–157 [G]
40. Birmingham CL, Beumont PJV: Medical Management of Eating Disorders: A Practical Handbook for Healthcare Professionals. Cambridge, UK, Cambridge University Press, 2004 [G]
41. Mehler PS, Andersen AE: Eating Disorders: A Guide to Medical Care and Complications. Baltimore, Johns Hopkins University Press, 1999 [G]
42. Powers PS, Bannon YS: Medical comorbidity of anorexia nervosa, bulimia nervosa, and binge eating disorder, in Clinical Handbook of Eating Disorders: An Integrated Approach. Edited by Brewerton TD. New York, Marcel Dekker, 2004, pp 231–256 [G]
43. Miller KK, Grinspoon SK, Ciampa J, Hier J, Herzog D, Klibanski A: Medical findings in outpatients with anorexia nervosa. Arch Intern Med 2005; 165:561–566 [G]
44. Faine MP: Recognition and management of eating disorders in the dental office. Dent Clin North Am 2003; 47:395–410 [F]
45. Powers PS: Initial assessment and early treatment options for anorexia nervosa and bulimia nervosa. Psychiatr Clin North Am 1996; 19:639–655 [F]
46. Hebebrand J, Himmelmann GW, Heseker H, Schafer H, Remschmidt H: Use of percentiles for the body mass index in anorexia nervosa: diagnostic, epidemiological, and therapeutic considerations. Int J Eat Disord 1996; 19:359–369 [D]
47. Yates A, Edman J, Aruguete M: Ethnic differences in BMI and body/self-dissatisfaction among whites, Asian subgroups, Pacific Islanders, and African-Americans. J Adolesc Health 2004; 34:300–307 [G]
48. Lear SA, Toma M, Birmingham CL, Frohlich JJ: Modification of the relationship between simple anthropometric indices and risk factors by ethnic background. Metabolism 2003; 52:1295–1301 [C]
49. Yeung LP, Wong AC, Wang X, Birmingham CL, Lewicka S, Chanoine JP: Different relationship between anthropometric markers and umbilical cord plasma leptin in Asian and Caucasian neonates. Pediatr Res 2003; 53:1019–1024 [G]
50. Lear SA, Chen MM, Frohlich JJ, Birmingham CL: The relationship between waist circumference and metabolic risk factors: cohorts of European and Chinese descent. Metabolism 2002; 51:1427–1432 [D]
51. Chanoine JP, Yeung LP, Wong AC, Birmingham CL: Immunoreactive ghrelin in human cord blood: relation to anthropometry, leptin, and growth hormone. J Pediatr Gastroenterol Nutr 2002; 35:282–286 [G]

52. Birmingham CL: Book review: Report of the Task Force on the Treatment of Obesity. Health Services and Promotion Branch, Department of National Health and Welfare, Ottawa. Can Med Assoc J 1992; 146:1389 [G]
53. Mehler PS: Diagnosis and care of patients with anorexia nervosa in primary care settings. Ann Intern Med 2001; 134:1048–1059 [G]
54. Cooke RA, Chambers JB, Singh R, Todd GJ, Smeeton NC, Treasure J, Treasure T: QT interval in anorexia nervosa. Br Heart J 1994; 72:69–73 [C]
55. Mont L, Castro J, Herreros B, Pare C, Azqueta M, Magrina J, Puig J, Toro J, Brugada J: Reversibility of cardiac abnormalities in adolescents with anorexia nervosa after weight recovery. J Am Acad Child Adolesc Psychiatry 2003; 42:808–813 [C]
56. Franzoni F, Mataloni E, Femia R, Galetta F: Effect of oral potassium supplementation on QT dispersion in anorexia nervosa. Acta Paediatr 2002; 91:653–656 [A]
57. Powers PS, Schocken DD, Feld J, Holloway JD, Boyd FR: Cardiac function during weight restoration in anorexia nervosa. Int J Eat Disord 1991; 10:521 [C]
58. Frolich J, von Gontard A, Lehmkuhl G, Pfeiffer E, Lehmkuhl U: Pericardial effusions in anorexia nervosa. Eur Child Adolesc Psychiatry 2001; 10:54–57 [G]
59. Prousky JE: Pellagra may be a rare secondary complication of anorexia nervosa: a systematic review of the literature. Altern Med Rev 2003; 8:180–185 [F]
60. Winston AP, Jamieson CP, Madira W, Gatward NM, Palmer RL: Prevalence of thiamin deficiency in anorexia nervosa. Int J Eat Disord 2000; 28:451–454 [D]
61. Waldholtz BD: Gastrointestinal complaints and function in patients with eating disorders, in Eating Disorders: A Guide to Medical Care and Complications. Edited by Mehler PS, Andersen AE. Baltimore, Johns Hopkins University Press, 1999, pp 86–99 [G]
62. Brown RF, Bartrop R, Beumont P, Birmingham CL: Bacterial infections in anorexia nervosa: delayed recognition increases complications. Int J Eat Disord 2005; 37:261–265 [D]
63. Strumia R: Dermatologic signs in patients with eating disorders. Am J Clin Dermatol 2005; 6:165–173 [G]
64. Glorio R, Allevato M, De Pablo A, Abbruzzese M, Carmona L, Savarin M, Ibarra M, Busso C, Mordoh A, Llopis C, Haas R, Bello M, Woscoff A: Prevalence of cutaneous manifestations in 200 patients with eating disorders. Int J Dermatol 2000; 39:348–353 [C]
65. Birmingham CL, Tan AO: Respiratory muscle weakness and anorexia nervosa. Int J Eat Disord 2003; 33:230–233 [G]
66. Frank GK, Kaye WH, Greer P, Meltzer CC, Price JC: Regional cerebral blood flow after recovery from bulimia nervosa. Psychiatry Res 2000; 100:31–39 [D]
67. Doraiswamy PM, Krishnan KR, Figiel GS, Husain MM, Boyko OB, Rockwell WJ, Ellinwood EH Jr: A brain magnetic resonance imaging study of pituitary gland morphology in anorexia nervosa and bulimia. Biol Psychiatry 1990; 28:110–116 [D]
68. Hoffman GW, Ellinwood EH Jr, Rockwell WJ, Herfkens RJ, Nishita JK, Guthrie LF: Brain T1 measured by magnetic resonance imaging in bulimia. Biol Psychiatry 1990; 27:116–119 [G]
69. Hoffman GW, Ellinwood EH Jr, Rockwell WJ, Herfkens RJ, Nishita JK, Guthrie LF: Cerebral atrophy in bulimia. Biol Psychiatry 1989; 25:894–902 [G]
70. Andersen AE, Woodward PJ, LaFrance N: Bone mineral density of eating disorder subgroups. Int J Eat Disord 1995; 18:335–342 [D]
71. Nova E, Lopez-Vidriero I, Varela P, Toro O, Casas JJ, Marcos AA: Indicators of nutritional status in restricting-type anorexia nervosa patients: a 1-year follow-up study. Clin Nutr 2004; 23:1353–1359 [C]
72. Wyatt RJ, Farrell M, Berry PL, Forristal J, Maloney MJ, West CD: Reduced alternative complement pathway control protein levels in anorexia nervosa: response to parenteral alimentation. Am J Clin Nutr 1982; 35:973–980 [C]
73. Birmingham CL, Puddicombe D, Hlynsky J: Hypomagnesemia during refeeding in anorexia nervosa. Eat Weight Disord 2004; 9:236–237 [C]

74. Birmingham CL, Alothman AF, Goldner EM: Anorexia nervosa: refeeding and hypophosphatemia. Int J Eat Disord 1996; 20:211–213 [G]
75. Boag F, Weerakoon J, Ginsburg J, Havard CW, Dandona P: Diminished creatinine clearance in anorexia nervosa: reversal with weight gain. J Clin Pathol 1985; 38:60–63 [C]
76. Duncan A, Phillips IJ: Evaluation of thin-layer chromatography methods for laxative detection. Ann Clin Biochem 2001; 38:64–66 [G]
77. Turner J, Batik M, Palmer LJ, Forbes D, McDermott BM: Detection and importance of laxative use in adolescents with anorexia nervosa. J Am Acad Child Adolesc Psychiatry 2000; 39:378–385 [G]
78. Wildman P, Lilenfeld LR, Marcus MD: Axis I comorbidity onset and parasuicide in women with eating disorders. Int J Eat Disord 2004; 35:190–197 [D]
79. Casper RC, Hedeker D, McClough JF: Personality dimensions in eating disorders and their relevance for subtyping. J Am Acad Child Adolesc Psychiatry 1992; 31:830–840 [D]
80. Hudson JI, Hudson RA, Pope HG Jr: Psychiatric comorbidity and eating disorders, in AED Review of Eating Disorders, Part 1. Edited by Wonderlich S, Mitchell J, de Zwann M, Steiger H. Oxford, UK, Radcliffe, 2005 [G]
81. Thompson-Brenner H, Westen D: A naturalistic study of psychotherapy for bulimia nervosa, part 1: comorbidity and treatment outcomes. J Nerv Ment Dis 2005; 193:573–584 [G]
82. Kaye WH, Bulik CM, Thornton L, Barbarich N, Masters K: Comorbidity of anxiety disorders with anorexia and bulimia nervosa. Am J Psychiatry 2004; 161:2215–2221 [C]
83. Levitt JL, Sansone RA, Cohn L: Self-Harm Behavior and Eating Disorders: Dynamics, Assessment and Treatment. New York, Brunner-Routledge, 2004 [G]
84. American Psychiatric Association: Practice guideline for the assessment and treatment of patients with suicidal behaviors. Am J Psychiatry 2003; 160(11 suppl):1–60 [G]
85. Dare C, Eisler I, Russell G, Treasure J, Dodge L: Psychological therapies for adults with anorexia nervosa: randomised controlled trial of out-patient treatments. Br J Psychiatry 2001; 178:216–221 [A–]
86. Eisler I, Dare C, Hodes M, Russell G, Dodge E, Le GD: Family therapy for adolescent anorexia nervosa: the results of a controlled comparison of two family interventions. J Child Psychol Psychiatry 2000; 41:727–736 [A–]
87. Lock J: Treating adolescents with eating disorders in the family context: empirical and theoretical considerations. Child Adolesc Psychiatr Clin N Am 2002; 11:331–342 [G]
88. Gorin AA, Le GD, Stone AA: Effectiveness of spouse involvement in cognitive behavioral therapy for binge eating disorder. Int J Eat Disord 2003; 33:421–433 [A–]
89. le Grange D, Lock J, Dymek M: Family-based therapy for adolescents with bulimia nervosa. Am J Psychother 2003; 57:237–251 [G]
89a. Minuchin S, Rosman BL, Baker L: Psychosomatic Families: Anorexia Nervosa in Context. Cambridge, MA, Harvard University Press, 1978 [G]
90. Michel DM, Willard SG: An overview of family evaluation and therapy for anorexia nervosa, bulimia nervosa, and binge eating disorder, in Clinical Handbook of Eating Disorders: An Integrated Approach. Edited by Brewerton TD. New York, Marcel Dekker, 2004, pp 425–448 [G]
91. Bussolotti D, Fernandez-Aranda F, Solano R, Jimenez-Murcia S, Turon V, Vallejo J: Marital status and eating disorders: an analysis of its relevance. J Psychosom Res 2002; 53:1139–1145 [C]
92. Lock J, Le Grande D, Agras WS, Dare C: Treatment Manual for Anorexia Nervosa: A Family Based Approach. New York, Guilford, 2002 [G]
93. le Grange D, Binford R, Loeb KL: Manualized family-based treatment for anorexia nervosa: a case series. J Am Acad Child Adolesc Psychiatry 2005; 44:41–46 [G]
94. Golden NH, Jacobson MS, Schebendach J, Solanto MV, Hertz SM, Shenker IR: Resumption of menses in anorexia nervosa. Arch Pediatr Adolesc Med 1997; 151:16–21 [C]

95. Frisch RE, McArthur JW: Difference between postpartum and nutritional amenorrhea. Science 1979; 203:921–923 [F]
96. Frisch RE, McArthur JW: Menstrual cycles: fatness as a determinant of minimum weight for height necessary for their maintenance or onset. Science 1974; 185:949–951 [F]
97. Katzman DK, Zipursky RB: Adolescents with anorexia nervosa: the impact of the disorder on bones and brains. Ann N Y Acad Sci 1997; 817:127–137 [F]
98. Katzman DK, Zipursky RB, Lambe EK, Mikulis DJ: A longitudinal magnetic resonance imaging study of brain changes in adolescents with anorexia nervosa. Arch Pediatr Adolesc Med 1997; 151:793–797 [C]
99. Lambe EK, Katzman DK, Mikulis DJ, Kennedy SH, Zipursky RB: Cerebral gray matter volume deficits after weight recovery from anorexia nervosa. Arch Gen Psychiatry 1997; 54:537–542 [C]
100. La Via M, Kaye WH, Andersen A, Bowers W, Brandt HA, Brewerton TD, Costin C, Hill L, Lilenfeld L, McGilley B, Powers PS, Pryor T, Yager J, Zucker ML: Anorexia nervosa: criteria for levels of care. Paper presented at the annual meeting of the Eating Disorders Research Society, Cambridge, Mass, November 5–7, 1998 [G]
101. Olmsted MP, Kaplan AS, Rockert W: Relative efficacy of a 4-day versus a 5-day day hospital program. Int J Eat Disord 2003; 34:441–449 [C]
102. Appelbaum PS, Rumpf T: Civil commitment of the anorexic patient. Gen Hosp Psychiatry 1998; 20:225–230 [G]
103. Watson TL, Bowers WA, Andersen AE: Involuntary treatment of eating disorders. Am J Psychiatry 2000; 157:1806–1810 [D]
104. Maxmen JS, Siberfarb PM, Ferrell RB: Anorexia nervosa: practical initial management in a general hospital. JAMA 1974; 229:801–803 [G]
105. Palmer RL, Treasure J: Providing specialised services for anorexia nervosa. Br J Psychiatry 1999; 175:306–309 [D]
106. Kaye WH, Kaplan AS, Zucker ML: Treating eating-disorder patients in a managed care environment: contemporary American issues and Canadian response. Psychiatr Clin North Am 1996; 19:793–810 [F]
107. Kaplan AS, Olmsted MP: Partial hospitalization, in Handbook of Treatment for Eating Disorders, 2nd ed. Edited by Garner DM, Garfinkel PE. New York, Guilford, 1997, pp 354–360 [G]
108. Andersen AE: Practical Comprehensive Treatment of Anorexia Nervosa and Bulimia. Baltimore, Johns Hopkins University Press, 1985 [G]
109. Owen W, Halmi KA: Medical evaluation and management of anorexia nervosa, in Treatment of Psychiatric Disorders: A Task Force Report of the American Psychiatric Association, vol. 1. Washington, DC, American Psychiatric Association, 1989, pp 517–519 [G]
110. Golden NH, Meyer W: Nutritional rehabilitation of anorexia nervosa: goals and dangers. Int J Adolesc Med Health 2004; 16:131–144 [F]
111. Kaye WH, Gwirtsman HE, Obarzanek E, George DT: Relative importance of calorie intake needed to gain weight and level of physical activity in anorexia nervosa. Am J Clin Nutr 1988; 47:989–994 [C]
112. Reiff DW, Reiff KKL: Set Point in Eating Disorders: Nutrition Therapy in the Recovery Process. Gaithersburg, MD, Aspen, 1992 [G]
113. Guarda AS, Heinberg LJ: Effective weight gain in step down partial hospitalization program for eating disorders. Paper presented at the annual meeting of the Academy for Eating Disorders, San Diego, June 11–12, 1999 [G]
114. Okamoto A, Yamashita T, Nagoshi Y, Masui Y, Wada Y, Kashima A, Arii I, Nakamura M, Fukui K: A behavior therapy program combined with liquid nutrition designed for anorexia nervosa. Psychiatry Clin Neurosci 2002; 56:515–520 [A]

115. Piran N, Kaplan AS: A Day Hospital Group Treatment Program for Anorexia Nervosa and Bulimia Nervosa. Brunner/Mazel Eating Disorders Monograph Series, No. 3. New York, Brunner-Routledge, 1990 [G]
116. Hsu LK: Eating Disorders. New York, Guilford Press, 1990 [G]
117. Miller SP, Redlich AD, Steiner H: The stress response in anorexia nervosa. Child Psychiatry Hum Dev 2003; 33:295–306 [D]
118. Kohn MR, Golden NH, Shenker IR: Cardiac arrest and delirium: presentations of the refeeding syndrome in severely malnourished adolescents with anorexia nervosa. J Adolesc Health 1998; 22:239–243 [G]
119. Solomon SM, Kirby DF: The refeeding syndrome: a review. JPEN J Parenter Enteral Nutr 1990; 14:90–97 [F]
120. Ornstein RM, Golden NH, Jacobson MS, Shenker IR: Hypophosphatemia during nutritional rehabilitation in anorexia nervosa: implications for refeeding and monitoring. J Adolesc Health 2003; 32:83–88 [G]
121. Robb AS, Silber TJ, Orrell-Valente JK, Valadez-Meltzer A, Ellis N, Dadson MJ, Chatoor I: Supplemental nocturnal nasogastric refeeding for better short-term outcome in hospitalized adolescent girls with anorexia nervosa. Am J Psychiatry 2002; 159:1347–1353 [B]
122. Beumont P, Carney T: Can psychiatric terminology be translated into legal regulation? the anorexia nervosa example. Aust N Z J Psychiatry 2004; 38:819–829 [G]
123. Russell GF: Involuntary treatment in anorexia nervosa. Psychiatr Clin North Am 2001; 24:337–349 [G]
124. Goldner E: Treatment refusal in anorexia nervosa. Int J Eat Disord 1989; 8:297–306 [F]
125. Strober M: Managing the chronic, treatment-resistant patient with anorexia nervosa. Int J Eat Disord 2004; 36:245–255 [G]
126. Robin AL, Siegel PT, Moye AW, Gilroy M, Dennis AB, Sikand A: A controlled comparison of family versus individual therapy for adolescents with anorexia nervosa. J Am Acad Child Adolesc Psychiatry 1999; 38:1482–1489 [A–]
127. Danziger Y, Carel CA, Tyano S, Mimouni M: Is psychotherapy mandatory during the acute refeeding period in the treatment of anorexia nervosa? J Adolesc Health Care 1989; 10:328–331 [B]
128. McDermott C, Agras WS, Crow SJ, Halmi K, Mitchell JE, Bryson S: Participant recruitment for an anorexia nervosa treatment study. Int J Eat Disord 2004; 35:33–41 [G]
129. Lock J, Agras WS, Bryson S, Kraemer HC: A comparison of short- and long-term family therapy for adolescent anorexia nervosa. J Am Acad Child Adolesc Psychiatry 2005; 44:632–639 [A–]
130. Geist R, Heinmaa M, Stephens D, Davis R, Katzman DK: Comparison of family therapy and family group psychoeducation in adolescents with anorexia nervosa. Can J Psychiatry 2000; 45:173–178 [A–]
131. Fennig S, Fennig S, Roe D: Physical recovery in anorexia nervosa: is this the sole purpose of a child and adolescent medical-psychiatric unit? Gen Hosp Psychiatry 2002; 24:87–92 [G]
132. Lowe B, Zipfel S, Buchholz C, Dupont Y, Reas DL, Herzog W: Long-term outcome of anorexia nervosa in a prospective 21-year follow-up study. Psychol Med 2001; 31:881–890 [C]
133. Steinhausen HC, Seidel R, Winkler MC: Evaluation of treatment and intermediate and long-term outcome of adolescent eating disorders. Psychol Med 2000; 30:1089–1098 [C]
134. Fassino S, Piero A, Levi M, Gramaglia C, Amianto F, Leombruni P, Abbate DG: Psychological treatment of eating disorders: a review of the literature. Panminerva Med 2004; 46:189–198 [F]
135. Gowers S, Bryant-Waugh R: Management of child and adolescent eating disorders: the current evidence base and future directions. J Child Psychol Psychiatry 2004; 45:63–83 [F]
136. Pike KM, Walsh BT, Vitousek K, Wilson GT, Bauer J: Cognitive behavior therapy in the posthospitalization treatment of anorexia nervosa. Am J Psychiatry 2003; 160:2046–2049 [A–]

137. Fernandez-Aranda F, Bel M, Jimenez S, Vinuales M, Turon J, Vallejo J: Outpatient group therapy for anorexia nervosa: a preliminary study. Eat Weight Disord 1998; 3:1–6 [B]
138. Walsh BT, Kaplan AS, Attia E, Carter J, Devlin MJ, Olmsted M, Pike KM, Woodside B, Parides M: Fluoxetine vs placebo to prevent relapse in anorexia nervosa: primary outcome of drug on time to relapse in 93 weight restored subjects. Paper presented at the 11th annual meeting of the Eating Disorders Research Society, Toronto, Canada, September 29–October 1, 2005 [A]
139. Garner DM: Individual psychotherapy for anorexia nervosa. J Psychiatr Res 1985; 19:423–433 [F]
140. Hall A, Crisp AH: Brief psychotherapy in the treatment of anorexia nervosa: outcome at one year. Br J Psychiatry 1987; 151:185–191 [A–]
141. Zerbe KJ: The Body Betrayed: Women, Eating Disorders, and Treatment. Washington, DC, American Psychiatric Press, 1993 [G]
142. Zerbe KJ: Whose body is it anyway? understanding and treating psychosomatic aspects of eating disorders. Bull Menninger Clin 1993; 57:161–177 [F]
143. Schwartz HJ: Bulimia: Psychoanalytic Treatment and Theory. Madison, CT, International Universities Press, 1990 [G]
144. Zerbe KJ, Marsh SR, Coyne L: Comorbidity in an inpatient eating disordered population: clinical characteristics and treatment implications. Psychiatr Hosp 1993; 24:3–8 [D]
145. Wilson CP, Mintz IL (eds): Psychosomatic Symptoms: Psychoanalytic Treatment of the Underlying Personality Disorder. Northvale, NJ, Jason Aronson, 1989 [F]
146. Brody S: The Development of Anorexia Nervosa: The Hunger Artists. Madison, CT, International Universities Press, 2002 [F]
147. Bloom C, Gitter A, Gutwill S: Eating Problems: A Feminist Psychoanalytic Treatment Model. New York, Basic Books, 1994 [G]
148. Dare C, Crowther C: Living dangerously: psychoanalytic psychotherapy of anorexia nervosa, in Handbook of Eating Disorders: Theory, Treatment, and Research. Edited by Szmukler G, Dare C, Treasure J. London, Wiley, 1995, pp 293–308 [G]
149. Bruch H, Czyewski DSM: Conversations With Anorexics. New York, Basic Books, 1988 [G]
150. Crisp AH: Anorexia: Let Me Be. East Sussex, UK, Lawrence Erlbaum Associates, 1995 [G]
151. Reindl SM: Sensing the Self: Women's Recovery From Bulimia. Cambridge, MA, Harvard University Press, 2001 [F]
152. Steiner H: Defense styles in eating disorders. Int J Eat Disord 1990; 9:141–151 [D]
153. Thompson-Brenner H, Westen D: A naturalistic study of psychotherapy for bulimia nervosa, part 2: therapeutic interventions and outcome in the community. J Nerv Ment Dis 2005; 193:585–595 [G]
154. Russell GF, Szmukler GI, Dare C, Eisler I: An evaluation of family therapy in anorexia nervosa and bulimia nervosa. Arch Gen Psychiatry 1987; 44:1047–1056 [A]
155. Eisler I, Dare C, Russell GF, Szmukler G, le Grange D, Dodge E: Family and individual therapy in anorexia nervosa: a 5-year follow-up. Arch Gen Psychiatry 1997; 54:1025–1030 [B]
156. Zerbe KJ: Knowable secrets: transference and countertransference manifestations in eating disordered patients, in Treating Eating Disorders: Ethical, Legal, and Personal Issues. Edited by Vandereycken W, Beumont PJV. New York, New York University Press, 1998, pp 30–55 [G]
157. Zunino N, Agoos E, Davis WN: The impact of therapist gender on the treatment of bulimic women. Int J Eat Disord 1991; 10:253–263 [E]
158. Zerbe KJ: Integrating feminist and psychodynamic principles in the treatment of an eating disorder patient: implications for using countertransference responses. Bull Menninger Clin 1995; 59:160–176 [G]
159. Yager J: Management of patients with intractable eating disorders, in Eating Disorders and Obesity: A Comprehensive Handbook, 2nd ed. Edited by Fairburn CG, Brownell KD. New York, Guilford, 2002, pp 345–349 [G]

160. Andersen AE, Corson PW: Characteristics of an ideal psychotherapist for eating-disordered patients. Psychiatr Clin North Am 2001; 24:351–358, xii [G]
161. Betan E, Heim AK, Zittel CC, Westen D: Countertransference phenomena and personality pathology in clinical practice: an empirical investigation. Am J Psychiatry 2005; 162:890–898 [G]
162. Bradley R, Heim AK, Westen D: Transference patterns in the psychotherapy of personality disorders: empirical investigation. Br J Psychiatry 2005; 186:342–349 [C]
163. Steinhausen HC: The outcome of anorexia nervosa in the 20th century. Am J Psychiatry 2002; 159:1284–1293 [E]
164. Katzman MA, Waller G: Implications of therapist gender in the treatment of eating disorders: daring to ask the question, in The Burden of the Therapist. Edited by Vandereycken W. London, Athelone Press, 1998, pp 56–79 [G]
165. Waller G, Katzman MA: Female or male therapist for women with eating disorders? a pilot study of expert opinions. Int J Eat Disord 1997; 22:111–114 [G]
166. Kaplan AS, Fallon P: Therapeutic boundaries in the treatment of patients with eating disorders. Paper presented at the 4th London International Conference on Eating Disorders, April 20–22, 1999 [G]
167. Johnson CL, Sansone RA: Integrating the twelve-step approach with traditional psychotherapy for the treatment of eating disorders. Int J Eat Disord 1993; 14:121–134 [G]
168. Yager J, Landsverk J, Edelstein CK: Help seeking and satisfaction with care in 641 women with eating disorders, I: patterns of utilization, attributed change, and perceived efficacy of treatment. J Nerv Ment Dis 1989; 177:632–637 [G]
169. Zerbe KJ: Feminist psychodynamic psychotherapy of eating disorders: theoretic integration informing clinical practice. Psychiatr Clin North Am 1996; 19:811–827 [F]
170. Dare C: The starving and the greedy. J Child Psychotherapy 1993; 19:3–22 [F]
171. Hornyak LM, Baker EK: Experiential Therapies for Eating Disorders. New York, Guilford Press, 1989 [G]
172. Breden AK: Occupational therapy and the treatment of eating disorders. Occupational Therapy in Health Care 1992; 8:49–68 [G]
173. Lim PY: Occupational therapy with eating disorders: a study on treatment approaches. Br J Occupational Therapy 1994; 57:309–314 [G]
174. Attia E, Haiman C, Walsh BT, Flater SR: Does fluoxetine augment the inpatient treatment of anorexia nervosa? Am J Psychiatry 1998; 155:548–551 [A]
175. Strober M, Pataki C, Freeman R, DeAntonio M: No effect of adjunctive fluoxetine on eating behavior or weight phobia during the inpatient treatment of anorexia nervosa: an historical case-control study. J Child Adolesc Psychopharmacol 1999; 9:195–201 [D]
176. Fassino S, Leombruni P, Daga G, Brustolin A, Migliaretti G, Cavallo F, Rovera G: Efficacy of citalopram in anorexia nervosa: a pilot study. Eur Neuropsychopharmacol 2002; 12:453–459 [A–]
177. Kaye WH, Nagata T, Weltzin TE, Hsu LK, Sokol MS, McConaha C, Plotnicov KH, Weise J, Deep D: Double-blind placebo-controlled administration of fluoxetine in restricting- and restricting-purging-type anorexia nervosa. Biol Psychiatry 2001; 49:644–652 [A]
178. Delgado PL, Moreno FA, Onate L, Gelenberg AJ: Sequential catecholamine and serotonin depletion in mirtazapine-treated depressed patients. Int J Neuropsychopharmacol 2002; 5:63–66 [B]
179. Delgado PL, Miller HL, Salomon RM, Licinio J, Krystal JH, Moreno FA, Heninger GR, Charney DS: Tryptophan-depletion challenge in depressed patients treated with desipramine or fluoxetine: implications for the role of serotonin in the mechanism of antidepressant action. Biol Psychiatry 1999; 46:212–220 [B]
180. Medical Economics: 2005 Physicians' Desk Reference, 59th ed. Montvale, NJ, Thompson Healthcare, 2004 [G]

181. Horne RL, Ferguson JM, Pope HG Jr, Hudson JI, Lineberry CG, Ascher J, Cato A: Treatment of bulimia with bupropion: a multicenter controlled trial. J Clin Psychiatry 1988; 49:262–266 [A]
182. Demers JC, Malone M: Serotonin syndrome induced by fluvoxamine and mirtazapine. Ann Pharmacother 2001; 35:1217–1220 [G]
183. Brent DA: Antidepressants and pediatric depression: the risk of doing nothing. N Engl J Med 2004; 351:1598–1601 [G]
184. Newman TB: A black-box warning for antidepressants in children? N Engl J Med 2004; 351:1595–1598 [G]
185. Lock J, Walker LR, Rickert VI, Katzman DK: Suicidality in adolescents being treated with antidepressant medications and the black box label: position paper of the Society for Adolescent Medicine. J Adolesc Health 2005; 36:92–93 [G]
186. Katzman DK, Walker LR, Rickert VI, Lock J: The authors reply. J Adolesc Health 2005; 36:454–456 [G]
187. U.S. Food and Drug Administration: FDA launches a multi-pronged strategy to strengthen safeguards for children treatment with antidepressant medications, 2004. http://www.fda.gov/ bbs/topics/news/2004/NEW01124.html. Accessed November 11, 2004 [G]
188. Sarles RM: Joint meeting of the Psychopharmacologic Drugs Advisory Committee and the Pediatric Advisory Committee. Academy of Child and Adolescent Psychiatry, 2004. http://www.aacap.org/Announcements/AACAP_Comment.html [G]
189. American Psychiatric Association, American Academy of Child and Adolescent Psychiatry: Physicians Med Guide: the use of medication in treating child and adolescent depression: information for physicians. 2004. http://www.parentsmedguide.org/physiciansmedguide.htm#17 [G]
190. Barbarich NC, McConaha CW, Gaskill J, La VM, Frank GK, Achenbach S, Plotnicov KH, Kaye WH: An open trial of olanzapine in anorexia nervosa. J Clin Psychiatry 2004; 65:1480–1482 [B]
191. Malina A, Gaskill J, McConaha C, Frank GK, Lavia M, Scholar L, Kaye WH: Olanzapine treatment of anorexia nervosa: a retrospective study. Int J Eat Disord 2003; 33:234–237 [G]
192. Powers PS, Santana CA, Bannon YS: Olanzapine in the treatment of anorexia nervosa: an open label trial. Int J Eat Disord 2002; 32:146–154 [B]
193. Mehler C, Wewetzer C, Schulze U, Warnke A, Theisen F, Dittmann RW: Olanzapine in children and adolescents with chronic anorexia nervosa: a study of five cases. Eur Child Adolesc Psychiatry 2001; 10:151–157 [G]
194. Mondraty N, Birmingham CL, Touyz S, Sundakov V, Chapman L, Beumont P: Randomized controlled trial of olanzapine in the treatment of cognitions in anorexia nervosa. Australas Psychiatry 2005; 13:72–75 [A]
195. Kaye WH: Atypicals in the treatment of anorexia nervosa. Paper presented at the Broadening the Horizon of Atypical Antipsychotic Applications symposium, New York, 2004. http://www.medscape.com/viewprogram/3137 [G]
196. Bosanac P, Norman T, Burrows G, Beumont P: Serotonergic and dopaminergic systems in anorexia nervosa: a role for atypical antipsychotics? Aust N Z J Psychiatry 2005; 39:146–153 [F]
197. Powers PP: Quetiapine in the treatment of anorexia nervosa: a pilot study. Int J Eat Disord (in press) [B]
198. Cassano GB, Miniati M, Pini S, Rotondo A, Banti S, Borri C, Camilleri V, Mauri M: Six-month open trial of haloperidol as an adjunctive treatment for anorexia nervosa: a preliminary report. Int J Eat Disord 2003; 33:172–177 [B]
199. Garfinkel PE, Garner DM: Anorexia Nervosa: A Multidimensional Perspective. New York, Brunner/Mazel, 1982 [G]

200. Garfinkel PE, Garner DM: The Role of Drug Treatments for Eating Disorders. New York, Brunner/Mazel, 1987 [G]
201. Wells LA, Logan KM: Pharmacologic treatment of eating disorders: review of selected literature and recommendations. Psychosomatics 1987; 28:470–479 [F]
202. Robinson E, Bachrach LK, Katzman DK: Use of hormone replacement therapy to reduce the risk of osteopenia in adolescent girls with anorexia nervosa. J Adolesc Health 2000; 26:343–348 [G]
203. Golden NH, Lanzkowsky L, Schebendach J, Palestro CJ, Jacobson MS, Shenker IR: The effect of estrogen-progestin treatment on bone mineral density in anorexia nervosa. J Pediatr Adolesc Gynecol 2002; 15:135–143 [C]
204. Klibanski A, Biller BM, Schoenfeld DA, Herzog DB, Saxe VC: The effects of estrogen administration on trabecular bone loss in young women with anorexia nervosa. J Clin Endocrinol Metab 1995; 80:898–904 [B]
205. Emans SJ, Goldstein DP: Pediatric and Adolescent Gynecology, 3rd ed. Boston, Little, Brown, 1990 [G]
206. Odvina CV, Zerwekh JE, Rao DS, Maalouf N, Gottschalk FA, Pak CY: Severely suppressed bone turnover: a potential complication of alendronate therapy. J Clin Endocrinol Metab 2005; 90:1294–1301 [G]
207. Golden NH: Osteopenia and osteoporosis in anorexia nervosa. Adolesc Med 2003; 14:97–108 [G]
208. Laessle RG, Zoettle C, Pirke KM: Meta-analysis of treatment studies for bulimia. Int J Eat Disord 1987; 6:647–654 [E]
209. Anderson CB, Joyce PR, Carter FA, McIntosh VV, Bulik CM: The effect of cognitive-behavioral therapy for bulimia nervosa on temperament and character as measured by the temperament and character inventory. Compr Psychiatry 2002; 43:182–188 [G]
210. Bulik CM, Sullivan PF, Carter FA, McIntosh VV, Joyce PR: Predictors of rapid and sustained response to cognitive-behavioral therapy for bulimia nervosa. Int J Eat Disord 1999; 26:137–144 [G]
211. Mitchell JE, Halmi K, Wilson GT, Agras WS, Kraemer H, Crow S: A randomized secondary treatment study of women with bulimia nervosa who fail to respond to CBT. Int J Eat Disord 2002; 32:271–281 [A]
212. Agras WS, Walsh T, Fairburn CG, Wilson GT, Kraemer HC: A multicenter comparison of cognitive-behavioral therapy and interpersonal psychotherapy for bulimia nervosa. Arch Gen Psychiatry 2000; 57:459–466 [A–]
213. Rock CL, Curran-Celentano J: Nutritional management of eating disorders. Psychiatr Clin North Am 1996; 19:701–713 [G]
214. Thackwray DE, Smith MC, Bodfish JW, Meyers AW: A comparison of behavioral and cognitive-behavioral interventions for bulimia nervosa. J Consult Clin Psychol 1993; 61:639–645 [A–]
215. Westen D, Novotny CM, Thompson-Brenner H: The empirical status of empirically supported psychotherapies: assumptions, findings, and reporting in controlled clinical trials. Psychol Bull 2004; 130:631–663 [G]
216. Thompson-Brenner H, Glass S, Westen D: A multidimensional meta-analysis of psychotherapy for bulimia nervosa. Clinical Psychology: Science and Practice 2003; 10:269–287 [E]
217. Farrell E: Lost for Words: The Psychoanalysis of Anorexia and Bulimia. New York, Other Press, 2000 [G]
218. Petrucelli J, Stuart C: Hungers and Compulsions: The Psychodynamic Treatment of Eating Disorders and Addictions. Northvale, NJ, Jason Aronson, 2001 [G]
219. Zerbe KJ: The crucial role of psychodynamic understanding in the treatment of eating disorders. Psychiatr Clin North Am 2001; 24:305–313 [G]

220. Carter JC, Olmsted MP, Kaplan AS, McCabe RE, Mills JS, Aime A: Self-help for bulimia nervosa: a randomized controlled trial. Am J Psychiatry 2003; 160:973–978 [A–]
221. Schmidt U, Tiller J, Treasure J: Self-treatment of bulimia nervosa: a pilot study. Int J Eat Disord 1993; 13:273–277 [B]
222. Thiels C, Schmidt U, Treasure J, Garthe R, Troop N: Guided self-change for bulimia nervosa incorporating use of a self-care manual. Am J Psychiatry 1998; 155:947–953 [A–]
223. Rorty M, Yager J, Rossotto E: Why and how do women recover from bulimia nervosa? the subjective appraisals of forty women recovered for a year or more. Int J Eat Disord 1993; 14:249–260 [D]
224. Goldstein DJ, Wilson MG, Thompson VL, Potvin JH, Rampey AH Jr: Long-term fluoxetine treatment of bulimia nervosa: Fluoxetine Bulimia Nervosa Research Group. Br J Psychiatry 1995; 166:660–666 [A]
225. Kotler LA, Devlin MJ, Davies M, Walsh BT: An open trial of fluoxetine for adolescents with bulimia nervosa. J Child Adolesc Psychopharmacol 2003; 13:329–335 [G]
226. Romano SJ, Halmi KA, Sarkar NP, Koke SC, Lee JS: A placebo-controlled study of fluoxetine in continued treatment of bulimia nervosa after successful acute fluoxetine treatment. Am J Psychiatry 2002; 159:96–102 [A]
227. Milano W, Petrella C, Sabatino C, Capasso A: Treatment of bulimia nervosa with sertraline: a randomized controlled trial. Adv Ther 2004; 21:232–237 [A]
228. Mitchell JE, Peterson CB, Myers T, Wonderlich S: Combining pharmacotherapy and psychotherapy in the treatment of patients with eating disorders. Psychiatr Clin North Am 2001; 24:315–323 [F]
229. Pederson KJ, Roerig JL, Mitchell JE: Towards the pharmacotherapy of eating disorders. Expert Opin Pharmacother 2003; 4:1659–1678 [F]
230. Fluoxetine Bulimia Nervosa Collaborative Study Group: Fluoxetine in the treatment of bulimia nervosa: a multicenter, placebo-controlled, double-blind trial. Arch Gen Psychiatry 1992; 49:139–147 [A]
231. Bacaltchuk J, Hay P: Antidepressants versus placebo for people with bulimia nervosa. Cochrane Database Syst Rev 2003; CD003391 [E]
232. Raymond NC, Mitchell JE, Fallon P, Katzman MA: A collaborative approach to the use of medication, in Feminist Perspectives on Eating Disorders. Edited by Fallon P, Katzman MA, Wooley SC. New York, Guilford Press, 1994, pp 231–250 [G]
233. Pope HG Jr, Hudson JI, Jonas JM, Yurgelun-Todd D: Bulimia treated with imipramine: a placebo-controlled, double-blind study. Am J Psychiatry 1983; 140:554–558 [A]
234. Hughes PL, Wells LA, Cunningham CJ, Ilstrup DM: Treating bulimia with desipramine: a double-blind, placebo-controlled study. Arch Gen Psychiatry 1986; 43:182–186 [A]
235. Mitchell JE, Groat R: A placebo-controlled, double-blind trial of amitriptyline in bulimia. J Clin Psychopharmacol 1984; 4:186–193 [A]
236. Agras WS, Dorian B, Kirkley BG, Arnow B, Bachman J: Imipramine in the treatment of bulimia: a double-blind controlled study. Int J Eat Disord 1987; 6:29–38 [A]
237. Barlow J, Blouin J, Blouin A, Perez E: Treatment of bulimia with desipramine: a double-blind crossover study. Can J Psychiatry 1988; 33:129–133 [A]
238. Blouin AG, Blouin JH, Perez EL, Bushnik T, Zuro C, Mulder E: Treatment of bulimia with fenfluramine and desipramine. J Clin Psychopharmacol 1988; 8:261–269 [A]
239. Fallon BA, Walsh BT, Sadik C, Saoud JB, Lukasik V: Outcome and clinical course in inpatient bulimic women: a 2- to 9-year follow-up study. J Clin Psychiatry 1991; 52:272–278 [C]
240. Walsh BT, Hadigan CM, Devlin MJ, Gladis M, Roose SP: Long-term outcome of antidepressant treatment for bulimia nervosa. Am J Psychiatry 1991; 148:1206–1212 [A]
241. Hsu LK, Clement L, Santhouse R, Ju ES: Treatment of bulimia nervosa with lithium carbonate: a controlled study. J Nerv Ment Dis 1991; 179:351–355 [A]

242. Hedges DW, Reimherr FW, Hoopes SP, Rosenthal NR, Kamin M, Karim R, Capece JA: Treatment of bulimia nervosa with topiramate in a randomized, double-blind, placebo-controlled trial, part 2: improvement in psychiatric measures. J Clin Psychiatry 2003; 64:1449–1454 [A]
243. Hoopes SP, Reimherr FW, Hedges DW, Rosenthal NR, Kamin M, Karim R, Capece JA, Karvois D: Treatment of bulimia nervosa with topiramate in a randomized, double-blind, placebo-controlled trial, part 1: improvement in binge and purge measures. J Clin Psychiatry 2003; 64:1335–1341 [A]
244. Findling RL, McNamara NK, Youngstrom EA, Stansbrey R, Gracious BL, Reed MD, Calabrese JR: Double-blind 18-month trial of lithium versus divalproex maintenance treatment in pediatric bipolar disorder. J Am Acad Child Adolesc Psychiatry 2005; 44:409–417 [A]
245. Rana M, Khanzode L, Karnik N, Saxena K, Chang K, Steiner H: Divalproex sodium in the treatment of pediatric psychiatric disorders. Expert Rev Neurother 2005; 5:165–176 [G]
246. French JA, Kanner AM, Bautista J, Abou-Khalil B, Browne T, Harden CL, Theodore WH, Bazil C, Stern J, Schachter SC, Bergen D, Hirtz D, Montouris GD, Nespeca M, Gidal B, Marks WJ Jr, Turk WR, Fischer JH, Bourgeois B, Wilner A, Faught RE Jr, Sachdeo RC, Beydoun A, Glauser TA: Efficacy and tolerability of the new antiepileptic drugs, I: treatment of new onset epilepsy. Report of the Therapeutics and Technology Assessment Subcommittee and Quality Standards Subcommittee of the American Academy of Neurology and the American Epilepsy Society. Neurology 2004; 62:1252–1260 [G]
247. Drimmer EJ: Stimulant treatment of bulimia nervosa with and without attention-deficit disorder: three case reports. Nutrition 2003; 19:76–77 [G]
248. Schweickert LA, Strober M, Moskowitz A: Efficacy of methylphenidate in bulimia nervosa comorbid with attention-deficit hyperactivity disorder: a case report. Int J Eat Disord 1997; 21:299–301 [G]
249. Sokol MS, Gray NS, Goldstein A, Kaye WH: Methylphenidate treatment for bulimia nervosa associated with a cluster B personality disorder. Int J Eat Disord 1999; 25:233–237 [G]
250. Walsh BT, Agras WS, Devlin MJ, Fairburn CG, Wilson GT, Kahn C, Chally MK: Fluoxetine for bulimia nervosa following poor response to psychotherapy. Am J Psychiatry 2000; 157:1332–1334 [A]
251. Walsh BT, Wilson GT, Loeb KL, Devlin MJ, Pike KM, Roose SP, Fleiss J, Waternaux C: Medication and psychotherapy in the treatment of bulimia nervosa. Am J Psychiatry 1997; 154:523–531 [G]
252. Agras WS: Pharmacotherapy of bulimia nervosa and binge eating disorder: longer-term outcomes. Psychopharmacol Bull 1997; 33:433–436 [F]
253. Mitchell JE, Pyle RL, Eckert ED, Hatsukami D, Pomeroy C, Zimmerman R: A comparison study of antidepressants and structured intensive group psychotherapy in the treatment of bulimia nervosa. Arch Gen Psychiatry 1990; 47:149–157 [A–]
254. Agras WS, Rossiter EM, Arnow B, Schneider JA, Telch CF, Raeburn SD, Bruce B, Perl M, Koran LM: Pharmacologic and cognitive-behavioral treatment for bulimia nervosa: a controlled comparison. Am J Psychiatry 1992; 149:82–87 [A–]
255. Goldbloom DS, Olmsted M, Davis R, Clewes J, Heinmaa M, Rockert W, Shaw B: A randomized controlled trial of fluoxetine and cognitive behavioral therapy for bulimia nervosa: short-term outcome. Behav Res Ther 1997; 35:803–811 [A–]
256. Nakash-Eisikovits O, Dierberger A, Westen D: A multidimensional meta-analysis of pharmacotherapy for bulimia nervosa: summarizing the range of outcomes in controlled clinical trials. Harv Rev Psychiatry 2002; 10:193–211 [E]

257. Braun DL, Sunday SR, Fornari VM, Halmi KA: Bright light therapy decreases winter binge frequency in women with bulimia nervosa: a double-blind, placebo-controlled study. Compr Psychiatry 1999; 40:442–448 [A]
258. Blouin AG, Blouin JH, Iversen H, Carter J, Goldstein C, Goldfield G, Perez E: Light therapy in bulimia nervosa: a double-blind, placebo-controlled study. Psychiatry Res 1996; 60:1–9 [A]
259. Lam RW, Goldner EM, Solyom L, Remick RA: A controlled study of light therapy for bulimia nervosa. Am J Psychiatry 1994; 151:744–750 [B]
260. Hausmann A, Mangweth B, Walpoth M, Hoertnagel C, Kramer-Reinstadler K, Rupp CI, Hinterhuber H: Repetitive transcranial magnetic stimulation (rTMS) in the double-blind treatment of a depressed patient suffering from bulimia nervosa: a case report. Int J Neuropsychopharmacol 2004; 7:371–373 [G]
261. Brewerton TD, Nihad Z, Malloy M, Risch SC, George MS: Transcranial magnetic stimulation (TMS) in a woman with major depression and bulimia nervosa. Eighth Annual New York International Conference on Eating Disorders. New York, April 24–26, Abstract #195, 1998 [G]
262. Norring C, Palmer RL: EDNOS: Eating Disorders Not Otherwise Specified. Scientific and Clinical Perspectives on the Other Eating Disorders. New York, Brunner-Routledge, 2005 [G]
263. Fairburn CG, Bohn K: Eating disorder NOS (EDNOS): an example of the troublesome "not otherwise specified" (NOS) category in DSM-IV. Behav Res Ther 2005; 43:691–701 [G]
264. Roerig JL, Mitchell JE, de Zwaan M, Wonderlich SA, Kamran S, Engbloom S, Burgard M, Lancaster K: The eating disorders medicine cabinet revisited: a clinician's guide to appetite suppressants and diuretics. Int J Eat Disord 2003; 33:443–457 [G]
265. Willard SG, McDermott BE, Woodhouse LM: Lipoplasty in the bulimic patient. Plast Reconstr Surg 1996; 98:276–278 [G]
266. Segal A, Kinoshita KD, Larino MA: Post-surgical refusal to eat: anorexia nervosa, bulimia nervosa or a new eating disorder? a case series. Obes Surg 2004; 14:353–360 [G]
267. Herzog DB, Hopkins JD, Burns CD: A follow-up study of 33 subdiagnostic eating disordered women. Int J Eat Disord 1993; 14:261–267 [C]
268. Wonderlich SA, de Zwaan M, Mitchell JE, Peterson C, Crow S: Psychological and dietary treatments of binge eating disorder: conceptual implications. Int J Eat Disord 2003; 34(suppl):S58-S73 [F]
269. Grilo CM: Treatment of obesity: an integrative model, in Body Image, Eating Disorders, and Obesity: An Integrative Guide for Assessment and Treatment. Edited by Thompson JK. Washington, DC, American Psychological Association, 1996, pp 389–424 [G]
270. Marcus MD: Obese patients with binge-eating disorder, in The Management of Eating Disorders and Obesity. Edited by Goldstein DJ. Totowa, NJ, Humana Press, 1999, pp 125–138 [G]
271. Agras WS, Telch CF, Arnow B, Eldredge K, Marnell M: One-year follow-up of cognitive-behavioral therapy for obese individuals with binge eating disorder. J Consult Clin Psychol 1997; 65:343–347 [C]
272. Wilfley DE, Welch RR, Stein RI, Spurrell EB, Cohen LR, Saelens BE, Dounchis JZ, Frank MA, Wiseman CV, Matt GE: A randomized comparison of group cognitive-behavioral therapy and group interpersonal psychotherapy for the treatment of overweight individuals with binge-eating disorder. Arch Gen Psychiatry 2002; 59:713–721 [B]
273. Carter JC, Fairburn CG: Cognitive-behavioral self-help for binge eating disorder: a controlled effectiveness study. J Consult Clin Psychol 1998; 66:616–623 [A–]
274. Ghaderi A, Scott B: Pure and guided self-help for full and sub-threshold bulimia nervosa and binge eating disorder. Br J Clin Psychol 2003; 42:257–269 [B]
275. Loeb KL, Wilson GT, Gilbert JS, Labouvie E: Guided and unguided self-help for binge eating. Behav Res Ther 2000; 38:259–272 [B]

276. Peterson CB, Mitchell JE, Engbloom S, Nugent S, Mussell MP, Miller JP: Group cognitive-behavioral treatment of binge eating disorder: a comparison of therapist-led versus self-help formats. Int J Eat Disord 1998; 24:125–136 [B]
277. Grilo CM, Masheb RM: A randomized controlled comparison of guided self-help cognitive behavioral therapy and behavioral weight loss for binge eating disorder. Behav Res Ther 2005; 43:1509–1525 [A–]
278. Polivy J, Herman CP: Dieting and binging: a causal analysis. Am Psychol 1985; 40:193–201 [F]
279. Keys A, Brozek J, Henschel A, Mickelsen O, Taylor HL: The Biology of Human Starvation. Minneapolis, University of Minnesota Press, 1950 [G]
280. Carrier KM, Steinhardt MA, Bowman S: Rethinking traditional weight management programs: a 3-year follow-up evaluation of a new approach. J Psychol 1993; 128:517–535 [D]
281. Ciliska D: Beyond Dieting: Psychoeducational Interventions for Chronically Obese Women. New York, Brunner/Mazel, 1990 [G]
282. Kaplan AS, Ciliska D: The relationship between eating disorders and obesity: psychopathologic and treatment considerations. Psychiatr Ann 1999; 29:197–202 [B]
283. Stice E, Presnell K, Spangler D: Risk factors for binge eating onset in adolescent girls: a 2-year prospective investigation. Health Psychol 2002; 21:131–138 [C]
284. Appolinario JC, Bacaltchuk J, Sichieri R, Claudino AM, Godoy-Matos A, Morgan C, Zanella MT, Coutinho W: A randomized, double-blind, placebo-controlled study of sibutramine in the treatment of binge-eating disorder. Arch Gen Psychiatry 2003; 60:1109–1116 [A]
285. Jordan J, Scholze J, Matiba B, Wirth A, Hauner H, Sharma AM: Influence of sibutramine on blood pressure: evidence from placebo-controlled trials. Int J Obes (Lond) 2005; 29:509–516 [E]
286. McElroy SL, Arnold LM, Shapira NA, Keck PE Jr, Rosenthal NR, Karim MR, Kamin M, Hudson JI: Topiramate in the treatment of binge eating disorder associated with obesity: a randomized, placebo-controlled trial. Am J Psychiatry 2003; 160:255–261 [A]
287. McElroy SL, Shapira NA, Arnold LM, Keck PE, Rosenthal NR, Wu SC, Capece JA, Fazzio L, Hudson JI: Topiramate in the long-term treatment of binge-eating disorder associated with obesity. J Clin Psychiatry 2004; 65:1463–1469 [B]
288. McElroy SL, Kotwal R, Hudson JI, Nelson EB, Keck PE: Zonisamide in the treatment of binge-eating disorder: an open-label, prospective trial. J Clin Psychiatry 2004; 65:50–56 [B]
289. Stunkard A, Berkowitz R, Tanrikut C, Reiss E, Young L: D-Fenfluramine treatment of binge eating disorder. Am J Psychiatry 1996; 153:1455–1459 [A]
290. Agras WS, Telch CF, Arnow B, Eldredge K, Wilfley DE, Raeburn SD, Henderson S, Marnell M: Weight loss cognitive-behavioral and desipramine treatments in binge-eating disorder: an addictive design. Behav Ther 1994; 25:225–238 [A–]
291. Marcus MD, Wing RR, Ewing L, Kern E, McDermott M, Gooding W: A double-blind, placebo-controlled trial of fluoxetine plus behavior modification in the treatment of obese binge-eaters and non-binge-eaters. Am J Psychiatry 1990; 147:876–881 [A]
292. Laederach-Hofmann K, Graf C, Horber F, Lippuner K, Lederer S, Michel R, Schneider M: Imipramine and diet counseling with psychological support in the treatment of obese binge eaters: a randomized, placebo-controlled double-blind study. Int J Eat Disord 1999; 26:231–244 [A]
293. Grilo CM, Masheb RM, Wilson GT: Efficacy of cognitive behavioral therapy and fluoxetine for the treatment of binge eating disorder: a randomized double-blind placebo-controlled comparison. Biol Psychiatry 2005; 57:301–309 [A]
294. Devlin MJ, Goldfein JA, Petkova E, Jiang H, Raizman PS, Wolk S, Mayer L, Carino J, Bellace D, Kamenetz C, Dobrow I, Walsh BT: Cognitive behavioral therapy and fluoxetine as adjuncts to group behavioral therapy for binge eating disorder. Obes Res 2005; 13:1077–1088 [A]

295. Grilo CM, Masheb RM, Salant SL: Cognitive behavioral therapy guided self-help and orlistat for the treatment of binge eating disorder: a randomized, double-blind, placebo-controlled trial. Biol Psychiatry 2005; 57:1193–1201 [A]
296. de Zwaan J, Burgard MA, Schenck CH, Mitchell JE: Night time eating: a review of the literature. Eur Eating Disorders Rev 2003; 11:7–24 [F]
297. Stunkard AJ, Grace WJ, Wolff HG: The night-eating syndrome: a pattern of food intake among certain obese patients. Am J Med 1955; 19:78–86 [G]
298. Lu ML, Shen WW: Sleep-related eating disorder induced by risperidone. J Clin Psychiatry 2004; 65:273–274 [G]
299. Khazaal Y, Krenz S, Zullino DF: Bupropion-induced somnambulism. Addict Biol 2003; 8:359–362 [G]
300. Paquet V, Strul J, Servais L, Pelc I, Fossion P: Sleep-related eating disorder induced by olanzapine. J Clin Psychiatry 2002; 63:597 [G]
301. Pawlow LA, O'Neil PM, Malcolm RJ: Night eating syndrome: effects of brief relaxation training on stress, mood, hunger, and eating patterns. Int J Obes Relat Metab Disord 2003; 27:970–978 [A–]
302. O'Reardon JP, Stunkard AJ, Allison KC: Clinical trial of sertraline in the treatment of night eating syndrome. Int J Eat Disord 2004; 35:16–26 [B]
303. O'Reardon J, Allison K, Martino N, Stunkard A: A randomized, placebo-controlled trial of sertraline in the treatment of night eating syndrome. Obes Res 2004; 12:A64 [A]
304. Yager J: Patients with chronic, recalcitrant eating disorders, in Special Problems in Managing Eating Disorders. Edited by Yager J, Gwirtsman HE, Edelstein CK. Washington, DC, American Psychiatric Press, 1992, pp 205–231 [G]
305. Kerr A, Lesaca M, Kaplan AS: Continuing care groups for chronic anorexia nervosa, in Group Psychotherapy for Eating Disorders. Edited by Harper-Giuffre H, MacKenzie KR. Washington, DC, American Psychiatric Press, 1992, pp 261–272 [G]
306. Maine M, Kelly J: The Body Myth: Adult Women and the Pressure To Be Perfect. Hoboken, NJ, Wiley, 2005 [G]
307. Tanofsky MB, Wilfley DE, Spurrell EB, Welch R, Brownell KD: Comparison of men and women with binge eating disorder. Int J Eat Disord 1997; 21:49–54 [C]
308. Bulik CM, Klump KL, Thornton L, Kaplan AS, Devlin B, Fichter MM, Halmi KA, Strober M, Woodside DB, Crow S, Mitchell JE, Rotondo A, Mauri M, Cassano GB, Keel PK, Berrettini WH, Kaye WH: Alcohol use disorder comorbidity in eating disorders: a multicenter study. J Clin Psychiatry 2004; 65:1000–1006 [C]
309. Holderness CC, Brooks-Gunn J, Warren MP: Co-morbidity of eating disorders and substance abuse: review of the literature. Int J Eat Disord 1994; 16:1–34 [F]
310. Herzog DB, Keller MB, Sacks NR, Yeh CJ, Lavori PW: Psychiatric comorbidity in treatment-seeking anorexics and bulimics. J Am Acad Child Adolesc Psychiatry 1992; 31:810–818 [D]
311. Bulik CM, Sullivan P, Epstein L, McKee M, Kaye W, Dahl R, Weltzin T: Drug use in women with anorexia and bulimia nervosa. Int J Eat Disord 1992; 11:214–225 [D]
312. Bulik CM, Sullivan PF, Fear JL, Pickering A, Dawn A, McCullin M: Fertility and reproduction in women with anorexia nervosa: a controlled study. J Clin Psychiatry 1999; 60:130–135 [B]
313. Wilfley DE, Friedman MA, Dounchis JZ, Stein RI, Welch RR, Ball SA: Comorbid psychopathology in binge eating disorder: relation to eating disorder severity at baseline and following treatment. J Consult Clin Psychol 2000; 68:641–649 [C]
314. Wonderlich SA, Mitchell JE: Eating disorders and comorbidity: empirical, conceptual, and clinical implications. Psychopharmacol Bull 1997; 33:381–390 [F]
315. Hatsukami D, Mitchell JE, Eckert ED, Pyle R: Characteristics of patients with bulimia only, bulimia with affective disorder, and bulimia with substance abuse problems. Addict Behav 1986; 11:399–406 [D]

316. Solano R, Aitken A, Lopez C, Vallejo J, Fernandez-Aranda F: Self-injurious behaviour in eating disorders. Eur Eating Disorders Rev 2005; 13:3–10 [D]
317. Dansky BS, Brewerton TD, Kilpatrick DG: Comorbidity of bulimia nervosa and alcohol use disorders: results from the National Women's Study. Int J Eat Disord 2000; 27:180–190 [G]
318. Collins S, King M: Ten-year follow-up of 50 patients with bulimia nervosa. Br J Psychiatry 1994; 164:80–87 [C]
319. Mitchell JE, Pyle R, Eckert ED, Hatsukami D: The influence of prior alcohol and drug abuse problems on bulimia nervosa treatment outcome. Addict Behav 1990; 15:169–173 [D]
320. Strasser TJ, Pike KM, Walsh BT: The impact of prior substance abuse on treatment outcome for bulimia nervosa. Addict Behav 1992; 17:387–395 [C]
321. Keel PK, Dorer DJ, Eddy KT, Franko D, Charatan DL, Herzog DB: Predictors of mortality in eating disorders. Arch Gen Psychiatry 2003; 60:179–183 [C]
322. Westermeyer J, Specker S: Social resources and social function in comorbid eating and substance disorder: a matched-pairs study. Am J Addict 1999; 8:332–336 [D]
323. Halmi KA, Eckert E, Marchi P, Sampugnaro V, Apple R, Cohen J: Comorbidity of psychiatric diagnoses in anorexia nervosa. Arch Gen Psychiatry 1991; 48:712–718 [C]
324. Herzog DB, Nussbaum KM, Marmor AK: Comorbidity and outcome in eating disorders. Psychiatr Clin North Am 1996; 19:843–859 [F]
325. Hudson JI, Pope HG Jr, Jonas JM, Yurgelun-Todd D: Phenomenologic relationship of eating disorders to major affective disorder. Psychiatry Res 1983; 9:345–354 [D]
326. Cooper PJ: Eating disorders and their relationship to mood and anxiety disorders, in Eating Disorders and Obesity: A Comprehensive Handbook. Edited by Brownell KD, Fairburn CG. New York, Guilford, 1995, pp 159–164 [G]
327. Edelstein CK, Yager J: Eating disorders and affective disorders, in Special Problems in Managing Eating Disorders. Edited by Yager J, Gwirtsman HE, Edelstein CK. Washington, DC, American Psychiatric Press, 1992, pp 15–50 [G]
328. Cooper PJ, Fairburn CG: The depressive symptoms of bulimia nervosa. Br J Psychiatry 1986; 148:268–274 [G]
329. Keel PK, Mitchell JE: Outcome in bulimia nervosa. Am J Psychiatry 1997; 154:313–321 [F]
330. Godart NT, Flament MF, Curt F, Perdereau F, Lang F, Venisse JL, Halfon O, Bizouard P, Loas G, Corcos M, Jeammet P, Fermanian J: Anxiety disorders in subjects seeking treatment for eating disorders: a DSM-IV controlled study. Psychiatry Res 2003; 117:245–258 [D]
331. Braun DL, Sunday SR, Halmi KA: Psychiatric comorbidity in patients with eating disorders. Psychol Med 1994; 24:859–867 [C]
332. Dansky BS, Brewerton TD, Kilpatrick DG, O'Neil PM: The National Women's Study: relationship of victimization and posttraumatic stress disorder to bulimia nervosa. Int J Eat Disord 1997; 21:213–228 [D]
333. Brewerton TD: Eating disorders, victimization and comorbidity: principles of treatment, in Clinical Handbook of Eating Disorders: An Integrated Approach. Edited by Brewerton TD. New York, Marcel Dekker, 2004, pp 509–546 [G]
334. Telch CF, Stice E: Psychiatric comorbidity in women with binge eating disorder: prevalence rates from a non-treatment-seeking sample. J Consult Clin Psychol 1998; 66:768–776 [D]
335. Yanovski SZ, Nelson JE, Dubbert BK, Spitzer RL: Association of binge eating disorder and psychiatric comorbidity in obese subjects. Am J Psychiatry 1993; 150:1472–1479 [D]
336. Brody ML, Walsh BT, Devlin MJ: Binge eating disorder: reliability and validity of a new diagnostic category. J Consult Clin Psychol 1994; 62:381–386 [G]
337. Mussell MP, Mitchell JE, de Zwaan M, Crosby RD, Seim HC, Crow SJ: Clinical characteristics associated with binge eating in obese females: a descriptive study. Int J Obes Relat Metab Disord 1996; 20:324–331 [D]

338. Hudson JI, Pope HG Jr, Wurtman J, Yurgelun-Todd D, Mark S, Rosenthal NE: Bulimia in obese individuals: relationship to normal-weight bulimia. J Nerv Ment Dis 1988; 176:144–152 [D]
339. Marcus MD, Wing RR, Ewing L, Kern E, Gooding W, McDermott M: Psychiatric disorders among obese binge eaters. Int J Eat Disord 1990; 9:69–70 [D]
340. Bulik CM, Sullivan PF, Kendler KS: Medical and psychiatric morbidity in obese women with and without binge eating. Int J Eat Disord 2002; 32:72–78 [D]
341. Bulik CM, Sullivan PF, Fear JL, Joyce PR: Eating disorders and antecedent anxiety disorders: a controlled study. Acta Psychiatr Scand 1997; 96:101–107 [B]
342. Serpell L, Hirani V, Willoughby K, Neiderman M, Lask B: Personality or pathology? Obsessive-compulsive features in children and adolescents with anorexia nervosa [abstract]. Int J Eat Disord 2004; 35:425 [G]
343. Wonderlich SA, Crosby RD, Mitchell JE, Thompson KM, Redlin J, Demuth G, Smyth J, Haseltine B: Eating disturbance and sexual trauma in childhood and adulthood. Int J Eat Disord 2001; 30:401–412 [C]
344. Schoemaker C, Smit F, Bijl RV, Vollebergh WA: Bulimia nervosa following psychological and multiple child abuse: support for the self-medication hypothesis in a population-based cohort study. Int J Eat Disord 2002; 32:381–388 [C]
345. Dohm FA, Striegel-Moore RH, Wilfley DE, Pike KM, Hook J, Fairburn CG: Self-harm and substance use in a community sample of black and white women with binge eating disorder or bulimia nervosa. Int J Eat Disord 2002; 32:389–400 [C]
346. Wonderlich SA, Brewerton TD, Jocic Z, Dansky BS, Abbott DW: Relationship of childhood sexual abuse and eating disorders. J Am Acad Child Adolesc Psychiatry 1997; 36:1107–1115 [F]
347. Connors ME, Morse W: Sexual abuse and eating disorders: a review. Int J Eat Disord 1993; 13:1–11 [F]
348. Goldner EM, Srikameswaran S, Schroeder ML, Livesley WJ, Birmingham CL: Dimensional assessment of personality pathology in patients with eating disorders. Psychiatry Res 1999; 85:151–159 [D]
349. Grilo CM, Sanislow CA, Skodol AE, Gunderson JG, Stout RL, Shea MT, Zanarini MC, Bender DS, Morey LC, Dyck IR, McGlashan TH: Do eating disorders co-occur with personality disorders? comparison groups matter. Int J Eat Disord 2003; 33:155–164 [C]
350. Diaz-Marsa M, Carrasco JL, Saiz J: A study of temperament and personality in anorexia and bulimia nervosa. J Personal Disord 2000; 14:352–359 [D]
351. Casper RC, Troiani M: Family functioning in anorexia nervosa differs by subtype. Int J Eat Disord 2001; 30:338–342 [D]
352. Fahy TA, Eisler I, Russell GF: Personality disorder and treatment response in bulimia nervosa. Br J Psychiatry 1993; 162:765–770 [B]
353. Westen D, Thompson-Brenner H, Peart J: Personality and eating disorders, in Annual Review of Eating Disorders, Part 2. Edited by Wonderlich S, Mitchell J, de Zwaan M, Steiger H. Oxford, UK, Radcliffe (in press) [F]
354. Herzog DB, Keller MB, Lavori PW, Kenny GM, Sacks NR: The prevalence of personality disorders in 210 women with eating disorders. J Clin Psychiatry 1992; 53:147–152 [G]
355. Bulik CM, Sullivan PF, Joyce PR, Carter FA: Temperament, character, and personality disorder in bulimia nervosa. J Nerv Ment Dis 1995; 183:593–598 [B]
356. Johnson C, Tobin D, Enright A: Prevalence and clinical characteristics of borderline patients in an eating-disordered population. J Clin Psychiatry 1989; 50:9–15 [D]
357. Vitousek K, Manke F: Personality variables and disorders in anorexia nervosa and bulimia nervosa. J Abnorm Psychol 1994; 103:137–147 [G]
358. Wonderlich SA: Personality and eating disorders, in Eating Disorders and Obesity: A Comprehensive Textbook. Edited by Brownell KD, Fairburn CG. New York, Guilford, 1995, pp 171–176 [G]

359. Wonderlich SA, Mitchell JE: Eating disorders and personality disorders, in Special Problems in Managing Eating Disorders. Edited by Yager J, Gwirtsman HE, Edelstein CK. Washington, DC, American Psychiatric Press, 1992, pp 51–86 [G]
360. Wonderlich SA, Swift WJ: Borderline versus other personality disorders in the eating disorders: clinical description. Int J Eat Disord 1990; 9:629–638 [G]
361. Sansone RA, Levitt JL, Sansone LA: The prevalence of personality disorders among those with eating disorders. Eating Disorders: The Journal of Treatment and Prevention 2005; 13:7–21 [E]
362. Johnson C, Tobin DL, Dennis A: Differences in treatment outcome between borderline and non-borderline bulimics at one-year follow-up. Int J Eat Disord 1990; 9:617–627 [B]
363. Westen D, Harnden-Fischer J: Personality profiles in eating disorders: rethinking the distinction between axis I and axis II. Am J Psychiatry 2001; 158:547–562 [G]
364. Ames-Frankel J, Devlin MJ, Walsh BT, Strasser TJ, Sadik C, Oldham JM, Roose SP: Personality disorder diagnoses in patients with bulimia nervosa: clinical correlates and changes with treatment. J Clin Psychiatry 1992; 53:90–96 [C]
365. Thompson-Brenner H, Westen D: Personality subtypes in eating disorders: validation of a classification in a naturalistic sample. Br J Psychiatry 2005; 186:516–524 [G]
366. Affenito SG, Adams CH: Are eating disorders more prevalent in females with type 1 diabetes mellitus when the impact of insulin omission is considered? Nutr Rev 2001; 59:179–182 [C]
367. Herpertz S, Albus C, Wagener R, Kocnar M, Wagner R, Henning A, Best F, Foerster H, Schulze SB, Thomas W, Kohle K, Mann K, Senf W: Comorbidity of diabetes and eating disorders: does diabetes control reflect disturbed eating behavior? Diabetes Care 1998; 21:1110–1116 [C]
368. Crow SJ, Keel PK, Kendall D: Eating disorders and insulin-dependent diabetes mellitus. Psychosomatics 1998; 39:233–243 [F]
368a. Verrotti A, Catino M, De Luca FA, Morgese G, Chiarelli F: Eating disorders in adolescents with type 1 diabetes mellitus. Acta Diabetol 1999; 36:21–25 [F]
369. Rydall AC, Rodin GM, Olmsted MP, Devenyi RG, Daneman D: Disordered eating behavior and microvascular complications in young women with insulin-dependent diabetes mellitus. N Engl J Med 1997; 336:1849–1854 [C]
370. Nielsen S, Emborg C, Molbak AG: Mortality in concurrent type 1 diabetes and anorexia nervosa. Diabetes Care 2002; 25:309–312 [G]
371. Rodin G, Daneman D, DeGroot J: The interaction of chronic medical illness and eating disorders, in Medical Issues and the Eating Disorders: The Interface. Brunner/Mazel Eating Disorders Monograph Series, No. 7. Edited by Kaplan AS, Garfinkel PE. New York, Brunner/Mazel, 1993, pp 176–192 [G]
372. Yager J, Young RT: Eating disorders and diabetes mellitus, in Special Problems in Managing Eating Disorders. Edited by Yager J, Gwirtsman HE, Edelstein CK. Washington, DC, American Psychiatric Press, 1992, pp 185–203 [G]
373. Takii M, Uchigata Y, Komaki G, Nozaki T, Kawai H, Iwamoto Y, Kubo C: An integrated inpatient therapy for type 1 diabetic females with bulimia nervosa: a 3-year follow-up study. J Psychosom Res 2003; 55:349–356 [B]
374. Herpertz S, Albus C, Kielmann R, Hagemann-Patt H, Lichtblau K, Kohle K, Mann K, Senf W: Comorbidity of diabetes mellitus and eating disorders: a follow-up study. J Psychosom Res 2001; 51:673–678 [G]
375. Powers PS: Management of patients with comorbid medical conditions, in Handbook of Treatment for Eating Disorders. Edited by Garner DM, Garfinkel PE. New York, Guilford, 1997, pp 424–436 [G]
376. Brinch M, Isager T, Tolstrup K: Anorexia nervosa and motherhood: reproduction pattern and mothering behavior of 50 women. Acta Psychiatr Scand 1988; 77:611–617 [C]

377. Rand CWS, Willis DC, Koldau JM: Pregnancy after anorexia nervosa. Int J Eat Disord 1987; 6:671–674 [G]
378. Stewart DE, Raskin J, Garfinkel PE, MacDonald OL, Robinson GE: Anorexia nervosa, bulimia, and pregnancy. Am J Obstet Gynecol 1987; 157:1194–1198 [C]
379. Treasure JL, Russell GF: Intrauterine growth and neonatal weight gain in babies of women with anorexia nervosa. Br Med J (Clin Res Ed) 1988; 296:1038 [B]
380. Kouba S, Hallstrom T, Lindholm C, Hirschberg AL: Pregnancy and neonatal outcomes in women with eating disorders. Obstet Gynecol 2005; 105:255–260 [D]
381. Franko DL, Blais MA, Becker AE, Delinsky SS, Greenwood DN, Flores AT, Ekeblad ER, Eddy KT, Herzog DB: Pregnancy complications and neonatal outcomes in women with eating disorders. Am J Psychiatry 2001; 158:1461–1466 [C]
382. Carmichael SL, Shaw GM, Schaffer DM, Laurent C, Selvin S: Dieting behaviors and risk of neural tube defects. Am J Epidemiol 2003; 158:1127–1131 [D]
383. Carter FA, McIntosh VV, Joyce PR, Frampton CM, Bulik CM: Bulimia nervosa, childbirth, and psychopathology. J Psychosom Res 2003; 55:357–361 [C]
384. Blais MA, Becker AE, Burwell RA, Flores AT, Nussbaum KM, Greenwood DN, Ekeblad ER, Herzog DB: Pregnancy: outcome and impact on symptomatology in a cohort of eating-disordered women. Int J Eat Disord 2000; 27:140–149 [C]
385. Sollid CP, Wisborg K, Hjort J, Secher NJ: Eating disorder that was diagnosed before pregnancy and pregnancy outcome. Am J Obstet Gynecol 2004; 190:206–210 [D]
386. Agras WS, Hammer LD, McNicholas F: A prospective study of the influence of eating-disordered mothers on their children. Int J Eat Disord 1999; 25:253–262 [C]
387. Russell GF, Treasure J, Eisler I: Mothers with anorexia nervosa who underfeed their children: their recognition and management. Psychol Med 1998; 28:93–108 [D]
388. Stein A, Woolley H, Cooper SD, Fairburn CG: An observational study of mothers with eating disorders and their infants. J Child Psychol Psychiatry 1994; 35:733–748 [C]
389. Morgan JF, McCluskey SE, Brunton JN, Hubert LJ: Polycystic ovarian morphology and bulimia nervosa: a 9-year follow-up study. Fertil Steril 2002; 77:928–931 [C]
390. Carlat DJ, Camargo CA Jr, Herzog DB: Eating disorders in males: a report on 135 patients. Am J Psychiatry 1997; 154:1127–1132 [G]
391. Andersen AE (ed): Males With Eating Disorders. Brunner/Mazel Eating Disorders Monograph Series, No. 4. Philadelphia, Brunner/Mazel, 1990 [G]
392. Fichter M, Krenn H: Eating disorders in males, in Handbook of Eating Disorders, 2nd ed. Edited by Treasure J, Schmidt U, van Furth E. West Sussex, UK, Wiley, 2003, pp 369–384 [G]
393. Braun DL, Sunday SR, Huang A, Halmi KA: More males seek treatment for eating disorders. Int J Eat Disord 1999; 25:415–424 [C]
394. Striegel-Moore RH, Garvin V, Dohm FA, Rosenheck RA: Eating disorders in a national sample of hospitalized female and male veterans: detection rates and psychiatric comorbidity. Int J Eat Disord 1999; 25:405–414 [D]
395. Woodside DB, Garfinkel PE, Lin E, Goering P, Kaplan AS, Goldbloom DS, Kennedy SH: Comparisons of men with full or partial eating disorders, men without eating disorders, and women with eating disorders in the community. Am J Psychiatry 2001; 158:570–574 [D]
396. Ackard DM, Neumark-Sztainer D, Hannan PJ, French S, Story M: Binge and purge behavior among adolescents: associations with sexual and physical abuse in a nationally representative sample: the Commonwealth Fund survey. Child Abuse Negl 2001; 25:771–785 [G]
397. Fernandez-Aranda F, Aitken A, Badia L, Giménez D, Collier D, Treasure J: Personality and psychopathological traits of males with an eating disorder. Eur Eating Disorders Rev 2004; 12:367–374 [D]
398. Powers PS, Spratt EG: Males and females with eating disorders. J Treatment and Prevention 1994; 2:197–214 [D]

399. Andersen AE: Gender-related aspects of eating disorders: a guide to practice. J Gend Specif Med 1999; 2:47–54 [F]
400. Barry DT, Grilo CM, Masheb RM: Gender differences in patients with binge eating disorder. Int J Eat Disord 2002; 31:63–70 [G]
401. Grant JE, Kim SW, Eckert ED: Body dysmorphic disorder in patients with anorexia nervosa: prevalence, clinical features, and delusionality of body image. Int J Eat Disord 2002; 32:291–300 [G]
402. Phillips KA, Diaz SF: Gender differences in body dysmorphic disorder. J Nerv Ment Dis 1997; 185:570–577 [G]
403. Perugi G, Akiskal HS, Giannotti D, Frare F, Di Vaio S, Cassano GB: Gender-related differences in body dysmorphic disorder (dysmorphophobia). J Nerv Ment Dis 1997; 185:578–582 [G]
404. Grant JE, Phillips KA: Is anorexia nervosa a subtype of body dysmorphic disorder? probably not, but read on. Harv Rev Psychiatry 2004; 12:123–126 [G]
405. Woodside DB, Bulik CM, Thornton L, Klump KL, Tozzi F, Fichter MM, Halmi KA, Kaplan AS, Strober M, Devlin B, Bacanu SA, Ganjei K, Crow S, Mitchell J, Rotondo A, Mauri M, Cassano G, Keel P, Berrettini WH, Kaye WH: Personality in men with eating disorders. J Psychosom Res 2004; 57:273–278 [D]
406. Arnow B, Sanders M, Steiner H: Pre-pubertal vs post-pubertal anorexia nervosa: psychological characteristics. Clin Child Psychol and Psychiatry 1999; 4:403–416 [G]
407. Lask B, Bryant-Waugh R: Childhood Onset Anorexia Nervosa and Related Eating Disorders. Hillsdale, NJ, Lawrence Erlbaum Associates, 1993 [G]
408. Cooper PJ, Watkins B, Bryant-Waugh R, Lask B: The nosological status of early onset anorexia nervosa. Psychol Med 2002; 32:873–880 [D]
409. Golden NH, Kreitzer P, Jacobson MS, Chasalow FI, Schebendach J, Freedman SM, Shenker IR: Disturbances in growth hormone secretion and action in adolescents with anorexia nervosa. J Pediatr 1994; 125:655–660 [D]
410. Nussbaum M, Baird D, Sonnenblick M, Cowan K, Shenker IR: Short stature in anorexia nervosa patients. J Adolesc Health Care 1985; 6:453–455 [D]
411. Pfeiffer RJ, Lucas AR, Ilstrup DM: Effect of anorexia nervosa on linear growth. Clin Pediatr (Phila) 1986; 25:7–12 [G]
412. Misra M, Aggarwal A, Miller KK, Almazan C, Worley M, Soyka LA, Herzog DB, Klibanski A: Effects of anorexia nervosa on clinical, hematologic, biochemical, and bone density parameters in community-dwelling adolescent girls. Pediatrics 2004; 114:1574–1583 [D]
413. Bachrach LK, Guido D, Katzman D, Litt IF, Marcus R: Decreased bone density in adolescent girls with anorexia nervosa. Pediatrics 1990; 86:440–447 [C]
414. Bachrach LK, Katzman DK, Litt IF, Guido D, Marcus R: Recovery from osteopenia in adolescent girls with anorexia nervosa. J Clin Endocrinol Metab 1991; 72:602–606 [B]
415. Sokol MS: Infection-triggered anorexia nervosa in children: clinical description of four cases. J Child Adolesc Psychopharmacol 2000; 10:133–145 [B]
416. Swedo SE, Leonard HL, Rapoport JL: The pediatric autoimmune neuropsychiatric disorders associated with streptococcal infection (PANDAS) subgroup: separating fact from fiction. Pediatrics 2004; 113:907–911 [F]
417. Zerbe K: Eating disorders in middle and later life: a neglected problem. Primary Psychiatry 2003; 10:80–83 [F]
418. Zerbe K: Eating disorders in midlife and beyond: transition and transformation at a crucial developmental stage. Psychoanal Psychother 2002; 19:9–19 [G]
419. Zerbe K, Domnitei D: Eating disorders at middle age, parts 1 and 2. Eating Disorders Review 2004; 15:1–2 [F]

420. Forman ME, Davis WN: Characteristics of middle-aged women in inpatient treatment for eating disorders. Eating Disorders: The Journal of Treatment and Prevention 2005; 13:231–243 [B]
421. Lucas AR, Crowson CS, O'Fallon WM, Melton LJ III: The ups and downs of anorexia nervosa. Int J Eat Disord 1999; 26:397–405 [G]
422. Gupta MA: Concerns about aging and a drive for thinness: a factor in the biopsychosocial model of eating disorders? Int J Eat Disord 1995; 18:351–357 [B]
423. Boast N, Coker E, Wakeling A: Anorexia nervosa of late onset. Br J Psychiatry 1992; 160:257–260 [G]
424. Becker AE: New global perspectives on eating disorders. Cult Med Psychiatry 2004; 28:433–437 [G]
425. Hoek HW, van Harten PN, Hermans KM, Katzman MA, Matroos GE, Susser ES: The incidence of anorexia nervosa on Curacao. Am J Psychiatry 2005; 162:748–752 [G]
426. Katzman MA, Hermans KM, Van Hoeken D, Hoek HW: Not your "typical island woman": anorexia nervosa is reported only in subcultures in Curacao. Cult Med Psychiatry 2004; 28:463–492 [G]
427. Nasser M, Katzman MA, Gordon RA (eds): Eating Disorders and Cultures in Transition. New York, Taylor & Francis, 2001 [G]
428. Popkin BM, Gordon-Larsen P: The nutrition transition: worldwide obesity dynamics and their determinants. Int J Obes Relat Metab Disord 2004; 28(suppl 3):S2–S9 [E]
429. Becker AE, Burwell RA, Gilman SE, Herzog DB, Hamburg P: Eating behaviours and attitudes following prolonged exposure to television among ethnic Fijian adolescent girls. Br J Psychiatry 2002; 180:509–514 [C]
430. Becker AE: Eating disorders and social transition. Primary Psychiatry 2003; 10:75–79 [F]
431. Tsai G: Eating disorders in the Far East. Eat Weight Disord 2000; 5:183–197 [E]
432. Gordon RA: Eating Disorders: Anatomy of a Social Epidemic, 2nd ed. Oxford, UK, Blackwell, 2000 [G]
433. Katzman MA, Lee S: Beyond body image: the integration of feminist and transcultural theories in the understanding of self starvation. Int J Eat Disord 1997; 22:385–394 [F]
434. le Grange D, Louw J, Breen A, Katzman MA: The meaning of "self-starvation" in impoverished black adolescents in South Africa. Cult Med Psychiatry 2004; 28:439–461 [G]
435. Lee S, Ho TP, Hsu LK: Fat phobic and non-fat phobic anorexia nervosa: a comparative study of 70 Chinese patients in Hong Kong. Psychol Med 1993; 23:999–1017 [D]
436. Ramacciotti CE, Dell'Osso L, Paoli RA, Ciapparelli A, Coli E, Kaplan AS, Garfinkel PE: Characteristics of eating disorder patients without a drive for thinness. Int J Eat Disord 2002; 32:206–212 [G]
437. Stephens NM, Schumaker JF, Sibiya TE: Eating disorders and dieting behavior among Australian and Swazi university students. J Soc Psychol 1999; 139:153–158 [G]
438. Sjostedt JP, Schumaker JF, Nathawat SS: Eating disorders among Indian and Australian university students. J Soc Psychol 1998; 138:351–357 [G]
439. Johnson C, Powers PS, Dick R: Athletes and eating disorders: the National Collegiate Athletic Association study. Int J Eat Disord 1999; 26:179–188 [G]
440. Sherman RT, Thompson RA: The female athlete triad. J Sch Nurs 2004; 20:197–202 [G]
441. Thompson RA, Sherman RT: Helping Athletes With Eating Disorders. Champaign, IL, Human Kinetics, 1993 [G]
442. Williamson DA, Netemeyer RG, Jackman LP, Anderson DA, Funsch CL, Rabalais JY: Structural equation modeling of risk factors for the development of eating disorder symptoms in female athletes. Int J Eat Disord 1995; 17:387–393 [E]
443. Fulkerson JA, Keel PK, Leon GR, Dorr T: Eating-disordered behaviors and personality characteristics of high school athletes and nonathletes. Int J Eat Disord 1999; 26:73–79 [D]

444. Davison KK, Earnest MB, Birch LL: Participation in aesthetic sports and girls' weight concerns at ages 5 and 7 years. Int J Eat Disord 2002; 31:312–317 [D]
445. Smolak L, Murnen SK, Ruble AE: Female athletes and eating problems: a meta-analysis. Int J Eat Disord 2000; 27:371–380 [E]
446. Davis C, Kennedy SH, Ravelski E, Dionne M: The role of physical activity in the development and maintenance of eating disorders. Psychol Med 1994; 24:957–967 [B]
447. Davis C, Katzman DK, Kirsh C: Compulsive physical activity in adolescents with anorexia nervosa: a psychobehavioral spiral of pathology. J Nerv Ment Dis 1999; 187:336–342 [G]
448. Klein DA, Bennett AS, Schebendach J, Foltin RW, Devlin MJ, Walsh BT: Exercise "addiction" in anorexia nervosa: model development and pilot data. CNS Spectr 2004; 9:531–537 [G]
449. Otis CL, Drinkwater B, Johnson M, Loucks A, Wilmore J: American College of Sports Medicine position stand: the female athlete triad. Med Sci Sports Exerc 1997; 29:i–ix [G]
450. Beals KA, Manore MM: Disorders of the female athlete triad among collegiate athletes. Int J Sport Nutr Exerc Metab 2002; 12:281–293 [G]
451. Raglin JS, Wilson GS: Overtraining in athletes, in Emotions in Sport. Edited by Hanin YL. Champaign, IL, Human Kinetics, 1999, pp 191–207 [G]
452. Yates A: Athletes, eating disorders, and the overtraining syndrome, in Activity Anorexia: Theory, Research, and Treatment. Edited by Epling WF, Pierce WD. Hillsdale, NJ, Lawrence Erlbaum Associates, 1996, pp 179–188 [G]
453. Hebebrand J, Exner C, Hebebrand K, Holtkamp C, Casper RC, Remschmidt H, Herpertz-Dahlmann B, Klingenspor M: Hyperactivity in patients with anorexia nervosa and in semi-starved rats: evidence for a pivotal role of hypoleptinemia. Physiol Behav 2003; 79:25–37 [G]
454. Epling WF, Pierce WD (eds): Activity Anorexia: Theory, Research, and Treatment. Hillsdale, NJ, Lawrence Erlbaum Associates, 1996 [G]
455. Mann T, Nolen-Hoeksema S, Huang K, Burgard D, Wright A, Hanson K: Are two interventions worse than none? joint primary and secondary prevention of eating disorders in college females. Health Psychol 1997; 16:215–225 [B]
456. Shisslak CM, Crago M, Estes LS, Gray N: Content and method of developmentally appropriate prevention programs, in The Developmental Psychopathology of Eating Disorders: Implications for Research, Prevention, and Treatment. Edited by Smolak L, Levine MP, Striegel-Moore R. Mahwah, NJ, Lawrence Erlbaum Associates, 1996, pp 341–363 [E]
457. Glenn AA, Pollard JW, Denovcheck JA, Smith AF: Eating disorders on campus: a procedure for community intervention. J Couns Dev 1986; 65:163–165 [G]
458. Coll KM: Mandatory psychiatric withdrawal from public colleges and universities: a review of potential legal violations and appropriate use. J College Student Psychotherapy 1991; 5:91–98 [E]
459. Steiner H, Kwan W, Shaffer TG, Walker S, Miller S, Sagar A, Lock J: Risk and protective factors for juvenile eating disorders. Eur Child Adolesc Psychiatry 2003; 12(suppl 1):I38–I46 [F]
460. Leonard S, Steiger H, Kao A: Childhood and adulthood abuse in bulimic and nonbulimic women: prevalences and psychological correlates. Int J Eat Disord 2003; 33:397–405 [D]
461. Anderluh MB, Tchanturia K, Rabe-Hesketh S, Treasure J: Childhood obsessive-compulsive personality traits in adult women with eating disorders: defining a broader eating disorder phenotype. Am J Psychiatry 2003; 160:242–247 [D]
462. Scourfield J: Anorexia by proxy: are the children of anorexic mothers an at-risk group? Int J Eat Disord 1995; 18:371–374 [G]
463. Ward A, Ramsay R, Turnbull S, Steele M, Steele H, Treasure J: Attachment in anorexia nervosa: a transgenerational perspective. Br J Med Psychol 2001; 74:497–505 [G]
464. Seigel K, Hetta J: Exercise and eating disorder symptoms among young females. Eat Weight Disord 2001; 6:32–39 [D]

465. Klump KL, Ringham RM, Marcus MD, Kaye WH: A family history/family study approach to examining the nature of eating disorder risk in ballet dancers: evidence for gene-environment combinations? Paper presented at the annual meeting of the Eating Disorders Research Society, Albuquerque, November 29–December 2, 2001 [D]
466. Powers PS, Schocken DD, Boyd FR: Comparison of habitual runners and anorexia nervosa patients. Int J Eat Disord 1998; 23:133–143 [G]
467. Choi PY, Pope HG Jr, Olivardia R: Muscle dysmorphia: a new syndrome in weightlifters. Br J Sports Med 2002; 36:375–376 [G]
468. Pope HG Jr, Gruber AJ, Choi P, Olivardia R, Phillips KA: Muscle dysmorphia: an underrecognized form of body dysmorphic disorder. Psychosomatics 1997; 38:548–557 [G]
469. Morgan JF: From Charles Atlas to Adonis complex: fat is more than a feminist issue. Lancet 2000; 356:1372–1373 [G]
470. Pope HG Jr, Phillips KA, Olivardia R: The Adonis Complex: The Secret Crisis of Male Body Obsession. New York, Free Press, 2000 [G]
471. Stice E, Shaw H: Eating disorder prevention programs: a meta-analytic review. Psychol Bull 2004; 130:206–227 [E]
472. Matusek JA, Wendt SJ, Wiseman CV: Dissonance thin-ideal and didactic healthy behavior eating disorder prevention programs: results from a controlled trial. Int J Eat Disord 2004; 36:376–388 [A–]
473. Elliot DL, Goldberg L, Moe EL, Defrancesco CA, Durham MB, Hix-Small H: Preventing substance use and disordered eating: initial outcomes of the ATHENA (Athletes Targeting Healthy Exercise and Nutrition Alternatives) program. Arch Pediatr Adolesc Med 2004; 158:1043–1049 [A–]
474. Stice E, Trost A, Chase A: Healthy weight control and dissonance-based eating disorder prevention programs: results from a controlled trial. Int J Eat Disord 2003; 33:10–21 [A–]
475. Shisslak CM, Crago M, Neal ME, Swain B: Primary prevention of eating disorders. J Consult Clin Psychol 1987; 55:660–667 [G]
476. Bulik CM, Sullivan PF, Fear J, Pickering A: Predictors of the development of bulimia nervosa in women with anorexia nervosa. J Nerv Ment Dis 1997; 185:704–707 [G]
477. Tozzi F, Thornton LM, Klump KL, Fichter MM, Halmi KA, Kaplan AS, Strober M, Woodside DB, Crow S, Mitchell J, Rotondo A, Mauri M, Cassano G, Keel P, Plotnicov KH, Pollice C, Lilenfeld LR, Berrettini WH, Bulik CM, Kaye WH: Symptom fluctuation in eating disorders: correlates of diagnostic crossover. Am J Psychiatry 2005; 162:732–740 [C]
478. Strober M, Freeman R, Morrell W: Atypical anorexia nervosa: separation from typical cases in course and outcome in a long-term prospective study. Int J Eat Disord 1999; 25:135–142 [C]
479. Wolk SL, Loeb KL, Walsh BT: Assessment of patients with anorexia nervosa: interview versus self-report. Int J Eat Disord 2005; 37:92–99 [G]
480. Beumont PJ, George GC, Smart DE: "Dieters" and "vomiters and purgers" in anorexia nervosa. Psychol Med 1976; 6:617–622 [C]
481. Casper RC, Eckert ED, Halmi KA, Goldberg SC, Davis JM: Bulimia: its incidence and clinical importance in patients with anorexia nervosa. Arch Gen Psychiatry 1980; 37:1030–1035 [C]
482. Garfinkel PE, Moldofsky H, Garner DM: The heterogeneity of anorexia nervosa: bulimia as a distinct subgroup. Arch Gen Psychiatry 1980; 37:1036–1040 [C]
483. Kassett JA, Gwirtsman HE, Kaye WH, Brandt HA, Jimerson DC: Pattern of onset of bulimic symptoms in anorexia nervosa. Am J Psychiatry 1988; 145:1287–1288 [C]
484. Bunnell DW, Shenker IR, Nussbaum MP, Jacobson MS, Cooper P, Phil D: Subclinical versus formal eating disorders: differentiating psychological features. Int J Eat Disord 1990; 9:357–362 [D]
485. Goss K, Gilbert P: Eating disorders, shame and pride: a cognitive-behavioural functional analysis, in Body Shame: Conceptualization, Research, and Treatment. Edited by Gilbert P, Miles J. East Sussex, UK, Brunner/Routledge, 2002, pp 219–255 [G]

486. Favaro A, Ferrara S, Santonastaso P: Impulsive and compulsive self-injurious behavior and eating disorders: an epidemiological study, in Self-Harm Behavior and Eating Disorders: Dynamics, Assessment, and Treatment. Edited by Levitt JL, Sansone RA, Cohn L. New York, Brunner/Routledge, 2004, pp 31–44 [G]
487. Favaro A, Santonastaso P: Different types of self-injurious behavior in bulimia nervosa. Compr Psychiatry 1999; 40:57–60 [G]
488. McDermott BM, Batik M, Roberts L, Gibbon P: Parent and child report of family functioning in a clinical child and adolescent eating disorders sample. Aust N Z J Psychiatry 2002; 36:509–514 [G]
489. Neumark-Sztainer D, Story M, Hannan PJ, Beuhring T, Resnick MD: Disordered eating among adolescents: associations with sexual/physical abuse and other familial/psychosocial factors. Int J Eat Disord 2000; 28:249–258 [C]
490. Klump KL, Bulik CM, Pollice C, Halmi KA, Fichter MM, Berrettini WH, Devlin B, Strober M, Kaplan A, Woodside DB, Treasure J, Shabbout M, Lilenfeld LR, Plotnicov KH, Kaye WH: Temperament and character in women with anorexia nervosa. J Nerv Ment Dis 2000; 188:559–567 [D]
491. Paul T, Schroeter K, Dahme B, Nutzinger DO: Self-injurious behavior in women with eating disorders. Am J Psychiatry 2002; 159:408–411 [G]
492. Brewerton TD, Dansky BS, Kilpatrick DG, O'Neil PM: Bulimia nervosa, PTSD and "forgetting": results from the National Women's Study, in Trauma and Memory. Edited by Williams LM, Banyard VL. Durham, NC, Sage, 1999, pp 127–138 [G]
493. Casper RC, Davis JM: On the course of anorexia nervosa. Am J Psychiatry 1977; 134:974–978 [C]
494. Garfinkel PE, Kaplan AS: Starvation-based perpetuating mechanisms in anorexia nervosa and bulimia. Int J Eat Disord 1985; 4:651–655 [E]
495. Sutandar-Pinnock K, Blake WD, Carter JC, Olmsted MP, Kaplan AS: Perfectionism in anorexia nervosa: a 6- to 24-month follow-up study. Int J Eat Disord 2003; 33:225–229 [C]
496. Fichter MM: Starvation-related endocrine changes, in Psychobiology and Treatment of Anorexia Nervosa and Bulimia (American Psychopathological Association Series). Edited by Halmi KA. Washington, DC, American Psychiatric Association, 1993, pp 193–210 [G]
497. Fichter MM, Pirke KM, Pollinger J, Wolfram G, Brunner E: Disturbances in the hypothalamo-pituitary-adrenal and other neuroendocrine axes in bulimia. Biol Psychiatry 1990; 27:1021–1037 [D]
498. Vestergaard P, Emborg C, Stoving RK, Hagen C, Mosekilde L, Brixen K: Fractures in patients with anorexia nervosa, bulimia nervosa, and other eating disorders: a nationwide register study. Int J Eat Disord 2002; 32:301–308 [C]
499. Rigotti NA, Neer RM, Skates SJ, Herzog DB, Nussbaum SR: The clinical course of osteoporosis in anorexia nervosa: a longitudinal study of cortical bone mass. JAMA 1991; 265:1133–1138 [C]
500. Hartman D, Crisp A, Rooney B, Rackow C, Atkinson R, Patel S: Bone density of women who have recovered from anorexia nervosa. Int J Eat Disord 2000; 28:107–112 [D]
501. Modan-Moses D, Yaroslavsky A, Novikov I, Segev S, Toledano A, Miterany E, Stein D: Stunting of growth as a major feature of anorexia nervosa in male adolescents. Pediatrics 2003; 111:270–276 [C]
502. Lantzouni E, Frank GR, Golden NH, Shenker RI: Reversibility of growth stunting in early onset anorexia nervosa: a prospective study. J Adolesc Health 2002; 31:162–165 [C]
503. Isner JM, Roberts WC, Heymsfield SB, Yager J: Anorexia nervosa and sudden death. Ann Intern Med 1985; 102:49–52 [G]
504. Beumont PJ, Kopec-Schrader EM, Lennerts W: Eating disorder patients at a NSW teaching hospital: a comparison with state-wide data. Aust N Z J Psychiatry 1995; 29:96–103 [G]

505. de Zwaan M, Mitchell JE: Medical complications of anorexia nervosa and bulimia nervosa, in Medical Issues and the Eating Disorders: The Interface. Brunner/Mazel Eating Disorders Monograph Series, No. 7. Edited by Kaplan AS, Garfinkel PE. New York, Brunner/Mazel, 1993, pp 60–100 [G]
506. Halmi KA: Anorexia nervosa and bulimia. Annu Rev Med 1987; 38:373–380 [F]
507. Herzog DB, Copeland PM: Eating disorders. N Engl J Med 1985; 313:295–303 [F]
508. Swayze VW, Andersen AE, Andreasen NC, Arndt S, Sato Y, Ziebell S: Brain tissue volume segmentation in patients with anorexia nervosa before and after weight normalization. Int J Eat Disord 2003; 33:33–44 [D]
509. Katzman DK, Lambe EK, Mikulis DJ, Ridgley JN, Goldbloom DS, Zipursky RB: Cerebral gray matter and white matter volume deficits in adolescent girls with anorexia nervosa. J Pediatr 1996; 129:794–803 [D]
510. Kingston K, Szmukler G, Andrewes D, Tress B, Desmond P: Neuropsychological and structural brain changes in anorexia nervosa before and after refeeding. Psychol Med 1996; 26:15–28 [C]
511. Katzman DK, Christensen B, Young AR, Zipursky RB: Starving the brain: structural abnormalities and cognitive impairment in adolescents with anorexia nervosa. Semin Clin Neuropsychiatry 2001; 6:146–152 [F]
512. Powers PS, Tyson IB, Stevens BA, Heal AV: Total body potassium and serum potassium among eating disorder patients. Int J Eat Disord 1995; 18:269–276 [G]
513. Wolfe BE, Metzger ED, Levine JM, Jimerson DC: Laboratory screening for electrolyte abnormalities and anemia in bulimia nervosa: a controlled study. Int J Eat Disord 2001; 30:288–293 [D]
514. Mitchell JE, Pyle RL, Eckert ED, Hatsukami D, Lentz R: Electrolyte and other physiological abnormalities in patients with bulimia. Psychol Med 1983; 13:273–278 [G]
515. Kaplan AS: Hyperamylasemia and bulimia: a clinical review. Int J Eat Disord 1987; 6:537–543 [G]
516. Hoek HW, van Hoeken D: Review of the prevalence and incidence of eating disorders. Int J Eat Disord 2003; 34:383–396 [F]
517. Walters EE, Kendler KS: Anorexia nervosa and anorexic-like syndromes in a population-based female twin sample. Am J Psychiatry 1995; 152:64–71 [D]
518. Garfinkel PE, Lin E, Goering P, Spegg C, Goldbloom DS, Kennedy S, Kaplan AS, Woodside DB: Bulimia nervosa in a Canadian community sample: prevalence and comparison of subgroups. Am J Psychiatry 1995; 152:1052–1058 [C]
519. Kendler KS, MacLean C, Neale M, Kessler R, Heath A, Eaves L: The genetic epidemiology of bulimia nervosa. Am J Psychiatry 1991; 148:1627–1637 [G]
520. Keel PK, Heatherton TF, Dorer DJ, Joiner TE, Haedt A: How has bulimia nervosa changed over time? results from a cross-sectional and longitudinal study in college students: 1982, 1992, and 2002. Paper presented at the annual meeting of the Eating Disorders Research Society, Amsterdam, October 7–9, 2004 [C]
521. Keel PK, Klump KL: Are eating disorders culture-bound syndromes? implications for conceptualizing their etiology. Psychol Bull 2003; 129:747–769 [E]
522. Striegel-Moore RH, Dohm FA, Kraemer HC, Taylor CB, Daniels S, Crawford PB, Schreiber GB: Eating disorders in white and black women. Am J Psychiatry 2003; 160:1326–1331 [G]
523. Neumark-Sztainer D, Croll J, Story M, Hannan PJ, French SA, Perry C: Ethnic/racial differences in weight-related concerns and behaviors among adolescent girls and boys: findings from Project EAT. J Psychosom Res 2002; 53:963–974 [D]
524. Crago M, Shisslak CM, Estes LS: Eating disturbances among American minority groups: a review. Int J Eat Disord 1996; 19:239–248 [F]
525. Striegel-Moore RH, Schreiber GB, Pike KM, Wilfley DE, Rodin J: Drive for thinness in black and white preadolescent girls. Int J Eat Disord 1995; 18:59–69 [G]

526. Hermes SF, Keel PK: The influence of puberty and ethnicity on awareness and internalization of the thin ideal. Int J Eat Disord 2003; 33:465–467 [G]
527. Striegel-Moore RH, Schreiber GB, Lo A, Crawford P, Obarzanek E, Rodin J: Eating disorder symptoms in a cohort of 11- to 16-year-old black and white girls: the NHLBI Growth and Health Study. Int J Eat Disord 2000; 27:49–66 [C]
528. Kjelsas E, Bjornstrom C, Gotestam KG: Prevalence of eating disorders in female and male adolescents (14-15 years). Eat Behav 2004; 5:13–25 [G]
529. Maekawa H: The factors and process of weight and shape concerns in Japanese female adolescents. Paper presented at the International Conference on Eating Disorders, Orlando, Fla, April 29–May 2, 2004 [G]
530. Bell CA, Adair LS, Popkin BM: Ethnic differences in the association between body mass index and hypertension. Am J Epidemiol 2002; 155:346–353 [C]
531. Lee S, Lee AM: Disordered eating in three communities of China: a comparative study of female high school students in Hong Kong, Shenzhen, and rural Hunan. Int J Eat Disord 2000; 27:317–327 [G]
532. Lee S: Eating disorders are becoming more common in the East too. BMJ 2000; 321:1023 [G]
533. Lai KY: Anorexia nervosa in Chinese adolescents: does culture make a difference? J Adolesc 2000; 23:561–568 [C]
534. Nobakht M, Dezhkam M: An epidemiological study of eating disorders in Iran. Int J Eat Disord 2000; 28:265–271 [G]
535. le Grange D, Telch CF, Tibbs J: Eating attitudes and behaviors in 1,435 South African Caucasian and non-Caucasian college students. Am J Psychiatry 1998; 155:250–254 [G]
536. Mangweth B, Hudson JI, Pope HG, Hausmann A, De Col C, Laird NM, Beibl W, Tsuang MT: Family study of the aggregation of eating disorders and mood disorders. Psychol Med 2003; 33:1319–1323 [D]
537. Strober M, Freeman R, Lampert C, Diamond J, Kaye W: Males with anorexia nervosa: a controlled study of eating disorders in first-degree relatives. Int J Eat Disord 2001; 29:263–269 [D]
538. Lilenfeld LR, Kaye WH, Greeno CG, Merikangas KR, Plotnicov K, Pollice C, Rao R, Strober M, Bulik CM, Nagy L: A controlled family study of anorexia nervosa and bulimia nervosa: psychiatric disorders in first-degree relatives and effects of proband comorbidity. Arch Gen Psychiatry 1998; 55:603–610 [D]
539. Strober M, Freeman R, Lampert C, Diamond J, Kaye W: Controlled family study of anorexia nervosa and bulimia nervosa: evidence of shared liability and transmission of partial syndromes. Am J Psychiatry 2000; 157:393–401 [D]
540. Lilenfeld LR, Kaye WH, Greeno CG, Merikangas KR, Plotnicov K, Pollice C, Rao R, Strober M, Bulik CM, Nagy L: Psychiatric disorders in women with bulimia nervosa and their first-degree relatives: effects of comorbid substance dependence. Int J Eat Disord 1997; 22:253–264 [D]
541. Lilenfeld LR, Stein D, Bulik CM, Strober M, Plotnicov K, Pollice C, Rao R, Merikangas KR, Nagy L, Kaye WH: Personality traits among currently eating disordered, recovered and never ill first-degree female relatives of bulimic and control women. Psychol Med 2000; 30:1399–1410 [D]
542. Becker AE, Burwell RA, Navara K, Gilman SE: Binge eating and binge eating disorder in a small-scale, indigenous society: the view from Fiji. Int J Eat Disord 2003; 34:423–431 [C]
543. Godart NT, Flament MF, Perdereau F, Jeammet P: Comorbidity between eating disorders and anxiety disorders: a review. Int J Eat Disord 2002; 32:253–270 [F]
544. Srinivasagam NM, Kaye WH, Plotnicov KH, Greeno C, Weltzin TE, Rao R: Persistent perfectionism, symmetry, and exactness after long-term recovery from anorexia nervosa. Am J Psychiatry 1995; 152:1630–1634 [C]

545. Franko DL, Dorer DJ, Keel PK, Jackson S, Manzo MP, Herzog DB: How do eating disorders and alcohol use disorder influence each other? Int J Eat Disord 2005; 38:200–207 [C]
546. Ilkjaer K, Kortegaard L, Hoerder K, Joergensen J, Kyvik K, Gillberg C: Personality disorders in a total population twin cohort with eating disorders. Compr Psychiatry 2004; 45:261–267 [D]
547. Skodol AE, Oldham JM, Hyler SE, Kellman HD, Doidge N, Davies M: Comorbidity of DSM-III-R eating disorders and personality disorders. Int J Eat Disord 1993; 14:403–416 [D]
548. Vize CM, Cooper PJ: Sexual abuse in patients with eating disorder, patients with depression, and normal controls: a comparative study. Br J Psychiatry 1995; 167:80–85 [D]
549. Deep AL, Lilenfeld LR, Plotnicov KH, Pollice C, Kaye WH: Sexual abuse in eating disorder subtypes and control women: the role of comorbid substance dependence in bulimia nervosa. Int J Eat Disord 1999; 25:1–10 [D]
550. Brewerton TD: Psychological trauma and eating disorders, in AED Review of Eating Disorders, Part 1. Edited by Wonderlich S, Mitchell J, de Zwann M, Steiger H. Oxford, UK, Radcliffe, 2005, pp 137–154 [F]
551. Johnson JG, Cohen P, Kasen S, Brook JS: Childhood adversities associated with risk for eating disorders or weight problems during adolescence or early adulthood. Am J Psychiatry 2002; 159:394–400 [C]
552. Herpertz-Dahlmann B, Muller B, Herpertz S, Heussen N, Hebebrand J, Remschmidt H: Prospective 10-year follow-up in adolescent anorexia nervosa: course, outcome, psychiatric comorbidity, and psychosocial adaptation. J Child Psychol Psychiatry 2001; 42:603–612 [C]
553. Eckert ED, Halmi KA, Marchi P, Grove W, Crosby R: Ten-year follow-up of anorexia nervosa: clinical course and outcome. Psychol Med 1995; 25:143–156 [B]
554. Bulik CM, Sullivan PF, Fear JL, Pickering A: Outcome of anorexia nervosa: eating attitudes, personality, and parental bonding. Int J Eat Disord 2000; 28:139–147 [D]
555. Eddy KT, Keel PK, Dorer DJ, Delinsky SS, Franko DL, Herzog DB: Longitudinal comparison of anorexia nervosa subtypes. Int J Eat Disord 2002; 31:191–201 [C]
556. Fisher M: The course and outcome of eating disorders in adults and in adolescents: a review. Adolesc Med 2003; 14:149–158 [F]
557. Kreipe RE, Churchill BH, Strauss J: Long-term outcome of adolescents with anorexia nervosa. Arch Pediatr Adolesc Med 1989; 143:1322–1327 [C]
558. Harris EC, Barraclough B: Excess mortality of mental disorder. Br J Psychiatry 1998; 173:11–53 [F]
559. Nielsen S, Moller-Madsen S, Isager T, Jorgensen J, Pagsberg K, Theander S: Standardized mortality in eating disorders: a quantitative summary of previously published and new evidence. J Psychosom Res 1998; 44:413–434 [F]
560. Reas DL, Kjelsas E, Heggestad T, Eriksen L, Nielsen S, Gjertsen F, Gotestam KG: Characteristics of anorexia nervosa-related deaths in Norway (1992–2000): data from the National Patient Register and the Causes of Death Register. Int J Eat Disord 2005; 37:181–187 [G]
561. Sullivan PF: Mortality in anorexia nervosa. Am J Psychiatry 1995; 152:1073–1074 [E]
562. Keel PK, Mitchell JE, Miller KB, Davis TL, Crow SJ: Long-term outcome of bulimia nervosa. Arch Gen Psychiatry 1999; 56:63–69 [C]
563. Nielsen S: Epidemiology and mortality of eating disorders. Psychiatr Clin North Am 2001; 24:201–214, vii–viii [F]
564. Drewnowski A, Yee DK, Krahn DD: Dieting and Bulimia: A Continuum of Behaviors. Washington, DC, American Psychiatric Press, 1989 [G]
565. Yager J, Landsverk J, Edelstein CK: A 20-month follow-up study of 628 women with eating disorders, I: course and severity. Am J Psychiatry 1987; 144:1172–1177 [B]
566. Hsu LK, Sobkiewicz TA: Bulimia nervosa: a four- to six-year follow-up study. Psychol Med 1989; 19:1035–1038 [B]
567. Fairburn CG, Cooper Z, Doll HA, Norman P, O'Connor M: The natural course of bulimia nervosa and binge eating disorder in young women. Arch Gen Psychiatry 2000; 57:659–665 [C]

568. Herzog DB, Dorer DJ, Keel PK, Selwyn SE, Ekeblad ER, Flores AT, Greenwood DN, Burwell RA, Keller MB: Recovery and relapse in anorexia and bulimia nervosa: a 7.5-year follow-up study. J Am Acad Child Adolesc Psychiatry 1999; 38:829–837 [C]
569. Fichter MM, Quadflieg N: Six-year course of bulimia nervosa. Int J Eat Disord 1997; 22:361–384 [C]
570. Quadflieg N, Fichter MM: The course and outcome of bulimia nervosa. Eur Child Adolesc Psychiatry 2003; 12(suppl 1):I99–I109 [C]
571. Crow SJ, Thuras P, Keel PK, Mitchell JE: Long-term menstrual and reproductive function in patients with bulimia nervosa. Am J Psychiatry 2002; 159:1048–1050 [C]
572. Keel PK, Mitchell JE, Davis TL, Crow SJ: Long-term impact of treatment in women diagnosed with bulimia nervosa. Int J Eat Disord 2002; 31:151–158 [C]
573. Reas DL, Schoemaker C, Zipfel S, Williamson DA: Prognostic value of duration of illness and early intervention in bulimia nervosa: a systematic review of the outcome literature. Int J Eat Disord 2001; 30:1–10 [F]
574. Milos G, Spindler A, Ruggiero G, Klaghofer R, Schnyder U: Comorbidity of obsessive-compulsive disorders and duration of eating disorders. Int J Eat Disord 2002; 31:284–289 [G]
575. Grilo CM, Sanislow CA, Shea MT, Skodol AE, Stout RL, Pagano ME, Yen S, McGlashan TH: The natural course of bulimia nervosa and eating disorder not otherwise specified is not influenced by personality disorders. Int J Eat Disord 2003; 34:319–330 [C]
576. Fairburn CG, Stice E, Cooper Z, Doll HA, Norman PA, O'Connor ME: Understanding persistence in bulimia nervosa: a 5-year naturalistic study. J Consult Clin Psychol 2003; 71:103–109 [C]
577. Franko DL, Keel PK, Dorer DJ, Blais MA, Delinsky SS, Eddy KT, Charat V, Renn R, Herzog DB: What predicts suicide attempts in women with eating disorders? Psychol Med 2004; 34:843–853 [C]
578. Spitzer RL, Devlin MJ, Walsh BT, Hasin D: Binge eating disorder: a multisite field trial of the diagnostic criteria. Int J Eat Disord 1992; 11:191–203 [D]
579. Dingemans AE, Bruna MJ, van Furth EF: Binge eating disorder: a review. Int J Obes Relat Metab Disord 2002; 26:299–307 [F]
580. Marcus MD, Kalarchian MA: Binge eating in children and adolescents. Int J Eat Disord 2003; 34(suppl):S47–S57 [F]
581. Specker S, de Zwaan M, Raymond N, Mitchell J: Psychopathology in subgroups of obese women with and without binge eating disorder. Compr Psychiatry 1994; 35:185–190 [D]
582. Cachelin FM, Striegel-Moore RH, Elder KA, Pike KM, Wilfley DE, Fairburn CG: Natural course of a community sample of women with binge eating disorder. Int J Eat Disord 1999; 25:45–54 [C]
583. Fichter MM, Quadflieg N, Gnutzmann A: Binge eating disorder: treatment outcome over a 6-year course. J Psychosom Res 1998; 44:385–405 [C]
584. Stunkard AJ, Allison KC: Binge eating disorder: disorder or marker? Int J Eat Disord 2003; 34(suppl):S107–S116 [F]
585. Raymond NC, de Zwaan M, Mitchell JE, Ackard D, Thuras P: Effect of a very low calorie diet on the diagnostic category of individuals with binge eating disorder. Int J Eat Disord 2002; 31:49–56 [B]
586. Sherwood NE, Jeffery RW, Wing RR: Binge status as a predictor of weight loss treatment outcome. Int J Obes Relat Metab Disord 1999; 23:485–493 [B]
587. Bulik CM, Sullivan PF, Kendler KS: Heritability of binge-eating and broadly defined bulimia nervosa. Biol Psychiatry 1998; 44:1210–1218 [E]
588. Bulik CM, Sullivan PF, Wade TD, Kendler KS: Twin studies of eating disorders: a review. Int J Eat Disord 2000; 27:1–20 [F]
589. Kendler KS: Twin studies of psychiatric illness: an update. Arch Gen Psychiatry 2001; 58:1005–1014 [E]

590. Klump KL, Holly A, Iacono WG, McGue M, Willson LE: Physical similarity and twin resemblance for eating attitudes and behaviors: a test of the equal environments assumption. Behav Genet 2000; 30:51–58 [G]
591. Wade TD, Bulik CM, Neale M, Kendler KS: Anorexia nervosa and major depression: shared genetic and environmental risk factors. Am J Psychiatry 2000; 157:469–471 [D]
592. Grice DE, Halmi KA, Fichter MM, Strober M, Woodside DB, Treasure JT, Kaplan AS, Magistretti PJ, Goldman D, Bulik CM, Kaye WH, Berrettini WH: Evidence for a susceptibility gene for anorexia nervosa on chromosome 1. Am J Hum Genet 2002; 70:787–792 [G]
593. Bulik CM, Devlin B, Bacanu SA, Thornton L, Klump KL, Fichter MM, Halmi KA, Kaplan AS, Strober M, Woodside DB, Bergen AW, Ganjei JK, Crow S, Mitchell J, Rotondo A, Mauri M, Cassano G, Keel P, Berrettini WH, Kaye WH: Significant linkage on chromosome 10p in families with bulimia nervosa. Am J Hum Genet 2003; 72:200–207 [G]
594. Devlin B, Bacanu SA, Klump KL, Bulik CM, Fichter MM, Halmi KA, Kaplan AS, Strober M, Treasure J, Woodside DB, Berrettini WH, Kaye WH: Linkage analysis of anorexia nervosa incorporating behavioral covariates. Hum Mol Genet 2002; 11:689–696 [G]
595. Hinney A, Remschmidt H, Hebebrand J: Candidate gene polymorphisms in eating disorders. Eur J Pharmacol 2000; 410:147–159 [F]
596. Gorwood P, Kipman A, Foulon C: The human genetics of anorexia nervosa. Eur J Pharmacol 2003; 480:163–170 [E]
597. Urwin RE, Nunn KP: Epistatic interaction between the monoamine oxidase A and serotonin transporter genes in anorexia nervosa. Eur J Hum Genet 2005; 13:370–375 [F]
598. Bergen AW, van den Bree MB, Yeager M, Welch R, Ganjei JK, Haque K, Bacanu S, Berrettini WH, Grice DE, Goldman D, Bulik CM, Klump K, Fichter M, Halmi K, Kaplan A, Strober M, Treasure J, Woodside B, Kaye WH: Candidate genes for anorexia nervosa in the 1p33-36 linkage region: serotonin 1D and delta opioid receptor loci exhibit significant association to anorexia nervosa. Mol Psychiatry 2003; 8:397–406 [D]
599. Birmingham CL, Gutierrez E, Jonat L, Beumont P: Randomized controlled trial of warming in anorexia nervosa. Int J Eat Disord 2004; 35:234–238 [A–]
600. Hill K, Bucuvalas J, McClain C, Kryscio R, Martini RT, Alfaro MP, Maloney M: Pilot study of growth hormone administration during the refeeding of malnourished anorexia nervosa patients. J Child Adolesc Psychopharmacol 2000; 10:3–8 [A]
601. Kaye WH, Weltzin TE, Hsu LK, Bulik CM: An open trial of fluoxetine in patients with anorexia nervosa. J Clin Psychiatry 1991; 52:464–471 [G]
602. Winter TA, O'Keefe SJ, Callanan M, Marks T: The effect of severe undernutrition and subsequent refeeding on whole-body metabolism and protein synthesis in human subjects. JPEN J Parenter Enteral Nutr 2005; 29:221–228 [D]
603. Levine JA, Eberhardt NL, Jensen MD: Role of nonexercise activity thermogenesis in resistance to fat gain in humans. Science 1999; 283:212–214 [B]
604. Van Wymelbeke V, Brondel L, Marcel Brun J, Rigaud D: Factors associated with the increase in resting energy expenditure during refeeding in malnourished anorexia nervosa patients. Am J Clin Nutr 2004; 80:1469–1477 [C]
605. Willer MG, Thuras P, Crow SJ: Implications of the changing utilization of hospitalization to treat anorexia nervosa. Am J Psychiatry 2005; 162:2374–2376 [F]
606. Baran SA, Weltzin TE, Kaye WH: Low discharge weight and outcome in anorexia nervosa. Am J Psychiatry 1995; 152:1070–1072 [C]
607. Commerford MC, Licinio J, Halmi KA: Guidelines for Discharging Eating Disorder Patients. Eating Disorders: The Journal of Treatment and Prevention 1997; 5:69–74 [G]
608. Andersen AE: Using medical information psychotherapeutically, in Eating Disorders: A Guide to Medical Care and Complications. Edited by Mehler PS, Andersen AE. Baltimore, Johns Hopkins University Press, 1999, pp 192–201 [G]

609. Bell L: What can we learn from consumer studies and qualitative research in the treatment of eating disorders? Eat Weight Disord 2003; 8:181–187 [F]
610. Prochaska JO, DiClemente CC: Stages of change in the modification of problem behaviors. Prog Behav Modif 1992; 28:183–218 [G]
611. Rieger E, Touyz S, Schotte D, Beumont P, Russell J, Clarke S, Kohn M, Griffiths R: Development of an instrument to assess readiness to recover in anorexia nervosa. Int J Eat Disord 2000; 28:387–396 [G]
612. Rieger E, Touyz SW, Beumont PJ: The Anorexia Nervosa Stages of Change Questionnaire (ANSOCQ): information regarding its psychometric properties. Int J Eat Disord 2002; 32:24–38 [G]
613. Geller J, Cockell SJ, Drab DL: Assessing readiness for change in the eating disorders: the psychometric properties of the Readiness and Motivation Interview. Psychol Assess. 2001; 13:189–198 [G]
614. Geller J, Drab D: The Readiness and Motivation Interview: a symptom-specific measure of readiness for change in the eating disorders. Eur Eating Disorders Rev 1999; 7:259–278 [G]
615. Geller J, Drab-Hudson D, Whisenhunt B, Srikameswaran S: Readiness to change dietary restrictions predicts outcomes in the eating disorders. Eating Disorders: The Journal of Treatment and Prevention 2004; 12:209–224 [C]
616. Jordan PJ, Redding CA, Troop NA, Treasure J, Serpell L: Developing a stage of change measure for assessing recovery from anorexia nervosa. Eat Behav 2003; 3:365–385 [G]
617. Geller J: Estimating readiness for change in anorexia nervosa: comparing clients, clinicians, and research assessors. Int J Eat Disord 2002; 31:251–260 [C]
618. Anzai N, Lindsey-Dudley K, Bidwell RJ: Inpatient and partial hospital treatment for adolescent eating disorders. Child Adolesc Psychiatr Clin N Am 2002; 11:279–309 [G]
619. Wolfe BE, Gimby LB: Caring for the hospitalized patient with an eating disorder. Nurs Clin North Am 2003; 38:75–99 [G]
620. Agras WS: Eating Disorders: Management of Obesity, Bulimia and Anorexia Nervosa. Oxford, UK, Pergamon, 1987 [F]
621. Nusbaum JG, Drever E: Inpatient survey of nursing care measures for treatment of patients with anorexia nervosa. Issues Ment Health Nurs 1990; 11:175–184 [G]
622. Touyz SW, Beumont PJ, Glaun D, Phillips T, Cowie I: A comparison of lenient and strict operant conditioning programmes in refeeding patients with anorexia nervosa. Br J Psychiatry 1984; 144:517–520 [F]
623. Thien V, Thomas A, Markin D, Birmingham CL: Pilot study of a graded exercise program for the treatment of anorexia nervosa. Int J Eat Disord 2000; 28:101–106 [A]
624. Beumont PJ, Arthur B, Russell JD, Touyz SW: Excessive physical activity in dieting disorder patients: proposals for a supervised exercise program. Int J Eat Disord 1994; 15:21–36 [F]
625. Russell JD, Mira M, Allen BJ, Stewart PJ, Vizzard J, Arthur B, Beumont PJ: Effect of refeeding and exercise in restoration of body protein in anorexia nervosa. Basic Life Sci 1993; 60:207–210 [C]
626. Zuercher JNC: Efficacy of voluntary nasogastric tube feeding in female inpatients with anorexia nervosa. JPEN J Parenter Enteral Nutr 2003; 27:268–276 [G]
627. Imbierowicz K, Braks K, Jacoby GE, Geiser F, Conrad R, Schilling G, Liedtke R: High-caloric supplements in anorexia treatment. Int J Eat Disord 2002; 32:135–145 [B]
628. Silber TJ, Robb AS, Orrell-Valente JK, Ellis N, Valadez-Meltzer A, Dadson MJ: Nocturnal nasogastric refeeding for hospitalized adolescent boys with anorexia nervosa. J Dev Behav Pediatr 2004; 25:415–418 [C]
629. Halvorsen I, Andersen A, Heyerdahl S: Good outcome of adolescent onset anorexia nervosa after systematic treatment: intermediate to long-term follow-up of a representative county-sample. Eur Child Adolesc Psychiatry 2004; 13:295–306 [C]

630. Ro O, Martinsen EW, Hoffart A, Rosenvinge JH: Short-term follow-up of adults with long standing anorexia nervosa or non-specified eating disorder after inpatient treatment. Eat Weight Disord 2004; 9:62–68 [C]
631. Castro J, Gila A, Puig J, Rodriguez S, Toro J: Predictors of rehospitalization after total weight recovery in adolescents with anorexia nervosa. Int J Eat Disord 2004; 36:22–30 [C]
632. Johnson CL, Taylor C: Working with difficult-to-treat eating disorders using an integration of twelve-step and traditional psychotherapies. Psychiatr Clin North Am 1996; 19:829–841 [F]
633. Gwirtsman HE, Guze BH, Yager J, Gainsley B: Fluoxetine treatment of anorexia nervosa: an open clinical trial. J Clin Psychiatry 1990; 51:378–382 [G]
634. Bergh C, Eriksson M, Lindberg G, Sodersten P: Selective serotonin reuptake inhibitors in anorexia. Lancet 1996; 348:1459–1460 [B]
635. Halmi KA, Eckert E, LaDu TJ, Cohen J: Anorexia nervosa: treatment efficacy of cyproheptadine and amitriptyline. Arch Gen Psychiatry 1986; 43:177–181 [A]
636. Lacey JH, Crisp AH: Hunger, food intake and weight: the impact of clomipramine on a refeeding anorexia nervosa population. Postgrad Med J 1980; 56(suppl 1):79–85 [A]
637. Powers PS, Bannon Y, Eubanks R: Anorexia nervosa and quetiapine: effect on weight and psychopathology. Paper presented at the 157th annual meeting of the American Psychiatric Association, New York, May 1–6, 2004 [C]
638. Vandereycken W, Pierloot R: Pimozide combined with behavior therapy in the short-term treatment of anorexia nervosa: a double-blind placebo-controlled cross-over study. Acta Psychiatr Scand 1982; 66:445–450 [A]
639. Gross HA, Ebert MH, Faden VB, Goldberg SC, Nee LE, Kaye WH: A double-blind controlled trial of lithium carbonate primary anorexia nervosa. J Clin Psychopharmacol 1981; 1:376–381 [A]
640. Treasure JL, Russell GF, Fogelman I, Murby B: Reversible bone loss in anorexia nervosa. Br Med J (Clin Res Ed) 1987; 295:474–475 [D]
641. Grinspoon S, Thomas L, Miller K, Herzog D, Klibanski A: Effects of recombinant human IGF-I and oral contraceptive administration on bone density in anorexia nervosa. J Clin Endocrinol Metab 2002; 87:2883–2891 [A–]
642. Golden NH, Iglesias EA, Jacobson MS, Carey D, Meyer W, Schebendach J, Hertz S, Shenker IR: Alendronate for the treatment of osteopenia in anorexia nervosa: a randomized, double-blind, placebo-controlled trial. J Clin Endocrinol Metab 2005; 90:3179–3185 [A]
643. Fairburn CG, Jones R, Peveler RC, Hope RA, O'Connor M: Psychotherapy and bulimia nervosa: longer-term effects of interpersonal psychotherapy, behavior therapy, and cognitive behavior therapy. Arch Gen Psychiatry 1993; 50:419–428 [A–]
644. Fairburn CG, Marcus MD, Wilson GT: Cognitive-behavioral therapy for binge eating and bulimia nervosa: a comprehensive treatment manual, in Binge Eating: Nature, Assessment, and Treatment. Edited by Fairburn CG, Wilson GT. New York, Guilford, 1993, pp 361–404 [G]
645. Garner DM, Rockert W, Davis R, Garner MV, Olmsted MP, Eagle M: Comparison of cognitive-behavioral and supportive-expressive therapy for bulimia nervosa. Am J Psychiatry 1993; 150:37–46 [B]
646. Mitchell JE, Pyle RL, Pomeroy C, Zollman M, Crosby R, Seim H, Eckert ED, Zimmerman R: Cognitive-behavioral group psychotherapy of bulimia nervosa: importance of logistical variables. Int J Eat Disord 1993; 14:277–287 [B]
647. Vandereycken W: The addiction model in eating disorders: some critical remarks and a selected bibliography. Int J Eat Disord 1990; 9:95–102 [G]
648. Bulik CM, Sullivan PF, Carter FA, McIntosh VV, Joyce PR: The role of exposure with response prevention in the cognitive-behavioural therapy for bulimia nervosa. Psychol Med 1998; 28:611–623 [A–]
649. Bulik CM, Sullivan PF, Joyce PR, Carter FA, McIntosh VV: Predictors of 1-year treatment outcome in bulimia nervosa. Compr Psychiatry 1998; 39:206–214 [G]

650. Davis R, McVey G, Heinmaa M, Rockert W, Kennedy S: Sequencing of cognitive-behavioral treatments for bulimia nervosa. Int J Eat Disord 1999; 25:361–374 [G]
651. Hay PJ, Bacaltchuk J, Stefano S: Psychotherapy for bulimia nervosa and binging. Cochrane Database Syst Rev 2004; CD000562 [B]
652. Hsu LK, Rand W, Sullivan S, Liu DW, Mulliken B, McDonagh B, Kaye WH: Cognitive therapy, nutritional therapy and their combination in the treatment of bulimia nervosa. Psychol Med 2001; 31:871–879 [A]
653. Wilson GT, Fairburn CC, Agras WS, Walsh BT, Kraemer H: Cognitive-behavioral therapy for bulimia nervosa: time course and mechanisms of change. J Consult Clin Psychol 2002; 70:267–274 [G]
654. Wilson GT, Loeb KL, Walsh BT, Labouvie E, Petkova E, Liu X, Waternaux C: Psychological versus pharmacological treatments of bulimia nervosa: predictors and processes of change. J Consult Clin Psychol 1999; 67:451–459 [C]
655. Agras WS, Schneider JA, Arnow B, Raeburn SD, Telch CF: Cognitive-behavioral and response-prevention treatments for bulimia nervosa. J Consult Clin Psychol 1989; 57:215–221 [A–]
656. Fairburn CG: Cognitive behavioral treatment for bulimia, in Handbook of Psychotherapy for Anorexia Nervosa and Bulimia. Edited by Garner DM, Garfinkel PE. New York, Guilford, 1985, pp 160–192 [G]
657. Fairburn CG, Kirk J, O'Connor M, Cooper PJ: A comparison of two psychological treatments for bulimia nervosa. Behav Res Ther 1985; 24:629–643 [B]
658. Fairburn C: A cognitive behavioural approach to the treatment of bulimia. Psychol Med 1981; 11:707–711 [B]
659. Fairburn CG, Norman PA, Welch SL, O'Connor ME, Doll HA, Peveler RC: A prospective study of outcome in bulimia nervosa and the long-term effects of three psychological treatments. Arch Gen Psychiatry 1995; 52:304–312 [A–]
660. Fairburn CG, Jones R, Peveler RC, Carr SJ, Solomon RA, O'Connor ME, Burton J, Hope RA: Three psychological treatments for bulimia nervosa: a comparative trial. Arch Gen Psychiatry 1991; 48:463–469 [A–]
661. Wilson GT, Eldredge KL, Smith D, Niles B: Cognitive-behavioral treatment with and without response prevention for bulimia. Behav Res Ther 1991; 29:575–583 [A–]
662. Wilson GT, Rossiter E, Kleifield EI, Lindholm L: Cognitive-behavioral treatment of bulimia nervosa: a controlled evaluation. Behav Res Ther 1986; 24:277–288 [B]
663. Lacey JH: Bulimia nervosa, binge eating, and psychogenic vomiting: a controlled treatment study and long term outcome. Br Med J (Clin Res Ed) 1983; 286:1609–1613 [B]
664. Connors ME, Johnson CL, Stuckey MK: Treatment of bulimia with brief psychoeducational group therapy. Am J Psychiatry 1984; 141:1512–1516 [B]
665. Freeman CP, Barry F, Dunkeld-Turnbull J, Henderson A: Controlled trial of psychotherapy for bulimia nervosa. Br Med J (Clin Res Ed) 1988; 296:521–525 [A–]
666. Kirkley BG, Schneider JA, Agras WS, Bachman JA: Comparison of two group treatments for bulimia. J Consult Clin Psychol 1985; 53:43–48 [A–]
667. Lee NF, Rush AJ: Cognitive-behavioral group therapy for bulimia. Int J Eat Disord 1986; 5:599–615 [A–]
668. Ordman AM, Kirschenbaum DS: Cognitive-behavioral therapy for bulimia: an initial outcome study. J Consult Clin Psychol 1985; 53:305–313 [A–]
669. Beck AT, Steer RA, Garbin MG: Psychometric properties of the BDI: twenty-five years of evaluation. Clin Psychol Rev 1988; 8:77–100 [G]
670. Hamilton M: A rating scale for depression. J Neurol Neurosurg Psychiatry 1960; 23:56–62 [D]
671. Lock J: Adjusting cognitive behavior therapy for adolescents with bulimia nervosa: results of a case series. Am J Psychother 2005; 59:267–281[G]

672. Schapman-Williams AM, Lock J, Couturier J: Cognitive-behavioral therapy for adolescents with binge eating syndromes: a case series. Int J Eat Disord (in press) [G]
673. Root MPP: Persistent, disordered eating as a gender-specific, post-traumatic stress response to sexual assault. Psychotherapy 1991; 28:96–102 [G]
674. Laessle RG, Tuschl RJ, Kotthaus BC, Pirke KM: A comparison of the validity of three scales for the assessment of dietary restraint. J Abnorm Psychol 1989; 98:504–507 [E]
675. Leitenberg H, Rosen JC, Gross J, Nudelman S, Vara LS: Exposure plus response-prevention treatment of bulimia nervosa. J Consult Clin Psychol 1988; 56:535–541 [A–]
676. Johnson C: Diagnostic survey for eating disorders in initial consultation for patients with bulimia and anorexia nervosa, in Handbook of Psychotherapy for Anorexia Nervosa and Bulimia. Edited by Garner DM, Garfinkel PE. New York, Guilford, 1985, pp 19–51 [G]
677. Safer DL, Telch CF, Agras WS: Dialectical behavior therapy for bulimia nervosa. Am J Psychiatry 2001; 158:632–634 [A–]
678. Favazza AR, DeRosear L, Conterio K: Self-mutilation and eating disorders. Suicide Life Threat Behav 1989; 19:352–361 [G]
679. Esplen MJ, Garfinkel PE, Olmsted M, Gallop RM, Kennedy S: A randomized controlled trial of guided imagery in bulimia nervosa. Psychol Med 1998; 28:1347–1357 [A–]
680. Oesterheld JR, McKenna MS, Gould NB: Group psychotherapy of bulimia: a critical review. Int J Group Psychother 1987; 37:163–184 [F]
681. Chen E, Touyz SW, Beumont PJ, Fairburn CG, Griffiths R, Butow P, Russell J, Schotte DE, Gertler R, Basten C: Comparison of group and individual cognitive-behavioral therapy for patients with bulimia nervosa. Int J Eat Disord 2003; 33:241–254 [A]
682. Schwartz RC, Barett MJ, Saba G: Family Therapy for Bulimia. New York, Guilford, 1985 [G]
683. Malenbaum R, Herzog D, Eisenthal S, Wyshak G: Overeaters Anonymous. Int J Eat Disord 1988; 7:139–144 [G]
684. Cooper PJ, Coker S, Fleming C: Self-help for bulimia nervosa: a preliminary report. Int J Eat Disord 1994; 16:401–404 [B]
685. Cooper PJ, Coker S, Fleming C: An evaluation of the efficacy of supervised cognitive behavioral self-help bulimia nervosa. J Psychosom Res 1996; 40:281–287 [B]
686. Treasure J, Schmidt U, Troop N, Tiller J, Todd G, Keilen M, Dodge E: Sequential treatment for bulimia nervosa incorporating a self-care manual. Br J Psychiatry 1995; 167:1–5 [B]
687. Treasure J, Schmidt U, Troop N, Tiller J, Todd G, Keilen M, Dodge E: First step in managing bulimia nervosa: controlled trial of therapeutic manual. BMJ 1994; 308:686–689 [B]
688. Thiels C, Schmidt U, Treasure J, Garthe R: Four-year follow-up of guided self-change for bulimia nervosa. Eat Weight Disord 2003; 8:212–217 [G]
689. Mitchell JE, Fletcher L, Hanson K, Mussell MP, Seim H, Crosby R, Al Banna M: The relative efficacy of fluoxetine and manual-based self-help in the treatment of outpatients with bulimia nervosa. J Clin Psychopharmacol 2001; 21:298–304 [A–]
690. Perkins S, Schmidt U: Self-help for eating disorders, in AED Review of Eating Disorders, Part 1. Edited by Wonderlich S, Mitchell JE, de Zwaan M, Steiger H. Oxford, UK, Radcliffe, 2005, pp 87–104 [G]
691. Agras WS: Cognitive Behavior Therapy Treatment Manual for Bulimia Nervosa. Stanford, CA, Stanford University School of Medicine, Department of Psychiatry and Behavioral Sciences, 1991 [G]
692. Agras WS, Apple R: Overcoming Eating Disorders: Therapist's Guide. San Antonio, Psychological Corp (Harcourt), 1998 [G]
693. Apple R, Agras WS: Overcoming Eating Disorders: Client Workbook. San Antonio, Psychological Corp (Harcourt), 1998 [G]
694. Boutacoff LI, Zollman M, Mitchell JE: Healthy Eating: A Meal Planning System: Group Treatment Manual. Minneapolis, University of Minnesota Hospital and Clinic, Department of Psychiatry, 1989 [G]

695. Mitchell JE: Bulimia Nervosa: Individual Treatment Manual. Eating Disorders Program Staff. Minneapolis, University of Minnesota Hospital and Clinic, Department of Psychiatry, 1989 [G]
696. Mitchell JE: Bulimia Nervosa: Group Treatment Manual. Eating Disorders Program Staff. Minneapolis, University of Minnesota Hospital and Clinic, Department of Psychiatry, 1991 [G]
697. Walsh BT, Stewart JW, Roose SP, Gladis M, Glassman AH: Treatment of bulimia with phenelzine: a double-blind, placebo-controlled study. Arch Gen Psychiatry 1984; 41:1105–1109 [A]
698. Goldstein DJ, Wilson MG, Ascroft RC, Al Banna M: Effectiveness of fluoxetine therapy in bulimia nervosa regardless of comorbid depression. Int J Eat Disord 1999; 25:19–27 [G]
699. Alger SA, Schwalberg MD, Bigaouette JM, Michalek AV, Howard LJ: Effect of a tricyclic antidepressant and opiate antagonist on binge-eating behavior in normoweight bulimic and obese, binge-eating subjects. Am J Clin Nutr 1991; 53:865–871 [A]
700. Fahy TA, Eisler I, Russell GF: A placebo-controlled trial of D-fenfluramine in bulimia nervosa. Br J Psychiatry 1993; 162:597–603 [B]
701. Fichter MM, Kruger R, Rief W, Holland R, Dohne J: Fluvoxamine in prevention of relapse in bulimia nervosa: effects on eating-specific psychopathology. J Clin Psychopharmacol 1996; 16:9–18 [A]
702. Fichter MM, Leibl K, Rief W, Brunner E, Schmidt-Auberger S, Engel RR: Fluoxetine versus placebo: a double-blind study with bulimic inpatients undergoing intensive psychotherapy. Pharmacopsychiatry 1991; 24:1–7 [A]
703. Freeman CP, Morris JE, Cheshire KE, Davies M, Hamson M: A double-blind controlled trial of fluoxetine versus placebo for bulimia nervosa, in Proceedings of the Third International Conference on Eating Disorders. New York, 1988 [A]
704. Igoin-Apfelbaum L, Apfelbaum M: Naltrexone and bulimic symptoms. Lancet 1987; 2:1087–1088 [A]
705. Jonas JM, Gold MS: Naltrexone reverses bulimic symptoms. Lancet 1986; 1:807 [G]
706. Jonas JM, Gold MS: Treatment of antidepressant-resistant bulimia with naltrexone. Int J Eat Disord 1986; 16:306–309 [B]
707. Mitchell JE, Christenson G, Jennings J, Huber M, Thomas B, Pomeroy C, Morley J: A placebo-controlled, double-blind crossover study of naltrexone hydrochloride in outpatients with normal weight bulimia. J Clin Psychopharmacol 1989; 9:94–97 [A]
708. Pope HG Jr, Keck PE Jr, McElroy SL, Hudson JI: A placebo-controlled study of trazodone in bulimia nervosa. J Clin Psychopharmacol 1989; 9:254–259 [A]
709. Rothschild R, Quitkin HM, Quitkin FM, Stewart JW, Ocepek-Welikson K, McGrath PJ, Tricamo E: A double-blind placebo-controlled comparison of phenelzine and imipramine in the treatment of bulimia in atypical depressives. Int J Eat Disord 1994; 15:1–9 [A]
710. Sabine EJ, Yonace A, Farrington AJ, Barratt KH, Wakeling A: Bulimia nervosa: a placebo-controlled double-blind therapeutic trial of mianserin. Br J Clin Pharmacol 1983; 15(suppl 2):195S–202S [A]
711. Bacaltchuk J, Hay P, Trefiglio R: Antidepressants versus psychological treatments and their combination for bulimia nervosa. Cochrane Database Syst Rev 2001; CD003385 [E]
712. Bacaltchuk J, Trefiglio RP, Oliveira IR, Hay P, Lima MS, Mari JJ: Combination of antidepressants and psychological treatments for bulimia nervosa: a systematic review. Acta Psychiatr Scand 2000; 101:256–264 [E]
713. Bacaltchuk J, Trefiglio RP, de Oliveira IR, Lima MS, Mari JJ: Antidepressants versus psychotherapy for bulimia nervosa: a systematic review. J Clin Pharm Ther 1999; 24:23–31 [E]
714. Fassino S, Daga GA, Boggio S, Garzaro L, Piero A: Use of reboxetine in bulimia nervosa: a pilot study. J Psychopharmacol 2004; 18:423–428 [C]
715. Schmidt U, Cooper PJ, Essers H, Freeman CP, Holland RL, Palmer RL, Shur E, Russell GF, Bowler C, Coker S, Geddes JR, Mackenzie F, Munro J, Newton R, Tiller J, Tattersall

ML, Vize C, Webster J: Fluvoxamine and graded psychotherapy in the treatment of bulimia nervosa: a randomized, double-blind, placebo-controlled, multicenter study of short-term and long-term pharmacotherapy combined with a stepped care approach to psychotherapy. J Clin Psychopharmacol 2004; 24:549–552 [A]
716. Kennedy SH, Piran N, Warsh JJ, Prendergast P, Mainprize E, Whynot C, Garfinkel PE: A trial of isocarboxazid in the treatment of bulimia nervosa. J Clin Psychopharmacol 1988; 8:391–396 [A]
717. Carruba MO, Cuzzolaro M, Riva L, Bosello O, Liberti S, Castra R, Dalle GR, Santonastaso P, Garosi V, Nisoli E: Efficacy and tolerability of moclobemide in bulimia nervosa: a placebo-controlled trial. Int Clin Psychopharmacol 2001; 16:27–32 [A]
718. Marrazzi MA, Wroblewski JM, Kinzie J, Luby ED: High-dose naltrexone and liver function safety. Am J Addict 1997; 6:21–29 [B]
719. Faris PL, Kim SW, Meller WH, Goodale RL, Oakman SA, Hofbauer RD, Marshall AM, Daughters RS, Banerjee-Stevens D, Eckert ED, Hartman BK: Effect of decreasing afferent vagal activity with ondansetron on symptoms of bulimia nervosa: a randomised, double-blind trial. Lancet 2000; 355:792–797 [A]
720. Kaplan AS, Garfinkel PE, Darby PL, Garner DM: Carbamazepine in the treatment of bulimia. Am J Psychiatry 1983; 140:1225–1226 [A]
721. Leitenberg H, Rosen JC, Wolf J, Vara LS, Detzer MJ, Srebnik D: Comparison of cognitive-behavior therapy and desipramine in the treatment of bulimia nervosa. Behav Res Ther 1994; 32:37–45 [A–]
722. Olmsted MP, Kaplan AS, Rockert W: Rate and prediction of relapse in bulimia nervosa. Am J Psychiatry 1994; 151:738–743 [C]
723. de Zwaan M, Mitchell JE, Mussell MP, Crosby RD: Does CBT improve outcomes in obese binge eaters participating in a very low-calorie diet treatment? Paper presented at the annual meeting of the Eating Disorders Research Society, Pittsburgh, November 15–17, 1996 [B]
724. Telch CF, Agras WS: The effects of a very low calorie diet on binge eating. Behavior Therapy 1993; 24:177–193 [B]
725. Wadden TA, Foster GD, Letizia KA: Response of obese binge eaters to treatment by behavior therapy combined with very low calorie diet. J Consult Clin Psychol 1992; 60:808–811 [A–]
726. Yanovski SZ, Gormally JF, Leser MS, Gwirtsman HE, Yanovski JA: Binge eating disorder affects outcome of comprehensive very-low calorie diet treatment. Obes Res 1994; 2:205–212 [B]
727. Marcus MD, Wing RR: Cognitive treatment of binge eating, V: behavioral weight control in the treatment of binge eating disorder (letter). Ann Behav Med 1995; 17:S090 [A–]
728. Reeves RS, McPherson RS, Nichaman MZ, Harrist RB, Foreyt JP, Goodrick GK: Nutrient intake of obese female binge eaters. J Am Diet Assoc 2001; 101:209–215 [A–]
729. Gladis MM, Wadden TA, Vogt R, Foster G, Kuehnel RH, Bartlett SJ: Behavioral treatment of obese binge eaters: do they need different care? J Psychosom Res 1998; 44:375–384 [B]
730. Linde JA, Jeffery RW, Levy RL, Sherwood NE, Utter J, Pronk NP, Boyle RG: Binge eating disorder, weight control self-efficacy, and depression in overweight men and women. Int J Obes Relat Metab Disord 2004; 28:418–425 [A–]
731. Pendleton VR, Goodrick GK, Poston WS, Reeves RS, Foreyt JP: Exercise augments the effects of cognitive-behavioral therapy in the treatment of binge eating. Int J Eat Disord 2002; 31:172–184 [B]
732. Wadden TA, Foster GD, Sarwer DB, Anderson DA, Gladis M, Sanderson RS, Letchak RV, Berkowitz RI, Phelan S: Dieting and the development of eating disorders in obese women: results of a randomized controlled trial. Am J Clin Nutr 2004; 80:560–568 [A–]
733. Agras WS, Telch CF, Arnow B, Eldredge K, Detzer MJ, Henderson J, Marnell M: Does interpersonal therapy help patients with binge eating disorder who fail to respond to cognitive-behavioral therapy? J Consult Clin Psychol 1995; 63:356–360 [B]

734. Eldredge KL, Agras WS, Arnow B, Telch CF, Bell S, Castonguay L, Marnell M: The effects of extending cognitive-behavioral therapy for binge eating disorder among initial treatment nonresponders. Int J Eat Disord 1999; 21:352 [B]
735. Smith DE, Marcus MD, Kaye W: Cognitive-behavioral treatment of obese binge eaters. Int J Eat Disord 1992; 12:257–262 [B]
736. Telch CF, Agras WS, Rossiter EM, Wilfley D, Kenardy J: Group cognitive-behavioral treatment for the nonpurging bulimic: an initial evaluation. J Consult Clin Psychol 1990; 58:629–635 [B]
737. Wilfley DE, Agras WS, Telch CF, Rossiter EM, Schneider JA, Cole AG, Sifford LA, Raeburn SD: Group cognitive-behavioral therapy and group interpersonal psychotherapy for the nonpurging bulimic individual: a controlled comparison. J Consult Clin Psychol 1993; 61:296–305 [A–]
738. Telch CF, Agras WS, Linehan MM: Dialectical behavior therapy for binge eating disorder. J Consult Clin Psychol 2001; 69:1061–1065 [A–]
739. Riva G, Bacchetta M, Cesa G, Conti S, Molinari E: Six-month follow-up of in-patient experiential cognitive therapy for binge eating disorders. Cyberpsychol Behav 2003; 6:251–258 [A–]
740. Riva G, Bacchetta M, Baruffi M, Molinari E: Virtual-reality-based multidimensional therapy for the treatment of body image disturbances in binge eating disorders: a preliminary controlled study. IEEE Trans Inf Technol Biomed 2002; 6:224–234 [B]
741. Tanco S, Linden W, Earle T: Well-being and morbid obesity in women: a controlled therapy evaluation. Int J Eat Disord 1998; 23:325–339 [A–]
742. Bacon L, Stern JS, Van Loan MD, Keim NL: Size acceptance and intuitive eating improve health for obese, female chronic dieters. J Am Diet Assoc 2005; 105:929–936 [A–]
743. Goodrick GK, Poston WS, Kimball KT, Reeves RS, Foreyt JP: Nondieting versus dieting treatment for overweight binge-eating women. J Consult Clin Psychol 1998; 66:363–368 [A–]
744. McElroy SL, Hudson JI, Malhotra S, Welge JA, Nelson EB, Keck PE Jr: Citalopram in the treatment of binge-eating disorder: a placebo-controlled trial. J Clin Psychiatry 2003; 64:807–813 [A]
745. Arnold LM, McElroy SL, Hudson JI, Welge JA, Bennett AJ, Keck PE: A placebo-controlled, randomized trial of fluoxetine in the treatment of binge-eating disorder. J Clin Psychiatry 2002; 63:1028–1033 [A]
746. Hudson JI, McElroy SL, Raymond NC, Crow S, Keck PE Jr, Carter WP, Mitchell JE, Strakowski SM, Pope HG Jr, Coleman BS, Jonas JM: Fluvoxamine in the treatment of binge-eating disorder: a multicenter placebo-controlled, double-blind trial. Am J Psychiatry 1998; 155:1756–1762 [A]
747. McElroy SL, Casuto LS, Nelson EB, Lake KA, Soutullo CA, Keck PE Jr, Hudson JI: Placebo-controlled trial of sertraline in the treatment of binge eating disorder. Am J Psychiatry 2000; 157:1004–1006 [A]
748. McCann UD, Agras WS: Successful treatment of nonpurging bulimia nervosa with desipramine: a double-blind, placebo-controlled study. Am J Psychiatry 1990; 147:1509–1513 [A]
749. Pearlstein T, Spurell E, Hohlstein LA, Gurney V, Read J, Fuchs C, Keller MB: A double-blind, placebo-controlled trial of fluvoxamine in binge eating disorder: a high placebo response. Arch Women Ment Health 2003; 6:147–151 [A]
750. Malhotra S, King KH, Welge JA, Brusman-Lovins L, McElroy SL: Venlafaxine treatment of binge-eating disorder associated with obesity: a series of 35 patients. J Clin Psychiatry 2002; 63:802–806 [G]
751. Hirschfeld RM: Long-term side effects of SSRIs: sexual dysfunction and weight gain. J Clin Psychiatry 2003; 64(suppl 18):20–24 [F]

752. Mitchell JE, Gosnell BA, Roerig JL, de Zwaan M, Wonderlich SA, Crosby RD, Burgard MA, Wambach BN: Effects of sibutramine on binge eating, hunger, and fullness in a laboratory human feeding paradigm. Obes Res 2003; 11:599–602 [A]
753. Abenhaim L, Moride Y, Brenot F, Rich S, Benichou J, Kurz X, Higenbottam T, Oakley C, Wouters E, Aubier M, Simonneau G, Begaud B: Appetite-suppressant drugs and the risk of primary pulmonary hypertension. International Primary Pulmonary Hypertension Study Group. N Engl J Med 1996; 335:609–616 [D]
754. Connolly HM, Crary JL, McGoon MD, Hensrud DD, Edwards BS, Edwards WD, Schaff HV: Valvular heart disease associated with fenfluramine-phentermine. N Engl J Med 1997; 337:581–588 [C]
755. Graham DJ, Green L: Further cases of valvular heart disease associated with fenfluramine-phentermine. N Engl J Med 1997; 337:635 [G]
756. Mark EJ, Patalas ED, Chang HT, Evans RJ, Kessler SC: Fatal pulmonary hypertension associated with short-term use of fenfluramine and phentermine. N Engl J Med 1997; 337:602–606 [G]
757. Shapira NA, Goldsmith TD, McElroy SL: Treatment of binge-eating disorder with topiramate: a clinical case series. J Clin Psychiatry 2000; 61:368–372 [G]
758. Appolinario JC, Fontenelle LF, Papelbaum M, Bueno JR, Coutinho W: Topiramate use in obese patients with binge eating disorder: an open study. Can J Psychiatry 2002; 47:271–273 [B]
759. Ricca V, Mannucci E, Mezzani B, Moretti S, Di Bernardo M, Bertelli M, Rotella CM, Faravelli C: Fluoxetine and fluvoxamine combined with individual cognitive-behaviour therapy in binge eating disorder: a one-year follow-up study. Psychother Psychosom 2001; 70:298–306 [A–]
760. O'Reardon JO, Allison KC, Martino NS, Lundgren JD, Heo M, Stunkard AJ: A randomized placebo-controlled trial of sertraline in the treatment of the night eating syndrome. Am J Psychiatry (in press) [A]
761. Winkelman JW: Treatment of nocturnal eating syndrome and sleep-related eating disorder with topiramate. Sleep Med 2003; 4:243–246 [G]
762. Schenck CH, Mahowald MW: Combined bupropion-levodopa-trazodone therapy of sleep-related eating and sleep disruption in two adults with chemical dependency. Sleep 2000; 23:587–588 [G]
763. Schenck CH, Hurwitz TD, O'Connor KA, Mahowald MW: Additional categories of sleep-related eating disorders and the current status of treatment. Sleep 1993; 16:457–466 [G]
764. Maj M, Halmi K, Lopez-Ibor JJ, Sartorius N (eds): Eating Disorders: WPA Series Evidence and Experience in Psychiatry, vol 6. West Sussex, UK, Wiley, 2003 [G]
765. Strober M: The future of treatment research in anorexia nervosa. Int J Eat Disord 2005; 37(suppl): S90–S94 [G]

GUIDELINE WATCH: PRACTICE GUIDELINE FOR THE TREATMENT OF PATIENTS WITH BORDERLINE PERSONALITY DISORDER

John M. Oldham, M.D., M.S.

Since the 2001 publication of APA's *Practice Guideline for the Treatment of Patients With Borderline Personality Disorder* (1), more studies have been published on borderline personality disorder (BPD) than on any other personality disorder (2, 3). New analyses of the validity of the DSM-IV-TR criteria–defined construct of BPD have been published, new data on the prevalence of BPD are available, risk factors for and biological characteristics of BPD are being elucidated, and new studies on the treatment of BPD have been carried out. This guideline watch highlights the most important of these developments.

DEFINITION, DIAGNOSTIC STABILITY, AND LONGITUDINAL COURSE

Definition

With an eye toward DSM-V, careful examination of axis II is occurring. This has, in part, included comparing the relative merits of categorical systems such as DSM-IV-TR and dimensional systems such as the five-factor model (4). This debate is as yet unresolved. However, recent studies have analyzed the nine DSM-IV criteria that define BPD and have concluded that, as defined, BPD appears to reflect a statistically coherent construct (5, 6). Utilization of a polythetic system requiring five out of nine criteria to make a categorical BPD diagnosis inevitably results in extensive heterogeneity within and between BPD populations being treated

---

The American Psychiatric Association (APA) practice guidelines are developed by expert work groups using an explicit methodology that includes rigorous review of available evidence, broad peer review of iterative drafts, and formal approval by the APA Assembly and Board of Trustees. APA practice guidelines are intended to assist psychiatrists in clinical decision making. They are not intended to be a standard of care. The ultimate judgment regarding a particular clinical procedure or treatment plan must be made by the psychiatrist in light of the clinical data presented by the patient and the diagnostic and treatment options available. Guideline watches summarize significant developments in practice since publication of an APA practice guideline. Watches may be authored and reviewed by experts associated with the original guideline development effort and are approved for publication by APA's Executive Committee on Practice Guidelines. Thus, watches represent opinion of the authors and approval of the Executive Committee but not policy of the APA. This guideline watch was published in March 2005. Suggested citation: Oldham JM: *Guideline Watch: Practice Guideline for the Treatment of Patients With Borderline Personality Disorder.* Arlington, VA: American Psychiatric Association, 2005. Available online at http://www.psych.org/psych_pract/treatg/pg/prac_guide.cfm.

or studied. Increased attention is being focused on how to set the appropriate diagnostic "cut-off point" (i.e., the minimum number of criteria required to make the diagnosis). Also under discussion is whether some core criteria should be essential or whether all criteria should be weighted equally in establishing a diagnosis. New data also emphasize the importance of evaluating the degree of functional impairment in patients with BPD (7). A dimensional approach can be used to measure overall levels of dysfunction (8). Alternatively, the DSM criteria can be assessed in a dimensional fashion to capture functional impairment (9). However, even with proposed dimensional approaches, a discrete diagnostic threshold would need to be established in terms of illness severity and need for treatment (10).

A number of recent studies have examined the boundaries between BPD and selected axis I conditions. Since some patients with BPD may benefit from mood-stabilizing medications, the overlap between BPD and bipolar II disorder has been of particular interest (11–13). Although some individuals with BPD will also have a co-occurring bipolar disorder, the majority of the evidence to date supports BPD as an independent diagnosis rather than an attenuated form of a mood disorder (14–16). Similarly, though patients with BPD frequently have a history of trauma, the diagnosis is not considered a variant of posttraumatic stress disorder (PTSD) (17, 18). Of continuing interest is the identification of early precursors of BPD, such as a possible association between a history of childhood attention deficit hyperactivity disorder (ADHD) symptoms and diagnosis of BPD in adulthood (19).

Diagnostic stability and longitudinal course

New prospective longitudinal studies evaluating the long-term stability of BPD have been published. Results of the NIMH Collaborative Longitudinal Personality Disorders Study indicate that at 2 years after BPD diagnosis, only 44% of the patients retain the diagnosis (20). The McLean Hospital group has reported a 6-year follow-up of borderline patients in which 74% of the patients met criteria for remission over the entire follow-up period (21). Longer-term results have been published by Canadian researchers indicating that only 8% of the total borderline patient group still met diagnostic criteria at 27-year follow-up (22, 23). High rates of remission are speculated to relate to a number of factors, such as treatment effectiveness and/or fluctuating severity of comorbid axis I conditions. BPD has been shown to be significantly associated with major depressive disorder (MDD) and PTSD longitudinally (24). Somewhat counterintuitively, however, when BPD and MDD were followed over time, improvement in MDD was not followed by improvement in BPD; instead, improvement in MDD was more often predicted by prior improvement in BPD (25). Thus, the primary determinants of change in patients with BPD may not be related to comorbid axis I psychopathology (26). Other suggested contributions to high rates of remission of BPD over time include diminished impulsivity with increased age (27), social learning, and stress-reducing life adjustments such as avoidance of interpersonal intimacy (22). It should be noted that the concept of remission of BPD reflects dropping below the DSM-IV-TR threshold on the continuum of criteria defining the disorder, yet significant problems relating to the personality structure and organization can continue even if the diagnostic threshold has not been met.

EPIDEMIOLOGY, BIOLOGY, AND ETIOLOGY

To date, few population-based studies of personality disorders have been carried out. Torgersen (28) tabulated the results of eight epidemiological studies, including the large Norwegian study done by his own group; the mean prevalence of BPD across all studies was 1.2%. In Torgersen et al.'s study of 2,053 individuals in Norway, BPD was found to be equally prevalent among males and females (29). Although it is widely perceived that treatment populations of patients with BPD consist predominantly of females, published studies are in fact contradictory on this point (30). Prevalence of BPD in treatment populations remains much higher than in the general population, and a recent study of a primary care population reported BPD to be fourfold higher than in the general population (31).

New studies are examining the multiple etiologies of BPD, based on the clear relevance of genetic, neurobiological, and psychosocial factors (32, 33). Although the magnitude of the heritability of BPD is thought to be significant (34), genetic risk factors specific to BPD have not been identified. One promising approach may be the study of underlying traits, such as novelty seeking (35) or impulsivity (36). Among the environmental contributions to the etiology of BPD, the role of childhood abuse remains prominent (37), particularly severe abuse (38) and sustained abuse (39).

Deficits in cognitive functioning, such as decision making (40), conflict resolution (41), and "effortful control" (41, 42), are being reported. These deficits are thought to be mediated in the frontal lobe, although not all studies have found frontal lobe impairment in cognitive functioning (43). A number of studies have suggested reduced central nervous system serotonin levels in borderline patients and other patients who demonstrate impulsive-aggressive behavior, but such behavioral disinhibition may reflect dysfunction in multiple monoaminergic systems and may not be specific to BPD (44).

Brain imaging studies of patients with BPD suggest irregularities in both structure and function (44–46). Limbic studies have found reduced volume in the amygdala and hippocampus (47, 48), altered amygdala activation (49, 50), and hippocampal hypometabolism (51). Frontal lobe studies suggest dysfunction of the dorsolateral and medial prefrontal cortex in connection with memories of abandonment (52), of the medial orbital frontal cortex in connection with diminished regulation of impulsive behavior (53), and of the prefrontal cortex under resting conditions (51). In addition, decreased binding of a serotonin precursor has been reported in the medial prefrontal cortex and anterior cingulate cortex in patients with BPD (54). Taken together, these studies suggest abnormalities in prefrontal, corticostriatal, and limbic networks perhaps related to lowered serotonin neurotransmission and behavioral disinhibition (55). Although findings from brain imaging studies are "not ready for prime time" to guide treatment planning for patients with BPD, these techniques may well have relevance in the future for individualized prediction of treatment outcome (46).

TREATMENT

Evidence and opinion continue to support the recommendation of the 2001 guideline that psychotherapy represents the primary, or core, treatment for this disorder and that adjunctive, symptom-targeted pharmacotherapy can be helpful. For personality disorders in general, studies of psychotherapy report its effectiveness (56, 57). Persuasive data from randomized, controlled trials (RCTs) of BPD suggest that more than one type of psychotherapy is effective, and additional studies are under way. Dialectical behavior therapy (DBT) has been shown in an RCT to be effective for borderline symptoms in patients with comorbid BPD and substance abuse, though no improvement was shown for the substance abuse itself (58). In another RCT, in patients with BPD and comorbid opiate use, DBT was compared with comprehensive validation therapy (CVT). Both types of treatment were effective. There were fewer dropouts in the CVT group, and the maintenance of gains was greater in the DBT group (59). Studies of DBT by diverse research groups are being published, including a study of female veterans with BPD that compared 6 months of DBT with treatment as usual and reported improvement in the DBT group compared with the control group (60). Another study from the Netherlands that compared 12 months of outpatient DBT with treatment as usual showed better treatment retention, reduced self-mutilation, and reduced self-damaging impulsivity in the DBT group (61). An intriguing inpatient RCT that compared 3 months of inpatient DBT with treatment as usual in the community demonstrated significant gains in the DBT group compared with the control group, including reduced self-injury, dissociation, depression, and anxiety, and improved interpersonal functioning and social adjustment (62).

Promising new psychotherapies for BPD are being piloted in open trials. These include interpersonal therapy (63); cognitive therapy (64); cognitive analytic therapy (CAT), a fusion of cognitive and psychodynamic therapy (65, 66); and systems training for emotional predictability and problem solving (STEPPS), a cognitive-behavioral systems–based form of time-limited group treatment for patients with BPD (67). In an ongoing study comparing transference-focused psychotherapy (TFP) with DBT and supportive psychotherapy, TFP appeared to be beneficial (68), although the comparative analysis of the other two treatments has yet to be completed. The efficacy of TFP is also being assessed in a large multicenter study comparing TFP with schema therapy for patients with BPD (69).

A number of recent studies have focused on the benefits of pharmacotherapy for patients with BPD. An RCT that compared patients receiving fluvoxamine with a control group showed robust, long-lasting reduction in rapid mood shifts only in the treatment group (70). Another RCT that compared olanzapine with placebo in borderline patients showed improvement in global functioning in the medication group compared with the placebo group (71). Another RCT studied three groups of BPD patients—one group receiving fluoxetine, a second group receiving olanzapine, and a third receiving a combination of both; all three interventions led to substantial improvement, though a significantly greater rate of improvement in clinician-rated depression and impulsive aggression was seen in the olanzapine and the combination groups (72). Also, double-blind, placebo-controlled trials demonstrated benefit of divalproex sodium for patients with BPD (73) and for patients with cluster B personality disorders who demonstrate impulsive aggression (74). A number of case reports and noncontrolled medication trials have also been published (75–81).

All in all, the database is growing, and further evidence is accumulating that BPD is a condition that can be effectively treated by a combination of psychotherapy and symptom-targeted pharmacotherapy. Further research is needed to validate the approach taken by the 2001 guideline to select one of three different medication algorithms on the basis of the predominance of cognitive-perceptual symptoms, affective dysregulation symptoms, or impulse dyscontrol symptoms. One retrospective report from the NIMH Collaborative Longitudinal Personality Disorders Study produced mixed results on this question (82).

REFERENCES

1. American Psychiatric Association: Practice guideline for the treatment of patients with borderline personality disorder. Am J Psychiatry 2001; 158:1–52
2. Trull TJ, Stepp SD, Durrett CA: Research on borderline personality disorder: an update. Current Opinion in Psychiatry 2003; 16:77–82
3. Skodol AE: Manifestations, clinical diagnosis, and comorbidity, in The American Psychiatric Publishing Textbook of Personality Disorders. Edited by Oldham JM, Skodol AE, Bender DS. Washington, DC, American Psychiatric Publishing, 2005, pp 57–87
4. Simonsen E, Widiger TA: Limitations of existing diagnostic categories. Launch Conference on Personality Disorders, Washington, DC, December 2–3, 2004
5. Sanislow CA, Grilo CM, Morey LC, Bender DS, Skodol AE, Gunderson JG, Shea MT, Stout RL, Zanarini MC, McGlashan TH: Confirmatory factor analysis of DSM-IV criteria for borderline personality disorder: findings from the Collaborative Longitudinal Personality Disorders Study. Am J Psychiatry 2002; 159:284–290

6. Morey LC, Skodol AE, Grilo CM, Sanislow CA, Zanarini MC, Shea MT, Gunderson JG, McGlashan TH: Temporal coherence of criteria for four personality disorders. J Personal Disord 2004; 18:394–398
7. Skodol AE, Gunderson JG, McGlashan TH, Dyck IR, Stout RL, Bender DS, Grilo CM, Shea MT, Zanarini MC, Morey LC, Sanislow CA, Oldham JM: Functional impairment in patients with schizotypal, borderline, avoidant, or obsessive-compulsive personality disorder. Am J Psychiatry 2002; 159:276–283
8. Trull TJ, Widiger TA, Lynam DR, Costa PT Jr: Borderline personality disorder from the perspective of general personality functioning. J Abnorm Psychol 2003; 112:193–202
9. Skodol AE, Oldham JM, Bender DS, Dyck IR, Stout RL, Morey LC, Shea MT, Zanarini MC, Sanislow CA, Grilo CM, McGlashan TH, Gunderson JG: Dimensional representations of DSM-IV personality disorders: relationships to functional impairment. Am J Psychiatry 2005; 162:1919–1925
10. Rothschild L, Cleland C, Haslam N, Zimmerman M: A taxometric study of borderline personality disorder. J Abnorm Psychol 2003; 112:657–666
11. Deltito J, Martin L, Riefkohl J, Austria B, Kissilenko A, Corless CM: Do patients with borderline personality disorder belong to the bipolar spectrum? J Affect Disord 2001; 67:221–228
12. Henry C, Mitropoulou V, New AS, Koenigsberg HW, Silverman J, Siever LJ: Affective instability and impulsivity in borderline personality and bipolar II disorders: similarities and differences. J Psychiatr Res 2001; 35:307–312
13. Smith DJ, Muir WJ, Blackwood DH: Is borderline personality disorder part of the bipolar spectrum? Harv Rev Psychiatry 2004; 12:133–139
14. Koenigsberg HW, Harvey PD, Mitropoulou V, Schmeidler J, New AS, Goodman M, Silverman JM, Serby M, Schopick F, Siever LJ: Characterizing affective instability in borderline personality disorder. Am J Psychiatry 2002; 159:784–788
15. Magill CA: The boundary between borderline personality disorder and bipolar disorder: current concepts and challenges. Can J Psychiatry 2004; 49:551–556
16. Paris J: Borderline or bipolar? Distinguishing borderline personality disorder from bipolar spectrum disorders. Harv Rev Psychiatry 2004; 12:140–145
17. Golier JA, Yehuda R, Bierer LM, Mitropoulou V, New AS, Schmeidler J, Silverman JM, Siever LJ: The relationship of borderline personality disorder to posttraumatic stress disorder and traumatic events. Am J Psychiatry 2003; 160:2018–2024
18. Zlotnick C, Johnson DM, Yen S, Battle CL, Sanislow CA, Skodol AE, Grilo CM, McGlashan TH, Gunderson JG, Bender DS, Zanarini MC, Shea MT: Clinical features and impairment in women with Borderline Personality Disorder (BPD) with Posttraumatic Stress Disorder (PTSD), BPD without PTSD, and other personality disorders with PTSD. J Nerv Ment Dis 2003; 191:706–713
19. Fossati A, Novella L, Donati D, Donini M, Maffei C: History of childhood attention deficit/hyperactivity disorder symptoms and borderline personality disorder: a controlled study. Compr Psychiatry 2002; 43:369–377
20. Grilo CM, Shea MT, Sanislow CA, Skodol AE, Gunderson JG, Stout RL, Pagano ME, Yen S: Two-year stability and change of schizotypal, borderline, avoidant, and obsessive-compulsive personality disorders. J Consult Clin Psychol (in press)
21. Zanarini MC, Frankenburg FR, Hennen J, Silk KR: The longitudinal course of borderline psychopathology: 6-year prospective follow-up of the phenomenology of borderline personality disorder. Am J Psychiatry 2003; 160:274–283
22. Paris J: Implications of long-term outcome research for the management of patients with borderline personality disorder. Harv Rev Psychiatry 2002; 10:315–323
23. Paris J, Zweig-Frank H: A 27-year follow-up of patients with borderline personality disorders. Psychiatr Q 2000; 71:291–307

24. Shea MT, Stout RL, Yen S, Pagano ME, Skodol AE, Morey LC, Gunderson JG, McGlashan TH, Grilo CM, Sanislow CA, Bender DS, Zanarini MC: Associations in the course of personality disorders and axis I disorders over time. J Abnorm Psychol 2004; 113:499–508
25. Gunderson JG, Morey LC, Stout RL, Skodol AE, Shea MT, McGlashan TH, Zanarini MC, Grilo CM, Sanislow CA, Yen S, Daversa MT, Bender DS: Major depressive disorder and borderline personality disorder revisited: longitudinal interactions. J Clin Psychiatry 2004; 65:1049–1056
26. Warner MB, Morey LC, Finch JF, Gunderson JG, Skodol AE, Sanislow CA, Shea MT, McGlashan TH, Grilo CM: The longitudinal relationship of personality traits and disorders. J Abnorm Psychol 2004; 113:217–227
27. Stevenson J, Meares R, Comerford A: Diminished impulsivity in older patients with borderline personality disorder. Am J Psychiatry 2003; 160:165–166
28. Torgersen S: Epidemiology, in The American Psychiatric Publishing Textbook of Personality Disorders. Edited by Oldham JM, Skodol AE, Bender DS. Washington, DC, American Psychiatric Publishing, 2005, pp 129–141
29. Torgersen S, Kringlen E, Cramer V: The prevalence of personality disorders in a community sample. Arch Gen Psychiatry 2001; 58:590–596
30. Zlotnick C, Rothschild L, Zimmerman M: The role of gender in the clinical presentation of patients with borderline personality disorder. J Personal Disord 2002; 16:277–282
31. Gross R, Olfson M, Gameroff M, Shea S, Feder A, Fuentes M, Lantigua R, Weissman MM: Borderline personality disorder in primary care. Arch Intern Med 2002; 162:53–60
32. Skodol AE, Siever LJ, Livesley WJ, Gunderson JG, Pfohl B, Widiger TA: The borderline diagnosis II: biology, genetics, and clinical course. Biol Psychiatry 2002; 51:951–963
33. Siever LJ, Torgersen S, Gunderson JG, Livesley WJ, Kendler KS: The borderline diagnosis III: identifying endophenotypes for genetic studies. Biol Psychiatry 2002; 51:964–968
34. Torgersen S, Lygren S, Oien PA, Skre I, Onstad S, Edvardsen J, Tambs K, Kringlen E: A twin study of personality disorders. Compr Psychiatry 2000; 41:416–425
35. Cloninger CR: Genetics, in The American Psychiatric Publishing Textbook of Personality Disorders. Edited by Oldham JM, Skodol AE, Bender DS. Washington, DC, American Psychiatric Publishing, 2005, pp 143–154
36. New AS, Siever LJ: Neurobiology and genetics of borderline personality disorder. Psychiatric Annals 2002; 32:329–336
37. Trull TJ: Structural relations between borderline personality disorder features and putative etiological correlates. J Abnorm Psychol 2001; 110:471–481
38. Zanarini MC, Yong L, Frankenburg FR, Hennen J, Reich DB, Marino MF, Vujanovic AA: Severity of reported childhood sexual abuse and its relationship to severity of borderline psychopathology and psychosocial impairment among borderline inpatients. J Nerv Ment Dis 2002; 190:381–387
39. Rinne T, de Kloet ER, Wouters L, Goekoop JG, DeRijk RH, van den BW: Hyperresponsiveness of hypothalamic-pituitary-adrenal axis to combined dexamethasone/corticotropin-releasing hormone challenge in female borderline personality disorder subjects with a history of sustained childhood abuse. Biol Psychiatry 2002; 52:1102–1112
40. Bazanis E, Rogers RD, Dowson JH, Taylor P, Meux C, Staley C, Nevinson-Andrews D, Taylor C, Robbins TW, Sahakian BJ: Neurocognitive deficits in decision-making and planning of patients with DSM-III-R borderline personality disorder. Psychol Med 2002; 32:1395–1405
41. Posner MI, Rothbart MK, Vizueta N, Levy KN, Evans DE, Thomas KM, Clarkin JF: Attentional mechanisms of borderline personality disorder. Proc Natl Acad Sci USA 2002; 99:16366–16370

42. Lenzenweger MF, Clarkin JF, Fertuck EA, Kernberg OF: Executive neurocognitive functioning and neurobehavioral systems indicators in borderline personality disorder: a preliminary study. J Personal Disord 2004; 18:421–438
43. Kunert HJ, Druecke HW, Sass H, Herpertz SC: Frontal lobe dysfunctions in borderline personality disorder? Neuropsychological findings. J Personal Disord 2003; 17:497–509
44. Coccaro EF, Siever LJ: Neurobiology, in The American Psychiatric Publishing Textbook of Personality Disorders. Edited by Oldham JM, Skodol AE, Bender DS. Washington, DC, American Psychiatric Publishing, 2005, pp 155–169
45. Nahas Z, Molnar C, George MS: Brain imaging, in The American Psychiatric Publishing Textbook of Personality Disorders. Edited by Oldham JM, Skodol AE, Bender DS. Washington, DC, American Psychiatric Publishing, 2005, pp 623–639
46. Etkin A, Pittenger CJ, Kandel ER: Biology in the service of psychotherapy, in The American Psychiatric Publishing Textbook of Personality Disorders. Edited by Oldham JM, Skodol AE, Bender DS. Washington, DC, American Psychiatric Publishing, 2005, pp 669–682
47. Schmahl CG, Vermetten E, Elzinga BM, Douglas BJ: Magnetic resonance imaging of hippocampal and amygdala volume in women with childhood abuse and borderline personality disorder. Psychiatry Res 2003; 122:193–198
48. Rusch N, van Elst LT, Ludaescher P, Wilke M, Huppertz HJ, Thiel T, Schmahl C, Bohus M, Lieb K, Hesslinger B, Hennig J, Ebert D: A voxel-based morphometric MRI study in female patients with borderline personality disorder. Neuroimage 2003; 20:385–392
49. Herpertz SC, Dietrich TM, Wenning B, Krings T, Erberich SG, Willmes K, Thron A, Sass H: Evidence of abnormal amygdala functioning in borderline personality disorder: a functional MRI study. Biol Psychiatry 2001; 50:292–298
50. Donegan NH, Sanislow CA, Blumberg HP, Fulbright RK, Lacadie C, Skudlarski P, Gore JC, Olson IR, McGlashan TH, Wexler BE: Amygdala hyperreactivity in borderline personality disorder: implications for emotional dysregulation. Biol Psychiatry 2003; 54:1284–1293
51. Juengling FD, Schmahl C, Hesslinger B, Ebert D, Bremner JD, Gostomzyk J, Bohus M, Lieb K: Positron emission tomography in female patients with borderline personality disorder. J Psychiatr Res 2003; 37:109–115
52. Schmahl CG, Elzinga BM, Vermetten E, Sanislow C, McGlashan TH, Bremner JD: Neural correlates of memories of abandonment in women with and without borderline personality disorder. Biol Psychiatry 2003; 54:142–151
53. Soloff PH, Meltzer CC, Becker C, Greer PJ, Kelly TM, Constantine D: Impulsivity and prefrontal hypometabolism in borderline personality disorder. Psychiatry Res 2003; 123:153–163
54. Leyton M, Okazawa H, Diksic M, Paris J, Rosa P, Mzengeza S, Young SN, Blier P, Benkelfat C: Brain regional alpha-[^{11}C]methyl-L-tryptophan trapping in impulsive subjects with borderline personality disorder. Am J Psychiatry 2001; 158:775–782
55. Johnson PA, Hurley RA, Benkelfat C, Herpertz SC, Taber KH: Understanding emotion regulation in borderline personality disorder: contributions of neuroimaging. J Neuropsychiatry Clin Neurosci 2003; 15:397–402
56. Leichsenring F, Leibing E: The effectiveness of psychodynamic therapy and cognitive behavior therapy in the treatment of personality disorders: a meta-analysis. Am J Psychiatry 2003; 160:1223–1232
57. Leichsenring F, Rabung S, Leibing E: The efficacy of short-term psychodynamic psychotherapy in specific psychiatric disorders: a meta-analysis. Arch Gen Psychiatry 2004; 61:1208–1216
58. van den Bosch LM, Verheul R, Schippers GM, van den BW: Dialectical behavior therapy of borderline patients with and without substance use problems: implementation and long-term effects. Addict Behav 2002; 27:911–923
59. Linehan MM, Dimeff LA, Reynolds SK, Comtois KA, Welch SS, Heagerty P, Kivlahan DR: Dialectical behavior therapy versus comprehensive validation therapy plus 12-step for

the treatment of opioid dependent women meeting criteria for borderline personality disorder. Drug Alcohol Depend 2002; 67:13–26
60. Koons C, Robins CJ, Tweed JL, Lynch TR, Gonzalez AM, Morse JQ, Bishop GK, Butterfield MI, Bastian LA: Efficacy of dialectical behavior therapy in women veterans with borderline personality disorder. Behavior Therapy 2001; 32:371–390
61. Verheul R, van den Bosch LM, Koeter MW, De Ridder MA, Stijnen T, van den BW: Dialectical behaviour therapy for women with borderline personality disorder: 12-month, randomised clinical trial in the Netherlands. Br J Psychiatry 2003; 182:135–140
62. Bohus M, Haaf B, Simms T, Limberger MF, Schmahl C, Unckel C, Lieb K, Linehan MM: Effectiveness of inpatient dialectical behavioral therapy for borderline personality disorder: a controlled trial. Behav Res Ther 2004; 42:487–499
63. Markowitz JC: Interpersonal therapy, in The American Psychiatric Publishing Textbook of Personality Disorders. Edited by Oldham JM, Skodol AE, Bender DS. Washington, DC, American Psychiatric Publishing, 2005, pp 321–334
64. Brown GK, Newman CF, Charlesworth SE, Crits-Christoph P, Beck AT: An open clinical trial of cognitive therapy for borderline personality disorder. J Personal Disord 2004; 18:257–271
65. Ryle A, Golynkina K: Effectiveness of time-limited cognitive analytic therapy of borderline personality disorder: factors associated with outcome. Br J Med Psychol 2000; 73(Pt 2): 197–210
66. Ryle A: The contribution of cognitive analytic therapy to the treatment of borderline personality disorder. J Personal Disord 2004; 18:3–35
67. Blum N, Pfohl B, John DS, Monahan P, Black DW: STEPPS: a cognitive-behavioral systems–based group treatment for outpatients with borderline personality disorder—a preliminary report. Compr Psychiatry 2002; 43:301–310
68. Clarkin JF, Foelsch PA, Levy KN, Hull JW, Delaney JC, Kernberg OF: The development of a psychodynamic treatment for patients with borderline personality disorder: a preliminary study of behavioral change. J Personal Disord 2001; 15:487–495
69. Young J, Klosko J: Schema therapy, in The American Psychiatric Publishing Textbook of Personality Disorders. Edited by Oldham JM, Skodol AE, Bender DS. Washington, DC, American Psychiatric Publishing, 2005, pp 289–306
70. Rinne T, van den BW, Wouters L, van Dyck R: SSRI treatment of borderline personality disorder: a randomized, placebo-controlled clinical trial for female patients with borderline personality disorder. Am J Psychiatry 2002; 159:2048–2054
71. Bogenschutz MP, Nurnberg HG: Olanzapine versus placebo in the treatment of borderline personality disorder. J Clin Psychiatry 2001; 65:104–109
72. Zanarini MC, Frankenburg FR, Parachini EA: A preliminary, randomized trial of fluoxetine, olanzapine, and the olanzapine-fluoxetine combination in women with borderline personality disorder. J Clin Psychiatry 2004; 65:903–907
73. Hollander E, Allen A, Lopez RP, Bienstock CA, Grossman R, Siever LJ, Merkatz L, Stein DJ: A preliminary double-blind, placebo-controlled trial of divalproex sodium in borderline personality disorder. J Clin Psychiatry 2001; 62:199–203
74. Hollander E, Tracy KA, Swann AC, Coccaro EF, McElroy SL, Wozniak P, Sommerville KW, Nemeroff CB: Divalproex in the treatment of impulsive aggression: efficacy in cluster B personality disorders. Neuropsychopharmacology 2003; 28:1186–1197
75. Cassano P, Lattanzi L, Pini S, Dell'Osso L, Battistini G, Cassano GB: Topiramate for self-mutilation in a patient with borderline personality disorder. Bipolar Disord 2001; 3:161
76. Hilger E, Barnas C, Kasper S: Quetiapine in the treatment of borderline personality disorder. World J Biol Psychiatry 2003; 4:42–44
77. Rizvi ST: Lamotrigine and borderline personality disorder. J Child Adolesc Psychopharmacol 2002; 12:365–366

78. Rocca P, Marchiaro L, Cocuzza E, Bogetto F: Treatment of borderline personality disorder with risperidone. J Clin Psychiatry 2002; 63:241–244
79. Philipsen A, Richter H, Schmahl C, Peters J, Rusch N, Bohus M, Lieb K: Clonidine in acute aversive inner tension and self-injurious behavior in female patients with borderline personality disorder. J Clin Psychiatry 2004; 65:1414–1419
80. Pascual JC, Oller S, Soler J, Barrachina J, Alvarez E, Perez V: Ziprasidone in the acute treatment of borderline personality disorder in psychiatric emergency services. J Clin Psychiatry 2004; 65:1281–1282
81. Nickel MK, Nickel C, Mitterlehner FO, Tritt K, Lahmann C, Leiberich PK, Rother WK, Loew TH: Topiramate treatment of aggression in female borderline personality disorder patients: a double-blind, placebo-controlled study. J Clin Psychiatry 2004; 65:1515–1519
82. Oldham JM, Bender DS, Skodol AE, Dyck IR, Sanislow CA, Yen S, Grilo CM, Shea MT, Zanarini MC, Gunderson EJ, McGlashan TH: Testing an APA practice guideline: symptom-targeted medication utilization for patients with borderline personality disorder. J Psychiatr Pract 2004; 10:156–161

PRACTICE GUIDELINE FOR THE

Treatment of Patients With Borderline Personality Disorder

WORK GROUP ON BORDERLINE PERSONALITY DISORDER

John M. Oldham, M.D., Chair
Glen O. Gabbard, M.D.
Marcia K. Goin, M.D., Ph.D.
John Gunderson, M.D.
Paul Soloff, M.D.
David Spiegel, M.D.
Michael Stone, M.D.
Katharine A. Phillips, M.D. (Consultant)

Originally published in October 2001. A guideline watch, summarizing significant developments in the scientific literature since publication of this guideline, may be available in the Psychiatric Practice section of the APA web site at www.psych.org.

CONTENTS

Guide to Using This Practice Guideline 1237

Introduction 1238

Development Process 1239

Part A: Treatment Recommendations for Patients With Borderline Personality Disorder 1241

I. Executive Summary of Recommendations 1241
   A. Coding System 1241
   B. General Considerations 1241
   C. Summary of Recommendations 1241

II. Formulation and Implementation of a Treatment Plan 1244
   A. The Initial Assessment 1245
   B. Principles of Psychiatric Management 1246
   C. Principles of Treatment Selection 1250
   D. Specific Treatment Strategies for the Clinical Features of Borderline Personality Disorder 1252

III. Special Features Influencing Treatment 1263
   A. Comorbidity 1263
   B. Problematic Substance Use 1264
   C. Violent Behavior and Antisocial Traits 1264
   D. Chronic Self-Destructive Behavior 1265
   E. Childhood Trauma and PTSD 1266
   F. Dissociative Features 1267
   G. Psychosocial Stressors 1268
   H. Gender 1269
   I. Cultural Factors 1269
   J. Age 1269

IV. Risk Management Issues 1270
   A. General Considerations 1270
   B. Suicide 1270
   C. Anger, Impulsivity, and Violence 1271
   D. Boundary Violations 1272

Part B: Background Information and Review of Available Evidence 1272

V. Disease Definition, Epidemiology, and Natural History 1272
  A. Definition and Core Clinical Features 1272
  B. Assessment 1274
  C. Differential Diagnosis 1275
  D. Epidemiology 1275
  E. Natural History and Course 1276

VI. Review and Synthesis of Available Evidence 1276
  A. Issues in Interpreting the Literature 1276
  B. Review of Psychotherapy and Other Psychosocial Treatments 1277
  C. Review of Pharmacotherapy and Other Somatic Treatments 1287

Part C: Future Research Needs 1299

VII. Psychotherapy 1299

VIII. Pharmacotherapy and Other Somatic Treatments 1300

Appendixes: Psychopharmacological Treatment Algorithms 1301

Individuals and Organizations That Submitted Comments 1304

References 1305

GUIDE TO USING THIS PRACTICE GUIDELINE

This practice guideline offers treatment recommendations based on available evidence and clinical consensus to help psychiatrists develop plans for the care of adult patients with borderline personality disorder. This guideline contains many sections, not all of which will be equally useful for all readers. The following guide is designed to help readers find the sections that will be most useful to them.

Part A contains the treatment recommendations for patients with borderline personality disorder. Section I is the summary of treatment recommendations, which includes the main treatment recommendations along with codes that indicate the degree of clinical confidence in each recommendation. Section II is a guide to the formulation and implementation of a treatment plan for the individual patient. This section includes all of the treatment recommendations. Section III, "Special Features Influencing Treatment," discusses a range of clinical considerations that could alter the general recommendations discussed in section II. Section IV addresses risk management issues that should be considered when treating patients with borderline personality disorder.

Part B, "Background Information and Review of Available Evidence," presents, in detail, the evidence underlying the treatment recommendations of Part A. Section V provides an overview of DSM-IV-TR criteria, prevalence rates for borderline personality disorder, and general information on its natural history and course. Section VI is a structured review and synthesis of published literature regarding the available treatments for borderline personality disorder.

Part C, "Future Research Needs," draws from the previous sections to summarize those areas in which better research data are needed to guide clinical decisions.

To share feedback on this or other published APA practice guidelines, a form is available at http://www.psych.org/psych_pract/pg/reviewform.cfm.

INTRODUCTION

This practice guideline summarizes data regarding the care of patients with borderline personality disorder.

Borderline personality disorder is the most common personality disorder in clinical settings, and it is present in cultures around the world. However, this disorder is often incorrectly diagnosed or underdiagnosed in clinical practice. Borderline personality disorder causes marked distress and impairment in social, occupational, and role functioning, and it is associated with high rates of self-destructive behavior (e.g., suicide attempts) and completed suicide.

The essential feature of borderline personality disorder is a pervasive pattern of instability of interpersonal relationships, affects, and self-image, as well as marked impulsivity. These characteristics begin by early adulthood and are present in a variety of contexts. The diagnostic criteria are shown in Table 1. For the diagnosis to be given, five of nine criteria must be present. The polythetic nature of the criteria set reflects the heterogeneity of the disorder. The core features of borderline personality disorder can also be conceptualized as consisting of a number of psychopathological dimensions (e.g., impulsivity, affective instability). A more complete description of the disorder, including its clinical features, assessment, differential diagnosis, epidemiology, and natural history and course, is provided in Part B of this guideline.

This guideline reviews the treatment that patients with borderline personality disorder may need. Psychiatrists care for patients in many different settings and serve a variety of functions and thus should either provide or recommend the appropriate treatment for patients with borderline personality disorder. In addition, many patients have comorbid conditions that may need treatment. Therefore, psychiatrists caring for patients with borderline personality disorder should consider, but not be limited to, treatments recommended in this guideline.

TABLE 1. Diagnostic Criteria for Borderline Personality Disorder

A pervasive pattern of instability of interpersonal relationships, self-image, and affects, and marked impulsivity beginning by early adulthood and present in a variety of contexts, as indicated by five (or more) of the following:

1) Frantic efforts to avoid real or imagined abandonment[a]
2) A pattern of unstable and intense interpersonal relationships characterized by alternating between extremes of idealization and devaluation
3) Identity disturbance: markedly and persistently unstable self-image or sense of self
4) Impulsivity in at least two areas that are potentially self-damaging (e.g., spending, sex, substance abuse, reckless driving, binge eating)[a]
5) Recurrent suicidal behavior, gestures, or threats, or self-mutilating behavior
6) Affective instability due to a marked reactivity of mood (e.g., intense episodic dysphoria, irritability, or anxiety usually lasting a few hours and only rarely more than a few days)
7) Chronic feelings of emptiness
8) Inappropriate, intense anger or difficulty controlling anger (e.g., frequent displays of temper, constant anger, recurrent physical fights)
9) Transient, stress-related paranoid ideation or severe dissociative symptoms

Source. Reprinted from *Diagnostic and Statistical Manual of Mental Disorders,* 4th Edition, Text Revision. Washington, DC, American Psychiatric Association, 2000. Copyright © 2000, American Psychiatric Association.

[a]Excluding suicidal or self-mutilating behavior (covered in criterion 5).

DEVELOPMENT PROCESS

This document is a practical guide to the management of patients—primarily adults over the age of 18—with borderline personality disorder and represents a synthesis of current scientific knowledge and rational clinical practice. This guideline strives to be as free as possible of bias toward any theoretical approach to treatment.

This practice guideline was developed under the auspices of the Steering Committee on Practice Guidelines. The process is detailed in a document available from the APA Department of Quality Improvement and Psychiatric Services: the "APA Guideline Development Process." Key features of the process include the following:

- a comprehensive literature review and development of evidence tables;
- initial drafting by a work group that included psychiatrists with clinical and research expertise in borderline personality disorder;
- the production of multiple drafts with widespread review, in which 13 organizations and more than 60 individuals submitted significant comments;
- approval by the APA Assembly and Board of Trustees;
- planned revisions at regular intervals.

A computerized search of the relevant literature from MEDLINE and PsycINFO was conducted.

The first literature search was conducted by searching MEDLINE for the period from 1966 to December 1998 and used the keywords "borderline personality disorder," "therapy," "drug therapy," "psychotherapy," "pharmacotherapy," "psychopharmacology," "group psychotherapy," "hysteroid dysphoria," "parasuicidal," "emotionally unstable," and "treatment." A total of 1,562 citations were found.

The literature search conducted by using PsycINFO covered the period from 1967 to November 1998 and used the keywords "borderline personality disorder," "hysteroid dysphoria," "parasuicidal," "emotionally unstable," "therapy," "treatment," "psychopharmacology," "pharmacotherapy," "borderline states," "cognitive therapy," "drug therapy," "electroconvulsive shock therapy," "family therapy," "group therapy," "insulin shock therapy," "milieu therapy," "occupational therapy," "psychoanalysis," and "somatic treatment." A total of 2,460 citations were found.

An additional literature search was conducted by using MEDLINE for the period from 1990 to 1999 and the key words "self mutilation" and "mental retardation." A total of 182 citations were found.

Additional, less formal literature searches were conducted by APA staff and individual members of the work group on borderline personality disorder.

The recommendations are based on the best available data and clinical consensus. The summary of treatment recommendations is keyed according to the level of confidence with which each recommendation is made. In addition, each reference is followed by a letter code in brackets that indicates the nature of the supporting evidence.

PART A:
TREATMENT RECOMMENDATIONS FOR PATIENTS WITH BORDERLINE PERSONALITY DISORDER

I. EXECUTIVE SUMMARY OF RECOMMENDATIONS

A. CODING SYSTEM

Each recommendation is identified as falling into one of three categories of endorsement, indicated by a bracketed Roman numeral following the statement. The three categories represent varying levels of clinical confidence regarding the recommendation:

[I] Recommended with substantial clinical confidence.
[II] Recommended with moderate clinical confidence.
[III] May be recommended on the basis of individual circumstances.

B. GENERAL CONSIDERATIONS

Borderline personality disorder is the most common personality disorder in clinical settings. It is characterized by marked distress and functional impairment, and it is associated with high rates of self-destructive behavior (e.g., suicide attempts) and completed suicide. The care of patients with borderline personality disorder involves a comprehensive array of approaches. This guideline presents treatment options and addresses factors that need to be considered when treating a patient with borderline personality disorder.

C. SUMMARY OF RECOMMENDATIONS

1. The initial assessment

The psychiatrist first performs an initial assessment of the patient to determine the treatment setting [I]. Because suicidal ideation and suicide attempts are common, safety issues should be given priority, and a thorough safety evaluation should be done. This evaluation, as well as consideration of other clinical factors, will determine the necessary treatment setting (e.g., outpatient or inpatient). A more comprehensive evaluation of the patient should then be completed [I]. It is important at the outset of treatment to establish a clear and explicit treatment framework [I], which includes establishing agreement with the patient about the treatment goals.

2. Psychiatric management

Psychiatric management forms the foundation of treatment for all patients. The primary treatment for borderline personality disorder is psychotherapy, complemented by symptom-targeted pharmacotherapy [I]. In addition, psychiatric management consists of a broad array of ongoing activities and interventions that should be instituted by the psychiatrist for all patients with borderline personality disorder [I]. Regardless of the specific primary and adjunctive treatment modalities selected, it is important to continue providing psychiatric management throughout the course of treatment. The components of psychiatric management for patients with borderline personality disorder include responding to crises and monitoring the patient's safety, establishing and maintaining a therapeutic framework and alliance, providing education about borderline personality disorder and its treatment, coordinating treatment provided by multiple clinicians, monitoring the patient's progress, and reassessing the effectiveness of the treatment plan. The psychiatrist must also be aware of and manage potential problems involving splitting (see Section II.B.6.a) and boundaries (see Section II.B.6.b).

3. Principles of treatment selection

a) Type

Certain types of psychotherapy (as well as other psychosocial modalities) and certain psychotropic medications are effective in the treatment of borderline personality disorder [I]. Although it has not been empirically established that one approach is more effective than another, clinical experience suggests that most patients with borderline personality disorder will need extended psychotherapy to attain and maintain lasting improvement in their personality, interpersonal problems, and overall functioning [II]. Pharmacotherapy often has an important adjunctive role, especially for diminution of symptoms such as affective instability, impulsivity, psychotic-like symptoms, and self-destructive behavior [I]. No studies have compared a combination of psychotherapy and pharmacotherapy to either treatment alone, but clinical experience indicates that many patients will benefit most from a combination of these treatments [II].

b) Focus

Treatment planning should address borderline personality disorder as well as comorbid axis I and axis II disorders, with priority established according to risk or predominant symptoms [I].

c) Flexibility

Because comorbid disorders are often present and each patient's history is unique, and because of the heterogeneous nature of borderline personality disorder, the treatment plan needs to be flexible, adapted to the needs of the individual patient [I]. Flexibility is also needed to respond to the changing characteristics of patients over time.

d) Role of patient preference

Treatment should be a collaborative process between patient and clinician(s), and patient preference is an important factor to consider when developing an individual treatment plan [I].

e) Multiple- versus single-clinician treatment

Treatment by a single clinician and treatment by more than one clinician are both viable approaches [II]. Treatment by multiple clinicians has potential advantages but may become fragmented; good collaboration among treatment team members and clarity of roles are essential [I].

4. Specific treatment strategies

a) Psychotherapy

Two psychotherapeutic approaches have been shown in randomized controlled trials to have efficacy: psychoanalytic/psychodynamic therapy and dialectical behavior therapy [I]. The treatment provided in these trials has three key features: weekly meetings with an individual therapist, one or more weekly group sessions, and meetings of therapists for consultation/supervision. No results are available from direct comparisons of these two approaches to suggest which patients may respond better to which type of treatment. Although brief therapy for borderline personality disorder has not been systematically examined, studies of more extended treatment suggest that substantial improvement may not occur until after approximately 1 year of psychotherapeutic intervention has been provided; many patients require even longer treatment.

Clinical experience suggests that there are a number of common features that help guide the psychotherapist, regardless of the specific type of therapy used [I]. These features include building a strong therapeutic alliance and monitoring self-destructive and suicidal behaviors. Some therapists create a hierarchy of priorities to consider in the treatment (e.g., first focusing on suicidal behavior). Other valuable interventions include validating the patient's suffering and experience as well as helping the patient take responsibility for his or her actions. Because patients with borderline personality disorder may exhibit a broad array of strengths and weaknesses, flexibility is a crucial aspect of effective therapy. Other components of effective therapy for patients with borderline personality disorder include managing feelings (in both patient and therapist), promoting reflection rather than impulsive action, diminishing the patient's tendency to engage in splitting, and setting limits on any self-destructive behaviors.

Individual psychodynamic psychotherapy without concomitant group therapy or other partial hospital modalities has some empirical support [II]. The literature on group therapy or group skills training for patients with borderline personality disorder is limited but indicates that this treatment may be helpful [II]. Group approaches are usually used in combination with individual therapy and other types of treatment. The published literature on couples therapy is limited but suggests that it may be a useful and, at times, essential adjunctive treatment modality. However, it is not recommended as the only form of treatment for patients with borderline personality disorder [II]. While data on family therapy are also limited, they suggest that a psychoeducational approach may be beneficial [II]. Published clinical reports differ in their recommendations about the appropriateness of family therapy and family involvement in the treatment; family therapy is not recommended as the only form of treatment for patients with borderline personality disorder [II].

b) Pharmacotherapy and other somatic treatments

Pharmacotherapy is used to treat state symptoms during periods of acute decompensation as well as trait vulnerabilities. Symptoms exhibited by patients with borderline personality disorder often fall within three behavioral dimensions—affective dysregulation, impulsive-behavioral dyscontrol, and cognitive-perceptual difficulties—for which specific pharmacological treatment strategies can be used.

(i) Treatment of affective dysregulation symptoms

Patients with borderline personality disorder displaying this dimension exhibit mood lability, rejection sensitivity, inappropriate intense anger, depressive "mood crashes," or outbursts of temper. These symptoms should be treated initially with a selective serotonin reuptake inhibitor (SSRI) or related antidepressant such as venlafaxine [I]. Studies of tricyclic antidepressants have produced inconsistent results. When affective dysregulation appears as anxiety, treatment with an SSRI may be insufficient, and addition of a benzodiazepine should be considered, although research on these medications in patients with borderline personality disorder is limited, and their use carries some potential risk [III].

When affective dysregulation appears as disinhibited anger that coexists with other affective symptoms, SSRIs are also the treatment of choice [II]. Clinical experience suggests that for patients with severe behavioral dyscontrol, low-dose neuroleptics can be added to the regimen for rapid response and improvement of affective symptoms [II].

Although the efficacy of monoamine oxidase inhibitors (MAOIs) for affective dysregulation in patients with borderline personality disorder has strong empirical support, MAOIs are not a first-line treatment because of the risk of serious side effects and the difficulties with adherence to required dietary restrictions [I]. Mood stabilizers (lithium, valproate, carbamazepine) are another second-line (or adjunctive) treatment for affective dysregulation, although studies of these approaches are limited [II]. There is a paucity of data on the efficacy of electroconvulsive therapy (ECT) for treatment of affective dysregulation symptoms in patients with borderline personality disorder. Clinical experience suggests that while ECT may sometimes be indicated for patients with comorbid severe axis I depression that is resistant to pharmacotherapy, affective features of borderline personality disorder are unlikely to respond to ECT [II].

An algorithm depicting steps that can be taken in treating symptoms of affective dysregulation in patients with borderline personality disorder is shown in Appendix 1.

(ii) Treatment of impulsive-behavioral dyscontrol symptoms

Patients with borderline personality disorder displaying this dimension exhibit impulsive aggression, self-mutilation, or self-damaging behavior (e.g., promiscuous sex, substance abuse, reckless spending). As seen in Appendix 2, SSRIs are the initial treatment of choice [I]. When behavioral dyscontrol poses a serious threat to the patient's safety, it may be necessary to add a low-dose neuroleptic to the SSRI [II]. Clinical experience suggests that partial efficacy of an SSRI may be enhanced by adding lithium [II]. If an SSRI is ineffective, switching to an MAOI may be considered [II]. Use of valproate or carbamazepine may also be considered for impulse control, although there are few studies of these treatments for impulsive aggression in patients with borderline personality disorder [II]. Preliminary evidence suggests that atypical neuroleptics may have some efficacy for impulsivity in patients with borderline personality disorder [II].

(iii) Treatment of cognitive-perceptual symptoms

Patients with borderline personality disorder displaying this dimension exhibit suspiciousness, referential thinking, paranoid ideation, illusions, derealization, depersonalization, or hallucination-like symptoms. As seen in Appendix 3, low-dose neuroleptics are the treatment of choice for these symptoms [I]. These medications may improve not only psychotic-like symptoms but also depressed mood, impulsivity, and anger/hostility. If response is suboptimal, the dose should be increased to a range suitable for treating axis I disorders [II].

5. Special features influencing treatment

Treatment planning and implementation should reflect consideration of the following characteristics: comorbidity with axis I and other axis II disorders, problematic substance use, violent behavior and antisocial traits, chronic self-destructive behavior, trauma and posttraumatic stress disorder (PTSD), dissociative features, psychosocial stressors, gender, age, and cultural factors [I].

6. Risk management issues

Attention to risk management issues is important [I]. Risk management considerations include the need for collaboration and communication with any other treating clinicians as well as the need for careful and adequate documentation. Any problems with transference and countertransference should be attended to, and consultation with a colleague should be considered for unusually high-risk patients. Standard guidelines for terminating treatment should be followed in all cases. Psychoeducation about the disorder is often appropriate and helpful. Other clinical features requiring particular consideration of risk management issues are the risk of suicide, the potential for boundary violations, and the potential for angry, impulsive, or violent behavior.

II. FORMULATION AND IMPLEMENTATION OF A TREATMENT PLAN

When the psychiatrist first meets with a patient who may have borderline personality disorder, a number of important issues related to differential diagnosis, etiology, the formulation, and treatment planning need to be considered. The psychiatrist performs an initial assessment to determine the treatment setting, completes a comprehensive evaluation (including differential diagnosis), and works with the patient to mutually establish the treatment framework. The psychiatrist also attends to a number of principles of psychiatric management that form the foundation of care for patients with borderline personality disorder. The psychiatrist next considers several principles of treatment selection (e.g., type, focus, number of clinicians to involve). Finally, the psychiatrist selects specific treatment strategies for the clinical features of borderline personality disorder.

A. THE INITIAL ASSESSMENT

1. Initial assessment and determination of the treatment setting

The psychiatrist first performs an initial assessment of the patient and determines the treatment setting (e.g., inpatient or outpatient). Since patients with borderline personality disorder commonly experience suicidal ideation (and 8%–10% commit suicide), safety issues should be given priority in the initial assessment (see Section II.B.1, "Responding to Crises and Safety Monitoring," for a further discussion of this issue). A thorough safety evaluation should be done before a decision can be reached about whether outpatient, inpatient, or another level of care (e.g., partial hospitalization or residential care) is needed. Presented here are some of the more common indications for particular levels of care. However, this list is not intended to be exhaustive. Since indications for level of care are difficult to empirically investigate and studies are lacking, these recommendations are derived primarily from expert clinical opinion.

Indications for partial hospitalization (or brief inpatient hospitalization if partial hospitalization is not available) include the following:

- Dangerous, impulsive behavior unable to be managed with outpatient treatment
- Nonadherence with outpatient treatment and a deteriorating clinical picture
- Complex comorbidity that requires more intensive clinical assessment of response to treatment
- Symptoms of sufficient severity to interfere with functioning, work, or family life that are unresponsive to outpatient treatment

Indications for brief inpatient hospitalization include the following:

- Imminent danger to others
- Loss of control of suicidal impulses or serious suicide attempt
- Transient psychotic episodes associated with loss of impulse control or impaired judgment
- Symptoms of sufficient severity to interfere with functioning, work, or family life that are unresponsive to outpatient treatment and partial hospitalization

Indications for extended inpatient hospitalization include the following:

- Persistent and severe suicidality, self-destructiveness, or nonadherence to outpatient treatment or partial hospitalization
- Comorbid refractory axis I disorder (e.g., eating disorder, mood disorder) that presents a potential threat to life
- Comorbid substance abuse or dependence that is severe and unresponsive to outpatient treatment or partial hospitalization
- Continued risk of assaultive behavior toward others despite brief hospitalization
- Symptoms of sufficient severity to interfere with functioning, work, or family life that are unresponsive to outpatient treatment, partial hospitalization, and brief hospitalization

2. Comprehensive evaluation

Once an initial assessment has been done and the treatment setting determined, a more comprehensive evaluation should be completed as soon as clinically feasible. Such an evaluation includes assessing the presence of comorbid disorders, degree and type of functional impairment, needs and goals, intrapsychic conflicts and defenses, developmental progress and arrests, adaptive and maladaptive coping styles, psychosocial stressors, and strengths in the face of stressors (see Part B, Section V.B, "Assessment"). The psychiatrist should attempt to understand the biological, interpersonal, familial, social, and cultural factors that affect the patient (3).

Special attention should be paid to the differential diagnosis of borderline personality disorder versus axis I conditions (see Part B, Sections V.A.2, "Comorbidity," and V.C, "Differential Diagnosis"). Treatment planning should address comorbid disorders from axis I (e.g., substance use disorders, depressive disorders, PTSD) and axis II as well as borderline personality disorder, with priority established according to risk or predominant symptoms. When priority is given to treating comorbid conditions (e.g., substance abuse, depression, PTSD, or an eating disorder), it may be helpful to caution patients or their families about the expected rate of response or extent of improvement. The prognosis for treatment of these axis I disorders is often poorer when borderline personality disorder is present. It is usually better to anticipate realistic problems than to encourage unrealistically high hopes.

3. Establishing the treatment framework

It is important at the outset of treatment to establish a clear and explicit treatment framework. This is sometimes called "contract setting." While this process is generally applicable to the treatment of all patients, regardless of diagnosis, such an agreement is particularly important for patients with borderline personality disorder. The clinician and the patient can then refer to this agreement later in the treatment if the patient challenges it.

Patients and clinicians should establish agreements about goals of treatment sessions (e.g., symptom reduction, personal growth, improvement in functioning) and what role each is expected to perform to achieve these goals. Patients, for example, are expected to report on such issues as conflicts, dysfunction, and impending life changes. Clinicians are expected to offer understanding, explanations for treatment interventions, undistracted attention, and respectful, compassionate attitudes, with judicious feedback to patients that can help them attain their goals. In addition, it is essential for patients and clinicians to work toward establishing agreements about 1) when, where, and with what frequency sessions will be held; 2) a plan for crises management; 3) clarification of the clinician's after-hours availability; and 4) the fee, billing, and payment schedule.

B. PRINCIPLES OF PSYCHIATRIC MANAGEMENT

Psychiatric management forms the foundation of psychiatric treatment for patients with borderline personality disorder. It consists of an array of ongoing activities and interventions that should be instituted for all patients. These include providing education about borderline personality disorder, facilitating adherence to a psychotherapeutic or psychopharmacological regimen that is satisfactory to both the patient and psychiatrist, and attempting to help the patient solve practical problems, giving advice and guidance when needed.

Specific components of psychiatric management are discussed here as well as additional important issues—such as the potential for splitting and boundary problems—that may complicate treatment and of which the clinician must be aware and manage.

1. Responding to crises and safety monitoring

Psychiatrists should assume that crises, such as interpersonal crises or self-destructive behavior, will occur. Psychiatrists may wish to establish an explicit understanding about what they expect a patient to do during crises and may want to be explicit about what the patient can expect from them. While some clinicians believe that this is of critical importance (4, 5), others believe that this approach is too inflexible and potentially adversarial. From the latter perspective, there is often a tension between the psychiatrist's role in helping patients to understand their behavior and the psychiatrist's role in ensuring patients' safety and in managing problematic behaviors. This tension may be particularly prominent when the psychiatrist is using a psychodynamic approach that relies heavily on interpretation and exploration. Regardless of the psychotherapeutic strategy, however, the psychiatrist has a fundamental responsibility to monitor this tension as part of the treatment process.

Patients with borderline personality disorder commonly experience suicidal ideation and are prone to make suicide attempts or engage in self-injurious behavior (e.g., cutting). Monitoring patients' safety is a critically important task. It is important that psychiatrists always evaluate indicators of self-injurious or suicidal ideas and reformulate the treatment plan as appropriate. Serious self-harm can occur if the potential danger is ignored or minimized. Before intervening to prevent self-endangering behaviors, the psychiatrist should first assess the potential danger, the patient's motivations, and to what extent the patient can manage his or her safety without external interventions (6). When the patient's safety is judged to be at serious risk, hospitalization may be indicated. Even in the context of appropriate treatment, some patients with borderline personality disorder will commit suicide.

2. Establishing and maintaining a therapeutic framework and alliance

Patients with borderline personality disorder have difficulty developing and sustaining trusting relationships. This issue may be a focus of treatment as well as a significant barrier to the development of the treatment alliance necessary to carry out the treatment plan. Therefore, the psychiatrist should pay particular attention to ascertaining that the patient agrees with and accepts the treatment plan; adherence or agreement cannot be assumed. Agreements should be explicit.

The first aspect of alliance building, referred to earlier as "contract setting," is establishing an agreement about respective roles and responsibilities and treatment goals. The next aspect of alliance building is to encourage patients to be actively engaged in the treatment, both in their tasks (e.g., monitoring medication effects or noting and reflecting on their feelings) and in the relationship (e.g., disclosing reactions or wishes to the clinician). This can be accomplished by focusing attention on whether the patient 1) understands and accepts what the psychiatrist says and 2) seems to feel understood and accepted by the psychiatrist. Techniques such as confrontation or interpretation may be appropriate over the long term after a "working alliance" (collaboration over a task) has been established. Psychotherapeutic approaches are often helpful in developing a working alliance for a pharmacotherapy component of the treatment plan. Reciprocally, the experience of being helped by medication that the psychiatrist prescribed can help a patient develop trust in his or her psychotherapeutic interventions.

3. Providing education about the disorder and its treatment

Psychoeducational methods often are helpful and generally are welcomed by patients and, when appropriate, their families. At an appropriate point in treatment, patients should be familiarized with the diagnosis, including its expected course, responsiveness to treatment, and, when appropriate, pathogenic factors. Many patients with borderline personality disorder profit from ongoing education about self-care (e.g., safe sex, potential legal problems, balanced diet). Formal psychoeducational approaches may include having the patient read the text of DSM-IV-TR or books on borderline personality disorder written for laypersons. Some clinicians prefer to frame psychoeducational discussions in everyday terms and use the patient's own language to negotiate a shared understanding of the major areas of difficulty without turning to a text or manual. More extensive psychoeducational intervention, consisting of workshops, lectures, or seminars, may also be helpful.

Families or others—especially those who are younger—living with individuals with borderline personality disorder will also often benefit from psychoeducation about the disorder, its course, and its treatment. It is wise to introduce information about pathogenic issues that may involve family members with sensitivity to the information's likely effects (e.g., it may evoke undesirable reactions of guilt, anger, or defensiveness). Psychoeducation for families should be distinguished from family therapy, which is sometimes a desirable part of the treatment plan and sometimes not, depending on the patient's history and status of current relationships.

4. Coordinating the treatment effort

Providing optimal treatment for patients with borderline personality disorder who may be dangerously self-destructive frequently requires a treatment team that involves several clinicians. If the team members work collaboratively, the overall treatment will usually be enhanced by being better able to help patients contain their acting out (via fight or flight) and their projections onto others. It is essential that ongoing coordination of the overall treatment plan is assured by clear role definitions, plans for management of crises, and regular communication among the clinicians.

The team members must also have a clear agreement about which clinician is assuming the primary overall responsibility for the patient's safety and treatment. This individual serves as a gatekeeper for the appropriate level of care (whether it be hospitalization, residential treatment, or day hospitalization), oversees the family involvement, makes decisions regarding which potential treatment modalities are useful or should be discontinued, helps assess the impact of medications, and monitors the patient's safety. Because of the diversity of knowledge and expertise required for this oversight function, a psychiatrist is usually optimal for this role.

5. Monitoring and reassessing the patient's clinical status and treatment plan

With all forms of treatment, it is important to monitor the treatment's effectiveness in an ongoing way. Often the course of treatment is uneven, with periodic setbacks (e.g., at times of stress). Such setbacks do not necessarily indicate that the treatment is ineffective. Nonetheless, ultimate improvement should be a reasonably expected outcome.

a) Recognizing functional regression

Patients with borderline personality disorder sometimes regress early in treatment as they begin to engage in the treatment process, getting somewhat worse before they get better. However, sustained deterioration is a problem that requires attention. Examples of such regressive phenomena include dysfunctional behavior (e.g., cessation of work, increased suicidality, onset of compulsive overeating) or immature behavior. This may occur when patients believe that they no longer need to be as responsible for taking care of themselves, thinking that their needs can and will now be met by those providing treatment.

Clinicians should be prepared to recognize this effect and then explore with patients whether their hope for such care is realistic and, if so, whether it is good for their long-term welfare. When the decline of functioning is sustained, it may mean that the focus of treatment needs to shift from exploration to other strategies (e.g., behavioral modification, vocational counseling, family education, or limit-setting). Of special significance is that such declines in function are likely to occur when patients with borderline personality disorder have reductions in the intensity or amount of support they receive, such as moving to a less intensive level of care. Clinicians need to be alert to the fact that such regressions may reflect the need to add support or structure temporarily to the treatment by way of easing the transition to less intensive treatment. Regressions may also occur when patients perceive particularly sympathetic, nurturant, or protective inclinations in those who are providing their care. Under these circumstances, clinicians need to clarify that these inclinations do not signify a readiness to take on a parenting role.

b) Treating symptoms that reappear despite continued pharmacotherapy

An issue that frequently requires assessment and response by psychiatrists is the sustained return of symptoms, the previous remission of which had been attributed, at least in part, to medications (although placebo effects may also have been involved). Assessment of such symptom "breakthroughs" requires knowledge of the patient's symptom presentation before the use of medication. Has the full symptom presentation returned? Are the current symptoms sustained over time, or do they reflect transitory and reactive moods in response to an interpersonal crisis? Medications can modulate the intensity of affective, cognitive, and impulsive symptoms, but they should not be expected to extinguish feelings of anger, sadness, and pain in response to separations, rejections, or other life stressors. When situational precipitants are identified, the clinician's primary focus should be to facilitate improved coping. Frequent medication changes in pursuit of improving transient mood states are unnecessary and generally ineffective. The patient should not be given the erroneous message that emotional responses to life events are merely biologic symptoms to be regulated by medications.

c) Obtaining consultations

Clinicians with overall or primary responsibilities for patients with borderline personality disorder should have a low threshold for seeking consultation because of 1) the high frequency of countertransference reactions and medicolegal liability complications; 2) the high frequency of complicated multitreater, multimodality treatments; and 3) the particularly high level of inference, subjectivity, and life/death significance that clinical judgments involve. The principle that should guide whether a consultation is obtained is that improvement (e.g., less distress, more adaptive behaviors, greater trust) is to be expected during treatment. Thus, failure to show improvement in targeted goals by 6–12 months should raise considerations of introducing changes in the treatment. When a patient continues to do poorly after the treatment has been modified, consultation is indicated as a way of introducing and implementing treatment changes. When a consultant believes that the existing treatment cannot be improved, this offers support for continuing this treatment.

6. Special issues

a) Splitting

The phenomenon of "splitting" signifies an inability to reconcile alternative or opposing perceptions or feelings within the self or others, which is characteristic of borderline personality disorder. As a result, patients with borderline personality disorder tend to see people or situations in "black or white," "all or nothing," "good or bad" terms. In clinical settings, this phenomenon may be evident in their polarized but alternating views of others as either idealized (i.e., "all good") or devalued (i.e., "all bad"). When they perceive primary clinicians as "all bad" (usually prompted by feeling frustrated), this may precipitate flight from treatment. When splitting threatens continuation of the treatment, clinicians should be prepared to examine the transference and countertransference and consider altering treatment. This can be done by offering increased support, by seeking consultation, or by otherwise suggesting changes in the treatment. Clinicians should always arrange to communicate regularly about their patients to avoid splitting within the treatment team (i.e., one clinician or treatment is idealized while another is devalued). Integration of the clinicians helps patients integrate their internal splits.

b) Boundaries

Clinicians/therapists vary considerably in their tolerance for patient behaviors (e.g., phone calls, silences) and in their expectations of the patient (e.g., promptness, personal disclosures, homework between sessions). It is important to be explicit about these issues, thereby establishing "boundaries" around the treatment relationship and task. It is also important to be consistent with agreed-upon boundaries. Although patients may agree to such boundaries, some patients with borderline personality disorder will attempt to cross them (e.g., request between-session contacts or seek a personal, nonprofessional relationship). It remains the therapist's responsibility to monitor and sustain the treatment boundaries. Certain situations—e.g., practicing in a small community, rural area, or military setting—may complicate the task of maintaining treatment boundaries (7).

To diminish the problems associated with boundary issues, clinicians should be alert to their occurrence. Clinicians should then be proactive in exploring the meaning of the boundary crossing—whether it originated in their own behavior or that of the patient. After efforts are made to examine the meaning, whether the outcome is satisfactory or not, clinicians should restate their expectations about the treatment boundaries and their rationale. If the patient keeps testing the agreed-upon framework of therapy, clinicians should explicate its rationale. An example of this rationale is, "There are times when I may not answer your personal questions if I think it would be better for us to know why you've inquired." If a patient continues to challenge the framework despite exploration and clarification, a limit will eventually need to be set. An example of setting a limit is, "You recall that we agreed that if you feel suicidal, then you will go to an emergency room. If you cannot do this then your treatment may need to be changed."

When a boundary is crossed by the clinician/therapist, it is called a boundary "violation." The boundary can usually be restored with comments like the following: "If I were to call you every time I'm worried, your safety might come to depend too much on my intuition," or "Whenever I tell you something about my personal life, it limits our opportunity to understand more about what you imagine in the absence of knowing." When therapists find themselves making exceptions to their usual treatment boundaries, it is important to examine their motives (see Section IV, "Risk Management Issues"). It often signals the need for consultation or supervision.

Any consideration of sexual boundary violations by therapists must begin with a caveat: Patients can never be blamed for ethical transgressions by their therapists. It is the therapist's responsibility to act ethically, no matter how the patient may behave. Nevertheless, specific transference-countertransference enactments are at high risk for occurring with patients with borderline personality disorder. If a patient has experienced neglect and abuse in childhood, he or she may wish for the therapist to provide the love the patient missed from parents. Therapists may have rescue fantasies that lead them to collude with the patient's wish for the therapist to offer that love. This collusion in some cases leads to physical contact and even inappropriate physical contact between therapist and patient. Clinicians should be alert to these dynamics and seek consultation or personal psychotherapy or both whenever there is a risk of a boundary violation. Sexual interactions between a therapist and a patient are always unethical. When this type of boundary violation occurs, the therapist should immediately refer the patient to another therapist and seek consultation or personal psychotherapy.

C. PRINCIPLES OF TREATMENT SELECTION

1. Type

Certain types of psychotherapy (as well as other psychosocial modalities) and certain psychotropic medications are effective for the treatment of borderline personality disorder. Although it has not been empirically established that one approach is more effective than another, clinical experience suggests that most patients with borderline personality disorder will need some form of extended psychotherapy in order to resolve interpersonal problems and attain and maintain lasting improvements in their personality and overall functioning. Pharmacotherapy often has an important adjunctive role, especially for diminution of targeted symptoms such as affective instability, impulsivity, psychotic-like symptoms, and self-destructive behavior. However, pharmacotherapy is unlikely to have substantial effects on some interpersonal problems and some of the other primary features of the disorder. Although no studies have compared a combination of psychotherapy and pharmacotherapy with either treatment alone, clinical experience indicates that many patients will benefit most from a combination of psychotherapy and pharmacotherapy.

2. Focus

Patients with borderline personality disorder frequently have comorbid axis I and other axis II conditions. The nature of certain borderline characteristics often complicates the treatment provided, even when treatment is focused on a comorbid axis I condition. For example, chronic self-destructive behaviors in response to perceived abandonment, marked impulsivity, or difficulties in establishing a therapeutic alliance have been referred to as "therapy-interfering behaviors." Treatment planning should address comorbid axis I and axis II disorders as well as borderline personality disorder, with priority established according to risk or predominant symptoms. The coexisting presence of borderline personality disorder with axis I disorders is associated with a poorer outcome of a number of axis I conditions. Treatment should usually be focused on both axis I and axis II disorders to facilitate the treatment of axis I conditions as well as address problematic, treatment-interfering personality features of borderline personality disorder itself. For patients with axis I conditions and coexisting borderline traits who do not meet full criteria for borderline personality disorder, it may be sufficient to focus treatment on the axis I conditions alone, although the therapy should be monitored and the focus changed to include the borderline traits if necessary to ensure the success of the treatment.

3. Flexibility

Features of borderline personality disorder are of a heterogeneous nature. Some patients, for example, display prominent affective instability, whereas others exhibit marked impulsivity or antisocial traits. The many possible combinations of comorbid axis I and axis II disorders further contribute to the heterogeneity of the clinical picture. Because of this heterogeneity, and because of each patient's unique history, the treatment plan needs to be flexible, adapted to the needs of the individual patient. Flexibility is also needed to respond to the changing characteristics of patients over time (e.g., at one point, the treatment focus may be on safety, whereas at another, it may be on improving relationships and functioning at work). Similarly, the psychiatrist may need to use different treatment modalities or refer the patient for adjunctive treatments (e.g., behavioral, supportive, or psychodynamic psychotherapy) at different times during the treatment.

4. Role of patient preference

Successful treatment is a collaborative process between the patient and the clinician. Patient preference is an important factor to consider when developing an individual treatment plan. The psychiatrist should explain and discuss the range of treatments available for the patient's condition, the modalities he or she recommends, and the rationale for having selected them. He or she should take time to elicit the patient's views about this provisional treatment plan and modify it to the extent feasible to take into account the patient's views and preferences. The hazard of nonadherence makes it worthwhile to spend whatever time may be required to gain the patient's assent to a viable treatment plan and his or her agreement to collaborate with the clinician(s) before any therapy is instituted.

5. Multiple- versus single-clinician treatment

Treatment can be provided by more than one clinician, each performing separate treatment tasks, or by a single clinician performing multiple tasks; both are viable approaches to treating borderline personality disorder. When there are multiple clinicians on the treatment team, they may be involved in a number of tasks, including individual psychotherapy, pharmacotherapy, group therapy, family therapy, or couples therapy or be involved as administrators on an inpatient unit, partial hospital setting, halfway house, or other living situation. Such treatment has a number of potential advantages. For example, it brings more types of expertise to the patient's treatment, and multiple clinicians may better contain the patient's self-destructive tendencies. However, because of patients' propensity for engaging in "splitting" (i.e., seeing one clinician as "good" and another as "bad") as well as the real-world difficulties of maintaining good collaboration with all other clinicians, the treatment has the potential to become fragmented. For this type of treatment to be successful, good collaboration of the entire treatment team and clarity of roles are essential (7). Regardless of whether treatment involves multiple clinicians or a single therapist, its effectiveness should be monitored over time, and it should be changed if the patient is not improving.

D. SPECIFIC TREATMENT STRATEGIES FOR THE CLINICAL FEATURES OF BORDERLINE PERSONALITY DISORDER

Although there is a long clinical tradition of treating borderline personality disorder, there are no well-designed studies comparing pharmacotherapy with psychotherapy. Nor are there any systematic investigations of the effects of combined medication and psychotherapy to either modality alone. Hence, in this section we will consider psychotherapy and pharmacotherapy separately, knowing that in clinical practice the two treatments are frequently combined. Indeed, many of the pharmacotherapy studies included patients with borderline personality disorder who were also in psychotherapy, and many patients in psychotherapy studies were also taking medication. A good deal of clinical wisdom supports the notion that carefully focused pharmacotherapy may enhance the patient's capacity to engage in psychotherapy.

1. Psychotherapy

Two psychotherapeutic approaches have been shown to have efficacy in randomized controlled trials: psychoanalytic/psychodynamic therapy and dialectical behavior therapy. We emphasize that these are psychotherapeutic *approaches* because the trials that have demonstrated efficacy (8–10) have involved sophisticated therapeutic programs rather than simply the provision of individual psychotherapy. Both approaches have three key features: 1) weekly meetings with an individual therapist, 2) one or more weekly group sessions, and 3) meetings between therapists for consultation/supervision. No results are available from direct comparisons of the two approaches to suggest which patients may respond better to which modality.

Psychoanalytic/psychodynamic therapy and dialectical behavior therapy are described in more detail in Part B of this guideline (see Section VI.B, "Review of Psychotherapy and Other Psychosocial Treatments"). One characteristic of both dialectical behavior therapy and psychoanalytic/psychodynamic therapy involves the length of treatment. Although brief therapy has not been systematically tested for patients with borderline personality disorder, the studies of extended treatment suggest that substantial improvement may not occur until after approximately 1 year of psychotherapeutic intervention has been provided and that many patients require even longer treatment.

In addition, clinical experience suggests that there are a number of "common features" that help guide the psychotherapist who is treating a patient with borderline personality disorder, regardless of the specific type of therapy used. The psychotherapist must emphasize the building of a strong therapeutic alliance with the patient to withstand the frequent affective storms within the treatment (11, 12). This process of building a positive working relationship is greatly enhanced by careful attention to specific goals for the treatment that both patient and therapist view as reasonable and attainable. Consolidation of a therapeutic alliance is facilitated as well by the establishment of clear boundaries within and around the treatment. Clinicians may find it useful to keep in mind that often patients will attempt to redefine, cross, or even violate boundaries as a test to see whether the treatment situation is safe enough for them to reveal their feelings to the therapist. Regular meeting times with firm expectation of attendance and participation are important as well as an understanding of the relative contributions of patient and therapist to the treatment process (12).

Therapists need to be active, interactive, and responsive to the patient. Self-destructive and suicidal behaviors need to be actively monitored. As seen in Figure 1, some therapists create a hierarchy of priorities to be considered in the treatment. For example, practitioners of dialectical behavior therapy (5) might consider suicidal behaviors first, followed by behaviors that interfere with therapy and then behaviors that interfere with quality of life. Practitioners of psychoanalytic or psychodynamic therapy (4, 13) might construct a similar hierarchy.

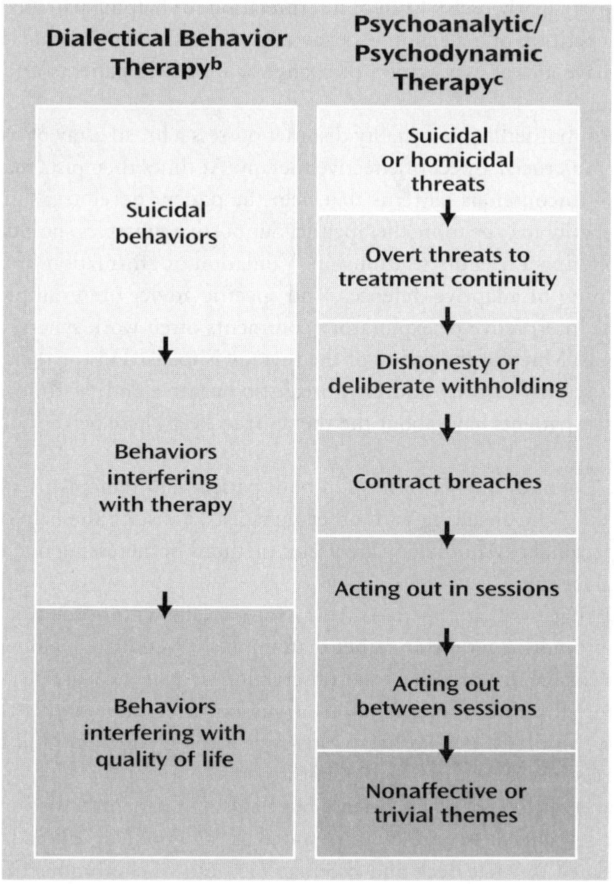

FIGURE 1. Treatment Priorities of Two Psychotherapeutic Approaches for Patients With Borderline Personality Disorder.[a]

[a]Specific behaviors that practitioners of each approach may encounter in patients with borderline personality disorder are presented, with those of highest priority sitting atop the "ladder"; treatment priority lessens as one goes down the ladder.

[b]As described by Linehan et al. (5).

[c]As described by Kernberg et al. (4) and Clarkin et al. (13).

Many patients with borderline personality disorder have experienced considerable childhood neglect and abuse, so an empathic validation of the reality of that mistreatment and the suffering it has caused is a valuable intervention (12, 14–17). This process of empathizing with the patient's experience is also valuable in building a stronger therapeutic alliance (11) and paving the way for interpretive comments.

While validating patients' suffering, therapists must also help them take appropriate responsibility for their actions. Many patients with borderline personality disorder who have experienced trauma in the past blame themselves. Effective therapy helps patients realize that while they were not responsible for the neglect and abuse they experienced in childhood, they *are* currently responsible for controlling and preventing self-destructive patterns in the present. Psychotherapy can become derailed if there is too much focus on past trauma instead of attention to current functioning and problems in relating to others. Most therapists believe that interventions like interpretation, confrontation, and clarification should focus more on here-and-now situations than on the distant past (18). Interpretations of the here and now as it links to events in the past is a particularly useful form of interpretation for helping patients learn about the tendency toward repetition of maladaptive behavior patterns throughout their lives. Moreover, therapists must have a clear expectation of change as they help patients understand the origins of their suffering.

Because patients with borderline personality disorder possess a broad array of strengths and weaknesses, flexibility is a crucial aspect of effective therapy. At times therapists may be able to offer interpretations of unconscious patterns that help the patient develop insight. At other times, support and empathy may be more therapeutic. Supportive strategies should not be misconstrued as simply offering a friendly relationship. Validation or affirmation of the patient's experience, strengthening of adaptive defenses, and specific advice are examples of useful supportive approaches. Interpretive or exploratory comments often work synergistically with supportive interventions. Much of the action of the therapy is focused in the therapeutic relationship, and therapists must directly address unrealistic negative and, at times, unrealistic positive perceptions that patients have about the therapist to keep these perceptions from disrupting the treatment.

Appropriate management of intense feelings in both patient and therapist is a cornerstone of good psychotherapy (15). Consulting with other therapists, enlisting the help of a supervisor, and engaging in personal psychotherapy are useful methods of increasing one's capacity to contain these powerful feelings.

Clinical experience suggests that effective therapy for patients with borderline personality disorder also involves promoting reflection rather than impulsive action. Therapists should encourage the patient to engage in a process of self-observation to generate a greater understanding of how behaviors originate from internal motivations and affect states rather than coming from "out of the blue." Similarly, psychotherapy involves helping patients think through the consequences of their actions so that their judgment improves.

As previously noted, splitting is a major defense mechanism of patients with borderline personality disorder. The self and others are often regarded as "all good" or "all bad." This phenomenon is closely related to what Beck and Freeman (19) call "dichotomous thinking" and what Linehan (17) refers to as "all or none thinking." Psychotherapy must be geared to helping the patient begin to experience the shades of gray between the extremes and integrate the positive and negative aspects of the self and others. A major thrust of psychotherapy is to help patients recognize that their perception of others, including the therapist, is a *representation* rather than how they really are.

Because of the potential for impulsive behavior, therapists must be comfortable with setting limits on self-destructive behaviors. Similarly, at times therapists may need to convey to patients the limits of the therapist's own capacities. For example, therapists may need to lay out what they see as the necessary conditions to make therapy viable, with the understanding that the particular therapy may not be able to continue if the patient cannot adhere to minimal conditions that make psychotherapy possible.

Individual psychodynamic therapy without concomitant group therapy or other partial hospital modalities has some empirical support (20, 21). These studies, which used nonrandomized waiting list control conditions and "pre-post" comparisons, suggested that twice-weekly psychodynamic therapy for 1 year may be helpful for many patients with borderline personality disorder. In these studies, as in the randomized controlled trials, the therapists met regularly for group consultation.

There is a large clinical literature describing psychoanalytic/psychodynamic individual therapy for patients with borderline personality disorder (12, 14, 15, 18, 22–38). Most of these clinical reports document the difficult transference and countertransference aspects of the treatment, but they also provide considerable encouragement regarding the ultimate treatability of borderline personality disorder. Therapists who persevere describe substantial improvement in well-suited patients. Some of these skilled clinicians have reported success with the use of psychoanalysis four or five times weekly (22, 24, 34, 39). These cases may have involved "higher level" patients with borderline personality disorder who more likely fit into the Kernberg category of borderline personality organization (a broader theoretical rubric that describes a specific intrapsychic structural organization [27]). Some exceptional patients who do meet criteria for borderline personality disorder may be analyzable in the hands of gifted and well-trained clinicians, but most psychotherapists and psychoanalysts agree that psychoanalytic psychotherapy, at a frequency of one to three times a week face-to-face with the patient, is a more suitable treatment than psychoanalysis.

The limited literature on group therapy for patients with borderline personality disorder indicates that group treatment is not harmful and may be helpful, but it does not provide evidence of any clear advantage over individual psychotherapy. In general, group therapy is usually used in combination with individual therapy and other types of treatment, reflecting clinical wisdom that the combination is more effective than group therapy alone. Studies of combined individual dynamic therapy plus group therapy suggest that nonspecified components of combined interventions may have the greatest therapeutic power (40). Clinical experience suggests that a relatively homogeneous group of patients with borderline personality disorder is generally recommended for group therapy, although patients with dependent, schizoid, and narcissistic personality disorders or chronic depression also mix well with patients with borderline personality disorder (12). It is generally recommended that patients with antisocial personality disorder, untreated substance abuse, or psychosis not be included in groups designed for patients with borderline personality disorder.

The published literature on couples therapy with patients with borderline personality disorder consists only of reported clinical experience and case reports. This clinical literature suggests that couples therapy may be a useful and at times essential adjunctive treatment modality, since inherent in the very nature of the illness is the potential for chaotic interpersonal relationships. However, couples therapy is not recommended as the only form of treatment for patients with borderline personality disorder. Clinical experience suggests that it is relatively contraindicated when either partner is unable to listen to the other's criticisms or complaints without becoming too enraged, terrified, or despairing (41).

There is only one published study of family therapy for patients with borderline personality disorder (12), which found that a psychoeducational approach could greatly enhance communication and diminish conflict about independence. Published clinical reports differ in their recommendations about the appropriateness of family therapy and family involvement in the treatment. Whereas some clinicians recommend removing the patient's treatment from the family setting and not attempting family therapy (12), others recommend working with the patient and family together (42).

Clinical experience suggests that family work is most apt to be helpful and can be of critical importance when patients with borderline personality disorder have significant involvement with, or are financially dependent on, the family. Failure to enlist family support is a common reason for treatment dropout. The decision about whether to work with the family should depend on the degree of pathology within the family and strengths and weaknesses of the family members. Clinical experience suggests that a psychoeducational approach may lay the groundwork for the small subset of families for whom subsequent dynamic family therapy may be effective. Family therapy is not recommended as the only form of treatment for patients with borderline personality disorder.

2. Pharmacotherapy and other somatic treatments

A pharmacological approach to the treatment of borderline personality disorder is based upon evidence that some personality dimensions of patients appear to be mediated by dysregulation of neurotransmitter physiology and are responsive to medication (43). Pharmacotherapy is used to treat state symptoms during periods of acute decompensation as well as trait vulnerabilities. Although medications are widely used to treat patients who have borderline personality disorder, the Food and Drug Administration has not approved any medications specifically for the treatment of this disorder.

Pharmacotherapy may be guided by a set of basic assumptions that provide the theoretical rationale and empirical basis for choosing specific treatments. First, borderline personality disorder is a chronic disorder. Pharmacotherapy has demonstrated significant efficacy in many studies in diminishing symptom severity and optimizing functioning. However, cure is not a realistic goal—medications do not cure character. Second, borderline personality disorder is characterized by a number of dimensions; treatment is symptom-specific, directed at particular behavioral dimensions, rather than the disorder as a whole. Third, affective dysregulation and impulsive aggression are dimensions that require particular attention because they are risk factors for suicidal behavior, self-injury, and assaultiveness and are thus given high priority in selecting pharmacological agents. Fourth, pharmacotherapy targets the neurotransmitter basis of behavioral dimensions, affecting both acute symptomatic expression (e.g., anger treated with dopamine-blocking agents) and chronic vulnerability (e.g., temperamental impulsivity treated with serotonergic agents). Last, symptoms common to both axis I and II disorders may respond similarly to the same medication.

Symptoms exhibited within three behavioral dimensions seen in patients with borderline personality disorder are targeted for pharmacotherapy: affective dysregulation, impulsive-behavioral dyscontrol, and cognitive-perceptual difficulties.

a) Treatment of affective dysregulation symptoms

Affective dysregulation in patients with borderline personality disorder is manifested by symptoms such as mood lability, rejection sensitivity, inappropriate intense anger, depressive "mood crashes," and temper outbursts. As seen in Table 2, patients displaying these features should be treated initially with one of the SSRIs, since this recommendation has strong empirical support (44–49). SSRIs have a broad spectrum of therapeutic effects, are relatively safe in overdose (compared with the tricyclic antidepressants or MAOIs), and have a favorable side effect profile, which supports treatment adherence. For example, fluoxetine has been found to improve depressed mood, mood lability, rejection sensitivity, impulsive behavior, self-mutilation, hostility, and even psychotic features. Research trials of SSRIs for treatment of borderline personality disorder have ranged in duration from 6 to 14 weeks for acute treatment studies, with continuation studies lasting up to 12 months. Some patients have retained improvement with maintenance treatment of 1–3 years. Studies have been reported with fluoxetine (in doses of 20–80 mg/day), sertraline (in doses of 100–200 mg/day), and the mixed norepinephrine/serotonin reuptake blocker venlafaxine (in doses of up to 400 mg/day) (45). A reasonable trial of an SSRI for treatment of patients with borderline personality disorder is at least 12 weeks.

Empirical trials of tricyclic antidepressants have produced inconsistent results (50, 51). Patients with comorbid major depression and borderline personality disorder have shown improvement following treatment with tricyclic antidepressants. However, in one placebo-controlled study, amitriptyline had a paradoxical effect in patients with borderline personality disorder, increasing suicidal ideation, paranoid thinking, and assaultiveness (50).

Since affective dysregulation is a dimension of temperament in patients with borderline personality disorder and not an acute illness, the duration of continuation and maintenance phases of pharmacotherapy cannot presently be defined. Significant improvement in the quality of the patient's coping skills and interpersonal relationships may be required before medication can be discontinued. Clinical experience suggests caution in discontinuing a successful antidepressant trial, especially if prior medication trials have failed. In the event of a suboptimal response to an SSRI, consideration should be given to switching to a second SSRI or related antidepressant. In one study of patients with borderline personality disorder (45), one-half of the patients who failed to respond to fluoxetine subsequently responded to sertraline.

When affective dysregulation appears as anxiety, an SSRI may be insufficient. At this point, the use of a benzodiazepine should be considered, although there is little systematic research on the use of these medications in patients with borderline personality disorder. Use of benzodiazepines may be problematic, given the risk of abuse, tolerance, and even behavioral toxicity. Despite clinical use of benzodiazepines (52), the short-acting benzodiazepine alprazolam was associated in one study with serious behavioral dyscontrol (53). Case reports demonstrate some utility for the long half-life benzodiazepine clonazepam (54). Clinical experience suggests that this medication, if used over the longer term, is best used adjunctively with an SSRI.

In theory, buspirone may treat anxiety or impulsive aggression without the risk of abuse or tolerance. However, the absence of an immediate effect generally makes this drug less acceptable to patients with borderline personality disorder. Currently, there are no published data on the use of buspirone for the treatment of affective dysregulation symptoms in patients with borderline personality disorder.

When affective dysregulation appears as disinhibited anger that coexists with other affective symptoms, SSRIs are the treatment of first choice. Fluoxetine has been shown to be effective for anger in patients with borderline personality disorder independent of its effects on depressed mood (44). Effects of fluoxetine on anger and impulsivity may appear within days, much earlier than antidepressant effects. Clinical experience suggests that in patients with severe behavioral dyscontrol, low-dose neuroleptics can be added to the regimen for a rapid response; they may also improve affective symptoms (50). Augmentation with neuroleptics should be considered before trying an MAOI, which requires more patient cooperation and adherence.

The efficacy of MAOIs for affective dysregulation symptoms in patients with borderline personality disorder has strong empirical support (55, 56). However, they are not a first-line treatment because of concerns about adherence to required dietary restrictions and because of their more problematic side effects. The effectiveness of MAOIs is supported by randomized controlled studies in patients with a primary diagnosis of borderline personality disorder as well as syndromes (e.g., atypical depression) in which the diagnosis of borderline personality disorder is considered secondary (57). MAOI antidepressants have demonstrated efficacy for impulsivity, mood reactivity, rejection sensitivity, anger, and hostility. They may also be effective for atypical depression and "hysteroid dysphoria." If a psychiatrist wishes to use an MAOI as a second-line treatment for symptoms of affective dysregulation, care should be taken to allow an adequate washout period after discontinuing SSRIs, particularly those with a long half-life.

Mood stabilizers are another second-line (or adjunctive) treatment for affective dysregulation symptoms in patients with borderline personality disorder. Lithium carbonate, carbamazepine, and valproate have been used for treatment of mood instability in patients with an axis II disorder, but there is a surprising paucity of empirical support for their use in borderline per-

TABLE 2. Psychopharmacological Treatment Recommendations for Affective Dysregulation Symptoms in Patients With Borderline Personality Disorder

Drug Class	Specific Medications Studied	Symptoms for Which Medication Is Recommended	Strength of Evidence[a]	Issues
SSRIs and related antidepressants	Fluoxetine, sertraline, venlafaxine[b]	Depressed mood, mood lability, rejection sensitivity, anxiety, impulsivity, self-mutilation, anger/hostility, psychoticism, and poor global functioning	A	Relatively safe in overdose; favorable side effect profile; evidence obtained from acute (6–14 weeks), continuation (up to 12 months), and maintenance (1–3 years) treatment trials; second SSRI trial may still be effective if first trial fails ("salvage strategy," strength of evidence=C)
MAOIs	Phenelzine, tranylcypromine	Mood reactivity, rejection sensitivity, impulsivity, irritability, anger/hostility, atypical depression, hysteroid dysphoria	B	Second-line treatment after SSRI failure; complete elimination of initial SSRI required before MAOI treatment; adherence to required dietary restrictions problematic; effective for atypical depression only when borderline personality disorder is secondary, not primary, diagnosis
Mood stabilizers	Lithium carbonate	Mood lability, mood swings, anger, suicidality, impulsivity, poor global functioning	C	Can be used as primary or adjunctive treatment (overlaps with treatment of impulsive-behavioral domain); narrow margin of safety in overdose; blood level monitoring required; risk of hypothyroidism; to date, best studied of the mood stabilizers in treatment of personality disorders, but older literature focuses on reduction of impulsive behavior
	Carbamazepine	Suicidality, anxiety, anger, impulsivity	C	Efficacy in patients exhibiting hysteroid dysphoria; can precipitate melancholic depression; risk of bone marrow suppression; blood draws required to monitor WBC count
	Valproate	Global symptom severity, depressed mood, anger, impulsivity, rejection sensitivity, irritability, agitation, aggression, anxiety	C	Paucity of research support for this indication despite widespread use; blood draws required to monitor liver function
Benzodiazepines[c]	Alprazolam, clonazepam	Refractory anxiety, impulsivity, agitation	C	Risk of abuse, tolerance; alprazolam associated with behavioral dyscontrol
Neuroleptics[c]	Haloperidol	Behavioral dyscontrol, anger/hostility, assault, self-injury	A	Rapid onset of effect provides immediate control of behavior

[a]Ratings used by Jobson and Potter (2): A=supported by two or more randomized, placebo-controlled, double-blind trials; B=supported by at least one randomized, placebo-controlled, double-blind trial; C=supported by open-label studies, case reports, and studies that do not meet standards of randomized, placebo-controlled, double-blind trials. See text for specific supporting studies.

[b]A mixed norepinephrine/serotonin reuptake blocker.

[c]Agents primarily used as adjunctive treatment.

sonality disorder, although studies are currently under way. Lithium carbonate has the most research support in randomized controlled trials studying patients with personality disorders (although not specifically borderline personality disorder). However, these studies focused primarily on impulsivity and aggression rather than mood regulation (58–60). Nonetheless, lithium may be helpful for mood lability as a primary presentation in patients with a personality disorder (61). Lithium has the disadvantage of a narrow margin of safety in overdose and the risk of hypothyroidism with long-term use.

Carbamazepine has demonstrated efficacy for impulsivity, anger, suicidality, and anxiety in patients with borderline personality disorder and hysteroid dysphoria (62). However, a small, controlled study of patients with borderline personality disorder with no axis I affective disorder found no significant benefit for carbamazepine (63). Carbamazepine has been reported to precipitate melancholic depression in patients with borderline personality disorder who have a history of this disorder (64), and it has the potential to cause bone marrow suppression.

Valproate demonstrated modest efficacy for depressed mood in patients with borderline personality disorder in one small, randomized, controlled trial (65). Open-label case reports suggest that this medication may also decrease agitation, aggression, anxiety, impulsivity, rejection sensitivity, anger, and irritability in patients with borderline personality disorder (66). Although the use of carbamazepine and valproate is widespread, psychiatrists should be aware of the lack of solid research support for their use in patients with borderline personality disorder.

Although there is a paucity of data on the efficacy of ECT for patients with borderline personality disorder, much of the available data suggest that depressed patients with a personality disorder generally have a poorer outcome with ECT than depressed patients without a personality disorder. Clinical experience suggests that while ECT may sometimes be indicated for patients with borderline personality disorder and severe axis I depression that has been resistant to pharmacotherapy, affective features of the borderline diagnosis are unlikely to respond to ECT.

b) Treatment of impulsive-behavioral dyscontrol symptoms

As seen in Table 3, SSRIs are the treatment of choice for impulsive, disinhibited behavior in patients with borderline personality disorder. Randomized controlled trials and open-label studies with fluoxetine and sertraline have shown that their effect on impulsive behavior is independent of their effect on depression and anxiety (67). The effect of SSRIs on impulsivity may appear earlier than the effect on depression, with onset of action within days in some reports. Similarly, discontinuation of an SSRI following successful treatment may result in the reemergence of impulsive aggression within days. Clinical experience suggests that the duration of treatment following improvement of impulsive aggression should be determined by the clinical state of the patient, including his or her risk of exposure to life stressors and progress in learning coping skills. When the target for treatment is a trait vulnerability, a predetermined limit on treatment duration cannot be set.

When behavioral dyscontrol poses a serious threat to the patient's safety, it may be necessary to add a low-dose neuroleptic to the SSRI. Although this combination has not been studied, randomized controlled trials of neuroleptics alone have demonstrated their efficacy for impulsivity in patients with borderline personality disorder. The effect is rapid in onset, often within hours with oral use (and more rapidly when given intramuscularly), providing immediate control of escalating impulsive-aggressive behavior.

If an SSRI is ineffective, a trial of another SSRI or related antidepressant may be considered, although there are no published studies of this approach with impulsivity as a target symptom.

Clinical experience suggests that partial efficacy of an SSRI may be enhanced by adding lithium carbonate, although this combination has not been studied in patients with borderline personality disorder. Nonetheless, studies in impulsive adults and adolescents with criminal behavior (who were not selected for having borderline personality disorder) demonstrate that lithium alone is effective for impulsive-aggressive symptoms (58–60). If an SSRI is ineffective,

TABLE 3. Psychopharmacological Treatment Recommendations for Impulsive-Behavioral Dyscontrol Symptoms in Patients With Borderline Personality Disorder

Drug Class	Specific Medications Studied	Symptoms for Which Medication Is Recommended	Strength of Evidence[a]	Issues
SSRIs and related antidepressants	Fluoxetine, sertraline	Impulsive aggression, anger, irritability, self-injurious behavior, poor global functioning	A	Effects on anger and impulsive aggression may appear earlier and independently of effects on depressed mood and anxiety; no published literature on second "salvage" trials if first trial fails to reduce impulsive behavior
MAOIs	Phenelzine, tranylcypromine	Anger, irritability; impulsivity in patients with hysteroid dysphoria	A	Second-line treatment after SSRI failure; complete elimination of initial SSRI required before MAOI treatment; adherence to required dietary restrictions problematic
Mood stabilizers	Lithium carbonate	Impulsive aggression in patients with related personality disorders, impulsive behavior in patients with borderline personality disorder	A	Can be used as primary or adjunctive treatment (overlaps with treatment of affective dysregulation domain); older literature does not address borderline personality disorder; toxicity a concern in overdose; blood monitoring necessary; risk of hypothyroidism with long-term use
	Carbamazepine	Impulsivity in patients with hysteroid dysphoria	C	Risk of precipitating melancholic depression reported; blood monitoring required
	Valproate	Impulsive aggression, agitation; for adolescents with disruptive behavior disorders: tension, anxiety, chronic temper outbursts, poor global functioning	C	Paucity of research support for this indication despite widespread use; one randomized, placebo-controlled, double-blind trial is under way
Atypical neuroleptics	Clozapine	Severe self-mutilation, psychoticism	C	Risk of agranulocytosis renders clozapine treatment a last resort for this indication; blood monitoring required
Typical neuroleptics (low-dose)[b]	Haloperidol	Acute anger, hostility, assaultiveness, self-injury	A	Nonspecific effects on impulsivity as adjunctive agent; more specific effects on anger; rapid onset of effect provides immediate control of escalating impulsive symptoms

[a]Ratings used by Jobson and Potter (2): A=supported by two or more randomized, placebo-controlled, double-blind trials; B=supported by at least one randomized, placebo-controlled, double-blind trial; C=supported by open-label studies, case reports, and studies that do not meet standards of randomized, placebo-controlled, double-blind trials. See text for specific supporting studies.

[b]Agents primarily used as adjunctive treatment.

switching to an MAOI antidepressant may be considered, although it is critical to have an adequate washout period. In a placebo-controlled crossover study of women with borderline personality disorder and hysteroid dysphoria, tranylcypromine was effective for the treatment of impulsive behavior (55). In another randomized controlled trial, phenelzine was effective for the treatment of anger and irritability (56, 68). On the basis of these findings, MAOIs are recommended for treatment of impulsivity, anger, and irritability in patients with borderline personality disorder. Combining MAOIs with valproate would also appear to be rational for selected patients, although there are no studies of these combinations.

Although the use of MAOIs in patients with borderline personality disorder is supported by randomized controlled trials, because of safety considerations many clinicians prefer to use mood stabilizers for treatment of impulsive behavior. The use of carbamazepine or valproate for impulse control in patients with borderline personality disorder appears to be widespread in clinical practice, although empirical evidence for their efficacy for impulsive aggression is limited and inconclusive. Carbamazepine has been shown to decrease behavioral impulsivity in patients with borderline personality disorder and hysteroid dysphoria. However, in a small controlled study that excluded patients with an affective disorder (63), carbamazepine proved no better than placebo for impulsivity in borderline personality disorder. Support for the use of valproate for impulsivity in borderline personality disorder is derived only from case reports, one small randomized control study, and one open-label trial in which impulsivity significantly improved (65, 66, 69, 70). Preliminary evidence suggests that the atypical neuroleptics may have some efficacy for impulsivity in patients with borderline personality disorder, especially severe self-mutilation and other impulsive behaviors arising from psychotic thinking. One open-label trial (71) and one case report (72) support the use of clozapine for this indication. The difficulties and risks involved in using clozapine (e.g., neutropenia) generally warrant its use only after other treatments have failed. The newer atypical neuroleptics have fewer risks, but there are few published data on their efficacy. Further investigation is warranted for their use as a treatment for refractory impulsive aggression in patients with borderline personality disorder.

Opioid antagonists (e.g., naltrexone) are sometimes used in an attempt to decrease self-injurious behavior in patients with borderline personality disorder. However, empirical support for this approach is very preliminary, since their efficacy has been demonstrated only in case reports and small case series.

c) Treatment of cognitive-perceptual symptoms

As seen in Table 4, low-dose neuroleptics are the treatment of choice for these symptoms. This recommendation is strongly supported by randomized, double-blind controlled studies and open-label trials involving a variety of neuroleptics in both inpatient and outpatient settings and in adult and adolescent populations (50, 51, 55, 73–78).

Low-dose neuroleptics appear to have a broad spectrum of efficacy in acute use, improving not only psychotic-like symptoms but also depressed mood, impulsivity, and anger/hostility. Treatment effects appear within days to several weeks. Patients with cognitive symptoms as a primary complaint respond best to the use of low-dose neuroleptics. Patients with borderline personality disorder with prominent affective dysregulation and labile, depressive moods, in whom cognitive-perceptual distortions are secondary mood-congruent features, may do less well with neuroleptics alone. In this case, treatments more effective for affective dysregulation should be considered. Duration of treatment may be guided by the length of treatment trials in the literature, which are generally up to 12 weeks. Prolonged use of neuroleptic medication alone in patients with borderline personality disorder (i.e., up to 22 weeks in one study) has been associated with progressive nonadherence and dropout from treatment (68, 79). There is currently a paucity of research on the use of neuroleptic medication as long-term maintenance therapy for patients with borderline personality disorder, although many clinicians regularly use low-dose neuroleptics to help patients manage their vulnerability to disruptive anger. One

TABLE 4. Psychopharmacological Treatment Recommendations for Cognitive-Perceptual Symptoms in Patients With Borderline Personality Disorder

Drug Class	Specific Medications Studied	Symptoms for Which Medication Is Recommended	Strength of Evidence[a]	Issues
Typical neuroleptics (low-dose)	Haloperidol, perphenazine, thiothixene, thioridazine, flupentixol, loxapine, chlorpromazine, trifluoperazine	Ideas of reference, illusions, and paranoid ideation (and associated anger/hostility); global symptom severity, depressed mood, anxiety, impulsivity, recurrent suicidal behavior	A	Effects demonstrated in short-term studies (e.g., 5–16 weeks); poor tolerance over longer trials (e.g., 22 weeks) with increased akinesia, depression; reduction of recurrent parasuicidal behaviors reported in one long-term (6-month) study; risk of tardive dyskinesia with maintenance treatment
Atypical neuroleptics	Clozapine, olanzapine, risperidone	In theory, same as for typical neuroleptics as well as self-mutilation and severe, neuroleptic-resistant psychoticism	C	No published randomized, placebo-controlled, double-blind trials in support of this indication despite widespread use; risk of agranulocytosis renders clozapine treatment a last resort for this indication
SSRIs[b]		Irritability, anger/hostility, depressed mood, impulsive aggression	A	Especially effective if affective symptoms are present; overlaps with treatment of affective dysregulation and impulsive-behavioral dyscontrol domains
MAOIs[b]		Same as for SSRIs	A	Adherence to required dietary restrictions problematic

[a]Ratings used by Jobson and Potter (2): A=supported by two or more randomized, placebo-controlled, double-blind trials; B=supported by at least one randomized, placebo-controlled, double-blind trial; C=supported by open-label studies, case reports, and studies that do not meet standards of randomized, placebo-controlled, double-blind trials. See text for specific supporting studies.

[b]Agents primarily used as adjunctive treatment.

longer-term study (80) found that a depot neuroleptic was effective for recurrent parasuicidal behaviors in patients with borderline personality disorder. The risk of tardive dyskinesia must be weighed carefully against perceived prophylactic benefit if maintenance strategies are considered (although this risk may be lessened by the use of atypical neuroleptics).

If response to treatment with low-dose neuroleptics is suboptimal after 4 to 6 weeks, the dose should be increased into a range suitable for treating axis I disorders and continued for a second trial period of 4–6 weeks. A suboptimal response at this point should prompt rereview of the etiology of the cognitive-perceptual symptoms. If the symptom presentation is truly part of a nonaffective presentation, atypical neuroleptics may be considered. Although there are no published randomized controlled trials of atypical neuroleptics in patients with borderline personality disorder, open-label trials and case studies support the use of clozapine for patients with severe, refractory psychotic symptoms "of an atypical nature" or for severe self-mutilation (71, 72, 81). However, clozapine is best used in patients with refractory borderline personality disorder, given the risk of agranulocytosis. Studies are currently under way with olanzapine and risperidone (82, 83). The generally favorable side effect profiles of risperidone and olanzapine, compared with those of traditional neuroleptics, indicate that these medications warrant careful empirical trials. As yet, there are no published data on the efficacy of quetiapine for borderline personality disorder.

Neuroleptics are often effective for anger and hostility regardless of whether these symptoms occur in the context of cognitive-perceptual symptoms or other types of symptoms. It is important to note that both MAOI and SSRI antidepressants have also been shown in randomized controlled trials to be effective for irritability and anger in some patients with borderline personality disorder with cognitive-perceptual symptoms.

III. SPECIAL FEATURES INFLUENCING TREATMENT

A. COMORBIDITY

Other disorders may be comorbid with borderline personality disorder, such as mood disorders, substance-related disorders, eating disorders (notably, bulimia), PTSD, other anxiety disorders, dissociative identity disorder, and attention-deficit/hyperactivity disorder (ADHD) (see Section V.A.2, "Comorbidity," and refer to relevant APA Practice Guidelines [84–88]). These disorders can complicate the clinical picture and need to be addressed in treatment. Depression, often with atypical features, is particularly common in patients with borderline personality disorder (89, 90). Depressive features may meet criteria for major depressive disorder or dysthymic disorder, or they may be a manifestation of the borderline personality disorder itself. Although this distinction can be difficult to make, depressive features that appear particularly characteristic of borderline personality disorder are emptiness, self-condemnation, abandonment fears, hopelessness, self-destructiveness, and repeated suicidal gestures (91, 92). Depressive features that appear to be due to borderline personality disorder may respond to treatment approaches described in this practice guideline. Depressive features that meet criteria for major depression (especially if prominent neurovegetative symptoms are present) should be treated by using standard treatment approaches for major depression (see the APA *Practice Guideline for the Treatment of Patients With Major Depressive Disorder* [84; included in this volume]) in combination with treatment targeted at the borderline personality disorder. Available evidence suggests that SSRIs and MAOIs are more effective than tricyclic antidepressants for depressive features in patients with borderline personality disorder (although safety issues must be particularly carefully considered when using MAOIs).

B. PROBLEMATIC SUBSTANCE USE

Substance use disorders are common in patients with borderline personality disorder. The presence of substance use has major implications for treatment, since patients with borderline personality disorder who abuse substances generally have a poor outcome and are at greatly higher risk for suicide and for death or injury resulting from accidents. Persons with borderline personality disorder often abuse substances in an impulsive fashion that contributes to lowering the threshold for other self-destructive behavior such as body mutilation, sexual promiscuity, or provocative behavior that incites assault (including homicidal assault).

Patients with borderline personality disorder who abuse substances are seldom candid and forthcoming about the nature and extent of their abuse, especially in the early phases of therapy. For this reason, therapists should inquire specifically about substance abuse at the beginning of treatment and educate patients about the risks involved.

Vigorous treatment of any substance use disorder is essential in working with patients with borderline personality disorder (87). Depending on the severity of the alcohol abuse, if outpatient treatment is ineffective, inpatient treatment may be needed for detoxification and participation in various alcohol-treatment interventions. Participation in Alcoholics Anonymous is often helpful on both an inpatient and an outpatient basis. Clinical experience suggests that the use of disulfiram may occasionally be helpful as adjunctive treatment for patients with borderline personality disorder who use alcohol, but it must be used with caution because of the risk of impulsivity or nonadherence. Other medications effective for the treatment of alcohol abuse or dependence (e.g., naltrexone) may also be considered. Twelve-step programs are also available for persons abusing narcotics or cocaine. Opioid antagonists (e.g., naltrexone) are effective in treating opiate overdoses and are occasionally used in an attempt to decrease opiate abuse. However, they require diligent patient adherence, and there is little empirical support for the effectiveness of this approach for addiction.

Drug counseling may be a useful component of treatment. However, except perhaps for mild marijuana use, psychotherapy alone is generally ineffective for treating substance use disorders.

To the extent that various substances may be abused in order to mask depression, anxiety, and other related states, clinical experience suggests that prescribed medications—antidepressants (especially SSRIs) or nonhabituating anxiolytics such as buspirone—may help to alleviate the underlying symptoms, thus lessening the temptation to resort to the use of alcohol or drugs.

C. VIOLENT BEHAVIOR AND ANTISOCIAL TRAITS

Some patients with borderline personality disorder engage in violent behaviors. Violence may take such forms as hurling objects at family members—or at therapists—during moments of intense anger or frustration. Others may commit physical assaults. Some patients with borderline personality disorder are physically abusive toward their children. Patients with antisocial traits may engage in robbery, burglary, and car theft. Acts of this sort are often associated with an arrest record.

Therapeutic strategies optimal for dealing with antisocial features vary, depending on the severity of these features, and range from minor interventions to broader and more complex strategies suitable for a clinical picture in which antisociality is a major factor.

When antisocial features are mild (e.g., occasional shoplifting at times of severe stress), clinical experience suggests that individual cognitive therapy may be successful (e.g., encouraging the patient to weigh the risks versus the benefits—and the short-term versus the long-term consequences—of various antisocial choices the patient had been contemplating as well as identifying alternative coping strategies). This becomes in effect a psychoeducative approach in which the patient is helped to understand the advantages, in the long term, of socially appropriate alternatives (93).

When more severe antisocial features are present, residential treatment may be indicated. This may take the form of the "therapeutic community" as described by Losel (94) and by Dolan et al. (95). Various forms of group therapy are a mainstay of this approach. When episodic outbursts of violent behavior are present, the use of mood-stabilizing medications or an SSRI may be indicated (59, 96).

When antisocial features are even more severe and become dominant, and when the threat of violence is imminent, psychotherapy of any type may prove ineffective. In this situation hospitalization (involuntary, if necessary) may be required to help the patient regain control and, in cases in which a specific threat has been communicated by the patient, to reduce the risk to the potential victim(s).

Clinicians should be aware that some patients with borderline personality disorder with antisocial comorbidity may not be good candidates for therapy. This is especially true when the clinical picture is dominated by psychopathic traits (as described by Hare [97]) of the intensely narcissistic type: grandiosity, conning, lack of remorse, lying, and manipulativeness. Similarly, when underlying motives of jealousy or of revenge are of extreme intensity, therapy may prove ineffective (93).

D. CHRONIC SELF-DESTRUCTIVE BEHAVIOR

A primary feature of borderline personality disorder is impulsive self-destructive behavior, including reckless driving and spending, shoplifting, bingeing and purging, substance abuse, risky sexual behavior, self-mutilation, and suicide attempts. This behavior is thought to reflect the difficulties patients with borderline personality disorder have with modulation and containment of intense emotions or impulses. Some clinicians who are expert in the treatment of borderline personality disorder (4, 17) suggest that the psychotherapist should approach each session with a hierarchy of priorities in mind (as exhibited in Figure 1). In other words, suicidal and self-destructive behaviors would be addressed as the highest priorities, with an effort to evaluate the patient's risk for these behaviors and help the patient find ways to maintain safety. Alternatives to self-mutilation, for example, can be considered (12, 17), and insights might be offered about the meaning of self-defeating behavior. SSRIs might also be prescribed for the self-mutilating patient.

Most experts agree that some type of limit-setting is necessary at times in the treatment of patients with borderline personality disorder. Because patients engage in so many self-destructive and self-defeating behaviors, clinicians may find themselves spending a great deal of the therapy setting limits on the patient's behaviors. The risk in these situations is that therapists may become entrenched in a countertransference posture of policing the patient's behavior to the point that treatment goals are lost and the therapeutic alliance is compromised. Waldinger (18) has suggested that limit-setting should be targeted at a subgroup of behaviors, namely, those that are destructive to the patient, the therapist, or the therapy. Limit-setting is not necessarily an ultimatum involving a threat to discontinue the treatment. Therapists can indicate to the patient that certain conditions are necessary to make treatment viable.

It is also useful for psychiatrists to help the patient think through the consequences of chronic self-destructive behaviors. In this way the behavior may gradually shift from being ego syntonic to ego dystonic (i.e., the behavior becomes more distressing to the patient as he or she becomes more reflective about the adverse consequences). The patient and therapist can then form a stronger therapeutic alliance around strategies to control the behavior.

If self-destructive behaviors are relentless and out of control, and especially if patients are not willing to work on controlling such behaviors, patients may need referral to a more intensive level of care before they are able to resume outpatient treatment. Consultation may also be useful.

E. CHILDHOOD TRAUMA AND PTSD

Childhood trauma is a common although not universal feature of borderline personality disorder (98–104). Recognizing trauma-related aspects of the patient's affective instability, damaged self-image, relationship problems, fears of abandonment, self-injurious behavior, and impulsiveness is important and can facilitate psychotherapy in a variety of ways.

1. Threats to the therapeutic alliance

Recognizing a trauma history, if present, can help the therapist and patient understand current distortions in the patient's view of self and others as an understandable residual of prior life experiences that would produce mistrust. Anger, impulsiveness, and self-defeating behavior in relationships take on different meanings when understood as, in part, displaced responses to abusive early life experiences. Discounting a trauma history has the potential to undermine the therapeutic alliance and the progress of treatment. It can also hamper patients' ability to integrate and come to terms with the trauma. Not integrating traumatic material into the treatment can lead patients to experience the therapy as a form of collusion with the abuser.

2. Issues with transference

Many traumatized patients expect others, including their therapists, to be malevolent, for example, inflicting harm in the guise of providing help, analogous to a parent or other caretaker exploiting and abusing a child. This core transference mistrust may become an ongoing issue to be worked on during psychotherapy.

3. Determining appropriate treatment focus

Decisions about whether and when to focus on trauma, if present, during treatment should be based on the patient's agitation, stability, fragility, evidence of psychotic symptoms, and potential for self-harm or disruption of current vocational, family, or other roles. It is generally thought that working through the residue of trauma is best done at a later phase of treatment, after solidifying the therapeutic alliance, achieving stabilization of symptoms, and establishing an understanding of the patient's history and psychological structures (8).

4. Working through traumatic memories

In the later phase of treatment, one component of effective psychotherapy for patients with a trauma history involves exposure to, managing affect related to, and cognitively restructuring memories of the traumatic experience. This involves grief work (105), acknowledging, bearing, and putting into perspective the residue of traumatic experiences (106). This process helps to reduce the unbidden, intrusive, and alien nature of traumatic memories and differentiates affect associated with the trauma from that elicited by current relationships.

5. Importance of group support and therapy

For patients with borderline personality disorder who have experienced trauma, group work can be particularly helpful in providing support and understanding from other trauma survivors as well as a milieu in which they can gain understanding about their self-defeating behaviors and interpersonal relationship patterns. Some patients with borderline personality disorder can be less defensive receiving feedback from peers, and at certain points in therapy this may be the only place they feel understood and safe.

6. Risk of reenactment or revictimization

The vulnerability of traumatized patients to revictimization, or their deliberate incurring of risk and reenactment of early trauma, has implications for patient safety and management of the transference. The therapist should address the possibility of current or future harm to the patient.

7. Treating PTSD-like symptoms

Even when full criteria for comorbid PTSD are not present, patients with borderline personality disorder may experience PTSD-like symptoms. For example, symptoms such as intrusion, avoidance, and hyperarousal may emerge during psychotherapy. Awareness of the trauma-related nature of these symptoms can facilitate both psychotherapeutic and pharmacological efforts in symptom relief.

8. Reassignment of blame

Victims of trauma, especially early in life, typically blame themselves inappropriately for traumatic events over which they had no control (107). This may happen because the trauma was experienced during a developmental period when the child was unable to appreciate independent causation and therefore assumed he or she was responsible. Many adults blame themselves so that they avoid reexperiencing the helplessness associated with trauma. It is important in therapy to listen to a patient's guilt and sense of responsibility for past trauma and, when appropriate, to clarify the patient's lack of responsibility for past trauma as well as the importance of taking responsibility for present life circumstances.

9. Use of eye movement therapy

Eye movement desensitization and reprocessing (108) has been presented as a treatment for trauma symptoms. It involves having patients discuss a traumatic memory and then move their eyes back and forth rapidly as though they were in rapid eye movement sleep. The specific effect of the eye movements has not been established, and the treatment may mainly involve exposure to and working through trauma-related cognition and affect (109, 110). This therapy is currently under investigation. There is currently no evidence of specific efficacy for this treatment in patients with borderline personality disorder.

10. Accuracy of distant memories

Ignoring or discounting a trauma history can undermine the therapeutic alliance by aligning the therapist with individuals in the patient's past who either inflicted harm or ignored it. On the other hand, memories of remote traumatic experiences may contain inaccuracies. Dissociative symptoms may complicate retrieval of traumatic memories in patients with borderline personality disorder (111, 112). The affect may be correct even when the details about events are wrong (113). Furthermore, confrontation of family members regarding possible abusive activity is likely to produce substantial emotional response and family disruption. Thus, the approach to traumatic origins of symptoms should be open-ended, sensitive to both the effects of possible trauma and the fallibility of memory.

F. DISSOCIATIVE FEATURES

There is considerable comorbidity between borderline personality disorder and various dissociative symptoms and disorders (100, 114–117). Transient dissociative symptoms, including depersonalization, derealization, and loss of reality testing, are not uncommon and may contribute to the psychotic-like symptoms that patients with borderline personality disorder may experience. The percentage of patients with borderline personality disorder who also have dissociative identity disorder is unknown, but it is estimated that one-third of patients with dissociative identity disorder also have borderline personality disorder (118). Dissociative symptoms and dissociative identity disorder may appear as or exacerbate other borderline personality disorder characteristics, including identity disturbance, impulsivity, recurrent suicidal behavior, and affective instability. Thus, to manage these symptoms, identification of and attention to comorbid dissociative identity disorder or prominent dissociative symptoms is mandated. This includes the following:

- Exploring the extent of the dissociative symptoms
- Exploring current issues that may lead to dissociative episodes
- Clarifying the nature of dissociative symptoms and distinguishing them from malingering or deception on the one hand and psychotic symptoms on the other
- Teaching the patient how to access and learn to control dissociation, including the possible use of hypnosis in patients with full dissociative disorder
- Working through any possible posttraumatic symptoms associated with the dissociative symptoms
- Facilitating integration of dissociated identities or personality states and integrating amnesic episodes by explaining to patients that the problem is one of fragmentation of personality structure elements; practicing with the patient more fluid transitions among various identities and personality states
- Working through transference issues related to trauma and feelings about controlling dissociative symptoms
- Consolidating and stabilizing gains by providing positive reinforcement for integrated function and consistent response to dissociative components of the personality structure
- Supporting the patient in case of relapse

When borderline personality disorder and dissociative identity disorder coexist, clinical reports suggest that hypnosis may be useful for identifying and controlling dissociative symptoms (119–121). These symptoms can be reconceptualized as uncontrolled hypnotic-like states that can be elicited and modulated with hypnosis, both as a technique in therapy and as a self-hypnotic exercise to be practiced by patients under the therapist's supervision.

A crucial element in working through issues of transference/countertransference and limit-setting is the extent to which the patient is consciously aware and in control of mental states in which impulsive behavior or strong emotions are experienced. Treatment of comorbid dissociative symptoms can help to delineate the areas of available control and expand the patient's repertoire of adaptive symptom-control skills.

G. PSYCHOSOCIAL STRESSORS

In borderline personality disorder, stress may be a contributing factor in the disorder's etiology and a precipitant of symptomatic exacerbation (122). Physical or sexual abuse is not uncommon during childhood for these patients; histories of other forms of trauma, such as verbal abuse or neglect (123) and early parental separation or loss (124), are frequently elicited as well. In addition, most patients with borderline personality disorder are acutely sensitive to psychosocial stressors, particularly interpersonal stressors. Self-esteem is often fragile, and patients seek to shore up their sense of self by "borrowing" a stable, established identity from another (usually idealized) person. Relationships are intense, and everyday distractions or inattention can be interpreted as abandonment, resulting in panic-like anxiety, impulsive self-destructive acts, excessive anger, paranoia, or dissociative episodes. These sensitivities are important in therapy, since regardless of the type of treatment, once a therapeutic relationship has developed, it will take on this overdetermined, intense quality. The psychiatrist should be alert, nimble, flexible, and on the lookout for ways in which the limits of the therapeutic relationship may stimulate anxiety-driven reactions in the patient—reactions that may be confrontational, depressive, or invisible until revealed by self-destructive or impulsive acting out.

H. GENDER

Borderline personality disorder is diagnosed predominantly in women, with an estimated gender ratio of 3:1. The disorder may be missed in men, who may instead receive diagnoses of antisocial or narcissistic personality disorder. Men should be as carefully assessed for borderline personality disorder as women. The diagnostic assessment of the patient should include a detailed inquiry regarding reproductive life history, including sexual practices and birth control.

Most treatment studies of borderline personality disorder primarily involve women. There has been little systematic investigation of gender differences in treatment response.

The treatment of pregnant and nursing women raises specific concerns regarding the use of psychotropic medications. The potential risks, which are highest during the first trimester of pregnancy, have been reviewed elsewhere (125). When treating women with borderline personality disorder who are pregnant or nursing, the risks of treatment with medication must be carefully weighed against the potential risks and benefits of alternative treatment (e.g., psychotherapy alone) as well as the risk to the woman if the borderline personality disorder and comorbid conditions are not treated (125, 126). These potential risks and benefits should be discussed with the patient.

Because anticonvulsants are associated with a potential risk of birth defects, and the risk of birth defects from other psychotropic medications is unknown, psychiatrists should encourage careful contraceptive practices for all female patients of childbearing age who are receiving pharmacological treatment. Since carbamazepine can increase the metabolism of birth control pills, the dosage of oral contraceptives may need to be adjusted accordingly. Whenever possible, planned pregnancy should be pursued in consultation with the psychiatrist so that options, including maintenance of pharmacological treatment or discontinuation of these agents, can be thoughtfully pursued. For patients who become pregnant while on a maintenance regimen of psychiatric medications, a consultation for further consideration of the relative risks of continuing or discontinuing medications should also be considered (127, 128).

Gender issues, including psychotropic medication use during pregnancy, that are associated with certain comorbid conditions are discussed in other APA Practice Guidelines (84–86).

I. CULTURAL FACTORS

Borderline personality disorder has been reported in many cultures around the world (129). The cultural context of a patient's presentation should be considered. Cultural factors may hamper the accurate assessment of borderline personality disorder. An appreciation by the clinician of cultural variables is critical in making an accurate diagnosis. Clinicians should be especially careful to avoid cultural bias when applying the diagnostic criteria and evaluating sexual behavior, expressions of emotion, or impulsiveness, which may have different norms in different cultures.

Ethnic groups may differ in their response to psychotropic medications. Although inconclusive, some studies have suggested that Asian patients may require lower doses of haloperidol and have higher serum levels of haloperidol after oral administration than Caucasian patients (130). Psychiatrists should be aware of this possibility when administering neuroleptic medication to Asian patients. Some studies also suggest that ethnic groups may differ in their response to antidepressant medications (131, 132).

J. AGE

Because the personality of adolescents is still developing, the diagnosis of borderline personality disorder should be made with care in this age group. Borderline personality disorder may be present in the elderly, although later in life a majority of individuals with this disorder attain greater stability in functioning. Virtually no treatment studies have been done in adolescents or elderly persons with borderline personality disorder. Although treatments effective in adults would be expected to be efficacious in these age groups, research that demonstrates this efficacy is needed, especially in adolescents. It should be kept in mind that elderly patients are particularly prone to certain medication side effects (e.g., orthostatic hypotension and anticholinergic effects) and therefore may tolerate certain medications less well than younger adults.

IV. RISK MANAGEMENT ISSUES

A. GENERAL CONSIDERATIONS

When treating patients with any mental disorder, attention to risk management issues is important and often enhances patient care. Attention to these issues is particularly important when treating patients with borderline personality disorder, given the potential for self-injury, violent behavior, and suicide, as well as impulsivity, splitting, problems with the therapeutic alliance, and transference and countertransference problems (e.g., the mobilization of intense feelings in the clinician). The following are general risk management considerations for patients with borderline personality disorder:

- Good collaboration and communication with other clinicians who are also treating the patient are necessary.
- Attention should be paid to careful and adequate documentation, including assessment of risk, communication with other clinicians, the decision-making process, and the rationale for the treatment used.
- Attention should be paid to any transference and countertransference problems that have the potential to cloud good clinical judgment. The clinician should be especially aware of the potential for splitting to occur and should resist taking on the role of the "all good" or rescuing clinician. In this regard, close collaboration and communication with other team members are important. Keep in mind that different perspectives of different clinicians can be valid, since the patient may act differently with different clinicians.
- Consultation with a colleague should be considered and may be useful for unusually high-risk patients (e.g., when suicide risk is very high), when the patient is not improving, or when it is unclear what the best treatment approach might be. It is important to document the consultation (i.e., that the consultation has occurred, what the recommendations were, whether the recommendations were followed or not, and, if the clinician made a different treatment decision, why the recommendations were not followed).
- Termination of treatment with a patient with borderline personality disorder must be managed with care. Standard guidelines for terminating psychiatric treatment should be followed, even if it is the patient's decision to terminate treatment (133). Careful attention must be paid to timing, transfer, and discussion with the patient. If the treatment termination process is unusually difficult or complex, obtaining a consultation should be considered.
- Psychoeducation about the disorder is often appropriate and helpful from both a clinical and risk management perspective. When appropriate, family members should be included, with attention to confidentiality issues. Psychoeducation should include discussion of the risks inherent in the disorder and the uncertainties of the treatment outcome.

B. SUICIDE

Suicidal threats, gestures, and attempts are very common among patients with borderline personality disorder, and 8%–10% commit suicide. Managing suicide risk therefore poses important clinical and medicolegal challenges for clinicians. However, it can be difficult to address suicide risk in these patients for a number of reasons. First, suicidality can be acute, chronic, or both, and responses to these types of suicidality differ in some ways. Second, given the tendency of patients with borderline personality disorder to be chronically suicidal and to engage in self-destructive behaviors, it can be difficult to discern when a patient is at imminent risk of making a serious suicide attempt. Third, even with careful attention to suicide risk, it is often difficult to predict serious self-harm or suicide, since this behavior can occur impulsively and without warning. Fourth, given the potential for difficulties in forming a good therapeutic alliance, it may be difficult to work collaboratively with the patient to protect him or her from serious self-harm or suicide. Last, even with good treatment, some patients will commit suicide. The following are risk management considerations for suicidal behavior in patients with borderline personality disorder:

- Monitor patients carefully for suicide risk and document this assessment; be aware that feelings of rejection, fears of abandonment, or a change in the treatment may precipitate suicidal ideation or attempts.
- Take suicide threats seriously and address them with the patient. Taking action (e.g., hospitalization) in an attempt to protect the patient from serious self-harm is indicated for acute suicide risk.
- Chronic suicidality without acute risk needs to be addressed in therapy (e.g., focusing on the interpersonal context of the suicidal feelings and addressing the need for the patient to take responsibility for his or her actions). If a patient with chronic suicidality becomes acutely suicidal, the clinician should take action in an attempt to prevent suicide.
- Actively treat comorbid axis I disorders, with particular attention to those that may contribute to or increase the risk of suicide (e.g., major depression, bipolar disorder, alcohol or drug abuse/dependence).
- If acute suicidality is present and not responding to the therapeutic approaches being used, consultation with a colleague should be considered.
- Consider involving the family (if otherwise clinically appropriate and with adequate attention to confidentiality issues) when patients are chronically suicidal. For acute suicidality, involve the family or significant others if their involvement will potentially protect the patient from harm.
- A promise to keep oneself safe (e.g., a "suicide contract") should not be used as a substitute for a careful and thorough clinical evaluation of the patient's suicidality with accompanying documentation. However, some experienced clinicians carefully attend to and intentionally utilize the negotiation of the therapeutic alliance, including discussion of the patient's responsibility to keep himself or herself safe, as a way to monitor and minimize the risk of suicide.

C. ANGER, IMPULSIVITY, AND VIOLENCE

Anger and impulsivity are hallmarks of borderline personality disorder and can be directed at others, including the clinician. This is particularly likely to occur when there is a disruption in the patient's relationships or when he or she feels abandoned (e.g., there is a change in clinicians) or when the patient feels betrayed, unjustly accused, or seriously misunderstood and blamed by the clinician or a significant other. Even with close monitoring and attention to these issues in the treatment, it is difficult to predict their occurrence. Another complicating factor is that the patient's anger or behavior may produce anger in the therapist, which has the potential to adversely affect clinical judgment. The following are risk management considerations for anger, impulsivity, and violence in patients with borderline personality disorder:

- Monitor the patient carefully for impulsive or violent behavior, which is difficult to predict and can occur even with appropriate treatment.
- Address abandonment/rejection issues, anger, and impulsivity in the treatment.
- Arrange for adequate coverage when away; carefully communicate this to the patient and document coverage.
- If the patient makes threats toward others (including the clinician) or exhibits threatening behavior, the clinician may need to take action to protect self or others.

D. BOUNDARY VIOLATIONS

With patients with borderline personality disorder there is a risk of boundary crossings and violations. The following are risk management considerations for boundary issues with patients with borderline personality disorder:

- Monitor carefully and explore countertransference feelings toward the patient.
- Be alert to deviations from the usual way of practicing, which may be signs of countertransference problems—e.g., appointments at unusual hours, longer-than-usual appointments, doing special favors for the patient.
- Always avoid boundary violations, such as the development of a personal friendship outside of the professional situation or a sexual relationship with the patient.
- Get a consultation if there are striking deviations from the usual manner of practice.

PART B: BACKGROUND INFORMATION AND REVIEW OF AVAILABLE EVIDENCE

V. DISEASE DEFINITION, EPIDEMIOLOGY, AND NATURAL HISTORY

A. DEFINITION AND CORE CLINICAL FEATURES

The essential feature of borderline personality disorder is a pervasive pattern of instability of interpersonal relationships, affects, and self-image, as well as marked impulsivity that begins by early adulthood and appears in a variety of contexts. These characteristics are severe and persistent enough to result in clinically significant impairment in social, occupational, or other important areas of functioning. Common and important features of borderline personality disorder are a severely impaired capacity for attachment and predictably maladaptive behavior in response to separation. Individuals with this disorder are very sensitive to abandonment and make frantic efforts to avoid real or perceived abandonment. They often experience intense abandonment fears and anger in reaction to even realistic time-limited separation. Efforts to avoid abandonment may include inappropriate rage, unfair accusations, and impulsive behaviors such as self-mutilation or suicidal behaviors, which often elicit a guilty or fearful protective response from others.

The relationships of individuals with borderline personality disorder tend to be unstable, intense, and stormy. Their views of others may suddenly and dramatically shift, alternating between extremes of idealization and devaluation, or seeing others as beneficent and nurturing and then as cruel, punitive, and rejecting. These shifts are particularly likely to occur in response to disillusionment with a significant other or when a sustaining relationship is threatened or lost.

The disorder is usually characterized by identity disturbance, which consists of markedly and persistently unstable self-image or sense of self. Self-image (goals, values, type of friends, vocational goals) may suddenly and dramatically shift. Individuals with this disorder usually feel bad or evil, but they may also feel that they do not exist at all, especially when feeling unsupported and alone.

Many individuals with borderline personality disorder are impulsive in one or more potentially self-damaging areas, such as spending money irresponsibly, gambling, engaging in unsafe sexual behavior, abusing drugs or alcohol, driving recklessly, or binge eating. Self-mutilation (e.g., cutting or burning) and recurrent suicidal behaviors, gestures, or threats are common. These self-destructive acts are often precipitated by potential separation from others, perceived or actual rejection or abandonment, or the expectation from others that they assume more responsibility.

Affective instability is another common feature of the disorder. This consists of marked mood reactivity (e.g., intense episodic dysphoria, irritability, or anxiety that usually lasts for a few hours and only rarely for more than a few days). The usual dysphoric mood of these individuals is often punctuated by anger, panic, or despair and is only infrequently relieved by periods of well-being. These episodes may be triggered by the individual's extreme reactivity to interpersonal stressors. Individuals with this disorder also typically have chronic feelings of emptiness. Many experience inappropriate, intense anger or have difficulty controlling their anger. For example, they may lose their temper, feel constant anger, have verbal outbursts, or engage in physical fights. This anger may be triggered by their perception that an important person is neglectful, withholding, uncaring, or abandoning. Expressions of anger may be followed by feelings of being evil or by feelings of shame and guilt. During periods of extreme stress (e.g., perceived or actual abandonment), these individuals may experience transient paranoid ideation or severe dissociative symptoms (e.g., depersonalization).

It is not necessary for an individual to have all of the above features for borderline personality disorder to be diagnosed. As indicated in Table 1, the diagnosis is given if at least five of the nine diagnostic criteria are present.

1. Associated features

Transient psychotic-like symptoms (e.g., hearing their name called) may occur at times of stress. These episodes usually last for minutes or hours and are generally of insufficient duration or severity to warrant an additional diagnosis. Another common associated feature is a tendency for these individuals to undermine themselves when a goal is about to be reached (e.g., severely regressing after a discussion of how well therapy is going). Individuals with this disorder may feel more secure with transitional objects (e.g., a pet or inanimate object) than with interpersonal relationships. Despite their significant relationship problems, they may deny that they are responsible for such problems and may instead blame others for their difficulties.

Physical and sexual abuse, neglect, hostile conflict, and early parental loss or separation are more common in the childhood histories of those with borderline personality disorder than in those without the disorder.

2. Comorbidity

Axis I disorders and other axis II disorders are often comorbid with borderline personality disorder. Among the most common comorbid axis I disorders are mood disorders, substance-related disorders, eating disorders (notably bulimia), PTSD, panic disorder, and ADHD. Such axis I comorbidity can complicate and worsen the course of borderline personality disorder. Commonly co-occurring axis II disorders are antisocial, avoidant, histrionic, narcissistic, and schizotypal personality disorders.

3. Complications

Borderline personality disorder is characterized by notable distress and functional impairment. A majority of patients attempt suicide. Completed suicide occurs in 8%–10% of individuals with this disorder, a rate that is approximately 50 times higher than in the general population. Risk of suicide appears to be highest when patients are in their 20s as well as in the presence of co-occurring mood disorders or substance-related disorders (87). Physical handicaps may result from self-inflicted injury or failed suicide attempts. These individuals often have notable difficulty with occupational, academic, or role functioning. Their functioning may deteriorate in unstructured work or school situations, and recurrent job loss and interrupted education are common. Difficulties in relationships, as well as divorce, are also common.

The social cost for patients with borderline personality disorder and their families is substantial. Longitudinal studies of patients with borderline personality disorder indicate that even though these patients may gradually attain functional roles 10–15 years after admission to psychiatric facilities, still only about one-half will have stable, full-time employment or stable marriages (40, 134). Recent data indicate that patients with borderline personality disorder show greater lifetime utilization of most major categories of medication and of most types of psychotherapy than do patients with schizotypal, avoidant, or obsessive-compulsive personality disorder or patients with major depressive disorder (135).

B. ASSESSMENT

A skilled clinical interview is the mainstay of diagnosing borderline personality disorder. This approach should be complemented by knowledge of the DSM criteria and a longitudinal view of the clinical picture. The additional use of assessment instruments can be useful, especially when the diagnosis is unclear. Use of such instruments must be accompanied by clinical judgment.

Certain assessment issues relevant to all personality disorders should be considered when diagnosing borderline personality disorder. For the diagnosis to be made, the personality traits must cause subjective distress or significant impairment in functioning. The traits must also deviate markedly from the culturally expected and accepted range, or norm, and this deviation must be manifested in more than one of the following areas: cognition, affectivity, control over impulses, and ways of relating to others. Therefore, multiple domains of experience and behavior (i.e., cognition, affect, intrapsychic experience, and interpersonal interaction) must be assessed to determine whether borderline traits are distressing or impairing. The clinician should also ascertain that the personality traits are of early onset, pervasive, and enduring; they should not be transient or present in only one situation or in response to only one specific trigger. It is important that borderline personality disorder be assessed as carefully in men as in women.

The ego-syntonicity of the personality traits may complicate the assessment process; the use of multiple sources of information (e.g., medical records and informants who know the patient well) can be particularly helpful in establishing the diagnosis if the patient's self-awareness is limited. Given the high comorbidity of axis I disorders with borderline personality disorder, it is important to do a full axis I evaluation. An attempt should be made to distinguish axis I states (e.g., mood disorder) from borderline personality disorder, which can be a complex process. Useful approaches are to obtain a description of the patient's personality traits and coping styles when prominent axis I symptoms are absent and to use information provided by people who have known the patient without an axis I disorder. If axis I disorders are present, both the axis I disorders and borderline personality disorder should be diagnosed.

Because the personality of children and adolescents is still developing, borderline personality disorder should be diagnosed with care in this age group. Often, the presence of the disorder does not become clear until late adolescence or adulthood.

When assessing a patient with borderline personality disorder, the clinician should carefully look for the presence of risk-taking and impulsive behaviors, mood disturbance and reactivity, risk of suicide, risk of violence to persons or property, substance abuse, the patient's ability to care for himself/herself or others (e.g., children), financial resources, psychosocial stressors, and psychosocial supports (e.g., family and friends).

C. DIFFERENTIAL DIAGNOSIS

Borderline personality disorder often co-occurs with mood disorders, and when criteria for both are met, both should be diagnosed. However, some features of borderline personality disorder may overlap with those of mood disorders, complicating the differential diagnostic assessment. For example, the affective instability and impulsivity of borderline personality disorder may mimic features of bipolar disorder, especially bipolar II disorder. However, in borderline personality disorder, the mood swings are often triggered by interpersonal stressors (e.g., rejection), and a particular mood is usually less sustained than in bipolar disorder. Depressive features may meet criteria for major depressive disorder or may be features of the borderline personality disorder itself. Depressive features that appear particularly characteristic of borderline personality disorder are emptiness, self-condemnation, abandonment fears, self-destructiveness, and hopelessness (91, 92). It can be particularly difficult to differentiate dysthymic disorder from borderline personality disorder, given that chronic dysphoria is so common in individuals with borderline personality disorder. However, the presence of the aforementioned affective features (e.g., mood swings triggered by interpersonal stressors) should prompt consideration of the diagnosis of borderline personality disorder. In addition, the other features of borderline personality disorder (e.g., identity disturbance, chronic self-destructive behaviors, frantic efforts to avoid abandonment) are generally not characteristic of axis I mood disorders. In other cases, what appear to be features of borderline personality disorder may constitute symptoms of an axis I disorder (e.g., bipolar disorder). A more in-depth consideration of the differential diagnosis or treatment of the presumed axis I condition may help clarify such questions.

PTSD is a common comorbid condition in patients with borderline personality disorder and, when present, should be diagnosed. However, a history of trauma is often characteristic of patients with borderline personality disorder and does not necessarily warrant an additional diagnosis of PTSD. PTSD should be diagnosed only when full criteria for the disorder are met. PTSD is characterized by rapid-onset symptoms that occur, usually in adulthood, in reaction to exposure to a recognizable and extreme stressor; in contrast, borderline personality disorder consists of the early-onset, enduring personality traits described elsewhere in this guideline.

Although borderline personality disorder may be comorbid with dissociative identity disorder, the latter (unlike borderline personality disorder) is characterized by the presence of two or more distinct identities or personality states that alternate, manifesting different patterns of behavior.

D. EPIDEMIOLOGY

Borderline personality disorder is the most common personality disorder in clinical settings. It is present in 10% of individuals seen in outpatient mental health clinics, 15%–20% of psychiatric inpatients, and 30%–60% of clinical populations with a personality disorder. It occurs in an estimated 2% of the general population (1, 136).

Borderline personality disorder is diagnosed predominantly in women, with an estimated gender ratio of 3:1. The disorder is present in cultures around the world. It is approximately five times more common among first-degree biological relatives of those with the disorder than in the general population. There is also a greater familial risk for substance-related disorders, antisocial personality disorder, and mood disorders.

E. NATURAL HISTORY AND COURSE

Long-term follow-up studies of treated patients with borderline personality disorder indicate that the course is variable. Early adulthood is often characterized by chronic instability, with episodes of serious affective and impulsive dyscontrol and high levels of use of health and mental health resources. Later in life, a majority of individuals attain greater stability in social and occupational functioning.

In the largest follow-up study to date (137), about one-third of patients with borderline personality disorder had recovered by the follow-up evaluation, having solidified their identity during the intervening years and having replaced their tendency toward self-damaging acts, inordinate anger, and stormy relationships with more mature and more modulated behavior patterns. Longitudinal studies of hospitalized patients with borderline personality disorder indicate that even though they may gradually attain functional roles 10–15 years after admission to psychiatric facilities, only about one-half of the women and one-quarter of the men will have attained enduring success in intimacy (as indicated by marriage or long-term sexual partnership) (137). One-half to three-quarters will have by that time achieved stable full-time employment. These studies concentrated on patients with borderline personality disorder from middle-class or upper-middle-class families. Patients with borderline personality disorder from backgrounds of poverty have substantially lower success rates in the spheres of intimacy and work. Despite these somewhat favorable outcomes, the suicide rate among patients with borderline personality disorder is high—approximately 9%. The risk of suicide appears highest in the young-adult years.

VI. REVIEW AND SYNTHESIS OF AVAILABLE EVIDENCE

A. ISSUES IN INTERPRETING THE LITERATURE

The following issues should be considered when interpreting the literature presented in this guideline on the efficacy of treatments for borderline personality disorder. Virtually all of the studies involved adults with borderline personality disorder. While the results may be applicable to adolescents, there is a paucity of research that has examined the efficiency of these treatments for this age group. Although some of these treatments have been evaluated through randomized, placebo-controlled trials—the gold standard for determining treatment efficacy— information for other treatments is available only from case reports, case series, or retrospective studies, which limits the conclusions that can be drawn about treatment efficacy.

Another consideration is that efficacy studies (e.g., placebo-controlled trials) have notable strengths but also some limitations. Although such studies are necessary to establish that a particular treatment is effective, there may be limits to how generalizable the study findings are. For example, inclusion and exclusion criteria result in particular types of patients being involved in a study. When reviewing the data presented in this guideline, clinicians should consider how similar their patient is to the population included in a particular study. This is particularly important because of the heterogeneous nature of borderline personality disorder symptoms. Some studies, for example, select patients with marked impulsivity, whereas others include patients with prominent affective features. In addition, many studies have been relatively short-term; longer-term treatment outcome studies are needed.

Another issue to consider is that some studies are done in specialized research settings with more expertise and training in the treatment modality than is generally available in the community. In addition, the amount of treatment provided in a study may be greater than is actually available in the community.

When evaluating studies of psychosocial treatments that consist of multiple elements, such as psychodynamic psychotherapy, it may be difficult to know which elements are responsible for the treatment outcome. Another factor to consider is that patients in certain studies of psychosocial treatment were also taking prescription medication, and no steps were taken to control for these effects. Conversely, patients in some studies of medication efficacy also received psychotherapy, and no steps were taken to control for these effects. Therefore, the literature on the efficacy of any one particular treatment is often confounded by the presence of other simultaneous treatments. It can be difficult, then, to isolate the impact of a single modality in most treatment efficacy studies involving patients with borderline personality disorder.

In clinical practice, a combination of treatment approaches is often used and appropriate. Few data are available on the complex treatment regimens often required by the realities of clinical practice (e.g., the use of multiple medications simultaneously). Many clinically important and complex treatment questions have not been (and are unlikely to ever be) addressed in research studies. For such questions, clinical consensus is the best available guide.

B. REVIEW OF PSYCHOTHERAPY AND OTHER PSYCHOSOCIAL TREATMENTS

1. Psychodynamic psychotherapy

Psychodynamic psychotherapy has been defined as a therapy that involves careful attention to the therapist-patient interaction with, when indicated, thoughtfully timed interpretation of transference and resistance embedded in a sophisticated appreciation of the therapist's contribution to the two-person field. Psychodynamic psychotherapy draws from three major theoretical perspectives: ego psychology, object relations, and self psychology. Most therapeutic approaches to patients with borderline personality disorder do not adhere strictly to only one of these theoretical frameworks. The approach of Stevenson and Meares (20, 138), for example, encompasses the self-psychological ideas of Kohut and the object relations ideas of Winnicott, whereas the technique of Kernberg et al. (4, 13, 28) is based on an amalgamation of ego psychology and object relations theory.

a) Definition and goals

Psychodynamic psychotherapy is usually conceptualized as operating on an exploratory-supportive (also called expressive-supportive) continuum of interventions (Figure 2). At the more exploratory end of the continuum, the goals of psychodynamic psychotherapy with patients with borderline personality disorder are to make unconscious patterns more consciously available, to increase affect tolerance, to build a capacity to delay impulsive action, to provide insight into relationship problems, and to develop reflective functioning so that there is greater appreciation of internal motivation in self and others. From the standpoint of object relations theory, one major goal is to integrate split-off aspects of self and object representations so that the patient's perspective is more balanced (e.g., seeing others as simultaneously having both positive and negative qualities). From a self-psychological perspective, a major goal is to strengthen the self so that there is less fragmentation and a greater sense of cohesion or wholeness in the patient's self-experience. On the supportive end of the continuum, the goals involve strengthening of defenses, the shoring up of self-esteem, the validation of feelings, the internalization of the therapeutic relationship, and creation of a greater capacity to cope with disturbing feelings.

Interpretation	Confrontation	Clarification	Encouragement to Elaborate	Empathic Validation	Advice and Praise	Affirmation
Linking a patient's feeling, thought, behavior, or symptom to its unconscious meaning or origin	Addressing issues the patient does not want to accept or wishes to avoid	Reformulating what the patient says into a more coherent view of what is meant	Requesting more information from the patient	Demonstrating empathy with the patient's internal state	Prescribing and reinforcing certain activities of benefit to the patient	Supporting the patient's comments or behaviors
Exploratory						**Supportive**

FIGURE 2. The Exploratory-Supportive Intervention Continuum of Psychodynamic Psychotherapy.
Source. Adapted from Gabbard (139).

Of these interventions, only interpretation is unique to the psychodynamic approach. The more exploratory interventions (interpretation, confrontation, and clarification) may be focused on either transference or extratransference issues.

(i) Interpretation

Among the most exploratory forms of treatment, interpretation is regarded as the therapist's ultimate therapeutic tool. In its simplest form, interpretation involves making something conscious that was previously unconscious. An interpretation is an explanatory statement that links a feeling, thought, behavior, or symptom to its unconscious meaning or origin. For example, a therapist might make the following observation to a patient with borderline personality disorder: "I wonder if your tendency to undermine yourself when things are going better is a way to ensure that your treatment with me will continue."

(ii) Confrontation

This exploratory intervention addresses something the patient does not want to accept or identifies the patient's avoidance or minimization. A confrontation may be geared to clarifying how the patient's behavior affects others or reflects a denied or suppressed feeling. An example might be, "I think talking exclusively about your medication problems may be a way of avoiding any discussion with me about your painful feelings that make you feel suicidal."

(iii) Clarification

This intervention involves a reformulation or pulling together of the patient's verbalizations to convey a more coherent view of what is being communicated. A therapist might say, "It sounds like what you're saying is that in every relationship you have, no one seems to be adequately attuned to your needs."

(iv) Encouragement to elaborate

Closer to the center of the continuum are interventions that are characteristic of both supportive and exploratory therapies. Encouragement to elaborate may be broadly defined as a request for information about a topic brought up by the patient. Simple comments like "Tell me more about that" and "What do you mean when you say you feel 'empty'?" are examples of this intervention.

(v) Empathic validation

This intervention is a demonstration of the therapist's empathic attunement with the patient's internal state. This approach draws from self psychology, which emphasizes the value of empathy in strengthening the self. A typically validating comment is, "I can understand why you feel depressed about that," or, "It hurts when you're treated that way."

(vi) Advice and praise

This category includes two interventions that are linked by the fact that they both prescribe and reinforce certain activities. Advice involves direct suggestions to the patient regarding how to behave, while praise reinforces certain patient behaviors by expressing overt approval of them. An example of advice would be, "I don't think you should see that man again because you get beaten up every time you're with him." An example of praise would be, "I think you used excellent judgment in breaking off your relationship with that man."

(vii) Affirmation

This simple intervention involves succinct comments in support of the patient's comments or behaviors such as "Yes, I see what you mean" or "What a good idea."

Some patients with borderline personality disorder receive a highly exploratory or interpretive therapy that is focused on the transference relationship. This approach is sometimes called transference-focused psychotherapy (4, 140). Patients who lack good abstraction capacity and psychological mindedness may require a therapy that is primarily supportive, even though it is psychodynamically informed by a careful analysis of the patient's ego capacities, defenses, and weaknesses. Most psychotherapies involve both exploratory and supportive elements and include some, although not exclusive, focus on the transference. Hence, psychodynamic psychotherapy is often conceptualized as exploratory-supportive or expressive-supportive psychotherapy (16, 139, 141).

b) Efficacy

While there is a great deal of clinical literature on psychodynamic psychotherapy with patients who have borderline personality disorder, there are relatively few methodologically rigorous efficacy studies. One randomized controlled trial assessed the efficacy of psychoanalytically informed partial hospitalization treatment, of which dynamic therapy was the primary modality (9). In this study, 44 patients were randomly assigned to either the partial hospitalization program or general psychiatric care. Treatment in the partial hospitalization program consisted of weekly individual psychoanalytic psychotherapy, three-times-a-week group psychoanalytic psychotherapy, weekly expressive therapy informed by psychodrama, weekly community meetings, monthly meetings with a case administrator, and monthly medication review by a resident. The control group received general psychiatric care consisting of regular psychiatric review with a senior psychiatrist twice a month, inpatient admission as appropriate, outpatient and community follow-up, and no formal psychotherapy. The average length of stay in the partial hospitalization program was 1.5 years. Relative to the control group, the completers of the partial hospitalization program showed significant improvement: self-mutilation decreased, the proportion of patients who attempted suicide decreased from 95% before treatment to 5% after treatment, and patients improved in terms of state and trait anxiety, depression, global symptoms, social adjustment, and interpersonal problems. In the last 6 months of the study, the number of inpatient episodes and duration of inpatient length of stay dramatically increased for the control subjects, whereas these utilization variables remained stable for subjects in the partial hospitalization group.

One can conclude from this study that patients with borderline personality disorder treated with this program for 18 months showed significant improvement in terms of both symptoms and functioning. Reduction of symptoms and suicidal acts occurred after the first 6 months of treatment, but the differences in frequency and duration of inpatient treatment emerged only during the last 6 months of treatment. In addition, depressive symptoms were significantly reduced. Although the principal treatment received by subjects in the partial hospitalization group was psychoanalytic individual and group therapy, one cannot definitively attribute this group's better outcome to the type of therapy received, since the overall community support and social network within which these therapies took place may have exerted significant effects. Pharmacotherapy received was similar in the two treatment groups, but subjects in the partial hospitalization program had a greater amount of psychotherapy than did the control subjects. In a subsequent report (10), patients who had received partial hospitalization treatment not only maintained their substantial gains at an 18-month follow-up evaluation but also showed statistically significant continued improvement on most measures, whereas the control group showed only limited change during the same period.

A study from Australia of twice-weekly psychodynamic therapy (20) prospectively compared the year before 12 months of psychodynamic therapy was given with the year after the therapy was received for a group of poorly functioning outpatients with borderline personality disorder. Among the 30 completers, there were significant reductions in violent behavior, use of illegal drugs, number of medical visits, self-harm, time away from work, severity of global symptoms, number of DSM-III symptoms of borderline personality disorder, number of hospital admissions, and time spent as an inpatient. Although this study did not include a control group, there were dramatic improvements in patients that support the value of the yearlong treatment intervention.

In another study (21), this same group of 30 patients who received psychodynamic therapy was compared with 30 control subjects drawn from an outpatient waiting list who then received treatment as usual, consisting of supportive therapy, cognitive therapy, and crisis intervention. The control subjects were assessed at baseline and at varying intervals, with an average follow-up duration of 17.1 months. In this nonrandomized controlled study, the group receiving psychodynamic therapy had a significantly better outcome than the control subjects (i.e., fewer subjects in the treatment versus the control group still met DSM-III criteria for borderline personality disorder), even though the group that received psychodynamic therapy was more severely ill at baseline. This study suggests that psychodynamic therapy is efficacious, but the investigation has a number of limitations, including the lack of randomization, different follow-up durations for different subjects, nonblind assessment of outcome, and lack of detail about the amount of treatment received by the control subjects. Without more data on the amount of treatment received, it is unclear whether the better outcome of the subjects who received dynamic therapy was due to the type of therapy or the greater amount of treatment received.

c) Cost-effectiveness

The investigators of the Australian study also did a preliminary cost-benefit analysis (138) in which they compared the direct cost of treatment for the 12 months preceding psychodynamic therapy with the direct cost of treatment for the 12 months following this therapy. In Australian dollars, the cost of the treatment for all patients decreased from $684,346 to $41,424. Including psychotherapy in the cost of treatment, there was a total savings per patient of $8,431 per year. This cost-effectiveness was accounted for almost entirely by a decrease in the number of hospital days. Without a control group, however, one cannot definitively conclude that the cost savings were the result of the psychotherapy.

d) Length and frequency of treatment

Most clinical reports of psychodynamic psychotherapy involving patients with borderline personality disorder refer to the treatment duration as "extended" or "long term." However, there are only limited data about how much therapy is adequate or optimal. In the aforementioned randomized controlled trial of psychoanalytically focused partial hospitalization treatment (9), the effect of psychotherapy on reducing hospitalization was not significant until after the patients had been in therapy for more than 12 months. There are no studies demonstrating that brief therapy or psychotherapy less than twice a week is helpful for patients with borderline personality disorder. Howard and colleagues (142), to study the psychotherapeutic dose-effect relationship, conducted a meta-analysis comprising 2,431 subjects from 15 patient groups spanning 30 years. One study they examined in detail involved a group of 151 patients evaluated by self-report and by chart review; 28 of these patients had a borderline personality disorder diagnosis. Whereas 50% of patients with anxiety or depression improved in 8–13 sessions, the same degree of improvement occurred after 13–26 sessions for "borderline psychotic" patients according to self-ratings (the same degree of improvement occurred after 26–52 sessions according to chart ratings by researchers [143]). Seventy-five percent of patients with borderline personality disorder had improved by 1 year (52 sessions) and 87%–95% by 2 years (104 sessions). While this study confirms the conventional wisdom that more therapy is needed for patients with borderline personality disorder than for patients with an axis I disorder, it is unclear whether raters were blind to diagnosis. It appears that a standardized diagnostic assessment and standard threshold for improvement were not used, there are no data on treatment dropouts, and little information is provided about the type of therapy or the therapists except that they were predominantly psychodynamically oriented. What can be concluded is that in a naturalistic setting outpatients who are clinically diagnosed as "borderline psychotic" will likely need more extended therapy than will depressed or anxious patients.

e) Adverse effects

While no adverse effects were reported in the aforementioned studies, psychodynamic psychotherapy has the potential to disorganize some patients if the focus is too exploratory or if there is too much emphasis on transference without an adequately strong alliance. Intensive dynamic psychotherapy may also activate strong dependency wishes in the patient as transference wishes and feelings develop in the context of the treatment. It is the exploration of such dependency that is often essential to help the patient to achieve independence. This dependence may elicit countertransference problems in the therapist, which can lead to inappropriate or ineffective treatment. The most serious examples of this include unnecessary increases in the frequency or duration of treatment or transgression of professional boundaries.

f) Implementation issues

(i) Difficulties with adherence

Most studies report a high dropout rate from dynamic psychotherapy among patients with borderline personality disorder. However, this is true for almost all approaches to the treatment of these patients, and it has not been demonstrated to be any higher for dynamic therapy. It does, however, emphasize the paramount importance of adequate attention to the therapeutic alliance as well as to transference and countertransference issues.

(ii) Need for therapist flexibility

Early in the treatment, and periodically in the later stages, a therapist who is also functioning as primary clinician may need to take a major role in management issues, including limit-setting, attending to suicidality, addressing pharmacotherapy, and helping to arrange hospitalization. A stance in which the therapist only explores the patient's internal experience and does not become involved in management of life issues may lead to adverse outcomes for some patients.

(iii) Importance of judicious transference interpretation

Excessive transference interpretation or confrontation early in treatment may increase the risk that the patient will drop out of therapy. One process study of psychoanalytic therapy with patients with borderline personality disorder (11) found that for some patients, transference interpretation is a "high-risk, high-gain" phenomenon in that it may improve the therapeutic alliance but also may cause substantial deterioration in that alliance. Therapists must use transference interpretation judiciously on the basis of their sense of the state of the alliance and the patient's capacity to hear and reflect on observations about the therapeutic relationship. A series of empathic and supportive comments often paves the way for an effective transference interpretation. Other patients may be able to use transference interpretation effectively without this much preparatory work.

(iv) Role of therapist training and competency
Psychodynamic therapy for patients with borderline personality disorder is uncommonly demanding. Consultation from an experienced colleague is highly recommended for all therapists during the course of the therapy. In some situations, personal psychotherapy can help the clinician develop skills to manage the intense transference/countertransference interactions that are characteristic of these treatments.

2. Cognitive behavior therapy

a) Definition and goals

Although cognitive behavior therapy has been widely used and described in the clinical literature, it has more often been used to treat axis I conditions (e.g., anxiety or depressive disorders) than personality disorders. Cognitive behavior therapy assumes that maladaptive and distorted beliefs and cognitive processes underlie symptoms and dysfunctional affect or behavior and that these beliefs are behaviorally reinforced. It generally involves attention to a set of dysfunctional automatic thoughts or deeply ingrained belief systems (often referred to as schemas), along with learning and practicing new, nonmaladaptive behaviors. Utilization of cognitive behavior methods in the treatment of the personality disorders has been described (19), but because persistent dysfunctional belief systems in patients with personality disorders are usually "structuralized" (i.e., built into the patient's usual cognitive organization), substantial time and effort are required to produce lasting change. Modifications of standard approaches (e.g., schema-focused cognitive therapy, complex cognitive therapy, or dialectical behavior therapy) are often recommended in treating certain features typical of the personality disorders. However, other than dialectical behavior therapy (17, 144–147), these modifications have not been studied.

b) Efficacy

Most published reports of cognitive behavior treatment for patients with borderline personality disorder are uncontrolled clinical or single case studies. Recently, however, several controlled studies have been done, particularly of a form of cognitive behavior therapy called dialectical behavior therapy. Dialectical behavior therapy consists of approximately 1 year of manual-guided therapy (involving 1 hour of weekly individual therapy for 1 year and 2.5 hours of group skills training per week for either 6 or 12 months) along with a requirement for all therapists in a study or program to meet weekly as a group. Linehan and colleagues (8) reported a randomized controlled trial of dialectical behavior therapy involving patients with borderline personality disorder whose symptoms included "parasuicidal" behavior (defined as any intentional acute self-injurious behavior with or without suicide intent). Control subjects in this study received "treatment as usual" (defined as "alternative therapy referrals, usually by the original referral source, from which they could choose"). Of the 44 study completers, 22 received dialectical behavior therapy, and 22 received treatment as usual; patients were assessed at 4, 8, and 12 months. At pretreatment, 13 of the control subjects had been receiving individual psychotherapy, and 9 had not. Patients who received dialectical behavior therapy had less parasuicidal behavior, reduced medical risk due to parasuicidal acts, fewer hospital admissions, fewer psychiatric hospital days, and a greater capacity to stay with the same therapist than did the control subjects. Both groups improved with respect to depression, suicidal ideation, hopelessness, or reasons for living; there were no group differences on these variables. Because there were substantial dropout rates overall (30%) and the number of study completers in each group was small, it is unclear how generalizable these results are. Nonetheless, this study is a promising first report of a manualized regimen of cognitive behavior treatment for a specific type of patient with borderline personality disorder.

A second cohort of patients was subsequently studied; the same study design was used (148). In this report, there were 26 intent-to-treat patients (13 received dialectical behavior therapy, and 13 received treatment as usual). One patient who received dialectical behavior therapy committed suicide late in the study, and 3 patients receiving dialectical behavior therapy and 1 patient receiving treatment as usual dropped out. Nine of the 13 control patients were already receiving individual psychotherapy at the beginning of the study or entered such treatment during the study. Patients who received dialectical behavior therapy had greater reduction in trait anger and greater improvement in Global Assessment Scale scores.

One year after termination of their previously described study (8), the Linehan group reevaluated their patient group (5). After 1 year, the greater reduction in parasuicide rates and in severity of suicide attempts seen in the dialectical behavior therapy group relative to the control subjects did not persist, although there were significantly fewer psychiatric hospital days for the dialectical behavior therapy group during the follow-up year. These findings suggest that although dialectical behavior therapy produces a greater reduction in parasuicidal behavior than treatment as usual, the durability of this advantage is unclear.

In a subsequent report, Linehan and colleagues (149) compared dialectical behavior therapy with treatment as usual in patients with borderline personality disorder with drug dependence. Only 18 of the 28 intent-to-treat patients completed the study (7 who received dialectical behavior therapy and 11 given treatment as usual). Patients receiving dialectical behavior therapy had more drug- and alcohol-abstinent days after 4, 8, and 16 months. All patients had reduced parasuicidal behavior as well as state and trait anger; there was no difference between the groups. This study, too, involved small numbers of patients and had substantial dropout rates, but it represents an important attempt to evaluate the impact of dialectical behavior therapy with severely ill patients with borderline personality disorder and comorbid substance abuse.

In all of these studies, it is difficult to ascertain whether the improvement reported for patients receiving dialectical behavior therapy derived from specific ingredients of dialectical behavior therapy or whether nonspecific factors such as either the greater time spent with the patients or therapist bias contributed to the results. In a small study in which skills training alone was compared with a no-skills training control condition, no difference was found between the groups (unpublished 1993 study of M.M. Linehan and H.L. Heard). The researchers concluded that the specific features of individual dialectical behavior therapy are necessary for patients to show greater improvement than control groups. Linehan and Heard (150) reported that more time with therapists does not account for improved outcome. Nonetheless, other special features of dialectical behavior therapy, such as the requirement for all therapists to meet weekly as a group, could contribute to the results.

Springer et al. (151) used an inpatient group therapy version of dialectical behavior therapy for patients with personality disorders, 13 of whom had borderline personality disorder. The patients with borderline personality disorder exhibited improvement in depression, hopelessness, and suicidal ideation, but the improvement was not greater than it was for a control group. In this study, compared with control subjects, patients receiving the dialectical behavior therapy treatment showed a paradoxical increase in parasuicidal acting out during the brief hospitalization (average length of stay was 12.6 days).

Barley and colleagues (152) compared dialectical behavior therapy received by patients with borderline personality disorder on a specialized personality disorder inpatient unit with treatment as usual on a similar-sized inpatient unit. They found that the use of dialectical behavior therapy was associated with reduced parasuicidal behavior. It is unclear whether improvement was due to dialectical behavior therapy per se or to other elements of the specialized unit.

Perris (153) reported preliminary findings from a small uncontrolled, naturalistic follow-up study of 13 patients with borderline personality disorder who received cognitive behavior therapy similar to dialectical behavior therapy. Twelve patients were evaluated at a 2-year follow-up point, and all patients maintained the normalization of functioning that had been evident at the end of the study treatment.

Other controlled studies reported in the literature of cognitive behavior approaches are difficult to interpret because of small patient group sizes or because the studies focused on mixed types of personality disorders without specifying borderline cohorts (154–156).

In summary, there are a number of studies in the literature suggesting that cognitive behavior therapy approaches may be effective for patients with borderline personality disorder. Most of these studies involved dialectical behavior therapy and were carried out by Linehan and her group. Replication studies by other groups in other centers are needed to confirm the validity and generalizability of these findings.

c) Cost-effectiveness

Published data are not available on the cost-effectiveness of cognitive behavior approaches for treatment of borderline personality disorder, although Linehan and colleagues (8) reported that patients receiving dialectical behavior therapy had fewer psychiatric inpatient days and psychiatric hospital admissions than did control subjects.

d) Length and frequency of treatment

Short-term cognitive therapy involving 16–20 sessions has been described as a generic treatment approach; however, the patient characteristics thought to be necessary for a successful treatment outcome are not typical of patients with personality disorders (147). Instead, longer forms of treatment, such as "schema-focused cognitive therapy" (147), "complex cognitive therapy" (144), or dialectical behavior therapy (17), are usually recommended.

The standard length of dialectical behavior therapy is approximately 1 year for the most commonly administered phase of the treatment. It involves 1 hour of individual therapy per week, more than 2 hours of group skills training per week (for either 6 or 12 months), and 1 hour of group process for the therapists per week. Other versions of dialectical behavior therapy, such as that administered in a brief inpatient setting (151), may be useful but are not necessarily more effective than other forms of inpatient treatment.

e) Adverse effects

Although there are no reports of adverse effects of cognitive behavior therapy, including dialectical behavior therapy, as administered on an outpatient basis, one inpatient study (151) reported a paradoxical increase in parasuicidal acting out in the dialectical behavior therapy group compared with the control group—a finding thought perhaps to be due to the contagion effect within a closed, intensive milieu.

f) Implementation issues

Many components of cognitive behavior therapy are similar to elements of psychodynamic psychotherapy, although they may have different labels. For example, as Linehan (17) pointed out, focusing on "therapy-interfering behavior" is similar to the psychodynamic emphasis on transference behaviors. Similarly, the notion of validation resembles that of empathy. Beck and Freeman (19) noted that cognitive therapists and psychoanalysts have the common goal of identifying and modifying "core" personality disorder problems. However, psychodynamic therapists view these core problems as having important unconscious roots that are not available to the patient, whereas cognitive therapists view them as largely in the realm of awareness. It is not clear how successfully psychiatrists who have not been trained in cognitive behavior therapy can implement manual-based cognitive behavior approaches.

Although dialectical behavior therapy has been well described in the literature for many years, it is not clear how difficult it is to teach to new therapists in settings other than that where it was developed. Variable results in other settings could be due to a number of factors, such as less enthusiasm for the method among therapists, differences in therapist training in dialectical behavior therapy, and different patient populations. Although the Linehan group has developed training programs for therapists, certain characteristics recommended in dialectical behavior therapy (e.g., "a matter-of-fact, somewhat irreverent, and at times outrageous attitude about current and previous parasuicidal and other dysfunctional behaviors" [17]) may be more effective when carried out by therapists who are comfortable with this particular style.

3. Group therapy

a) Goals

The goals of group therapy are consistent with those of individual psychotherapy and include stabilization of the patient, management of impulsiveness and other symptoms, and examination and management of transference and countertransference reactions. Groups provide special opportunities for provision of additional social support, interpersonal learning, and diffusion of the intensity of transference issues through interaction with other group members and the therapists. In addition, the presence of other patients provides opportunities for patient-based limit-setting and for altruistic interactions in which patients can consolidate their gains in the process of helping others.

b) Efficacy

Some uncontrolled studies suggest that group treatment (157), including process-focused groups in a therapeutic community setting (158), may be helpful for patients with borderline personality disorder. However, these studies had no true control condition, and the efficacy of the group treatment is unclear, given the complexity of the treatment received. Another small chart review study of an "incest group" for patients with borderline personality disorder (159) suggested shorter subsequent inpatient stays and fewer outpatient visits for treated patients than for control subjects. A randomized trial (160) involving patients with borderline personality disorder showed equivalent results with group versus individual dynamically oriented psychotherapy, but the small sample size and high dropout rate make the results inconclusive. Wilberg et al. (161) did a naturalistic follow-up study of two cohorts of patients with borderline personality disorder. This quasi-experimental, nonrandomized study showed that patients with borderline personality disorder discharged from a day program with continuing outpatient group therapy (N=12) did better than those who did not have group therapy (N=31). They had better global health and lower global severity index symptoms, lower Health-Sickness Rating Scale scores, lower SCL-90 scores, lower rehospitalization rates, fewer suicide attempts, and less substance abuse. There were, however, important differences between the two comparison groups that could account for outcome differences.

Perhaps the most interesting aspect of group therapy is the use of groups to consolidate and maintain improvement from the inpatient stay. Linehan and colleagues (8) combined individual and group therapy, making the specific effect of the group component unclear. They reported that, contrary to expectations, the addition of group skills training to individual dialectical behavior therapy did not improve clinical outcome. For those patients with borderline personality disorder who have experienced shame or have become isolated as a result of trauma, including those with comorbid PTSD, group therapy with others who have experienced trauma can be helpful. Such groups provide a milieu in which their current emotional reactions and self-defeating behaviors can be seen and understood. Groups may also provide a context in which patients may initiate healthy risk-taking in relationships. Group treatment has also been included in studies of psychodynamic psychotherapy; although the overall treatment program was effective, the effectiveness of the group therapy component is unknown (9, 162). Clinical wisdom indicates for many patients combined group and individual psychotherapy is more effective than either treatment alone.

c) Cost-effectiveness

Group psychotherapy is substantially less expensive than individual therapy because of the favorable therapist-patient ratio. Marziali and Monroe-Blum (163) calculated that group psychotherapy for borderline personality disorder costs about one-sixth as much as individual psychotherapy, assuming that the fee for individual therapy is only slightly higher than that for group therapy. However, this potential saving is tempered by the fact that most treatment regimens for borderline personality disorder combine group interventions with individual therapy.

d) Length and frequency of treatment

Groups generally meet once a week, although in inpatient settings sessions may occur daily. In some studies, groups are time-limited—for example, 12 weekly sessions—whereas in other studies they continue for a year or more.

e) Adverse effects

Acute distress from exposure to emotionally arousing group issues has been reported. Other potential risks of treating patients with borderline personality disorder in group settings include shared resistance to therapeutic work, hostile or other destructive interactions among patients, intensification of transference problems, and symptom "contagion."

f) Implementation issues

Groups take considerable effort to set up and require a group of patients with similar problems and willingness to participate in group treatment. Patients in group therapy must agree to confidentiality regarding the information shared by other patients and to clear guidelines regarding contact with other members outside the group setting. It is critical that there be no "secrets" and that all interactions among group members be discussed in the group, especially information regarding threats of harm to self or others.

4. Couples therapy

a) Goals

The usual goal of couples therapy is to stabilize and strengthen the relationship between the partners or to clarify the nonviability of the relationship. An alternative or additional goal for some is to educate and clarify for the spouse or partner of the patient with borderline personality disorder the process that is taking place within the relationship. Partners of patients with borderline personality disorder may struggle to accommodate the patient's alternating patterns of idealization and depreciation as well as other interpersonal behaviors. As a result, spouses may become dysphoric and self-doubting; they may also become overly attentive and exhibit reaction formation. The goal of treatment is to explore and change these maladaptive reactions and problematic interactions between partners.

b) Efficacy

The literature on the effectiveness of couples therapy for patients with borderline personality disorder is limited to clinical experience and case reports. In some cases, the psychopathology and potential mutual interdependence of each partner may serve a homeostatic function (164–166). Improvement can occur in the relationship when there is recognition of the psychological deficits of both parties. The therapeutic task is to provide an environment in which each spouse can develop self-awareness within the context of the relationship.

c) Adverse effects

One report (41) described an escalation of symptoms when traditional marital therapy was used with a couple who both were diagnosed with borderline personality disorder. Clinical experience would indicate the need for careful psychiatric evaluation of the spouse. When severe character pathology is present in both, the clinician will need to use a multidimensional approach, providing a holding environment for both partners while working toward individuation and intrapsychic growth. Because the spouse's own interpersonal needs or behavioral patterns may, however pathological, serve a homeostatic function within the marriage, couples therapy has the potential to further destabilize the relationship.

d) Implementation issues

At times, it might be helpful for the primary clinician to meet with the spouse or partner and evaluate his or her strengths and weaknesses. It is important to recognize the contingencies of the extent of the partner's loyalty and his or her understanding of what can be expected from the patient with borderline personality disorder before recommending couples therapy. Couples therapy with patients with borderline personality disorder requires considerable understanding of borderline personality disorder and the attendant problems and compensations that such individuals bring to relationships.

5. Family therapy

a) Goals

Relationships in the families of patients with borderline personality disorder are often turbulent and chaotic. The goal of family therapy is to increase family members' understanding of borderline personality disorder, improve relationships between the patient and family members, and enhance the overall functioning of the family.

b) Efficacy

The published literature on family therapy with patients with borderline personality disorder consists of case reports (167–170) and one published study (12) that found a psychoeducational approach could improve communication, diminish alienation and burden, and diminish conflicts over separation and independence. The clinical literature suggests that family therapy may be useful for some patients—in particular, those who are still dependent on or significantly involved with their families. Some clinicians report the efficacy of dynamically based therapy, whereas others support the efficacy of a psychoeducational approach in which the focus is on educating the family about the diagnosis, improving communication, diminishing hostility and guilt, and diminishing the burden of the illness.

c) Adverse effects

Some clinicians report that traditional dynamically based family therapy has the potential to end prematurely and have a poor outcome, since patients may alienate their family members or leave the treatment themselves because they feel misunderstood (171) when family involvement is indicated. A psychoeducational approach appears to be less likely to have such adverse effects; however, even psychoeducational approaches can upset family members who wish to avoid knowledge about the illness or involvement in the family member's treatment.

d) Implementation issues

Traditional dynamically based family therapy requires considerable training and sufficient experience with patients with borderline personality disorder to appreciate their problems and conflicts and to be judicious in the selection of appropriate families.

C. REVIEW OF PHARMACOTHERAPY AND OTHER SOMATIC TREATMENTS

1. SSRI antidepressants

a) Goals

In borderline personality disorder, SSRIs are used to treat symptoms of affective dysregulation and impulsive-behavioral dyscontrol, particularly depressed mood, anger, and impulsive aggression, including self-mutilation.

b) Efficacy

Early case reports and small open-label trials with fluoxetine, sertraline, and venlafaxine (a mixed norepinephrine/serotonin reuptake blocker) indicated significant efficacy for symptoms of affective dysregulation, impulsive-behavioral dyscontrol, and cognitive-perceptual difficulties in patients with borderline personality disorder (44–49, 67). Aggression, irritability, depressed mood, and self-mutilation responded to fluoxetine (up to 80 mg/day), venlafaxine (up to 400 mg/day), or sertraline (up to 200 mg/day) in trials of 8–12 weeks (45). An unexpected finding in some of these early reports was that improvement in impulsive behavior appeared rapidly, often within the first week of treatment, and disappeared as quickly with discontinuation or nonadherence. Improvement in impulsive aggression appeared to be independent of effects on depression and anxiety and occurred whether or not the patient had comorbid major depressive disorder (67). Nonresponse to one SSRI did not predict poor response to all SSRIs. For example, some patients who did not respond to fluoxetine, 80 mg/day, responded to a subsequent trial of sertraline. Similarly, patients who did not respond to sertraline, paroxetine, or fluoxetine subsequently responded to venlafaxine. In one study, higher doses and a longer trial (24 weeks) with sertraline converted half of sertraline nonresponders to responders (45).

Three double-blind, placebo-controlled studies have been conducted. Salzman and colleagues (44) conducted a 12-week trial of fluoxetine (20–60 mg/day) in 27 relatively high-functioning subjects (mean Global Assessment Scale score of 74) with borderline personality disorder or borderline traits. Other axis I or axis II comorbid diagnoses were absent, as were recent suicidal behavior, self-mutilation, substance abuse, and current severe aggressive behavior (i.e., behaviors typical of patients with borderline personality disorder seeking treatment). This strategy diminishes generalizability to more seriously ill patients but has the advantage of allowing for a test of efficacy in the absence of comorbidity. For the 22 subjects who completed the study (13 given fluoxetine and 9 who received placebo), significant reduction in symptoms of anger and depression and improvement in global functioning were reported for subjects given fluoxetine compared with those given placebo. Improvement in anger was independent of improvement in depressed mood. Improvement was modest, with no subject improving more than 20% on any measure. In addition, a large placebo response was noted.

Markovitz (45) studied 17 patients (9 given fluoxetine, 80 mg/day, and 8 given placebo) for 14 weeks. This patient group was noteworthy for the high rate of comorbid axis I mood disorders (10 with major depression and 6 with bipolar disorder), anxiety disorders, and somatic complaints (e.g., headaches, premenstrual syndrome, irritable bowel syndrome). While this group is more typical of an impaired borderline personality disorder patient population, comorbidity with affective and anxiety disorders confounds interpretation of results. Patients receiving fluoxetine improved significantly more than those given placebo in depression, anxiety, and global symptoms. Measures of impulsive aggression were not included in this study. Some patients with premenstrual syndrome and headaches noted improvement in these somatic presentations with fluoxetine, whereas none improved with placebo.

A double-blind, placebo-controlled study by Coccaro and Kavoussi (67) focused attention on impulsive aggression as a dimensional construct (i.e., a symptom domain found across personality disorders but especially characteristic of borderline personality disorder). Forty subjects with prominent impulsive aggression in the context of a personality disorder, one-third of whom had borderline personality disorder, participated. There was a high rate of comorbidity with dysthymic disorder or depressive disorder not otherwise specified; subjects with major depression and bipolar disorder were excluded. Anxiety disorders, as well as alcohol and drug abuse, were common. In this 12-week, double-blind, placebo-controlled trial, fluoxetine (20–60 mg/day) was more effective than placebo for treatment of verbal aggression and aggression against objects. Improvement was significant by week 10, with improvement in irritability appearing by week 6. Global improvement, favoring fluoxetine, was significant by week 4. As in the open-label trials and the aforementioned Salzman et al. study (44), these investigators found that the effects on aggression and irritability did not appear as a result of improvement in mood or anxiety symptoms.

In summary, these three randomized, double-blind, placebo-controlled studies show efficacy for fluoxetine for affective symptoms—specifically, depressed mood (44, 45), anger (44), and anxiety (45, 67)—although effects on anger and depressed mood appear quantitatively modest. Efficacy has also been demonstrated for impulsive-behavioral symptoms—specifically, verbal and indirect aggression (67)—and global symptom severity (44, 45, 67). Effects on impulsive aggression (67) and anger (44) were independent of effects on affective symptoms, including depressed mood (44, 67) and anxiety (67). Although the three published double-blind, placebo-controlled trials used fluoxetine, open-label studies and clinical experience suggest potential usefulness for other SSRIs.

c) Side effects

The side effect profile of the SSRIs is favorable compared with that of older tricyclic, heterocyclic, or MAOI antidepressants, including low risk in overdose. Side effects reported in these studies are consistent with routine clinical usage.

d) Implementation issues

The SSRI antidepressants may be used in their customary antidepressant dose ranges and durations (e.g., fluoxetine, 20–80 mg/day; sertraline, 100–200 mg/day). One investigator used very high doses of sertraline (200–600 mg/day) for nonresponders, with some improved efficacy (45). At these high doses, peripheral tremor was noted. There are no published studies of continuation and maintenance strategies with SSRIs, although anecdotal reports suggest continuation of improvement in impulsive aggression and self-mutilation for up to several years while the medication is taken and rapid return of symptoms upon discontinuation (49, 172, 173). The duration of treatment is therefore a clinical judgment that depends on the patient's clinical status and medication tolerance at any point in time.

2. Tricyclic and heterocyclic antidepressants

a) Goals

In borderline personality disorder, antidepressants are used for affective dysregulation, manifested most commonly by depressed mood, irritability, and mood lability. Evaluation of antidepressant trials in the treatment of borderline personality disorder must take into account the presence of comorbid axis I mood disorders, which are common in patients with borderline personality disorder. Studies in which there is a preponderance of comorbid axis I depression would be expected to demonstrate a favorable response to antidepressant treatments but may not reflect the pharmacological responsiveness of borderline personality disorder.

b) Efficacy

Double-blind, placebo-controlled trials of tricyclic antidepressants in borderline personality disorder have used amitriptyline, imipramine, and desipramine in both inpatient and outpatient settings. Mianserin, a tetracyclic antidepressant not available in the United States, has been used in an outpatient setting. Most of these studies were parallel comparisons with another medication and placebo. A 5-week inpatient study of patients with borderline personality disorder that compared amitriptyline (mean dose=149 mg/day) with haloperidol and placebo found that amitriptyline decreased depressive symptoms and indirect hostility and enhanced attitudes about self-control compared with placebo (51). It is interesting to note that amitriptyline was not effective for the "core" depressive features of the Hamilton Depression Rating Scale but rather was effective for the seven "associated" symptoms of diurnal variation, depersonalization, paranoid symptoms, obsessive-compulsive symptoms, helplessness, hopelessness, and worthlessness. Patients who had major depression were not more likely to respond. Schizotypal symptoms and paranoia predicted a poor response to amitriptyline.

A small crossover study comparing desipramine (mean dose=162.5 mg/day) with lithium carbonate (mean dose=985.7 mg/day) and placebo in outpatients with borderline personality disorder and minimal axis I mood comorbidity found no significant differences between desipramine and placebo in improvement of affective symptoms, anger, or suicidal symptoms or in therapist or patient perceptions of improvement after 3 and 6 weeks (61).

A small open-label study that assessed the use of amoxapine (an antidepressant with neuroleptic properties) in patients with borderline personality disorder with or without schizotypal personality disorder found that it was not effective for patients with only borderline personality disorder (174). However, it was effective for patients with borderline personality disorder and comorbid schizotypal personality disorder, who had more severe symptoms. This latter group had improvement in cognitive-perceptual, depressive, and global symptoms (174).

In outpatients with a primary diagnosis of atypical depression (which required a current diagnosis of major, minor, or intermittent depression plus associated atypical features) and borderline personality disorder as a secondary diagnosis, imipramine (200 mg/day) produced global improvement in 35% of patients with comorbid borderline personality disorder. In contrast, phenelzine had a 92% response rate in the same sample (57). The presence of borderline personality disorder symptoms predicted a negative global response to imipramine but a positive global response to phenelzine.

One longer-term study was conducted in patients hospitalized for a suicide attempt who were diagnosed with borderline personality disorder or histrionic personality disorder but not axis I depression (175). In this 6-month, double-blind, placebo-controlled study of a low dose of mianserin (30 mg/day), no antidepressant or prophylactic efficacy was found for mianserin compared with placebo for mood symptoms or recurrence of suicidal acts. (The same investigators did demonstrate efficacy against recurrent suicidal acts in this high-risk population with a depot neuroleptic, flupentixol [80].)

These data suggest that the utility of tricyclic antidepressants in patients with borderline personality disorder is highly questionable. When a clear diagnosis of comorbid major depression can be made, SSRIs are the treatment of choice. When atypical depression is present, the MAOIs have demonstrated superior efficacy to tricyclic antidepressants; however, they must be used with great caution given the high risk of toxicity. (Although the SSRIs have not been extensively studied in atypical depression, at least one double-blind study has indicated comparable efficacy for fluoxetine and phenelzine for the treatment of atypical depression [176].) The efficacy of SSRIs in borderline personality disorder and their favorable safety profile argue for their empirical use in patients with borderline personality disorder with atypical depression.

At best, the response to tricyclic antidepressants (e.g., imipramine) in patients with borderline personality disorder appears modest. The possibility of behavioral toxicity and the known lethality of tricyclic antidepressants in overdose support the preferential use of an SSRI or related antidepressant for patients with borderline personality disorder.

c) Side effects

Common side effects of tricyclic antidepressants include sedation, constipation, dry mouth, and weight gain. The toxicity of tricyclic antidepressants in overdose, including death, indicates that they should be used with caution in patients at risk for suicide. Patients with cardiac conduction abnormalities may experience a fatal arrhythmia with tricyclic antidepressant treatment. For some inpatients with borderline personality disorder, treatment with amitriptyline has paradoxically been associated with behavioral toxicity, consisting of increased suicide threats, paranoid ideation, demanding and assaultive behaviors, and an apparent disinhibition of impulsive behavior (50, 177).

d) Implementation issues

Other antidepressants are generally preferred over the tricyclic antidepressants for patients with borderline personality disorder. If tricyclic antidepressants are used, the patient should be carefully monitored for signs of toxicity and paradoxical worsening. Doses used in published studies were in the range of 150–250 mg/day of amitriptyline, imipramine, or desipramine. Blood levels may be a useful guide to whether the dose is adequate or toxicity is present.

3. MAOI antidepressants

a) Goals

MAOIs are used to treat affective symptoms, hostility, and impulsivity related to mood symptoms in patients with borderline personality disorder.

b) Efficacy

MAOIs have been studied in patients with borderline personality disorder in three placebo-controlled acute treatment trials (55–57). In an outpatient study of phenelzine versus imipramine that selected patients with atypical depression (with borderline personality disorder as a secondary comorbid condition), global improvement occurred in 92% of patients given 60 mg/day of phenelzine compared with 35% of patients given 200 mg/day of imipramine (57). In a study of tranylcypromine, trifluoperazine, alprazolam, and carbamazepine in which borderline personality disorder was a primary diagnosis but comorbid with hysteroid dysphoria (55), tranylcypromine (40 mg/day) improved a broad spectrum of mood symptoms, including depression, anger, rejection sensitivity, and capacity for pleasure. Cowdry and Gardner (55) noted that "the MAOI proved to be the most effective psychopharmacological agent overall, with clear effects on mood and less prominent effects on behavioral control." Tranylcypromine also significantly decreased impulsivity and suicidality, with a near significant effect on behavioral dyscontrol. When borderline personality disorder is the primary diagnosis, with no selection for atypical depression or hysteroid dysphoria, results are clearly less favorable. Soloff and colleagues (56) studied borderline personality disorder inpatients with comorbid major depression (53%), hysteroid dysphoria (44%), and atypical depression (46%); the patient group was not selected for presence of a depressive disorder. Phenelzine was effective for self-rated anger and hostility but had no specific efficacy, compared with placebo or haloperidol, for atypical depression or hysteroid dysphoria. These three acute trials were 5–6 weeks in duration. A 16-week continuation study of the responding patients in a follow-up study (68) showed some continuing modest improvement over placebo beyond the acute 5-week trial for depression and irritability. Phenelzine appeared to be activating, which was considered favorable in the clinical setting.

On balance, these studies suggest that MAOIs are often helpful for atypical depressive symptoms, anger, hostility, and impulsivity in patients with borderline personality disorder. These effects appear to be independent of a current mood disorder diagnosis (56), although one study found a nonsignificantly higher rate of MAOI response for patients with a past history of major depression or bipolar II disorder (55).

c) Side effects

Phenelzine can cause weight gain (56) and can be difficult to tolerate. Other side effects include orthostatic hypotension (55). Fatal hypertensive crises are the most serious potential side effect of MAOIs, although no study reported any hypertensive crises due to violation of the tyramine dietary restriction. The initial clinical picture of MAOI poisoning is one of agitation, delirium, hallucinations, hyperreflexia, tachycardia, tachypnea, dilated pupils, diaphoresis, and, often, convulsions. Hyperpyrexia is one of the most serious problems (178).

d) Implementation issues

Doses of phenelzine and tranylcypromine used in published studies ranged from 60 to 90 mg/day and 10 to 60 mg/day, respectively. Experienced clinicians may vary doses according to their usual practice in treating depressive or anxiety disorders. Adherence to a tyramine-free diet is critically important and requires careful patient instruction, ideally supplemented by a printed guide to tyramine-rich foods and medication interactions, especially over-the-counter decongestants found in common cold and allergy remedies. Given the impulsivity of patients with borderline personality disorder, it is helpful to review in detail the potential for serious medical consequences of nonadherence to dietary restrictions, the symptoms of hypertensive crisis, and an emergency treatment plan in case of a hypertensive crisis. Patients must be instructed to discontinue an SSRI long enough in advance of instituting MAOI therapy to avoid precipitating a serotonin syndrome.

4. Lithium carbonate and anticonvulsant mood stabilizers

a) Goals

Lithium carbonate and the anticonvulsant mood stabilizers carbamazepine and divalproex sodium are used to treat symptoms of behavioral dyscontrol in borderline personality disorder, with possible efficacy for symptoms of affective dysregulation.

b) Efficacy

The efficacy of lithium carbonate for bipolar disorder led to treatment trials in patients with personality disorders characterized by mood dysregulation and impulsive aggression. Rifkin and colleagues (179, 180) demonstrated improvement in mood swings in 21 patients with emotionally unstable character disorder, a DSM-I diagnosis characterized by brief but nonreactive mood swings, both depressive and hypomanic, in the context of a chronically maladaptive personality resembling "hysterical character." In this placebo-controlled crossover study (each medication was taken for 6 weeks), there was decreased variation in mood (i.e., fewer "mood swings") and global improvement in 14 of 21 patients during lithium treatment. Subsequent case reports demonstrated that lithium had mood-stabilizing and antiaggressive effects in patients with borderline personality disorder (181, 182).

One double-blind, placebo-controlled crossover study compared lithium with desipramine in 17 patients with borderline personality disorder (61). All patients took lithium for 6 weeks (mean dose=985.7 mg/day) and received concurrent psychotherapy. Among 10 patients completing both lithium and placebo treatments, therapists' blind ratings indicated greater improvement during the lithium trial, although patients' self-ratings did not reflect significant differences between lithium and placebo. The authors noted that therapists were favorably impressed by decreases in impulsivity during the lithium trial, an improvement not fully appreciated by the patients themselves. There has never been a double-blind, placebo-controlled trial of the antiaggressive effects of lithium carbonate in patients with borderline personality disorder selected for histories of impulsive aggression.

The anticonvulsant mood stabilizer carbamazepine has been studied in two double-blind, placebo-controlled studies that used very different patient groups, resulting in inconsistent findings. Gardner and Cowdry (55, 62), in a crossover trial, studied female outpatients with borderline personality disorder and comorbid hysteroid dysphoria along with extensive histories of behavioral dyscontrol. Patients underwent a 6-week trial of carbamazepine (mean dose= 820 mg/day) and continued receiving psychotherapy. Patients had decreased frequency and severity of behavioral dyscontrol during the carbamazepine trial. Among all patients, there were significantly fewer suicide attempts or other major dyscontrol episodes along with improvement in anxiety, anger, and euphoria (by a physician's assessment only) with carbamazepine treatment compared with placebo.

De la Fuente and Lotstra (63) failed to replicate these findings, although this may be due to their small study group size (N=20). These investigators conducted a double-blind, placebo-controlled trial of carbamazepine in inpatients with a primary diagnosis of borderline personality disorder. Patients with any comorbid axis I disorder, a history of epilepsy, or EEG abnormalities were excluded. Unlike in the Cowdry and Gardner study (55), patients were not selected for histories of behavioral dyscontrol. There were no significant differences between carbamazepine and placebo on measures of affective or cognitive-perceptual symptoms, impulsive-behavioral "acting out," or global symptoms.

Divalproex sodium has been used in open-label trials targeting the agitation and aggression of patients with borderline personality disorder in a state hospital setting (70) and mood instability and impulsivity in an outpatient clinic (66). Wilcox (70) reported a 68% decrease in time spent in seclusion as well as improvement in anxiety, tension, and global symptoms among 30 patients with borderline personality disorder receiving divalproex sodium (with dose titrated to a level of 100 mg/ml) for 6 weeks in a state hospital. Patients did not have "psychiatric comorbid conditions" (by clinical assessment), although 5 had an EEG abnormality (but no seizure disorders); concurrent psychotropic medications were allowed. An abnormal EEG predicted improvement with divalproex sodium. The author noted that both the antiaggressive and antianxiety effects of divalproex sodium appeared instrumental in decreasing agitation and time spent in seclusion.

An open-label study by Stein and colleagues (66) enrolled 11 cooperative outpatients with borderline personality disorder, all of whom had been in psychotherapy for a minimum of 8 weeks and were free of other medications before starting divalproex sodium treatment, which was titrated to levels of 50–100 mg/ml. Among the 8 patients who completed the study, 4 responded in terms of global improvement and observed irritability; physician ratings of mood, anxiety, anger, impulsivity, and rejection sensitivity; and patient ratings of global improvement. There were no significant changes in measures specific for depression and anxiety, but baseline depression and anxiety scores were low in this population.

Kavoussi and Coccaro (69) also reported significant improvement in impulsive aggression and irritability after 4 weeks of treatment with divalproex sodium in 10 patients with impulsive aggression in the context of a cluster B personality disorder, 5 of whom (4 completers) had borderline personality disorder. Among the 8 patients who completed the 8-week trial, 6 had a 50% or greater reduction in aggression and irritability. All patients had not responded to a previous trial with fluoxetine (up to 60 mg/day for 8 weeks).

Only one small, randomized controlled trial of divalproex has been reported that involved patients with borderline personality disorder (65). Among 12 patients randomly assigned to divalproex, only 6 completed a 10-week trial, 5 of whom responded in terms of global measures. There was improvement in depression, albeit not statistically significant, and aggression was unchanged. None of the 4 patients randomly assigned to placebo completed the study.

In summary, preliminary evidence suggests that lithium carbonate and the mood stabilizers carbamazepine and divalproex may be useful in treating behavioral dyscontrol and affective dysregulation in some patients with borderline personality disorder, although further studies are needed. The only report on the newer anticonvulsants (i.e., gabapentin, lamotrigine, topiramate) in borderline personality disorder is a case series in which three of eight patients had a good response to lamotrigine (183). Because of the paucity of evidence concerning these agents, careful consideration of the risks and benefits is recommended when using such medications pending the publication of findings from systematic studies.

c) Side effects

Although lithium commonly causes side effects, most are minor or can be reduced or eliminated by lowering the dose or changing the dosage schedule. More common side effects include polyuria, polydipsia, weight gain, cognitive problems (e.g., dulling, poor concentration), tremor, sedation or lethargy, and gastrointestinal distress (e.g., nausea). Lithium may also have renal effects and may cause hypothyroidism. Lithium is potentially fatal in overdose and should be used with caution in patients at risk of suicide.

Carbamazepine's most common side effects include neurological symptoms (e.g., diplopia), blurred vision, fatigue, nausea, and ataxia. Other side effects include skin rash, mild leukopenia or thrombocytopenia, and hyponatremia. Rare, idiosyncratic, but potentially fatal side effects include agranulocytosis, aplastic anemia, hepatic failure, exfoliative dermatitis, and pancreatitis. Carbamazepine may be fatal in overdose. In studies of patients with borderline personality disorder, carbamazepine has been reported to cause melancholic depression (64).

Common dose-related side effects of valproate include gastrointestinal distress (e.g., nausea), benign hepatic transaminase elevations, tremor, sedation, and weight gain. With long-term use, women may be at risk of developing polycystic ovaries or hyperandrogenism. Mild, asymptomatic leukopenia and thrombocytopenia occur less frequently. Rare, idiosyncratic, but potentially fatal adverse events include hepatic failure, pancreatitis, and agranulocytosis.

d) Implementation issues

Full guidelines for the use of these medications can be found in the APA *Practice Guideline for the Treatment of Patients With Bipolar Disorder* (85; included in this volume). Lithium carbonate and the anticonvulsant mood stabilizers are used in their full therapeutic doses, with plasma levels guiding dosing. Routine precautions observed for the use of these medications in other disorders also apply to their use in borderline personality disorder, e.g., plasma level monitoring of thyroid and kidney function with prolonged lithium use, periodic measure of WBC count with carbamazepine therapy, and hematological and liver function tests for divalproex sodium.

5. Anxiolytic agents

a) Goals

Anxiolytic medications are used to treat the many manifestations of anxiety in patients with borderline personality disorder, both as an acute and as a chronic symptom.

b) Efficacy

Despite widespread use, there is a paucity of studies investigating the use of anxiolytic medications in borderline personality disorder. Cowdry and Gardner (55) included alprazolam in their double-blind, placebo-controlled, crossover study of outpatients with borderline personality disorder, comorbid hysteroid dysphoria, and extensive histories of behavioral dyscontrol. Use of alprazolam (mean dose=4.7 mg/day) was associated with greater suicidality and episodes of serious behavioral dyscontrol (drug overdoses, self-mutilation, and throwing a chair at a child). This occurred in 7 (58%) of 12 patients taking alprazolam compared with 1 (8%) of 13 patients receiving placebo. However, in a small number of patients (N=3), alprazolam was noted to be helpful for anxiety in carefully selected patients with borderline personality disorder (52). Case reports suggest that clonazepam is helpful as an adjunctive agent in the treatment of impulsivity, violent outbursts, and anxiety in a variety of disorders, including borderline personality disorder (54).

Although clinicians have presented preliminary experiences with nonbenzodiazepine anxiolytics in patients with borderline personality disorder (e.g., buspirone) (184), there are currently no published studies of these anxiolytics in borderline personality disorder.

c) Side effects

Behavioral disinhibition, resulting in impulsive and assaultive behaviors, has been reported with alprazolam in patients with borderline personality disorder. Benzodiazepines, in general, should be used with care because of the potential for abuse and the development of pharmacological tolerance with prolonged use. These are particular risks in patients with a history of substance use.

d) Implementation issues

In the absence of clear evidence-based recommendations, dose and duration of treatment must be guided by clinical need and judgment, keeping in mind the potential for abuse and pharmacological tolerance.

6. Opiate antagonists

a) Goals

It has been suggested that the relative subjective numbing and physical analgesia that patients with borderline personality disorder often feel during episodes of self-mutilation, as well as the reported sense of relative well-being afterward, might be due to release of endogenous opiates (185–187). Opiate antagonists have been employed in an attempt to block mutilation-induced analgesia and euphoria and thereby reduce self-injurious behavior in patients with borderline personality disorder.

b) Efficacy

Clinical case reports (188) and several small case series have assessed the efficacy of opiate antagonists for self-injurious behavior, and two suggested some improvement in this behavior (189, 190). One small, double-blind study involving female patients with borderline personality disorder with a history of self-injurious behavior who underwent a stress challenge showed no effect of opiate receptor blockade with naloxone on cold pressor pain perception or mood ratings (191). While the stress level may not have been high enough to mimic clinical situations, the study does not support the theory that opiate antagonism plays a role in reducing self-injurious behavior.

Despite the few promising clinical case reports, these reports are very preliminary, and there is no clear evidence from well-controlled trials indicating that opiate antagonists are effective in reducing self-injurious behavior among patients with borderline personality disorder.

c) Side effects

Nausea and diarrhea are occasionally reported (190).

d) Implementation issues

In published reports, the typical dose of naltrexone was 50 mg/day. No time limit for treatment emerges from the literature, but the effect is presumably reversed when the medication stops.

7. Neuroleptics

a) Goals

The primary goal of treatment with neuroleptics in borderline personality disorder is to reduce acute symptom severity in all symptom domains, particularly schizotypal symptoms, psychosis, anger, and hostility.

b) Efficacy

Early clinical experience with neuroleptics targeted the "micropsychotic" or schizotypal symptoms of borderline personality disorder. However, affective symptoms (mood, anxiety, anger) and somatic complaints also improved with low doses of haloperidol, perphenazine, and thiothixene. An open-label trial of thioridazine (mean dose=92 mg/day) led to marked improvement in impulsive-behavioral symptoms, global symptom severity, and overall borderline psychopathology (78). Similar findings were reported for adolescents with borderline personality disorder treated with flupentixol (mean dose=3 mg/day) (77), with improvement in impulsivity, depression, and global functioning.

Systematic, parallel studies that compared neuroleptics without a placebo control condition also reported a broad spectrum of efficacy. Leone (73) found that loxapine succinate (mean dose=14.5 mg/day) or chlorpromazine (mean dose=110 mg/day) improved depressed mood, anxiety, anger/hostility, and suspiciousness. Serban and Siegel (74) reported that thiothixene (mean dose=9.4 mg/day, SD=7.6) or haloperidol (mean dose=3.0 mg/day, SD=0.8) produced improvement in anxiety, depression, derealization, paranoia (ideas of reference), general symptoms, and a global measure of borderline psychopathology.

Subsequent double-blind, placebo-controlled trials also suggested a broad spectrum of efficacy for low-dose neuroleptics in the treatment of borderline personality disorder. Acute symptom severity improved in cognitive-perceptual, affective, and impulsive-behavioral symptom domains, although efficacy for schizotypal symptoms, psychoticism, anger, and hostility was most consistently noted.

Many of the double-blind, placebo-controlled studies of neuroleptics in borderline personality disorder are noteworthy for biases in sample selection that strongly affected outcomes. In a study of patients with borderline or schizotypal personality disorder and at least one psychotic symptom (which biased the sample toward cognitive-perceptual symptoms), thiothixene (mean dose=8.7 mg/day for up to 12 weeks) was more effective than placebo for psychotic cluster symptoms—specifically illusions and ideas of reference—and self-rated obsessive-compulsive and phobic anxiety symptoms but not depression or global functioning (75). The more severely symptomatic patients were at baseline (e.g., in terms of illusions, ideas of reference, or obsessive-compulsive and phobic anxiety symptoms), the better they responded to thiothixene (75).

Cowdry and Gardner (55) conducted a complex, placebo-controlled, four-drug crossover study in borderline personality disorder outpatients with trifluoperazine (mean dose=7.8 mg/day). Patients were required to meet criteria for hysteroid dysphoria and have a history of extensive behavioral dyscontrol, introducing a bias toward affective and impulsive-behavioral symptoms. All patients were receiving psychotherapy. Those patients who were able to keep taking trifluoperazine for 3 weeks or longer (7 of 12 patients) had improved mood, with significant improvement over placebo on physician ratings of depression, anxiety, rejection sensitivity, and suicidality.

Soloff and colleagues (50, 51) studied acutely ill inpatients, comparing haloperidol with amitriptyline and placebo in a 5-week trial. Patients who received haloperidol (mean dose=4.8 mg/day) improved significantly more than those receiving placebo across all symptom domains (50), including global measures, self- and observer-rated depression, anger and hostility, schizotypal symptoms, psychoticism, and impulsive behaviors (51). Haloperidol was as effective as amitriptyline for depressive symptoms.

However, a second study by the same group (56) that used the same design but compared haloperidol with phenelzine and placebo failed to replicate the broad-spectrum efficacy of haloperidol (mean dose=3.9 mg/day). Efficacy for haloperidol was limited to hostile belligerence and impulsive-aggressive behaviors, and placebo effects were powerful. Patients in this study had milder symptoms, especially in the cognitive-perceptual and impulsive-behavioral symptom domains, than patients in the first study.

Cornelius and colleagues (68) followed a subset of the aforementioned group who had responded to haloperidol, phenelzine, or placebo for 16 weeks following acute treatment. Patients' intolerance of the medication, a high dropout rate, and nonadherence were decisive factors in this study. The attrition rates at 22 weeks were 87.5% for haloperidol, 65.7% for phenelzine, and 58.1% for placebo. Further significant improvement with haloperidol treatment (compared with placebo) occurred only for irritability (with improvement for hostility that was not statistically significant). Depressive symptoms significantly worsened with haloperidol treatment over time, which was attributed, in part, to the side effect of akinesia. Clinical improvement was modest and of limited clinical importance.

Montgomery and Montgomery (80) controlled for nonadherence by using depot flupentixol decanoate, 20 mg once a month, in a continuation study of recurrently parasuicidal patients with borderline personality disorder and histrionic personality disorder. Over a 6-month period, patients receiving flupentixol had a significant decrease in suicidal behaviors compared with the placebo group. Significant differences emerged by the fourth month and were sustained through 6 months of treatment. This important study awaits replication.

The introduction of the newer atypical neuroleptics increases clinicians' options for treating borderline personality disorder. To date, findings from only two small open-label trials have been published, both with clozapine. Frankenburg and Zanarini (81) reported that clozapine (mean dose=253.3 mg/day, SD=163.7) improved positive and negative psychotic symptoms and global functioning (but not depression or other symptoms) in 15 patients with borderline personality disorder and comorbid axis I psychotic disorder not otherwise specified who had not responded to (or were intolerant of) other neuroleptics. Improvement was modest but statistically significant. Patients were recruited from a larger study of patients with treatment-resistant psychotic disorders, raising the question of whether their psychotic symptoms were truly part of their borderline personality disorder.

These concerns were addressed by Benedetti and colleagues (71), who excluded all patients with axis I psychotic disorders from their cohort of patients with refractory borderline personality disorder. Target symptoms included "psychotic-like" symptoms that are more typical of borderline personality disorder. Patients had not responded to at least 4 months of prior treatment with medication and psychotherapy. In a 4-month, open-label trial of 12 patients treated with clozapine (mean dose=43.8 mg/day, SD=18.8) and concurrent psychotherapy, a low dose of clozapine improved symptoms in all domains—cognitive-perceptual, affective, and impulsive-behavioral.

Despite a lack of data, clinicians are increasingly using olanzapine, risperidone, and quetiapine for patients with borderline personality disorder. These medications have less risk than clozapine and may be better tolerated than the typical neuroleptics. Schulz and colleagues (83) presented preliminary data from a double-blind, placebo-controlled, 8-week trial of risperidone in 27 patients with borderline personality disorder who received an average dose of 2.5 mg/day (to a maximum of 4 mg/day). On global measures of functioning, there was no significant difference between risperidone and placebo, although the authors noted that risperidone-treated patients were "diverging from the placebo group" in paranoia, psychoticism, interpersonal sensitivity, and phobic anxiety (83). The same group conducted an 8-week, open-label study of olanzapine in patients with borderline personality disorder and comorbid dysthymia (82). Patients received an average dose of 7.5 mg/day (range=2.5–10 mg/day). Among the 11 completers, significant improvement was reported across all domains, with particular improvement noted in depression, interpersonal sensitivity, psychoticism, anxiety, and anger/hostility. These medications require further investigation in double-blind studies.

In summary, neuroleptics are the best-studied psychotropic medications for borderline personality disorder. The literature supports the use of low-dose neuroleptics for the acute management of global symptom severity, with specific efficacy for schizotypal symptoms and psychoticism, anger, and hostility. Relief of global symptom severity in the acute setting may be due, in part, to nonspecific "tranquilizer" effects of neuroleptics, whereas symptom-specific actions against psychoticism, anger, and hostility may relate more directly to dopaminergic blockade. Acute treatment effects of neuroleptic drugs in borderline personality disorder tend to be modest but clinically and statistically significant.

Two studies that addressed continuation and maintenance treatment of a patient with borderline personality disorder with neuroleptics had contradictory results. The Montgomery and Montgomery study (80) reported efficacy for recurrent parasuicidal behaviors, whereas the Cornelius et al. study (68) suggested very modest utility for only irritability and hostility. More controlled trials are needed to investigate low-dose neuroleptics in continuation and maintenance treatment.

c) Side effects

Dropout rates in neuroleptic trials in borderline outpatients range from 13.7% for a 6-week trial (73) to 48.3% for a 12-week trial (75) to 87.5% for a 22-week continuation study (68). In acute studies, patient nonadherence is often due to typical medication side effects, e.g., extrapyramidal symptoms, akathisia, sedation, and hypotension. Patients with borderline personality disorder who have experienced relief of acute symptoms with low-dose neuroleptics may not tolerate the side effects of the drug with longer-term treatment. The risk of tardive dyskinesia must be considered in any decision to continue neuroleptic medication over the long term. Thioridazine has been associated with cardiac rhythm disturbances related to widening of the Q-T interval and should be avoided. In the case of clozapine, the risk of agranulocytosis is especially problematic. While the newer atypical neuroleptics promise a more favorable side effect profile, evidence of efficacy in borderline personality disorder is still awaited. Neuroleptics should be given in the context of a supportive doctor-patient relationship in which side effects and nonadherence are addressed frequently.

d) Implementation issues

All studies have used a low dose and demonstrated beneficial effects within several weeks. With the exception of one study that used a depot neuroleptic (flupentixol, which is not available in the United States), all medications were given orally and daily. Acute treatment studies are a good model for acute clinical care and typically range from 5 to 12 weeks in duration. There is insufficient evidence to make a strong recommendation concerning continuation and maintenance therapies. At present, this is best left to the clinician's judgment after carefully weighing the risks and benefits for the individual patient. CBC monitoring must be done if clozapine is used.

8. ECT

a) Goals

The goal of ECT in patients with borderline personality disorder is to decrease depressive symptoms in individuals with a comorbid axis I mood disorder, which is present in as many as one-half of hospitalized patients with borderline personality disorder.

b) Efficacy

Most of the clinical and empirical literature that describes experience with ECT in patients with major depression comorbid with personality disorders does not report results specifically for borderline personality disorder. Although studies that used a naturalistic design have had inconsistent findings, patients with major depression and a comorbid personality disorder were generally less responsive to somatic treatments than patients with major depression alone.

In one naturalistic follow-up study (based on chart review), there was no significant difference in recovery rates for 10 patients with major depressive disorder and a personality disorder (40% recovery) compared with 41 patients with major depressive disorder alone (65.9% recovery) (192). In another study, involving 1,471 depressed inpatients, depressed patients with a personality disorder were 50% less likely to be recovered at hospital discharge than depressed patients without a personality disorder (193).

Several uncontrolled studies found that outcome was dependent on the time of assessment. In one small study (194), there were no significant differences in immediate response to ECT between depressed subjects with or without a personality disorder; however, at a 6-month follow-up evaluation, the patients with a personality disorder had more rehospitalizations and more severe depression symptoms. Conversely, in another uncontrolled study of inpatients with major depression (195), compared with depressed patients without a personality disorder, those with a personality disorder had a poorer outcome in terms of depression and social functioning immediately following treatment. However, after 6 and 12 weeks of follow-up, there were no differences between the two groups in terms of depression and social functioning. The number of rehospitalizations did not differ between groups at the 6-month and 12-month follow-up evaluations.

In another small study (N=16) (196–198) that used the self-rated Millon Clinical Multiaxial Inventory—II and assessed borderline personality disorder, there was significant improvement in avoidant, histrionic, aggressive/sadistic, and schizotypal personality traits with ECT. Improvements were noted in passive-aggressive and borderline personality traits that did not reach statistical significance. The presence of pretreatment borderline traits predicted poorer outcome with ECT (198).

Although the results of these studies appear somewhat divergent, most found that patients with major depression and a personality disorder have a less favorable outcome with ECT than depressed patients without a personality disorder.

c) Adverse effects

Because ECT is not recommended for borderline personality disorder per se, adverse effects are not described here and can be found in the APA *Practice Guideline for the Treatment of Patients With Major Depressive Disorder* (84; included in this volume).

d) Implementation issues

The affective dysregulation, low self-esteem, pessimism, chronic suicidality, and self-mutilation of patients with borderline personality disorder are often misconstrued as axis I depression. Clinical experience suggests that, not infrequently, these characterological manifestations of borderline personality disorder are treated with ECT, often resulting in a poor outcome. Although there is a paucity of ECT studies involving patients with borderline personality disorder, a recommendation for ECT in these patients with comorbid major depression should be guided by the presence and severity of verifiable neurovegetative symptoms, e.g., sleep disturbance, appetite disturbance, weight change, low energy, and anhedonia. These symptoms should ideally be confirmed by outside observers, as they provide an objective way to assess treatment response. Perhaps the greatest challenge for the clinician is not when to institute ECT in the depressed patient with borderline personality disorder but when to stop. As the neurovegetative symptoms of major depression resolve, many patients continue to have borderline features that clinical experience suggests are unresponsive to ECT. Knowledge of the patient's personality functioning before the onset of major depression is critical to knowing when the "baseline" has been achieved. Many patients with borderline personality disorder who are considered nonresponsive to ECT because of persistence of depressive features are, in fact, already in remission from their axis I depression but continue to experience chronic characterological depressive features.

Notable progress has been made in our understanding of borderline personality disorder and its treatment. However, there are many remaining questions regarding treatments with demonstrated efficacy, including how to optimally use them to achieve the best health outcomes for patients with borderline personality disorder. In addition, many therapeutic modalities have received little empirical investigation for borderline personality disorder and require further study. The efficacy of various treatments also needs to be studied in populations such as adolescents, the elderly, forensic populations, and patients in long-term institutional settings. The following is a sample of the types of research questions that require further study.

PART C: FUTURE RESEARCH NEEDS

VII. PSYCHOTHERAPY

Many aspects of psychotherapy in the treatment of borderline personality disorder require further investigation. For example, further controlled treatment studies of psychodynamic psychotherapy, dialectical behavior therapy, and other forms of cognitive behavior therapy are needed, particularly in outpatient settings. In addition, psychotherapeutic interventions that have received less investigation, such as group therapy, couples therapy, and family interventions, require study. The following are some specific questions that need to be addressed by future research:

- What is the relative efficacy of different psychotherapeutic approaches? Which types of patients respond to which types of psychotherapy?
- What components of dialectical behavior therapy and psychodynamic psychotherapy are responsible for their efficacy? What common elements of these treatments are responsible for their efficacy?

- What are the indications for use of psychodynamic psychotherapy and dialectical behavior therapy? How does the presence of certain clinical features (e.g., prominent self-destructive behavior or dissociative features) affect response to these treatments?
- To what extent is a good outcome due to the unique components of these treatments versus the amount of treatment received?
- How effective are psychodynamic psychotherapy and dialectical behavior therapy when used in the community rather than in specialized treatment settings, and how can these treatments be optimally implemented in community settings?
- What is the optimal duration of psychotherapy for patients with borderline personality disorder?
- Is there a model of brief psychotherapy (12–30 sessions) that is effective for borderline personality disorder?
- What are the optimal frequencies of psychotherapeutic contact for different psychotherapies during different stages of treatment?
- What is the relative efficacy of psychotherapy versus pharmacotherapy for patients with borderline personality disorder? Do certain patients respond better to one treatment modality than to the other?
- What is the relative efficacy of a combination of psychotherapy and pharmacotherapy versus either treatment modality alone?

VIII. PHARMACOTHERAPY AND OTHER SOMATIC TREATMENTS

Many aspects of pharmacotherapy in the treatment of borderline personality disorder also require investigation. Further controlled treatment studies of medications—in particular, those that have received relatively little investigation (for example, atypical neuroleptics)—are needed. Studies of continuation and maintenance treatment as well as treatment discontinuation are especially needed, as are systematic studies of treatment sequences and algorithms. The following are some specific questions that need to be addressed by future research:

- What is the relative efficacy of different pharmacological approaches for the behavioral dimensions of borderline personality disorder?
- What is the relative efficacy of different pharmacological augmentation and combination strategies, and what is their efficacy compared with treatment with single agents?
- How does the presence of certain clinical features (for example, prominent self-destructive behavior or dissociative features) affect response to pharmacotherapy?
- What is the minimal dose and duration of an adequate trial for different medications in patients with borderline personality disorder?
- What is the optimal duration of different types of medication treatment?
- What are the indications for discontinuation of effective pharmacological treatment?
- Are atypical neuroleptics or typical neuroleptics more effective or better tolerated in patients with borderline personality disorder?
- How efficacious are mood stabilizers for patients with borderline personality disorder, and which patients are most likely to benefit from this treatment? Are certain mood stabilizers more effective than others?
- What role should ECT have in the treatment of patients with refractory or severe borderline personality disorder?

APPENDIXES:
PSYCHOPHARMACOLOGICAL TREATMENT ALGORITHMS

APPENDIX 1
PSYCHOPHARMACOLOGICAL TREATMENT OF AFFECTIVE DYSREGULATION SYMPTOMS IN PATIENTS WITH BORDERLINE PERSONALITY DISORDER[a].

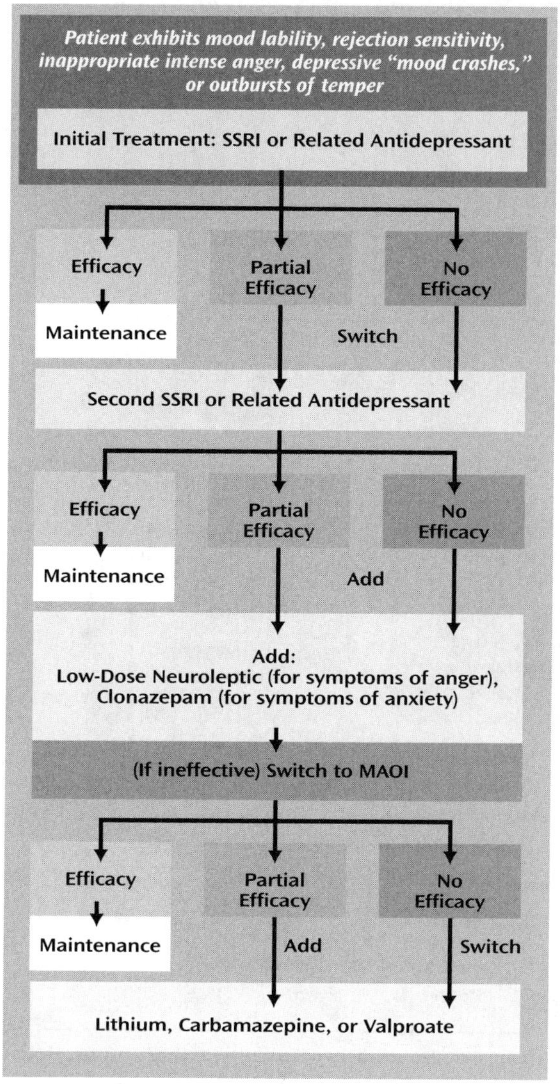

[a]Algorithm based on clinical judgment that uses evidence currently in the literature, following the format of the International Psychopharmacology Algorithm Project (2). The first step in the algorithm is generally supported by the best empirical evidence. Recommendations may not be applicable to all patients or take individual needs into account. The empirical research studies on which these recommendations are based may be "first trials" involving previously untreated patients and may not take into account previous patient nonresponse to one, two, or even three levels of the algorithm (i.e., patients who, by definition, have more refractory disorders). There are no empirical trials of the complete algorithm.

APPENDIX 2
PSYCHOPHARMACOLOGICAL TREATMENT OF IMPULSIVE-BEHAVIORAL DYSCONTROL SYMPTOMS IN PATIENTS WITH BORDERLINE PERSONALITY DISORDER[a].

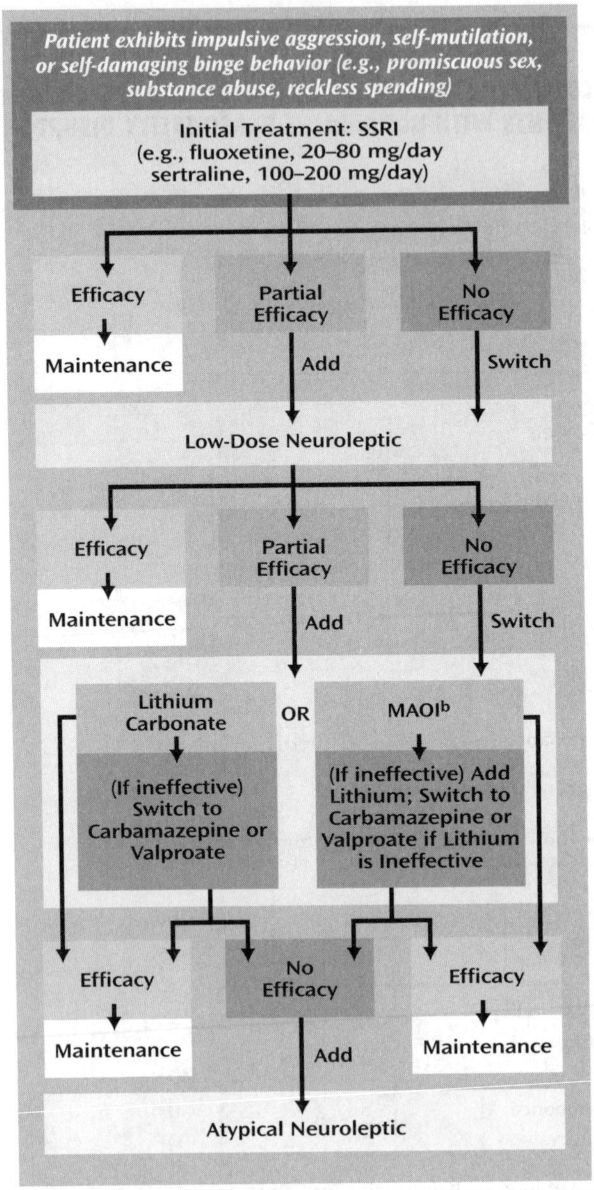

[a]Algorithm based on clinical judgment that uses evidence currently in the literature, following the format of the International Psychopharmacology Algorithm Project (2). The first step in the algorithm is generally supported by the best empirical evidence. Recommendations may not be applicable to all patients or take individual needs into account. The empirical research studies on which these recommendations are based may be "first trials" involving previously untreated patients and may not take into account previous patient nonresponse to one, two, or even three levels of the algorithm (i.e., patients who, by definition, have more refractory disorders). There are no empirical trials of the complete algorithm.

[b]SSRI treatment must be discontinued and followed with an adequate washout period before initiating treatment with an MAOI.

APPENDIX 3
PSYCHOPHARMACOLOGICAL TREATMENT OF COGNITIVE-PERCEPTUAL SYMPTOMS IN PATIENTS WITH BORDERLINE PERSONALITY DISORDER[a].

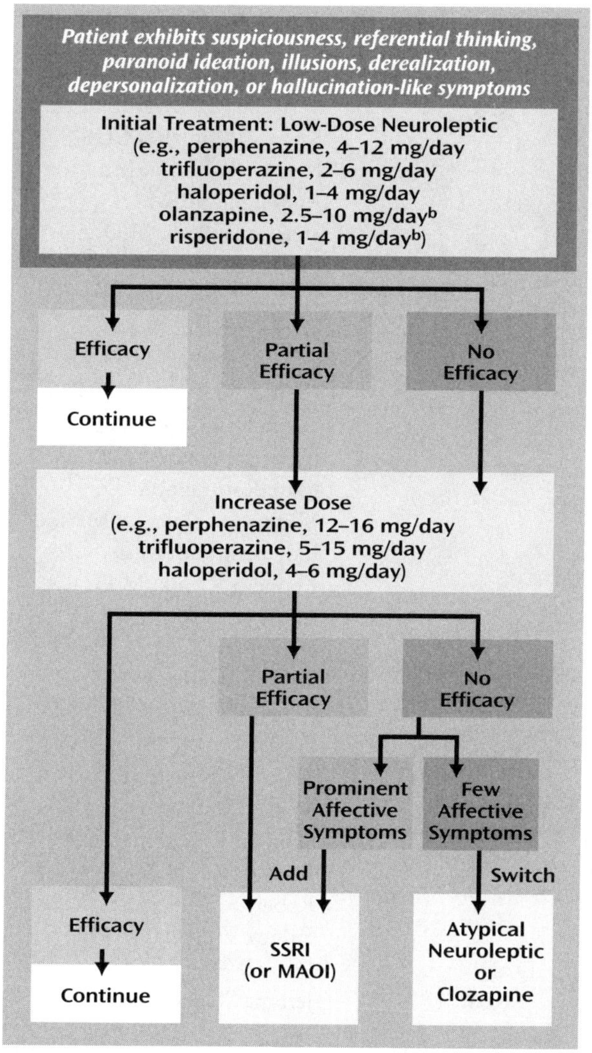

[a]Algorithm based on clinical judgment that uses evidence currently in the literature, following the format of the International Psychopharmacology Algorithm Project (2). The first step in the algorithm is generally supported by the best empirical evidence. Recommendations may not be applicable to all patients or take individual needs into account. The empirical research studies on which these recommendations are based may be "first trials" involving previously untreated patients and may not take into account previous patient nonresponse to one, two, or even three levels of the algorithm (i.e., patients who, by definition, have more refractory disorders). There are no empirical trials of the complete algorithm.

[b]The generally favorable side effect profiles of the newer atypical neuroleptic medications compared with those of conventional neuroleptics underscore the need for careful empirical trials of these newer medications in the treatment of patients with borderline personality disorder.

INDIVIDUALS AND ORGANIZATIONS THAT SUBMITTED COMMENTS

Gerald Adler, M.D.
Hagop Akiskal, M.D.
Deborah Antai-Otong, M.S., R.N., P.M.H.N.P., C.S.
Lorna Benjamin, Ph.D.
Sandra Smith Bjork, R.N., J.D.
Nashaat N. Boutros, M.D.
Daniel Buie, M.D.
Kenneth Busch, M.D.
Carlyle H. Chan, M.D.
Richard D. Chessick, M.D., Ph.D.
Diego Cohen, M.D.
Nancy Collins, R.N., M.P.H.
Alv A. Dahl, M.D.
Dave M. Davis, M.D.
Diana Dell, M.D.
Anita S. Everett, M.D.
Robert Findling, M.D.
Douglas H. Finestone, M.D.
Arnold Goldberg, M.D.
William M. Greenberg, M.D.
Elliot A. Harris, M.D.
Al Herzog, M.D.
Eric Hollander, M.D.
Patricia Hoffman Judd, Ph.D.
Morten Kjolbye, M.D.
Ronald Koegler, M.D.
Paul S. Links, M.D.
Cesare Maffei, M.D.
Paul Markovitz, M.D., Ph.D.
John C. Markowitz, M.D.
James F. Masterson, M.D.
William Meissner, M.D.
Robert Michels, M.D.
Mary D. Moller, M.S.N., C.S., P.M.H.N.P.
Richard Munich, M.D.
Nathan A. Munn, M.D.
Andrei Novac, M.D.
Stefano Pallanti, M.D.
Joel Paris, M.D.
Jane L. Pearson, Ph.D.
Gary Peterson, M.D.
Eric M. Plakun, M.D.
Charles W. Portney, M.D.
Lawrence H. Rockland, M.D.
Barbara Rosenfeld, M.D.
Marc Rothman, M.D.
Marian Scheinholtz, M.S., O.T.R.L.
Judy Sigmund, M.D.
Kenneth R. Silk, M.D.
Andrew E. Skodol, M.D.
Robert Stern, M.D., Ph.D.
Nada L. Stotland, M.D., M.P.H.
Richard T. Suchinsky, M.D.
Peter J. Sukin, M.D.
Arthur Summer, M.D.
Marijo Tamburrino, M.D.
William R. Tatomer, M.D.
Per Vaglum, M.D.
Robert S. Wallerstein, M.D.
Sidney Weissman, M.D.
Drew Westen, Ph.D.
Jerome Winer, M.D.

American Academy of Ophthalmology
American College of Obstetrics and Gynecology
American College of Radiology
American Occupational Therapy Association
American Psychiatric Nurses Association
American Psychoanalytic Association
Commonwealth of Virginia Department of Mental Health, Mental Retardation and Substance Abuse Services
Illinois Psychiatric Society
International Society for the Study of Personality Disorders
New Jersey Psychiatric Association
Norwegian Psychiatric Association
Royal Australian and New Zealand College of Psychiatrists

REFERENCES

The following coding system is used to indicate the nature of the supporting evidence in the references:

[A] *Randomized clinical trial.* A study of an intervention in which subjects are prospectively followed over time; there are treatment and control groups; subjects are randomly assigned to the two groups; both the subjects and the investigators are blind to the assignments.

[B] *Clinical trial.* A prospective study in which an intervention is made and the results of that intervention are tracked longitudinally; study does not meet standards for a randomized clinical trial.

[C] *Cohort or longitudinal study.* A study in which subjects are prospectively followed over time without any specific intervention.

[D] *Case-control study.* A study in which a group of patients and a group of control subjects are identified in the present and information about them is pursued retrospectively or backward in time.

[E] *Review with secondary data analysis.* A structured analytic review of existing data, e.g., a meta-analysis or a decision analysis.

[F] *Review.* A qualitative review and discussion of previously published literature without a quantitative synthesis of the data.

[G] *Other.* Textbooks, expert opinion, case reports, and other reports not included above.

1. American Psychiatric Association: Diagnostic and Statistical Manual of Mental Disorders, 4th ed, Text Revision (DSM-IV-TR). Washington, DC, APA, 2000 [G]
2. Jobson KO, Potter WZ: International Psychopharmacology Algorithm Project report. Psychopharmacol Bull 1995; 31:457–507 [F]
3. American Psychiatric Association: Practice Guideline for Psychiatric Evaluation of Adults. Am J Psychiatry 1995; 152(Nov suppl) [G]
4. Kernberg OF, Selzer M, Koenigsberg H, Carr A, Appelbaum A: Psychodynamic Psychotherapy of Borderline Patients. New York, Basic Books, 1989 [G]
5. Linehan MM, Heard HL, Armstrong HE: Naturalistic follow-up of a behavioral treatment for chronically parasuicidal borderline patients. Arch Gen Psychiatry 1993; 50:971–974; correction, 1994; 51:422 [A]
6. Kjelsberg E, Eikeseth PH, Dahl AA: Suicide in borderline patients—predictive factors. Acta Psychiatr Scand 1991; 84:283–287 [D]
7. Sederer LI, Ellison J, Keyes C: Guidelines for prescribing psychiatrists in consultative, collaborative, and supervisory relationships. Psychiatr Serv 1998; 49:1197–1202 [F]
8. Linehan MM, Armstrong HE, Suarez A, Allmon D, Heard HL: Cognitive-behavioral treatment of chronically parasuicidal borderline patients. Arch Gen Psychiatry 1991; 48:1060–1064 [A]
9. Bateman A, Fonagy P: Effectiveness of partial hospitalization in the treatment of borderline personality disorder: a randomized controlled trial. Am J Psychiatry 1999; 156:1563–1569 [A]
10. Bateman A, Fonagy P: Treatment of borderline personality disorder with psychoanalytically oriented partial hospitalization: an 18-month follow-up. Am J Psychiatry 2001; 158:36–42 [A]
11. Gabbard GO, Horwitz L, Allen JG, Frieswyk S, Newsom G, Colson DB, Coyne L: Transference interpretation in the psychotherapy of borderline patients: a high-risk, high-gain phenomenon. Harv Rev Psychiatry 1994; 2:59–69 [B]
12. Gunderson JG: Borderline Personality Disorder: A Clinical Guide. Washington, DC, American Psychiatric Press, 2001 [G]

13. Clarkin JF, Yeomans FE, Kernberg OF: Psychotherapy for Borderline Personality. New York, John Wiley & Sons, 1999 [G]
14. Adler G: Borderline Psychopathology and Its Treatment. New York, Jason Aronson, 1985 [G]
15. Gabbard GO, Wilkinson SM: Management of Countertransference With Borderline Patients. Washington, DC, American Psychiatric Press, 1994 [G]
16. Horwitz L, Gabbard GO, Allen JG: Borderline Personality Disorder: Tailoring the Psychotherapy to the Patient. Washington, DC, American Psychiatric Press, 1996 [B]
17. Linehan MM: Cognitive-Behavioral Treatment of Borderline Personality Disorder. New York, Guilford, 1993 [G]
18. Waldinger RJ: Intensive psychodynamic therapy with borderline patients: an overview. Am J Psychiatry 1987; 144:267–274 [G]
19. Beck AT, Freeman AM: Cognitive Therapy of Personality Disorders. New York, Guilford, 1990 [G]
20. Stevenson J, Meares R: An outcome study of psychotherapy for patients with borderline personality disorder. Am J Psychiatry 1992; 149:358–362 [B]
21. Meares R, Stevenson J, Comerford A: Psychotherapy with borderline patients, I: a comparison between treated and untreated cohorts. Aust N Z J Psychiatry 1999; 33:467–472 [B]
22. Boyer LB: Working with a borderline patient. Psychoanal Q 1977; 46:386–424 [G]
23. Chessick RD: Intensive Psychotherapy of the Borderline Patient. New York, Jason Aronson, 1977 [G]
24. Grotstein JS: The analysis of a borderline patient, in Technical Factors in the Treatment of the Severely Disturbed Patient. Edited by Giovacchini PL, Boyer LB. New York, Jason Aronson, 1982, pp 261–288 [G]
25. Grotstein JS, Solomon MF, Lang JA: The Borderline Patient: Emerging Concepts in Diagnosis, Psychodynamics, and Treatment. Hillsdale, NJ, Analytic Press, 1987 [G]
26. Gunderson JG: Borderline Personality Disorder. Washington, DC, American Psychiatric Press, 1984
27. Kernberg OF: Borderline Conditions and Pathological Narcissism. New York, Jason Aronson, 1975 [G]
28. Kernberg OF: Severe Personality Disorders: Psychotherapeutic Strategies. New Haven, Conn, Yale University Press, 1984 [G]
29. Masterson JF: Psychotherapy of the Borderline Adult: A Developmental Approach. New York, Brunner/Mazel, 1976 [G]
30. Masterson JF: The Personality Disorders: A New Look at the Developmental Self and Object Relations Approach. Phoenix, Ariz, Zeig, Tucker, 2000 [G]
31. Meares R: Metaphor of Play: Disruption and Restoration in the Borderline Experience. Northvale, NJ, Jason Aronson, 1993 [G]
32. Meares R: Intimacy and Alienation: Memory, Trauma, and Personal Being. New York, Routledge, 2000 [G]
33. Meissner WW: The Borderline Spectrum: Differential Diagnosis and Developmental Issues. New York, Jason Aronson, 1984 [G]
34. Meissner WW: Treatment of Patients in the Borderline Spectrum. Northvale, NJ, Jason Aronson, 1988 [G]
35. Rinsley DB: Developmental Pathogenesis and Treatment of Borderline and Narcissistic Personalities. Northvale, NJ, Jason Aronson, 1989 [G]
36. Searles HF: My Work With Borderline Patients. Northvale, NJ, Jason Aronson, 1986 [G]
37. Stone MH: The Borderline Syndromes: Constitution, Personality, and Adaptation. New York, McGraw-Hill, 1980 [G]
38. Waldinger RJ, Gunderson JG: Effective Psychotherapy With Borderline Patients: Case Studies. Washington, DC, American Psychiatric Press, 1987 [D]

39. Abend SM, Porder MS, Willick MS: Borderline Patients: Psychoanalytic Perspectives. Madison, Conn, International Universities Press, 1983 [G]
40. McGlashan TH: The Chestnut Lodge follow-up study, III: long-term outcome of borderline personalities. Arch Gen Psychiatry 1986; 43:20–30 [C]
41. Seeman M, Edwardes-Evans B: Marital therapy with borderline patients: is it beneficial? J Clin Psychiatry 1979; 40:308–312 [G]
42. Shapiro ER: Family dynamics and borderline personality disorder, in Handbook of Borderline Disorders. Edited by Silver D, Rosenbluth M. Madison, Conn, International Universities Press, 1992, pp 471–493 [G]
43. Siever LJ, Trestman R: The serotonin system and aggressive personality disorder. Int Clin Psychopharmacol 1993; 8:33–39 [F]
44. Salzman C, Wolfson AN, Schatzberg A, Looper J, Henke R, Albanese M, Schwartz J, Miyawaki E: Effect of fluoxetine on anger in symptomatic volunteers with borderline personality disorder. J Clin Psychopharmacol 1995; 15:23–29 [A]
45. Markovitz P: Pharmacotherapy of impulsivity, aggression, and related disorders, in Impulsivity and Aggression. Edited by Hollander E, Stein DJ. New York, John Wiley & Sons, 1995, pp 263–287 [B]
46. Cornelius JR, Soloff PH, Perel JM, Ulrich RF: Fluoxetine trial in borderline personality disorder. Psychopharmacol Bull 1990; 26:151–154 [B]
47. Kavoussi RJ, Liu J, Coccaro EF: An open trial of sertraline in personality disordered patients with impulsive aggression. J Clin Psychiatry 1994; 55:137–141 [B]
48. Markovitz PJ, Calabrese JR, Charles SC, Meltzer HY: Fluoxetine in the treatment of borderline and schizotypal personality disorders. Am J Psychiatry 1991; 148:1064–1067 [B]
49. Norden MJ: Fluoxetine in borderline personality disorder. Prog Neuropsychopharmacol Biol Psychiatry 1989; 13:885–893 [G]
50. Soloff PH, George A, Nathan RS, Schulz PM, Ulrich RF, Perel JM: Progress in pharmacotherapy of borderline disorders: a double-blind study of amitriptyline, haloperidol, and placebo. Arch Gen Psychiatry 1986; 43:691–697 [A]
51. Soloff PH, George A, Nathan S, Schulz PM, Cornelius JR, Herring J, Perel JM: Amitriptyline versus haloperidol in borderlines: final outcomes and predictors of response. J Clin Psychopharmacol 1989; 9:238–246 [A]
52. Faltus FJ: The positive effect of alprazolam in the treatment of three patients with borderline personality disorder. Am J Psychiatry 1984; 141:802–803 [G]
53. Gardner DL, Cowdry RW: Alprazolam-induced dyscontrol in borderline personality disorder. Am J Psychiatry 1985; 142:98–100 [A]
54. Freinhar JP, Alvarez WA: Clonazepam: a novel therapeutic adjunct. Int J Psychiatry Med 1985; 15:321–328 [G]
55. Cowdry RW, Gardner DL: Pharmacotherapy of borderline personality disorder: alprazolam, carbamazepine, trifluoperazine, and tranylcypromine. Arch Gen Psychiatry 1988; 45:111–119 [A]
56. Soloff PH, Cornelius J, George A, Nathan S, Perel JM, Ulrich RF: Efficacy of phenelzine and haloperidol in borderline personality disorder. Arch Gen Psychiatry 1993; 50:377–385 [A]
57. Parsons B, Quitkin FM, McGrath PJ, Stewart JW, Tricamo E, Ocepek-Welikson K, Harrison W, Rabkin JG, Wager SG, Nunes E: Phenelzine, imipramine, and placebo in borderline patients meeting criteria for atypical depression. Psychopharmacol Bull 1989; 25:524–534 [A]
58. Sheard MH: Lithium in the treatment of aggression. J Nerv Ment Dis 1975; 160:108–118 [B]
59. Sheard MH, Marini JL, Bridges CI, Wagner E: The effect of lithium on impulsive aggressive behavior in man. Am J Psychiatry 1976; 133:1409–1413 [A]
60. Tupin JP, Smith DB, Clanon TL, Kim LI, Nugent A, Groupe A: The long-term use of lithium in aggressive prisoners. Compr Psychiatry 1973; 14:311–317 [B]

61. Links P, Steiner M, Boiago I, Irwin D: Lithium therapy for borderline patients: preliminary findings. J Personal Disord 1990; 4:173–181 [A]
62. Gardner DL, Cowdry RW: Positive effects of carbamazepine on behavioral dyscontrol in borderline personality disorder. Am J Psychiatry 1986; 143:519–522 [A]
63. De la Fuente J, Lotstra F: A trial of carbamazepine in borderline personality disorder. Eur Neuropsychopharmacol 1994; 4:479–486 [A]
64. Gardner DL, Cowdry RW: Development of melancholia during carbamazepine treatment in borderline personality disorder. J Clin Psychopharmacol 1986; 6:236–239 [A]
65. Hollander E, Allen A, Lopez RP, Bienstock C, Grossman R, Siever L, Margolin L, Stein D: A preliminary double-blind, placebo-controlled trial of divalproex sodium in borderline personality disorder. J Clin Psychiatry 2001; 62:199–203 [A]
66. Stein DJ, Simeon D, Frenkel M, Islam MN, Hollander E: An open trial of valproate in borderline personality disorder. J Clin Psychiatry 1995; 56:506–510 [B]
67. Coccaro EF, Kavoussi RJ: Fluoxetine and impulsive aggressive behavior in personality-disordered subjects. Arch Gen Psychiatry 1997; 54:1081–1088 [A]
68. Cornelius JR, Soloff PH, Perel JM, Ulrich RF: Continuation pharmacotherapy of borderline personality disorder with haloperidol and phenelzine. Am J Psychiatry 1993; 150: 1843–1848 [A]
69. Kavoussi RJ, Coccaro EF: Divalproex sodium for impulsive aggressive behavior in patients with personality disorder. J Clin Psychiatry 1998; 59:676–680 [B]
70. Wilcox J: Divalproex sodium in the treatment of aggressive behavior. Ann Clin Psychiatry 1994; 6:17–20 [B]
71. Benedetti F, Sforzini L, Colombo C, Maffei C, Smeraldi E: Low-dose clozapine in acute and continuation treatment of severe borderline personality disorder. J Clin Psychiatry 1998; 59:103–107 [B]
72. Chengappa KN, Baker RW: The successful use of clozapine in ameliorating severe self mutilation in a patient with borderline personality disorder. J Personal Disord 1995; 9:76–82 [G]
73. Leone N: Response of borderline patients to loxapine and chlorpromazine. J Clin Psychiatry 1982; 43:148–150 [A]
74. Serban G, Siegel S: Response of borderline and schizotypal patients to small doses of thiothixene and haloperidol. Am J Psychiatry 1984; 141:1455–1458 [A]
75. Goldberg S, Schulz C, Schulz P, Resnick R, Hamer R, Friedel R: Borderline and schizotypal personality disorder treated with low-dose thiothixene vs placebo. Arch Gen Psychiatry 1986; 43:680–686 [A]
76. Goldberg S: Prediction of change in borderline personality disorder. Psychopharmacol Bull 1989; 25:550–555 [E]
77. Kutcher S, Papatheodorou G, Reiter S, Gardner D: The successful pharmacological treatment of adolescents and young adults with borderline personality disorder: a preliminary open trial of flupenthixol. J Psychiatry Neurosci 1995; 20:113–118 [B]
78. Teicher M, Glod C, Aaronson S, Gunter P, Schatzberg A, Cole J: Open assessment of the safety and efficacy of thioridazine in the treatment of patients with borderline personality disorder. Psychopharmacol Bull 1989; 25:535–549 [B]
79. Kelly T, Soloff PH, Cornelius JR, George A, Lis J: Can we study (treat) borderline patients: attrition from research and open treatment. J Personal Disord 1992; 6:417–433 [A]
80. Montgomery SA, Montgomery D: Pharmacological prevention of suicidal behaviour. J Affect Disord 1982; 4:291–298 [A]
81. Frankenburg F, Zanarini MC: Clozapine treatment of borderline patients: a preliminary study. Compr Psychiatry 1993; 34:402–405 [B]
82. Schulz S, Camlin KL, Berry SA, Jesberger JA: Olanzapine safety and efficacy in patients with borderline personality disorder and comorbid dysthymia. Biol Psychiatry 1999; 46: 1429–1435 [B]

83. Schulz SC, Camlin KL, Berry S, Friedman L: Risperidone for borderline personality disorder: a double blind study, in Proceedings of the 39th Annual Meeting of the American College of Neuropsychopharmacology. Nashville, Tenn, ACNP, 1999 [A]
84. American Psychiatric Association: Practice Guideline for the Treatment of Patients With Major Depressive Disorder (Revision). Am J Psychiatry 2000; 157(April suppl) [G]
85. American Psychiatric Association: Practice Guideline for the Treatment of Patients With Bipolar Disorder (Revision). Am J Psychiatry 2002; 159(April suppl) [G]
86. American Psychiatric Association: Practice Guideline for the Treatment of Patients With Eating Disorders (Revision). Am J Psychiatry 2000; 157(Jan suppl) [G]
87. American Psychiatric Association: Practice Guideline for the Treatment of Patients With Substance Use Disorders: Alcohol, Cocaine, Opioids. Am J Psychiatry 1995; 152(Nov suppl) [G]
88. American Psychiatric Association: Practice Guideline for the Treatment of Patients With Panic Disorder. Am J Psychiatry 1998; 155(May suppl) [G]
89. Soloff P, Cornelius J, George A: Relationship between axis I and axis II disorders: implications for treatment. Psychopharmacol Bull 1991; 27:23–30 [F]
90. Soloff PH, George A, Nathan RS, Schulz PM: Characterizing depression in borderline patients. J Clin Psychiatry 1987; 48:155–157 [E]
91. Rogers JH, Widiger TA, Krupp A: Aspects of depression associated with borderline personality disorder. Am J Psychiatry 1995; 152:268–270 [D]
92. Gunderson JG, Phillips KA: A current view of the interface between borderline personality disorder and depression. Am J Psychiatry 1991; 148:967–975 [F]
93. Stone MH: Abnormalities of Personality: Within and Beyond the Realm of Treatment. New York, WW Norton, 1993 [G]
94. Losel F: Management of psychopaths, in Psychopathy: Theory, Research and Implications for Society. Edited by Cooke DJ, Forth AE, Hare RD. Boston, Kluwer, 1998, pp 303–354 [G]
95. Dolan BM, Evans C, Wilson J: Therapeutic community treatment for personality disordered adults: changes in neurotic symptomatology on follow-up. Int J Soc Psychiatry 1992; 38:243–250 [B]
96. Coccaro EF, Kavoussi RJ, Sheline YI, Lish JD, Csernansky JG: Impulsive aggression in personality disorder correlates with tritiated paroxetine binding in the platelet. Arch Gen Psychiatry 1996; 53:531–536 [G]
97. Hare RD: The Hare Psychopathy Checklist—Revised. North Tonawanda, NY, Mental Health Systems, 1991 [G]
98. Gunderson JG, Sabo AN: The phenomenological and conceptual interface between borderline personality disorder and PTSD. Am J Psychiatry 1993; 150:19–27 [F]
99. Gunderson JG, Chu JA: Treatment implications of past trauma in borderline personality disorder. Harv Rev Psychiatry 1993; 1:75–81 [F]
100. Paris J, Zweig-Frank H: Dissociation in patients with borderline personality disorder (letter). Am J Psychiatry 1997; 154:137–138 [F]
101. Resnick HS, Kilpatrick DG, Dansky BS, Saunders BE, Best CL: Prevalence of civilian trauma and posttraumatic stress disorder in a representative national sample of women. J Consult Clin Psychol 1993; 61:984–991 [D]
102. Davidson JR, Hughes D, Blazer DG, George LK: Post-traumatic stress disorder in the community: an epidemiological study. Psychol Med 1991; 21:713–721 [D]
103. Ogata SN, Silk KR, Goodrich S, Lohr NE, Westen D, Hill EM: Childhood sexual and physical abuse in adult patients with borderline personality disorder. Am J Psychiatry 1990; 147:1008–1013 [D]
104. Fossati A, Madeddu F, Maffei C: Borderline personality disorder and childhood sexual abuse: a meta-analytic study. J Personal Disord 1999; 13:268–280 [E]

105. Lindemann E: Symptomatology and management of acute grief (1944). Am J Psychiatry 1994; 151(June suppl):155–160 [G]
106. Spiegel D: Vietnam grief work using hypnosis. Am J Clin Hypn 1981; 24:33–40 [B]
107. Butler LD, Duran REF, Jasiukaitis P, Kopan C, Spiegel D: Hypnotizability and traumatic experience: a diathesis-stress model of dissociative symptomatology (festschrift). Am J Psychiatry 1996; 153(July suppl):42–63 [F]
108. Shapiro F: Eye movement desensitization and reprocessing (EMDR) and the anxiety disorders: clinical and research implications of an integrated psychotherapy treatment. J Anxiety Disord 1999; 13:35–67 [F]
109. Wilson SA, Becker LA, Tinker RH: Eye movement desensitization and reprocessing (EMDR) treatment for psychologically traumatized individuals. J Consult Clin Psychol 1995; 63:928–937 [A]
110. Wilson SA, Becker LA, Tinker RH: Fifteen-month follow-up of eye movement desensitization and reprocessing (EMDR) treatment for posttraumatic stress disorder and psychological trauma. J Consult Clin Psychol 1997; 65:1047–1056 [B]
111. Jones B, Heard H, Startup M, Swales M, Williams JM, Jones RS: Autobiographical memory and dissociation in borderline personality disorder. Psychol Med 1999; 29:1397–1404 [D]
112. Chu JA, Dill DL: Dissociative symptoms in relation to childhood physical and sexual abuse. Am J Psychiatry 1990; 147:887–892 [D]
113. Neisser U, Fivush R (eds): The Remembering Self: Construction and Accuracy in the Self-Narrative. New York, Cambridge University Press, 1994 [G]
114. Saxe GN, van der Kolk BA, Berkowitz R, Chinman G, Hall K, Lieberg G, Schwartz J: Dissociative disorders in psychiatric inpatients. Am J Psychiatry 1993; 150:1037–1042 [D]
115. Galletly C: Borderline-dissociation comorbidity (letter). Am J Psychiatry 1997; 154:1629 [G]
116. Brodsky BS, Cloitre M, Dulit RA: Relationship of dissociation to self-mutilation and childhood abuse in borderline personality disorder. Am J Psychiatry 1995; 152:1788–1792 [D]
117. Ross CA, Miller SD, Reagor P, Bjornson L, Fraser GA, Anderson G: Structured interview data on 102 cases of multiple personality disorder from four centers. Am J Psychiatry 1990; 147:596–601 [D]
118. Braun BG, Sacks RG: The development of multiple personality disorder: predisposing, precipitating, and perpetuating factors, in Childhood Antecedents of Multiple Personality. Edited by Kluft RP. Washington, DC, American Psychiatric Press, 1985, pp 37–64 [F]
119. Kluft RP: The use of hypnosis with dissociative disorders. Psychiatr Med 1992; 10:31–46 [F]
120. Spiegel D, Maldonado J: Dissociative disorders, in The American Psychiatric Press Textbook of Psychiatry, 3rd ed. Edited by Hales RE, Yudofsky S, Talbott JA. Washington, DC, American Psychiatric Press, 1999, pp 711–737 [F]
121. Spiegel D: Dissociative Disorders: A Clinical Review. Lutherville, Md, Sidran Press, 1996, pp 1156–1172 [G]
122. Paris J, Zelkowitz P, Guzder J, Joseph S, Feldman R: Neuropsychological factors associated with borderline pathology in children. J Am Acad Child Adolesc Psychiatry 1999; 38:770–774 [D]
123. Zanarini MC, Williams AA, Lewis RE, Reich RB, Vera SC, Marino MF, Levin A, Yong L, Frankenburg FR: Reported pathological childhood experiences associated with the development of borderline personality disorder. Am J Psychiatry 1997; 154:1101–1106 [D]
124. Paris J: The etiology of borderline personality disorder: a biopsychosocial approach. Psychiatry 1994; 57:316–325 [F]
125. Altshuler LL, Cohen L, Szuba MP, Burt VK, Gitlin M, Mintz J: Pharmacologic management of psychiatric illness during pregnancy: dilemmas and guidelines. Am J Psychiatry 1996; 153:592–606 [F]
126. Cohen LS, Heller VL, Rosenbaum JF: Treatment guidelines for psychotropic drug use in pregnancy. Psychosomatics 1989; 30:25–33 [G]

127. Cohen L: Approach to the patient with psychiatric disorders during pregnancy, in The MGH Guide to Psychiatry and Primary Care. New York, McGraw-Hill, 1998, pp 311–317 [F]
128. Omtzigt JG, Los FJ, Grobbee DE, Pijpers L, Jahoda MG, Brandenburg H, Stewart PA, Gaillard HL, Sachs ES, Wladimiroff JW: The risk of spina bifida aperta after first-trimester exposure to valproate in a prenatal cohort. Neurology 1992; 42:119–125 [G]
129. Loranger AW, Sartorius N, Andreoli A, Berger P, Buchheim P, Channabasavanna SM, Coid B, Dahl A, Diekstra RFW, Ferguson B, Jacobsberg LB, Mombour W, Pull C, Ono Y, Regier DA: The International Personality Disorder Examination: the World Health Organization/Alcohol, Drug Abuse, and Mental Health Administration International Pilot Study of Personality Disorders. Arch Gen Psychiatry 1994; 51:215–224 [B]
130. Kissling W (ed): Guidelines for Neuroleptic Relapse Prevention in Schizophrenia. Berlin, Springer-Verlag, 1991 [G]
131. Marcos LR, Cancro R: Pharmacotherapy of Hispanic depressed patients: clinical observations. Am J Psychother 1982; 36:505–512 [F]
132. Escobar JI, Tuason VB: Antidepressant agents: a cross-cultural study. Psychopharmacol Bull 1980; 16:49–52 [F]
133. Klein JI, Macbeth JE, Onek JN: Legal Issues in the Private Practice of Psychiatry. Washington, DC, American Psychiatric Press, 1994 [G]
134. Paris J, Brown R, Nowlis D: Long-term follow-up of borderline patients in a general hospital. Compr Psychiatry 1987; 28:530–535 [D]
135. Bender DS, Dolan RT, Skodol AE, Sanislow CA, Dyck IR, McGlashan TH, Shea MT, Zanarini MC, Oldham JM, Gunderson JG: Treatment utilization by patients with personality disorders. Am J Psychiatry 2001; 158:295–302 [C]
136. Phillips KA, Gunderson JG: Personality disorders, in The American Psychiatric Press Textbook of Psychiatry, 3rd ed. Edited by Hales RE, Yudofsky SC, Talbott JA. Washington, DC, American Psychiatric Press, 1999, pp 795–823 [G]
137. Stone MH: Long-Term Follow-Up Study of Borderline Patients: The Fate of Borderlines. New York, Guilford, 1990 [C]
138. Stevenson J, Meares R: Psychotherapy with borderline patients, II: a preliminary cost benefit study. Aust N Z J Psychiatry 1999; 33:473–477 [B]
139. Gabbard GO: Psychodynamic Psychiatry in Clinical Practice, 3rd ed. Washington, DC, American Psychiatric Press, 2000 [G]
140. Clarkin JF, Yeomans F, Kernberg OF: Psychodynamic Psychotherapy of Borderline Personality Organization: A Treatment Manual. New York, John Wiley & Sons, 1998 [G]
141. Wallerstein RW: Forty-Two Lives in Treatment. New York, Guilford, 1986 [D]
142. Howard KI, Kopta SM, Krause MS, Orlinsky DE: The dose-effect relationship in psychotherapy. Am Psychol 1986; 41:159–164 [D]
143. Gabbard GO: Borderline Personality Disorder and Rational Managed Care Policy. Psychoanal Inquiry Suppl 1997, pp 17–28 [G]
144. Beck JS: Complex cognitive therapy treatment for personality disorder patients. Bull Menninger Clin 1998; 62:170–194 [G]
145. Layden MA, Newman CF, Freeman A, Morse SB: Cognitive Therapy of Borderline Personality Disorder. Boston, Allyn & Bacon, 1993 [G]
146. Millon T: On the genesis and prevalence of the borderline personality disorder: a social learning thesis. J Personal Disord 1987; 1:354–372 [G]
147. Young JE: Cognitive Therapy for Personality Disorders: A Schema-Focused Approach. Sarasota, Fla, Professional Resource Exchange, 1990 [G]
148. Linehan MM, Tutek DA, Heard HL, Armstrong HE: Interpersonal outcome of cognitive behavioral treatment for chronically suicidal borderline patients. Am J Psychiatry 1994; 151:1771–1776 [B]

149. Linehan MM, Schmidt H III, Dimeff LA, Craft JC, Kanter J, Comtois KA: Dialectical behavior therapy for patients with borderline personality disorder and drug-dependence. Am J Addict 1999; 8:279–292 [A]
150. Linehan MM, Heard HL: Impact of treatment accessibility on clinical course of parasuicidal patients (letter). Arch Gen Psychiatry 1993; 50:157–158 [G]
151. Springer T, Lohr NE, Buchtel HA, Silk KR: A preliminary report of short-term cognitive-behavioral group therapy for inpatients with personality disorders. J Psychother Pract Res 1995; 5:57–71 [A]
152. Barley W, Buie SE, Peterson EW, Hollingsworth A, Griva M, Hickerson S, Lawson J, Bailey B: Development of an inpatient cognitive-behavioral treatment program for borderline personality disorder. J Personal Disord 1993; 7:232–240 [B]
153. Perris C: Cognitive therapy in the treatment of patients with borderline personality disorders. Acta Psychiatr Scand Suppl 1994; 379:69–72 [F]
154. Liberman RP, Eckman T: Behavior therapy vs insight-oriented therapy for repeated suicide attempters. Arch Gen Psychiatry 1981; 38:1126–1130 [A]
155. Salkovskis PM, Atha C, Storer D: Cognitive-behavioural problem solving in the treatment of patients who repeatedly attempt suicide: a controlled trial. Br J Psychiatry 1990; 157: 871–876 [A]
156. Evans K, Tyrer P, Catalan J, Schmidt U, Davidson K, Dent J, Tata P, Thornton S, Barber J, Thompson S: Manual-assisted cognitive-behaviour therapy (MACT): a randomized controlled trial of a brief intervention with bibliotherapy in the treatment of recurrent deliberate self-harm. Psychol Med 1999; 29:19–25 [A]
157. Greene LR, Cole MB: Level and form of psychopathology and the structure of group therapy. Int J Group Psychother 1991; 41:499–521 [B]
158. Hafner RJ, Holme G: The influence of a therapeutic community on psychiatric disorder. J Clin Psychol 1996; 52:461–468 [C]
159. Goodwin JM, Wilson N, Connell V: Natural history of severe symptoms in borderline women treated in an incest group. Dissociation 1994; 5:221–226 [D]
160. Marziali E, Munroe-Blum H, McCleary L: The contribution of group cohesion and group alliance to the outcome of group psychotherapy. Int J Group Psychother 1997; 47:475–497 [A]
161. Wilberg T, Friis S, Karterud S, Mehlum L, Urnes O, Vaglum P: Outpatient group psychotherapy: a valuable continuation treatment for patients with borderline personality disorder treated in a day hospital? a 3-year follow-up study. Nord Psykiatr Tidsskr 1998; 52:213–222 [B]
162. Higgitt A, Fonagy P: Psychotherapy in borderline and narcissistic personality disorder. Br J Psychiatry 1992; 161:23–43 [F]
163. Marziali E, Monroe-Blum H: Interpersonal Group Psychotherapy for Borderline Personality Disorder. New York, Basic Books, 1994 [A]
164. Koch A, Ingram T: The treatment of borderline personality disorder within a distressed relationship. J Marital Fam Ther 1985; 11:373–380 [G]
165. Weddige R: The hidden psychotherapeutic dilemma: spouse of the borderline. Am J Psychother 1986; 40:52–61 [G]
166. McCormack C: The borderline/schizoid marriage: the holding environment as an essential treatment construct. J Marital Fam Ther 1989; 15:299–309 [G]
167. Jones SA: Family therapy with borderline and narcissistic patients. Bull Menninger Clin 1987; 51:285–295 [G]
168. Clarkin JF, Marziali E, Munroe-Blum H: Group and family treatments for borderline personality disorder. Hosp Community Psychiatry 1991; 42:1038–1043 [F]
169. Villeneuve C, Roux N: Family therapy and some personality disorders in adolescence. Adolesc Psychiatry 1995; 20:365–380 [G]

170. Gunderson JG, Berkowitz C, Ruiz-Sancho A: Families of borderline patients: a psychoeducational approach. Bull Menninger Clin 1997; 61:446–457 [G]
171. Gunderson JG, Kerr J, Englund DW: The families of borderlines: a comparative study. Arch Gen Psychiatry 1980; 37:27–33 [D]
172. Markovitz P, Wagner S: Venlafaxine in the treatment of borderline personality disorder. Psychopharmacol Bull 1995; 31:773–777 [B]
173. Coccaro EF, Astill JL, Herbert JL, Schut AG: Fluoxetine treatment of impulsive aggression in DSM-III-R personality disorder patients (letter). J Clin Psychopharmacol 1990; 10:373–375 [G]
174. Jensen HV, Andersen J: An open, noncomparative study of amoxapine in borderline disorders. Acta Psychiatr Scand 1989; 79:89–93 [B]
175. Montgomery SA, Roy D, Montgomery DB: The prevention of recurrent suicidal acts. Br J Clin Pharmacol 1983; 15(suppl 2):183S–188S [A]
176. Pande AC, Birkett M, Fechner-Bates S, Haskett RF, Greden JF: Fluoxetine versus phenelzine in atypical depression. Biol Psychiatry 1996; 40:1017–1020 [A]
177. Soloff PH, George A, Nathan RS, Schulz PM, Perel JM: Behavioral dyscontrol in borderline patients treated with amitriptyline. Psychopharmacol Bull 1987; 23:177–181 [A]
178. Shader RI, DiMascio A: Psychotropic Drug Side Effects. Baltimore, Williams & Wilkins, 1970 [G]
179. Rifkin A, Levitan SJ, Galewski J, Klein DF: Emotionally unstable character disorder—a follow-up study, I: description of patients and outcome. Biol Psychiatry 1972; 4:65–79 [C]
180. Rifkin A, Levitan SJ, Galewski J, Klein DF: Emotionally unstable character disorder—a follow-up study, II: prediction of outcome. Biol Psychiatry 1972; 4:81–88 [C]
181. Shader RI, Jackson AH, Dodes LM: The antiaggressive effects of lithium in man. Psychopharmacologia 1974; 40:17–24 [G]
182. LaWall JS, Wesselius CL: The use of lithium carbonate in borderline patients. J Psychiatr Treatment and Evaluation 1982; 4:265–267 [G]
183. Pinto OC, Akiskal HS: Lamotrigine as a promising approach to borderline personality: an open case series without concurrent DSM-IV major mood disorder. J Affect Disord 1998; 51:333–343 [B]
184. Wolf M, Grayden T, Carreon D, Cosgro M, Summers D, Leino R, Goldstein J, Kim S: Psychotherapy and buspirone in borderline patients, in 1990 Annual Meeting New Research Program and Abstracts. Washington, DC, American Psychiatric Association, 1990, p 244 [B]
185. Winchel RM, Stanley M: Self-injurious behavior: a review of the behavior and biology of self-mutilation. Am J Psychiatry 1991; 148:306–317 [F]
186. van der Kolk BA, Greenberg MS, Orr SP, Pitman RK: Endogenous opioids, stress induced analgesia, and posttraumatic stress disorder. Psychopharmacol Bull 1989; 25:417–421 [F]
187. Konicki PE, Schulz SC: Rationale for clinical trials of opiate antagonists in treating patients with personality disorders and self-injurious behavior. Psychopharmacol Bull 1989; 25:556–563 [E]
188. McGee M: Cessation of self-mutilation in a patient with borderline personality disorder treated with naltrexone. J Clin Psychiatry 1997; 58:32–33 [E]
189. Sonne S, Rubey R, Brady K, Malcolm R, Morris T: Naltrexone treatment of self-injurious thoughts and behaviors. J Nerv Ment Dis 1996; 184:192–195 [B]
190. Roth AS, Ostroff RB, Hoffman RE: Naltrexone as a treatment for repetitive self-injurious behaviour: an open-label trial. J Clin Psychiatry 1996; 57:233–237 [B]
191. Russ M, Roth SD, Kakuma T, Harrison K, Hull JW: Pain perception in self-injurious borderline patients: naloxone effects. Biol Psychiatry 1994; 35:207–209 [B]
192. Black DW, Bell S, Hulbert J, Nasrallah A: The importance of axis II in patients with major depression: a controlled study. J Affect Disord 1988; 14:115–122 [D]

193. Black DW, Goldstein RB, Nasrallah A, Winokur G: The prediction of recovery using a multivariate model in 1471 depressed inpatients. Eur Arch Psychiatry Clin Neurosci 1991; 241:41–45 [E]
194. Zimmerman M, Coryell W, Pfohl B, Corenthal C, Stangl D: ECT response in depressed patients with and without a DSM-III personality disorder. Am J Psychiatry 1986; 143: 1030–1032 [B]
195. Pfohl B, Stangl D, Zimmerman M: The implications of DSM-III personality disorders for patients with major depression. J Affect Disord 1984; 7:309–318 [B]
196. Casey P, Butler E: The effects of personality on response to ECT in major depression. J Personal Disord 1995; 9:134–142 [B]
197. Casey P, Meagher D, Butler E: Personality, functioning, and recovery from major depression. J Nerv Ment Dis 1996; 184:240–245 [B]
198. Blais MA, Matthews J, Schouten R, O'Keefe SM, Summergrad P: Stability and predictive value of self-report personality traits pre- and post-electroconvulsive therapy: a preliminary study. Compr Psychiatry 1998; 39:231–235 [B]

PRACTICE GUIDELINE FOR THE Assessment and Treatment of Patients With Suicidal Behaviors

WORK GROUP ON SUICIDAL BEHAVIORS

Douglas G. Jacobs, M.D., Chair

Ross J. Baldessarini, M.D.
Yeates Conwell, M.D.
Jan A. Fawcett, M.D.
Leslie Horton, M.D., Ph.D.
Herbert Meltzer, M.D.
Cynthia R. Pfeffer, M.D.
Robert I. Simon, M.D.

Originally published in November 2003. A guideline watch, summarizing significant developments in the scientific literature since publication of this guideline, may be available in the Psychiatric Practice section of the APA web site at www.psych.org.

CONTENTS

Guide to Using This Practice Guideline 1319

Development Process 1320

Part A: Assessment, Treatment, and Risk Management Recommendations 1321

I. Executive Summary of Recommendations 1321
   A. Definitions and General Principles 1321
   B. Suicide Assessment 1322
   C. Estimation of Suicide Risk 1324
   D. Psychiatric Management 1324
   E. Specific Treatment Modalities 1326

II. Assessment of Patients With Suicidal Behaviors 1328
   A. Overview 1328
   B. Conduct a Thorough Psychiatric Evaluation 1329
   C. Specifically Inquire About Suicidal Thoughts, Plans, and Behaviors 1331
   D. Establish a Multiaxial Diagnosis 1335
   E. Estimate Suicide Risk 1336
   F. Additional Considerations When Evaluating Patients in Specific Treatment Settings 1359

III. Psychiatric Management 1362
   A. Establish and Maintain a Therapeutic Alliance 1362
   B. Attend to the Patient's Safety 1363
   C. Determine a Treatment Setting 1364
   D. Develop a Plan of Treatment 1367
   E. Coordinate Care and Collaborate With Other Clinicians 1368
   F. Promote Adherence to the Treatment Plan 1369
   G. Provide Education to the Patient and Family 1369
   H. Reassess Safety and Suicide Risk 1370
   I. Monitor Psychiatric Status and Response to Treatment 1373
   J. Obtain Consultation, if Indicated 1373

IV. Specific Treatment Modalities 1373
   A. Somatic Therapies 1373
   B. Psychotherapies 1377

V. Documentation and Risk Management 1378
   A. General Risk Management and Documentation Issues Specific to Suicide 1378
   B. Suicide Contracts: Usefulness and Limitations 1379
   C. Communication With Significant Others 1380

D. Management of Suicide in One's Practice ... 1381
E. Mental Health Interventions for Surviving Family and Friends After a Suicide ... 1382

Part B: Background Information and Review of Available Evidence ... 1383

VI. Review and Synthesis of Available Evidence ... 1383
A. Factors Altering Risk of Suicide and Attempted Suicide ... 1383
B. Psychiatric Assessment Techniques ... 1437
C. Special Issues ... 1440
D. Somatic Therapies ... 1442
E. Psychotherapies ... 1451

Part C: Future Research Needs ... 1454

Individuals and Organizations That Submitted Comments ... 1456

References ... 1457

GUIDE TO USING THIS PRACTICE GUIDELINE

Practice Guideline for the Assessment and Treatment of Patients With Suicidal Behaviors consists of three parts (Parts A, B, and C) and many sections, not all of which will be equally useful for all readers. The following guide is designed to help readers find the sections that will be most useful to them.

Part A, "Assessment, Treatment, and Risk Management Recommendations," is published as a supplement to the *American Journal of Psychiatry* and contains the general and specific recommendations for the assessment and treatment of patients with suicidal behaviors. Section I summarizes the key recommendations of the guideline and codes each recommendation according to the degree of clinical confidence with which the recommendation is made. Section II discusses the assessment of the patient, including a consideration of factors influencing suicide risk. Section III discusses psychiatric management, Section IV discusses specific treatment modalities, and Section V addresses documentation and risk management issues.

Part B, "Background Information and Review of Available Evidence," and Part C, "Future Research Needs," are not included in the *American Journal of Psychiatry* supplement but are provided with Part A in the complete guideline, which is available in print format from American Psychiatric Publishing, Inc., and online through the American Psychiatric Association (http://www.psych.org). Part B provides an overview of suicide, including general information on its natural history, course, and epidemiology. It also provides a structured review and synthesis of the evidence that underlies the recommendations made in Part A. Part C draws from the previous sections and summarizes areas for which more research data are needed to guide clinical decisions.

To share feedback on this or other published APA practice guidelines, a form is available at http://www.psych.org/psych_pract/pg/reviewform.cfm.

DEVELOPMENT PROCESS

This practice guideline was developed under the auspices of the Steering Committee on Practice Guidelines. The development process is detailed in the document "APA Guideline Development Process," which is available from the APA Department of Quality Improvement and Psychiatric Services. Key features of this process include the following:

- A comprehensive literature review
- Development of evidence tables
- Initial drafting of the guideline by a work group that included psychiatrists with clinical and research expertise in suicide and suicidality
- Production of multiple revised drafts with widespread review; six organizations and more than 60 individuals submitted significant comments
- Approval by the APA Assembly and Board of Trustees
- Planned revisions at regular intervals

Relevant literature was identified through a computerized search of PubMed for the period from 1966 to 2002. Keywords used were "suicides," "suicide," "attempted suicide," "attempted suicides," "parasuicide," "parasuicides," "self-harm," "self-harming," "suicide, attempted," "suicidal attempt," and "suicidal attempts." A total of 34,851 citations were found. After limiting these references to literature published in English that included abstracts, 17,589 articles were screened by using title and abstract information. Additional, less formal literature searches were conducted by APA staff and individual members of the work group on suicidal behaviors through the use of PubMed, PsycINFO, and Social Sciences Citation Index. Sources of funding were not considered when reviewing the literature.

This document represents a synthesis of current scientific knowledge and rational clinical practice on the assessment and treatment of adult patients with suicidal behaviors. It strives to be as free as possible of bias toward any theoretical approach to treatment. In order for the reader to appreciate the evidence base behind the guideline recommendations and the weight that should be given to each recommendation, the summary of treatment recommendations is keyed according to the level of confidence with which each recommendation is made. Each rating of clinical confidence considers the strength of the available evidence and is based on the best available data. When evidence is limited, the level of confidence also incorporates clinical consensus with regard to a particular clinical decision. In the listing of cited references, each reference is followed by a letter code in brackets that indicates the nature of the supporting evidence.

PART A: ASSESSMENT, TREATMENT, AND RISK MANAGEMENT RECOMMENDATIONS

I. EXECUTIVE SUMMARY OF RECOMMENDATIONS

A. DEFINITIONS AND GENERAL PRINCIPLES

1. Coding system

Each recommendation is identified as falling into one of three categories of endorsement, indicated by a bracketed Roman numeral following the statement. The three categories represent varying levels of clinical confidence regarding the recommendation:

[I] Recommended with substantial clinical confidence.
[II] Recommended with moderate clinical confidence.
[III] May be recommended on the basis of individual circumstances.

2. Definitions of terms

In this guideline, the following terms will be used:

- Suicide—self-inflicted death with evidence (either explicit or implicit) that the person intended to die.
- Suicide attempt—self-injurious behavior with a nonfatal outcome accompanied by evidence (either explicit or implicit) that the person intended to die.
- Aborted suicide attempt—potentially self-injurious behavior with evidence (either explicit or implicit) that the person intended to die but stopped the attempt before physical damage occurred.
- Suicidal ideation—thoughts of serving as the agent of one's own death. Suicidal ideation may vary in seriousness depending on the specificity of suicide plans and the degree of suicidal intent.
- Suicidal intent—subjective expectation and desire for a self-destructive act to end in death.
- Lethality of suicidal behavior—objective danger to life associated with a suicide method or action. Note that lethality is distinct from and may not always coincide with an individual's expectation of what is medically dangerous.
- Deliberate self-harm—willful self-inflicting of painful, destructive, or injurious acts without intent to die.

A detailed exposition of definitions relating to suicide has been provided by O'Carroll et al. (1).

B. SUICIDE ASSESSMENT

The psychiatric evaluation is the essential element of the suicide assessment process [I]. During the evaluation, the psychiatrist obtains information about the patient's psychiatric and other medical history and current mental state (e.g., through direct questioning and observation about suicidal thinking and behavior as well as through collateral history, if indicated). This information enables the psychiatrist to 1) identify specific factors and features that may generally increase or decrease risk for suicide or other suicidal behaviors and that may serve as modifiable targets for both acute and ongoing interventions, 2) address the patient's immediate safety and determine the most appropriate setting for treatment, and 3) develop a multiaxial differential diagnosis to further guide planning of treatment. The breadth and depth of the psychiatric evaluation aimed specifically at assessing suicide risk will vary with setting; ability or willingness of the patient to provide information; and availability of information from previous contacts with the patient or from other sources, including other mental health professionals, medical records, and family members. Although suicide assessment scales have been developed for research purposes, they lack the predictive validity necessary for use in routine clinical practice. Therefore, suicide assessment scales may be used as aids to suicide assessment but should not be used as predictive instruments or as substitutes for a thorough clinical evaluation [I].

Table 1 presents important domains of a suicide assessment, including the patient's current presentation, individual strengths and weaknesses, history, and psychosocial situation. Information may come from the patient directly or from other sources, including family members, friends, and others in the patient's support network, such as community residence staff or members of the patient's military command. Such individuals may be able to provide information about the patient's current mental state, activities, and psychosocial crises and may also have observed behavior or been privy to communications from the patient that suggest suicidal ideation, plans, or intentions. Contact with such individuals may also provide opportunity for the psychiatrist to attempt to fortify the patient's social support network. This goal often can be accomplished without the psychiatrist's revealing private or confidential information about the patient. In clinical circumstances in which sharing information is important to maintain the safety of the patient or others, it is permissible and even critical to share such information without the patient's consent [I].

It is important to recognize that in many clinical situations not all of the information described in this section may be possible to obtain. It may be necessary to focus initially on those elements judged to be most relevant and to continue the evaluation during subsequent contacts with the patient.

When communicating with the patient, it is important to remember that simply asking about suicidal ideation does not ensure that accurate or complete information will be received. Cultural or religious beliefs about death or suicide, for example, may influence a patient's willingness to speak about suicide during the assessment process as well as the patient's likelihood of acting on suicidal ideas. Consequently, the psychiatrist may wish to explore the patient's cultural and religious beliefs, particularly as they relate to death and to suicide [II].

It is important for the psychiatrist to focus on the nature, frequency, depth, timing, and persistence of suicidal ideation [I]. If ideation is present, request more detail about the presence or absence of specific plans for suicide, including any steps taken to enact plans or prepare for death [I]. If other aspects of the clinical presentation seem inconsistent with an initial denial of suicidal thoughts, additional questioning of the patient may be indicated [II].

Where there is a history of suicide attempts, aborted attempts, or other self-harming behavior, it is important to obtain as much detail as possible about the timing, intent, method, and consequences of such behaviors [I]. It is also useful to determine the life context in which they occurred and whether they occurred in association with intoxication or chronic use of alcohol or other substances [II]. For individuals in previous or current psychiatric treatment, it is helpful to determine the strength and stability of the therapeutic relationship(s) [II].

TABLE 1. Characteristics Evaluated in the Psychiatric Assessment of Patients With Suicidal Behavior

Current presentation of suicidality
Suicidal or self-harming thoughts, plans, behaviors, and intent
Specific methods considered for suicide, including their lethality and the patient's expectation about lethality, as well as whether firearms are accessible
Evidence of hopelessness, impulsiveness, anhedonia, panic attacks, or anxiety
Reasons for living and plans for the future
Alcohol or other substance use associated with the current presentation
Thoughts, plans, or intentions of violence toward others
Psychiatric illnesses
Current signs and symptoms of psychiatric disorders with particular attention to mood disorders (primarily major depressive disorder or mixed episodes), schizophrenia, substance use disorders, anxiety disorders, and personality disorders (primarily borderline and antisocial personality disorders)
Previous psychiatric diagnoses and treatments, including illness onset and course and psychiatric hospitalizations, as well as treatment for substance use disorders
History
Previous suicide attempts, aborted suicide attempts, or other self-harming behaviors
Previous or current medical diagnoses and treatments, including surgeries or hospitalizations
Family history of suicide or suicide attempts or a family history of mental illness, including substance abuse
Psychosocial situation
Acute psychosocial crises and chronic psychosocial stressors, which may include actual or perceived interpersonal losses, financial difficulties or changes in socioeconomic status, family discord, domestic violence, and past or current sexual or physical abuse or neglect
Employment status, living situation (including whether or not there are infants or children in the home), and presence or absence of external supports
Family constellation and quality of family relationships
Cultural or religious beliefs about death or suicide
Individual strengths and vulnerabilities
Coping skills
Personality traits
Past responses to stress
Capacity for reality testing
Ability to tolerate psychological pain and satisfy psychological needs

If the patient reports a specific method for suicide, it is important for the psychiatrist to ascertain the patient's expectation about its lethality, for if actual lethality exceeds what is expected, the patient's risk for accidental suicide may be high even if intent is low [I]. In general, the psychiatrist should assign a higher level of risk to patients who have high degrees of suicidal intent or describe more detailed and specific suicide plans, particularly those involving violent and irreversible methods [I]. If the patient has access to a firearm, the psychiatrist is advised to discuss with and recommend to the patient or a significant other the importance of restricting access to, securing, or removing this and other weapons [I].

Documenting the suicide assessment is essential [I]. Typically, suicide assessment and its documentation occur after an initial evaluation or, for patients in ongoing treatment, when suicidal ideation or behaviors emerge or when there is significant worsening or dramatic and unanticipated improvement in the patient's condition. For inpatients, reevaluation also typically occurs with changes in the level of precautions or observations, when passes are issued, and during evaluation for discharge. As with the level of detail of the suicide assessment, the extent of documentation at each of these times varies with the clinical circumstances. Communications with other caregivers and with the family or significant others should also be documented [I]. When the patient or others have been given specific instructions about firearms or other weapons, this communication should also be noted in the record [I].

C. ESTIMATION OF SUICIDE RISK

Suicide and suicidal behaviors cause severe personal, social, and economic consequences. Despite the severity of these consequences, suicide and suicidal behaviors are statistically rare, even in populations at risk. For example, although suicidal ideation and attempts are associated with increased suicide risk, most individuals with suicidal thoughts or attempts will never die by suicide. It is estimated that attempts and ideation occur in approximately 0.7% and 5.6% of the general U.S. population per year, respectively (2). In comparison, in the United States, the annual incidence of suicide in the general population is approximately 10.7 suicides for every 100,000 persons, or 0.0107% of the total population per year (3). This rarity of suicide, even in groups known to be at higher risk than the general population, contributes to the impossibility of predicting suicide.

The statistical rarity of suicide also makes it impossible to predict on the basis of risk factors either alone or in combination. For the psychiatrist, knowing that a particular factor (e.g., major depressive disorder, hopelessness, substance use) increases a patient's relative risk for suicide may affect the treatment plan, including determination of a treatment setting. At the same time, knowledge of risk factors will not permit the psychiatrist to predict when or if a specific patient will die by suicide. This does not mean that the psychiatrist should ignore risk factors or view suicidal patients as untreatable. On the contrary, an initial goal of the psychiatrist should be to estimate the patient's risk through knowledgeable assessment of risk and protective factors, with a primary and ongoing goal of reducing suicide risk [I].

Some factors may increase or decrease risk for suicide; others may be more relevant to risk for suicide attempts or other self-injurious behaviors, which are in turn associated with potential morbidity as well as increased suicide risk. In weighing risk and protective factors for an individual patient, consideration may be given to 1) the presence of psychiatric illness; 2) specific psychiatric symptoms such as hopelessness, anxiety, agitation, or intense suicidal ideation; 3) unique circumstances such as psychosocial stressors and availability of methods; and 4) other relevant clinical factors such as genetics and medical, psychological, or psychodynamic issues [I].

It is important to recognize that many of these factors are not simply present or absent but instead may vary in severity. Others, such as psychological or psychodynamic issues, may contribute to risk in some individuals but not in others or may be relevant only when they occur in combination with particular psychosocial stressors.

Once factors are identified, the psychiatrist can determine if they are modifiable. Past history, family history, and demographic characteristics are examples of nonmodifiable factors. Financial difficulties or unemployment can also be difficult to modify, at least in the short term. While immutable factors are important to identify, they cannot be the focus of intervention. Rather, to decrease a patient's suicide risk, the treatment should attempt to mitigate or strengthen those risk and protective factors that can be modified [I]. For example, the psychiatrist may attend to patient safety, address associated psychological or social problems and stressors, augment social support networks, and treat associated psychiatric disorders (such as mood disorders, psychotic disorders, substance use disorders, and personality disorders) or symptoms (such as severe anxiety, agitation, or insomnia).

D. PSYCHIATRIC MANAGEMENT

Psychiatric management consists of a broad array of therapeutic interventions that should be instituted for patients with suicidal thoughts, plans, or behaviors [I]. Psychiatric management includes determining a setting for treatment and supervision, attending to patient safety, and working to establish a cooperative and collaborative physician-patient relationship. For patients in ongoing treatment, psychiatric management also includes establishing and maintaining a therapeutic alliance; coordinating treatment provided by multiple clinicians; monitoring the patient's progress and response to the treatment plan; and conducting ongoing assessments of the patient's safety, psychiatric status, and level of functioning. Additionally, psychiatric management may include encouraging treatment adherence and providing education to the patient and, when indicated, family members and significant others.

Patients with suicidal thoughts, plans, or behaviors should generally be treated in the setting that is least restrictive yet most likely to be safe and effective [I]. Treatment settings and conditions include a continuum of possible levels of care, from involuntary inpatient hospitalization through partial hospital and intensive outpatient programs to occasional ambulatory visits. Choice of specific treatment setting depends not only on the psychiatrist's estimate of the patient's current suicide risk and potential for dangerousness to others, but also on other aspects of the patient's current status, including 1) medical and psychiatric comorbidity; 2) strength and availability of a psychosocial support network; and 3) ability to provide adequate self-care, give reliable feedback to the psychiatrist, and cooperate with treatment. In addition, the benefits of intensive interventions such as hospitalization must be weighed against their possible negative effects (e.g., disruption of employment, financial and other psychosocial stress, social stigma).

For some individuals, self-injurious behaviors may occur on a recurring or even chronic basis. Although such behaviors may occur without evidence of suicidal intent, this may not always be the case. Even when individuals have had repeated contacts with the health care system, each act should be reassessed in the context of the current situation [I].

In treating suicidal patients, particularly those with severe or recurring suicidality or self-injurious behavior, the psychiatrist should be aware of his or her own emotions and reactions that may interfere with the patient's care [I]. For difficult-to-treat patients, consultation or supervision from a colleague may help in affirming the appropriateness of the treatment plan, suggesting alternative therapeutic approaches, or monitoring and dealing with countertransference issues [I].

The suicide prevention contract, or "no-harm contract," is commonly used in clinical practice but should not be considered as a substitute for a careful clinical assessment [I]. A patient's willingness (or reluctance) to enter into an oral or a written suicide prevention contract should not be viewed as an absolute indicator of suitability for discharge (or hospitalization) [I]. In addition, such contracts are not recommended for use with patients who are agitated, psychotic, impulsive, or under the influence of an intoxicating substance [II]. Furthermore, since suicide prevention contracts are dependent on an established physician-patient relationship, they are not recommended for use in emergency settings or with newly admitted or unknown inpatients [II].

Despite best efforts at suicide assessment and treatment, suicides can and do occur in clinical practice. In fact, significant proportions of individuals who die by suicide have seen a physician within several months of death and may have received specific mental health treatment. Death of a patient by suicide will often have a significant effect on the treating psychiatrist and may result in increased stress and loss of professional self-esteem. When the suicide of a patient occurs, the psychiatrist may find it helpful to seek support from colleagues and obtain consultation or supervision to enable him or her to continue to treat other patients effectively and respond to the inquiries or mental health needs of survivors [II]. Consultation with an attorney or a risk manager may also be useful [II]. The psychiatrist should be aware that patient confidentiality extends beyond the patient's death and that the usual provisions relating to medical records still apply. Any additional documentation included in the medical record after the patient's death should be dated contemporaneously, not backdated, and previous entries should not be altered [I]. Depending on the circumstances, conversations with family members may be appropriate and can allay grief [II]. In the aftermath of a loved one's suicide, family members themselves are more vulnerable to physical and psychological disorders and should be helped to obtain psychiatric intervention, although not necessarily by the same psychiatrist who treated the individual who died by suicide [II].

E. SPECIFIC TREATMENT MODALITIES

In developing a plan of treatment that addresses suicidal thoughts or behaviors, the psychiatrist should consider the potential benefits of somatic therapies as well as the potential benefits of psychosocial interventions, including the psychotherapies [I]. Clinical experience indicates that many patients with suicidal thoughts, plans, or behaviors will benefit most from a combination of these treatments [II]. The psychiatrist should address the modifiable risk factors identified in the initial psychiatric evaluation and make ongoing assessments during the course of treatment [I]. In general, therapeutic approaches should target specific axis I and axis II psychiatric disorders; specific associated symptoms such as depression, agitation, anxiety, or insomnia; or the predominant psychodynamic or psychosocial stressor [I]. While the goal of pharmacologic treatment may be acute symptom relief, including acute relief of suicidality or acute treatment of a specific diagnosis, the treatment goals of psychosocial interventions may be broader and longer term, including achieving improvements in interpersonal relationships, coping skills, psychosocial functioning, and management of affects. Since treatment should be a collaborative process between the patient and clinician(s), the patient's preferences are important to consider when developing an individual treatment plan [I].

1. Somatic interventions

Evidence for a lowering of suicide rates with antidepressant treatment is inconclusive. However, the documented efficacy of antidepressants in treating acute depressive episodes and their long-term benefit in patients with recurrent forms of severe anxiety or depressive disorders support their use in individuals with these disorders who are experiencing suicidal thoughts or behaviors [II]. It is advisable to select an antidepressant with a low risk of lethality on acute overdose, such as a selective serotonin reuptake inhibitor (SSRI) or other newer antidepressant, and to prescribe conservative quantities, especially for patients who are not well-known [I]. For patients with prominent insomnia, a sedating antidepressant or an adjunctive hypnotic agent can be considered [II]. Since antidepressant effects may not be observed for days to weeks after treatment has started, patients should be monitored closely early in treatment and educated about this probable delay in symptom relief [I].

To treat symptoms such as severe insomnia, agitation, panic attacks, or psychic anxiety, benzodiazepines may be indicated on a short-term basis [II], with long-acting agents often being preferred over short-acting agents [II]. The benefits of benzodiazepine treatment should be weighed against their occasional tendency to produce disinhibition and their potential for interactions with other sedatives, including alcohol [I]. Alternatively, other medications that may be used for their calming effects in highly anxious and agitated patients include trazodone, low doses of some second-generation antipsychotics, and some anticonvulsants such as gabapentin or divalproex [III]. If benzodiazepines are being discontinued after prolonged use, their doses should be reduced gradually and the patient monitored for increasing symptoms of anxiety, agitation, depression, or suicidality [II].

There is strong evidence that long-term maintenance treatment with lithium salts is associated with major reductions in the risk of both suicide and suicide attempts in patients with bipolar disorder, and there is moderate evidence for similar risk reductions in patients with recurrent major depressive disorder [I]. Specific anticonvulsants have been shown to be efficacious in treating episodes of mania (i.e., divalproex) or bipolar depression (i.e., lamotrigine), but there is no clear evidence that their use alters rates of suicide or suicidal behaviors [II]. Consequently, when deciding between lithium and other first-line agents for treatment of patients with bipolar disorder, the efficacy of lithium in decreasing suicidal behavior should be taken into consideration when weighing the benefits and risks of treatment with each medication. In addition, if lithium is prescribed, the potential toxicity of lithium in overdose should be taken into consideration when deciding on the quantity of lithium to give with each prescription [I].

Clozapine treatment is associated with significant decreases in rates of suicide attempts and perhaps suicide for individuals with schizophrenia and schizoaffective disorder. Thus, clozapine treatment should be given serious consideration for psychotic patients with frequent suicidal ideation, attempts, or both [I]. However, the benefits of clozapine treatment need to be weighed against the risk of adverse effects, including potentially fatal agranulocytosis and myocarditis, which has generally led clozapine to be reserved for use when psychotic symptoms have not responded to other antipsychotic medications. If treatment is indicated with an antipsychotic other than clozapine, the other second-generation antipsychotics (e.g., risperidone, olanzapine, quetiapine, ziprasidone, aripiprazole) are preferred over the first-generation antipsychotic agents [I].

ECT has established efficacy in patients with severe depressive illness, with or without psychotic features. Since ECT is associated with a rapid and robust antidepressant response as well as a rapid diminution in associated suicidal thoughts, ECT may be recommended as a treatment for severe episodes of major depression that are accompanied by suicidal thoughts or behaviors [I]. Under certain clinical circumstances, ECT may also be used to treat suicidal patients with schizophrenia, schizoaffective disorder, or mixed or manic episodes of bipolar disorder [II]. Regardless of diagnosis, ECT is especially indicated for patients with catatonic features or for whom a delay in treatment response is considered life threatening [I]. ECT may also be indicated for suicidal individuals during pregnancy and for those who have already failed to tolerate or respond to trials of medication [II]. Since there is no evidence of a long-term reduction of suicide risk with ECT, continuation or maintenance treatment with pharmacotherapy or with ECT is recommended after an acute ECT course [I].

2. Psychosocial interventions

Psychotherapies and other psychosocial interventions play an important role in the treatment of individuals with suicidal thoughts and behaviors [II]. A substantial body of evidence supports the efficacy of psychotherapy in the treatment of specific disorders, such as nonpsychotic major depressive disorder and borderline personality disorder, which are associated with increased suicide risk. For example, interpersonal psychotherapy and cognitive behavior therapy have been found to be effective in clinical trials for the treatment of depression. Therefore, psychotherapies such as interpersonal psychotherapy and cognitive behavior therapy may be considered appropriate treatments for suicidal behavior, particularly when it occurs in the context of depression [II]. In addition, cognitive behavior therapy may be used to decrease two important risk factors for suicide: hopelessness [II] and suicide attempts in depressed outpatients [III]. For patients with a diagnosis of borderline personality disorder, psychodynamic therapy and dialectical behavior therapy may be appropriate treatments for suicidal behaviors [II], because modest evidence has shown these therapies to be associated with decreased self-injurious behaviors, including suicide attempts. Although not targeted specifically to suicide or suicidal behaviors, other psychosocial treatments may also be helpful in reducing symptoms and improving functioning in individuals with psychotic disorders and in treating alcohol and other substance use disorders that are themselves associated with increased rates of suicide and suicidal behaviors [II]. For patients who have attempted suicide or engaged in self-harming behaviors without suicidal intent, specific psychosocial interventions such as rapid intervention; follow-up outreach; problem-solving therapy; brief psychological treatment; or family, couples, or group therapies may be useful despite limited evidence for their efficacy [III].

TABLE 2. Circumstances in Which a Suicide Assessment May Be Indicated Clinically

- Emergency department or crisis evaluation
- Intake evaluation (on either an inpatient or an outpatient basis)
- Before a change in observation status or treatment setting (e.g., discontinuation of one-to-one observation, discharge from inpatient setting)
- Abrupt change in clinical presentation (either precipitous worsening or sudden, dramatic improvement)
- Lack of improvement or gradual worsening despite treatment
- Anticipation or experience of a significant interpersonal loss or psychosocial stressor (e.g., divorce, financial loss, legal problems, personal shame or humiliation)
- Onset of a physical illness (particularly if life threatening, disfiguring, or associated with severe pain or loss of executive functioning)

II. ASSESSMENT OF PATIENTS WITH SUICIDAL BEHAVIORS

A. OVERVIEW

The assessment of the suicidal patient is an ongoing process that comprises many interconnected elements (Table 1). In addition, there are a number of points during patients' evaluation and treatment at which a suicide assessment may be indicated (Table 2).

The ability of the psychiatrist to connect with the patient, establish rapport, and demonstrate empathy is an important ingredient of the assessment process. For suicidal patients who are followed on an ongoing basis, the doctor-patient relationship will provide the base from which risk and protective factors continue to be identified and from which therapeutic interventions, such as psychotherapies and pharmacotherapies, are offered.

At the core of the suicide assessment, the psychiatric evaluation will provide information about the patient's history, current circumstances, and mental state and will include direct questioning about suicidal thinking and behaviors. This evaluation, in turn, will enable the psychiatrist to identify specific factors and features that may increase or decrease the potential risk for suicide or other suicidal behaviors. These factors and features may include developmental, biomedical, psychopathologic, psychodynamic, and psychosocial aspects of the patient's current presentation and history, all of which may serve as modifiable targets for both acute and ongoing interventions. Such information will also be important in addressing the patient's immediate safety, determining the most appropriate setting for treatment, and developing a multiaxial differential diagnosis that will further guide the planning of treatment.

Although the approach to the suicidal patient is common to all individuals regardless of diagnosis or clinical presentation, the breadth and depth of the psychiatric evaluation will vary with the setting of the assessment; the ability or willingness of the patient to provide information; and the availability of information from previous contacts with the patient or from other sources, including other mental health professionals, medical records, and family members. Since the approach to assessment does vary to some degree in the assessment of suicidal children and adolescents, the psychiatrist who evaluates youths may wish to review the American Academy of Child and Adolescent Psychiatry's *Practice Parameter for the Assessment and Treatment of Children and Adolescents With Suicidal Behavior* (4). In some circumstances, the urgency of the situation or the presence of substance intoxication may necessitate making a decision to facilitate patient safety (e.g., instituting hospitalization or one-to-one observation) before all relevant information has been obtained. Furthermore, when working with a team of other professionals, the psychiatrist may not obtain all information him- or herself but will need to provide leadership for the assessment process so that necessary information is obtained and integrated into a final assessment. Since the patient may minimize the severity or even the existence of his or her difficulties, other individuals may be valuable resources for the psychiatrist in providing information about the patient's current mental state, activities, and psychosocial crises. Such individuals may include the patient's family members and friends but may also include other physicians, other medical or mental health professionals, teachers or other school personnel, members of the patient's military command, and staff from supervised housing programs or other settings where the patient resides.

B. CONDUCT A THOROUGH PSYCHIATRIC EVALUATION

The psychiatric evaluation is the core element of the suicide risk assessment. This section provides an overview of the key aspects of the psychiatric evaluation as they relate to the assessment of patients with suicidal behaviors. Although the factors that are associated with an increased or decreased risk of suicide differ from the factors associated with an increased or decreased risk of suicide attempts, it is important to identify factors modulating the risk of any suicidal behaviors. Additional details on specific risk factors that should be identified during the assessment are discussed in Sections II.E, "Estimate Suicide Risk," and III.H, "Reassess Safety and Suicide Risk." For further discussion of other aspects of the psychiatric evaluation, the psychiatrist is referred to the American Psychiatric Association's *Practice Guideline for Psychiatric Evaluation of Adults* (5) (included in this volume). Additional information on details of the suicide assessment process is reviewed elsewhere (6, 7).

1. Identify specific psychiatric signs and symptoms

It is important to identify specific psychiatric signs and symptoms that are correlated with an increased risk of suicide or other suicidal behaviors. Symptoms that have been associated with suicide attempts or with suicide include aggression, violence toward others, impulsiveness, hopelessness, and agitation. Psychic anxiety, which has been defined as subjective feelings of anxiety, fearfulness, or apprehension whether or not focused on specific concerns, has also been associated with an increased risk of suicide, as have anhedonia, global insomnia, and panic attacks. In addition, identifying other psychiatric signs and symptoms (e.g., psychosis, depression) will aid in determining whether the patient has a psychiatric syndrome that should also be a focus of treatment.

2. Assess past suicidal behavior, including intent of self-injurious acts

A history of past suicide attempts is one of the most significant risk factors for suicide, and this risk may be increased by more serious, more frequent, or more recent attempts. Therefore, it is important for the psychiatrist to inquire about past suicide attempts and self-destructive behaviors, including specific questioning about aborted suicide attempts. Examples of the latter would include putting a gun to one's head but not firing it, driving to a bridge but not jumping, or creating a noose but not using it. For each attempt or aborted attempt, the psychiatrist should try to obtain details about the precipitants, timing, intent, and consequences as well as the attempt's medical severity. The patient's consumption of alcohol and drugs before the attempt should also be ascertained, since intoxication can facilitate impulsive suicide attempts but can also be a component of a more serious suicide plan. In understanding the issues that culminated in the suicide attempt, interpersonal aspects of the attempt should also be delineated. Examples might include the dynamic or interpersonal issues leading up to the attempt, significant persons present at the time of the attempt, persons to whom the attempt was communicated, and how the attempt was averted. It is also important to determine the patient's thoughts about the attempt, such as his or her own perception of the chosen method's lethality, ambivalence toward living, visualization of death, degree of premeditation, persistence of suicidal ideation, and reaction to the attempt. It is also helpful to inquire about past risk-taking behaviors such as unsafe sexual practices and reckless driving.

3. Review past treatment history and treatment relationships

A review of the patient's treatment history is another crucial element of the suicide risk assessment. A thorough treatment history can serve as a systematic method for gaining information on comorbid diagnoses, prior hospitalizations, suicidal ideation, or previous suicide attempts. Obtaining a history of medical treatment can help in identifying medically serious suicide attempts as well as in identifying past or current medical diagnoses that may be associated with augmented suicide risk.

Many patients who are being assessed for suicidality will already be in treatment, either with other psychiatrists or mental health professionals or with primary care physicians or medical specialists. Contacts with such caregivers can provide a great deal of relevant information and help in determining a setting and/or plan for treatment. With patients who are currently in treatment, it is also important to gauge the strength and stability of the therapeutic relationships, because a positive therapeutic alliance has been suggested to be protective against suicidal behaviors. On the other hand, a patient with a suicide attempt or suicidal ideation who does not have a reliable therapeutic alliance may represent an increased risk for suicide, which would need to be addressed accordingly.

4. Identify family history of suicide, mental illness, and dysfunction

Identifying family history is particularly important during the psychiatric evaluation. The psychiatrist should specifically inquire about the presence of suicide and suicide attempts as well as a family history of any psychiatric hospitalizations or mental illness, including substance use disorders. When suicides have occurred in first-degree relatives, it is often helpful to learn more about the circumstances, including the patient's involvement and the patient's and relative's ages at the time of the suicide.

The patient's childhood and current family milieu are also relevant, since many aspects of family dysfunction may be linked to self-destructive behaviors. Such factors include a history of family conflict or separation, parental legal trouble, family substance use, domestic violence, and physical and/or sexual abuse.

5. Identify current psychosocial situation and nature of crisis

An assessment of the patient's current psychosocial situation is important to detect acute psychosocial crises or chronic psychosocial stressors that may augment suicide risk (e.g., financial or legal difficulties; interpersonal conflicts or losses; stressors in gay, lesbian, or bisexual youths; housing problems; job loss; educational failure). Other significant precipitants may include perceived losses or recent or impending humiliation. An understanding of the patient's psychosocial situation is also essential in helping the patient to mobilize external supports, which can have a protective influence on suicide risk.

6. Appreciate psychological strengths and vulnerabilities of the individual patient

In estimating suicide risk and formulating a treatment plan, the clinician needs to appreciate the strengths and vulnerabilities of the individual patient. Particular strengths and vulnerabilities may include such factors as coping skills, personality traits, thinking style, and developmental and psychological needs. For example, in addition to serving as state-dependent symptoms, hopelessness, aggression, and impulsivity may also constitute traits, greater degrees of which may be associated with an increased risk for suicidal behaviors. Increased suicide risk has also been seen in individuals who exhibit thought constriction or polarized (either-or) thinking as well in individuals with closed-mindedness (i.e., a narrowed scope and intensity of interests). Perfectionism with excessively high self-expectation is another factor that has been noted in clinical practice to be a possible contributor to suicide risk. In weighing the strengths and vulnerabilities of the individual patient, it is also helpful to determine the patient's tendency to engage in risk-taking behaviors as well as the patient's past responses to stress, including the capacity for reality testing and the ability to tolerate rejection, subjective loneliness, or psychological pain when his or her unique psychological needs are not met.

C. SPECIFICALLY INQUIRE ABOUT SUICIDAL THOUGHTS, PLANS, AND BEHAVIORS

In general, the more an individual has thought about suicide, has made specific plans for suicide, and intends to act on those plans, the greater will be his or her risk. Thus, as part of the suicide assessment it is essential to inquire specifically about the patient's suicidal thoughts, plans, behaviors, and intent. Although such questions will often flow naturally from discussion of the patient's current situation, this will not invariably be true. The exact wording of questions and the extent of questioning will also differ with the clinical situation. Examples of issues that the psychiatrist may wish to address in this portion of the suicide assessment are given in Table 3.

1. Elicit the presence or absence of suicidal ideation

Inquiring about suicidal ideation is an essential component of the suicide assessment. Although some fear that raising the topic of suicide will "plant" the issue in the patient's mind, this is not the case. In fact, broaching the issue of suicidal ideation may be a relief for the suicidal patient by opening an avenue for discussion and giving him or her an opportunity to feel understood.

In asking about suicidal ideas, it is often helpful to begin with questions that address the patient's feelings about living, such as, "How does life seem to you at this point?" or "Have you ever felt that life was not worth living?" or "Did you ever wish you could go to sleep and just not wake up?" If the patient's response reflects dissatisfaction with life or a desire to escape it, this response can lead naturally into more specific questions about whether the patient has had thoughts of death or suicide. When such thoughts are elicited, it is important to focus on the nature, frequency, extent, and timing of them and to understand the interpersonal, situational, and symptomatic context in which they are occurring.

Even if the patient initially denies thoughts of death or suicide, the psychiatrist should consider asking additional questions. Examples might include asking about plans for the future or about recent acts or thoughts of self-harm. Regardless of the approach to the interview, not all individuals will report having suicidal ideas even when such thoughts are present. Thus, depending on the clinical circumstances, it may be important for the psychiatrist to speak with family members or friends to determine whether they have observed behavior (e.g., recent purchase of a gun) or have been privy to thoughts that suggest suicidal ideation (see Section V.C, "Communication With Significant Others"). In addition, patients who are initially interviewed when they are intoxicated with alcohol or other substances should be reassessed for suicidality once the intoxication has resolved.

2. Elicit the presence or absence of a suicide plan

If suicidal ideation is present, the psychiatrist will next probe for more detailed information about specific plans for suicide and any steps that have been taken toward enacting those plans. Although some suicidal acts can occur impulsively with little or no planning, more detailed plans are generally associated with a greater suicide risk. Violent and irreversible methods, such as firearms, jumping, and motor vehicle accidents, require particular attention. However, the patient's belief about the lethality of the method may be as important as the actual lethality of the method itself.

TABLE 3. Questions That May Be Helpful in Inquiring About Specific Aspects of Suicidal Thoughts, Plans, and Behaviors

Begin with questions that address the patient's feelings about living

- Have you ever felt that life was not worth living?
- Did you ever wish you could go to sleep and just not wake up?

Follow up with specific questions that ask about thoughts of death, self-harm, or suicide

- Is death something you've thought about recently?
- Have things ever reached the point that you've thought of harming yourself?

For individuals who have thoughts of self-harm or suicide

- When did you first notice such thoughts?
- What led up to the thoughts (e.g., interpersonal and psychosocial precipitants, including real or imagined losses; specific symptoms such as mood changes, anhedonia, hopelessness, anxiety, agitation, psychosis)?
- How often have those thoughts occurred (including frequency, obsessional quality, controllability)?
- How close have you come to acting on those thoughts?
- How likely do you think it is that you will act on them in the future?
- Have you ever started to harm (or kill) yourself but stopped before doing something (e.g., holding knife or gun to your body but stopping before acting, going to edge of bridge but not jumping)?
- What do you envision happening if you actually killed yourself (e.g., escape, reunion with significant other, rebirth, reactions of others)?
- Have you made a specific plan to harm or kill yourself? (If so, what does the plan include?)
- Do you have guns or other weapons available to you?
- Have you made any particular preparations (e.g., purchasing specific items, writing a note or a will, making financial arrangements, taking steps to avoid discovery, rehearsing the plan)?
- Have you spoken to anyone about your plans?
- How does the future look to you?
- What things would lead you to feel more (or less) hopeful about the future (e.g., treatment, reconciliation of relationship, resolution of stressors)?
- What things would make it more (or less) likely that you would try to kill yourself?
- What things in your life would lead you to want to escape from life or be dead?
- What things in your life make you want to go on living?
- If you began to have thoughts of harming or killing yourself again, what would you do?

TABLE 3. Questions That May Be Helpful in Inquiring About Specific Aspects of Suicidal Thoughts, Plans, and Behaviors *(continued)*

For individuals who have attempted suicide or engaged in self-damaging action(s), parallel questions to those in the previous section can address the prior attempt(s). Additional questions can be asked in general terms or can refer to the specific method used and may include:

- Can you describe what happened (e.g., circumstances, precipitants, view of future, use of alcohol or other substances, method, intent, seriousness of injury)?
- What thoughts were you having beforehand that led up to the attempt?
- What did you think would happen (e.g., going to sleep versus injury versus dying, getting a reaction out of a particular person)?
- Were other people present at the time?
- Did you seek help afterward yourself, or did someone get help for you?
- Had you planned to be discovered, or were you found accidentally?
- How did you feel afterward (e.g., relief versus regret at being alive)?
- Did you receive treatment afterward (e.g., medical versus psychiatric, emergency department versus inpatient versus outpatient)?
- Has your view of things changed, or is anything different for you since the attempt?
- Are there other times in the past when you've tried to harm (or kill) yourself?

For individuals with repeated suicidal thoughts or attempts

- About how often have you tried to harm (or kill) yourself?
- When was the most recent time?
- Can you describe your thoughts at the time that you were thinking most seriously about suicide?
- When was your most serious attempt at harming or killing yourself?
- What led up to it, and what happened afterward?

For individuals with psychosis, ask specifically about hallucinations and delusions

- Can you describe the voices (e.g., single versus multiple, male versus female, internal versus external, recognizable versus nonrecognizable)?
- What do the voices say (e.g., positive remarks versus negative remarks versus threats)? (If the remarks are commands, determine if they are for harmless versus harmful acts; ask for examples)?
- How do you cope with (or respond to) the voices?
- Have you ever done what the voices ask you to do? (What led you to obey the voices? If you tried to resist them, what made it difficult?)
- Have there been times when the voices told you to hurt or kill yourself? (How often? What happened?)
- Are you worried about having a serious illness or that your body is rotting?
- Are you concerned about your financial situation even when others tell you there's nothing to worry about?
- Are there things that you've been feeling guilty about or blaming yourself for?

TABLE 3. **Questions That May Be Helpful in Inquiring About Specific Aspects of Suicidal Thoughts, Plans, and Behaviors** ***(continued)***

Consider assessing the patient's potential to harm others in addition to him- or herself

- Are there others who you think may be responsible for what you're experiencing (e.g., persecutory ideas, passivity experiences)? Are you having any thoughts of harming them?
- Are there other people you would want to die with you?
- Are there others who you think would be unable to go on without you?

If the patient does not report a plan, the psychiatrist can ask whether there are certain conditions under which the patient would consider suicide (e.g., divorce, going to jail, housing loss) or whether it is likely that such a plan will be formed or acted on in the near future. If the patient reports that he or she is unlikely to act on the suicidal thoughts, the psychiatrist should determine what factors are contributing to that expectation, as such questioning can identify protective factors.

Whether or not a plan is present, if a patient has acknowledged suicidal ideation, there should be a specific inquiry about the presence or absence of a firearm in the home or workplace. It is also helpful to ask whether there have been recent changes in access to firearms or other weapons, including recent purchases or altered arrangements for storage. If the patient has access to a firearm, the psychiatrist is advised to discuss with and recommend to the patient or a significant other the importance of restricting access to, securing, or removing this and other weapons. Such discussions should be documented in the medical record, including any instructions that have been given to the patient and significant others about firearms or other weapons.

3. Assess the degree of suicidality, including suicidal intent and lethality of plan

Regardless of whether the patient has developed a suicide plan, the patient's level of suicidal intent should be explored. Suicidal intent reflects the intensity of a patient's wish to die and can be assessed by determining the patient's motivation for suicide as well as the seriousness and extent of his or her aim to die, including any associated behaviors or planning for suicide. If the patient has developed a suicide plan, it is important to assess its lethality. The lethality of the plan can be ascertained through questions about the method, the patient's knowledge and skill concerning its use, and the absence of intervening persons or protective circumstances. In general, the greater and clearer the intent, the higher the risk for suicide will be. Thus, even a patient with a low-lethality suicide plan or attempt may be at high risk in the future if intentions are strong and the patient believes that the chosen method will be fatal. At the same time, a patient with low suicidal intent may still die from suicide by erroneously believing that a particular method is not lethal.

4. Understand the relevance and limitations of suicide assessment scales

Although a number of suicide assessment scales have been developed for use in research and are described more fully in Part B of the guideline, their clinical utility is limited. Self-report rating scales may sometimes assist in opening communication with the patient about particular feelings or experiences. In addition, the content of suicide rating scales, such as the Scale for Suicide Ideation (8) and the Suicide Intent Scale (9), may be helpful to psychiatrists in developing a thorough line of questioning about suicide and suicidal behaviors. However, existing suicide assessment scales suffer from high false positive and false negative rates and have very low positive predictive values (10). As a result, such rating scales cannot substitute for thoughtful and clinically appropriate evaluation and are not recommended for clinical estimations of suicide risk.

D. ESTABLISH A MULTIAXIAL DIAGNOSIS

In conceptualizing suicide risk, it is important for the psychiatrist to develop a multiaxial differential diagnosis over the course of the psychiatric evaluation. Studies have shown that more than 90% of individuals who die by suicide satisfy the criteria for one or more psychiatric disorders. Thus, the psychiatrist should determine whether a patient has a primary axis I or axis II diagnosis. Suicide and other suicidal behaviors are also more likely to occur in individuals with more than one psychiatric diagnosis. As a result, it is important to note other current or past axis I or axis II diagnoses, including those that may currently be in remission.

Identification of physical illness (axis III) is essential since such diagnoses may also be associated with an increased risk of suicide as well as with an increased risk of other suicidal behaviors.

For some individuals, this increase in risk may result from increased rates of comorbid psychiatric illness or from the direct physiological effects of physical illness or its treatment. Physical illnesses may also be a source of social and/or psychological stress, which in turn may augment risk.

Also crucial in determining suicide risk is the recognition of psychosocial stressors (axis IV), which may be either acute or chronic. Certain stressors, such as sudden unemployment, interpersonal loss, social isolation, and dysfunctional relationships, can increase the likelihood of suicide attempts as well as increase the risk of suicide. At the same time, it is important to note that life events have different meanings for different individuals. Thus, in determining whether a particular stressor may confer risk for suicidal behavior, it is necessary to consider the perceived importance and meaning of the life event for the individual patient.

As the final component of the multiaxial diagnosis, the patient's baseline and current levels of functioning are important to assess (axis V). Also, the clinician should assess the relative change in the patient's level of functioning and the patient's view of and feelings about his or her functioning. Although suicidal ideation and/or suicide attempts are reflected in the Global Assessment of Functioning (GAF) scoring recommendations, it should be noted that there is no agreed-on correlation between a GAF score and level of suicide risk.

E. ESTIMATE SUICIDE RISK

The goal of the suicide risk assessment is to identify factors that may increase or decrease a patient's level of suicide risk, to estimate an overall level of suicide risk, and to develop a treatment plan that addresses patient safety and modifiable contributors to suicide risk. The assessment is comprehensive in scope, integrating knowledge of the patient's specific risk factors; clinical history, including psychopathological development; and interaction with the clinician. The estimation of suicide risk, at the culmination of the suicide assessment, is the quintessential clinical judgment, since no study has identified one specific risk factor or set of risk factors as specifically predictive of suicide or other suicidal behavior.

Table 4 provides a list of factors that have been associated with increased suicide risk, and Table 5 lists factors that have been associated with protective effects. While risk factors are typically additive (i.e., the patient's level of risk increases with the number of risk factors), they may also interact in a synergistic fashion. For example, the combined risk associated with comorbid depression and physical illness may be greater than the sum of the risk associated with each in isolation. At the same time, certain risk factors, such as a recent suicide attempt (especially one of high lethality), access to a firearm, and the presence of a suicide note, should be considered serious in and of themselves, regardless of whether other risk factors are present.

The effect on suicide risk of some risk factors, such as particular life events or psychological strengths and vulnerabilities, will vary on an individual basis. Risk factors must also be assessed in context, as certain risk factors are more applicable to particular diagnostic groups, while others carry more general risk. Finally, it should be kept in mind that, because of the low rate of suicide in the population, only a small fraction of individuals with a particular risk factor will die from suicide.

Risk factors for suicide attempts, which overlap with but are not identical to risk factors for suicide, will also be identified in the assessment process. These factors should also be addressed in the treatment planning process, since suicide attempts themselves are associated with morbidity in addition to the added risk that they confer for suicide.

1. Demographic factors

In epidemiologic studies, a number of demographic factors have been associated with increased rates of suicide. However, these demographic characteristics apply to a very broad population of people and cannot be considered alone. Instead, such demographic parameters must be considered within the context of other interacting factors that may influence individual risk.

TABLE 4. Factors Associated With an Increased Risk for Suicide

Suicidal thoughts/behaviors	
Suicidal ideas (current or previous)	
Suicidal plans (current or previous)	
Suicide attempts (including aborted or interrupted attempts)	
Lethality of suicidal plans or attempts	
Suicidal intent	
Psychiatric diagnoses	
Major depressive disorder	
Bipolar disorder (primarily in depressive or mixed episodes)	
Schizophrenia	
Anorexia nervosa	
Alcohol use disorder	
Other substance use disorders	
Cluster B personality disorders (particularly borderline personality disorder)	
Comorbidity of axis I and/or axis II disorders	
Physical illnesses	
Diseases of the nervous system	
Multiple sclerosis	
Huntington's disease	
Brain and spinal cord injury	
Seizure disorders	
Malignant neoplasms	
HIV/AIDS	
Peptic ulcer disease	
Chronic obstructive pulmonary disease, especially in men	
Chronic hemodialysis-treated renal failure	
Systemic lupus erythematosus	
Pain syndromes	
Functional impairment	
Psychosocial features	
Recent lack of social support (including living alone)	
Unemployment	
Drop in socioeconomic status	
Poor relationship with family[a]	
Domestic partner violence[b]	
Recent stressful life event	
Childhood traumas	
Sexual abuse	
Physical abuse	
Genetic and familial effects	
Family history of suicide (particularly in first-degree relatives)	
Family history of mental illness, including substance use disorders	

TABLE 4. Factors Associated With an Increased Risk for Suicide *(continued)*

Psychological features
Hopelessness
Psychic pain[a]
Severe or unremitting anxiety
Panic attacks
Shame or humiliation[a]
Psychological turmoil[a]
Decreased self-esteem[a]
Extreme narcissistic vulnerability[a]
Behavioral features
Impulsiveness
Aggression, including violence against others
Agitation
Cognitive features
Loss of executive function[b]
Thought constriction (tunnel vision)
Polarized thinking
Closed-mindedness
Demographic features
Male gender[c]
Widowed, divorced, or single marital status, particularly for men
Elderly age group (age group with greatest proportionate risk for suicide)
Adolescent and young adult age groups (age groups with highest numbers of suicides)
White race
Gay, lesbian, or bisexual orientation[b]
Additional features
Access to firearms
Substance intoxication (in the absence of a formal substance use disorder diagnosis)
Unstable or poor therapeutic relationship[a]

[a]Association with increased rate of suicide is based on clinical experience rather than formal research evidence.

[b]Associated with increased rate of suicide attempts, but no evidence is available on suicide rates per se.

[c]For suicidal attempts, females have increased risk, compared with males.

a) Age

Suicide rates differ dramatically by age. In addition, age-related psychosocial stressors and family or developmental issues may influence suicide risk. The age of the patient can also be of relevance to psychiatric diagnosis, since specific disorders vary in their typical ages of onset.

Between age 10 and 24 years, suicide rates in the general population of the United States rise sharply to approximately 13 per 100,000 in the 20- to 24-year-old age group before essentially plateauing through midlife. After age 70, rates again rise to a high of almost 20 per 100,000 in those over age 80 (Figure 1). These overall figures can be misleading, however, since the age distribution of suicide rates varies as a function of gender as well as with race and ethnicity. For example, among male African Americans and American Indians/Alaska Natives, sui-

TABLE 5. Factors Associated With Protective Effects for Suicide

- Children in the home[a]
- Sense of responsibility to family[b]
- Pregnancy
- Religiosity
- Life satisfaction
- Reality testing ability[b]
- Positive coping skills[b]
- Positive problem-solving skills[b]
- Positive social support
- Positive therapeutic relationship[b]

[a]Except among those with postpartum psychosis or mood disorder.

[b]Association with decreased rate of suicide is based on clinical experience rather than formal research evidence.

cide rates rise dramatically during adolescence, peak in young adulthood, and then fall through mid- and later life. Thus, in adolescence and young adulthood, the suicide rates of African American men are comparable with those of white men, although overall, African American males are half as likely to die from suicide as white males. While suicide rates in many age groups have remained relatively stable over the last 50 years, the rate among adolescents and young adults has increased dramatically, and the rate among the elderly has decreased. Among the 14- to 25-year-old age group, suicide is now the third leading cause of death, with rates that are triple those in the 1950s (12).

Suicide rates are higher in older adults than at any other point in the life course. In 2000 in the United States there were approximately 5,300 suicides among individuals over age 65, a rate of 15.3 per 100,000. Whereas older adults made up 12.6% of the population, they accounted for 18.1% of suicides. In addition, the high suicide rate in those over age 65 is largely a reflection of the high suicide rate in white men, which reaches almost 60 per 100,000 by age 85. While rates in Asian men also increase after age 65 and rates in Asian women increase dramatically after age 80, the rate for all other women is generally flat in late life.

Thoughts of death are also more common in older than in younger adults, but paradoxically, as people age they are less likely to endorse suicidal ideation per se (13). Attempted suicide is also less frequent among persons in later life than among younger age groups (14). Whereas the ratio of attempted suicides to suicides in adolescents may be as high as 200:1, there are as few as one to four attempts for each suicide in later life (15). However, the self-destructive acts that do occur in older people are more lethal. This greater lethality is a function of several factors, including reduced physical resilience (greater physical illness burden), greater social isolation (diminished likelihood of rescue), and a greater determination to die (15). Suicidal elders give fewer warnings to others of their plans, use more violent and potentially deadly methods, and apply those methods with greater planning and resolve (15, 16). Therefore, compared with a suicide attempt in a younger person, a suicide attempt in an older person confers a higher level of future suicide risk.

b) Gender

In virtually all countries that report suicide statistics to the World Health Organization, suicide risk increases with age in both sexes, and rates for men in older adulthood are generally higher than those for women (17). One exception is China, where the suicide rate of women is much greater than that of men (18). In the United States, death by suicide is more frequent in men than in women, with the suicide rate in males approximately four times that in females (Figure 1). In the psychiatric population, these gender differences are also present but are less prominent.

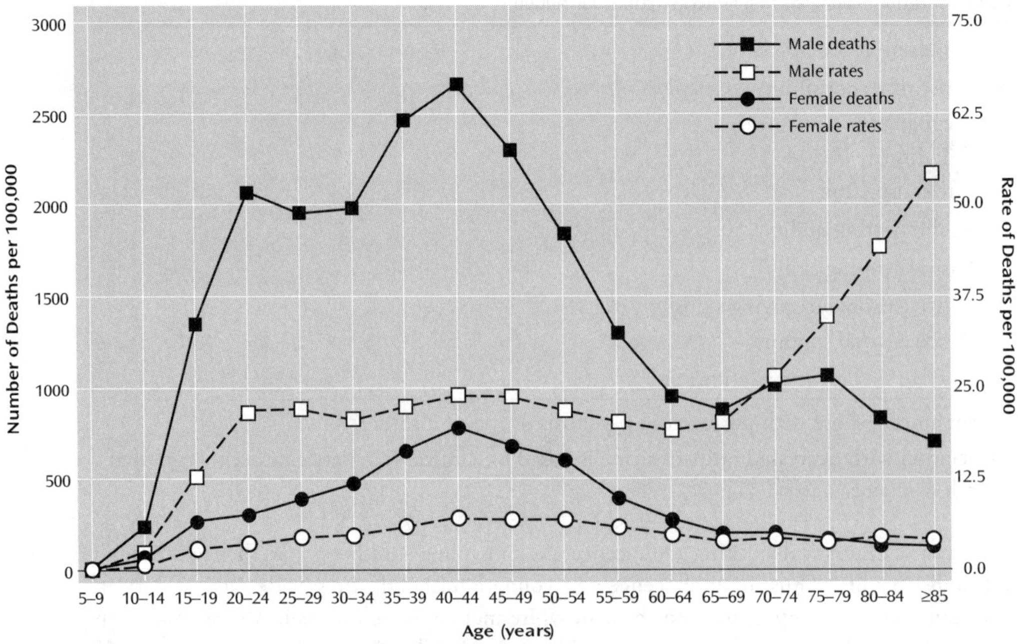

FIGURE 1. Number and Rate of Deaths by Suicide in Males and Females in the United States in 2000, by Age Group[a]

[a]Includes deaths by suicide injury (ICD-10 codes X60–X84, Y87.0). From the Web-Based Injury Statistics Query and Reporting System, National Center for Injury Prevention and Control, Centers for Disease Control and Prevention (11).

In terms of murder-suicide, the male predominance is more pronounced, with identified typologies including young men with prominent sexual jealousy and elderly men with ailing spouses (19, 20). From age 65 on, there are progressive increases in suicide rates for white men and for Asian men as well as for men overall. With the exception of high suicide rates in Asian women over age 80, women in the United States are at highest risk in midlife (11).

A number of factors may contribute to these gender differences in suicide risk (21). Men who are depressed are more likely to have comorbid alcohol and/or substance abuse problems than women, which places the men at higher risk. Men are also less likely to seek and accept help or treatment. Women, meanwhile, have factors that protect them against suicide. In addition to their lower rates of alcohol and substance abuse, women are less impulsive, more socially embedded, and more willing to seek help. Among African American women, rates of suicide are remarkably low, a fact that has been attributed to the protective factors of religion and extended kin networks (22). At the same time, women have higher rates of depression (23) and respond to unemployment with greater and longer-lasting increases in suicide rates than do men (24).

Overall, for women in the general population, pregnancy is a time of significantly reduced suicide risk (25). Women with young children in the home are also less likely to kill themselves (26). Nonetheless, women with a history of depression or suicide attempts are at greater risk for poor outcomes postpartum. Although suicide is most likely to occur in the first month after delivery, risk continues throughout the postpartum period. Teenagers, women of lower socioeconomic status, and women hospitalized with postpartum psychiatric disorders may be at particularly increased risk postpartum (27, 28).

Women tend to choose less lethal suicide methods than men do (e.g., overdose or wrist cutting versus firearms or hanging). Such differences may in part account for the reversal in the gender ratio for suicide attempters, with women being reported to attempt suicide three times as often as men (29). This female predominance among suicide attempters varies with age, however, and in older adults the ratio of women to men among suicide attempters approaches 1:1 (11, 30). Rates of suicidal ideation and attempts are also increased in individuals with borderline personality disorder and in those with a history of domestic violence or physical and/or sexual abuse, all of which are more common among women (31–36). In addition, the likelihood of suicide attempts may vary with the phase of the menstrual cycle (37, 38).

c) Race, ethnicity, and culture

Variations in suicide rates across racial and ethnic groups have been mentioned earlier in the discussion of the influences of age and gender on suicide risk. Overall, however, in the United States, age-adjusted rates for suicide in whites and in non-Hispanic Native Americans are approximately double those observed in Hispanics, non-Hispanic African Americans, and Asian-Pacific Islanders (12.1 and 13.6 per 100,000 versus 6.1, 5.8, and 6.0 per 100,000, respectively) (11). For immigrant groups, in general, suicide rates tend to mirror the rates in the country of origin and converge toward the rate in the host country over time (39–41).

In the United States, racial and ethnic differences are also seen in the rates of suicide across the lifespan, with the highest suicide rates occurring in those over age 65 among non-Hispanic whites, Hispanics, and Asian-Pacific Islanders (11). In contrast, among Native Americans and African Americans, the highest suicide rates occur during adolescence and young adulthood (11). Such figures may be deceptive, however, since each of these groups exhibits a striking degree of heterogeneity that is rarely addressed in compilations of suicide rates.

Racial and ethnic differences in culture, religious beliefs, and societal position may influence not only the actual rates of suicide but also the views of death and suicide held by members of a particular group. For some groups, suicide can be considered a traditionally accepted way of dealing with shame, distress, and/or physical illness (42). In addition, cultural values about conveying suicidal ideas may differ; in some cultures, for example, suicidal ideation may be considered a disgraceful or private matter that should be denied. Cultural differences, particularly in immigrants and in Native Americans and Alaska Natives, may generate acculturative stresses that in turn may contribute to suicidality (43, 44). Thus, knowledge of and sensitivity to common contributors to suicide in different racial and ethnic groups as well as cultural differences in beliefs about death and views of suicide are important when making clinical estimates of suicide risk and implementing plans to address suicide risk.

d) Marital status

Suicide risk also varies with marital status, with the suicide rate of single persons being twice that of those who are married. Divorced, separated, or widowed individuals have rates four to five times higher than married individuals (45, 46). Variations in suicide rates with marital status may reflect differing rates of baseline psychiatric illness but may also be associated with psychological or health variations. The presence of another person in the household may also serve as a protective factor by decreasing social isolation, engendering a sense of responsibility toward others, and increasing the likelihood of discovery after a suicide attempt. For women, the presence of children in the home may provide an additional protective effect (26, 47). It is also important to note that although married adults have lower rates of suicide overall, young married couples may have increased risk, and the presence of a high-conflict or violent marriage can be a precipitant rather than a protective factor for suicide.

e) Sexual orientation

Although no studies have examined rates of suicide among gay, lesbian, and bisexual individuals, available evidence suggests that they may have an increased risk for suicidal behaviors. Many recent studies involving diverse sample populations and research methods have consistently found that gay, lesbian, and bisexual youths have a higher risk of suicide attempts than matched heterosexual comparison groups (48–53). The female-to-male ratio for reported suicide attempts in the general population is reversed in lesbian and gay youths, with more males than females attempting suicide (48). While some risk factors leading to suicide, such as psychiatric and substance use disorders, are shared by both gay, lesbian, and bisexual youths and heterosexual youths, others are unique to being gay, lesbian, or bisexual (e.g., disclosure of sexual orientation to friends and family, experience of homophobia and harassment, and gender nonconformity). Aggressive treatment of psychiatric and substance use disorders, open and nonjudgmental support, and promotion of healthy psychosocial adjustment may help to decrease the risk for suicide in gay, lesbian, and bisexual youths and adults.

f) Occupation

Occupational groups differ in a number of factors contributing to suicide risk. These factors include demographics (e.g., race, gender, socioeconomic class, marital status), occupational stress (54, 55), psychiatric morbidity (56), and occupationally associated opportunities for suicide (56, 57). Physicians have been consistently found to be at higher risk for suicide than persons in other occupations including professionals (57, 58). After basic demographic correlates of suicide across 32 occupations were controlled, risk was found to be highest among dentists and physicians (with multivariate logistic regression odds ratios of 5.43 and 2.31, respectively) and was also increased among nurses, social workers, artists, mathematicians, and scientists (54). Although evidence is more varied, farmers may be at somewhat higher risk, whereas risk in police officers generally does not appear to differ from that of age- and sex-matched comparison subjects (54, 57).

2. Major psychiatric syndromes

The presence of a psychiatric disorder is probably the most significant risk factor for suicide. Psychological autopsy studies have consistently shown that more than 90% of persons who die from suicide satisfy the criteria for one or more psychiatric disorders (59, 60). The psychological autopsy method involves a retrospective investigation of the deceased person, within several months of death, and uses psychological information gathered from personal documents; police, medical, and coroner records; and interviews with family members, friends, co-workers, school associates, and health care providers to classify equivocal deaths or establish diagnoses that were likely present at the time of suicide (61–63).

In addition to there being high rates of psychiatric disorder among persons who die by suicide, almost all psychiatric disorders with the exception of mental retardation have been shown to increase suicide risk as measured by standardized mortality ratios (SMRs) (64) (Table 6). An SMR reflects the relative mortality from suicide in individuals with a particular risk factor, compared with the general population. Thus, the SMR will be equal to 1.0 when the number of observed suicide deaths is equivalent to the number of expected deaths by suicide in an age- and sex-matched group in the general population. Values of the SMR for suicide that are greater than 1.0 indicate an increased risk of suicide, whereas values less than 1.0 indicate a decreased risk (i.e., a protective effect). It is also important to note that SMRs do not correspond precisely to the incidence or prevalence of suicide and may vary in their reliability depending on the number of suicides in the sample, the time period of the study, and the representativeness of the study population. Thus, SMRs should be viewed as estimates of relative risk and not as reflections of absolute risk for individuals with a particular disorder. It is equally necessary to appreciate distinctions in risk across disorders and variations in risk at differing points in the illness course in the effort to differentiate high-risk patients within an overall at-risk population identified in terms of standardized mortality.

a) Mood disorders

Study after study has confirmed that the presence of a major mood disorder is a significant risk factor for suicide. Not surprisingly, mood disorders, primarily in depressive phases, are the diagnoses most often found in suicide deaths (59, 65–67). Although most suicides in individuals

TABLE 6. Risk of Suicide in Persons With Previous Suicide Attempts and Psychiatric Disorders[a]

Condition	Number of Studies	Standardized Mortality Ratio (SMR)[b]	Annual Suicide Rate (%)	Estimated Lifetime Suicide Rate (%)
Previous suicide attempts	9	38.4	0.549	27.5
Psychiatric disorders				
Eating disorders	15	23.1		
Major depression	23	20.4	0.292	14.6
Sedative abuse	3	20.3		
Mixed drug abuse	4	19.2	0.275	14.7
Bipolar disorder	15	15.0	0.310	15.5
Opioid abuse	10	14.0		
Dysthymia	9	12.1	0.173	8.6
Obsessive-compulsive disorder	3	11.5	0.143	8.2
Panic disorder	9	10.0	0.160	7.2
Schizophrenia	38	8.45	0.121	6.0
Personality disorders	5	7.08	0.101	5.1
Alcohol abuse	35	5.86	0.084	4.2
Pediatric psychiatric disorders	11	4.73		
Cannabis abuse	1	3.85		
Neuroses	8	3.72		
Mental retardation	5	0.88		

[a]Based on a meta-analysis by Harris and Barraclough (64) of 249 reports published between 1966 and 1993. Table adapted with permission.

[b]The SMR is the ratio of the observed mortality to the expected mortality and approximates the risk of mortality resulting from suicide in the presence of a particular condition. For the general population, the value of the SMR is 1.0, with an annual suicide rate of 0.014% per year and a lifetime rate of 0.72%.

with bipolar disorder occur during depressive episodes, mixed episodes are also associated with increased risk (68–70). Suicidal ideation and attempts are also more common during mixed episodes than in mania (71).

When viewed from the standpoint of lifetime risk, mood disorders are associated with an increased risk of mortality that has been estimated to range from a 12-fold increase in risk with dysthymia to a 20-fold increase in risk with major depression (64). Lifetime suicide risk in bipolar disorder has generally been found to be similar to that in unipolar major depression (69, 72). However, several longitudinal studies of patients followed after an index hospitalization have demonstrated suicide risks in patients with major depressive disorder that are greater than those in patients with either bipolar I disorder or bipolar II disorder (73–75).

Particularly for younger patients, suicides are more likely to occur early in the course of illness (68, 73, 75, 76). Nonetheless, risk persists throughout life in major depressive disorder as well as in bipolar disorder (73, 74). Suicide risk also increases in a graduated fashion with illness severity as reflected by the level of required treatment. Lifetime suicide rates in psychiatric outpatients ranged from 0.7% for those without an affective disorder to 2.2% for those with affective disorders, whereas lifetime suicide rates for individuals requiring hospitalization ranged from 4% for those whose admission for depression was not prompted by suicidal behavior or risk to 8.6% for those whose admission was the result of suicidality (77). Illness severity may also be an indicator of risk for suicide attempts (75, 78).

Among patients with mood disorders, lifetime risk also depends on the presence of other psychiatric symptoms or behaviors, some of which are modifiable with treatment. For example, patients with mood disorders who died by suicide within 1 year of initial evaluation were more likely to have panic attacks, severe psychic anxiety, diminished concentration, global insomnia, moderate alcohol abuse, and severe loss of pleasure or interest in activities (79). At later time points, hopelessness has been associated with increased suicide risk in mood disorder patients (78, 79). Suicidal ideation and a history of suicide attempts also augment risk (74, 79). Comorbid anxiety, alcohol use, and substance use are common in patients with mood disorders and may also increase the risk of suicide and suicide attempts (see Sections II.E.2.f, "Alcohol Use Disorders," and II.E.2.g, "Other Substance Use Disorders"). Although a greater risk for suicide or suicidal behaviors among patients with psychotic mood disorders has been seen in some studies (80–83), this relationship has not been found in other studies (84–88).

b) Schizophrenia

Compared to the risk in the general population, the risk of suicide in patients with schizophrenia is estimated to be about 8.5-fold higher (64), with even greater increments in risk in patients who have been hospitalized (89). Although earlier research suggested a 10%–15% lifetime risk of suicide among patients with schizophrenia (90–93), such estimates were likely inflated by biases in the patient populations and length of follow-up. More recent estimates suggest a lifetime risk of suicide in schizophrenia of about 4% (94).

Suicide may occur more frequently during the early years of the illness, with the time immediately after hospital discharge being a period of heightened risk (83, 89, 90, 95–98). However, risk continues throughout life (99, 100) and appears to be increased in those with a chronic illness course (83, 89, 101), multiple psychiatric hospitalizations (89, 95), or a previous suicide attempt (89, 90, 95, 100). Other consistently identified factors that confer an increased risk of suicide in patients with schizophrenia include male sex (83, 89, 90, 95, 102, 103), younger age (<30 years) (83, 90, 102), and social isolation (97, 104).

In individuals with schizophrenia or schizoaffective disorder, psychotic symptoms are often present at the time of a suicide attempt or suicide (105–107). However, command hallucinations seem to account for a relatively small percentage of suicides, and there is limited evidence on whether they increase suicide risk. Nonetheless, they may act as a precipitant to a suicide attempt or to suicide in some individuals (106, 108) (see Section II.E.3.c, "Command Hallucinations"). Suicide in patients with schizophrenia may be more likely to occur during periods of improvement after relapse or during periods of depressed mood (83, 89, 90, 95, 100, 109–111), including what has been termed postpsychotic depression (112, 113). Also, patients with schizoaffective disorder appear to be at greater risk for suicide than those with schizophrenia (114).

Suicide risk may paradoxically be increased in those who have insight into the implications of having a schizophrenic illness, particularly if this insight is coupled with a feeling of hopelessness. Suicide risk is also increased in those who recognize a loss of previous abilities and are pessimistic about the benefits of treatment in restoring those abilities (93, 101, 115). This pattern is consistent with the increased risk of suicide observed in individuals with schizophrenia who had a history of good premorbid and intellectual functioning (83, 89, 103) as well as with the decreased risk of suicide in patients with prominent negative symptoms (83, 89, 103, 116).

Suicidal ideation and suicide attempts are common among individuals with schizophrenia and need to be identified and addressed in the assessment process. In series of hospitalized or longitudinally followed patients with schizophrenia, 40%–53% reported having suicidal ideation at some point in their lives and 23%–55% reported prior suicide attempts (80, 93, 108, 117). For individuals with schizoaffective disorder, these figures are likely to be even higher (80). Patients often reported that suicide attempts were precipitated by depression, stressors, or psychotic symptoms (108). In addition, suicide attempts among individuals with schizophrenia or schizoaffective disorder were often medically serious and associated with a high degree of intent (108), both of which would confer greater future risk for suicide.

c) Anxiety disorders

Although studies of lifetime suicide risk in anxiety disorders are more limited than for mood disorders, evidence suggests anxiety disorders are associated with a six- to 10-fold increase in suicide risk (64, 118, 119). Among persons who die from suicide, rates of anxiety disorders appear to be lower than rates of mood disorders, with one psychological autopsy study identifying an anxiety disorder in only 11% of persons who died from suicide (120). However, the prevalence of anxiety disorders may be underestimated because of the masking of anxiety by affective disorders and by alcohol use (121).

Of the anxiety disorders, panic disorder has been studied in the most detail. In psychological autopsy studies, panic disorder is present in about 1% of persons who die from suicide (120), whereas other studies of panic disorder show an SMR for suicide that is about 10 times that of the general population (64). As with anxiety disorders in general, comorbid depression, alcohol use, or axis II disorders are often present in individuals with panic disorder who die by suicide (122, 123).

Suicidal ideation and suicide attempts are common in individuals with anxiety disorders, but their rates vary with the patient population and with the presence of comorbid diagnoses. In panic disorder, for example, reported rates of prior suicide attempts range from 0% to 42% (124–129). In other anxiety disorders, the relative risks of suicidal ideation and suicide attempts also appear to be increased (118, 130). In addition, in patients with major depression, the presence of a comorbid anxiety disorder appears to increase the risk of suicidal ideation or suicide attempts (131, 132). Less clear, however, is whether anxiety disorders are associated with an increased risk for suicide and other suicidal behaviors in the absence of comorbid diagnoses (130, 132–136) or whether the observed increases in risk can be accounted for solely on the basis of comorbid disorders (127, 137). Nonetheless, suicide risk may be diminished by identifying masked anxiety symptoms and anxiety disorders that are misdiagnosed as medical illness as well as by explicitly assessing and treating comorbid psychiatric diagnoses in individuals with anxiety disorders.

d) Eating disorders

Eating disorders, particularly anorexia nervosa, are a likely risk factor for suicide as well as being associated with an increased risk of mortality in general (64, 138, 139). Exact risk is difficult to determine, however, as data on rates of suicide in eating disorders may be subject to underreporting bias (140). Suicide attempts are also common, particularly in individuals with bingeing and purging behaviors and in those with comorbid mood disorders, aggression, or impulsivity (141, 142). Conversely, suicide attempters may have increased rates of abnormal eating behaviors (142). The role of comorbid diagnoses in increasing the risk of suicidal behaviors remains to be delineated. It is also not clear whether the self-imposed morbidity and mortality associated with severe caloric restriction or bingeing and purging should be viewed as a self-injurious or suicidal behavior. Regardless, clinicians conducting a suicide risk assessment should be attentive to the presence of eating disorders and especially the co-occurrence of eating disorders with behaviors or symptoms such as deliberate self-harm or depression.

e) Attention deficit hyperactivity disorder

The relationship between attention deficit hyperactivity disorder (ADHD) and suicidal behavior is unclear, with some studies indicating an association between the diagnosis of ADHD and suicide attempts or completions (143, 144) and other studies indicating no such connection (145, 146). However, individuals with ADHD, combined type, may be at greater risk than those with ADHD, inattentive type, perhaps because of an increased level of impulsivity in the combined type of the disorder (144). In addition, the presence of ADHD may increase suicide risk through comorbidity with conduct disorder, substance abuse, and/or depressive disorder (143).

f) Alcohol use disorders

Alcoholism is associated with an increased risk for suicide, with suicide mortality rates for alcoholics that are approximately six times those of the general population (64, 94). In fact, abuse of substances including alcohol may be the second most frequent psychiatric precursor to suicide (147). Although suicide rates among alcoholics are higher in Europe and older literature indicated a lifetime risk for suicide in the 11%–15% range, recent literature suggests the lifetime risk of suicide among alcoholics in the United States is as low as 3.4% (148). In addition, in psychological autopsy studies, alcohol abuse or dependence is present in 25%–50% of those who died by suicide (59, 149–151).

Several factors, including recent or impending interpersonal losses and comorbid psychiatric disorders, have been specifically linked to suicide in alcoholic individuals. The loss or disruption of a close interpersonal relationship or the threatened loss of such a relationship may be both a consequence of alcohol-related behavior and a precipitant to suicide (110, 152–154). Suicide is also more likely to occur among alcoholics who suffer from depressive episodes than in persons with major depression or alcoholism alone. In addition, studies have found major depressive episodes in half to three-fourths of alcoholics who die by suicide (67, 120, 149, 152, 155–157). As a result, psychiatrists should systematically rule out the presence of a comorbid depressive disorder and not simply assume that depressive symptoms result from alcohol use or its psychosocial consequences.

Whereas full-time employment appears to be a protective factor in alcoholics, factors that increase suicide risk include communications of suicidal intent, prior suicide attempts, continued or heavier drinking, recent unemployment, living alone, poor social support, legal and financial difficulties, serious medical illness, other psychiatric disorders, personality disturbance, and other substance use (64, 149, 152, 154, 156, 158, 159). In terms of gender, alcoholic men are more likely to die by suicide, but female alcoholics appear to have a greater standardized mortality due to suicide than men (64), indicating an increased risk of suicide in alcoholics regardless of gender. While the likelihood of a suicidal outcome increases with the total number of risk factors (149, 160), not all of these factors suggest an immediate risk. In fact, in contrast to suicide in depressed and schizophrenic patients, suicide in alcoholics appears to be a relatively late sequela of the disease (161), with communications of suicidal intent usually being of several years' duration and health, economic, and social functioning showing a gradual deterioration (149).

In addition to being associated with an increased risk of suicide, alcohol use disorders are associated with a greater likelihood of suicide attempts (162, 163). For suicide attempts among alcoholics, greater rates are associated with female sex, younger age, lower economic status, early onset of heavy drinking and alcohol-related problems, consumption of greater amounts of alcohol when drinking, and having a first- or second-degree relative who abused alcohol (164–167). The risk of suicide attempts among alcoholics is also increased by the presence of a comorbid psychiatric diagnosis, particularly major depression, other substance use disorders, antisocial personality disorder, or an anxiety disorder (165–171).

Thus, individuals with alcohol use disorders are at increased risk for suicide attempts as well as for suicide. Family histories of alcoholism and comorbid psychiatric disorders, particularly mood disorders and other substance use disorders, are frequent in alcoholics who die by suicide and who attempt suicide. Interpersonal loss and other adverse life events are commonly noted to precede suicide in alcoholics. These factors may act as precipitants, or, conversely, alcohol use disorders may have a deteriorating effect on the lives of alcoholics and culminate in suicide. Together, however, these findings suggest the need to identify and address comorbid psychiatric diagnoses, family history, and psychosocial factors, including recent interpersonal losses, as part of the suicide assessment of persons with alcohol use disorders.

g) Other substance use disorders

Although the role of alcoholism in suicide has been widely studied and recognized, abuse of other substances is also associated with increased rates of suicide (172). Substance use disorders are particularly common among adolescents and young adults who die by suicide (110, 145, 173, 174). In fact, it has been suggested that the spread of substance abuse may have contributed to the two- to fourfold increase in youth suicide since 1970 (147). For many individuals, substance abuse and alcoholism are co-occurring, making it difficult to distinguish the contributions of each to rates of suicide (153, 172, 173). In addition, other comorbid psychiatric disorders, particularly mood disorders and personality disorders, may add to the risk of suicide in patients with substance use disorders (145, 173–175).

Substance use disorders also seem to make an independent contribution to the likelihood of making a suicide attempt (176, 177). In addition, a history of suicide attempts is common among individuals with substance use disorders (31, 178–180). Even after other factors, including comorbid psychiatric disorders and demographic characteristics, are controlled, it is the number of substances used, rather than the type of substance, that appears to be important (176). As with suicide in individuals with alcohol use disorders, the loss of a significant personal relationship is a common precipitant for a suicide attempt (179). Suicide attempts are also more likely in individuals with substance abuse who also have higher childhood trauma scores for emotional neglect (180, 181). Moreover, a substance use disorder may complicate mood disorders (182), increasing susceptibility to treatment resistance, increasing psychological impairment, and contributing to an elevated risk for suicide attempts. Thus, it is important to identify patterns of substance use during the psychiatric evaluation and to note comorbid psychiatric diagnoses or psychosocial factors that may also affect the likelihood of suicidal behaviors among individuals with substance use disorders.

h) Personality disorders

Diagnoses of personality disorders have been associated with an increased risk for suicide, with estimated lifetime rates of suicide ranging from 3% to 9% (183–185). Compared with the general population, individuals with personality disorders have an estimated risk for suicide that is about seven times greater (64). Specific increases in suicide risk have been associated with borderline and antisocial personality disorders, with possible increases in risk associated with avoidant and schizoid personality disorders (186). Psychological autopsy studies have shown personality disorders to be present in approximately one-third of those who die by suicide (174, 183, 186, 187). Among psychiatric outpatients, personality disorders are present in about one-half of patients who die by suicide (78, 188).

In individuals with personality disorders, suicide risk may also be increased by a number of other factors, including unemployment, financial difficulty, family discord, and other interpersonal conflicts or loss (189, 190). In individuals with borderline personality disorder, in particular, impulsivity may also increase suicide risk (185).

Although comorbid diagnoses do not account for the full increase in suicide risk with personality disorders (184, 185), comorbid diagnoses are frequent and augment suicide risk. In fact, for individuals with personality disorders, concurrent depressive symptoms or substance use disorders are seen in nearly all individuals who die by suicide (187).

Among individuals who attempt suicide, diagnoses of personality disorders are also common, with overall rates of about 40% (31, 177, 184). Individuals with personality disorders tend to attempt suicide more often than individuals with other diagnoses (191–193), with 40%–90% of individuals with personality disorders making a suicide attempt during their lifetime (184). Comorbid psychiatric diagnoses, including mood disorders and substance use disorders, are quite prevalent among suicide attempters with personality disorders and independently contribute to risk (131, 184, 191, 192, 194, 195). Impulsivity has also been shown to increase the risk of suicide attempts in some (196, 197) but not all studies (191). Rates of suicide attempts in those with personality disorder may also vary with treatment setting, with greater risk in individuals who are receiving acute inpatient treatment (198).

Of personality disorder diagnoses, borderline personality disorder and antisocial personality disorder confer an added risk of suicide attempts (31, 177, 191, 193). In individuals with borderline personality disorder, there is some evidence of increased risk being associated with the number and severity of symptoms (195). Among female suicide attempters, rates of borderline personality disorder are higher than among male suicide attempters (199, 200). These findings suggest that personality disorders, particularly borderline personality disorder and antisocial personality disorder, should be identified and addressed as part of the suicide assessment process.

i) Comorbidity

As discussed in preceding sections, comorbid psychiatric diagnoses (most commonly, major depression, borderline and antisocial personality disorders, and alcohol and other substance use disorders) increase suicide risk and are often present in individuals who die by suicide (13, 59, 120, 174, 201). Comorbid medical diagnoses may also increase suicide risk, as will be discussed in Section II.E.5, "Physical Illness." In general, the greater the number of comorbid diagnoses that are present, the greater will be the increase in risk. Furthermore, even in the absence of a formal comorbid diagnosis, suicide is more likely to occur when there are high levels of additional psychiatric symptoms (67, 185, 202–204).

In patients with a mood disorder, either bipolar disorder or major depression, the risk of suicide is particularly increased in the presence of comorbid alcohol or substance use (68, 205–207), with some studies suggesting that males are at additional risk (68, 205). Comorbid alcohol use may also increase suicide risk in patients with schizophrenia (107). In addition, suicide in schizophrenia may be more likely to occur during periods of depression (83, 90, 109–113). In anxiety disorders and particularly in panic disorder, individuals who die by suicide often have experienced comorbid depression, alcohol use, or axis II disorders (122, 123). Similarly, when suicide occurs in individuals with eating disorders, it is often associated with a comorbid mood disorder or substance use disorder (138).

For individuals with alcohol use disorders, major depression is found in half to three-fourths of individuals who die by suicide (67, 120, 149, 152, 155–157), and alcoholics who suffer from depressive episodes are more likely to die from suicide than persons with major depression or alcoholism alone. Serious medical illness and other psychiatric disorders, including personality disturbance and other substance use disorders, also increase suicide risk in alcoholics (64, 149, 152, 154, 156, 158, 159). For many individuals, substance abuse and alcoholism are co-occurring, making it difficult to distinguish the contributions of each to rates of suicide (153, 172, 173, 208). Furthermore, it appears to be the number of substances used, rather than the specific substance, that determines risk (176).

Individuals who die by suicide and who abuse or are dependent on substances other than alcohol are typically adolescents or young adults. Comorbid mood disorders are commonly seen in both males and females (66, 145, 204). In addition, borderline personality disorder is relatively frequent in females with substance use disorders (175), whereas young males with substance use disorders who die by suicide more commonly have comorbid antisocial personality disorder (120, 159, 173, 204). The presence of ADHD may increase suicide risk through comorbidity with conduct disorder, substance abuse, and/or depressive disorder (143). For individuals with personality disorders, concurrent depressive symptoms or substance use disorders augment suicide risk (184, 185, 209, 210) and are seen in nearly all suicides (187).

Comorbid diagnoses are also essential to identify and address because of their role in increasing the risk of suicide attempts (199). Furthermore, the likelihood of a suicide attempt appears to increase with an increasing number of comorbid diagnoses (166, 176, 177, 211). In addition, the number and severity of symptoms may play a role in increasing risk, regardless of whether the full criteria for a separate diagnosis are met. The specific comorbid disorders that augment the risk of suicide attempts are similar to those that are commonly seen to augment the risk of suicide and include comorbid depression (129, 131, 193, 195, 197, 211), alcohol and other substance use disorders (31, 129, 167, 168, 170, 180, 182, 191, 199, 211–214), anxiety disorders (127, 130–135, 137, 211, 215), and personality disorders (184, 191), particularly borderline personality disorder (31, 195, 200) and antisocial personality disorder (165, 204, 216). Thus, given the evidence that comorbidity increases the risks for suicide and for suicide attempts, the suicide risk assessment should give strong consideration to all current and previous psychiatric diagnoses.

3. Specific psychiatric symptoms

a) Anxiety

Anxiety appears to increase the risk for suicide (79, 217, 218). Specifically implicated has been severe psychic anxiety consisting of subjective feelings of fearfulness or apprehension, whether or not the feelings are focused on specific concerns. Clinical observation suggests that anxious patients may be more inclined to act on suicidal impulses than individuals whose depressive symptoms include psychomotor slowing. Studies of suicide in patients with affective disorders have shown that those who died by suicide within the first year after contact were more likely to have severe psychic anxiety or panic attacks (79, 219). In an inpatient sample, severe anxiety, agitation, or both were found in four-fifths of patients in the week preceding suicide (218). Similar associations of anxiety with suicide attempts have been noted in some (212) but not all (220) studies. Since severe anxiety does seem to increase suicide risk, at least in some subgroups of patients, anxiety should be viewed as an often hidden but potentially modifiable risk factor for suicide (109). Once identified, symptoms of anxiety can be addressed with psychotherapeutic approaches and can also respond rapidly to aggressive short-term treatment with benzodiazepines, second-generation antipsychotic medications, and possibly anticonvulsant medications.

b) Hopelessness

Hopelessness is well established as a psychological dimension that is associated with increased suicide risk (10, 78, 79, 217, 221–223). Hopelessness may vary in degree from having a negative expectation for the future to being devoid of hope and despairing for the future. In general, patients with high levels of hopelessness have an increased risk for future suicide (78, 221–225). However, among patients with alcohol use disorders, the presence of hopelessness may not confer additional risk (226, 227). For patients with depression, hopelessness has been suggested to be the factor that explains why some patients choose suicide, whereas others do not (222). Hopelessness also contributes to an increased likelihood of suicidal ideation (192, 228) and suicide attempts (197, 212, 229–231) as well as an increased level of suicidal intent (197, 232, 233).

Hopelessness often occurs in concert with depression as a "state-dependent" characteristic, but some individuals experience hopelessness on a primary and more enduring basis (221). High baseline levels of hopelessness have also been associated with an increased likelihood of suicidal behaviors (234). However, patients experiencing similar levels of depression may have differing levels of hopelessness (222), and this difference, in turn, may affect their likelihood of developing suicidal thoughts (228). Whatever the source or conceptualization of hopelessness, interventions that reduce hopelessness may be able to reduce the potential for suicide (10, 222, 235–237).

c) Command hallucinations

Command hallucinations, which order patients to carry out tasks or actions, can occur in individuals with psychotic disorders, primarily schizophrenia (238). Evidence for the association of command hallucinations with suicide is extremely limited (102, 239). The presence of auditory command hallucinations in inpatients does not appear to increase the likelihood of assaultiveness or of suicidal ideation or behavior over that associated with auditory hallucinations alone (240). Furthermore, in patients who do experience auditory command hallucinations, reported rates of compliance with commands vary widely from 40% to 84% (106, 241–244). Variables that have been associated with a propensity to obey command hallucinations include being able to identify the hallucinatory voice, having more severe psychotic disturbance, having a less dangerous command, and experiencing the commands for the first time or outside of a hospital environment (241, 242, 245). Thus, at least for some individuals, suicidal behaviors can occur in response to hallucinated commands, and individuals with prior suicide attempts may be particularly susceptible (106). Consequently, in the psychiatric evaluation, it is important to identify auditory command hallucinations, assess them in the context of other clinical features, and address them as part of the treatment planning process.

d) Impulsiveness and aggression

Impulsivity, hostility, and aggression may act individually or together to increase suicide risk. For example, many studies provide moderately strong evidence for the roles of impulsivity and hostility-related affects and behavior in suicide across diagnostic groups (89, 217, 246–248). Multiple other studies have also demonstrated increased levels of impulsivity and aggression in individuals with a history of attempted suicide (31, 193, 197, 212, 220, 249–252). Many patients with borderline personality disorder exhibit self-mutilating behaviors, and, overall, such behaviors are associated with increased impulsivity (251). However, for many self-mutilating patients, these behaviors are premeditated rather than impulsive (253). Consequently, self-mutilatory behaviors alone should not be regarded as an indicator of high impulsivity. Moreover, measures of aggression and impulsivity are not highly correlated (253), making aggression a poor marker of impulsivity as well. Thus, impulsivity, hostility, aggression, and self-mutilating behaviors should be considered independently in the psychiatric evaluation as well as in estimating suicide risk.

4. Other aspects of psychiatric history

a) Alcohol intoxication

In addition to the increased suicide risk conferred by alcohol abuse or dependence, intoxication itself appears to play a role in alcoholic as well as nonalcoholic populations (254). Autopsies have found alcohol to be present in 20%–50% of all persons who die by suicide (121, 255). Those who consume alcohol before suicide are more likely to have experienced a recent breakup of an interpersonal relationship but less likely to have sought help before death (255). They are also more likely to have chosen a firearm as a suicide method (151, 256, 257). Alcohol intoxication at the time of suicide may also be more common in younger individuals (154, 255, 258), in men (121, 255), and in individuals without any lifetime history of psychiatric treatment (154). Among suicide attempters who later died by suicide, alcohol appeared to contribute to death in more than a third (259). In addition, a study of the interaction of employment and weekly patterns of suicide emphasizes the role of intoxication in suicides and indicates that employment may be a stabilizing factor that curbs heavy drinking during the work week (260), thereby decreasing rates of suicide. Consequently, in some subsets of patients, alcohol consumption appears to contribute to the decision to die by suicide (255).

Alcohol use is also a common prelude to suicide attempts (258). Some estimates show that more than 50% of individuals have used alcohol just before their suicide attempt. Among alcoholics, heavier drinking adds to risk (64, 149, 165). Suicide attempts that involve alcohol are more likely to be impulsive (258). Indeed, the majority of acutely intoxicated alcoholics either did not remember the reason for their attempt or had done it on a sudden impulse (258). Thus, alcohol consumption may make intervention more difficult by simultaneously limiting the communication of intent (255, 261), increasing impulsivity, decreasing inhibition, and impairing judgment (262).

Alcohol use in conjunction with attempted suicide is more common in men than in women (258), although among younger attempters, females may be more likely than males to consume alcohol (258). Alcohol use in conjunction with a suicide attempt has also been associated with repeated suicide attempts and future suicide (263). In some individuals, intentionally drinking to overcome ambivalence about suicide may signify serious suicidal intent. Thus, since intoxication is a risk factor for suicide attempts as well as for suicide, the clinician should inquire about a patient's drinking habits and consider the effect of alcohol intoxication when estimating suicide risk.

b) Past suicide attempts

Individuals who have made a suicide attempt constitute a distinct but overlapping population with those who die by suicide. As with individuals who die by suicide, a high preponderance of suicide attempters have one or more axis I or II diagnoses, with major depression and alcohol dependence observed most commonly for axis I and borderline personality disorder observed most commonly for axis II (199, 200, 264). However, suicide attempts are about 10–20 times more prevalent than suicide (265), with lifetime prevalence ranging from 0.7% to 6% per 100,000 in a random sample of U.S. adults (2). Although a substantial percentage of individuals will die on their initial suicide attempt (266), a past suicide attempt is one of the major risk factors for future suicide attempts (164, 267) and for future suicide (64, 78, 79, 266, 268–271).

After a suicide attempt, there can be significant mortality from both natural and unnatural causes (259, 272). A suicide attempt by any method is associated with a 38-fold increase in suicide risk, a rate that is higher than that associated with any psychiatric disorder (64). Depending on the length of the follow-up, from 6% to 27.5% of those who attempt suicide will ultimately die by suicide (64, 273), and similar results have been suggested for acts of deliberate self-harm (274). Some studies have found that suicide risk appears to be particularly high during the first year after a suicide attempt (259, 275). An additional increase in risk may be associated with aborted suicide attempts (276, 277) or repeated suicide attempts (64, 259, 263, 272, 274, 278). Thus, the increase in suicide mortality subsequent to attempted suicide emphasizes the need for aftercare planning in this heterogeneous population.

In the context of a suicide attempt, a number of other factors are associated with increases in suicide risk. For example, risk is augmented by medical and psychiatric comorbidity, particularly comorbid depression, alcohol abuse, or a long-standing medical illness (64). Low levels of social cohesion may also increase risk (64). Risk of later suicide in males, particularly younger males, appears to be two to four times greater than that in females after a suicide attempt (275). In addition, serious suicide attempts are associated with a higher risk of eventual suicide, as are having high intent (164), taking measures to avoid discovery, and using more lethal methods that resulted in physical injuries (263).

Given this increased likelihood of additional suicide attempts and suicide deaths after a suicide attempt or aborted suicide attempt, psychiatric evaluation should be incorporated into emergency medical assessments of suicide attempters (279) and the importance of follow-up should be emphasized (2, 280).

c) History of childhood physical and/or sexual abuse

A history of childhood abuse has been associated with increased rates of suicidal behaviors in multiple studies. Rates of suicide in individuals with a history of childhood abuse have not been widely studied, but available evidence suggests that suicide rates are increased at least 10-fold in those with a history of childhood abuse (36). In addition, a number of studies have demonstrated that individuals with a history of childhood abuse have an increased risk of suicide attempts (230, 281–283), suggesting that risk of later suicide will also be increased. Rates of suicide attempts are increased in individuals who report experiencing childhood physical abuse (196, 250, 284–290) as well as in individuals who report experiencing childhood sexual abuse (33, 35, 36, 164, 196, 250, 284, 285, 288–294). Rates of suicidal ideation are similarly increased in individuals with a childhood history of abuse (284).

Since many traumatized individuals have experienced both sexual and physical abuse during childhood, it is often difficult to establish the specific contributions of each form of abuse to the risk of suicide and other suicidal behaviors. In addition, the duration and severity of childhood abuse vary across individuals and can also influence risk. It appears, however, that the risk of suicide attempts is greater in individuals who have experienced both physical and sexual abuse in childhood (288) and that greater levels of risk are associated with increasing abuse severity (285, 286, 291).

Childhood trauma can also be associated with increased self-injurious behaviors, including self-cutting and self-mutilation, without associated suicidal intent. Sexual abuse may be a particular risk factor for such behaviors, which can often become repetitive (164). Indeed, deliberate self-harm is common in patients with posttraumatic stress disorder and other traumatic disorders and serves to reduce internal tension and provide nonverbal communication about their self-hate and intense distress (295). As a result, inquiring about the motivations of self-injurious behavior may help to inform estimates of suicide risk.

Gender may also influence the risk of suicidal behaviors in those with a history of childhood abuse. This influence, in part, relates to differences in the prevalence of childhood abuse between men and women, with rates of childhood physical abuse being higher in men and rates of childhood sexual abuse being higher in women (288). However, in individuals who have a history of childhood sexual abuse, the risk of a suicide attempt may be greater in men than in women (33).

Given the significant rates of childhood physical and/or sexual abuse, particularly among psychiatric patient populations (35, 284, 288, 292), and the increased risk for suicidal behaviors that such abuse confers, it important to assess for a history of physical abuse and sexual abuse as part of the psychiatric evaluation. In addition, the duration and severity of childhood abuse should be determined, as these factors will also influence risk.

d) History of domestic partner violence

Domestic partner violence has been associated with increased rates of suicide attempts and suicidal ideation; however, there is no information about its effects on risk for suicide per se. The risk for suicide attempts in individuals who have experienced recent domestic partner violence has been estimated to be four- to eightfold greater than the risk for individuals without such experiences (34, 296–300). Conversely, among women presenting with suicide attempts, there is a severalfold increase in their risk for experiencing domestic partner violence (230, 301).

Although much more commonly experienced by women, domestic partner violence is also experienced by men and can increase their risk for suicide attempts (302). Men with a history of domestic violence toward their partners may also be at increased risk for suicide (303). Furthermore, domestic violence in the home may increase the risk for suicide attempts among children who are witnesses to such violence (281).

Given the clear increase in risk for suicide attempts in individuals experiencing domestic partner violence and the likely association of suicide attempts with an increased risk for suicide, it is important to specifically ask about domestic partner violence as a part of the suicide assessment. Such inquiry may also help to identify individuals in addition to the identified patient who may be at increased risk for suicidal behaviors.

e) Treatment history

Multiple studies have shown that greater treatment intensity is associated with greater rates of eventual suicide (64, 77, 198). Although hospitalization generally occurs because a patient has a more severe illness and is deemed to be at increased risk for suicide, for some patients, hospitalization could conceivably result in increased distress and thus an increase in suicide risk. Thus, as a general rule, a past history of treatment, including a past history of hospitalization, should be viewed as a marker that alerts the clinician to increased suicide risk.

Temporally, the risk for suicide appears to be greatest after changes in treatment setting or intensity (304), with recently admitted and recently discharged inpatients showing increased risk (64, 72, 91, 95, 305–308). This increase in rates of suicide after hospital discharge is seen across diagnostic categories and has been observed in individuals with major depressive disorder, bipolar disorder, schizophrenia, and borderline personality disorder. Rates decline with time since discharge but may remain high for as long as several years (91, 306, 309). Similar findings are seen with suicide attempts, which are also more frequent in the period after hospitalization (267, 305, 308). These observations suggest a need for close follow-up during the period immediately after discharge.

f) Illness course and severity

In some psychiatric disorders, suicide risk is greater at certain points in the illness or episode course. For example, in the course of major depressive disorder, suicidality tends to occur early, often before a diagnosis has been made or treatment has begun (304, 310–312). In patients with major depressive disorder (73, 313), as well as in those with bipolar disorder (73, 74, 305) or schizophrenia (83), suicide has been noted to be more likely during the first few episodes, early in the illness (314, 315). After a suicide attempt, the risk for suicide is also greatest initially, with most suicides occurring in the first year after the attempt (275). Although risks of suicide and suicide attempts later in the illness course are less than they are earlier on, these risks remain greater than those for the general population (74, 100, 316–318). These findings highlight the need for early identification of these disorders and for therapeutic approaches that will treat the illness while simultaneously promoting longer-term treatment adherence.

Risk may also vary with severity of symptoms. For example, higher levels of depression have been associated with increased risk of suicide in at least one study (319), whereas greater numbers of symptoms of borderline personality disorder have been associated with an increased risk for suicide attempts (195). In addition, higher levels of suicidal ideation and subjective hopelessness also increase risk for suicide (78) and suicide attempts (31). In contrast, higher levels of negative symptoms have been associated with decreased suicide risk in individuals with schizophrenia (320). It is also important to recognize that other factors such as age will modulate the effects of symptom severity on risk. With older adults, for example, milder symptoms may be associated with greater risk than moderate symptoms in younger adults (207, 321). Consequently, clinicians should consider the severity of a patient's illness and psychiatric symptoms in the context of other patient-specific factors when assessing suicide risk.

5. Physical illness

Identification of medical illness (axis III) is also an essential part of the assessment process. Such diagnoses will need to be considered in developing a plan of treatment, and they may influence suicide risk in several ways. First, specific medical disorders may themselves be associated with an increased risk for suicide. Alternatively, the physiological effects of illness or its treatment may lead to the development of psychiatric syndromes such as depression, which may also increase suicide risk. Physical illnesses are also a source of social and/or psychological stress, which in turn augments risk. Physical illnesses such as hepatitis C or sexually transmitted diseases may signal an increased likelihood of impulsive behaviors or comorbid substance use disorders that may in turn be associated with greater risk for suicidal behaviors. Finally, when physical illness is present, psychiatric signs and symptoms may be ascribed to comorbid medical conditions, delaying recognition and treatment of the psychiatric disorder.

Data from clinical cohort and record linkage studies indicate clearly that medical illness is associated with increased likelihood of suicide (Table 7). Not surprisingly, disorders of the nervous system are associated with an elevated risk for suicide. The association between seizure disorders and increased suicide risk is particularly strong and consistently observed (64, 322–328). Presumably because of its close association with impulsivity, mood disorders, and psychosis, temporal lobe epilepsy is associated with increased risk in most (322, 327, 328) but not all (325) studies. Suicide attempts are also more common among individuals with epilepsy (329–

TABLE 7. Risk of Suicide in Persons With Physical Disorders[a]

Disorder	Number of Studies	Standardized Mortality Ratio (SMR)[b]
AIDS	1	6.58
Epilepsy	12	5.11
Spinal cord injury	1	3.82
Brain injury	5	3.50
Huntington's chorea	4	2.90
Cancer	1	1.80

[a]Based on a meta-analysis by Harris and Barraclough (64) of 249 reports published between 1966 and 1993. Table adapted with permission.

[b]The SMR is the ratio of the observed mortality to the expected mortality and approximates the risk of mortality resulting from suicide in the presence of a particular disorder.

331). Other neurological disorders that are associated with increased risk for suicide include multiple sclerosis, Huntington's disease, and brain and spinal cord injury (25, 323, 332–334).

Other medical disorders that have also been associated with an increased risk for suicide include HIV/AIDS (25, 335, 336), malignancies (especially of the head and neck) (25, 333, 337, 338), peptic ulcer disease (25), systemic lupus erythematosus (25), chronic hemodialysis-treated renal failure (339), heart disease (337), and, in men, chronic obstructive pulmonary disease and prostate disease (337). In contrast, studies have not demonstrated increased suicide risk in patients with amyotrophic lateral sclerosis (ALS), blindness, cerebrovascular disease, hypertension, rheumatoid arthritis, or diabetes mellitus (25, 337).

Beyond the physical illness itself, functional impairments (321, 333, 338), pain (340–342), disfigurement, increased dependence on others, and decreases in sight (333) and hearing increase suicide risk. Furthermore, in many instances, the risk for suicide associated with a medical disorder is mediated by psychiatric symptoms or illness (321, 342, 343). Indeed, suicidality is rarely seen in individuals with serious physical illness in the absence of clinically significant mood disturbance. Finally, the risk for suicide or suicide attempts may also be affected by characteristics of the individual patient, including gender, coping style, availability of social supports, presence of psychosocial stressors, previous history of suicidal behaviors, and the image and meaning to the individual of the illness itself.

6. Family history

In individuals with a history of suicide among relatives, the risk of suicidal behaviors is increased, apparently through genetic as well as environmental effects. An increased relative risk for suicide or suicide attempts in close relatives of suicidal subjects has been demonstrated repeatedly (31, 82, 202, 214, 312, 344–364). Overall, it appears that the risk of suicidal behaviors among family members of suicidal individuals is about 4.5 times that observed in relatives of nonsuicidal subjects (365–368; R. Baldessarini, personal communication, 2002). Furthermore, this increase in the risk of suicidal behaviors among family members seems, at least in part, to be independent of genetic contributions from comorbid psychiatric diagnoses (355, 361, 367, 368).

Twin studies also provide strong support for the role of a specific genetic factor for suicidal behaviors (365, 368, 369), since there is substantially higher concordance of suicide and suicide attempts in identical twins, compared with fraternal twin pairs (370–375). Adoption studies substantiate the genetic aspect of suicide risk in that there is a greater risk of suicidal behavior among biologic than among adopted relatives of individuals with suicidal behavior or depression (376–378).

Despite the fact that family, twin, and adoption methods provide highly suggestive evidence of heritable factors in risk of suicide as well as some evidence for nonlethal suicidal behavior, the mode of transmission of this genetic risk remains obscure. Thus far, molecular genetic approaches have not yielded consistent or unambiguous evidence of a specific genetic basis for suicide risk (16). In addition, genetic associations with suicide risk may be confounded by the heritability of other factors such as mood disorders or substance use disorder that are also associated with increased risk for suicidal behaviors.

7. Psychosocial factors

a) Employment

Unemployment has long been associated with increased rates of suicide (379, 380). In recent case-control and longitudinal studies, higher rates of unemployment have been consistently noted in suicide attempters (78, 149, 361, 381–383) and in persons who died by suicide (24, 190, 384, 385). Compared with individuals in control groups, unemployed persons have a two- to fourfold greater risk for suicide. Risk is particularly elevated in those under age 45 and in the years closest to job loss, with even greater and longer-lasting effects noted in women (24). Parallel increases in rates of suicide and suicide attempts are also seen in socioeconomically deprived geographical areas, which have larger numbers of unemployed people (386).

For many individuals, unemployment occurs concomitantly with other factors that affect the risk of suicidal behaviors. For example, with job loss, financial and marital difficulties may increase. Alternatively, factors such as psychiatric illness (380) or adverse childhood experiences (361) may affect rates of suicidal behaviors but also influence the likelihood of gaining and maintaining employment. Thus, while unemployment appears to be associated with some independent increase in risk, a substantial fraction of the increase in risk for suicidal behaviors among unemployed persons can be accounted for by co-occurring factors (361, 381, 384, 385).

Among individuals with alcohol use disorders, particularly those under age 45, unemployment is one of a number of stressors that is a common precipitant to suicide (149, 382, 387). Even in those without substance use disorders, unemployment may result in increased drinking, which in turn may precipitate self-destructive behavior (154). Conversely, in those with substance use disorders, full-time employment protects against suicidal behaviors, a finding that may in part relate to decreases in use of alcohol or other substances during the work week (260). Thus, unemployment may serve as a risk factor for suicide, whereas employment may have protective effects on suicide risks.

b) Religious beliefs

The likelihood of suicide may also vary with religious beliefs as well as with the extent of involvement in religious activities. In general, individuals are less likely to act on suicidal thoughts when they have a strong religious faith and believe that suicide is morally wrong or sinful. Similar findings of low suicide rates are found in cultures with strong religious beliefs that the body is sacred and not to be damaged intentionally. In the United States, Catholics have the lowest rate of suicide, followed by Jews, then Protestants (388). Among other religious groups, Islamic tradition has consistently regarded suicide as morally wrong, and some Islamic countries have legal sanctions for attempted suicide (389, 390). In some countries, suicide rates among Muslims appear to be greater than those among Hindus (391, 392), although suicide rates across countries do not appear to vary with the proportion of Muslims in the population (393).

Additional evidence suggests that it is the strength of the religious beliefs and not the specific religion per se that alters suicide rates (43, 394–398). In the African American community, for example, religion is viewed as a source of social solidarity and hope (22). Religious involvement may also help to buffer acculturative stress, which is associated with depression and suicidal ideation (43). The religious belief system itself and the practice of spiritual techniques may also decrease suicide risk by acting as a coping mechanism and providing a source of hope and purpose.

Although protective effects can be afforded by religious beliefs, this is not invariably the case. For example, suicide may be more likely to occur among cultures in which death by suicide is a traditionally accepted way of dealing with distress or in religions that deemphasize the boundaries between the living and the dead. Particularly for adolescents, belief in an afterlife may lead to suicide in an effort to rejoin a deceased loved one. Thus, it is important to gain an understanding of the specific religious beliefs and religious involvement of individuals and also to inquire how these religious beliefs relate to thoughts and conceptions of suicide.

c) Psychosocial support

The presence of a social support system is another factor that may reduce suicide risk (399, 400). Consequently, communicating with members of the patient's support network may be important in assessing and helping to strengthen social supports (see Section V.C, "Communication With Significant Others"). Although social supports typically include family members or friends, individuals may also receive support from other sources. For example, those in the military and those who belong to religious, community, or self-help organizations may receive support through these affiliations.

In addition to determining whether a support system is present, the clinician should assess the patient's perception of available social supports. Individuals who report having more friends and less subjective loneliness are less likely to have suicidal ideation or engage in suicidal behaviors (401). By the same token, if other social supports are not available, living alone may increase suicide risk (149, 385, 402), although this is not invariably true (343, 403, 404). Family discord, other relationship problems, and social isolation may also increase risk (403, 405, 406). Risk of suicidal behaviors may also increase when an individual rightly or wrongly fears that an interpersonal loss will occur (149). Thus, in estimating suicide risk, the clinician should assess the patient's support network as well as his or her perception of available social supports.

d) Reasons for living, including children in the home

An additional protective factor against suicidal behaviors is the ability to cite reasons for living (231, 407), which reflects the patient's degree of optimism about life. A sense of responsibility to family, particularly children, is a commonly cited reason for living that makes suicide a less viable option to escape from pain. The presence of children in the home as well as the number of children appear to decrease the risk for suicide in women (26, 47). Although less well-studied, a smaller effect on suicide potential may also be present in men who have children under age 18 within the home (408). Thus, knowledge of the patient's specific reasons for living, including information about whether there are children in the home, can help inform estimates of suicide risk.

e) Individual psychological strengths and vulnerabilities

Estimates of suicide risk should also incorporate an assessment of the patient's strengths and vulnerabilities as an individual. For example, healthy and well-developed coping skills may buffer stressful life events, decreasing the likelihood of suicidal actions (409). Conversely, lifelong patterns of problematic coping skills are common among those who die by suicide (410). Such factors may be particularly important in patients with substance use or personality disorders, for whom heightened suicide risk may be associated with life stressors or interpersonal loss.

In addition to the diagnosis of categorical axis II disorders, as discussed elsewhere, dimensional and trait approaches to personality can also inform estimates of suicide risk. Although the positive correlation value of individual personality traits with suicide is low, increased suicide risk may be associated with antisocial traits (411) as well as with hostility, helplessness/dependency, and social disengagement/self-consciousness (246).

Extensive clinical literature and clinical consensus support the role of psychodynamics in assessing a patient's risk for suicidal behavior (409, 410, 412–419). Suicide may have multiple motivations such as anger turned inward or a wish of death toward others that is redirected toward the self. Other motivations include revenge, reunion, or rebirth. Another key psychodynamic concept is the interpretation of suicide as rooted in a triad of motivations: the wish to die, the wish to kill, and the wish to be killed (415). Other clinicians have conceptualized these motivations as escape (the wish to die), anger or revenge (the wish to kill), and guilt (the wish to be killed). The presence of one or several of these motivations can inform the psychiatrist about a patient's suicide risk.

Object relations theories offer important concepts for psychodynamic formulations of suicide. Suicidal behavior has been associated with poor object relations, the inability to maintain a stable, accurate, and emotionally balanced memory of the people in one's life (413). In some cases the wish to destroy the lives of the survivors is a powerful motivator (415, 420). For other individuals, a sadistic internal object is so tormenting that the only possible outcome is to submit to the tormentor through suicide (416, 417).

Other important psychodynamic concepts for the clinician to assess are shame, worthlessness, and impaired self-esteem. Early disturbance in parent-child relationships through failure of empathy or traumatic loss can result in an increased vulnerability to later injuries of self-esteem. These patients are vulnerable to narcissistic injuries, which can trigger psychic pain or uncontrollable negative affects. In these situations some patients may experience thoughts of death as peaceful, believing that their personal reality is emotionally intolerable and that it is possible to end pain by stopping consciousness.

Suicidal individuals are often ambivalent about making a suicidal action. As a result, suicide is less likely if an individual sees alternative strategies to address psychological pain (410). However, certain traits and cognitive styles limit this ability to recognize other options. For example, thought constriction and polarized, all-or-nothing thinking are characterized by rigid thinking and an inability to consider different options and may increase the likelihood of suicide (410, 421–423). Individuals who are high in neuroticism and low in "openness to experience" (affectively blunted and preferring the familiar, practical, and concrete) may also be at greater risk for suicide (424). Perfectionism with excessively high self-expectation is another factor that has been noted in clinical practice to be a possible contributor to suicide risk (425). As already discussed, pessimism and hopelessness may also act in a trait-dependent fashion and further influence individual risk.

In estimating suicide risk it is therefore important for the clinician to appreciate the contributions of patients' individual traits, early or traumatic history, ability to manage affects including psychological pain, past response to stress, current object relations, and ability to use external resources during crises. Identifying these issues may help the psychiatrist in assessing suicide risk. In addition, gaining an empathic understanding of the patient's unique motivations for suicide in the context of past experiences will aid in developing rapport as well as in formulating and implementing a psychotherapeutic plan to reduce suicide risk (410, 412, 421, 426).

8. Degree of suicidality

a) Presence, extent, and persistence of suicidal ideation

Suicidal ideation is an important determinant of risk because it precedes suicide. Moreover, suicidal ideation is common, with an estimated annual incidence of 5.6% (2) and estimated lifetime prevalence of 13.5% (427). Since the majority of individuals with suicidal ideation will not die by suicide, the clinician should consider factors that may increase risk among individuals with suicidal ideation. Although current suicidal ideation increases suicide risk (78, 79), death from suicide is even more strongly correlated with the worst previous suicidal ideation (273, 428). Thus, during the suicide assessment, it is important to determine the presence, magnitude, and persistence of current as well as past suicidal ideation.

In addition to reporting suicidal ideation per se, patients may report thoughts of death that may be nonspecific ("life is not worth living") or specific ("I wish I were dead"). These reports should also be assessed through further questioning since they may serve as a prelude to later development of suicidal ideas or may reflect a sense of pessimism and hopelessness about the future (see Section II.E.3.b, "Hopelessness" [p. 870]). At the same time, individuals with suicidal ideation will often deny such ideas even when asked directly (218, 429–431). Given these associations of suicide with suicidal ideation, the presence of suicidal ideation indicates a need for aggressive intervention. At the same time, since as many as a quarter of suicide attempts occur impulsively (432), the absence of suicidal ideation does not eliminate risk for suicidal behaviors.

b) Presence of a suicide plan and availability of a method

Determining whether or not the patient has developed a suicide plan is a key part of assessing suicide risk. For many patients, the formation of a suicide plan precedes a suicidal act, typically within 1 year of the onset of suicidal ideation (427). A suicide plan entails more than simply a reference to a particular method of harm and includes at least several of the following elements: timing, availability of method, setting, and actions made in furtherance of the plan (procuring a method, "scoping out" the setting, rehearsing the plan in any way). The more detailed and specific the suicide plan, the greater will be the level of risk. Plans that use lethal methods or are formulated to avoid detection are particularly indicative of high risk (433). Access to suicide methods, particularly lethal methods, also increases suicide risk. Even in the absence of a specific suicide plan, impulsive actions may end in suicide if lethal methods are readily accessible. Thus, it is important to determine access to methods for any patient who is at risk for suicide or displays suicidal ideation.

In the United States, geographic variations in rates of firearm suicide parallel variations in the rates of gun ownership (434). Although individuals may opt for a different suicide method when a particular method is otherwise unavailable, studies show some decreases in overall suicide rates with restrictions in access to lethal suicide methods (e.g., domestic gas and paracetamol) (435–437). Men are most likely to use firearms in suicidal acts, but other specific populations at increased risk of using firearms include African Americans, elderly persons, and married women. In adolescents and possibly in other age groups, the presence of firearms may be an independent risk factor for suicide (438). Consequently, if the patient has access to a firearm, the psychiatrist is advised to discuss with and recommend to the patient or a significant other the importance of restricting access to, securing, or removing this and other weapons.

In addition to addressing access to firearms, clinicians should recognize the potential lethality of other suicide methods to which the patient may have access. As with restrictions for firearms, it is important for the psychiatrist to work with the patient, family members, and other social support persons in restricting the patient's access to potentially lethal suicide methods, particularly during periods of enhanced risk. Removal of such methods from a patient's presence does not remove the risk for suicide, but it removes the potential for the patient to impulsively gain access to the means with which to carry out a suicidal wish.

c) Lethality and intent of self-destructive behavior

Suicidal intent refers to the patient's subjective expectation and desire to die as a result of a self-inflicted injury. This expectation may or may not correspond to the lethality of an attempt, which represents the medical likelihood that death will result from use of a given method. For example, some patients may make a nonlethal attempt with the intention of being saved and getting help, whereas others may make a nonlethal attempt, thinking it will kill them. From the standpoint of suicide risk assessment, the strength of the patient's intent to die and his or her subjective belief about the lethality of a method are more relevant than the objective lethality of the chosen method (439, 440). The presence of a suicide note also indicates intensification of a suicidal idea and/or plan and generally signifies premeditation and greater suicidal intent. Regardless of whether the patient has attempted suicide or is displaying suicidal ideation, the clinician should assess the timing and content of any suicide note and discuss its meaning with the patient. The more specifically a note refers to actual suicide or steps to be taken after death, the greater the associated increase in suicidal intent and risk. Factors separating suicide attempters who go on to make future fatal versus nonfatal attempts include an initial attempt with high intent (164, 441), having taken measures to avoid discovery (224), and having used more lethal methods that resulted in physical injuries (263), all of which indicate a greater degree of suicidal intent. Consequently, suicidal intent should be assessed in any patient with suicidal ideation. In addition, for any patient who has made a prior suicide attempt, the level of intent at the time of the suicide attempt should be determined.

F. ADDITIONAL CONSIDERATIONS WHEN EVALUATING PATIENTS IN SPECIFIC TREATMENT SETTINGS

1. Inpatient settings

Patients are often admitted to an inpatient unit in the midst of an acute suicidal crisis with either overt suicidal behavior or intense suicidal ideation. Even when a patient who is not in an acute suicidal crisis is admitted, the symptoms and disorders that typically lead to psychiatric hospitalization are associated with an increased suicide risk. There do not appear to be specific risk factors that are unique to the inpatient setting, with about half of inpatient suicides in a recent study involving individuals with prior suicide attempts and about half occurring in individuals with psychosis (218). Inpatient suicides also cannot be predicted by the reason for hospitalization, since fewer than half of the patients who die by suicide in the hospital were admitted with suicidal ideation and only a quarter were admitted after a suicide attempt. However, extreme agitation or anxiety (218) or a rapidly fluctuating course (442) is common before suicide. Thus, it is important to conduct a suicide risk assessment, as discussed earlier, when individuals are admitted for inpatient treatment, when changes in observation status or treatment setting occur, when there are significant changes in the patient's clinical condition, or when acute psychosocial stressors come to light in the course of the hospitalization. For patients with repeated hospitalizations for suicidality, each suicidal crisis must be treated as new with each admission and assessed accordingly.

2. Outpatient settings

An initial evaluation of a patient in an office-based setting should be comprehensive and include a suicide assessment. The intensity and depth of the suicide assessment will depend on the patient's clinical presentation. In following outpatients over time, the psychiatrist should be aware that suicidality may wax and wane in the course of treatment. Sudden changes in clinical status, which may include worsening or precipitous and unexpected improvements in reported symptoms, require that suicidality be reconsidered. Furthermore, risk may also be increased by the lack of a reliable therapeutic alliance, by the patient's unwillingness to engage in psychotherapy or adhere to medication treatment, or by inadequate family or social supports. Again, however, the frequency, intensity, and depth of the suicide assessment will depend on the patient's clinical state, past history, and other factors, including individual strengths, vulnerabilities, and stressors that will simultaneously influence risk. These factors will also be important in judging when family members or other significant support persons may need to be contacted.

3. Emergency settings

Regardless of the patient's presenting problem, the suicide assessment is an integral part of the psychiatric evaluation in an emergency setting. As in the inpatient setting, substantial numbers of individuals present to emergency settings with suicidal ideation or after having made a suicide attempt (443–447). Even when suicidality is not a part of the initial presentation, the majority of individuals seen in emergency psychiatric settings have diagnoses that are associated with an increased risk of suicide (268, 269, 271, 275, 448).

As the suicide assessment proceeds, the psychiatrist should be alert for previously unrecognized symptoms of trauma or toxicity resulting from ingestions. Ambivalence is a key element in individuals presenting with suicidality, and individuals may simultaneously seek help yet withhold information about recent ingestions (449) or self-induced trauma. Thus, in addition to initially assessing the patient's vital signs, the psychiatrist should investigate any changes in the patient's physical condition or level of consciousness that may develop during the course of the evaluation. For patients who are administered medications in the emergency area or who have concomitant alcohol or substance use, serial monitoring of vital signs is important to detect adverse events or signs of substance withdrawal.

Simultaneous presentation with intoxication and suicidality is common in emergency settings (444, 450–454) and requires some modification in the assessment process. Depending on the severity of the intoxication, medical intervention may be needed before psychiatric assessment begins. Also, it is often necessary to maintain the patient in a safe setting until the intoxication resolves and a thorough suicide assessment can be done. In this regard, some institutions find it helpful to quantify the level of intoxication (with serum alcohol levels or breath alcohol measurements), since some individuals may not show physical symptoms of intoxication despite substantially elevated blood alcohol concentrations (455). At some facilities, short-term observation beds are available in the emergency area or elsewhere for monitoring and serial assessments of intoxicated individuals who present with suicidality. At other facilities, such observation may need to be carried out in a more typical medical or psychiatric inpatient setting.

Although obtaining collateral information is useful with all suicidal individuals, in the emergency setting such information is particularly important to obtain from involved family members, from those who live with the patient, and from professionals who are currently treating the patient. Patients in emergency settings may not always share all of the potentially relevant aspects of their recent symptoms and their past psychiatric history, including treatment adherence. In addition, most psychiatrists who evaluate patients in emergency settings do not have the benefit of knowing and working with the patient on a longitudinal basis. Corroboration of history is particularly important when aspects of the clinical picture do not correspond to other aspects of the patient's history or mental state. Examples include patients who deny suicidal ideas and request discharge yet who made a highly lethal suicide attempt with clear suicidal intent or those who request admission on the basis of command hallucinations while seeming relaxed and jovial and without appearing to respond to internal stimuli.

The process by which the patient arrived at the emergency department can provide helpful information about his or her insight into having an illness or needing treatment. Typically, individuals who are self-referred have greater insight than those who are brought to the hospital by police or who reluctantly arrive with family members. For individuals who are brought to the emergency department by police (or as a result of a legally defined process such as an emergency petition), it is particularly important to address the reasons for the referral in estimating suicide risk.

4. Long-term care facilities

When evaluating patients in long-term care facilities, psychiatrists and staff should be aware of the varied forms that suicidality may take in such settings. In particular, it is important to recognize that indirect self-destructive acts are found among both men and women with chronic medical conditions (456–459) and are a common manifestation of suicide in institutional settings (460). Despite these occurrences, suicide rates in long-term care facilities are generally lower than expected (460, 461), perhaps as a result of greater supervision and residents' limited access to potentially lethal means and physical inability to carry out the act as well as underreporting or misattribution of self-destructive behaviors to accident or natural death (66).

Risk factors for suicide and other self-destructive behaviors are similar to those assessed in other settings of care. For example, 90% or more of randomly sampled residents of long-term care facilities have been shown to have a diagnosable psychiatric illness (462, 463), with the prevalence of depression in nursing homes estimated to range from 15% to 50% (66). Physical illness, functional impairment, and pain are associated with increased risk for suicide and are ubiquitous factors in long-term care facilities. Hopelessness (228) and personality styles that impede adaptation to a dependent role in the institutional setting also play a role (464).

When treating individuals in long-term care facilities, the psychiatrist should be mindful of the need for follow-up assessments, even when initial evaluation does not show evidence of depression or increased risk for suicide or other self-injurious behaviors. To facilitate early intervention, safety and suicide risk should be reassessed with significant changes in behavior, psychiatric symptoms, medical status, and/or level of functional disability. Psychiatrists can also play a critical role in educating long-term care providers about risk factors and warning signs for suicide in residents under their care.

5. Jail and correctional facilities

In jails, prisons, and other correctional facilities, most initial mental health assessments are not done by psychiatrists (465, 466); however, psychiatrists are often asked to perform urgent suicide assessments for individuals identified as being at risk. The actual rates of suicide in jails and in prisons are somewhat controversial, and reported rates depend on the method by which they are calculated (467). The U.S. Department of Justice Bureau of Justice Statistics reported that the rate of suicide per 100,000 prison inmates was 14 during 1999, compared with 55 per 100,000 jail inmates (468). However, reported rates are generally based on the average daily census of the facility. Since jails are local facilities used for the confinement of persons awaiting trial and those convicted of minor crimes, whereas prisons are usually under state control and are used to confine persons serving sentences for serious crimes, jails have a much more rapid turnover of detainees than prisons. This turnover results in a higher reported rate of suicides per 100,000 incarcerated persons in jails relative to prisons, since annual jail admissions are more than 20 times the average daily jail census, whereas the annual number of persons admitted to prisons nationwide is about 50% of the average daily prison census. Reported suicide rates in jails are also elevated relative to those in prisons because the majority of suicides in jail occur during the first 24 hours of incarceration (469, 470).

The importance of identification and assessment of individuals at increased risk for suicide is underscored by the fact that suicide is one of the leading causes of death in correctional settings. For example, from July 1, 1998, to June 30, 1999, natural causes other than AIDS barely led suicide as the leading cause of death in jails. Between 1995 and 1999, suicide was the third leading cause of death in prisons, after natural causes other than AIDS and deaths due to AIDS (468). In relative terms, suicides among youths in juvenile detention and correctional facilities are about four times more frequent, suicide rates for men in jails are about nine to 15 times greater, and the suicide rate in prisons is about one-and-a-half times greater than the suicide rate in the general population (471).

Factors that increase risk in other populations are very prevalent and contribute to increased risk in correctional populations (472, 473). Persons who die by suicide in jails have been consistently shown to be young, white, single, intoxicated individuals with a history of substance abuse (470, 474–476). Suicide in correctional facilities generally occurs by hanging, with bed clothing most commonly used (470, 474, 476–478). It is not clear whether first-time nonviolent offenders (474, 476) or violent offenders (473, 477) are at greater risk. Most (473, 474, 476, 479) but not all (480) investigators have reported that isolation may increase suicide in correctional facilities and should be avoided. While inmates may become suicidal anytime during their incarceration, there are times when the risks of suicidal behavior may be heightened. Experience has shown that suicidal behaviors increase immediately on entry into the facility, after new legal complications with the inmate's case (e.g., denial of parole), after inmates receive bad news about loved ones at home, or after sexual assault or other trauma (471).

There is little doubt that successful implementation of suicide prevention programs results in a significantly decreased suicide rate in correctional facilities (469, 481–483). Consequently, the standards of the National Commission on Correctional Health Care (NCCHC) require jails and prisons to have a written policy and defined procedures for identifying and responding to suicidal inmates, including procedures for training, identification, monitoring, referral, evaluation, housing, communication, intervention, notification, reporting, review, and critical incident stress debriefing (484, 485). Other useful resources include a widely used instrument for suicide screening (486) and the detailed discussions of specific approaches to suicidal detainees that are provided in a later NCCHC publication (487).

III. PSYCHIATRIC MANAGEMENT

Psychiatric management consists of a broad array of interventions and approaches that should be instituted by psychiatrists for all patients with suicidal behaviors. Psychiatric management serves as the framework by which the patient and psychiatrist will collaborate in the ongoing processes of assessing and monitoring the patient's clinical status, choosing among specific treatments, and coordinating the various treatment components. Psychiatric management includes establishing and maintaining a therapeutic alliance; attending to the patient's safety; and determining the patient's psychiatric status, level of functioning, and clinical needs to arrive at a plan and setting for treatment. For individuals with suicidal behaviors, such treatment planning will encompass interventions targeted to suicidality per se as well as therapeutic approaches designed to address psychosocial or interpersonal difficulties and any axis I and axis II disorders that may be present. Once a plan of treatment has been established with the patient, additional goals of psychiatric management include facilitating treatment adherence and providing education to patients and, when indicated, family members and significant others.

A. ESTABLISH AND MAINTAIN A THERAPEUTIC ALLIANCE

Beginning with the initial encounter with the patient, the psychiatrist should attempt to build trust, establish mutual respect, and develop a therapeutic relationship with the patient. Suicidal ideation and behaviors can be explored and addressed within the context of this cooperative doctor-patient relationship, with the ultimate goal of reducing suicide risk. This relationship also provides a context in which additional psychiatric symptoms or syndromes can be evaluated and treated. At the same time, the psychiatrist should recognize that an individual who is determined to die may not be motivated to develop a cooperative doctor-patient relationship and indeed may view the psychiatrist as an adversary. Appreciating the patient's relationship to and with significant others can help inform the clinician about the patient's potential to form a strong therapeutic relationship. In addition, the therapeutic alliance can be enhanced by paying careful attention to the concerns of patients and their family members as well as their wishes for treatment. Empathy (488, 489) and understanding of the suicidal individual (488–491) are also important in establishing a therapeutic psychiatrist-patient relationship, helping the patient feel emotionally supported, and increasing the patient's sense of possible choices other than suicide (492). In this manner, a positive and cooperative psychotherapeutic relationship can be an invaluable and even life-sustaining force for suicidal patients.

In caring for potentially suicidal patients, the psychiatrist will need to manage the often competing goals of encouraging the patient's independence yet simultaneously addressing safety. In addition, the psychiatrist should be aware of his or her own emotions and reactions to the suicidal patient that may influence the patient's care (488). Psychiatrists should acknowledge the unique place that they may hold in a patient's life, often seeming to be the only source of stability or consistency. At the same time, the clinician must guard against falling into the role of constant savior (490, 491). Suicidal patients may wish to be taken care of unconditionally (493, 494) or alternatively, to assign others the responsibility for keeping them alive (490). Therapists who are drawn into the role of savior with suicidal patients often operate on the conscious or unconscious assumption that they can provide the love and concern that others have not, thus magically transforming the patient's wish to die into a desire to live (420, 490). Under such circumstances, or if the therapist uses defensive reaction formation to deny hostile feelings toward the patient, the therapist may go to great lengths to assure the patient that he or she has only positive feelings about the patient and will do whatever is necessary to save the patient's life. In the worst-case scenario, this need to demonstrate one's caring may contribute to boundary crossings or outright boundary violations (495). Also, by producing false or unrealistic hopes, the psychiatrist may ultimately disappoint the patient by not fulfilling those expectations. Thus, the psychiatrist must remember that taking responsibility for a patient's care is not the same as taking responsibility for a patient's life.

Suicidal patients can also activate a clinician's own latent emotions about death and suicide, leading to a number of defensive responses on the part of the clinician (426). On one hand, there is a potential to develop countertransference hate and anger at suicidal patients (496) that may be manifested by rejecting behavior on the part of the clinician (488). At the other extreme, the clinician may avoid patients who bring up his or her own anxieties surrounding suicide (426, 490). Clinicians may also overestimate the patient's capabilities, creating unrealistic and overwhelming expectations for the patient. Conversely, they may become enveloped by the patient's sense of hopelessness and despair and become discouraged about the progress of treatment and the patient's capacity to improve (488). Thus, management of the therapeutic alliance should include an awareness of transference and countertransference issues, regardless of the theoretical approach used for psychotherapy and regardless of whether these issues are directly addressed in treatment. In this regard, the use of consultation with a senior colleague with experience and some expertise in the management of suicidal patients may be helpful. It is also important to keep in mind that the course and conduct of treatment may be influenced by gender and cultural differences between patients and therapists as well as by cultural differences between patients and other aspects of the care delivery system.

B. ATTEND TO THE PATIENT'S SAFETY

Although it is impossible to prevent all self-injurious actions including actual suicide, it is critically important to attend to the patient's safety and work to minimize self-endangering behaviors throughout the evaluation and treatment process. The preceding sections have discussed an orderly process for assessing the patient, estimating suicide risk, and then instituting interventions to target that risk. In actual practice, however, some interventions may be needed to address the patient's safety while the initial evaluation proceeds. For example, in emergency or inpatient settings, specific interventions may include ordering observation of the patient on a one-to-one basis or by continuous closed-circuit television monitoring, removing potentially hazardous items from the patient's room, and securing the patient's belongings (since purses and backpacks may contain weapons, cigarette lighters or matches, and medications or other potentially toxic substances). If restraints are indicated, continuous observation is also recommended (497, 498). Some institutions screen patients for potentially dangerous items by searching patients or scanning them with metal detectors (499). In addition, some institutions have policies prohibiting any guns in emergency areas, since police or security officers' weapons may be taken by suicidal patients. In other circumstances, such as with agitated, uncooperative, intoxicated, or medically ill patients, significant time may elapse before it will be possible to complete a full psychiatric evaluation, including a suicide assessment. Under such conditions, the psychiatrist will need to use the information that is available to make a clinical judgment, with steps being taken to enhance the patient's safety in the interim.

C. DETERMINE A TREATMENT SETTING

Treatment settings include a continuum of possible levels of care, from involuntary hospitalizations to partial hospital and intensive outpatient programs to more typical ambulatory settings. In general, patients should be treated in the setting that is least restrictive yet most likely to prove safe and effective. In addition, the optimal treatment setting and the patient's ability to benefit from a different level of care should be reevaluated on an ongoing basis throughout the course of treatment.

The choice of an appropriate site of treatment will generally occur after the psychiatrist evaluates the patient's clinical condition, including specific psychiatric disorder(s) and symptoms (e.g., hopelessness, impulsiveness, anxiety), symptom severity, level of functioning, available support system, and activities that give the patient a reason to live. The psychiatrist should also consider whether or not the current suicidality is related to an interpersonal crisis such as a recent separation, loss of a loved one, or other trauma. The estimate of suicide risk will obviously be an important component of the choice of treatment setting, and the potential for dangerousness to others should also be taken into consideration. Under some clinical circumstances, a decision for hospitalization may need to be made on the basis of high potential dangerousness to self or others, even if additional history is unavailable or if the patient is unable to cooperate with the psychiatric evaluation (e.g., in the presence of extreme agitation, psychosis, or catatonia). At the same time, the benefits of intensive interventions such as hospitalization must be weighed against their possible negative effects (e.g., disruption of employment, financial and other psychosocial stress, persistent societal stigma). Other aspects to be incorporated into the determination of a treatment setting include the patient's ability to provide adequate self-care, understand the risks and benefits of various treatment approaches, understand what to do in a crisis (e.g., contact family members or other support persons, contact the psychiatrist, seek emergency care), give reliable feedback to the psychiatrist, and cooperate with treatment planning and implementation. Consequently, choice of a specific treatment setting will not depend entirely on the estimate of suicide risk but rather will rely on the balance between these various elements. An overview of factors to consider in determining a setting for treatment is provided in Table 8.

Hospitalization should always be viewed as a possible intervention and should be considered whenever the patient's safety is in question. Hospitalization, by itself, is not a treatment. Rather, it is a treatment setting that may facilitate the evaluation and treatment of a suicidal person. In addition, inpatient settings can implement approaches such as constant observation, seclusion, or physical or pharmacological restraint that may restrict an individual's ability to act on suicidal impulses. Although such interventions may delay suicide and permit initiation of treatment approaches, there is no empirical evidence that these methods reduce the incidence of suicide in the long term (77, 500, 501). In addition, hospitals must balance requirements for security against the patient's need to prepare to return to independent living in the community. Since patients cannot be continuously observed or restrained, they can and do die by suicide while hospitalized. In fact, it is estimated that approximately 1,500 inpatient suicides occur in the United States each year, with about a third of these occurring while patients are on one-to-one observation or every-15-minute checks (218).

Although no guidelines regarding hospitalization decisions can be absolute, inpatient care is usually indicated for individuals who are considered to pose a serious threat of harm to themselves or others. Other indications for hospitalization include factors based on illness (e.g., symptom severity, violent or uncontrollable behavior) and those based on the intensity of services needed (e.g., a need for continuous skilled observation; complicated medication trials, particularly for an elderly or a medically fragile patient; ECT; clinical tests or diagnostic evaluation that cannot be performed on an outpatient basis). Severely ill individuals may require hospitalization if they cannot be maintained safely in a less restrictive environment or if they lack adequate structure and social support outside of a hospital setting. More intensive treatment will also be called for whenever there is a new, acute presentation that is not part of a repetitive pattern. Additionally, those patients who have complicating psychiatric or general medical conditions or who have not re-

TABLE 8. Guidelines for Selecting a Treatment Setting for Patients at Risk for Suicide or Suicidal Behaviors

Admission generally indicated

After a suicide attempt or aborted suicide attempt if:

- Patient is psychotic
- Attempt was violent, near-lethal, or premeditated
- Precautions were taken to avoid rescue or discovery
- Persistent plan and/or intent is present
- Distress is increased or patient regrets surviving
- Patient is male, older than age 45 years, especially with new onset of psychiatric illness or suicidal thinking
- Patient has limited family and/or social support, including lack of stable living situation
- Current impulsive behavior, severe agitation, poor judgment, or refusal of help is evident
- Patient has change in mental status with a metabolic, toxic, infectious, or other etiology requiring further workup in a structured setting

In the presence of suicidal ideation with:

- Specific plan with high lethality
- High suicidal intent

Admission may be necessary

After a suicide attempt or aborted suicide attempt, except in circumstances for which admission is generally indicated

In the presence of suicidal ideation with:

- Psychosis
- Major psychiatric disorder
- Past attempts, particularly if medically serious
- Possibly contributing medical condition (e.g., acute neurological disorder, cancer, infection)
- Lack of response to or inability to cooperate with partial hospital or outpatient treatment
- Need for supervised setting for medication trial or ECT
- Need for skilled observation, clinical tests, or diagnostic assessments that require a structured setting
- Limited family and/or social support, including lack of stable living situation
- Lack of an ongoing clinician-patient relationship or lack of access to timely outpatient follow-up

In the absence of suicide attempts or reported suicidal ideation/plan/intent but evidence from the psychiatric evaluation and/or history from others suggests a high level of suicide risk and a recent acute increase in risk

Release from emergency department with follow-up recommendations may be possible

After a suicide attempt or in the presence of suicidal ideation/plan when:

- Suicidality is a reaction to precipitating events (e.g., exam failure, relationship difficulties), particularly if the patient's view of situation has changed since coming to emergency department
- Plan/method and intent have low lethality
- Patient has stable and supportive living situation
- Patient is able to cooperate with recommendations for follow-up, with treater contacted, if possible, if patient is currently in treatment

Outpatient treatment may be more beneficial than hospitalization

Patient has chronic suicidal ideation and/or self-injury without prior medically serious attempts, if a safe and supportive living situation is available and outpatient psychiatric care is ongoing sponded adequately to outpatient treatment may need to be hospitalized. Inpatient care may also be necessary at lower levels of suicide risk in geographic areas where partial hospital or intensive outpatient programs are not readily accessible. If the clinician is not the patient's regular health care provider, does not have an ongoing relationship with the patient, or otherwise does not know the patient well and does not have access to the patient's history or medical records, hospitalization may be necessary until further data can be collected. More intensive treatment may also be necessary even for patients with lesser degrees of suicidality if the patient lacks a strong psychosocial support system, is unable to gain timely access to outpatient care, has limited insight into the need for treatment, or is unable to adhere to recommendations for ambulatory follow-up.

The hospital length of stay should similarly be determined by the ability of the patient to receive the needed care safely in a less intensive environment. In addition, before the patient is transitioned to a less restrictive setting, the patient's condition should show evidence of being improved and more stable both in the estimated level of suicide risk and in the symptoms of any associated psychiatric disorders.

Less intensive treatment may be more appropriate if suicidal ideation or attempts are part of a chronic, repetitive cycle and the patient is aware of the chronicity. For such patients, suicidal ideation may be a characteristic response to disappointment or a way to cope with psychological distress. If the patient has a history of suicidal ideation without suicidal intent and an ongoing doctor-patient relationship, the benefits of continued treatment outside the hospital may outweigh the possible detrimental effects of hospitalization even in the presence of serious psychiatric symptoms.

When considering hospitalization, the risk of suicide is not the only factor to take into account. Patients may feel humiliated or frightened in the hospital rather than experience a sense of emotional relief. Hospitalization can also be associated with realistic life stressors, including the social and financial burdens of having received inpatient treatment. For some patients, treatment in a restrictive setting such as an inpatient unit may foster dependency and a regressive, vicious cycle of intensifying suicidal thoughts requiring ever more restrictive care. Such individuals, most notably those with personality disorders, suffer chronic morbidity if they are never supportively challenged to bear painful feelings. In addition, some patients may gain positive reinforcement from hospitalization and repeatedly harm themselves with the goal of regaining admission. Psychiatric hospitalization may also arouse unrealistic expectations in patients, family members, therapists, and medical and nursing staff members. Often, a plea for hospitalization comes from a sense of exasperation on the part of an individual involved with the patient's situation. When hospital treatment does not meet these unrealistic expectations, the associated disillusionment may contribute to hopelessness and have a negative effect on future therapeutic relationships. The inpatient admission process itself may also cause the patient to mistrust mental health professionals, particularly when hospitalization occurs on an involuntary basis. Thus, the clinician's key responsibility is to weigh the risks and benefits of hospitalization before and during admission (especially around decisions related to therapeutic passes and privilege levels) and ultimately when contemplating discharge (502). Moreover, a person's right to privacy and self-determination (which includes the right to be treated in the least restrictive environment) must be balanced against the issue of potential dangerousness to self or others.

If hospitalization is indicated, the psychiatrist must next decide whether it should occur on a voluntary or involuntary basis. This decision will also depend on multiple factors, including the estimated level of risk to the patient and others, the patient's level of insight and willingness to seek care, and the legal criteria for involuntary hospitalization in that jurisdiction. In general, patients at imminent risk for suicide will satisfy the criteria for involuntary hospitalization; however, the specific commitment criteria vary from state to state (503), and in some states, willingness to enter a hospital voluntarily may preclude involuntary admission. To that end, psychiatrists should be familiar with their specific state statutes regarding involuntary hospitalization.

Patients who are not assessed to be at imminent risk for suicide and who do not require inpatient treatment for other reasons may be suitable for treatment on an outpatient basis. Outpatient treatment may vary in its intensity from infrequent office visits for stable patients to more frequent office visits (up to several times per week) to intensive outpatient or partial hospital treatment. Either of the latter settings may function as a "step-down" from inpatient treatment or as a "step-up" from outpatient therapy, if once- or twice-a-week therapy is insufficient to maintain the patient's stabilization. For patients at significant risk for suicide in these treatment programs, a member of the treatment team must be available to respond to emergencies by telephone, beeper, or other means of contact. In military settings, "unit watch" protocols may be activated to look after the patient between treatment sessions. For patients who continue to be followed by an outside therapist or psychiatrist while in a partial hospital or intensive outpatient treatment program, regular communication among treating professionals is important. Communication with significant others is also helpful, and appropriate supervision and supports should be available and may include a plan for continued after-hours monitoring. If such supervision is not possible, a higher level of care (i.e., inpatient admission) may be needed to maintain the patient's safety even at lower levels of suicide risk. Worsening of a patient's condition, with a concomitant increase in the risk of suicide, requires the careful assessment of the patient's risk for suicide and possible hospitalization. Discharge planning should include appropriate continuing treatment to maintain stability gains and to continue monitoring of suicide risk.

Under some circumstances, individuals who are not currently engaged in outpatient treatment may be referred for care after a suicide attempt or emergency department visit in which suicidality was at issue. Since adherence is often a problem when individuals are referred for outpatient follow-up from emergency departments (448, 504), it may be helpful to discuss the referral with the patient during the course of the interview and if possible arrange a specific appointment time (505–507). When determining a treatment setting in emergency situations, it is also important to consider the potential effects of countertransference and lack of knowledge about suicidality on clinical decision making, since individuals who present with suicidal ideas or attempts may engender a broad range of countertherapeutic reactions in medical professionals, including antipathy, anger, helplessness, and indifference (445, 450, 508–510).

D. DEVELOP A PLAN OF TREATMENT

Individuals with suicidal thoughts, plans, or behaviors may benefit from a variety of treatments. If the patient is at risk for suicide, a plan that integrates a range of biological and psychosocial therapies may increase the likelihood of a successful outcome. Choosing among possible treatments requires knowledge of the potential beneficial and adverse effects of each option along with information about the patient's preferences. In addition, treatment decisions should be continually reassessed as new information becomes available, the patient's clinical status changes, or both. For patients in ongoing treatment, this may mean that existing treatment plans will require modification as suicidal ideas or behaviors emerge or wane. Thus, treatment planning is an iterative process in which the psychiatrist works with the patient to implement and modify treatments over time, depending on the patient's responses and preferences. Depending on the clinical circumstances, it may be important for the treatment planning process to include family members or other significant supports (e.g., military unit personnel, community residence or adult home providers, case management staff). More detail on the specific therapeutic approaches discussed subsequently can be found in APA practice guidelines that discuss treatment of specific psychiatric disorders (all included in this volume), including major depressive disorder (511), bipolar disorder (512), schizophrenia (513), panic disorder (514), and borderline personality disorder (515).

Psychiatrists should be cautioned against developing a treatment plan in which the stated goal is to "eliminate" suicide risk; this is impossible to do for the reasons already discussed. Instead, the goals of treatment should include a comprehensive approach to treatment with the major focus directed at reducing risk. Since individuals with suicidal behaviors often have axis I and axis II disorders, reducing risk frequently involves treating an associated psychiatric illness. Given the high rates of comorbid alcohol and substance use among individuals with suicidal behaviors, it is particularly important to address substance use disorders in the treatment plan (516). Medical disorders and treatments for those disorders will also need to be considered in developing a plan of treatment for the patient with suicidal behaviors.

In the early stages of treatment, more intense follow-up may be needed to provide support for the patient as well as to monitor and rapidly institute treatment for relevant symptoms such as anxiety, insomnia, or hopelessness. In addition, it is during the early stages of illness that denial of symptoms and lack of insight into the need for treatment are likely to be most prominent, and, therefore, specific education and supportive psychotherapy are required to target these issues. Appreciating the patient's past responses to stress, vulnerability to life-threatening affects, available external resources, death fantasies, and capacity for reality testing may help the clinician to weigh the strengths and vulnerabilities of the individual patient (412) and may aid in the planning of treatment. For patients treated in ambulatory settings, it is also important for the psychiatrist to review with the patient guidelines for managing exacerbations of suicidal tendencies or other symptoms that may occur between scheduled sessions and could contribute to increased suicide risk.

E. COORDINATE CARE AND COLLABORATE WITH OTHER CLINICIANS

Providing optimal treatment for patients with suicidal behaviors frequently involves a multidisciplinary treatment team that includes several mental health professionals. While ongoing coordination of the overall treatment plan is generally easier to implement in inpatient or partial hospital settings as opposed to less integrated ambulatory settings, useful strategies for coordination in any treatment setting include clear role definitions, regular communication among team members, and advance planning for management of crises. It is also helpful to clarify with the patient that a number of individuals will be involved in his or her care and to outline the specific roles of each. In this regard, it is important for patients to understand that treatment team members assist the psychiatrist in many respects and may supply clinical information that will influence decisions about the level of precautions, readiness for discharge, medications, and other aspects of treatment planning.

Many patients have ongoing medical illnesses for which they receive care from one or more physicians. Particularly for individuals whose medical disorders or treatments interface with their psychiatric symptoms or treatments, it is helpful to communicate with the patient's primary care physician as well as with any specialists who are actively involved in the patient's care.

In inpatient settings, the treatment team generally consists of a psychiatrist, nurses, social workers, psychologists, and other mental health workers, with the psychiatrist acting as the team leader. In this capacity, with input from the other members of the treatment team, the psychiatrist will make the critical decisions regarding the patient's care. Such decisions include but are not limited to the patient's diagnosis, specific medications, level of precautions, passes, discharge, and follow-up treatment plan. Given the key roles and observations of other treatment team members in such decisions, the psychiatrist should encourage open communication among the staff members regarding historical and clinical features of the patient.

In an outpatient setting, there may also be other professionals involved in the care of the patient. In some instances, the patient may be referred to individuals with expertise in symptom-specific treatments (e.g., cognitive behavior therapy for hopelessness or dialectical behavior therapy for recurrent suicidal behavior). In other instances, the psychiatrist may be providing primarily psychopharmacologic management, with another psychiatrist or other mental health professional conducting the psychotherapy. During visits with the patient, it is important for the psychiatrist to review the patient's response to all aspects of the treatment. In addition, it is useful for the psychiatrist to communicate with the therapist and to establish guidelines or expectations as to when and under what conditions the therapist and the psychiatrist should be contacted in the event of a significant clinical change in the patient. Moreover, if the psychiatrist has direct supervisory responsibilities for the therapist, the level of communication should be increased and may include a chart review.

F. PROMOTE ADHERENCE TO THE TREATMENT PLAN

The successful treatment of many psychiatric disorders requires close adherence to treatment plans, in some cases for long or indefinite durations. With individuals whose clinical symptoms include suicidal thoughts, plans, or behaviors, it is particularly important that management be optimized through regular adherence with the treatment plan. Facilitating adherence begins with the initial establishing of the physician-patient relationship and the collaborative development of a plan of care that is attentive to the needs and preferences of the individual patient. Within the therapeutic relationship the psychiatrist should create an atmosphere in which the patient can feel free to discuss what he or she experiences as positive or negative in the treatment process. Side effects or requirements of treatment are common causes of nonadherence. Other common contributors include financial constraints, scheduling or transportation difficulties, perceived differences of opinion with the clinician, and misunderstandings about the recommended plan of treatment or dosing of medications. Especially while symptomatic, patients may be poorly motivated, less able to care for themselves, or unduly pessimistic about their chances of recovery with treatment, or they may suffer from memory deficits or psychosis. In some instances, psychiatric disorders are associated with reductions in insight about having an illness or needing treatment, making adherence less likely. Particularly during maintenance phases of treatment, when symptoms are less salient, patients may tend to undervalue the benefits of treatment and instead focus on its burdens. The psychiatrist should recognize these possibilities, encourage the patient to articulate any concerns regarding adherence, and emphasize the importance of adherence for successful treatment and for minimizing the risk of future suicidal behaviors (306). Specific components of a message to the patient that have been shown to improve adherence include 1) when and how often to take the medicine, 2) the fact that some medications may take several weeks before beneficial effects may be noticed, 3) the need to take medication even after feeling better, 4) the need to consult with the doctor before discontinuing medication, and 5) what to do if problems or questions arise (517).

To facilitate adherence, it is helpful to reassess the treatment plan on a regular basis in collaboration with the patient and attempt to modify it in accord with the patient's preferences and needs. Some patients, particularly elderly patients, have been shown to have improved adherence when both the complexity of medication regimens and the costs of treatments are minimized. When a patient does not appear for appointments or is nonadherent in other ways, outreach, including telephone calls, may be helpful in reengaging the patient in treatment. This outreach can be carried out by the psychiatrist or other designated team members in consultation with the psychiatrist. For patients in an involuntary outpatient treatment program, the judicial system may also be involved in outreach efforts. Severe or persistent problems of nonadherence may represent psychological conflicts or psychopathology, for which psychotherapy should be considered. Educating patients about medications, aspects of suicidality, and specific psychiatric disorders and their management can be useful. When family members or other supportive individuals are involved (e.g., military command personnel, supported housing staff), they can also benefit from education and can be encouraged to play a helpful role in improving adherence.

G. PROVIDE EDUCATION TO THE PATIENT AND FAMILY

Most patients can benefit from education about the symptoms and disorders being treated as well as about the therapeutic approaches employed as part of the treatment plan. When appropriate, and with the patient's permission, education should also be provided to involved family members. Understanding that psychiatric disorders are real illnesses and that effective treatments are both necessary and available may be crucial for patients who attribute their illness to a moral defect or for family members who are convinced that there is nothing wrong with the patient. Patients and family members can also benefit from an understanding of the role of psychosocial stressors and other disruptions in precipitating or exacerbating suicidality or symptoms of psychiatric disorders. Education regarding available treatment options will help patients make informed decisions, anticipate side effects, and adhere to treatments. Patients also need to be advised that improvement is not linear and that recovery may be uneven. Certain patients or family members may become overwhelmed or devastated by a recurrence of symptoms or a temporary worsening of symptoms after the initiation of treatment. Since suicidal patients tend to be overly critical of themselves, a recurrence or worsening of symptoms may be seen as evidence of personal failure; they need to be reassured that this can be part of the recovery process.

It is also useful to have an open discussion with the patient about the phenomenon of suicide. When there has been a family history of suicide, some patients will feel that it is their fate to die from suicide as well. The age at which a family member died or the specific anniversary of the family member's death may take on special significance for some patients. Education for the patient and the family should emphasize that a family history of suicide may increase risk of suicide, but it does not make suicide inevitable. It can be helpful to educate the patient and involved family members about how to identify symptoms, such as insomnia, hopelessness, anxiety, or depression, that may herald a worsening of the patient's clinical condition. In addition, patients and family members should be encouraged to think about other symptoms, specific to the individual patient, that have been associated with suicidality in the past. Furthermore, patients and family members should be aware that thoughts of suicide may return and that they should inform the psychiatrist or a significant other as soon as possible if that occurs. There should also be an open discussion about what to do in the event of an emergency and how to obtain emergency services. Under some circumstances, this discussion may include an explanation of methods for involving the police to facilitate an involuntary evaluation.

Some family members, particularly those of patients with borderline personality disorder, mistakenly view suicide attempts or communications of suicidal intent as "manipulative" or "attention-seeking" behaviors. Thus, it is important to provide family members with education about the lifetime risks of suicide in such patients and to help family members learn ways to respond in a helpful and positive manner when the patient is experiencing a suicidal crisis.

H. REASSESS SAFETY AND SUICIDE RISK

The waxing and waning nature of suicidality is one of the difficult challenges in the care of the suicidal patient and often requires that suicide assessments be repeated over time (Table 2). Although a full suicide assessment is not required at each encounter with the patient, the psychiatrist should use reasonable judgment in determining the extent of the repeat assessment needed to estimate the patient's current suicide risk. In inpatient settings, repeat suicide assessments should occur at critical stages of treatment (e.g., with a change in level of privilege, abrupt change in mental state, and before discharge). When a reassessment is done, the psychiatrist often finds that a patient who initially reported suicidal ideation with lethal intent no longer reports suicidal ideation at a subsequent visit. As stated earlier, it is not possible to predict which individuals with recent suicidal ideation will experience it again nor which patients will deny suicidal ideation even when it is present. Nonetheless, if a patient is assessed as being at high risk for suicide, a plan to address this risk must be implemented and documented. This plan may include changes in the setting of care or level of observation, changes in medication therapy or psychotherapy, or both kinds of changes.

Patients with a recent onset of severe suicidal ideation should be treated with particular caution. For those experiencing suicidal ideation in the context of an underlying depressive disorder, it can be useful to monitor other depressive symptoms. The psychiatrist also needs to be mindful of other symptoms that may be associated with increased suicide risk, such as hopelessness, anxiety, insomnia, or command hallucinations. Behaviors that may be associated with an acute increase in risk include giving away possessions, readying legal or financial affairs (e.g., finalizing a will, assigning a power of attorney), or communicating suicidal intentions or "goodbye" messages.

Patients who are responding to ongoing treatment or who are in remission with continuation or maintenance treatment should be assessed for suicide risk when there is evidence of an abrupt clinical change, a relapse or recurrence, or some major adverse life event. In this context, the new emergence of suicidality should be responded to by an alteration of the treatment plan. The nature of this alteration depends on the clinical situation and can include a change in treatment setting or level of observation, increased visits, a change of medication or psychotherapeutic approach, inclusion of a significant other person, and consultation. With changes in clinical status or as new information becomes available, the psychiatrist must also be prepared to reevaluate the patient's psychiatric diagnosis and also evaluate the nature and strength of the therapeutic alliance.

1. Patients in a suicidal crisis

There will be times when a patient in ongoing treatment is in an acute suicidal crisis and the psychiatrist has to respond immediately. There may be communications directly from the patient, the family, or significant others, including employers or co-workers. In urgent situations, it may be necessary to have telephone calls traced or involve the police. The challenge for the psychiatrist is not only to evaluate the extent of the emergency but also to assess the content of the communication and its source. To better assess the situation, it is critical to speak with the patient directly, if at all possible. In addition, the psychiatrist should remain mindful of issues relating to confidentiality and breach confidentiality only to the extent needed to address the patient's safety (see also Section V.C, "Communication With Significant Others").

Under some circumstances, the psychiatrist may need to refer a suicidal patient to an emergency department for evaluation or hospitalization. When doing so, it is important for the psychiatrist to communicate with the psychiatric evaluator in the emergency department. Although such communication may not always be possible because of the exigencies of the emergency situation, such contact does provide hospital personnel with the context for the emergency. Particularly when a patient is brought to the hospital by police, it is not unusual for the patient to minimize the symptoms and reasons for the referral after arriving in the emergency setting. Adequate information about the reasons for the emergency department referral and about the patient's previous and recent history can be crucial in helping the emergency department evaluator determine a safe and appropriate setting for treatment. When hospitalization is recommended by the referring psychiatrist, the reasons for that recommendation should similarly be communicated to the emergency department evaluator who will be making the final determination about the need for hospital admission.

2. Patients with chronic suicidality

For some individuals, self-injurious behaviors and/or suicidality are chronic and repetitive, resulting in frequent contacts with the health care system for assessment of suicide potential. It is important to recognize that self-injurious behaviors may or may not be associated with suicidal intent (518). Although self-injurious behaviors are sometimes characterized as "gestures" aimed at achieving secondary gains (e.g., receiving attention, avoiding responsibility through hospitalization), patients' motivations for such behaviors are quite different. For example, without having any desire for death, individuals may intentionally injure themselves to express anger, relieve anxiety or tension, generate a feeling of "normality or self-control," terminate a state of depersonalization, or distract or punish themselves (519, 520). Conceptualizing such behaviors as "gestures" is also problematic because suicide attempts may be downplayed when associated with minimal self-harm. Self-destructive acting out can also result in accidentally lethal self-destructive behaviors even in the absence of suicidal intent. Furthermore, a past or current history of nonlethal self-injurious behaviors does not preclude development of suicidal ideas, plans, or attempts with serious intent and lethality (521). In fact, among suicide attempters with suicidal intent, those who also had histories of self-injurious behaviors without suicidal intent were more likely to underestimate the objective lethality of their attempt and to have symptoms associated with greater suicide risk (251). Thus, in assessing chronic self-injurious behaviors, it is important to determine whether suicidal intent is present with self-injury and, if so, to what extent and with what frequency. In addition, an absence of suicidal intent or a minimal degree of self-injury should not lead the psychiatrist to overlook other evidence of increased suicide risk.

For patients who are prone to chronic self-injurious behavior, each act needs to be assessed in the context of the current situation; there is not a single response to self-injurious behaviors that can be recommended. For example, there are times when outpatient management is most appropriate; under other circumstances, hospitalization may be indicated. In general, for such individuals, hospitalization should be used for short-term stabilization, since prolonged hospital stays may potentiate dependency, regression, and acting-out behaviors. When chronic self-injurious behaviors are present, behavioral techniques such as dialectical behavior therapy can be helpful (522, 523). In addition, at times when care of the patient is being transitioned to another clinician, the risk of suicidal behaviors may increase.

Diagnostically, severe personality disorders, particularly borderline (521) and antisocial personality disorders, predominate among patients who exhibit chronic self-injurious behaviors without associated suicidal intent. Such individuals may also have higher rates of comorbid panic disorder and posttraumatic stress disorder (524). Patients with schizoaffective disorder, bipolar disorder, and schizophrenia may also be represented, but more often such patients have ongoing thoughts of suicide or repeated suicide attempts in the presence of suicidal intent. There is evidence that the presence of comorbid personality disorders or substance use disorders not only increases suicide risk in these individuals but also decreases treatment response. For example, patients with a combination of affective disorder and personality disorder are prone to frequent suicidal crises, difficulties with mood instability and impulse control, and problems with treatment adherence. Consequently, for patients whose nonadherence contributes to a chronic risk for suicide, psychiatrists should be familiar with statutes on involuntary outpatient treatment, if it is applicable in their jurisdiction (525).

When treating chronically suicidal individuals, it is important for the psychiatrist to monitor his or her own feelings, including countertransference reactions. Careful attention to the treatment relationship and the psychosocial context of the patient is also critical. Consistency and limit-setting are often needed, but the latter needs to be established on the basis of clinical judgment and should not be framed in punitive terms. Helping patients develop skills for coping with self-injurious impulses is often a valuable part of treatment.

In outlining a detailed treatment plan, it is helpful to incorporate input from the patient and significant others, when clinically appropriate. During periods of crisis, disagreements may occur about the need for hospitalization. In some circumstances, the psychiatrist may view hospitalization as essential, whereas the patient or family members may not. Alternatively, the patient, family members, or other involved persons may demand hospitalization when outpatient management may seem more appropriate. When such disagreements occur, power struggles are best avoided. Instead, gaining a deeper understanding of the conflicting viewpoints will often lead to a successful resolution. In addition, educational efforts with the patient and others should discuss the fact that risk in chronically suicidal individuals will be increased on an ongoing basis. Thus, the risk of suicide outside of the hospital must be balanced against the potentially detrimental effects of hospitalization (see Section III.C, "Determine a Treatment Setting").

I. MONITOR PSYCHIATRIC STATUS AND RESPONSE TO TREATMENT

In addition to reassessing the patient's safety and degree of suicidality, it is equally important for the psychiatrist to monitor the patient's psychiatric status and response to treatment. This is particularly the case during the early phases of treatment, since some medications, particularly antidepressants, may take several weeks to reach therapeutic benefit. Also, with the exception of suicides in persons with alcoholism, suicides tend to occur early in the course of most psychiatric disorders, when individuals are least likely to have insight into having an illness and are least likely to adhere to treatment. Moreover, clinical observations suggest that there may be an early increase in suicide risk as depressive symptoms begin to lift but before they are fully resolved. Thus, ongoing monitoring of the patient's clinical condition is needed to determine the patient's symptoms and response to treatment (e.g., determining the optimal dose of a drug and evaluating its efficacy). Often the course of treatment is uneven, with periodic setbacks, for example, at times of stress. Such setbacks do not necessarily indicate that the treatment is ineffective. Nonetheless, ultimate improvement should be a reasonably expected outcome. Furthermore, as treatment progresses, different features and symptoms of the patient's illness may emerge or subside. Significant changes in a patient's psychiatric status or the emergence of new symptoms may indicate a need for a diagnostic reevaluation, a change in treatment plan, or both. Such modifications may include a change in treatment setting, medication, or frequency of visits; involvement of significant others; referral for additional treatments (e.g., dialectical behavior therapy, ECT) that are targeted at specific symptoms or syndromes; and consultation.

J. OBTAIN CONSULTATION, IF INDICATED

In treating suicidal patients, particularly those with severe or chronic suicidality, consultation may be helpful from a number of standpoints. The use of consultation or supervision from a colleague may be of help in monitoring and addressing countertransference issues. Since clinical judgments regarding assessment and treatment issues with suicidal patients may be quite difficult, input from other colleagues may be important in affirming the appropriateness of the treatment plan or suggesting other possible therapeutic approaches. For complex clinical presentations in which alcohol or other substance use disorders might be present, referral to a psychiatrist specializing in the treatment of addictive disorders may be helpful for consultation, management, or involvement in a program of recovery. However, in the context of a suicidal crisis, psychiatrists need to be careful in referring a long-term patient for consultation. Some patients may perceive such a referral as the first step to termination of therapy and may need to be reassured that the referral is only for consultation.

IV. SPECIFIC TREATMENT MODALITIES

A. SOMATIC THERAPIES

For the purposes of this practice guideline, psychiatrists should be familiar with specific psychotropic medicines that have been found to be useful in the care of the suicidal patient. In general, somatic therapies such as antidepressants, antipsychotics, or mood-stabilizing agents will be targeted to specific axis I and/or axis II psychiatric disorders. However, early use of supplemental medicines, including sedative-anxiolytics or low doses of second-generation antipsychotics, may also be helpful to rapidly address agitation, anxiety, and insomnia, which are additional risk factors for suicide.

1. Antidepressants

A mainstay of the treatment of suicidal patients suffering from acute, recurrent, and chronic depressive illness is the administration of antidepressant medication in an adequate dose (526). Antidepressants also have demonstrated efficacy in the treatment of anxiety disorders (526). They have also been used successfully in treating suicidal patients with comorbid depression and substance use disorders (527). Remarkably, however, there is relatively limited evidence that antidepressant treatment reduces risk (69, 526, 528–533). On the basis of a large number of short-term randomized, placebo-controlled trials for acute major depression (534–546) that were subjected to meta-analysis (533), antidepressant treatment has not been shown to reduce rates of suicide or suicide attempts. Studies using data on antidepressants from Food and Drug Administration clinical trial databases also do not show differences in rates of suicide or suicide attempts with antidepressant treatment (546–548). However, reductions in risk might not be observed as readily over short time periods or in studies in which suicidality was used as an exclusion criterion. Furthermore, long-term studies with relevant data are rare and too small to support any conclusions (526). However, since the late 1980s, suicide rates in several countries, regions, or subpopulations have fallen appreciably (69, 531, 532, 549, 550), coinciding with the increasing clinical use of nontricyclic and non–monoamine oxidase inhibitor (non-MAOI) antidepressants in adequate doses and perhaps providing indirect evidence for a role of antidepressant treatment in the treatment of suicidal behaviors.

After publication of several case reports suggesting that SSRI antidepressants might be associated with increased risks of aggressive or impulsive acts, including suicide (551–553), a number of investigators retrospectively analyzed clinical trial data to determine whether suicidality and/or suicide rates are increased with SSRI treatment (537, 548, 554, 555). These studies did not show evidence that suicide or suicidality is increased by treatment with specific types of antidepressants. At the same time, these medications are prescribed in order to treat disorders that may have anxiety, agitation, and suicidality as part of the illness course, making it difficult to distinguish the etiology of symptoms that emerge in the course of treatment. Thus, as treatment begins, it is important to determine baseline levels of symptoms and then to observe patients for symptoms such as anxiety, agitation, or sleep disturbance as well as for the development of mixed states or psychosis, all of which may increase their subjective sense of distress and increase suicide risk. In addition, antidepressant therapy typically involves a substantial delay before clinically obvious improvements occur. During initial, partial recovery, it is possible that suicidal impulses as well as the energy to act on them may increase. Patients should be forewarned of this likely delay in treatment effects and should be given encouragement and monitored especially closely in the initial days and weeks of treatment. If full response to treatment is not observed, adjustments in medication dosage or a change to a different antidepressant medication may be necessary. Nontricyclic, non-MAOI antidepressants are relatively safe and present virtually negligible risks of lethality on overdose (526). Nevertheless, it is wise to request that conservative quantities of medication be dispensed for suicidal patients, especially for patients who are not well known. Although the tricyclic antidepressants and MAOIs are much more toxic in overdose and more limited in their use, they may still be valuable in treating individuals with suicidal behaviors and depressive disorders who have not responded to treatment with SSRIs or other newer antidepressants (526, 556, 557). Overall, from a clinical perspective, the strong association between clinical depression and suicide and the availability of reasonably effective and quite safe antidepressants support their use, in adequate doses and for an adequate duration, as part of a comprehensive program of care for potentially suicidal patients, including long-term use in patients with recurrent forms of depressive or severe anxiety disorders.

2. Lithium

There is strong and consistent evidence in patients with recurring bipolar disorder and major depressive disorder that long-term maintenance treatment with lithium salts is associated with major reductions in risk of both suicide and suicide attempts (69, 558–565). A recent meta-analysis (563) of available studies of suicide rates with versus without long-term lithium maintenance treatment (76, 534, 559, 565–595) found a highly statistically significant decrease in suicidal acts (i.e., suicide or suicide attempts) of almost 14-fold. For suicide, lithium maintenance treatment was associated with an 80%–90% decrease in risk, whereas the reduction in suicide attempt rates was more than 90%. Although suicide rates during lithium treatment are still greater than those in the general population, maintenance therapy with lithium for bipolar disorder patients is associated with substantial and significant reductions in suicide risk, compared to non-lithium-treated bipolar disorder patients. As with antidepressants, the potential lethality of lithium in overdose (596) should be taken into consideration when deciding on the quantity of lithium to give with each prescription. However, given the long-term benefits of lithium in reducing risks of suicidal behaviors, the potential for overdose effects should not preclude treatment of suicidal patients with lithium when it is clinically indicated.

3. "Mood-stabilizing" anticonvulsant agents

Despite the increased use and antimanic efficacy of specific anticonvulsant and antipsychotic agents (e.g., divalproex, olanzapine), their long-term effectiveness in protecting against recurrent mood episodes is less well established. Moreover, there is no established evidence of a reduced risk of suicidal behavior with any other "mood-stabilizing" anticonvulsants. Although treatment with these agents may be associated with some decrease in suicidal behaviors, lithium treatment is still associated with a greater diminution in rates of suicidal acts than treatment with carbamazepine or divalproex (592, 597, 598). Consequently, when deciding between lithium and other first-line agents for treatment of patients with bipolar disorder, the efficacy of lithium in decreasing suicidal behavior should be taken into consideration when weighing the benefits and risks of treatment with each medication.

4. Antipsychotic agents

Analogous to the use of antidepressants for patients with depression, the antipsychotic medications have been the mainstay of somatic treatment for suicidal patients with psychotic disorders. First-generation antipsychotic agents are highly effective in treating delusions and hallucinations as well as agitation, aggression, and confusion and may also have some beneficial actions in major affective disorders. Their potential effects in limiting suicidal risk in psychotic patients are unknown, although annual rates of suicide associated with schizophrenia have not fallen appreciably since their introduction (599–602).

Particularly in highly agitated patients, the beneficial effects of first-generation and modern antipsychotics may serve to reduce suicide risk (603). However, use of older neuroleptic agents may also be associated with adverse effects, including extrapyramidal neurological side effects and possible worsening of depression as a result of induction of akathisia (603–606). Given the fact that treatment of psychotic disorders with second-generation antipsychotic agents is associated with lower risks of some, particularly extrapyramidal-neurological, adverse effects (512, 513, 596), use of first-generation antipsychotics in individuals with suicidal behaviors currently is usually reserved for those needing the enhanced treatment adherence afforded by depot forms of medication or those whose psychosis has not responded to a second-generation antipsychotic, or when economic considerations are compelling.

In the United States, the second-generation antipsychotic medications, such as aripiprazole, clozapine, olanzapine, quetiapine, risperidone, and ziprasidone, are now used to treat the majority of individuals with schizophrenia or schizoaffective disorder. In addition to their use as first-line agents in the treatment of schizophrenia, the second-generation antipsychotic agents may also be indicated for use in individuals with other psychotic disorders as well as in patients with bipolar disorder, particularly during manic episodes. Among the second-generation antipsychotic agents, clozapine has generally been reserved for use when psychotic symptoms have not responded to other antipsychotic medications. As for effects on suicide attempts and suicide, clozapine is the best studied of any of the antipsychotic agents. Reductions in the rates of suicide attempts and suicides have been reported in specific studies of patients with schizophrenia treated with clozapine (607) as well as in registry studies (533, 606, 608–613), which may include patients with other psychotic diagnoses. Earlier studies could not eliminate the possibility that suicide rates were decreased by a nonspecific effect of increased clinical contact due to hematologic monitoring during clozapine therapy. However, significant reductions in suicide attempts and hospitalization for suicidality were also seen in a more recent blinded study comparing clozapine and olanzapine (603). The reduction of suicide attempts in both groups, compared to the rate in the year preceding the study, suggests that olanzapine may also offer some protection against suicide attempts. These findings suggest that use of clozapine might be considered earlier in the treatment of individuals with schizophrenia or schizoaffective disorders. At the same time, the potential benefits of treatment with clozapine need to be weighed against the potential for adverse effects with long-term clozapine treatment, including agranulocytosis, myocarditis, weight gain, and glucose dysregulation. Further study is needed to determine whether clozapine can reduce suicide risk in patients with other diagnoses or whether other second-generation antipsychotic drugs may reduce suicide risk in schizophrenia in comparison with one another or with first-generation antipsychotic drugs.

5. Antianxiety agents

Since anxiety is a significant and modifiable risk factor for suicide, utilization of antianxiety agents may have the potential to decrease this risk. More specifically, before accompanying depression has resolved, acute suicide risk may be associated with severe psychic anxiety, panic attacks, agitation, and severe insomnia (79). Although these symptoms may be reduced by aggressive short-term benzodiazepine treatment (lasting 1–4 weeks), research on suicide risk with antianxiety treatment is quite limited, with no clinical trial of antianxiety treatment showing short- or long-term antisuicide effects. However, a recent analysis of data obtained in controlled trials of treatments for anxiety disorders showed no significant differences in rates of suicidal behavior between those treated with active agents and those taking placebo (118).

To minimize severe recurrent (rebound) anxiety/agitation, long-acting benzodiazepines may be preferable to short-acting ones. At the same time, long-acting benzodiazepines may be more likely to cause daytime sedation. Psychiatrists should also keep in mind that benzodiazepines occasionally disinhibit aggressive and dangerous behaviors and enhance impulsivity, particularly in patients with borderline personality disorder (614, 615). For patients treated with benzodiazepines on a chronic basis, discontinuation of the benzodiazepine may be associated with an increase in suicide risk (616). As alternatives to benzodiazepines, second-generation antipsychotic medications or anticonvulsant medications such as divalproex or gabapentin may be helpful, although no specific research information on their potential to limit anxiety is available. Persistent, severe insomnia is also a modifiable risk factor for suicide and can be addressed with the use of benzodiazepines or sedating second-generation antipsychotics (617–619). Choice of a sedating antidepressant can also be considered for depressed patients with prominent insomnia.

6. ECT

ECT is sometimes used to treat patients who are acutely suicidal, and available evidence suggests that ECT reduces short-term suicidal ideation (620–622). The efficacy of ECT is best established in patients with severe depressive illness, but ECT may also be used in treating individuals with manic or mixed episodes of bipolar disorder, schizoaffective disorder, or schizophrenia, under certain clinical circumstances (623). ECT is especially likely to be considered for patients for whom a delay in treatment response is considered life-threatening. Such patients may include individuals who are refusing to eat because of psychosis or depressive symptoms as well as those with catatonic features or prominent psychosis. ECT may also be indicated for suicidal individuals during pregnancy and for those who have already failed to tolerate or respond to trials of medication. Although ECT is often raised as a possible treatment for chronically suicidal individuals with borderline personality disorder, ECT in such patients should target comorbid disorders that may be present, particularly comorbid major depressive disorder. In the absence of another indication for use, ECT is not indicated for the treatment of suicidality in borderline personality disorder. For further details on the clinical use of ECT, including the pre-ECT evaluation, the informed consent process, the numbers of treatments generally given, and the technical aspects of ECT administration, the reader is referred to APA's 2001 report, *The Practice of Electroconvulsive Therapy: Recommendations for Treatment, Training, and Privileging: A Task Force Report of the American Psychiatric Association* (623). Since there is no evidence for long-term or sustained reduction of suicide risk after an acute course of ECT, close clinical supervision and additional treatment with psychotropic medications are usually required during subsequent weeks and months.

B. PSYCHOTHERAPIES

In addition to pharmacotherapies and ECT, psychotherapies play a central role in the management of suicidal behavior in clinical practice. Although few rigorous studies have directly examined whether these interventions reduce suicide morbidity or mortality per se, clinical consensus suggests that psychosocial interventions and specific psychotherapeutic approaches are of benefit to the suicidal patient. Furthermore, in recent years, studies of psychotherapy have demonstrated its efficacy in treating disorders such as depression and borderline personality disorder that are associated with increased suicide risk. For example, cognitive behavior therapy, psychodynamic therapy, and interpersonal psychotherapy have been found effective in clinical trials for the treatment of these disorders (511, 515). A small randomized, controlled trial of psychoanalytically oriented partial hospital treatment for individuals with borderline personality disorder showed a beneficial effect on suicide attempts and self-harming behaviors during treatment and follow-up (624, 625). These observations as well as clinical experience lend support to the use of such psychotherapeutic approaches in the treatment of suicidal ideation and behaviors.

A number of other specific and nonspecific interventions have been assessed in small methodologically sound, randomized, controlled trials involving individuals with suicidal ideation or attempts as well as other forms of deliberate self-harm (626, 627). Dialectical behavior therapy has been studied for effects in a narrow range of potentially suicidal patients, particularly chronically suicidal or self-harming women with personality disorders. By targeting deficits in specific skills, such as emotional regulation, impulse control, anger management, and interpersonal assertiveness, dialectical behavior therapy may be effective in reducing suicide attempts when applied over longer time frames, especially for patients with personality disorders. There is also some preliminary evidence that cognitive and behavioral psychotherapy may reduce the incidence of suicide attempts in depressed outpatients (236, 626). However, other forms of cognitive behavior therapy that include a problem-solving component have shown mixed results (524, 628–632), suggesting the need for additional study. Other nonspecific interventions have been studied in relatively small samples and have similarly shown mixed results. Most of these studies are limited in the size and scope of the patient population and provide only narrow support for an effect on suicidal behaviors (633).

V. DOCUMENTATION AND RISK MANAGEMENT

A. GENERAL RISK MANAGEMENT AND DOCUMENTATION ISSUES SPECIFIC TO SUICIDE

Risk management is an important component of psychiatric practice, especially in the assessment and management of patients at risk for suicide. Clinically based risk management is patient centered and supports the therapeutic alliance and the treatment process. The most frequent lawsuits, settlements, and verdicts against psychiatrists are for patients' suicides. Thus, when treating a patient with suicidal behaviors, it is important to be aware of and pay attention to certain general risk management considerations, which are summarized in Table 9.

Documentation of patient care is a cornerstone of medical practice, but it is also essential to risk management (634, 635). If a malpractice claim is brought against the psychiatrist, documentation of suicide risk assessments assists the court in evaluating the many clinical complexities and ambiguities that exist in the treatment and management of patients at suicide risk. The failure to document suicide risk assessments and interventions may give the court reason to conclude they were not done. For patients who are hospitalized, it is also important to document the aspects of the risk assessment that justify inpatient treatment, particularly when it is occurring on an involuntary basis (636). Thus, it is crucial for the suicide risk assessment to be documented in the medical record.

Despite the time burdens faced by the psychiatrist, documentation is best done just after the suicide assessment is completed. Reference to the reason for the assessment (e.g., relapse, worsening, a reversal in the patient's life) will set the context for the evaluation. Subsequent discussion reviews the factors that may contribute to increased shorter-term or longer-term suicide risk as well as the reasoning process that went into the assessment. Clinical conclusions and any changes in the treatment plan should also be noted, along with the rationale for such actions. If other interventions or actions were considered but rejected, that reasoning should be recorded as well.

Consider the example of a patient who was in remission after a prior hospitalization for a suicide attempt but who recently had a relapse or a recurrent episode. The psychiatrist may document that suicidal ideation is present but that there is no evidence of a specific plan or specific symptoms that would augment risk (i.e., agitation, severe anxiety, severe insomnia). It may also be noted that the patient is under increased stress and is in some distress but is responsive to support. On the basis of the patient's willingness to accept help and the lack of evidence of acute suicide risk factors, continued outpatient management may be reasonable, with changes in the treatment plan, such as increasing the frequency of visits, perhaps increasing anxiolytic medication doses temporarily, and perhaps talking with a supportive relative or friend to obtain more information and to solidify the patient's support system.

In all settings, the psychiatrist should be aware that suicide risk assessment is a process and never simply an isolated event. Specific points at which reassessment may be indicated have been detailed in Table 2. On inpatient units, important points of documentation of assessment occur at admission, changes in the level of precautions or observations, transitions between treatment units, the issuance of passes, marked changes in the clinical condition of the patient, and evaluation for discharge (637). In particular, the determination of the level of suicide precautions (one-to-one versus every-15-minute checks, etc.) should be based on the patient's clinical presentation and be supported by a clinical rationale. Because care in inpatient settings is generally delivered by a multidisciplinary treatment team, it is important for the psychiatrist either to review the patient's records regularly or to communicate verbally with staff throughout the patient's hospital stay. At the time of the patient's discharge from the hospital, risk-benefit assessments for both continued hospitalization and discharge should be documented, and follow-up arrangements for the patient's outpatient care should be recorded.

TABLE 9. General Risk Management and Documentation Considerations in the Assessment and Management of Patients at Risk for Suicide

Good collaboration, communication, and alliance between clinician and patient
Careful and attentive documentation, including:
• Risk assessments
• Record of decision-making processes
• Descriptions of changes in treatment
• Record of communications with other clinicians
• Record of telephone calls from patients or family members
• Prescription log or copies of actual prescriptions
• Medical records of previous treatment, if available, particularly treatment related to past suicide attempts
Critical junctures for documentation:
• At first psychiatric assessment or admission
• With occurrence of any suicidal behavior or ideation
• Whenever there is any noteworthy clinical change
• For inpatients, before increasing privileges or giving passes and before discharge
Monitoring issues of transference and countertransference in order to optimize clinical judgment
Consultation, a second opinion, or both should be considered when necessary
Careful termination (with appropriate documentation)
Firearms
• If present, document instructions given to the patient and significant others
• If absent, document as a pertinent negative
Planning for coverage

In outpatient settings, the process of suicide risk assessment and documentation typically occurs during the initial interview; at the emergence or reemergence of suicidal ideation, plans, or behavior; and when there are other significant changes in the patient's condition. Revisions of the treatment plan are appropriately noted at these times. For patients in psychoanalysis or modified psychoanalytic treatment, the psychiatrist may elect to follow the charting recommendations of the psychoanalytic subspecialty practice guideline (638).

B. SUICIDE CONTRACTS: USEFULNESS AND LIMITATIONS

As originally designed, the suicide prevention contract, which is sometimes known as a no-harm contract, was intended to facilitate management of the patient at suicide risk (639). Although in the era of managed care, suicide prevention contracts are increasingly being used with patients at risk for suicide, the patient's willingness (or reluctance) to enter into a suicide prevention contract should not be viewed as an absolute indicator of suitability for discharge (or hospitalization). In addition, since the utility of the suicide prevention contract is based on subjective belief rather than objective evidence, it is overvalued as a clinical or risk management technique. Furthermore, the suicide prevention contract is not a legal document and cannot be used as exculpatory evidence in the event of litigation (640). Thus, the suicide prevention contract cannot and should not take the place of a thorough suicide risk assessment (637).

Although suicide prevention contracts are commonly used in clinical practice (429), no studies have shown their effectiveness in reducing suicide. In fact, studies of suicide attempters and of inpatients who died by suicide have shown that a significant number had a suicide prevention contract in place at the time of their suicidal act (212, 218, 430). Consequently, although verbal and written suicide prevention contracts have each been proposed as aids to assessing the therapeutic alliance, their limitations should also be clearly understood (641). Relying on suicide prevention contracts may reflect the clinician's understandable but not necessarily effective attempt to control the inevitable anxiety associated with treating patients at suicide risk. At the same time, undue reliance on a patient's suicide prevention contract may falsely lower clinical vigilance without altering the patient's suicidal state.

Some clinicians gauge the patient's suicidal intent by his or her willingness to formalize the alliance by a written or an oral contract. For example, when discussing a suicide prevention contract, some patients will state openly that they cannot be sure that they can (or will want to) call the psychiatrist or other treatment team members if self-destructive impulses threaten. Patients who reject a suicide prevention contract are communicating that they see the therapeutic alliance as suboptimal or that they feel unable to adhere to such a contract. Consequently, patients who refuse to commit to contracts against suicide put the clinician on notice that the therapeutic alliance and the level of suicide risk should be reassessed. An alternative approach to suicide prevention contracts proposed by Miller et al. (642) relies on the basic tenets of informed consent and includes discussion of the risks and benefits of treatment and management options with the patient as a means of assessing his or her ability to develop and maintain a therapeutic alliance. In inpatient settings such discussions can emphasize the availability of the clinical staff and be used as a way to educate the patient about options for dealing with suicidal impulses.

Regardless of their potential advantages, suicide prevention contracts are only as reliable as the state of the therapeutic alliance. Thus, with a new patient, the psychiatrist may not have had sufficient time to make an adequate assessment or to evaluate the patient's capacity to form a therapeutic alliance, creating little or no basis for relying on a suicide prevention contract. As a result, the use of suicide prevention contracts in emergency settings or with newly admitted and unknown inpatients is not recommended. Furthermore, patients in crisis may not be able to adhere to a contract because of the severity of their illness. Suicide prevention contracts are also ill-advised with agitated, psychotic, or impulsive patients or when the patient is under the influence of an intoxicating substance. For these individuals, as for all patients presenting with suicidal behaviors, the psychiatrist must be ever mindful of the need for ongoing suicide assessments.

C. COMMUNICATION WITH SIGNIFICANT OTHERS

The confidential nature of the doctor-patient relationship is a fundamental aspect of the psychotherapeutic process. Consequently, the psychiatrist will need to manage the tension between this requirement and the wish to act in the patient's best interest. The default position is to maintain confidentiality unless the patient gives consent to a specific intervention or communication. However, in maintaining a safe environment for the patient, significant others may need to be contacted to furnish historical information or carry out specific tasks such as removing firearms from the home. If the psychiatrist determines that the patient is (or is likely to become) dangerous to him- or herself or to others and the patient will not consent to interventions that aim to reduce those risks, then the psychiatrist is justified in attenuating confidentiality to the extent needed to address the safety of the patient and others. More specifically, the 2001 edition of *The Principles of Medical Ethics With Annotations Especially Applicable to Psychiatry* states: "[P]sychiatrists at times may find it necessary, in order to protect the patient or the community from imminent danger, to reveal confidential information disclosed by the patient" (Section IV, Annotation 8) (643). As with many situations involving the suicidal patient, such decisions require much clinical judgment in weighing the effects of breaching confidentiality on the therapeutic relationship against the potential safety risks for the patient or others. It should also be noted that the psychiatrist can listen to information provided by friends or family without violating confidentiality by disclosing information about the patient to the informant. In addition, in an emergency situation, necessary information about the patient can be communicated with police and with emergency personnel, including medical staff and emergency medical technicians.

D. MANAGEMENT OF SUICIDE IN ONE'S PRACTICE

Because psychiatrists work with individuals who are by definition at increased risk for suicide, suicides can and do occur in clinical practice despite the best efforts at suicide assessment and treatment (489, 491). At least half of psychiatrists can expect in the course of their practice that one of their patients will die from suicide (644, 645). A patient's suicide is among the most difficult professional experiences encountered by a psychiatrist. It can lead to symptoms of posttraumatic stress disorder, shock, anger, grief, guilt, isolation, shame, diminished self-esteem, and concern about reactions of colleagues (646, 647). In one study (644), approximately half of the psychiatrists who had lost a patient to suicide experienced stress levels comparable with those of persons recovering from a parent's death. The significant effects of a patient's suicide on the psychiatrist, especially posttraumatic stress responses (644), suggest that support for the psychiatrist and a review of events leading to the suicide are warranted. Specific training may also be useful in helping the psychiatrist deal with the aftermath of a patient's suicide (644). In addition to receiving support from colleagues after a patient's suicide, some psychiatrists find it helpful to seek consultation or supervision to enable them to continue to respond effectively in working with other patients.

After a patient's suicide, clinicians may experience conflicting roles and concerns. However, a number of steps can be taken to facilitate the aftercare process. Many psychiatrists find it helpful to consult with a colleague or with an attorney. In addition, the psychiatrist should ensure that the patient's records are complete. Any additional documentation included in the medical record after the patient's death should be dated contemporaneously, not backdated, and previous entries should not be altered.

Conversations with family members can be appropriate and can allay grief and assist devastated family members in obtaining help after a suicide. This recommendation is based primarily on humanitarian concerns for survivors, but this approach may also have a powerful, though incidental, risk management aspect. Nonetheless, attorneys advise clinicians in two very different ways on the issue of suicide aftercare. After a bad outcome, some attorneys recommend that the case be sealed and no communication be established with the family, except through the attorney. Other attorneys encourage judicious communication or consultation, if indicated. If this approach is taken, the psychiatrist should concentrate on addressing the feelings of the family members rather than specific details of the patient's care. In addition, in speaking with survivors, care must be exercised not to reveal confidential information about the patient and not to make self-incriminating or self-exonerating statements, since these statements may further distress the family and provide a spur to litigation. The individuals who lived with the patient before the suicide not only currently experience intense emotional pain but also shared it with the patient before death. Thus, a number of lawsuits are filed because of the clinician's refusal to express, in any way, feelings of condolence, sadness, sympathy, or regret for the patient's death. A number of states have statutes that prohibit statements, writings, or benevolent human expressions of sympathy such as condolences and regrets from being admissible as evidence of an admission of liability in a civil action (648). However, statutes often distinguish between the part of a statement that is an expression of sympathy and the part of a statement that expresses fault, e.g., in the case of an automobile accident, "I'm sorry you were hurt" (inadmissible as evidence of liability) versus "I was using my cell phone and just didn't see you coming" (admissible as evidence of liability). Consequently, it may be useful for psychiatrists to know whether an apology statute is applicable within their jurisdiction and, if so, to know the specific provisions of the statute. The individual psychiatrist must use his or her clinical judgment to decide whether attending the patient's funeral would be appropriate. It may also be helpful to include a risk manager in this decision process.

Many occasions arise in which information is requested after a patient's death. As a general rule, written authorization should be obtained from the executor or administrator of the deceased patient's estate before releasing a copy of the medical records. If the estate has been settled and an executor or administrator no longer exists, a copy of the medical records should be released only to properly appointed legal representatives (649).

E. MENTAL HEALTH INTERVENTIONS FOR SURVIVING FAMILY AND FRIENDS AFTER A SUICIDE

The survivors of suicide are more vulnerable to physical and psychological disorders and are at increased risk of suicide themselves (see Section II.E.6, "Family History"). Although there are relatively few systematic studies of adult bereavement after suicide, existing studies suggest that emotional, social, and physical conditions of survivors are significantly changed after the suicide of a relative. Within 6 months after a suicide, 45% of bereaved adults report mental deterioration, with physical deterioration in 20% (650). Symptoms of depression, posttraumatic stress, guilt, and shame as well as somatic complaints are prevalent during that period and are more severe among parents of deceased children (650–652). While the majority of bereaved adults within 6 months after a suicide acknowledge a need for intervention, only approximately 25% seek psychiatric treatment (650). Despite this low rate of treatment, the majority of bereaved adults adapt well in the long term (653, 654).

The most comprehensive data on bereavement after suicide exist for youths. These data indicate that within 6 months after the suicide of a friend or sibling, symptoms of major depressive and posttraumatic stress disorders are prevalent among bereaved youths (145, 651, 655). The long-term outcomes, up to 18 months, of adolescents whose friends had died by suicide suggest the incidence of major depressive disorder is higher in those who had depression before the friend's suicide, intermediate in those who developed depression immediately after the suicide, and lowest in those who were not depressed immediately after the suicide (656). Those who became depressed after the death were closer to the friend who died by suicide, showed more intense grief, and had more intense exposure to the suicide. Within 6 years of the suicide of a friend, adolescents with syndromal levels of traumatic grief were five times more likely to report suicidal ideation than those without traumatic grief (657). However, there was no greater incidence of suicide attempts among adolescents with a friend who had died by suicide than among adolescents who did not know someone who died by suicide. Adolescent siblings of youths who died by suicide had a sevenfold increased risk for developing major depressive disorder within 6 months (651). However, in a related 3-year follow-up of siblings of adolescents who died by suicide, the siblings suffered more significant grief than the friends of the adolescents who died by suicide, although the rates of psychiatric disorders in follow-up were similar to those for adolescents who did not have a friend or sibling who died by suicide (651).

These studies suggest an increased risk of psychiatric symptoms and impairment after the suicide of a relative. As a result, psychiatric intervention should be offered to family members shortly after the death and maintained to reduce risk for psychiatric impairment. Such intervention is particularly important for youths and for those who witnessed the suicide or were at the scene of the death. The goals of psychiatric intervention include the identification and treatment of major depressive and posttraumatic stress disorders as well as related symptoms (658, 659). Longer-term follow-up with evaluation and intervention for adolescents bereaved after the suicide of a relative or friend is also indicated to decrease the risk for recurrent depression and other morbidities (660). Furthermore, a family approach to evaluation and intervention is needed for those who are bereaved after an adolescent's suicide. Evaluation and treatment of grief may be similarly important in reducing risk for suicidal ideation among youths who are bereaved as a result of the suicide of a person who is emotionally important to them. For all family members and close friends of individuals who die by suicide, referral to a survivor support group can be helpful.

PART B:
BACKGROUND INFORMATION AND REVIEW OF AVAILABLE EVIDENCE

VI. REVIEW AND SYNTHESIS OF AVAILABLE EVIDENCE

A. FACTORS ALTERING RISK OF SUICIDE AND ATTEMPTED SUICIDE

1. Demographic factors

a) Age

As shown in Table 10, suicide rates vary with age, gender, and race or ethnicity. Annual rates in the general U.S. population rise sharply in adolescence and young adulthood, plateau through midlife, then rise again in individuals over age 65. The increased rates of suicide in youths are even more dramatic in some ethnic and racial subgroups of the population. For example, the suicide rate among American Indian males between ages 15 and 34 years averaged about 36 per 100,000 during the period from 1979 to 1993, whereas Alaska Native males between ages 14 and 19 years had an even more dramatic rate, at 120 per 100,000 (661). Black male youths, who were historically at low risk for suicide, now have a suicide rate comparable to their white peers. Although the suicide rate in adolescents, like the overall U.S. suicide rate, has dropped in the past decade, the relative suicide risk of youths remains high, and this has been attributed to increases in alcohol and substance abuse (662), breakdown in extended family and intergenerational support, and increased availability of firearms, especially for young African American males (663).

Individuals over age 65 are disproportionately represented among those who die by suicide. Compared with suicide rates in men ages 55 to 64 years, suicide rates in men over age 85 are two- to threefold higher for all races except African Americans. For elderly women, suicide rates are relatively unchanged with increasing age, with the exception of Asian women over age 85, whose suicide rate increases threefold from middle age.

Overall suicide rates among those over age 65 have decreased substantially over the course of the last century, with a further decrease over the past decade. Although the reasons for the decline are unknown, a variety of mechanisms have been postulated, including improved access to social and health care resources by older adults with the implementation of Social Security and Medicare legislation and the more widespread use of safe and effective antidepressant medications (664). The incidence of suicide among elderly persons may increase again, however, as the large, post–World War II baby boom generation continues to age. Relative to age groups born in earlier or later periods, baby boomers have been distinguished by suicide rates that have been comparatively higher at all ages (665). Of additional concern is the fact that elders are the fastest growing segment of the U.S. population. Thus, as large numbers of this high-risk cohort enter the phase of life associated with greatest risk, the absolute number of suicides among older adults may increase dramatically (666).

TABLE 10. Suicide Rates in the United States by Age, Gender, and Race or Ethnicity[a]

	Non-Hispanic White		Non-Hispanic Black		Hispanic		Asian/Pacific Islander		American Indian/Alaska Native	
Age (years)	Male	Female	Male	Female	Male	Female	Male	Female	Male	Female
<15	0.93	0.25	0.79	0.12	0.44	0.15	0.24	0.25	1.78	0.36
15–24	18.98	3.25	14.66	2.32	13.23	2.21	10.86	3.29	36.81	8.78
25–34	23.89	5.34	16.96	2.76	13.66	1.94	12.81	3.86	34.37	12.52
35–44	26.42	7.74	13.67	2.81	12.69	2.69	9.44	3.15	34.04	9.10
45–54	25.71	7.98	11.75	2.60	12.75	3.15	10.86	3.25	21.63	5.81
55–64	22.09	6.41	8.02	1.60	10.88	1.37	9.75	3.92	23.54	1.38
65–74	25.15	4.65	11.06	0.95	14.52	1.55	9.75	3.57	21.39	0.00
75–84	41.29	4.24	12.16	2.40	21.59	1.73	25.10	7.72	4.91	0.00
>84	60.68	4.63	12.04	0.46	21.68	0.74	38.24	9.34	0.00	0.00

[a]Suicide rates per 100,000 in the United States in the year 2000 for ICD-10 codes X60–X84, Y87.0. From the Web-Based Injury Statistics Query and Reporting System, National Center for Injury Prevention and Control, Centers for Disease Control and Prevention (11).

Suicidal ideation and suicide attempts are more frequent in younger age groups than in later life (14). Kuo et al. (29), using prospectively gathered data from the Epidemiologic Catchment Area (ECA) survey, found a progressive decrease in the annual incidences of suicidal ideation and suicide attempts with increasing age. Compared with the rate in individuals over age 65, the rate of suicide attempts was 10-fold greater in those ages 18 to 29 years, at approximately 310 per 100,000 person-years. The rate of suicidal ideation in individuals ages 18 to 29 was approximately 630 per 100,000 person-years, a rate that was sixfold greater than that in those over age 65. Duberstein et al. (13), in a study of adults age 50 years and older, also found that people are less likely to report suicidal ideation as they age.

In other studies, estimates of the prevalence of suicidal ideation in older adults have varied with the population sampled and the site, time frame, and study methods. Lish and colleagues (667) found that 7.3% of an older sample in Department of Veterans Affairs (VA) primary care practices had thoughts of suicide, and elders with a history of mental health treatment were at far greater risk. Callahan and colleagues (668) used a far more stringent definition of suicidal ideation, limited ascertainment to within the past week, and required the ideation to include a specific suicide plan. They found that 0.7%–1.2% of elders in primary care had suicidal ideation, all of whom had a simultaneous mood disorder. Skoog et al. (669), in a survey of nondemented Swedes age 85 years and older, inquired about the presence of both active and passive suicidal ideation in the month preceding the interview. They found that 16% of the subjects had thoughts of suicide. Again, the rate was higher in subjects with mental disorder, in those taking anxiolytic and neuroleptic agents, and in those with significant physical illness. Among community-dwelling Floridians 60 years of age and older, less than 6% reported ever having had suicidal thoughts in a study by Schwab et al. (670), while in the Berlin Aging Study (671) 21% of subjects over age 70 reported having had suicidal ideation. Again, psychiatric illness was present in virtually all subjects, suggesting a need for careful screening for psychiatric disorder in elders with suicidal ideation.

b) Gender

In the United States, epidemiologic data show that suicide is more frequent in men than in women. For example, data from the National Center for Health Statistics for the year 2000 showed an age-adjusted suicide rate for males that was approximately 4.5-fold that for females (18.08 per 100,000 and 4.03 per 100,000, respectively) (11). This differential is comparable to the male-to-female ratio for suicide found in the National Longitudinal Mortality Study for the years 1979 to 1989 (672). Within the U.S. population, males are disproportionately represented among deaths by suicide in all racial and ethnic groups, with rates that range from more than 5.5-fold greater than that for females among African Americans and Hispanics to threefold greater than that for females among Asian/Pacific Islanders. This is not the case in other parts of the world, however. For example, in China the suicide rate for women is 25% higher than that for men (18).

The male-to-female predominance in suicide in the United States persists across the lifespan. Adolescent and young adult males are about 5.5 times more likely to die from suicide than females, whereas in midlife the male-to-female ratio is approximately 3.5 to 1. After about age 65, however, there is a steadily widening male-to-female ratio of suicide rates in all groups except Asians, with differences of more than 10-fold after age 80.

Differences in suicide risk with gender may be explained in part by factors that contribute to risk in general but that are present to differing degrees in men and in women. For example, men are less likely than women to seek help, admit the severity of their symptoms, or accept treatment, increasing their likelihood of suicide. In contrast, women tend to be less impulsive, have more social support, and have lower rates of comorbid alcohol and substance use disorders, all of which may have a protective effect (21). Among African American women, the potential protective factors of religion and extended kin networks have been suggested as possible explanations for this group's very low rate of suicide (22).

Despite their lower rate of suicide, women have higher rates of depressive illness than men (23, 673). Furthermore, in a 10-year follow-up study using data from the National Longitudinal Mortality Study, unemployment was associated with a greater and longer-lasting effect on the suicide rate of women compared to men (24). Compared to men, women also have an increased likelihood of having been physically or sexually abused, which may also increase the risk for suicide (36). The relative lethality of the suicide methods chosen by women remains less than those chosen by men; however, the recent, more frequent use of firearms among women suggests that this distinction may be diminishing (11, 674).

Suicide rates have also been examined in pregnant women and during the postpartum period. Dannenberg et al. (675) reviewed New York City medical examiner records of 293 pregnant or recently pregnant women ages 15 to 44 years who died of injury during a 4-year period. Of these, 15 died by suicide, a rate that was not significantly different from the expected age- and race-specific rates in the general population. However, Marzuk et al. (676) analyzed autopsy data from female residents of New York City who were of childbearing age and found the standardized mortality rate for suicide during pregnancy to be one-third the expected rate. Appleby (677), using retrospective population data for England and Wales from 1973 to 1984, also noted decreased rates of suicide among pregnant women and among women during the first year after childbirth, with SMRs of 0.05 and 0.17, respectively. In contrast to decreased suicide rates for women in general during pregnancy and the puerperium, Appleby et al. (27) subsequently found an extremely high suicide rate among women who had been psychiatrically hospitalized during the postpartum period. In this study of 1,567 women admitted to Danish psychiatric hospitals within the first year after childbirth, the SMR for suicide within 1 year was more than 70 times the expected rate. Although risk was greatest within the first month postpartum, it persisted throughout the initial year after childbirth. In addition, women who died by suicide after childbirth often used violent methods. Thus, although evidence is limited, women with severe postpartum psychiatric disturbances appear to be at significantly increased risk during the initial year after childbirth. Other groups with a particularly increased postpartum risk include teenagers and women of lower socioeconomic status (27, 28). For women as a group, however, a protective effect seems to be present during pregnancy and the postpartum period (25).

In terms of suicide attempts, women in the United States are reported to attempt suicide three times as often as men. This female predominance of suicide attempters varies with age, however, and in older adults the ratio of female-to-male suicide attempters approaches 1:1 (11). Similar trends are observed in the incidence of suicidal ideation. For example, Kuo et al. (29), using data from 3,481 prospectively followed individuals from the Baltimore ECA study, found that females ages 18 to 29 years had a higher incidence of suicidal ideation and suicide attempts than their male peers. However, this female-to-male predominance in suicidal ideation and suicide attempts was not observed for older age groups or for the sample as a whole.

As noted earlier, women are more likely to have experienced domestic violence or physical or sexual abuse, all of which have been associated with higher rates of suicidal ideation and suicide attempts (32–34). In a study of psychosocial outcomes in 1,991 same-sex twin pairs, Nelson et al. (35) found that childhood sexual abuse was three times more common in women and was associated with an increased risk of attempting suicide. Borderline personality disorder is also present more often in women (515) and is itself associated with increased rates of suicidal ideation, suicide, suicide attempts, and other self-injurious behaviors. In addition, borderline personality disorder is particularly common in women who have experienced childhood sexual abuse, physical abuse, or both (31). As a result, physical and sexual abuse and domestic violence should be given particular consideration in the assessment and treatment of women with suicidal ideation, suicide attempts, and other self-injurious behaviors.

c) Race, ethnicity, and culture

Race, ethnicity, and culture are all associated with variations in rates of suicide. In the United States for the year 2000, the overall age-adjusted rates of suicide were highest in Native Americans and non-Hispanic whites, at 13.6 and 12.1 per 100,000, respectively (11). In contrast, the age-adjusted rate of suicide in Hispanics was substantially less, at 6.13 per 100,000, and was similar to the rates for non-Hispanic African Americans and Asian/Pacific Islanders, at 5.8 and 6.0 per 100,000, respectively.

For immigrant groups, suicide rates in general tend to mirror rates in the countries of origin, with trends converging toward the host country over time (40, 41). In a large epidemiological study, Singh and Siahpush (39) found that between 1979 and 1989, foreign-born men in the United States were 52% less likely to die by suicide than native-born men, but the difference narrowed in the older age cohorts. Data for immigrant women were not statistically significant because of the small number of deaths.

In the United States, racial and ethnic differences are also seen in the rates of suicide across the lifespan (Table 10). Among European-American non-Hispanic whites, Hispanics, and Asian/Pacific Islanders, the highest suicide rates occur during the senior years, in those over age 65. In contrast, among Native Americans and African Americans, the highest suicide rates occur during adolescence and young adulthood. For example, in Native American and African American males ages 15 to 24, suicide rates in the year 2000 were 36.81 and 14.66 per 100,000, respectively. Young African American men have been described as being caught in a cycle of drug abuse, criminal activity, and self-devaluation and may view an early death as inevitable or as an alternative to the wearying struggle that life has become (678). Additional risk factors for suicide in young African American males include substance abuse (662, 679), presence of a firearm (663), and in particular the combination of cocaine abuse and the presence of a firearm (679). Suicidal ideation and suicide attempts are also common in urban African American young adults, with 6-month prevalences of 1.9% and 0.4%, respectively (680).

In contrast to young African American males, African American women have a very low rate of suicide. Gibbs (22) attributes this low rate to the protective factors of religion, including the role of religion in the civil rights movement, women's central involvement in the church, and strong values for endurance in the face of adversity. Women-dominated kinship networks are also believed to be protective, providing flexible roles, resource sharing, and social support (681).

Although black women are less likely to die from suicide than white women, they attempt suicide and express negative emotional states such as hopelessness and depression just as frequently. In addition, both black men and black women are less likely than their white counterparts to pursue professional counseling in the face of depression or other mental illness. Instead, African Americans are more likely to view depression as a "personal weakness" that can be successfully treated with prayer and faith alone some or almost all of the time (682). When depression is discussed, it may be described in different terms such as having "the blues" or "the aching misery" or "being down" (678). Consequently, sensitivity to language and beliefs about illness are important in recognizing depression and other risk factors for suicide among African Americans.

Among Native Americans (American Indians and Alaska Natives), suicide also is predominately an epidemic of the young and is the second leading cause of death for Native Americans between ages 15 and 24 years. As with other racial and ethnic groups, Native American and Alaska Natives are a very heterogeneous population, with different tribal identities, varying degrees of urbanization, different levels of tribal organization, and diverse approaches to historical and cultural integration. For example, in a study of three groups of Native Americans in New Mexico, the Apache had the highest suicide rate (43.3 per 100,000) and the highest degree of acculturation but also had the lowest degree of social integration and generally viewed religion as unimportant (683). In contrast, the Navajo had the lowest suicide rate (12.0 per 100,000) and the lowest level of acculturation but had moderate social integration and were organized into bands with a strong matrilineal clan influence. In the third group, the Pueblo, the subgroup with the most acculturation, had a higher suicide rate than the most traditional subgroup, again suggesting an effect of acculturation on suicide risk. Acculturation has also been proposed as a contributor to the extremely high suicide rate in Alaska Native youths, which in one study approached 120 per 100,000 (661). Theories to explain these high rates tend to rely on family disintegration, social disruption, and alcohol use (684), as well as rapid social and cultural changes associated with intensive energy development projects in the Arctic and the resulting stress of acculturation. In contrast, in Hawaiian youths, the relationship between acculturation and suicidal behavior is less clear, with increased numbers of suicide attempts in those with stronger Hawaiian cultural affiliation (685).

Research on suicide among Hispanics in the United States is limited and rarely differentiates among different Hispanic groups. In addition, many individuals of Hispanic origin are undocumented workers who are not represented in census data or epidemiological studies. Large-scale grouping of diverse ethnic groups also obscures intracultural variations in important social and economic categories. For example, Cuban American women and Mexican Americans and Puerto Ricans of both genders were reported to have lower than expected suicide rates, relative to 1-year prevalence of major depression, than were whites, blacks, and Cuban American males (23). In terms of suicidal ideation, higher levels have been reported in Central American immigrants experiencing heightened levels of acculturative stress (43). In addition, lifetime age- and gender-adjusted rates of suicidal ideation were significantly lower for Mexican Americans born in Mexico (4.5%) than for Mexican Americans born in the United States (13%) or for non-Latino whites (19.2%) (686). Similarly, rates of suicide attempt were lower among Mexican Americans born in Mexico (1.6%) and higher among both Mexican Americans born in the United States (4.8%) and non-Latino whites (4.4%). The rate of suicide attempt is also elevated among Hispanic youths, who had higher numbers of reported suicide attempts compared to non-Hispanic youths in a nationwide survey of high school students (687).

The suicide rate for Asians overall is the lowest of all of the major American ethnic groups, but Asian Americans themselves have diverse ethnic backgrounds, languages, and cultures. Some groups, such as the Japanese, have been in the United States for generations. Others, such as the Chinese, include both recent immigrants and descendants of 19th-century immigrants, whereas the Vietnamese have arrived in large numbers only since the 1960s. These individuals bring with them attitudes toward coping and suicide from their home countries, which can influence the circumstances of suicidal behavior (688). In Japan, for example, suicide is permissible or even appropriate in particular contexts, and ritual suicide has been an honorable solution to certain social dilemmas. For example, the disgrace of bankruptcy in Japan can shame the family for generations, making suicide a preferable way to resolve debt. When it is culturally important for a man to be physically healthy and able to support his family, suicide may be viewed as an option if a serious physical illness impairs his ability to function. For example, in Hawaii, 20.5% of suicides by Japanese American men occurred in individuals with health problems, in contrast to only 11.8% of suicides by Caucasian men and 3.0% by Hawaiian men (42). In addition, for individuals who come from a culture in which mental illness is highly stigmatized, receipt of a psychiatric diagnosis may increase the risk for suicide. Although Chinese societies have not generally codified suicide as socially acceptable, more recent suicide rates in China are quite high, particularly in women and in rural settings, where use of agricultural poisons is a common suicide method (18).

In the United States, acculturation and acculturative stress may be a contributor to suicide risk among Asian Americans. For most Asian Americans, the family unit is central to identity. Children are socialized into awareness that their individual actions reflect upon the entire family, including extended family members (689). While this feature may impede a family's willingness to seek treatment for a troubled relative, the strong sense of family as a support and source of obligation protects against suicide as well. At the same time, family conflict as a reason for suicide is more common in Eastern societies (42). For example, if a young woman from a traditional society experiences conflicts with her in-laws that have no apparent solution, the woman may be more likely to view suicide as an option than would someone from a different family system in which close family relationships are not as imperative. Transition to the individualistic, communication-oriented U.S.

society is a major and stressful change for many families (44). The group most at risk appears to be traditionalists who live in tight-knit groups resistant to acculturative processes. They appear to function relatively well until their elderly years, when the culture clash between the values of the larger society and the Confucian tradition of strong family identity results in alienation of elders and contributes to suicide in the style of the old country (44). For example, a major factor in the high suicide rate of elderly Asian/Pacific Islander women was reported to be the failure of younger family members to provide support for their elderly parents, especially widowed mothers (690). Such deaths occurred predominantly by hanging, which was traditionally seen as an act of revenge, since someone who died by hanging was believed to return to haunt the living as a ghost (690).

In summary, race, ethnicity, and culture may all influence population-based rates of suicide and suicide attempts. Of equal importance to the clinician, however, each of these factors may modify suicide risk within the individual. Views of death and cultural beliefs regarding suicide can vary widely, even among members of apparently homogeneous racial, ethnic, or cultural groups. Thus, as part of the assessment and treatment planning process, it can be helpful for the psychiatrist to explore the patient's beliefs about death and suicide and the role of cultural and family dynamics in these beliefs.

d) Marital status

Marital status has been correlated with variations in suicide mortality in a number of studies. Smith et al. (691) used data from the U.S. National Center for Health Statistics for the years 1979 to 1981 to calculate age-adjusted suicide rates for each marital status. Regardless of age or racial group, the suicide rate was consistently lowest in married individuals. An intermediate rate was seen in those who had never been married, with a relative risk that was about twice that in married individuals. The highest suicide rate was found for divorced or widowed individuals, with a relative risk that was about threefold greater than that in married individuals. Whereas divorced women had a higher age-adjusted suicide rate than widowed women, the opposite was true among men, with a particularly striking rate of suicide in young widowed men.

Kposowa (672) applied Cox proportional hazards regression models to data from the 1979–1989 follow-up of the National Longitudinal Mortality Study and made adjustments for age, sex, race, education, family income, and region of residence to estimate the effect of marital status on suicide risk. Although in this sample being single or widowed had no significant effect on suicide risk, divorced and separated persons had suicide rates that were more than twice that of married persons. Stratification of the sample by sex showed that the effect of marital status on suicide rates occurred only among men.

Luoma and Pearson (46) also examined whether marital status is associated with variations in suicide rates. Suicide rates broken down by race, 5-year age groups, sex, and marital status were calculated by using data compiled from the U.S. National Center for Health Statistics Multiple-Cause-of-Death Files for the years 1991 to 1996. Widowed white and African American men under age 50 were found to have substantial elevations in suicide rates, with 17-fold and ninefold higher rates, respectively, compared with married men under age 50. At younger ages, for women as well as for men, being widowed was associated with a higher suicide rate, compared with being married.

Using data from the National Suicide Prevention Project in Finland, Heikkinen et al. (402) investigated age-related variations in marital status as well as other social factors in a sample of 1,067 individuals who died by suicide during a 1-year period and for whom relevant data were available. Compared with the general population, individuals who died by suicide were more commonly divorced, widowed, or never married. Among individuals under age 50 who died by suicide, more males than females had never been married. Among those over age 50, more women than men were widowed.

Other data from Finland obtained through the Finnish Population Register and cause-of-death files also suggest that the rate of suicide is elevated among widowed individuals (45). Among

95,647 persons who were widowed during 1972–1976 and followed up to the end of 1976, 7,635 deaths were observed, of which 144 were due to suicide. During the initial month of bereavement, men had a much greater increase in suicide mortality than women (17.2-fold versus 4.5-fold), but this disproportionate ratio primarily resulted from occurrences of homicide-suicide. In the remaining first year of bereavement, men had a 3.1-fold increase in suicide mortality and women a 2.2-fold increase, and rates remained higher than expected throughout the follow-up period.

Overall, these studies suggest that married individuals have a significantly lower rate of suicide than unmarried individuals. In addition, elevations in the suicide rate are especially striking for widowed men in general and young widowed men in particular. What remains unclear is whether this protective effect of marriage on the suicide rate relates to specific benefits of marriage, such as a greater likelihood of social integration. In contrast, the decrease in social integration and the psychological experience of loss with widowhood and with divorce may increase the tendency for suicide. The suicide rate among divorced individuals could also be higher because individuals who stay married have a greater likelihood of stable mental health at baseline. Other confounding factors, such as differences in substance use or socioeconomic status with marital status, could play additional roles that should be considered in the assessment process.

e) Sexual orientation

It remains unclear whether suicide rates in gay, lesbian, and bisexual individuals differ from the suicide rate among heterosexual individuals. One psychological autopsy study compared gay males to all other similarly aged males in the sample and did not find any characteristics that distinguished the two groups (692). However, research on suicide among gay, lesbian, and bisexual individuals is particularly complex because of many factors, including small sample sizes, difficulties in achieving random sampling, problems in obtaining baseline prevalences, and problems in reliability of postmortem reports of sexual orientation. In addition, individuals may choose not to disclose their sexual orientation to researchers or may engage in same-sex behavior but not identify themselves as gay or lesbian.

The risks for suicide attempts and suicidal ideation in gay, lesbian, and bisexual individuals have been assessed by using several approaches. Fergusson et al. (51), analyzing longitudinal data gathered on a New Zealand birth cohort, found that those who identified themselves as gay, lesbian, and bisexual or reported having a same-sex partner since the age of 16 had elevated rates of suicidal ideation (odds ratio=5.4) and suicide attempts (odds ratio=6.2). A study by Cochran and Mays (50) examined lifetime prevalences of suicide-related symptoms among men with same-gender partners and found that approximately one-half (53.2%) of the men reported experiencing at least one suicide-related symptom in their lifetime, with a suicide attempt reported by 19.3%. In contrast, in men with female partners only, 33.2% had at least one suicide-related symptom and 3.6% reported a suicide attempt. Corresponding figures for those with no sexual partners were 28.1% and 0.5%, respectively. Using the population-based Vietnam Era Twin Registry, Herrell et al. (52) identified a subsample of 103 middle-aged male twin pairs in which one of the twins from each pair reported having a male sexual partner after age 18 while the other did not. Suicide attempts were more common in the men with same-gender sexual orientation, with 15% reporting a suicide attempt, compared with only 4% of their twin brothers. In the Twin Registry sample as a whole, which included 16 twin pairs concordant for having a male sexual partner after age 18 and 6,434 twin pairs concordant for having no adult same-gender partners, the men with same-gender sexual orientation had more than a fourfold increase in suicidal ideation and more than a 6.5-fold increase in suicide attempts.

Gay, lesbian, and bisexual youths may be at particular risk for suicidal behaviors. Paul et al. (53), in a study of a large urban population–based telephone probability sample of gay men, found that 21% had made a suicide plan and 12% had attempted suicide. Of the latter, almost one-half had made multiple attempts, and most had made their first attempt before age 25. The importance of sexual orientation to suicidal behaviors in youths is also highlighted by the findings of a statewide population-based study of public high school students by Remafedi et al. (48). In this study, suicide attempts were reported by 28.1% of bisexual/homosexual males, 20.5% of bisexual/homosexual females, 14.5% of heterosexual females, and 4.2% of heterosexual males. For males, but not for females, a bisexual/homosexual orientation was associated with suicidal intent (odds ratio=3.61) and with suicide attempts (odds ratio=7.10).

Thus, although evidence is limited, there is clearly an elevated risk for suicide attempts among cohorts of gay, lesbian, and bisexual individuals that is particularly striking among youths. In addition to addressing risk factors such as psychiatric and substance use disorders in the assessment and treatment planning processes, it is also important for the clinician to address stresses that are unique to being gay, lesbian, or bisexual (e.g., disclosure of sexual orientation to friends and family, homophobia, harassment, and gender nonconformity). Since suicide attempts themselves increase the risk for later suicide, it is presumed that suicide rates may also be increased in gay, lesbian, and bisexual individuals. However, this hypothesis remains to be tested empirically.

f) Occupation

Occupational groups differ in a number of factors contributing to suicide risk. These factors include demographics (e.g., race, gender, socioeconomic class, and marital status), occupational stress, psychiatric morbidity, and occupationally associated opportunities for suicide. Although many studies have reported increased rates of suicide in specific occupational groups, most have not controlled for other suicide risk factors. In one study, however, that controlled for basic demographic correlates of suicide across 32 occupations (54), risk was found to be highest among dentists and physicians, compared with the rest of the working-age population, with multivariate logistic regression odds ratios of 5.43 and 2.31, respectively. The odds of suicide were also significantly higher in nurses (1.58 times the risk), social workers (1.52 times the risk), mathematicians and scientists (1.47 times the risk), and artists (1.30 times the risk). Rates of suicide among physicians have also been found to be elevated, compared with rates for other white male professionals, with white male physicians having a 70% greater proportionate mortality ratio for suicide (58). In well-designed epidemiological studies, police officers have generally not been found to be at higher risk for suicide than age- and sex-matched comparison subjects (54, 57).

Factors that may play a role in the increased suicide rates in specific professions may include occupational stresses, as is seen in helping professionals (54), or social isolation, as is seen in sheepherders, who had the highest suicide rate of 22 occupational groups studied in Washington State (56). Although data are inconsistent, additional work stress may occur with infrequent role sets such as female laborers or pilots (55, 57) or in nontraditional occupations (693). In some occupations, suicide rates may be influenced by greater access to lethal methods such as medications or chemicals, as in health care professionals, scientists, and agricultural workers (57).

Differential rates of psychiatric illness may be present in some occupations and may predate employment. Artists, for example, have higher rates of psychiatric morbidity and suicide than the general population. Highly educated people with depressive disorders also have a higher suicide rate. Among physicians, such individuals may tend to specialize in psychiatry (56).

In general, specific occupations do seem to be associated with an increased risk for suicide, but more research is needed to distinguish occupational from nonoccupational stressors (56) and to determine whether it is the occupation itself or associated factors such as psychiatric morbidity that affect suicide risk.

2. Major psychiatric syndromes

a) Mood disorders

Major depressive disorder and other depressive syndromes are the most commonly and most consistently identified axis I diagnoses in individuals who die by suicide (694, 695). For example, Robins et al. (60) found that among 134 persons who died by suicide, 98% were psychiatrically ill and most had depression or chronic alcoholism. Barraclough et al. (65), in a similar study, found that of 100 individuals who died by suicide, 93% were mentally ill and 85% had either depression or alcoholism. Henriksson et al. (59), using psychological autopsy methods to investigate current mental disorders among a random sample of 229 persons who died by suicide during a 1-year period in Finland, found that 93% of those persons had received at least one axis I diagnosis and that 59% had a depressive disorder.

In patients with bipolar disorder who die by suicide, the majority are experiencing either a depressive or mixed episode of illness (69, 72, 315). For example, Isometsa et al. (68) noted that among 31 patients with bipolar disorder identified in a group of 1,397 persons who died by suicide in Finland in a 12-month period, 79% died while in a major depressive episode and 11% while in a mixed state. In a study of more than 300 patients who were discontinued from lithium treatment, Baldessarini et al. (696) found that the majority of suicidal acts occurred either during a major depressive episode (73%) or during a dysphoric-mixed episode (16%).

In addition to being highly prevalent in individuals who die from suicide, mood disorders have long been associated with an increased risk for suicide. For example, in 1970, Guze and Robins (697) reviewed 17 studies that assessed the risk of suicide in individuals with primary affective disorders and calculated the frequency of suicide as a percentage of all deaths. High suicide rates were found, with the ultimate risk of suicide estimated to be about 15%, or approximately 30 times that seen in the general population. For major depression, review of the literature suggests that overall rates of suicide mortality range from 5% to 26% and are about twice as high for men as for women (694). However, these studies generally assessed severely ill patient populations and individuals early in the course of their illness, when suicide rates are known to be highest.

Several investigators have subsequently reexamined these estimates of lifetime suicide risk in individuals with mood disorders. For example, Inskip et al. (94), using cohort-based curve-fitting techniques and data from previous studies, estimated the lifetime risk for suicide in mood disorders to be 6%. In addition, Bostwick and Pankratz (77) used data from prior studies to calculate case fatality prevalences (the ratio of suicides to the total number of subjects) to determine suicide risks for three groups of patients with affective disorders—outpatients, inpatients, and suicidal inpatients. With this method, which provides a less biased estimate of risk, they found a gradation in suicide risk that varied with treatment setting as well as with hospitalization for suicidality. For example, in patients with mood disorders who were previously hospitalized for suicidality, the estimated lifetime prevalence of suicide was 8.6%, compared to a lifetime risk of 4% for those with a psychiatric hospitalization for any reason. For mixed inpatient/outpatient populations, the prevalence of suicide was 2.2%, whereas for the populations without affective illness, it was less than 0.5%. For individuals with major depressive disorder, Blair-West et al. (205) used age- and gender-stratified calculations to arrive at comparable estimates for lifetime suicide risk of 3.4%, with a lifetime risk for males more than six times than for females (6.8% versus 1.1%).

Harris and Barraclough (64), in their meta-analysis of suicide as an outcome in psychiatric illness, assessed relative suicide risk in mood disorder by calculating SMRs. Their analysis used data from published English-language studies that had mean or median follow-up periods of at least 2 years and that provided sufficient data to calculate ratios of observed to expected numbers of suicides. For patients with major depressive disorder, 23 studies that included a total of 351 suicides among more than 8,000 patients yielded an SMR of 20.35, or a 20-fold increase in risk. A key finding was that risk in patients with major depressive disorder was highest immediately after hospital discharge (698, 699). For patients with bipolar disorder, data from 15 studies including a total of 93 suicides among 3,700 subjects yielded an SMR for suicide of 15.05. Although patients with dysthymia also had an elevated SMR for suicide, of 12.12, the nine studies that contributed to this estimate were extremely heterogeneous in their findings and most had extremely small samples, which raises some question about the validity of this approximation.

Several studies have examined rates of suicide in longitudinal follow-up in individuals hospitalized for mood disorder. Hoyer et al. (75) used data from the Danish Psychiatric Case Register to determine SMRs for suicide among 54,103 patients (19,638 male and 34,465 female patients) who had an initial admission to a Danish psychiatric hospital between 1973 and 1993 and who received a mood disorder diagnosis. During the study period, 29% of the patients died, and of those, suicide occurred in 20%. Standardized mortalities for suicide were comparable for patients with ICD-8 diagnoses of unipolar major depression, psychotic reactive depression, and bipolar disorder, with SMRs of 19.33, 18.67, and 18.09, respectively. In contrast, the SMR for suicide in patients with neurotic depression was significantly less, at 10.51. In all diagnostic subgroups and regardless of age and gender, the risk of suicide was greatest during the first year after the initial admission, decreased over the subsequent 5 years, and then stabilized. Overall, the risk for suicide was comparable in men and women, except in patients with bipolar disorder, for whom the SMR for suicide was somewhat greater in women than in men (20.31 versus 18.09).

In a similarly designed study using data from a Swedish inpatient register, Osby et al. (73) obtained the date and cause of death for patients hospitalized between 1973 and 1995 with a diagnosis of bipolar disorder (N=15,386) or unipolar depressive disorder (N=39,182). SMRs for suicide were found to be significantly increased in women and in patients with a unipolar depressive disorder diagnosis (15.0 for male bipolar disorder patients, 20.9 for male unipolar depressive disorder patients, 22.4 for female bipolar disorder patients, and 27.0 for female unipolar depressive disorder patients). Suicide mortality was more pronounced in younger individuals and with shorter intervals from the index hospitalization. Although SMRs decreased in all age groups with increasing time of follow-up, some suicide risk persisted even at long follow-up intervals.

Baxter and Appleby (188) used the Salford (U.K.) Psychiatric Case Register to identify 7,921 individuals who had received psychiatric or mental health care and determined their mortality rates (estimated as rate ratios) over a follow-up period of up to 18 years. Among individuals with affective disorders, there was a 12.2-fold elevation in observed suicide mortality in men, compared to expected mortality based on population rates. For women, the relative increase in suicide mortality was even greater, with a 16.3-fold elevation.

Angst et al. (74) followed a sample of 406 hospitalized patients with mood disorders (220 with bipolar disorder and 186 with unipolar depressive disorder) on a prospective basis for 22 years or more and found an overall standardized mortality rate for suicide of 18.04, comparable to the SMRs found in the Swedish and Danish longitudinal follow-up studies. Sixty-one percent of the sample had manifested psychotic symptoms at least once over their lifetime, suggesting that this was a particularly ill group of patients. The suicide rate was greatest near the age of illness onset; however, from ages 30 to 70 years, the rate was remarkably constant, suggesting a persistence of risk throughout the illness course. The suicide mortality in women was greater than that in men (SMR of 21.87 for women, compared to 13.49 for men), in part reflecting the greater rate of suicide for men in the general population. Patients with unipolar depressive disorder had a significantly higher rate of suicide than patients with bipolar I disorder or bipolar II disorder, with an SMR for suicide of 26.7, compared with 12.3 for bipolar disorder patients. The SMR for suicide did not differ significantly between bipolar I disorder patients and bipolar II disorder patients.

Some evidence suggests that in individuals with mood disorders, the rate of suicide may be increasing over time. For example, Harris and Barraclough (64) noted that the suicide risk for patients with major depression in cohorts treated before 1970 was increased by 17-fold in contrast to a 36-fold increase in risk for cohorts treated after 1970. In the study described earlier, Hoyer et al. (75) noted an increase in both the absolute and relative risks for suicide over the 20-year study time period, and they suggested that the increase may have been related to changes in the health care delivery system and the availability of psychiatric inpatient services.

In addition, Baldessarini et al. (563) observed that the annualized rates of suicide and suicide attempts in patients with major affective disorders appear to have risen across the decades since 1970. This trend was sustained and statistically significant for both suicides and suicide attempts, as well as for treated and untreated samples considered separately. Although this apparent secular trend could reflect increased recruitment of more severely ill patients to more recent studies or increased reporting of suicidal behaviors, the percentage reduction of suicide risk with lithium treatment did not decline across the years, suggesting that the patient populations are in fact comparable and that the prevention of suicide in major affective disorders is becoming increasingly challenging (558). Furthermore, suicide attempts that do occur in individuals with major mood disorders may be more lethal than suicide attempts by individuals in the general population. The reported ratio of suicide attempts to deaths from suicide averages between 3:1 and 5:1 among persons with mood disorders, whereas in the general population the suicide attempt rate has been estimated to be about 10–20 times (average, 18 times) greater than the suicide rate, or about 0.3% per year (700).

For individuals with mood disorders, it is also important to note factors that are particularly associated with increased risk. Fawcett et al. (79, 313) determined time-related predictors of suicide in a sample of 954 psychiatric inpatients in the NIMH Collaborative Program on the Psychobiology of Depression, about one-third of whom had bipolar disorder and the rest of whom had other mood disorders. During the initial 10 years of follow-up, 34 patients died by suicide, an overall rate that was extremely low, at 0.36% per year. The first year of follow-up was the time of highest risk, with 38% of suicides occurring during that period. Within 1 year of admission, six factors were associated with suicide: panic attacks, severe psychic anxiety, diminished concentration, global insomnia, moderate alcohol abuse, and anhedonia. The three factors associated with suicide that occurred after 1 year were severe hopelessness, suicidal ideation, and history of previous suicide attempts. By 14 years, among individuals for whom follow-up information was available, 36 had died by suicide, 120 had attempted suicide, and 373 had no recorded suicide attempt (247). Analysis at that time point showed that patients who died by suicide and patients with suicide attempts shared core characteristics, including a history of previous suicide attempts, alcohol and substance abuse, impulsivity, and psychic turmoil within a cycling/mixed bipolar disorder. In contrast to suicide within 12 months of intake, which was predicted by clinical variables, suicide beyond 12 months was prospectively predicted by temperament attributes, such as higher levels of impulsivity and assertiveness. Stressful life events (701), executive dysfunction (702), and higher levels of depression (10, 78, 221, 222, 703) may also be associated with greater risk, as may an awareness of the discrepancies between a previously envisioned "normal" future and the patient's likely degree of future chronic disability (273).

In summary, mood disorders are consistently identified as conferring a significant increase in the risk for suicide as well as for suicide attempts. However, among individuals with mood disorders, a variety of factors commonly modify that risk and should be taken into consideration during the assessment and treatment planning processes. These factors include the specific mood disorder diagnosis and duration of illness, the type and severity of the mood episode, the prior history of treatment, the presence of comorbid diagnoses or specific psychiatric symptoms such as severe anxiety or agitation, and the occurrence of significant psychosocial stressors. It is important to note, however, that this increased risk of suicidal behaviors among individuals with mood disorders has been consistently shown to be modifiable with treatment (see Section VI.D, "Somatic Therapies").

b) Schizophrenia

Schizophrenia has also been associated with an increase risk of suicide in multiple studies. Harris and Barraclough (172), for example, analyzed data from 38 studies that had follow-up periods of up to 60 years. Acknowledging that some heterogeneity in the diagnosis of schizophrenia across studies was likely as a result of changes in diagnostic criteria, the authors noted 1,176 suicides among more than 30,000 patients with schizophrenia, yielding an SMR for suicide in schizophrenia of 8.45. Baxter and Appleby (188), in a case registry study of long-term suicide risk in the United Kingdom, found an even higher 14-fold increase in rate ratios for suicide among individuals with schizophrenia. In contrast, using cohort-based curve-fitting techniques and data from 29 studies of mortality in schizophrenia, Inskip et al. (94) estimated the lifetime risk for suicide as 4%.

In addition to assessing suicide rates among patients with schizophrenia, longitudinal follow-up studies have also examined factors associated with increased risk of suicide. Black et al. (98) found that suicide occurred in 14 of 688 schizophrenia patients (2%) who were admitted to an Iowa psychiatric hospital over a 10-year period, with the majority of deaths occurring within 2 years of hospital discharge. Although women were found to be at relatively greater risk, the numbers of suicides significantly exceeded expected rates for both male and female patients. Nyman and Jonsson (101) found that suicide occurred in 10 of 110 (9%) young patients with schizophrenia who were hospitalized between 1964 and 1967 and followed for up to 17 years. In this group, suicide was associated with a more chronic course as well as with social and financial dependency. Dingman and McGlashan (103) longitudinally followed 163 Chestnut Lodge patients with a diagnosis of schizophrenia and noted that the 13 patients who died by suicide were predominantly male and had a later onset of illness, less chronic illness, better premorbid functioning, and a greater ability for abstract and conceptual thinking. At a later follow-up (mean=19 years), 6.4% of the Chestnut Lodge sample had died by suicide, and this group had exhibited fewer negative symptoms but more severe delusions and suspiciousness at index admission than those who did not die by suicide (93). A group of young psychotic patients who had not exhibited a chronic course was followed after discharge from an index hospitalization by Westermeyer et al. (83), who found that 36 patients died by suicide and 550 did not. Suicide occurred in about 9% of individuals with schizophrenia and was more likely during the early years of their illness, particularly within 6 years of initial hospitalization. At greater risk for suicide were unmarried white male patients with chronic symptoms, relatively high IQs, and a gradual onset of illness.

De Hert et al. (89) studied outcomes for 870 patients (536 men and 334 women) with schizophrenia (87%) or schizoaffective disorder (13%) after a mean duration of follow-up of 11.4 years. Sixty-three individuals died by suicide, yielding a suicide rate of 635 per 100,000 per year and an SMR for suicide of 39.7. The frequency of suicide in men was twice that in women, although the SMR and the age at the time of suicide did not differ significantly between the sexes. Of the suicides, 33 (52.4%) occurred while the patient was hospitalized (although only nine actually took place in the hospital) and 12 (19.1%) occurred during the first 6 months after discharge. When the patients who died by suicide were compared with an age- and sex-matched group of 63 patients from the remaining sample, a number of differences between the groups were observed. Those who died by suicide were more likely to have a family history of suicide, had had more and shorter hospitalizations and more past suicide attempts, and were more likely to have used a highly lethal method in prior suicide attempts. They also had higher total WAIS IQ scores and were more likely to have been psychotic or depressed or to have suffered a major loss in the 6 months before death or follow-up. Compared with control subjects, the patients who died by suicide were also less likely to have received community-based care and were less likely to have had a useful daily activity, remission of symptoms, or an early onset of prominent negative symptoms.

Among individuals with schizophrenia who die by suicide, a number of demographic factors seem to be present more often than in living control subjects. In a cohort of 9,156 patients with schizophrenia, Rossau and Mortensen (95) individually matched 10 control subjects to each of 508 individuals who were admitted to Danish hospitals between 1970 and 1987 and who later died by suicide. They found suicide risk to be particularly high during the first 5 days after discharge, with some excess suicides during temporary hospital leaves. Increases in risk were also associated with multiple psychiatric admissions during the previous year, previous suicide attempts, previous diagnosis of depression, male sex, and previous admissions to general hospitals for physical disorders. Breier and Astrachan (102) compared 20 schizophrenia patients who died by suicide with a randomly selected sex-matched group of nonsuicidal schizophrenia patients and a group of persons without schizophrenia who died by suicide. Patients with schizophrenia who died by suicide were more likely to be men and tended to be young, white, and never married. In contrast to the persons without schizophrenia who died by suicide, the schizophrenia patients who died by suicide tended not to show a temporal relationship of suicide with suicide attempts or stressful life events.

Among individuals who died by suicide, comparisons have also been made between those with schizophrenia and those with other diagnoses. Heila et al. (100) used psychological autopsy data for 1,397 individuals who died by suicide over a 1-year period in Finland and compared the 92 individuals with schizophrenia (7%) to the remainder of the sample. They found that suicide occurred at any point during the course of schizophrenia and over a large age range. In addition, among the individuals with schizophrenia, 71% had a history of suicide attempts, and, particularly in women, active illness and depressive symptoms were often observed immediately before the suicide. Significant life events, however, were seen less often before suicide in individuals with schizophrenia than in those with other diagnoses (46% and 83%, respectively).

Other studies have found suicidal ideation and suicide attempts to be common among individuals with schizophrenia. For example, in the Chestnut Lodge sample, over an average of 19 years of follow-up, 40% of the patients with schizophrenia spectrum disorders reported suicidal ideation since their initial hospitalization, and 23% reported at least one suicide attempt (93). Radomsky et al. (80) evaluated lifetime rates of suicidal behavior among 1,048 consecutively admitted psychiatric inpatients with DSM-III-R psychotic disorders. Of the 454 individuals with a diagnosis of schizophrenia, 27.3% reported at least one lifetime suicide attempt, with an additional 26.4% reporting suicidal ideation only. For the 159 patients with schizoaffective disorder, 42.8% and 27% reported suicide attempts and suicidal ideation, respectively. Roy et al. (117) found that 55% of a series of 127 consecutively admitted patients with chronic schizophrenia had previously made a suicide attempt. Harkavy-Friedman et al. (108), in a sample of 104 individuals with schizophrenia or schizoaffective disorder, found that 33% had made a suicide attempt, with 60% of those reporting multiple attempts. Attempts were often medically serious, requiring medical inpatient care in 57% of cases and emergency medical evaluation in an additional 11%, and were associated with strong suicidal intent (in the 76% of patients for whom this information was available). As with suicide in schizophrenia, initial suicide attempts tended to occur early during the course of the illness.

A number of specific factors appear to increase the likelihood of a suicide attempt among individuals with schizophrenia. For example, in the study by Roy et al. (117), those who had attempted suicide had significantly more psychiatric admissions and were more likely to have experienced a major depressive episode or received antidepressant treatment, compared with those who had not attempted suicide. Young et al. (704), in a longitudinal study of 96 individuals with recent-onset schizophrenia who were followed for a 1-year period, noted that depression was moderately correlated with concurrent suicidality but was not independently associated with future suicidality, whereas the presence of suicidal ideation even at low levels increased the risk for significant suicidal ideation or a suicide attempt during the subsequent 3 months. In their sample, Harkavy-Friedman et al. (108) found that suicide attempts were reported to be precipitated by depression (27%), loss of a significant other or other stressful life event (24%), being bothered by psychotic symptoms (11%), and responding to command hallucinations (4%). In a subsequent study of 100 individuals with schizophrenia, Harkavy-Friedman et al. (106) found that 8% of suicide attempts were associated with command auditory hallucinations for suicide and that individuals with previous suicide attempts were at particularly increased risk. In a prospective study of 333 patients with chronic schizophrenia (705), multivariate analysis suggested that current and lifetime suicide attempts and suicidal ideation were associated with hopelessness and possibly with greater levels of insight or higher cognitive functioning. Increased insight, specifically awareness of delusions and negative symptoms, has also been noted in individuals with schizophrenia who experience recurrent suicidal thoughts and behaviors (706).

In summary, an increase in the risks of suicide and suicide attempts is seen in individuals with schizophrenia and should be taken into consideration in the assessment and treatment planning process. Additional factors that modify risk include the duration of illness, the patient's insight into the illness's implications, the patient's history of treatment, and the presence of comorbid diagnoses or specific psychiatric symptoms, such as depression, hopelessness, or negative symptoms. As with mood disorders, however, increasing evidence also suggests that the risk of suicidal behaviors among individuals with schizophrenia can be modifiable with treatment (see Section VI.D, "Somatic Therapies").

c) Anxiety disorders

Data on lifetime rates of suicide among patients with anxiety disorders are limited but suggest that these diagnoses are associated with an increase in suicide risk. At the same time, it is not clear whether anxiety disorders represent an independent risk factor for suicide or whether this increased risk is attributable to the presence of depressive disorders or substance use disorders, which commonly co-occur with anxiety disorders.

Among broadly defined groups of individuals with anxiety disorders, increased rates of suicide have been seen in several studies. Khan et al. (118) used the U.S. Food and Drug Administration (FDA) database to assess the risk of suicide among patients who were participating in recent clinical trials of antianxiety medications and had diagnoses of panic disorder, social phobia, generalized anxiety disorder, posttraumatic stress disorder, or obsessive-compulsive disorder. Among the 20,076 patients, 12 died by suicide, yielding a suicide risk among patients with anxiety disorders of 193 per 100,000 patients, or at least 10-fold higher than that in the general population. This finding is particularly striking since the patients were receiving treatment and since current suicidality is generally an exclusion criterion for clinical trials. Allgulander (119) also noted an increased risk of suicide in individuals with anxiety disorders. Data on 9,912 patients with anxiety neurosis in the Swedish National Psychiatric Case Register between 1973 and 1983 yielded SMRs for suicide before age 45 of 6.7 and 4.9 for men and women, respectively. Suicide risk was highest within 3 months of discharge and was two- to threefold less than the risk in individuals with depressive neurosis.

Several studies have examined characteristics of patients with panic attacks or panic disorder who have died by suicide. Henriksson et al. (707) used data on suicides in Finland in a 1-year period to examine the relationship between panic disorder and suicide. All of the 17 persons with a current diagnosis of panic disorder who died by suicide—1.22% of the 1,397 suicides in Finland in the 1-year period—also had another axis I disorder, most often major depression. A substance use disorder was found in one-half of these individuals, with almost one-half of those persons also receiving an axis II diagnosis. These results are in accord with those of a study by Barraclough et al. (65), which found a principal diagnosis of either alcoholism or depression in virtually all persons who died by suicide and who had had a panic attack in the week before death.

Two smaller follow-up studies of patients with panic disorder yielded similar conclusions. Noyes et al. (122) found that 4% (three of 74) of patients with panic disorder followed up after 7 years had died by suicide, with an additional 7% (five of 74) having made a serious suicide attempt. Comorbid diagnoses, particularly major depression and axis II disorders, were more likely to be present in those who died by suicide and in serious suicide attempters. Coryell et al. (123) found that 35 years after an index admission, approximately 20% of 113 patients with panic disorder had died by suicide and that alcoholism and secondary depression may have had a role in those deaths.

Rates of suicidal ideation and suicide attempts are also increased in individuals with anxiety disorders, but again, comorbid diagnoses may play a role in mediating this effect. In a random sample of 18,011 adults from five U.S. communities derived from the ECA study, Weissman et al. (125) found that the presence of suicidal ideation and suicide attempts varied. Levels were highest among subjects with a lifetime diagnosis of panic disorder, followed by those who had panic attacks but not panic disorder and those with other DSM-III disorders but not panic attacks or panic disorder; lower levels were found in individuals with no prior panic attacks or DSM-III diagnoses. Weissman et al. also found that 20% of the subjects with panic disorder and 12% of those with panic attacks had made suicide attempts. Furthermore, this increase in risk was not solely attributable to comorbid diagnoses, since the lifetime rate of suicide attempts for persons with uncomplicated panic disorder was consistently higher than that for persons with no psychiatric disorder (7% and 1%, respectively) (708). This conclusion contrasted with the findings of Hornig and McNally (137), who reanalyzed the ECA data with the effects of comorbid disorders and sociodemographic variables controlled in the aggregate rather than singly. Using both stepwise and backward logistic regression analyses, they did not find panic disorder to be associated with a significant increase in risk for suicide attempts beyond that predicted by the presence of other disorders.

Other investigators have assessed other populations to determine whether panic attacks or panic disorder is associated with increases in suicidal behaviors. Pilowsky et al. (130), in a study of 1,580 adolescents in an urban public school system, found that suicidal ideation was three times more likely and a history of suicide attempts twice as likely in individuals with panic attacks, even after the effects of demographic factors, major depression, and substance use were controlled. Fleet et al. (136) assessed 441 consecutive patients who presented to an emergency department with chest pain and who underwent a structured psychiatric interview. Of the total sample, 108 (25%) met the DSM-III-R criteria for panic disorder. The investigators found that more of those with panic disorder had experienced suicidal ideation during the preceding week than of those without panic disorder (25% and 5%, respectively), even after controlling for the effect of coexisting major depression. In addition, of the 44 patients (10% of the sample) who had experienced suicidal ideation during the preceding week, 60% met the DSM-III-R criteria for panic disorder (709). Thus, in both of these populations, panic attacks or panic disorder was a significant risk factor for suicidal ideation or suicide attempts, independent of comorbid disorders.

Other studies have assessed psychiatric outpatients with panic disorder and have demonstrated substantial variability in its effect on suicidality. Cox et al. (124), for example, used the suicide questions from the ECA study to assess 106 patients with panic disorder and found that 31% of the patients reported suicidal ideation and 18% reported a history of suicide attempts. Very few individuals with suicidal ideation reported actual suicide attempts within the preceding year. However, when suicide attempts did occur, they were predominantly in the context of depressed mood. In a sample of 100 outpatients with panic disorder, Lepine et al. (129) found that 42% had a prior suicide attempt. Suicide attempters were more likely to be female or unmarried, and 88% of the patients met the DSM-III-R criteria for at least one additional diagnosis, predominantly major depressive disorder (52%) or substance use disorder (31%). Warshaw et al. (127) followed 498 patients with panic disorder and found a 6% risk of suicidal behaviors over a 5-year period. Being married or having children were protective factors, whereas mood disorders, substance use, eating disorders, personality disorders, female sex, and a prior history of suicide attempts were associated with increased risk. In the absence of other risk factors, the risk of a suicide attempt in persons with panic disorder was minimal. King et al. (126) studied 346 depressed outpatients and found a significant difference in the frequency of suicide attempts in those with a history of panic attacks compared with those without such a history (26.9% and 16.8%, respectively). Paradoxically, however, depressed patients with a history of infrequent panic attacks had a higher incidence of suicide attempts than those with panic disorder (32.3% and 21.5%, respectively). Friedman et al. (710) assessed 293 patients with panic disorder, of whom 59 had comorbid borderline personality disorder. A past history of suicide attempts was reported by 25% of the patients with comorbid borderline personality disorder and by 2% of those without that comorbidity. In contrast, Beck et al. (128) found that none of the 73 patients with primary panic disorder in a study of 900 consecutive psychiatric outpatients reported having made a prior suicide attempt.

Other anxiety disorders, although less well studied, may also influence suicide attempts or suicidal ideation. For example, in recent clinical trials of new antianxiety medications that included patients with a broad range of diagnoses, the risk of suicide attempts was increased relative to the general population, with attempts occurring in 28 of 20,076 patients, for an annualized risk of 1,350 per 100,000 patients (118). Cox et al. (124) found that of 41 outpatients with a diagnosis of social phobia, 14 (34%) had experienced suicidal ideation and two (5%) had made a suicide attempt within the prior year, although five (12%) had at least one lifetime suicide attempt. Oquendo et al. (131) assessed 156 inpatients with a diagnosis of major depressive episode and found that those with comorbid posttraumatic stress disorder were more likely to have attempted suicide, a finding that was more prominent in women than in men and that was independent of the presence of borderline personality disorder. Schaffer et al. (132) retrospectively reviewed the assessments of 533 patients with major depression and found that suicidal ideation was present in 57.8%. Suicidal ideation was more likely to be present in the 43.2% of the sample that had a lifetime anxiety disorder, and this association was independent of either age or severity of depressive symptoms. In contrast, in a study of 272 inpatients with at least one major depressive episode, Placidi et al. (220) found that rates of panic disorder did not differ between the 143 patients who had attempted suicide and the 129 patients who had not. In fact, agitation, psychic anxiety, and hypochondriasis were more severe in the nonattempter group, and these effects were independent of severity of aggression and impulsivity. However, rates of comorbid borderline personality disorder were much greater in those who attempted suicide, which may have contributed to these findings.

Even subsyndromal anxiety symptoms may contribute to an increase in risk. For example, Marshall et al. (135) found that rates of suicidal ideation increased linearly and significantly with an increasing number of subthreshold symptoms of posttraumatic stress disorder. They reported that for the 2,608 of 9,358 individuals who were screened in 1997 as part of National Anxiety Disorders Screening Day and who reported at least one symptom of posttraumatic stress disorder of at least 1 month's duration, the risk of suicidal ideation was increased, even after controlling for the effect of comorbid major depressive disorder.

Anxiety disorders may be overrepresented among individuals with suicidal ideation or suicide attempts. Pirkis et al. (383) analyzed data from 10,641 respondents in the Australian National Survey of Mental Health and Wellbeing and found that the relative risk of anxiety disorder was increased 3.5-fold in individuals with suicidal ideation in the prior year and increased sevenfold in those with a suicide attempt in the prior year.

Thus, available evidence suggests that anxiety disorders, particularly panic disorder, may be associated with increased rates of suicidal ideation, suicide attempts, and suicide. It remains unclear whether panic attacks and panic disorder represent independent risk factors for suicide or whether elevations in suicidality associated with these disorders are simply a reflection of comorbidity with other disorders such as depression, substance use disorders, or personality disorders. Nonetheless, individuals with anxiety disorders warrant explicit evaluation and follow-up for comorbid diagnoses and for suicide risk. Psychiatrists should also be alert for masked anxiety symptoms and for anxiety disorders that are misdiagnosed as physical illnesses.

d) Eating disorders

Studies point to eating disorders in general as a risk factor for death and as a likely risk factor for suicide. For example, Harris and Barraclough (64) calculated SMRs for suicide using data from 15 studies and found a 23.1-fold increase in risk in patients with eating disorders. Herzog et al. (138), in an 11-year longitudinal study of 246 women with eating disorders, noted a crude mortality rate of 5.1% and an SMR for death by any cause of 9.6. Three of the women died by suicide, yielding a significantly elevated SMR for suicide of 58.1.

The risk associated with specific eating disorders is less clear. Eckert et al. (139), in a similar longitudinal study, examined the clinical course and outcome of anorexia nervosa in 76 severely ill females. Although none of the deaths were attributed to suicide, by the time of 10-year follow-up, five subjects (6.6%) had died, yielding an almost 13-fold increase in mortality.

Coren and Hewitt (140) extracted data from all death certificates in the United States registered with the National Center for Health Statistics from 1986 through 1990. Of 5.5 million females who died in that period, 571 had anorexia nervosa listed as an underlying cause or accompanying condition of death. Of these, 1.4% died by suicide, compared to 4.1% of a matched control sample, suggesting that the risk of suicide in persons with anorexia nervosa is, if anything, lower than that in control subjects. However, substantial underreporting bias may be present, since personnel recording information on death certificates may not recognize anorexia as a contributory comorbid condition.

Eating disorders, particularly bulimia nervosa, have also been associated with an increased rate of suicide attempts, and, conversely, suicide attempters may have an increased rate of abnormal eating behaviors. Kent et al. (141) compared 48 women who were referred for psychiatric assessment after an act of deliberate self-poisoning with 50 control subjects who were evaluated in a hospital emergency department after a minor accidental injury. Even after controlling for the effect of differences in rates of depression, the investigators found that disordered eating behaviors were significantly more prevalent in the self-poisoning group. Compared to the general community, for whom surveys suggest rates of bulimia nervosa of 1%–2%, four subjects (8%) in the self-poisoning group met the diagnostic criteria for bulimia nervosa. Thus, awareness of eating disorders may be important in evaluating patients after a suicide attempt.

By the same token, suicide attempts may be more likely in women with eating disorders. Using anonymous survey data gathered from 3,630 girls in grades 6 through 12 in the upper Midwest, Thompson et al. (142) found that eating disturbances and aggressive behavior were significantly associated with substance use and with attempted suicide. In addition, adolescents reporting disturbed eating behaviors were three times more likely to report suicidal behaviors than were other respondents.

In summary, individuals with eating disorders may be at increased risk for suicidal behaviors. Anorexia nervosa seems more likely to be a potential risk factor for suicide, whereas bingeing, purging, and bulimia may be more likely to be associated with suicide attempts. The role of comorbid diagnoses in increasing the risk of suicidal behaviors remains unclear. Also unclear is whether the self-imposed morbidity and mortality associated with severe caloric restriction or bingeing and purging should be viewed as a self-injurious or suicidal behavior. Regardless, clinicians conducting suicide risk assessment should be attentive to the presence of eating disorders and especially the co-occurrence of eating disorders with other psychiatric disorders or symptoms such as depression or deliberate self-harm.

e) ADHD

The relationship between ADHD and suicidal behavior is unclear, with some but not all studies indicating an association between the diagnosis of ADHD and suicide attempts or suicide. To identify psychiatric risk factors for adolescent suicide, Brent et al. (145) used psychological autopsy data to match 67 adolescents who died by suicide to community control subjects. At the time of death, 89.6% of those who died by suicide had a psychiatric disorder, with major depression, bipolar disorder–mixed episode, substance use disorder, and conduct disorder seen at increased rates relative to the rates for the community control subjects. In contrast, the rate of ADHD in those who died by suicide was 13.4% and did not differ from the rate in the control subjects (145). Similarly, in a case-control study of adolescent suicide attempters, ADHD was actually less likely in those who attempted suicide than in the control subjects (146).

In a group of subjects between ages 17 and 28 years, Murphy et al. (144) compared 60 subjects with ADHD, combined type, to 36 subjects with ADHD, predominantly inattentive type, and to 64 community control subjects. A higher proportion of the group with ADHD, combined type (15%), reported attempting suicide, compared with the group with ADHD, predominantly inattentive type (2.8%), and the control group (0%). Compared to the control group, both ADHD groups had greater amounts of psychological distress, received more prescriptions for psychiatric medication and more types of psychiatric services, and had a higher prevalence of alcohol/cannabis use disorders and learning disorders. The groups did not differ in comorbidity of conduct disorder, major depressive disorder, or anxiety disorders. Patients with the combined type of ADHD are clinically more likely to present with distractible and impulsive behavior, whereas patients with the predominantly inattentive type of ADHD are more likely to present with problems of staring, daydreaming, confusion, passivity, withdrawal, and sluggishness or hypoactivity. These differences in clinical features may account for the differences in the numbers of suicide attempts in the two subgroups.

Nasser and Overholser (143) examined the lethality of suicidal behavior in 60 hospitalized adolescent inpatients who had recently attempted suicide. The subjects were divided into three equal groups on the basis of the qualities of their suicidal acts (nonlethal, low-lethal, and high-lethal). The groups did not differ significantly in terms of hopelessness, depression, substance abuse, and self-esteem or in diagnoses of major depression, adjustment disorder, substance abuse, and bipolar disorder. However, the group of high-lethal attempters included four individuals with a diagnosis of major depressive episode and comorbid ADHD. Thus, it may be the comorbidity of ADHD with other disorders that increases the relative lethality of suicide attempts.

In summary, evidence for an independent association between ADHD and risk for suicide or attempted suicide appears weak. Individuals with ADHD, combined type, seem to be at greater risk than those with ADHD, predominantly inattentive type, perhaps because of an increased level of impulsivity. In addition, there may be a relationship between ADHD and suicide risk that relates to comorbidity with conduct disorder, substance abuse, and/or depressive disorder. Given the frequent occurrence of ADHD in patients with other psychiatric disorders, it is important for psychiatrists to be aware that comorbid ADHD may augment the risk of suicidal behaviors.

f) Alcohol use disorders

The presence of an alcohol use disorder increases suicide risk. Estimates based on computerized curve fitting of data from 27 studies have suggested a 7% lifetime risk of suicide in individuals with alcohol dependence (94). Other approximations of lifetime suicide risk have ranged from 3.4% to as high as 15% (148, 157) but vary by country and depend on the definition of alcoholism used. In fact, the vast majority of studies have not used the DSM-IV criteria for alcohol use disorders, making comparisons across studies difficult. As a result, descriptions of studies in this document will use the diagnostic terms employed by the study authors.

Harris and Barraclough (64) used data from 32 publications, including findings for more than 45,000 individuals with follow-up periods for up to 30 years, to calculate an SMR for suicide of 5.86 among persons with alcohol abuse or dependence. The overall suicide rate for women with alcohol abuse or dependence was about 20 times the expected rate, whereas the rate for men was only about four times the expected rate. Beck et al. (227) also found a risk of suicide in alcoholics that was about fivefold greater than in nonalcoholics in a sample of 413 patients hospitalized for a suicide attempt and prospectively followed for 5–10 years. They also noted that the timing of suicides was spread throughout the follow-up, with no particular period of increased risk.

The association between alcohol use disorders and suicide is also demonstrated by psychological autopsy studies, which show alcohol use disorders to be common among individuals who die by suicide. For example, Henriksson et al. (59), in a random sample of 229 Finnish suicide deaths during a 1-year period, found that alcohol dependence was present in 43% of cases. In the United States, Conner et al. (150) found that 39% of 141 individuals who died by suicide over a 2.5-year period had had a history of alcohol use disorder.

Significant rates of alcohol use were also seen in a sample of youth suicides that included older adolescents. Brent et al. (151) examined death certificates and coroners' reports for all suicides, undetermined causes of death, and questionable accidents for 10- to 19-year-old residents of Allegheny County, Pennsylvania, from 1960 to 1983. Altogether, 159 definite suicides and 38 likely suicides were noted, but the suicide rate increased markedly over the study period, particularly among white males ages 15–19 years. During the study period there was also a 3.6-fold increase in the percentage of suicides with detectable blood alcohol levels (12.9% in 1968–1972, compared to 46.0% in 1978–1983). In addition, the rate of suicide by firearms increased much faster than that by other methods (2.5-fold and 1.7-fold, respectively), and persons who died by suicide with firearms were almost five times more likely to have been drinking than individuals who used other suicide methods.

A number of factors have been specifically observed with suicide in individuals with alcohol use disorders (153). Murphy et al. (152), in a study of 50 alcoholics who died by suicide, found that 26% had experienced interpersonal loss within 6 weeks of their death. These findings were comparable to those in a prior group of 31 alcoholics who died by suicides, one-third of whom had experienced the loss of a close interpersonal relationship within 6 weeks of the suicide. An earlier study by Murphy and Robins (156) also found a high proportion of recent interpersonal disruptions, as did a study of suicides in San Diego by Rich et al. (67). To identify other factors associated with increased risk for suicide among alcoholics, a subsequent study by Murphy et al. (149) pooled these two similar groups of alcoholics who died by suicide and compared them to two control samples of white male alcoholics, one from a psychiatric patient population and one from the ECA community-based population. Clinical features that were significantly more frequent among those who died by suicide than among the control subjects included current alcohol use, poor social support, serious physical illness, unemployment, living alone, and having made a suicidal communication. Eighty-three percent of the alcoholics who died by suicide had four or more of the seven risk factors.

Pirkola et al. (154) also examined factors associated with increased likelihood of suicide among alcohol misusers. They found that alcohol misusers who died by suicide (N=349) were more likely to be young, male, and divorced or separated, compared with individuals who did not misuse alcohol in the several months preceding their suicide (N=648). Alcohol misusers were also more likely to be intoxicated with alcohol at the time of death or to have died from an overdose of medications. Those with alcohol misuse had also experienced more adverse life events close to the time of their suicide despite having better psychosocial adjustment earlier in their lifetime. For example, alcoholics who died by suicide had more often worked but were also more likely to be recently unemployed.

A number of studies have identified comorbid disorders as being common among individuals with alcohol use disorders who die by suicide. In a series of 1,312 alcoholics admitted to a Swedish psychiatric hospital between 1949 and 1969 and followed through 1980, Berglund (157) found that alcoholics who died by suicide had a higher rate of depressive and dysphoric symptoms than alcoholics who died of other causes or who were alive at the end of the follow-up period. Murphy et al. (152) also found that concurrent depression was present in most but not all of their sample of alcoholics who died by suicide, suggesting that depression was neither a necessary nor a sufficient precondition for suicide. In a later study, Murphy et al. (149) found that major depressive episodes were significantly more frequent among alcoholics who died by suicide than among alcoholic control subjects and also found that 58% of the alcoholics who died by suicide had comorbid major depression.

Shaffer et al. (159) compared 120 individuals under age 20 who died by suicide to 147 age-, sex-, and ethnicity-matched community control subjects and found that 59% of the subjects who died by suicide and 23% of the control subjects met the DSM-III criteria for a psychiatric diagnosis based on information obtained from the subject's parents. When information from multiple informants was obtained, 91% of the subjects who died by suicide met the criteria for a DSM-III psychiatric diagnosis. In addition, with increasing age, there was an increased prevalence of a psychiatric diagnosis in general and of a substance and/or alcohol use disorder in particular. Previous suicide attempts and mood disorders were risk factors for suicide in both male and female subjects, whereas substance and/or alcohol abuse occurred exclusively in males and was present in 62% of 18- to 19-year-old subjects who died by suicide.

Even in individuals whose alcohol use disorder has remitted, suicide risk may still be increased but is likely to be influenced by comorbid disorders. Conner et al. (150) analyzed data from a community sample of 141 individuals who died by suicide and found that 39% (N=55) had a history of alcohol misuse. Compared with those who were actively using alcohol, those with remitted alcohol use disorders were predominantly younger individuals with psychotic disorders or older individuals with major depression.

In addition to being associated with an increased risk of suicide, alcohol use disorder is associated with a greater likelihood of suicide attempts. For example, Petronis et al. (163) analyzed data from 13,673 participants in the ECA survey and found that active alcoholism was associated with an 18-fold increase in the relative odds of making a suicide attempt. Gomberg (162) compared 301 women admitted to 21 alcohol treatment facilities to an equal number of age-matched nonalcoholic women from the community. Alcoholic women were far more likely to have attempted suicide (40%, compared with 8.8% of nonalcoholic women), and suicide attempts were particularly likely among alcoholic women under age 40. Alcoholic women who had attempted suicide were more likely to have used other drugs, and they reported significantly more tension, explosiveness, indecisiveness, fearfulness/anxiety, and difficulty concentrating and getting up in the morning.

Among alcoholics, differences also have been noted between those who attempt suicide and those who do not. Roy et al. (165), for example, performed a case-control study to determine the differences between alcoholic suicide attempters and alcoholic nonattempters. Of the 298 alcoholic patients studied, 19% had attempted suicide. Compared with the nonattempters, the attempters were significantly more likely to be female, to be young, and to have a lower economic status. They also were more likely to have first- or second-degree relatives who abused alcohol, to consume a greater amount of alcohol when drinking, and to have begun heavy drinking and experienced the onset of alcohol-related problems at an earlier age.

In addition, comorbid diagnoses are frequently identified among alcoholics who attempt suicide. Roy et al. (165), for example, found the most common comorbid psychiatric diagnoses among alcoholic suicide attempters to be major depression, antisocial personality disorder, substance abuse, panic disorder, and generalized anxiety disorder. Hesselbrock et al. (166), in a sample of 321 inpatients (231 men, 90 women) in alcoholism treatment centers, found that suicide attempters typically had multiple psychiatric diagnoses (e.g., depression, antisocial personality disorder, and substance abuse) and more severe psychiatric symptoms than nonattempters. Two-thirds of alcoholics who attempted suicide had a lifetime diagnosis of major depressive disorder, and most reported symptoms of depression within 2 weeks of the interview. Alcoholic suicide attempters tended to have a parental history of alcoholism, to have begun abusing alcohol at an early age, and to have abused other substances in addition to alcohol.

Preuss et al. (167), using data for 3,190 alcohol-dependent individuals from the Collaborative Study on the Genetics of Alcoholism, found that alcohol-dependent individuals with a history of suicide attempts were more likely to be dependant on other substances and more likely to have other psychiatric disorders. In addition, subjects with suicide attempts had a more severe course of alcohol dependence and more first-degree relatives with suicide attempts. In a subsequent study that followed 1,237 alcohol-dependent subjects over 5 years, Preuss et al. (168) found that the 56 alcohol-dependent subjects with suicide attempts during the follow-up period were more likely to have a diagnosis of a substance-induced psychiatric disorder or be dependent on other drugs. Furthermore, among 371 alcohol-dependent individuals who had made a suicide attempt and also had had an episode of depression, the 145 individuals (39.1%) with alcohol-independent mood disturbance had a greater number of prior suicide attempts and were more likely to have an independent panic disorder but reported a less severe history of alcohol dependence and were less likely to have been drinking during their most severe attempt (169). These findings suggest that in taking a clinical history in suicide attempters it is useful to identify comorbid depression but also to determine whether depressive episodes are alcohol induced or not.

That the presence of prior attempts is predictive of future attempts also highlights a need for taking a thorough history of past suicidal behaviors. Preuss et al. (168) followed 1,237 alcohol-dependent subjects over 5 years and found that the 56 alcohol-dependent subjects with suicide attempts during the follow-up period were more likely to have made prior attempts than subjects with no suicide attempts. Persons with comorbid major depression and alcohol use have higher rates of suicidal symptoms than those with either alone. Cornelius et al. (170) compared 107 patients with both major depression and alcohol dependence to 497 nondepressed alcoholics and 5,625 nonalcoholic patients with major depression assessed at the same psychiatric facility using a semistructured initial evaluation form. Depressed alcoholics had a significantly greater degree of suicidality, as reflected by a global measure that included wishes for death, suicidal ideation, and suicidal behaviors. They also differed significantly from the nonalcoholic depressed patients in having lower self-esteem and greater impulsivity and functional impairment.

In a subsequent study, Cornelius et al. (171) found that among psychiatrically hospitalized alcoholics with major depression, almost 40% had made a suicide attempt in the week before admission, with 70% having made a suicide attempt at some point in their lifetime. There was a significant association between recent suicidal behavior and recent heavy drinking, with most subjects also reporting drinking more heavily than usual on the day of their suicide attempt. In addition, these suicide attempts were usually impulsive. Suicidal ideation, however, was not increased by more recent heavy alcohol use, suggesting that alcohol increases suicidal attempts by increasing the likelihood of acting on suicidal ideation.

In summary, alcohol use disorders are associated with increased risks of suicide and suicide attempts. Conversely, rates of alcohol use disorders are elevated among those who die by suicide as well as among suicide attempters. The common occurrence of comorbid psychiatric symptoms and diagnoses suggests a need for thorough assessment and treatment of such complicating factors in users of alcohol. Also, the frequent presence of psychosocial stressors including unemployment and interpersonal losses should also be taken into consideration in the assessment and treatment planning process.

g) Other substance use disorders

As with disorders of alcohol use, other substance use disorders may be associated with an increased risk of suicide. Harris and Barraclough (172) noted that the SMRs for suicide varied widely across studies and that calculations were often confounded by the subjects' simultaneous use of multiple substances and by the difficulties in distinguishing accidental overdoses from suicide. Nonetheless, their meta-analysis of published literature found that substance use disorders were associated with a substantial increase in suicide risk. The SMRs for suicide were 14.0 for those with opioid abuse or dependence; 20.3 for those with sedative, hypnotic, or anxiolytic abuse or dependence; and 19.2 for individuals with mixed substance abuse or dependence.

Among individuals with substance use disorders, suicide may be more likely in the presence of comorbid diagnoses such as mood disorders. For example, in a study comparing 67 adolescents who died by suicide to 67 demographically matched community control subjects, Brent et al. (145) found that substance abuse conferred more significant risk when it was comorbid with affective illness than when it was present alone (odds ratio of 17.0 and 3.3, respectively). Lesage et al. (174) compared 75 male subjects ages 18–35 years who died by suicide to a group of 75 demographically matched living control subjects and found significantly greater rates of DSM-III-R psychoactive substance dependence among the subjects who died by suicide (22.7% versus 2.7%). They also found that comorbid major depression or borderline personality disorder was common among those with substance dependence who died by suicide.

In psychological autopsy studies, diagnoses of substance use disorders are particularly common among individuals under age 30 who die by suicide. For example, Fowler et al. (173) studied a subset of 128 individuals from the San Diego Suicide Study (67) who were under 30 years old and found that 53% had a diagnosis of substance abuse. Of this group, about one-half had an additional psychiatric diagnosis such as atypical depression, atypical psychosis, or adjustment disorder with depression. Despite the young age of the study sample, substance abuse was typically a chronic condition that had been present for an average of 9 years. Abuse of multiple substances was the norm, with marijuana, alcohol, and cocaine being the most frequently abused substances. Other data from the San Diego Suicide Study sample as a whole (110) showed that most substance users abused alcohol as well as other substances, with relatively small numbers of "pure" alcoholics or "pure" substance users. They also noted that interpersonal conflicts or loss occurred more frequently near the time of death for substance abusers with and without depression than for persons with mood disorders alone.

Although the majority of persons with substance use disorders who die by suicide are male, it is important to recognize that men and women with substance use disorders may differ in their characteristics and their risk for suicide. Pirkola et al. (175) used data from a nationwide psychological autopsy study in Finland to study the characteristics of a sample of 172 men and 57 women who died by suicide and had a DSM-III-R diagnosis of psychoactive substance dependence. They found that women were more likely than men to have abused or been dependent on prescribed medication. In addition, women were more likely than men to have a substance use disorder preceded by a comorbid axis I disorder (45% and 18%, respectively). Borderline personality disorder, previous suicide attempts, and suicidal communications were more common in women age 40 years or younger. In addition, alcohol-dependent women died at a younger age than women with nonalcohol substance dependence and also died at a younger age than men with either alcohol dependence or nonalcohol substance dependence.

Available evidence suggests that suicide attempts are common in substance users and that substance use disorders are associated with an increased risk of suicide attempts. Borges et al. (176) used data from the U.S. National Comorbidity Survey, a nationally representative sample of 8,098 persons age 15–54 years that was carried out in 1990–1992, to examine whether retrospectively reported substance use, abuse, and dependence are predictors of the onset of suicidal behavior. After controlling for the effects of sociodemographic factors and comorbid psychiatric disorders, the investigators found that subsequent suicide attempts were predicted by use of alcohol, heroin, or inhalants. Current substance use, rather than a history of use, increased the likelihood of suicidal behavior, with the number of substances used being more important than the types of substances used. In addition, among those with suicidal ideation, current substance use, abuse, and dependence were significant risk factors for unplanned suicide attempts.

Rossow and Lauritzen (178) assessed the self-reported prevalences of nonfatal overdoses and suicide attempts in 2,051 individuals who were being treated for substance abuse. Almost one-half (45.5%) reported having had one or more life-threatening overdoses, and nearly one-third (32.7%) reported one or more suicide attempts. Suicide attempts were more often reported among those who had overdosed, and the number of life-threatening overdoses and number of suicide attempts were positively and moderately associated. Individuals who had exhibited both life-threatening behaviors also showed higher rates of HIV risk-taking behaviors, poor social functioning, and use of multiple substances. Suicide attempters also had more symptoms of depression and anxiety as measured by the Global Assessment Scale. Thus, there is substantial covariation between suicide attempts and drug overdoses in individuals with substance use disorders that is also associated with other risk-taking behaviors and poor social integration.

Individuals with substance use disorders also have an increased likelihood of making a suicide attempt, compared to control subjects. Beautrais et al. (177) compared 302 individuals who had made medically serious suicide attempts to 1,028 control subjects who were randomly selected from local electoral rolls. Overall, those who had made a serious suicide attempt had high rates of substance use disorders (odds ratio=2.6). Furthermore, of those with a serious suicide attempt, 16.2% met the DSM-III-R criteria for cannabis abuse/dependence at the time of the attempt, compared with 1.9% of the control subjects (181). Mann et al. (31), in a study of 347 consecutive admissions to a university psychiatric hospital, found that the 184 patients who had made a prior suicide attempt had a greater likelihood of past substance use disorder or alcoholism. Johnsson and Fridell (179) assessed 125 substance abusers 5 years after hospitalization for detoxification and short-term rehabilitation. Although seven patients were dead at the time of follow-up, none of the deaths were from suicide. Of 92 interviewed subjects, nearly one-half the group (45%) reported having attempted suicide at some point in their lives, with about 50% of that group having attempted suicide with prescribed psychotropic drugs such as antidepressants or sedatives. Only a few of the suicide attempts were made by using the individual's primary substance of abuse. The most common reasons given for suicide attempts were the loss of a person whom they loved and feelings of loneliness. Compared to those who had never made a suicide attempt, the suicide attempters were more likely to have had childhood psychiatric hospitalizations or experienced loss of significant others in childhood. They also were more likely to experience depressive moods or other psychiatric comorbidity.

The combination of cocaine use plus alcohol use also appears to increase the risk of suicide attempts. Cornelius et al. (711) found that of 41 consecutively admitted depressed alcoholic inpatients, 16 had made a suicide attempt and 10 had used cocaine during the week before their hospitalization. The proportion of patients making a suicide attempt in the week before admission was greater in those who had used cocaine than in those who had not (70% and 32%, respectively). Suicidal ideation was also more prevalent in the depressed alcoholics who also used cocaine. Roy (180) studied the characteristics of cocaine-dependent patients in a substance abuse treatment center and compared the 130 individuals who had never attempted suicide with the 84 individuals who had made prior suicide attempts (a mean of 2.1 prior attempts). Compared with nonattempters, attempters were more likely to be female and to have a lifetime history of alcohol dependence (58.3%, compared with 34.6% for nonattempters) and a family history of suicidal behavior (25%, compared with 5.4% for nonattempters). Attempters also had significantly higher childhood trauma scores for emotional abuse, physical abuse, sexual abuse, emotional neglect, and physical neglect than the nonattempters; however, these scores were not corrected for the differences in the gender ratios in the two groups. Thus, suicide attempts are common among individuals seeking treatment for cocaine dependence, and factors that seem to augment risk are similar to those for other groups of suicide attempters.

In summary, studies indicate that substance use is a significant risk factor for suicide attempts and suicide. This is particularly true in younger individuals, leading some researchers to hypothesize that increasing suicide rates among youths may be related to increasing rates of substance use. Individuals with chronic substance use disorders, those who have experienced life-threatening nonsuicidal overdoses, and those who abuse multiple substances, including alcohol, may be at even greater risk. Moreover, substance use disorders may complicate mood disorders (182), increasing susceptibility to treatment-resistant illness and psychological impairment, and on that basis may contribute to an elevated risk for suicide and for suicide attempts. As a result, it is important to evaluate individuals with suicidality in the context of substance use for the presence of comorbid mood disorders as well as other comorbid psychiatric diagnoses. The evaluation should also be aimed toward identifying patterns of recent substance use and psychosocial factors such as recent interpersonal loss or history of childhood trauma that may also affect the likelihood of suicidal behaviors among substance users.

h) Personality disorders

Although personality disorders are often comorbid with substance use disorders and with other psychiatric diagnoses, they also appear to confer an independent risk for suicide. In addition, among individuals with personality disorders, the rate of suicide may be equivalent to rates in individuals with other major psychiatric syndromes. For example, in a meta-analysis of 14 case-control samples and nine longitudinal samples of patients with personality disorders, Linehan et al. (184) found rates of suicide that were between 4% and 8%. For patients with borderline personality disorder, studies have shown suicide rates ranging from 3% to 9% (183). Harris and Barraclough (64) also found suicide risk to be increased, calculating an SMR for suicide of 7.08 among individuals with personality disorder. However, the majority of patients included in their analysis were male and from a Veterans Administration study, raising questions about the representativeness of the population. Baxter and Appleby (188), in a large case registry study of long-term suicide risk in the United Kingdom, found even higher risks for suicide among individuals with personality disorder diagnoses, with a 12.8-fold elevation of risk in men and a 20.9-fold elevation of risk in women with personality disorders.

In a longitudinal follow-up study of individuals with personality disorders, Stone et al. (185) found that 18 of the 196 patients who were able to be located had died by suicide by 16.5 years. Compared to a suicide rate of 8.5% for the borderline personality group as a whole, those with alcohol problems had a twofold increase in the rate (19%), with a 38% rate of suicide among women who had a combination of alcoholism, major affective disorder, and borderline personality disorder. Other factors that appeared to contribute to suicide in individuals with borderline personality disorder were continuing alcohol abuse, impulsivity, and a history of parental brutality, specifically sexual molestation.

Psychological autopsy studies also show significant rates of personality disorder diagnoses among individuals who die by suicide. Duberstein and Conwell (186) reviewed case-based and cohort studies on suicide in individuals with personality disorders and found that approximately 30%–40% of suicides occur in individuals with personality disorders, with increased risk conferred by the presence of borderline, antisocial, and possibly avoidant and schizoid personality disorder diagnoses.

In a random sample of all persons who died by suicide in Finland within a 1-year period, Isometsa et al. (187) found that 29% of the subjects (N=67) had an axis II disorder. All individuals with a personality disorder also had at least one axis I diagnosis, which in 95% included a depressive syndrome, a substance use disorder, or both. Individuals with cluster B personality disorders were more likely to have substance use disorders and to have had a previous suicide attempt and were less likely to have had a health care contact during their final 3 months of life. In the same group of subjects, Heikkinen et al. (190) examined data on recent life events for 56 subjects with personality disorder who died by suicide and matched those subjects to control subjects who did not have a personality disorder diagnosis. Those with a personality disorder were more likely to have experienced one or more stressful life events in the last 3 months of life as well as in the week preceding the suicide. Specifically, of those with a personality disorder, 70% had a significant event in the week before suicide, with job problems, family discord, unemployment, and financial difficulty reported most commonly. Thus, these findings suggest that individuals with personality disorders who die from suicide have high rates of comorbid depression and substance use as well as high rates of significant life stressors that precede suicide.

The increased risk of suicide with personality disorders seems to be a particular factor that contributes to risk in young adults. Lesage et al. (174) compared 75 young men who died by suicide to a demographically matched group of men in the community and found that the 6-month prevalence of borderline personality disorder was substantially increased among those who died by suicide (28.0% versus 4.0%). In a study of adolescents and young adults who had been admitted to a regional poisoning treatment center because of deliberate self-poisoning or self-injury, Hawton et al. (384) compared 62 individuals who died by suicide or possible suicide to 124 matched control subjects and found that an increased risk of death was associated with the presence of a personality disorder (odds ratio=2.1).

Suicide attempts may also be more likely to occur in individuals with personality disorders than in those with other diagnoses. In a review of the topic, Linehan et al. (184) noted that suicide attempts are estimated to occur in 40%–90% of individuals with personality disorders. Soloff et al. (193) examined data for 84 patients who met the DSM-III-R criteria for borderline personality disorder and found that 61 patients (72.6%) had a lifetime history of suicide attempts, with an average of more than three attempts per patient. Risk factors for suicide attempts in patients with borderline personality disorder included older age, prior suicide attempts, antisocial personality, impulsive actions, and a depressed mood, but not comorbid mood disorder or substance use disorder. Ahrens and Haug (194), in a case-control study of 226 patients with a personality disorder who were admitted to a psychiatric hospital, found that patients with a personality disorder (including, but not limited to, borderline personality disorder) were more likely than other hospitalized patients to have had a suicide attempt immediately before admission, with persistent clinically relevant suicidal behavior within the first 24 hours after admission (39% versus 24%). Furthermore, in patients with a personality disorder, suicidality was not related to the presence of a specific mood disorder, since only 3% of the patients with personality disorder met the criteria for a major affective syndrome. However, the rates of reported suicide attempts in individuals with personality disorder diagnoses varied with the treatment setting. Pirkis et al. (198), in a study of suicide attempts by psychiatric patients under active treatment, observed a rate of suicide attempts in acute inpatients that was 10-fold greater than those for individuals in community-based and for individuals in long-stay inpatient care (22.7 attempts per 1,000 episode-days, compared with 2.3 and 2.1 attempts per 1,000 episode-days, respectively).

Conversely, among individuals who attempt suicide, personality disorders are commonly observed. Mann et al. (31), in a study of 347 consecutive patients who were admitted to a university psychiatric hospital, found that comorbid borderline personality disorder was more common among the 184 patients who had attempted suicide than among those with no prior suicide attempts. Beautrais et al. (177) compared 302 consecutive individuals who made serious suicide attempts with 1,028 randomly selected comparison subjects. Multiple logistic regression showed that those who made suicide attempts had a high rate of conduct disorder or antisocial personality disorder (odds ratio=3.7, 95% confidence interval=2.1–6.5). Thus, both borderline personality disorder and antisocial personality disorder appear to occur more frequently among suicide attempters. In a study of consecutive patients who had attempted suicide, Suominen et al. (191) compared 65 patients who did not have a personality disorder diagnosis to 46 patients who received a diagnosis of personality disorder. Of those with a diagnosis, 74% had a cluster B personality disorder and 46% had a diagnosis of borderline personality disorder. Individuals with a personality disorder were more likely to have attempted suicide in the past (78%, compared to 57% of those without a personality disorder diagnosis) and were more likely to have had psychiatric treatment in their lifetime (85% versus 57%); however, those with and without personality disorders did not differ in their degree of intent, hopelessness, somatic severity, or impulsiveness. Personality disorders were associated with a high degree of comorbidity, with comorbid alcohol dependence being particularly common and associated with greater difficulty in pursuing follow-up.

A number of additional factors may act as contributors to risk for suicide attempts among individuals with personality disorders. Brodsky et al. (196) analyzed data for 214 inpatients with a diagnosis of borderline personality disorder according to a structured clinical interview and examined the relationship between the specific DSM-IV criteria for borderline personality disorder and measures of suicidal behavior. After excluding self-destructive behavior and controlling for the effects of lifetime diagnoses of depressive disorder and substance abuse, they found that impulsivity was the only characteristic of borderline personality disorder that was associated with a higher number of suicide attempts. In addition, the number of previous suicide attempts was associated with having a history of substance abuse.

Comorbid mood disorders are also common among suicide attempters with personality disorder diagnoses. For example, Van Gastel et al. (192), in a study of 338 depressed psychiatric inpatients, found significantly more suicide attempts and more suicidal ideation among those with a comorbid personality disorder diagnosis than among depressed inpatients without a personality disorder. In addition, Oquendo et al. (131) found that among 156 inpatients with a diagnosis of a major depressive episode, having a history of suicide attempts was independently related to the presence of a cluster B personality disorder and to PTSD.

Corbitt et al. (195) also examined the effects of comorbid borderline personality disorder in 102 individuals with mood disorders and found that the 30 patients with major depressive disorder and comorbid borderline personality disorder were just as likely to have made a highly lethal suicide attempt as the 72 patients with major depressive disorder alone. However, those with comorbid borderline personality disorder were more likely to have a history of multiple serious suicide attempts, and past suicidal behavior was better predicted by the number of personality disorder symptoms than by the number of depressive symptoms. Thus, they suggested that the severity as well as the presence of comorbid cluster B personality disorder symptoms should be ascertained in assessing the risk of suicide attempts in patients with major depressive disorder.

Soloff et al. (197) compared the characteristics of suicide attempts in 77 inpatients with major depressive episodes to suicide attempts in 81 patients with borderline personality disorder, 49 of whom had a concomitant major depressive episode. Compared to patients with borderline personality disorder alone, all of the depressed patients had more severe observer-rated depression and lower levels of functioning. Patients with borderline personality disorder had higher rates of impulsivity, regardless of whether depression was also present. However, the diagnostic groups did not differ in their subjective intent to die, their degree of objective planning for death, the violence of the suicide method, or the degree of physical damage in the attempt as measured by the Beck Suicide Intent Scale.

In summary, individuals with personality disorders, and particularly those with a diagnosis of borderline personality disorder or antisocial personality disorder, have increased risks for suicide and for suicide attempts. These risks appear to be further augmented by the presence of comorbid disorders such as major depression, PTSD, and substance use disorders. The severity of symptoms such as impulsivity may also play a role in increasing risk, suggesting that such factors should be identified and addressed in the assessment and treatment of individuals with personality disorders.

3. Specific psychiatric symptoms

a) Anxiety

Anxiety has been suggested to increase the risk of suicide even when a specific anxiety disorder is not present. In a review of 46 cohort or case-control studies that used standardized or structured assessments of psychological dimensions to assess psychological vulnerability to suicide, Conner et al. (217) noted anxiety to be one of five constructs that is consistently associated with suicide. Busch et al. (218) reviewed the charts of 76 patients who died by suicide while in the hospital or immediately after discharge and found that 79% (N=60) met the criteria for severe or extreme anxiety and/or agitation according to Schedule for Affective Disorders and Schizophrenia ratings. In addition, Fawcett et al. (79), in a study of 954 psychiatric patients with major affective disorders, found that panic attacks and severe psychic anxiety were factors associated with suicide within 1 year of index evaluation. In these studies, the anxiety levels associated with suicide often took the form of anxious ruminations, panic attacks, or agitation and were in the severe range (i.e., severe anxiety most of the time).

With respect to the effect of anxiety on the risk of suicide attempts, the findings are more mixed. For example, Hall et al. (212) studied the characteristics of 100 patients who made a severe suicide attempt and found that severe anxiety and panic attacks were among the factors that were associated with the attempt. However, Placidi et al. (220), in a study of 272 inpatients with at least one major depressive episode, found that agitation and psychic anxiety were more severe in those who had not reported making a past suicide attempt.

Thus, although the relationship between anxiety and suicide attempts is unclear, and specific measures of anxiety have not been found to be predictive of suicide (78), severe anxiety does seem to increase suicide risk at least in some subgroups of patients. In particular, psychic anxiety, which may not be obvious to the clinician, should be specifically assessed, since such symptoms can respond rapidly to aggressive short-term treatment with benzodiazepines, second-generation antipsychotic medications, and possibly anticonvulsant medications (109).

b) Hopelessness

Hopelessness has been consistently identified as a factor associated with an increased risk of suicide, independent of diagnosis (217). Many studies that have assessed hopelessness have used the Beck Hopelessness Scale (712), which is described further in Section VI.B.1, "Rating Scales." For example, Beck et al. (222) followed 207 patients who were hospitalized for suicidal ideation but who had not made a recent suicide attempt to identify predictors of later suicide. After a follow-up period of 5–10 years, 14 individuals (6.9%) had died by suicide. Although a score of 10 or more on the Beck Hopelessness Scale correctly identified 91% of the patients who eventually died by suicide, there was significant overidentification of at-risk patients, with a false positive rate of 88%. The group who died by suicide also had a higher mean score on clinicians' ratings of hopelessness (223).

A later longitudinal study that included 1,958 consecutive psychiatric outpatients examined whether the level of hopelessness at intake could predict eventual suicide (221). In this patient population, those with a suicide death scored significantly higher on both the Beck Hopelessness Scale and the Beck Depression Inventory. Although a Beck Hopelessness Scale score of 10 or more was associated with an 11-fold increase in the likelihood of suicide, the specificity was again low. Since a high level of hopelessness is common in psychiatric patients, applying this Beck Hopelessness Scale cutoff to a larger population would identify 100 patients as being at risk for every one or two eventual suicides (713).

In a subsequent study that included an expanded sample of 6,891 psychiatric outpatients seen between 1975 and 1995 and followed for up to 20 years (with a median length of follow-up of 10 years), Brown et al. (78) used survival analysis to identify factors associated with increased risk for suicide. Along with higher levels of suicidal ideation and depression, hopelessness was identified as a risk factor for suicide, with patients who scored above 8 on the Beck Hopelessness Scale being at four times greater risk for suicide in a given year than those with lower scores.

The effect of hopelessness on suicide risk may vary by diagnosis, however. Fawcett et al. (79), in a longitudinal follow-up study of 954 patients with major affective disorder, found that severe hopelessness was one of several factors associated with an increased risk of suicide more than 1 year after the index assessment. However, among subjects who met the criteria for alcohol or substance abuse at any time, those who were not pervasively hopeless had the highest suicide risk at 5-year follow-up (226). This pattern is consistent with the findings of Beck et al. (227), who followed 161 alcohol-abusing patients for 7–12 years after they were hospitalized for a suicide attempt. Comparison of the 18 individuals who died by suicide to the remainder of the group failed to show a relationship between suicide and either hopelessness or depression.

Hopelessness at the termination of treatment may also reflect an increased risk for suicide. Dahlsgaard et al. (236) compared 17 cognitive therapy outpatients with mood disorder who died by suicide with a matching group of 17 outpatients who did not. Although the sample was small, those who died by suicide had higher levels of hopelessness at the end of treatment and were more likely to have ended treatment prematurely.

In addition to being a risk factor for suicide, hopelessness is more prominent in individuals who have reported previous suicide attempts, compared to individuals without such a history. Cohen et al. (229), for example, found greater levels of hopelessness in the 43 suicide attempters among 184 individuals with a first admission for psychosis. Hall et al. (212), in a study of 100 patients who had made severe suicide attempts, also noted feelings of hopelessness to be associated with suicidal behavior. Among 84 inpatients with DSM-III-R major depression, Malone et al. (230) found that the 45 individuals who had made a suicide attempt had higher subjective ratings of hopelessness and depression severity and that these ratings were inversely correlated with "reasons for living." In a study comparing 148 low-income African American women who had made a suicide attempt to 137 demographically similar women who presented for general medical care, Kaslow et al. (230) found hopelessness to be associated with a nearly eightfold increase in the risk of a suicide attempt in a univariate analysis. In a multivariate logistic regression analysis, hopelessness was independently associated with an increased risk of suicidal behaviors. Van Gastel et al. (192) also found that hopelessness was associated with suicidal ideation among 338 depressed inpatients and that the presence of a comorbid personality disorder was associated with additional increases in suicidal ideation and suicide attempts.

Across diagnostic groups, hopelessness appears to relate to the seriousness of suicidal ideation and intent. Soloff et al. (197) assessed the relationship of hopelessness to suicide attempts in inpatients with major depressive disorder (N=77) as well as in inpatients with borderline personality disorder alone (N=32) or in combination with major depressive disorder (N=49). Across groups, increased hopelessness was associated with an increased number of suicide attempts as well as an increase in the lethal intent associated with attempts. In addition, in patients with both disorders, higher levels of hopelessness were associated with objective planning of suicide attempts, which would further enhance risk. In a sample of 384 individuals who had attempted suicide, Weissman et al. (233) found that hopelessness contributed to the severity of suicidal intent in those with substance use disorders (N=86) as well as in those without substance use disorders (N=298).

Other evidence suggests that the level of hopelessness cannot be considered independently of other factors. For example, Uncapher et al. (228) analyzed data for 60 institutionalized elderly men and found that the relationship between hopelessness and suicidal ideation varied with the level of depressive symptoms and was most pronounced at moderate or higher levels of depression. Mendonca and Holden (232) assessed 97 outpatients and found the strongest predictors of the seriousness of current suicidal inclinations (as measured by the Beck Scale of Suicidal Ideation) to be hopelessness (as measured by the Beck Hopelessness Scale) and "unusual thinking" (defined as a state of cognitive distress with confused, disorganized thinking, including "trouble concentrating" and "mind going blank").

Furthermore, cross-sectional assessments of hopelessness may not necessarily be as relevant to risk as the level of hopelessness at baseline when the individual is not depressed. Young et al. (234), in a longitudinal study of 316 individuals, found that the baseline level of hopelessness was a better predictor of suicide attempts than either the level of hopelessness when depressed or the relative change in hopelessness from baseline levels during depression.

In summary, hopelessness is well established as a psychological dimension that is associated with an increased risk for suicide and suicide attempts and an increased level of suicidal intent. This relationship between hopelessness and suicidality holds true across diagnostic groups, with the possible exception of individuals with alcohol use disorder. These findings suggest the importance of inquiring about current levels of hopelessness as well as inquiring about usual levels of optimism about life and plans for the future. They also suggest the use of interventions to reduce hopelessness as a part of treatment.

c) Command hallucinations

Although command hallucinations have been regarded clinically as being associated with increased suicide risk, there is limited evidence that addresses this question. In addition, those studies that are available have included relatively small numbers of patients, making it difficult to detect differences in rates of suicide or suicide attempts between patient groups. Furthermore, in psychological autopsy studies, it is impossible to determine whether command hallucinations were present immediately before death or may have contributed to suicide.

Two small studies have noted whether command hallucinations had been present on index assessment in individuals who later died by suicide. Breier and Astrachan (102) described 20 schizophrenia patients who died from suicide and found that none had previously reported hallucinated suicidal commands. In contrast, Zisook et al. (239) found that command hallucinations, which were often violent in content, had been reported by 46 of 106 outpatients with schizophrenia, including the two patients who died by suicide during the study.

Other studies have tried to determine the rates at which patients follow command hallucinations and the factors that contribute to following or resisting such commands. For example, Junginger (241) used a semistructured psychiatric interview and hospital chart review to obtain information on 51 psychiatric inpatients and outpatients, all of whom had experienced recent command hallucinations. Of these subjects, 39.2% reported that they had followed the commands, 47.1% reported that they did not follow the commands, and 13.7% were unable to recall their response. Patients with hallucination-related delusions and identifiable hallucinatory voices were more likely to follow the commands than patients who were unable to identify the voices that they heard. In a subsequent study of 93 psychiatric inpatients who had a history of at least one command hallucination, the most recent command hallucination reported by the subject was rated for level of dangerousness and level of compliance with the command (242). Of the 93 subjects, 52 (56%) reported at least partial compliance with their most recent command hallucination, and 40 (43%) reported full compliance. Individuals who experienced less dangerous commands or who could identify the hallucinated voice reported higher levels of compliance, although reported compliance with more dangerous commands was not uncommon. Commands experienced in the hospital were less dangerous than those experienced elsewhere, tended to be specific to the hospital environment, and were less likely to be followed. Based on these self-reports, the authors concluded that psychiatric patients who experience command hallucinations are at risk for dangerous behavior and that a patient's ability to identify the hallucinated voice is a fairly reliable predictor of subsequent compliance. Also, the level of dangerousness that results from compliance with command hallucinations may be a function of the patient's environment.

Erkwoh et al. (245) used a 24-item questionnaire to assess the psychopathological characteristics of command hallucinations in 31 patients with schizophrenia. Like Junginger, they found that following the commands was predicted by recognizing the voice. In addition, patients were more likely to comply with commands from hallucinations that they viewed as "real" and that produced an emotional response during the hallucination.

Kasper et al. (243) compared 27 psychotic patients with command hallucinations to 27 patients with other hallucinations and 30 patients with other psychotic symptoms. Although the groups did not differ in aggressive or violent behavior or in most nonhallucinatory symptoms, 84% of the patients with command hallucinations had recently obeyed them, even during their hospital stays. Among those with command hallucinations, almost one-half had heard and attempted to obey messages of self-harm during the previous month. Rogers et al. (244), in a study of 65 forensic inpatients with psychotic disorders, also found that a significant number of individuals (44%) often responded to command hallucinations with unquestioning obedience.

These findings, that significant numbers of individuals comply with at least some hallucinated commands, are in contrast with the findings of Hellerstein et al. (240). Among 789 consecutive inpatients admitted over a 2-year period, they found that 19.1% had auditory hallucinations within 2 weeks of hospital admission, and, of these, 38.4% heard commands to behave violently or self-destructively. It is not surprising that hallucinations were more common in the 159 patients with schizophrenia, with 50.3% experiencing auditory hallucinations and 18.2% experiencing command hallucinations. Among 167 patients with affective disorder, rates of auditory and command hallucinations were 13.2% and 4.2%, respectively. The presence of auditory hallucinations was significantly associated with use of maximal observation and seclusion. However, patients with command hallucinations were not significantly different from patients without command hallucinations on demographic and behavioral variables, including suicidal ideation or behavior and assaultiveness. This finding suggests that command hallucinations alone may not imply a greater risk for acute, life-threatening behavior. In addition, consistent with the findings of Goodwin et al. (714), these findings imply that many patients are able to ignore or resist command hallucinations.

The most specific assessment of the role of command hallucinations in suicidal behaviors is that of Harkavy-Friedman et al. (106). They interviewed 100 individuals with schizophrenia or schizoaffective disorder who were hospitalized on an inpatient research unit about their experiences with command auditory hallucinations as well as about suicide attempts. Suicide attempts were reported by 33% of the sample, and the relative frequency of individuals with command hallucinations did not statistically differ between those who had and those who had not reported a suicide attempt (30% and 18%, respectively). Command hallucinations were present in 22% of the sample as a whole, and, of these, 45% had made at least one suicide attempt. Among individuals with command hallucinations who had made a suicide attempt, however, 80% had at least one attempt in response to the hallucinations. Thus, these findings suggest that for some individuals, particularly those with prior suicide attempts, suicidal behavior may occur in the context of auditory command hallucinations.

In summary, study findings are inconsistent about whether patients with command hallucinations are likely to obey them. Patients who recognize the hallucinated voices or view them as real or benevolent may be more likely to follow their directives. In addition, patients with prior suicide attempts may be more likely to follow suicidal commands. In terms of suicide risk, per se, patients with command hallucinations may not be at greater risk than other severely psychotic patients. However, existing studies include too few subjects to draw strong conclusions. In addition, since some patients do seem to act in response to auditory command hallucinations, it is important to identify such hallucinations, assess them in the context of other clinical features, and address them as part of the treatment planning process.

d) Impulsiveness and aggression

Factors such as impulsivity, hostility, and aggression may act individually or together to increase suicide risk. For example, many studies have provided moderately strong evidence for the roles of impulsivity and hostility-related affects and behavior in suicide (217, 246). In particular, impulsivity and aggression have been shown to be associated with suicide in patients with schizophrenia as well as in those with mood disorder. For example, De Hert et al. (89) compared 63 patients who died by suicide and 63 control subjects from a consecutive admission series of patients with a diagnosis of schizophrenia, all of whom were under age 30 on admission. In this sample, impulsive acting-out behavior was associated with an increased likelihood of suicide (odds ratio=6.4). Among 529 patients with affective illness who were followed naturalistically for up to 14 years and who either attempted suicide or died by suicide, Maser et al. (247) also found that impulsivity was a core characteristic of patients with suicidal behaviors. In fact, beyond 12 months, higher levels of impulsivity and assertiveness were the best prospective predictors of suicide.

Angst and Clayton (248) found a significant effect of premorbid aggression on the risk of suicide attempts or suicide. To assess the effect of personality traits on suicidal behaviors, they administered the Freiberg Personality Inventory to 6,315 Swiss army conscripts. Twelve years later, 185 of these individuals were identified as receiving psychiatric treatment during that time period, and a record review was conducted to establish a blind diagnosis and assess measures of suicidality and mortality in a subgroup of 87 of those individuals. Those who made suicide attempts or died by suicide were found to have scored higher on aggression than control subjects. In contrast, subjects with suicidal ideation alone scored lower on aggression, suggesting a role for premorbid aggression in suicidal behaviors.

Multiple other studies have demonstrated increased levels of impulsivity and aggression in individuals with a history of attempted suicide. For example, Mann et al. (31), in a study of 347 consecutive patients admitted to a university psychiatric hospital, found that rates of lifetime aggression and impulsivity were greater in the 184 patients who had attempted suicide than in those without a history of suicide attempts. Hall et al. (212) found that the recent onset of impulsive behavior was an excellent predictor of suicidal behavior in 100 patients who had made a severe suicide attempt. Kotler et al. (249) compared 46 patients with PTSD to 42 non-PTSD anxiety disorder patients and 50 healthy control subjects and found that impulsivity was positively correlated with the risk of suicidal behavior in the PTSD group.

Impulsivity and aggression have also been associated with suicide attempts among patients with mood disorders. Brodsky et al. (250), in a study of 136 depressed adult inpatients, found that individuals with at least one prior suicide attempt had significantly higher scores on measures of impulsivity and aggression than individuals without reported suicide attempts. Placidi et al. (220) analyzed data for 272 inpatients with at least one major depressive episode and found significant increases in measures of aggression and impulsivity in those with a history of suicide attempts, compared to those without suicide attempts. Finally, in a study of 44 individuals with a DSM-III-R diagnosis of bipolar disorder, Oquendo et al. (252) found that suicide attempters were more likely to have more lifetime aggression than nonattempters, although lifetime rates of impulsivity were not increased among those with a prior suicide attempt.

Suicide attempters with borderline personality disorder similarly have been reported to exhibit increased levels of aggression and impulsivity. Soloff et al. (197) compared 32 inpatients with borderline personality disorder alone and 77 inpatients with major depressive episode alone to 49 patients with both diagnoses and found that a greater number of suicide attempts was associated with a diagnosis of borderline personality disorder or with increases in either hopelessness or impulsive aggression. Soloff et al. (193) studied the characteristics of 84 patients with borderline personality disorder, of whom 61 had a lifetime history of suicide attempts (72.6%), with an average of 3.39 (SD=2.87) attempts per patient. Those with a history of suicide attempts were found to have had more impulsive actions than patients who had never attempted suicide.

Many individuals with borderline personality disorder and other cluster B personality disorders have a history of suicide attempts, but they may also have a history of self-mutilatory behaviors. However, it is important to recognize that these three characteristics define overlapping but not identical groups of individuals. Stanley et al. (251) compared 30 suicide attempters with a cluster B personality disorder and a history of self-mutilation to a matched group of 23 suicide attempters with a cluster B personality disorder but no history of self-mutilation. Individuals with a history of self-mutilation had higher levels of impulsivity and aggression than those without such a history. Herpertz et al. (253) examined characteristics of self-mutilatory behaviors and found that an ongoing tendency for behavioral dyscontrol was present only in patients exhibiting impulsive self-mutilatory behaviors and not in those with premeditated self-mutilatory behaviors. Thus, although self-mutilatory behaviors and impulsivity share many associated features and antecedents and are common among individuals with borderline personality disorder or histories of physical or sexual abuse, self-mutilatory behavior cannot be regarded as synonymous with impulsivity. In a similar fashion, the presence of other risk-taking behaviors such as reckless driving or unsafe sexual practices is not necessarily a reflection of increased impulsivity per se. Nonetheless, the presence of impulsivity, violence, risk-taking, or self-mutilatory behaviors requires a careful assessment and plan of treatment to address these clinical characteristics and minimize their effect on the risk of suicide and suicide attempts.

4. Other aspects of psychiatric history

a) Alcohol intoxication

Intoxication with alcohol and/or with other substances is often found in individuals who have died by suicide, independent of whether they meet the diagnostic criteria for a substance use disorder. Hayward et al. (255) reviewed coroners' records for 515 consecutive suicides in Western Australia and found that 35.8% of the persons who died by suicide had a nonzero blood alcohol level, with 24.5% being moderately to significantly impaired by alcohol at the time of death. Alcohol consumption before suicide was more prevalent in younger individuals, with 44.8% of teenagers and 35.1% of those age 20–24 years having used alcohol, in contrast to 25.9% of individuals over age 45 years. In addition, those with nonzero blood alcohol levels were more likely to have experienced a breakup in a relationship but less likely to have a history of psychiatric illness or treatment.

As part of the National Suicide Prevention Project in Finland (1987–1988), Ohberg et al. (121) conducted toxicological screening in 1,348 consecutive suicides in a 1-year period and found alcohol use before suicide in 35.9% of the sample. Alcohol was present in men twice as often as in women, whereas prescribed medications, which were found on toxicological screening in 41.6% of suicides overall, were more commonly noted in women.

Brent et al. (151), in a study of suicides in 10- to 19-year-old residents of Allegheny County, Pennsylvania, from 1960 to 1983, found that the proportion of persons who died by suicide with detectable blood alcohol levels rose from 12.9% in 1968–1972 to 46.0% in 1978–1983. In addition, individuals who used a firearm for suicide were 4.9 times more likely to have been drinking than individuals who used other suicide methods.

That intoxication increases the likelihood of suicide is also suggested by the role of employment in modulating suicide risk among alcohol users. Specifically, Pirkola et al. (260) found that alcohol misusers who were employed were more likely to have died by suicide on a weekend than those who were unemployed, suggesting that alcohol use per se contributes to risk, perhaps by increasing impulsivity.

Alcohol intoxication is also a common concomitant of suicide attempts. Borges et al. (715) assessed measures of alcohol intoxication in 40 emergency department patients who had attempted suicide and compared them to 372 patients who presented to the emergency department because of animal bites or workplace or recreational accidents. Patients with suicide attempts were significantly more likely to be under the influence of alcohol, as measured by breath alcohol testing or by self-report of alcohol consumption in the preceding 6 hours. In a study of 325 individuals with deliberate self-poisoning who presented to a Brisbane hospital over a 12-month period, McGrath (453) found that almost one-third had consumed alcohol before their suicide attempt. Varadaraj and Mendonca (454) found similar rates of intoxication in a study of 158 emergency department patients who had attempted suicide by overdose, with 41% consuming alcohol prior to the attempt and 29% having serum alcohol levels above 80 mg/dl.

Individuals who have made a suicide attempt while intoxicated are also at increased risk of later suicide. A study by Suokas and Lonnqvist (258) included data for 1,018 individuals who made a total of 1,207 suicide attempts and were evaluated in the emergency department of a Helsinki, Finland, hospital in a single year. Of these patients, 62% had recently consumed alcohol. Suicide attempts that occurred while intoxicated were more likely to be impulsive. After 5.5 years of follow-up, suicide had occurred in 3.3% of those who had used alcohol with their index suicide attempt. The majority of deaths occurred within the initial year of follow-up, yielding a 51-fold increase in risk of suicide, compared to the general population in the initial year, and a 17-fold increase in risk for the follow-up period as a whole. These findings suggest a need for careful follow-up of intoxicated individuals who present with a suicide attempt. In addition, they suggest a need to determine whether prior suicide attempts occurred in the context of intoxication.

b) Past suicide attempts

A substantial percentage of individuals will die on their initial attempt at suicide. For example, Isometsa and Lonnqvist (266) found that 56% of the 1,397 individuals in the Finnish psychological autopsy study had died with their first suicide attempt and that this pattern was particularly evident in males (62%, compared with 38% of females). In addition, however, individuals with nonfatal suicide attempts have an increased likelihood of later suicide. From a public health standpoint, this finding is particularly important, given the high occurrence of attempted suicide, which in recent decades has had annual rates ranging from 2.6 to 1,100 per 100,000, with lifetime prevalence rates ranging from 720 to 5,930 per 100,000 (2, 518).

Multiple studies have indicated that suicide attempts increase the risk of subsequent suicide. In fact, depending on the length of the follow-up period, from 6% to 10% of those who attempt suicide will ultimately die by suicide. For example, in follow-up studies of patients seen in psychiatric emergency settings after a suicide attempt, 4%–12% die by suicide within 5 years (268, 269, 275). In a 14-year follow-up of 1,018 deliberate self-poisoning patients, Suokas et al. (271) found a 6.7% rate of suicide overall, with the rate in men approximately twice that in women. Among 1,573 individuals who had been hospitalized after attempted suicide and followed up 4–11 years later, Nordstrom et al. (275) found an overall mortality of 11%, with a suicide risk of 6%. Tejedor et al. (272), in a 10-year follow-up of 150 patients admitted to a psychiatric department after a suicide attempt, found an even higher mortality rate from suicide (12%) as well as from natural causes (10%). Furthermore, in a meta-analysis of literature on psychiatric disorders and suicide, Harris and Barraclough (64) found that attempted suicide had a relative risk of later suicide that was greater than that of any psychiatric disorder. Compared to the general population, patients who attempted suicide were at 38 times greater risk of suicide, with the majority of evidence suggesting that this increase in suicide risk is related to the recency of the suicide attempt. This effect has also been noted by Nordstrom et al. (275), who found the greatest risk for suicide during the first year after an attempt. In addition, among the 1,397 individuals in the Finnish psychological autopsy study, Isometsa et al. (266) found that a nonfatal suicide attempt had occurred in 19% of the males and 39% of the females in the year preceding their suicide. In contrast, Fawcett et al. (79) found that among patients with a major affective disorder, a history of previous suicide attempts was associated with suicide that occurred more than 1 year after index hospital admission.

Other factors may also modulate suicide risk following a suicide attempt. Harris and Barraclough (64) found that risk for suicide after an attempt varied with measures of social cohesion and was increased by the presence of long-standing physical illness or a history of multiple previous attempts or prior psychiatric treatment. Risk of suicide following a suicide attempt may also vary with gender, since Nordstrom et al. (275) found a twofold increase in suicide risk in males, compared with females, with the risk for younger male attempters being four times that for younger females.

Other investigators have examined factors associated with subsequent suicide attempts following an index suicide attempt. Hjelmeland (164), for example, studied 1,220 patients who had attempted suicide and compared those who had a repeated attempt within 12 months to those who did not. Although there were no gender differences between repeaters and nonrepeaters, repeaters were more likely to be unmarried, to be unemployed, to abuse alcohol, and to report their own psychiatric problems as their main concern. Repeaters were also more likely to have had a history of sexual abuse, a criminal record, a recent address change, or a relative or friend who had attempted suicide. Others have confirmed an increased risk of repeated suicide attempts in individuals with multiple prior attempts (272, 278). Aborted suicide attempts are also common among those who attempt suicide (276).

Given this increased likelihood of suicide or additional suicide attempts, particularly in the first few years after a suicide attempt, assessment and treatment of suicide attempters should be an integral part of risk reduction. All too often, however, suicide attempters do not receive a psychiatric assessment or follow-up care (2, 279, 280). Thus, in addition to a thorough psychiatric assessment, determining a patient's history of suicide attempts (including aborted suicide attempts) yields information that is important in estimating the level of suicide risk of an individual patient. Additional factors such as psychiatric diagnosis, comorbid alcohol abuse, physical illness, or psychosocial stressors may augment risk following a suicide attempt. Furthermore, the significant mortality observed in suicide attempters underscores the need for careful aftercare planning for suicide attempters.

c) History of childhood physical and/or sexual abuse

Multiple studies have examined the association between childhood abuse and suicidal behaviors, although few have examined the effect of childhood abuse on risk for suicide per se. Plunkett et al. (36), however, assessed 183 young people who had experienced childhood sexual abuse and individuals from a nonabused comparison group 9 years after study intake. Those who had experienced childhood sexual abuse had a suicide rate that was 10.7–13.0 times the national rate, whereas no suicides occurred in the control group.

The bulk of studies have assessed the effects of childhood abuse on suicidal ideation and suicide attempts, both of which are common among individuals reporting childhood abuse. For example, in the study by Plunkett et al. (36), 43% of the 183 young people who had experienced childhood sexual abuse had thought of suicide, whereas 32% had made a suicide attempt.

Other studies have examined the effect of childhood abuse on the risk of suicidal ideation and suicide attempts. Fergusson et al. (286), in an 18-year longitudinal study of a birth cohort of 1,265 New Zealand children, found that those reporting childhood sexual abuse had higher rates of suicidal behaviors than those not reporting such abuse. In addition, the extent of childhood sexual abuse was consistently correlated with risk, with the highest risk of suicidal behaviors in those whose childhood sexual abuse involved intercourse. Even after controlling for the effects of confounding variables, the investigators found that those who reported harsh or abusive childhood experiences were also at increased risk for suicide attempts (282).

Brown et al. (294) followed a cohort of 776 randomly selected children over a 17-year period to adulthood and found that adolescents and young adults with a history of childhood maltreatment were three times more likely to become suicidal than individuals without such a history. Again, the effects of childhood sexual abuse on suicidal behavior were greater than the effects of other forms of abuse, with the risk of repeated suicide attempts being eight times greater for youths with a history of sexual abuse.

Several Australian investigators have used data from twin pairs to assess the effect of childhood abuse on the risk of suicidal ideation or suicide attempts. In structured telephone interviews with 5,995 Australian twins, Dinwiddie et al. (292) found that the 5.9% of women and 2.5% of men who reported a history of childhood sexual abuse were more likely to report suicidal ideation or prior suicide attempts. Nelson et al. (35), using data from 1,991 Australian twin pairs, found even greater rates of childhood sexual abuse (16.7% of women and 5.4% of men) but confirmed that a history of childhood sexual abuse significantly increased risk for suicide attempts, with the greatest risk associated with sexual abuse that involved intercourse. Even in twin pairs who were discordant for childhood sexual abuse, both twins had increased rates for many adverse outcomes, probably as a result of shared family background risk factors. Nonetheless, the twin who reported experiencing childhood sexual abuse had an even greater risk of a subsequent suicide attempt than the co-twin, which suggests an independent contribution of childhood sexual abuse to the risk for suicidal behaviors.

In contrast to the authors of the longitudinal studies described earlier, Romans et al. (291) selected a random community sample of New Zealand women and compared those who reported having been sexually abused as children to those who did not report such abuse. The presence of self-harming behaviors was associated with sexual abuse in childhood and was most marked in individuals who were subjected to more intrusive and frequent abuse.

Cross-sectional assessments of nonpsychiatric populations in the United States have also found associations between suicide attempts and childhood abuse, particularly childhood sexual abuse. Among the 2,918 respondents in the Duke University ECA study, Davidson et al. (293) found that subjects reporting a history of sexual assault also reported higher lifetime rates of suicide attempts than individuals without such a history. In women, a history of sexual trauma before age 16 was a particularly strong correlate of suicide attempts. Among U.S. women physicians (N=4,501), data from a nationally distributed questionnaire showed that the 4.7% of respondents with a history of childhood sexual abuse were more likely to report a history of suicide attempts (287). Kaslow et al. (230) compared 148 low-income African American women who presented to the hospital following a suicide attempt to a similar group of 137 women who presented for general medical care and found a threefold greater risk of childhood maltreatment among suicide attempters. Molnar et al. (33) analyzed data for 5,877 individuals from the National Comorbidity Survey and found that individuals with a history of sexual abuse were more likely to attempt suicide than those without such a history. This risk differed by sex, with a two- to fourfold increase in risk among women and a four- to 11-fold increase in risk among men. Dube et al. (281), in a sample of 17,337 adults (mean age=56 years), also found that the risk of suicide attempts was increased in those who had experienced childhood abuse. They observed this risk to be augmented by multiple other factors, including parental separation or divorce, witnessing of domestic violence, and living with substance abusing, mentally ill, or criminal household members.

In addition to the augmentation of suicide risk associated with sexual abuse, risk appears to be further increased among individuals who have experienced multiple forms of abuse. Anderson et al. (289) examined the association between childhood abuse and adult suicidal behavior in a sample of low-income African American women. Compared to the women who did not report experiencing any emotional, physical, or sexual childhood abuse, those who experienced one, two, or three forms of abuse were, respectively, 1.83, 2.29, or 7.75 times more likely to attempt suicide. In addition, women who reported all three types of abuse were more likely to attempt suicide than women who reported one or two types of abuse.

Childhood abuse is particularly frequent among individuals with psychiatric diagnoses and appears to increase the likelihood of suicide attempts even after the effects of psychiatric comorbidity are controlled. For example, in a study of 251 psychiatric outpatients (68 men and 183 women), Kaplan et al. (284) found that 51% of the subjects had reported experiencing childhood abuse, with 15% reporting sexual abuse alone, 17% reporting physical abuse alone, and 18% reporting a combination of physical and sexual abuse during childhood. Abusive experiences in adulthood were reported by 38% of the subjects, with physical abuse alone in 21%, sexual abuse alone in 8%, and both physical and sexual abuse in 9%. Compared to control subjects without a history of abuse, subjects with a history of abuse were more likely to have been suicidal at a younger age and to have made multiple suicide attempts. Among patients with a history of abuse, suicide attempters could be distinguished from nonattempters on the basis of higher levels of dissociation, depression, and somatization. In analyzing data from the National Comorbidity Survey, Molnar et al. (33) also found that those with a comorbid psychiatric disorder were younger at the time of their first suicide attempt than those without concomitant psychiatric illness. In addition, a history of childhood sexual abuse remained a risk factor for attempting suicide even after adjustment for the effect of a lifetime psychiatric diagnosis.

The presence of childhood physical and/or sexual abuse has also been associated with an increased likelihood of suicidality in studies of patients with specific psychiatric diagnoses. For example, Brodsky et al. (196), in a study of 214 inpatients with a diagnosis of borderline personality disorder, found that the number of lifetime suicide attempts was correlated with a history of childhood abuse. Van der Kolk et al. (285) assessed 74 individuals with personality disorders or bipolar II disorder and found that histories of childhood sexual and physical abuse were highly significant predictors of self-cutting and suicide attempts. During a follow-up period that averaged 4 years, the patients who continued being self-destructive were those with the most severe histories of separation and neglect and those with past sexual abuse.

For individuals with major depressive disorder, evidence in the literature is more complex. Brodsky et al. (250) found that adults with major depressive disorder who had a history of childhood physical or sexual abuse were more likely to have made a suicide attempt than those who did not report an abuse history, even after adjustment for the effects of impulsivity, aggression history, and presence of borderline personality disorder. Zlotnick et al. (716), in a study of 235 outpatients with major depression, found substantial rates of diagnostic comorbidity, primarily with borderline personality disorder and PTSD. After controlling for the effects of the presence of these diagnoses, however, they did not find an independent contribution of childhood sexual abuse to the likelihood of suicide attempts.

Childhood abuse is also prevalent among individuals with substance use disorders and, again, is associated with increased rates of suicide attempts. In a group of 481 male and 321 female alcoholic inpatients (age 19–57 years), Windle et al. (288) found a high prevalence of reported childhood abuse. For women, the rates of physical abuse only, sexual abuse only, and dual abuse were 10%, 26%, and 23%, respectively, whereas for men the corresponding rates were 19%, 7%, and 5%, respectively. For both sexes, a reported history of childhood abuse was associated with a higher rate of suicide attempts, with an even larger effect associated with a history of both physical and sexual abuse. Roy (290) examined abuse histories in a consecutive series of 100 male cocaine-dependent patients and found that the 34 patients who had attempted suicide reported significantly higher scores for childhood emotional abuse, physical abuse, sexual abuse, and emotional and physical neglect than the 66 patients who had never made a suicide attempt.

In addition to increasing risk for suicide attempts within community samples and across subgroups of psychiatric patients, the presence of a childhood abuse history in individuals who have made a suicide attempt should alert the psychiatrist to a further increase in the risk of repeated attempts (284). Elliott et al. (717) compared 65 patients hospitalized for a medically serious suicide attempt to 32 patients seen in the emergency room for a suicide attempt but who were not medically hospitalized. Those with attempts that were not medically serious had higher rates of previous sexual and physical abuse as well as higher rates of traumatic life events and borderline personality disorder. Hjelmeland (164) also found that patients in a Norwegian county who required medical treatment after an initial suicide attempt were more likely to have a repeated suicide attempt during 6 years of follow-up if they had a history of being sexually abused.

In summary, there is consistent evidence, in multiple samples studied with multiple study designs, that a history of abuse augments the risk for later suicidal ideation and suicide attempts. The effect of abuse on suicide per se has been less well studied, but the few findings that are available suggest that abuse increases suicide risk. Childhood abuse and particularly childhood sexual abuse appear to be associated with greater increases in risk than childhood physical abuse or abuse during adulthood. Individuals who have experienced multiple forms of abuse are at particularly increased risk of suicidal ideation and behaviors. Although a history of abuse is common in individuals with suicide attempts and in individuals with a psychiatric diagnosis, the contribution of childhood abuse to the risk of suicidal behaviors seems to be independent of the effects of psychiatric diagnoses. Consequently, in patients who have attempted suicide as well as in those presenting for any type of psychiatric treatment, it is important to inquire about childhood and adult experiences of physical, sexual, or emotional abuse and to incorporate this information into the risk assessment and treatment planning process.

d) History of domestic partner violence

Although studies have not directly assessed the effects of domestic partner violence on risk for suicide, domestic partner violence has been associated with increased rates of suicide attempts and suicidal ideation. For example, after adjustment for the effects of sociodemographic characteristics and alcohol use in a nationally representative sample of 5,238 U.S. adults, Simon et al. (298) found that being physically assaulted was associated with suicidal ideation or behavior (odds ratio=2.7) and that this pattern was particularly true for individuals who sustained injury (odds ratio=3.4) or were assaulted by a relative or intimate partner (odds ratio=7.7). McCauley et al. (300) surveyed 1,952 respondents in a primary medical care practice and found that 5.5% had experienced domestic violence in the year before presentation. Compared with women who had not recently experienced domestic violence, those with recent experiences of such violence were four times more likely to have attempted suicide. Among women physicians (N=4,501 respondents) who responded to the Women Physicians' Health Study questionnaire, suicide attempts were significantly more prevalent among the 3.7% of respondents with a history of domestic partner violence (34).

Domestic partner violence is particularly a risk factor for suicide attempts among women in low-income urban environments. In a group of 648 women, most of whom were young and unemployed and had an annual household income of less than $10,000, Abbott et al. (299) found that among the 418 women with a current male partner, 11.7% reported being recently assaulted, threatened, or intimidated by their partner. For the entire sample, the cumulative lifetime prevalence of exposure to domestic violence was 54.2%. Women with any exposure to domestic partner violence had an increased rate of suicide attempts, compared to women without such exposure (26% and 8%, respectively). Kaslow et al. (230) compared 148 low-income African American women who presented to the hospital after a suicide attempt to a similar group of 137 women who presented for general medical care. Women who presented with a suicide attempt had a greater likelihood of having experienced either physical or nonphysical partner abuse (odds ratios=2.5 and 2.8, respectively). Thompson et al. (301), in a sample of low-income, inner-city women, found that suicide attempters (N=119) were approximately three times more likely to experience significant physical partner abuse, nonphysical abuse, and PTSD than nonattempters (N=85). In addition, increased suicidality in individuals who were experiencing physical partner abuse appeared to depend on the presence of PTSD rather than the independent contribution to risk of the abuse.

Increased risk for suicide attempts is also seen in battered women presenting to emergency department settings or to women's shelters. Muelleman et al. (296) surveyed 4,501 women between age 19 and 65 years who presented to 10 hospital-based emergency departments in two cities serving inner city, urban, and suburban populations. Of these, 266 (5.9%) had definite or probable battering injuries and an additional 266 (5.9%) were currently in a physically abusive relationship but did not present with evidence of a battering injury. Compared to the 3,969 women (88.2%) who were not currently in a physically abusive relationship, women in physically abusive relationships were more likely to present to the emergency department after an attempted suicide. In a cross-sectional study of 203 women seeking refuge in battered women's shelters, Wingood et al. (297) found, after controlling for the effects of sociodemographic characteristics, that women experiencing both sexual and physical abuse were more likely to have attempted suicide than women experiencing physical abuse alone.

Although much more commonly experienced by women, domestic partner violence also affects men. Ernst et al. (302) surveyed 233 men and 283 women who presented to an inner-city emergency department for past and current histories of domestic partner violence and found that such experiences were associated with increased rates of suicidal ideation in both sexes. It is important to note that men with a history of domestic violence toward their partners may also be at increased risk for suicide. Conner et al. (303), for example, noted that one-half of the 42 male alcoholics who died by suicide and were originally described by Murphy et al. (149) had a history of domestic violence.

Domestic violence in the home may also affect the risk for suicide attempts among those who witness that violence. Dube et al. (281) examined the relationship to suicide attempts of eight adverse childhood experiences, including witnessing domestic violence, in 17,337 adults (mean age=56 years) and found that childhood exposure to parental domestic violence increased the risk of later suicide attempts.

Thus, although data on suicide risk per se are not available, there is clear evidence that domestic partner violence is associated with an increased risk of suicide attempts. In addition, although evidence is more limited, individuals who become violent with their partners or who observe domestic partner violence may also be at increased risk for suicidal behaviors. Since a past or current history of domestic partner violence is often overlooked, even in settings such as emergency departments where it is quite prevalent, it is important to specifically ask about domestic partner violence as a part of the suicide assessment.

e) Treatment history

A past history of treatment of mental illness, including a past history of hospitalization, should be viewed as a marker that alerts the clinician to an increase in suicide risk (64, 198). Furthermore, greater treatment intensity is associated with a higher rate of eventual suicide. For example, Bostwick and Pankratz (77) used meta-analytic techniques to calculate suicide risks for outpatients, inpatients, or suicidal inpatients and found a hierarchy in suicide risk among patients with affective disorders. The estimated lifetime prevalence of suicide in those ever hospitalized for suicidality was 8.6%, compared to a lifetime suicide rate of 4.0% for all hospitalized patients. For mixed inpatient/outpatient populations, the lifetime suicide prevalence was even lower, at 2.2%, whereas for the population without affective illness, it was less than 0.5%. A similar phenomenon was noted by Simon and VonKorff (718) among patients treated for depression in a large health plan in western Washington State. Computerized discharge diagnoses, outpatient visit diagnoses, and outpatient prescription records were used to identify all enrollees who received treatment for depression during a 3-year period. During the study period, 35,546 individuals received some treatment for depression and accounted for 62,159 person-years of follow-up. Thirty-six individuals (4.2% of all deaths) were classified as having definitely or possibly died by suicide, yielding an overall suicide mortality rate of 59 per 100,000 person-years, with the rate for men more than threefold higher than the rate for women. Patients who received any inpatient psychiatric treatment had a risk for suicide of 224 per 100,000 person-years, with suicide rates among those who received outpatient specialty mental health treatment and those treated with antidepressant medications in primary care of 64 and 43 per 100,000 person-years, respectively. No patient with a diagnosis of depression who was treated only in primary care and who did not receive antidepressant medication died by suicide.

In terms of suicide attempts, Pirkis et al. (198) analyzed data for 12,229 patients in 13,632 episodes of care and found that the risk of suicide attempts was 10-fold higher in acute inpatient settings, compared with longer-stay inpatient or community-based settings (5.4 attempts per 1,000 episode-days, compared with 0.6 and 0.5 attempts per 1,000 episode-days, respectively). Thus, the rate of suicidality is increased in individuals with prior inpatient treatment, although it is not clear whether the rate is higher because the patients have more severe illnesses (and are deemed to be at increased risk for suicide) or because hospitalization increases suicide risk by increasing emotional or psychosocial distress.

Temporally, the risk for suicide appears to be greatest after changes in treatment setting or intensity (304). Recently admitted and recently discharged inpatients show particularly increased risks (64, 72), and this pattern is seen across diagnostic categories (91, 95, 305–308). Rates decline with time since discharge but may remain high for as long as several years (91, 306, 309). For example, Pirkis and Burgess (309) systematically reviewed the literature on suicide and health care contacts and found that up to 41% of those in the general population who die by suicide may have had psychiatric inpatient care in the year before death, with up to 9% dying by suicide within 1 day of discharge. Appleby et al. (304) compared individuals who died by suicide within 5 years of discharge from psychiatric inpatient care to surviving demographically matched patients and found that those who died by suicide were more likely to have had their care reduced at the final appointment in the community before death (odds ratio=3.7).

Black et al. (91) assessed 5,412 patients admitted to the University of Iowa Psychiatric Hospital and found that 331 died over a 9-year follow-up period. Ninety-nine percent of all premature deaths occurred during the initial 2 years after discharge, with the risk for premature death being greatest among women and the young. Over the initial 2-year period, 29% of deaths were by suicide and suicide occurred at a rate that was more than 50 times the expected rate for the group as a whole.

Roy (96) compared 90 psychiatric patients who had attempted suicide (53 male patients and 37 female patients) to a group of 90 matched control subjects who had not attempted suicide. Of the 75 patients who had died by suicide as outpatients, 58% had seen a psychiatrist within the previous week, 81% had been admitted in their last episode of contact, and 44% of those who had been inpatients attempted suicide within 1 month of discharge.

Goldacre et al. (307) determined the risk of suicide within a year of psychiatric discharge in a population-based study in Oxford, U.K., and found that SMRs for suicide in the first 28 days after discharge from inpatient care were 213 and 134 for male and female patients, respectively. The rate of suicide in the first 28 days after discharge was 7.1 times higher for male patients and 3.0 times higher for female patients than the rate during the remaining 48 weeks of the first year after discharge.

More recently, Appleby et al. (306) analyzed data for 10,040 individuals in the United Kingdom who died by suicide over a 2-year period and found that 2,370 (24%) had been in contact with mental health services in the 12 months before death. Of these, 358 (16%) were psychiatric inpatients at the time of death, and one-fifth of those patients were being monitored with special observation procedures. An additional 519 suicides (24%) occurred within 3 months of hospital discharge, with the highest number occurring in the first week. Rossau and Mortensen (95) found that 508 suicides occurred among 9,156 patients who were admitted to psychiatric hospitals in Denmark between 1970 and 1987 and who received a diagnosis of schizophrenia for the first time. Suicide risk was particularly high during the first 5 days after discharge, and risk was also increased in individuals with multiple admissions during the prior year.

Similar findings have been reported for suicide attempts, which are also more frequent in the period following hospitalization. Oquendo et al. (267) followed 136 patients after hospitalization for major depressive disorder and found that 15% of the subjects made a suicide attempt within 2 years, with more than 50% of attempts occurring within the first 5 months of follow-up.

Given that the intensity of past treatment is associated with risk for suicide and suicide attempts, the treatment history is an important part of the assessment process. In addition, these observations suggest specific points in the course of treatment (e.g., hospital discharge or other changes in treatment setting) at which risk of suicidal behaviors may be particularly increased. Awareness of these factors will allow the psychiatrist to take them into consideration in developing a plan of treatment with the patient.

f) Illness course and severity

In some psychiatric disorders, suicide risk is greater at certain points in the illness or episode course. Multiple studies have shown that suicidality tends to occur early in the course of affective disorder, often before diagnosis or before treatment has begun (310, 719). These observations emphasize the importance of early identification of these disorders and early implementation of effective interventions.

Appleby et al. (304) compared individuals who died by suicide within 5 years of discharge from psychiatric inpatient care to surviving demographically matched patients and found that suicide was more likely in those whose index hospitalization was at the beginning of their illness (odds ratio=2.0). Bradvik and Berglund (317) followed 1,206 inpatients who had received a discharge diagnosis of severe depression/melancholia between 1956 and 1969. At the time of the initial follow-up in 1984, 22% had died by suicide, whereas by the second follow-up in 1998, an additional 4% had died by suicide. Although mortality due to suicide declined with time, the standardized mortality was still increased late in the course of depressive illness (SMR=1.3). Osby et al. (73) identified all patients in Sweden with a hospital diagnosis of bipolar disorder (N=15,386) or unipolar depressive disorder (N=39,182) between 1973 and 1995 and determined the date and cause of death using national registries. They found that the SMR for suicide was especially high for younger patients during the first years after initial diagnosis, although an increasing SMR was found for female patients with major depressive disorder over the course of the study. Fawcett et al. (313) found that for the 954 patients with major affective disorder in the NIMH Collaborative Program on the Psychobiology of Depression, 32% of the 25 suicides occurred within 6 months and 52% occurred within 1 year of entry into the study.

Suicide has been noted to be more likely early in the illness course in individuals with schizophrenia. Westermeyer et al. (83), for example, compared 36 patients with schizophrenia who died by suicide to a similar group of patients who did not die by suicide and found that individuals with schizophrenia and other psychotic disorders were especially vulnerable to suicide within the first 6 years of their initial hospitalization. Suicides were present throughout the course of schizophrenia in the National Suicide Prevention Project in Finland (100).

Although patients' risks for suicide and suicide attempts later in the illness course are less than those earlier on, their risks remain greater than those in the general population (74, 100, 316, 317). Angst et al. (74) followed 406 hospitalized patients with affective disorder for 22 years or more and found that the suicide rate was most elevated at the age of onset but that, from age 30 to 70 years, the suicide rate was remarkably constant despite the different courses of illness. Ahrens et al. (316) examined the illness course of 310 patients with mood disorder, 98 of whom had made a suicide attempt, and found no significant correlation between age and suicide attempts, suggesting that the rate of suicide attempts was not declining as the patient aged and the illness progressed. Malone et al. (312) analyzed data for 100 inpatients during a major depressive episode and noted that the first 3 months after the onset of a major depressive episode and the first 5 years after the lifetime onset of major depressive disorder represented the highest-risk period for attempted suicide, independent of the severity or duration of depression.

Risk for suicide may also vary with the severity of symptoms. For example, Brown et al. (78) prospectively followed 6,891 psychiatric outpatients and found that in the 49 (1%) who died by suicide the severity of depression, hopelessness, and suicide ideation were significant risk factors. In contrast, in individuals with schizophrenia, low levels of negative symptoms have been associated with increased suicide risk (93).

It is also important to recognize that other factors such as age modulate the effects of symptom severity on risk. With older adults, for example, milder symptoms may be associated with greater risk than moderate symptoms in younger adults (66). Waern et al. (207) analyzed data for 85 individuals over 65 years of age who had died by suicide and 153 randomly selected living comparison subjects and found that elevated suicide risk was associated with minor as well as major depressive disorder.

In terms of attempted suicide, Mann et al. (31) followed 347 consecutive patients after admission to a university hospital and found that the objective severity of current depression or psychosis did not distinguish the 184 patients who had attempted suicide from those who had never attempted suicide. However, those who had attempted suicide reported higher levels of subjective depression and suicidal ideation and fewer reasons for living. Corbitt et al. (195), using data from structured interviews of 102 psychiatric inpatients, found that past suicidal behavior was better predicted by the number of criteria for borderline personality disorder and other cluster B personality disorders that were met than by depressive symptoms.

That the risk for suicidality may be associated with symptom or illness severity suggests that it is important to determine the magnitude and not simply the presence of risk factors as part of the assessment process. In addition, when estimating risk and implementing a plan of treatment to address risk, variations in risk with illness course may need to be considered in the context of other patient-specific factors.

5. Physical illness

Considerable evidence derived from a variety of sources supports a link between physical illness and suicide (Table 7). Methods used to establish this relationship have included record linkage and prospective cohort studies of clinical samples with specific physical illnesses, as well as retrospective examinations of the prevalence of specific physical illnesses in samples of individuals who took their own lives.

Harris and Barraclough (25) conducted a comprehensive, systematic literature review and meta-analysis to determine the suicide risk associated with 63 specific physical disorders that had been posited to influence this risk. They did not include reports of epilepsy, conceding that the evidence base was already strong for its association with suicide. Their review yielded 235 reports that met the specific criteria for consideration, from which data were abstracted to enable calculation of pooled SMRs for each condition. The authors concluded that the disorders demonstrating significantly increased risk for suicide included HIV/AIDS, Huntington's disease, malignant neoplasm, multiple sclerosis, peptic ulcer disease, chronic hemodialysis-treated renal failure, spinal cord injury, and systemic lupus erythematosus. The data were insufficient to conclude whether amputation, valve replacement, intestinal diseases, cirrhosis, Parkinson's disease, or systemic sclerosis conferred an increased risk for suicide. Surprising findings included the association of amyotrophic lateral sclerosis, blindness, stroke, diabetes mellitus, rheumatoid arthritis, and hypertension with only average risk that was no greater than that in the general population. Pregnancy and the puerperium were associated with a statistically reduced risk for suicide. Although the authors were unable to examine the influence of mental disorders or other mediating or moderating effects, many of the disorders associated with increased risk are also associated with mental disorders (e.g., multiple sclerosis with depression and peptic ulcer disease with alcohol abuse). Therefore, when the influence of comorbid psychiatric illness is accounted for, the independent risk associated with physical illness may be less.

Quan and colleagues (337) reported results of a record linkage study conducted in Alberta, Canada, that was designed to establish whether specific illnesses distinguish persons who died by suicide from comparison subjects who died in accidents. In univariate statistical analyses comparing 822 persons age 55 years and older who died by suicide with 944 subjects of similar age who died in motor vehicle accidents, those who died by suicide were more likely to have had malignant neoplasm, arteriosclerotic heart disease, chronic obstructive pulmonary disease, peptic ulcer disease, prostate disorders, depression, and other psychiatric diagnoses. In multivariate analyses in which the effects of demographic and health characteristics were controlled, arteriosclerotic heart disease and peptic ulcer disease did not differentiate the groups. Among the physical illnesses, only malignant neoplasm and prostate disorders (excluding prostate cancer) remained significant predictors, along with chronic obstructive pulmonary disease in married (but not single) men.

Grabbe and colleagues (338) used data from the National Mortality Followback Survey to identify health status variables related to suicide in older persons, compared with natural deaths and deaths from injury. In comparing suicides with injury deaths, they found that malignant neoplasm, but not lung conditions, was associated with increased risk. The presence of a stroke, paradoxically, appeared to lower risk. The study reinforced the powerful influence of cancer.

Other studies have also specifically looked for associations between suicide and central nervous system disorders that are known to increase the rates of depressive syndromes. Stenager et al. (334), for example, found that patients with a diagnosis of multiple sclerosis after age 40 were at no greater risk for suicide than control subjects, but that men and women who received this diagnosis before age 40 were at approximately three times and two times greater risk, respectively. Stenager et al. (720) also cross-referenced data for all patients discharged with a diagnosis of a cerebrovascular accident in selected areas of Denmark between 1973 and 1990 with death records and found 140 suicides among almost 38,000 patients with a history of cerebrovascular accident and increased suicide risks for both men and women with this diagnosis in all age groups. In general, risk for suicide was higher in women than in men and in age groups under age 60 years, compared to older adults. The group at highest risk was women under age 50 with a stroke, who had a risk for suicide almost 14 times greater than that for women of similar age in the general population. These data provide additional support for an association between suicide and cerebrovascular disease, particularly among younger and middle-aged stroke patients.

Evidence for increased suicide risk in people with epilepsy is similarly strong. Stenager and Stenager (323) examined all published reports concerning the link between suicide and neurologic disorders in order to critically evaluate the strength of the evidence. They identified a variety of common methodologic problems in this body of research, including sources of bias in selection of cases, inadequate definition of control samples, imprecise definitions of disease, inadequate sample sizes, absent or imprecise definitions of suicidal behavior, and inadequate follow-up intervals. Nonetheless, they concluded that sufficiently rigorous studies of patients with multiple sclerosis, patients with spinal cord injury, and selected groups of patients with epilepsy did establish increased risk in these conditions. The most rigorous studies examining risk associated with epilepsy were conducted by White and colleagues in 1979 (324). They followed 2,099 patients with epilepsy who had been committed for institutional care and treatment and compared their risk for suicide with that in an age- and sex-standardized control population. They found that individuals with epilepsy were at 5.4 times higher risk for suicide than the control subjects.

Rafnsson et al. (326) analyzed data for 224 individuals who first received a diagnosis of unprovoked seizures in Iceland between 1960 and 1964 and who were followed for up to 25 years. Among men, the relative risk of dying by suicide was almost six times the expected risk in the general population, and the rates of death from accidents, poisoning, and violence were about three times the expected rates.

Nilsson et al. (325) used data from the Swedish National Cause of Death Register to determine causes of death among 6,880 patients with a diagnosis of epilepsy registered in the Stockholm County In-Patient Register. In a comparison of 26 individuals who died by suicide and 23 individuals suspected of having died by suicide with 171 living control subjects, individuals with an onset of epilepsy before age 18 had a higher risk for suicide than those with comorbid psychiatric diagnoses or those treated with antipsychotics. However, unlike other studies, this study did not find a specific association with particular types of epilepsy, including temporal lobe seizures.

Suicide attempts also appear to be increased in frequency among patients with epilepsy, compared to the general population. Hawton et al. (330) analyzed data for patients admitted after deliberate self-poisoning or self-injury over a 2-year period and found that the number of patients with epilepsy was five times higher than general population prevalence rates. Mendez et al. (329) compared 175 outpatients with epilepsy to a group of 70 comparably disabled outpatients and found that prior suicide attempts were reported by 30% of the patients with epilepsy, compared to only 7% of the control subjects. Rates of depression were similarly increased among the patients with epilepsy (55%, compared with 30% of the control subjects). In a subsequent study, Mendez et al. (331) compared 62 patients with epilepsy to 62 patients with schizophrenia and to 62 patients with both diagnoses and found that suicidal behaviors were more common among individuals with epilepsy.

The association between terminal physical illnesses and suicide is complex. Brown and colleagues (721) found that 34 of 44 terminally ill patients receiving palliative care had never wished for an early death. All of the 10 patients who had wished for an early death were found to have clinical depressive illness, but only three reported suicidal ideation. Chochinov and colleagues (342) interviewed 200 patients who had terminal cancer to determine their psychiatric status and whether they had thoughts of death. Almost 45% had wished for an early death, but in only 8.5% were the thoughts serious and persistent. Predictors of desire for death included pain, a low level of family support, and clinically significant depression. Diagnosable depressive illness was found in almost 60% of those with a desire to die and in 8% of those without a desire to die.

Other features of physical illness that may augment the likelihood of suicidal ideation or suicide include functional impairments (338), pain (340, 341), disfigurement, increased dependence on others, and decreases in sight and hearing (321, 333). Waern et al. (333) compared consecutive records of people who had died by suicide (46 men and 39 women) with those of living control participants selected from the tax register (84 men and 69 women) in Gothenburg, Sweden. In addition to neurological disorders and malignant disease, which were associated with three- to fourfold increases in suicide risk, visual impairment and serious physical illness of any type were also associated with increased risk, with odds ratios of 7.0 and 6.4, respectively. Although the number of women in the sample was small, the risk appeared to be greater among men, particularly in those with a high burden of physical illness. Conwell et al. (321) also found physical illness burden and functional limitations to be more common among individuals seen in primary care settings who die by suicide. They compared 196 patients age 60 years and older from a group practice of general internal medicine (N=115) or family medicine (N=81) to 42 individuals age 60 years and older who had visited a primary care provider and who died by suicide within 30 days of their visit. Those who died by suicide were significantly more likely than control subjects to have had a depressive illness, greater functional impairment, or a larger burden of physical illness.

While several studies have shown that people with HIV and AIDS are at high risk for suicide, the data on the extent of that risk vary. In particular, suicide risk among people with HIV/AIDS is likely to relate to other comorbid factors such as substance abuse and other psychiatric diagnoses, stigma, social isolation, and lack of support (722), as well as the direct effects of HIV on the brain (335, 723). Even at the time of HIV serum antibody testing, suicidal ideation is highly prevalent, being noted by about 30% of individuals and diminishing over time after notification of test results (724). Nonetheless, elevations in the suicide rate are present among persons with AIDS and range from seven to 36 times the rates in comparable age- and sex-matched populations (335, 336, 725). For example, Marzuk et al. (335) studied suicide rates in 1985 in New York City and found a rate of 18.75 per 100,000 person-years for men age 20–59 years without a known diagnosis of AIDS, compared to 680.56 per 100,000 person-years for those with a known diagnosis of AIDS, a 36-fold increase in relative risk. Cote et al. (336) used public-access AIDS surveillance data and National Center for Health Statistics multiple-cause mortality data for the period from 1987 through 1989 to identify suicides among persons with AIDS and found that all but one of the persons who died by suicide were male. Compared to demographically similar men in the general population, men with AIDS had a rate of suicide that was 7.4-fold higher, at 165 per 100,000 person-years of observation. Cote et al. also noted that the suicide risk for persons with AIDS decreased significantly from 1987 to 1989, suggesting that the rate of suicide associated with AIDS may be decreasing.

In summary, physical illnesses are associated with increased risk for suicide. The strength of the evidence for malignant neoplasms, central nervous system disorders, peptic ulcer disease, and HIV/AIDS is strong. Although the evidence is less compelling, indications are that a range of other conditions may also be associated with suicide and suicidal behaviors. It is probable that mood and substance use disorders, either as precipitants or sequelae, account in part for the increased SMRs for suicide ascribed to specific physical conditions in the literature. However, further study is needed to determine the role of social and psychological factors as mediators or moderators of the relationship between physical illness and suicide. As a result, in assessing suicide risk among individuals with physical illness, consideration should be given to the presence of comorbid mood symptoms as well as to the functional effects of the illness.

6. Family history

Findings from at least three types of studies suggests that risk for suicide has a familial and probably genetic contribution. These include: 1) strong and consistent findings that risk for suicidal behavior is much higher among first-degree relatives of individuals with suicide attempts or deaths than in the general population, 2) higher concordance for suicidal behavior among identical versus fraternal twins, and 3) greater risk of suicidal behavior among biological versus adoptive relatives of persons adopted early in life who later died by suicide (365–368). These familial associations appear to be accounted for only partly by familial risks for major affective illness or other clinical risk factors for suicide. Recent efforts to specify molecular genetic markers that segregate or associate with suicidal behavior, including those relating to the serotonin (5-hydroxytryptamine [5-HT]) neurotransmission system, have yielded inconsistent findings that are not easily interpreted (17, 366, 368).

a) Family studies

Evidence from family studies of suicide was recently summarized by Turecki (368). In addition to studies showing increased rates of suicidal behaviors among family members of suicidal individuals (31, 82, 360–364), at least 20 reports of controlled comparisons involving more than 11,000 subjects have been published (202, 214, 312, 344–359). The pooled overall relative risk of suicidal behavior in first-degree relatives of suicidal probands compared to control or population risks, weighted by the number of subjects in each study, was 4.48 (95% CI=3.71–5.25), indicating a nearly 4.5-fold excess of risk of suicidal behavior among relatives of suicidal subjects, compared to nonsuicidal subjects (R. Baldessarini, personal communication, 2002).

Across studies, reported estimates of relative risk for suicidal behavior within families vary greatly, depending in part on the types of behavior included (suicide, suicide attempts of varying lethality, or both) and their defining criteria, the prevalence of psychiatric risk factors for suicide among the control subjects, the closeness of kinship (first-degree relatives, including parents and siblings, with or without second-degree relatives), and differences in sample size. Such studies, while demonstrating a powerful association, do not prove genetic risk nor rule out shared environmental factors. Moreover, it remains to be proved that the relationship for suicide is separable from the well-known heritability of leading risk factors for suicide, including major affective illness. Nevertheless, the findings from pooled family studies strongly support the conclusion that overall risk for suicidal behavior is at least four times greater among close relatives of suicidal persons than among unrelated persons.

b) Twin studies

A powerful method of separating risks that result from shared environments from risks that result from genetic factors is to compare the rate of concordance (index condition appearing in both twins) for a condition between identical, or monozygotic (single-egg), twins and fraternal, or dizygotic (two-egg), twins. Risks for dizygotic twins should be similar to those found among other first-degree family members in family studies. Seven such twin studies pertaining to suicide were identified in the research literature (365, 370–375) and reviewed by Roy et al. (365, 369) and Turecki (368). None of the studies involved samples of twins raised separately from early life, and, thus, the confounding effects of shared environments were possible. Moreover, the size and statistical power of these studies varied markedly, from an analysis of a single monozygotic twin-pair (373) to a study of an entire Australian national twin registry involving more than 1,500 monozygotic and nearly 1,200 dizygotic twin-pairs (375). When the data from all seven twin studies were pooled, the overall concordance rate for suicide or suicide attempts, weighted for the numbers of subjects involved, was 23.5% (401 of 1,704) for monozygotic twin-pairs and 0.135% (two of 1,486) for dizygotic twin-pairs, for a highly significant 175-fold increase in pooled relative risk in the monozygotic twin-pairs (R. Baldessarini, personal communication, 2002). Given the low frequency of suicidal behavior found among fraternal co-twins, this relative risk is likely to be a quantitatively unstable estimate. Nevertheless, its magnitude strongly supports a genetic contribution to suicidal behavior. A highly significant fourfold excess of risk in identical twins remained, even after statistical corrections for depressive and other psychiatric morbidity associated with suicide (375). Therefore, twin studies add strong support for the heritability of suicide risk that is separate from the heritability of risk factors such as mood disorders but that is still likely to be influenced by environmental factors.

c) Adoption studies

A less commonly employed technique to separate genetic from shared environmental factors is to study outcomes for persons adopted from their biological families very early in life. For the study of suicide, this approach has been reported only three times, and each study used the same Danish health and vital statistics registers that included data for 5,483 adoptions in greater Copenhagen between 1924 and 1947 (376–378). When data for suicide were pooled across all studies, to include affectively as well as psychotically ill probands (376, 378), there was an approximately fivefold greater risk among biological than among adoptive relatives (20 of 543 subjects [3.68%] versus two of 263 subjects [0.76%]).

Later, the same American and Danish collaborators (378) compared all adoptees identified as having an affective spectrum disorder (N=71) with matched control adoptees without such disorders (N=71). The index disorders included not only DSM-III major depression and bipolar disorder but also milder "neurotic" depressions and a condition ("affect reaction") marked by affective instability that may resemble some forms of personality disorder in current classifications. In relatives of affectively ill adopted probands, there was a significant, approximately sevenfold greater risk for suicide in biological relatives, compared with adopted relatives (15 of 387 subjects [3.88%] versus one of 180 subjects [0.56%]). Further analysis of the suicide rate for biological relatives, compared with control subjects, also yielded a highly significant 13.3-fold difference (15 of 387 subjects [3.88%] versus one of 344 subjects [0.29%]) (378). In striking contrast, however, when suicide attempts were considered separately, there was a 1.16-fold lower but nonsignificant risk in the biological relatives, compared with the adoptive relatives, of affectively ill adopted probands (13 of 387 subjects [3.36%] versus seven of 180 subjects [3.89%]). A similar comparison of the rate of suicide attempts in biological relatives of adopted probands and in matched but not affectively ill control subjects showed a modest 2.89-fold difference that failed to reach significance (13 of 387 subjects [3.36%] versus four of 344 subjects [1.16%]). Among relatives of index adoptees with a diagnosis of schizophrenia, there was a nonsignificant 2.67-fold greater risk for suicide in biological relatives, compared with adoptive relatives (five of 156 subjects [3.20%] versus one of 83 subjects [1.20%]) (376).

Matched comparison of 57 early-adopted individuals who died by suicide with other adoptees lacking evidence of suicide or psychiatric illnesses also showed a great excess risk of suicide in biological over adoptive relatives (12 of 269 subjects [4.46%] versus none of 148 subjects [0.00%]) (378). Risk of suicide was approximately sixfold greater in relatives of suicidal probands compared to relatives of matched, nonsuicidal control subjects (12 of 269 subjects [4.46%] versus two of 269 subjects [0.74%]). However, this study did not consider the possible coincident heritability of clinical risk factors for suicide, such as major affective illnesses and substance use disorders.

Overall, these adoption studies indicate a greater risk of suicide, but not of suicide attempts, among biological relatives of suicidal probands, compared with adoptive relatives. They also show greater risk among biological relatives of probands, compared with control subjects, that is consistent with the hypothesis that suicidality is heritable. Given the broader range of severity and lethality of suicide attempts and the greater likelihood of environmentally determined actions in many instances, the heritability of suicide may well be much greater than that of suicide attempts.

7. Psychosocial factors

a) Employment

Unemployment has long been associated with increased rates of suicide (379, 380, 726). Furthermore, the link between suicide and unemployment has been confirmed by a recent study that used U.S. National Longitudinal Mortality Study data to assess whether unemployed individuals were at greater risk for suicide than employed persons (24). At 2-year follow-up, unemployed men were two to three times more likely to have died by suicide, compared with employed men. Living alone, being divorced, and having lower socioeconomic status increased the suicide risk. At or beyond 4 years of follow-up, however, there was no statistical association between unemployment and suicide for men. For women, the relationship between suicide and unemployment was even stronger and longer-lasting. Unemployed women had a much higher risk for suicide at each year of follow-up than employed women. Unemployed women continued to show an elevated risk at 9-year follow-up, by which time they were three times as likely to die by suicide as employed women. As with men, younger unemployed women were more at risk than women over age 45 years. While the number of women who died by suicide was small, the results remain significant and powerful. While in the past men were considered most at risk for suicide after becoming unemployed, it is now known that women are at an even greater risk and for a longer period of time. The relationship between unemployment, suicide, and psychiatric disorders remains unclear. Persons with psychiatric disorders may be more likely to quit jobs or to be fired as well as more likely to die by suicide (727).

Areas with socioeconomic deprivation also have larger numbers of unemployed people, and these differences have been used to examine effects of unemployment on rates of suicide and suicide attempts. Hawton et al. (386), for example, analyzed data for different wards, or communities, within Oxford, England, and found that wards with the highest socioeconomic deprivation were associated with the highest rates of suicide attempts. Individuals who attempted suicide, both men and women, were more likely to be unemployed, living alone, and having problems with housing. For men, but not for women, a strong association was also found between the rate of suicide attempts and socioeconomic deprivation. Men living in less deprived areas who had financial problems were even more likely to attempt suicide, suggesting that the dissonance between one's own financial status and that of the neighborhood may affect risk. Unemployment and financial problems can affect suicide in other ways as well. Alcohol consumption and marital conflict, each of which increases with financial difficulties or unemployment, may also contribute to increased risk for suicidal behaviors.

Political context and large-scale economic changes can also influence suicide and may provide clues about the effect of employment status on suicide rates. During times of war, for example, suicide rates decline (728), whereas increased suicide rates are found in political systems associated with violence or social movements. Areas of the former Soviet Union with high levels of sociopolitical oppression (i.e., Baltic States) have had higher suicide rates than other regions with less oppression (729). From an economic standpoint, research on the business cycle and suicide has relied primarily on unemployment rates, but other indicators include growth rates of the gross domestic product, the Ayres index of industrial activity, change in the stock market index, and the rate of new dwelling construction (730). Especially for men, the data suggest that the greater the prosperity, the lower the suicide rate, and, conversely, the greater the trend toward recession, the greater the suicide rate. During periods of high unemployment, such as the Great Depression, the relationship of unemployment to suicide is strengthened (731). However, studies using the Ayres index of industrial activity and monthly suicide trends have suggested that large swings in industrial production, such as those that occurred during the 1930s, are needed to influence the suicide rate (732).

In summary, it is important to ascertain the patient's employment status as part of the assessment process, since unemployment may increase suicide risk, whereas employment may offer some protection against suicide and suicide attempts. However, a patient's job status should also be considered in terms of other psychosocial stressors that may be related to job loss, such as financial or marital difficulties. In addition, there is often a complex interplay between employment status and psychiatric illness, including substance use disorder, that may influence treatment planning.

b) Religious beliefs

Limited evidence points to religion as a protective factor against suicide. Pescosolido and Giorgianna (733) used suicide rates from the National Center for Health Statistics, data on affiliation rates in various Christian denominations from the National Council of Churches, and data on Jewish affiliation from the American Jewish Yearbook to determine whether suicide rates differ according to religious affiliation. They found that religion affected suicide rates, with Catholicism, Evangelical Protestantism, and membership in Church of the Nazarenes being associated with lower rates and Jewish affiliation producing a small but inconsistent protective effect. In contrast, various denominations of mainstream Protestantism tended to be associated with increased suicide rates.

Within specific religious denominations, the strength of religious belief may also play a role. Maris (394) compared suicide rates among Catholics and Protestants in Chicago between 1966 and 1968. Scores on church attendance, perception of religiosity, and influence of religion were negatively associated with suicidal ideation. After controlling for the effects of confounding variables such as sex, marital status, and socioeconomic status, Maris found that the perceived influence of religion was the most significant correlate of suicidal ideation. In immigrants from Central America, infrequent church attendance and low levels of perceived influence of religion were related to high levels of suicidal ideation (43). Thus, religious involvement may serve as a protective factor against suicide, either by helping to buffer acculturative stress (43) or by enhancing social networks and support (733).

In summary, some evidence suggests that religious beliefs and the strength of those beliefs may offer protective effects in relation to suicide risk. At the same time, these protective effects neither are specific to particular religious denominations nor are invariably present. Indeed, for some individuals, religious beliefs or beliefs about death may increase rather than decrease the likelihood of acting on suicidal thoughts. Consequently, the clinician may wish to gain an understanding of the patient's specific religious beliefs and the depth of the patient's religiosity as well as determine the ways in which these beliefs influence the patient's conceptions of death and suicide.

c) Psychosocial support

Although it is often difficult to distinguish perceived from objective measures of social support, available data strongly suggest that the presence of a social network is a powerful and independent predictor of suicide risk. In particular, those who have (or perceive themselves to have) supportive interpersonal relationships are at lower risk for suicide than those without such actual or perceived supports. Rubenowitz et al. (405) used the psychological autopsy method to compare 85 persons age 65 years and older who died by suicide with 153 age- and sex-matched living persons selected from the tax roster in Gothenburg, Sweden. In addition to identifying a powerful influence of psychiatric disorders, they found that family discord was a significant risk factor for those who died by suicide (odds ratio≈19). Further, being active in a social club was a significant protective factor for both men and women. Another recent psychological autopsy study compared 53 individuals age 55 years and older who had either died by suicide or made a serious suicide attempt with 269 matched control subjects (403). Psychiatric illness was again a powerful predictor of suicide case status, but, in addition, those who died by suicide had significantly fewer social interactions and significantly more relationship problems, compared to the control subjects. Turvey and colleagues (400) used data from the Established Populations for Epidemiologic Studies in the Elderly database to identify 21 elderly persons who died by suicide over a 10-year follow-up period and compared those subjects to 420 control subjects matched for age, sex, and study site. In addition to depressive symptoms, poor perceived health status, and poor sleep quality, the absence of a relative or friend in whom to confide was a significant risk factor for late-life suicide. Finally, Miller (399) compared 30 men age 60 years and older who died by suicide with 30 men, matched on age, race, marital status, and county of residence, who died of natural causes. He reported that the control subjects were significantly more likely to have had a confidante and that the subjects who died by suicide had significantly fewer visits with friends and relatives. Thus, while social support is a complex construct and the data on this factor come primarily from elderly populations, decreases in measures of social support appear to increase suicide risk, and, conversely, increases in social support may serve as a protective factor in relation to suicide.

d) Reasons for living, including children in the home

An additional protective factor against suicide is the ability to cite reasons for living, which often reflect the patient's degree of optimism about life. Malone et al. (231) assessed 84 patients, 45 of whom had attempted suicide, to determine whether "reasons for living" might protect or restrain patients with major depression from making a suicide attempt. Depressed patients who had not attempted suicide were found to have expressed more feelings of responsibility toward their families, more fear of social disapproval, more moral objections to suicide, greater survival and coping skills, and a greater fear of suicide than the depressed patients who had attempted suicide. Although objective severity of depression and quantity of recent life events did not differ between the two groups, scores for hopelessness, subjective depression, and suicidal ideation were significantly higher for the suicide attempters.

Particularly in women, the presence of children in the home is an additional factor that appears to protect against suicide. Hoyer and Lund (26) used data from the Norwegian Central Bureau of Statistics to prospectively follow 989,949 women over a 15-year period. During that time there were 1,190 deaths from suicide, with parous women of all ages having lower relative risks than nonparous women (relative risk=0.4–0.8, depending on age). For both premenopausal and postmenopausal women, a strong linear decrease in relative risk for suicide was found with an increasing number of children.

Consequently, during the assessment and treatment planning process, clinicians should discuss reasons for living with at-risk patients and the need to develop coping skills that may serve as protective factors during periods of high risk for suicide.

e) Individual psychological strengths and vulnerabilities

A number of personality traits and characteristics have been associated with suicide and suicidal risk and behaviors. Conner et al. (217) reviewed the literature on psychological vulnerabilities to suicide, including 46 publications describing 35 distinct case-control or cohort samples, and found no evidence for a link between suicide and guilt or inwardly directed anger. They did find that suicide was consistently associated with five constructs—impulsivity/aggression, depression, hopelessness, anxiety, and self-consciousness/social disengagement. Although other factors often moderate the relationships between these variables and suicide, they are not always interpretable in the literature because of measurement and definitional issues. Nonetheless, psychological vulnerabilities likely influence suicide risk by exacerbating other psychiatric or social risk factors in individual patients.

A number of other concepts have also been explored in relating suicide to individual vulnerabilities. For example, Duberstein (423) used questionnaires to assess personality dimensions in 81 depressed patients over age 50 and found that individuals who reported lower levels of openness to new experiences were less likely to report suicidal ideation. These findings are consistent with other work, suggesting that elderly persons tend to deny suicidality, whereas younger persons tend to exaggerate it. These findings may also provide support for the protective role of expressing suicidal ideation. Thus, when closed-minded people do come into contact with treatment services, their psychiatric symptoms may not be as obvious and their need for treatment may not be appreciated.

Hughes and Neimeyer (422) assessed 79 hospitalized psychiatric patients, 91% of whom had a principal diagnosis that included depression, and examined the utility of several cognitive variables as predictors of suicidal ideation. Level of pessimism, as measured by the Hopelessness Scale, was the best predictor of subsequent suicidal ideation and was reliably related to placement on either one-to-one observation or every-15-minute checks for suicide precautions. In addition, hopelessness, self-negativity, polarization (all-or-nothing thinking), and poor problem-solving performance were associated with suicidal ideation, whereas self-evaluated problem-solving ability was not. A low level of constriction was related to the intensity of subsequent suicidal ideation and to later suicide attempts.

Josepho and Plutchik (409) investigated the relationship between interpersonal problems, coping styles, and suicide attempts in 71 adult psychiatric inpatients. Patients who were hospitalized after a suicide attempt had more interpersonal problems and also had distinct patterns of coping methods, including more use of suppression and substitution and less use of replacement. These coping styles were also associated with higher scores on a rating of suicide risk. After controlling for the effect of interpersonal problems, the authors found that greater suppression, less minimization, and less replacement were significantly related to increased suicide risk scores. The higher the risk score, the greater the likelihood that the patient was admitted to the hospital secondary to a suicide attempt. Depressed patients also had higher suicide risk scale scores.

Stravynski and Boyer (401) collected data from 19,724 persons who returned the Quebec Health Survey and tested whether there was an association between loneliness and suicidal thoughts or behaviors in the general population. A significant correlation was found between experiencing suicidal ideation or attempting suicide and living alone, having no friends, or feeling alone, with psychological distress being the strongest correlate of suicidal ideation. Of individuals who were severely distressed and very lonely, 25% reported serious suicidal ideation or actions. Overall, thoughts of suicide were reported by 3.1% of the population, and 0.9% had attempted suicide.

Maser et al. (247) examined the correlations between suicide and clinical and personality factors in 955 depressed patients who were followed over 14 years as part of the NIMH Collaborative Program on the Psychobiology of Depression. During that time, 3.8% died by suicide and 12.6% attempted suicide. Suicide within 12 months of intake to the study was associated with clinical variables, including emotional turmoil plus depression in the index episode, a history of both alcohol and drug use disorders, and meeting the criteria for antisocial personality disorder. Additional predictors included hopelessness, delusions of grandeur, indecisiveness, definite delusions or hallucinations during the index episode, reduced functional role, dissatisfaction with life, or any prior history of serious suicide attempts as of the intake episode. Beyond 1 year after intake, suicide was associated with temperamental factors, including high levels of impulsivity and shyness and low sanguinity scores. Suicide attempters and those who died by suicide shared core characteristics, including previous attempts, impulsivity, substance abuse, and psychic turmoil within a cycling/mixed bipolar disorder.

Kaslow et al. (413) conducted an empirical study of the psychodynamics of suicide among 52 patients hospitalized for a suicide attempt and 47 psychiatrically hospitalized control subjects with no history of suicidal behaviors. Overall, 49% of the subjects had depression, 25% had substance use disorders, and 63% had a cluster B personality disorder. Individuals who had attempted suicide were significantly more likely to report childhood loss combined with adulthood loss. Furthermore, they had more impairment in their object relations and viewed relationships in a more negative manner, showing lower levels of individuation and separation. Although self-directed anger was associated with homicidal ideation, there was little support for the psychodynamic concepts that depression, self-directed anger, or ego functioning would be associated with having made a suicide attempt.

In a group of 438 undergraduate college students who ranged in age from 16 to 65 years, Boudewyn and Liem (734) compared low and high scorers on a chronic self-destructiveness scale that measured behaviors such as chronic gambling or unsafe sexual behaviors that had a potential for later negative consequences. Overall, those scoring high in self-destructiveness were younger and reported more childhood and adulthood maltreatment, lower self-esteem, greater depression, greater externality, less need for control in interpersonal relationships, and more frequent suicidal and self-injurious thoughts and acts. These findings suggest that other manifestations of self-destructiveness should be assessed in the individual evaluation of the suicidal patient and that childhood and adult maltreatment should be specifically identified and addressed in the treatment planning process.

Together with extensive clinical observations on individual strengths and vulnerabilities as they relate to suicidality (410, 412, 420, 426), research on various psychological dimensions has demonstrated the need to include such features in assessing suicide risk. In particular, personality traits such as aggression, impulsivity, social disengagement and subjective loneliness, hopelessness, anxiety, low self-esteem (and protective narcissism), dependence, ambivalence, and depression may increase risk for suicidal behaviors. Thinking styles such as closed-mindedness or polarized (either-or) thinking may also augment risk. If dilemmas are seen only in black-and-white terms, with fewer perceived options, patients may see no solution to their problems other than suicide. In addition to personality traits and thinking style, an individual's psychological needs, when not met, can cause intense psychological pain, contributing to a suicidal state. Early trauma and loss may thwart the development of healthy coping skills. In addition, individual perceptions of interpersonal supports, particularly subjective perceptions of loneliness, may also contribute to suicide risk. Thus, in weighing the strengths and vulnerabilities of the individual patient and developing and implementing a plan of treatment, it is helpful to assess the patient's past response to stress, vulnerability to life-threatening affects, available external resources, perceived sense of loneliness, fantasies about death, and capacity for reality testing and for tolerating psychological pain.

8. Degree of suicidality

a) Presence, extent, and persistence of suicidal ideation

Suicidal ideation is common, with an estimated annual incidence of 5.6% (2). Kessler et al. (427) examined the lifetime prevalence of suicidal ideation and suicide attempts in a sample of 5,877 individuals age 15–54 years as part of the National Comorbidity Survey. The estimated lifetime prevalences of suicidal ideation, plans, and attempts were 13.5%, 3.9%, and 4.6%, respectively. The cumulative probability of moving from suicidal ideation to an unplanned attempt was 26%. The corresponding cumulative probability for transitioning from suicidal ideation to suicidal plans was 34%, with a 72% cumulative probability for going from a suicide plan to an attempt. About 90% of unplanned attempts and 60% of planned first attempts occurred within 1 year of the onset of suicidal ideation, suggesting a need for aggressive aftercare and attention to potentially modifiable risk factors in individuals with suicidal ideation.

Longitudinal studies also demonstrate an increased risk of eventual suicide in patients with suicidal ideation. Among 6,891 psychiatric outpatients who were followed for up to 20 years, Brown et al. (78) found that patients' scores on clinician-administered measures of current suicidal ideation and depression were most closely associated with eventual suicide. Fawcett et al. (79), using a case-control method to determine time-related predictors of suicide among 954 patients with major affective disorder, examined suicidal ideation as one possible predictor of actual suicide over a 10-year period. They found that the presence of suicidal ideation was associated with an increased risk for suicide on a long-term basis but not within the first year after study entry.

Others have examined the association between eventual suicide and suicidal ideation at its worst using the Scale for Suicide Ideation–Worst (SSI–W) (428). In a group of 3,701 outpatients in which there were 30 suicides, patients who scored in the high-risk category on the SSI–W had a rate of later suicide that was 14 times greater than that of the patients in the low-risk category. After controlling for the effects of other factors, the investigators found that only the SSI–W score, and not the scores on measures of current suicidal ideation or hopelessness, was associated with future suicide (428). Consistent with the findings of Clark and Fawcett (273), the authors concluded that retrospective report of suicidal ideation at its worst may be a better predictor of suicide than currently reported suicidal ideation.

Intuitively, since suicidal ideas would be expected to precede suicidal intent or suicidal acts, they may serve as a guide for clinicians in identifying and addressing suicide risk. These studies also suggest that past as well as current suicidal ideation is relevant to the assessment process. However, since the vast majority of individuals with suicidal ideation do not die by suicide, additional factors are likely to be modulating suicide risk even in individuals with suicidal ideas.

b) Presence of a suicide plan and availability of a method

As noted earlier, about one-third of individuals with suicidal ideas go on to develop a suicide plan, and about three-quarters of those with a plan eventually make a suicide attempt. Other individuals, however, go on to attempt suicide in an unplanned manner. Thus, the presence of a suicide plan signifies that the risk of a later attempt is increased, but it by no means indicates that an attempt will occur or even the time frame within which an attempt may occur. By the same token, the absence of a suicide plan does not eliminate suicide risk. In general, however, the presence of a specific plan involving an available method is associated with a greater degree of risk for suicide. In addition, availability of methods with relatively high levels of lethality may increase the likelihood that a suicide attempt, either planned or impulsive, will result in suicide.

A number of studies have examined population-based trends in suicide rates as they relate to the availability of specific methods for suicide. Ohberg et al. (735), for example, evaluated trends in suicide rates and availability of methods used for suicide in Finland from 1947 to 1990. For both sexes, the overall suicide rate in Finland rose significantly in that time period, but method-specific rates of suicide varied. For example, the rate of suicide by using the highly lethal pesticide parathion decreased after its availability was restricted, but this decrease was offset by an increased rate of suicide by other methods. Before 1962, most suicides occurred by hanging or drowning, but after 1963, there was a rapid increase in the use of firearms. Coincident with increases in the availability of antidepressants and neuroleptics, the rates of suicide by overdose of these medications increased. There was a high number of overdoses of tricyclic antidepressants, which accounted for most of the deaths attributed to antidepressants. On the other hand, the number of overdose deaths attributed to nontricyclic antidepressants decreased, despite increased availability, and the number of overdose deaths attributed to barbiturates remained stable despite reduction in their availability.

Gunnell et al. (436) investigated method-specific trends in suicide between 1950 and 1975 in England and Wales. In the 1950s and early 1960s, domestic gas poisoning was the most frequently used method of suicide among men and women, accounting for one-half of all suicides. Changes in domestic gas supply and manufacture resulted in a reduction in its carbon monoxide content and thus lethality, and overall suicide rates declined in men and women of all ages. In women and younger men (younger than age 55 years), the effects of these reductions on overall suicide rates were partially offset by a rise in the rates of drug overdose deaths, but there were no immediate increases in the use of other suicide methods. In older men, a reduction in the rate of suicide by gassing was accompanied by only a slight increase in the rate of suicide by overdose as well as reductions in rates of suicide by using all other methods.

Marzuk et al. (437) investigated the relationship between the availability of lethal methods of injury and suicide rates by prospectively classifying lethal methods according to their accessibility in the five counties of New York City over a 4-year period and then comparing the age- and gender-adjusted method-specific suicide rates of the counties. During the study period, there were a total of 2,820 suicides, a rate of 9.81 per 100,000 persons. The study found marked differences in overall crude suicide rates among the five counties, which ranged from 15.27 per 100,000 persons in Manhattan to 5.58 per 100,000 persons in Staten Island. The counties had similar suicide rates involving methods that were equally accessible to all persons in each county (e.g., hanging, laceration, suffocation, and burns) as well as methods that were accessible to a smaller but similar proportion of the population in each county (e.g., firearms and drowning in waterways). Virtually all of the differences in overall suicide risk among the counties were explained by methods that were differentially available, such as fall from height, overdose of prescription drugs, and carbon monoxide poisoning (explained by access to private parking). The availability of a greater variety of alternative lethal methods in some counties did not suppress the rates of use of other methods, and a relative lack of the availability of a specific method did not result in a comparative increase in the rates of use of alternative methods that were available, as the substitution hypothesis would have predicted. Thus, restriction of the availability of a method may reduce its use for suicide, but other methods may tend to be used instead. At the same time, the accessibility to and lethality of particular methods of suicide may have definite effects on the overall suicide rate.

In the United States, firearms constitute the most common method for suicide (736, 737). Fox et al. (738) used mortality data for 1979–1994 from the Wisconsin Center for Health Statistics and the U.S. Census Bureau population estimates for Wisconsin to describe trends for firearm-related suicides in that state. During that period, there were an average of 588 suicides annually, with firearms eclipsing all other methods combined as the most common method of suicide in the 1980s. Between 1981 and 1992, the proportion of firearm suicides increased from 48% to 57%. While the overall suicide rate remained unchanged over the period, the firearm suicide rate increased 17% in all sex, race, and age categories. Among males, the firearm-related suicide rate rose by 13% during the study period, while the rate of suicide by all other methods combined fell 12%. In comparison, among females, the firearm-related suicide rate rose 20%, and the rate of suicide by all other methods fell 26%.

Kaplan and Geling (434) investigated the sociodemographic and geographic patterns of firearm suicides in the United States using mortality data from the National Center for Health Statistics Mortality detail files and death certificate files reported by each state from 1989 to 1993. During this time period, 59.2% of the 139,566 suicides were by firearms. Married persons had the lowest rate of any form of suicide across all race, sex, and age groups. The adjusted odds of using firearms increased with age among men and decreased with age among women. Widowed men and married women had the highest odds of using firearms, and the odds of using a firearm for suicide were also high among those without college education, those who had lived in nonmetropolitan areas, and those who had lived in the East South Central and West South Central geographic divisions. Rates of nonfirearm suicides were higher than firearm suicides everywhere but in the regions of the South. Thus, the likelihood of firearm suicide varied significantly across sociodemographic and geographic subgroups of the U.S. population and paralleled variations in gun ownership, suggesting that regional cultural factors may account for differential rates in suicidal behavior involving firearms.

In addition to population-based data on firearm availability and suicide risk, some data also suggest an effect at an individual level. Brent et al. (438) performed a case-control study to determine the relationship between the presence of guns in the home, the type of gun, the method of storage, and the risk of suicide among adolescents. Forty-seven adolescents from the community who died by suicide were compared with two control groups from a psychiatric hospital: 47 patients who attempted suicide but survived and 47 patients who had never attempted suicide. The study found that guns were twice as likely to be found in the homes of those who died by suicide as in the homes of the suicide attempters or psychiatric control subjects. There was no significant difference in association with suicide between handguns and long guns, and there was no difference in the methods of storage of firearms among the groups. The authors concluded that the availability of guns in the home, independent of the type of firearm or storage method, appears to increase the risk for suicide, at least among adolescents.

In summary, the presence of a suicide plan and the availability of a method for suicide increase risk and are important issues to address as part of the suicide assessment. Since firearm-related suicides account for a significant fraction of suicides in the United States, the presence and availability of firearms are also an important line of inquiry in a suicide risk assessment. A debate remains over whether a reduction in the availability of a particular method of suicide reduces overall risk, although most evidence indicates that restrictions on the availability of particular types of popular methods result in a lower overall suicide rate. At the individual level, reducing access to specific suicide methods may also be indicated. See Section II.C.2, "Elicit the Presence or Absence of a Suicide Plan," for additional discussion of inquiries, removal, and documentation issues related to firearms and the suicidal patient.

c) Lethality and intent of self-destructive behavior

In addition to being increased by the presence of suicidal ideation, a suicide plan, or an available suicide method, suicide risk is also influenced by the patient's subjective expectation and desire to die as a result of a self-inflicted injury. This factor has generally been termed suicidal intent, although the patient's subjective expectation may or may not correspond to the lethality of an attempt made by using a given method. Other facets of a suicide plan or attempt that are often considered when estimating suicidal intent include the severity and potential lethality of the suicide attempt or aborted suicide attempt, the patient's degree of premeditation, whether precautions were taken to avoid intervention or discovery, and whether the patient's intentions were communicated to others (263, 433, 440).

Several studies have longitudinally assessed the influence of suicidal intent on later suicide risk. In a group of 500 patients who had completed a scale measuring suicidal intent after an episode of self-injury, Pierce (441) found that the seven individuals who had died by suicide by the time of a 5-year follow-up tended to have high suicidal intent scores at the time of their initial self-injury. In addition, individuals with increasing levels of suicidal intent with repeated self-injury appeared to be at greater risk for further repetition of self-injury (739). Suokas et al. (271) also conducted a longitudinal assessment of the effect of suicidal intent on suicide risk. They found that 68 (6.7%) of 1,018 deliberate self-poisoning patients had died by suicide by 14-year follow-up. Risk factors for suicide included being male, having previous psychiatric treatment or suicide attempts, having a somatic disease, and having a genuine intent to die at the time of the index self-poisoning.

Thus, for any patient with suicidal ideation, it is important to determine suicidal intent as part of the assessment process. In addition, for any patient who has made a prior suicide attempt, the level of intent at the time of the previous attempt should be determined.

9. Weighting of risk factors in suicide prediction

As noted previously, it is impossible to accurately predict suicide. Nevertheless, given the large number of risk factors and protective factors that can affect the likelihood of suicide, a number of statistical models have been developed to attempt to pinpoint which patients may be at greatest risk. In a longitudinal study by Pokorny (160) that followed 4,800 subjects (4,691 males and 109 females) over a 5-year period, stepwise discriminant analysis was used to select a weighted combination of predictive variables from the identified high-risk characteristics, i.e., being a white male; being single; having a diagnosis of affective disorder, schizophrenia, or alcoholism; having made a previous suicide attempt; or having personality disorder-related traits such as manipulativeness and hostility. This method was able to correctly identify 30 of the 67 subjects who died by suicide but also falsely predicted suicide in 773 individuals. Thus, while it may be possible to identify a high-risk group of patients who warrant more detailed clinical screening, it may not be possible to identify the particular individuals at greatest risk.

Goldstein et al. (740) also used a statistical model that incorporated multiple risk factors for suicide and applied it in a group of 1,906 patients with affective disorders who were admitted to a tertiary care hospital and were followed longitudinally. The identified risk factors included the number of prior suicide attempts, the presence of suicidal ideation on admission, gender, outcome at discharge, and a diagnosis of either bipolar affective disorder (manic or mixed type) or, in individuals with a family history of mania, unipolar depressive disorder. The full statistical model, however, was unable to identify any of the patients who died by suicide, highlighting the difficulty of estimating suicide risk with such methods.

In general, statistical models may be valuable in the epidemiological and research arenas by identifying factors that distinguish high-risk populations of patients. They can also suggest clinically important risk factors that, if identified, are potentially amenable to treatment. However, given the low base rates of suicide in the population, accurate prediction of suicide remains impossible, regardless of the complexity of the statistical model used. Consequently, the psychiatric assessment, in combination with clinical judgment, is still the best tool for assessing suicide risk. In addition, intervention must be based not on the simple presence of risk factors as identified by statistical models but on the interaction of those factors with the individual patient's personal and clinical manifestations and the clinician's assessment of the patient's risk at that particular point in time.

B. PSYCHIATRIC ASSESSMENT TECHNIQUES

1. Rating scales

A wide variety of self-report and clinician-administered scales are available that measure various aspects of suicidal thoughts and behaviors as well as symptoms associated with suicide. These scales are reliable and have adequate concurrent validity, and they may have application as research tools. However, their usefulness and generalizability in clinical practice are questionable. Most of the scales have been tested in nonrepresentative samples composed of college students or psychiatric patients and have not been adequately tested in important subpopulations of patients, such as elderly patients, minority group patients, and patients in common clinical settings, including emergency departments or primary care practices. Few of these scales have been tested in prospective studies, and those that have been tested have shown very low positive predictive validity and high rates of false positive findings. As a result, for the practicing clinician, these rating scales are primarily of value in learning to develop a thorough line of questioning about suicide (see Section II.C.4, "Understand the Relevance and Limitations of Suicide Assessment Scales"). It is for this reason that the specific rating scales will be reviewed briefly here. In addition, information about the scales may be helpful in interpreting the findings of other studies discussed in this guideline.

The Scale for Suicide Ideation (8) is a 19-item, clinician-administered scale that takes approximately 10 minutes to administer and was designed to quantify the intensity of current and conscious suicidal intent by assessing the extent and characteristics of suicidal thoughts; the patient's attitude toward suicidal thoughts; the wish to die; motivations, deterrents, and plans for a suicide attempt; and feelings of control and courage about a suicide attempt. Although standardized for use with adult psychiatric patients, the Scale for Suicide Ideation has been used in a variety of settings and has high levels of internal consistency and interrater reliability. Scores on the Scale for Suicide Ideation have been correlated with the self-harm item of the Beck Depression Inventory and have been shown to discriminate between depressed outpatients and patients hospitalized for suicidal ideation, despite similar levels of depression in the two groups (8), suggesting that the scale measures something above and beyond depression alone. Although the Scale for Suicide Ideation is one of the few instruments with a demonstrated positive predictive validity for suicide, its positive predictive value is only 3%, and it has a high rate of false positive findings (78). A number of modified versions of the Scale for Suicide Ideation exist, including a 21-item self-report version (741) and a measure of suicidal ideation at its worst, the SSI–W, which is also a 19-item, clinician-administered instrument (428).

The Suicide Behavior Questionnaire (SBQ) is a self-report measure of suicidal thoughts and behaviors that is significantly correlated with the Scale for Suicide Ideation (10). The original four-item version has adequate internal consistency, high test-retest reliability, and takes less than 5 minutes to complete. A 14-item revised version (SBQ-14) is a more comprehensive measure of suicidal attempts, ideation, and acts and includes items on suicidal ideation, future suicidal ideation, past suicide threats, future suicide attempts, and the likelihood of dying by suicide in the future. Although the SBQ has high internal reliability and an ability to differentiate between clinical and nonclinical samples (10), the positive predictive validity of the SBQ is not known.

The Suicide Intent Scale (9) is a 20-item clinician-administered scale that has high internal and interrater reliabilities and that quantifies a patient's perceptions and verbal and nonverbal behaviors before and during a recent suicide attempt. It includes questions about circumstances surrounding an attempt, the method and setting of the attempt, the patient's perception of the lethality of the method, expectations about the probability of rescue, premeditation of the attempt, and the purpose of the attempt. Although scores on the Suicide Intent Scale are associated with the lethality of the method, the scale is unable to distinguish between those who attempted suicide and those who aborted their suicide attempts, and it does not predict death by suicide (10).

The Reasons for Living Inventory (407) is a self-report instrument that takes approximately 10 minutes to administer and uses 48 Likert-type scale items to assess beliefs and expectations that would keep one from acting on suicidal ideas. This scale has high internal validity and reliability and moderately high test-retest reliability. It is moderately correlated with the Scale for Suicide Ideation and the Beck Hopelessness Scale and is able to differentiate between inpatients and control subjects as well as between suicide attempters and those with suicidal ideation alone (10).

A number of other scales have been devised to assess suicidality. Among them are the Risk-Rescue Rating, which assesses lethality of a suicide attempt and the level of suicidal intent (433), and the Suicide Assessment Scale, which assesses suicidality over time in the five areas of affect, bodily state, control and coping, emotional reactivity, and suicidal thoughts and behaviors (742). Other more general rating scales include items that have also been used in assessing suicide risk. For example, the Thematic Apperception Test has been used to indicate dichotomous thinking as a risk factor for suicide (743), and the General Health Questionnaire includes a subset of four items that can be used to assess suicidal ideation (744). Based on the theory that psychological pain (or psychache) may be related to suicide, Shneidman (745) developed a psychological pain assessment scale that uses pictures to assess the patient's unmet psychological needs, providing a measure of the introspective experience of negative emotions that may relate to suicidality. By using the scale to explore a patient's perception of psychological pain, clinicians may be able to identify the patient's coping mechanisms and ego strengths. Use of this scale may also help the clinician assess the patient's mental anguish and address the psychological needs that the patient views as important and unmet.

In addition, because depression and hopelessness are risk factors for suicide, corresponding rating scales are often used as indicators of suicide risk. The Beck Hopelessness Scale is a self-report measure consisting of 20 true-false statements that assess positive and negative beliefs about the future that are present during the week before administration (712). The Beck Hopelessness Scale demonstrates high internal validity, adequate test-retest reliability, and moderate to high correlations with clinicians' rating of hopelessness (10). In addition, it is one of the only scales that has demonstrated positive predictive validity (10). In a 10-year prospective study of hospitalized patients with suicidal ideation, the Beck Hopelessness Scale was able to distinguish those who died by suicide and those who did not (222). Nonetheless, its positive predictive value is only 1% (78, 713), and its rate of false positive findings is high (221).

The most frequently used depression scales for suicide assessment are the Hamilton Depression Rating Scale and the Beck Depression Inventory. As measured by these scales, higher levels of depression have been associated with suicide in long-term studies of psychiatric outpatients (78, 221). In addition to being associated with the overall Beck Depression Inventory score, suicide has also been associated with specific inventory items. For example, the Beck Depression Inventory item that measures pessimism has been shown to differentiate between patients who die by suicide and those who do not (222), and the suicide item, which has possible responses on a 4-point scale ranging from "no thoughts of killing myself" to "would kill myself if I had the chance," is also associated with increased suicide risk (10). The corresponding suicide item in the Hamilton Depression Rating Scale measures suicidal behavior on a scale of 0 (absent) to 4 (attempts suicide), has high interrater reliability, and is similarly associated with increased suicide risk (10).

Thus, there are a variety of rating scales that are useful for research purposes and that may be helpful to clinicians in tracking clinical symptoms over time and in developing a thorough line of questioning about suicide and suicidal behaviors. At the same time, because of their high rates of false positive and false negative findings and their low positive predictive values, these rating scales cannot be recommended for use in clinical practice in estimating suicide risk.

2. Biological markers

Multiple studies, reviewed elsewhere (366, 746, 747), have suggested that suicidal behaviors may be associated with alterations in serotonergic function. As a result, a number of biological markers of serotonergic function, including cerebrospinal fluid (CSF) levels of monoamine metabolites such as 5-hydroxyindoleacetic acid (5-HIAA), have been suggested for use in assessing suicide risk. Traskman et al. (748) compared suicide attempters (N=30) to normal control subjects (N=45) and found that the attempters, particularly those who had made more violent suicide attempts, had significantly lower CSF 5-HIAA levels that were independent of psychiatric diagnosis. Subsequent longitudinal follow-up of 129 individuals after a suicide attempt showed that 20% of those with CSF 5-HIAA levels below the median had died by suicide within 1 year (748). Serotonergic function, as measured by the response of prolactin to the specific serotonin releaser and uptake inhibitor *d*-fenfluramine, was also found to be blunted in medication-free patients with DSM-IV schizophrenia who had attempted suicide, compared with nonattempters and healthy control subjects (749).

Hyperactivity of the hypothalamic-pituitary-adrenal (HPA) axis has been associated with suicide since 1965, when Bunney and Fawcett (750) reported three suicides occurring in patients with very high levels of urine 17-hydroxycorticosteroids. Subsequent literature has shown evidence of hypertrophic adrenal glands (751–753) and elevated levels of brain corticotropin-releasing hormone (754, 755) in individuals who died by suicide. The dexamethasone test (DST) has also been used to study whether HPA dysfunction is associated with a type of depressive illness that is likely to end in suicide. In 234 inpatients with unipolar depression, 96 had abnormal DST results, and of these, four died by suicide, in contrast to one suicide death in the group with normal DST results (756). In a subsequent longitudinal study of hospitalized patients with either major depressive disorder or the depressed type of schizoaffective disorder, survival analyses in the 32 patients with abnormal DST results showed an estimated risk for eventual suicide of 26.8%, in contrast to an estimated risk of 2.9% in the 46 patients with normal DST results (757).

On the basis of a series of population studies (758) and a study by Ellison and Morrison (759) showing associations between low cholesterol levels and increased rates of suicide and violent death, cholesterol levels have also been suggested as a putative biological marker for suicidal behaviors. Fawcett et al. (760) reported decreased mean levels of cholesterol in a sample of 47 inpatients who died by suicide. However, Tsai et al. (82) did not find decreased cholesterol levels in a chart-review study of 43 bipolar disorder patients who died by suicide. A case-control study found significantly lower mean cholesterol levels in a group of 100 psychiatric inpatients who had attempted suicide, compared with a matched group of patients hospitalized for physical illness (761). No correlation existed between cholesterol levels and ratings of depression or suicidal intent, and a significant negative correlation between cholesterol levels and self-reported levels of impulsivity was seen across the groups. In a group of 783 outpatients consecutively admitted to a lithium clinic, Bocchetta et al. (762) found a significantly higher likelihood of a history of violent suicide attempts and of suicide in first-degree relatives among men in the lowest quartile of cholesterol levels, compared with men with higher cholesterol levels. Alvarez (763) also reported an association of violent, but not nonviolent, suicide attempts with low cholesterol levels. However, the clinical importance of these findings is unclear, since the use of statin drugs to reduce cholesterol does not appear to be associated with any increase in violence, aggressiveness, unhappiness, accidents, or suicide (764).

Overall, a great deal of evidence suggests that specific biological markers may relate to suicidal behaviors, perhaps through links to impulsivity or aggression. Nevertheless, while intriguing and potentially useful in further understanding the biological underpinnings of suicidal behaviors, none of these putative biological markers are sensitive or specific enough to recommend their use in routine screening or in clinical practice.

C. SPECIAL ISSUES

1. Homicide-suicide

Homicide-suicide, which has often been referred to in the literature as murder-suicide, is relatively uncommon yet essential to keep in mind when assessing individuals at risk for suicidal ideation or behaviors. Suicide is an act of violence toward one's self that may also be an expression of anger or other-directed violence toward another person. After reviewing the literature on risk factors for suicide and for violence, Plutchik (765) proposed a theoretical model that numerically weights a series of variables in order to systematically relate suicide risk to the risk of violence. Of 37 variables noted to be risk factors for violence, 23 were also risk factors for suicide. Another 17 variables were identified as protective factors that decreased the risks of both suicide and violence. Thus, some correlates of suicidal behavior are also associated with violence, an overlap that may contribute to homicide-suicides.

Epidemiologically, homicide-suicide occupies a distinct but overlapping domain with suicide, domestic homicide, and mass murder (20). Although definitions of homicide-suicide vary (20, 766, 767), in general, the two acts occur in close temporal proximity, often with the suicide occurring within seconds or minutes of the homicide. The annual incidence in the United States is difficult to determine but has been estimated to be 0.2–0.9 per 100,000 persons, without significant changes over the past several decades (19, 20). It is likely that about 1.5% of all suicides and 5% of all homicides in the United States occur in the context of homicide-suicide. Homicide-suicide between spouses or lovers represents the majority of homicide-suicides in the United States (19, 766–768), and shooting is the method used in almost all cases (768).

The principal perpetrators of homicide-suicide are young men with intense sexual jealousy or despairing elderly men with ailing spouses (19, 767, 768). In the latter group, associated symptoms of depression are often compounded by financial stressors, resulting in despair (768). Histories of violence and domestic abuse are common (19, 768), as is substance use (19, 768, 769), although perpetrators tend to be less deviant and have less previous criminal involvement than the typical homicide perpetrator (768). Ninety percent of all homicide-suicide incidents involve only one victim, and the principal victims are female sexual partners or consanguineous relatives, usually children (20, 768). Although infanticide is an extremely rare phenomenon (766), mothers who develop postpartum psychosis need to be assessed for suicidal and homicidal impulses directed toward their newborn or other children (27). The risk is especially high in the first postnatal year, when the suicide risk is increased 70-fold (27). Under all of these circumstances, the common theme is the perpetrator's overvalued attachment to a relationship, which leads him or her to destroy the relationship if it is threatened by real or imagined dissolution.

The management of patients assessed to have both suicidal and homicidal impulses should parallel that for either type of risk alone. In particular, in addition to identifying risk factors and protective factors, careful attention should be given to previous hospitalizations, psychosocial stressors, past and current interpersonal relationships, and comorbid factors such as the use of alcohol or other substances. It is also crucial to inquire about firearms and to address the issue with the patient and others if firearms are accessible (see Sections II.E.8.b, "Presence of a Suicide Plan and Availability of a Method," and V.C, "Communication With Significant Others"). Although the legal duty for psychiatrists to warn and protect endangered third parties varies in each state, clinical interventions should endeavor to protect endangered third parties whenever possible.

As for psychopharmacologic management, questions have been raised about the effects of fluoxetine and other serotonin reuptake inhibitor (SRI) antidepressants on violence and suicide. Tardiff et al. (770) analyzed data from the New York City medical examiner's office on all 127 homicide-suicides that took place in that city from 1990 to 1998. Only three of the perpetrators (2.4%) were taking antidepressants. Given the fact that SRIs were widely prescribed in the 1990s, this finding provides no support for the view that SRI treatment is associated with violence or suicide.

In summary, data on homicide-suicide are limited but suggest that patients who present with a recent suicide attempt, have a suicide plan, or voice suicidal ideation should be evaluated for their risk of violent or homicidal behavior. Similarly, patients who present with recent violent behavior or homicidal ideation should be evaluated for suicidal behavior. Clinicians should also assess whether obsessive or delusional jealousy or paranoia is present, especially if such symptoms are comorbid with depression in a patient with a history of domestic abuse. In addition, in older individuals, clinicians should assess for signs of depression or dependency in a spouse whose partner's medical condition is deteriorating. Although less common among homicide-suicide perpetrators, mothers with postpartum psychosis or depression also require careful assessment. Key interventions include treating the mental illness, removing firearms and other lethal methods, and providing assistance with psychosocial supports and social services.

2. Suicide pacts

Suicide pacts, defined as a mutual arrangement between two people to kill themselves at the same time, account for a very small percentage of suicides (0.3%–2.4%, depending on the study) (771–773). As with homicide-suicides, the majority of suicide pact deaths occur in married couples. Social isolation is common, and rates of psychiatric illness, particularly depression, are high in one or both decedents (771–773). Other risk factors also parallel risks for suicide, in general, suggesting that the best approach to detection of suicide pacts is a thorough suicide assessment with attention to psychiatric and psychosocial factors.

3. Deliberate self-harm

Deliberate self-harm is a phenomenon related to but distinct from attempted suicide. Although deliberate self-harm behavior can encompass suicide attempts, it also includes self-mutilation, such as burning, cutting, and hair pulling, that is not associated with fatal intentions (520). Three categories of self-mutilation have been described. Major self-mutilation is infrequent and is usually associated with psychosis or intoxication. Stereotypic self-mutilation is repetitive and driven by a biologic imperative to harm the self. Superficial to moderate self-mutilators use self-harming behaviors as a way to relieve tension, release anger, regain self-control, escape from misery, or terminate a state of depersonalization (520). Extreme forms of self-harm are very rare and often accompany religious or sexual delusions in patients with prominent psychosis or depression (520). Individuals with a history of deliberate and particularly repetitive self-harm also show significantly greater degrees of impulsiveness (774) and are likely to have a diagnosis of borderline personality disorder (521). In addition, repetitive self-mutilators who become depressed and demoralized over their inability to stop the behavior may be at increased risk for suicide attempts (520).

From a clinical standpoint, it is essential to recognize that a past or current history of nonlethal self-harming behaviors does not preclude development of suicidal ideation or plans or preclude suicide attempts with serious intent and lethality. For example, Soloff et al. (521) examined aspects of self-mutilation and suicidal behavior in 108 patients with borderline personality disorder and found evidence of self-mutilation in 63% and suicide attempts in 75.7% of the patients. Compared to patients without self-mutilation, those with self-mutilation were significantly younger and had more serious suicidal ideation, more recent suicide attempts, and more symptoms, including psychosis and depersonalization.

Stanley et al. (251) compared 30 suicide attempters with cluster B personality disorders and a history of self-mutilation to 23 matched suicide attempters with cluster B personality disorders but no prior self-mutilation. While the two groups did not differ in the objective lethality of their suicide attempts, those with a history of self-mutilation perceived their suicide attempts as less lethal, with a greater likelihood of rescue and with less certainty of death. Suicide attempters with a history of self-mutilation had significantly higher levels of other symptoms, such as depression, hopelessness, aggression, anxiety, and impulsivity, that are associated with an increased risk of suicide. Furthermore, self-mutilators had higher and more persistent levels of suicidal ideation than those without a history of self-mutilation. These findings highlight the importance of distinguishing self-mutilatory behaviors from other, more lethal forms of deliberate self-harm. In addition, they underscore the need for a thorough suicide assessment and an appreciation of the multiple determinants of suicide risk in individuals with histories of repetitive deliberate self-harm.

D. SOMATIC THERAPIES

Evidence for reduction of suicidal risk with specific forms of psychiatric treatment is very limited. The most secure research support pertains to psychopharmacological treatments for major affective and psychotic disorders, but even this evidence should be considered preliminary. Moreover, support for reduced suicide risk with psychopharmacological treatment is limited to lithium in various forms of recurrent major affective disorders and clozapine in chronic psychotic illnesses. Support for reduction of suicide risk with antidepressants and mood-stabilizing anticonvulsants is very limited and is at best only suggestive and inconclusive.

1. Pharmacotherapy

a) Antidepressants

A growing number of antidepressant drugs have been shown to be clinically effective in the treatment of acute, recurrent, and chronic depressive illness and a number of anxiety disorders (526). Moreover, nontricyclic, non-SRI antidepressants are relatively safe and present virtually negligible risks of lethality on overdose (526). Since suicidal behavior is strongly associated with depressive illnesses and some forms of anxiety, treatment with antidepressants should plausibly be associated with reduced suicide rates. However, the available evidence remains surprisingly inconclusive that any type of antidepressant or antianxiety treatment is associated with lowering of risk for suicidal behavior (69, 526, 528–532, 563).

Specific types of antidepressants vary greatly in their potential lethality on overdose and relative safety for use by potentially suicidal patients. All tricyclic antidepressants and monoamine oxidase inhibitors (MAOIs) are potentially lethal on acute overdose (526, 556, 557), contributing to their currently limited clinical use, particularly for potentially suicidal patients. Most newer antidepressants, including bupropion, mirtazapine, and nefazodone, and the SRIs have very low lethality in acute overdose (526). The finding of Kapur et al. (557) that tricyclic antidepressants were associated with greater rates of suicide than the nontricyclic antidepressants fluoxetine and trazodone was likely due to the differential toxicity of these agents in overdose, since rates of suicide attempts among patients taking either of the two types of medication were comparable. With the preferential use of nontricyclic, non-MAOI antidepressants by primary care physicians as well as psychiatrists (526), antidepressant overdoses are less often associated with suicide than they were formerly (775, 776), although methods of suicide also may be shifting from overdoses to more lethal alternatives (735, 777).

Coincident with wide clinical acceptance of the safer, nontricyclic, non-MAOI antidepressants since the late 1980s, suicide rates in several countries, regions, or subpopulations have fallen appreciably (69, 531, 532, 549, 550), although international average suicide rates have remained relatively flat for many years, and rates have risen in some subgroups (69, 529, 775, 778, 779). Even stable suicide rates, however, may suggest some improvement in suicide prevention in view of the epidemiological evidence of rising incidence (or greater recognition and diagnosis) of major affective illnesses over the past several decades (694, 780, 781). Since multiple studies have suggested that many depressed individuals do not receive psychiatric intervention or effective antidepressant treatment prior to suicide (206, 267, 578, 782–784), further decreases in suicide rates might occur as a result of improved recognition and treatment of depression.

Longitudinal follow-up data also suggest that long-term antidepressant treatment is associated with a decreased risk of suicide. Angst et al. (74) followed 406 patients with affective disorders for 34 to 38 years after an index psychiatric hospitalization and found that standardized mortality rates for suicide were significantly lower in patients with unipolar depressive disorder as well as in patients with bipolar disorder during long-term treatment with antidepressants alone, with a neuroleptic, or with lithium in combination with antidepressants and/or neuroleptics. This lowering of suicide mortality was particularly striking in light of the fact that the treated patients were more severely ill than the patients who did not receive long-term medication therapy.

Data from one double-blind placebo-controlled study (785) suggested that suicide attempts may also be reduced by long-term antidepressant treatment. In a 1-year trial in nondepressed individuals with repeated suicide attempts, paroxetine treatment was associated with a decreased likelihood of an additional suicide attempt. Although many of the patients in the study met the criteria for a cluster B personality disorder, paroxetine was significantly more effective in those who met fewer of those criteria.

More specific information is available from therapeutic trials of antidepressants in depressed subjects, including data on suicides and serious suicide attempts. These findings were recently evaluated in a meta-analysis (533, 562) based on 13 pertinent reports that appeared between 1974 and 2000 and had data suitable for analysis (534–546). A majority of the studies (eight of 13) involved double-blind designs and random assignment to treatment with a then-experimental or standard antidepressant, to placebo treatment, or to an untreated comparison condition in a total of 37 separate treatment arms; several of the studies included pooled data from multiple trials. A total of 258,547 patient-subjects were included, with a total of 189,817 person-years of risk exposure encompassing short-term efficacy trials as well as reasonably long-term treatment trials. Based on these reports, pooled rates of suicide or suicide attempts by type of treatment suggested that antidepressant treatment is associated with a substantial, approximately fourfold lowering of risk for suicidal behaviors (533). However, owing mainly to the large variance in outcomes between studies, none of the effects of antidepressants in reducing rates of suicidal behaviors reached statistical significance. When comparisons were made among specific types of antidepressants, there was a substantial difference between tricyclic and SRI antidepressants, suggesting the possible superiority of tricyclics, but this effect also failed to reach statistical significance.

Using data from studies in the FDA database of controlled clinical trials for antidepressant treatment of depressed patients, Khan et al. (548) used meta-analysis to compare rates of suicide in patients treated with SRI antidepressants, non-SRI antidepressants, or placebo and found no significant differences across treatment groups. This result is consistent with the finding from many comparisons and meta-analyses that SRIs and other newer antidepressants have usually proved to be effective in placebo-controlled trials and seemed indistinguishable from tricyclic antidepressants in efficacy based on measures other than suicidal behaviors (526, 786).

After publication of several case reports suggesting that SRI antidepressants might be associated with increased risks of aggressive or impulsive acts, including suicide (551–553, 787), a number of investigators retrospectively analyzed clinical trial data to determine whether rates of suicide and suicidal behaviors are increased with SRI treatment (533, 537, 548, 554, 555, 788). These studies did not show evidence that suicide or suicidal behaviors are increased by treatment with specific types of antidepressants. Nonetheless, the safe and effective use of antidepressant treatment for an increasingly wide range of psychiatric disorders should include due regard to early adverse reactions to any antidepressant. These reactions may include increased anxiety, restless agitation, disturbed sleep, and mixed or psychotic bipolar episodes—all of which represent heightened subjective distress in already disturbed patients that might increase the risk of impulsive or aggressive behaviors in some vulnerable individuals. At the same time, these medications are prescribed in order to treat disorders that may have anxiety, agitation, and suicidality as part of the illness course, making it difficult to distinguish the etiology of symptoms that emerge in the course of treatment.

The evidence supporting an expected lowering of the risk for suicidal behavior during antidepressant treatment is limited to findings for patients with a diagnosis of major depression and is, at best, only suggestive. At the same time, existing studies in the literature are limited by the short-term nature of many trials, the widely varying rates of suicide and suicidal acts across trials, inclusion of some patients with probably unrepresentatively high pretreatment suicide risk, and, in other studies, efforts to screen out patients deemed to be at increased suicide risk. Nonetheless, from a clinical perspective, the strong association between clinical depression and suicide and the availability of reasonably effective and very safe antidepressants support the use of an antidepressant in an adequate dose and for an adequate duration as part of a comprehensive program of care for potentially suicidal patients, including long-term use in patients with recurrent forms of depressive or severe anxiety disorders.

b) Lithium

On the basis of present knowledge about pharmacological interventions and risk of suicidal behaviors, prophylactic treatment with lithium salts of patients with recurrent major affective disorders is supported by the strongest available evidence of major reductions in suicide risk of any currently employed psychiatric treatment (528, 559–563, 565, 789). In contrast to antidepressants, and similar to clozapine for schizophrenia, lithium typically is used in relatively structured settings, including specialized programs for affective disorders, lithium clinics, and prolonged maintenance therapy. This practice pattern may itself contribute to the reduction of suicide risk as a result of close, medically supervised monitoring of long-term treatment. Several decades of clinical and research experience with long-term maintenance treatment in recurrent major affective disorders encouraged the development of controlled and naturalistic studies with large numbers of patients given therapeutic dosages of lithium for several years. Studies reporting on the relationship of lithium treatment and suicide in patients with bipolar disorder and other major affective disorders have consistently found much lower rates of suicide and suicide attempts during lithium maintenance treatment than without it (562, 563, 565, 789).

A recent meta-analysis of studies of suicide rates with and without long-term lithium maintenance treatment (563) updated other reviews of this topic (314, 315, 528, 558, 560, 562, 564, 565, 700, 790, 791) and found 34 reports for the period from 1970 through 2002 by computerized and other literature searching (76, 534, 559, 565–595). These studies included 67 treatment arms or conditions (42 with and 25 without lithium treatment). The total number of patients was 16,221 (corrected for appearance of some subjects in both treatment conditions), and treatment lasted an average of 3.36 years with lithium therapy (N=15,323 subjects, for 51,485 person-years of risk-exposure) and 5.88 years without lithium maintenance treatment

(N=2,168, for 12,748 person-years of exposure), with an overall time at risk (weighted by the number of subjects per study) of 3.76 years.

Meta-analysis yielded an overall estimated rate for all suicidal acts (including suicide attempts) from all identified studies of 3.10% per year without lithium treatment, compared to 0.21% per year with lithium treatment, a 14.8-fold (93.2%) reduction that was highly statistically significant. Moreover, the finding of lower rates of suicide and suicide attempts was consistently seen in all 25 sets of observations except one, an early study with a small sample size and relatively short time of exposure to lithium treatment in which no suicidal acts were observed with or without lithium treatment (566).

For suicides considered separately, pooled rates were 0.942% per year without lithium treatment, compared to 0.174% per year with lithium treatment. The corresponding figures for suicide attempts considered separately were 4.65% per year and 0.312% per year, respectively. Thus, long-term lithium treatment was associated with a 5.43-fold reduction in the risk of suicide and a 14.9-fold reduction in the risk of suicide attempts (563).

The apparent sparing of risk of suicide and suicide attempts was very similar in patients with a diagnosis of bipolar disorder and in those with other recurrent major affective disorders, although patients with unipolar depressive disorder were evaluated separately in only two relatively small studies involving a total of 121 patients that found a reduction in risk of suicidal acts from 1.33% per year to nil (563, 575). In addition, a comparison of subjects with bipolar I disorder (N=263) and those with bipolar II disorder (N=153) found a somewhat greater sparing of suicidal risk in the patients with bipolar II disorder (from 1.70% to 0.305% per year, compared to a reduction from 2.73% to 0.898% per year in bipolar I disorder patients) (563).

Despite these striking reductions in risk, it is also important to note that lithium maintenance treatment does not provide complete protection against suicide. The overall rate of suicide during lithium treatment was 0.174% per year, which was much lower than the untreated risk of 0.942% per year but was still 10.5 times higher than the average international rate of 0.0166% per year in the general population (700, 792). In contrast, the rate of suicide attempts during lithium treatment was very close to the estimated risk for the general population, and the total pooled rate of all suicidal acts with lithium treatment, remarkably, was 33% lower than the estimated general population risk. This striking finding may be plausible in that much of the risk of suicidal behavior in the general population represents untreated affective illness and because suicide attempts are far more common than deaths by suicide. In addition, these observations may suggest a relatively greater effect of lithium treatment on suicide attempts than on suicide, although the variability in relationship to general population risks may also reflect variance in the samples available for the analysis of rates of suicide and suicide attempts.

These studies have several notable limitations, including a potential lack of control over random assignment and retention of subjects in some treatment trials, inclusion of some patients with probably unrepresentatively high pretreatment suicide risk, and the presence in several trials of potential effects of treatment discontinuation (565), which can contribute to an excess of early recurrence of affective illness (315, 791, 793, 794), with sharply increased suicide risk (315, 700). However, there was no evidence that the time at risk influenced the annualized computed rate of suicide or suicide attempts. Finding a reduction of suicide risk during lithium treatment also might involve biased self-selection, since patients who remain in any form of maintenance treatment for many months are more likely to be treatment adherent and conceivably also less likely to become suicidal. However, it is not feasible to evaluate any long-term treatment in nonadherent patients. Moreover, several of the reported studies involved either the same persons observed with and without lithium treatment or random assignment to treatment options, minimizing the effects of self-selection bias. Results of these studies were consistent with the overall findings of marked reductions of risk of suicidal behaviors during lithium treatment (565).

If lithium is indeed effective in preventing suicide in broadly defined recurrent major affective syndromes, as it appears to be, it seems likely that this effect operates through reduction of risk or severity of recurrences in depression or mixed dysphoric-agitated states (69, 315, 700). An additional factor may be reduction of impulsivity or of aggressive and hostile behavior with lithium facilitation of the central serotonergic neurotransmission system (226, 366, 526, 795), although this hypothesis is inconsistent with evidence that the antiserotonergic agent clozapine may reduce suicide risk in schizophrenia (603, 796) and the lack of evidence for a beneficial effect of SRI antidepressants on suicidal behavior (533, 563). An additional nonspecific but potentially important benefit of lithium treatment may arise from the supportive, long-term therapeutic relationships associated with the typically structured and relatively closely medically monitored maintenance treatment of patients with recurrent major mood disorders who are being treated with lithium.

c) "Mood-stabilizing" anticonvulsant agents

Evidence for a protective effect against suicide of putative "mood-stabilizing" agents other than lithium is extremely limited. Reports from a long-term collaborative German study that involved random assignment of patients with bipolar disorder and schizoaffective disorder to 2 years of treatment with either lithium or carbamazepine found no suicidal acts with lithium but substantial remaining risk with carbamazepine (592, 597). A recent study by Goodwin et al. (598) analyzed computerized records of 20,878 patients with a diagnosis of bipolar disorder (60,518 person-years of follow-up) in two major integrated health plans who were treated with lithium, divalproex, or carbamazepine. Approximately 27% of the person-years of exposure were to lithium alone, 22% were to carbamazepine or divalproex alone, and 47% had no exposure to any of the three medications. After adjustment for potential confounds, including age, gender, health plan, year of diagnosis, physical illness comorbidity, and use of other psychotropic medications, the authors found that the risk of suicide was 2.7 times higher during treatment with divalproex or carbamazepine than during treatment with lithium. For suicide attempts, the risk during divalproex or carbamazepine treatment was 1.9 times higher for attempts resulting in inpatient care and 1.7 times higher for attempts resulting in emergency department care, compared to risk during lithium treatment. Thus, in patients treated for bipolar disorder, risk for suicide attempts and for suicide was significantly lower during lithium treatment than during treatment with carbamazepine or divalproex.

No studies have addressed the risks of suicide attempts or suicide during treatment with other proposed mood-stabilizing agents. Given the widespread and growing use of divalproex, lamotrigine, oxcarbazepine, topiramate, and other anticonvulsants, often instead of lithium, it is extremely important to include measures of mortality risk and suicidal behavior in long-term studies of the effectiveness of these and other potential treatments for bipolar disorder. Such information may eventually allow an approximate ranking of the effectiveness of specific agents against the risk of suicidal behavior.

d) Antipsychotic agents

First-generation antipsychotic agents such as fluphenazine, thiothixene, and haloperidol are highly effective in treating delusions and hallucinations. However, it is not known whether or to what extent they may have beneficial effects in limiting suicide risk in psychotic patients. In the United States, the annual rate of suicide associated with schizophrenia has not fallen appreciably since the introduction of neuroleptics in the late 1950s (599–602), suggesting that first-generation antipsychotics have a limited effect on suicide risk.

Some first-generation antipsychotic agents may also have beneficial actions in major affective disorders. Virtually all antipsychotic agents are highly and rapidly effective in mania, and antipsychotic drugs may also have beneficial effects in some patients with major depression, with or without psychotic features (596). While these benefits may reflect nonspecific improvements in agitation, insomnia, and other distressing symptoms rather than specific antidepressant effects, they may nevertheless reduce suicide risk in highly agitated patients, especially those with psychotic forms of depression and mixed bipolar states. On the other hand, haloperidol and perhaps some other first-generation antipsychotics may worsen depression in patients with chronic psychotic disorders as well as in those with major affective disorders, with or without psychotic features (112, 797). Although not well studied, the potentially distressing adverse effect of akathisia may actually increase risk of suicidal and other impulsive or violent acts (604, 605). Thus, because of the other advantages of second-generation antipsychotic agents in treating psychotic disorders (513) and perhaps manic, mixed, and depressive phases of bipolar disorder (512), use of first-generation antipsychotics in individuals with suicidal behaviors should generally be reserved for those needing the enhanced treatment adherence afforded by depot forms of medication.

Of all antipsychotics, clozapine is, by far, the best studied for specific beneficial effects on suicidal behaviors. As the prototype second-generation antipsychotic agent, clozapine differs from first-generation antipsychotics in several respects, including a markedly lesser propensity to induce adverse extrapyramidal neurological effects (596). Clozapine has particular utility in the substantial subgroup of patients with schizophrenia who poorly tolerate (798) or do not respond adequately to first-generation agents (799) and perhaps to other antipsychotics (596). In addition, clozapine may have beneficial effects on cognition in psychotic patients (800, 801), can improve social and occupational functioning (513), may limit the risk of abusing alcohol and other substances (802, 803), and may also decrease impulsive and aggressive behaviors (804–806).

Evidence for the effect of clozapine on the risk of suicidal behaviors comes from clinical trials involving patients with schizophrenia and schizoaffective disorder as well as from registry studies, which include all patients treated with clozapine regardless of diagnosis. Data from the clozapine national registry, for example, indicated a 75%–82% reduction in mortality, which is primarily attributable to a decrease in suicide risk (608, 609). An additional analysis of these registry data found a 67% reduction in risk for suicide attempts (607). Reduced annual risk of suicide was also found in clozapine-treated patients, compared to those given other antipsychotic agents, in the Texas State Mental Health System (609) as well as in the United Kingdom (610).

Sernyak et al. (611) used data on patients treated within the VA system and compared all patients over a 4-year period who initiated treatment with clozapine while hospitalized (N=1,415) to a control group of patients with schizophrenia who were matched to the clozapine-treated patients by using propensity scoring (N=2,830). Over the follow-up period, the patients who had been treated with clozapine at the index hospitalization experienced a lower rate of mortality, due to lower rates of respiratory disorders. However, the rate of suicide did not differ between the groups, although there was a nonsignificant trend for fewer suicides among those treated with clozapine. In addition, since patients were not treated with clozapine throughout the follow-up period, potential effects of clozapine on suicidality may have been less pronounced (612, 613).

The effects of clozapine on suicidal ideation and suicide attempts relative to patients' own baseline levels of suicidality were first examined in a retrospective study of 88 patients with chronic, neuroleptic-resistant DSM-III-R schizophrenia (N=55) or schizoaffective disorder (N=33) and a mean duration of illness of 14 years (607). Clozapine monotherapy with a mean daily dose of 500 mg was initiated in the hospital, and suicidality was assessed over a mean follow-up period of 3.5 years. At follow-up, improvements in symptoms of depression and hopelessness were noted, and the percentage of patients with no suicidal thoughts, plans, or attempts had increased from 53% at baseline to 88% with clozapine treatment. Compared to the 2-year period before initiation of clozapine, there was also a decrease in the relative lethality of suicide attempts and a 12.8-fold decrease in the annualized number of suicide attempts.

Other studies have compared clozapine-treated patients to patients treated with first-generation antipsychotics. Glazer and Dickson (807), for example, found a 57% lower risk of suicide attempts among schizophrenia patients treated with clozapine, compared with those treated with haloperidol (606). In another study, Spivak et al. (808) compared 30 patients with chronic, treatment-resistant schizophrenia who had been maintained on clozapine for at least 1 year with an equal number of patients who had been treated with first-generation antipsychotics for similar lengths of time (808). They found that clozapine treatment was associated with significant reductions in ratings of impulsiveness and aggressiveness, along with fewer suicide attempts.

In the International Suicide Prevention Trial (InterSePT), a 2-year, multicenter randomized, controlled study with an open-label design with masked ratings, the effects of clozapine (N=479) were compared to those of olanzapine (N=477) in patients with DSM-IV schizophrenia (N=609) or schizoaffective disorder (N=371). Only 27% of the patients had an illness that was refractory to prior treatment, but all were deemed to be at unusually high risk for suicide, on the basis of having current suicidal ideation or having made a suicide attempt during the previous 3 years. The prestudy rate of suicide attempts in this group was 21% per year, or about four times that of broader samples of patients with schizophrenia (603, 606, 607). Although only patients receiving clozapine had blood drawn to monitor white blood cell counts, all patients were seen weekly for 6 months, then biweekly for an additional 18 months to minimize bias from the clozapine-treated patients' more frequent contact with health care staff. Primary endpoints, determined by blinded raters and certified by a three-member independent, blinded, expert Suicide Monitoring Board, included suicide attempts (including those that led to death), hospitalizations to prevent suicide, and a rating of "much worse suicidality" compared to baseline. Patients randomly assigned to receive clozapine showed a significantly longer time to a suicide event as defined previously, with a significant reduction in the rate of all suicidal events. In addition, fewer clozapine-treated patients required hospitalization or other clinical interventions intended to minimize suicidal behavior or were given an antidepressant or a sedative. The significant advantage of clozapine was evident in patients with schizoaffective disorder as well as those with schizophrenia. In addition, patients with more prestudy risk factors showed a relatively greater reduction in the rate of suicidal behavior. Furthermore, the greater effectiveness of clozapine was not due to superiority in treating positive or negative symptoms as rated at endpoint. Very few of these high-risk subjects died of suicide during the study (eight of 956 [0.837%] within 2 years), and the risk of suicide was nonsignificantly greater with clozapine than olanzapine (1.044% and 0.629%, respectively). The rate of suicide attempts was significantly less during clozapine treatment than during olanzapine treatment (7.7% and 13.8%, respectively, without correction for exposure times). However, the rate of suicide attempts during treatment with olanzapine was approximately half that found among these high-risk patients before the trial, suggesting that olanzapine treatment was associated with some beneficial effects on the risk of suicidal behaviors.

Overall, studies of the risk of suicidal behaviors during treatment with clozapine or other antipsychotic agents in chronically psychotic patients have involved nearly 134,000 subjects treated with clozapine and 123,000 given other antipsychotic agents (809). Although the selection of high-risk subjects in the InterSePT study (603) resulted in a great degree of heterogeneity in the frequencies of suicidal acts across studies, together these results indicate substantial superiority of clozapine over other antipsychotic agents in preventing suicidal acts in patients with schizophrenia and schizoaffective disorders. For other disorders, such as otherwise treatment-resistant bipolar disorder, no information is available about the effects of clozapine on risk of suicidal behaviors.

In clinical practice, the evident advantage of clozapine in reducing the rate of suicide attempts and perhaps the rate of suicide must be weighed against the risks of death from agranulocytosis, cardiomyopathy, myocarditis, and rare atypical forms of a syndrome similar to neuroleptic malignant syndrome (596). Other potential side effects of clozapine, including seizures, weight gain, hyperlipidemia, and type II diabetes, may also adversely affect longevity. Thus, in deciding whether to institute or continue clozapine treatment in patients with psychosis who are at risk for suicidal behaviors, the clinician will need to weigh the advantages and disadvantages of clozapine therapy for the individual patient.

For other second-generation antipsychotic agents, with the exception of perhaps olanzapine as discussed earlier, there is little direct evidence of an effect on suicidal behaviors. For the InterSePT study, olanzapine was chosen as the comparator because of its use in treating schizophrenia as well as limited evidence that it might have a superior effect in reducing suicidal behaviors, compared with haloperidol (810). There is also some evidence that the second-generation antipsychotic agents, including olanzapine and risperidone, may have mood-elevating or mood-stabilizing actions in addition to the ubiquitous antimanic effects of virtually all antipsychotics (112). These observations have led to the inference that second-generation antipsychotics also may have greater utility than first-generation agents in minimizing suicidal behaviors (811).

Compared to first-generation antipsychotics, the second-generation agents are less likely to be associated with nonadherence that results from extrapyramidal side effects and more likely to be associated with stable or improved cognition and higher levels of social and occupational functioning (801). Thus, there are general reasons for preferring to use second-generation antipsychotic drugs rather than first-generation antipsychotic drugs to reduce the risk for suicide in patients with schizophrenia. At the same time, it remains to be shown whether specific second-generation antipsychotic agents differ from each other or from first-generation antipsychotics in relative protective effects against suicidal behavior.

e) Antianxiety agents

Some patients who die by suicide have symptoms of severe psychic anxiety, panic, agitation, or severe insomnia close to the time of the suicidal act (79, 217, 218). Such persons may also abuse alcohol or other substances, perhaps in an attempt at "self-medication" for otherwise intolerably distressing symptoms. Since antianxiety agents can limit such symptoms, they also hold the possibility of reducing short-term suicide risk. Several agents, including benzodiazepines, buspirone, older sedatives, many antidepresssants, low doses of some second-generation antipsychotics, and some mood-altering anticonvulsants, may have calming effects in highly anxious and agitated patients and so might be expected to limit suicide risk. However, research addressing this plausible expectation is limited and inconclusive. No clinical trial has demonstrated short- or long-term effects on suicidal behavior of any type of antianxiety treatment. However, a recent analysis of data obtained in controlled trials of treatments for anxiety disorders found no significant differences in rates of suicidal behavior between those treated with active agents and those treated with placebo (118).

In treating potentially suicidal patients, benzodiazepines are often avoided because of concerns about their potential for inducing dependency (812), respiratory depression, or disinhibition, as has been observed in some patients with borderline personality disorder or mental retardation (614, 615, 813–815). Nevertheless, the risk of disinhibition appears small (816). In addition, benzodiazepines can limit psychic distress in depressed patients and improve sleep and may thereby potentiate the clinical benefits of antidepressant therapy (617–619). Whether such benefits are associated with reduced suicide risk remains unproved, however. In contrast, removal of a benzodiazepine during treatment may be associated with increased risk of suicidal behavior (817). Thus, decisions about initiating or continuing benzodiazepines in suicidal patients should consider these risks and benefits as they relate to the individual patient.

In summary, it is clinically appropriate to provide treatments aimed at reducing anxiety, psychic distress, agitation, and insomnia, regardless of the primary diagnosis, as part of a comprehensive effort to limit suicide risk, and antianxiety agents may have a useful empirical role in such situations, when employed with due regard to their risk of disinhibiting impulsive or aggressive behavior (219).

2. ECT

Prominent suicidality is widely considered a clinical indication for ECT (511, 512, 623). Much of the rationale for this practice is indirect and based primarily on the established and superior efficacy of ECT in treating severe depression that is often associated with suicidal ideation and behaviors (623). ECT affords a more rapid and robust clinical antidepressant response than psychopharmacological, psychosocial, or other treatments, especially in severe, acute major depression, with or without psychotic features (623).

Only four studies have directly assessed the short-term effects of ECT on "suicidality" defined as apparent suicidal thinking. Rich et al. (620) analyzed depression and suicide ratings in a study designed primarily to measure treatment response with increasing numbers of alternate-day, right unilateral ECT. Suicide ratings, based on one item of the Hamilton Depression Rating Scale, improved maximally within 1 week and improved significantly more rapidly than measures of mood or lack of energy or interests. Similarly rapid and robust declines in suicide ratings were found in a naturalistic study of depressed patients with medication-resistant bipolar disorder who were given ECT with pharmacotherapy (818). Prudic and Sackeim (621) also found rapid and marked short-term reductions of suicidality with ECT in 148 depressed patients, reductions that even exceeded those in other Hamilton Depression Rating Scale items, especially, but not only, among the 49% of individuals considered clinically responsive to ECT. In data from a larger sample of 405 ECT-treated depressed patients recently analyzed by Kellner et al. (622), 58% of the patients were considered suicidal on the basis of suicidal ideation or suicide plans or attempts. The patients were treated with bitemporal ECT, and after a single treatment, suicidality was considered to have resolved in one-third of these suicidal patients, in two-thirds after three treatments, and in 95% by the end of a clinically determined series of ECT treatments (averaging just over seven treatments in the acute course).

These studies were limited by reliance on a single item from one rating scale. In addition, examination of the effects of ECT on suicidality was incidental to the primary aims of the studies, and any changes in suicidality associated with ECT were possibly incidental to the antidepressant effects of ECT. Moreover, no data directly address the effects of ECT on suicidal behavior or suicide fatalities. Nevertheless, and consistent with impressions arising from clinical experience, available studies indicate that acute treatment with ECT is associated with frequent and rapid reductions in apparent suicidality, possibly even before major improvements in other symptoms of depression.

As a means of evaluating possible long-term benefits of ECT on suicidal risk, several studies have examined rates of suicide in different treatment eras, before and after the introduction of ECT (and other treatments), with follow-up periods as long as 10 years. A recent meta-analysis, which calculated suicide rates from published literature for patients with mood disorder who were followed naturalistically for at least 6 months after an index hospitalization, indicated a 41% decrease in suicide rates, from 1.33% to 0.770% per year, between the pre-ECT years and later years when ECT and then antidepressants were in widespread use (819). However, interpretation of this information for possible effects of ECT is obscured by uncertain reliability in identifying persons who died by suicide in different eras and by the effect of multiple therapeutic developments across the decades included in the analysis.

In an earlier study comparing clinically matched samples of depressed patients from a Monroe County, New York, psychiatric case register, Babigian and Guttmacher (820) assessed the effect of ECT on mortality at 5-year follow-up between 1960 and 1975 for 1,587 patients treated with ECT and 1,587 who did not receive ECT. The groups did not differ in risk for suicidal behavior or in overall mortality, but their comparison may be confounded by the selection of patients with severe symptoms for treatment with ECT. Additional studies involving ECT were reviewed by Tanney (821), Prudic and Sackeim (621), and Sharma (822). These studies were primarily nonrandomized, uncontrolled, retrospective clinical observations from relatively small case series. It is not surprising that they also failed to find evidence of enduring effects on suicide rates after short-term ECT.

The available data thus suggest rapid short-term benefits against suicidal thinking but do not provide evidence of a sustained reduction of suicide risk following short-term ECT, despite its superior effectiveness in severe depression (623). Similar to the situation with antidepressant therapy, there is still very little information arising from systematically applied and evaluated long-term treatment with ECT comparable to the data available for maintenance treatment with lithium and clozapine, and it is not reasonable to expect long-term effects on suicide risk from time-limited treatment interventions of any kind. In short, it remains to be tested whether long-term use of maintenance ECT or short-term ECT followed by long-term antidepressant or mood-stabilizing treatment may affect long-term risk of suicidal behavior.

E. PSYCHOTHERAPIES

In addition to pharmacotherapies and ECT, psychotherapies play a central role in the management of suicidal behavior in clinical practice. Although few rigorous studies have directly examined whether these interventions reduce suicide morbidity or mortality per se, clinical consensus suggests that psychosocial interventions and specific psychotherapeutic approaches are beneficial to the suicidal patient. Furthermore, in recent years, studies of psychotherapies have demonstrated their efficacy in treating disorders such as depression and borderline personality disorder that are associated with increased suicide risk (511, 515, 823–830). The apparent superiority of combination treatment with psychotherapy and pharmacotherapy in individuals with depression also suggests a need for further study of such combination treatment in individuals with suicidal behaviors (824, 826–830). Other psychosocial interventions may also be of value in treating suicidal patients, particularly given their utility in minimizing symptoms and risk of relapse in patients with bipolar disorder and patients with schizophrenia (512, 513, 831).

1. Psychodynamic and psychoanalytic psychotherapies

In patients with suicidal behaviors, experience with psychodynamically and psychoanalytically oriented psychotherapies is extensive and lends support to the use of such approaches in clinical practice. Research data on the effects of these therapies in suicidal patients are more limited but supportive. For example, Bateman and Fonagy (624, 625) randomly assigned 44 patients with borderline personality disorder, diagnosed according to standardized criteria, to either a standard psychiatric care group or a partially hospitalized group who received individual and group psychoanalytic psychotherapy for a maximum of 18 months. At the end of the treatment period, as well as at 6-, 12-, and 18-month follow-ups, patients assigned to the psychoanalytically oriented partial hospitalization group had significantly lower numbers of self-mutilatory acts and were more likely to have refrained entirely from self-mutilatory behavior in the preceding 6 months. In the partial hospitalization group, similar highly significant reductions were seen in the number of suicide attempts and in the number of patients who had made a suicide attempt during the follow-up period. During and after the treatment, parallel persistent improvements were seen in other outcome measures, including fewer inpatient days, reductions in depressive symptoms, and improved social and interpersonal functioning in the psychoanalytically treated group. These data demonstrate the efficacy of psychoanalytically oriented partial hospital treatment in patients with borderline personality disorder. Further, they show that such treatment can improve factors such as depression and interpersonal functioning that modify suicide risk and can simultaneously diminish a range of self-harming and suicidal behaviors.

Stevenson and Meares (832) studied a group of 30 poorly functioning outpatients with borderline personality disorder and found that twice-weekly psychodynamic therapy resulted in significant reductions in self-harm behaviors as well as in improved overall outcomes, compared to the year preceding treatment. In addition, the 30 patients treated with twice-weekly psychodynamic therapy also had better outcomes and fewer self-harming behaviors relative to a group of control subjects who received treatment as usual (833). Thus, although limited by small samples and lack of random assignment to the control condition, these studies also suggest a benefit of psychodynamic approaches in reducing self-harming behaviors among individuals with borderline personality disorder.

Clarkin et al. (834) developed a modified form of psychodynamic treatment called Transference Focused Psychotherapy and used this approach to treat 23 female patients with a diagnosis of DSM-IV borderline personality disorder. Twice-weekly treatment with Transference Focused Psychotherapy was associated with significant decreases on measures of suicidality, self-injurious behavior, and medical and psychiatric service utilization, relative to baseline levels. In addition, compared to the year preceding treatment, there was a significant decrease in the number of patients who made suicide attempts and in the medical risk and severity of physical injury associated with self-harming behaviors. Although again limited by a small sample as well as by the lack of a control group, these findings coincide with clinical impressions of benefit to suicidal patients treated with psychoanalytic and psychodynamic approaches.

2. Cognitive behavior therapy

Given the evidence for the effectiveness of cognitive behavior therapy in treating depression and related symptoms such as hopelessness (511, 825, 835–837), it might be expected to also be of benefit in the treatment of suicidal behaviors. Again, however, evidence from randomized trials is extremely limited. In a randomized clinical trial involving 20 patients, Salkovskis et al. (628) examined whether individuals at high risk for repeated suicide attempts were more improved by treatment as usual or by a cognitive behavior intervention that focused on teaching problem-solving techniques. At the end of treatment and at follow-up up to 1 year later, the group randomly assigned to the problem-solving treatment showed significantly more improvement than control subjects on ratings of depression, hopelessness, and suicidal ideation, and over 6 months of follow-up, there was some evidence for a decrease in suicide attempts. Although the sample was small, these findings provide some evidence for the benefit of cognitive behavior interventions in reducing suicidal ideation and behaviors in patients at high risk for repeated suicide attempts.

3. Dialectical behavior therapy

Dialectical behavior therapy, a psychosocial treatment for borderline personality disorder that combines individual psychotherapy with group practice of behavioral skills, has also been studied in a randomized fashion with respect to its effects on self-injurious behaviors. Linehan et al. (522, 838) randomly assigned 39 women who had a history of self-injurious behavior and met the criteria for borderline personality disorder to 1 year of dialectical behavior therapy or treatment as usual. During the year of treatment, as well as during the initial 6 months of follow-up, the patients treated with dialectical behavior therapy had fewer incidents of self-injurious behavior and those that did occur were less medically severe. Functioning, as measured by the Global Assessment Scale, and social adjustment were also better in the group treated with dialectical behavior therapy. After 1 year, the group treated with dialectical behavior therapy continued to require significantly fewer psychiatric hospital days, but the benefits of the intervention in reducing the number and severity of suicide attempts were no longer apparent. In a subsequent study, Linehan et al. (523) compared dialectical behavior therapy to treatment as usual in a group of patients with borderline personality disorder and comorbid substance dependence. Patients treated with dialectical behavior therapy had more days of substance abstinence at follow-up intervals of up to 16 months. In terms of self-harming behaviors, dialectical behavior therapy showed no benefits over treatment as usual, although patients in both groups experienced reductions in self-injury. An additional prospective study (839) evaluated 24 female patients with borderline personality disorder who were treated with dialectical behavior therapy in a 3-month inpatient treatment program and continued in outpatient treatment with dialectical behavior therapy. Compared to ratings at the time of hospital admission, a significant decrease in the frequency of self-injury was noted 1 month after discharge that coincided with improvements in ratings of depression, dissociation, anxiety, and global stress.

Additional evidence for the effects of dialectical behavior therapy in treating women with borderline personality disorder comes from a randomized clinical trial conducted by Verheul et al. (840). In this study, 58 women with borderline personality disorder were assigned to 12 months of treatment with either dialectical behavior therapy or treatment as usual. Particularly in patients with a history of frequent self-mutilation, dialectical behavior therapy was associated with greater reductions in suicidal, self-mutilating, and self-damaging impulsive behaviors, compared to usual treatment.

Taken together, the data from these trials suggest the possible utility of dialectical behavior therapy in treating suicidal and self-injurious behaviors in individuals with borderline personality disorder. However, the sample sizes in these trials were small, and it is not clear whether the patients were representative of those seen in usual clinical practice. Larger samples are also needed to determine whether some patients may be prone to paradoxical increases in self-injurious behavior with dialectical behavior therapy (841). Finally, since no data are available on the utility of dialectical behavior therapy in the treatment of patients with diagnoses other than borderline personality disorder, further study is needed before recommending dialectical behavior therapy for routine use in the treatment of individuals with suicidal behaviors.

4. Other psychosocial interventions

As noted earlier, psychosocial interventions other than psychotherapies have shown clear efficacy in the treatment of a number of psychiatric disorders. To date, however, randomized clinical trials and longitudinal studies of various psychosocial treatments have produced conflicting results in individuals at risk for suicidal behaviors. Most interventions have focused on the treatment of individuals identified at the time of an index suicide attempt. For example, van der Sande et al. (842) compared the clinical efficacy of an intensive psychosocial intervention with treatment as usual in 274 randomly assigned individuals who presented for medical treatment after attempting suicide. At 12-month follow-up, the authors found no difference in the number of repeat suicide attempts in patients receiving treatment as usual, compared to those given intensive psychosocial treatment, which consisted of brief admission to a crisis-intervention unit and problem-solving aftercare. In contrast, in a randomized trial that compared brief psychological treatment to treatment as usual in 119 individuals seen in an emergency department for self-poisoning, Guthrie et al. (843) found significant decreases in suicidal ideation and in additional self-harm. Also, in a study of 120 suicide attempters, Welu (844) found a statistically significant reduction in suicide attempts in those who were randomly assigned to a 4-month follow-up outreach program, compared with those randomly assigned to receive treatment as usual.

The three studies just described (842–844) were included in an extensive review and meta-analysis of randomized clinical trials of psychosocial interventions for the treatment of patients with deliberate self-harm by Hawton et al. (627, 633). The interventions considered in the meta-analysis were diverse and included problem-solving therapy, dialectical behavior therapy, home-based family therapy, provision of an emergency card to quickly gain access to care, and intensive intervention plus outreach. While promising results were noted for problem-solving therapy and provision of an emergency card, as well as for dialectical behavior therapy, the sample sizes were too small and the studies too underpowered to detect clinically significant differences in effects on repetition of deliberate self-harm. Thus, a number of psychosocial interventions have been targeted to individuals who have made suicide attempts or engaged in other self-harming behaviors; however, current evidence from randomized clinical trials is too limited to support reliable conclusions about the efficacy of these approaches in individuals with suicidal behaviors.

In addition to specifically targeting suicidal behaviors, psychosocial interventions may indirectly decrease rates of suicide attempts by enhancing the treatment of the patient's underlying diagnosis. Rucci et al. (595) treated 175 patients with bipolar I disorder for a 2-year period using primarily lithium pharmacotherapy and either psychotherapy specific to bipolar disorder, which included help in regularizing daily routines, or nonspecific intensive clinical management involving regular visits with empathic clinicians. Before patients entered the trial, the rate of suicide attempts was 1.05 per 100 person-months. During the acute treatment phase, patients experienced a threefold reduction in the rate of suicide attempts, with a 17.5-fold reduction during maintenance treatment, suggesting that treatment in a maximally supportive environment could significantly reduce suicidal behaviors in high-risk patients with bipolar disorder. During the follow-up period, fewer suicide attempts occurred in patients treated with psychotherapy specific to bipolar disorder; however, because of the low numbers of suicide attempts during treatment, it was not possible to determine whether the two psychosocial interventions were statistically different in their effectiveness. Nonetheless, these findings suggest that combinations of psychosocial interventions and pharmacotherapy offer promise in diminishing risk of suicidal behaviors in at-risk individuals.

PART C: FUTURE RESEARCH NEEDS

In assessing and caring for patients with suicidal ideas and behaviors, multiple questions remain to be answered and would benefit from additional research. These future research directions can be divided into three major categories: delineating the neurobiological underpinnings of suicide and other suicidal behaviors, more precisely defining the factors that affect short-term and longer-term risk for suicide and other suicidal behaviors, and determining the most effective interventions for diminishing such risks.

In terms of the underlying neurobiology of suicide and other suicidal behaviors, a great deal of work has already focused on the role of the serotonergic neurotransmitter system in suicide attempts and in suicide (366). Additional research has suggested an association between suicide and hyperactivity of the HPA axis (757, 845), while still other work has suggested a correlation between suicidal behaviors and serum cholesterol levels (758, 759, 846). In keeping with the remarkable recent advances in molecular genetics, there has also been intense interest in seeking associations between candidate genes (primarily relating to serotonergic function) and suicide risk. Although polygenic inheritance is suspected, a specific genetic model for suicidal behaviors remains elusive (17, 368). Furthermore, while the biological markers described earlier are potentially useful in understanding the biological underpinnings of suicidal behaviors, none are sufficiently sensitive or specific enough to recommend their use in routine screening or in clinical practice. Additional work is clearly needed to identify specific genes, biological markers, or imaging findings that are indicative of a particularly high risk for suicide or suicidal behaviors. Availability of such markers would allow at-risk individuals to be identified and treated more readily, presumably decreasing their risk for suicide. In addition, identification of more homogenous groups of at-risk individuals might permit more precise targeting of treatments to address underlying neurobiological abnormalities.

Many studies have already examined particular risk and protective factors for suicide and suicidal behaviors; however, more information is needed. Specifically, future research should focus on determining factors that are associated with modifying short-term risk (days to weeks), compared with intermediate-term risk (weeks to months) or longer-term or lifetime risks. In addition to strengthening the existing evidence base on the multiple factors already reviewed, future research should also address the effects of multiple co-occurring risk factors as well as the relative contributions of different factors to the overall risk of suicide or other suicidal behaviors. For example, studies of the relationship between physical illness and suicide are needed to determine the contributions of social and psychological factors to suicide in patients with physical illnesses. Similarly, with increased rates of suicide in specific occupational groups, more research is needed to determine whether suicide risk relates to preexisting factors such as psychiatric illness or to specific occupational stressors and/or characteristics such as access to lethal methods. In addition, data for individuals who die from suicide should be clearly distinguished and analyzed separately from data for individuals exhibiting other suicidal behaviors, since the two groups almost certainly constitute distinct although overlapping populations. Furthermore, given the low population rates of suicide and other suicidal behaviors, all studies of risk factors will need to have adequate statistical power in order to draw meaningful conclusions from their results. The ultimate goals of these avenues of research would include an improved ability to estimate suicidal risk in the clinical context. Such findings may also permit development of a reliable scale for suicide assessment that would have greater positive predictive value and might be usable for clinical screening of at-risk individuals at the initiation of treatment or for ongoing assessments of risk during treatment.

Rather than simply identifying associations between suicide and static risk factors such as demographic variables, research should have the specific goal of identifying factors that may be modifiable with interventions. In addition, future research should provide information on rates of suicide and other suicidal behaviors in clinically important subgroups of at-risk individuals that could serve as a baseline for studies of specific interventions to decrease risk. Although most efforts in the past have been aimed at decreasing the effects of suicide risk factors, research should also develop approaches to increase the effects of factors that protect against suicide. Finally, an improved understanding of risk factors for suicidal behaviors may suggest selective or population-based approaches to suicide prevention that could then be subjected to empirical testing.

In terms of treatment, studies with lithium and with clozapine have clearly demonstrated that interventions are capable of reducing the likelihood of suicide and of other suicidal behaviors. Additional research with these agents should focus on delineating factors such as serum levels that may correlate with improved response and on defining the patient populations in which these medications are most likely to be effective (e.g., patients grouped by diagnoses and diagnostic subtypes, associated clinical symptoms, treatment histories, and estimated level of suicide risk). Clinical trials are also needed to determine whether similar benefits are seen with other second-generation antipsychotic medications or with anticonvulsant medications (e.g., divalproex, lamotrigine, carbamazepine, oxcarbazepine, and topiramate). Pharmacoepidemiologic studies may provide additional information to complement the results of clinical trials.

With ECT, it remains to be tested whether long-term reduction of suicide or other suicidal behaviors can be accomplished by long-term use of maintenance ECT or by an acute course of ECT followed by long-term antidepressant or mood-stabilizing treatment. If other somatic treatments such as transcranial magnetic stimulation or vagal nerve stimulation continue to show promise in the treatment of depressive and/or psychotic disorders, their ability to affect the risk for suicide and other suicidal behaviors should also be examined.

Clinical trials with psychotherapy should not only examine the effects of specific psychotherapeutic approaches in reducing the rate of suicide and other suicidal behaviors but should also aim to identify specific aspects of those psychotherapeutic approaches that are associated with beneficial outcomes. Additional studies should compare combined treatment with psychotherapy and pharmacotherapy to treatment with either form of therapy alone. Studies in clinically important patient subgroups, such as those with chronic suicidality or with comorbid physical diagnoses or substance use, are also essential.

The effects of other interventions should also be examined, including comparisons of approaches such as hospitalization that have been inadequately tested but are assumed to be "best practice." Given the frequent use of suicide prevention contracts in clinical practice, their safety and effectiveness should be assessed in a methodologically rigorous fashion in key subgroups of patients. Other possible interventions might be designed to improve treatment adherence, continuity of care, or access to emergency services.

When designing studies of pharmacotherapies, psychotherapies, and other interventions, consideration should be given to targeting particular factors or time periods that are associated with increased risk (e.g., immediately after hospital discharge or after a serious interpersonal loss). As with studies of specific risk factors, intervention studies should have adequate statistical power. They should clearly distinguish between effects on suicide and effects on other suicidal behaviors and should also be designed to give information about treatment effects over specific time periods of risk (e.g., immediate versus lifetime). In addition, they should attempt to determine whether effects on suicidal behaviors occur as a result of or are independent from effects of treatments on associated psychiatric disorders. Finally, they should establish the duration and intensity of treatment that produce optimal benefits to suicidal patients.

INDIVIDUALS AND ORGANIZATIONS THAT SUBMITTED COMMENTS

Aaron T. Beck, M.D.
Carl Bell, M.D.
Lanny Berman, M.D.
Romano Biancoli, Ph.D.
Dan Blazer, M.D.
Bruce Bongar, Ph.D.
Jeff Bridge, Ph.D.
Robert S. Brown, Sr., Ph.D., M.D.
William T. Carpenter, Jr., M.D.
Ken Certa, M.D.
Paula Clayton, M.D.
Jack R. Cornelius, M.D., M.P.H.
Robert R. Cummings, M.D.
Glenn W. Currier, M.D., M.P.H.
William Dalsey, M.D.
Jose de Leon, M.D.
Lisa Dixon, M.D., M.P.H.
Paul Duberstein, Ph.D.
Jill M. Harkavy-Friedman, Ph.D.
Glen Gabbard, M.D.
Jeffrey Geller, M.D., M.P.H.
Sukhmani K. Gill, M.D.
Leslie Hartley Gise, M.D.
Allen I. Green, M.D.
William M. Greenberg, M.D.
Herbert Hendin, M.D.
Robert M.A. Hirschfeld, M.D.
Kay Redfield Jamison, Ph.D.
Jeffrey Janofsky, M.D.
Jack Krasuski, M.D.
Anthony Lehman, M.D.
John T. Maltsberger, M.D.
J. John Mann, M.D.
Peter M. Marzuk, M.D.
Marlin Mattson, M.D.
Thomas H. McGlashan, M.D.
Joseph P. Merlino, M.D.
Jeffrey L. Metzner, M.D.
Alexander Miller, M.D.
Michael Craig Miller, M.D.
George E. Murphy, M.D.
Maria A. Oquendo, M.D.
Jane Pearson, Ph.D.
Debra A. Pinals, M.D.
Harold Alan Pincus, M.D.
Eric Plakun, M.D.
Charles W. Portney, M.D.
Victor I. Reus, M.D.
Charles L. Rich, M.D.
Carl Salzman, M.D.
Moisy Shopper, M.D.
Stephen F. Signer, M.D.
Joseph S. Silverman, M.D.
Barbara H. Stanley, Ph.D.
Robert Stern, M.D., Ph.D.
Nada Stotland, M.D., M.P.H.
Nicholas E. Stratas, M.D.
Howard S. Sudak, M.D.

William R. Tatomer, M.D.
Bryce Templeton, M.D., M.Ed.
Leonardo Tondo, M.D.
Edward A. Volkman, M.D.
Joan Wheelis, M.D.

American Academy of Psychiatry and the Law
American Academy of Psychoanalysis and Dynamic Psychiatry
American Association for Emergency Psychiatry
American Association for Geriatric Psychiatry
American College of Emergency Physicians
American Foundation for Suicide Prevention
American Psychoanalytic Association
Professional Risk Management Services

Acknowledgment
Amy S. Bloom, M.P.H., assisted in research and development of this guideline.

REFERENCES

The following coding system is used to indicate the nature of the supporting evidence in the references:

[A] *Randomized, double-blind clinical trial.* A study of an intervention in which subjects are prospectively followed over time; there are treatment and control groups; subjects are randomly assigned to the two groups; both the subjects and the investigators are blind to the assignments.
[A–] *Randomized clinical trial.* Same as [A] but not double-blind.
[B] *Clinical trial.* A prospective study in which an intervention is made and the results of that intervention are tracked longitudinally; study does not meet standards for a randomized clinical trial.
[C] *Cohort or longitudinal study.* A study in which subjects are prospectively followed over time without any specific intervention.
[D] *Control study.* A study in which a group of patients and a group of control subjects are identified in the present and information about them is pursued retrospectively or backward in time.
[E] *Review with secondary data analysis.* A structured analytic review of existing data, e.g., a meta-analysis or a decision analysis.
[F] *Review.* A qualitative review and discussion of previously published literature without a quantitative synthesis of the data.
[G] *Other.* Textbooks, expert opinion, case reports, and other reports not included above.

1. O'Carroll PW, Berman AL, Maris RW, Moscicki EK, Tanney BL, Silverman MM: Beyond the Tower of Babel: a nomenclature for suicidology. Suicide Life Threat Behav 1996; 26:237–252 [G]
2. Crosby AE, Cheltenham MP, Sacks JJ: Incidence of suicidal ideation and behavior in the United States, 1994. Suicide Life Threat Behav 1999; 29:131–140 [G]
3. Minino AM, Arias E, Kochanek KD, Murphy SL, Smith BL: Deaths: Final Data for 2000. National Vital Statistics Reports, vol 50, no 15. DHHS Publication PHS 2002-1120. Hyattsville, Md, National Center for Health Statistics, 2002 [G]

4. American Academy of Child and Adolescent Psychiatry: Practice Parameter for the Assessment and Treatment of Children and Adolescents With Suicidal Behavior. J Am Acad Child Adolesc Psychiatry 2001; 40:24S–51S [G]
5. American Psychiatric Association: Practice guideline for psychiatric evaluation of adults. Am J Psychiatry 1995; 152(Nov suppl):63–80 [G]
6. Shea SC: The Practical Art of Suicide Assessment: A Guide for Mental Health Professionals and Substance Abuse Counselors. New York, John Wiley & Sons, 2002 [G]
7. Jacobs DG (ed): The Harvard Medical School Guide to Suicide Assessment and Intervention. San Francisco, Jossey-Bass, 1998 [G]
8. Beck AT, Kovacs M, Weissman A: Assessment of suicidal intention: the Scale for Suicide Ideation. J Consult Clin Psychol 1979; 47:343–352 [G]
9. Beck AT, Schuyler D, Herman I: Development of suicidal intent scales, in The Prevention of Suicide. Edited by Beck AT, Resnik H, Lettieri DJ. Bowie, Md, Charles Press, 1974, pp 45–56 [G]
10. Brown GK: A Review of Suicide Assessment Measures for Intervention Research With Adults and Older Adults. Rockville, Md, National Institute of Mental Health, 2002. http://www.nimh. nih.gov/research/adultsuicide.pdf [F]
11. Web-Based Injury Statistics Query and Reporting System, National Center for Injury Prevention and Control, Centers for Disease Control and Prevention: Fatal injury data for 2000. http://www.cdc.gov/ncipc/wisqars/default.htm [G]
12. Anderson RN: Deaths: Leading Causes for 1999. National Vital Statistics Reports, vol 49, no 11. Hyattsville, Md, National Center for Health Statistics, 2001 [G]
13. Duberstein PR, Conwell Y, Seidlitz L, Lyness JM, Cox C, Caine ED: Age and suicidal ideation in older depressed inpatients. Am J Geriatr Psychiatry 1999; 7:289–296 [D]
14. Moscicki EK: Identification of suicide risk factors using epidemiologic studies. Psychiatr Clin North Am 1997; 20:499–517 [F]
15. Conwell Y, Duberstein PR, Cox C, Herrmann J, Forbes N, Caine ED: Age differences in behaviors leading to completed suicide. Am J Geriatr Psychiatry 1998; 6:122–126 [D]
16. Frierson RL: Suicide attempts by the old and the very old. Arch Intern Med 1991; 151:141–144 [E]
17. Institute of Medicine: Reducing Suicide: A National Imperative. Washington, DC, National Academies Press, 2002. http://books.nap.edu/books/0309083214/html/index.html [G]
18. Phillips MR, Li X, Zhang Y: Suicide rates in China, 1995–99. Lancet 2002; 359:835–840 [G]
19. Cohen D, Llorente M, Eisdorfer C: Homicide-suicide in older persons. Am J Psychiatry 1998; 155:390–396 [G]
20. Marzuk PM, Tardiff K, Hirsch CS: The epidemiology of murder-suicide. JAMA 1992; 267:3179–3183 [F]
21. Murphy GE: Why women are less likely than men to commit suicide. Compr Psychiatry 1998; 39:165–175 [F]
22. Gibbs JT: African-American suicide: a cultural paradox. Suicide Life Threat Behav 1997; 27:68–79 [F]
23. Oquendo MA, Ellis SP, Greenwald S, Malone KM, Weissman MM, Mann JJ: Ethnic and sex differences in suicide rates relative to major depression in the United States. Am J Psychiatry 2001; 158:1652–1658 [G]
24. Kposowa AJ: Unemployment and suicide: a cohort analysis of social factors predicting suicide in the US National Longitudinal Mortality Study. Psychol Med 2001; 31:127–138 [C]
25. Harris EC, Barraclough BM: Suicide as an outcome for medical disorders. Medicine (Baltimore) 1994; 73:281–296 [E]
26. Hoyer G, Lund E: Suicide among women related to number of children in marriage. Arch Gen Psychiatry 1993; 50:134–137 [C]

27. Appleby L, Mortensen PB, Faragher EB: Suicide and other causes of mortality after post-partum psychiatric admission. Br J Psychiatry 1998; 173:209–211 [D]
28. Yonkers KA, Ramin SM, Rush AJ, Navarrete CA, Carmody T, March D, Heartwell SF, Leveno KJ: Onset and persistence of postpartum depression in an inner-city maternal health clinic system. Am J Psychiatry 2001; 158:1856–1863 [C]
29. Kuo WH, Gallo JJ, Tien AY: Incidence of suicide ideation and attempts in adults: the 13-year follow-up of a community sample in Baltimore, Maryland. Psychol Med 2001; 31:1181–1191 [C]
30. Lawrence D, Almeida OP, Hulse GK, Jablensky AV, D'Arcy C, Holman J: Suicide and attempted suicide among older adults in Western Australia. Psychol Med 2000; 30:813–821 [G]
31. Mann JJ, Waternaux C, Haas GL, Malone KM: Toward a clinical model of suicidal behavior in psychiatric patients. Am J Psychiatry 1999; 156:181–189 [G]
32. Wunderlich U, Bronisch T, Wittchen HU, Carter R: Gender differences in adolescents and young adults with suicidal behaviour. Acta Psychiatr Scand 2001; 104:332–339 [G]
33. Molnar BE, Berkman LF, Buka SL: Psychopathology, childhood sexual abuse and other childhood adversities: relative links to subsequent suicidal behaviour in the US. Psychol Med 2001; 31:965–977 [G]
34. Doyle JP, Frank E, Saltzman LE, McMahon PM, Fielding BD: Domestic violence and sexual abuse in women physicians: associated medical, psychiatric, and professional difficulties. J Womens Health Gend Based Med 1999; 8:955–965 [G]
35. Nelson EC, Heath AC, Madden PA, Cooper ML, Dinwiddie SH, Bucholz KK, Glowinski A, McLaughlin T, Dunne MP, Statham DJ, Martin NG: Association between self-reported childhood sexual abuse and adverse psychosocial outcomes: results from a twin study. Arch Gen Psychiatry 2002; 59:139–145 [G]
36. Plunkett A, O'Toole B, Swanston H, Oates RK, Shrimpton S, Parkinson P: Suicide risk following child sexual abuse. Ambul Pediatr 2001; 1:262–266 [D]
37. Baca-Garcia E, Diaz-Sastre C, de Leon J, Saiz-Ruiz J: The relationship between menstrual cycle phases and suicide attempts. Psychosom Med 2000; 62:50–60 [D]
38. Baca-Garcia E, Sanchez-Gonzalez A, Gonzalez Diaz-Corralero P, Gonzalez Garcia I, de Leon J: Menstrual cycle and profiles of suicidal behaviour. Acta Psychiatr Scand 1998; 97:32–35 [G]
39. Singh GK, Siahpush M: All-cause and cause-specific mortality of immigrants and native born in the United States. Am J Public Health 2001; 91:392–399 [G]
40. Kliewer EV, Ward RH: Convergence of immigrant suicide rates to those in the destination country. Am J Epidemiol 1988; 127:640–653 [G]
41. Sainsbury P: Suicide in London: An Ecological Study. London, Chapman and Hall, 1955 [G]
42. Tseng W: Handbook of Cultural Psychiatry. San Diego, Academic Press, 2001 [G]
43. Hovey JD: Acculturative stress, depression, and suicidal ideation among Central American immigrants. Suicide Life Threat Behav 2000; 30:125–139 [C]
44. Committee on Cultural Psychiatry, Group for the Advancement of Psychiatry: Suicide and Ethnicity in the United States. New York, Brunner/Mazel, 1989 [G]
45. Kaprio J, Koskenvuo M, Rita H: Mortality after bereavement: a prospective study of 95,647 widowed persons. Am J Public Health 1987; 77:283–287 [C]
46. Luoma JB, Pearson JL: Suicide and marital status in the United States, 1991–1996: is widowhood a risk factor? Am J Public Health 2002; 92:1518–1522 [G]
47. Clark DC, Fawcett J: The relation of parenthood to suicide. Arch Gen Psychiatry 1994; 51:160 [F]
48. Remafedi G, French S, Story M, Resnick MD, Blum R: The relationship between suicide risk and sexual orientation: results of a population-based study. Am J Public Health 1998; 88:57–60 [C]

49. Garofalo R, Wolf RC, Wissow LS, Woods ER, Goodman E: Sexual orientation and risk of suicide attempts among a representative sample of youth. Arch Pediatr Adolesc Med 1999; 153:487–493 [C]
50. Cochran SD, Mays VM: Lifetime prevalence of suicide symptoms and affective disorders among men reporting same-sex sexual partners: results from NHANES III. Am J Public Health 2000; 90:573–578 [G]
51. Fergusson DM, Horwood LJ, Beautrais AL: Is sexual orientation related to mental health problems and suicidality in young people? Arch Gen Psychiatry 1999; 56:876–880 [C]
52. Herrell R, Goldberg J, True WR, Ramakrishnan V, Lyons M, Eisen S, Tsuang MT: Sexual orientation and suicidality: a co-twin control study in adult men. Arch Gen Psychiatry 1999; 56:867–874 [D]
53. Paul JP, Catania J, Pollack L, Moskowitz J, Canchola J, Mills T, Binson D, Stall R: Suicide attempts among gay and bisexual men: lifetime prevalence and antecedents. Am J Public Health 2002; 92:1338–1345 [G]
54. Stack S: Occupation and suicide. Soc Sci Q 2001; 82:384–396 [E]
55. Stack S: Gender and suicide risk among laborers. Arch Suicide Res 1995; 1:19–26 [G]
56. Wasserman I: Economy, Work, Occupation, and Suicide. New York, Guilford, 1992 [G]
57. Boxer PA, Burnett C, Swanson N: Suicide and occupation: a review of the literature. J Occup Environ Med 1995; 37:442–452 [F]
58. Frank E, Biola H, Burnett CA: Mortality rates and causes among US physicians. Am J Prev Med 2000; 19:155–159 [G]
59. Henriksson MM, Aro HM, Marttunen MJ, Heikkinen ME, Isometsa ET, Kuoppasalmi KI, Lonnqvist JK: Mental disorders and comorbidity in suicide. Am J Psychiatry 1993; 150:935–940 [C]
60. Robins E, Murphy GE, Wilkinson RH, Gassner S, Kayes J: Some clinical considerations in the prevention of suicide based on a study of 134 successful suicides. Am J Public Health 1959; 49:888–899 [C]
61. Clark DC, Horton-Deutsch SL: Assessment in absentia: the value of the psychological autopsy method for studying antecedents of suicide and predicting future suicides, in Assessment and Prediction of Suicide. Edited by Maris RW, Berman AL, Maltsberger JT, Yufit RI. New York, Guilford, 1992, pp 144–182 [G]
62. Jacobs DG, Klein-Benheim M: The psychological autopsy: a useful tool for determining proximate causation in suicide cases. Bull Am Acad Psychiatry Law 1995; 23:1–18 [G]
63. Jacobs DG, Klein ME: The expanding role of psychological autopsies: a review of the literature and two case examples, in Suicidology: Essays in Honor of Edwin S. Shneidman. Edited by Leenaars AA. Northvale, NJ, Jason Aronson, 1993, pp 209–247 [G]
64. Harris EC, Barraclough B: Suicide as an outcome for mental disorders: a meta-analysis. Br J Psychiatry 1997; 170:205–228 [E]
65. Barraclough B, Bunch J, Nelson B, Sainsbury P: A hundred cases of suicide: clinical aspects. Br J Psychiatry 1974; 125:355–373 [C]
66. Conwell Y, Duberstein PR, Cox C, Herrmann JH, Forbes NT, Caine ED: Relationships of age and axis I diagnoses in victims of completed suicide: a psychological autopsy study. Am J Psychiatry 1996; 153:1001–1008 [D]
67. Rich CL, Young D, Fowler RC: San Diego suicide study. I. young vs old subjects. Arch Gen Psychiatry 1986; 43:577–582 [G]
68. Isometsa ET, Henriksson MM, Aro HM, Lonnqvist JK: Suicide in bipolar disorder in Finland. Am J Psychiatry 1994; 151:1020–1024 [C]
69. Tondo L, Isacsson G, Baldessarini RJ: Suicidal behaviour in bipolar disorder: risk and prevention. CNS Drugs 2003; 17:491–511 [F]
70. Strakowski SM, McElroy SL, Keck PE Jr, West SA: Suicidality among patients with mixed and manic bipolar disorder. Am J Psychiatry 1996; 153:674–676 [G]

71. Goldberg JF, Garno JL, Portera L, Leon AC, Kocsis JH, Whiteside JE: Correlates of suicidal ideation in dysphoric mania. J Affect Disord 1999; 56:75–81 [D]
72. Jamison KR: Suicide and manic-depressive illness: an overview and personal account, in The Harvard Medical School Guide to Suicide Assessment and Intervention. Edited by Jacobs DG. San Francisco, Jossey-Bass, 1998, pp 251–269 [G/F]
73. Osby U, Brandt L, Correia N, Ekbom A, Sparen P: Excess mortality in bipolar and unipolar disorder in Sweden. Arch Gen Psychiatry 2001; 58:844–850 [D]
74. Angst F, Stassen HH, Clayton PJ, Angst J: Mortality of patients with mood disorders: follow-up over 34–38 years. J Affect Disord 2002; 68:167–181 [D]
75. Hoyer EH, Mortensen PB, Olesen AV: Mortality and causes of death in a total national sample of patients with affective disorders admitted for the first time between 1973 and 1993. Br J Psychiatry 2000; 176:76–82 [C]
76. Sharma R, Markar HR: Mortality in affective disorder. J Affect Disord 1994; 31:91–96 [G]
77. Bostwick JM, Pankratz VS: Affective disorders and suicide risk: a reexamination. Am J Psychiatry 2000; 157:1925–1932 [F]
78. Brown GK, Beck AT, Steer RA, Grisham JR: Risk factors for suicide in psychiatric outpatients: a 20-year prospective study. J Consult Clin Psychol 2000; 68:371–377 [C]
79. Fawcett J, Scheftner WA, Fogg L, Clark DC, Young MA, Hedeker D, Gibbons R: Time-related predictors of suicide in major affective disorder. Am J Psychiatry 1990; 147:1189–1194 [D]
80. Radomsky ED, Haas GL, Mann JJ, Sweeney JA: Suicidal behavior in patients with schizophrenia and other psychotic disorders. Am J Psychiatry 1999; 156:1590–1595 [G]
81. Roose SP, Glassman AH, Walsh BT, Woodring S, Vital-Herne J: Depression, delusions, and suicide. Am J Psychiatry 1983; 140:1159–1162 [D]
82. Tsai SY, Kuo CJ, Chen CC, Lee HC: Risk factors for completed suicide in bipolar disorder. J Clin Psychiatry 2002; 63:469–476 [C]
83. Westermeyer JF, Harrow M, Marengo JT: Risk for suicide in schizophrenia and other psychotic and nonpsychotic disorders. J Nerv Ment Dis 1991; 179:259–266 [C]
84. Black DW, Winokur G, Nasrallah A: Effect of psychosis on suicide risk in 1,593 patients with unipolar and bipolar affective disorders. Am J Psychiatry 1988; 145:849–852 [C]
85. Coryell W, Tsuang MT: Primary unipolar depression and the prognostic importance of delusions. Arch Gen Psychiatry 1982; 39:1181–1184 [G]
86. Grunebaum MF, Oquendo MA, Harkavy-Friedman JM, Ellis SP, Li S, Haas GL, Malone KM, Mann JJ: Delusions and suicidality. Am J Psychiatry 2001; 158:742–747 [G]
87. Kaplan KJ, Harrow M: Positive and negative symptoms as risk factors for later suicidal activity in schizophrenics versus depressives. Suicide Life Threat Behav 1996; 26:105–121 [C]
88. Serretti A, Lattuada E, Cusin C, Gasperini M, Smeraldi E: Clinical and demographic features of psychotic and nonpsychotic depression. Compr Psychiatry 1999; 40:358–362 [D]
89. De Hert M, McKenzie K, Peuskens J: Risk factors for suicide in young people suffering from schizophrenia: a long-term follow-up study. Schizophr Res 2001; 47:127–134 [D]
90. Tsuang MT, Fleming JA, Simpson JC: Suicide and schizophrenia, in The Harvard Medical School Guide to Suicide Assessment and Intervention. Edited by Jacobs DG. San Francisco, Jossey-Bass, 1998, pp 287–299 [G]
91. Black DW, Warrack G, Winokur G: Excess mortality among psychiatric patients: the Iowa Record-Linkage Study. JAMA 1985; 253:58–61 [C]
92. Allebeck P: Schizophrenia: a life-shortening disease. Schizophr Bull 1989; 15:81–89 [F]
93. Fenton WS, McGlashan TH, Victor BJ, Blyler CR: Symptoms, subtype, and suicidality in patients with schizophrenia spectrum disorders. Am J Psychiatry 1997; 154:199–204 [C]
94. Inskip HM, Harris EC, Barraclough B: Lifetime risk of suicide for affective disorder, alcoholism and schizophrenia. Br J Psychiatry 1998; 172:35–37 [F]

95. Rossau CD, Mortensen PB: Risk factors for suicide in patients with schizophrenia: nested case-control study. Br J Psychiatry 1997; 171:355–359 [D]
96. Roy A: Risk factors for suicide in psychiatric patients. Arch Gen Psychiatry 1982; 39:1089–1095 [D]
97. Drake RE, Gates C, Whitaker A, Cotton PG: Suicide among schizophrenics: a review. Compr Psychiatry 1985; 26:90–100 [F]
98. Black DW, Winokur G, Warrack G: Suicide in schizophrenia: the Iowa Record Linkage Study. J Clin Psychiatry 1985; 46:14–17 [C]
99. Miles CP: Conditions predisposing to suicide: a review. J Nerv Ment Dis 1977; 164:231–246 [F]
100. Heila H, Isometsa ET, Henriksson MM, Heikkinen ME, Marttunen MJ, Lonnqvist JK: Suicide and schizophrenia: a nationwide psychological autopsy study on age- and sex-specific clinical characteristics of 92 suicide victims with schizophrenia. Am J Psychiatry 1997; 154:1235–1242 [C]
101. Nyman AK, Jonsson H: Patterns of self-destructive behaviour in schizophrenia. Acta Psychiatr Scand 1986; 73:252–262 [C]
102. Breier A, Astrachan BM: Characterization of schizophrenic patients who commit suicide. Am J Psychiatry 1984; 141:206–209 [D]
103. Dingman CW, McGlashan TH: Discriminating characteristics of suicides: Chestnut Lodge follow-up sample including patients with affective disorder, schizophrenia and schizoaffective disorder. Acta Psychiatr Scand 1986; 74:91–97 [D]
104. Roy A: Suicide in schizophrenia, in Suicide. Edited by Roy A. Baltimore, Williams & Wilkins, 1986, pp 97–112 [G]
105. Kaplan KJ, Harrow M: Psychosis and functioning as risk factors for later suicidal activity among schizophrenia and schizoaffective patients: a disease-based interactive model. Suicide Life Threat Behav 1999; 29:10–24 [C]
106. Harkavy-Friedman JM, Kimhy D, Nelson EA, Venarde DF, Malaspina D, Mann JJ: Suicide attempts in schizophrenia: the role of command auditory hallucinations for suicide. J Clin Psychiatry 2003; 64:871–874 [D]
107. Heila H, Isometsa ET, Henriksson MM, Heikkinen ME, Marttunen MJ, Lonnqvist JK: Suicide victims with schizophrenia in different treatment phases and adequacy of antipsychotic medication. J Clin Psychiatry 1999; 60:200–208 [G]
108. Harkavy-Friedman JM, Restifo K, Malaspina D, Kaufmann CA, Amador XF, Yale SA, Gorman JM: Suicidal behavior in schizophrenia: characteristics of individuals who had and had not attempted suicide. Am J Psychiatry 1999; 156:1276–1278 [D]
109. Fawcett J, Clark DC, Busch K: Assessing and treating the patient at risk for suicide. Giornale Italiano di Suicidologia 1993; 3:9–23 [C]
110. Rich CL, Motooka MS, Fowler RC, Young D: Suicide by psychotics. Biol Psychiatry 1988; 24:595–601 [C]
111. Drake RE, Gates C, Cotton PG, Whitaker A: Suicide among schizophrenics: who is at risk? J Nerv Ment Dis 1984; 172:613–617 [E]
112. Siris SG: Depression in schizophrenia: perspective in the era of "atypical" antipsychotic agents. Am J Psychiatry 2000; 157:1379–1389 [F]
113. McGlashan TH, Carpenter WT Jr: Postpsychotic depression in schizophrenia. Arch Gen Psychiatry 1976; 33:231–239 [G]
114. Meltzer HY: Suicidality in schizophrenia: a review of the evidence for risk factors and treatment options. Curr Psychiatry Rep 2002; 4:279–283 [F]
115. Virkkunen M: Attitude to psychiatric treatment before suicide in schizophrenia and paranoid psychoses. Br J Psychiatry 1976; 128:47–49 [D]
116. Fenton WS, McGlashan TH: Natural history of schizophrenia subtypes. I. longitudinal study of paranoid, hebephrenic, and undifferentiated schizophrenia. Arch Gen Psychiatry 1991; 48:969–977 [C]

117. Roy A, Mazonson A, Pickar D: Attempted suicide in chronic schizophrenia. Br J Psychiatry 1984; 144:303–306 [D]
118. Khan A, Leventhal RM, Khan S, Brown WA: Suicide risk in patients with anxiety disorders: a meta-analysis of the FDA database. J Affect Disord 2002; 68:183–190 [E]
119. Allgulander C: Suicide and mortality patterns in anxiety neurosis and depressive neurosis. Arch Gen Psychiatry 1994; 51:708–712 [G]
120. Lonnqvist JK, Henriksson MM, Isometsa ET, Marttunen MJ, Heikkinen ME, Aro HM, Kuoppasalmi KI: Mental disorders and suicide prevention. Psychiatry Clin Neurosci 1995; 49(suppl 1):S111–S116 [C]
121. Ohberg A, Vuori E, Ojanpera I, Lonngvist J: Alcohol and drugs in suicides. Br J Psychiatry 1996; 169:75–80 [C]
122. Noyes R Jr, Christiansen J, Clancy J, Garvey MJ, Suelzer M, Anderson DJ: Predictors of serious suicide attempts among patients with panic disorder. Compr Psychiatry 1991; 32:261–267 [C]
123. Coryell W, Noyes R, Clancy J: Excess mortality in panic disorder: a comparison with primary unipolar depression. Arch Gen Psychiatry 1982; 39:701–703 [G]
124. Cox BJ, Direnfeld DM, Swinson RP, Norton GR: Suicidal ideation and suicide attempts in panic disorder and social phobia. Am J Psychiatry 1994; 151:882–887 [D]
125. Weissman MM, Klerman GL, Markowitz JS, Ouellette R: Suicidal ideation and suicide attempts in panic disorder and attacks. N Engl J Med 1989; 321:1209–1214 [D]
126. King MK, Schmaling KB, Cowley DS, Dunner DL: Suicide attempt history in depressed patients with and without a history of panic attacks. Compr Psychiatry 1995; 36:25–30 [G]
127. Warshaw MG, Dolan RT, Keller MB: Suicidal behavior in patients with current or past panic disorder: five years of prospective data from the Harvard/Brown Anxiety Research Program. Am J Psychiatry 2000; 157:1876–1878 [C]
128. Beck AT, Steer RA, Sanderson WC, Skeie TM: Panic disorder and suicidal ideation and behavior: discrepant findings in psychiatric outpatients. Am J Psychiatry 1991; 148:1195–1199 [G]
129. Lepine JP, Chignon JM, Teherani M: Suicide attempts in patients with panic disorder. Arch Gen Psychiatry 1993; 50:144–149 [G]
130. Pilowsky DJ, Wu LT, Anthony JC: Panic attacks and suicide attempts in mid-adolescence. Am J Psychiatry 1999; 156:1545–1549 [G]
131. Oquendo MA, Friend JM, Halberstam B, Brodsky BS, Burke AK, Grunebaum MF, Malone KM, Mann JJ: Association of comorbid posttraumatic stress disorder and major depression with greater risk for suicidal behavior. Am J Psychiatry 2003; 160:580–582 [G]
132. Schaffer A, Levitt AJ, Bagby RM, Kennedy SH, Levitan RD, Joffe RT: Suicidal ideation in major depression: sex differences and impact of comorbid anxiety. Can J Psychiatry 2000; 45:822–826 [G]
133. Noyes R Jr: Suicide and panic disorder: a review. J Affect Disord 1991; 22:1–11 [F]
134. Weissman MM, Klerman GL, Johnson J: Panic disorder and suicidal ideation. Am J Psychiatry 1992; 149:1411–1412 [G]
135. Marshall RD, Olfson M, Hellman F, Blanco C, Guardino M, Struening EL: Comorbidity, impairment, and suicidality in subthreshold PTSD. Am J Psychiatry 2001; 158:1467–1473 [G]
136. Fleet RP, Dupuis G, Marchand A, Burelle D, Arsenault A, Beitman BD: Panic disorder in emergency department chest pain patients: prevalence, comorbidity, suicidal ideation, and physician recognition. Am J Med 1996; 101:371–380 [G]
137. Hornig CD, McNally RJ: Panic disorder and suicide attempt: a reanalysis of data from the Epidemiologic Catchment Area study. Br J Psychiatry 1995; 167:76–79 [E]
138. Herzog DB, Greenwood DN, Dorer DJ, Flores AT, Ekeblad ER, Richards A, Blais MA, Keller MB: Mortality in eating disorders: a descriptive study. Int J Eat Disord 2000; 28:20–26 [C]
139. Eckert ED, Halmi KA, Marchi P, Grove W, Crosby R: Ten-year follow-up of anorexia nervosa: clinical course and outcome. Psychol Med 1995; 25:143–156 [C]

140. Coren S, Hewitt PL: Is anorexia nervosa associated with elevated rates of suicide? Am J Public Health 1998; 88:1206–1207 [D]
141. Kent A, Goddard KL, van den Berk PA, Raphael FJ, McCluskey SE, Lacey JH: Eating disorder in women admitted to hospital following deliberate self-poisoning. Acta Psychiatr Scand 1997; 95:140–144 [D]
142. Thompson KM, Wonderlich SA, Crosby RD, Mitchell JE: The neglected link between eating disturbances and aggressive behavior in girls. J Am Acad Child Adolesc Psychiatry 1999; 38:1277–1284 [D]
143. Nasser EH, Overholser JC: Assessing varying degrees of lethality in depressed adolescent suicide attempters. Acta Psychiatr Scand 1999; 99:423–431 [C]
144. Murphy KR, Barkley RA, Bush T: Young adults with attention deficit hyperactivity disorder: subtype differences in comorbidity, educational, and clinical history. J Nerv Ment Dis 2002; 190:147–157 [D]
145. Brent DA, Perper JA, Moritz G, Allman C, Friend A, Roth C, Schweers J, Balach L, Baugher M: Psychiatric risk factors for adolescent suicide: a case-control study. J Am Acad Child Adolesc Psychiatry 1993; 32:521–529 [D]
146. Brent DA, Johnson B, Bartle S, Bridge J, Rather C, Matta J, Connolly J, Constantine D: Personality disorder, tendency to impulsive violence, and suicidal behavior in adolescents. J Am Acad Child Adolesc Psychiatry 1993; 32:69–75 [D]
147. Murphy GE: Psychiatric aspects of suicidal behaviour: substance abuse, in The International Handbook of Suicide and Attempted Suicide. Edited by Hawton K, van Heeringen K. Chichester, England, John Wiley & Sons, 2000, pp 135–146 [F]
148. Murphy GE, Wetzel RD: The lifetime risk of suicide in alcoholism. Arch Gen Psychiatry 1990; 47:383–392 [F]
149. Murphy GE, Wetzel RD, Robins E, McEvoy L: Multiple risk factors predict suicide in alcoholism. Arch Gen Psychiatry 1992; 49:459–463 [C]
150. Conner KR, Duberstein PR, Conwell Y, Herrmann JH Jr, Cox C, Barrington DS, Caine ED: After the drinking stops: completed suicide in individuals with remitted alcohol use disorders. J Psychoactive Drugs 2000; 32:333–337 [G]
151. Brent DA, Perper JA, Allman CJ: Alcohol, firearms, and suicide among youth: temporal trends in Allegheny County, Pennsylvania, 1960 to 1983. JAMA 1987; 257:3369–3372 [G]
152. Murphy GE, Armstrong JW Jr, Hermele SL, Fischer JR, Clendenin WW: Suicide and alcoholism: interpersonal loss confirmed as a predictor. Arch Gen Psychiatry 1979; 36:65–69 [C]
153. Murphy GE: Suicide and substance abuse. Arch Gen Psychiatry 1988; 45:593–594 [G]
154. Pirkola SP, Isometsa ET, Heikkinen ME, Lonnqvist JK: Suicides of alcohol misusers and non-misusers in a nationwide population. Alcohol Alcohol 2000; 35:70–75 [C]
155. Beskow J: Suicide and mental disorder in Swedish men. Acta Psychiatr Scand Suppl 1979; 277:1–138 [E]
156. Murphy GE, Robins E: Social factors in suicide. JAMA 1967; 199:303–308 [D]
157. Berglund M: Suicide in alcoholism: a prospective study of 88 suicides. I. the multidimensional diagnosis at first admission. Arch Gen Psychiatry 1984; 41:888–891 [C]
158. Rich CL, Fowler RC, Fogarty LA, Young D: San Diego Suicide Study. III. relationships between diagnoses and stressors. Arch Gen Psychiatry 1988; 45:589–592 [G]
159. Shaffer D, Gould MS, Fisher P, Trautman P, Moreau D, Kleinman M, Flory M: Psychiatric diagnosis in child and adolescent suicide. Arch Gen Psychiatry 1996; 53:339–348 [D]
160. Pokorny AD: Prediction of suicide in psychiatric patients: report of a prospective study. Arch Gen Psychiatry 1983; 40:249–257 [D]
161. Hirschfeld RM, Russell JM: Assessment and treatment of suicidal patients. N Engl J Med 1997; 337:910–915 [G]
162. Gomberg ES: Suicide risk among women with alcohol problems. Am J Public Health 1989; 79:1363–1365 [D]

163. Petronis KR, Samuels JF, Moscicki EK, Anthony JC: An epidemiologic investigation of potential risk factors for suicide attempts. Soc Psychiatry Psychiatr Epidemiol 1990; 25:193–199 [E]
164. Hjelmeland H: Repetition of parasuicide: a predictive study. Suicide Life Threat Behav 1996; 26:395–404 [C]
165. Roy A, Lamparski D, DeJong J, Moore V, Linnoila M: Characteristics of alcoholics who attempt suicide. Am J Psychiatry 1990; 147:761–765 [D]
166. Hesselbrock M, Hesselbrock V, Syzmanski K, Weidenman M: Suicide attempts and alcoholism. J Stud Alcohol 1988; 49:436–442 [D]
167. Preuss UW, Schuckit MA, Smith TL, Danko GP, Buckman K, Bierut L, Bucholz KK, Hesselbrock MN, Hesselbrock VM, Reich T: Comparison of 3190 alcohol-dependent individuals with and without suicide attempts. Alcohol Clin Exp Res 2002; 26:471–477 [D]
168. Preuss UW, Schuckit MA, Smith TL, Danko GP, Bucholz KK, Hesselbrock MN, Hesselbrock V, Kramer JR: Predictors and correlates of suicide attempts over 5 years in 1,237 alcohol-dependent men and women. Am J Psychiatry 2003; 160:56–63 [C]
169. Preuss UW, Schuckit MA, Smith TL, Danko GR, Dasher AC, Hesselbrock MN, Hesselbrock VM, Nurnberger JI Jr: A comparison of alcohol-induced and independent depression in alcoholics with histories of suicide attempts. J Stud Alcohol 2002; 63:498–502 [G]
170. Cornelius JR, Salloum IM, Mezzich J, Cornelius MD, Fabrega H Jr, Ehler JG, Ulrich RF, Thase ME, Mann JJ: Disproportionate suicidality in patients with comorbid major depression and alcoholism. Am J Psychiatry 1995; 152:358–364 [D]
171. Cornelius JR, Salloum IM, Day NL, Thase ME, Mann JJ: Patterns of suicidality and alcohol use in alcoholics with major depression. Alcohol Clin Exp Res 1996; 20:1451–1455 [G]
172. Harris EC, Barraclough B: Excess mortality of mental disorder. Br J Psychiatry 1998; 173:11–53 [E]
173. Fowler RC, Rich CL, Young D: San Diego Suicide Study. II. substance abuse in young cases. Arch Gen Psychiatry 1986; 43:962–965 [D]
174. Lesage AD, Boyer R, Grunberg F, Vanier C, Morissette R, Menard-Buteau C, Loyer M: Suicide and mental disorders: a case-control study of young men. Am J Psychiatry 1994; 151:1063–1068 [D]
175. Pirkola SP, Isometsa ET, Heikkinen ME, Henriksson MM, Marttunen MJ, Lonnqvist JK: Female psychoactive substance-dependent suicide victims differ from male—results from a nationwide psychological autopsy study. Compr Psychiatry 1999; 40:101–107 [C]
176. Borges G, Walters EE, Kessler RC: Associations of substance use, abuse, and dependence with subsequent suicidal behavior. Am J Epidemiol 2000; 151:781–789 [C]
177. Beautrais AL, Joyce PR, Mulder RT, Fergusson DM, Deavoll BJ, Nightingale SK: Prevalence and comorbidity of mental disorders in persons making serious suicide attempts: a case-control study. Am J Psychiatry 1996; 153:1009–1014 [D]
178. Rossow I, Lauritzen G: Balancing on the edge of death: suicide attempts and life-threatening overdoses among drug addicts. Addiction 1999; 94:209–219 [G]
179. Johnsson E, Fridell M: Suicide attempts in a cohort of drug abusers: a 5-year follow-up study. Acta Psychiatr Scand 1997; 96:362–366 [C]
180. Roy A: Characteristics of cocaine-dependent patients who attempt suicide. Am J Psychiatry 2001; 158:1215–1219 [D]
181. Beautrais AL, Joyce PR, Mulder RT: Cannabis abuse and serious suicide attempts. Addiction 1999; 94:1155–1164 [D]
182. Goldberg JF, Singer TM, Garno JL: Suicidality and substance abuse in affective disorders. J Clin Psychiatry 2001; 62:35–43 [F]
183. Bronisch T: The typology of personality disorders—diagnostic problems and their relevance for suicidal behavior. Crisis 1996; 17:55–58 [F]

184. Linehan MM, Rizvi SL, Welch SS, Page B: Psychiatric aspects of suicidal behaviour: personality disorders, in The International Handbook of Suicide and Attempted Suicide. Edited by Hawton K, van Heeringen K. Chichester, England, John Wiley & Sons, 2000, pp 147–178 [G]
185. Stone MH, Stone DK, Hurt SW: Natural history of borderline patients treated by intensive hospitalization. Psychiatr Clin North Am 1987; 10:185–206 [C]
186. Duberstein PR, Conwell Y: Personality disorders and completed suicide: a methodological and conceptual review. Clin Psychol Sci Pract 1997; 4:359–376 [E]
187. Isometsa ET, Henriksson MM, Heikkinen ME, Aro HM, Marttunen MJ, Kuoppasalmi KI, Lonnqvist JK: Suicide among subjects with personality disorders. Am J Psychiatry 1996; 153:667–673 [C]
188. Baxter D, Appleby L: Case register study of suicide risk in mental disorders. Br J Psychiatry 1999; 175:322–326 [C]
189. Heikkinen ME, Isometsa ET, Henriksson MM, Marttunen MJ: Psychosocial factors and completed suicide in personality disorders. Acta Psychiatr Scand 1997; 95:49–57 [C]
190. Heikkinen ME, Henriksson MM, Isometsa ET, Marttunen MJ, Aro HM, Lonnqvist JK: Recent life events and suicide in personality disorders. J Nerv Ment Dis 1997; 185:373–381 [D]
191. Suominen KH, Isometsa ET, Henriksson MM, Ostamo AI, Lonnqvist JK: Suicide attempts and personality disorder. Acta Psychiatr Scand 2000; 102:118–125 [C]
192. Van Gastel A, Schotte C, Maes M: The prediction of suicidal intent in depressed patients. Acta Psychiatr Scand 1997; 96:254–259 [C]
193. Soloff PH, Lis JA, Kelly T, Cornelius J, Ulrich R: Risk factors for suicidal behavior in borderline personality disorder. Am J Psychiatry 1994; 151:1316–1323 [G]
194. Ahrens B, Haug HJ: Suicidality in hospitalized patients with a primary diagnosis of personality disorder. Crisis 1996; 17:59–63 [D]
195. Corbitt EM, Malone KM, Haas GL, Mann JJ: Suicidal behavior in patients with major depression and comorbid personality disorders. J Affect Disord 1996; 39:61–72 [D]
196. Brodsky BS, Malone KM, Ellis SP, Dulit RA, Mann JJ: Characteristics of borderline personality disorder associated with suicidal behavior. Am J Psychiatry 1997; 154:1715–1719 [C]
197. Soloff PH, Lynch KG, Kelly TM, Malone KM, Mann JJ: Characteristics of suicide attempts of patients with major depressive episode and borderline personality disorder: a comparative study. Am J Psychiatry 2000; 157:601–608 [D]
198. Pirkis J, Burgess P, Jolley D: Suicide attempts by psychiatric patients in acute inpatient, long-stay inpatient and community care. Soc Psychiatry Psychiatr Epidemiol 1999; 34:634–644 [G]
199. Suominen K, Henriksson M, Suokas J, Isometsa E, Ostamo A, Lonnqvist J: Mental disorders and comorbidity in attempted suicide. Acta Psychiatr Scand 1996; 94:234–240 [C]
200. Persson ML, Runeson BS, Wasserman D: Diagnoses, psychosocial stressors and adaptive functioning in attempted suicide. Ann Clin Psychiatry 1999; 11:119–128 [D]
201. Pirkola SP, Isometsa ET, Henriksson MM, Heikkinen ME, Marttunen MJ, Lonnqvist JK: The treatment received by substance-dependent male and female suicide victims. Acta Psychiatr Scand 1999; 99:207–213 [C]
202. Shafii M, Carrigan S, Whittinghill JR, Derrick A: Psychological autopsy of completed suicide in children and adolescents. Am J Psychiatry 1985; 142:1061–1064 [D]
203. Brent DA, Perper JA, Goldstein CE, Kolko DJ: Risk factors for adolescent suicide: a comparison of adolescent suicide victims with suicidal inpatients. Arch Gen Psychiatry 1988; 45:581–588 [G]
204. Rich CL, Runeson BS: Similarities in diagnostic comorbidity between suicide among young people in Sweden and the United States. Acta Psychiatr Scand 1992; 86:335–339 [C]
205. Blair-West GW, Cantor CH, Mellsop GW, Eyeson-Annan ML: Lifetime suicide risk in major depression: sex and age determinants. J Affect Disord 1999; 55:171–178 [G]

206. Isometsa ET, Henriksson MM, Aro HM, Heikkinen ME, Kuoppasalmi KI, Lonnqvist JK: Suicide in major depression. Am J Psychiatry 1994; 151:530–536 [D]
207. Waern M, Runeson BS, Allebeck P, Beskow J, Rubenowitz E, Skoog I, Wilhelmsson K: Mental disorder in elderly suicides: a case-control study. Am J Psychiatry 2002; 159:450–455 [D]
208. Berglund M, Ojehagen A: The influence of alcohol drinking and alcohol use disorders on psychiatric disorders and suicidal behavior. Alcohol Clin Exp Res 1998; 22:333S–345S [G]
209. Stone MH: The course of borderline personality disorder, in American Psychiatric Press Review of Psychiatry, vol 8. Edited by Tasman A, Hales RE, Frances AJ. Washington, DC, American Psychiatric Press, 1989, pp 103–122 [G]
210. McGlashan TH: The Chestnut Lodge follow-up study. III. long-term outcome of borderline personalities. Arch Gen Psychiatry 1986; 43:20–30 [C]
211. Wunderlich U, Bronisch T, Wittchen HU: Comorbidity patterns in adolescents and young adults with suicide attempts. Eur Arch Psychiatry Clin Neurosci 1998; 248:87–95 [G]
212. Hall RC, Platt DE, Hall RC: Suicide risk assessment: a review of risk factors for suicide in 100 patients who made severe suicide attempts: evaluation of suicide risk in a time of managed care. Psychosomatics 1999; 40:18–27 [C]
213. Tondo L, Baldessarini RJ, Hennen J, Minnai GP, Salis P, Scamonatti L, Masia M, Ghiani C, Mannu P: Suicide attempts in major affective disorder patients with comorbid substance use disorders. J Clin Psychiatry 1999; 60(suppl 2):63–69 [G]
214. Potash JB, Kane HS, Chiu YF, Simpson SG, MacKinnon DF, McInnis MG, McMahon FJ, DePaulo JR Jr: Attempted suicide and alcoholism in bipolar disorder: clinical and familial relationships. Am J Psychiatry 2000; 157:2048–2050 [G]
215. Rudd MD, Dahm PF, Rajab MH: Diagnostic comorbidity in persons with suicidal ideation and behavior. Am J Psychiatry 1993; 150:928–934 [G]
216. Goodwin RD, Hamilton SP: Lifetime comorbidity of antisocial personality disorder and anxiety disorders among adults in the community. Psychiatry Res 2003; 117:159–166 [G]
217. Conner KR, Duberstein PR, Conwell Y, Seidlitz L, Caine ED: Psychological vulnerability to completed suicide: a review of empirical studies. Suicide Life Threat Behav 2001; 31:367–385 [F]
218. Busch KA, Fawcett J, Jacobs DG: Clinical correlates of inpatient suicide. J Clin Psychiatry 2003; 64:14–19 [C]
219. Fawcett J: Predictors of early suicide: identification and appropriate intervention. J Clin Psychiatry 1988; 49(suppl):7–8 [C]
220. Placidi GP, Oquendo MA, Malone KM, Brodsky B, Ellis SP, Mann JJ: Anxiety in major depression: relationship to suicide attempts. Am J Psychiatry 2000; 157:1614–1618 [D]
221. Beck AT, Brown G, Berchick RJ, Stewart BL, Steer RA: Relationship between hopelessness and ultimate suicide: a replication with psychiatric outpatients. Am J Psychiatry 1990; 147:190–195 [C]
222. Beck AT, Steer RA, Kovacs M, Garrison B: Hopelessness and eventual suicide: a 10-year prospective study of patients hospitalized with suicidal ideation. Am J Psychiatry 1985; 142:559–563 [C]
223. Beck AT, Brown G, Steer RA: Prediction of eventual suicide in psychiatric inpatients by clinical ratings of hopelessness. J Consult Clin Psychol 1989; 57:309–310 [C]
224. Beck AT, Steer RA: Clinical predictors of eventual suicide: a 5- to 10-year prospective study of suicide attempters. J Affect Disord 1989; 17:203–209 [C]
225. Beck AT, Steer RA, Beck JS, Newman CF: Hopelessness, depression, suicidal ideation, and clinical diagnosis of depression. Suicide Life Threat Behav 1993; 23:139–145 [D]
226. Young MA, Fogg LF, Scheftner WA, Fawcett JA: Interactions of risk factors in predicting suicide. Am J Psychiatry 1994; 151:434–435 [C]

227. Beck AT, Steer RA, Trexler LD: Alcohol abuse and eventual suicide: a 5- to 10-year prospective study of alcohol-abusing suicide attempters. J Stud Alcohol 1989; 50:202–209 [C]
228. Uncapher H, Gallagher-Thompson D, Osgood NJ, Bongar B: Hopelessness and suicidal ideation in older adults. Gerontologist 1998; 38:62–70 [D]
229. Cohen S, Lavelle J, Rich CL, Bromet E: Rates and correlates of suicide attempts in first-admission psychotic patients. Acta Psychiatr Scand 1994; 90:167–171 [G]
230. Kaslow N, Thompson M, Meadows L, Chance S, Puett R, Hollins L, Jessee S, Kellermann A: Risk factors for suicide attempts among African American women. Depress Anxiety 2000; 12:13–20 [D]
231. Malone KM, Oquendo MA, Haas GL, Ellis SP, Li S, Mann JJ: Protective factors against suicidal acts in major depression: reasons for living. Am J Psychiatry 2000; 157:1084–1088 [D]
232. Mendonca JD, Holden RR: Interaction of affective and cognitive impairments in the suicidal state: a brief elaboration. Acta Psychiatr Scand 1998; 97:149–152 [C]
233. Weissman AN, Beck AT, Kovacs M: Drug abuse, hopelessness, and suicidal behavior. Int J Addict 1979; 14:451–464 [D]
234. Young MA, Fogg LF, Scheftner W, Fawcett J, Akiskal H, Maser J: Stable trait components of hopelessness: baseline and sensitivity to depression. J Abnorm Psychol 1996; 105:155–165 [G]
235. Rush AJ, Beck AT, Kovacs M, Weissenburger J, Hollon SD: Comparison of the effects of cognitive therapy and pharmacotherapy on hopelessness and self-concept. Am J Psychiatry 1982; 139:862–866 [G]
236. Dahlsgaard KK, Beck AT, Brown GK: Inadequate response to therapy as a predictor of suicide. Suicide Life Threat Behavior 1998; 28:197–204 [D]
237. Nordentoft M, Jeppesen P, Abel M, Kassow P, Petersen L, Thorup A, Krarup G, Hemmingsen R, Jorgensen P: OPUS study: suicidal behaviour, suicidal ideation and hopelessness among patients with first-episode psychosis. One-year follow-up of a randomised controlled trial. Br J Psychiatry Suppl 2002; 43:S98–S106 [A–]
238. Resnick P: Command Hallucination Questionnaire. Cleveland, Case Western Reserve University, 1992 [G]
239. Zisook S, Byrd D, Kuck J, Jeste DV: Command hallucinations in outpatients with schizophrenia. J Clin Psychiatry 1995; 56:462–465 [G]
240. Hellerstein D, Frosch W, Koenigsberg HW: The clinical significance of command hallucinations. Am J Psychiatry 1987; 144:219–221 [G]
241. Junginger J: Predicting compliance with command hallucinations. Am J Psychiatry 1990; 147:245–247 [D]
242. Junginger J: Command hallucinations and the prediction of dangerousness. Psychiatr Serv 1995; 46:911–914 [D]
243. Kasper ME, Rogers R, Adams PA: Dangerousness and command hallucinations: an investigation of psychotic inpatients. Bull Am Acad Psychiatry Law 1996; 24:219–224 [D]
244. Rogers R, Gillis JR, Turner RE, Frise-Smith T: The clinical presentation of command hallucinations in a forensic population. Am J Psychiatry 1990; 147:1304–1307 [D]
245. Erkwoh R, Willmes K, Eming-Erdmann A, Kunert HJ: Command hallucinations: who obeys and who resists when? Psychopathology 2002; 35:272–279 [G]
246. Duberstein P, Seidlitz L, Conwell Y: Reconsidering the role of hostility in completed suicide: a lifecourse perspective, in Psychoanalytic Perspectives on Developmental Psychology. Edited by Bornstein RF, Masling J. Washington, DC, American Psychological Association, 1996, pp 257–323 [G]
247. Maser JD, Akiskal HS, Schettler P, Scheftner W, Mueller T, Endicott J, Solomon D, Clayton P: Can temperament identify affectively ill patients who engage in lethal or near-lethal suicidal behavior? a 14-year prospective study. Suicide Life Threat Behav 2002; 32:10–32 [C]
248. Angst J, Clayton P: Premorbid personality of depressive, bipolar, and schizophrenic patients with special reference to suicidal issues. Compr Psychiatry 1986; 27:511–532 [C]

249. Kotler M, Iancu I, Efroni R, Amir M: Anger, impulsivity, social support, and suicide risk in patients with posttraumatic stress disorder. J Nerv Ment Dis 2001; 189:162–167 [D]
250. Brodsky BS, Oquendo M, Ellis SP, Haas GL, Malone KM, Mann JJ: The relationship of childhood abuse to impulsivity and suicidal behavior in adults with major depression. Am J Psychiatry 2001; 158:1871–1877 [D]
251. Stanley B, Gameroff MJ, Michalsen V, Mann JJ: Are suicide attempters who self-mutilate a unique population? Am J Psychiatry 2001; 158:427–432 [D]
252. Oquendo MA, Waternaux C, Brodsky B, Parsons B, Haas GL, Malone KM, Mann JJ: Suicidal behavior in bipolar mood disorder: clinical characteristics of attempters and nonattempters. J Affect Disord 2000; 59:107–117 [G]
253. Herpertz S, Steinmeyer SM, Marx D, Oidtmann A, Sass H: The significance of aggression and impulsivity for self-mutilative behavior. Pharmacopsychiatry 1995; 28(suppl 2):64–72 [D]
254. Frances RJ, Franklin J, Flavin DK: Suicide and alcoholism. Am J Drug Alcohol Abuse 1987; 13:327–341 [G]
255. Hayward L, Zubrick SR, Silburn S: Blood alcohol levels in suicide cases. J Epidemiol Community Health 1992; 46:256–260 [C]
256. Brent DA, Perper JA, Moritz G, Baugher M, Schweers J, Roth C: Firearms and adolescent suicide: a community case-control study. Am J Dis Child 1993; 147:1066–1071 [D]
257. Hlady WG, Middaugh JP: Suicides in Alaska: firearms and alcohol. Am J Public Health 1988; 78:179–180 [G]
258. Suokas J, Lonnqvist J: Suicide attempts in which alcohol is involved: a special group in general hospital emergency rooms. Acta Psychiatr Scand 1995; 91:36–40 [D]
259. Ostamo A, Lonnqvist J: Excess mortality of suicide attempters. Soc Psychiatry Psychiatr Epidemiol 2001; 36:29–35 [C]
260. Pirkola S, Isometsa E, Heikkinen M, Lonnqvist J: Employment status influences the weekly patterns of suicide among alcohol misusers. Alcohol Clin Exp Res 1997; 21:1704–1706 [C]
261. Suominen KH, Isometsa ET, Henriksson MM, Ostamo AI, Lonnqvist JK: Treatment received by alcohol-dependent suicide attempters. Acta Psychiatr Scand 1999; 99:214–219 [C]
262. Marzuk PM, Mann JJ: Suicide and substance abuse. Psychiatr Ann 1988; 18:639–645 [G]
263. Arensman E, Kerkhof JF: Classification of attempted suicide: a review of empirical studies, 1963–1993. Suicide Life Threat Behav 1996; 26:46–67 [F]
264. Ferreira de Castro E, Cunha MA, Pimenta F, Costa I: Parasuicide and mental disorders. Acta Psychiatr Scand 1998; 97:25–31 [D]
265. Isacsson G, Rich CL: Management of patients who deliberately harm themselves. Br Med J 2001; 322:213–215 [F]
266. Isometsa ET, Lonnqvist JK: Suicide attempts preceding completed suicide. Br J Psychiatry 1998; 173:531–535 [C]
267. Oquendo MA, Kamali M, Ellis SP, Grunebaum MF, Malone KM, Brodsky BS, Sackeim HA, Mann JJ: Adequacy of antidepressant treatment after discharge and the occurrence of suicidal acts in major depression: a prospective study. Am J Psychiatry 2002; 159:1746–1751 [C]
268. Ekeberg O, Ellingsen O, Jacobsen D: Suicide and other causes of death in a five-year follow-up of patients treated for self-poisoning in Oslo. Acta Psychiatr Scand 1991; 83:432–437 [C]
269. Nielsen B, Wang AG, Brille-Brahe U: Attempted suicide in Denmark. IV. a five-year follow-up. Acta Psychiatr Scand 1990; 81:250–254 [C]
270. Nordstrom P, Asberg M, Aberg-Wistedt A, Nordin C: Attempted suicide predicts suicide risk in mood disorders. Acta Psychiatr Scand 1995; 92:345–350 [C]
271. Suokas J, Suominen K, Isometsa E, Ostamo A, Lonnqvist J: Long-term risk factors for suicide mortality after attempted suicide—findings of a 14-year follow-up study. Acta Psychiatr Scand 2001; 104:117–121 [C]
272. Tejedor MC, Diaz A, Castillon JJ, Pericay JM: Attempted suicide: repetition and survival—findings of a follow-up study. Acta Psychiatr Scand 1999; 100:205–211 [C]

273. Clark DC, Fawcett J: An empirically based model of suicide risk assessment for patients with affective disorder, in Suicide and Clinical Practice. Edited by Jacobs D. Washington, DC, American Psychiatric Press, 1992, pp 16–48 [G]
274. de Moore GM, Robertson AR: Suicide in the 18 years after deliberate self-harm: a prospective study. Br J Psychiatry 1996; 169:489–494 [C]
275. Nordstrom P, Samuelsson M, Asberg M: Survival analysis of suicide risk after attempted suicide. Acta Psychiatr Scand 1995; 91:336–340 [C]
276. Barber ME, Marzuk PM, Leon AC, Portera L: Aborted suicide attempts: a new classification of suicidal behavior. Am J Psychiatry 1998; 155:385–389 [F]
277. Marzuk PM, Tardiff K, Leon AC, Portera L, Weiner C: The prevalence of aborted suicide attempts among psychiatric in-patients. Acta Psychiatr Scand 1997; 96:492–496 [C]
278. Hall DJ, O'Brien F, Stark C, Pelosi A, Smith H: Thirteen-year follow-up of deliberate self-harm, using linked data. Br J Psychiatry 1998; 172:239–242 [C]
279. Hickey L, Hawton K, Fagg J, Weitzel H: Deliberate self-harm patients who leave the accident and emergency department without a psychiatric assessment: a neglected population at risk of suicide. J Psychosom Res 2001; 50:87–93 [C]
280. Jauregui J, Martinez ML, Rubio G, Santo-Domingo J: Patients who attempted suicide and failed to attend mental health centres. Eur Psychiatry 1999; 14:205–209 [D]
281. Dube SR, Anda RF, Felitti VJ, Chapman DP, Williamson DF, Giles WH: Childhood abuse, household dysfunction, and the risk of attempted suicide throughout the life span: findings from the Adverse Childhood Experiences Study. JAMA 2001; 286:3089–3096 [C]
282. Fergusson DM, Lynskey MT: Physical punishment/maltreatment during childhood and adjustment in young adulthood. Child Abuse Negl 1997; 21:617–630 [C]
283. Felitti VJ, Anda RF, Nordenberg D, Williamson DF, Spitz AM, Edwards V, Koss MP, Marks JS: Relationship of childhood abuse and household dysfunction to many of the leading causes of death in adults: the Adverse Childhood Experiences (ACE) Study. Am J Prev Med 1998; 14:245–258 [G]
284. Kaplan M, Asnis GM, Lipschitz DS, Chorney P: Suicidal behavior and abuse in psychiatric outpatients. Compr Psychiatry 1995; 36:229–235 [D]
285. van der Kolk BA, Perry JC, Herman JL: Childhood origins of self-destructive behavior. Am J Psychiatry 1991; 148:1665–1671 [C]
286. Fergusson DM, Horwood LJ, Lynskey MT: Childhood sexual abuse and psychiatric disorder in young adulthood. II. psychiatric outcomes of childhood sexual abuse. J Am Acad Child Adolesc Psychiatry 1996; 35:1365–1374 [C]
287. Frank E, Dingle AD: Self-reported depression and suicide attempts among US women physicians. Am J Psychiatry 1999; 156:1887–1894 [G]
288. Windle M, Windle RC, Scheidt DM, Miller GB: Physical and sexual abuse and associated mental disorders among alcoholic inpatients. Am J Psychiatry 1995; 152:1322–1328 [D]
289. Anderson PL, Tiro JA, Price AW, Bender MA, Kaslow NJ: Additive impact of childhood emotional, physical, and sexual abuse on suicide attempts among low-income African American women. Suicide Life Threat Behav 2002; 32:131–138 [G]
290. Roy A: Childhood trauma and suicidal behavior in male cocaine dependent patients. Suicide Life Threat Behav 2001; 31:194–196 [G]
291. Romans SE, Martin JL, Anderson JC, Herbison GP, Mullen PE: Sexual abuse in childhood and deliberate self-harm. Am J Psychiatry 1995; 152:1336–1342 [D]
292. Dinwiddie S, Heath AC, Dunne MP, Bucholz KK, Madden PA, Slutske WS, Bierut LJ, Statham DB, Martin NG: Early sexual abuse and lifetime psychopathology: a co-twin-control study. Psychol Med 2000; 30:41–52 [D]
293. Davidson JR, Hughes DC, George LK, Blazer DG: The association of sexual assault and attempted suicide within the community. Arch Gen Psychiatry 1996; 53:550–555 [D]

294. Brown J, Cohen P, Johnson JG, Smailes EM: Childhood abuse and neglect: specificity of effects on adolescent and young adult depression and suicidality. J Am Acad Child Adolesc Psychiatry 1999; 38:1490–1496 [C]
295. Chu JA: Trauma and suicide, in The Harvard Medical School Guide to Suicide Assessment and Intervention. Edited by Jacobs D. San Francisco, Jossey-Bass, 1998, pp 332–354 [F]
296. Muelleman RL, Lenaghan PA, Pakieser RA: Nonbattering presentations to the ED of women in physically abusive relationships. Am J Emerg Med 1998; 16:128–131 [G]
297. Wingood GM, DiClemente RJ, Raj A: Adverse consequences of intimate partner abuse among women in non-urban domestic violence shelters. Am J Prev Med 2000; 19:270–275 [G]
298. Simon TR, Anderso M, Thompson MP, Crosby A, Sacks JJ: Assault victimization and suicidal ideation or behavior within a national sample of US adults. Suicide Life Threat Behav 2002; 32:42–50 [G]
299. Abbott J, Johnson R, Koziol-McLain J, Lowenstein SR: Domestic violence against women: incidence and prevalence in an emergency department population. JAMA 1995; 273:1763–1767 [G]
300. McCauley J, Kern DE, Kolodner K, Dill L, Schroeder AF, DeChant HK, Ryden J, Bass EB, Derogatis LR: The "battering syndrome": prevalence and clinical characteristics of domestic violence in primary care internal medicine practices. Ann Intern Med 1995; 123:737–746 [D]
301. Thompson MP, Kaslow NJ, Kingree JB, Puett R, Thompson NJ, Meadows L: Partner abuse and posttraumatic stress disorder as risk factors for suicide attempts in a sample of low-income, inner-city women. J Trauma Stress 1999; 12:59–72 [D]
302. Ernst AA, Nick TG, Weiss SJ, Houry D, Mills T: Domestic violence in an inner-city ED. Ann Emerg Med 1997; 30:190–197 [G]
303. Conner KR, Duberstein PR, Conwell Y: Domestic violence, separation, and suicide in young men with early onset alcoholism: reanalyses of Murphy's data. Suicide Life Threat Behav 2000; 30:354–359 [G]
304. Appleby L, Dennehy JA, Thomas CS, Faragher EB, Lewis G: Aftercare and clinical characteristics of people with mental illness who commit suicide: a case-control study. Lancet 1999; 353:1397–1400 [D]
305. Sachs GS, Yan LJ, Swann AC, Allen MH: Integration of suicide prevention into outpatient management of bipolar disorder. J Clin Psychiatry 2001; 62(suppl 25):3–11 [F]
306. Appleby L, Shaw J, Amos T, McDonnell R, Harris C, McCann K, Kiernan K, Davies S, Bickley H, Parsons R: Suicide within 12 months of contact with mental health services: national clinical survey. Br Med J 1999; 318:1235–1239 [G]
307. Goldacre M, Seagroatt V, Hawton K: Suicide after discharge from psychiatric inpatient care. Lancet 1993; 342:283–286 [E]
308. Roy A: Suicide in chronic schizophrenia. Br J Psychiatry 1982; 141:171–177 [D]
309. Pirkis J, Burgess P: Suicide and recency of health care contacts: a systematic review. Br J Psychiatry 1998; 173:462–474 [E]
310. Himmelhoch JM: Lest treatment abet suicide. J Clin Psychiatry 1987; 48(suppl):44–54 [F]
311. Bradvik L, Berglund M: Treatment and suicide in severe depression: a case-control study of antidepressant therapy at last contact before suicide. J ECT 2000; 16:399–408 [D]
312. Malone KM, Haas GL, Sweeney JA, Mann JJ: Major depression and the risk of attempted suicide. J Affect Disord 1995; 34:173–185 [G]
313. Fawcett J, Scheftner W, Clark D, Hedeker D, Gibbons R, Coryell W: Clinical predictors of suicide in patients with major affective disorders: a controlled prospective study. Am J Psychiatry 1987; 144:35–40 [D]
314. Baldessarini RJ, Tondo L: Antisuicidal effect of lithium treatment in major mood disorders, in The Harvard Medical School Guide to Suicide Assessment and Intervention. Edited by Jacobs DG. San Francisco, Jossey-Bass, 1998, pp 355–371 [F]

315. Tondo L, Baldessarini RJ, Hennen J, Floris G, Silvetti F, Tohen M: Lithium treatment and risk of suicidal behavior in bipolar disorder patients. J Clin Psychiatry 1998; 59:405–414 [B]
316. Ahrens B, Berghofer A, Wolf T, Muller-Oerlinghausen B: Suicide attempts, age and duration of illness in recurrent affective disorders. J Affect Disord 1995; 36:43–49 [E]
317. Bradvik L, Berglund M: Late mortality in severe depression. Acta Psychiatr Scand 2001; 103:111–116 [C]
318. Clark DC, Gibbons RD, Fawcett J, Scheftner WA: What is the mechanism by which suicide attempts predispose to later suicide attempts? a mathematical model. J Abnorm Psychol 1989; 98:42–49 [G]
319. Hagnell O, Rorsman B: Suicide in the Lundby study: a comparative investigation of clinical aspects. Neuropsychobiology 1979; 5:61–73 [D]
320. Fenton WS, McGlashan TH: Natural history of schizophrenia subtypes. II. positive and negative symptoms and long-term course. Arch Gen Psychiatry 1991; 48:978–986 [C]
321. Conwell Y, Lyness JM, Duberstein P, Cox C, Seidlitz L, DiGiorgio A, Caine ED: Completed suicide among older patients in primary care practices: a controlled study. J Am Geriatr Soc 2000; 48:23–29 [D]
322. Conwell Y, Henderson R, Caine E: Suicide and neurological illness. Neurolog 1995; 1:284–294 [F]
323. Stenager EN, Stenager E: Suicide and patients with neurologic diseases: methodologic problems. Arch Neurol 1992; 49:1296–1303 [E]
324. White SJ, McLean AE, Howland C: Anticonvulsant drugs and cancer: a cohort study in patients with severe epilepsy. Lancet 1979; 2:458–461 [C]
325. Nilsson L, Ahlbom A, Farahmand BY, Asberg M, Tomson T: Risk factors for suicide in epilepsy: a case control study. Epilepsia 2002; 43:644–651 [D]
326. Rafnsson V, Olafsson E, Hauser WA, Gudmundsson G: Cause-specific mortality in adults with unprovoked seizures: a population-based incidence cohort study. Neuroepidemiology 2001; 20:232–236 [G]
327. Fukuchi T, Kanemoto K, Kato M, Ishida S, Yuasa S, Kawasaki J, Suzuki S, Onuma T: Death in epilepsy with special attention to suicide cases. Epilepsy Res 2002; 51:233–236 [D]
328. Barraclough BM: The suicide rate of epilepsy. Acta Psychiatr Scand 1987; 76:339–345 [F]
329. Mendez MF, Cummings JL, Benson DF: Depression in epilepsy: significance and phenomenology. Arch Neurol 1986; 43:766–770 [D]
330. Hawton K, Fagg J, Marsack P: Association between epilepsy and attempted suicide. J Neurol Neurosurg Psychiatry 1980; 43:168–170 [G]
331. Mendez MF, Grau R, Doss RC, Taylor JL: Schizophrenia in epilepsy: seizure and psychosis variables. Neurology 1993; 43:1073–1077 [G]
332. Arciniegas DB, Anderson CA: Suicide in neurologic illness. Curr Treat Options Neurol 2002; 4:457–468 [G]
333. Waern M, Rubenowitz E, Runeson B, Skoog I, Wilhelmson K, Allebeck P: Burden of illness and suicide in elderly people: case-control study. Br Med J 2002; 324:1355 [D]
334. Stenager EN, Stenager E, Koch-Henriksen N, Bronnum-Hansen H, Hyllested K, Jensen K, Bille-Brahe U: Suicide and multiple sclerosis: an epidemiological investigation. J Neurol Neurosurg Psychiatry 1992; 55:542–545 [C]
335. Marzuk PM, Tierney H, Tardiff K, Gross EM, Morgan EB, Hsu MA, Mann JJ: Increased risk of suicide in persons with AIDS. JAMA 1988; 259:1333–1337 [E]
336. Cote TR, Biggar RJ, Dannenberg AL: Risk of suicide among persons with AIDS: a national assessment. JAMA 1992; 268:2066–2068 [G]
337. Quan H, Arboleda-Florez J, Fick GH, Stuart HL, Love EJ: Association between physical illness and suicide among the elderly. Soc Psychiatry Psychiatr Epidemiol 2002; 37:190–197 [D]

338. Grabbe L, Demi A, Camann MA, Potter L: The health status of elderly persons in the last year of life: a comparison of deaths by suicide, injury, and natural causes. Am J Public Health 1997; 87:434–437 [D]
339. Whitlock FA: Suicide and physical illness, in Suicide. Edited by Roy A. Baltimore, Williams & Wilkins, 1986, pp 151–170 [G]
340. Fishbain DA, Goldberg M, Rosomoff RS, Rosomoff H: Completed suicide in chronic pain. Clin J Pain 1991; 7:29–36 [E]
341. Fishbain DA: The association of chronic pain and suicide. Semin Clin Neuropsychiatry 1999; 4:221–227 [F]
342. Chochinov HM, Wilson KG, Enns M, Mowchun N, Lander S, Levitt M, Clinch JJ: Desire for death in the terminally ill. Am J Psychiatry 1995; 152:1185–1191 [C]
343. Cattell H, Jolley DJ: One hundred cases of suicide in elderly people. Br J Psychiatry 1995; 166:451–457 [G]
344. Woodruff RAJ, Clayton PJ, Guze SB: Suicide attempts and psychiatric diagnosis. Dis Nerv Syst 1972; 33:617–621 [G]
345. Roy A: Family history of suicide. Arch Gen Psychiatry 1983; 40:971–974 [D]
346. Tsuang MT: Risk of suicide in the relatives of schizophrenics, manics, depressives, and controls. J Clin Psychiatry 1983; 44:396–400 [D]
347. Linkowski P, de Maertelaer V, Mendlewicz J: Suicidal behavior in major depressive illness. Acta Psychiatr Scand 1985; 72:233–238 [G]
348. Runeson B, Beskow J: Borderline personality disorder in young Swedish suicides. J Nerv Ment Dis 1991; 179:153–156 [G]
349. Pfeffer CR, Normandin L, Kakuma T: Suicidal children grow up: suicidal behavior and psychiatric disorders among relatives. J Am Acad Child Adolesc Psychiatry 1994; 33:1087–1097 [D]
350. Brent DA, Bridge J, Johnson BA, Connolly B: Suicidal behavior runs in families: a controlled family study of adolescent suicide victims. Arch Gen Psychiatry 1996; 53:1145–1152 [D]
351. Gould MS, Fisher P, Parides M, Flory M, Shaffer D: Psychosocial risk factors of child and adolescent completed suicide. Arch Gen Psychiatry 1996; 53:1155–1162 [D]
352. Johnson BA, Brent DA, Bridge J, Connolly J: The familial aggregation of adolescent suicide attempts. Acta Psychiatr Scand 1998; 97:18–24 [D]
353. Foster T, Gillispie K, Patterson C: Risk factors for suicide independent of DSM-III-R axis I disorder: case-control psychological autopsy study in Northern Ireland. Br J Psychiatry 1999; 175:175–179 [D]
354. Cavazzoni P, Grof P, Zvolsky P, Alda M: A family study of suicidal behavior in bipolar-spectrum disorders. Bipolar Disord 1999; 1:27–28 [G]
355. Vijayakumar L, Rajkumar S: Are risk factors for suicide universal? a case-control study in India. Acta Psychiatr Scand 1999; 99:407–411 [D]
356. Cheng AT, Jenkins R: Psychosocial and psychiatric risk factors for suicide: case-control psychological autopsy study. Br J Psychiatry 2000; 177:360–365 [D]
357. Powell J, Geddes J, Hawton K: Suicide in psychiatric hospital inpatients: risk factors and their predictive power. Br J Psychiatry 2000; 176:266–272 [D]
358. Roy A: Relation of family history of suicide to suicide attempts in alcoholics. Am J Psychiatry 2000; 157:2050–2051 [G]
359. Brent DA, Oquendo M, Birmaher B, Greenhill L, Kolko D, Stanley B, Zelazny J, Brodsky B, Bridge J, Ellis S, Salazar JO, Mann JJ: Familial pathways to early-onset suicide attempt: risk for suicidal behavior in offspring of mood-disordered suicide attempters. Arch Gen Psychiatry 2002; 59:801–807 [C]
360. Egeland JA, Sussex JN: Suicide and family loading for affective disorders. JAMA 1985; 254:915–918 [G]

361. Fu Q, Heath AC, Bucholz KK, Nelson EC, Glowinski AL, Goldberg J, Lyons MJ, Tsuang MT, Jacob T, True MR, Eisen SA: A twin study of genetic and environmental influences on suicidality in men. Psychol Med 2002; 32:11–24 [G]
362. Grossman DC, Milligan BC, Deyo RA: Risk factors for suicide attempts among Navajo adolescents. Am J Public Health 1991; 81:870–874 [G]
363. Reynolds P, Eaton P: Multiple attempters of suicide presenting at an emergency department. Can J Psychiatry 1986; 31:328–330 [G]
364. Runeson BS: History of suicidal behaviour in the families of young suicides. Acta Psychiatr Scand 1998; 98:497–501 [G]
365. Roy A, Nielsen D, Rylander G, Sarchiapone M, Segal N: Genetics of suicide in depression. J Clin Psychiatry 1999; 60(suppl 2):12–17 [F]
366. Mann JJ, Brent DA, Arango V: The neurobiology and genetics of suicide and attempted suicide: a focus on the serotonergic system. Neuropsychopharmacology 2001; 24:467–477 [F]
367. McGuffin P, Marusic A, Farmer A: What can psychiatric genetics offer suicidology? Crisis 2001; 22:61–65 [E]
368. Turecki G: Suicidal behavior: is there a genetic predisposition? Bipolar Disord 2001; 3:335–349 [F]
369. Roy A, Rylander G, Sarchiapone M: Genetics of suicides: family studies and molecular genetics. Ann N Y Acad Sci 1997; 836:135–157 [F]
370. Kallman F, Anastasio M: Twin studies on the psychopathology of suicide. J Nerv Ment Dis 1947; 105:40–55 [G]
371. Haberlandt W: Aportacion a la genetica del suicidio (Contribution to the genetics of suicide). Folia Clin Int (Barc) 1967; 17:319–322 [F]
372. Juel-Nielsen N, Videbech T: A twin study of suicide. Acta Genet Med Gemellol (Roma) 1970; 19:307–310 [G]
373. Zair K: A suicidal family. Br J Psychiatry 1981; 189:68–69 [G]
374. Roy A, Segal NL, Centerwall BS, Robinette CD: Suicide in twins. Arch Gen Psychiatry 1991; 48:29–32 [C]
375. Statham DJ, Heath AC, Madden PA, Bucholz KK, Bierut L, Dinwiddie SH, Slutske WS, Dunne MP, Martin NG: Suicidal behaviour: an epidemiological and genetic study. Psychol Med 1998; 28:839–855 [G]
376. Kety SS, Rosenthal D, Wender PH, Schulsinger F: The types and prevalence of mental illness in the biological and adoptive families of adopted schizophrenics. J Psychiatr Res 1968; 6(suppl 1):345–362 [D]
377. Schulsinger F, Kety SS, Rosenthal D, Wender R: A family study of suicide, in Origins, Prevention, and Treatment of Affective Disorders. Edited by Schou M, Stromgren E. New York, Academic Press, 1979, pp 277–287 [G]
378. Wender PH, Kety SS, Rosenthal D, Schulsinger F, Ortmann J, Lunde I: Psychiatric disorders in the biological and adoptive families of adopted individuals with affective disorders. Arch Gen Psychiatry 1986; 43:923–929 [D]
379. Durkheim E: Suicide: A Study in Sociology. New York, Free Press, 1951 [G]
380. Platt S: Unemployment and suicidal behaviour: a review of the literature. Soc Sci Med 1984; 19:93–115 [F]
381. Beautrais AL, Joyce PR, Mulder RT: Unemployment and serious suicide attempts. Psychol Med 1998; 28:209–218 [D]
382. Owens D, Dennis M, Read S, Davis N: Outcome of deliberate self-poisoning: an examination of risk factors for repetition. Br J Psychiatry 1994; 165:797–801 [C]
383. Pirkis J, Burgess P, Dunt D: Suicidal ideation and suicide attempts among Australian adults. Crisis 2000; 21:16–25 [G]

384. Hawton K, Fagg J, Platt S, Hawkins M: Factors associated with suicide after parasuicide in young people. Br Med J 1993; 306:1641–1644 [D]
385. Johansson SE, Sundquist J: Unemployment is an important risk factor for suicide in contemporary Sweden: an 11-year follow-up study of a cross-sectional sample of 37,789 people. Public Health 1997; 111:41–45 [C]
386. Hawton K, Harriss L, Hodder K, Simkin S, Gunnell D: The influence of the economic and social environment on deliberate self-harm and suicide: an ecological and person-based study. Psychol Med 2001; 31:827–836 [D]
387. Conner KR, Duberstein PR, Conwell Y: Age-related patterns of factors associated with completed suicide in men with alcohol dependence. Am J Addict 1999; 8:312–318 [G]
388. Tsuang MT, Simpson JC, Fleming JA: Epidemiology of suicide. Int Rev Psychiatry 1992; 4:117–129 [E]
389. Khan MM, Reza H: The pattern of suicide in Pakistan. Crisis 2000; 21:31–35 [G]
390. Kamal Z, Lowenthal KM: Suicide beliefs and behaviour among young Muslims and Hindus in the UK. Ment Health Relig Cult 2002; 5:111–118 [D]
391. Ineichen B: The influence of religion on the suicide rate: Islam and Hinduism compared. Ment Health Relig Cult 1998; 1:31–36 [G]
392. Simpson ME, Conklin GH: Socioeconomic development, suicide, and religion. Social Forces 1989; 67:945–964 [G]
393. Lester D: Islam and suicide. Psychol Rep 2000; 87:692 [G]
394. Maris RW: Pathways to Suicide: A Survey of Self-Destructive Behaviors. Baltimore, Johns Hopkins University Press, 1981 [G]
395. Hilton SC, Fellingham GW, Lyon JL: Suicide rates and religious commitment in young adult males in Utah. Am J Epidemiol 2002; 155:413–419 [G]
396. Neeleman J, Wessely S, Lewis G: Suicide acceptability in African- and white Americans: the role of religion. J Nerv Ment Dis 1998; 186:12–16 [G]
397. Neeleman J, Halpern D, Leon D, Lewis G: Tolerance of suicide, religion and suicide rates: an ecological and individual study in 19 Western countries. Psychol Med 1997; 27:1165–1171 [G]
398. Nisbet PA, Duberstein PR, Conwell Y, Seidlitz L: The effect of participation in religious activities on suicide versus natural death in adults 50 and older. J Nerv Ment Dis 2000; 188:543–546 [D]
399. Miller M: Geriatric suicide: the Arizona study. Gerontologist 1978; 18:488–495 [D]
400. Turvey CL, Conwell Y, Jones MP, Phillips C, Simonsick E, Pearson JL, Wallace R: Risk factors for late-life suicide: a prospective, community-based study. Am J Geriatr Psychiatry 2002; 10:398–406 [C]
401. Stravynski A, Boyer R: Loneliness in relation to suicide ideation and parasuicide: a population-wide study. Suicide Life Threat Behav 2001; 31:32–40 [C]
402. Heikkinen ME, Isometsa ET, Marttunen MJ, Aro HM, Lonnqvist JK: Social factors in suicide. Br J Psychiatry 1995; 167:747–753 [C]
403. Beautrais AL: A case control study of suicide and attempted suicide in older adults. Suicide Life Threat Behav 2002; 32:1–9 [D]
404. Phillips MR, Yang G, Zhang Y, Wang L, Ji H, Zhou M: Risk factors for suicide in China: a national case-control psychological autopsy study. Lancet 2002; 360:1728–1736 [D]
405. Rubenowitz E, Waern M, Wilhelmson K, Allebeck P: Life events and psychosocial factors in elderly suicides—a case-control study. Psychol Med 2001; 31:1193–1202 [D]
406. Beautrais AL: Suicides and serious suicide attempts: two populations or one? Psychol Med 2001; 31:837–845 [D]
407. Linehan MM, Goodstein JL, Nielsen SL, Chiles JA: Reasons for staying alive when you are thinking of killing yourself: the reasons for living inventory. J Consult Clin Psychol 1983; 51:276–286 [D]

408. Wenz FV: Family constellation factors and parent suicide potential. J Nerv Ment Dis 1982; 170:270–274 [G]
409. Josepho SA, Plutchik R: Stress, coping, and suicide risk in psychiatric inpatients. Suicide Life Threat Behav 1994; 24:48–57 [D]
410. Shneidman ES: Overview: a multidimensional approach to suicide, in Suicide: Understanding and Responding. Edited by Jacobs D, Brown HN. Madison, Conn, International Universities Press, 1989, pp 1–30 [G]
411. Marttunen MJ, Aro HM, Henriksson MM, Lonnqvist JK: Antisocial behaviour in adolescent suicide. Acta Psychiatr Scand 1994; 89:167–173 [G]
412. Maltsberger JT: Suicide danger: clinical estimation and decision. Suicide Life Threat Behav 1988; 18:47–54 [G]
413. Kaslow NJ, Reviere SL, Chance SE, Rogers JH, Hatcher CA, Wasserman F, Smith L, Jessee S, James ME, Seelig B: An empirical study of the psychodynamics of suicide. J Am Psychoanal Assoc 1998; 46:777–796 [D]
414. Gabbard GO: Psychodynamic psychotherapy of borderline personality disorder: a contemporary approach. Bull Menninger Clin 2001; 65:41–57 [G]
415. Menninger K: Psychoanalytic aspects of suicide. Int J Psychoanal 1933; 14:376–390 [G]
416. Asch SS: Suicide and the hidden executioner. Int Rev Psychoanal 1980; 7:51–60 [G]
417. Meissner WW: Psychotherapy and the Paranoid Process. Northvale, NJ, Jason Aronson, 1986 [G]
418. Fenichel O: The Psychoanalytic Theory of Neurosis. New York, WW Norton, 1945 [G]
419. Dorpat TL: Suicide, loss, and mourning. Suicide Life Threat Behav 1973; 3:213–224 [G]
420. Gabbard GO: Psychodynamic Psychiatry in Clinical Practice, 3rd ed. Washington, DC, American Psychiatric Press, 2000 [G]
421. Shneidman ES: Suicide as psychache: a clinical approach to self-destructive behavior. J Nerv Ment Dis 1993; 181:147–149 [G]
422. Hughes SL, Neimeyer RA: Cognitive predictors of suicide risk among hospitalized psychiatric patients: a prospective study. Death Stud 1993; 17:103–124 [C]
423. Duberstein PR: Are closed-minded people more open to the idea of killing themselves? Suicide Life Threat Behav 2001; 31:9–14 [C]
424. Duberstein PR, Conwell Y, Caine ED: Age differences in the personality characteristics of suicide completers: preliminary findings from a psychological autopsy study. Psychiatry 1994; 57:213–224 [D]
425. Shulman E: Vulnerability factors in Sylvia Plath's suicide. Death Stud 1998; 22:597–613 [G]
426. Birtchnell J: Psychotherapeutic considerations in the management of the suicidal patient. Am J Psychother 1983; 37:24–36 [G]
427. Kessler RC, Borges G, Walters EE: Prevalence of and risk factors for lifetime suicide attempts in the National Comorbidity Survey. Arch Gen Psychiatry 1999; 56:617–626 [C]
428. Beck AT, Brown GK, Steer RA, Dahlsgaard KK, Grisham JR: Suicide ideation at its worst point: a predictor of eventual suicide in psychiatric outpatients. Suicide Life Threat Behav 1999; 29:1–9 [C]
429. Kroll J: Use of no-suicide contracts by psychiatrists in Minnesota. Am J Psychiatry 2000; 157:1684–1686 [C]
430. Drew BL: Self-harm behavior and no-suicide contracting in psychiatric inpatient settings. Arch Psychiatr Nurs 2001; 15:99–106 [C]
431. Robins E: The Final Months: A Study of the Lives of 134 Persons Who Committed Suicide. New York, Oxford University Press, 1981 [G]
432. Simon OR, Swann AC, Powell KE, Potter LB, Kresnow MJ, O'Carroll PW: Characteristics of impulsive suicide attempts and attempters. Suicide Life Threat Behav 2001; 32:49–59 [D]
433. Weissman A, Worden JW: Risk-rescue rating in suicide assessment. Arch Gen Psychiatry 1972; 26:553–560 [G]

434. Kaplan MS, Geling O: Sociodemographic and geographic patterns of firearm suicide in the United States, 1989–1993. Health Place 1999; 5:179–185 [F]
435. Hawton K, Townsend E, Deeks J, Appleby L, Gunnell D, Bennewith O, Cooper J: Effects of legislation restricting pack sizes of paracetamol and salicylate on self poisoning in the United Kingdom: before and after study. Br Med J 2001; 322:1203–1207 [C]
436. Gunnell D, Middleton N, Frankel S: Method availability and the prevention of suicide: a re-analysis of secular trends in England and Wales 1950–1975. Soc Psychiatry Psychiatr Epidemiol 2000; 35:437–443 [C]
437. Marzuk PM, Leon AC, Tardiff K, Morgan EB, Stajic M, Mann JJ: The effect of access to lethal methods of injury on suicide rates. Arch Gen Psychiatry 1992; 49:451–458 [C]
438. Brent DA, Perper JA, Allman CJ, Moritz GM, Wartella ME, Zelenak JP: The presence and accessibility of firearms in the homes of adolescent suicides: a case-control study. JAMA 1991; 266:2989–2995 [D]
439. Beck AT, Beck R, Kovacs M: Classification of suicidal behaviors. I. quantifying intent and medical lethality. Am J Psychiatry 1975; 132:285–287 [G]
440. Beck AT, Weissman A, Lester D, Trexler L: Classification of suicidal behaviors. II. dimensions of suicidal intent. Arch Gen Psychiatry 1976; 33:835–837 [G]
441. Pierce DW: The predictive validation of a suicide intent scale: a five year follow-up. Br J Psychiatry 1981; 139:391–396 [C]
442. Sharma V, Persad E, Kueneman K: A closer look at inpatient suicide. J Affect Disord 1998; 47:123–129 [D]
443. Myers DH, Neal CD: Suicide in psychiatric patients. Br J Psychiatry 1978; 133:38–44 [G]
444. Breslow RE, Klinger BI, Erickson BJ: Acute intoxication and substance abuse among patients presenting to a psychiatric emergency service. Gen Hosp Psychiatry 1996; 18:183–191 [G]
445. Jacobs D: Evaluation and care of suicidal behavior in emergency settings. Int J Psychiatry Med 1982; 12:295–310 [F]
446. Schnyder U, Valach L: Suicide attempters in a psychiatric emergency room population. Gen Hosp Psychiatry 1997; 19:119–129 [G]
447. Szuster RR, Schanbacher BL, McCann SC: Characteristics of psychiatric emergency room patients with alcohol- or drug-induced disorders. Hosp Community Psychiatry 1990; 41:1342–1345 [G]
448. Hillard JR, Ramm D, Zung WW, Holland JM: Suicide in a psychiatric emergency room population. Am J Psychiatry 1983; 140:459–462 [C]
449. Skelton H, Dann LM, Ong RT, Hamilton T, Ilett KF: Drug screening of patients who deliberately harm themselves admitted to the emergency department. Ther Drug Monit 1998; 20:98–103 [G]
450. Dennis M, Beach M, Evans PA, Winston A, Friedman T: An examination of the accident and emergency management of deliberate self harm. J Accid Emerg Med 1997; 14:311–315 [G]
451. Dhossche DM: Suicidal behavior in psychiatric emergency room patients. South Med J 2000; 93:310–314 [G]
452. Hawley CJ, James DV, Birkett PL, Baldwin DS, de Ruiter MJ, Priest RG: Suicidal ideation as a presenting complaint: associated diagnoses and characteristics in a casualty population. Br J Psychiatry 1991; 159:232–238 [G]
453. McGrath J: A survey of deliberate self-poisoning. Med J Aust 1989; 150:317–318, 320–321, 324 [G]
454. Varadaraj R, Mendonca J: A survey of blood-alcohol levels in self-poisoning cases. Adv Alcohol Subst Abuse 1987; 7:63–69 [G]
455. Simon RI, Goetz S: Forensic issues in the psychiatric emergency department. Psychiatr Clin North Am 1999; 22:851–864 [G]

456. Kastenbaum R, Mishara BL: Premature death and self-injurious behavior in old age. Geriatrics 1971; 26:71–81 [C]
457. Nelson FL, Farberow NL: The development of an Indirect Self-Destructive Behaviour Scale for use with chronically ill medical patients. Int J Soc Psychiatry 1982; 28:5–14 [C]
458. Draper B, Brodaty H, Low LF: Types of nursing home residents with self-destructive behaviours: analysis of the Harmful Behaviours Scale. Int J Geriatr Psychiatry 2002; 17:670–675 [G]
459. Draper B, Brodaty H, Low LF, Richards V, Paton H, Lie D: Self-destructive behaviors in nursing home residents. J Am Geriatr Soc 2002; 50:354–358 [G]
460. Osgood NJ, Brant BA: Suicidal behavior in long-term care facilities. Suicide Life Threat Behav 1990; 20:113–122 [G]
461. Abrams RC, Young RC, Holt JH, Alexopoulos GS: Suicide in New York City nursing homes: 1980–1986. Am J Psychiatry 1988; 145:1487–1488 [G]
462. Rovner BW, Kafonek S, Filipp L, Lucas MJ, Folstein MF: Prevalence of mental illness in a community nursing home. Am J Psychiatry 1986; 143:1446–1449 [G]
463. Tariot PN, Podgorski CA, Blazina L, Leibovici A: Mental disorders in the nursing home: another perspective. Am J Psychiatry 1993; 150:1063–1069 [G]
464. Nelson FL, Farberow NL: Indirect self-destructive behavior in the elderly nursing home patient. J Gerontol 1980; 35:949–957 [G]
465. American Psychiatric Association: Psychiatric Services in Jails and Prisons, 2nd ed. Washington, DC, American Psychiatric Association, 2000 [G]
466. Metzner JL, Miller RD, Kleinsasser D: Mental health screening and evaluation within prisons. Bull Am Acad Psychiatry Law 1994; 22:451–457 [F]
467. Metzner JL: Class action litigation in correctional psychiatry. J Am Acad Psychiatry Law 2002; 30:19–29 [F]
468. Maruschak LM: HIV in Prisons and Jails, 1999. Bureau of Justice Statistics Bulletin NCJ 187456. Washington, DC, US Department of Justice, Bureau of Justice Statistics, July 2001 [E]
469. Hayes LM: Prison Suicide: An Overview and Guide to Prevention. Washington, DC, US Department of Justice, National Institute of Corrections, 1995 [G]
470. McKee GR: Lethal vs nonlethal suicide attempts in jail. Psychol Rep 1998; 82:611–614 [G]
471. Bell CC: Correctional psychiatry, in Kaplan and Sadock's Comprehensive Textbook of Psychiatry, 8th ed. Edited by Sadock BJ, Sadock VA. Philadelphia, Lippincott Williams & Wilkins (in press) [G]
472. Metzner JL: An introduction to correctional psychiatry, part I. J Am Acad Psychiatry Law 1997; 25:375–381 [F]
473. Marcus P, Alcabes P: Characteristics of suicides by inmates in an urban jail. Hosp Community Psychiatry 1993; 44:256–261 [C]
474. Hayes LM, Kajden B: And Darkness Closes In...A National Study of Jail Suicides: Final Report to the National Institute of Corrections. Washington, DC, National Center on Institutions and Alternatives, 1981 [E]
475. Salive ME, Smith GS, Brewer TF: Suicide mortality in the Maryland state prison system, 1979 through 1987. JAMA 1989; 262:365–369 [G]
476. Hayes LM: National study of jail suicides: seven years later. Psychiatr Q 1989; 60:7–29 [F]
477. Dooley E: Prison suicide in England and Wales, 1972–87. Br J Psychiatry 1990; 156:40–45 [G]
478. Wobeser WL, Datema J, Bechard B, Ford P: Causes of death among people in custody in Ontario, 1990–1999. Can Med Assoc J 2002; 167:1109–1113 [G]
479. Bonner RL: Isolation, seclusion, and psychosocial vulnerability as risk factors for suicide behind bars, in Assessment and Prediction of Suicide. Edited by Berman AL, Maris RW, Maltsberger JT, Yufit RI. New York, Guilford, 2002, pp 398–419 [F]
480. Felthous AR: Does "isolation" cause jail suicides? J Am Acad Psychiatry Law 1997; 25:285–294 [F]

481. Cox JF, Landsberg G, Paravati MP: The essential components of a crisis intervention program for local jails: the New York Local Forensic Suicide Prevention Crisis Service Model. Psychiatr Q 1989; 60:103–117 [F]
482. Freeman A, Alaimo C: Prevention of suicide in a large urban jail. Psychiatr Ann 2001; 31:447–452 [F]
483. Rowan JR, Hayes LM: Training Curriculum on Suicide Detection and Prevention in Jails and Lockups. Washington, DC, National Institute of Corrections, 1995 [G]
484. National Commission on Correctional Health Care: Standards for Health Services in Jails. Chicago, National Commission on Correctional Health Care, 1996 [G]
485. National Commission on Correctional Health Care: Standards for Health Services in Prisons. Chicago, National Commission on Correctional Health Care, 1997 [G]
486. Sherman LG, Morschauser PC: Screening for suicide risk in inmates. Psychiatr Q 1989; 60:119–138 [F]
487. National Commission on Correctional Health Care: Correctional Mental Health Care: Standards and Guidelines for Delivering Services. Chicago, National Commission on Correctional Health Care, 1999 [G]
488. Havens LL: The anatomy of a suicide. N Engl J Med 1965; 272:401–406 [G]
489. Jacobs D: Psychotherapy with suicidal patients: the empathic method, in Suicide: Understanding and Responding. Edited by Jacobs D, Brown HN. Madison, Conn, International Universities Press, 1989, pp 329–342 [G]
490. Hendin H: Psychotherapy and suicide. Am J Psychother 1981; 35:469–480 [G]
491. Schwartz D, Flinn DE, Slawson PF: Treatment of the suicidal character. Am J Psychother 1974; 28:194–207 [G]
492. Shneidman E: Psychotherapy with suicidal patients, in Specialized Techniques in Individual Psychotherapy. Edited by Karasu TB, Bellak L. New York, Brunner/Mazel, 1980, pp 304–313 [G]
493. Richmond J, Eyman JR: Psychotherapy of suicide: individual, group, and family approaches, in Understanding Suicide: The State of the Art. Edited by Lester D. Philadelphia, Charles C Thomas, 1990, pp 139–158 [G]
494. Smith K, Eyman J: Ego structure and object differentiation in suicidal patients, in Primitive Mental States and the Rorschach. Edited by Lerner HD, Lerner PM. New York, International Universities Press, 1988, pp 175–202 [G]
495. Gabbard G, Lester E: Boundaries and Boundary Violations in Psychoanalysis. New York, Basic Books, 1995 [G]
496. Maltsberger JT, Buie DH: The devices of suicide. Int Rev Psychoanal 1980; 7:61–71 [G]
497. Jacobs D: Evaluation and management of the violent patient in emergency settings. Psychiatr Clin North Am 1983; 6:259–269 [G]
498. American Psychiatric Association, American Psychiatric Nurses Association, National Association of Psychiatric Health Systems: Learning From Each Other: Success Stories and Ideas for Reducing Restraint/Seclusion in Behavioral Health. Arlington, Va, American Psychiatric Association, 2003. http://www.psych. org/clin_res/learningfromeachother.cfm [G]
499. McCulloch LE, McNiel DE, Binder RL, Hatcher C: Effects of a weapon screening procedure in a psychiatric emergency room. Hosp Community Psychiatry 1986; 37:837–838 [G]
500. Paris J: Chronic suicidality among patients with borderline personality disorder. Psychiatr Serv 2002; 53:738–742 [E]
501. Waterhouse J, Platt S: General hospital admission in the management of parasuicide: a randomised controlled trial. Br J Psychiatry 1990; 156:236–242 [A–]
502. Bongar B, Maris RW, Berman AL, Litman RE, Silverman MM: Inpatient standards of care and the suicidal patient, part I: general clinical formulations and legal considerations. Suicide Life Threat Behav 1993; 23:245–256 [G]

503. McCormick JJ, Currier GW: Emergency medicine and mental health law. Top Emerg Med 1999; 21:28–37 [G]
504. Stewart SE, Manion IG, Davidson S, Cloutier P: Suicidal children and adolescents with first emergency room presentations: predictors of six-month outcome. J Am Acad Child Adolesc Psychiatry 2001; 40:580–587 [G]
505. Craig TJ, Huffine CL, Brooks M: Completion of referral to psychiatric services by inner city residents. Arch Gen Psychiatry 1974; 31:353–357 [B]
506. Knesper DJ: A study of referral failures for potentially suicidal patients: a method of medical care evaluation. Hosp Community Psychiatry 1982; 33:49–52 [G]
507. Jellinek M: Referrals from a psychiatric emergency room: relationship of compliance to demographic and interview variables. Am J Psychiatry 1978; 135:209–213 [G]
508. Dressler DM, Prusoff B, Mark H, Shapiro D: Clinician attitudes toward the suicide attempter. J Nerv Ment Dis 1975; 160:146–155 [G]
509. Gillig PM, Hillard JR, Deddens JA, Bell J, Combs HE: Clinicians' self-reported reactions to psychiatric emergency patients: effect on treatment decisions. Psychiatr Q 1990; 61:155–162 [G]
510. Rotheram-Borus MJ, Piacentini J, Cantwell C, Belin TR, Song J: The 18-month impact of an emergency room intervention for adolescent female suicide attempters. J Consult Clin Psychol 2000; 68:1081–1093 [C]
511. American Psychiatric Association: Practice guideline for the treatment of patients with major depressive disorder (revision). Am J Psychiatry 2000; 157(April suppl):1–45 [G]
512. American Psychiatric Association: Practice guideline for the treatment of patients with bipolar disorder (revision). Am J Psychiatry 2002; 159(April suppl):1–50 [G]
513. American Psychiatric Association: Practice guideline for the treatment of patients with schizophrenia. Am J Psychiatry 1997; 154(April suppl):1–63 [G]
514. American Psychiatric Association: Practice guideline for the treatment of patients with panic disorder. Am J Psychiatry 1998; 155(May suppl):1–34 [G]
515. American Psychiatric Association: Practice guideline for the treatment of patients with borderline personality disorder. Am J Psychiatry 2001; 158(Oct suppl):1–52 [G]
516. Cornelius JR, Salloum IM, Lynch K, Clark DB, Mann JJ: Treating the substance-abusing suicidal patient. Ann N Y Acad Sci 2001; 932:78–90 [E]
517. Lin EH, Von Korff M, Katon W, Bush T, Simon GE, Walker E, Robinson P: The role of the primary care physician in patients' adherence to antidepressant therapy. Med Care 1995; 33:67–74 [B]
518. Welch SS: A review of the literature on the epidemiology of parasuicide in the general population. Psychiatr Serv 2001; 52:368–375 [F]
519. Brown MZ, Comtois KA, Linehan MM: Reasons for suicide attempts and nonsuicidal self-injury in women with borderline personality disorder. J Abnorm Psychol 2002; 111:198–202 [G]
520. Favazza A: Self-mutilation, in The Harvard Medical School Guide to Suicide Assessment and Intervention. Edited by Jacobs DG. San Francisco, Jossey-Bass, 1998, pp 125–145 [F]
521. Soloff PH, Lis JA, Kelly T, Cornelius J, Ulrich R: Self-mutilation and suicidal behavior in borderline personality disorder. J Personal Disord 1994; 8:257–267 [D/E]
522. Linehan MM, Armstrong HE, Suarez A, Allmon D, Heard HL: Cognitive-behavioral treatment of chronically parasuicidal borderline patients. Arch Gen Psychiatry 1991; 48:1060–1064 [A–]
523. Linehan MM, Schmidt H III, Dimeff LA, Craft JC, Kanter J, Comtois KA: Dialectical behavior therapy for patients with borderline personality disorder and drug-dependence. Am J Addict 1999; 8:279–292 [A]
524. Rudd MD, Joiner T, Rajab MH: Relationships among suicide ideators, attempters, and multiple attempters in a young-adult sample. J Abnorm Psychol 1996; 105:541–550 [C]

525. Gerbasi JB, Bonnie RJ, Binder RL: Resource document on mandatory outpatient treatment. J Am Acad Psychiatry Law 2000; 28:127–144 [F]
526. Baldessarini RJ: Drugs and the treatment of psychiatric disorders: antidepressant and antianxiety agents, in Goodman and Gilman's The Pharmacological Basis of Therapeutics, 10th ed. Edited by Hardman JG, Limbird LE, Gilman AG. New York, McGraw-Hill, 2001, pp 485–520 [G]
527. Cornelius JR, Salloum IM, Thase ME, Haskett RF, Daley DC, Jones-Barlock A, Upsher C, Perel JM: Fluoxetine versus placebo in depressed alcoholic cocaine abusers. Psychopharmacol Bull 1998; 34:117–121 [A]
528. Malone KM: Pharmacotherapy of affectively ill suicidal patients. Psychiatr Clin North Am 1997; 20:613–625 [G]
529. Angst J, Sellaro R, Angst F: Long-term outcome and mortality of treated vs untreated bipolar and depressed patients: a preliminary report. Int J Psychiatr Clin Pract 1998; 2:115–119 [D]
530. Müller-Oerlinghausen B, Berghofer A: Antidepressants and suicidal risk. J Clin Psychiatry 1999; 60(suppl 2):94–99 [F]
531. Carlsten A, Waern M, Ekedahl A, Ranstam J: Antidepressant medication and suicide in Sweden. Pharmacoepidemiol Drug Saf 2001; 10:525–530 [G]
532. Joyce PR: Improvements in the recognition and treatment of depression and decreasing suicide rates. N Z Med J 2001; 114:535–536 [G]
533. Baldessarini RJ, Hennen J, Kwok KW, Ioanitescu DO, Ragade J, Tondo L, Simhandl C: Suicidal risk and assessment and antidepressant treatment: a meta-analysis (unpublished manuscript). Mailman Research Center, McLean Hospital, Belmont, Mass, 2002 [E]
534. Prien RF, Klett CJ, Caffey CM: Lithium prophylaxis in recurrent affective illness. Am J Psychiatry 1974; 131:198–203 [B]
535. Avery D, Winokur G: Suicide, attempted suicide, and relapse rates in depression. Arch Gen Psychiatry 1978; 35:749–753 [C]
536. Rouillon F, Phillips R, Serrurier D, Ansart E, Gérard MJ: Rechutes de dépression unipolaire et efficacité de la maprotiline (RECURRENCE OF UNIPOLAR DEPRESSION AND EFFICACY OF MAPROTILINE). L'Éncephale 1989; 15:527–534 [A]
537. Beasley CM Jr, Dornseif BE, Bosomworth JC, Sayler ME, Rampey AHJ, Heiligenstein JH, Thompson VL, Murphy DJ, Masica DN: Fluoxetine and suicide: a meta-analysis of controlled trials of treatment for depression. Br Med J 1991; 303:685–692 [E]
538. Jick H, Ulcickas M, Dean A: Comparison of frequencies of suicidal tendencies among patients receiving fluoxetine, lofepramine, mianserin, or trazodone. Pharmacotherapy 1992; 12:451–454 [G]
539. Möller H-J, Steinmeyer EM: Are serotonergic reuptake inhibitors more potent in reducing suicidality? an empirical study on paroxetine. Eur Neuropsychopharmacol 1994; 4:55–59 [A]
540. Jick SS, Dean AD, Jick H: Antidepressants and suicide. Br Med J 1995; 310:215–218 [C/D]
541. Montgomery SA, Dunner DL, Dunbar GC: Reduction of suicidal thoughts with paroxetine in comparison with reference antidepressants and placebo. Eur Neuropsychopharmacol 1995; 5:5–13 [E]
542. Warshaw MG, Keller MB: The relationships between fluoxetine use and suicidal behavior in 654 subjects with anxiety disorders. J Clin Psychiatry 1996; 57:158–166 [C]
543. Kasper S: The place of milnacipran in the treatment of depression. Hum Psychopharmacol 1997; 12(suppl):135–141 [F]
544. Mucci M: Reboxetine: a review of antidepressant tolerability. J Psychopharmacol 1997; 11(suppl 4):S33–S37 [B]
545. Leon AC, Keller MB, Warshaw MG, Mueller TI, Solomon DA, Coryell W, Endicott J: Prospective study of fluoxetine treatment and suicidal behavior in affectively ill subjects. Am J Psychiatry 1999; 156:195–201 [C]

546. Khan A, Warner HA, Brown WA: Symptom reduction and suicide risk in patients treated with placebo in antidepressant clinical trials: an analysis of the Food and Drug Administration database. Arch Gen Psychiatry 2000; 57:311–317 [G]
547. Khan A, Khan SR, Leventhal RM, Brown WA: Symptom reduction and suicide risk among patients treated with placebo in antipsychotic clinical trials: an analysis of the Food and Drug Administration database. Am J Psychiatry 2001; 158:1449–1454 [C]
548. Khan A, Khan S, Kolts R, Brown WA: Suicide rates in clinical trials of SSRIs, other antidepressants, and placebo: analysis of FDA reports. Am J Psychiatry 2003; 160:790–792 [E]
549. Ohberg A, Vuori E, Klaukka T, Lonnqvist J: Antidepressants and suicide mortality. J Affect Disord 1998; 50:225–233 [F]
550. Isacsson G, Holmgren P, Druid H, Bergman U: Psychotropics and suicide prevention: implications from toxicological screening of 5,281 suicides in Sweden 1992–1994. Br J Psychiatry 1999; 174:259–265 [G]
551. Rothschild AJ, Locke CA: Re-exposure to fluoxetine after serious suicide attempts by three patients: the role of akathisia. J Clin Psychiatry 1992; 52:491–492 [G]
552. Teicher MH, Glod C, Cole JO: Emergence of intense suicidal preoccupation during fluoxetine treatment. Am J Psychiatry 1990; 147:207–210 [E]
553. Healy D, Langmaak C, Savage M: Suicide in the course of the treatment of depression. J Psychopharmacol 1999; 13:94–99 [F]
554. Tollefson GD, Rampey AH, Beasley CM, Enas GG, Potvin JH: Absence of a relationship between adverse events and suicidality during pharmacotherapy for depression. J Clin Psychopharmacol 1994; 14:163–169 [E]
555. Beasley CM Jr, Potvin JH, Masica DN, Wheadon DE, Dornseif BE, Genduso LA: Fluoxetine: no association with suicidality in obsessive-compulsive disorder. J Affect Disord 1992; 24:1–10 [A]
556. Cassidy S, Henry J: Fatal toxicity of antidepressant drugs in overdose. Br Med J 1987; 295:1021–1024 [G]
557. Kapur S, Mieczkowski T, Mann JJ: Antidepressant medications and the relative risk of suicide attempt and suicide. JAMA 1992; 268:3441–3445 [E]
558. Baldessarini RJ, Tondo L, Hennen J: Treating the suicidal patient with bipolar disorder: reducing suicide risk with lithium. Ann N Y Acad Sci 2001; 932:24–38 [E]
559. Coppen A, Standish-Barry H, Bailey J, Houston G, Silcocks P, Hermon S: Does lithium reduce mortality of recurrent mood disorders? J Affect Disord 1991; 23:1–7 [C]
560. Crundwell JK: Lithium and its potential benefit in reducing increased mortality rates due to suicide. Lithium 1994; 5:193–204 [C]
561. Nilsson A: Lithium therapy and suicide risk. J Clin Psychiatry 1999; 60(suppl 2):85–88 [C]
562. Baldessarini RJ, Tondo L, Hennen J, Viguera AC: Is lithium still worth using? an update of selected recent research. Harv Rev Psychiatry 2002; 10:59–75 [E]
563. Baldessarini RJ, Tondo L, Hennen J: Lithium treatment and suicide risk in major affective disorders: update and new findings. J Clin Psychiatry 2003; 64(suppl 5):44–52 [E]
564. Tondo L, Ghiani C, Albert M: Pharmacologic interventions in suicide prevention. J Clin Psychiatry 2001; 62:51–55 [F]
565. Tondo L, Hennen J, Baldessarini RJ: Lower suicide risk with long-term lithium treatment in major affective illness: a meta-analysis. Acta Psychiatr Scand 2001; 104:163–172 [E]
566. Baastrup PC, Poulsen JC, Schou M, Thomsen K, Amdisen A: Prophylactic lithium: double-blind discontinuation in manic-depressive and recurrent-depressive disorders. Lancet 1970; 1:326–330 [A]
567. Bech P, Vendsborg PB, Rafaelsen O: Lithium maintenance treatment of manic-melancholic patients: its role in the daily routine. Acta Psychiatr Scand 1976; 53:70–81 [G]
568. Kay DWK, Petterson U: Manic-depressive illness. Acta Psychiatr Scand 1977; 269(suppl): 55–60 [G]

569. Poole AJ, James HD, Hughes WC: Treatment experiences in the lithium clinic at St. Thomas' Hospital. J R Soc Med 1978; 71:890–894 [C]
570. Glen AIM, Dodd M, Hulme EB, Kreitman N: Mortality on lithium. Neuropsychobiology 1979; 5:167–173 [G]
571. Ahlfors UG, Baastrup PC, Dencker SJ, Elgen K, Lingjærde O, Pedersen V, Schou M, Aaskoven O: Flupentixol decanoate in recurrent manic-depressive illness: a comparison with lithium. Acta Psychiatr Scand 1981; 64:226–237 [A–]
572. Venkoba-Rao A, Hariharasubramanian N, Parvathi-Devi S, Sugumar A, Srinivasan V: Lithium prophylaxis in affective disorder. Indian J Psychiatry 1982; 23:22–23 [C]
573. Hanus K, Zalpetálek M: Suicidal activity of patients with affective disorders in the course of lithium prophylaxis. Ceskoslovenská Psychiatrie 1984; 80:97–100 [C]
574. Norton B, Whalley LH: Mortality of a lithium treatment population. Br J Psychiatry 1984; 145:277–282 [C]
575. Lepkifker E, Horesh N, Floru S: Long-term lithium prophylaxis in recurrent unipolar depression: a controversial indication. Acta Psychiatr Belg 1985; 85:434–443 [C]
576. Jamison KR: Suicide and bipolar disorders. Ann N Y Acad Sci 1986; 487:301–315 [F]
577. Page C, Benaim S, Lappin F: A long-term retrospective follow-up study of patients treated with prophylactic lithium carbonate. Br J Psychiatry 1987; 150:175–179 [C]
578. Schou M, Weeke A: Did manic-depressive patients who committed suicide receive prophylactic or continuation treatment at the time? Br J Psychiatry 1988; 153:324–327 [G]
579. Wehr TS, Sack DA, Rosenthal NE, Cowdry RW: Rapid cycling affective disorder: contributing factors and treatment responses in 51 patients. Am J Psychiatry 1988; 145:179–184 [G]
580. Nilsson AR, Axelsson R: Lithium discontinuers: clinical characteristics and outcome. Acta Psychiatr Scand 1990; 82:433–438 [C]
581. O'Connell R, Mayo JA, Flatow L, Cuthbertson VB, O'Brien NE: Outcome of bipolar disorder on long-term treatment with lithium. Br J Psychiatry 1991; 159:123–129 [B]
582. Vestergaard P, Aagaard J: Five-year mortality in lithium-treated manic-depressive patients. J Affect Disord 1991; 21:33–38 [C]
583. Modestin J, Schwartzenbach F: Effect of psychopharmacotherapy on suicide risk in discharged psychiatric inpatients. Acta Psychiatr Scand 1992; 85:173–175 [D]
584. Müller-Oerlinghausen B, Müser-Causemann B, Volk J: Suicides and parasuicides in a high-risk patient group on and off lithium long-term medication. J Affect Disord 1992; 25:261–270 [C]
585. Rihmer Z, Rutz W, Barsi J: Suicide rate, prevalence of diagnosed depression and prevalence of working physicians in Hungary. Acta Psychiatr Scand 1993; 88:391–394 [G]
586. Felber W, Kyber A: Suizide und parasuizide während und ausserhalb einer lithium prophylaxe, in Ziele und Ergebnisse der Medikamentosen Prophylaxe Affektiver Psychosen. Edited by Müller-Oerlinghausen B, Berghöfer A. Stuttgart, Germany, G Thieme Verlag, 1994, pp 53–59 [G]
587. Lenz G, Ahrens B, Denk BE, Müller-Oerlinghausen B, Schatzberger-Topitz A, Simhandl C, Wancata J: Mortalität nach ausschneiden aus der lithiumambulanz (Increased mortality after drop-out from lithium clinic), in Ziele und Ergebnisse der Medicamentösen Prophylaxe Affecktiver Psychosen. Edited by Müller-Oerlinghausen B, Berghöfer A. Stuttgart, Germany, G Theme Verlag, 1994, pp 49–52 [G]
588. Müller-Oerlinghausen B: Die "IGSLI" Studie zur mortalität lithium behandelter patienten mit affektiven psychosen, in Ziele und Ergebnisse der Medikamentosen Prophylaxe Affektiver Psychosen. Edited by Müller-Oerlinghausen B, Berghöfer A. Stuttgart, Germany, G Thieme Verlag, 1994, pp 35–40 [F]
589. Ahrens B, Müller-Oerlinghausen B, Schou M, Wolf T, Alda M, Grof E, Grof P, Simhandl C, Thau K, Vestergaard P, Wolf R, Möller HJ: Excess cardiovascular and suicide mortality of affective disorders may be reduced by lithium prophylaxis. J Affect Disord 1995; 33:67–75 [E]

590. Koukopoulos A, Reginaldi D, Minnai G, Serra G, Pani L, Johnson FN: The long-term prophylaxis of affective disorders, in Depression and Mania: From Neurobiology to Treatment. Edited by Gessa G, Fratta W, Pani L, Serra G. New York, Raven Press, 1995, pp 127–147 [G]
591. Nilsson A: Mortality in recurrent mood disorders during periods on and off lithium: a complete population study in 362 patients. Pharmacopsychiatry 1995; 28:8–13 [C]
592. Thies-Flechtner K, Müller-Oerlinghausen B, Seibert W, Walther A, Greil W: Effect of prophylactic treatment on suicide risk in patients with major affective disorders. Pharmacopsychiatry 1996; 29:103–107 [A–]
593. Bocchetta A, Ardau R, Burrai C, Chillotti C, Quesada G, Del Zompo M: Suicidal behavior on and off lithium prophylaxis in a group of patients with prior suicide attempts. J Clin Psychopharmacol 1998; 18:384–389 [C]
594. Coppen A, Farmer R: Suicide mortality in patients on lithium maintenance therapy. J Affect Disord 1988; 50:261–267 [C]
595. Rucci P, Frank E, Kostelnik B, Fagiolini A, Mallinger AG, Swartz HA, Thase ME, Siegel L, Wilson D, Kupfer DJ: Suicide attempts in patients with bipolar I disorder during acute and maintenance phases of intensive treatment with pharmacotherapy and adjunctive psychotherapy. Am J Psychiatry 2002; 159:1160–1164 [B]
596. Baldessarini RJ, Tarazi FI: Drugs and the treatment of psychiatric disorders: psychosis and mania, in Goodman and Gilman's The Pharmacological Basis of Therapeutics, 10th ed. Edited by Hardman JG, Limbird LE, Gilman AG. New York, McGraw-Hill, 2001, pp 485–520 [G]
597. Greil W, Kleindienst N: The comparative prophylactic efficacy of lithium and carbamazepine in patients with bipolar I disorder. Int Clin Psychopharmacol 1999; 14:277–281 [C/A–]
598. Goodwin F, Fireman B, Simon G, Hunkeler E, Lee J, Revicki D: Suicide risk in bipolar disorder during treatment with lithium, divalproex, and carbamazepine. JAMA (in press) [D]
599. Beisser AR, Blanchette JE: A study of suicide in a mental hospital. Dis Nerv Syst 1961; 22:365–369 [B]
600. Cohen S, Leonard CV, Farberow NL, Shneidman ES: Tranquilizers and suicide in the schizophrenic patient. Arch Gen Psychiatry 1964; 11:312–321 [C]
601. Ciompi L: Late suicide in former mental patients. Psychiatr Clin (Basel) 1976; 9:59–63 [D]
602. Palmer DD, Henter ID, Wyatt RJ: Do antipsychotic medications decrease the risk of suicide in patients with schizophrenia? J Clin Psychiatry 1999; 60(suppl 2):100–103 [F]
603. Meltzer H, Alphs L, Green A, Altamura A, Anand R, Bertoldi A, Bourgeois M, Chouinard G, Islam M, Kane J, Krishnan R, Lindenmayer J-P, Potkin S: Clozapine treatment for suicidality in schizophrenia: International Suicide Prevention Trial (InterSePT). Arch Gen Psychiatry 2003; 60:82–91 [A–]
604. Shear MK, Frances A, Weiden P: Suicide associated with akathisia and depot fluphenazine treatment. J Clin Psychopharmacol 1983; 3:235–236 [C]
605. Drake RE, Ehrlich J: Suicide attempts associated with akathisia. Am J Psychiatry 1985; 142:499–501 [C]
606. Glazer WM: Formulary decisions and health economics. J Clin Psychiatry 1998; 59(suppl 19):23–29 [C]
607. Meltzer HY, Okayli G: Reduction of suicidality during clozapine treatment of neuroleptic-resistant schizophrenia: impact on risk-benefit assessment. Am J Psychiatry 1995; 152:183–190 [D]
608. Walker AM, Lanza LL, Arellano F, Rothman KJ: Mortality in current and former users of clozapine. Epidemiology 1997; 8:671–677 [D]
609. Reid WH, Mason M, Hogan T: Suicide prevention effects associated with clozapine therapy in schizophrenia and schizoaffective disorder. Psychiatr Serv 1998; 49:1029–1033 [C]

610. Munro J, O'Sullivan D, Andrews C, Arana A, Mortimer A, Kerwin R: Active monitoring of 12,760 clozapine recipients in the UK and Ireland: beyond pharmacovigilance. Br J Psychiatry 1999; 175:576–580 [E]
611. Sernyak MJ, Desai R, Stolar M, Rosenheck R: Impact of clozapine on completed suicide. Am J Psychiatry 2001; 158:931–937 [D]
612. Ertugrul A: Clozapine and suicide (letter). Am J Psychiatry 2002; 159:323 [G]
613. Meltzer H: Clozapine and suicide (letter). Am J Psychiatry 2002; 159:323–324 [G]
614. Cowdry RW, Gardner DL: Pharmacotherapy of borderline personality disorder: alprazolam, carbamazepine, trifluoperazine, and tranylcypromine. Arch Gen Psychiatry 1988; 45:111–119 [A]
615. Gardner DL, Cowdry RW: Alprazolam-induced dyscontrol in borderline personality disorder. Am J Psychiatry 1985; 142:98–100 [G]
616. Gaertner I, Gilot C, Heidrich P, Gaertner HJ: A case control study on psychopharmacotherapy before suicide committed by 61 psychiatric inpatients. Pharmacopsychiatry 2002; 35:37–43 [D]
617. Londborg PD, Smith WT, Glaudin V, Painter JR: Short-term cotherapy with clonazepam and fluoxetine: anxiety, sleep disturbance and core symptoms of depression. J Affect Disord 2000; 61:73–79 [A]
618. Smith WT, Londborg PD, Glaudin V, Painter JR: Short-term augmentation of fluoxetine with clonazepam in the treatment of depression: a double-blind study. Am J Psychiatry 1998; 155:1339–1345 [A]
619. Smith WT, Londborg PD, Glaudin V, Painter JR: Is extended clonazepam cotherapy of fluoxetine effective for outpatients with major depression? J Affect Disord 2002; 70:251–259 [A–]
620. Rich CL, Spiker DG, Jewell SW, Neil JF: Response of energy and suicidal ideation to ECT. J Clin Psychiatry 1986; 47:31–32 [C]
621. Prudic J, Sackeim HA: Electroconvulsive therapy and suicide risk. J Clin Psychiatry 1999; 60(suppl 2):104–110 [C]
622. Kellner CH, Fink M, Knapp R, Petrides G, Husain M, Rummans T, Rasmussen K, Mueller M, O'Connor K, Smith G, Bernstein H, Biggs M, Bailine S, Rush AJ: Bilateral ECT rapidly relieves suicidality: findings from phase I of the CORE ECT study. Am J Psychiatry (submitted) [A]
623. American Psychiatric Association: The Practice of Electroconvulsive Therapy: Recommendations for Treatment, Training, and Privileging: A Task Force Report of the American Psychiatric Association, 2nd ed. Washington, DC, American Psychiatric Press, 2001 [G]
624. Bateman A, Fonagy P: Effectiveness of partial hospitalization in the treatment of borderline personality disorder: a randomized controlled trial. Am J Psychiatry 1999; 156:1563–1569 [A–]
625. Bateman A, Fonagy P: Treatment of borderline personality disorder with psychoanalytically oriented partial hospitalization: an 18-month follow-up. Am J Psychiatry 2001; 158:36–42 [C/A–]
626. Linehan MM: Behavioral treatments of suicidal behaviors: definitional obfuscation and treatment outcomes. Ann N Y Acad Sci 1997; 836:302–328 [F]
627. Hawton K, Arensman E, Townsend E, Bremner S, Feldman E, Goldney R, Gunnell D, Hazell P, van Heeringen K, House A, Owens D, Sakinofsky I, Traskman-Bendz L: Deliberate self harm: systematic review of efficacy of psychosocial and pharmacological treatments in preventing repetition. Br Med J 1998; 317:441–447 [F]
628. Salkovskis PM, Atha C, Storer D: Cognitive-behavioural problem solving in the treatment of patients who repeatedly attempt suicide: a controlled trial. Br J Psychiatry 1990; 157:871–876 [A]
629. Patsiokas AT, Clum GA: Effects of psychotherapeutic strategies in the treatment of suicide attempters. Psychother Theory Res Pract Train 1985; 22:281–290 [A]

630. Liberman RP, Eckman T: Behavior therapy vs insight-oriented therapy for repeated suicide attempters. Arch Gen Psychiatry 1981; 38:1126–1130 [A]
631. Hawton K, McKeown S, Day A, Martin P, O'Connor M, Yule J: Evaluation of out-patient counselling compared with general practitioner care following overdoses. Psychol Med 1987; 17:751–761 [A]
632. Townsend E, Hawton K, Altman DG, Arensman E, Gunnell D, Hazell P, House A, van Heeringen K: The efficacy of problem-solving treatments after deliberate self-harm: meta-analysis of randomized controlled trials with respect to depression, hopelessness and improvement in problems. Psychol Med 2001; 31:979–988 [E]
633. Hawton K, Townsend E, Arensman E, Gunnell D, Hazell P, House A, van Heeringen K: Psychosocial versus pharmacological treatments for deliberate self harm. Cochrane Database Syst Rev 2000;CD001764 [E]
634. Simon RI: Assessing and Managing Suicide Risk: Guidelines for Clinical Risk Management. Arlington, Va, American Psychiatric Publishing (in press) [G]
635. Gutheil TJ, Applebaum PS: Clinical Handbook of Psychiatry and the Law, 3rd ed. Philadelphia, Lippincott Williams & Wilkins, 2000 [G]
636. Austin KM, Moline ME, Williams GT: Confronting Malpractice: Legal and Ethical Dilemmas in Psychotherapy. Newbury Park, Calif, Sage Publications, 1990 [G]
637. Simon RI: Taking the "sue" out of suicide. Psychiatr Ann 2000; 30:399–407 [G]
638. American Psychoanalytic Association: Charting psychoanalysis. J Am Psychoanal Assoc 1997; 45:656–672 [G]
639. Miller M: Suicide-prevention contacts: advantages, disadvantages, and an alternative approach, in The Harvard Medical School Guide to Suicide Assessment and Intervention. Edited by Jacobs D. San Francisco, Jossey-Bass, 1998, pp 463–481 [G]
640. Simon RI: The suicide prevention contract: clinical, legal, and risk management issues. J Am Acad Psychiatry Law 1999; 27:445–450 [F]
641. Stanford EJ, Goetz RR, Bloom JD: The no harm contract in the emergency assessment of suicidal risk. J Clin Psychiatry 1994; 55:344–348 [F]
642. Miller MC, Jacobs DG, Gutheil TG: Talisman or taboo: the controversy of the suicide-prevention contract. Harv Rev Psychiatry 1998; 6:78–87 [C]
643. American Psychiatric Association: The Principles of Medical Ethics With Annotations Especially Applicable to Psychiatry. Washington, DC, American Psychiatric Publishing, 2001 [G]
644. Chemtob CM, Hamada RS, Bauer G, Kinney B, Torigoe RY: Patients' suicides: frequency and impact on psychiatrists. Am J Psychiatry 1988; 145:224–228 [G]
645. Rubenstein HJ: Psychotherapists' Experiences of Patient Suicide (doctoral dissertation). New York, City University of New York, Department of Psychology, 2002 [G]
646. Hendin H, Lipschitz A, Maltsberger JT, Haas AP, Wynecoop S: Therapists' reactions to patients' suicides. Am J Psychiatry 2000; 157:2022–2027 [G]
647. Gitlin MJ: A psychiatrist's reaction to a patient's suicide. Am J Psychiatry 1999; 156:1630–1634 [G]
648. Slovenko R: Psychiatry in Law. New York, Brunner-Rutledge, 2002 [G]
649. Simon RI: Clinical Psychiatry and the Law, 2nd ed. Washington, DC, American Psychiatric Press, 1992, p 80 [G]
650. Saarinen PI, Viinamaeki H, Hintikka J, Lehtonen J, Lonnqvist J: Psychological symptoms of close relatives of suicide victims. Eur J Psychiatry 1999; 13:33–39 [C]
651. Brent DA, Moritz G, Bridge J, Perper J, Canobbio R: The impact of adolescent suicide on siblings and parents: a longitudinal follow-up. Suicide Life Threat Behav 1996; 26:253–259 [D]
652. Seguin M, Lesage A, Kiely MC: Parental bereavement after suicide and accident: a comparative study. Suicide Life Threat Behav 1995; 25:489–492 [C]
653. Shepherd D, Barraclough BM: The aftermath of suicide. Br Med J 1974; 2:600–603 [C]

654. Saarinen PI, Hintikka J, Viinamaki H, Lehtonen J, Lonnqvist J: Is it possible to adapt to the suicide of a close individual? results of a 10-year prospective follow-up study. Int J Soc Psychiatry 2000; 46:182–190 [C]
655. Brent DA, Perper JA, Moritz G, Allman CJ, Roth C, Schweers J, Balach L: The validity of diagnoses obtained through the psychological autopsy procedure in adolescent suicide victims: use of family history. Acta Psychiatr Scand 1993; 87:118–122 [G]
656. Brent DA, Perper JA, Moritz G, Liotus L, Schweers J, Canobbio R: Major depression or uncomplicated bereavement? a follow-up of youth exposed to suicide. J Am Acad Child Adolesc Psychiatry 1994; 33:231–239 [D]
657. Prigerson HG, Bridge J, Maciejewski PK, Beery LC, Rosenheck RA, Jacobs SC, Bierhals AJ, Kupfer DJ, Brent DA: Influence of traumatic grief on suicidal ideation among young adults. Am J Psychiatry 1999; 156:1994–1995 [G]
658. Callahan J: Predictors and correlates of bereavement in suicide support group participants. Suicide Life Threat Behavior 2000; 30:104–124 [C]
659. Zisook S, Chentsova-Dutton Y, Shuchter SR: PTSD following bereavement. Ann Clin Psychiatry 1998; 10:157–163 [C]
660. Brent DA, Moritz G, Bridge J, Perper J, Canobbio R: Long-term impact of exposure to suicide: a three-year controlled follow-up. J Am Acad Child Adolesc Psychiatry 1996; 35:646–653 [C]
661. Gessner BD: Temporal trends and geographic patterns of teen suicide in Alaska, 1979–1993. Suicide Life Threat Behav 1997; 27:264–273 [C]
662. Garlow SJ: Age, gender, and ethnicity differences in patterns of cocaine and ethanol use preceding suicide. Am J Psychiatry 2002; 159:615–619 [C]
663. Joe S, Kaplan MS: Firearm-related suicide among young African-American males. Psychiatr Serv 2002; 53:332–334 [C]
664. Conwell Y: Suicide in the elderly. Crisis 1992; 13:6–8 [G]
665. Blazer DG, Bachar JR, Manton KG: Suicide in late life: review and commentary. J Am Geriatr Soc 1986; 34:519–525 [F]
666. Haas AP, Hendin H: Suicide among older people: projections for the future. Suicide Life Threat Behav 1983; 13:147–154 [C]
667. Lish JD, Zimmerman M, Farber NJ, Lush DT, Kuzma MA, Plescia G: Suicide screening in a primary care setting at a Veterans Affairs medical center. Psychosomatics 1996; 37:413–424 [D]
668. Callahan CM, Hendrie HC, Nienaber NA, Tierney WM: Suicidal ideation among older primary care patients. J Am Geriatr Soc 1996; 44:1205–1209 [C]
669. Skoog I, Aevarsson O, Beskow J, Larsson L, Palsson S, Waern M, Landahl S, Ostling S: Suicidal feelings in a population sample of nondemented 85-year-olds. Am J Psychiatry 1996; 153:1015–1020 [D]
670. Schwab JJ, Warheit GJ, Holzer CE III: Suicidal ideation and behavior in a general population. Dis Nerv Syst 1972; 33:745–748 [G]
671. Linden M, Barnow S: 1997 IPA/Bayer Research Awards in Psychogeriatrics. The wish to die in very old persons near the end of life: a psychiatric problem? Results from the Berlin Aging Study. Int Psychogeriatr 1997; 9:291–307 [G]
672. Kposowa AJ: Marital status and suicide in the National Longitudinal Mortality Study. J Epidemiol Community Health 2000; 54:254–261 [G]
673. Kessler RC, Berglund P, Demler O, Jin R, Koretz D, Merikangas KR, Rush AJ, Walters EE, Wang PS: The epidemiology of major depressive disorder: results from the National Comorbidity Survey Replication (NCS-R). JAMA 2003; 289:3095–3105 [G]
674. Cutright P, Fernquist RM: Firearms and suicide: the American experience, 1926–1996. Death Stud 2000; 24:705–719 [G]

675. Dannenberg AL, Carter DM, Lawson HW, Ashton DM, Dorfman SF, Graham EH: Homicide and other injuries as causes of maternal death in New York City, 1987 through 1991. Am J Obstet Gynecol 1995; 172:1557–1564 [G]
676. Marzuk PM, Tardiff K, Leon AC, Hirsch CS, Portera L, Hartwell N, Iqbal MI: Lower risk of suicide during pregnancy. Am J Psychiatry 1997; 154:122–123 [G]
677. Appleby L: Suicide during pregnancy and in the first postnatal year. BMJ 1991; 302:137–140 [C]
678. Poussaint A, Alexander A: Lay My Burden Down. Boston, Beacon Press, 2000 [G]
679. Joe S, Kaplan MS: Suicide among African American men. Suicide Life Threat Behav 2001; 31(suppl):106–121 [F]
680. Ialongo N, McCreary BK, Pearson JL, Koenig AL, Wagner BM, Schmidt NB, Poduska J, Kellam SG: Suicidal behavior among urban, African American young adults. Suicide Life Threat Behav 2002; 32:256–271 [G]
681. Nisbet PA: Protective factors for suicidal black females. Suicide Life Threat Behav 1996; 26:325–341 [C]
682. National Mental Health Association: Clincial Depression and African Americans (fact sheet). Alexandria, Va, National Mental Health Association, 2000 [G]
683. Van Winkle NW, May PA: Native American suicide in New Mexico, 1957–1979: a comparative study. Human Organization 1986; 45:296–309 [G]
684. Klausner SZ, Foulks EF: Eskimo Capitalists: Oil, Politics, and Alcohol. Totowa, NJ, Allanheld, Osmun, 1982 [G]
685. Yuen NY, Nahulu LB, Hishinuma ES, Miyamoto RH: Cultural identification and attempted suicide in Native Hawaiian adolescents. J Am Acad Child Adolesc Psychiatry 2000; 39:360–367 [G]
686. Sorenson SB, Golding JM: Prevalence of suicide attempts in a Mexican-American population: prevention implications of immigration and cultural issues. Suicide Life Threat Behav 1988; 18:322–333 [G]
687. Grunbaum JA, Kann L, Kinchen SA, Williams B, Ross JG, Lowry R, Kolbe L: Youth risk behavior surveillance—United States, 2001. MMWR Surveill Summ 2002; 51:1–62 [G]
688. Lester D: Differences in the epidemiology of suicide in Asian Americans by nation of origin. Omega 1994; 29:89–93 [G]
689. Lee E: Asian American families: an overview, in Ethnicity and Family Therapy. Edited by McGoldrick M, Giordano J, Pearce JK. New York, Guilford, 1996, pp 227–248 [G]
690. Shiang J, Blinn R, Bongar B, Stephens B, Allison D, Schatzberg A: Suicide in San Francisco, CA: a comparison of Caucasian and Asian groups, 1987–1994. Suicide Life Threat Behav 1997; 27:80–91 [C]
691. Smith JC, Mercy JA, Conn JM: Marital status and the risk of suicide. Am J Public Health 1988; 78:78–80 [G]
692. Rich CL, Fowler RC, Young D, Blenkush M: San Diego suicide study: comparison of gay to straight males. Suicide Life Threat Behav 1986; 16:448–457 [G]
693. Stack S: The effect of female participation in the labor force on suicide: a time series analysis. Sociol Forum 1987; 2:257–277 [G]
694. Clark DC, Goebel-Fabbri AE: Lifetime risk of suicide in major affective disorders, in The Harvard Medical School Guide to Suicide Assessment and Intervention. Edited by Jacobs DG. San Francisco, Jossey-Bass, 1999, pp 270–286 [F]
695. Sher L, Oquendo MA, Mann JJ: Risk of suicide in mood disorders. Clinical Neuroscience Research 2001; 1:337–344 [C]
696. Baldessarini RJ, Tondo L, Hennen J: Effects of lithium treatment and its discontinuation on suicidal behavior in bipolar manic-depressive disorders. J Clin Psychiatry 1999; 60(suppl 2):77–84 [E]

697. Guze SB, Robins E: Suicide and primary affective disorders. Br J Psychiatry 1970; 117:437–438 [G]
698. Perris C, d'Elia G: A study of bipolar (manic-depressive) and unipolar recurrent depressive psychoses: X. mortality, suicide, and life-cycles. Acta Psychiatr Scand Suppl 1966; 194:172–189 [G]
699. Buchholtz-Hansen PE, Wang AG, Kragh-Sorensen P: Mortality in major affective disorder: relationship to subtype of depression. The Danish University Antidepressant Group. Acta Psychiatr Scand 1993; 87:329–335 [C]
700. Tondo L, Baldessarini RJ: Reduced suicide risk during lithium maintenance treatment. J Clin Psychiatry 2000; 61(suppl 9):97–104 [F]
701. Isometsa E, Heikkinen M, Henriksson M, Aro H, Lonnqvist J: Recent life events and completed suicide in bipolar affective disorder: a comparison with major depressive suicides. J Affect Disord 1995; 33:99–106 [D]
702. Keilp JG, Sackeim HA, Brodsky BS, Oquendo MA, Malone KM, Mann JJ: Neuropsychological dysfunction in depressed suicide attempters. Am J Psychiatry 2001; 158:735–741 [D]
703. Gladstone GL, Mitchell PB, Parker G, Wilhelm K, Austin MP, Eyers K: Indicators of suicide over 10 years in a specialist mood disorders unit sample. J Clin Psychiatry 2001; 62:945–951 [C]
704. Young AS, Nuechterlein KH, Mintz J, Ventura J, Gitlin M, Liberman RP: Suicidal ideation and suicide attempts in recent-onset schizophrenia. Schizophr Bull 1998; 24:629–634 [C]
705. Kim CH, Jayathilake K, Meltzer HY: Hopelessness, neurocognitive function, and insight in schizophrenia: relationship to suicidal behavior. Schizophr Res 2003; 60:71–80 [D]
706. Amador XF, Friedman JH, Kasapis C, Yale SA, Flaum M, Gorman JM: Suicidal behavior in schizophrenia and its relationship to awareness of illness. Am J Psychiatry 1996; 153:1185–1188 [G]
707. Henriksson MM, Isometsa ET, Kuoppasalmi KI, Heikkinen ME, Marttunen MJ, Lonnqvist JK: Panic disorder in completed suicide. J Clin Psychiatry 1996; 57:275–281 [G]
708. Johnson J, Weissman MM, Klerman GL: Panic disorder, comorbidity, and suicide attempts. Arch Gen Psychiatry 1990; 47:805–808 [G]
709. Fleet RP, Dupuis G, Kaczorowski J, Marchand A, Beitman BD: Suicidal ideation in emergency department chest pain patients: panic disorder a risk factor. Am J Emerg Med 1997; 15:345–349 [G]
710. Friedman S, Jones JC, Chernen L, Barlow DH: Suicidal ideation and suicide attempts among patients with panic disorder: a survey of two outpatient clinics. Am J Psychiatry 1992; 149:680–685 [D]
711. Cornelius JR, Thase ME, Salloum IM, Cornelius MD, Black A, Mann JJ: Cocaine use associated with increased suicidal behavior in depressed alcoholics. Addict Behav 1998; 23:119–121 [D]
712. Beck AT, Weissman A, Lester D, Trexler L: The measurement of pessimism: the hopelessness scale. J Consult Clin Psychol 1974; 42:861–865 [G]
713. Tomasson K: Hopelessness as a predictor of suicide. Am J Psychiatry 1990; 147:1577–1578 [G]
714. Goodwin DW, Alderson P, Rosenthal R: Clinical significance of hallucinations in psychiatric disorders: a study of 116 hallucinatory patients. Arch Gen Psychiatry 1971; 24:76–80 [G]
715. Borges G, Rosovsky H: Suicide attempts and alcohol consumption in an emergency room sample. J Stud Alcohol 1996; 57:543–548 [D]
716. Zlotnick C, Mattia J, Zimmerman M: Clinical features of survivors of sexual abuse with major depression. Child Abuse Negl 2001; 25:357–367 [D]
717. Elliott AJ, Pages KP, Russo J, Wilson LG, Roy-Byrne PP: A profile of medically serious suicide attempts. J Clin Psychiatry 1996; 57:567–571 [D]
718. Simon GE, VonKorff M: Suicide mortality among patients treated for depression in an insured population. Am J Epidemiol 1998; 147:155–160 [G]
719. Jamison KR: Night Falls Fast: Understanding Suicide. New York, Knopf, 1999 [G]

720. Stenager EN, Madsen C, Stenager E, Boldsen J: Suicide in patients with stroke: epidemiological study. BMJ 1998; 316:1206 [D]
721. Brown JH, Henteleff P, Barakat S, Rowe CJ: Is it normal for terminally ill patients to desire death? Am J Psychiatry 1986; 143:208–211 [G]
722. Kalichman SC, Heckman T, Kochman A, Sikkema K, Bergholte J: Depression and thoughts of suicide among middle-aged and older persons living with HIV-AIDS. Psychiatr Serv 2000; 51:903–907 [G]
723. Marzuk PM, Tardiff K, Leon AC, Hirsch CS, Hartwell N, Portera L, Iqbal MI: HIV seroprevalence among suicide victims in New York City, 1991–1993. Am J Psychiatry 1997; 154:1720–1725 [G]
724. Perry S, Jacobsberg L, Fishman B: Suicidal ideation and HIV testing. JAMA 1990; 263:679–682 [C]
725. Clark D: Suicide risk and persons with AIDS. Suicide Research Digest 1992; 6:12–13 [G]
726. Breault KD: Beyond the quick and dirty: reply to Girard. AJS 1988; 93:1479–1486 [G]
727. Platt S, Micciolo R, Tansella M: Suicide and unemployment in Italy: description, analysis and interpretation of recent trends. Soc Sci Med 1992; 34:1191–1201 [G]
728. Lester D: The effect of war on suicide rates: a study of France from 1826 to 1913. Eur Arch Psychiatry Clin Neurosci 1993; 242:248–249 [G]
729. Varnik A, Wasserman D: Suicides in the former Soviet republics. Acta Psychiatr Scand 1992; 86:76–78 [G]
730. Stack S: Suicide: a 15-year review of the sociological literature. Part II: modernization and social integration perspectives. Suicide Life Threat Behav 2000; 30:163–176 [F]
731. Sainsbury P, Jenkins J, Levey A: The social correlates of suicide in Europe, in The Suicide Syndrome. Edited by Farmer R, Hirsch S. London, Croom and Helm, 1980, pp 38–53 [G]
732. Wasserman IM: Political business cycles, presidential elections, and suicide and mortality patterns. Am Sociol Rev 1983; 48:711–720 [G]
733. Pescosolido BA, Georgianna S: Durkheim, suicide, and religion: toward a network theory of suicide. Am Sociol Rev 1989; 54:33–48 [G]
734. Boudewyn AC, Liem JH: Psychological, interpersonal, and behavioral correlates of chronic self-destructiveness: an exploratory study. Psychol Rep 1995; 77:1283–1297 [D]
735. Ohberg A, Lonnqvist J, Sarna S, Vuori E: Trends and availability of suicide methods in Finland: proposals for restrictive measures. Br J Psychiatry 1995; 166:35–43 [G]
736. Ikeda RM, Gorwitz R, James SP, Powell KE, Mercy JA: Trends in fatal firearm-related injuries, United States, 1962–1993. Am J Prev Med 1997; 13:396–400 [C]
737. Krug EG, Powell KE, Dahlberg LL: Firearm-related deaths in the United States and 35 other high- and upper-middle-income countries. Int J Epidemiol 1998; 27:214–221 [C]
738. Fox J, Stahlsmith L, Nashold R, Remington P: Increasing use of firearms in completed suicides in Wisconsin, 1979–1994. Wis Med J 1996; 95:283–285 [F]
739. Pierce D: Suicidal intent and repeated self-harm. Psychol Med 1984; 14:655–659 [C]
740. Goldstein RB, Black DW, Nasrallah A, Winokur G: The prediction of suicide: sensitivity, specificity, and predictive value of a multivariate model applied to suicide among 1906 patients with affective disorders. Arch Gen Psychiatry 1991; 48:418–422 [C]
741. Beck AT, Steer RA, Ranieri WF: Scale for Suicide Ideation: psychometric properties of a self-report version. J Clin Psychol 1988; 44:499–505 [G]
742. Nimeus A, Alsen M, Traeskman-Bendz L: The Suicide Assessment Scale: an instrument assessing suicide risk of suicide attempters. Eur Psychiatry 2000; 15:416–423 [C]
743. Litinsky AM, Haslam N: Dichotomous thinking as a sign of suicide risk on the TAT. J Pers Assess 1998; 71:368–378 [D]
744. Watson D, Goldney R, Fisher L, Merritt M: The measurement of suicidal ideation. Crisis 2001; 22:12–14 [C]

745. Shneidman ES: The Psychological Pain Assessment Scale. Suicide Life Threat Behav 1999; 29:287–294 [G]
746. Mann JJ: The neurobiology of suicide. Nat Med 1998; 4:25–30 [G]
747. Verona E, Patrick CJ: Suicide risk in externalizing syndromes: tempermental and neurobiological underpinnings, in Suicide Science: Expanding the Boundaries. Edited by Joiner TE, Rudd D. Boston, Kluwer Academic, 2000, pp 137–173 [F]
748. Traskman L, Asberg M, Bertilsson L, Sjostrand L: Monoamine metabolites in CSF and suicidal behavior. Arch Gen Psychiatry 1981; 38:631–636 [D]
749. Correa H, Duval F, Mokrani MC, Bailey P, Tremeau F, Staner L, Diep TS, Crocq MA, Macher JP: Serotonergic function and suicidal behavior in schizophrenia. Schizophr Res 2002; 56:75–85 [B]
750. Bunney WEJ, Fawcett JA: The possibility of a biochemical test for suicidal potential. Arch Gen Psychiatry 1965; 13:232–238 [G]
751. Dumser T, Barocka A, Schubert E: Weight of adrenal glands may be increased in persons who commit suicide. Am J Forensic Med Pathol 1998; 19:72–76 [D]
752. Szigethy E, Conwell Y, Forbes NT, Cox C, Caine ED: Adrenal weight and morphology in victims of completed suicide. Biol Psychiatry 1994; 36:374–380 [D]
753. Dorovini-Zis K, Zis AP: Increased adrenal weight in victims of violent suicide. Am J Psychiatry 1987; 144:1214–1215 [D]
754. Nemeroff CB, Owens MJ, Bissette G, Andorn AC, Stanley M: Reduced corticotropin releasing factor binding sites in the frontal cortex of suicide victims. Arch Gen Psychiatry 1988; 45:577–579 [D]
755. Austin MC, Janosky JE, Murphy HA: Increased corticotropin-releasing hormone immunoreactivity in monoamine-containing pontine nuclei of depressed suicide men. Mol Psychiatry 2003; 8:324–332 [D]
756. Coryell W, Schlesser MA: Suicide and the dexamethasone suppression test in unipolar depression. Am J Psychiatry 1981; 138:1120–1121 [B]
757. Coryell W, Schlesser M: The dexamethasone suppression test and suicide prediction. Am J Psychiatry 2001; 158:748–753 [C]
758. Partonen T, Haukka J, Virtamo J, Taylor PR, Lonnqvist J: Association of low serum total cholesterol with major depression and suicide. Br J Psychiatry 1999; 175:259–262 [C]
759. Ellison LF, Morrison HI: Low serum cholesterol concentration and risk of suicide. Epidemiology 2001; 12:168–172 [C]
760. Fawcett J, Busch KA, Jacobs D, Kravitz HM, Fogg L: Suicide: a four-pathway clinical-biochemical model. Ann N Y Acad Sci 1997; 836:288–301 [E]
761. Garland M, Hickey D, Corvin A, Golden J, Fitzpatrick P, Cunningham S, Walsh N: Total serum cholesterol in relation to psychological correlates in parasuicide. Br J Psychiatry 2000; 177:77–83 [A]
762. Bocchetta A, Chillotti C, Carboni G, Oi A, Ponti M, Del Zompo M: Association of personal and familial suicide risk with low serum cholesterol concentration in male lithium patients. Acta Psychiatr Scand 2001; 104:37–41 [D]
763. Alvarez JC, Cremniter D, Gluck N, Quintin P, Leboyer M, Berlin I, Therond P, Spreux-Varoquaux O: Low serum cholesterol in violent but not in non-violent suicide attempters. Psychiatry Res 2000; 95:103–108 [D]
764. Manfredini R, Caracciolo S, Salmi R, Boari B, Tomelli A, Gallerani M: The association of low serum cholesterol with depression and suicidal behaviours: new hypotheses for the missing link. J Int Med Res 2000; 28:247–257 [E]
765. Plutchik R: Outward and inward directed aggressiveness: the interaction between violence and suicidality. Pharmacopsychiatry 1995; 28(suppl 2):47–57 [F]
766. Nock MK, Marzuk PM: Murder-suicide: phenomenology and clinical implications, in The Harvard Medical School Guide to Suicide Assessment and Intervention. Edited by Jacobs DG. San Francisco, Jossey-Bass, 1999, pp 188–209 [G]

767. Berman AL: Dyadic death: a typology. Suicide Life Threat Behav 1996; 26:342–350 [G]
768. Allen NH: Homicide followed by suicide: Los Angeles, 1970–1979. Suicide Life Threat Behav 1983; 13:155–165 [E]
769. Trezza GR, Popp SM: The substance user at risk of harm to self or others: assessment and treatment issues. J Clin Psychol 2000; 56:1193–1205 [F]
770. Tardiff K, Marzuk PM, Leon AC: Role of antidepressants in murder and suicide. Am J Psychiatry 2002; 159:1248–1249 [G]
771. Fishbain DA, D'Achille L, Barsky S, Aldrich TE: A controlled study of suicide pacts. J Clin Psychiatry 1984; 45:154–157 [D]
772. Brown M, King E, Barraclough B: Nine suicide pacts: a clinical study of a consecutive series 1974–93. Br J Psychiatry 1995; 167:448–451 [D]
773. Brown M, Barraclough B: Epidemiology of suicide pacts in England and Wales, 1988–92. BMJ 1997; 315:286–287 [C]
774. Evans J, Platts H, Liebenau A: Impulsiveness and deliberate self-harm: a comparison of "first-timers" and "repeaters." Acta Psychiatr Scand 1996; 93:378–380 [C]
775. Isacsson G, Holmgren P, Druid H, Bergman U: The utilization of antidepressants—a key issue in the prevention of suicide. An analysis of 5,281 suicides in Sweden 1992–94. Acta Psychiatr Scand 1997; 96:94–100 [E]
776. Frey R, Schreinzer D, Stimpfl T, Vycudilik W, Berzlanovich A, Kasper S: Suicide by antidepressant intoxication identified at autopsy in Vienna from 1991–1997: the favourable consequences of the increasing use of SSRIs. Eur Neuropsychopharmacol 2000; 10:133–142 [G]
777. Freemantle N, House A, Song F, Mason JM, Sheldon TA: Prescribing selective serotonin reuptake inhibitors as strategy for prevention of suicide. Br Med J 1994; 309:249–253 [F]
778. Mäkinen IH, Wasserman D: Suicide prevention and cultural resistance: stability in suicide ranking of European countries, 1970–88. Ital J Suicidology 1997; 7:73–85 [G]
779. Rihmer Z, Belso N, Kalmár S: Antidepressants and suicide prevention in Hungary. Acta Psychiatr Scand 2001; 103:238–239 [G]
780. Monk M: Epidemiology of suicide. Epidemiol Rev 1987; 9:51–69 [F]
781. Klerman GL, Weissman MM: Increasing rate of depression. JAMA 1989; 261:2229–2235 [G]
782. Andersen UA, Andersen M, Rosholm JU, Gram LF: Psychopharmacological treatment and psychiatric morbidity in 390 cases of suicide with special focus on affective disorders. Acta Psychiatr Scand 2001; 104:458–465 [G]
783. Oquendo MA, Malone KM, Ellis SP, Sackeim HA, Mann JJ: Inadequacy of antidepressant treatment for patients with major depression who are at risk for suicidal behavior. Am J Psychiatry 1999; 156:190–194 [D]
784. Suominen KH, Isometsa ET, Henriksson MM, Ostamo AI, Lonnqvist JK: Inadequate treatment for major depression both before and after attempted suicide. Am J Psychiatry 1998; 155:1778–1780 [G]
785. Verkes RJ, van der Mast RC, Hengeveld MW, Tuyl JP, Zwinderman AH, van Kempen GM: Reduction by paroxetine of suicidal behavior in patients with repeated suicide attempts but not major depression. Am J Psychiatry 1998; 155:543–547 [A]
786. Hirschfeld RMA: Efficacy of SSRIs and newer antidepressants in severe depression: comparison with TCAs. J Clin Psychiatry 1999; 60:326–335 [E]
787. Mann JJ, Kapur S: The emergence of suicidal ideation and behavior during antidepressant pharmacotherapy. Arch Gen Psychiatry 1991; 48:1027–1033 [F]
788. Letizia C, Kapik B, Flanders WD: Suicidal risk during controlled clinical investigations of fluvoxamine. J Clin Psychiatry 1996; 57:415–421 [E]
789. Tondo L, Baldessarini RJ, Floris G: Long-term clinical effectiveness of lithium maintenance treatment in types I and II bipolar disorders. Br J Psychiatry Suppl 2001; 41:s184–s190 [C]
790. Baldessarini RJ, Jamison KR: Effects of medical interventions on suicidal behavior: summary and conclusions. J Clin Psychiatry 1999; 60(suppl 2):117–122 [G]

791. Baldessarini RJ, Tondo L, Viguera AC: Effects of discontinuing lithium maintenance treatment. Bipolar Disord 1999; 1:17–24 [C]
792. Diekstra RF: The epidemiology of suicide and parasuicide. Acta Psychiatr Scand Suppl 1993; 371:9–20 [G]
793. Faedda GL, Tondo L, Baldessarini RJ, Suppes T, Tohen M: Outcome after rapid vs gradual discontinuation of lithium treatment in bipolar disorders. Arch Gen Psychiatry 1993; 50:448–455 [C]
794. Viguera AC, Nonacs R, Cohen LS, Tondo L, Murray A, Baldessarini RJ: Risk of recurrence of bipolar disorder in pregnant and nonpregnant women after discontinuing lithium maintenance. Am J Psychiatry 2000; 157:179–184 [G]
795. Wickham EA, Reed JV: Lithium for the control of aggressive and self-mutilating behaviour. Int Clin Psychopharmacol 1987; 2:181–190 [F]
796. Meltzer HY, Anand R, Alphs L: Reducing suicide risk in schizophrenia: focus on the role of clozapine. CNS Drugs 2000; 14:355–365 [F]
797. Van Putten T, May RP: "Akinetic depression" in schizophrenia. Arch Gen Psychiatry 1978; 35:1101–1107 [G]
798. Claghorn J, Honigfeld G, Abuzzahab FS Sr, Wang R, Steinbook R, Tuason V, Klerman G: The risks and benefits of clozapine versus chlorpromazine. J Clin Psychopharmacol 1987; 7:377–384 [A]
799. Kane J, Honigfeld G, Singer J, Meltzer H: Clozapine for the treatment-resistant schizophrenic: a double-blind comparison with chlorpromazine. Arch Gen Psychiatry 1988; 45:789–796 [A]
800. Hagger C, Buckley P, Kenny JT, Friedman L, Ubogy D, Meltzer HY: Improvement in cognitive functions and psychiatric symptoms in treatment-refractory schizophrenic patients receiving clozapine. Biol Psychiatry 1993; 34:702–712 [B]
801. Meltzer HY, McGurk SR: The effects of clozapine, risperidone, and olanzapine on cognitive function in schizophrenia. Schizophr Bull 1999; 25:233–255 [E]
802. Green AI, Burgess ES, Dawson R, Zimmet SV, Strous RD: Alcohol and cannabis use in schizophrenia: effects of clozapine vs risperidone. Schizophr Res 2003; 60:81–85 [G]
803. Kavanagh DJ, McGrath J, Saunders JB, Dore G, Clark D: Substance misuse in patients with schizophrenia: epidemiology and management. Drugs 2002; 62:743–755 [F]
804. Citrome L, Volavka J, Czobor P, Sheitman B, Lindenmayer JP, McEvoy J, Cooper TB, Chakos M, Lieberman JA: Effects of clozapine, olanzapine, risperidone, and haloperidol on hostility among patients with schizophrenia. Psychiatr Serv 2001; 52:1510–1514 [A]
805. Brieden T, Ujeyl M, Naber D: Psychopharmacological treatment of aggression in schizophrenic patients. Pharmacopsychiatry 2002; 35:83–89 [F]
806. Chengappa KN, Vasile J, Levine J, Ulrich R, Baker R, Gopalani A, Schooler N: Clozapine: its impact on aggressive behavior among patients in a state psychiatric hospital. Schizophr Res 2002; 53:1–6 [G]
807. Glazer WM, Dickson RA: Clozapine reduces violence and persistent aggression in schizophrenia. J Clin Psychiatry 1998; 59(suppl 3):8–14 [D]
808. Spivak B, Roitman S, Vered Y, Mester R, Graff E, Talmon Y, Guy N, Gonen N, Weizman A: Diminished suicidal and aggressive behavior, high plasma norepinephrine levels, and serum triglyceride levels in chronic neuroleptic-resistant schizophrenic patients maintained on clozapine. Clin Neuropharmacol 1998; 21:245–250 [D]
809. Baldessarini RJ, Hennen J: Effects of clozapine treatment on suicide risk in psychotic patients: a meta-analysis (unpublished manuscript). Mailman Research Center, McLean Hospital, Belmont, Mass, 2003 [E]
810. Beasley CM, Dellva MA, Tamura RN, Morgenstern H, Glazer WM, Ferguson K, Tollefson GD: Randomised double-blind comparison of the incidence of tardive dyskinesia in patients with schizophrenia during long-term treatment with olanzapine or haloperidol. Br J Psychiatry 1999; 174:23–30 [A]

811. Keck PE Jr, Strakowski SM, McElroy SL: The efficacy of atypical antipsychotics in the treatment of depressive symptoms, hostility, and suicidality in patients with schizophrenia. J Clin Psychiatry 2000; 61(suppl 3):4–9 [F]
812. Salzman C: Addiction to benzodiazepines. Psychiatr Q 1998; 69:251–261 [F]
813. Dietch JT, Jennings RK: Aggressive dyscontrol in patients treated with benzodiazepines. J Clin Psychiatry 1988; 49:184–188 [F]
814. O'Sullivan GH, Noshirvani H, Basoglu M, Marks IM, Swinson R, Kuch K, Kirby M: Safety and side-effects of alprazolam: controlled study in agoraphobia with panic disorder. Br J Psychiatry 1994; 165:79–86 [A–]
815. Kalachnik JE, Hanzel TE, Sevenich R, Harder SR: Benzodiazepine behavioral side effects: review and implications for individuals with mental retardation. Am J Ment Retard 2002; 107:376–410 [F]
816. Rothschild AJ, Shindul R, Viguera A, Murray M, Brewster S: Comparison of the frequency of behavioral disinhibition on alprazolam, clonazepam, or no benzodiazepine in hospitalized psychiatric patients. J Clin Psychopharmacol 2000; 20:7–11 [G]
817. Joughin N, Tata P, Collins M, Hooper C, Falkowski J: In-patient withdrawal from long-term benzodiazepine use. Br J Addict 1991; 86:449–455 [G]
818. Ciapparelli A, Dell'Osso L, Tundo A, Pini S, Chiavacci MC, Di Sacco I, Cassano GB: Electroconvulsive therapy in medication-nonresponsive patients with mixed mania and bipolar depression. J Clin Psychiatry 2001; 62:552–555 [C]
819. O'Leary D, Paykel E, Todd C, Vardulaki K: Suicide in primary affective disorders revisited: a systematic review by treatment era. J Clin Psychiatry 2001; 62:804–811 [E]
820. Babigian HM, Guttmacher LB: Epidemiologic considerations in electroconvulsive therapy. Arch Gen Psychiatry 1984; 41:246–253 [C]
821. Tanney BL: Electroconvulsive therapy and suicide. Suicide Life Threat Behav 1986; 16:198–222 [F]
822. Sharma V: The effect of electroconvulsive therapy on suicide risk in patients with mood disorders. Can J Psychiatry 2001; 46:704–709 [F]
823. Jarrett RB, Kraft D, Doyle J, Foster BM, Eaves GG, Silver PC: Preventing recurrent depression using cognitive therapy with and without a continuation phase: a randomized clinical trial. Arch Gen Psychiatry 2001; 58:381–388 [B]
824. Hirschfeld RM, Dunner DL, Keitner G, Klein DN, Koran LM, Kornstein SG, Markowitz JC, Miller I, Nemeroff CB, Ninan PT, Rush AJ, Schatzberg AF, Thase ME, Trivedi MH, Borian FE, Crits-Christoph P, Keller MB: Does psychosocial functioning improve independent of depressive symptoms? a comparison of nefazodone, psychotherapy, and their combination. Biol Psychiatry 2002; 51:123–133 [A–]
825. DeRubeis RJ, Gelfand LA, Tang TZ, Simons AD: Medications versus cognitive behavior therapy for severely depressed outpatients: mega-analysis of four randomized comparisons. Am J Psychiatry 1999; 156:1007–1013 [E]
826. Frank E, Grochocinski VJ, Spanier CA, Buysse DJ, Cherry CR, Houck PR, Stapf DM, Kupfer DJ: Interpersonal psychotherapy and antidepressant medication: evaluation of a sequential treatment strategy in women with recurrent major depression. J Clin Psychiatry 2000; 61:51–57 [B]
827. Keller MB, McCullough JP, Klein DN, Arnow B, Dunner DL, Gelenberg AJ, Markowitz JC, Nemeroff CB, Russell JM, Thase ME, Trivedi MH, Zajecka J: A comparison of nefazodone, the cognitive behavioral-analysis system of psychotherapy, and their combination for the treatment of chronic depression. N Engl J Med 2000; 342:1462–1470 [A–]
828. Paykel ES, Scott J, Teasdale JD, Johnson AL, Garland A, Moore R, Jenaway A, Cornwall PL, Hayhurst H, Abbott R, Pope M: Prevention of relapse in residual depression by cognitive therapy: a controlled trial. Arch Gen Psychiatry 1999; 56:829–835 [A–]

829. Reynolds CF III, Frank E, Perel JM, Imber SD, Cornes C, Miller MD, Mazumdar S, Houck PR, Dew MA, Stack JA, Pollock BG, Kupfer DJ: Nortriptyline and interpersonal psychotherapy as maintenance therapies for recurrent major depression: a randomized controlled trial in patients older than 59 years. JAMA 1999; 281:39–45 [A]
830. Thase ME, Greenhouse JB, Frank E, Reynolds CF, III, Pilkonis PA, Hurley K, Grochocinski V, Kupfer DJ: Treatment of major depression with psychotherapy or psychotherapy-pharmacotherapy combinations. Arch Gen Psychiatry 1997; 54:1009–1015 [E]
831. Colom F, Vieta E, Martinez-Aran A, Reinares M, Goikolea JM, Benabarre A, Torrent C, Comes M, Corbella B, Parramon G, Corominas J: A randomized trial on the efficacy of group psychoeducation in the prophylaxis of recurrences in bipolar patients whose disease is in remission. Arch Gen Psychiatry 2003; 60:402–407 [A–]
832. Stevenson J, Meares R: An outcome study of psychotherapy for patients with borderline personality disorder. Am J Psychiatry 1992; 149:358–362 [B]
833. Meares R, Stevenson J, Comerford A: Psychotherapy with borderline patients: I. a comparison between treated and untreated cohorts. Aust N Z J Psychiatry 1999; 33:467–472 [B]
834. Clarkin JF, Foelsch PA, Levy KN, Hull JW, Delaney JC, Kernberg OF: The development of a psychodynamic treatment for patients with borderline personality disorder: a preliminary study of behavioral change. J Personal Disord 2001; 15:487–495 [B]
835. Gloaguen V, Cottraux J, Cucherat M, Blackburn IM: A meta-analysis of the effects of cognitive therapy in depressed patients. J Affect Disord 1998; 49:59–72 [E]
836. Dobson KS: A meta-analysis of the efficacy of cognitive therapy for depression. J Consult Clin Psychol 1989; 57:414–419 [E]
837. Gaffan EA, Tsaousis I, Kemp-Wheeler SM: Researcher allegiance and meta-analysis: the case of cognitive therapy for depression. J Consult Clin Psychol 1995; 63:966–980 [E]
838. Linehan MM, Heard HL, Armstrong HE: Naturalistic follow-up of a behavioral treatment for chronically parasuicidal borderline patients. Arch Gen Psychiatry 1993; 50:971–974 [A]
839. Bohus M, Haaf B, Stiglmayr C, Pohl U, Bohme R, Linehan M: Evaluation of inpatient dialectical-behavioral therapy for borderline personality disorder—a prospective study. Behav Res Ther 2000; 38:875–887 [B]
840. Verheul R, Van Den Bosch LM, Koeter MW, De Ridder MA, Stijnen T, Van Den Brink: Dialectical behaviour therapy for women with borderline personality disorder: 12-month, randomised clinical trial in The Netherlands. Br J Psychiatry 2003; 182:135–140 [A–]
841. Barley W, Buie SE, Peterson EW, Hollingsworth A, Griva M, Hickerson S, Lawson J, Bailey B: Development of an inpatient cognitive-behavioral treatment program for borderline personality disorder. J Personal Disord 1993; 7:232–240 [B]
842. van der Sande R, van Rooijen L, Buskens E, Allart E: Intensive in-patient and community intervention versus routine care after attempted suicide. a randomised controlled intervention study. Br J Psychiatry 1997; 171:35–41 [A]
843. Guthrie E, Kapur N, Mackway-Jones K, Chew-Graham C, Moorey J, Mendel E, Marino-Francis F, Sanderson S, Turpin C, Boddy G, Tomenson B: Randomised controlled trial of brief psychological intervention after deliberate self poisoning. BMJ 2001; 323:135–138 [A]
844. Welu TC: A follow-up program for suicide attempters: evaluation of effectiveness. Suicide Life Threat Behav 1977; 7:17–20 [A]
845. Lopez JF, Vazquez DM, Chalmers DT, Watson SJ: Regulation of 5-HT receptors and the hypothalamic-pituitary-adrenal axis: implications for the neurobiology of suicide. Ann N Y Acad Sci 1997; 836:106–134 [F]
846. Lester D: Serum cholesterol levels and suicide: a meta-analysis. Suicide Life Threat Behav 2002; 32:333–346 [E]

APPENDIX

Practice Guideline Development Process

I. BACKGROUND AND DEFINITION

The American Psychiatric Association (APA) began developing practice guidelines in 1991. *Practice guidelines* are defined as systematically developed documents in a standardized format that present patient care strategies to assist psychiatrists in clinical decision making. Although APA guidelines may be used for a variety of reasons, their primary purpose is to assist psychiatrists in their care of patients.

Both the American Medical Association (AMA) and the Institute of Medicine (IOM) have sought to define the key features necessary to ensure that practice guidelines are of high quality. The AMA's attributes apply to the development process, stating that practice parameters or guidelines should 1) be developed by or in conjunction with physician organizations, 2) explicitly describe the methodology and process used in their development, 3) assist practitioner and patient decisions about appropriate health care for specific clinical circumstances, 4) be based on current professional knowledge and reviewed and revised at regular intervals, and 5) be widely disseminated. The IOM's attributes are criteria for evaluating the finished product; these criteria include 1) validity, based on the strength of the evidence, expert judgment, and estimates of health and cost outcomes compared with alternative practices; 2) reliability and reproducibility; 3) clinical applicability and flexibility; 4) clarity; 5) attention to multidisciplinary concerns; 6) timely updates; and 7) documentation. Taken together, the IOM and AMA prescriptives have essentially set national standards for guideline efforts.

II. TOPIC SELECTION

APA's Steering Committee on Practice Guidelines oversees development of APA guidelines. The Steering Committee selects topics for practice guidelines according to the following criteria:

1. Degree of public importance (prevalence and seriousness)
2. Relevance to psychiatric practice
3. Availability of information and relevant data
4. Availability of work already done that would be useful in the development of a practice guideline
5. An area in which increased psychiatric attention and involvement would be helpful for the field

III. CONTRIBUTORS

Each APA practice guideline is developed by a work group of psychiatrists in active clinical practice, including academicians or researchers who spend a significant percentage of their time in the clinical care of patients. Work group members are selected on the basis of their knowledge and experience in the topic area, their commitment to the integrity of the guideline development process as outlined by the AMA and IOM, and their representativeness of the diversity of American psychiatry.

Many experts in psychiatric treatment, particularly in the area of psychopharmacology, have significant research activities funded by the pharmaceutical industry. Recognizing this, APA has implemented a number of mechanisms to minimize the potential for producing recommendations that are biased because of conflicts of interest from contributors. On appointment, work group members are asked to disclose potential conflicts of interest, and these disclosures are reviewed by the work group chair and the APA Executive Committee on Practice Guidelines. Work group members are asked to decline participation if they feel there are conflicts of interest or biases that could impact their ability to maintain scientific objectivity. At an initial meeting, work group members are also asked to disclose potential conflicts of interest with each other. This transparency helps the group to evaluate and, as necessary, dissent with each other's work during evidence review and draft development. The following statement appears in every practice guideline to clarify this point:

This practice guideline has been developed by psychiatrists who are in active clinical practice. In addition, some contributors are primarily involved in research or other academic endeavors. It is possible that through such activities some contributors, including work group members and reviewers, have received income related to treatments discussed in this guideline. A number of mechanisms are in place to minimize the potential for producing biased recommendations due to conflicts of interest. Work group members are selected on the basis of their expertise and integrity. Any work group member or reviewer who has a potential conflict of interest that may bias (or appear to bias) his or her work is asked to disclose this to the Steering Committee on Practice Guidelines and the work group. Iterative guideline drafts are reviewed by the Steering Committee, other experts, allied organizations, APA members, and the APA Assembly and Board of Trustees; substantial revisions address or integrate the comments of these multiple reviewers. The development of the APA practice guidelines is not financially supported by any commercial organization.

Potential bias is also minimized by iterative broad review of guideline drafts, as described in Section VI of this document. Finally, no commercial organizations provide support for the development of the APA practice guidelines.

APA is listed as the "author" of practice guidelines, with individual contributions and reviewers acknowledged. Final editorial responsibility for practice guidelines rests with the Steering Committee and the Department of Quality Improvement and Psychiatric Services.

IV. EVIDENCE BASE

The evidence base for practice guidelines is derived from two sources: research studies and clinical consensus. Where gaps exist in the research data, evidence is derived from clinical consensus, obtained through broad review of multiple drafts of each guideline (see Section VI). Both research data and clinical consensus vary in their validity and reliability for different clinical situations; guidelines state explicitly the nature of the supporting evidence for specific recommendations so that readers can make their own judgments regarding the utility of the recommendations. The following coding system is used for this purpose:

[A] *Randomized, double-blind clinical trial.* A study of an intervention in which subjects are prospectively followed over time; there are treatment and control groups; subjects are randomly assigned to the two groups; and both the subjects and the investigators are "blind" to the assignments.

[A–] *Randomized clinical trial.* Same as above but not double blind.

[B] *Clinical trial.* A prospective study in which an intervention is made and the results of that intervention are tracked longitudinally. Does not meet standards for a randomized clinical trial.

[C] *Cohort or longitudinal study.* A study in which subjects are prospectively followed over time without any specific intervention.

[D] *Control study.* A study in which a group of patients and a group of control subjects are identified in the present and information about them is pursued retrospectively or backward in time.

[E] *Review with secondary data analysis.* A structured analytic review of existing data, e.g., a meta-analysis or a decision analysis.

[F] *Review.* A qualitative review and discussion of previously published literature without a quantitative synthesis of the data.

[G] *Other.* Opinion-like essays, case reports, and other reports not categorized above.

The literature review process is explicitly described in every guideline, including statements concerning

1. Basic search strategy (e.g., keywords, time period covered, research methodologies considered)
2. Sources used for identifying studies (e.g., review articles, texts, abstracting and indexing services, Index Medicus, Science Citation Index, computer search services)
3. Criteria for selecting publications (e.g., how many relevant publications were identified, whether all were reviewed, whether only prospective studies were selected)
4. Review methods (e.g., whether publications were reviewed in their entirety or in abstract)
5. Methods for cataloging reported outcomes (e.g., study design, sample characteristics, relevant findings)

The literature review will include other guidelines addressing the same topic, when available. The work group constructs evidence tables to illustrate the data regarding risks and benefits for each treatment and to evaluate the quality of the data. These tables facilitate group discussion of the evidence and agreement on treatment recommendations before guideline text is written. Evidence tables do not appear in the guideline; however, they are retained by APA to document the development process in case queries are received and to inform revisions of the guideline.

V. FORMAT

Each practice guideline follows a standardized format, with variations as appropriate (e.g., format for a guideline about psychiatric evaluation or a procedure may vary from format for a guideline about a specific illness).

Since the 2000 revision of the guideline on major depressive disorder, the general outline for all guidelines and revisions has been as follows:

Part A. Treatment Recommendations
- I. Executive Summary of Recommendations
- II. Formulation and Implementation of a Treatment Plan
- III. Specific Clinical Features Influencing the Treatment Plan

Part B. Background Information and Review of Available Evidence
- IV. Disease Definition, Epidemiology, and Natural History
- V. Review and Synthesis of Available Evidence

Part C. Future Research Needs

Individuals and Organizations That Submitted Comments

References

Section I provides an overview of the organization and scope of recommendations contained in subsequent sections. Each recommendation is identified as falling into one of three categories of endorsement:

[I] Recommended with substantial clinical confidence.
[II] Recommended with moderate clinical confidence.
[III] May be recommended on the basis of individual circumstances.

Section II presents a synthesis of the information discussed in Section V, directed at providing a framework for clinical decision making for the individual patient.

Section III addresses psychiatric, general medical, and demographic factors influencing treatment, including comorbidities. Relevant ethnic, cross-cultural, social, or extrinsic factors (e.g., cultural mores, family, support system, living situation, health care beliefs) that could potentially preclude or modify the practical application of guidelines and may play a role in health care decisions are emphasized.

Section IV presents the characteristics of the illness using current DSM criteria. Differential diagnosis, appropriate diagnostic procedures, aspects of the epidemiology and natural history with important treatment implications, and issues concerning special patient characteristics are outlined in this section.

Section V presents a review of the available data on all potential treatments, organized according to three broad categories: 1) psychiatric management, 2) psychosocial interventions, and 3) somatic interventions. For each treatment, this information is presented in a standard format:

a. Goals of treatment
b. Efficacy data
c. Side effects and safety
d. Implementation issues (e.g., patient selection, laboratory testing, dosing, frequency, duration)

Part C identifies directions for further research.

Individuals and organizations that submitted substantive comments on guideline drafts are acknowledged.

Last, all cited references are listed.

VI. REVIEW, DISSEMINATION, AND UPDATES

Each practice guideline is extensively reviewed at multiple draft stages. Draft 1 is reviewed by the Steering Committee. Draft 2 is reviewed by approximately 50 reviewers with expertise in the topic, representatives of allied organizations, the APA Assembly, District Branches, the Joint Reference Committee, the Board of Trustees, the Council on Quality Care, other components related to the subject area, and any APA member by request. Draft 3 is reviewed and approved for publication by the Assembly and the Board of Trustees.

The development process may be summarized as follows:

Step 1: The Steering Committee on Practice Guidelines selects about five individuals to serve as the work group chair and members.

Step 2: The work group chair and Department of Quality Improvement and Psychiatric Services staff develop a preliminary outline, to be continuously revised and refined throughout subsequent steps in the development process.

Step 3: A literature search is conducted by APA and/or the work group. Relevant articles from the search are obtained, in abstract or in entirety. The work group reviews these articles, codes them for study design, and constructs evidence tables for each treatment.

Step 4: Draft 1 is written based on evidence tables and outline.

Step 5: Draft 1 is circulated to the work group and Steering Committee for review and comment.

Step 6: Draft 2 is written based on comments received.

Step 7: Draft 2 is circulated for general review.

Step 8: Draft 3 is written based on comments received.

Step 9: Draft 3 is submitted to the formal APA review and approval process (Council on Quality Improvement, Assembly, Board of Trustees).

After final approval by the Assembly and Board of Trustees, each practice guideline is widely disseminated. Practice guidelines are made available to all psychiatrists in a variety of ways, including publication in *The American Journal of Psychiatry*. Each practice guideline is revised at regular intervals to reflect new knowledge in the field.

To help maintain currency of guideline recommendations, in 2004 the Steering Committee on Practice Guidelines began publishing "guideline watches," brief articles that highlight significant developments relevant to specific guidelines. As they are completed, watches are made available online in the Psychiatric Practice section of the APA web site at http://www.psych.org. Watches are also included in guideline compendiums available from American Psychiatric Publishing, Inc.

INDEX

*Page numbers printed in **boldface** type refer to tables or figures.*

A

AA (Alcoholics Anonymous), 301, 320, 331–332, 349, 386–387, 396, 444, 606, 1264
Abacavir, **204,** 252
Abdominal pain
  naltrexone-induced, 437
  in serotonin syndrome, 808
Abnormal Involuntary Movement Scale (AIMS), 27, 580
Abstinence from substances of abuse, 304, 305
  alcohol, 379
  cocaine, 397–398
  opioids, 399
  in 12-step programs, 331
ABT 431, for cocaine dependence, 448
Abuse/assault
  borderline personality disorder and, 215, 1020, 1045, 1225, 1254, 1266–1267, 1273
  eating disorders and, 1021, 1155, 1164
  of elderly persons, 124, 127
  sexual
    gender and, 1035
    HIV and, 194, 215, 221, 235
    initial assessment of victims of, 1014, 1018, 1019–1020
    posttraumatic stress disorder and, 215, 221, 1014, 1030, 1036, 1057
  substance use disorders and, 335–336
  suicide risk in persons with history of, 1351–1352, 1386, 1417–1419
Acamprosate
  for alcohol dependence, 301, 324, 378, 383–384, 439–440
    naltrexone and, 384
  dosage of, 384
  for mania, 891
  side effects of, 440
Access to care
  for HIV/AIDS, 236–237
  for schizophrenia among homeless persons, 610
  for substance use disorders, 321
Access to Community Care and Effective Services and Supports (ACCESS), 610, 611
Access to medical records, 39
Acne, lithium-induced, 662, 882–883
Acquired immunodeficiency syndrome. *See* Human immunodeficiency virus/acquired immunodeficiency syndrome
Activities of daily living, assessment of, 31
Activity scheduling, for depression, 817
Acupuncture
  for cocaine dependence, 395–396, 448
  for persons with HIV/AIDS, 229, 261
  for smoking cessation, 300, 368, 370, 430
Acute stress disorder (ASD), 1003–1070
  adaptive functioning in, 1026, 1027
  comorbidity with, 1020–1021, 1026–1027
  development of practice guideline for, 1008–1009
  diagnostic criteria for, 1015–1016, **1016,** 1039–1043, **1040–1042**
  differential diagnosis of, 1043–1045, **1046–1047**
  epidemiology of, 1045–1051
  factors affecting response to treatment for, 1029
  features associated with, 1043
  future research needs related to, 1067–1070
    early interventions/posttrauma treatment, 1067–1068
    generalization of research trials to clinical populations, 1069
    identification of risk factors, 1068
    pharmacotherapies and psychotherapies, 1069
    subthreshold and complex disorders, 1068
    treatment of specific symptoms, 1069
  initial assessment of, 1011, 1014–1021

Acute stress disorder (ASD) *(continued)*
initial assessment of *(continued)*
approach to patient, 1014–1015
clinical domains of, 1018, **1020**
comorbid conditions, 1020–1021
crime victims and legal system involvement, 1019–1020
exposure to traumatic event and diagnosis, 1015–1016
military and war-related traumatic event history, 1019
psychiatric history and evaluation, 1016–1018
interpreting literature on treatments for, 1051–1052
introduction to, 1010
natural history and course of, 1051
pharmacotherapy for, 1013, 1030–1031, 1063–1067
benzodiazepines, 1031, 1066
monoamine oxidase inhibitors, 1013, 1031, 1065–1066
nefazodone, 1064
other medications, 1066–1067
selective serotonin reuptake inhibitors, 1013, 1028, 1030, 1063–1064
trazodone, 1065
tricyclic antidepressants, 1013, 1031, 1065
prevalence of, 1048
principles of treatment selection for, 1012–1013, 1026–1029
choice of initial treatment modality, 1027–1028
lack of response to initial treatment, 1028–1029
treatment goals, 1012, 1026–1027
psychiatric management of, 1012, 1021–1026
coordination of care, 1023–1024, 1036
education of patient/family, 1024
enhancing treatment adherence, 1024–1025
monitoring treatment response, 1024
physical health and functional impairments, 1026
psychosocial effects of disorder, 1025–1026
suicide/violence risk assessment, 1021–1022
therapeutic alliance, 1023
treatment setting, 1022
psychosocial interventions for, 1013–1014, 1031–1034, 1052–1063
cognitive behavior therapy, 1014, 1028, 1031–1032, 1053–1057
early intervention strategies, 1061–1063
eye movement desensitization and reprocessing, 1014, 1028, 1032, 1057–1059
other psychotherapies, 1063
psychodynamic psychotherapy, 1014, 1033, 1052
psychoeducation, 1024, 1034
psychological debriefing, 1013, 1028, 1033–1034
risk factors for, 1068
safe environment for treatment of, 1015, 1023
subthreshold, 1068
summary of treatment recommendations for, 1011–1014
temporal relationship to traumatic stressor, 1043
Acyclovir, **209**
Adefovir, **204**
S-Adenosylmethionine (SAM-e), 246
Adherence to treatment
for acute stress disorder and posttraumatic stress disorder, 1024–1025
antiretroviral therapy for HIV/AIDS, 171, 175, 203, 217
enhancement of, 249, **250**
factors affecting, 249
for bipolar disorder, 864–865
for depression, 781
for panic disorder, 958
for schizophrenia, 581–582, 609
for substance use disorders, 319, 320
dual-diagnosis patients, 338, 340
smoking cessation, 366–367
for suicidal behavior, 1369
Adjustment disorder
in HIV/AIDS, 196, 222, 258
among traumatized persons, **1047**
Administrative issues, 38, 40
Adolescents
antidepressants for, suicide risk and, 748–749, 934–936
benzodiazepines for, 87
bereavement after suicide of friend, 1382
bipolar disorder in, 874–875, 880
somatic treatment of, 905–906

borderline personality disorder in, 1269–1270
eating disorders in, 1108, 1110, 1156–1157
HIV/AIDS in, 196, 208–210
psychiatric management of, 222, 259
panic disorder in, 984–985
schizophrenia in, 603
substance use disorders in, 354–355, 414
smoking, 417
suicidal behavior in, 1339, 1383, **1384**, 1385, 1387, 1390–1391
"Adonis complex," 1160
Adoption studies, of suicidal behavior, 1428
α-Adrenergic agonists, for posttraumatic stress disorder, 1013, 1031
β-Adrenergic blockers
for aggressive behavior, 609, 660–661
for akathisia, 649, 660
for alcohol withdrawal, 381, 436
interaction with antipsychotics, 635
for panic disorder, 975
for persons with schizophrenia, 573, 593, 601, 609, 660–661
for posttraumatic stress disorder, 1013, 1031
side effects of, 120
depression, 793, 799
for social anxiety disorder, 346
for tachycardia, 653
use in dementia, 114, 142
Adult Children of Alcoholics, 387
Adult psychiatric evaluation, 1–44
in dementia, 122
development of practice guideline for, 5
domains of, 12–23
developmental, psychosocial, and sociocultural history, 18–19, **19**
family history, 20
general medical history, 17–18
history of present illness, 12, 16
legal history, 19–20
mental status examination, 21–23
occupational and military history, 19
past psychiatric history, 17
physical examination, 20–21
questions related to, **13–16**
reason for evaluation, 12
review of systems, 20
substance abuse history, 17
future research needs related to, 42–44
diagnosis and formulation, 43
diagnostic testing, 43–44
interviewing approaches, 42–43
rating scales, 43
introduction to, 6
legal and administrative issues in institutions, 40
methods of obtaining information for, 23–35
collateral sources, 25
diagnostic tests, 31–34, **33**
patient interview, 23–25
physical examination, 34
structured interviews, questionnaires, and rating scales, 25–31, **26–30**
working with multidisciplinary teams, 34–35
privacy and confidentiality in, 7, 8, 11, 38–39
process of, 35–38
clinical formulation, 35
cultural formulation, 35–36, **36**
diagnosis, 36–37
initial treatment plan, 37–38
risk assessment, 36
systems issues, 38
treatment-related legal and administrative issues, 38, 40
purpose of, 7–10
clinical consultation, 9
emergency evaluation, 8–9
general psychiatric evaluation, 7
other consultations, 9–10
sites of, 10–12
general medical settings, 11
inpatient settings, 10
other settings, 12
outpatient settings, 10–11
in special populations, 40–42
elderly and/or medically ill persons, 40–41
homeless persons, 41
incarcerated persons, 41
persons with mental retardation, 41–42
third-party payers and, 39
Advance directives, 40, 128, 218, 590
Affect
assessment of, 21
flat or inappropriate, in schizophrenia, 623, 625
Affective disorders. *See* Mood disorders
Affective dysregulation, in borderline personality disorder, 1273
pharmacotherapy for, 1243–1244, 1256–1259, **1258**, **1301**

A-FRAMES model, for substance use disorders, 316, 333
Aftercare
for schizophrenia, 584
for substance use disorders, 314
alcohol dependence, 387–388, 445
Age at onset
of Alzheimer's disease, 118
of bipolar disorder, 880
of depression, 802
of frontal lobe dementias, 120
of panic disorder, 955
of Parkinson's disease, 119
of schizophrenia, 627
of vascular dementia, 119
Age/aging. *See also* Adolescents; Children; Elderly persons
acute stress disorder, posttraumatic stress disorder and, 1034, 1045, 1048
borderline personality disorder and, 1269–1270
cognitive decline due to, 117
delirium and, 92–93
dementia and, 117, 126, 153
eating disorders and, 1156–1157
HIV/AIDS and, 226
substance use disorders and, 354–356
suicide risk and, 1338–1339, 1383–1385, **1384**
Agency for Health Care Policy and Research, 122
A Clinical Practice Guideline for Treating Tobacco Use and Dependence, 372–373
Aggressive/violent behavior
benzodiazepine-induced, 87
bipolar disorder and, 870
borderline personality disorder and, 1244, 1264–1265, 1271–1272, 1273
dementia and, 122, 123
evaluation of person exhibiting, 24–25
patient restraint or seclusion for, 609
pharmacotherapy for, 609
β-blockers, 609, 660–661
posttraumatic stress disorder and, 1021–1022, 1038
rating scale for, **30**
schizophrenia and, 573, 578, 585, 608–609
substance use disorders and, 335–336
suicidality and, 1329, 1350, 1413–1414
"talking down" techniques for, 609
Agitation
catatonic, 789
causes of, 137
definition of, 137
in delirium, 72
in dementia, 113–114, 116, 119, 122, 123
anticonvulsants for, 114, 141–142
antipsychotics for, 113–114, 138–140
benzodiazepines for, 114, 140–141
goals of treatment for, 137
other agents for, 142
principles of treatment for, 137–138
drug-induced
aripiprazole, 647
psychostimulants, 144
selective serotonin reuptake inhibitors, 144
evaluation of person exhibiting, 24–25
rating scale for, **30**
in schizophrenia, 593
emergency treatment of, 589–590
suicidality and, 1329
Agnosia, 116, 118
Agoraphobia
behavioral exposure for, 961
panic disorder with, 954–955
Agranulocytosis, drug-induced
carbamazepine, 887, 1293
chlorpromazine, 632
clozapine, 114, 139, 242, 340, 612, 635, 636–638, 1263
mirtazapine, **796**, 809
treatment of, 638
valproate, 886, 1294
AIDS. *See* Human immunodeficiency virus/acquired immunodeficiency syndrome
AIDS Dementia Rating Scale, **210**
AIDS Litigation Project, 247
AIMS (Abnormal Involuntary Movement Scale), **27**, 580
Akathisia, drug-induced
antipsychotics, 85, 114, 138, 139, 241, 593, 648, 649–650
aggression and, 609
aripiprazole, 842
olanzapine, 642, 845
quetiapine, 644
risperidone, 649
ziprasidone, 842
clinical features of, 649
in persons with anorexia nervosa, 1121
vs. psychotic agitation, 649
selective serotonin reuptake inhibitors, 144, 808
treatment of, **594**, 649–650

Akinesia, antipsychotic-induced, 648
Akinetic depression, 648
Al-Anon, 332, 387, 445
Alateen, 332, 387
Alcohol interactions
with cocaine, 393
with disulfiram, 383, 438
Alcohol use disorders, 301, 377–391, 434–445. *See also* Substance use disorders
in children and adolescents, 354–355
clinical features influencing treatment for, 388–391
medical comorbidity, 389–390
pregnancy, 352, 390–391
psychiatric comorbidity, 388–389
cognitive impairment and, 390
course of, 377
detoxification from, 299
efficacy of treatments for, 377–378
in elderly persons, 356
epidemiology of, 377, 418–419
gender differences in, 353–354
goals of treatment for, 377
intoxication, 300, 335
breath, blood, or urine testing for, 317
management of, 379
suicide and, 1350–1351, 1415
legal issues related to
driving under the influence of alcohol, 315, 317, 416
mandated treatment, 315
medical comorbidity with, 319, **351**, 389–390
HIV/AIDS, 246
laboratory testing for, 319
treatment effects of, 389–390
natural history and course of, 415
neurological complications of, 390
occupations associated with, 307
in pregnancy, 352, 390–391
fetal alcohol spectrum disorder, 390–391
psychiatric comorbidity with, 336–337, 388–389, 419
anxiety disorders, 346, 388, 389
bipolar disorder, 336, 389, 871
borderline personality disorder, 1264
delirium, 76
dementia, 120
depression, 335, 336, 388–389, 790
eating disorders, 348, 1152
pathological gambling, 349
posttraumatic stress disorder, 346
schizophrenia, 340, 389
social anxiety disorder, 346
suicidal behavior, 334–335, 388, **1343**, 1346, 1348, 1350–1351, 1355, 1401–1404, 1415
treatment effects of, 388–389
psychosocial interventions for, 301, 385–388, 442–445
aftercare, 387–388
behavior therapy, 386
brief therapies, 386
cognitive behavior therapy, 385, 442
family therapy, 331, 387
interpersonal therapy, 386
marital therapy, 387
psychodynamic psychotherapy, 386
relapse prevention, 379, 385, 443
self-guided therapies, 387
self-help groups and 12-step programs, 331–332, 386–387
psychotropic drug use in persons with
antidepressants, 342
antipsychotics, 340
benzodiazepines, 346
screening instruments for, **28**, 307
sleep disturbances and, 336
smoking cessation and, 367
somatic treatments for, 301, 379–385, 435–442
acamprosate, 301, 324, 378, 383–384, 439–440
disulfiram, 301, 324, 378, 383, 438–439
in dual-diagnosis patients, 339, 341
in persons with HIV/AIDS, 246
for intoxication, 379
lithium, 385
naltrexone, 301, 324, 378, 382, 436–438
ondansetron, 385, 440–442
in patients with psychiatric comorbidity, 339
selective serotonin reuptake inhibitors, 384, 440–442
tricyclic antidepressants, 384
for withdrawal syndromes, 379–382, 435–436
treatment settings for, 299, 378–379, 434–435
unemployment and, 1355
Alcohol Use Disorders Identification Test (AUDIT), 307, 605

Alcohol withdrawal
assessment instruments for, 379
complications of, 301, 379
course of, 301
delirium tremens during, 379
electroencephalogram in, 74
goals of treatment for, 379
management of, **81**, 301
onset of symptoms of, 301, 379
opioid withdrawal concurrent with, 302
repeated episodes of, 379
schizophrenia and, 585
seizures during, 75, 379
prophylaxis for, 381
somatic treatments for, 301, 379–382, 435–436
anticonvulsants, 381, 435–436
antipsychotics, 381
benzodiazepines, 72, 86, 87, 90, 301, 380–381, 435–436
β-blockers, 381, 436
clonidine, 381, 436
intravenous ethanol, 382
thiamine, 301, 380, 390
supportive treatment for, 379–380
symptoms of, 301, 379
Alcoholics Anonymous (AA), 301, 320, 331–332, 349, 386–387, 396, 444, 606, 1264
Allergic reactions
to antipsychotics, 631
to carbamazepine, 887
Alogia, 625
Alopecia, drug-induced
lithium, 662, 882
valproate, 885
Alprazolam
for alcohol withdrawal, 436
for borderline personality disorder, 1294
for depression with anxiety symptoms, 790
extended-release, 936, 937
interaction with ritonavir, 244
for panic disorder, 936, 937, 970
discontinuation of, 971
dosage of, 972
length of treatment with, 972–973
vs. propranolol, 975
side effects of, 1294
use in opioid-dependent patients, 410
Alternative and complementary medicine, for HIV/AIDS, 229, 246
Alzheimer's Association, 126, 127, 148, 153
Safe Return Program, 124
Alzheimer's disease, 118. *See also* Dementia
age at onset of, 118
apolipoprotein E4 genotype and, 122, 126, 154
assessing and monitoring psychiatric status in, 122–123
behavioral disturbances in, 118
cognitive deficits in, 118
course of, 117, 118
depression and, 122, 143
among caregivers, 151
diagnosis of, 118
family history of, 154
functional neuroimaging in, 44
gender distribution of, 153
home care for, 150–151
introduction to, 109
monitoring psychiatric status in, 122
neuroimaging in, 101
neuropathology of, 118
onset and course of, 117, 118
pharmacotherapy for, 112–115, 130–147
cholinesterase inhibitors, 102, 112–113, 131–133, 147, 148
ergoloid mesylates, 136
other agents, 113, 136–137
selegiline, 113, 135, 148, 149
vitamin E, 102, 113, 134, 148, 149, 154
prevalence of, 117
prevention of, 102
protective factors against, 126
risk factors for, 126
somatic treatments for, 102, 112–115, 130–148
for cognitive and functional losses, 112–113, 131–137
for depression, 114–115, 142–145
for psychosis and agitation, 113–114, 137–142
for sleep disturbances, 115, 146–147
stroke and, 119
subtypes of, 118
suicidality and, 123
support groups for, 126, 127
vascular dementia and, 119
wandering in, 118, 124
Amantadine
for cocaine dependence/withdrawal, 394, 447
in methadone-maintained patients, 397

dosage of, 145
for extrapyramidal symptoms, **594**, 649
for hyperprolactinemia, 656
for neuroleptic malignant syndrome, 652
for persons with dementia, 115, 143, 145
for sexual dysfunction, **796**, 808
side effects of, 144
American Academy of Child and Adolescent Psychiatry
Practice Parameter for the Assessment and Treatment of Children and Adolescents With Substance Use Disorders, 354
Practice Parameter for the Assessment and Treatment of Children and Adolescents With Suicidal Behavior, 1328
Practice Parameters for the Assessment and Treatment of Children and Adolescents With Anxiety Disorders, 984
Practice Parameters for the Assessment and Treatment of Children and Adolescents With Posttraumatic Stress Disorder, 1008
American Academy of Neurology, practice guideline for dementia, 122
American Psychiatric Association (APA)
Handbook of Psychiatric Measures, 580
Practice Guideline for Psychiatric Evaluation of Adults, 122, 779, 863, 956, 984, 1018
Practice Guideline for the Assessment and Treatment of Patients With Suicidal Behaviors, 36, 335, 608, 1021
Practice Guideline for the Treatment of Patients With Acute Stress Disorder and Posttraumatic Stress Disorder, 347, 1007
Practice Guideline for the Treatment of Patients With Bipolar Disorder, 344, 662, 778, 841, 862, 1294
Practice Guideline for the Treatment of Patients With Borderline Personality Disorder, 349
Practice Guideline for the Treatment of Patients With Delirium, 208
Practice Guideline for the Treatment of Patients With Eating Disorders, 349
Practice Guideline for the Treatment of Patients With HIV/AIDS, 352, 876
Practice Guideline for the Treatment of Patients With Major Depressive Disorder, 143, 342, 747, 856, 861, 892, 903, 1263, 1298
Practice Guideline for the Treatment of Patients With Panic Disorder, 940
Practice Guideline for the Treatment of Patients With Schizophrenia, 340
Practice Guideline for the Treatment of Patients With Substance Use Disorders, 17
The Practice of Electroconvulsive Therapy: Recommendations for Treatment, Training, and Privileging, 595, 751, 1377
recommendations for use of antidepressants in pediatric patients, 935
on suicide risk related to antidepressant use in children, 749, 935
Task Force on Benzodiazepine Dependence, Toxicity, and Abuse, 971
American Society of Addiction Medicine (ASAM), 310, 311, 312
Americans with Disabilities Act, 218
Amiloride, 882
Amitriptyline
for acute stress disorder, 1031
for anorexia nervosa, 1174
for borderline personality disorder, 1257, 1289, 1290
for bulimia nervosa, 1177
contraindicated in persons with dementia, 114, 145
dosage of, 774
for HIV-associated neuropathy, 261
for insomnia during opioid withdrawal, 408
for posttraumatic stress disorder, 1031, 1065
side effects of, 144
Amnestic disorders, 117. *See also* Memory impairment
Amobarbital, for catatonia, 789
Amoxapine
for borderline personality disorder, 1290
dosage of, 774
side effects of, **795**
extrapyramidal effects, 807
use in Parkinson's disease, 799
Amphetamine
abuse and dependence on, 393, 420
schizophrenia and, 625
replacement therapy for cocaine dependence, 395, 448
Amphotericin B, **209**
Amprenavir, **204**
Anabolic steroid abuse, 308, 335, 1160
Anesthesia-assisted rapid opioid detoxification (AROD), 302

Angiotensin-converting enzyme inhibitors, interaction with lithium, 876
Anhedonia
schizophrenia and, 625
suicidality and, 1329
Anorexia nervosa. *See also* Eating disorders
body dysmorphic disorder and, 1156
bupropion contraindicated in, 369, 429, 1112
chronicity of, 1151–1152, 1164–1165
clinical features of, 1160–1162
diagnostic criteria for, 1119, **1119**
epidemiology of, 1163
family interventions for, 1110, 1140, 1171–1172
future research needs related to, 1181–1183
genetic factors and, 1167–1168
goals of treatment for, 1108, 1134
hormone replacement therapy for, 1113, 1145, 1174–1175
laboratory abnormalities in, 1162
medications for, 1112–1113, 1143–1145, 1173–1175
natural history and course of, 1164–1166
nutritional rehabilitation for, 1108–1110, 1134–1138, 1169
personality disorders and, 1153
physical complications of, **1123–1125,** 1162
prevalence of, 1163
psychodynamic issues in, 1161
psychosocial interventions for, 1110–1111, 1138–1143
relapse prevention for, 1112–1113, 1173
substance use disorders and, 1152
subtypes of, 1161
suicidality and, 1345, 1400
support groups for, 349, 1111, 1114, 1141–1142, 1172
therapeutic alliance for treatment of, 1116–1118
treatment settings for, 1106–1108, 1129–1134, **1131–1133,** 1169, 1170–1171
Anorexia Nervosa Stages of Change Questionnaire, 1170
Anorexics and Bulimics Anonymous, 1111, 1141
Anoxia, delirium induced by, **81**
Antiarrhythmic agents, interaction with tricyclic antidepressants, 806
Antibody testing for HIV infection, 194, 212–213, 231
Anticholinergic agents
for antipsychotic overdose, 635
avoiding in persons with dementia, 114
delirium induced by, 72, **81**, 87, 654
for extrapyramidal side effects, 594, **594,** 649–650
toxicity of, 654
water intoxication and, 609
Anticholinergic effects of drugs
amantadine, 144
antidepressants, 114, 144, 429, **795,** 806–807, 952, 968
antipsychotics, 85, 114, 138, **592,** 614, 631, 654
aripiprazole, 647
clozapine, 636, 654
diphenhydramine, 115
in elderly persons, 112
olanzapine, 642
opiates, 88
ziprasidone, 645
Anticonvulsants
for alcohol withdrawal, 301, 435–436
for antidepressant augmentation, 784
for antipsychotic augmentation, 602
for behavioral symptoms of dementia, 114, 141–142
for bipolar disorder
in children and adolescents, 874, 905–906
depressive episodes, 860, 867–868, 893–894
maintenance treatment, 844–845, 861, 868
manic episodes, 843, 859–860, 866–867, 885–889
rapid cycling, 868, 897
for borderline personality disorder, 1226, 1243, 1244, **1258,** 1259, **1260,** 1261, 1292–1294
for cocaine dependence, 448
interaction with oral contraceptives, 871
for panic disorder, 974
for persons with HIV/AIDS, 196, 243–244, 256
for persons with schizophrenia, 657
for posttraumatic stress disorder, 1013, 1031, 1066
in pregnancy, 872, 873, 1269
prophylaxis for alcohol withdrawal seizures, 381
side effects of, 141, 142
for suicidal persons, 1326, 1375, 1446

Antidepressants, **774,** 803–813. *See also specific drugs and classes*
for acute stress disorder, 1013, 1030–1031
for alcohol dependence, 384
augmentation of, 751–752, 784, 812, 823
for bipolar disorder, 844, 860, 868, 895–896
in dual-diagnosis patients, 345
blood levels of, 811
for borderline personality disorder, 1243, 1244, 1256–1257, **1258,** 1259–1261, **1260, 1262,** 1287–1292
for children and adolescents, 793
suicide risk and, 748–749, 934–936
choice of, 752, 772, 783, **783**
for cocaine dependence, 447
for depression
in acute phase, 772–775, 782–785
with atypical features, 772–773, 789–790
combined with psychotherapy, 751, 772, 777, 782, 786, 820
in continuation phase, 751–752, 787, 820–821
in dual-diagnosis patients, 338, 342–343, 388–389, 790
with dysthymia, 791
as initial primary treatment, 772
in maintenance phase, 751–752, **777,** 777–778, 787, 821–822
with psychotic features, 750, 752, 789
discontinuation of, 778, 788, 821
dosage of, 752, 773, **774,** 783, 810
drug interactions with
antipsychotics, 635, 658
antiretroviral agents, 174
carbamazepine, 888
for dysthymia, 791
for eating disorders, 1153
anorexia nervosa, 1112, 1143–1144, 1173–1174
binge eating disorder, 1115–1116, 1150, 1180–1181
bulimia nervosa, 1114–1115, 1147–1148, 1177–1178
efficacy of, 772, 783, 804–805
for elderly persons, 752–753, 793–794, 875
failure to respond to, 751–752, 775, **776,** 784–785, 811–813
future research needs related to, 822
gender-related response to, 752
goals of treatment with, 803–804
implementation of, 783–784, 810–811
new drugs, 749–750
overdose of, 811, 1442
for panic disorder, 934, 936–937, 965–969, 973–974, 979
combined with benzodiazepines, 938
in dual-diagnosis patients, 345
patient monitoring during treatment with, 783, 785
for persons with concurrent medical conditions, 783, 797–799
asthma, 797
cardiac disease, 797–798
cardiovascular disease, 144, 783
dementia, 102, 114, 143–145, 798
epilepsy, 798
glaucoma, 798
hepatitis C, 176–177
HIV/AIDS, 174, 195, 196, 220, 240–241, 254–255
hypertension, 798–799
obstructive uropathy, 799
Parkinson's disease, 799
for persons with schizophrenia, 573, 576, 577, 594, 601, 607, 614, 657–659
for posttraumatic stress disorder, 1013, 1030–1031, 1063–1066
in pregnancy, 794–797
side effects of, 144, 658, 806–810
in elderly persons, 794
hypomania or mania, 866, 897, 935
management of, **775, 795–796**
for smoking cessation, 430
for suicidal behavior, 1326, 1374, 1442–1444
suicide risk associated with, 748–749, 934–936
switching between, 784, 812
washout times for, 784, **784**
time to clinical response to, 784, 811
Antidepressants, tricyclic (TCAs). *See also specific drugs*
for acute stress disorder, 1031
for alcohol dependence, 384
blood levels of, 811
for borderline personality disorder, 1257, 1289–1290
combined with monoamine oxidase inhibitors, 812
for depression
in bipolar disorder, 896
in dual-diagnosis patients, 342–343, 388

Antidepressants, tricyclic (TCAs) *(continued)*
dosage of, **774**, 968–969, 1290
drug interactions with, 807
antiarrhythmic agents, 806
antihypertensive agents, 798
disulfiram, 439
diuretics, 798–799
ritonavir, 241
selective serotonin reuptake inhibitors, 807, 812
selegiline, 135
efficacy of, 752, 804
for elderly persons, 968
neonatal withdrawal from, 796
for obsessive-compulsive disorder, in dual-diagnosis patients, 346
overdose of, 144, 345, 346, 369, 429, 811, 968, 1290, 1434, 1442
for panic disorder, 934, 937, 952, 967–969, 979
in dual-diagnosis patients, 345
maintenance treatment, 937
for persons with concurrent medical conditions, 783
cardiac disease, 144, 797
dementia, 114, 145, 798
HIV/AIDS, 241, 254, 255
for persons with schizophrenia, 607, 658
for posttraumatic stress disorder, 1013, 1031, 1065
in pregnancy, 796, 872
side effects of, 144, 429, **795–796**, 806–807, 968, 1290
for suicidal behavior, 1374
use in persons with eating disorders, 1112, 1114, 1143–1144, 1147, 1174, 1177–1178, 1180
Antiemetics, for opioid withdrawal symptoms, 408
Antihistamines, interaction with nefazodone, 809
Antihypertensive drugs, interaction with antidepressants, 798–799
Antimicrobial agents
interaction with carbamazepine, 888
side effects of, **209**
Antioxidants, for HIV-related cognitive disorders, 253
Antiparkinsonian drugs, 594, **594**, 649
prophylactic, 594, 650
Antipsychotics, **589**, 628–657. *See also specific drugs*
for acute stress disorder, 1031
administration routes for, 72, 85, 140, 632
during alcohol withdrawal, 301
for alcohol withdrawal, 381
for anorexia nervosa, 1112, 1144, 1174
augmentation of, 602
for bipolar disorder, 1376
in children and adolescents, 906
depressive episodes, 843, 860, 896
in dual-diagnosis patients, 344
maintenance treatment, 845, 861, 869, 900
manic or mixed episodes, 842–843, 859–860, 866–867
for borderline personality disorder, 1244, **1258**, 1259, **1260**, 1261–1263, **1262**, 1295–1298
for cocaine intoxication, 394
combinations of, 659
continuous intravenous infusion of, 86, 90
for delirium, 62, 72, 84–86, 90
combined with benzodiazepines, 72, 86, 87, 90–91
in elderly patients, 72, 93
goals and efficacy of, 84
in HIV/AIDS, 253–254
for dementia, 102, 113–114, 138–140, 148
in Parkinson's disease, 150
for sleep disturbances, 146–147
use in long-term care facilities, 115, 151–152
discussing risks and benefits of, 573, 588
dosage of, 85, 114, 139–140, 573, **589**, 592–593, 632–634
drug interactions with, 635
anticonvulsants, 657
antidepressants, 635, 658
antiretroviral agents, 221, 242
carbamazepine, 888
nicotine, 340
selective serotonin reuptake inhibitors, 607
tricyclic antidepressants, 807
for elderly persons, 72, 85, 93, 614, 875
"extrapyramidal symptom threshold" for, 575, 593, 599, 648
half-lives of, **589**
high-potency, 633
intramuscular, 609, 632, 633
laboratory studies before initiation of, 588

long-acting injectable preparations of, 140, 573, 592, 632
dosage of, 634
for dual-diagnosis patients, 340
low-potency, 633
overdose of, 634–635
for panic disorder, 975
for persons with HIV/AIDS, 175, 195, 196, 221–222, 241–242, 253–254, 258
for posttraumatic stress disorder, 1013, 1031
in pregnancy, 613, 872–873
receptor affinity of, 632–633
for schizophrenia, 573–576, 628–657, 1375
in acute phase, 573, 588–593, **589–592**, 629–630
advance directives for use of, 590
aggressive behavior, 609
clozapine, 576
combinations of, 659
in dual-diagnosis patients, 340–341, 449, 606
duration of trial of, 576
electroconvulsive therapy and, 594
emergency treatment, 589–590
evaluating response to, 576
lack of response to, **591**, 593, 601–602
patient ambivalence about, 581
patient refusal of, 589–590
in pregnancy, 613
for relapse prevention, 575, 599–601, 603–604
in stabilization phase, 574, 595, 630
in stable phase, 574–576, **591**, 599–600, 603–604, 630–631
second-generation, 588, **589**, 590–591, 628, 635–647
aripiprazole, 646–647
clozapine, 635–639
olanzapine, 641–643
quetiapine, 643–644
risperidone, 639–641
ziprasidone, 644–646
selection of, 139, 573, 590–591, **590–591**
sensitivity to, in Lewy body disease, 119
side effects of, 85, 102, 113–114, 138–139, 241, 344, 574–575, 588, 591–593, **592**, 600, 628–629, 631–632, 647–657, 1297
allergic and dermatological effects, 631
anticholinergic and antiadrenergic effects, 85, 114, 138, **592**, 614, 631, 654
cardiovascular effects, 72, 85, 114, 138, 590, 616, 631, 653–654
diabetes, 575
dysphoria, 606, 607
in elderly persons, 614
extrapyramidal effects, 85, 114, 138–139, **592**, 592–593, 648–651
hematological effects, 85, 114, 139, 632
hepatic effects, 85, 631
for high-potency and low-potency drugs, 633
hyperprolactinemia, 614, 615
metabolic effects, 178, 631
monitoring for, 574–575
neuroleptic malignant syndrome, 85, 114, 139, 631, 651–652
neurological effects, 647–652
ophthalmological effects, 631–632
orthostatic hypotension, 85, 114, 138, 592, **592**, 614, 631, 633, 653
pathophysiology of, 629
polydipsia and water intoxication, 609–610, 625
QTc interval prolongation, 72, 85, 86, 90, **592**, 616, 653–654
sedation, 85, 113, 114, 138, 139, 592, **592**, 614, 631, 652
seizures, 85, 114, 138, 631
sexual dysfunction, 631, 656–657
tachycardia, 85, 86, 631, 653
weight gain and metabolic abnormalities, 102, 575, **592**, 614, 631, 654–655
for suicidal persons, 1326, 1375–1376, 1446–1449
Antiretroviral therapy, 170–172, 202–203. *See also specific drugs and classes*
adherence to, 171, 175, 203, 217, 248–249, **250**
combination, 170, 238
cost of, 203
directly observed, 171
drug interactions with, 171–172, **172**, 195
antidepressants, 174
antipsychotics, 221, 242
benzodiazepines, 195, 221, 238, 244
carbamazepine, 888
cytochrome P450–related, 171, **238**, 238–241, **239**, 244, 245, 261
methadone, 171, 245–246, 351
St. John's wort, 750
sildenafil, 241, 261
valproate, 243
drugs for, 170, 202, **204**

Antiretroviral therapy *(continued)*
goal of, 202
for HIV-associated dementia, 250–252
lack of response to, 203
for pediatric patients, 196, 259
penetration of blood-brain barrier by, 173, 251
for postexposure prophylaxis, 194, 213–214, 234
recommended regimens for, 170–171
to reduce perinatal HIV transmission, 170, 233–234
resistance to, 170, 171, 203
side effects of, 203, 208, **209**, 220
central nervous system effects, 172
metabolic syndrome and lipodystrophy, 171, 177–178
timing of, 170
viral replication cycle targets for, **201**, 202
for women, 225
Antisocial features, in borderline personality disorder, 1264–1265
Antisocial personality disorder (ASPD)
substance use disorders and, 349
pathological gambling and, 350
suicide and, 1347, 1348, 1408, 1409
Anxiety
dementia and, 116, 122
drug-induced
benzodiazepines, 87, 140
cocaine withdrawal, 394
naltrexone, 404
selective serotonin reuptake inhibitors, 966
selegiline, 135
suicidality and, 1329, 1349, 1399, 1409–1410
Anxiety disorders. *See also specific anxiety disorders*
acute stress disorder and posttraumatic stress disorder, 1003–1070
bipolar disorder and, 871
depression and, 790–791
eating disorders and, 1153, 1164
hepatitis C and, **176**
in HIV/AIDS, 195, 221, 244, 257–258
panic disorder, 933–987
prevalence of, 345
rating scales for, **29**
substance use disorders and, 336, 345–347
among adolescents, 355
assessment of, 345
integrated treatments for, 338, 345–347
pathological gambling and, 350
pharmacotherapy for, 389
prevalence of, 345
suicidal behavior and, **1343**, 1345, 1397–1399
APA. *See* American Psychiatric Association
Apathy, in dementia, 115, 119, 122, 143
Aphasia
in delirium, 73
in dementia, 116, 118
Aplastic anemia, carbamazepine-induced, 887, 1293
Apolipoprotein E4 genotype (*APOE4*), 122, 126, 154
Appearance, assessment of, 21
Appetite changes, drug-induced. *See also* Weight changes
cocaine, 394, 397
fluoxetine-olanzapine combination, 843
olanzapine, 845, 890
psychostimulants, 144
valproate, 885
Apraxia, in dementia, 116, 118, 119
Aricept. *See* Donepezil
Aripiprazole, 588, **589**, 646–647
for bipolar disorder
in dual-diagnosis patients, 344
manic episodes, 842, 891
dosage of, **589**, 647, 842
efficacy of, 646–647
implementing treatment with, 647
receptor affinity of, 646
for schizoaffective disorder, 646–647
for schizophrenia, 646–647
side effects of, **592**, 647, 842
suppression of prolactin release, 615
AROD (anesthesia-assisted rapid opioid detoxification), 302
Arrhythmias
in anorexia nervosa, **1123**
in bulimia nervosa, **1126**
drug-induced
antidepressants, 144, **795**, 806
antipsychotics, 85, 86, 614
cocaine, 301, 393, 397
LAAM, 401
lithium, 882
psychostimulants, 144
trazodone, 798, 809
electroconvulsive therapy–induced, 664

Art therapy, 112, 130
ASAM (American Society of Addiction Medicine), 310, 311, 312
ASD. *See* Acute stress disorder
ASPD (antisocial personality disorder)
substance use disorders and, 349
pathological gambling and, 350
suicide and, 1347, 1348, 1408, 1409
Aspirin
for dementia, 136
for stroke prevention, 150
Assault victims. *See* Abuse/assault
Assertive community treatment, for schizophrenia, 576, 578, 596, 617
Assessment
of acute stress disorder and posttraumatic stress disorder, 1011, 1014–1021, **1020**
adult psychiatric evaluation, 1–44
of bipolar disorder, 863
of borderline personality disorder, 1241, 1245–1246, 1274–1275
of delirium, 77–78, **80**
of dementia, 122–123
of depression, 779
of eating disorders, 1105–1106, 1119–1120, **1121**
functional, **16**, 31
in acute stress disorder and posttraumatic stress disorder, 1026, 1027, 1051
in bipolar disorder, 866
in borderline personality disorder, 1248, 1274
in dementia, 122
in depression, 780
in panic disorder, 956–957
in schizophrenia, 583, 598–599
in substance use disorders, 303, 305
of HIV/AIDS, 202, **202, 203**
of language competence, 7
of mental status, **15–16,** 21–23
for nicotine dependence, **360,** 360–362
of patients with schizophrenia, 572–573, 584–585, **586–587,** 596
of substance use disorders, 297, 303, 306–310
of suicidal behavior, 1322–1324, **1323, 1328,** 1328–1362, 1437–1440
Assessment and Treatment of Patients With Coexisting Mental Illness and Alcohol and Other Drug Abuse, 17
Assessment instruments, 25–31
Abnormal Involuntary Movement Scale, **27,** 580
AIDS Dementia Rating Scale, **210**
Alcohol Use Disorders Identification Test, 307, 605
Anorexia Nervosa Stages of Change Questionnaire, 1170
Bayley Scales of Infant Development, 259
Beck Depression Inventory, **28,** 1057, 1438–1439
Beck Hopelessness Scale, 1410, 1438
Brief Psychiatric Rating Scale, **30,** 580
Brief Symptom Inventory, 260
Bulimia Test—Revised, **1121**
CAGE Questionnaire, **28,** 307
Center for Epidemiologic Studies Depression Scale, 256
Clinical Assessment of Confusion–A, 78
Clinical Global Impression Scale, **26**
Clinical Global Impression Scale for Bipolar Illness, 889
Clinical Institute Narcotic Assessment, 405
Clinical Institute Withdrawal Assessment of Alcohol Scale, Revised, 379
Clinician-Administered PTSD Scale, 1018, 1054, 1055
Composite International Diagnostic Interview, 1045, 1048
Confusion Assessment Method, 78
Confusion Assessment Method for the Intensive Care Unit, 61
Confusion Rating Scale, 78
Dartmouth Assessment of Lifestyle Instrument, 605
Delirium Observation Screening Scale, 61
Delirium Rating Scale, **27,** 61, 62, 78, 84, 254
Delirium Scale, 78
Delirium Symptom Interview, 78
Diagnostic Interview Schedule, 1045
Diagnostic Survey for Eating Disorders, **1121**
Drug Abuse Screening Test, 307
Eating Attitudes Test, **1121**
Eating Disorder Examination, **1121**
Eating Disorders Examination—Questionnaire, **1121**
Eating Disorders Inventory–2, **1121**
Eating Disorders Questionnaire, **1121**
Executive Interview Test, **219**
Fagerström Test for Nicotine Dependence, 360, **360,** 368

Assessment instruments *(continued)*
Finger Tapping Test, **210**
Freiberg Personality Inventory, 1413
General Health Questionnaire, 1438
Geriatric Depression Scale, **29**
Global Accessibility Rating Scale, 78
Global Assessment of Functioning Scale, **26**
Hamilton Anxiety Rating Scale, **29,** 968
Hamilton Depression Rating Scale, **28,** 255, 258, 816, 817, 893, 894, 1289, 1438–1439
Harvard Trauma Questionnaire, 1050
HIV Dementia Scale, 173, 174, **219**
Hopkins Symptom Checklist–25, 1050
Impact of Event Scale, 1018, 1057, 1058, 1059
International HIV Dementia Scale, 173
Inventory of Depressive Symptomatology, 894
McCarthy Scales of Children's Abilities, 259
MCV Nursing Delirium Rating Scale, 78
Memorial Delirium Assessment Scale, 78
Mental Alteration Test, **219**
Millon Clinical Multiaxial Inventory–II, 1298
Mini-Mental State Exam, **27,** 84, 101, 122, 174, 219
Mississippi PTSD Rating Scale, 1057
Montgomery-Åsberg Depression Rating Scale, 893
Mood Disorder Questionnaire, 841, 866
NEECHAM Confusion Scale, 78
Organic Brain Syndrome Scale, 78
Overt Aggression Scale—Modified, **30**
Patient Health Questionnaire, **29**
Positive and Negative Syndrome Scale, **30,** 580
PTSD Checklist, 1018
Quality of Life Enjoyment & Satisfaction Questionnaire, **26**
Questionnaire on Eating and Weight Patterns, **1121**
Quick Inventory of Depression Symptomatology—Self-Report, **28**
Rating Scale for Extrapyramidal Side Effects, **27**
Readiness and Motivation Interview, 1170
Reasons for Living Inventory, 1438
Risk-Rescue Rating, 1438
Saskatoon Delirium Checklist, 78
Scale for Suicide Ideation, 1335, 1437
Scale for Suicide Ideation–Worst, 1433, 1437
Scale for the Assessment of Negative Symptoms, 659
Scale for the Assessment of Positive Symptoms, 659
Schedule for Affective Disorders and Schizophrenia, 1409
Simpson-Angus Extrapyramidal Symptom Rating Scale, **27**
Social and Occupational Functioning Assessment Scale, **26**
Spielberger State-Trait Anxiety Inventory, 976
Structured Clinical Interview for DSM-IV, 580
Structured Interview for PTSD, 1018
Suicide Assessment Scale, 1438
Suicide Behavior Questionnaire, 1437–1438
Suicide Intent Scale, 1335, 1438
Thematic Apperception Test, 1438
Trail Making Test, 174, **210**
Wechsler Intelligence Scale for Children, 259
Yale-Brown Obsessive Compulsive Scale, **29**
Yale-Brown-Cornell Eating Disorder Scale, **1121**
Young Mania Rating Scale, **29,** 889, 893, 906
Zung Anxiety Scale, 976
Asterixis, 74
Asthenia, drug-induced
duloxetine, 749
fluoxetine-olanzapine combination, 843
Asthma medications, interactions with antidepressants, 797
Ataxia
delirium and, 74
drug-induced
benzodiazepines, 86, 140, 660, 937, 970
carbamazepine, 141, 843, 887, 1293
valproate, 141
Atenolol
for alcohol withdrawal, 381
for tachycardia, 653
Athletes, eating disorders in, 1158
Atomoxetine
for attention-deficit/hyperactivity disorder, 750
in dual-diagnosis patients, 348
for depression, 750
hepatotoxicity of, 750
Attentional problems, in schizophrenia, 623

Attention-deficit/hyperactivity disorder (ADHD)
atomoxetine for, 750
bipolar disorder and, 871, 874–875, 880
borderline personality disorder and, 1224
bulimia nervosa and, 1114
in HIV-infected children, 259
psychostimulants for
in dual-diagnosis patients, 348
lack of association with substance use disorders in adulthood, 348, 355
stimulant abuse in, 324
substance use disorders and, 336, 347–348
among adolescents, 355
cocaine dependence, 397
pathological gambling and, 350
suicidality and, 1345, 1400–1401
AUDIT (Alcohol Use Disorders Identification Test), 307, 605
Australian National Survey of Mental Health and Wellbeing, 1399
Autonomic dysfunction, in neuroleptic malignant syndrome, 651
Aversion therapy, for substance use disorders, 329
alcohol dependence, 386, 443
nicotine dependence, 370, 433
Avoidant personality disorder
depression and, 792
eating disorders and, 1153, 1154, 1164
panic disorder and, 983
Avolition, in schizophrenia, 623, 625

B

Baclofen, for cocaine dependence, 395, 448
Barbiturates
delirium induced by, 76
drug interactions with
antipsychotics, 625
tricyclic antidepressants, 807
prophylaxis for alcohol withdrawal seizures, 381
Barotrauma, cocaine-induced, 397
Battered women, suicide risk among, 1352, 1419–1421
Bayley Scales of Infant Development, 259
BDD (body dysmorphic disorder), anorexia nervosa and, 1156
Beck Depression Inventory, **28,** 1057, 1438–1439
Beck Hopelessness Scale, 1410, 1438
Behavior, assessment, 21
Behavior therapy. *See also* Cognitive behavior therapy
for acute stress disorder and posttraumatic stress disorder, 1053–1055
for aggression in persons with schizophrenia, 609
for dementia, 112, 129
for depression, 817
in bipolar disorder, 903
double depression, 791
for substance use disorders, 298, 315, 325, 328
alcohol dependence, 386, 443
cocaine dependence, 396, 449–450
in depression, 344
in group format, 330
nicotine dependence, 368, 370, 432–433
opioid dependence, 408–409, 463–465
Behavioral contracting
for substance use disorders, 331
suicide prevention contracts, 1325, 1379–1380, 1455–1456
Behavioral disinhibition/dyscontrol
benzodiazepine-induced, 86, 87, 140–141, 660, 1294
in borderline personality disorder, pharmacotherapy for, 1244, 1259–1261, **1260, 1302**
in dementia, 116, 119, 122
frontal lobe dementias, 119
sexual, medroxyprogesterone for, 114, 142
Behavioral disturbances
in Alzheimer's disease, 118
in schizophrenia, 623
Behavioral family systems therapy (BFST), for anorexia nervosa, 1172
Behavioral self-control training
for depression, 817
for substance use disorders, 298, 315, 333
alcohol dependence, 442
Belief modification, for schizophrenia, 669
Benefits of using practice guidelines, x
Benzodiazepines. *See also specific drugs*
abuse or dependence on, 660, 790, 1449
for agitation, 647
for akathisia, 649, 650
for alcohol or sedative-hypnotic withdrawal, 72, 86, 87, 90, 301, 380–381, 435–436
for antidepressant augmentation, 751
for antipsychotic augmentation, 602
for borderline personality disorder, 1243, 1257, **1258,** 1294

Benzodiazepines *(continued)*
for catatonia, 573, 604, 660, 789
for children, 87
for cocaine intoxication, 301, 394
contraindications to, 87
for delirium, 62, 72, 84, 86–87, 90–91, 92
combined with antipsychotics, 72, 86, 87, 90–91
goals and efficacy of, 86
dependence on, 86, 141
discontinuation of, 141, 1326
dosage of, 972
drug interactions with, 87
buprenorphine, 404, 460
carbamazepine, 888
clozapine, 639
nefazodone, 809
protease inhibitors, 195, 221, 238, 241, 244
for elderly persons, 86–87, 356, 875, 971
for emergency treatment of acute psychosis, 589, 660
fear of addiction to, 971
hepatic metabolism of, 92
for mania, 860, 867, 892
for neuroleptic malignant syndrome, 652
overdose of, 322
flumazenil for, 322–323
for panic disorder, 936, 937, 952, 953, 969–973
cognitive behavior therapy during discontinuation of, 962
combined with antidepressants, 938
in dual-diagnosis patients, 345–346
for early symptom control, combined with another treatment modality, 980–981
length of treatment with, 972–973
for persons with anorexia nervosa, 1112
for persons with dementia, 114, 115, 140–141, 146, 147
for persons with depression, 790
for persons with HIV/AIDS, 195–196, 221, 244
for persons with posttraumatic stress disorder, 1013
for persons with schizophrenia, 573, 576, 589, 593, 601, 659–660
aggressive behavior, 609
antipsychotic augmentation, 660
for posttraumatic stress disorder, 1031, 1066
in pregnancy, 613, 873
side effects of, 86–87, 114, 120, 140–141, 660, 970–971, 1294
for sleep disturbances, 115, 146, 147, 259
during opioid withdrawal, 408
for suicidal persons, 1326, 1376, 1449
use in dual-diagnosis patients, 344, 347, 349, 389
use in opioid-dependent patients, 410
use in persons with hepatic disease, 87, 92, 381
use in persons with obstructive uropathy, 799
withdrawal from, 86, 141, 660, 971
neonatal, 873
opioid withdrawal concurrent with, 302
Benztropine mesylate
delirium induced by, 87
for extrapyramidal symptoms, **594**, 649
Bereavement
depression and, 792
HIV/AIDS and, 227
suicide and, 1389–1390
after suicide of family member or friend, 1382
traumatic, 1021
group therapy for, 1060
Beta-blockers. *See* β-Adrenergic blockers
Bethanechol, **795**, 806
BFST (behavioral family systems therapy), for anorexia nervosa, 1172
Binge eating disorder. *See also* Eating disorders
future research needs related to, 1181–1183
medications for, 1115–1116, 1150, 1180–1181
natural history and course of, 1167
nutritional rehabilitation/counseling for, 1115, 1149, 1179
psychosocial interventions for, 1115, 1150, 1179–1180
psychotherapy combined with medications for, 1116, 1151, 1181
research diagnostic criteria for, 1149
substance use disorders and, 1152
Biofeedback, for posttraumatic stress disorder, 1053
Biological markers for suicide, 1439–1440, 1454
Bipolar disorder, 841–908
acute treatment for, 842–844, 859–861, 866–868, 881–897, 907
depressive episodes, 843–844, 860, 867–868, 892–897, 907
manic or mixed episodes, 842–843, 859–860, 866–867, 881–892, 907
rapid cycling, 860–861, 868, 897, 907

age at onset of, 880
in children and adolescents, 874–875
somatic treatment of, 905–906
definition of, 876–877
development of practice guideline for, 857
diagnostic criteria for, 876–877
hypomanic episode, **879**
major depressive episode, **878**
manic episode, **877**
mixed episode, **880**
summary of manic and depressive symptom criteria, **881**
educational resources for, **908**
in elderly persons, 875, 880
epidemiology of, 880
family history of, 797
future research needs related to, 906–908
acute treatment, 907
general treatment principles, 907
maintenance treatment, 908
psychosocial interventions, 908
goals of treatment for, 862
guide to using practice guideline for, 855
guideline watch for, 841–846
acute treatment of depressive episodes, 843–844
acute treatment of manic or mixed episodes, 842–843
maintenance treatment, 844–845
psychiatric management, 841–846
psychosocial interventions, 845–846
heritability of, 880
introduction to, 856
maintenance treatment for, 844–845, 861, 868–869, 898–901, 908
antipsychotics, 845, 861, 900
carbamazepine, 868, 900
in children and adolescents, 874
electroconvulsive therapy, 861, 869, 901
lamotrigine, 844, 861, 868, 900
lithium, 844, 845, 861, 868, 898–899
olanzapine, 845
oxcarbazepine, 868
psychosocial therapies, 904
valproate, 845, 861, 868, 899–900
medical comorbidity with, 875–876
HIV/AIDS, 175, 243–244, 256
natural history and course of, 877–879
in postpartum period, 873
prevalence of, 841
psychiatric features influencing treatment of, 869–871
catatonia, 870
comorbid psychiatric conditions, 871
eating disorders, 1163
panic disorder, 982
psychosis, 869–870
risk of suicide, homicide, or violence, 870
substance use disorders, 306, 336, 344–345, 870–871
among adolescents, 355, 875
alcohol dependence, 389
cocaine dependence, 397
nicotine dependence, 345
psychiatric management of, 841, 859, 862–866
addressing early signs of relapse, 865–866
diagnostic evaluation, 863
enhancing treatment compliance, 864–865
functional assessment, 866
monitoring treatment response, 864
patient/family education, 864
stressors and regular activity and sleep patterns, 865
suicide risk assessment, **863**, 863–864
therapeutic alliance, 864
treatment setting, 864
psychosocial interventions for, 845–846, 867–869, 901–905, 908
for comorbid disorders and psychosocial consequences, 904–905
for depression, 867–868, 903–904
efficacy of, 902–903
maintenance treatment, 866, 869, 904
for mania, 867, 903
psychosocial morbidity in, 879
rapid cycling, 860–861, 868, 897
relapses of, 861, 865–866
postpartum, 873
relationship to borderline personality disorder, 1224
screening for, 841, 863
sociodemographic features influencing treatment of, 871–875
in children and adolescents, 874–875
cross-cultural issues, 874
in elderly persons, 875
gender, 871, 877, 880
pregnancy, 871–874
somatic treatment for acute depressive episodes in, 843–844, 860, 867–868, 892–897

Bipolar disorder *(continued)*
somatic treatment for acute depressive episodes in *(continued)*
antipsychotics, 843–844, 896
bupropion, 860, 895–896
carbamazepine, 893
citalopram, 895
electroconvulsive therapy, 860, 867, 868, 896
fluoxetine, 895
lamotrigine, 844, 860, 867, 893–894
lithium, 867, 892
moclobemide, 895
novel treatments, 896–897
paroxetine, 844, 860, 895
topiramate, 894
tranylcypromine, 894
tricyclic antidepressants, 896
valproate, 893
venlafaxine, 844, 896
somatic treatment for acute manic or mixed episodes in, 842–843, 859–860, 866–867, 881–892
antipsychotics, 842–843, 859–860, 866–867
mood stabilizers and, 842, 845, 859–861, 866, 891
aripiprazole, 842
benzodiazepines, 860, 867, 892
calcium channel blockers, 892
carbamazepine, 843, 859, 860, 866, 887–888
chlorpromazine, 890–891
clozapine, 891
combination therapy, 891
electroconvulsive therapy, 860, 867, 891
gabapentin, 889
lamotrigine, 889
lithium, 859, 866, 881–885
novel treatments, 891–892
olanzapine, 842, 859, 866, 867, 889–890
oxcarbazepine, 859, 860, 867, 889
phenytoin, 889
quetiapine, 842–843
risperidone, 842, 867, 891
valproate, 842, 859, 866, 885–887
ziprasidone, 842, 866, 891
somatic treatment for rapid cycling in, 860–861, 868, 897
suicidality and, 335, 863–864, 870, 878–879, 1343, **1343**, 1392–1394
summary of treatment recommendations for, 859–860
treatment plan for, 861–862
Bisexuality
HIV/AIDS and, 225
substance use disorders and, 357
suicide and, 1341–1342, 1390–1391
Bisphosphonates, use in anorexia nervosa, 1113, 1145, 1175
Blood alcohol level, **33**
Blood transfusion, HIV transmission via, 199
BMI (body mass index), 1106, 1122, 1163, 1169
Board-and-care homes, for persons with schizophrenia, 620
Body dysmorphic disorder (BDD), anorexia nervosa and, 1156
Body mass index (BMI), 1106, 1122, 1163, 1169
Bone abnormalities
anorexia nervosa and, 1113, **1125**, 1145, 1157, 1162, 1175
bulimia nervosa and, **1127**
valproate-induced, 885
Bone marrow suppression, drug-induced
antiretroviral agents, 203, 221
carbamazepine, 141, 243
clozapine, 221
valproate, 141, 142, 886
Borderline personality disorder (BPD), 1223–1300
assessment of, 1241, 1245–1246, 1274–1275
comprehensive evaluation, 1246
level of care, 1245
treatment framework, 1245
brain imaging in, 1225
chronic self-destructive behavior in, 1244, 1254, 1265–1266
clinical features of, 1248, 1272–1273
associated features, 1273
core features, 1272–1273
functional impairment, 1248, 1274
comorbidity with, 1224, 1263–1264, 1273–1274
depression, 792, 1224, 1263–1264
eating disorders, 1153–1154, 1164
HIV/AIDS, 228
posttraumatic stress disorder, 1224, 1266–1267

substance use disorders, 349, 1264
suicidality, 1238, 1244, 1247, 1253, **1253,** 1270–1271, 1274, 1327, 1341, 1347–1348, 1386, 1399, 1407–1409
complications of, 1274
development of practice guideline for, 1239
diagnostic criteria for, 1223–1224, 1238, **1238**
differential diagnosis of, 1275
dissociative features of, 1267–1268
electroconvulsive therapy for, 1243–1244, 1259, 1298–1299, 1300
epidemiology of, 1224–1225, 1275–1276
family history of, 1275
features influencing treatment for, 1244
future research needs related to, 1299–1300
pharmacotherapy and other somatic treatments, 1300
psychotherapy, 1299–1300
guide to using practice guideline for, 1237
guideline watch for, 1223–1226
biology, 1225
definition, 1223–1224
diagnostic stability and longitudinal course, 1224
epidemiology, 1224–1225
etiology, 1225
treatment, 1225–1226
impact of childhood trauma and posttraumatic stress disorder on treatment of, 215, 1020, 1045, 1225, 1254, 1266–1267, 1273
accuracy of distant memories, 1267
eye movement therapy, 1267
group support and therapy, 1266
reassignment of blame, 1267
risk of reenactment/revictimization, 1267
threats to therapeutic alliance, 1266
transference issues, 1266
treating posttraumatic symptoms, 1267
treatment focus, 1266
working through traumatic memories, 1266
interpreting literature on treatment of, 1276–1277
introduction to, 1238
natural history and course of, 1224, 1276
pharmacotherapy for, 1226, 1243–1244, 1256–1263, 1287–1298, 1300
for affective dysregulation symptoms, 1243–1244, 1256–1259, **1258, 1301**
algorithms for, **1301–1303**
antipsychotics, 1244, **1258,** 1259, **1260,** 1261–1263, **1262,** 1295–1298
anxiolytics, 1243, 1257, **1258,** 1294
for cognitive-perceptual symptoms, 1244, 1261–1263, **1262, 1303**
for impulsive-behavioral dyscontrol symptoms, 1244, 1259–1261, **1260, 1302**
monoamine oxidase inhibitors, 1243, 1244, 1257, **1258, 1260,** 1261, **1262,** 1291–1292
mood stabilizers, 1243, 1244, 1257–1259, **1258, 1260,** 1261, 1292–1294
opiate antagonists, 1261, 1295–1296
selective serotonin reuptake inhibitors, 1243, 1244, 1256, 1257, **1258,** 1259, **1260, 1262,** 1287–1289
tricyclic and heterocyclic antidepressants, 1257, 1289–1290
in pregnancy, 1269
prevalence of, 1275
principles of treatment selection for, 1242, 1250–1252
flexibility, 1251
focus, 1251
multiple- vs. single-clinician treatment, 1251–1252
patient preference, 1251
type, 1250–1251
psychiatric management of, 1241–1242, 1246–1250
boundary issues, 1249–1250, 1253, 1272
consultations, 1249
coordination of care, 1248
crisis response and safety monitoring, 1246–1247
monitoring clinical status and treatment plan, 1248
patient/family education, 1247–1248
recognizing functional regression, 1248
splitting, 1249, 1254
therapeutic alliance, 1243, 1247
treating symptoms that reappear during pharmacotherapy, 1249
psychosocial stressors and, 1268

Borderline personality disorder (BPD) *(continued)*
psychotherapy for, 1225–1226, 1242–1243, 1252–1256, 1277–1287, 1299–1300
cognitive behavior therapy/dialectical behavior therapy, 228, 1225–1226, 1282–1284, 1452–1453
couples therapy, 1243, 1255, 1286–1287
family therapy, 1243, 1255–1256, 1287
group therapy, 1243, 1255, 1285–1286
hierarchy of priorities for, 1253, **1253**
psychodynamic psychotherapy, 1243, 1252, **1253**, 1255, 1277–1282, **1278**, 1451–1452
Transference-Focused Psychotherapy, 1226, 1452
relationship to bipolar disorder, 1224
remission of, 1224
risk management issues in, 1244, 1270–1272
anger, impulsivity, and violence, 1244, 1264–1265, 1271–1272
boundary violations, 1249, 1250, 1253, 1272
suicide, 1238, 1244, 1247, 1253, 1270–1271, 1274
sociodemographic factors and, 1269–1270
age, 1269–1270
cultural factors, 1269
gender, 1224–1225, 1269, 1275
summary of treatment recommendations for, 1241–1244
treatment plan for, 1244–1245
treatment settings for, 1245–1246
with violent behavior and antisocial traits, 1244, 1264–1265, 1271–1272
Boundary issues
in treatment of borderline personality disorder, 1249–1250, 1253, 1272
in treatment of suicidal patients, 1363
BPD. *See* Borderline personality disorder
BPRS (Brief Psychiatric Rating Scale), **30**, 580, 633, 659
Bradycardia
drug-induced
β-blockers, 142
cholinesterase inhibitors, 87, 132
electroconvulsive therapy–induced, 664
Bradykinesia
antipsychotic-induced, 648
in Parkinson's disease, 119
Brain imaging, **33**, 43, 44
in borderline personality disorder, 1225
in delirium, 78
in dementia, 122
Alzheimer's disease, 101
Pick's disease, 120
Brain injury
dementia and, 120
due to falls, 123
seizures and, 75
suicide risk and, 1354
Brain tumor, 120
electroconvulsive therapy for persons with, 664
Breast cancer
antipsychotics for women with, 615
hyperprolactinemia and, 656
Breast-feeding, maternal drug use during, 873–874
Breath testing for substance abuse, 317
smoking, 361
Breathing exercises
in HIV/AIDS, 229
for posttraumatic stress disorder, 1053
Breathing retraining, in panic disorder, 960
Brief interventions
for substance use disorders, 298, 315, 325, 332–333
in adolescents, 355
alcohol dependence, 386, 444–445
marijuana dependence, 392
nicotine dependence, 370, 432
for suicidal behavior, 1327
Brief Psychiatric Rating Scale (BPRS), **30**, 580, 633, 659
Brief Symptom Inventory, 260
Bright light therapy
for bulimia nervosa, 1115, 1148
for depression with seasonal exacerbations, 792, 814–815, 823
side effects of, 815
for sleep disturbances in dementia, 146
Brofaromine
for acute stress disorder or posttraumatic stress disorder, 1031
for panic disorder, 973
Bromocriptine
for cocaine dependence/withdrawal, 394
in attention-deficit/hyperactivity disorder, 397
dosage of, 145
for hyperprolactinemia, 656

for neuroleptic malignant syndrome, 652
for night eating syndrome, 1181
for persons with dementia, 115, 143, 145
side effects of, 144
Bronchodilators, interaction with monoamine oxidase inhibitors, 797
Bulimia nervosa. *See also* Eating disorders
bupropion contraindicated in, 369, 429
clinical features of, 1160–1162
diagnostic criteria for, **1120**
epidemiology of, 1163
family interventions for, 1114, 1146, 1176–1177
future research needs related to, 1181–1183
genetic factors and, 1167–1168
goals of treatment for, 1113, 1145
group therapy for, 1176
laboratory abnormalities in, 1163
medications for, 1114, 1147–1148, 1177–1178
natural history and course of, 1166
nutritional rehabilitation/counseling for, 1113, 1145
other somatic treatments for, 1148
personality disorders and, 1153
physical complications of, **1126–1127,** 1162
posttraumatic stress disorder and, 1153
predictors of outcome in, 1166
prevalence of, 1163
psychodynamic issues in, 1161
psychosocial interventions for, 1113–1114, 1145–1147, 1175–1177
psychotherapy combined with medications for, 1115, 1148, 1178–1179
relapse prevention for, 1114
substance use disorders and, 338, 348–349, 1152
suicidality and, 1400
support groups for, 349, 1111, 1114, 1146–1147, 1177
treatment settings for, 1106–1108, 1129–1134, **1131–1133**
Bulimia Test—Revised (BULIT-R), **1121**
BULIT-R (Bulimia Test—Revised), **1121**
Buprenorphine, 455–460
abuse of, 456
for cocaine dependence, 448
formulations of, 455–456
interaction with benzodiazepines, 404, 460
maintenance therapy for opioid dependence, 302, 304, 323, 403–404, 456–458
combined with naloxone, 403
compared with methadone, 403
daily use of, 456–457
dosage and administration of, 403
in HIV-infected persons, 245
less-than-daily use of, 457–458
in patients with comorbid cocaine dependence, 395
in pregnancy, 411
regulations governing administration of, 359, 401
settings for, 401, 403
mechanism of action of, 403
for opioid withdrawal, 302, 323, 400, 407, 458–459
overdose of, 404
side effects of, 404, 459–460
sublingual, 401, 403, 455, 456
withdrawal from, 405
Bupropion
for attention-deficit/hyperactivity disorder, in dual-diagnosis patients, 348
for cocaine dependence, 395, 447
contraindicated in eating disorders, 369, 429, 1112, 1144
for depression, 772, 783
with atypical features, 789, 790
in bipolar disorder, 860, 868, 895–896
dosage of, 145, **774**
efficacy of, 805
interaction with clozapine, 658
overdose of, 1442
for panic disorder, 974
for persons with concurrent medical conditions
cardiac disease, 798
dementia, 114, 115, 143, 145, 798
glaucoma, 798
HIV/AIDS, 174, 241
obstructive uropathy, 799
Parkinson's disease, 799
in pregnancy, 872
side effects of, 144, 369, 429, **795,** 809
for smoking cessation, 300, 324, 369, 427–429
in adolescents, 355
in depression, 343, 375
dosage of, 369, 429
efficacy of, 427–429
goals of, 427
implementation of, 429

Bupropion *(continued)*
for smoking cessation *(continued)*
in patients with medical conditions, 376
in pregnancy, 377
in schizophrenia, 341, 428–429
sustained release, **774**
Burn patients, 74, 75
Buspirone
for antidepressant augmentation, 751
for borderline personality disorder, 1257, 1294
dosage and administration of, 142
for dual-diagnosis patients, 389
with anxiety, 346
with depression, 343
interaction with selective serotonin reuptake inhibitors, 142
for panic disorder, 976
for persons with dementia, 114, 142, 148
for persons with HIV/AIDS, 244, 257
for posttraumatic stress disorder, 1066
side effects of, 142
for smoking cessation, 370, 430
Butyrophenones. *See* Antipsychotics

C

CA (Cocaine Anonymous), 332, 396, 450, 451
CAC-A (Clinical Assessment of Confusion–A), 78
Caffeine
interaction with clozapine, 638
smoking cessation and, 367
CAGE Questionnaire, **28**, 307
Calcium channel blockers
drug interactions with
carbamazepine, 888
oxcarbazepine, 889
for mania, 892
for panic disorder, 975
Calcium supplementation, in anorexia nervosa, 1112, 1113, 1145, 1174
CAM (Confusion Assessment Method), 78
Cancer
adverse effects of chemotherapy for, **209**
benzodiazepines for patients with, 87
delirium and, 74
smoking-related, 376
substance use disorders and, **351**
suicide risk and, 1354, 1424
Cannabis. *See* Marijuana use disorders
Capacity to consent to treatment, 9, 38
Carbamazepine
for alcohol withdrawal, 381, 435–436
for bipolar disorder
acute manic or mixed episodes, 843, 859, 860, 866, 887–888
in children and adolescents, 874, 906
depressive episodes, 893
in dual-diagnosis patients, 344, 389
alcohol dependence, 871
maintenance treatment, 868, 899, 900
for borderline personality disorder, 1243, 1244, **1258**, 1259, **1260**, 1261, 1292–1294
in breast milk, 874
for bulimia nervosa, 1178
for cocaine dependence, 395, 448
dosage of, 141, 843, 888
drug interactions with, 888
antipsychotics, 625
clozapine, 639, 657
lamotrigine, 888, 894
oral contraceptives, 871
tricyclic antidepressants, 807
implementation of, 888
laboratory monitoring during treatment with, 142
monitoring during therapy with, 888
overdose of, 887–888, 1293
for panic disorder, 974
patient evaluation before initiation of, 888
for persons with dementia, 114, 141–142, 148
for persons with HIV/AIDS, 243, 256
for persons with schizophrenia, 657
for posttraumatic stress disorder, 1013, 1031, 1066
in pregnancy, 872, 873, 1269
side effects of, 141, 142, 243, 843, 887, 1293
for suicidal persons, 1446
Carbidopa
for HIV-related cognitive disorders, 253
for night eating syndrome, 1181
Carbon disulfide, 341
Cardiomyopathy, clozapine-induced, 635, 637
Cardiotomy, delirium after, 75
Cardiovascular disease
alcohol dependence and, 389
drug use in
antidepressants, 144, 783, 797–798, 968, 1290

antipsychotics, 614, 616
ziprasidone, 646
electroconvulsive therapy for persons with, 814
schizophrenia and, 615
smoking-related, 376
suicide risk and, 1354
Cardiovascular effects
of anorexia nervosa, **1123**
of bulimia nervosa, **1126**
of drugs
antidepressants, 144, 345, 429, **795**, 806, 952, 968
antipsychotics, 72, 85, 114, 138, 590, 616, 631, 653–654
aripiprazole, 647
carbamazepine, 887
clozapine, 635, 636, 637, 638
cocaine, 393–394, 397
LAAM, 401
lithium, 882
monoamine oxidase inhibitors, 144, 798, 810
protease inhibitors, 177–178
quetiapine, 644
risperidone, 640
substances of abuse, **351**
thioridazine, 616, 631, 1297
trazodone, 144, 809
ziprasidone, 645, 646
of electroconvulsive therapy, 664, 814
of panic attacks, 975
Cardiovascular shock, in serotonin syndrome, 808
CARE (Ryan White Comprehensive AIDS Resources Emergency) Act, 236
Case formulation, 35–36
Case management
goals of, 315
for schizophrenia, 341, 583, 673
for substance use disorders, 298, 315, 321, 341
for traumatized persons, 1013, 1014
CAT (cognitive analytic therapy), for borderline personality disorder, 1226
Catalepsy, 789
Cataracts
assessment for, **587**
quetiapine-induced, 644
Catastrophic reactions, in dementia, 116
Catatonia
benzodiazepines for, 573, 604, 660, 789
clinical features of, 789
depression with, 789
electroconvulsive therapy for, 594
mania with, 870
schizophrenia with, 604, 623, 625
CBT. *See* Cognitive behavior therapy
CD4 cells in HIV/AIDS, 197, 201, 202, 251–253
CDC. *See* Centers for Disease Control and Prevention
Center for Epidemiologic Studies Depression Scale (CES-D Scale), 256
Center for Substance Abuse Treatment, 403
Centers for Disease Control and Prevention (CDC), 748
growth charts, 1109, 1135
Tobacco Information and Prevention Source, 321
Cerebral blood flow, in delirium, 62
Cerebrovascular disease
cocaine and, 394, 397
dementia and, 150
Alzheimer's disease, 119
risperidone-induced, 616, 640
vascular dementia, 118–119
risk factors for, 126
seizures and, 75
suicide risk and, 1424–1425
use of electroconvulsive therapy in, 89
CES-D Scale (Center for Epidemiologic Studies Depression Scale), 256
CGI (Clinical Global Impression) Scale, **26**
Chelation agents, for Alzheimer's disease, 131, 137
Chest X-ray, **33**
Child abuse. *See also* Abuse/assault
substance use disorders and, 335–336
suicide risk in persons with history of, 1351–1352, 1386, 1417–1419
Child custody evaluations, 9
Children. *See also* Adolescents
antidepressants for, suicide risk and, 748–749, 934–936
benzodiazepines for, 87
bipolar disorder in, 874–875, 880
somatic treatment of, 905–906
HIV/AIDS in, 196, 208–210, 259
perinatal transmission of, 200, 233–234
psychiatric management of, 222
sexual abuse and, 235

Children *(continued)*
panic disorder in, 984–985
prenatal drug exposures of
alcohol, 390–391
antidepressants, 796, 872
antipsychotics, 613, 872–873
benzodiazepines, 613
buprenorphine, 411
bupropion, 377
cocaine, 398
marijuana, 392–393
methadone, 411
mood stabilizers, 613, 871–873
nicotine, 352, 376–377
opioids, 352, 411
schizophrenia in, 603
school refusal among, 985
sexually transmitted diseases in, 235
substance use disorders in, 354–355
suicidal behavior in, 1339, 1383, **1384,** 1385
whose parents have died from AIDS, 227
Chlamydial infection, 200
Chloral hydrate, for sleep disturbances, 115, 146, 147
Chlordiazepoxide
for alcohol withdrawal, 380, 435
in pregnancy, 873
Chlorpromazine, **589**
for borderline personality disorder, **1262,** 1295
for delirium, 84, 86, 254
dosage of, **589,** 633
interaction with nicotine, 340
for mania, 890–891
for persons with anorexia nervosa, 1112
for persons with HIV/AIDS, 241, 242, 254
side effects of, 138
hematological, 632
jaundice, 631
ophthalmological, 631
sedation, 652
Cholesterol levels, suicide and, 1439–1440
Cholinergic agonists, for antipsychotic augmentation, 602
Cholinesterase inhibitors
combined with vitamin E, 134
for delirium, 62, 87–88, 91
for dementia, 102, 112–113, 131–133, 147, 148
dosage and administration of, 88, 133
for persons with schizophrenia, 661
side effects of, 87–88, 102, 112, 132–133
Cimetidine, 885
drug interactions with
antipsychotics, 635, 638
carbamazepine, 888
Citalopram
for aggression in persons with schizophrenia, 609
for anorexia nervosa, 1143, 1173
for binge eating disorder, 1180
for bipolar depression, 895
dosage of, **774,** 937, 966
for elderly persons, 752
for panic disorder, 937, 966
for persons with HIV/AIDS, 177, 241
for persons with schizophrenia, 658
for posttraumatic stress disorder, 1064
in pregnancy, 872
S-enantiomer of (*See* Escitalopram)
Clinical Assessment of Confusion–A (CAC-A), 78
Clinical consultation, 9
Clinical formulation, 35–36
cultural, 35–36, **36**
future research needs related to, 43
risk assessment, 36
Clinical Global Impression (CGI) Scale, **26,** 894, 964, 967
Clinical Global Impression Scale for Bipolar Illness, 889, 905
Clinical Institute Narcotic Assessment, 405
Clinical Institute Withdrawal Assessment of Alcohol Scale, Revised, 379
Clinician-Administered PTSD Scale, 1018, 1054
Clomipramine
for anorexia nervosa, 1174
dosage of, **774,** 969
for obsessive-compulsive disorder, in dual-diagnosis patients, 346
for panic disorder, 968, 969
maintenance treatment, 937
for persons with schizophrenia, 658
Clonazepam
for akathisia, 649
for borderline personality disorder, 1294
for catatonia, 660
combined with haloperidol for schizophrenia, 660
discontinuation of, 937
dosage of, 937
for mania, 892
in HIV/AIDS, 256

for myoclonus, **795**, 807
for night eating syndrome, 1181
for panic disorder, 936, 937, 970
combined with sertraline, 938
dosage of, 972
for persons with dementia, 141
side effects of, 937
use in alcohol-dependent patients, 389
Clonidine
for alcohol withdrawal, 301, 381, 436
combined with haloperidol for schizophrenia, 662
contraindications to, 406
drug interactions with
antidepressants, 798
tricyclic antidepressants, 807
for opioid withdrawal, 302, 323, 400, 406, 462–463
with naltrexone, 302, 407
for panic disorder, 975–976
for posttraumatic stress disorder, 1031
for psychosis-induced polydipsia, 610
side effects of, 430, 463
for smoking cessation, 300, 369–370, 429–430
Clorazepate, use in opioid-dependent patients, 410
Clozapine, 588, **589**, 635–639
for bipolar disorder
maintenance treatment, 900
manic episodes, 843, 860, 891
for borderline personality disorder, **1260**, 1261, **1262**, 1263, 1296–1297
combined with glycine, 661
combined with other antipsychotics, 659
contraindications to, 616
for dementia, 138, 139
in Parkinson's disease, 138, 139, 150
dosage of, 140, **589**, 637, 638
drug interactions with, 638–639
antidepressants, 658
antiretroviral agents, 221, 241
carbamazepine, 639, 657
nicotine, 340
psychostimulants, 652
efficacy of, 635–636
half-life of, 638
implementing treatment with, 637–639
laboratory tests before initiation of, 637
for panic disorder, 975
for persons with HIV/AIDS, 221, 241
in pregnancy, 613, 873
receptor affinity of, 635
for schizophrenia, 576, 594, 602, 638
cognitive effects, 635
in dual-diagnosis patients, 340
alcohol dependence, 389
nicotine dependence, 375
negative symptoms, 604
positive symptoms, 635
psychosis-induced polydipsia, 609–610
to reduce suicide risk, 340, 608, 635, 1327, 1376, 1446–1447
for relapse prevention, 635–636
treatment-resistant, 635–636
side effects of, 114, 138, 139, 340, **592**, 636–637, 654
agranulocytosis, 114, 139, 242, 340, 612, 635, 636–638, 1263
anticholinergic effects, 636, 654
cardiovascular effects, 635, 636, 637, 638
fever, 636
monitoring for, 637–638
myocarditis and cardiomyopathy, 635, 637
priapism, 657
sedation, 636, 652
seizures, 138, 242, 340, 606, 635, 637
sialorrhea, 636
weight gain and metabolic effects, 636, 638, 654–655, 843
for tardive dyskinesia, 651
time to clinical effect of, 638
"Club drugs," 333–334
Coagulation disorders, 134
Cocaethylene, 393
Cocaine Anonymous (CA), 332, 396, 450, 451
Cocaine use disorders, 301–302, 393–398, 447–451
clinical features influencing treatment of, 397–398
medical comorbidity, **351**, 397
pregnancy, 352, 398
psychiatric comorbidity, 397
delirium and, 76
epidemiology of, 393, 420
in HIV/AIDS, 257
intoxication with, 301, 335, 393–394
posttraumatic stress disorder and, 346
in pregnancy, 352, 398

Cocaine use disorders *(continued)*
psychosocial interventions for, 302, 325, 396–397, 449–451
behavior therapies, 396, 449–450
cognitive behavior therapy, 396, 449
contingency management, 328
interpersonal therapy, 396, 450
psychodynamic psychotherapy, 396, 450
self-help groups and 12-step programs, 332, 396–397, 450–451
psychotropic drug use in persons with, antidepressants, 342, 343
schizophrenia and, 625
seizures and, 75
somatic treatments for, 302, 393–396, 447–449
acupuncture, 395–396, 448
to change subjective effects of cocaine, 395, 448
for cocaine dependence, 394–395, 447–448
in dual-diagnosis patients, 448–449
for intoxication, 393–394
in patient with co-occurring opioid dependence, 395
vaccine development, 395, 448
for withdrawal symptoms, 394
treatment settings for, 299, 393
Codeine, 245, 399
for night eating syndrome, 1181
Cognition enhancers. *See* Cholinesterase inhibitors
Cognitive analytic therapy (CAT), for borderline personality disorder, 1226
Cognitive assessment, 22–23
rating scales for, **27**
Cognitive behavior therapy (CBT). *See also* Behavior therapy
for acute stress disorder and posttraumatic stress disorder, 1014, 1028, 1031–1032, 1053–1057
for bipolar disorder, 903, 904
for borderline personality disorder, 1282–1284
adverse effects of, 1284
cost-effectiveness of, 1284
definition and goals of, 1282
efficacy of, 1282–1284
implementation of, 1284
length and frequency of, 1284
for depression, 751, 752, 775, 777, 785, 816–817
in children and adolescents, 749
double depression, 791
in older adults, 753
for eating disorders
anorexia nervosa, 1111, 1140, 1142, 1171
binge eating disorder, 1115, 1116, 1150, 1151, 1179–1181
bulimia nervosa, 1113–1114, 1115, 1146, 1148, 1175–1176, 1178
for panic disorder, 938, 940, 959, 960–962, **961**
during anxiolytic withdrawal, 962
approaches to, 960–961
combined with pharmacotherapy, 938–939, 979–980
factors affecting choice of, 977–980
in group format, 962, 964
length of treatment with, 953, 980
patient acceptance of, 962
in primary care settings, 939
for persons with HIV/AIDS, 174, 255, 256
for schizophrenia, 576, 597, 598, 602, 669
social skills training and, 615
for substance use disorders, 298, 315, 325, 327
in adolescents, 355
alcohol dependence, 385
with anxiety disorders, 345
with bipolar disorder, 345
with bulimia nervosa, 348
cocaine dependence, 396, 449
with depression, 344, 375
in group format, 330
marijuana dependence, 446
nicotine dependence, 370–371, 375, 433
with obsessive-compulsive disorder, 346
opioid dependence, 408, 463
with sleep disturbances, 336
for suicidal persons, 1327, 1377
Cognitive enhancers. *See* Cholinesterase inhibitors
Cognitive impairment
age-related cognitive decline, 117
in borderline personality disorder, pharmacotherapy for, 1244, 1261–1263, **1262, 1303**
in delirium, 72–73, 74, 117
in dementia, 74, 112–113, 116, 117, 119, 122, 131–137
Alzheimer's disease, 118
cholinesterase inhibitors for, 112–113, 131–133, 147, 148

ergoloid mesylates for, 113, 136, 150
frontal lobe dementias, 119–120
HIV-associated, 75, 120, 172, 173–174, 195, 205, **206**, 219–220, 250–253 (*See also* Dementia, HIV-associated)
other agents for, 113, 136–137
Parkinson's disease, 119, 150
selegiline for, 113, 135, 148, 149
vascular dementia, 119
vitamin E for, 102, 113, 134, 148, 149, 154
in depressive pseudodementia, 117, 143, 791
drug-induced
alcohol, 390
antipsychotics, 113, 648
benzodiazepines, 114, 660, 970
lithium, 662, 882, 1293
topiramate, 1180
tricyclic antidepressants, 144, 968
electroconvulsive therapy–induced, 89, 664, 813–814
in hepatitis C, 175–176
in mental retardation, 117
neuropsychological testing for, 32–33
in parkinsonism, 648
in schizophrenia, 117, 639, 642, 644, 661
Cognitive remediation and therapy, for schizophrenia, 673–674
Cognitive restructuring, for panic disorder, 960
Cognitive retraining, 112
Cognitive therapy
for bipolar disorder, 845
for borderline personality disorder, 1226
for dementia, 112, 129–130
for posttraumatic stress disorder, 1055
Cognitive-motor disorders, HIV-associated, 172–173, 205, **206**
Collaborative Study on the Genetics of Alcoholism, 1403
Collateral sources of patient information, 25
Coma, 75
drug-induced
opioids, 322
sedative-hypnotics, 322
COMBINE Study, 384
Community reinforcement approach (CRA), for substance use disorders, 298, 315, 329, 331
alcohol dependence, 386, 443
Community residential facilities
for persons with schizophrenia, 620–621
for persons with substance use disorders, 314
Community support resources
for dementia, 127
for HIV/AIDS, 247
Comorbidity
with acute stress disorder or posttraumatic stress disorder, 1020–1021, 1026–1027, 1036–1037
with alcohol use disorders, 319, 336–337, 388–390, 419
with bipolar disorder, 871, 875–876, 904–905
with borderline personality disorder, 1224, 1263–1264, 1273–1274
with cocaine use disorders, 397
with delirium, 92
with dementia, 149–150
with depression, 788–792, 797–799, 803
with eating disorders, 1152–1155, 1163–1164
with hepatitis C, 175, **176**
with HIV/AIDS, 195–196, 210–211, 219–223
with nicotine dependence, 335, 337, 350, 360, 374–376, 418
with opioid use disorders, **351**, 410
with panic disorder, 953, 983–984
with schizophrenia, 582–583, 625
with substance use disorders, 309–310, 318, 319, 336–350, 350–352, **351**, 413
with suicidal behavior, **1337**, 1342–1349, **1343**, 1391–1409
Competency
assessment of, 9, 38
delirium and, 91
Composite International Diagnostic Interview, 1045, 1050
Computed tomography (CT), **33**
in dementia, 122
in schizophrenia, 585
Computer-guided therapies, for substance use disorders, 333
Concentration problems
lithium-induced, 882, 1293
in schizophrenia, 623
Condoms, to minimize risk of HIV transmission, 213, **214**
Conduct disorder, 355
Confidentiality. *See also* Privacy
adult psychiatric evaluation and, 7, 8, 11, 38–39
of HIV status, 216, 247–248, 359

Confidentiality *(continued)*
after patient's suicide, 1325, 1381
related to acute stress disorder, posttraumatic stress disorder and legal system involvement, 1019
substance abuse treatment and, 358–359
Confrontational interventions, for substance use disorders, 331
Confusion
drug-induced
antipsychotics, 114, 138, 614
benzodiazepines, 140
bromocriptine, 144
carbamazepine, 141
lithium, 882
sedative-hypnotics, 322
tricyclic antidepressants, 807
electroconvulsive therapy–induced, 814
Confusion Assessment Method (CAM), 78
Confusion Assessment Method for the Intensive Care Unit, 61
Confusion Rating Scale (CRS), 78
Consent to treatment
assessing patient's capacity for, 9, 38
for delirium, 91
Constipation
drug-induced
antidepressants, 144, 429, **795**, 806, 968, 1290
antipsychotics, 138, 614, 654
buprenorphine, 460
clonidine, 430
clozapine, 654
duloxetine, 749
methadone, 455
nefazodone, 809
olanzapine, 654, 890
quetiapine, 654, 843
reboxetine, 809
management of, **795**, 807
use of antipsychotics in persons with, 616
Consultation
in psychiatric evaluation of adults, 9
in treatment of borderline personality disorder, 1249
in treatment of suicidal patients, 1373
Contingency contracting, for substance use disorders, 328–329
Contingency management, for substance use disorders, 298, 315, 328–329
cocaine dependence, 396, 449–450
in depression, 344
marijuana dependence, 328, 446, 447
nicotine dependence, 370, 432–433
opioid dependence, 408–409, 463–465
Continuing medical education, xii
Continuity of care
for eating disorders, 1107, 1130
for schizophrenia, 581, 595
Cooperative apartments, for persons with schizophrenia, 620
Coordination of care
for acute stress disorder or posttraumatic stress disorder, 1023–1024, 1036
for borderline personality disorder, 1248
for eating disorders, 1105, 1118–1119
for HIV/AIDS, 216
for panic disorder, 958
for substance use disorders, 321
for suicidal behavior, 1368–1369
Corneal opacities, antipsychotic-induced, 631
Correctional settings
administrative segregation in, 622–623
HIV/AIDS in, 229–230, 234
psychiatric evaluation in, 12, 41
schizophrenia in, 621–623
suicide risk in, 621, 1361–1362
Corticosteroids
mania induced by, 875, 876
in posttraumatic stress disorder, 1067
Co-trimoxazole, **209**
Counseling
of persons at risk for HIV/AIDS, 232, 248
of persons with schizophrenia, 597–598
Countertransference
cultural factors and, 36
in treatment of borderline personality disorder, 1244
in treatment of eating disorders, 1111, 1114
in treatment of suicidal patients, 1325, 1363, 1372
Couples therapy. *See* Marital/couples therapy
CRA (community reinforcement approach), for substance use disorders, 298, 315, 329, 331
alcohol dependence, 386, 443
Crack cocaine, 393. *See also* Cocaine use disorders
Cranial nerve palsies, 74
Creatine kinase, in neuroleptic malignant syndrome, 651, 652
Creutzfeldt-Jakob disease, 120

Criminal offenders. *See also* Incarcerated persons
legally mandated substance abuse treatment for, 315
Crisis intervention
in borderline personality disorder, 1246–1247
residential programs for schizophrenia, 578, 618–619, 620
for suicidal patient, 1371
Crossing the Quality Chasm, 6
Cross-National Collaborative Panic Study, 970
CRS (Confusion Rating Scale), 78
Cryptococcosis, 120
"Crystal Meth" Anonymous, 332
CT. *See* Computed tomography
Cue exposure therapy, for substance use disorders, 329
cocaine dependence, 450
nicotine dependence, 370, 433
opioid dependence, 465
Cultural factors. *See also* Race/ethnicity
acute stress disorder, posttraumatic stress disorder and, 1035–1036
bipolar disorder and, 874
borderline personality disorder and, 1269
depression and, 793
eating disorders and, 1157–1158
HIV/AIDS and, 223–225, **224**
panic disorder and, 986
schizophrenia and, 610
substance use disorders and, 356–357
suicidal behavior and, 1322, 1341, 1386–1389
Cultural formulation, 18, 35–36, **36**
Cultural humility, 36
Cultural identity, 35
Cutaneous effects
of anorexia nervosa, **1124**
of bulimia nervosa, **1126**
of drugs
antipsychotics, 631
antiretroviral agents, 203
carbamazepine, 887, 1293
lamotrigine, 844, 874, 893–894
lithium, 662, 882–883
Cyclooxygenase-2 inhibitors, interaction with lithium, 876
D-Cycloserine, **209**
for persons with schizophrenia, 602, 661
Cyclosporine, interaction with St. John's wort, 750
Cyclothymic disorder, 876
Cyproheptadine
for anorexia nervosa, 1174
for posttraumatic stress disorder, 1067
for sexual dysfunction, 657, **796,** 808
Cytochrome P450–related drug interactions
with antipsychotics
clozapine, 638–639
olanzapine, 643
quetiapine, 644
risperidone, 641
with antiretroviral agents, 171, **238,** 238–241, **239,** 244, 245, 261
with carbamazepine, 888
with St. John's wort, 750

D

Dance therapy, 130
Dangerousness
of HIV-infected persons, 248
of persons with schizophrenia, 609
Dantrolene, for neuroleptic malignant syndrome, 652
Dartmouth Assessment of Lifestyle Instrument, 605
Day treatment programs. *See also* Partial hospitalization
for acute stress disorder or posttraumatic stress disorder, 1022
for alcohol use disorders, 378
for dementia, 151
for eating disorders, 1134
for persons with HIV/AIDS, 247
for schizophrenia, 578, 619–620
DBT (dialectical behavior therapy)
for binge eating disorder, 1179
for borderline personality disorder, 228, 1225–1226, 1252, **1253**
Debriefing, psychological, of traumatized persons, 1013, 1028, 1033–1034, 1061–1062
Decubitus ulcers, 75
Deep tendon reflexes, 119
Deep vein thrombosis, clozapine-induced, 637
Dehydroepiandrosterone (DHEA), for persons with HIV/AIDS, 260
Delavirdine, 170, 171, **204**
drug interactions with, 238, **239**
Deliberate self-harm, 1321, 1441–1442. *See also* Self-injurious behavior; Suicidal behavior
Delirium, 61–93

Delirium *(continued)*
anticholinergic, 72, **81**, 87, 654, 807
assessment for, 77–78, **80**
diagnostic instruments, 61, 78
laboratory tests, 78, **80**
screening instruments, 78
symptom severity rating scales, 78
causes of, 73, 75–77
general medical condition, 75, **76**
heterogeneity of, 62
multiple etiologies, 76–77
reversible, **81**
substance use or withdrawal, 76, **77**
alcohol withdrawal, 301
unspecified etiology, 77
cerebral blood flow in, 62
clinical features influencing treatment of, 92–93
advanced age, 92–93
comorbid medical conditions, 92
comorbid psychiatric conditions, 92
competency and consent for treatment of, 91
course of, 75
definition and clinical features of, 71, 72–73
dementia and, 116, 149–150
detection of, 61
development of practice guideline for, 70
diagnostic criteria for, 73
differential diagnosis of, 74
dementia, 74, 116–117
drug-induced, 76, **77**, 86, 87, 88, 93, 114, 138, 144, 149–150, **795**
in elderly persons, 72, 75, 76–77, 92–93
electroconvulsive therapy–induced, 89
environmental and supportive interventions for, 71–72, 82–83, 90
features associated with, 74
follow-up care for, 82
guideline watch for, 61–62
detection, 61
management, 62
neuropathophysiologic models, 62
HIV-associated, 74, 75, 84, 92, 195, **207**, 208, 220
antipsychotics for, 253–254
hyperactive, hypoactive, and mixed forms of, 74
introduction to, 69
in liver disease, 92
in medically ill persons, 74–75, **76**
mortality related to, 75
patient/family education about, 82, 83
patient's emotional reaction to, 82
patient's memory of, 82
prevalence of, 74–75
prodromal symptoms of, 75
psychiatric management of, 62, 71, 79–82, 89–90
recovery from, 75
sensory impairments and, 83
sleep disturbances in, 62
somatic interventions for, 62, 72, 84–89
antipsychotics, 62, 72, 84–86, 90
benzodiazepines, 62, 72, 86–87, 90–91
choice of, 72, 90–91
cholinergics, 72, 87–88, 91
cholinesterase inhibitors, 62
electroconvulsive therapy, 88–89, 91
morphine and paralysis, 72, 88, 91
vitamins, 72, 88, 91
subclinical, 75
summary of treatment recommendations for, 71–72
terminal, 74
treatment plan for, 89–91
Delirium Observation Screening Scale, 61
Delirium Rating Scale (DRS), 27, 61, 62, 78, 84, 254
Delirium Scale (Dscale), 78
Delirium Symptom Interview (DSI), 78
Delirium tremens, 89, 379
Delta-9 tetrahydrocannabinol. *See* Marijuana use disorders
Delusions
in bipolar disorder, 869
cocaine-induced, 301
in delirium, 73, 74
in dementia, 116, 122, 148
in schizophrenia, 623, 625
Demeclocycline, for psychosis-induced polydipsia, 610
Dementia, 101–155
alcoholic, 390
of Alzheimer's type, 118 (*See also* Alzheimer's disease)
comorbidity with, 149–150
delirium, 116, 149–150
depression, 102, 114–115, 116, 122
general medical conditions, 149
Parkinson's disease, 150
stroke, 150, 616
course of, 117

definition of, 116
determining site and frequency of treatments for, 120–121
development of practice guideline for, 110
diagnosis of, 101
differential diagnosis of, 116–117
delirium, 74, 116–117
drug-induced, 120
due to other causes, 120
electroconvulsive therapy in persons with, 114, 145, 148, 798
features associated with, 116
guideline watch for, 101–102
diagnosis, 101
screening, 101
treatment, 102
HIV-associated, 75, 120, 172, 173–174, 195, 205, 219–220, 250–253
antiretroviral therapy for, 250–252
in children, 210
definitional criteria for, **206**
diagnosis of, 219
drugs that affect neurotransmitters for, 253
inflammatory mediators for, 252–253
management of, 219–220, 250–252
mania and, 207
nutritional therapies for, 253
prevalence of, 205
prevention of, 252
introduction to, 109
in Lewy body disease, 119
neuroimaging in, 101
in other progressive disorders, 120
in Parkinson's disease, 119
in Pick's disease and other frontal lobe dementias, 119–120
prevalence of, 117, 150
psychiatric management of, 111–112, 121–128
diagnostic evaluation and referral for medical care, 121–122
driving, 111–112, 124–125
financial and legal issues, 128
patient safety, 111–112, 123–124, 148
patient/family education, 112, 125–126
psychiatric assessment and monitoring, 122–123
sources of care and support, 127
therapeutic alliance, 121
wandering, 124
psychosocial treatments for, 112, 128–130
behavior-oriented approaches, 112, 129
cognition-oriented approaches, 112, 129–130
emotion-oriented approaches, 112, 129
goals of, 129
implementation of, 130
side effects of, 130
stimulation-oriented approaches, 112, 130
research directions related to, 154–155
reversibility of, 117
risk factors for, 126
screening for, 101
sociodemographic factors and, 153–154
age, 117, 153
ethnicity, 154
family history, 154
gender, 153
resource availability, 153
social support, 153
somatic treatments for elderly patients with, 102, 112–115, 130–147
for cognitive and functional losses, 112–113, 131–137
for depression, 114–115, 142–145
for psychosis and agitation, 113–114, 137–142
for sleep disturbances, 115, 146–147
special considerations for, 131
staging of, 117–118
summary of treatment recommendations for, 111–115
treatment plan for, 147–149
mildly impaired patients, 147–148
moderately impaired patients, 148
severely and profoundly impaired patients, 148–149
treatment settings for, 120–121, 150–153
day care, 151
home, 121, 150–151
inpatient medical/surgical services, 152
inpatient psychiatric units, 121, 153
long-term care, 115, 151–152
vascular (multi-infarct), 118–119
Dependent personality disorder
depression and, 792
panic disorder and, 983
Depersonalization, 22
in borderline personality disorder, 1244
L-Deprenyl. *See* Selegiline

Depression, 747–823. *See also* Antidepressants
acute phase management of, 772–777, **776**, 778, 782–786, 803–820
antidepressants, 747–750, 772–775, **774**, **775**, 782–785, **783**, **784**, 803–813
assessing adequacy of treatment response, 777, 786
choice of initial treatment modality, 772, **773**, 782
electroconvulsive therapy, 594–595, 750–751, 772, 782, 813–814
light therapy, 814–815
medications plus psychotherapy, 751, 772, 777, 782, 786, 820
psychotherapy, 751, 772, 775–776, 782, 785–786, 815–820
St. John's wort, 750, 815
age at onset of, 802
akinetic, 648
with atypical features, 772–773, 789–790
bipolar, 750, 778, 843–844, 860, 867–868, 892–897
among caregivers of patients with Alzheimer's disease, 151
with catatonic features, 789
in children and adolescents, 793
complications of, 803
continuation phase management of, 751–752, 777, 778, 787, 820–821
development of practice guideline for, 768
discontinuing treatment for, 778, 788, 821
double, 791, 800
drug-induced
carbamazepine, 1293
clonidine, 430
interferon, 176–177, 351–352
DSM-IV-TR criteria for, **801–802**
duration of episode of, 802
vs. dysthymia, 800
in elderly persons, 752–753, 793–794
electroconvulsive therapy for, 594–595, 750–751, 772, 777, 782, 784, 787, 789, 813–814, 822
epidemiology of, 800–802
family history of, 797, 800
functioning between episodes of, 802
future research needs related to, 822–823
antidepressants, 822
electroconvulsive therapy, 823
other treatment modalities, 823
psychotherapy, 823
guide to using practice guideline for, 767
guideline watch for, 747–753
continuation and maintenance treatment, 751–752
psychosocial treatments, 751
somatic treatments, 747–751
treatment in older adults, 752–753
maintenance phase management of, 751–752, 777, 777–778, 787, 821–822
medical comorbidity with, 797–799, 803
asthma, 797
cardiac disease, 797–798
dementia, 102, 114–115, 116, 122, 798
epilepsy, 798
glaucoma, 798
HIV/AIDS, 171, 174–175, 195, 220, 228, 240, 254–256
hypertension, 798–799
obstructive uropathy, 799
Parkinson's disease, 119, 150, 799
melancholic, 800
natural history and course of, 802–803
phases of treatment for, 778
postpartum, 797
in pregnancy, 794–797
prevalence of, 800
prodromal symptoms of, 802
vs. pseudodementia, 117, 143, 791
psychiatric comorbidity with, 788–792
anxiety disorders, 790–791
dementia, 102, 116, 122, 148, 149
Alzheimer's disease, 122, 143
Parkinson's disease, 119, 150
somatic treatments for, 114–115, 142–145
dysthymia, 791
eating disorders, 1152–1153, 1163
panic disorder, 790, 982
personality disorders, 792
borderline personality disorder, 1224, 1263–1264
posttraumatic stress disorder, 1021, 1026, 1037, 1044
schizophrenia, 577, 582, 594, 601, 606–607, 614, 625, 658
substance use disorders, 335, 341–344, 790
suicidal behavior, 335, 748, 779, 788–789, 803, 1342–1344, 1353, 1391–1394
psychiatric management of, 771, 779–781

addressing early signs of relapse, 781
diagnostic evaluation, 779
functional assessment, 780
monitoring patient's psychiatric status and safety, 781
patient/family education, 781
suicide risk assessment, 779, **780,** 788–789
therapeutic alliance, 780–781
treatment adherence, 781
treatment setting, 780
psychosocial interventions for, 751, 772, 775–776, 782, 785–786, 815–820
behavior therapy, 791, 817
cognitive behavior therapy, 751, 752, 775, 777, 785, 816–817
combined with pharmacotherapy, 751, 772, 777, 782, 786, 820
efficacy of, 816
family therapy, 819
goals of, 815–816
group therapy, 751, 819
interpersonal therapy, 777, 791, 817–818
marital therapy, 819
psychodynamic psychotherapy, 785, 792, 818
self-help groups, 819–820
with psychotic features, 750, 752, 789, 800
rating scales for, **28–29,** 255, 256
recurrence of, 802
early signs of, 781
risk factors for, **778**
seasonal, 792, 802–803
with seasonal pattern, 792, 802–803
severity of, 800
sociodemographic factors and, 792–797
bereavement, 792
children and adolescents, 793
cultural factors, 793
family distress, 793
family history, 797
gender, 794
older adults, 793–794
pregnancy, 794–797
psychosocial stressors, 792
substance use disorders and, 336, 341–344, 790
among adolescents, 355
alcohol dependence, 335, 336, 388–389
cocaine withdrawal, 394
nicotine dependence, 343, 375
pharmacotherapy for, 338, 342–343
prevalence of, 341
psychosocial treatments for, 343–344
after suicide of family member or friend, 1382
summary of treatment recommendations for, 771–778
among traumatized persons, 1021, 1026, 1037, 1044, **1046**
treatment plan for, 778–779
treatment settings for, 780
treatment-resistant, 750
Depressive pseudodementia, 117, 143, 791
Derealization, 22
in borderline personality disorder, 1244
Desferrioxamine, for Alzheimer's disease, 137
Desipramine
for bipolar depression, 896
blood levels of, 811
for borderline personality disorder, 1289, 1292
for bulimia nervosa, 1177, 1178
for depression, 772, 783
in older adults, 753
dosage of, 145, **774**
for panic disorder, 968
for persons with dementia, 145, 798
for persons with HIV/AIDS, 254
for persons with obstructive uropathy, 799
for persons with substance use disorders, 342
alcohol dependence, 384
attention-deficit/hyperactivity disorder and, 348
cocaine dependence, 395, 397, 447
side effects of, 144
Detoxification
from alcohol, 301
hospital-based programs for, 311
from multiple substances, 334, 410
from opioids, 302, 405–408
sleep disturbances after, 336
Detroit Area Survey of Trauma, 1045, 1048
Development of practice guidelines, ix–x
for acute stress disorder and posttraumatic stress disorder, 1008–1009
for bipolar disorder, 857
for borderline personality disorder, 1239
for delirium, 70
for dementia, 110
for depression, 768
for eating disorders, 1102
for HIV/AIDS, 192

Development of practice guidelines *(continued)*
for panic disorder, 950
process for, x, 1497–1503
background and definition, 1499
contributors, 1499–1500
evidence base, 1500–1501
format, 1501–1502
improvement of, xi–xii
review, dissemination, and updates, 1502–1503
topic selection, 1499
for psychiatric evaluation of adults, 5
reasons for, ix–x
for schizophrenia, 570
for substance use disorders, 296
for suicidal behavior, 1320
Developmental history, **14,** 18, **19**
Dexamethasone suppression test (DST), 1439
Dexfenfluramine
for binge eating disorder, 1150
interaction with selective serotonin reuptake inhibitors, 808
Dextroamphetamine
dosage of, 145
for erectile dysfunction, **795**
for persons with dementia, 143
for persons with HIV/AIDS, 174, 242, 253, 254, 255, 258, 260
side effects of, 144
Dextromethorphan, interaction with monoamine oxidase inhibitors, 973
DHEA (dehydroepiandrosterone), for persons with HIV/AIDS, 260
Diabetes insipidus, lithium-induced, 662
Diabetes mellitus. *See also* Glucose dysregulation
assessment for, **586**
drug-induced
antipsychotics, 575, 655, 843
antiretroviral agents, 203
eating disorders and, 1154
schizophrenia and, 615, 655
vascular dementia and, 126
Diabetic ketoacidosis, antipsychotic-induced, 655
Diagnosis, 36–37. *See also* Assessment; Assessment instruments; Laboratory testing
computerized approaches to, 43
future research needs related to, 43
Diagnostic and Statistical Manual of Mental Disorders (DSM-IV-TR), 37
acute stress disorder in, 1015, **1016,** 1039–1043, **1040–1042**
Alzheimer's disease in, 118
borderline personality disorder in, 1223, 1238, **1238**
delirium in, 73
eating disorders in, 1119
anorexia nervosa, **1119**
bulimia nervosa, **1120**
mood disorders in
hypomanic episode, **879**
major depressive episode and major depressive disorder, **801–802, 878**
manic episode, **877**
mixed episode, **880**
summary of manic and depressive symptom criteria for bipolar disorder, **881**
Outline for Cultural Formulation in, 18, 35–36, **36**
panic disorder in, 954
posttraumatic stress disorder in, 1015, **1017–1018,** 1039–1043, **1040–1042**
schizophrenia in, 623, **624**
substance dependence and abuse in, 306, **306, 307,** 412
vascular dementia in, 119
Diagnostic Interview Schedule (DIS), 1045
Diagnostic Survey for Eating Disorders (DSED), **1121**
Diagnostic tests, **16,** 31–34, **33.** *See also* Laboratory testing
future research needs related to, 43–44
Dialectical behavior therapy (DBT)
for binge eating disorder, 1179
for borderline personality disorder, 228, 1225–1226, 1252, **1253,** 1282–1284, 1452–1453
adverse effects of, 1284
cost-effectiveness of, 1284
efficacy of, 1282–1284
implementation of, 1284
length and frequency of, 1284
for suicidal persons, 1377, 1452–1453
Dialysis
delirium and, 74
for lithium intoxication, 883
suicide risk and, 1354, 1424
Diarrhea
drug-induced
acamprosate, 440
antiretroviral agents, 203

fluoxetine-olanzapine combination, 843
lithium, 844, 882
selective serotonin reuptake inhibitors, 807
valproate, 885
in serotonin syndrome, 808
Diazepam
for alcohol withdrawal, 380, 436
for catatonia, 789
for panic disorder, 970, 971
dosage of, 972
for persons with dementia, 140
for persons with schizophrenia, 660
in pregnancy, 873
use in opioid-dependent patients, 410
Didanosine, **204**
for children, 259
for HIV-associated dementia, 251–252
side effects of, **209**
Diet
monoamine oxidase inhibitor interaction with tyramine in, 114, 144, 810, 973, 1291
salt-restricted, effect on lithium excretion, 876
therapies for HIV/AIDS, 253
for weight gain in anorexia nervosa, 1109, 1136
vitamin and mineral supplementation, 1112, 1113, 1145
Differential diagnosis, 36–37
of acute stress disorder and posttraumatic stress disorder, 1043–1045, **1046–1047**
of borderline personality disorder, 1275
of delirium, 74
of dementia, 116–117
of extrapyramidal symptoms, 648
of HIV-associated neuropsychiatric syndromes, **207–210**, 208
of neuroleptic malignant syndrome, 652
of panic disorder, 954
of schizophrenia, 580
Digoxin, 93
drug interactions with
nefazodone, 809
St. John's wort, 750
Diphenhydramine
contraindicated for persons with dementia, 115, 147
for extrapyramidal symptoms, **594**
for insomnia during opioid withdrawal, 408
side effects of, 120
DIS (Diagnostic Interview Schedule), 1045
Disability
Americans with Disabilities Act, 218
HIV-associated, 218
Disability evaluations, 9
Disclosure of patient information, 39
about HIV status, 216, 247–248, 359
about substance abuse treatment, 359
about suicidal behavior, 1380
after patient's death, 1381
Disorganized schizophrenia, 604, 625
Disorientation, 73, 83
Dissociative disorders
borderline personality disorder and, 1267–1268
sexual abuse and, 215
Disulfiram
for alcohol dependence, 301, 324, 378, 383, 438–439
in dual-diagnosis patients, 339
borderline personality disorder, 1264
schizophrenia, 341
efficacy of, 438–439
goals of, 438
implementation of, 439
in persons with HIV/AIDS, 246
for cocaine dependence, 302, 395, 448
dosage of, 383, 438
drug interactions with, 383, 439
alcohol, 383, 438
psychosocial treatments to enhance effectiveness of, 326
side effects of, 383, 439
Diuretics
drug interactions with
antidepressants, 798–799
lithium, 876
hyponatremia induced by, 609
for lithium-induced polyuria and polydipsia, 882
Divalproex sodium. *See* Valproate
Dizziness, drug-induced
buspirone, 142
carbamazepine, 843
duloxetine, 749
olanzapine, 842, 890
quetiapine, 842, 843
reboxetine, 809
topiramate, 1180

Dizziness, drug-induced *(continued)*
tricyclic antidepressants, 806, 968
ziprasidone, 842
Docosahexaenoic acid, 662
Documentation
of adult psychiatric evaluation, 11
of care of suicidal patient, 1378
of schizophrenia treatment, 583–584
Domestic partner violence, suicide risk and history of, 1352, 1419–1421
Donepezil
for Alzheimer's disease, 102, 112–113, 131–133, 147, 148
for delirium, 62, 87
dosage of, 133
for persons with schizophrenia, 661
side effects of, 132
Dopaminergic agents
for cocaine dependence/withdrawal, 394, 447–448
for HIV-related cognitive disorders, 253
for hyperprolactinemia, 656
Double depression, 791, 800
Double Trouble, 387
Double-trouble groups, 387, 674
Down's syndrome, 126
"Downward drift," 319
Doxepin
dosage of, 774
for insomnia during opioid withdrawal, 408
Dreams, vivid, efavirenz-induced, 172
Driving
dementia and, 111–112, 124–125
under the influence of alcohol or drugs, 315, 317, 416
Dronabinol, for HIV-related wasting, 244
Drooling, clozapine-induced, 636
Droperidol
for aggressive behavior, 609
continuous infusion of, 86
for delirium, 72, 84, 85–86, 90
in HIV/AIDS, 254
for emergency treatment of acute psychosis, 590
side effects of, 85
QTc interval prolongation, 85, 590, 609, 616
Drowsiness, drug-induced
efavirenz, 172
selective serotonin reuptake inhibitors, 966
DRS (Delirium Rating Scale), **27**, 61, 62, 78, 84, 254
Drug Abuse Reporting Program, 451
Drug Abuse Screening Test, 307
Drug Abuse Treatment Outcome Study, 451–452
Drug Addiction Treatment Act of 2000, 359, 401
Drug interactions. *See also specific drugs*
with antipsychotics, 635
with antiretroviral agents, 171–172, **172**, 195–196, 238, **239**, 241, 242, 243, 245, 261
with carbamazepine, 888
with clozapine, 638–639
cytochrome P450–related, 171, 238, **239**
with disulfiram, 383, 439
with lithium, 876
with methadone, 402
with monoamine oxidase inhibitors, 144, 973
with nefazodone, 809
with olanzapine, 643
with quetiapine, 644
with risperidone, 641
with St. John's wort, 750, 815
with selective serotonin reuptake inhibitors, 144, 808
with selegiline, 135
in substance-abusing patients with co-occurring psychiatric disorders, 324
with tricyclic antidepressants, 807
with valproate, 887
"Drug-free programs," for opioid-dependent persons, 400
Dry mouth, drug-induced
antidepressants, 144, 429, **795**, 806, 968, 1290
antipsychotics, 138, 654
carbamazepine, 843
clonidine, 430
duloxetine, 749
fluoxetine-olanzapine combination, 843
lamotrigine, 893
management of, **795**, 806–807
mirtazapine, 809
monoamine oxidase inhibitors, 973
nefazodone, 809
olanzapine, 842, 845, 890
quetiapine, 654, 842, 843
reboxetine, 809
topiramate, 1180
trazodone, 142

Dscale (Delirium Scale), 78
DSED (Diagnostic Survey for Eating Disorders), **1121**
DSI (Delirium Symptom Interview), 78
DSM-IV-TR. *See Diagnostic and Statistical Manual of Mental Disorders*
DST (dexamethasone suppression test), 1439
Dual-diagnosis patients, 309–310, 319–320, 336–350. *See also* Substance use disorders
with anxiety disorders, 345–347
with attention-deficit/hyperactivity disorder, 347–348
with bipolar disorder, 335, 344–345
with delirium, 76, 77
with dementia, 120
with depression, 335, 341–344
with eating disorders, 348–349
hospitalization of, 311
integrated treatment of, 337–338, 345–347
management principles for, 336–337
with pathological gambling, 349–350
with personality disorders, 335, 349
pharmacotherapy for, 338–339
for psychiatric disorders, 338
for substance use disorders, 339
psychosocial treatments for, 339
risk of aggression and homicide in, 335–336
with schizophrenia, 339–341, 605–606
sleep disturbances in, 336
specialized care for, 321
suicide risk in, 334–335
treatment settings for, 337–338
Duloxetine, 747, 749–750
for anxiety, 750
dosage of, 749
efficacy of, 749
for pain, 749–750
side effects of, 749
Durable power of attorney, 40, 128, 218
Dysarthria, 73
Dysgraphia, 73
Dyskinesia, drug-induced. *See also* Tardive dyskinesia
bromocriptine, 144
olanzapine, 890
Dyslipidemia. *See* Hyperlipidemia
Dysnomia, 73
Dyspepsia, drug-induced
aripiprazole, 842
carbamazepine, 843
lithium, 882
topiramate, 1180
valproate, 885
Dysphoria, antipsychotic-induced, 606, 607
Dysthymia, 800
alcohol use disorders and, 336
depression and, 791
nicotine dependence and, 375
suicide and, **1343**
Dystonia
antipsychotic-induced, 241, 592, 648, 649
in HIV infection, 242
selective serotonin reuptake inhibitor–induced, 808
tardive, 651
treatment of, **594**, 649

E

EAPs (employee assistance programs), for substance use disorders, 314–315, 333
Early intervention, for schizophrenia, 671–672
Eating Attitudes Test (EAT), **1121**, 1158
Eating Disorder Examination (EDE), **1121**
Eating disorders, 1097–1183
assessment instruments for, **1121**
bupropion contraindicated in, 369, 429, 1112, 1144
chronicity of, 1151–1152, 1164–1167
clinical features of, 1160–1162
development of practice guideline for, 1102
diabetes and, 1154
eating disorder not otherwise specified, 1115–1116, 1149, 1167
binge eating disorder, 1115–1116, 1149, 1179–1181
night eating syndrome, 1116, 1151, 1181
epidemiology of, 1163–1164
future research needs related to, 1181–1183
genetic factors and, 1167–1168
guide to using practice guideline for, 1101
history of abuse in persons with, 1021, 1155, 1164
introduction to, 1103
laboratory abnormalities in, 1162–1163
laboratory assessments for persons with, **1128**
mortality rates in, 1165–1166
natural history and course of, 1164–1167
physical complications of, **1123–1127**, 1162
in pregnancy, 1154–1155

Eating disorders *(continued)*
prevalence of, 1163
psychiatric comorbidity with, 1152–1154, 1163–1164
anxiety disorders, 1153, 1164
bipolar disorder, 1163
depression, 1152–1153, 1163
personality disorders, 1153–1154, 1164
substance use disorders, 337, 348–349, 355, 1152, 1164
suicidality, 1106, **1131**, **1343**, 1345, 1399–1400
psychiatric management of, 1105–1106, 1116–1129
assessment/monitoring of medical condition, 1106, 1121–1122, **1123–1128**
assessment/monitoring of safety and psychiatric status, 1106, 1122
assessment/monitoring of symptoms and behaviors, 1105–1106, 1119–1120
coordination of care, 1105, 1118–1119
family assessment/treatment, 1106, 1122, 1129
therapeutic alliance, 1116–1118
psychodynamic issues in, 1161
self-help books and Internet resources on, **1117**
sociodemographic factors and, 1155–1160
age, 1156–1157
athletes, 1158
cultural factors, 1157–1158
high school and college students, 1158–1159
male gender, 1155–1156
risk and protective factors, 1159–1160
summary of treatment recommendations for, 1105–1116
support groups for, 349, 1111, 1114, 1141–1142, 1172, 1177
treatment of anorexia nervosa, 1108–1113, 1134–1145, 1169–1175
medications, 1112–1113, 1143–1145, 1173–1175
nutritional rehabilitation, 1108–1110, 1134–1138, 1169
other somatic treatments, 1174–1175
psychosocial interventions, 1110–1111, 1138–1143, 1170–1172
treatment of bulimia nervosa, 1113–1115, 1145–1149, 1175–1179
medications, 1114, 1147–1148, 1177–1178
nutritional rehabilitation/counseling, 1113, 1145
other somatic treatments, 1115, 1148
psychosocial interventions, 1113–1114, 1145–1147, 1175–1177
psychotherapy combined with medications, 1115, 1148, 1178–1179
treatment plan for, 1116–1151
treatment settings for, 1106–1108, 1129–1134
continuity of care, 1107, 1130
level of care guidelines, **1131–1133**
Eating Disorders Examination—Questionnaire (EDE-Q), **1121**
Eating Disorders Inventory–2 (EDI-2), **1121**
Eating Disorders Questionnaire (EDQ), **1121**
Ebstein's anomaly, lithium-induced, 872
ECA (Epidemiologic Catchment Area) study, 627, 800, 880, 955, 986, 1048, 1385, 1398, 1402, 1403, 1418
ECG. *See* Electrocardiogram
Echolalia/echopraxia, in catatonia, 789
Economic factors
dementia and, 128
HIV/AIDS and, 226
schizophrenia and, 628
substance use disorders and, 415, 416
"Ecstasy," 334
interaction with ritonavir, 240
ECT. *See* Electroconvulsive therapy
EDE (Eating Disorder Examination), **1121**
Edema, drug-induced
lithium, 662, 882
monoamine oxidase inhibitors, 810, 973
EDE-Q (Eating Disorders Examination—Questionnaire), **1121**
EDI-2 (Eating Disorders Inventory–2), **1121**
EDQ (Eating Disorders Questionnaire), **1121**
Education of patient/family
about acute stress disorder and posttraumatic stress disorder, 1024, 1034
about bipolar disorder, 846, 864, 903
about borderline personality disorder, 1247–1248
about delirium, 82, 83
about dementia, 112, 125–126
about depression, 781
about HIV-related neuropsychiatric syndromes, 174, 217

about nicotine dependence, 366
about panic disorder, 957–958, 960
about risk behaviors for HIV infection, 213, 232
about schizophrenia, 576, 582, 595, 673
about substance use disorders, 321
about suicidal behavior, 1369–1370
EEG (electroencephalogram)
in alcohol or sedative-hypnotic withdrawal, 74
in delirium, 74, 78
Efavirenz, 170–171, 172, 175, **204**, **209**
drug interactions with, 238, 246
side effects of, 171, 172, **209**
Effectiveness of Methadone Maintenance Treatment Study, 452
Eicosapentaenoic acid (EPA), for persons with schizophrenia, 662–663
Ejaculatory disturbances, antipsychotic-induced, 656–657
Elderly persons
abuse or neglect of, 124, 127
age-related cognitive decline in, 117
anorexia nervosa in, 1157
bipolar disorder in, 875, 880
borderline personality disorder in, 1269
delirium in, 72, 75, 76–77, 92–93
dementia in, 101–155
depression in, 752–753, 793–794
depressive pseudodementia in, 117, 143
drug use in, 112, 875
antidepressants, 875
antipsychotics, 72, 85, 93, 614, 875
benzodiazepines, 86–87, 356, 875, 971
lithium, 875
polypharmacy, 131
tricyclic antidepressants, 968
HIV/AIDS in, 226
panic disorder in, 985
psychiatric evaluation of, 40–41
schizophrenia in, 614–615, 627
substance use disorders in, 356
suicidal behavior in, 1339, 1383–1385, **1384**
use of restraints for, 93, 115, 151–152
Electrocardiogram (ECG), **33**, 798
lithium effects on, 882
monitoring in patients receiving
antipsychotics, 72, 90
clozapine, 638
ziprasidone, 646
Electroconvulsive therapy (ECT), 663–665
for bipolar disorder
in children and adolescents, 906
depressive episodes, 860, 867, 868, 896
maintenance treatment, 861, 869, 901
manic and mixed episodes, 860, 867, 891
for borderline personality disorder, 1243–1244, 1259, 1298–1299, 1300
for catatonia, 594
contraindications to, 664
for delirium, 88–89, 91
for depression, 594–595, 750–751, 772, 777, 782, 784, 787, 822
with catatonic features, 789
in dementia, 145
efficacy of, 813
in elderly persons, 794
with psychotic features, 789
treatment-resistant, 813
electrode placement for, 665, 750, 814
evaluation for, 814
future research needs related to, 822
in HIV/AIDS, 255
implementation of, 664–665, 814
informed consent for, 664–665
for neuroleptic malignant syndrome, 89, 91, 652
number and duration of treatments with, 665, 814
in pregnancy, 796, 873
for schizoaffective disorder, 663
for schizophrenia, 663–665
in acute phase, 594–595
efficacy of, 663–664
in stable phase, 601
treatment-resistant illness, 602
side effects of, 664, 813–814, 1298
cardiovascular effects, 664, 814
cognitive effects, 89, 664, 813–814
stimulus intensity for, 665, 751, 814
for suicidal persons, 1327, 1376–1377, 1449–1451, 1455
use in anorexia nervosa, 1112
use in persons with medical conditions, 89, 91
cardiac disease, 798
dementia, 114, 145, 148, 798
Parkinson's disease, 89, 799
Electroencephalogram (EEG)
in alcohol or sedative-hypnotic withdrawal, 74
in delirium, 74, 78

EMDR (eye movement desensitization and reprocessing)
for acute stress disorder and posttraumatic stress disorder, 1014, 1028, 1032, 1057–1059
for panic disorder, 938
for posttraumatic symptoms in borderline personality disorder, 1267
Emergency situations
history taking and confidentiality in, 7, 8
psychiatric evaluation of adults in, 8–9
suicide risk assessment in, 1328–1329, 1359–1360
Emotional lability
benzodiazepine-induced, 87
in borderline personality disorder, 1273
pharmacotherapy for, 1243–1244, 1256–1259, **1258**
in delirium, 74
Emotions Anonymous, 674
Emphysema, 625
Employee assistance programs (EAPs), for substance use disorders, 314–315, 333
Employment
history of, **14**, 19
postexposure prophylaxis for HIV exposure related to, 213–214, 234
substance use disorders and, 307–308
suicide risk and, 1342, 1346, 1355, 1428–1429
supported, for persons with schizophrenia, 576, 598, 668
Emtricitabine, 170
Enalapril, for psychosis-induced polydipsia, 610
Encephalopathy
hepatic, 87
HIV, 208, 210
Wernicke's, 74, **81**, 390
Endocrine abnormalities
alcohol dependence and, 389
anorexia nervosa and, **1123**
dementia and, 120
lithium-induced, 662, 882, 1293
Enfuvirtide, 171
Environmental interventions
for delirium, 71–72, 82–83, 90
for mania, 864
for schizophrenia, 574
EPA (eicosapentaenoic acid), for persons with schizophrenia, 662–663
Epidemiologic Catchment Area (ECA) study, 627, 800, 880, 955, 986, 1048, 1385, 1398, 1402, 1403, 1418
Epidemiology. *See also* Age/aging; Ethnicity; Gender; Prevalence
of acute stress disorder and posttraumatic stress disorder, 1045–1051
of bipolar disorder, 880
of borderline personality disorder, 1224–1225, 1275–1276
of depression, 800–802
of eating disorders, 1163–1164
of HIV/AIDS, 169–170, 197–198, **198**
of panic disorder, 955
of schizophrenia, 626–628
of substance use disorders, 415–420
alcohol use disorders, 377, 418–419
cocaine use, 393, 420
marijuana use disorders, 391, 419–420
nicotine dependence, 417–418
opioid dependence, 399, 420
of suicidal behavior, 1336–1342, **1337–1338**, 1383–1391, **1384**
Epilepsy. *See also* Seizures
antidepressants for persons with, 798
suicide risk among persons with, 1353, 1424, 1425
Epinephrine, interaction with tricyclic antidepressants, 807
EPS. *See* Extrapyramidal symptoms
Erectile dysfunction, drug-induced. *See also* Sexual dysfunction
antidepressants, **795**, 808, 810
antipsychotics, 656–657
Ergoloid mesylates
for dementia, 113, 136, 150
side effects of, 136
Ergot alkaloids, interaction with antiretroviral agents, 241
Erythromycin, interaction with clozapine, 638
Escitalopram, 747, 749
dosage of, 937
efficacy of, 749
for panic disorder, 937
Estrogen, for antidepressant augmentation, 751–752
Estrogen replacement therapy
for Alzheimer's disease, 126, 131, 136, 154
for anorexia nervosa, 1113, 1145, 1174–1175
Ethanol, for alcohol withdrawal, 382

Ethical issues
boundary violations
in treatment of borderline personality disorder, 1249–1250, 1253, 1272
in treatment of suicidal patients, 1363
in care of persons with HIV/AIDS, 247–248
confidentiality, 7, 8, 11, 38–39
in treatment of chronic anorexia nervosa, 1138
in treatment of suicidal patients, 1363, 1380
Ethnicity
acute stress disorder, posttraumatic stress disorder and, 1035–1036, 1049–1051
bipolar disorder and, 874
borderline personality disorder and, 1269
cytochrome P450 enzyme polymorphisms and, 1036
dementia and, 154
depression and, 793
eating disorders and, 1157–1158, 1163
HIV/AIDS and, 223–225, **224**
panic disorder and, 986
schizophrenia and, 611–612
substance use disorders and, 356–357
alcohol use, 418
marijuana use, 419
suicidal behavior and, 1341, **1384,** 1385, 1386–1389
Euphoria, benzodiazepine-induced, 87
Evidence Report on Treatment of Depression—Newer Pharmacotherapies, 804
Executive dysfunction, 32–33
in dementia, 116, 118, 119
in Parkinson's disease, 119
Executive Interview Test, **219**
Exercise
in Alzheimer's disease, 102
anorexia nervosa and, 1136, 1158
to assist with smoking cessation, 371, 433–434
for depression in older adults, 751, 753
in HIV/AIDS, 229
Exposure therapy
for acute stress disorder and posttraumatic stress disorder, 1014, 1053–1057
for bulimia nervosa, 1176
for panic disorder, 960–961
"Extrapyramidal symptom threshold" for antipsychotics, 575, 593, 599, 648
Extrapyramidal symptoms (EPS), 85, 114, 138–139, **592,** 592–593, 631, 648–651
Abnormal Involuntary Movement Scale for, **27,** 580
acute dystonia, 241, 648, 649
acute vs. chronic, 648
akathisia, 85, 114, 138, 139, 144, 241, 648, 649–650
antidepressants and, **795,** 807, 808
assessment for, **586**
differential diagnosis of, 648
with intravenous antipsychotics, 85, 90
monitoring for, 575
in neonates, 872–873
parkinsonism, 112, 119, 138, 144, 241, 648–649
in persons with anorexia nervosa, 11112
in persons with HIV/AIDS, 241–242
pharmacotherapy for, 594, **594,** 601, 650
prophylaxis for, 594, 650
risk factors for, 615
second-generation antipsychotics and, 138–139, 648
aripiprazole, 647, 842
clozapine, 635, 636
olanzapine, 642–643, 890
quetiapine, 644
risperidone, 640, 641, 648
ziprasidone, 645, 842
selective serotonin reuptake inhibitors and, 966
tardive dyskinesia, 85, 114, 139, 152, 242, 648, 650–651
tardive dystonia, 648
Eye movement desensitization and reprocessing (EMDR)
for acute stress disorder and posttraumatic stress disorder, 1014, 1028, 1032, 1057–1059
for panic disorder, 938
for posttraumatic symptoms in borderline personality disorder, 1267

F

Factitious disorder, 117
Fagerström Test for Nicotine Dependence, 360, **360,** 368
Falls
drug-associated, 114, 115, 134, 138, 140, 141, 806, 875
prevention of, 123–124

Family history, **15**, 20. *See also* Genetic factors
bipolar disorder and, 797
borderline personality disorder and, 1275
dementia and, 154
depression and, 797, 800
eating disorders and, 1163
panic disorder and, 955
schizophrenia and, 627
suicide and, 1330, 1354–1355, 1426–1428
Family interventions
for bipolar disorder, 845, 902
for borderline personality disorder, 1243, 1255–1256, 1287
for depression, 819
for eating disorders, 1106, 1122, 1129
anorexia nervosa, 1110, 1140, 1171–1172
bulimia nervosa, 1114, 1146, 1176–1177
for panic disorder, 964–965
after patient's suicide, 1325–1326, 1382
for schizophrenia, 578, 597, 620, 667–668
for substance use disorders, 298, 315, 330–331
in adolescents, 355
alcohol dependence, 387, 445
opioid dependence, 409
for suicidal behavior, 1327
theoretical orientations of, 331
Family studies, of suicidal behavior, 1427
Family/caregivers
of patient with delirium, 82, 83
of patient with dementia, 121, 124–128, 148–149, 150–151
of patient with depression, 793
of patient with HIV/AIDS, 218–219
of patient with schizophrenia, 574, 584, 588, 595
of patient with substance use disorder, 303, 357–358
self-help groups for, 332, 387, 445
Family-focused therapy, for bipolar disorder, 845, 902, 904
Famotidine, 885
Fasting blood glucose, **33**
Fat redistribution syndromes, antiretroviral agent–induced, 171, 177–178, 203
Fatigue
drug-induced
benzodiazepines, 970
buspirone, 142
carbamazepine, 887, 1293
cocaine withdrawal, 394
ondansetron, 441
topiramate, 1180
tricyclic antidepressants, 968
in HIV/AIDS, 196, 220, 222–223, 260
Female athlete trial, 1158
Fenfluramine
for binge eating disorder, 1180
for bulimia nervosa, 1150, 1178
interaction with selective serotonin reuptake inhibitors, 808
Fentanyl, 88
Fetal alcohol spectrum disorder, 390–391
Fetal drug exposure
alcohol, 390–391
antidepressants, 796, 872
antipsychotics, 613, 872–873
benzodiazepines, 613
buprenorphine, 411
bupropion, 377
cocaine, 398
marijuana, 392–393
methadone, 411
mood stabilizers, 613, 871–873
nicotine, 352, 376–377
opioids, 352, 411
Fever
antipsychotic-induced, 654
clozapine-induced, 636
delirium and, **81**
in neuroleptic malignant syndrome, 651
in serotonin syndrome, 808
Financial decision making, dementia and, 128
Finger Tapping Test, **210**
Firearm-related suicides, 1323, 1329, 1331, 1335, 1351, 1358, 1402, 1434–1436
Flooding, for posttraumatic stress disorder, 1053
Fludrocortisone, for orthostatic hypotension, **795**
Fluid management, during alcohol withdrawal, 301
Flumazenil, for benzodiazepine overdose, 322–323
Flunitrazepam, interaction with buprenorphine, 460
Fluoxetine
for acute stress disorder or posttraumatic stress disorder, 1030
for bipolar depression, 895
for borderline personality disorder, 1226, 1256, 1257, **1258**, 1259, **1260**, 1287–1289

for in children and adolescents, 749
cognitive behavior therapy and, 749
dosage of, 144, **774**, 936, 967, 1289
drug interactions with
antipsychotics, 607
carbamazepine, 888
clozapine, 638
for eating disorders
anorexia nervosa, 1143, 1173
binge eating disorder, 1116, 1180–1181
bulimia nervosa, 1114, 1147, 1177
for elderly persons, 752
neonatal withdrawal from, 796
for obsessive-compulsive disorder, 257
for panic disorder, 936, 937, 965
for persons with concurrent medical conditions
dementia, 144, 798
glaucoma, 798
HIV/AIDS, 254–255, 257
for persons with schizophrenia, 658
for persons with substance use disorders, 342
alcohol dependence, 441
cocaine dependence, 395, 447
for posttraumatic stress disorder, 1064
in pregnancy, 796, 872
for relapse prevention in anorexia nervosa, 1112
side effects of, 144
switching to monoamine oxidase inhibitor from, 808, 812
Fluoxetine-olanzapine combination, 750
for bipolar depression, 750, 843
side effects of, 843
Flupenthixol, for borderline personality disorder, **1262**, 1295, 1296
Fluphenazine, **589**
interaction with nicotine, 340
for schizophrenia, 660
dosage of, **589**, 633, 634
side effects of, 138
Fluphenazine decanoate
for dementia, 140
dosage of, 634
for dual-diagnosis patients, 340
for schizophrenia, 592, 630
dosage of, 634
Flurazepam, for sleep disturbances, 259
Flushing, in serotonin syndrome, 808
Fluvoxamine
for acute stress disorder or posttraumatic stress disorder, 1030
for binge eating disorder, 1180
for borderline personality disorder, 1226
dosage of, **774**, 967
drug interactions with
antipsychotics, 607
carbamazepine, 888
clozapine, 638
for panic disorder, 966, 968
for pathological gambling, 350
for persons with HIV/AIDS, 255
for persons with schizophrenia, 658
for posttraumatic stress disorder, 1064
withdrawal from, 966
Food interactions with monoamine oxidase inhibitors, 114, 144, 810
Forensic evaluation, 9, 38
Foscarnet, **209**
Foster care, for persons with schizophrenia, 620
Freiberg Personality Inventory, 1413
Frontal lobe dementias, 119–120
Functional adaptation skills training, in schizophrenia, 615
Functional assessment/impairments, **16**, 31
in acute stress disorder and posttraumatic stress disorder, 1026, 1027, 1051
in bipolar disorder, 866
in borderline personality disorder, 1248, 1274
in dementia, 122
in depression, 780
in panic disorder, 956–957
in schizophrenia, 583, 598–599
in substance use disorders, 303, 305
Fusion/entry inhibitors, for HIV/AIDS, 170

G

Gabapentin
for bipolar disorder, 889
in children and adolescents, 906
for panic disorder, 974
for persons with HIV/AIDS, 243–244
for sleep disturbances in alcohol-dependent patients, 336
for suicidal persons, 1326, 1376
GAF (Global Assessment of Functioning) Scale, **26**, 816, 817
Gait disturbances. *See also* Ataxia
in dementia, 116, 118, 119, 123
efavirenz-induced, 172
falls due to, 114, 115, 134, 138, 140, 141
safety precautions for persons with, 123–124

Galactorrhea, antipsychotic-induced, 85
Galantamine, for dementia, 102
Gamblers Anonymous, 350
Gambling, pathological
pharmacotherapy for, 350
substance use disorders and, 337, 349–350
Gamma-hydroxybutyrate (GHB), 334
Gamma-hydroxybutyric acid withdrawal delirium, 62
GARS (Global Accessibility Rating Scale), 78
Gastrointestinal disorders
anorexia nervosa and, **1123**
bulimia nervosa and, **1126**
drug-induced
acamprosate, 440
antidepressants, 144, 429, **795**, 806
antipsychotics, 138, 592, 614, 654
antiretroviral agents, 203
aripiprazole, 842
buprenorphine, 460
bupropion, 369, 429, 809
buspirone, 142
carbamazepine, 843, 887, 1293
cholinesterase inhibitors, 87, 112, 132
clonidine, 430
clozapine, 654
duloxetine, 749
ergoloid mesylates, 136
fluoxetine-olanzapine combination, 843
lithium, 662, 844, 882, 1293
methadone, 455
naltrexone, 404, 437, 438
nefazodone, 809
olanzapine, 654
ondansetron, 441
quetiapine, 654, 843
reboxetine, 809
risperidone, 842
selective serotonin reuptake inhibitors, 144, 807, 966
substances of abuse, **351**
topiramate, 1180
tricyclic antidepressants, 144
valproate, 141, 885, 1293
venlafaxine, 809
ziprasidone, 842
Gastrostomy tube placement, in anorexia nervosa, 1110, 1138
GDS (Geriatric Depression Scale), **29**
Gender
acute stress disorder, posttraumatic stress disorder and, 1035, 1045
alcohol use and, 418
Alzheimer's disease and, 126, 153
bipolar disorder and, 871, 877, 880
borderline personality disorder and, 1224–1225, 1269, 1275
depression and, 794
eating disorders and, 1155–1156
HIV/AIDS and, 198, 225
panic disorder and, 986
schizophrenia and, 612–613, 627
sexually transmitted diseases and, 351
substance use disorders and, 353–354
suicidal behavior and, 1339–1341, **1341**, **1384**, 1385–1386, 1387
General Health Questionnaire, 1438
Generalized anxiety disorder (GAD)
panic disorder and, 983
substance use disorders and, 346
pharmacotherapy for, 338, 346
Genetic factors, 43. *See also* Family history
Alzheimer's disease and, 122, 126, 154
bipolar disorder and, 880
eating disorders and, 1167–1168
HIV infection and, 197
panic disorder and, 955
schizophrenia and, 627
suicide risk and, 1354–1355
Genitourinary disorders, anorexia nervosa and, **1123**
Geriatric Depression Scale (GDS), **29**
Geriatric patients. *See* Elderly persons
Gestalt therapy, for substance use disorders, 330
GHB (gamma-hydroxybutyrate), 334
Ginkgo biloba
for dementia, 102, 131, 137
for erectile dysfunction, **795**
for persons with HIV/AIDS, 246
Glaucoma, drug use in persons with
antidepressants, 783, 798, 966, 968
antipsychotics, 616
Global Accessibility Rating Scale (GARS), 78
Global Assessment of Functioning (GAF) Scale, **26**, 816, 817
Glucose dysregulation, drug-induced. *See also* Diabetes mellitus
antipsychotics, 102, **592**, 655
antiretroviral agents, 203
assessment for, **586**
clozapine, 638, 655, 843
olanzapine, 643, 655, 843, 890
quetiapine, 644
risperidone, 640

Glycine, for persons with schizophrenia, 602, 661
Goals of treatment, 37
Gonorrhea, 200
Granisetron, for orgasmic dysfunction, **796**
Granulocyte colony stimulating factor, for agranulocytosis, 638
Grasp reflex, 119
Grief, traumatic, **1047**
Grimacing, in catatonia, 789
Group residences, for persons with schizophrenia, 620
Group therapy
for AIDS-related bereavement, 227
for bipolar disorder, 861, 869
for borderline personality disorder, 1243, 1255, 1285–1286
for bulimia nervosa, 1176
for depression, 751, 819–820
in HIV-infected persons, 255, 256
for panic disorder, 962, 964
for posttraumatic stress disorder, 1059–1061
for schizophrenia, 671
for substance use disorders, 298, 315, 330
in adolescents, 355
for suicidal behavior, 1327
for traumatized persons, 1014
GROW, 674
Growth hormone, for HIV-associated wasting, 196, 244
Guanethidine, interaction with antidepressants, 798
Guardianship, 91
Guideline watches, ix
for bipolar disorder, 841–846
for borderline personality disorder, 1223–1226
for delirium, 61–62
for dementia, 101–102
for depression, 747–753
for HIV/AIDS, 169–178
for panic disorder, 933–940
Guilt, among survivors after a suicide, 1382

H

Hair loss
anorexia nervosa and, **1124**
drug-induced
lithium, 662, 882
valproate, 885
Halfway houses
for schizophrenia, 620
for substance use disorders, 314
Hallucinations, 22
during alcohol withdrawal, 301
benzodiazepine-induced, 87
in bipolar disorder, 869
in borderline personality disorder, 1244
command, suicide and, 1349–1350, 1412–1413
in delirium, 73, 74
in dementia, 116, 122, 148
in Lewy body disease, 119
in schizophrenia, 623, 625
Hallucinogen abuse
aggressive behavior and, 335
delirium and, 76
Haloperidol, **589**
administration routes for, 72, 90
for alcohol withdrawal, 381
for anorexia nervosa, 1144, 1174
for borderline personality disorder, **1258, 1260, 1262,** 1295, 1296
combined with clonidine, 662
continuous infusion of, 86, 90
for delirium, 62, 72, 84, 85, 90
combined with lorazepam, 86, 87, 91
in HIV/AIDS, 254
dosage of, 72, 85, 87, 90, 140, **589,** 633, 634
for elderly patients, 85, 93
for emergency treatment of acute psychosis, 589, 590
hepatic metabolism of, 92
interaction with nicotine, 340
intramuscular, for aggressive behavior, 609
intravenous, 85, 90
for mania, 842
for persons with dementia, 139, 146
in pregnancy, 872
for schizophrenia, **589,** 609, 633, 634
combined with clonazepam, 660
vs. olanzapine, 641–642
vs. risperidone, 639–640
side effects of, 85, 90, 138, 241, **592**
QTc interval prolongation, 85, 653
tardive dyskinesia, 650–651
for sleep disturbances, 146
for suicidal persons, 1446, 1447
use in hepatic disease, 92

Haloperidol decanoate
dosage of, 634
for dual-diagnosis patients, 340
for schizophrenia, 592
Hamilton Anxiety Rating Scale (HARS), **29**, 968
Hamilton Depression Rating Scale (Ham-D), **28**, 255, 258, 816, 817, 893, 894, 1289, 1438
Handbook of Psychiatric Measures, 25, 580
HARS (Hamilton Anxiety Rating Scale), **29**, 968
Harvard Trauma Questionnaire, 1050
Head trauma
dementia and, 120
due to falls, 123
seizures and, 75
suicide risk and, 1354
Headache
drug-induced
antidepressants, **795**
buprenorphine, 460
bupropion, 369, 429, 809
buspirone, 142
lamotrigine, 893
monoamine oxidase inhibitors, 810
ondansetron, 441
selective serotonin reuptake inhibitors, 808, 966
topiramate, 1180
electroconvulsive therapy–induced, 664
Health care proxy, 40
Health care workers
HIV exposure of
postexposure prophylaxis for, 234
universal precautions for prevention of, 350
misuse of prescription medications by, 307
multidisciplinary teams, 34–35
stresses associated with treatment of HIV-infected persons, 230
Health insurance benefits, 39
Health Insurance Portability and Accountability Act (HIPAA), 39, 359, 584
Hearing-impaired persons, 24, 41
Hematological effects
of anorexia nervosa, **1123**
of drugs
alcohol, **351**
antipsychotics, 85, 114, 139, 632
antiretroviral agents, 221
carbamazepine, 141, 243, 887, 1293
chlorpromazine, 632
clozapine, 114, 139, 221, 242, 340, 612, 635, 636–638, 1263
mirtazapine, **796**, 809
treatment of, 638
valproate, 141, 142, 885, 886, 1294
Hemodialysis
for lithium intoxication, 883
suicide risk and, 1354, 1424
Hemoglobin A1c, **33**
Hepatic dysfunction
delirium and, 92
dementia and, 120
drug use in patients with
benzodiazepines, 87, 92, 381
carbamazepine, 871
haloperidol, 92
quetiapine, 644
selective serotonin reuptake inhibitors, 966
valproate, 871, 885
ziprasidone, 646
drug-induced
alcohol, 790
antipsychotics, 85, 631
atomoxetine, 750
benzodiazepines, 87
buprenorphine, 404, 459–460
carbamazepine, 887, 1293
disulfiram, 383, 439
naltrexone, 246, 382, 404, 437–438, 461–462
nefazodone, 342, 747–748, 933–934
olanzapine, 845, 890
tacrine, 87–88, 102, 112, 132–133
valproate, 141, 142, 175, 243, 885, 886, 1293, 1294
Hepatic encephalopathy, 87
Hepatitis
clozapine-induced, 637
schizophrenia and, 625
Hepatitis C virus infection
cognitive impairment in, 175–176
HIV/AIDS and, 175–177, 237–238
managing psychiatric consequences of treatment for, 176–177
interferon-induced depression, 176–177, 351–352
psychiatric comorbidity with, 175, **176**
substance use disorders and, 351
suicide risk and, 1353
Herbal remedies
for dementia, 102, 131, 137
for persons with HIV/AIDS, 229, 246
for smoking cessation, 430

Heroin. *See* Opioid use disorders
5-HIAA (5-hydroxyindoleacetic acid), 253, 1439
Hip fracture, 93, 123, 140
Hip surgery, 74, 75
HIPAA (Health Insurance Portability and Accountability Act), 39, 359, 584
History of present illness, 12, **13**, 16
History taking, 12–20
  confidentiality and, 7, 8
Histrionic personality disorder
  anorexia nervosa and, 1153
  HIV/AIDS and, 228
HIV antibody testing, 194, 212–213, 231
  legal issues related to, 247
  in pregnancy, 194, 213, 233
HIV Cost and Services Utilization Study, 236
HIV Dementia Scale, 173, 174, **219**
HIV disease. *See* Human immunodeficiency virus/acquired immunodeficiency syndrome
HIV encephalopathy, 208, 210
HIV/AIDS Mental Health Services Demonstration Program, 211, 226
Homatropine eyedrops, 87
Home care
  for dementia, 121, 150–151
  for schizophrenia, 578
Home test kits for HIV, 231
Homeless Emergency Liaison Project (Project HELP), 611
Homeless persons
  psychiatric evaluation of, 41
  schizophrenia among, 610–611
  substance use disorders among, 319
Homicidal behavior
  bipolar disorder and, 870
  homicide-suicide, 1440–1441
  substance use disorders and, 335–336
Homosexuality
  HIV/AIDS and, 225
  substance use disorders and, 357
  suicide and, 1341–1342, 1390–1391
Hopelessness
  Beck Hopelessness Scale, 1410, 1438
  suicidality and, 1329, 1349, 1410–411
Hopkins Symptom Checklist–25, 1050
Hormone replacement therapy (HRT)
  for Alzheimer's disease, 126, 131, 136, 154
  for anorexia nervosa, 1113, 1145, 1174–1175
Hospice care, for patients with dementia, 149
Hospitalization. *See also* Inpatient treatment settings; Partial hospitalization
  for acute stress disorder or posttraumatic stress disorder, 1022
  advance directives and, 40
  for borderline personality disorder, 1245
  constraints on services during, 40
  delirium during, 74–75
  for dementia, 121, 152–153
  for depression, 780
  for eating disorders, 1107–1108, 1129–1134, **1131–1133**, 1169, 1170–1171
  for panic disorder, 976
  of patients at risk for suicide, 779
  of persons with HIV/AIDS, 248
  psychiatric evaluation of adults during, 10, 11
  for schizophrenia, 578, 616–618
  for substance use disorders, 299, 311–312
    alcohol dependence, 378, 434–435
    nicotine dependence, 300
    opioid withdrawal, 400
  for suicidal behavior, 1364–1366, **1365**
  treatment of smokers on smoke-free wards during, 371–373
  voluntary vs. involuntary, 40
Housing options, for persons with schizophrenia, 578, 620–621
HPA (hypothalamic-pituitary-adrenal) axis hyperactivity, suicide and, 1439, 1454
HRT (hormone replacement therapy)
  for Alzheimer's disease, 126, 131, 136, 154
  for anorexia nervosa, 1113, 1145, 1174–1175
Human immunodeficiency virus/acquired immunodeficiency syndrome (HIV/AIDS), 169–264
  access to care for, 236–237
  age at diagnosis of, 226
  antiretroviral therapy for, 170–172, 202–203
    adherence to, 171, 175, 203, 217, 248–249, **250**
    combination, 170, 238
    cost of, 203
    directly observed, 171
    drug interactions with, 171–172, **172**, 238, **239**
    drugs for, 170, 202, **204**
    goal of, 202
    for HIV-associated dementia, 250–252
    lack of response to, 203
    metabolic syndrome and lipodystrophy due to, 177–178
    for pediatric patients, 196, 259
    penetration of blood-brain barrier, 172, 251

Human immunodeficiency virus/acquired immunodeficiency syndrome (HIV/AIDS) *(continued)*
antiretroviral therapy for *(continued)*
for postexposure prophylaxis, 194, 213–214, 234
recommended regimens for, 170–171
to reduce perinatal HIV transmission, 170, 233–234
resistance to, 170, 171, 203
side effects of, 171, 172, 177–178, 203, 208, **209**
timing of, 170
viral replication cycle targets for, 201, **202**
for women, 225
assessment and staging of, 202
AIDS-defining conditions, 202, **203**
case definition, 202, **202**
central nervous system effects of, 204–205, **208**
in children, 210
clinical features affecting treatment of, 226–229
bereavement, 227
personality disorders, 228
psychoneuroimmunology, 228–229
suicidality, 226–227
comorbidity with, 195–196, 210–211, 219–223
schizophrenia, 625
substance use disorders, 195, 220–221, 234–235, 245–246, 256–257, 350–352, **351,** 416
suicidal behavior, 226–227, 1354, 1424, 1426
course of, **200,** 200–201
development of practice guideline for, 192
epidemiology of, 169–170, 197–198, **198**
future research needs related to, 261
guideline watch for, 169–178
antiretroviral agents, 170–172
bipolar disorders and psychosis, 175
classification of neurocognitive impairment, 173–174
depression, 174–175
epidemiology, 169–170
hepatitis C, 175–177, **176**
HIV-associated cognitive-motor disorders, 172–173
metabolic syndrome and lipodystrophy, 177–178
hepatitis C virus coinfection and, 175–177, **176,** 237–238
immune response to, 197, 200–201
introduction to, 191
leal and ethical issues related to, 247–248
mortality from, 169–170, 198, **198**
neuropsychiatric syndromes in, 195–196, 205–210
adjustment disorders, 196, 222, 258
anxiety disorders, 195–196, 221, 257–258
in children, 222, 259
classification of neurocognitive impairment, 173–174
delirium, 74, 75, 84, 92, 195, **207,** 253–254
dementia, 75, 120, 172, 173–174, 195, 205, **206,** 250–253
depression, 174–175, 195, 254–256
differential diagnosis of, **207–210,** 208
evaluation of mental status alterations, **210**
HIV-associated cognitive-motor disorders, 172–173, 205, **206**
mania and psychosis, 175, 195, 206–207, 256, 258
medication-induced, 208, **209**
prevalence of, 210–211
pathogenesis of, **200,** 200–202, **201**
pathophysiology and virology of, 196–197
genetic mutations, 197
HIV replication cycle, **197**
HIV structure, **196**
HIV-2, 197
viral load, 201
in pediatric patients, 196, 208–210, 259
pharmacotherapy for persons with, 237–246
for alcohol dependence, 246
alternative/complementary agents, 229, 246
antidepressants, 240–241
antipsychotics, 241–242
anxiolytics and sedative-hypnotics, 244
for dementia, 250–252
drug interactions with antiretroviral agents, 238, **239**
for HIV-related wasting, 244–245
mood stabilizers, 175, 243–244
opiate analgesics, 245
for opioid dependence, 245–246
psychostimulants, 242
testosterone, 174, 245

psychiatric management of persons at high risk for, 194, 211–215, 230–235
assessment of risk behavior, 211–212, **212**, 230–231
counseling, 232, 248
HIV antibody testing, 194, 212–213, 231
patients with severe mental illness, 215, 235
patients with substance use disorders, 214–215, 232–233, 234–235
postexposure prophylaxis, 194, 213–214, 234
risk reduction strategies, 194, 213, **214**, 231–233
victims of sexual abuse or trauma, 215, 235
psychiatric management of persons with, 194–195, 215–223, 235–261
access to services, 236–237
adherence to antiretroviral therapy, 171, 203, 217, 248–249, **250**
for adjustment disorders, 196, 222, 258
for anxiety disorders, 195–196, 221, 257–258
for associated psychiatric disorders, 195–196, 216–217
collaboration and coordination of care, 216
for delirium, 195, 220, 253–254
for dementia/cognitive disorders, 195, **219**, 219–220, 250–253
for disorders of infancy, childhood, and adolescence, 222, 259
for HIV-associated syndromes with psychiatric implications, 222–223, 259–261
for mood disorders, 195, 220, 254–256, 876
pharmacological, 217–246
preparation for disability, death, and dying, 218
psychoeducation, 217
psychological and social/adaptive functioning, 217–218
psychosocial treatment, 246–247
for psychotic disorders, 196, 221–222, 258
risk reduction strategies, 217
role of religion/spirituality, 218
for sleep disorders, 195, 222, 258–259
sources of care/support for significant others/family, 218–219
for substance use disorders, 195, 220–221, 256–257
therapeutic alliance, 216
psychological complications of, 247
psychosocial treatment of, 246–247
resources for information about, **262–264**
seroconversion in, 200
sociodemographic factors and, 223–226
age, 226
economic factors, 226
gender, 198, 225
race/ethnicity, 223–225, **224**
sexual orientation, 225
urban vs. rural residence, 226
special treatment situations in, 229–230
alternative and complementary medicine, 229, 246
health care clinician issues, 230
institutional settings, 229–230
summary of treatment recommendations for, 193–196
testing for, **33**
transmission of, 170, 198–200
blood transfusion, 199
cofactors for, 200
counseling about, 248
injection drug use, 195, 199, 232–233
partner notification about, 248
perinatal exposure, 200, 233–234
sexual exposure, 198–199, **199**
universal precautions for protection against, 350
Huntington's disease
dementia in, 120
suicide risk and, 1354, 1424
use of electroconvulsive therapy in, 89
Hydergine. *See* Ergoloid mesylates
Hydrocephalus, 120
Hydrochlorothiazide, 882
Hydrocodone, 245
Hydromorphone, 399
5-Hydroxyindoleacetic acid (5-HIAA), 253, 1439
9-Hydroxyrisperidone, 640–641
Hydroxyzine, for insomnia during opioid withdrawal, 408
Hyperandrogenism, valproate-induced, 1294
Hypercalcemia, 120

Hypercatabolic conditions, delirium and, **81**, 88, 91
Hypereosinophilia, clozapine-induced, 637, 638
Hyperglycemia, drug-induced. *See also* Diabetes mellitus; Glucose dysregulation
  antipsychotics, 102, **592**, 655
  antiretroviral agents, 177
Hyperkinesia, risperidone-induced, 842
Hyperlipidemia, **586**
  drug-induced
    antipsychotics, 102, **592**, 656
    antiretroviral agents, 177–178, 203
    clozapine, 638, 656, 843
    olanzapine, 643, 656, 843
    quetiapine, 644
    risperidone, 640
  lipid-lowering medications for, 126
  vascular dementia and, 126
Hyperparathyroidism, lithium-induced, 882
Hyperprolactinemia
  antipsychotic-induced, **592**, 614, 615, 656
    aripiprazole, 647
    clozapine, 636
    olanzapine, 642, 890
    quetiapine, 644
    risperidone, 640, 656
    ziprasidone, 645
  assessment for, **586**
  long-term clinical consequences of, 656
  treatment of, 656
Hyperpyrexia, monoamine oxidase inhibitor–induced, 1291
Hyperreflexia
  delirium and, 74
  vascular dementia and, 119
Hypersalivation, cholinesterase inhibitor–induced, 87
Hypersensitivity reactions, to carbamazepine, 887
Hypertension, 1354
  antidepressants for persons with, 798–799
  delirium and, **81**
  drug-induced
    antidepressants, **795**
    cocaine, 301, 393
    in substance abusers, 319
    venlafaxine, 144, 145, 799, 809
  in neuroleptic malignant syndrome, 651
  vascular dementia and, 126
Hypertensive crisis, drug-induced
  monoamine oxidase inhibitors, **795**, 809–810, 973, 1291–1292
  selegiline, 135
Hyperthermia
  antipsychotic-induced, 654
  delirium and, **81**
  in neuroleptic malignant syndrome, 651
  in serotonin syndrome, 808
Hyperthyroidism, dementia and, 143
Hypnotherapy
  for acute stress disorder and posttraumatic stress disorder, 1014
  for smoking cessation, 333, 434
Hypoglycemia
  delirium and, 75, **81**
  dementia and, 120
Hypomania, 876
  diagnostic criteria for, **879**
  dysphoric, 878
  monoamine oxidase inhibitor–induced, 973
Hyponatremia
  drug-induced
    carbamazepine, 141, 887, 1293
    valproate, 142
  due to psychosis-induced polydipsia, 609, 625
Hypo-osmolality, carbamazepine-induced, 887
Hypotension, drug-induced
  antidepressants, **795**, 806, 968
  antipsychotics, 85, 114, 138, 592, **592**, 614, 631, 653
  aripiprazole, 647
  clonidine, 430
  clozapine, 636, 653
  in elderly persons, 112
  monoamine oxidase inhibitors, 144, 798, 810, 973, 1291
  nefazodone, 809
  nortriptyline, 429
  olanzapine, 642, 643, 890
  quetiapine, 644
  risperidone, 640, 641
  selegiline, 135
  in substance abusers, 319
  trazodone, 142, 144, 809
  ziprasidone, 645
Hypothalamic-pituitary-adrenal (HPA) axis hyperactivity, suicide and, 1439, 1454
Hypothyroidism
  dementia and, 120, 143
  lithium-induced, 882, 1293
Hypoxia, delirium induced by, **81**, 88

I

ICU (intensive care unit)
environment of, 83
psychosis in, 77
Illusions, 22
in borderline personality disorder, 1244
in delirium, 73, 74
Imagery, in HIV/AIDS, 229, 256
Imipramine
for acute stress disorder or posttraumatic stress disorder, 1031, 1065, 1967
for alcohol dependence, 384
for antipsychotic-induced retrograde ejaculation, 656
for bipolar depression, 896
blood levels of, 811
for borderline personality disorder, 1290, 1291
for bulimia nervosa, 1177
contraindicated in persons with dementia, 114, 143, 145
dosage of, **774**, 969
for dual-diagnosis patients, 342
for panic disorder, 967–969
cognitive behavior therapy and, 938–939, 964
maintenance treatment, 937
for persons with HIV/AIDS, 254, 255
for persons with schizophrenia, 658
side effects of, 144
Immigrants
schizophrenia among, 627
suicide among, 1387–1389
Immune function, anorexia nervosa and, **1123**
Impact of Event Scale, 1018, 1057, 1058, 1059
Implosion, for posttraumatic stress disorder, 1053
Impulsivity
in borderline personality disorder, 1272–1273
pharmacotherapy for, 1244, 1254, 1259–1261, **1260**, **1302**
suicidality and, 1329, 1350, 1413–1414
Incarcerated persons
administrative segregation of, 622–623
HIV/AIDS in, 229–230, 234
psychiatric evaluation of, 12, 41
schizophrenia among, 621–623
substance abuse treatment for, 315
therapeutic communities, 314
suicide among, 621
Incontinence, in Alzheimer's disease, 118
Incoordination, drug-induced
benzodiazepines, 87
lithium, 662, 882
sedative-hypnotic overdose, 322
Indinavir, **204**
cytochrome P450 enzyme inhibition by, **238**
for HIV postexposure prophylaxis, 234
interaction with venlafaxine, 241
Indomethacin, for Alzheimer's disease, 136
Infectious diseases
dementia and, 120
hepatitis C, 175–177, **176**
HIV/AIDS, 169–264
among injection drug users, 175–177, **176**
lamotrigine-induced, 893
opportunistic, in HIV/AIDS, 202, **203**, **208**
schizophrenia and, 615
Inflammatory mediators, for HIV-associated cognitive disorders, 252–253
Informed consent
assessing patient's capacity for, 9, 38
delirium and, 91
for electroconvulsive therapy, 664–665
HIV/AIDS and, 248
Injection drug use. *See also* Substance use disorders
HIV transmission via, 195, 199, 214–215, 234–235, 410, 416
strategies to reduce risk of, 195, 215, 232–233
medical disorders associated with, 350, **351**, 410
Inositol
for panic disorder, 975
for posttraumatic stress disorder, 1067
Inpatient treatment settings. *See also* Hospitalization
legal and administrative issues in, 40
prevalence of alcohol use disorders among patients in, 419
prevalence of HIV infection among patients in, 215
psychiatric evaluation of adults in, 10, 11
suicide risk assessment in, 1359
treatment of smokers on smoke-free wards in, 371–373
Insight, assessment of, 22
Insomnia. *See* Sleep disturbances

Integrated treatment, 34–35
of dual-diagnosis patients, 337–338, 345–347
of schizophrenia, 583
Intensive care unit (ICU)
environment of, 83
psychosis in, 77
Intensive outpatient programs, for substance use disorders, 312
Interactive group therapy, for substance use disorders, 330
Interferon
for HIV-associated cognitive dysfunction, 253
side effects of, 176, **209**, 253
depression, 176–177, 351–352
International HIV Dementia Scale, 173
International Suicide Prevention Trial (InterSePT), 1448, 1449
Interpersonal and social rhythm therapy, for bipolar disorder, 903, 904
Interpersonal relationships, in borderline personality disorder, 1272–1273
Interpersonal therapy (IPT)
for borderline personality disorder, 1226
for depression, 777, 817–818
in bipolar disorder, 903, 904
double depression, 791
in elderly persons, 752, 753
for eating disorders
anorexia nervosa, 1111, 1140, 1171
binge eating disorder, 1179
bulimia nervosa, 1113, 1146, 1175–1176
for persons with HIV/AIDS, 174, 195, 255, 817–818
for substance use disorders, 298, 315, 325, 330
in adolescents, 355
alcohol dependence, 386, 443–444
in bipolar disorder, 345
cocaine dependence, 396, 450
in depression, 344
in group format, 330
opioid dependence, 409, 465
for suicidal behavior, 1327
Interpreter services, 24
Interviews
for adult psychiatric evaluation, 23–25
with agitated or aggressive persons, 24–25
research on approaches to, 42–43
structured, 25
use of interpreters in, 24
Intoxication. *See also* Overdose of drug; Substance use disorders
aggressive behavior during, 335
with alcohol, 300, 335
breath, blood, or urine testing for, 317
management of, 379
suicide and, 1350–1351, 1415
with cocaine, 301, 393–394
with lithium, 883
management of, 318
with multiple substances, 318, 334, 409–410
with opioids, 302, 318, 322, 400, 405
pharmacological treatment of, 322–323
Intracranial pressure elevation, electroconvulsive therapy–induced, 814
Intrusions, monitoring in traumatized persons, 1063
Inventory of Depressive Symptomatology, 894
IPT. *See* Interpersonal therapy
Irritability
in Alzheimer's disease, 118
drug-induced
selective serotonin reuptake inhibitors, 966
selegiline, 135
Irritable bowel syndrome, 984
Isocarboxazid, 805
for bulimia nervosa, 1177
Isoniazid, **209**

J

Jails. *See* Correctional settings
Jaundice, antipsychotic-induced, 631
Jejunostomy tube placement, in anorexia nervosa, 1110, 1138
Jitteriness, bupropion-induced, 369
Joint Commission on Accreditation of Healthcare Organizations, 402
Judgment
assessment of, 23
problems with, in schizophrenia, 623

K

Kaposi's sarcoma, **209**
Kava kava, 246
Ketamine, 334
Korsakoff syndrome, 390

L

LAAM, for opioid dependence, 401–403, 455
  in HIV-infected persons, 221, 245
  regulations governing administration of, 359, 402
Labetalol, for cocaine intoxication, 394
Laboratory testing, 9, 31–32, **33**
  for delirium, 78, **80**
  for dementia, 122
  of donated blood for HIV, 199
  to evaluate mental status changes in HIV/AIDS, **210**
  future research needs related to, 43–44
  HIV antibody testing, 194, 212–213, 231, 247
  for medical comorbidity in persons with substance use disorders, 319
  of persons with eating disorders, **1128**
  of schizophrenic patient, 572–573, 585, **586–587**
  toxicology screening, 9, **33**, 309, 317–318
β-Lactam antibiotics, **209**
Lamivudine, 170, **204**
  for HIV postexposure prophylaxis, 234
  side effects of, **209**
Lamivudine-zidovudine, **204**
Lamotrigine
  for antidepressant augmentation, 751
  for bipolar disorder
    depressive episodes, 844, 860, 867, 868, 893–894
    in dual-diagnosis patients, 344–345
    maintenance treatment, 844, 861, 900
    manic episodes, 889
    rapid cycling, 897
  in breast milk, 874
  dosage of, 844, 894
  drug interactions with
    carbamazepine, 888, 894
    valproate, 887, 894
  for persons with HIV/AIDS, 243
  for posttraumatic stress disorder, 1013, 1066
  side effects of, 844, 893
Language abnormalities
  in delirium, 73
  in dementia, 116, 118, 119
Language competence, assessment, 7
Language interpretation services, 24
Laryngospasm, antipsychotic-induced, 649
Laxatives, **795**, 807
Learning disabilities, substance use disorders and, 336–337, 355
  prenatal marijuana exposure, 392–393
Legal history, **15**, 19–20
Legal issues
  acute stress disorder, posttraumatic stress disorder and legal system involvement, 1019–1020
  advance directives, 40, 128, 218, 590
  in care of persons with HIV/AIDS, 247–248
  in institutions, 40
  malingering, 1019–1020
  related to adult psychiatric evaluation, 9–10, 38, 40
  related to dementia, 128
    driving privileges, 125
  related to substance use disorders, 358–359
    confidentiality, 358–359
    driving under the influence of alcohol or drugs, 315, 317, 416
    legally mandated treatment, 315, 358
    regulation of agonist maintenance therapies for opioid-dependent persons, 359, 401, 402
  related to treatment of eating disorders, 1108, 1130
  seclusion or restraint of patient, 25
    in nursing homes, 115, 151–152
  wills, 128
Lethargy
  lithium-induced, 882, 1293
  in serotonin syndrome, 808
Leukocytosis, lithium-induced, 662, 882
Leukopenia. *See also* Agranulocytosis
  drug-induced
    antipsychotics, 632, 638
    carbamazepine, 887, 1293
    valproate, 885, 1294
  lithium for, 638
Levetiracetam, for mania, 891
Levodopa
  for HIV-related cognitive disorders, 253
  mania induced by, 875
  for night eating syndrome, 1181
Levodopa/carbidopa, for cocaine dependence, 448
Lewy body disease, 93
  cholinesterase inhibitors for, 102
  dementia due to, 119
    clozapine for, 138, 139
  prevalence of, 117, 119

Lewy inclusion bodies, 119
Life skills training, to prevent substance use disorders in children and adolescents, 355
Light therapy
for bulimia nervosa, 1115, 1148
for depression with seasonal exacerbations, 792, 814–815, 823
side effects of, 815
for sleep disturbances in dementia, 146
Light-headedness, drug-induced
buspirone, 142
efavirenz, 172
Limit setting
for persons with borderline personality disorder, 1265
for persons with schizophrenia, 609
for persons with substance use disorders, 317
Lipid-lowering medications, 126
Lipodystrophy, antiretroviral agent–induced, 171, 177–178, 203
Lithium
for antidepressant augmentation, 751, 784, 812, 823
for antipsychotic augmentation, 661–662
for bipolar disorder
antipsychotics and, 842, 845, 866, 891
in children and adolescents, 874, 905
depressive episodes, 860, 867, 892
in dual-diagnosis patients, 344
alcohol dependence, 385, 389, 871
cocaine dependence, 397
maintenance treatment, 844, 845, 861, 898–899
manic or mixed episodes, 859, 866, 881–885
rapid cycling, 861, 897
for borderline personality disorder, 1243, 1244, 1257–1259, **1258, 1260,** 1292–1294
in breast milk, 873
dosage of, 662, 884
drug interactions with, 876
antipsychotics, 662
for elderly persons, 875
implementation of, 884–885
for leukopenia, 638
monitoring during treatment with, 884–885
overdose of, 883–884, 1293, 1327
for pathological gambling, 350
patient evaluation before initiation of, 884
for persons with HIV/AIDS, 243, 256
for persons with schizophrenia, 609, 661–662
in pregnancy, 872, 873
side effects of, 74, 662, 844, 882–883, 1293
for suicidal persons, 1326–1327, 1375, 1444–1446
use in bulimia nervosa, 1114, 1148, 1178
use in dementia, 114, 142
use in Parkinson's disease, 799
Living environment, of patients with substance use disorder, 358
Living will, 218
Lobeline, for smoking cessation, 430
Lofexidine, for opioid withdrawal, 462
Long-term care
for dementia, 115, 121, 151–152
regulations for use of restraints and psychotropic drugs during, 115, 151–152
for schizophrenia, 618
suicide risk assessment of persons in, 1360–1361
Loose associations, in schizophrenia, 623
Lopinavir, 170
Lopinavir-ritonavir, **204**
Lorazepam
for akathisia, 649
for alcohol withdrawal, 380, 381, 435–436
for catatonia, 258, 660, 789
for delirium, 62, 84, 86, 87, 90, 92
combined with haloperidol, 86, 87, 91
in HIV/AIDS, 254
dosage and administration of, 87, 141, 147, 972
for emergency treatment of acute psychosis, 589, 660
for extrapyramidal symptoms, **594**
for mania, 892
metabolism of, 92
for neuroleptic malignant syndrome, 652
for panic disorder, 970, 972
for persons with dementia, 141, 146, 147
for persons with HIV/AIDS, 244, 254, 258
for persons with schizophrenia, 589
in pregnancy, 873
for sleep disturbances, 146, 147
toxicity of, 62
use in hepatic disease, 92
Loxapine, **589**
for borderline personality disorder, **1262,** 1295

combined with clozapine for schizophrenia, 659
dosage of, **589**
LSD (lysergic acid diethylamide), 625
Lumbar puncture, **33**, **210**
Lyme serology, **33**
Lysergic acid diethylamide (LSD), 625

M

Magnesium sulfate, prophylaxis for alcohol withdrawal seizures, 381
Magnetic resonance imaging (MRI), **33**
in dementia, 101, 122
functional, **33**
in schizophrenia, 585
Malingering, 117, 1019–1020
Mania. *See also* Bipolar disorder
acute treatment of, 842–843, 859–860, 866–867, 881–892
antidepressant-precipitated, 866, 897, 935
with catatonia, 870
in children and adolescents, 874–875, 880
diagnostic criteria for, **877**
drug-induced, 875
in dual-diagnosis patients, 344
in elderly persons, 875, 880
electroconvulsive therapy for, 860, 867, 891
in children and adolescents, 906
in HIV/AIDS, 175, 195, 206–207, 220, 256
with psychosis, 869–870
psychotherapy for, 903
rating scales for, 889
Mannerisms, in catatonia, 789
MAOIs. *See* Monoamine oxidase inhibitors
Maprotiline
dosage of, 774
for panic disorder, 968
Marijuana Anonymous, 332
Marijuana use disorders, 391–393, 446–447
aggressive behavior and, 335
epidemiology of, 391, 419–420
medical disorders associated with, 350
outpatient treatment for, 299
in pregnancy, 392–393
prevalence of, 391
psychosocial interventions for, 301, 446–447
behavior therapies, 328, 447
cognitive behavior therapy, 446
relapse prevention, 446
schizophrenia and, 625
somatic treatments for, 391–392, 446
suicide and, **1343**
treatment settings for, 391
withdrawal syndromes, 392
in adolescents, 355
Marital status, suicide and, 1341, 1389–1390
Marital/couples therapy
for borderline personality disorder, 1243, 1255, 1286–1287
for bulimia nervosa, 1176
for depression, 819
for panic disorder, 964–965
for substance use disorders, 298, 315, 330, 331
alcohol dependence, 387, 445
for suicidal behavior, 1327
Massage therapy, in HIV/AIDS, 229
Maternal Health Practices and Child Development Project, 392
McCarthy Scales of Children's Abilities, 259
M-CET (multiple-channel exposure therapy), 1054
MCV Nursing Delirium Rating Scale (MCV-NDRS), 78
MDAS (Memorial Delirium Assessment Scale), 78
MDMA (3,4-methylenedioxymethamphetamine), 334
interaction with ritonavir, 240
Mecamylamine, for nicotine dependence, 323, 370, 430
Medical conditions. *See also specific medical conditions*
acute stress disorder or posttraumatic stress disorder and, 1020, 1036–1037
bipolar disorder and, 875–876
delirium and, 74–75, **76**, 92
dementia and, 120, 149
depression and, 797–799, 803
eating disorders and, 1106, 1121–1122, **1123–1125**, 1154–1155
mental retardation and, 42
panic disorder and, 953, 983–984
posttraumatic stress disorder and, 1027
psychiatric evaluation of adults with, 40–41
schizophrenia and, 582–583, 615–616, 625
substance use disorders and, 319, 350–352, **351**
alcohol dependence, 319, **351**, 389–390
cocaine dependence, **351**, 397

Medical conditions *(continued)*
substance use disorders and *(continued)*
nicotine dependence, 350, **351**, 360, 375–376, 417
opioid dependence, **351**, 410
suicide and, **1337**, 1353–1354, **1354**, 1424–1426
use of electroconvulsive therapy in, 89, 91
Medical history, **14**, 17–18
Medical records, 11, 39
release of patient information from, 584
after patient's death, 1325, 1381
of schizophrenia treatment, 583–584
Medical settings, psychiatric evaluation of adults in, 11
Meditation, in HIV/AIDS, 229
Medroxyprogesterone, for disinhibited sexual behavior, 114, 142
Megestrol acetate, for HIV-related wasting, 244
Melancholia, 800
Melatonin
for Alzheimer's disease, 131, 137
for persons with HIV/AIDS, 246
for sleep disturbances in dementia, 146
Memantine, for dementia, 102
HIV-associated, 253
Memorial Delirium Assessment Scale (MDAS), 78
Memory impairment
in amnestic disorders, 117
in delirium, 73
in dementia, 116, 119
in depression, 117
drug-induced
benzodiazepines, 86, 140, 970
lithium, 882
electroconvulsive therapy–induced, 89, 664, 814
in Parkinson's disease, 119
Menstrual irregularities
in anorexia nervosa, 1108–1109, **1125**, 1162
in bulimia nervosa, **1127**
in female athlete trial, 1158
Mental Alteration Test, **219**
Mental retardation, 117
psychiatric evaluation of adults with, 41–42
suicide and, **1343**
Mental status changes, in serotonin syndrome, 808
Mental status examination, **15–16**, 21–23
Mentally Ill Chemical/Substance Abusers, 387
Meperidine
delirium induced by, 76, 87, 88, 93
drug interactions with
monoamine oxidase inhibitors, 144, 973
selegiline, 135
Mesoridazine, **589**
dosage of, **589**
side effects of, 631
QTc interval prolongation, 653
for sleep disturbances, 147
MET. *See* Motivational enhancement therapy
Metabolic syndrome, drug-induced
antipsychotics, 178
antiretroviral agents, 171, 177–178
Methadone, 451–455
drug interactions with, 402
interaction with antiretroviral agents, 171, 245–246, 351
limitations of, 326
maintenance therapy for opioid dependence, 302, 304, 323, 401–403, 451–454
antidepressant use during, 342–343
clinical trials of, 452–454
compared with buprenorphine, 403
dosage of, 402, 453
effectiveness of, 402
family therapy and, 331
in HIV-infected persons, 221, 245–246, 257
naturalistic/survey studies of, 451–452
number of persons receiving, 401
in pregnancy, 411
psychosocial treatments to enhance effectiveness of, 326
regulations governing administration of, 359, 401, 402
settings for, 401
supportive-expressive therapy and, 329–330, 408
withdrawal from, 405
for opioid withdrawal, 302, 323, 400, 405–406, 454–455
overdose of, 402–403
for pain, abuse of, 403
side effects of, 400, 455
Methadone Anonymous, 332
Methamphetamine abuse, 335, 393, 420
Methotrexate, **209**
N-Methyl-D-aspartate (NMDA) receptor agonists, for antipsychotic augmentation, 602

α-Methyldopa, interaction with antidepressants, 798
3,4-Methylenedioxymethamphetamine (MDMA), 334
interaction with ritonavir, 240
Methylphenidate
abuse of, 420
for attention-deficit/hyperactivity disorder
with comorbid bulimia nervosa, 1114, 1148
lack of association with substance use disorders in adulthood, 355
dosage of, 145
for erectile dysfunction, **795**
for persons with dementia, 143
for persons with HIV/AIDS, 242, 253, 255, 258, 260
replacement therapy for cocaine dependence, 395, 448
side effects of, 144
Metoclopramide, during refeeding in anorexia nervosa, 1112, 1144
Metoprolol, for persons with dementia, 142
Mexiletine, for HIV-associated neuropathy, 260–261
Mianserin, for borderline personality disorder, 1289, 1290
Midazolam, interaction with saquinavir, 238, 244
Mifepristone, for psychotic depression, 752
Migraine
panic disorder and, 984
selective serotonin reuptake inhibitor–induced, 808
Military history, **14**, 19
Millon Clinical Multiaxial Inventory–II, 1298
Mindfulness meditation, for panic disorder, 964
Mini-Mental State Exam (MMSE), **27**, 84, 101, 122, 174, 219
Miosis, opioid-induced, 322
Mirtazapine
dosage of, 774
efficacy of, 805
overdose of, 1442
for persons with HIV/AIDS, 174, 241
for posttraumatic stress disorder, 1064
in pregnancy, 872
side effects of, **795–796**, 809
use in anorexia nervosa, 1144
Mississippi PTSD Rating Scale, 1057
Misuse of substances, 303, 307–308, 324
prescription medications, 307
combining with "club drugs," 334
among elderly persons, 356
by health care workers, 307
opioid analgesics, 399
MMSE (Mini-Mental State Exam), **27**, 84, 101, 122, 174, 219
Moclobemide
for bipolar depression, 895
dosage of, **774**
for panic disorder, 973
for posttraumatic stress disorder, 1066
for smoking cessation, 430
Modafinil
for antipsychotic-induced sedation, 652
for cocaine dependence, 302, 395, 448
interaction with clozapine, 652
for patients with depression, 752
for persons with HIV/AIDS, 174
Molindone, **589**
combined with tyrosine, 662
dosage of, **589**
for persons with HIV/AIDS, 242, 254
Monoamine oxidase inhibitors (MAOIs). *See also specific drugs*
for acute stress disorder, 1031
for borderline personality disorder, 1243, 1244, 1257, **1258, 1260**, 1261, **1262**, 1291–1292
combined with tricyclic antidepressants, 812
for depression, 813
with anxiety symptoms, 790
with atypical features, 772–773, 783, 789, 790, 805
in bipolar disorder, 868, 894–895
dietary tyramine interactions with, 114, 144, 810, 973, 1291
dosage of, 145, **774**, 973
drug interactions with, 144, 973
bronchodilators, 797
diuretics, 798–799
St. John's wort, 815
selective serotonin reuptake inhibitors, 808
tricyclic antidepressants, 807
efficacy of, 805
overdose of, 1442
for panic disorder, 934, 937, 952, 973–974, 979
for posttraumatic stress disorder, 1013, 1031, 1065–1066

Monoamine oxidase inhibitors (MAOIs) *(continued)*
side effects of, 144, **795–796**, 809–810, 973, 1291–1292
for smoking cessation, 370, 430
for suicidal behavior, 1374
switching from other antidepressants to, 784, **784**, 808, 810, 812, 1257
use in persons with eating disorders, 1112, 1114, 1147–1148, 1177
use in persons with medical conditions
asthma, 797
cardiac disease, 798
dementia, 114, 145
obstructive uropathy, 799
Parkinson's disease, 799
use in persons with substance use disorders, 790
alcohol dependence, 388–389
opioid dependence, 410
Montgomery-Åsberg Depression Rating Scale, 893
Mood, assessment of, 21
Mood Disorder Questionnaire, 841, 863
Mood disorders. *See also* Bipolar disorder; Depression; Mania
hepatitis C and, **176**
HIV/AIDS and, 195, 220, 240, 243–244, 254–256
rating scales for, **28–29**
suicide and, 1342–1344, 1391–1394
Mood stabilizers. *See also specific drugs*
for bipolar disorder
acute treatment, 843–844, 859–860, 866–867, 881–894
antipsychotics and, 842, 845, 859–861, 866, 891
maintenance treatment, 844–845, 861, 868–869
for borderline personality disorder, 1243, 1244, 1257–1259, **1258, 1260,** 1261, 1292–1294
for persons with bulimia nervosa, 1114, 1148
for persons with HIV/AIDS, 175, 195, 220, 243–244, 256
for persons with schizophrenia, 573, 576, 593, 601, 609
in pregnancy and lactation, 613, 871–873
for suicidal persons, 1326–1327, 1375, 1444–1446
use in dual-diagnosis patients, 344–345
alcohol dependence, 389
Morphine, 245, 399
for delirium, 72, 88, 91
Mortality
AIDS-related, 169–170, 198, **198**
delirium and, 75
eating disorders and, 1165–1166
schizophrenia and, 626
from suicide (*See* Suicidal behavior)
Motivation to change
assessment of, 22
in management of substance use disorders, 316
smoking cessation, 363
Motivational enhancement therapy (MET), for substance use disorders, 298, 304, 315, 316, 328
in adolescents, 355
alcohol dependence, 385, 443
in depression, 344
marijuana dependence, 392, 446, 447
nicotine dependence, 370, 432
in schizophrenia, 341
Motor activity, assessment of, 21
Motor disturbances
in delirium, 74
in dementia, 116, 118
induced by antipsychotic withdrawal, 85
in Parkinson's disease, 119
MRI. *See* Magnetic resonance imaging
MRI (magnetic resonance imaging), in schizophrenia, 585
Multidisciplinary team treatment, 34–35
of borderline personality disorder, 1248
of eating disorders, 1105, 1118–1119
of schizophrenia, 583
Multi-infarct dementia. *See* Vascular dementia
Multiple sclerosis, 120, 875, 1354, 1424
Multiple-channel exposure therapy (M-CET), 1054
Muscle abnormalities
alcohol-related, 389–390
anorexia nervosa and, **1123**
bulimia nervosa and, **1127**
Music therapy, 130
Mutism, in Alzheimer's disease, 118
Mutual help groups. *See* Self-help groups
Myocarditis, clozapine-induced, 635, 637
Myoclonus
antidepressant-induced, **795**, 807, 810, 973
delirium and, 74

dementia and, 116, 118
in serotonin syndrome, 808

N

Nadolol, for persons with schizophrenia, 609, 661
Naloxone
administration routes for, 322
for borderline personality disorder, 1295
combined with buprenorphine, 403
dosage of, 322
for HIV-associated cognitive dysfunction, 253
for opioid overdose, 302, 322
Naltrexone
for alcohol dependence, 301, 324, 378, 382, 436–438
acamprosate and, 384
in dual-diagnosis patients, 339
borderline personality disorder, 1264
efficacy of, 436–437
goals of, 436
implementation of, 438
in persons with HIV/AIDS, 246
for binge eating disorder, 1181
for borderline personality disorder, 1261, 1295
for bulimia nervosa, 349, 1178
hepatotoxicity of, 246, 382
interaction with nonsteroidal anti-inflammatory drugs, 382
for maintenance treatment of opioid dependence, 302, 404, 460–462
efficacy of, 460–461
psychotherapy to enhance effectiveness of, 325–326
for nicotine dependence, 370, 430
for pathological gambling, 350
for psychosis-induced polydipsia, 610
side effects of, 404, 437–438, 461–462
NAMI (National Alliance for the Mentally Ill), 588, 597, 675–676, 869, **908**
Nar-Anon, 332
Narcissistic personality disorder
bulimia nervosa and, 1153
depression and, 792
Narcotics Anonymous, 332, 401, 409, 450, 606
Nasal irritation/bleeding, cocaine-induced, 397
Nasogastric feeding, in anorexia nervosa, 1110, 1138
National Alliance for Research on Schizophrenia and Affective Disorders, 675
National Alliance for the Mentally Ill (NAMI), 588, 597, 675–676, 869, **908**
National Comorbidity Survey, 336, 337, 1045, 1048, 1051, 1433
National Comorbidity Survey Replication, 416
National Depressive and Manic-Depressive Association, 674, 869, **908**
National Epidemiologic Survey on Alcohol and Related Conditions, 349, 377, 418, 419
National Foundation for Depressive Illness, **908**
National Household Survey on Drug Abuse, 2001, 419
National Institute of Drug Abuse Collaborative Cocaine Treatment Study, 396, 397, 450
National Institute of Mental Health (NIMH)
Collaborative Longitudinal Personality Disorders Study, 1224, 1226
Collaborative Program on the Psychobiology of Depression, 1394, 1423
Depression Information Program, **908**
Treatment of Depression Collaborative Research Program, 816, 817, 820
National Institute on Aging, 121–122, 148
National Longitudinal Mortality Study, 1386, 1389, 1429
National Mental Health Association, **908**
National Suicide Prevention Project (Finland), 1389
National Survey on Drug Use and Health, 2003, 393, 399, 419, 420
National Survey on Drug Use and Health, 2004, 418
Nausea and vomiting
drug-induced
antidepressants, 795
antipsychotics, 592
antiretroviral agents, 203
aripiprazole, 842
buprenorphine, 460
bupropion, 429
buspirone, 142
carbamazepine, 843, 887, 1293
cholinesterase inhibitors, 87, 112, 132
duloxetine, 749
ergoloid mesylates, 136
lamotrigine, 893
lithium, 882, 1293
naltrexone, 437
nefazodone, 809

Nausea and vomiting *(continued)*
drug-induced *(continued)*
risperidone, 842
selective serotonin reuptake inhibitors, 144, 807, 966
valproate, 845, 885, 1293
venlafaxine, 809
ziprasidone, 842
electroconvulsive therapy–induced, 664
NEECHAM Confusion Scale, 78
Needle exchange programs, 195, 215, 232–233, 351
Nefazodone
dosage of, 774
drug interactions with, 809
clozapine, 658
protease inhibitors, 241
for dual-diagnosis patients, 342
efficacy of, 805
overdose of, 1442
for panic disorder, 974
for persons with HIV/AIDS, 241, 255
for posttraumatic stress disorder, 1064
in pregnancy, 872
side effects of, 144, **795**, 809
hepatotoxicity, 342, 747–748, 933–934
Neglect of elderly persons, 124, 127
Nelfinavir, **204**
cytochrome P450 enzyme inhibition by, **238**
drug interactions with, **239**, 246
for HIV postexposure prophylaxis, 234
Neostigmine, for erectile dysfunction, **795**, 808
Nervousness, valproate-induced, 845
Neural tube defects, 872, 873
Neurofibrillary tangles, 118
Neuroimaging, **33**, 43, 44
in borderline personality disorder, 1225
in delirium, 78
in dementia, 122
Alzheimer's disease, 101
Pick's disease, 120
Neuroleptic malignant syndrome, 85, 114, 139, 631, 651–652
clinical features of, 651
differential diagnosis of, 652
electroconvulsive therapy for delirium in, 89, 91
lithium and, 662
mortality from, 652
in persons with HIV/AIDS, 242
prevalence of, 651
risk factors for, 652
second-generation antipsychotics and, 651
clozapine, 636
olanzapine, 642
quetiapine, 644
risperidone, 640
ziprasidone, 645
treatment of, 652
Neuroleptics. *See* Antipsychotics
Neurological disorders
anorexia nervosa and, **1123**
bipolar disorder and, 875
bulimia nervosa and, **1126**
delirium and, 74, **76**
dementia and, 118, 119, 120
HIV/AIDS and, 204–205
substance use disorders and, **351**
alcohol dependence, 390
use of electroconvulsive therapy in patients with, 89
Neuropathology
of Alzheimer's disease, 118
of Lewy body disease, 119
of Pick's disease, 120
Neuropsychological testing, 32–33, **33**
in HIV/AIDS, **210**
Neurosyphilis, 120
Neurovestibular symptom complex, efavirenz-induced, 172
Neutropenia, clozapine contraindicated in, 616
Nevirapine, 170, **204**
drug interactions with, 238, 246
for HIV-associated dementia, 252
Niacin deficiency, 120
Nicotinamide, 88
Nicotine
interaction with antipsychotics, 340
withdrawal from, 365–366, 414
Nicotine Anonymous, 332, 431
Nicotine dependence, 300, 359–377, 420–434. *See also* Smoking cessation
among adolescents, 417
approach to treatment of, 362–368
abrupt vs. gradual smoking cessation, 364, 434
detecting exacerbations of psychiatric symptoms, 366
education and adherence to treatment, 366–367
identifying withdrawal symptoms, 365–366

initial treatment strategies, 365
monitoring clinical status, 365–366
overcoming barriers to smoking cessation, 363–364
patient treatment preferences, 364
for patients who do not respond to initial treatment, 367–368
readiness and motivation for smoking cessation, 363
setting quit date, 364–365
therapeutic alliance, 362–363
timing of smoking cessation, 364
assessment for, **360**, 360–362
clinical features influencing treatment for, 373–377, 374
psychiatric comorbidity, 374–375
use of multiple substances, 333, 373–374
components of treatment for, 360
DSM-IV-TR criteria for, 412
epidemiology of, 417–418
factors affecting strength of, 417
medical comorbidity with, 350, **351**, 360, 375–376
natural history and course of, 414
outpatient treatment for, 299
in pregnancy, 352, 376–377
psychiatric comorbidity with, 335, 337, 374–375, 418
anxiety disorders, 345, 375
attention-deficit/hyperactivity disorder, 347, 375
bipolar disorder, 345, 375
depression, 343, 375
eating disorders, 348
pathological gambling, 349–350
schizophrenia, 339, 374–375, 625
smoking cessation and exacerbation of, 366
treatment effects of, 374–375
psychosocial interventions for, 300, 370–371, 431–434
behavior therapies, 370, 432–433
brief therapies, 370, 432
cognitive behavior therapy, 370–371, 433
in dual-diagnosis patients, 374
efficacy of, 431
exercise, 371, 433–434
goals of, 431
hypnotherapy, 333, 434
implementation of, 431–432
other therapies, 371, 434–434
physiological feedback, 371, 434
self-guided therapies, 371, 433
side effects of, 431
social support, 370, 432
stimulus control techniques, 371, 434
race/ethnicity and, 357
rates of tobacco use and risk of, **415**, 416
screening for medical comorbidity with, 319
in smokeless tobacco users, 361
somatic treatments for, 300, 368–370, 420–431
acupuncture, 300, 368, 369, 430
bupropion, 300, 324, 369, 427–429
clonidine, 300, 369–370, 429–430
nicotine replacement therapies, 300, 368–369, 421–426
nortriptyline, 300, 369, 429
other agents, 370, 430–431
telephone quitlines for, 321
treatment of smokers on smoke-free wards, 371–373
monitoring of symptoms, 372
patient education, 372
system issues, 372
for withdrawal symptoms, 372–373
treatment settings for, 362
among women, 353
Nicotine replacement therapies (NRTs), 300, 304, 323, 368–369, 421–426
for adolescents, 355
behavioral therapies to enhance effectiveness of, 326
for dual-diagnosis patients, 374
depression, 343
schizophrenia, 341, 374
duration of use of, 426
efficacy of, 369, 422–425
for elderly persons, 356
goals of, 421
implementation of, 426
lack of response to, 367
nicotine gum, 368–369, 421, 424, 425–426
nicotine lozenges, 368–369, 422, 424, 426
nicotine nasal spray, 369, 422, 424–425, 426
nicotine transdermal patch, 368, 421, 422–424, 425
nicotine vapor inhalers, 369, 422, 425, 426
for patients with medical conditions, 376
in pregnancy, 376
side effects of, 300, 425–426
for smokers on smoke-free wards, 373
for women, 353

Nifedipine, 810
Night eating syndrome, 1116, 1151, 1181
NIMH. *See* National Institute of Mental Health
Nimodipine
for HIV-associated cognitive dysfunction, 253
for rapid-cycling bipolar disorder, 892
"No-harm contracts" for suicide prevention, 1325, 1379–1380, 1455–1456
Nonnucleoside reverse transcriptase inhibitors, 170, 202, **204**, 238
Nonsteroidal anti-inflammatory drugs (NSAIDs)
Alzheimer's disease and, 126, 131, 132, 136, 154
drug interactions with
lithium, 876
naltrexone, 382
Norepinephrine, interaction with tricyclic antidepressants, 807
Nortriptyline
blood levels of, 811
for depression, 772, 783
in elderly persons, 752
dosage of, 145, **774**
overdose of, 369, 429
for persons with dementia, 145, 798
in pregnancy, 796
side effects of, 144, 429
for smoking cessation, 300, 369, 429
in depression, 343, 375
NRTs. *See* Nicotine replacement therapies
NSAIDs. *See* Nonsteroidal anti-inflammatory drugs
Nucleoside analogue reverse transcriptase inhibitors, 202, **204**
Nucleotide analogues, 202, **204**
Nursing homes
for patients with dementia, 115, 151–152
for patients with schizophrenia, 620
use of antipsychotics in, 115
use of restraints in, 115, 151–152
Nutritional deficiencies
anorexia nervosa and, 1112, 1113, 1145
delirium and, 72, 88, 91
dementia and, 120
HIV/AIDS and, 253
Nutritional rehabilitation/counseling
for anorexia nervosa, 1108–1110, 1134–1138, 1169
for binge eating disorder, 1115, 1149, 1179
for bulimia nervosa, 1113, 1145
Nystagmus, 74

O

OAS-M (Overt Aggression Scale—Modified), **30**
Obesity, antipsychotics and, 575, 616
OBRA (Omnibus Budget Reconciliation Act of 1987), 151
OBS (Organic Brain Syndrome Scale), 78
Observations, 34–35
Obsessive-compulsive disorder (OCD)
depression and, 791
eating disorders and, 1153, 1164
HIV/AIDS and, 257
panic disorder and, 983
schizophrenia and, 594, 601, 625
substance use disorders and, 346
suicide and, **1343**
Obsessive-compulsive personality disorder
depression and, 792
eating disorders and, 1153, 1164
panic disorder and, 983
Obstetric complications, schizophrenia and, 627
Obstructive uropathy, antidepressants for persons with, 799
Occupation
employee assistance programs and, 315–316
history of, **14**, 19
postexposure prophylaxis for HIV exposure related to, 213–214, 234
substance use disorders and, 307–308
suicide risk and, 1342, 1355, 1391
OCD. *See* Obsessive-compulsive disorder
Oculogyric crisis, antipsychotic-induced, 649
Office of National Drug Control Policy, 399, 420
Olanzapine, 138, 588, **589**, 641–643
for anorexia nervosa, 1112, 1144, 1174
for bipolar disorder
in children and adolescents, 906
depressive episodes, 843, 896
in dual-diagnosis patients, 344
maintenance treatment, 845
manic or mixed episodes, 842, 859, 866, 867, 889–890
mood stabilizers and, 842, 845, 891
for borderline personality disorder, 1226, **1262**, 1297
for delirium, 62, 72, 84, 90
for dementia, 139
dosage of, **589**, 642, 643, 890
drug interactions with, 643
nicotine, 340

efficacy of, 641–642
for emergency treatment of acute psychosis, 589
implementing treatment with, 642–643, 890
for persons with HIV/AIDS, 242
for posttraumatic stress disorder, 1031, 1066
in pregnancy, 873
receptor affinity of, 641
for schizophrenia, 641–643
in dual-diagnosis patients, 340
cocaine dependence, 449
neurocognitive deficits, 642
positive and negative symptoms, 641
to reduce suicide risk, 1448, 1449
treatment-resistant, 642
side effects of, 138–139, **592**, 642, 842, 843, 845, 890
priapism, 657
sedation, 652
tardive dyskinesia, 651
Olanzapine-fluoxetine combination, 750
for bipolar depression, 750, 843
Omega-3 fatty acids
for antidepressant augmentation, 751
for mania, 891
Omnibus Budget Reconciliation Act of 1987 (OBRA), 151
Ondansetron
for alcohol dependence, 385, 440–442
for bulimia nervosa, 1149, 1178
side effects of, 441
Online continuing medical education programs, xii
OPC-14117, for HIV-related cognitive disorders, 253
Ophthalmological effects of antipsychotics, 631–632, 644
assessment for, **587**
Opioid analgesics
for delirium with pain, 72, 88, 91
interaction with monoamine oxidase inhibitors, 144
nonmedical use of, 399
for persons with HIV/AIDS, 245
use in elderly persons, 356
Opioid antagonists. *See also* Naloxone; Naltrexone
for borderline personality disorder, 1294–1295
Opioid use disorders, 302–304, 399–411, 451–465
agonist maintenance therapies for, 302, 323, 326
buprenorphine, 302, 323
methadone, 302, 323
regulations governing administration of, 359, 401, 402
clinical features influencing treatment of, 409–411
medical comorbidity, **351**, 410
pregnancy, 352, 411
psychiatric comorbidity, 410
use of multiple substances, 318, 409–410
epidemiology of, 399, 420
goals of treatment for, 399–400
intoxication and overdose, 302, 318, 322, 400, 405
clinical features of, 322
management of, 405
with multiple substances, 318, 409–410
naloxone for, 302, 322
limited availability of treatment programs for, 399
medical comorbidity with, **351**, 410
HIV/AIDS, 245–246, 256–257, 350–352
laboratory testing for, 319
needle exchange programs for persons with, 195, 215, 232–233, 351
in pregnancy, 352, 411
psychosocial interventions for, 302, 325–326, 408–409, 463–465
behavior therapies, 408–409, 463–465
cognitive behavior therapy, 408, 463
contingency management, 328, 408–409, 463–465
family therapy, 409
interpersonal therapy, 409, 465
psychodynamic psychotherapy, 409, 465
relapse prevention, 408, 463
self-help groups and 12-step programs, 332, 401, 409
psychotropic drug use in persons with, 410
antidepressants, 342–343
somatic treatments for, 401–408, 451–463
for dependence and abuse, 401–404
buprenorphine, 302, 304, 323, 403–404, 455–460
LAAM, 401–403, 455
methadone, 302, 304, 323, 401–403, 451–455
naltrexone, 302, 323, 325–326, 404, 460–462

Opioid use disorders *(continued)*
somatic treatments for *(continued)*
for dependence and abuse *(continued)*
in patients with co-occurring cocaine dependence, 395
in pregnancy, 411
for intoxication, 323, 405
for withdrawal, 405–408, 462–463
suicide and, **1343**
treatment settings for, 400–401
Opioid withdrawal, 405–408, 462–463
anesthesia-assisted rapid opioid detoxification for, 302
buprenorphine for, 302, 323, 400, 407, 458–459
clonidine for, 302, 323, 400, 406, 462–463
clonidine-naltrexone for, 302, 407
concurrent with use/withdrawal from other substances, 302
inpatient treatment for, 400
lofexidine for, 462
management of, 302, 323
methadone for, 302, 323, 400, 405–406, 454–455
in neonates, 411
opioid tapering for, 405
other medications for, 408
pharmacological strategies for, 405
in pregnancy, 411
rating scales for, 405
Opisthotonos, antipsychotic-induced, 649
Optimism, after traumatic exposure, 1025–1026
Oral contraceptive interactions
with anticonvulsants, 871, 888, 889
with St. John's wort, 750
Organic Brain Syndrome Scale (OBS), 78
Orthopedic surgery, 75, 88
Orthostatic hypotension, drug-induced
antidepressants, **795**, 806, 968
antipsychotics, 85, 114, 138, 592, **592**, 614, 631, 653
aripiprazole, 647
clonidine, 430
clozapine, 636, 653
in elderly persons, 112
monoamine oxidase inhibitors, 144, 798, 810, 973, 1291
nefazodone, 809
nortriptyline, 429
olanzapine, 642, 643, 890
quetiapine, 644
risperidone, 640, 641
selegiline, 135
trazodone, 142, 144, 809
ziprasidone, 645
Osteoarthritis, antipsychotics for persons with, 614, 615
Osteopenia/osteoporosis
anorexia nervosa and, 1113, **1125**, 1145, 1157, 1162, 1175
bulimia nervosa and, **1127**
valproate-induced, 885
Outpatient treatment settings
for acute stress disorder or posttraumatic stress disorder, 1022
advantages of, 11
for eating disorders, 1107, 1108, **1131–1133**
for panic disorder, 951, 976
psychiatric evaluation of adults in, 10–11
for substance use disorders, 299, 312, 314–315
alcohol dependence, 378
nicotine dependence, 362
opioid dependence, 400–401
for suicidal behavior, **1365**, 1366–1367
suicide risk assessment in, 1359
Overdose of drug. *See also* Intoxication
antipsychotics, 634–635
benzodiazepines, 322
buprenorphine, 404
bupropion, 1442
carbamazepine, 887–888, 1293
lithium, 883–884, 1293, 1327
methadone, 402–403
mirtazapine, 1442
monoamine oxidase inhibitors, 1442
nefazodone, 1442
opioids, 302
opioids intoxication and overdose, 302, 318, 322, 400, 405
sedative-hypnotics, 322–323
selective serotonin reuptake inhibitors, 966, 1442
trazodone, 1443
tricyclic antidepressants, 144, 345, 346, 369, 429, 811, 968, 1290, 1434, 1442
valproate, 885, 886
Overeaters Anonymous, 349, 1111, 1114, 1141, 1147, 1177
Overt Aggression Scale—Modified (OAS-M), **30**
Oxandrolone, for HIV-associated wasting, 244, 260

Oxazepam, 87, 92
for alcohol withdrawal, 380, 381, 435, 436
for catatonia, 660
dosage and administration of, 141, 147
for persons with dementia, 141, 146, 147
for persons with HIV/AIDS, 244
for sleep disturbances, 146, 147
use in opioid-dependent patients, 410
Oxcarbazepine
for bipolar disorder
maintenance treatment, 868
manic episodes, 859, 860, 867, 889
drug interactions with
calcium channel blockers, 871, 889
oral contraceptives, 871, 889
Oxycodone, 245, 399
Oxymetholone, for HIV-associated wasting, 260

P

PACT (Program for Assertive Community Treatment), 576, 597, 666–667
Pain syndromes, HIV-associated, 196, 222–223, 260–261
in children, 259
opiates for, 245
Pancreatitis, drug-induced
carbamazepine, 887, 1293
clozapine, 637
valproate, 886, 1294
Panic attacks, 954–955
other anxiety disorders and, 983
substance abuse and, 982
Panic disorder, 933–987
age at onset of, 955
with agoraphobia, 954–955
choice of treatment modalities for, 952, 977–979
cross-sectional issues in evaluation of, 954
depression and, 790
development of practice guideline for, 950
diagnostic criteria for, 954
differential diagnosis of, 954
epidemiology of, 955
features associated with, 955
guideline watch for, 933–940
combining treatments, 938–939
drug efficacy, 936–937
FDA approvals and availability of generics, 936
maintenance treatment, 937
predictors of treatment response, 939
primary care treatment, 939
psychosocial treatment, 938
safety issues, 933–936
heritability of, 955
interpreting results from studies of treatments for, 959
measurement of outcomes, 959
study design and interpretation, 959
introduction to, 949
length of treatment for, 953, 980
longitudinal issues in evaluation of, 954
maintenance treatment of, 937
medical comorbidity with, 953, 983–984
natural history and course of, 954–955
pharmacotherapy for, 952, 965–976
anticonvulsants, 974
antipsychotics, 975
benzodiazepines, 936, 937, 952, 953, 969–973, 980–981
β-blockers, 975
bupropion, 974
buspirone, 976
calcium channel blockers, 975
clonidine, 975–976
combined with psychotherapy, 953, 964, 979–980
in dual-diagnosis patients, 345–346
factors affecting choice of drug for, 979
inositol, 975
monoamine oxidase inhibitors, 952, 973–974
nefazodone, 974
selective serotonin reuptake inhibitors, 952, 965–967
trazodone, 974
tricyclic antidepressants, 952, 967–969
venlafaxine, 974
psychiatric comorbidity with, 953
psychiatric features influencing treatment of, 953, 981–983
mood disorders, 982
other anxiety disorders, 983
personality disorders, 983
substance use disorders, 345–346, 982
suicidality, 981–982
psychiatric management of, 951–952, 955–958, 977
addressing early signs of relapse, 958
diagnostic evaluation, 956

Panic disorder *(continued)*
psychiatric management of *(continued)*
education of patient/family, 957–958
enhancing treatment compliance, 958
functional assessment, 956–957
monitoring patient's psychiatric status, 957
symptom evaluation, 956
therapeutic alliance, 957
working with other physicians, 958
psychosocial interventions for, 938, 959–965
cognitive behavior therapy, 952, 960–962, **961**
combined with pharmacotherapy, 953, 964
group therapy, 962, 964
marital and family therapy, 964–965
mindfulness meditation, 964
patient support groups, 965
psychodynamic psychotherapy, 962–963
relapses of, 958
research directions related to, 986–987
social phobia and, 939
sociodemographic factors influencing treatment of, 984–986
children and adolescents, 984–985
cultural issues, 986
elderly persons, 985–986
gender, 986
suicidality and, 934, 981–982, 1329, **1343**, 1345, 1397–1399
summary of treatment recommendations for, 951–953
treatment plan for, 951, 977–981
treatment settings for, 951, 976
primary care settings, 939
PANSS (Positive and Negative Syndrome Scale), **30**, 580, 659
Paralytic ileus, antipsychotics for persons with, 616
Paranoia, phencyclidine-induced, 310
Paranoid schizophrenia, 604, 625
Parenteral feeding, in anorexia nervosa, 1110, 1138
Parenting, assessing patient's capacity for, 36
Paresthesias, drug-induced
monoamine oxidase inhibitors, 810, 973
topiramate, 894, 1180
Parkinsonism
clinical features of, 648
drug-induced
antipsychotics, 112, 138, 241, 593, 648–650
in elderly persons, 112
prophylaxis for, **594**
selective serotonin reuptake inhibitors, 144, 808
in HIV/AIDS, 242
in Lewy body disease, 119
treatment of, **594**, 648–649
Parkinson's disease
age at onset of, 119
antidepressants for persons with, 799
clinical features of, 119
dementia due to, 119, 150
clozapine for, 138, 139, 150
depression and, 119, 150, 799
use of electroconvulsive therapy in, 89, 799
Paroxetine
for adjustment disorders, 258
for bipolar depression, 844, 860, 868, 895
dosage of, 144, **774**, 936, 967
drug interactions with
antipsychotics, 607
clozapine, 638
for panic disorder, 936, 966
cognitive therapy and, 964
combined with cognitive behavior therapy, 939
maintenance treatment, 937
for pathological gambling, 350
for persons with dementia, 144
for persons with hepatitis C, 177
for persons with HIV/AIDS, 254, 255, 258
for posttraumatic stress disorder, 1064
side effects of, 144
for suicidal persons, 1443
Partial hospitalization. *See also* Day treatment programs
for borderline personality disorder, 1245, 1377
for eating disorders, 1106, 1107, **1131–1133**, 1134, 1170–1171
for schizophrenia, 619
for substance use disorders, 299, 312
alcohol-related disorders, 378
Pathological gambling
pharmacotherapy for, 350
substance use disorders and, 337, 349–350
Patient Health Questionnaire (PHQ-9), **29**
PCP. *See* Phencyclidine
Pediatric patients. *See* Adolescents; Children

Pedigrees, 20
Pemoline
for erectile dysfunction, **795**
for persons with HIV/AIDS, 260
Pentamidine, **209**
Pentobarbital, prophylaxis for alcohol withdrawal seizures, 381
Pentoxifylline
for HIV-associated cognitive dysfunction, 253
for poststroke dementia, 150
Peptide T, for HIV-associated cognitive disorders, 252–253
Perceptual disturbances
assessment of, 22
in borderline personality disorder, pharmacotherapy for, 1244, 1261–1263, **1262, 1303**
in delirium, 73, 74
in schizophrenia, 623
Pergolide, for cocaine dependence, 448
Perinatal HIV transmission, 200, 233–234
Peripheral neuropathy
alcoholic, 390
in HIV/AIDS, 196, 203, 205, 244, 260–261
monoamine oxidase inhibitor–induced, 810
Perphenazine, **589**
for borderline personality disorder, **1262,** 1295
for dementia, 139
dosage of, 140, **589**
in pregnancy, 872
prophylactic antiparkinsonian medication with, 650
for schizophrenia, 639
side effects of, **592**
Personal history, 18–19, **19**
Personal therapy, for schizophrenia, 598, 670–671
Personality changes
in Alzheimer's disease, 118
in frontal lobe dementias, 119
Personality disorders. *See also specific personality disorders*
bipolar disorder and, 871
borderline personality disorder, 1223–1300
depression and, 792
eating disorders and, 1153–1154, 1164
hepatitis C and, **176**
HIV/AIDS and, 228
panic disorder and, 983
posttraumatic stress disorder and, 1045
substance use disorders and, 335, 336, 339, 349
suicide and, 335, **1343,** 1347–1348, 1407–1409
self-mutilation and, 1442
PET (positron emission tomography), **33,** 44
in dementia, 101, 122
Pet therapy, 112, 130
Pharmacotherapy. *See also specific drugs and classes*
for acute stress disorder and posttraumatic stress disorder, 1013, 1030–1031, 1063–1067, 1069
for aggressive behavior, 609
for bipolar disorder, 842–845, 859–861, 866–869, 881–901, 907–908
for borderline personality disorder, 1226, 1243–1244, 1256–1263, **1258, 1260, 1262,** 1287–1298, 1300, **1301–1303**
for delirium, 62, 72, 84–88, 90–91
for dementia, 102, 112–115, 130–147, 154–155
HIV-associated, 219
for depression, 747–750
in dual-diagnosis patients, 338–339
for eating disorders
anorexia nervosa, 1112–1113, 1143–1145, 1173–1175
binge eating disorder, 1115, 1150, 1151, 1180–1181
bulimia nervosa, 1114–1115, 1147–1148, 1177–1178
in elderly persons, 112
in long-term care facilities, 115, 151–152
for panic disorder, 952, 965–976, 979–980
for pathological gambling, 350
for persons with HIV/AIDS, 237–246
for schizophrenia, 573–576, 588–594, 599–604, 628–663
in acute phase, 573
in stabilization phase, 574
in stable phase, 574–576
for sleep disturbances, 115, 146–147
for substance use disorders, 298, 321–324 (*See also specific substances of abuse*)
alcohol dependence, 379–385, 435–442
cocaine dependence, 394–395
in dual-diagnosis patients, 339
nicotine dependence, 368–370, 420–430
opioid dependence, 401–404
opioid withdrawal, 405–408

Pharmacotherapy *(continued)*
for substance use disorders *(continued)*
relation of psychosocial treatments to, 325–327
for suicidal persons, 1326–1327, 1374–1376, 1442–1449, 1455
Phencyclidine (PCP)
aggressive behavior and, 335
paranoia and, 310
schizophrenia and, 625
Phenelzine, 805
for acute stress disorder or posttraumatic stress disorder, 1031
for borderline personality disorder, **1258, 1260**, 1291
for bulimia nervosa, 1177
dosage of, 145, **774**, 973, 1291
for panic disorder, 973
for persons with dementia, 144, 145
for posttraumatic stress disorder, 1065
side effects of, 144, 810
Phenobarbital
for alcohol withdrawal, 381, 435, 436
interaction with efavirenz, 171
Phenothiazines. *See* Antipsychotics
Phentermine, 1150, 1180
Phentolamine, for hypertensive crisis, **795**
Phenytoin
drug interactions with
clozapine, 639
quetiapine, 644
for HIV-related mania, 256
for mania, 889
Phobias, panic disorder and, 983, 985
Photosensitivity, antipsychotic-induced, 631
PHQ-9 (Patient Health Questionnaire), **29**
Physical examination, **15**, 20–21, 34
chaperones for, 34
restraint of patient for, 25
Physical illness. *See* Medical conditions
Physiological feedback, for smoking cessation, 371, 434
Physostigmine
for delirium, 72, 87, 91, 654
dosage and administration of, 88
side effects of, 87
Pick inclusion bodies, 120
Pick's disease, 119–120
Pigmentary retinopathies, antipsychotic-induced, 631
Pilocarpine, **795**, 806, 807
Pimozide
combined with clozapine for schizophrenia, 659
drug interactions with, 241, 242
side effects of, 616, 631
QTc interval prolongation, 616, 631, 653
Pindolol
for bipolar depression, 896
use in dementia, 142
Pioglitazone, for lipodystrophy, 178
Pneumonia, 75
Polycystic ovarian syndrome, valproate-induced, 885–886, 1294
Polydipsia
lithium-induced, 662, 882, 1293
psychosis-induced, 609–610, 625
Polypharmacy, in elderly persons, 131
Polysomnography, **33**
Polyunsaturated fatty acids, for persons with schizophrenia, 662–663
Polyuria, lithium-induced, 662, 882, 1293
PORT (Schizophrenia Patient Outcomes Research Team), 611–612
Positive and Negative Syndrome Scale (PANSS), **30**, 580, 659
Positron emission tomography (PET), **33**, 44
in dementia, 101, 122
Postcardiotomy delirium, 75
Postexposure prophylaxis for HIV, 194, 213–214, 234
Postoperative delirium, 74–75
Postpartum period
bipolar disorder in, 873
blues in, 796–797
depression in, 797
psychosis in, 797
suicide in, 1340, 1386
Posttraumatic stress disorder (PTSD), 1003–1070
adaptive functioning in, 1026, 1027
clinical features influencing treatment plan for, 1030, 1034–1039
age, 1034
aggressive behavior, 1038
comorbid conditions, 1036–1037
ethnic and cross-cultural factors, 1035–1036
gender, 1035
history of previous traumas, 215, 221, 1037–1038

self-injurious and suicidal behaviors, 1038–1039
comorbidity with, 1020–1021, 1026–1027, 1036–1037
borderline personality disorder, 1224, 1266–1267
depression, 1021, 1026, 1037, 1044
eating disorders, 1153
HIV/AIDS, 234, 257
panic disorder, 983
schizophrenia, 582
substance use disorders, 336, 346–347, 355, 1021, 1037, 1044
treatment of, 338–339, 347
suicidality, 1021–1022, 1037, 1038–1039, 1399, 1414
core clinical features of, 1039–1043
development of practice guideline for, 1008–1009
diagnostic criteria for, 1015–1016, **1017–1018,** 1039–1043, **1040–1042**
differential diagnosis of, 1043–1045, **1046–1047**
epidemiology of, 1045–1051
factors affecting response to treatment for, 1029
features associated with, 1043
future research needs related to, 1067–1070
early interventions/posttrauma treatment, 1067–1068
generalization of research trials to clinical populations, 1069
identification of risk factors, 1068
pharmacotherapies and psychotherapies, 1069
subthreshold and complex disorders, 1068
treatment of specific symptoms, 1069
guide to using practice guideline for, 1007
initial assessment of, 1011, 1014–1021
approach to patient, 1014–1015
clinical domains of, 1018, **1020**
comorbid conditions, 1020–1021
crime victims and legal system involvement, 1019–1020
exposure to traumatic event and diagnosis, 1015–1016
military and war-related traumatic event history, 1019
psychiatric history and evaluation, 1016–1018
interpreting literature on treatments for, 1051–1052
introduction to, 1010
natural history and course of, 1051
pharmacotherapy for, 1013, 1030–1031, 1063–1067, 1069
benzodiazepines, 1031, 1066
monoamine oxidase inhibitors, 1013, 1031, 1065–1066
nefazodone, 1064
other medications, 1066–1067
selective serotonin reuptake inhibitors, 1013, 1028, 1030, 1063–1064
trazodone, 1065
tricyclic antidepressants, 1013, 1031, 1065
prevalence of, 1048–1049
principles of treatment selection for, 1012–1013, 1026–1029
choice of initial treatment modality, 1027–1028
lack of response to initial treatment, 1028–1029
treatment goals, 1012, 1026–1027
psychiatric management of, 1012, 1021–1026
coordination of care, 1023–1024, 1036
education of patient/family, 1024
enhancing treatment adherence, 1024–1025
monitoring treatment response, 1024
physical health and functional impairments, 1026
psychosocial effects of disorder, 1025–1026
suicide/violence risk assessment, 1021–1022
therapeutic alliance, 1023
treatment setting, 1022
psychosocial interventions for, 1013–1014, 1031–1034, 1052–1063, 1069
cognitive behavior therapy, 1014, 1028, 1031–1032, 1053–1057
eye movement desensitization and reprocessing, 1014, 1028, 1032, 1057–1059
group psychotherapy, 1059–1061
individual psychotherapies, 1052–1059
monitoring of intrusions, 1063
other early strategies, 1061–1063
other psychotherapies, 1063
psychodynamic psychotherapy, 1014, 1033, 1052
psychoeducation, 1024, 1034

Posttraumatic stress disorder (PTSD) *(continued)*
psychosocial interventions for *(continued)*
psychological debriefing, 1013, 1028, 1033–1034, 1061–1062
written emotional disclosure, 1063
rating scales for, 1018
relapses of, 1027
risk factors for, 1068
safe environment for treatment of, 1015, 1023
screening for, 1014
subthreshold, 1068
after suicide of family member or friend, 1382
summary of treatment recommendations for, 1011–1014
temporal relationship to traumatic stressor, 1043
Postural hypotension. *See* Orthostatic hypotension
Postural instability, in Parkinson's disease, 119
Posturing, catatonic, 789
Practice Guideline for Psychiatric Evaluation of Adults, 122, 779, 863, 956, 984, 1018
Practice Guideline for the Assessment and Treatment of Patients With Suicidal Behaviors, 36, 335, 608, 1021
Practice Guideline for the Treatment of Patients With Acute Stress Disorder and Posttraumatic Stress Disorder, 347, 1007
Practice Guideline for the Treatment of Patients With Bipolar Disorder, 344, 662, 778, 841, 862, 1294
Practice Guideline for the Treatment of Patients With Borderline Personality Disorder, 349
Practice Guideline for the Treatment of Patients With Delirium, 208
Practice Guideline for the Treatment of Patients With Eating Disorders, 349
Practice Guideline for the Treatment of Patients With HIV/AIDS, 352, 876
Practice Guideline for the Treatment of Patients With Major Depressive Disorder, 143, 342, 747, 856, 861, 892, 903, 1263, 1298
Practice Guideline for the Treatment of Patients With Panic Disorder, 940
Practice Guideline for the Treatment of Patients With Schizophrenia, 340
Practice Guideline for the Treatment of Patients With Substance Use Disorders, 17
Practice Parameter for the Assessment and Treatment of Children and Adolescents With Substance Use Disorders, 354
Practice Parameter for the Assessment and Treatment of Children and Adolescents With Suicidal Behavior, 1328
Practice Parameters for the Assessment and Treatment of Children and Adolescents With Anxiety Disorders, 984
Practice Parameters for the Assessment and Treatment of Children and Adolescents With Posttraumatic Stress Disorder, 1008
Pramipexole
for bipolar depression, 844
for HIV-associated cognitive dysfunction, 253
Prayer, 229
Prazosin
interaction with antidepressants, 798
for posttraumatic stress disorder, 1031
Pregnancy
bipolar disorder in, 871–873
borderline personality disorder in, 1269
depression in, 794
eating disorders in, 1154–1155
electroconvulsive therapy in, 796, 873
HIV antibody testing in, 194, 213, 233
maternal-fetal HIV transmission in, 200, 233–234
medication use in
anticonvulsants, 1269
antidepressants, 794–797, 872
antipsychotics, 613, 872–873
benzodiazepines, 613, 873
buprenorphine, 411
bupropion, 377
methadone, 411
mood stabilizers, 613, 871–873
schizophrenia in, 613
substance use in, 300, 352–353, 467
alcohol, 352, 390–391
cocaine, 398
marijuana, 392–393
nicotine, 352, 376–377
opioids, 352, 411
suicide in, 1386
testing for, 33, 213, 573
Prevalence
of acute stress disorder, 1048
of alcohol use disorders among patients in inpatient treatment settings, 419
of Alzheimer's disease, 117
of anxiety disorders, 345
of bipolar disorder, 841, 880
of borderline personality disorder, 1275

of delirium, 74–75
of delirium among medically ill patients, 74–75
of dementia, 117, 150
of depression, 800
of HIV/AIDS, 169–170
among patients in inpatient treatment settings, 215
of HIV-associated neuropsychiatric syndromes, 205, 210–211
of Lewy body disease, 117, 119
of marijuana use disorders, 391
of neuroleptic malignant syndrome, 651
of panic disorder, 955
of posttraumatic stress disorder, 1048–1049
of schizophrenia, 627
of substance use disorders, 416
of tardive dyskinesia, 650
Prevention. *See also* Relapse prevention
of Alzheimer's disease, 102
of falls, 123–124
of HIV transmission, 194, 213, **214**, 217, 231–233
of HIV-associated dementia, 252
of stroke, 150
of substance use disorders in children and adolescents, 355
of suicide, 1325, 1379–1380, 1455–1456
Priapism, drug-induced
antipsychotics, 657
trazodone, 144, 794, **796**, 809
Primitive reflexes, 119
Principles of Medical Ethics: With Annotations Especially Applicable to Psychiatry, 584
PRISM-E Study, 356
Prisons. *See* Correctional settings
Privacy. *See also* Confidentiality
adult psychiatric evaluation and, 38–39
Health Insurance Portability and Accountability Act for protection of, 39, 359, 584
Problem-solving therapy
for depression, 751, 817
for suicidal behavior, 1327, 1377
Procarbazine, **209**
Procyclidine hydrochloride, for extrapyramidal side effects, 650
Program for AIDS Counseling and Education, 257
Program for Assertive Community Treatment (PACT), 576, 597, 666–667
Progressive muscle relaxation
for night eating syndrome, 1116, 1151, 1181
for posttraumatic stress disorder, 1053
Project HELP (Homeless Emergency Liaison Project), 611
Project MATCH, 385, 387, 444, 445
Prolactin elevation. *See* Hyperprolactinemia
Propoxyphene, 399
Propranolol
for aggression in persons with schizophrenia, 609
for akathisia, 649
for alcohol withdrawal, 381, 436
for cocaine withdrawal symptoms, 394
depression induced by, 799
for extrapyramidal symptoms, **594**
for panic disorder, 975
for posttraumatic stress disorder, 1031, 1067
for psychosis-induced polydipsia, 610
use in dementia, 142
PROSPECT study, 752
Prostatic hypertrophy, drug use in persons with
antidepressants, 783, 794, 799, 966, 968
antipsychotics, 616
Protease inhibitors, 202, **204**
cytochrome P450 enzyme inhibition by, 171, 238, **238**
drug interactions with, 171, 195–196, 238–240, **239**
benzodiazepines, 195, 221
carbamazepine, 888
methadone, 246
St. John's wort, 246, 750
sildenafil, 261
for HIV postexposure prophylaxis, 234
lipodystrophy and metabolic syndrome induced by, 171, 177–178
Protriptyline, **774**
Pruritus, carbamazepine-induced, 843
Pseudobulbar palsy, 119
Pseudodementia, depressive, 117, 143, 791
Psoriasis, lithium exacerbation of, 882
Psychiatric history, **13,** 17
Psychiatric management
of acute stress disorder and posttraumatic stress disorder, 1013
of bipolar disorder, 841, 859, 862–866
of borderline personality disorder, 1241–1242, 1246–1250
of delirium, 62, 71, 79–82, 89–90
of dementia, 111–112, 121–128

Psychiatric management *(continued)*
of depression, 771, 779–781
of eating disorders, 1105–1106, 1116–1129
of panic disorder, 951–952, 955–958, 977
of persons at high risk for HIV/AIDS, 194, 211–215, 230–235
of persons with HIV/AIDS, 194–195, 215–223, 235–261
of schizophrenia, 579–588
of substance use disorders, 298, 316–321
of suicidal behavior, 1324–1326, 1362–1373
Psychoanalysis, for suicidal persons, 1451–1452
Psychodrama therapy, for persons with substance use disorders, 330
Psychodynamic psychotherapy
for acute stress disorder and posttraumatic stress disorder, 1014, 1033, 1052
for borderline personality disorder, 1243, 1252, **1253**, 1255, 1277–1282, 1451–1452
adherence to, 1281
adverse effects of, 1281
cost-effectiveness of, 1280
efficacy of, 1279–1280
goals of, 1277–1279, **1278**
length and frequency of, 1280–1281
therapist flexibility for, 1281
therapist training and competency for, 1282
transference interpretation in, 1281
definition of, 1277
for depression, 785, 792, 818
for eating disorders
anorexia nervosa, 1111, 1138–1139, 1171
binge eating disorder, 1149
bulimia nervosa, 1113, 1146, 1175
for panic disorder, 938, 962–963
adverse effects of, 963
efficacy of, 963
goals of, 962–963
implementation of, 963
pharmacotherapy and, 964
for persons with HIV/AIDS, 174–175
for substance use disorders, 298, 315, 325, 329–330
in adolescents, 355
alcohol dependence, 386, 443–444
cocaine dependence, 396, 450
in depression, 344
opioid dependence, 409, 465
for suicidal persons, 1451–1452
theoretical perspectives of, 1277
Psychological debriefing, of traumatized persons, 1013, 1028, 1033–1034, 1061–1062
Psychoneuroimmunology, 228–229
Psychosis. *See also* Antipsychotics
in bipolar disorder, 869–870
in borderline personality disorder, 1244, 1273
in dementia, 113–114, 116, 118, 122, 137–142, 148, 149
Alzheimer's disease, 113–114, 137–142
anticonvulsants for, 114, 141–142
antipsychotics for, 113–114, 138–140
benzodiazepines for, 114, 140–141
goals of treatment for, 137
Lewy body disease, 119
other agents for, 142
Parkinson's disease, 119
principles of treatment for, 137–138
drug-induced
antiretroviral agents, 175
bromocriptine, 144
bupropion, 809
carbamazepine, 887
marijuana, 391
in hepatitis C, **176**
history of abuse in persons with, 1020
HIV/AIDS and, 175, 196, 206–207, 221–222, 258
in intensive care unit, 77
polydipsia induced by, 609–610
puerperal, 797
rating scales for, **30**
schizophrenia, 565–677
time from onset to first treatment of, 626
Psychosocial history, **14**, 18
Psychosocial interventions, 247
for acute stress disorder and posttraumatic stress disorder, 1013–1014, 1031–1034, 1052–1063, 1069
for bipolar disorder, 845–846, 861, 867–869, 901–905
for dementia, 112, 128–130
for depression, 751
for eating disorders
anorexia nervosa, 1110–1111, 1138–1143, 1170–1172
binge eating disorder, 1115, 1149–1151, 1179–1180
bulimia nervosa, 1113–1114, 1145–1147, 1175–1177
for HIV/AIDS, 246–247

for panic disorder, 938, 952, 959–965
for schizophrenia, 574, 575, 576, 596–599, 666–676
for substance use disorders, 298, 324–333
in adolescents, 355
alcohol dependence, 301, 385–388, 442–445
cocaine dependence, 396–397, 449–451
in dual-diagnosis patients, 339
anxiety disorders, 346–347
attention-deficit/hyperactivity disorder, 348
bipolar disorder, 345
depression, 343–344
schizophrenia, 341
marijuana dependence, 392, 446–447
nicotine dependence, 300, 370–371, 431–434
opioid dependence, 302, 325–326, 408–409, 463–465
relation to pharmacotherapy, 325–327
for suicidal persons, 1327, 1377, 1451–1454
Psychostimulants
abuse of, 324, 420
schizophrenia and, 625
for antidepressant augmentation, 784, 812
for antipsychotic-induced sedation, 652
for attention-deficit/hyperactivity disorder
in dual-diagnosis patients, 348
lack of association with substance use disorders in adulthood, 348, 355
dosage of, 145
for erectile dysfunction, **795**
interaction with clozapine, 652
occupations associated with misuse of, 308
for persons with dementia, 115, 143, 145
for persons with HIV/AIDS, 195, 196, 242, 253, 255, 258, 259, 260
replacement therapy for cocaine dependence, 395, 448
side effects of, 144
Psychotherapy. *See also specific types of psychotherapy*
for acute stress disorder and posttraumatic stress disorder, 1013–1014, 1028, 1031–1032, 1052–1063
for bipolar disorder, 845, 860, 861, 869, 902–905
for borderline personality disorder, 1225–1226, 1242–1243, 1252–1256, 1277–1287, 1299–1300
for dementia, 112, 129–130
for depression, 751, 752, 775–777, 782, 785–786, 815–820
in bipolar disorder, 903–904
combined with pharmacotherapy, 751, 772, 777, 782, 786
discontinuation of, 788
with dysthymia, 791
efficacy of, 816
future research needs related to, 822
goals of, 815–816
in persons with personality disorders, 792
for eating disorders
anorexia nervosa, 1110–1111, 1138–1143, 1170–1172
binge eating disorder, 1115, 1149–1151
bulimia nervosa, 1113–1115, 1145–1147, 1175–1176
for mania, 903
for panic disorder, 938–940, 952, 959–965
factors affecting choice of, 977–980
pharmacotherapy and, 953, 964, 979–980
for persons with HIV/AIDS, 174–175, 195, 217, 220, 221, 222, 246, 255–256
for schizophrenia, 597, 669–671
for substance use disorders, 298, 315, 325–331
in adolescents, 355
alcohol dependence, 385–387, 442–445
cocaine dependence, 396, 449–450
in dual-diagnosis patients, 339
depression, 343–344
marijuana dependence, 392
nicotine dependence, 370–371, 431–433
opioid dependence, 408–409, 463–465
relation of pharmacotherapy to, 325–327
for suicidal behavior, 1327, 1377, 1451–1453
Psychotherapy notes, 39
Psychotic depression, 789, 800
electroconvulsive therapy for, 789
fluoxetine-olanzapine combination for, 750
mifepristone for, 752
PTSD. *See* Posttraumatic stress disorder
PTSD Checklist, 1018
Puerperal psychosis, 797
Pulmonary disorders
anorexia nervosa and, **1124**
panic disorder and, 984
schizophrenia and, 615
substance use disorders and, **351**
cocaine, 397
smoking, 376

Pulmonary edema, due to opioid overdose, 322
Pulmonary embolism, clozapine-induced, 637

Q

QEWP (Questionnaire on Eating and Weight Patterns), **1121**
QIDS-SR (Quick Inventory of Depression Symptomatology—Self-Report), **28**
Q-LES-Q (Quality of Life Enjoyment & Satisfaction Questionnaire), **26**
QTc interval prolongation
  antipsychotic-induced, 72, 85, 86, 90, **592**, 616, 653–654
    droperidol, 85, 590, 609, 616
    in dual-diagnosis patients, 340
    haloperidol, 85, 86
    monitoring for, 72, 90
    pimozide, 616
    thioridazine, 616, 1297
    ziprasidone, 616
  assessment for, **586**
  drug use in patients with
    antidepressants, 144
    antipsychotics, 616
    ziprasidone, 646
  methadone-induced, 455
Quality of life, schizophrenia and, 598
Quality of Life Enjoyment & Satisfaction Questionnaire (Q-LES-Q), **26**
Questionnaire on Eating and Weight Patterns (QEWP), **1121**
Questionnaires, 25. *See also* Assessment instruments
Quetiapine, 138, 588, **589**, 643–644
  for anorexia nervosa, 1112, 1144, 1174
  for bipolar disorder
    depressive episodes, 843
    in dual-diagnosis patients, 344
    manic or mixed episodes, 842–843, 866, 891
  for borderline personality disorder, 1297
  for delirium, 62, 72, 84, 90
  for dementia, 139
  dosage of, **589**, 644, 842–843
  drug interactions with, 644
  efficacy of, 643–644
  half-life of, 644
  implementing treatment with, 644
  for posttraumatic stress disorder, 1031, 1066
  in pregnancy, 873
  receptor affinity of, 643
  for schizoaffective disorder, 643
  for schizophrenia, 643–644
    negative and positive symptoms, 643
    neurocognitive deficits, 644
    relapse prevention, 643
    treatment-resistant, 643
  for schizophreniform disorder, 643
  side effects of, 138–139, **592**, 644, 842, 843
    priapism, 657
    sedation, 652
    tardive dyskinesia, 651
Quick Inventory of Depression Symptomatology—Self-Report (QIDS-SR), **28**
Quick reference guides for practice guidelines, xii
Quinidine, interaction with risperidone, 641
Quinolones, **209**

R

Race/ethnicity
  acute stress disorder, posttraumatic stress disorder and, 1035–1036, 1049–1051
  bipolar disorder and, 874
  borderline personality disorder and, 1269
  cytochrome P450 enzyme polymorphisms and, 1036
  dementia and, 154
  depression and, 793
  eating disorders and, 1157–1158, 1163
  HIV/AIDS and, 223–225, **224**
  panic disorder and, 986
  schizophrenia and, 611–612
  substance use disorders and, 356–357
    alcohol use, 418
    marijuana use, 419
  suicidal behavior and, 1341, **1384**, 1385, 1386–1389
Ranitidine, 87, 93
Rape. *See* Sexual abuse/assault
Rash, drug-induced
  antiretroviral agents, 203
  carbamazepine, 887, 1293
  lamotrigine, 844, 874, 893–894
Rating Scale for Extrapyramidal Side Effects, **27**
Rating scales, 25–31, **26–30**. *See also* Assessment instruments; *specific rating scales*
  for aggression/agitation, **30**

for alcohol use disorders, **28**, 307
for anxiety disorders, **29**
for cognitive function, **27**
for delirium, **27**, 78
for depression, **28–29**, 255, 256
for eating disorders, **1121**
future research needs related to, 43
for mania, 889
for posttraumatic stress disorder, 1018
for schizophrenia, **30**, 580
for suicidal behavior, 36, 1335, 1437–1439
Rational Recovery, 387
Readiness and Motivation Interview, 1170
Reality orientation, 112, 129–130
Reality testing, impaired
in intoxication states, 335
in schizophrenia, 623
Reasons for Living Inventory, 1438
Reboxetine, 750
dosage of, **774**
efficacy of, 805
side effects of, **795**, 809
Recognition and Initial Assessment of Alzheimer's Disease and Related Dementias, 122
Recovery, Inc., 674
Recovery-oriented therapies, for persons with substance use disorders, 325, 341
Recreational therapy, 112, 130
Refeeding programs, for anorexia nervosa, 1109–1110, 1134–1137, 1169
Refeeding syndrome, in anorexia nervosa, 1110
Reflexes
in delirium, 74
primitive, 119
in vascular dementia, 119
Rehabilitation programs
for dementia, 155
for persons with HIV/AIDS, 247
Relapse prevention
in anorexia nervosa, 1112–1113, 1173
in bulimia nervosa, 1114
in schizophrenia, 575, 597–601, 603–604, 670
in substance use disorders, 298, 304, 315, 320–321
alcohol dependence, 379, 385, 443
with bulimia nervosa, 348
cognitive behavior therapy for, 327
with depression, 344
group therapy for, 330
marijuana dependence, 392, 446, 447
opioid dependence, 408, 463
pharmacotherapy for, 323–324
with posttraumatic stress disorder, 347
with schizophrenia, 341
Relaxation training
for night eating syndrome, 1116, 1151, 1181
for persons with HIV/AIDS, 256
for posttraumatic stress disorder, 1053, 1055
for substance use disorders, 329
nicotine dependence, 434
Religious beliefs
HIV/AIDS and, 218, 229
suicide risk and, 1322, 1341, 1355–1356, 1385, 1430
Reminiscence therapy, 112, 129
Remoxipride, 242
Renal dysfunction
delirium and, 74
dementia and, 120
drug use in patients with
acamprosate, 384
quetiapine, 644
drug-induced
antiretroviral agents, 203
carbamazepine, 887
lithium, 662, 882, 883, 1293
in serotonin syndrome, 808
Repetitive transcranial magnetic stimulation (rTMS)
for comorbid depression and bulimia nervosa, 1148–1149
for schizophrenia, 595, 665
Reproductive abnormalities
anorexia nervosa and, **1125**
bulimia nervosa and, **1127**
Residential treatment settings
for eating disorders, **1131–1133**
for schizophrenia, 578, 620–621
crisis programs, 618–619
for substance use disorders, 299, 312–313
in adolescents, 355
Resilience, after traumatic exposure, 1025–1026
Respiratory depression, drug-induced
antipsychotics, 634
benzodiazepines, 86, 244
opioids, 302, 322, 402, 455
Respiratory disorders
anorexia nervosa and, **1124**
panic disorder and, 984
schizophrenia and, 615
substance use disorders and, **351**

Respiratory disorders *(continued)*
substance use disorders and *(continued)*
cocaine, 397
smoking, 376
Respite care, for patient with dementia, 127, 148
Restlessness. *See also* Akathisia
psychostimulant-induced, 144
Restraint of patients
for aggressive behavior in schizophrenia, 609
elderly persons, 93
for interview or examination, 25
in long-term care facilities, 115, 151–152
Retinopathies, pigmentary, antipsychotic-induced, 631
Retrograde ejaculation, antipsychotic-induced, 656–657
Review of systems, **15,** 20
Rhabdomyolysis, in serotonin syndrome, 808
Rifabutin, interaction with efavirenz, 171
Rifampin, drug interactions with
clozapine, 639
efavirenz, 171
Rigidity
antipsychotic-induced, 241, 648
in neuroleptic malignant syndrome, 651
in Parkinson's disease, 119
Risk assessment, 36
for HIV infection, 211–212, **212,** 230–231
for suicide, 36, 779, **780, 863,** 863–864, 1021, 1324, 1336–1359, **1337–1338,** 1378–1379
Risk factors
for acute stress disorder or posttraumatic stress disorder, 1068
for dementia, 126
for depression recurrence, **778**
for HIV infection, 211–212, **212,** 230–231
for neuroleptic malignant syndrome, 652
for schizophrenia, 627
for stroke, 126
for suicide, 577–578, 607–608, 1324, 1336–1359, **1337–1338,** 1383–1437, 1454–1455
for tardive dyskinesia, 615, 650
for vascular dementia, 126
Risk management issues
in treatment of borderline personality disorder, 1244, 1270–1272
anger, impulsivity, and violence, 1244, 1264–1265, 1271–1272
boundary violations, 1249, 1250, 1253, 1272
suicide, 1238, 1244, 1247, 1253, 1270–1271, 1274
in treatment of suicidal persons, 1378–1382, **1379**
communication with significant others, 1380
documentation of patient care, 1378
management of suicide in one's practice, 1381
mental health interventions for surviving family and friends after a suicide, 1325–1326, 1382
suicide prevention contracts, 1325, 1379–1380, 1455–1456
suicide risk assessment, 1378–1379
Risk-reduction strategies
to minimize HIV transmission, 194, 213, **214,** 217, 231–233
for persons with substance use disorders, 304
Risk-Rescue Rating, 1438
Risks of using practice guidelines, x–xi
Risperidone, 588, **589,** 639–641
active metabolite of, 640–641
for bipolar disorder
in children and adolescents, 906
in dual-diagnosis patients, 344
manic episodes, 842, 867, 891
mood stabilizers and, 842, 891
for borderline personality disorder, **1262,** 1297
for delirium, 62, 72, 84, 90
in HIV/AIDS, 254
for dementia, 138, 139
stroke risk with, 616
dosage of, 140, **589,** 640, 842
drug interactions with, 641
efficacy of, 639–640
for emergency treatment of acute psychosis, 589–590
half-life of, 640, 641
implementing treatment with, 640–641
long-acting, injectable form of, 340, 592
for persons with anorexia nervosa, 1112
for persons with HIV/AIDS, 242, 254
for posttraumatic stress disorder, 1031, 1066
in pregnancy, 873
receptor affinity of, 639
for schizoaffective disorder, 639, 640
for schizophrenia, 592, 639–640
combined with clozapine, 659
in dual-diagnosis patients, 340
cocaine dependence, 449

hyperprolactinemia, 656
neurocognitive deficits, 639
positive and negative symptoms, 639
relapse prevention, 640
retrograde ejaculation, 656
treatment-resistant, 639–640
side effects of, 114, 138, 242, **592,** 640, 842
priapism, 657
sedation, 652
tardive dyskinesia, 650
Ritonavir, **204**
cytochrome P450 enzyme inhibition by, 171, 238, **238**
drug interactions with, 221, 238, **239,** 240, 241, 242, 244, 246, 261
Rivastigmine
for delirium, 62
for dementia, 102
Rosiglitazone, for lipodystrophy, 178
rTMS (repetitive transcranial magnetic stimulation)
for comorbid depression and bulimia nervosa, 1148–1149
for schizophrenia, 595, 665
Ruiz v. Estelle, 621
Rural areas, HIV/AIDS in, 226
Ryan White Comprehensive AIDS Resources Emergency (CARE) Act, 236

S

Safer sex practices, 213, **214,** 234, 248, 351
Safety issues
in borderline personality disorder, 1246–1247
in delirium, 62, 80–81
in dementia, 111–112, 123–124, 148
driving, 111–112, 124–125
falls, 114, 115, 123–124
wandering, 118, 124
in depression, 779, 781
interviews with agitated or aggressive persons, 24–25
in panic disorder, 933–936
in substance abusers, 317
suicide risk, 1363 (*See also* Suicidal behavior)
antidepressants and, 748–749, 934–936
assessment of, 36, 779, **780, 863,** 863–864, 1021, 1324, 1336–1359, **1337–1338,** 1378–1379
bipolar disorder and, **863,** 863–864
borderline personality disorder and, 1238, 1244, 1247
depression and, 779, **780,** 788–789
posttraumatic stress disorder and, **1021–1022**
schizophrenia and, 607–608
substance use disorders and, 334–335
suicide prevention contracts, 1325, 1379–1380, 1455–1456
St. John's wort
for depression, 750, 815
dosage of, 815
drug interactions with, 750, 815
antiretroviral agents, 246
for persons with HIV/AIDS, 246
SAM-e (*S*-adenosylmethionine), 246
SAMHSA (Substance Abuse and Mental Health Services Administration), 354, 357, 402, 596
San Diego Suicide Study, 1405
Saquinavir, **204**
cytochrome P450 enzyme inhibition by, **238**
drug interactions with, 261
midazolam, 238, 244
Saskatoon Delirium Checklist (SDC), 78
SBQ (Suicide Behavior Questionnaire), 1437–1438
Scale for Suicide Ideation, 1335, 1437
Scale for Suicide Ideation–Worst (SSI–W), 1433, 1437
Scale for the Assessment of Negative Symptoms, 659
Scale for the Assessment of Positive Symptoms, 659
Schedule for Affective Disorders and Schizophrenia, 1409
Schizoaffective disorder
aripiprazole for, 646–647
electroconvulsive therapy for, 663
lithium for, 662
quetiapine for, 643
risperidone for, 639, 640
ziprasidone for, 645
Schizophrenia, 565–677
acute phase treatment of, 572–574, 579, 584–595
adjunctive medications, 573, 593–594, **594**
antipsychotics, 573, 588–593, **589–592,** 629–630
assessment, 572–573, 584–585, **586–587**

Schizophrenia *(continued)*
acute phase treatment of *(continued)*
electroconvulsive therapy and other somatic therapies, 594–595
family involvement in, 574, 584, 588
psychiatric management, 585–588
psychosocial interventions, 574
adjunctive medications for, 573, 657–663
in acute phase, 573, 593–594, **594**
anticonvulsants, 657
antidepressants, 573, 576, 594, 601, 657–659
benzodiazepines, 573, 576, 589, 593, 601, 659–660
β-blockers, 573, 593, 601, 660–661
cognition enhancers, 661
glutamatergic agents, 602, 661
lithium, 661–662
monoaminergic agents, 662
mood stabilizers, 573, 576, 593, 601, 657, 661–662
polyunsaturated fatty acids, 662–663
in stable phase, 576, 601
to treat extrapyramidal symptoms, 594, **594**, 601
age at onset of, 627
antipsychotics for, **589**, 628–657, 1375 (*See also* Antipsychotics; *specific drugs*)
in acute phase, 573, 588–593, **590, 591**, 629–630
adherence to, 581–582, 609
administration routes for, 72, 85
advance directives about, 590
augmentation of, 602
clozapine to reduce suicide risk, 340, 608, 635, 1327, 1376, 1447–1448
combinations of, 659
discontinuation of, 575, 604
dosage of, 573, 575, **589**, 592–593, 632–634
drug interactions with, 635
in dual-diagnosis patients, 340–341, 449, 606
emergency treatment, 589–590
evaluating response to, 576
"extrapyramidal symptom threshold" for, 575, 593, 599
lack of response to, **591**, 593, **601–602**
patient ambivalence about, 581
patient refusal of, 589–590
for relapse prevention, 575, 599–601, 603–604
selection of, 590, **590**
side effects of, 574–575, 588, 591–593, **592**, 600, 628–629
in stabilization phase, 574, 595, 630
in stable phase, 574–576, **591**, 603–604, 630–631
antiretroviral therapy adherence in persons with, 175
catatonic, 604, 623, 625
in children and adolescents, 603
clinical features influencing treatment of, 602–616
concurrent medical conditions, 615–616
demographic and psychosocial variables, 610–615
cultural factors, 611
elderly patients, 614–615, 627
gender, 612–613, 627
homelessness, 610–611
pregnancy, 613
psychosocial stressors, 613–614
race, 611–612
psychiatric features, 602–610
aggressive behavior, 608–609
depressive symptoms, 606–607
first episode, 576–577, 602–604
psychosis-induced polydipsia, 609–610
substance use disorders, 605–606
subtypes and deficit symptoms, 604
suicide risk, 607–608
clinical features of, 623–625
disorganized symptoms, 625
duration of symptoms, 623
negative symptoms, 577, 598, 604, 625
positive symptoms, 625
prodromal symptoms, 603, 625–626, 670
remission of, 603
comorbidity with, 582–583, 625
depression, 577, 582, 594, 601, 606–607, 614, 625
medical conditions, 582–583, 615–616, 625
obsessive-compulsive disorder, 594, 601, 625
substance use disorders, 339–341, 573, 577, 582, 585, 605–606, 615, 625, 627
alcohol dependence, 340, 389
cocaine dependence, 397, 448–449
integrated treatments for, 339–340
nicotine dependence, 339, 374–375

pharmacotherapy for, 340–341
psychosocial treatments for, 339, 341
suicidal and aggressive behaviors, 573, 577–578, 585, 607–609, 623, **1343**, 1344, 1394–1397, 1446
summary of treatment recommendations for, 571–578
treatment plan for, 571
continuity of care for, 581, 595
development of practice guideline for, 570
diagnostic criteria for, 623, **624**
differential diagnosis of, 580
dementia, 117
disorganized, 604, 625
economic costs of, 628
in elderly persons, 614–615, 627
electroconvulsive therapy for, 594–595, 601, 602, 663–665
epidemiology of, 626–628
genetic factors in, 627
goals of treatment for, 571, 572, 574, 579, 584
guide to using practice guideline for, 569
housing options for persons with, 578, 620–621
maintenance treatment for, 575, 599–601
mortality related to, 626
natural history and course of, 625–626
early course, 626
premorbid phase, 625
prodromal phase, 603, 625–626, 670
psychotic phase, 626
paranoid, 604, 625
phases of treatment for, 579
predictors of long-term outcome of, 626
prevalence of, 627
psychiatric management of, 579–584
assessment and diagnosis, 571, 579–580
barriers to patient's participation, 572, 581
for comorbid conditions, 582–583
developing treatment plan, 580
documentation of, 583–584
family involvement, 574, 584, 588, 595, 667–668
first episode, 576–577, 602–604
integrated treatment, 583
negative symptoms, 577
patient/family education, 576, 582, 595
patient's social circumstances and functioning, 583
therapeutic alliance and treatment adherence, 572, 580–582, 630
psychosocial interventions for, 596–599, 666–676
in acute phase, 574, 585
case management, 341, 583, 673
cognitive behavior therapy, 576, 597, 669
cognitive remediation and therapy, 673–674
counseling, 597–598
early detection and intervention, 671–672
family interventions, 578, 597, 667–668
group therapies, 671
to improve functional status and quality of life, 598–599
for negative symptoms, 598
patient/family education, 576, 673
peer support and self-help groups, 599, 674–675
personal therapy, 598, 670–671
Program for Assertive Community Treatment, 576, 597, 666–667
for relapse prevention and reduction of symptom severity, 597–598, 670
relative organizations, 675–676
social skills training, 576, 669–670
in stabilization phase, 574, 595–596
in stable phase, 575, 576, 596–599
supported employment, 576, 598, 668
rating scales for, **30**, 580
relapse of, 574
antipsychotic dosage and, 575, 599–600, 630, 633–634
educating patient about signs of, 575
minimizing risk of, 575, 577, 599–601, 603–604
risk without maintenance treatment, 599, 600, 604, 630
treatment nonadherence and, 582
repetitive transcranial magnetic stimulation for, 595, 665
research directions related to, 676–677
residual, 604
risk factors for, 627
stabilization phase management of, 574, 579, 595–596, 630
stable phase management of, 574–576, 579, 596–601
adjunctive medications, 600
antipsychotics, 574–576, **591**, 599–600, 603–604, 630–631

Schizophrenia *(continued)*
stable phase management of *(continued)*
assessment, 596
electroconvulsive therapy, 600
psychosocial treatments, 596–599
subtypes of, 604, 625
treatment plan for, 571, 579, 580
treatment settings for, 578, 616–623
correctional settings, 621–623
crisis residential programs, 618–619
day treatment programs, 619–620
factors affecting choice of, **617**
hospitalization, 616–618
long-term hospitalization, 618
partial hospitalization, 619
treatment-resistant, **591,** 593, 601–602
clozapine for, 635–636
electroconvulsive therapy for, 602
olanzapine for, 642
quetiapine for, 643
risperidone for, 639–640
undifferentiated, 604, 625
Schizophrenia Patient Outcomes Research Team (PORT), 611–612
Schizophrenics Anonymous, 674
Schizophreniform disorder
aripiprazole for, 646
quetiapine for, 643
ziprasidone for, 645
School phobia, 985
School refusal, 985
Screening. *See also* Assessment instruments
for bipolar disorder, 841, 863
for delirium, 78
for dementia, 101
for posttraumatic stress disorder, 1014
for substance use disorders, 9, **33,** 307
toxicology, 9, **33,** 309, 317–318
SDC (Saskatoon Delirium Checklist), 78
Seasonal affective disorder, 792, 802–803
Secobarbital, prophylaxis for alcohol withdrawal seizures, 381
Secular Organizations for Sobriety, 332
Sedation, drug-induced
antidepressants, 144, 429, **795,** 807, 1290
antipsychotics, 85, 113, 114, 138, 139, 592, **592,** 614, 652
aripiprazole, 647
benzodiazepines, 86, 114, 140, 244, 660, 970
buprenorphine, 460
carbamazepine, 141
clonidine, 430
clozapine, 636, 652
in elderly persons, 112
lithium, 662, 882, 1293
methadone, 455
mirtazapine, 809
monoamine oxidase inhibitors, 810
nefazodone, 144, 809
olanzapine, 642, 643, 652
quetiapine, 644, 652, 843
risperidone, 652
trazodone, 142, 144, 809
valproate, 885, 1293
ziprasidone, 645
Sedative-hypnotics. *See also* Benzodiazepines
for elderly persons, 356
for opioid withdrawal symptoms, 408
overdose of, 322–323
for persons with HIV/AIDS, 244
for sleep disturbances, in dementia, 115, 146–147
withdrawal from, **81**
benzodiazepines for, 72, 86, 87
electroencephalogram in, 74
seizures during, 75
Seeking Safety, 347
Seizures
during alcohol withdrawal, 301, 379
antidepressants for persons with, 798
delirium and, 62, 75
dementia and, 116, 118
drug-induced
antidepressants, **795,** 798
antipsychotics, 85, 114, 138, 631
bupropion, 144, 369, 429, 809
clozapine, 138, 242, 340, 606, 635, 637
cocaine, 301, 394
olanzapine, 890
physostigmine, 87
suicide risk among persons with, 1353, 1424, 1425
Selective serotonin reuptake inhibitors (SSRIs). *See also specific drugs*
for alcohol dependence, 384, 440–442
efficacy of, 440–441
goals of, 440
implementation of, 441–442
for borderline personality disorder, 1243, 1244, 1256, 1257, **1258,** 1259, **1260, 1262,** 1287–1289
for depression, 772, 783

with atypical features, 773, 783, 789, 805
in bipolar disorder, 895
in dual-diagnosis patients, 342–343, 388–389
dosage of, 144, **774**, 967, 1289
drug interactions with, 144, 808
antipsychotics, 607, 635
buspirone, 142
clozapine, 638, 658
monoamine oxidase inhibitors, 808
selegiline, 135
tricyclic antidepressants, 807, 812
for eating disorders
anorexia nervosa, 1112, 1143, 1173
binge eating disorder, 1115, 1150, 1180–1181
bulimia nervosa, 1114, 1147, 1177–1178
night eating syndrome, 1116, 1151, 1181
efficacy of, 804–805
for elderly persons, 752
generic preparations of, 936
for obsessive-compulsive disorder, in dual-diagnosis patients, 346
overdose of, 966, 1442
for panic disorder, 934, 936–937, 952, 965–967, 979
combined with benzodiazepines, 938
in dual-diagnosis patients, 345
maintenance treatment, 937
for pathological gambling, 350
for persons with concurrent medical conditions
cardiac disease, 798
hepatitis C, 177
HIV/AIDS, 174, 195, 240, 253, 254–255
obstructive uropathy, 799
for persons with dementia, 114, 142, 144, 148
for persons with schizophrenia, 607, 658
aggressive behavior, 609
for posttraumatic stress disorder, 1013, 1028, 1030, 1063–1064
in dual-diagnosis patients, 347
suicidal behaviors, 1038
in pregnancy, 796, 872
side effects of, 144, 441, **795–796**, 807–808, 952, 966–967, 1289
hyponatremia, 609
sexual dysfunction, 144, 441, 442, 783, 794
suicide risk, 748, 1374
for smoking cessation, 370, 430
for social anxiety disorder, in dual-diagnosis patients, 346
for suicidal persons, 1442–1444
switching to monoamine oxidase inhibitor from, **784**, 808, 810, 812, 1257
withdrawal from, 966
Selegiline
for Alzheimer's disease, 113, 135, 148, 149
for cocaine dependence, 447
dosage of, 135
drug interactions with, 135
for HIV-associated cognitive dysfunction, 253
for Parkinson's disease, 799
for persons with schizophrenia, 658
side effects of, 135
for smoking cessation, 430
Selenium, for HIV-related cognitive disorders, 253
Self-control training
for depression, 817
for substance use disorders, 298, 315, 333
alcohol dependence, 442
Self-guided therapies, for substance use disorders, 298, 315, 333
alcohol dependence, 387
nicotine dependence, 371, 433
Self-help groups
for depression, 819–820
for eating disorders, 349, 1111, 1114, 1141–1142, 1146–1147, 1172, 1177
for schizophrenia, 599, 674–676
for substance use disorders, 331–332
in adolescents, 355
alcohol dependence, 331–332, 386–387, 444
cocaine dependence, 332, 396–397, 450, 451
for family members, 332
nicotine dependence, 332, 431
opioid dependence, 332, 401, 409
Self-injurious behavior
adolescent substance abuse and, 355
assessing risk for, 36
borderline personality disorder and, 1244, 1254, 1265–1266, 1273
chronic, 1325
deliberate self-harm, 1321, 1441–1442
eating disorders and, 1106, 1121
lethality and intent of, 1358–1359, 1436

Self-injurious behavior *(continued)*
posttraumatic stress disorder and, 1038–1039
suicidal, 1315–1456 (*See also* Suicidal behavior)
Self-Management and Recovery Training, 332
Self-mutilation, 1441–1442
Self-report scales, 25, 31. *See also* Assessment instruments
Senile plaques, 118
Sensory impairments
assessment for, 22
delirium and, 83
Sensory integration, 112, 129
D-Serine, for persons with schizophrenia, 602, 661
Serotonin
HIV/AIDS and, 253
suicidal behavior and, 1439
Serotonin syndrome, 142, **796**, 799, 808, 810, 973
Sertindole, 138
for dementia, 139
side effects of, 138–139
Sertraline
for borderline personality disorder, 1256, **1258**, 1259, **1260**, 1287–1289
dosage of, 144, **774**, 936, 967, 1289
for dual-diagnosis patients, 342
for eating disorders
binge eating disorder, 1180
bulimia nervosa, 1114, 1177
night eating syndrome, 1116, 1151, 1181
for elderly persons, 752, 753
interaction with clozapine, 638
neonatal withdrawal from, 796
for panic disorder, 936, 965–966
combined with clonazepam, 938
maintenance treatment, 937
for pathological gambling, 350
for persons with concurrent medical conditions
dementia, 102, 144, 798
glaucoma, 798
HIV/AIDS, 254, 255
for persons with schizophrenia, 658
for posttraumatic stress disorder, 1064
in pregnancy, 796
side effects of, 144
for trichotillomania, 258
Sexual abuse/assault
borderline personality disorder and, 215
eating disorders and, 1021, 1155, 1164
gender and, 1035
HIV and, 194, 215, 221, 235
initial assessment of victims of, 1014, 1018, 1019–1020
posttraumatic stress disorder and, 215, 221, 1014, 1030, 1036, 1057
suicide risk and, 1351–1352, 1386, 1417–1419
Sexual behavior/activity
compulsive, pathological gambling and, 349, 350
disinhibited, medroxyprogesterone for, 114
HIV transmission via, 170, 198–199, **199**
strategies to reduce risk of, 213, **214**, 231–232
substance use disorders and, 234
"survival sex," 235
safer sex practices, 213, **214**, 234, 248, 351
substance use disorders and, 350–352
Sexual development, eating disorders and, 1122, **1125**
Sexual dysfunction
drug-induced
antidepressants, **795–796**, 806, 968
antipsychotics, 631, 656–657
aripiprazole, 647
clozapine, 636, 656
methadone, 455
monoamine oxidase inhibitors, 810, 973
olanzapine, 642, 656
quetiapine, 644, 656
reboxetine, 809
risperidone, 640, 656
selective serotonin reuptake inhibitors, 144, 441, 442, 783, 794, **795–796**, 808, 952, 966
trazodone, 144, 794, **796**, 809
venlafaxine, 809
ziprasidone, 645
in HIV/AIDS, 196, 222–223, 261
Sexual orientation
HIV/AIDS and, 225
substance use disorders and, 357
suicidality and, 1341–1342, 1390–1391
Sexually transmitted diseases
in children, 235
cocaine use and, 397
dementia and, 120
gender differences in risk for, 351
HIV/AIDS transmission and, 200

Sialorrhea, clozapine-induced, 636
Sibutramine, for binge eating disorder, 1115, 1150, 1180
Side effects of drugs. *See also specific side effects*
acamprosate, 440
acyclovir, **209**
amantadine, 144
amitriptyline, 144
amphotericin B, **209**
antidepressants, 144, 658, **795–796**
antimicrobial agents, **209**
antipsychotics, 85, 102, 113–114, 138–139, 241, 344, 574–575, 588, 591–593, **592**, 600, 628–629, 631–632, 647–657, 1297
antiretroviral agents, 171, 172, 177–178, 208, **209**, 220
aripiprazole, **592**, 647, 842
benzodiazepines, 86–87, 114, 120, 140–141, 660, 970–971, 1294
β-blockers, 120
bromocriptine, 144
buprenorphine, 404, 459–460
bupropion, 144, 369, 429, 809
buspirone, 142
carbamazepine, 141, 142, 243, 843, 887, 1293
chlorpromazine, 138
cholinesterase inhibitors, 87–88, 102, 112, 132–133
clonazepam, 937
clonidine, 430, 463
clozapine, 114, 138, 139, 242, 340, **592**, 635, 636–637
co-trimoxazole, **209**
cycloserine, **209**
desipramine, 144
dextroamphetamine, 144
diphenhydramine, 120
disulfiram, 383
donepezil, 132
droperidol, 85
in elderly persons, 112, 875
ergoloid mesylates, 136
fluoxetine, 144
fluoxetine-olanzapine combination, 843
fluphenazine, 138
foscarnet, **209**
haloperidol, 85, 90, 138, 241
imipramine, 144
interferon, 176, **209**, 253, 351–352
isoniazid, **209**
LAAM, 401
β-lactam antibiotics, **209**
lamotrigine, 844, 893
lithium, 74, 662, 844, 882–883, 1293
mesoridazine, 631
methadone, 402, 455
methotrexate, **209**
methylphenidate, 144
mirtazapine, 809
monoamine oxidase inhibitors, 144, **795–796**, 809–810, 973, 1291
naltrexone, 246, 382, 404, 437–438, 461–462
nefazodone, 144, 342, 747–748, 809
nicotine replacement therapies, 300, 425–426
nortriptyline, 144, 429
olanzapine, 138–139, **592**, 642, 842, 843, 845, 890
ondansetron, 441
oxandrolone, 244
paroxetine, 144
pentamidine, **209**
perphenazine, **592**
phenelzine, 144
physostigmine, 87
pimozide, 616, 631
procarbazine, **209**
protease inhibitors, 171, 177–178
psychostimulants, 144
quetiapine, 138–139, **592**, 644, 842, 843
quinolones, **209**
reboxetine, 809
risperidone, 114, 138, 242, **592**, 640, 842
selective serotonin reuptake inhibitors, 144, 441, 952, 966–967, 1289
selegiline, 135
sertindole, 138–139
sertraline, 144
sulfonamides, **209**
tacrine, 87–88, 102, 112, 132–133
thiabendazole, **209**
thioridazine, 138, **592**, 616, 631
topiramate, 894, 1180
tranylcypromine, 144, 810
trazodone, 142, 144, 809
tricyclic antidepressants, 144, 968, 1290
valproate, 141, 142, 175, 243, 845, 885–886, 1293–1294
venlafaxine, 144, 809
vinblastine, **209**

Side effects of drugs *(continued)*
vincristine, **209**
vitamin E, 134
ziprasidone, **592**, 842
Sign language interpreters, 24, 41
Sildenafil
interaction with antiretroviral agents, 241, 261
for sexual dysfunction, **795–796**, 808
Simpson-Angus Extrapyramidal Symptom Rating Scale, **27**
Simulated presence therapy, 129
Single photon emission computed tomography (SPECT), **33**
in dementia, 101, 122
Sinusitis, cocaine-induced, 397
Sleep deprivation, for bipolar depression, 896
Sleep disturbances
bipolar disorder and, 865
delirium and, 62, 74
dementia and, 115, 116, 122, 146–147
drug-induced
antidepressants, **795**, 808, 968
antiretroviral agents, 172, 203
aripiprazole, 647, 842
benzodiazepines, 86, 87, 114
bupropion, 369, 429, 809
cocaine withdrawal, 394
duloxetine, 749
lithium, 845
monoamine oxidase inhibitors, 810, 973
psychostimulants, 144
reboxetine, 809
selective serotonin reuptake inhibitors, **966**
topiramate, 894
ziprasidone, 645
HIV/AIDS and, 195, 220, 222, 258–259
melatonin for, 146, 246
pharmacotherapy for, 115, 146–147
polysomnography studies in, **33**
substance use disorders and, 336
suicidality and, 1329
Smokeless tobacco, 353, 360, 361, 417
Smoking (tobacco). *See also* Nicotine dependence
among adolescents, 417
adverse health effects of, 350, **351**, 360, 375–376, 417
Alzheimer's disease risk and, 126
effects of secondhand smoke, 376
epidemiology of, 375, 417–418
heritability of, 417
history taking for, 307
interaction with antipsychotics, 340
clozapine, 639
olanzapine, 643
in pregnancy, 352, 376–377
preventing in children and adolescents, 355
race/ethnicity and, 357
treatment of smokers on smoke-free wards, 371–373
monitoring of symptoms, 372
patient education, 372
system issues, 372
for withdrawal symptoms, 372–373
water intoxication and, 609
Smoking cessation, 360, 420–434
abrupt vs. gradual, 364, 434
acupuncture for, 300, 368
among adolescents, 355
alcohol use and, 367
approach to, 362–368
assessment for, 361–362
behavior therapy for, 368
caffeine use and, 367
in dual-diagnosis patients, 374–375
depression, 375
other psychiatric disorders, 375
schizophrenia, 374–375
among elderly persons, 356
multiple attempts at, 361
nicotine withdrawal symptoms during, 365–366
outpatient treatment for, 299
overcoming barriers to, 363–364
in patients with medical disorders, 375–376
in pregnancy, 376–377
psychosocial interventions for, 300, 370–371, 431–434
behavior therapies, 370, 432–433
brief therapies, 370, 432
cognitive behavior therapy, 370–371, 433
efficacy of, 431
exercise, 371, 433–434
goals of, 431
hypnotherapy, 333, 434
implementation of, 431–432
other therapies, 371, 433–434
physiological feedback, 371, 434
self-guided therapies, 371, 433
self-help groups, 332, 431
social support, 370, 432
stimulus control techniques, 371, 434

quit date for, 364–365
readiness and motivation for, 363
relapses during attempts at, 367
somatic treatments for, 300, 368–370, 420–431
acupuncture, 300, 368, 369, 430
bupropion, 300, 324, 369, 427–429
clonidine, 300, 369–370, 429–430
in depression, 343
nicotine replacement therapies, 300, 368–369, 421–426
nortriptyline, 300, 369, 429
other agents, 370, 430–431
in schizophrenia, 341
telephone quitlines for, 321
timing of, 364
treatment settings for, 362
among women, 353
Snout reflex, 119
Sober houses, for substance use disorders, 314
Social and Occupational Functioning Assessment Scale (SOFAS), **26**
Social anxiety disorder
eating disorders and, 1153, 1164
panic disorder and, 939, 983
substance use disorders and, 337, 346
among adolescents, 355
pharmacotherapy for, 338
suicide and, 1399
Social functioning, in schizophrenia, 583, 598–599, 623
Social milieu, of patient with substance use disorder, 358
Social Security Disability Income, 341
Social skills training
in dementia, 112
in depression, 817
in schizophrenia, 576, 599, 669–670
cognitive behavior therapy and, 615
in substance use disorders, 298, 315, 327
alcohol dependence, 443
schizophrenia and, 341
Social support
for smoking cessation, 370, 432
suicide risk and, 1356, 1430–1431
Sociocultural history, **14**, 18–19
Sociodemographic factors
bipolar disorder, 871–875
borderline personality disorder and, 1269–1270
dementia and, 153–154
depression and, 792–797
eating disorders and, 1155–1160
HIV/AIDS and, 223–226
schizophrenia and, 610–615
substance use disorders and, 353–358
suicidal behavior and, 1336–1342, **1337–1338**, 1383–1391, **1384**
SOFAS (Social and Occupational Functioning Assessment Scale), **26**
Somatization disorder, posttraumatic, 1037
Somatotropin, for HIV-associated wasting, 244–245, 260
Somnolence, drug-induced
aripiprazole, 842
carbamazepine, 843
clonazepam, 937
duloxetine, 749
fluoxetine-olanzapine combination, 843
lithium, 844
olanzapine, 842, 845, 890
quetiapine, 842, 843
risperidone, 842
topiramate, 1180
ziprasidone, 842
SPECT (single photon emission computed tomography), **33**
in dementia, 101, 122
Speech
assessment of, 21
drug-induced disturbances of
benzodiazepines, 970
carbamazepine, 843
sedative-hypnotics, 322
Spielberger State-Trait Anxiety Inventory, 976
Spirituality. *See also* Religious beliefs
HIV/AIDS and, 218, 229
Splitting, in borderline personality disorder, 1249, 1254
SSI–W (Scale for Suicide Ideation–Worst), 1433
SSRIs. *See* Selective serotonin reuptake inhibitors
Standards of care, ix
Stavudine, **204**
for HIV-associated dementia, 252
side effects of, **209**
STEPPS (systems training for emotional predictability and problem solving), for borderline personality disorder, 1226
Stereotyped movements, in catatonia, 789
Stevens-Johnson syndrome, drug-induced
carbamazepine, 887, 1293
lamotrigine, 893–894

Stimulus control techniques, for smoking
cessation, 371, 434
Stress(ors)
acute stress disorder and posttraumatic stress disorder, 1003–1070
associated with treatment of HIV-infected persons, 230
bipolar disorder and, 865, 880, 902
borderline personality disorder and, 1268
dementia and, 116
depression and, 792
psychosocial, 18
schizophrenia and, 613–614
Stroke
cocaine-induced, 394, 397
dementia and, 150
Alzheimer's disease, 119
risperidone-induced, 616, 640
vascular dementia, 118–119
risk factors for, 126
seizures and, 75
suicide risk and, 1424–1425
use of electroconvulsive therapy in, 89
Structured Clinical Interview for DSM-IV, 580
Structured Interview for PTSD, 1018
Structured interviews, 25–31, **26–30**. *See also* Assessment instruments
Stupor, 75
in catatonia, 789
drug-induced
opioids, 322
sedative-hypnotics, 322
Subdural hematoma, 120
Substance Abuse and Mental Health Services Administration (SAMHSA), 354, 357, 402, 596
Substance misuse, 303, 307–308, 324, 1028
prescription medications, 307
combining with "club drugs," 334
among elderly persons, 356
by health care workers, 307
opioid analgesics, 399
Substance use disorders, 291–466. *See also specific substances of abuse*
acute interventions for, 303
alcohol use disorders, 301, 377–391, 434–445
antidepressants for persons with, 338, 342–343, 388–389, 790
antipsychotics for persons with, 340–341, 449, 606
assessment of, 297, 303, 306–310
childhood attention-deficit/hyperactivity disorder as risk factor for, 348
clinical features influencing treatment of, 300, 333–358
age, 354–356
children and adolescents, 354–355
elderly persons, 356
comorbid medical disorders, 350–352, **351**
co-occurring psychiatric disorders, 309–310, 318, 336–350, 416–417
anxiety disorders, 345–347
attention-deficit/hyperactivity disorder, 347–348
bipolar disorder, 336, 344–345, 870–871, 875, 880
borderline personality disorder, 349, 1264
delirium, 76, **77**
dementia, 120
depression, 336, 341–344, 790
eating disorders, 337, 348–349, 355, 1152, 1164
integrated treatment for, 337–338, 345–347
management principles for, 336–337
panic disorder, 345–346, 982
pathological gambling, 349–350
personality disorders, 349
pharmacotherapy for, 324, 338–339
posttraumatic stress disorder, 336, 346–347, 1021, 1037
psychosocial treatments for, 339
schizophrenia, 339–341, 573, 577, 582, 585, 605–606, 615, 625, 627
suicide risk and, 334–335, 1340, **1343**, 1346–1347, 1348, 1401–1406
family characteristics, 357–358
gay/lesbian/bisexual/transgender issues, 357
gender-related factors, 353–354
pregnancy, 300, 352–353
racial, ethnic, and cultural factors, 356–357
risk of aggression or homicide, 335–336
sleep disturbances, 336
social milieu and living environment, 358
use of multiple substances, 318, 333–334, 373–374, 409–410

cocaine use disorders, 301–302, 393–398, 447–451
development of practice guideline for, 296
DSM-IV-TR criteria for substance dependence and abuse, 306, **306, 307,** 412
duration of treatment for, 298
economic costs of, 415, 416
epidemiology of, 415–420
family/caregivers of patients with, 303
features associated with, 413–414
  cross-sectional features, 413
  longitudinal features, 413
functional impairments due to, 303, 305
future research needs related to, 465–467
goals of treatment for, 298, 304–305
  improved psychological, social, and adaptive functioning, 305
  reduced frequency/severity of substance use episodes, 305
  treatment retention and substance use reduction or abstinence, 304, 305
guide to using practice guideline for, 295
heterogeneity of patients with, 303
history of abuse in persons with, 1021
history taking in, 308–309
immediate interventions for, 303
intoxication and overdose, 318, 322–323
legal issues related to, 358–359
  confidentiality concerns, 358–359
  driving under the influence of alcohol or drugs, 315, 317, 416
  legally mandated treatment, 315, 358
  regulation of opioid agonist treatment, 359, 401, 402
marijuana use disorders, 301, 391–393, 446–447
medical comorbidity with, 319, 350–352, **351,** 413
  hepatitis C, **176,** 351
  HIV/AIDS, 195, 220–221, 234–235, 245–246, 256–257, 350–352, 416
    entry into treatment program for, 256
    LAAM treatment for, 221
    methadone maintenance for, 221, 257
    outcomes of psychiatric treatment of, 257
    pharmacotherapy for, 245–246, 257
    risk reduction strategies for, 194, 214–215
  tuberculosis, 352
morbidity and mortality associated with, 415
natural history and course of, 414–415
needle exchange programs for persons with, 195, 215, 232–233, 351
nicotine dependence, 300, 359–377, 420–434
occupations associated with, 307–308
opioid use disorders, 302–304, 399–411, 451–465
phases of treatment for, 303
in pregnancy, 300, 352–353, 467
prevention in children and adolescents, 355
psychiatric management of, 298, 316–321
  assessing safety and clinical status, 317–318
  establishing therapeutic framework and alliance, 316
  facilitating access to services and coordinating resources, 321
  facilitating treatment adherence and preventing relapse, 320–321
  managing intoxication, 318
  managing withdrawal, 318
  motivating change, 316
  providing education, 321
  reducing morbidity and sequelae, 319–320
psychosocial interventions for, 298, 324–333
  behavior therapies, 328–329
    aversion therapy, 329
    community reinforcement, 329
    contingency management, 328–329
    cue exposure, 329
    relaxation training, 329
  behavior therapy, 328
  brief therapies, 332–333
  cognitive behavior therapies, 327
  in dual-diagnosis patients, 339
    anxiety disorders, 346–347
    attention-deficit/hyperactivity disorder, 348
    bipolar disorder, 345
    depression, 343–344
    schizophrenia, 341
  family therapy, 330–331
  group therapy, 330
  hypnosis, 333
  interpersonal therapy, 330
  limitations of, 326
  motivational enhancement therapy, 328
  psychodynamic psychotherapy, 329–330

Substance use disorders *(continued)*
psychosocial interventions for, *(continued)*
relation to pharmacotherapy, 325–327
role of, 325
self-guided therapies, 333
self-help groups and 12-step programs, 331–332
rates of use and risk of dependence in, **415**, 416
relapses of, 415
prevention for, 298, 304, 315, 320–321
screening for, 9, **33**, 307
social stigma of, 330
somatic treatments for, 298, 321–324
abstinence-promoting and relapse prevention therapies, 323–324
agonist maintenance therapies, 323
antagonist therapies, 323
limitations of, 327
medications for co-occurring psychiatric conditions, 324
medications for intoxication states, 322–323
medications for withdrawal syndromes, 323
relation of psychosocial treatments to, 325–327
spectrum of, 303
summary of treatment recommendations for, 297–304
treatment plan for, 298
treatment settings for, 299, 310–316
aftercare, 314
case management, 315
community residential facilities, 314
employee assistance programs, 315–316
factors affecting choice of, 310
hospitals, 311–312
legally mandated treatment, 315
outpatient settings, 314–315
partial hospitalization and intensive outpatient programs, 312
residential treatment, 312–313
therapeutic communities, 313–314
withdrawal syndromes, 318, 323
aggression and, 335
Substance use history, **13**, 17, 307
Suck reflex, 119
Suicidal behavior, 1315–1456
among adolescents, 1339, 1383, **1384**, 1385, 1387, 1390–1391
adoption studies of, 1428
ambivalence about, 1357
antidepressant-related, 748–749, 934–936, 1374
anxiety disorders and, **1343**, 1345, 1397–1399
panic disorder, 934, 981–982, 1345, 1397–1399
posttraumatic stress disorder, 1021–1022, 1037, 1038–1039, 1399, 1414
social phobia, 1399
assessment of, 1322–1324, 1328–1362, 1437–1440
approach to, 1328–1329
biological markers, 1439–1440, 1454
children and adolescents, 1328
current psychosocial situation and nature of crisis, 1330
domains of, **1323**
in emergency settings, 1328–1329, 1359–1360
estimating suicide risk, 36, 779, **780, 863**, 863–864, 1021, 1324, 1336–1359, **1337–1338**, 1378–1379
family history, 1330
goal of, 1336
indications for, **1328**
individual psychological strengths and vulnerabilities, 1330–1331, 1356–1357, 1431–1433
in inpatient settings, 1359
inquiring about suicidal thoughts, plans, and behaviors, 1331–1335, **1332–1334**
in jail and correctional facilities, 1361–1362
in long-term care facilities, 1360–1361
multiaxial diagnosis, 1335–1336
in outpatient settings, 1359
overview of, 1328–1329
past suicide attempts, 1329–1330
past treatment history and treatment relationships, 1330
patients in suicidal crisis, 1371
patients with chronic suicidality, 1371–1372
psychiatric evaluation, 1329–1331
psychiatric signs and symptoms, 1329
rating scales, 36, 1335, 1437–1439
reassessments, 1370–1372
suicide plan, 1331, 1335, 1358

attention-deficit/hyperactivity disorder and, 1345, 1400–1401
chronic, 1371–1372
in correctional facilities, 621
cultural and religious beliefs about, 1322, 1341, 1355–1356
definitions related to, 1321
aborted suicide attempt, 1321
deliberate self-harm, 1321
lethality of suicidal behavior, 1321
suicidal ideation, 1321
suicidal intent, 1321
suicide, 1321
suicide attempt, 1321
dementia and, 114, 116, 122, 123, 143
development of practice guideline for, 1320
documentation and risk management issues for, 1378–1382, **1379**
communication with significant others, 1380
documentation of patient care, 1378
management of suicide in one's practice, 1381
mental health interventions for surviving family and friends after a suicide, 1325–1326, 1382
suicide prevention contracts, 1325, 1379–1380, 1455–1456
suicide risk assessment, 1378–1379
eating disorders and, 1106, **1131, 1343,** 1345, 1399–1400
electroconvulsive therapy for, 1327, 1376–1377, 1449–1451, 1455
establishing multiaxial diagnosis for, 1335–1336
family studies of, 1427
future research needs related to, 1454–1456
guide to using practice guideline for, 1319
history of, 1329–1330
HIV/AIDS and, 226–227, 1354, 1424, 1426
impact of patient suicide on treating psychiatrist, 1325
lethality of, 1321, 1335, 1340, 1358–1359, 1436
mood disorders and, 1342–1344, 1391–1394
bipolar disorder, 863–864, 870, 879–879, 1343, **1343,** 1392–1394
depression, 335, 748, 779, 788–789, 803, 1342–1344, **1343,** 1391–1394
motivations for, 1356–1357
personality disorders and, **1343,** 1347–1348, 1407–1409
antisocial personality disorder, 1347, 1348, 1408, 1409
borderline personality disorder, 1238, 1244, 1247, 1253, **1253,** 1274, 1327, 1347, 1348, 1386, 1407–1409
pharmacotherapy for, 1326–1327, 1374–1376, 1442–1449, 1455
anticonvulsant mood stabilizers, 1326, 1375, 1446
antidepressants, 1326, 1374, 1442–1444
antipsychotics, 1326, 1375–1376, 1446–1449
anxiolytics, 1326, 1376, 1449
lithium, 1326–1327, 1375, 1444–1446
in pregnancy and postpartum period, 1340, 1386
protective factors against, 1336, **1339,** 1429–1431
employment, 1355, 1429
marriage, 1341, 1389
psychosocial support, 1356, 1430–1431
reasons for living, including children in the home, 1356, 1431
religious beliefs, 1355–1356, 1430
psychiatric management of, 1324–1326, 1362–1373
adherence to treatment plan, 1369
boundary violations, 1363
consultation, 1373
coordination of care and collaboration with other physicians, 1368–1369
countertransference issues, 1325, 1363, 1372
interventions for family/friends after patient's suicide, 1325–1326, 1382
monitoring psychiatric status and response to treatment, 1373
patient safety, 1363
patient/family education, 1369–1370
reassessment of safety and suicide risk, 1370–1372
therapeutic alliance, 1362–1363, 1380
treatment plan, 1367–1368
treatment setting, 1325, 1364–1367, **1365**
psychodynamic factors and, 1356–1357
psychosocial interventions for, 1327, 1377, 1451–1454
cognitive behavior therapy, 1327, 1452
dialectical behavior therapy, 1377, 1452–1453

Suicidal behavior *(continued)*
psychosocial interventions for *(continued)*
other strategies, 1453–1454
psychodynamic and psychoanalytic psychotherapies, 1451–1452
rating scales for, 36, 1335, 1437–1439
risk factors for, 577–578, 607–608, 1324, 1336–1359, **1337–1338**, 1383–1437, 1454–1455
age, 1338–1339, 1383–1385, **1384**
alcohol intoxication, 1350–1351, 1415
anxiety, 1349, 1409–1410
command hallucinations, 1349–1350, 1412–1413
family history, 1330, 1354–1355, 1426–1428
gender, 1339–1341, **1340, 1384**, 1385–1386
history of childhood physical or sexual abuse, 1351–1352, 1386, 1417–1419
history of domestic partner violence, 1352, 1419–1421
hopelessness, 1349, 1410–1411
illness course and severity, 1353, 1422–1423
impulsivity and aggression, 1350, 1413–1414
individual psychological strengths and vulnerabilities, 1330–1331, 1356–1357, 1431–1433
lethality and intent of self-destructive behavior, 1358–1359, 1436
marital status, 1341, 1389–1390
occupation, 1342, 1391
past suicide attempts, 1329–1330, **1343**, 1351, 1416–1417
physical illness, **1337**, 1353–1354, **1354**, 1424–1426
presence, extent, and persistence of suicidal ideation, 1357–1358, 1433–1434
psychiatric comorbidity, **1337**, 1342–1349, **1343**, 1391–1409
race, ethnicity, and culture, 1341, **1384**, 1386–1389
sexual orientation, 1341–1342, 1390–1391
suicide plan and availability of method, 1331, 1335, 1358, 1434–1436
treatment history, 1330, 1352–1353, 1421–1422
unemployment, 1355, 1428–1429
weighting of, in suicide prediction, 1436–1437
schizophrenia and, 573, 577–578, 585, 607–608, 623, **1343**, 1344, 1394–1397
signs and symptoms associated with, 1329
special issues related to, 1440–1442
deliberate self-harm, 1441–1442
homicide-suicide, 1440–1441
suicide pacts, 1441
substance use disorders and, 334–335, 1340, **1343**, 1347, 1401–1406
among adolescents, 355
alcohol dependence, 334–335, 388, **1343**, 1346, 1401–1404
cocaine "crash," 394
summary of treatment recommendations for, 1321–1327
treatment settings for, 1325, 1364–1367, **1365**
twin studies of, 1354, 1427–1428
Suicide Assessment Scale, 1438
Suicide Behavior Questionnaire (SBQ), 1437–1438
Suicide Intent Scale, 1335, 1438
Suicide pacts, 1441
Suicide prevention contracts, 1325, 1379–1380, 1455–1456
Sulfonamides, **209**
Sulpiride, for schizophrenia, 659
"Sundowning," 116, 140
Supplemental Security Income, 341
Support groups. *See also* Self-help groups
for Alzheimer's disease, 126, 127
for bipolar disorder, 869
for eating disorders, 349, 1111, 1114, 1141–1142, 1146–1147, 1172, 1177
for HIV/AIDS, 229
for panic disorder, 965
for pathological gambling, 350
for schizophrenia, 599, 674–676
for substance use disorders, 331–332
for survivors of suicide victims, 1382
Supported employment, for persons with schizophrenia, 576, 598, 668
Supportive interventions
for delirium, 72, 83, 90
for traumatized persons, 1013, 1014
Supportive psychotherapy
for dementia, 112, 129
for HIV-related depression, 255, 256

Supportive-expressive psychotherapy, for methadone-maintained persons, 329–330, 408
Sweating
drug-induced
methadone, 455
reboxetine, 809
topiramate, 894
tricyclic antidepressants, 968
in serotonin syndrome, 808
Symbyax. *See* Fluoxetine-olanzapine combination
Syncope, drug-induced
monoamine oxidase inhibitors, 973
olanzapine, 890
Syphilis
dementia and, 120
HIV/AIDS and, 200
serologic tests for, **33**
Syringe exchange programs, 195, 215, 232–233, 351
Systematic desensitization, for posttraumatic stress disorder, 1053
Systems issues, 38
Systems training for emotional predictability and problem solving (STEPPS), for borderline personality disorder, 1226

T

T_3 (triiodothyronine), for antidepressant augmentation, 812, 897
T_4 (thyroxine)
in anorexia nervosa, 1162
for bipolar disorder, 897
Tachycardia
drug-induced
antipsychotics, 85, 86, 631, 653, 654
torsades de pointes, 85, 86, 616, 653
aripiprazole, 647
clozapine, 636, 653
cocaine, 301, 393
olanzapine, 642, 643, 890
psychostimulants, 144
quetiapine, 644
reboxetine, 809
risperidone, 640
tricyclic antidepressants, 144, 429, 806, 968
ziprasidone, 645
in neuroleptic malignant syndrome, 651
treatment of, 653
Tacrine
for Alzheimer's disease, 102, 112, 131–133, 147, 148
for delirium, 87, 91
dosage and administration of, 88, 133
side effects of, 87–88, 102, 112, 132–133
TADS (Treatment for Adolescents With Depression Study), 749
"Talking down" techniques, 609
Tardive dyskinesia, 85, 114, 139, 152, 242, 580, **592,** 650–651, 1297
amoxapine-induced, 807
assessment for, **586–587**
intermittent treatment strategies and, 600
prevalence of, 650
risk factors for, 615, 650
second-generation antipsychotics and, 650–651
selective serotonin reuptake inhibitor–induced, 808
severity of, 651
treatment of, 651
Tardive dystonia, 651
TCAs. *See* Antidepressants, tricyclic
Temazepam, 87, 92, 141
for persons with HIV/AIDS, 244
Tenofovir, 170
Teratogenic drugs. *See* Pregnancy, medication use in
Terminal delirium, 74
Terminal illness, suicide and, 1425
Testosterone, for persons with HIV/AIDS, 174, 195, 196, 223, 245, 254, 255, 259–260
Texas Medication Algorithm Project, 889
TFP (Transference-Focused Psychotherapy), for borderline personality disorder, 1226, 1452
Thalidomide, for persons with HIV/AIDS, 196, 245, 253, 260
The Practice of Electroconvulsive Therapy: Recommendations for Treatment, Training, and Privileging, 595, 751, 1377
The Principles of Medical Ethics With Annotations Especially Applicable to Psychiatry, 1380
Thematic Apperception Test, 1438
Theophylline interactions, with St. John's wort, 750
Therapeutic alliance
acute stress disorder or posttraumatic stress disorder and, 1023
bipolar disorder and, 864

Therapeutic alliance *(continued)*
borderline personality disorder and, 1243, 1247, 1266
cultural factors affecting, 36
delirium and, 82
dementia and, 111, 121
depression and, 780–781
eating disorders and, 1116–1118
HIV/AIDS and, 216
panic disorder and, 957
schizophrenia and, 572, 580–582
substance use disorders and, 316–317
nicotine dependence, 362–363
suicidal behavior and, 1362–1363, 1380
Therapeutic communities, 313–314
for borderline personality disorder, 1265, 1285
effectiveness of, 313
for incarcerated persons, 314, 401
modifications of traditional model of, 313
for opioid-dependent persons, 401
services available in, 313
structure of, 313
voluntary applicants to, 314
Thiabendazole, **209**
Thiamine, for alcohol withdrawal, 301, 380, 390
Thiamine deficiency, **81,** 88
dementia due to, 120
Thioridazine, **589**
for borderline personality disorder, **1262,** 1295
for dementia, 139
in Parkinson's disease, 150
dosage of, 140, **589,** 632
interaction with nicotine, 340
side effects of, 138, **592**
cardiovascular effects, 616, 631
hyperpigmentation, 631
ophthalmological, 631–632
QTc interval prolongation, 653, 1297
retrograde ejaculation, 656
for sleep disturbances, 147
Thiothixene, **589**
for borderline personality disorder, **1262,** 1295
dosage of, 140, **589**
in pregnancy, 872
Third-party payers, 39
Thought content, assessment of, 22
Thought disorder, in schizophrenia, 623
Thought processes, assessment of, 22
Thrombocytopenia, drug-induced
carbamazepine, 887, 1293
valproate, 885, 1294
Thyroid disorders, dementia and, 120, 143
Thyroid function tests, **33**
Thyroid hormone
for antidepressant augmentation, 751, 784, 812, 823, 897
for bipolar disorder, 897
Thyroxine (T_4)
in anorexia nervosa, 1162
for bipolar disorder, 897
Tiagabine, for cocaine dependence, 395, 448
Tobacco use. *See* Nicotine dependence; Smoking
α-Tocopherol. *See* Vitamin E
Topiramate
for binge eating disorder, 1116, 1150, 1180
for bipolar depression, 894
for bulimia nervosa, 1114, 1148, 1178
for cocaine dependence, 302, 448
interaction with oral contraceptives, 871
for persons with HIV/AIDS, 243
for posttraumatic stress disorder, 1013, 1031
side effects of, 894, 1180
Torsades de pointes, drug-induced
antipsychotics, 85, 86, 616, 653
methadone, 455
Torticollis, antipsychotic-induced, 649
Toxicology screening, 9, **33,** 309, 317–318
Toxin-induced delirium, 77
Trail Making Test, 174
Tramadol, 245
Transference, cultural factors and, 36
Transference-Focused Psychotherapy (TFP), for borderline personality disorder, 1226, 1452
Transgender patients, 357
Transplant surgery, 74
Tranylcypromine, 805
for bipolar depression, 894
for borderline personality disorder, **1258, 1260,** 1291
dosage of, 145, **774,** 894, 973, 1291
for panic disorder, 973
side effects of, 144, 810
Traumatized persons. *See also* Acute stress disorder; Posttraumatic stress disorder; Sexual abuse/assault
initial assessment of, 1013, 1014–1021
psychiatric diagnoses in, **1046–1047**
psychoeducation of, 1024, 1034

psychological debriefing of, 1013, 1028, 1033–1034, 1061–1062
resilience and optimism of, 1025–1026
suicide/violence risk among, 1021–1022
Trazodone
for bulimia nervosa, 1177
dosage of, 142, 145, 147, **774**
drug interactions with
antihypertensive agents, 798
diuretics, 798–799
efficacy of, 805
overdose of, 1443
for panic disorder, 974
for persons with dementia, 114, 115, 142, 145, 147, 148, 798
for persons with glaucoma, 798
for persons with obstructive uropathy, 799
for posttraumatic stress disorder, 1064
in pregnancy, 872
side effects of, 142, 144, **795–796,** 809
priapism, 144, 794
for sleep disturbances, 147, **795,** 808
in dual-diagnosis patients, 336, 343
during opioid withdrawal, 408
for suicidal persons, 1326
Treatment for Adolescents With Depression Study (TADS), 749
Treatment goals, 37
Treatment Outcome Prospective Study, 451
Treatment plan
for bipolar disorder, 861–862
for borderline personality disorder, 1244–1245
for delirium, 89–91
for dementia, 147–149
for depression, 778–779
for eating disorders, 1116–1151
initial, 37–38
for panic disorder, 951, 977–981
for persons at high risk for HIV/AIDS, 194, 211–215
for persons with HIV/AIDS, 194–195, 215–223
for schizophrenia, 571, 579, 580
for substance use disorders, 298
nicotine dependence, 365–366
for suicidal behavior, 1367–1368
Treatment settings, 10–12
for acute stress disorder or posttraumatic stress disorder, 1022
for bipolar disorder, 864
for borderline personality disorder, 1245–1246
for dementia, 120–121, 150–153
for depression, 780
for dual-diagnosis patients, 337–338
for eating disorders, 1106–1108, 1129–1134, 1169, 1170–1171
level of care guidelines, **1131–1133**
institutional, HIV-infected persons in, 229–230
for panic disorder, 951, 976
for schizophrenia, 578, 616–623
for substance use disorders, 299, 310–316
alcohol dependence, 299, 378–379, 434–435
cocaine dependence, 393
marijuana dependence, 391
nicotine dependence, 362
opioid dependence, 400–401
for suicidal patients, 1325, 1364–1367, **1365**
Tremor
delirium and, 74
drug-induced
bupropion, 809
lithium, 662, 844, 882, 1293
selective serotonin reuptake inhibitors, 966
topiramate, 894
valproate, 1293
ziprasidone, 842
in parkinsonism, 648
in Parkinson's disease, 119
in serotonin syndrome, 808
Triazolam, 115, 147
Trichotillomania, 258
Tricyclic antidepressants (TCAs). *See* Antidepressants, tricyclic
Trifluoperazine, **589**
for borderline personality disorder, **1262,** 1296
dosage of, 140, **589**
in pregnancy, 872
Trihexyphenidyl hydrochloride, for extrapyramidal symptoms, **594,** 650
Triiodothyronine (T_3), for antidepressant augmentation, 812, 897
Trimipramine, 774
TSF. *See* Twelve-step facilitation
Tuberculin skin testing, 319
Tuberculosis
schizophrenia and, 625
substance use disorders and, 352, 410

Twelve-step facilitation (TSF), for substance use disorders, 298, 300, 315, 332
alcohol dependence, 385, 437, 444
cocaine dependence, 396, 450
in depression, 344
Twelve-step–oriented programs
for eating disorders, 1111, 1114, 1141, 1147, 1150, 1172
for substance use disorders, 331–332
alcohol dependence, 385–387, 444
availability of, 332
cocaine dependence, 396–397, 450–451
opioid dependence, 409
in patients with borderline personality disorder, 1264
resistance to participation in, 332
spiritual tenets of, 332
use of psychiatric medications and, 338
Twin studies
of schizophrenia, 627
of suicide, 1354, 1427–1428
Tyramine in diet, interaction with monoamine oxidase inhibitors, 114, 144, 810, 973, 1291
Tyrosine, 662

U

Unemployment
alcohol use disorders and, 1355
suicide risk and, 1355, 1428–1429
Universal precautions, 350
Urban areas, HIV/AIDS in, 226
Urinary hesitancy or retention
drug-induced
antidepressants, 144, 429, **795**, 806, 809, 968
antipsychotics, 614, 654
clozapine, 654
management of, **795**, 806
psychotropic drug use in persons with
antidepressants, 783
antipsychotics, 616
Urine toxicology screening, 317–318
U.S. Drug Enforcement Agency, 359

V

Valerian root, 246
Validation therapy, 112, 129
Valproate
for aggression in persons with schizophrenia, 609
for alcohol withdrawal, 381, 436
for bipolar disorder
antipsychotics and, 842, 866, 891
in children and adolescents, 874, 905
depressive episodes, 893
in dual-diagnosis patients, 344, 389
alcohol dependence, 871
maintenance treatment, 845, 861, 899–900
manic or mixed episodes, 842, 859, 866, 885–887
rapid cycling, 861, 897
for borderline personality disorder, 1226, 1243, 1244, **1258**, 1259, **1260**, 1261, 1292–1294
in breast milk, 874
dosage of, 141, 886
drug interactions with, 887
antiretroviral agents, 243
carbamazepine, 888
lamotrigine, 887, 894
tricyclic antidepressants, 807
extended-release, 886
implementation of, 886–887
laboratory monitoring during treatment with, 142
for panic disorder, 974
for pathological gambling, 350
patient evaluation before initiation of, 886
for persons with dementia, 114, 141, 148
for persons with HIV/AIDS, 175, 243, 256
for persons with schizophrenia, 657
for posttraumatic stress disorder, 1013, 1031, 1066
in pregnancy, 872, 873
side effects of, 141, 142, 175, 243, 845, 885–886
for suicidal persons, 1326, 1376, 1446
toxicity/overdose of, 885, 886
use in bulimia nervosa, 1114, 1148
Vascular dementia, 118–119
age at onset of, 119
Alzheimer's disease and, 119
cholinesterase inhibitors for, 102
cognitive deficits in, 119
ergoloid mesylates for, 113, 136
onset and course of, 117, 118
risk factors for, 126
subtypes of, 119

Venlafaxine
for binge eating disorder, 1180
for borderline personality disorder, 1243, 1256, **1258**, 1287–1288
for depression, 772, 783
in bipolar disorder, 844, 868, 895, 896
dosage of, 145, **774**, 937
efficacy of, 805
extended release, **774**
interaction with indinavir, 241
for panic disorder, 936, 937, 974
for persons with dementia, 114, 145
for persons with HIV/AIDS, 174, 241, 255
in pregnancy, 872
side effects of, 144, **795–796**, 809
hypertension, 144, 145, 799
hyponatremia, 609
Ventricular fibrillation, antipsychotic-induced, 85, 86
Verapamil
for mania, 892
for panic disorder, 975
Vinblastine, **209**
Vincristine, **209**
Violence. *See* Aggressive/violent behavior
Visual changes, drug-induced
antidepressants, 144, 429, **795**, 806, 809, 968
antipsychotics, 654
carbamazepine, 843, 887, 1293
topiramate, 894
Visuoconstructional impairment, 73
Vitamin B deficiencies
delirium and, 72, 88, 91
dementia and, 120
HIV/AIDS and, 253
Vitamin D supplementation, in anorexia nervosa, 1112, 1113, 1145, 1174
Vitamin E
for Alzheimer's disease, 102, 113, 134, 148, 149, 154
vs. selegiline, 135
dosage of, 134
for HIV-related cognitive disorders, 253
side effects of, 134
for tardive dyskinesia, 651
Vitamin K deficiency, 134
Vitamin supplementation
for anorexia nervosa, 1112, 1113, 1145, 1174
for delirium, 72, 88, 91
for HIV/AIDS, 253

W

Wanderguard device, 124
Wandering, 118, 124
Warfarin interactions, with St. John's wort, 750
Washington v. Harper, 622
Wasting syndrome, HIV-associated, 196, 222–223, 244–245, 259–260
Water intoxication, 609, 625
Water restriction, for hyponatremia, 609
Weakness, drug-induced
benzodiazepines, 970
tricyclic antidepressants, 968
Wechsler Intelligence Scale for Children (WISC), 259
Weight changes, drug-induced
antidepressants, 144, **795**, 807, 808, 968, 1290
antipsychotics, 102, **592**, 614, 631, 654–655
aripiprazole, 647
carbamazepine, 887
clozapine, 636, 638, 654–655, 843
cocaine, 397
fluoxetine-olanzapine combination, 843
lithium, 662, 882, 1293
management of, 655
mirtazapine, 809
monoamine oxidase inhibitors, 810, 973, 1291
olanzapine, 642, 643, 655, 842, 843, 845, 890
quetiapine, 644, 842, 843
risperidone, 640, 655, 843
selective serotonin reuptake inhibitors, 144, 808
valproate, 885, 1293
Weight gain, in anorexia nervosa, 1109–1110, 1134–1137
Wernicke's encephalopathy, 74, **81**, 390
WHO (World Health Organization)
Determinants of Outcome Study, 627
Wills, 128
WISC (Wechsler Intelligence Scale for Children), 259
Women for Sobriety, 332, 387
Women Physicians' Health Study, 1420
World Health Organization (WHO)
Determinants of Outcome Study, 627

X

Xerostomia. *See* Dry mouth

Y

Yale-Brown Obsessive Compulsive Scale (Y-BOCS), **29**
Yale-Brown-Cornell Eating Disorder Scale (YBC-EDS), **1121**
YMRS (Young Mania Rating Scale), **29**, 889, 893, 906
Yohimbine, for sexual dysfunction, 657, **795**, 808
Young Mania Rating Scale (YMRS), **29**, 889, 893, 906

Z

Zalcitabine, **204**, **209**
Zidovudine, 170, **204**
  for children, 259
  dosage of, 251
  drug interactions with, 221, 243, 245
  for HIV postexposure prophylaxis, 234
  for HIV-associated dementia, 251–252
    prophylactic, 252
  to reduce perinatal HIV transmission, 233–234
  resistance to, 251
  side effects of, **209**
Zinc supplementation, in anorexia nervosa, 1112
Ziprasidone, 588, **589**, 644–646
  for agitation, 645
  for bipolar disorder
    in dual-diagnosis patients, 344
    manic episodes, 842, 866, 891
  contraindications to use of, 646
  for delirium, 62
  dosage of, **589**, 645, 842
  drug interactions with, 646
  efficacy of, 645
  for emergency treatment of acute psychosis, 589
  half-life of, 646
  implementing treatment with, 645–646
  intramuscular, for aggressive behavior, 609
  for persons with anorexia nervosa, 1112
  in pregnancy, 873
  receptor affinity of, 644
  for schizoaffective disorder, 645
  for schizophrenia, 609, 645–646
  for schizophreniform disorder, 645
  side effects of, **592**, 645, 842
    priapism, 657
    QTc interval prolongation, 616, 653–654
Zolpidem
  dosage of, 146, 147
  for persons with dementia, 115, 146, 147
  for sleep disturbances, 115, 146, 147
Zonisamide
  for binge eating disorder, 1116, 1150, 1180, 1181
  for mania, 891
Zung Anxiety Scale, 976